EGAN'S
Fundamentals of Respiratory Care

EGAN'S
Fundamentals of Respiratory Care

SENIOR EDITOR

Craig L. Scanlan
EdD, RRT

Professor
Department of Cardiopulmonary Sciences
School of Health Related Professions
University of Medicine and Dentistry of New Jersey
Newark, New Jersey

CONTRIBUTING EDITORS

Charles "Bud" Spearman
BS, RRT

Assistant Professor
Department of Respiratory Therapy
School of Allied Health Professions
Loma Linda University
Loma Linda, California

Richard L. Sheldon
MD, FCCP, FACP

Clinical Professor of Medicine
Loma Linda University School of Medicine
Loma Linda, California;
Medical Director, School of Respiratory Care
Crafton Hills College;
Beaver Medical Clinics, Inc
Redlands, California

PREVIOUS EDITIONS BY

Donald F. Egan
MD

formerly Chief, Pulmonary Disease Section,
Veteran's Administration Medical Center
Asheville, North Carolina

SIXTH EDITION

with 36 contributors and 821 illustrations

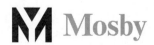

St. Louis Baltimore Boston Carlsbad Chicago Naples New York Philadelphia Portland
London Madrid Mexico City Singapore Sydney Tokyo Toronto Wiesbaden

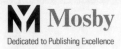
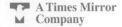

Acquisitions Editor: James F. Shanahan
Developmental Editor: Jennifer Roche
Project Manager: Gayle May Morris
Production: Diane B. Oehler, Publishers Services, Inc.
Editing: Jane Galati, Publishers Services, Inc.
Manufacturing Supervisor: Kathy Grone
Book and Cover Designer: Susan Lane
Cover Photograph: A color-enhanced bronchogram of the right lung
                     Biophoto Associates/Science Source

SIXTH EDITION

Printed in the United States of America
Composition by Black Dot Graphics
Printing/binding by Von Hoffmann Press

Mosby-Year Book, Inc.
11830 Westline Industrial Drive
St. Louis, Missouri 63146

International Standard Book Number 0-8016-7987-7

94 95 96 97 98 / 9 8 7 6 5 4 3 2 1

CONTRIBUTORS

Will D. Beachey, M.Ed., R.R.T.
Program Director,
Respiratory Therapy Program,
North Dakota School of Respiratory Therapy,
St. Alexius Medical Center University of Mary,
Bismarck, North Dakota

Christina Blazer, B.S., R.R.T.
Director of Cardiopulmonary Care,
Community Memorial Hospital,
Sidney, Montana

Robert L. Chatburn, R.R.T
Director
Pediatric Respiratory Care,
Rainbow Babies and Childrens Hospital,
Cleveland, Ohio

F. Herbert Douce, M.S., R.R.T.
Program Director,
Respiratory Therapy Program,
School of Allied Medical Professions,
The Ohio State University,
Columbus, Ohio

Richard D. Dunbar, M.D., F.A.C.P., F.A.C.R.
Associate Professor, School of Medicine,
Loma Linda University
Loma Linda, California;
Chief of Radiology,
Loma Linda Community Hospital,
Loma Linda, California

Crystal Dunlevy, Ed.D., R.R.T.
Director of Clinical Education,
Respiratory Therapy Program,
School of Allied Medical Professions,
The Ohio State University,
Columbus, Ohio

Linda Earl, R.R.T.
Clinical Instructor,
Respiratory Therapy Program,
UMDNJ/Camden County College,
Blackwood, New Jersey

Raymond S. Edge, Ed.D., R.R.T.
Dean,
School of Health Professions,
Maryville University,
St. Louis, Missouri

Alaa El-Gendy, M.D., R.R.T.
Resident Physician,
Internal Medicine,
University of Medicine and Dentistry of New Jersey,
Newark, New Jersey

Jim Fink, M.S., R.R.T.
Administrative Director,
Respiratory Care Department,
Edward Hines V.A. Hospital,
Hines, Illinois

William Goerlich, B.S., E.M.T.-P.
Program Director,
EMT-Paramedic Program,
Department of EMS and Trauma Education,
UMDNJ/Robert Wood Johnson University Hospital,
New Brunswick, New Jersey

G. Woodard Gross, M.A., R.R.T.
Program Director,
Respiratory Therapy Program,
UMDNJ/Camden County College,
Blackwood, New Jersey

Robin A. Harvan, Ed.D.
Associate Professor and Chair,
Department of Interdisciplinary Studies,
School of Health Related Professions,
University of Medicine and Dentistry of New Jersey,
Newark, New Jersey

Beaufort B. Longest, Jr., Ph.D.
Professor and Director,
Health Policy Institute,
Graduate School of Public Health,
University of Pittsburgh,
Pittsburgh, Pennsylvania

John H. Mathias II, B.S., R.R.T.
Regional Vice President,
Primedica,
Baltimore, Maryland

Patrick M. McDonald, M.A., R.C.P., R.R.T.
Western Regional Manager,
Primedica,
Marietta, Georgia

Tim Op't Holt, Ed.D., R.R.T.
Associate Professor,
Department of Cardiorespiratory Care,
College of Allied Health Professions,
University of South Alabama,
Mobile, Alabama

James A. Peters, M.D., Dr.P.H., R.R.T., R.D., F.A.C.P.M.
Medical Director,
Riverside-San Bernadino County Indian Health, Inc.,
Banning, California;
Associate Professor,
Loma Linda University,
Loma Linda, California

Barbara A. Peters, R.R.T.
Staff Respiratory Therapist,
Loma Linda University Medical Center,
Loma Linda, California

Alan M. Realey, B.A., R.R.T.
Director of Clinical Education,
Respiratory Therapy Program,
UMDNJ/Camden County College
Blackwood, New Jersey

Gregg L. Ruppel, M.Ed., R.R.T.
Director,
Pulmonary Function Laboratory,
St. Louis University Health Science Center,
St. Louis, Missouri

Craig L. Scanlan, Ed.D., R.R.T.
Professor,
Department of Cardiopulmonary Sciences,
School of Health Related Professions,
University of Medicine and Dentistry of New Jersey,
Newark, New Jersey

Norman Schussler, Ph.D., R.R.T.
Assistant Professor,
Coordinator of Clinical Education,
Division of Respiratory Therapy,
Florida A&M University,
Tallahassee, Florida

Richard L. Sheldon, M.D., F.A.C.P., F.C.C.P.
Pulmonary and Critical Care Medicine,
Beaver Medical Clinics,
Redlands, California;
Clinical Professor of Medicine,
Loma Linda University,
Loma Linda, California;
Medical Director,
Crafton Hills College
Respiratory Care Program,
Yucaipa, California;
Chief of Medicine and Director of Intensive Care
San Gorgonio Memorial Hospital,
Banning, California

Kim F. Simmons, M.H.S., R.R.T.
Director of Clinical Education,
Respiratory Therapy Program,
Department of Cardiopulmonary Sciences,
LSU Medical Center,
New Orleans, Louisianna

Catherine Smith, R.R.T.
Supervisor,
Infant Pulmonary Laboratory,
Respiratory Therapy Department,
Monmouth Medical Center,
Long Branch, New Jersey

Kathleen Smith–Wenning, R.R.T.
Clinical Instructor,
Respiratory Therapy Program,
Department of Cardiopulmonary Sciences,
School of Related Health Professions
University of Medicine and Dentistry of New Jersey,
Newark, New Jersey

Charles "Bud" Spearman, B.S., R.R.T.
Assistant Professor,
Department of Respiratory Therapy,
School of Allied Health Professions,
Loma Linda University,
Loma Linda, California

Halcyon St. Hill, Ed.D, M.T.(A.S.C.P.)
Director and Associate Professor,
Department of Medical Technology,
School of Allied Health,
Thomas Jefferson University,
Philadelphia, Pennsylvania

Robert E. St. John, M.S.N., R.N., R.R.T.
Pulmonary Clinical Nurse Specialist,
Jewish Hospital of St. Louis-BJC Health System,
St. Louis, Missouri;
Adjunct Assistant Professor of Nursing,
Jewish Hospital College of Nursing and Allied Health
St. Louis, Missouri

John V. Tesoriero, Ph.D.
Director of Research and Sponsored Programs,
Cathedral Healthcare Systems,
Newark, New Jersey

F. Robert Thalken, M.A., R.R.T.
Clincial Assistant Professor,
Respiratory Therapy Program,
Department of Cardiopulmonary Sciences,
School of Allied Health Sciences,
Indiana University School of Medicine
Indianapolis, Indiana

D. Theron Van Hooser, M.Ed., R.R.T.
Project Manager,
Ballard Medical Products
Salt Lake City, Utah

Robert L. Wilkins, M.A., R.R.T.
Coordinator of Clinical Education,
Department of Respiratory Therapy,
School of Allied Health Professions,
Loma Linda University,
Loma Linda, California

Kenneth A. Wyka, M.S., R.R.T.
Director of Clinical Education,
Respiratory Therapy Program,
Department of Cardiopulmonary Sciences,
School of Health Related Professions,
University of Medicine and Dentistry of New Jersey,
Newark, New Jersey

Robert L. Zanni, M.D.
Department of Pediatrics,
Monmouth Medical Center,
Long Branch, New Jersey

Since publication of the 5th edition of *Egan's Fundamentals of Respiratory Care,* technologic change in respiratory care has continued at a rapid pace. Particularly noteworthy during this period have been the many new clinical practice standards and protocols. Key national leadership organizations, such as the American Association for Respiratory Care (AARC) and American College of Chest Physicians (ACCP) have been instrumental in setting and updating standards relevant to the modern practice of respiratory care.

Both the content and organization of the 6th edition reflect these changes and advances. In terms of content, a new chapter on analysis of gas exchange has been added (Chapter 17). Several other chapters have been totally rewritten or significantly revised. The chapters on pulmonary function testing (Chapter 18) and humidity and aerosol therapy (Chapter 25) have been completely rewritten to better reflect both new technologic advances and recent practice guidelines. Synopsis of Cardiopulmonary Disease, Chapter 20, has been completely reorganized and contains expanded content on infectious and obstructive disorders. Chapter 23 (Emergency Life Support) has undergone major revision to assure consistency with the 1992 American Heart Association guidelines for CPR and emergency cardiac care. In addition, all chapters in Section 5 (Basic Therapeutics) have been revised to reflect applicable AARC Clinical Practice Guidelines.

In Section 6, (Acute and Critical Care), the entire framework for classifying ventilators is now consistent with the scheme developed by Chatburn and refined via the 1992 AARC Consensus Conference on Mechanical Ventilation. Also, the 5th edition chapter on Management and Monitoring has been expanded into three new chapters, with new content on initiating and discontinuing ventilatory support. Chapter 35 (Pediatric and Neonatal Respiratory Care) has also been expanded substantially, with new sections on surfactant replacement therapy and patient-triggered ventilation. Last, the chapter on Home Care, (Chapter 38), includes the newest JCAHO standards and has been broadened to provide more detail on areas such as noninvasive positive pressure ventilation.

In regard to organization, all general patient care content has been moved to the beginning of the text. In addition, the separate 5th edition chapters on general patient care and communications have been combined into a single chapter on Patient Safety, Communications, and Recordkeeping. Also, the revised chapter on computer applications now appears toward the front of the text along with other chapters on the technical aspects of respiratory care.

Sixth edition changes aimed at enhancing the practical utility of the text include ongoing emphasis on key terminology and reading level, and two important new features. All key terms are clearly identified when first introduced (by **boldfacing**), and are defined in the expanded text glossary. In addition, careful editing has brought the average reading level down to about the 12th grade.

Features new to the 6th edition include sections on equipment troubleshooting and the 'Mini Clinis.' Most chapters which review equipment application now provide guidelines on troubleshooting. Supplementing these guidelines are the dozens of Mini Clinis interspersed throughout the text. Mini Clinis are short exercises or scenarios designed to challenge readers to apply text content to practical problems. By carefully reviewing these Mini Clinis, readers should not only better understand how the content applies, but also see how expert reasoning is used to define and solve problems.

As with any compendium of foundation knowledge, the 6th edition of *Egan* is based on the efforts of many dedicated people. I am particularly proud to have worked with a fine cadre of contributing authors, without whose expertise this edition would simply not exist. In addition, I want to thank the dozens of individuals who made suggestions for improving the 5th edition. Although I was unable to respond to everyone, you can rest assured that all your thoughtful comments were incorporated into the 6th edition. Last, but certainly not least, I want to thank my students, past and present. It is you who provided the underlying motivation, intensity of purpose, and clarity of focus needed for me to continue the fine tradition begun by Dr. Egan over a quarter century ago.

Craig L. Scanlan

CONTENTS

SECTION 4

Assessment of Respiratory Disorders

16 Bedside Assessment of the Patient, 361

ROBERT L. WILKINS

17 Analysis of Gas Exchange, 391

THERON VAN HOOSER

18 Basic Pulmonary Function Measurements, 407

F. HERBERT DOUCE

19 Systematic Analysis of the Chest X-ray, 433

RICHARD L. SHELDON

20 Synopsis of Cardiopulmonary Disease, 451

CRAIG L. SCANLAN
GREGG L. RUPPEL
ALAA EL-GENDY

SECTION 5
Basic Therapeutics

21 Pharmacology for Respiratory Care, 506

JAMES A. PETERS
BARBARA A. PETERS

22 Airway Care, 540

KIM SIMMONS

23 Emergency Life Support, 581

CRAIG L. SCANLAN
WILLIAM GOERLICH

24 Production, Storage, and Delivery of Medical Gases, 633

ROBERT THALKEN

SECTION 7

Preventive and Long-Term Care

APPENDIXES

Foundations

of Respiratory

Care

1

Respiratory Care and the Health Care System

■

Beaufort B. Longest, Jr.
Craig L. Scanlan

CHAPTER LEARNING OBJECTIVES

1. Define the terms health, health services, and health care system;
2. List the factors that determine the health of the American population;
3. Identify the primary resources that support the U.S. health care system;
4. List the organizations that provide health services, and the role of respiratory care in those organizations;
5. List the organizations that provide the resources necessary to support the health care system (secondary providers), including those directly involved in respiratory care;
6. List the public and private organizations that regulate the primary and secondary health service providers, with an emphasis on those who oversee respiratory care;
7. Identify and describe the major problems confronting the U.S. health care system.

Respiratory care practitioners (RCPs) and students focus their main attention on applying their technical knowledge and skills to provide high-quality services. However, respiratory care is only part of a larger, dynamic health care system. Understanding the key elements of this system can help RCPs and students appreciate their professional role and contribute to providing better service.

HEALTH, HEALTH SERVICES, AND THE HEALTH CARE SYSTEM

Describing the modern health care system is a complex task. The scope of the subject is broad, and the system is constantly changing. As a useful starting point, we will define the meaning of the terms *health, health services,* and *health care system,* and then look at factors that affect the health of the population.

Health and health status

Health has been defined by the World Health Organization (WHO) as a state of "complete physical, mental, and social well-being and not merely the absence of disease." On the basis of this definition, the WHO strives to achieve an ambitious goal: that people in all countries have a level of health that will allow them to lead a socially and economically productive life.

The health or health status of a human being depends on many factors. These include basic biological and genetic traits, environmental conditions, and life-style. The WHO definition of health describes an

Adapted with permission from Longest BB Jr., Management practices for the health professional, ed 4, East Norwalk, Conn, 1990, Appleton & Lange.

ideal state—one that is impossible to measure—yet it provides a target that allows us to define a second important term.

Health services

Dictionaries generally define *service* as "an act of helpful activity." Thus *health services* are acts of helpful activity intended to maintain or improve health. Health is also partly determined by the type, quality, and timing of health services that people receive. Health services can be divided into three basic types:
1. Public health services: These are activities based in the community, such as communicable disease control and collection and analysis of health statistics.
2. Environmental health services: These often overlap with public health services. They include activities such as insect, rodent, and air pollution control.
3. Personal health services: These are services for individuals. Examples are promotion of health, prevention of illness, diagnosis, treatment, and rehabilitation.

Activities as different as the emergency room treatment of a child with croup, the drainage of a swamp in Louisiana during mosquito season, the dietary counseling of an obese member of a Health Maintenance Organization, and the creation of smoke-free workplaces are examples of health services.

In fulfilling their professional roles, RCPs generally work in the area of personal health services. Here they

have a variety of cardiopulmonary disorders. More recently, however, RCPs have been expanding their role by taking on more responsibility for promoting health and preventing disease. This role is discussed in detail in Chapter 36. As both health professionals and members of society at large, RCPs are more often acting as advocates in the areas of public and environmental health services.

Health care system

The *health care system* represents the combination of resources (such as money and people) and organizational systems needed to provide health services. Since providing health services is the purpose of the health care system, judgments about this system should consider the accessibility, quality, appropriateness, and efficiency of these services.

It is important to remember that the health care system and its services are not the only factors that affect the population's health. The environment in which people live, their life-styles, and their heredity have more effect on their health status than the health care system has. This does not mean the system is unimportant; after all, it provides treatment when disease occurs, even if it is caused by environmental, biologic, or behavioral factors. In this sense the health care system should be seen as a line of defense against untreated environmentally, biologically, and/or behaviorally caused illness and disease. Because prevention in these areas has not been adequate, the system is vital in maintaining and improving the health of the population. With this perspective as background, we now turn to a description of the health care system.

THE DYNAMICS OF THE HEALTH CARE SYSTEM

The resources and organizations needed to provide health services are described in the sections that follow. We will also consider the problems the system has as it tries to provide high-quality, appropriate, efficient, and accessible services. First, however, it is important to acknowledge the dynamic nature of the U.S. health care system.

The dynamism of this system is most obvious in the amount of money it consumes. In 1995, U.S. health costs will climb past *$1 trillion.* This is a dramatic increase from the $250 billion spent in 1980 and only $75 billion in 1970. Already, national health spending exceeds spending for education and defense combined. And, as health costs continue to take up more of the nation's resources, fewer resources are available for other uses. In 1995, health expenses will equal about 15% of gross domestic product (the total value of all goods and services produced in the country; also called the **GDP).** By the year 2000,

health costs are expected to be more than 18% of the GDP.[1]

These dramatic increases in spending reflect economic inflation and greater use of health services. But they also indicate growth and change in the system. Factors that contribute to the dynamic state of the health care system include social change, different priorities, new technology, more regulation of the system, changes in disease trends, new delivery methods, and new ways to pay for health care.

RESOURCES IN THE HEALTH CARE SYSTEM

The U.S. health care system requires an enormous amount and variety of resources. These basic "building blocks" of the system include money, people, **physical infrastructure,** and advances in technology.

Money

Figure 1-1 shows the trend of growth in total health expenditures. Figure 1-2 illustrates the source of these funds and the way they are now distributed.[2] They show that almost 90% of health spending is for personal health services. Most of that 90% pays for hospital care, physicians' services, and nursing home care. Spending for each of these types of services increased dramatically over the past three decades. For example, costs of hospital services in the United States increased by an average of nearly 12% a year between 1960 and 1991. For physicians' services in the same period the average increase was 11% per year. For nursing home services it was about 14%.[3]

Several factors have produced this dramatic increase in spending. Figure 1-3, page 4 sums up these factors for 1990–1992. During this period, 48% of the increased spending was caused by factors outside the health care system. Specifically, general price inflation accounted for 33% of the growth in health spending, and population growth and changes (such as aging of the population) accounted for 15% of the growth. The remaining 52% of the growth in spending was due to factors within the health care system itself. Three factors were most important. First, prices within the system increased at a faster rate than general inflation increased. Second, technological advances made more treatments and tests (an increase in the intensity of services) possible. Last, on average each person used more health care services.[3]

Personal health services are paid for in one of three basic ways:

1. Direct or "out-of-pocket" payment: Individuals pay for their care from their own funds.
2. Private insurance: Individuals or agents, such as employers, make contracts with insurers, who agree to pay for a specific set of services under specific conditions in return for **premium** pay-

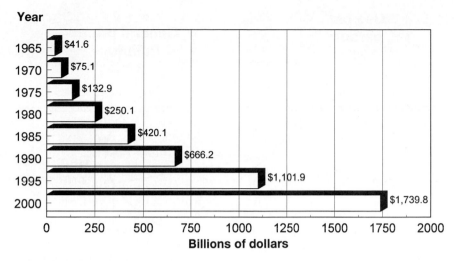

Fig. 1-1 Growth in total U.S. expenditures for health care, 1965 to 2000. (From Health Care Financing Administration, Office of the Actuary: Data from the Office of National Health Statistics.)

ments. Or a provider such as a health maintenance organization or an organization such as Blue Cross is prepaid, then makes contracts with providers to provide services to subscribers.

3. Government programs, mainly Medicare and Medicaid: In Medicare, the federal government pays for health care services to Social Security recipients over age 65. In Medicaid, federal and state funds are combined to pay for health care for welfare recipients and for people who qualify for the program under state law. In both Medi-

care and Medicaid providers of health service are paid on behalf of the **beneficiary** of the program. More is said about these two programs in a later section of this chapter.

The second and third types of payment—private insurance and government programs—are referred to as "third-party payments" because the people who provide the services are paid by someone other than the individual who receives the care. Although direct, out-of-pocket payment now accounts for less than 20% of personal health expenses, all money needed to

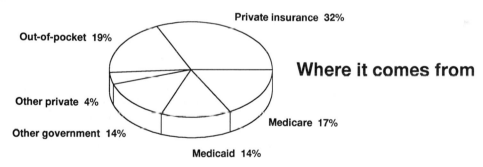

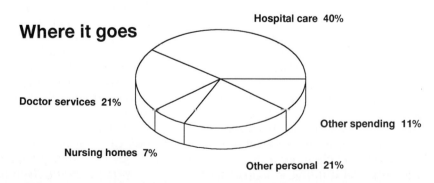

Fig. 1-2 The nation's health dollar: 1995. (From Health Care Financing Administration, Office of the Actuary: Data from the Office of National Health Statistics.)

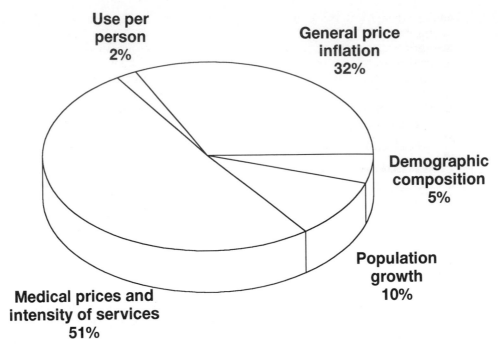

Fig. 1-3 Factors contributing to the 1990–1992 increase in personal health care spending. (From Congressional Research Service.)

support the health care system ultimately comes from the public.

People

Another basic building block of the health care system is its "people power." There currently are about 10 million health care workers in the United States, twice as many as in 1970!

This work force is not only large; it is also very diverse. According to the U.S. Department of Labor, there are over 700 different job categories in the health care industry. There are about 600,000 active physicians, including about 28,000 osteopaths (DOs). There are 1.7 million registered nurses, 172,000 pharmacists, and about 140,000 dentists. In addition, there are more than 3 million allied health care workers, made up of people who do more than 200 different kinds of work. These groups work in the fields of clinical laboratory technology, dental hygiene, dietetics, medical records administration, occupational therapy, physical therapy, radiologic technology, respiratory care, and speech-language pathology/audiology.[4]

About half of all health care workers, including most RCPs, work in hospitals. However, as health services change, more and more health personnel are finding challenging roles outside the traditional acute care hospital. This trend is likely to continue.

In terms of education and training, a large proportion of allied health professionals, including RCPs, train in either hospital programs or colleges and universities. In addition to the entry and graduation requirements of these educational programs, there are extensive regulations concerning credentials to ensure the competence of health care workers. **Credentialing** is a general term that refers to the recognition of individuals in particular occupations or professions. The two major forms of credentialing in the health fields are state licensure and voluntary certification.

Licensure is the process in which a government agency gives an individual permission to practice an occupation. Typically, a license is granted only after verifying that the applicant has demonstrated the minimum competency necessary to protect the public health, safety, or welfare. Because licensure is one of the police powers delegated to the states by the U.S. Constitution, licensure laws are normally made by state legislatures and enforced by specific state agencies, such as medical and nursing boards. In states where licensure laws govern an occupation, practicing in the field without a license is considered a crime, punishable by fines and/or imprisonment.

Licensure regulations are based on a practice act that defines (and limits) exactly what a professional can do. Two other forms of state credentialing are less restrictive. States that use *title protection* simply safeguard the use of a particular occupational or professional title. Alternatively, states may request or require practitioners to register with a governmental agency (*registration*). Neither title protection nor state registration necessarily involves a true practice act, and because both title protection and registration are voluntary, neither provides strong protection against unqualified or incompetent practice.

Certification is a voluntary nongovernmental process in which a private agency grants recognition to an individual who has met certain qualifications. Examples of qualifications are graduation from an approved educational program, completion of a specific amount of work experience, and acceptable performance on a qualifying examination(s). The term *registration* is often used interchangeably with *certification,* but it may also refer to a type of governmental credentialing. As a voluntary process, certification involves standards that may be and often are higher than the minimum standards specified for entry-level competency. However, certification generally does not prevent others from working in that occupation, as most forms of licensure do.

Both types of credentialing apply in respiratory care.[5] The primary method of assuring quality in respiratory care is voluntary certification, conducted by the National Board for Respiratory Care (**NBRC**). The NBRC is an independent national credentialing agency for individuals who work in respiratory care and related services. The NBRC is cooperatively sponsored by the American Association for Respiratory Care (**AARC**), the American College of Chest Physicians (ACCP), the American Society of Anesthesiologists (ASA), the American Thoracic Society (ATS), and the National Society for Cardiovascular Technology/Pulmonary Technology (NSCVT/NSPT). Representatives of these organizations make up the governing board of the NBRC, which assumes responsibility for all examination standards and policies through a standing committee.

The NBRC provides two levels of credentialing for RCPs: the entry-level credential, Certified Respiratory Therapy Technician (CRTT); and the advanced practitioner credential, Registered Respiratory Therapist (RRT). As of 1993, there were approximately 48,000 RRTs and 62,000 CRTTs credentialed by the NBRC.

In addition to the certification and registration of respiratory therapy practitioners, the NBRC provides credentialing in the areas of pulmonary function testing and neonatal/pediatric respiratory care. The NBRC also encourages professionals in the field to maintain and upgrade their skills through voluntary **recredentialing.** Both CRTTs and RRTs may demonstrate ongoing professional competency by retaking examinations. Individuals who pass these examinations are issued a certificate recognizing them as "recredentialed" practitioners.

Along with this private sector certification there has been recent growth in state credentialing of RCPs. As of late 1993, 36 states and Puerto Rico had set up credentialing regulations (Figure 1-4).[6] Of these 36 states, 29 have true practice acts; the rest have either title protection or registration. Licensure of RCPs is discussed further in Chapter 5.

Ideally, certification and licensure help ensure the availability of health care workers with acceptable levels of preparation. However, they can also limit the supply of health care workers and thus can increase the cost of this critical resource of the health care system.

Physical infrastructure

Another building block of the health care system is the nation's investment in the "bricks and mortar" of physical facilities. The most highly visible of these facilities are the nation's 6,600 hospitals. A hospital is "a health care institution which has an organized professional staff and medical staff and inpatient facilities, and which provides medical, nursing, and related services."[7] Various states have specific requirements for the licensure of hospitals; often they specify the types of services which they must supply. Chapter 2 contains information on the organization of hospitals and the role of respiratory care within them.

There are about 34 million admissions to hospitals a year. On any given day about 827,000 people are inpatients in the nation's hospitals. More than 388 million outpatient visits are made to these facilities every year. Hospitals differ in size and scope of services and have various ownership arrangements. There are 5,342 community acute care hospitals, 958 specialty hospitals (e.g., **psychiatric, rehabilitation, long-term care),** and 334 federal hospitals open only to military personnel, veterans, or native Americans. Of the 5,342 community hospitals, 3,175 of them are nongovernmental not-for-profit institutions, 1,429 are owned by state and local governments, and 738 are owned and operated as **for-profit** organizations.[8]

Another type of facility where health care services are provided is the nursing home. A nursing home is "an institution which provides continuous nursing and other services to patients who are not acutely ill, but who need nursing and personal services as inpatients. A nursing home has permanent facilities and an organized professional staff."[7] This category of health care facility is sometimes subdivided into skilled nursing facilities (SNFs), where on-site registered nurses supervise at least two nursing shifts per day, and intermediate care facilities (ICFs), where on-site registered nurses supervise only one shift per day.

There are almost 16,000 nursing homes in the United States, with more than 1.6 million licensed beds.[9] Spending on nursing home care has risen dramatically in the past three decades, from less than $1 billion in 1960 to about $75 billion at present. Spending for nursing home care is expected to reach $147 billion by the year 2000.[1]

In addition to the inpatient services provided by

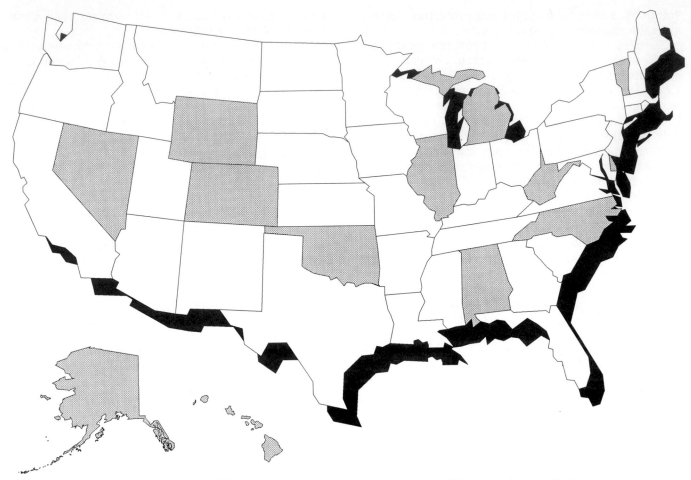

Fig. 1-4 Legal credentialing of respiratory care practitioners in the United States. Nonshaded states had legal credentialing mechanism as of 1993; shaded states did not (data from Konkle T: State credentialing update, AARC Times 17 (4):60–65, 1993.)

hospitals and nursing homes, more and more health care is being provided by outpatient and ambulatory care services. Hospitals are one of the major providers of ambulatory care services. Much ambulatory care is also provided in the private offices of physicians and dentists, including those associated with health maintenance organizations (HMOs). Increasingly, physicians have formed single- and multispecialty groups (three or more physicians formally associated to provide medical care, with shared offices, expenses, and income), often in large office complexes. There are also about 1,200 ambulatory surgery centers, 2,000 diagnostic imaging centers, and 3,000 medical laboratories aside from those in physicians' offices or hospitals.[10]

Technology

Another basic building block of the health care system is its remarkable technology. Technology has made organ transplantation and microscopic surgery possible. Advancing technology provides early diagnosis and improved treatment for many diseases and has

eradicated others. Of course, such advances have increased people's expectations. In addition, as expensive new technology has been adopted, the cost of health care has risen dramatically.

One aspect of technology is that as people live longer because of these advances, they need and use additional health services; the net effect is to drive up health costs. This situation becomes most difficult when there are limited dollars to spend. Recent efforts in health care reform are already focusing on the use and cost of technology. Among the changes likely to occur during the rest of this decade are the following:

- Those who develop medical technology will find an increasing demand for products and services which help lower or contain costs;
- Health professionals who use medical technology will have some restrictions on their use. Health care providers will be forced to make more careful decisions, based on efficiency, about what technology to provide. Research that evaluates the costs and benefits of various types of technology will guide decisions.

- Public and private payers will be less likely to pay for unnecessarily duplicated technology. The technologies they pay for will have been carefully screened to make sure the benefit they provide is worth the cost of providing it. However, because of policies intended to make health care accessible to everyone, payers are likely to be paying for the use of technology by more people.
- Patients and consumers will still have access to effective technology. In fact, more people will have such access, as the nation seeks to ensure that every citizen has basic health insurance coverage.

The health care system is structured from building blocks that include vast sums of money, many different categories of people with specialized training, a massive investment in physical facilities, and a growing supply of technological advances. In the next section, we turn our attention to some of the organizations that use these resources, and that convert resources into health services.

ORGANIZATIONS IN THE HEALTH CARE SYSTEM

Many kinds of organizations are part of the health care system. Although the diversity of these organizations defies easy categorization, five general groups can be identified. *Primary providers* include organizations such as hospitals, state and county health departments, HMOs, hospices, and nursing homes that provide health care services to individuals or groups of people. *Secondary providers* supply resources for the primary providers in the health care system. Examples of secondary providers are educational institutions that educate the system's work force, organizations such as Blue Cross plans and commercial insurance firms that help pay for health care services, and pharmaceutical and medical supply companies, among many others. *Regulators* are agencies that regulate the primary and secondary providers. They include federal and state government agencies and voluntary accrediting agencies. A fourth category of organizations are the *associations and professional societies* that represent the primary and secondary providers. The members of these organizations may be individual professionals (e.g., the American Medical Association or the American Association for Respiratory Care) or organizations such as hospitals (the American Hospital Association) or pharmaceutical manufacturers (Pharmaceutical Research & Manufacturers of America), who represent the interests of their members. The final category of health care organizations are *consumer groups*. Examples include the American Association of Retired Persons (AARP), Citizen Action, the National Council of Senior Citizens, Families U.S.A., and the Consortium for Citizens with Disabilities. Each of these

categories of health care organizations is examined in the following sections.

Organizations that provide health care services (primary providers)

Organizations in this category have one common characteristic: they all provide the means to deliver health care services directly to consumers. Within this broad category are agencies and facilities that specialize in preventative, curative, restorative, or continuing care.

One way to envision the diversity among primary providers is to consider clinical health care services as a continuum that extends from before birth to after death. In chronological order, primary providers include organizations such as the following:
- Prenatal ambulatory care facilities.
- Birthing facilities.
- Well-baby nurseries associated with the birthing facilities and centralized neonatal intensive care units (NICUs) in affiliated hospitals.
- Pediatric outpatient clinic services.
- Pediatric inpatient hospital facilities, including NICUs and pediatric ICUs (intensive care units).
- Child and adolescent psychiatric inpatient and outpatient facilities.
- Adult outpatient facilities.
- Adult inpatient hospital facilities, including cardiac care units, surgical intensive care units, monitored units, "transition" beds, and emergency departments.
- Cancer units (separate units that can provide radiation treatment and include short-stay recovery beds).
- Rehabilitation inpatient and outpatient facilities, including programs for orthopedic, neurological, cardiac, arthritis, speech, otologic, and other services.
- Psychiatric inpatient and outpatient facilities, including programs for psychotics, day programs, counseling services (adult and adolescent), and detoxification.
- Home health care facilities and programs, including programs for newborns, children, and adults.
- Skilled and intermediate nursing facilities.
- Adult day care facilities.
- Respite facilities for caregivers of homebound pediatric and adult patients, including services such as meals, visiting nurse and home health aides, electronic emergency call service, cleaning, and simple home maintenance.
- Hospice care facilities and associated family services, including grieving/psychological counseling, legal assistance, and financial counseling.[11]

The continuum of health care services outlined here has traditionally been provided by independent organizations, often in an uncoordinated and disjointed way. However, the health care system is undergoing a revolution in terms of how the primary provider organizations are related to each other. Vertical integration, in which many of the facilities listed here are joined into unified organizational arrangements, is reshaping the system.

Although their primary roles are still in acute care hospitals, RCPs are providing care throughout this continuum. Particularly important are the new and emerging roles RCPs are assuming in home and long-term care.

The American Association for Respiratory Care (AARC) defines respiratory home care as "those specific forms of respiratory care provided in the patient's place of residence by personnel trained in respiratory therapy working under medical supervision."[12] Among the key areas of home care are continuous oxygen therapy, long-term mechanical ventilation, and in-home continuation of planned pulmonary rehabilitation.

RCPs are also becoming increasingly involved in the nursing home setting. With the tendency for acute care hospitals to shorten patients' lengths of stay, many more individuals with severe, long-term illnesses are being cared for in skilled nursing facilities. For this reason, RCPs are being called on more frequently to provide patient care in this setting.

Organizations that provide resources for the health care system (secondary providers)

The organizations that provide resources used by the primary providers of health care are called *secondary providers*. They include educational institutions and programs, organizations that pay for care, and pharmaceutical and medical supply companies.

Educational Institutions

A wide variety of educational organizations and programs supply human resources to the health care system. Medical schools and nursing schools are the major examples, although many other institutions contribute vital resources to the health care system, including RCPs.

Medical education. The nation's physicians are educated in its 126 **allopathic** and 15 **osteopathic** medical schools. In addition, foreign medical graduates (**FMGs**) educated in other countries are an important source of physicians in the United States. Currently about 130,000, or about 22% of the 600,000 licensed physicians in the United States, are FMGs.[13]

The basic model of medical education is a 4-year postbaccalaureate program leading to the M.D. or D.O. degree, followed by several years of postgraduate training in a residency. The residency years are called postgraduate years and are numbered sequentially as PG-I, PG-II, and so on. The medical specialties determine the number of postgraduate years and the

specific clinical content in those years as the basis for certification in that specialty. For example, anesthesiology requires that PG-I be spent in a general residency and PG-II through PG-IV be spent in an anesthesiology residency program. The family practice specialty requires 3 years in a family practice residency. Neurological surgery requires 1 year of general residency and 5 years of neurological surgery residency. Residency programs receive **accreditation** from the Accreditation Council for Graduate Medical Education, which is composed of professional medical associations. Each specialty sets standards for its specialty training through its residency review committee.

Nursing education. The nation's registered nurses (RNs) are educated in 489 baccalaureate programs, 829 associate degree programs, and 152 hospital-based diploma programs.[14] After completing one of these approved programs, a nurse is registered by passing a state licensure examination (every state and the District of Columbia have mandatory licensing statutes). There are also master's degree and doctoral-level education programs that provide advanced training for nurses. Some of these graduate programs focus on education, research, or administration. Others provide specialized clinical training in areas such as public health, medical-surgical nursing, mental health, maternal and child health, or cardiovascular nursing. Other specialty training includes nurse anesthetists, nurse-midwives, and pediatric and family nurse practitioners. A pediatric nurse practitioner, for example, is a registered nurse who has received additional training that expands the nurse's role in the care of pediatric patients. Many nurses with advanced training are finding new roles in HMOs, ambulatory surgery centers, and home care programs providing care for elderly patients and chronically ill patients. RNs are also increasingly involved in utilization management and quality review roles in health care organizations.

Education in respiratory care. There are two levels of educational preparation in this field: the *technician* or entry level practitioner and the *therapist* or advanced level practitioner. Technician programs typically last one year and are sponsored primarily by postsecondary technical schools or two-year colleges. There are currently about 188 accredited technician programs in the United States. In 1993 these programs graduated some 4,400 entry level RCPs.

There are about 290 accredited therapist programs in the United States. These programs are sponsored mainly by two-year colleges and typically lead to an associate degree. About 10% of the therapist programs are sponsored by four-year colleges and universities and provide a baccalaureate degree upon completion. In 1993 these therapist programs graduated nearly 4,400 advanced level RCPs.

As with medical and nursing schools, the educational curriculum for RCPs typically starts with pre-clinical basic science courses. This is normally followed by or combined with intensive classroom, laboratory, and clinical study in the theory and application of respiratory care. Usually, all the classroom and laboratory instruction is provided by full-time faculty at the college, and the clinical experience takes place in hospitals affiliated with the program. After completing an accredited educational program of study, graduates are eligible for the applicable NBRC credentialing examination, and, where pertinent, for state licensure. Information on the accreditation of educational programs in respiratory care is provided in a later section of this chapter.

Organizations that pay for care (third-party payers)

A second important group of organizations that provide resources for the health care system are those that pay for health care. There are three categories of third-party payment or insurance in the United States. First are the voluntary, private health insurance plans, provided by either Blue Cross and Blue Shield, commercial insurance companies, or HMOs. Second are the government **entitlement** programs or "social health insurance." Worker's compensation insurance and the Medicare program are examples of this form of third-party payment. Last is public welfare, of which the Medicaid program is the most important example.[15]

Approximately 86% of the U.S. population has some form of health insurance coverage. About 74% of the population is covered by private health insurance (61% through employers and 13% by direct purchase of nongroup insurance). About 13% of the population has coverage through the Medicare program, 10% through the Medicaid program, and 4% through the military or veterans' program. Fourteen percent of the population, or over 35 million people, have no medical insurance. It should be noted that these percentages total more than 100% because some people have more than one type of health insurance coverage.[16]

More than 1,000 private health insurance companies provide health insurance policies. Several types of policies are available, including hospital/medical insurance, major medical expense insurance, Medicare supplemental insurance, disability income protection, dental expense insurance, and long-term care insurance. Prepaid health plans, HMOs in particular, are a rapidly growing segment of the private health insurance market in the United States. There are about 600 HMOs in the country today, which serve about 33 million people.

Medicare is the principal social health insurance program in the United States. Enacted into law as Title XVIII of the Social Security Act on July 30, 1965, Medicare is a federal program that is the single largest health insurer in the country. It covers those over the age of 65 as well as disabled individuals who are entitled to Social Security benefits and people with end-stage renal disease for a variety of hospital, physician, and other health care services.

The Medicare program includes two parts. Part A covers inpatient hospital care, very limited nursing home services, and some home health services. Medicare beneficiaries earn this coverage by contributing a payroll tax during their working years. At present, the tax is 1.45% of earnings for both the employer and the employee, for a total of 2.9% of annual income. Part B covers physician services, physician-ordered supplies and equipment, and certain ambulatory services such as hospital outpatient visits. Part B is voluntary, although about 97% of Part A beneficiaries choose to enroll in Part B. Part B of Medicare is paid for by a combination of enrollee monthly premiums ($41.10 in 1994), which cover about 25% of the costs, and general federal revenues, which pay for about 75% of the costs. Since Medicare covers only 50% of the total health care expenses of elderly people, more than 75% of them purchased supplemental, or "Medigap," health insurance plans in 1993.[17]

Because taxes from working people are used to provide services to elderly beneficiaries, Medicare operates as an intergenerational transfer program. Unfortunately, there is a basic weakness in this approach to financing an insurance program: There were five workers for each beneficiary when the program began. There will be only three workers per beneficiary in 2000, and only 1.9 by 2040.[18]

Medicaid, enacted along with Medicare on July 30, 1965, as Title XIX of the Social Security Act, became an important part of the existing federal-state social welfare structure. It was intended to provide health insurance coverage for preventive, acute, and long-term care for some of the nation's poorer citizens. This program currently covers about 25 million people, or 10% of the population. Through Medicaid, the federal government provides a subsidy to the states. This subsidy ranges from 50% to 83% of the program's total costs, depending upon the per capita income in the state. In return for this subsidy, the states administer their Medicaid programs under federal guidelines. These guidelines include the scope of services covered, the level of payments to health care service providers, and the eligibility requirements for coverage under the program.

Unlike Medicare, Medicaid is not an entitlement program. This means that Medicare recipients must prove their eligibility in accord with provisions of the program. Generally, requirements include being poor *and* aged, blind, disabled, pregnant, or the parent of a dependent child. Mothers and their dependent children are about 68% of those who receive Medicaid benefits, the elderly 13% (the impoverished elderly receive this coverage in addition to Medicare benefits), the blind and disabled 15%, and others 4%.[16]

Medicaid is the fastest-growing component of most state budgets, a fact that has led many states to try to reduce the growth of their Medicaid spending. They have followed various strategies to reduce these expenses. Examples of cost-cutting strategies are strict preadmission screening for hospital care, limiting the number of hospital days available for program participants, reducing the amount of payment to health care service providers (often to a point below their costs of producing the services), increasing the copayment requirements for optional services, raising the eligibility standards, and limiting the range of services covered by the program.

Pharmaceutical and Medical Supply Companies

A third category of resource-providing organizations are pharmaceutical and medical supply companies. National spending on the products of these organizations in 1995 totaled about $100 billion and could reach $150 billion by 2000.[1]

Pharmaceutical companies, such as Bristol Myers, Squibb, Merck, Pfizer, Eli Lilly, Upjohn, and Warner-Lambert, have been remarkably profitable enterprises. They have also made significant contributions to the quest for health. According to the Pharmaceutical Research & Manufacturers of America, there are now more than 30 anticancer drugs available in the United States and another 100 drugs to help treat and manage cancer are under development.

The companies that manufacture and distribute medical supplies are as diverse as their products, which range from cotton balls to very sophisticated imaging equipment. Firms such as Johnson & Johnson, Baxter International, Puritan-Bennett, Abbott Labs, and Bausch & Lomb make up this industry.

Organizations that regulate the primary and secondary providers

Several organizations and agencies regulate primary and secondary health care providers. They can be subdivided into two distinct groups: (1) federal and state government regulatory agencies and (2) voluntary accrediting organizations.

Federal and state government regulatory agencies

In many ways both federal and state governments try to influence the actions, behaviors, and decisions of primary and secondary health care providers. The purpose of this governmental intervention is to ensure that public objectives are met. In effect, government *regulates* the primary and secondary providers through five basic mechanisms:
1. Market entry restrictions,
2. Rate or price-setting controls on providers,
3. Provider quality controls,
4. Market-preserving controls, and
5. Social regulation.[19,20]

Regulations that restrict entry include those that license individual professionals (such as physicians, nurses, and RCPs) or organizations (such as hospitals and nursing homes). In addition to licensure regulations, state-operated Certificate of Need (**CON**) programs, in which new capital projects by health care providers (such as new buildings) must be approved by the state, are market entry restricting regulation.

A common example of rate or price regulation is government's control of the retail prices charged by public utilities such as those which sell natural gas or electricity. Although it is not classified as a public utility, the health care industry is also subject to certain price controls. Several states have established and continue to operate hospital cost-setting and rate-setting commissions. At the federal level, the government controls hospital reimbursement rates and physicians' fees for care of Medicare patients.

A third class of regulations are those intended to ensure that primary providers maintain acceptable levels of quality and that drug companies and equipment manufacturers meet safety and effectiveness standards. For example, the Food and Drug Administration ensures that new pharmaceuticals meet such standards. In addition, the Medical Device Amendment Act of 1976 places all medical devices under the authority of the Food and Drug Administration. Another example of the regulation of quality is the federal government's establishment of an elaborate system of Peer Review Organizations (PROs) to evaluate the quality and appropriateness of care given to Medicare beneficiaries.

Because the markets for health care services do not behave in truly competitive ways, the government establishes and enforces rules of conduct for market participants. These rules form a fourth class of regulation, market-preserving controls. Antitrust laws, which are intended to maintain conditions that permit markets to work well and fairly, are a good example of this type of regulation.

As the U.S. government moves toward managed competition as a central element of its health policy, a new era in market-preserving regulations is beginning. Managed competition is a strategy to stimulate the development of more vertically integrated networks of health service providers and more cost-conscious decision making by consumers. In theory these providers will compete with each other for large pools of insured people, keeping costs down while maintaining quality.

If it is to work well, managed competition will require much more activist regulation.[21,22] Regulations needed to make managed competition work include specifying minimum health insurance benefit packages, changes in the tax treatment of employer-provided health insurance, and new and less restrictive policies on eligibility for insurance coverage and ability to transfer that coverage.

The four types of regulation discussed here are all examples of economic regulation. The fifth class of regulations, termed *social regulation,* is somewhat different. The main purpose of this type of regulation is to achieve socially desirable results. Examples of these desirable results are nondiscrimination in providing health care services, assuring workplace safety, reducing environmental pollution, and decreasing spread of sexually transmitted diseases. Social regulation usually has an economic impact, but that impact is not the primary purpose of these regulations. Federal and state laws on environmental protection, workplace safety, disposal of medical waste, childhood immunization requirements, and mandatory reporting of communicable diseases are a few examples of social regulations.

Voluntary accrediting organizations

Many primary provider organizations seek voluntary accreditation as a way to improve their service and assure the public that they maintain high standards. In health care, no accrediting organization is more important than the Joint Commission on Accreditation of Healthcare Organizations (JCAHO). The Joint Commission began in 1918 as a program of the American College of Surgeons (ACS). This program used hospital surveys to help upgrade the quality of medical care.

In 1951, the ACS was joined by several other organizations, including the American Hospital Association (AHA) and the American Medical Association (AMA), in forming the Joint Commission. The JCAHO accredits various types of health service provider organizations. JCAHO accreditation is based on specific standards established by professional and technical advisory committees (PTACs). The importance of JCAHO standards for respiratory care services is discussed in detail in Chapter 2.

In addition to the accreditation of primary provider organizations by the Joint Commission, accreditation is widespread among the secondary providers that supply the human resources for the health care system. Educational accreditation is a process in which a private, nongovernmental organization reviews an educational institution or program of study with a set of established standards.

Up until 1993, educational programs for RCPs were accredited by the Committee on Allied Health Education (CAHEA), in collaboration with the Joint Review Committee for Respiratory Therapy Education (**JRCRTE**). CAHEA was a broad general agency that was sponsored mainly by the American Medical Association (AMA). In addition to respiratory care, CAHEA oversaw the accreditation process for about 25 other allied health fields through an umbrella review committee structure.[23] In a policy decision made in 1992, the AMA announced that it would no longer sponsor CAHEA but would support the development of an independent accrediting agency for allied health field workers. Under arrangements agreed to by its various collaborators, CAHEA began phasing out in 1993 and was replaced in 1994 by the Commission on Accreditation of Allied Health Education Programs, or CAAHEP. Review committees such as the JRCRTE continue to function under this new commission.

The JRCRTE is responsible for assuring that respiratory therapy educational programs follow accrediting standards, or *Essentials,* adopted by the American Medical Association.[24] Representatives of the JRCRTE visit educational programs for RCPs to judge applications for accreditation and make periodic reviews. In cooperation with CAAHEP, the JRCRTE publishes an annual listing of accredited educational programs for respiratory therapy technicians and respiratory therapists.

The JRCRTE is cooperatively sponsored by the American College of Chest Physicians (ACCP), the American Society of Anesthesiologists (ASA), and the American Thoracic Society (ATS). Along with a public member, representatives from these organizations act as members of the Committee, which, with the support of an executive office staff and many volunteer site visitors, has responsibility to review accreditation applications, conduct on-site evaluations of programs, and make accreditation recommendations to CAAHEP.

Organizations that represent primary and secondary providers

Primary provider organizations, such as hospitals and nursing homes, are represented by many associations. For example, most hospitals belong to the American Hospital Association (AHA). The AHA was established in 1898 to represent the interests of its member organizations in the nation's political process. Because of the diversity of the hospital industry, there are associations that represent subsets of hospitals. Examples include the Federation of American Health Systems, whose members are investor-owned hospitals. The Catholic Health Association and the Protestant Hospital Association are examples of hospitals with sectarian ownership and interests. The Council of Teaching Hospitals and the National Association of Children's Hospitals and Related Institutions represent institutions that have specialized purposes and interests.

The American Health Care Association (AHCA), established in 1949, is the largest association of long-term care providers in the United States. The Group Health Association of America (GHAA) is the association for all types of HMOs, and the Medical Group Management Association (MGMA) represents many of the nation's medical group practices.

Along with the associations that represent primary provider organizations, others associations have members who are individual practitioners. These associations serve the individual and collective interests of their members. The American Association for Respiratory Care (AARC) is an example of an organization that has individual professionals as its members. With over 30,000 members nationwide, the AARC represents the profession of respiratory care. The AARC promotes cooperation and communication between RCPs and the medical profession, hospitals, other health care organizations, service companies, and government organizations. The AARC also provides guidance and assistance to its members in the practice of respiratory care. This role is partly achieved through national and regional meetings, and through periodical publications, which include the AARC official scientific journal *Respiratory Care* and the *AARC Times,* a monthly professional interest magazine.

As shown in Figure 1-5, the AARC functions under the direction of a voluntary board of directors, elected by and accountable to the membership as a whole. An executive committee of the board, chaired by the president of the association, is responsible for overseeing the AARC central office, including its executive director. The executive director, in turn, oversees the day-to-day operations of the central office and its staff. Medical oversight of the AARC is provided through its board of medical advisers (**BOMA**), a group of physicians with expertise in the clinical, educational, or research aspects of pulmonary medicine.

According to its by-laws, decision making within the AARC occurs at two levels. Major policy and budgetary decisions are normally made by the board of directors. Decisions about other aspects of its operation are under the control of the general membership, either by direct vote (as in the election of officers) or through the association's representative body, called the house of delegates. Members of the AARC house of delegates are provided by affiliated state chapters of the association.

State chapters of the AARC have similar purposes and structures to the national association's, but their activities are limited to RCPs in their geographic locale. In some large states, such as New York and California, the state society is divided into regions, to promote better communication and coordination of services to meet local needs. In combination with the national AARC, these state affiliates provide a network of resources that promote and advance the practice of respiratory care.

Like the associations that represent primary provider organizations and individual practitioners, vari-

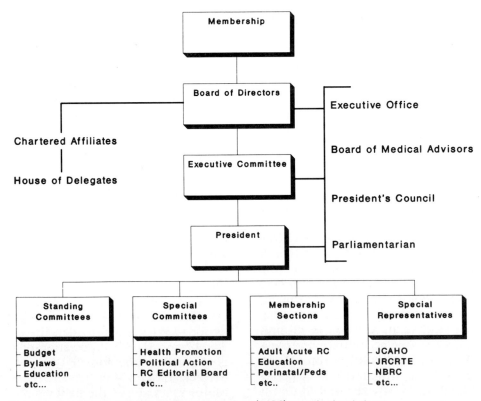

Fig. 1-5 American Association for Respiratory Care (AARC) organizational chart.

ous associations serve the secondary provider organizations. Examples include the Association of American Medical Colleges, Blue Cross and Blue Shield Association, Health Insurance Association of America, Pharmaceutical Research & Manufacturers of America, and the Industrial Biotechnology Association, among many others.

Consumer groups

The final type of organization in the health care system are those that directly represent consumer groups. Consumer groups with health care interests are quite varied, like the population from which their members are drawn. The American Association of Retired Persons (AARP) is a powerful association that has many of the nation's older citizens as members. Along with other consumer groups such as the National Council of Senior Citizens, AARP seeks to serve the interests of older citizens, including their health care interests. Other consumer-oriented associations are related to specific diseases, such as the American Cancer Society and the American Heart Association. Others represent the interests of broader groups of people. These include Citizen Action, Families U.S.A., and the Consortium for Citizens with Disabilities.

As individuals, consumers are remarkably diverse. Although they do not reflect the full diversity of the population of the United States, two demographic factors are very important to the health of consumers and the health care system: the changing age structure and the racial and ethnic diversity of the U.S. population. In 1990, about 32 million Americans were over the age of 65, and 13.5 million of them were over 75 years of age. By 2000, about 35.2 million will be over 65, with about 16.7 million of them over 75. By 2020, these numbers will increase to 52.7 million and 21 million.[1] Older people consume relatively more health care services, and their health care needs differ from those of younger people. They also are more likely to use long-term care services and community services intended to help them cope with various limitations in the activities of daily living.

The view of the United States as a great melting pot of people and cultures was always more myth than reality. Two groups in particular now challenge this view: African-Americans and Hispanic-Americans. Historically, African-Americans have had fewer opportunities for education and employment and less access to high-quality health care than the European-American majority. Among Hispanic-Americans, differences in language, geographic concentration, and cultural preferences are creating similar problems. Both groups are presently underserved by health care services. Growth in their numbers will worsen this problem, as does the fact that both groups are underrepresented in all of the health professions.

ISSUES FACING THE HEALTH CARE SYSTEM

The central problem facing the U.S. health care system is cost. This problem now threatens the very ability of the nation as a whole to pay its bills. In addition, rising health care costs are worsening the problem of access for those who lack either insurance or financial resources.

Rising costs can be illustrated by international comparisions. "By virtually all measures, U.S. health spending is the highest in the world. Over the past 10 years, whether in absolute dollar terms or relative to GDP, U.S. health care expenditures have increased faster than spending in other countries, and the gap between the United States and other major industrialized countries has increased."[25] Why are health care costs relatively high in the United States?

"It is not that we are sicker or suffer from more expensive illnesses. All the Western countries are afflicted by nearly the same constellation of illnesses at roughly the same rates; for example, heart disease, cancer, and strokes are the major killers in all of them. It is not that we are aging disproportionately; all of the Western countries have aging populations. And it is not that we have unique, more expensive technology. The same technology is available in all the Western countries—although, to be sure, it is more widely disseminated in the United States. Nor is our health care better; by all the usual, albeit crude, measures of health outcome—for example, life expectancy, infant mortality, childhood immunization rate—the United States does somewhat worse than most Western countries. The only plausible explanation lies in the system—in the way health care is paid for and delivered in this country. Clearly, our system is peculiarly inefficient and inflationary."[26]

In addition—and adding to the cost problem—the health care system continues to create both excesses and shortages of various resources. The population grossly underuses primary care and preventive services, while overusing certain high-technology services. Some of our citizens lack access to even basic health services; others are overtreated.

One of the results of these problems is a great pressure for change. As often happens in the United States, public pressure for change leads to new attempts to solve problems through changes in public policy. This process can be seen clearly in the political importance of the health care reform movement in the early 1990s.[21,27] This movement helped make health care policy one of the major issues of the 1992 presidential election. As a result, the government is now planning and may soon implement a major overhaul of the whole health care system. In general, this plan has two main goals: (1) to assure that all U.S. citizens have a basic minimum level of high-quality health care and (2) to decrease overall health care costs.

CHAPTER SUMMARY

Respiratory care is part of a large and changing health care system. The basic "building blocks" of this system are money, people, physical facilities, and technology. In addition, many types of organizations are part of the health care system. These organizations include primary providers, such as hospitals; secondary providers, such as insurance companies and educational institutions; regulators, mainly the government and voluntary accrediting agencies; associations and professional societies that represent primary providers, secondary providers, and consumer groups. Among these diverse groups and the public at large, rising cost is now considered the main problem facing the U.S. health care system. This problem threatens the ability of the nation to pay its bills and is worsening the growing problem of access to health care. As a result, major health care reforms are now under way. These reforms have two primary goals: to assure access and to decrease cost.

REFERENCES

1. Burner ST, Waldo DR, McKusic DR: National health expenditure projections through 2030, *Health Care Financing Rev* 14(1):1–29, 1992.
2. Sonnefeld ST et al: Projections of national health expenditures through the year 2000, *Health Care Financing Rev* 13(1):1–27, 1991.
3. United States House of Representatives, Committee on Ways and Means: *Health care resource book,* Washington, DC, 1993, US Government Printing Office.
4. O'Neil EH: *Health professions education for the future: schools in service to the nation,* San Francisco, 1993, Pew Health Professions Commission.
5. Mishoe SC: Current and future credentialing in respiratory therapy, *Respir Care* 25:345, 1980.
6. Konkle T: State credentialing update, *AARC Times* 17(4):60–65, 1993.
7. Slee VN, Slee DA: *Health care terms,* ed 2, St. Paul, Minn, 1991, Tringa Press.
8. American Hospital Association: *Hospital statistics,* Chicago, 1992, American Hospital Association.
9. Marion Merrel Dow: Marion Merrel Dow managed care digest: long-term care edition, Kansas City, 1991, Marion Merrel Dow.
10. Rakich JS, Longest BB Jr, Darr K: *Managing health services organizations,* ed 3, Baltimore, 1992, Health Professions Press.
11. Cummings KC, Abell RM: Loosing sight of the shore: how a future integrated American health care organization might look, *Health Care Manage Rev* 18(2):41–42, 1993.
12. American Association for Respiratory Care: Standards for respiratory therapy home care: an official statement by the American Association for Respiratory Care, *Respir Care* 24:1080–1082, 1979.
13. Mick SS, Moscovice I: Health care professionals. In Williams SJ, Torrens PR, editors: *Introduction to health services,* ed 4, Albany, NY, 1993, Delmar Publishers.
14. National League for Nursing: *Nursing data source 1991,* vol 1, New York, 1991, National League for Nursing.
15. Koch AL: Financing health services. In Williams SJ, Torrens PR, editors: *Introduction to health services,* ed 4, Albany, NY, 1993, Delmar Publishers.
16. De Lew N, Greenberg G, Kinchen K: A layman's guide to the U.S. health care system, *Health Care Financing Rev* 14(1):151–169, 1992.
17. Jensen D: Elderly out-of-pocket health care expenditures. Part I. Sources of liabilities, *Public Policy Institute of AARP Issue Brief* 16:1–13, April 1993.
18. United States House of Representatives, Committee on Ways and Means: *Overview of entitlement programs, 1991 green book,* Washington, DC, 1991, US Government Printing Office.
19. Bice, TW: *Health services planning and regulation.* In Williams SJ, Torrens PR, editors: *Introduction to health services,* ed 3, New York, 1988, John Wiley & Sons.
20. Williams SJ, Torrens PR: *Influencing, regulating, and monitoring the health care system,* In Williams SJ, Torrens PR, editors: *Introduction to health services,* ed 4, Albany, NY 1993, Delmar Publishers.
21. Starr P: *The logic of health-care reform: Transforming American medicine for the better,* Knoxville, Tenn, 1992, The Grand Rounds Press.
22. Starr P, Zelman WA: Bridge to compromise: competition under a budget, *Health Affairs* 12(suppl):7–23, 1993.
23. *Allied health education directory,* Chicago, 1992, American Medical Association.
24. Joint Review Committee for Respiratory Therapy Education: *Essentials and guidelines of an accredited educational program for the respiratory therapy technician and respiratory therapist,* Euless, Tex, 1986, Joint Review Committee for Respiratory Therapy Education.
25. Schieber GJ, Poullier JP, Greenwald LM: U.S. health expenditure performance: an international comparison and data update, *Health Care Financing Rev* 13(4):1–87, 1992.
26. Angell M: How much will health care reform cost? *N Engl J Med* 328(24):1778–1779, 1993.
27. Enthoven AC: The history and principles of managed competition, *Health Affairs* 12(suppl):24–48, 1993.

2

Modern Respiratory Care Services

■

Patrick M. McDonald

John H. Mathias

CHAPTER LEARNING OBJECTIVES

1. Outline the scope of services provided by a comprehensive respiratory care department in an acute care hospital;
2. Review organizational structure of a traditional respiratory care service;
3. Understand the key premises and concepts underlying the patient-focused model of hospital structure;
4. Classify the key roles and functions of various respiratory care personnel;
5. Describe the importance of written policies and procedures in the operation of a respiratory care service.
6. Differentiate between traditional prescription-driven respiratory therapy and the use of respiratory care protocols;
7. Define the importance of recordkeeping for both patient care documentation and accounting activities;
8. Describe the goals and outline the major procedures underlying a continuous quality improvement program.

The modern respiratory care service is a challenging and dynamic work setting. Technologic advances in medicine continue to create an ever-changing environment, with many rewarding opportunities for respiratory care practitioners (RCPs) nationwide. Despite advancements in technology, several aspects of respiratory care remain unchanged—total commitment to quality patient care and to the profession. Technologic advancements will never replace dedicated and committed professionals.

This chapter examines the basic structure and function of the RCP's work unit. While by no means covering respiratory care services in detail, we will identify and discuss the common and essential elements.

Over the past several years, hospitals and other health care facilities have faced an increasing number of patients with cardiopulmonary diseases. Technologic and educational advances continue to improve the quality of care. The techniques that have evolved for the treatment of these patients require highly educated and skilled professionals. In response to this need, respiratory care continues to grow.

Historically, respiratory care evolved from the hospital oxygen service. However, this modern technical profession bears little resemblance to these rudimentary beginnings. Today, RCPs undergo intensive medically supervised education and training, enabling them to provide very complex and sophisticated services. The importance of respiratory care personnel in assuring quality and cost-efficient care is evident in the use of these services. It is not unusual for a respiratory care service in a busy health care facility to provide some form of therapy to 25% or more of all patients admitted.

SCOPE AND ORGANIZATION OF RESPIRATORY CARE SERVICES

Financial pressures, governmental reforms and consumer demands are causing major changes in the structure and organization of both hospitals and their respiratory care services. We will first describe the traditional scope and organization of respiratory care services, as currently found in most hospitals. Following this review, we will describe some of the new, nontraditional ways these services are being delivered.

Traditional scope of services

The key services provided by a modern respiratory care service in a traditionally-organized, comprehensive hospital are outlined in the box on page 16. As is typical of a multipurpose department, these services often cut across established medical and administrative lines. This flexible approach to the organization and delivery of services is needed because patients in need of respiratory care can span all age groups and diagnoses.

The listing of services in the box is neither static nor all inclusive. Traditionally, the boundaries of respiratory care services have been flexible and responsive to changing needs and demands. Moreover, large differences in the range of services exist between facilities.

For example, in some organizations, efforts to contain costs and streamline administrative processes have resulted in the clustering of once separate departments into a single administrative structure, often called "cardiopulmonary services." In addition to traditional respiratory care, a comprehensive cardiopulmonary department may provide services in areas such as **electrocardiography, echocardiography,** cardiovascular catheterization, pulmonary function, stress testing, sleep disorders, and **hemodynamic** monitoring.

Services offered by a comprehensive respiratory care department

General therapeutic services

Therapeutic gas administration (O_2 and helium-oxygen mixtures)
Continuous aerosol and humidity therapy
Aerosol drug administration
Bronchial hygiene/chest physiotherapy
Incentive spirometry
Intermittent positive pressure breathing

Critical care services (adult, pediatric and neonatal)

Mechanical ventilation
Continuous positive airway pressure (CPAP)
Extracorporael membrane oxygenation*
Airway care
Patient transport

Emergency services

Cardiopulmonary resuscitation
Endotrachael intubation
Patient transport

Diagnostic services

Sputum collection (for cytologic/bacterial examination)
Arterial blood gas sampling and analysis
Hemodynamic monitoring
Pulmonary function testing
Bedside monitoring
　pulse oximetry
　end tidal CO_2 monitoring (capnometry)
　apnea monitoring
　transcutaneous O_2/CO_2 monitoring

Cardiac testing*
　EKG
　telemetry
　stress testing
　Holter monitoring
　echocardiography
Polysomnography (sleep studies)*
Metabolic studies (indirect calorimetry)*

Special procedures

Bronchoscopy (assist)*
Transtracheal aspiration (assist)*
Thoracentesis (assist)*

Educational services

Patient and family education*
Staff development and in-service education
Student clinical education (clinical affiliation)
Community education*

Pulmonary rehabilitation and home care

Home care discharge planning and follow-up
Outpatient pulmonary rehabilitation*

Support services

Equipment processing (cleaning, disinfection and sterilization)
Equipment maintenance (calibration, repair and preventive maintenance)
Supply inventory and stocking

Other services

Clinical research
Patient assessment

* Indicate special services not provided or available through all departments.

From facility to facility, there will be differences in the complexities, numbers, and types of services offered. It is essential that all departments maintain a philosophy of flexibility and cooperation with other health care disciplines to allow for future growth.

Service coverage

Therapeutic services

Local health care needs and available personnel determine the scope and coverage of therapeutic services. Ideally, therapeutic services should be available 24 hours a day, seven days a week. Most routine therapy is provided during the day and evening shifts. Nights and weekend coverage are usually less extensive, with priority given to critical and emergency care.

Diagnostic services

Unlike therapeutic services, most diagnostic or testing services can usually be scheduled in advance. Most departments maintain an appointment log to schedule patient testing based on diagnostic time standards. Efficiently run diagnostic services ensure that practitioner times correspond closely to scheduled tests. Although emergency requests can and do occur, physicians ordering diagnostic services should provide as much lead time as possible.

Facilities that have a high volume of diagnostic procedures may hire practitioners just to perform these services. However, with the advancement of technology and an ongoing effort to remain cost effective, most departments have developed sophisticated **cross-training programs.**

Cross-training prepares clinicians to provide services outside their profession's normal scope of practice. An example would be the RCP who also is certified as an IV therapist (usually a nursing skill). This individual is said to be cross-trained or **multicompetent.**

RCPs are uniquely qualified to be cross-trained to perform many services which were once provided solely by other health care personnel. The educational background and flexible hours of coverage provided by RCPs are two primary reasons for this evolution.

Some examples of services now performed by respiratory care as a result of cross-training include blood gas analysis, arterial punctures, pulmonary function testing, EEG, EKG, telemetry, Holter monitoring, Holter scanning, and Swan-Ganz monitoring. Cross-training practitioners to perform these services can contribute to increased productivity and improved availability of services.

Traditional administrative organization and personnel

A large, comprehensive respiratory care service normally includes some or all of personnel listed in the accompanying box.

In addition, some departments may have sleep technicians, echocardiographic personnel, pulmonary **rehabilitation,** and/or home care coordinators. In teaching hospitals, some RCPs may also be involved in clinical research activities. Obviously, the number and variety of personnel will vary according to the size of the health care facility and its scope of services.

Traditional organizational structure

Effective coordination of the activity of personnel requires some form of organizational structure. Figure 2-1 portrays a traditional organizational chart for a typical respiratory care service department, operating in a medium-to-large sized comprehensive acute care hospital.

Typically, overall policy-making responsibility for the organization is vested in a governing board of directors. Both the hospital administrative and medical staff function under the board of directors.

The administration oversees the traditional management functions of planning, supervising, controlling and budgeting. The director of the respiratory care service typically reports to a higher administrative official, such as a vice-president of clinical ser-

vices, who is responsible for several related ancillary service areas.

The medical staff structure is collegial in nature, typically organized into specialty departments, such as surgery, medicine, **pediatrics,** and **obstetrics** and **gynecology.** Typically, the medical staff leadership flows from an executive board or committee. The medical staff provides policy and administrative oversight over matters directly related to patient care.

On this side of the organization, the respiratory care department is typically responsible to a member of the medical staff who holds the title of medical director. Details on the critical role of the respiratory care medical director are provided in the following section.

In this representative organizational scheme, the respiratory care department is further divided into three major operational areas: clinical or therapeutic specialties, diagnostic services, and educational support. Variations in this structure are common, and again depend on the size and scope of services offered.

Ideally, a respiratory care service department should be an independent administrative unit, with a defined budget and managerial support stemming from the hospital administration. Thus, in administrative and fiscal matters, the department director works directly with the hospital administration.

The education services component of the depart-

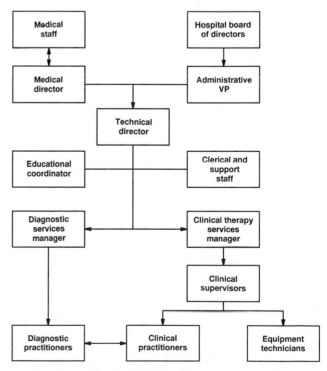

Fig. 2-1 Representative organizational chart for a respiratory care service department operating in a medium-to-large sized comprehensive acute care hospital. See text for details.

Typical personnel in a respiratory care service department
Medical director
Technical director/manager
Assistant director
Clinical supervisors
Staff respiratory care practitioners
Pulmonary function technicians
In-service/clinical instructors
Equipment technicians
Clerical staff

ment is particularly important in facilities affiliated with respiratory therapy educational programs. Even without such a relationship, ongoing staff development activities usually demand at least part-time oversight of the educational activities of the departments. In-service and **continuing education** are essential elements of any progressive department. **In-service education** normally extends beyond the bounds of the department staff, to include nurses, residents, and other professionals involved in respiratory care.

The medium to small community hospital will be primarily interested in the therapeutic and diagnostic functions of their respiratory care departments. A small hospital may be adequately served by a single medical director supervising both service areas and a modest pulmonary function laboratory.

In larger departments there may be an effective division of labor, with two or more associate medical directors. Here the duties may be divided, with one director responsible for service functions, another for the pulmonary laboratory, and perhaps yet another for critical care and clinical research projects. Large facilities may also have administrative section heads for each major subdivision of the department, such as adult critical care, neonatal/pediatric services, etc.

Classification of personnel

Most respiratory care services use officially recognized personnel categories in the development of job titles and clinical assignments. The accompanying box provides the current formal definitions used in the field.

This classification specifies two major levels of bedside personnel: therapists and the technicians. In some hospitals, there are clear differences between the responsibilities assumed by therapists and the technicians. On the other hand, due to factors such as local needs and personnel availability, the duties of the therapist and technician often overlap.

In many facilities all clinical personnel are classified as RCPs, with responsibilities and advancement based on a clinical career ladder approach (Table 2-1). This system provides career advancement opportunity for all department members and promotes professional growth for the respiratory care department as a whole.

Key roles and functions

Based on the prior descriptions of departmental structure and formal personnel classifications, we will provide a general overview of the roles and functions of the key personnel normally involved in providing respiratory care services. Rather than delineate job descriptions, we will highlight the key aspects of these important roles. For the respiratory therapy student, these descriptions should help clarify functional responsibilities within an affiliated department, while

---

Classification of respiratory care personnel

Respiratory therapy technician

A graduate of a school accredited by the Joint Review Committee for Respiratory Therapy Education (JRCRTE) designed to qualify the graduate for the entry-level examination of the National Board for Respiratory Care (NBRC). Usually, this means a 1-year program combining a curriculum of basic sciences with supervised clinical experience.

Respiratory therapist

A graduate of a JRCRTE-approved school designed to qualify the graduate for the registry examination of the NBRC. Usually, this means a 2- to 4-year program with advanced-level courses, leading to an associate or bachelor degree.

Certified respiratory therapy technician (CRTT)

A respiratory therapy technician who has successfully completed the technician (entry-level) certification examination of the NBRC.

Registered respiratory therapist (RRT)

A respiratory therapist who has successfully completed the registry (therapist) examination of the NBRC.

Credentialed respiratory care practitioner

An individual holding a legal credential issued by a state which officially recognizes the right to practice respiratory care. In some states, this credential is called a license. Most states use the NBRC certification exam as the basis for granting credentials to RCPs.

Certified pulmonary function technician (CPFT)

An individual, qualified by education and/or experience, who has successfully completed the pulmonary function certification examination of the NBRC.

Registered pulmonary function technologist (RPFT)

An individual, qualified by education and/or experience, and previously certified in pulmonary function technology, who has successfully completed the pulmonary function registry examination of the NBRC.

Respiratory therapy student

One who is enrolled in an accredited respiratory care educational program.

---

also showing what opportunities exist for job mobility within the field.

Medical director. The quality and strength of a respiratory care service depend first and foremost on the commitment of its medical director. The medical director must be a member of the medical staff who is interested in chest disease and who has had extensive training and clinical experience in this area.

Table 2-1 Career ladder approach to staffing

Title	Responsibilities	Criteria
Respiratory Care Practitioner I	Therapeutic gases	State license
	Continuous oxygen	Graduate of
	Medication nebulizers	JRCRTE-approved school
	MDI	Level I check-offs complete
	Bronchial hygiene	
	IPPB	
	CPR	
	Arterial blood drawing	
	Pulse oximetry	
Respiratory Care Practitioner II	Intubation	State license
	PFT	CRTT or equivalent
	Patient transport	Level II check-offs complete
	Airway care	
	Arterial lines	
	Hemodynamic monitoring	
	Bronchoscopy assisting	
	Mechanical ventilation	
Respiratory Care Practitioner III	Patient care-assessment	State license
	Neonatal care	RRT (supplemental)
	High-frequency ventilation	Level III check-offs complete
	Extracorporeal pump operation	
	Pulmonary rehabilitation	
	Indirect calorimetry	
	Clinical protocols	

Adapted from organizational structure, King Drew Medical Center, Los Angeles, California.

Historically, **anesthesiologists** were among the first medical directors of respiratory care. Over the last 25 years, however, medical direction by anesthesiologists has given way to primary oversight by pulmonary physicians.

Whether designated as a full or part-time position, being a respiratory care service medical director is a full-time responsibility. The medical director must be available for consultation and advice both to other physicians and to the respiratory care staff on a 24-hour basis.

The medical director of respiratory care is professionally responsible for the clinical function of the department. Typical responsibilities of a medical director are listed in the accompanying box. The medical director thus must have considerable authority in setting the policies and practices of respiratory care in the hospital. Of course, any major policy involving patient care or the relationships between the department and staff physicians must be approved by the hospital's medical board.

Typical responsibilities of the medical director of respiratory care

- Medical supervision of patients with respiratory diseases (including consultation and referral)
- General medical and respiratory intensive care
- Ambulatory care (including rehabilitation)
- Pulmonary function evaluation
- Development and approval of departmental clinical policies and procedures, including quality assurance activities
- Medical direction of the respiratory care in-service training and education program
- Education of medical and nursing staffs
- Participation in the selection and promotion of technical staff
- Participation in the preparation of the departmental budget

---

A challenge to both the medical and technical leadership of respiratory care services is provision of an increasingly better quality of patient service at lower cost. This is the current philosophy of cost containment and cost-effectiveness. The need for medical directors to possess administrative skills has long been recognized by those active in this work, but only recently has it been given significant emphasis. Physicians considering medical direction of a respiratory care services must be willing and ready to accept some administrative responsibilities.

Respiratory care services are provided on the orders of all staff physicians. Even though these services are ordered by other physicians, their quality and appropriateness are still the medical director's responsibility. For this reason, the medical director must oversee the development and implementation of the respiratory care service's quality assurance activities, as described later in this chapter.

Technical director. The efficiency of departmental operation depends on the quality of technical or managerial leadership. In most cases, the technical director of a respiratory care service must be well-trained in all aspects of respiratory care, and experienced in its clinical application. In addition to being proficient in therapeutic techniques and equipment function, however, the technical director must possess both leadership and managerial skills.

Although the position will probably have more prestige if the director is registered by the National Board for Respiratory Care, registration alone is not sufficient. There are many registered therapists who do not have the necessary leadership and management skills to assume this key role. No guideline exists to indicate the minimum experience needed for this position, but most technical directors have spent at least three years as bedside clinicians. Moreover, a technical director ideally should have demonstrated supervisory abilities, as acquired through two or more years in a supervisory role.

While the medical director is responsible for the overall quality of medical services provided by the department, the technical director oversees the daily operation and management of the service. The administrative authority of the position must be well understood and completely supported by the medical director, since the technical director is an important link between the medical director and the technical staff. Typical responsibilities of a technical director are listed in the accompanying box.

Assistant technical director. Given the technical director's scope of duties, one or more assistant technical directors may be needed, especially in larger departments. The assistant should possess technical skills at least equal to those of the technical director, but does not need as much administrative experience.

Typically, an assistant technical director serves a dual role. In the absence of the technical director, the assistant acts as the director of the department. On a daily basis, however, the assistant director commonly functions as the chief clinician and first line supervisor. The assistant director may also supervise the service in the respiratory care or intensive care unit, and consult with or advise staff practitioners in the management of difficult patients. The assistant director may also take an active role in the training and orientation of students and practitioners, and the evaluation of equipment. In teaching settings, the assistant director may also be involved in clinical research. Last, the assistant technical director may also coordinate the departmental quality assurance plan (covered later in this chapter).

Clinical supervisor. Clinical supervisors are responsible for the respiratory care service function during their particular segments of the day. Generally, they are directly responsible for the staff on their shifts.

Typical responsibilities of the technical director of respiratory care

- Assignment of staff according to departmental need
- Maintenance of payroll data on all personnel
- Development and application of a staff productivity system
- Preparation of the departmental budget
- Generation of departmental activity reports
- Justification of personnel needs
- Provision of advice and assistance to technical personnel
- Training and orientation of new practitioners
- Conducting quality assurance audits
- Evaluating equipment for purchase
- Development and implementation of special projects

Specific duties of these key personnel vary considerably from place to place. In response to general patient loads and specific area needs, clinical supervisors generally coordinate the work schedules of employees assigned to their shift, and make daily assignments of duties. Typically, clinical supervisors also coordinate emergency responses, and assist in clinical training or student supervision. Clinical supervisors may also assist staff personnel with common problems, and participate in service provision as needed.

Differences in activity between shifts means different supervisory responsibilities. For example, the day or evening supervisors might be primarily concerned with fulfilling requests for service, whereas the night clinical supervisor might be responsible for overseeing clerical work requiring technical knowledge. These supervisors must be flexible and adaptable, as well as mature, experienced, and totally supportive of the department's philosophy and purpose.

Clinical staff practitioners. The character of services provided by a respiratory care department depends on the quality of its practitioners. As the primary providers of bedside care, RCPs are expected to be technically proficient in the therapeutic modalities offered by the service, including a full knowledge of the indications, **contraindications** and hazards associated with these procedures. They must also know the basic maintenance procedures for equipment in the event of a malfunction. Because of close interaction with other health care professionals directly involved in the patient's care, RCPs also must understand the wide array of disorders that can affect the respiratory system.

However, technical proficiency and knowledge alone are not sufficient. RCPs also must be ethically sensitive to those aspects of care with which they are directly or indirectly involved, including the values and beliefs of patients and other health care providers. Often these human-oriented skills are just as important in determining patient outcomes as are technical knowledge and proficiency.

Education coordinator. Wherever respiratory care services are available, there should also be educational activities. These activities may vary from a series of periodic in-service or continuing education sessions to daily supervision of students enrolled in an accredited respiratory care educational program.

In places where the primary focus is on staff development, the educational coordinator assumes responsibility for regularly scheduled in-service workshops for the staff. Additional activities may include orientation sessions for new personnel, and the development of educational programs to introduce new techniques and skills.

In health care facilities where an affiliation with a formal educational program exists, educational staff supports the full-time program faculty by assisting in the bedside teaching and evaluation of students.

Whatever the focus, educational personnel must be well-trained, experienced, and able to transmit their knowledge to others. Capable RCPs should be given teaching roles if they are motivated to participate and are truly interested in providing quality educational experiences.

Equipment aides. Most departments employ one or more equipment aides. Equipment aides can fulfill many important tasks in an active respiratory care service that do not require the technical knowledge of a full-fledged RCP.

To make the most of valuable labor, nontechnical personnel can be employed and trained to perform duties such as the cleaning, **disinfection, sterilization,** and packaging of equipment; ordering, restocking, and delivery of supplies; simple equipment repair and maintenance; and basic clerical work. Many equipment aides are respiratory care students who work and learn on a part-time basis.

Nontraditional organization of services

There are two major concerns with the current traditional hospital structure: cost and quality. New, nontraditional ways of organizing services focus on both cost-efficiency and improved quality of patient care.

In terms of cost, hospitals are labor-intensive organizations. Typically, over 60% of a hospital's budget is devoted to personnel costs. Although driven by the large number of personnel a hospital usually employs, other factors contribute to these high personnel costs. First and foremost is the way traditional hospital services are delivered. For example, it is not unusual for 4–6 people to be involved with 20–30 different steps simply to draw a patient's blood and have it analyzed.

In terms of quality, the bureaucratic structure and specialized division of the hospital typically results in a fragmented approach to service delivery, with little essential teamwork and poor continuity of care.

To address these concerns, a new concept in hospital organization is evolving, called the *patient-focused hospital.* The five basic operating principles that underlie the operation of the patient-focused hospital are listed in the accompanying box.

The advantage of broadening the skills of providers was already discussed under the topic of cross-training. In terms of moving services, the patient-focused hospital will strive to have 80% or more of the personnel, equipment and supplies needed for patient care at the bedside or in the working unit. This would mean, for example, that RCPs (and radiographers, physical therapists, etc.) would be assigned to a patient care unit, and become part of that delivery team, as opposed to a member of a separate department. Moreover, when not providing respiratory care, this cross-trained individual might be starting IVs, performing phlebotomies, or conducting lab tests. Likewise, if the RCP is busy with one patient, the cross-trained nurse or physical therapist might provide basic respiratory care to another.

The patient-focused model also can simplify many of the processes normally required to provide patient care. Figure 2-2 compares the steps needed for a patient to receive a respiratory care treatment in the patient-focused model (with the RCP assigned as a unit team member) to those required in the traditional structure. Although the savings appears small (3 steps), multiplying the personnel time saved by thousands of similar procedures yields a large return. Of course, this frees up time that is better spent on direct patient care.

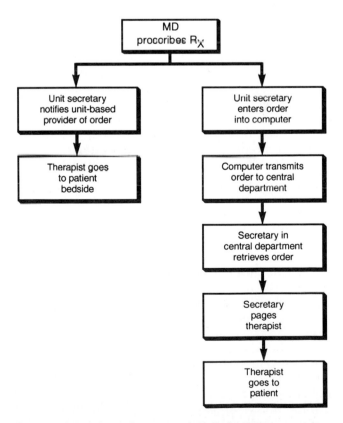

Fig. 2-2 Comparison of steps required for a patient to receive a nebulizer treatment in patient-focused (left) versus traditional hospital structure (right). (From: Snyder GM: Patient-focused hospitals: an opportunity for respiratory care practitioners, Respir Care 37(5):448–454, 1992.)

Basic operating principles in patient-focused hospital model

- Broadened skills of providers
- Move services closer to patient
- Simplify processes
- Streamline paperwork and eliminate duplication
- Focus patient populations

Source: Snyder GM: Patient-focused hospitals: an opportunity for respiratory care practitioners, Respir Care 37(5):448–454, 1992.

In terms of patient populations, the patient-focused approach emphasizes grouping of similar patients together. Of course, this structure already exists to some degree in most traditional hospitals (OB/Gyn, pediatrics, etc.). However, grouping in the patient-focused approach specifically aims to enhance quality by assuring that caregivers are adept at providing the particular type of services needed by that focused population.

Will the patient-focused model replace the traditionally organized hospital? If this new approach does in fact lower cost while simultaneously improving the quality of care, most hospitals will evolve in this direction. As yet, however, the jury is still out and it is simply too early to know.

DEPARTMENTAL OPERATION

Effective operation of a traditional respiratory care service must be guided by written policies and procedures and a clear delineation of patient care priorities. Written policies and procedures specify the scope and conduct of patient care services, including ways to respond to situations in which explicit instructions are lacking. Policy also must define service priority, according to patient need and medical staff expectations.

Policies and procedures

Of and by themselves, written policies and procedures do not assure quality. Obviously, policies and procedures must be carefully followed and executed by knowledgeable and dependable personnel. Nonetheless, without clear and explicit policies and procedures, consistent and high-quality care cannot be expected.

The respiratory care service policy and procedure manual specifies the scope and conduct of patient care services, as approved and regularly updated by the staff, under the guidance of the department's technical and medical directors.

Regarding specific procedures, the manual must specify who may perform the designated procedure, under what circumstances, and with what degree of supervision. Moreover, each procedure must describe the actions to be taken in case of adverse reactions. Last, the policy and procedure manual must provide guidance on how to respond to situations in which explicit instruction is lacking.

For staff and students, the department policy and procedure manual represents the primary technical and legal guide to service provision. Technically, these policies and procedures should represent state-of-the-art approaches to patients management, thereby providing a ready resource for effective clinical practice.

Legally, practitioners and students are obliged to follow these procedures under the conditions specified. Failure to follow the specifications can result in personal **liability,** especially if harm to a patient results from oversight or neglect (see Chapter 5).

Service priorities

Although there is no general rule for classifying patients according to need for respiratory care, the basic principles of **triage** must apply in establishing service priorities. The accompanying box suggests a priority scale to help respiratory care, medical, and nursing personnel set priorities of work assignments for respiratory care services.

This grouping represents a common-sense classification of patients from those most in need of attention to those least in need. The objective of such a scale is not to restrict the application of respiratory care services, but to enable the department to make maximum use of personnel. Proper assessment of the needs of patients determines the acuity of illness, such that the highest quality care can be given to those in greatest need.

Personnel requirements

The number of clinical personnel needed in a traditional respiratory care service varies according to the institution's bedsize, its **case mix,** and the utilization patterns of its attending physicians.

In determining manpower requirements, one must assess optimal workload per shift and monitor productivity levels. To create a uniform national system for collecting, reporting and comparing data, the American Association for Respiratory Care **(AARC)** has developed a series of uniform reporting guidelines. The AARC Uniform Reporting Manual identifies four primary areas of time usage for a respiratory care service (see box on page 23).

The uniform reporting system has now become the industry standard. It allows for an "apples-to-apples" comparison in an environment influenced by multiple factors. Total time for all clinical activities are calculated by multiplying each procedure by its assigned time standard. Then the user adds all the procedural

---

Suggested priorities of patient care
1. Emergency care (including resuscitation)
2. Continuous mechanical ventilation
3. Other intensive care services
4. Postoperative care
5. Oxygen administration
6. Prescheduled inpatient basic therapeutics
7. Elective inpatient diagnostic studies
8. Outpatient and ambulatory services

Areas of time usage for a respiratory care service

1. Clinical Activities With Time Standards
   Procedural activities which are consistent among surveyed hospitals. The time standards given to each procedure assumes one therapy or treatment per patient at a time, not multiple therapies on the same patient. The reporting system also assumes that the employee is doing only one activity at a time, not simultaneous administrations of therapy to more than one patient.
2. Clinical Activities Without Time Standards
   Activities that are unique to a specific hospital and may be difficult to project. Since most of these activities are billable, it is important to track and determine time requirements for each procedure. These activities can be useful in justifying staff and decision making regarding duty allocations.
3. Support Activities
   These activities include two major categories: Equipment and supplies, and management and supervisory.
   a. Equipment and Supplies—Activities dealing with equipment cleaning, maintenance, storage and acquisition.
   b. Management and Supervisory—These are fixed activities that do not vary as the volume of procedures performed increases or decreases. These activities must be closely controlled since they are usually not revenue-generating and will reduce the total productivity level for the department.
4. Non-Allocated Hours
   This area is designated for slack time which generally accounts for 6–8% of total time.

Source: AARC Uniform Reporting Manual, ed 3, Dallas, 1993, American Association for Respiratory Care.

---

times together to determine total work accomplished in hours.

The technical director can use workload hours as a means to estimate staffing needs on a per shift basis. It is important to note that the number of workload hours/FTE level varies from institution to institution. Determining optimal workloads and maintaining a balance of practitioners per shift to meet projected workload is key to achieving a productive department. The end result should be matching, as closely as possible, the number of personnel available per day to the anticipated workload.

Equipment and supplies

Health care reforms are increasing demands on provider institutions to contain costs. For this reason, both disposable supply and capital equipment expenditures are tightly controlled. In addition, all supplies and policies regarding their use are periodically reviewed to ensure the most cost-effective delivery of patient care.

In performing this review, the service manager must assess unit cost, disposable versus nondisposable product, specific need and application, and quality requirements. Policies governing disposable usage and the frequency an item should be replaced must be compared with current practice and literature. The manager's goal is to provide the least expensive cost per procedure without compromising the quality of patient care.

Of the major capital equipment, the largest and most expensive items are mechanical ventilators and pulmonary function testing equipment. Since there is no one "best" ventilator capable of serving all purposes, most departments select at least one primary general-duty system supplemented, as needed, by a smaller number of ventilators reserved for special duty, such as pediatric or **neonatal** application. This approach maintains consistency, lowers training costs, and reduces the likelihood of errors due to unfamiliarity with equipment.

The minimum equipment for the pulmonary laboratory consists of a spirometry system capable of measuring all standard lung volumes, capacities, and flows. Substantial long-term cost savings can be realized if such equipment provides computerized computation and reporting. Similarly, automated blood gas analysis equipment, besides providing more consistent results, saves personnel time in calibration, error determination, and troubleshooting.

Recordkeeping

Good records are the hallmark of a quality respiratory care service. Two general categories of records are maintained by a hospital and respiratory care service: patient records and financial (accounting) records. Patient records document the initiation, provision, and outcomes of the care provided by the respiratory care service. This information also provides a primary source of data for quality assurance monitoring (discussed in the next section). Financial records represent the business end of documentation, serving to ensure accurate patient billing and cost-accounting for services rendered.

Patient records

A patient's "chart" is the primary medical record. The chart represents the comprehensive, cumulative and legal documentation of the care provided throughout the hospital stay. Typical sections of a traditional patient record are listed in the box on page 24.

Admitting diagnosis and reimbursement. Under current methods of reimbursement for patient services, the admitting diagnosis of the patient is very important. Based on the admitting diagnosis, the

---

Typical sections of patient medical record
■ Admission data
■ History and physical information
■ Physicians' orders
■ Physician's progress notes
■ Nursing notes
■ Diagnostic test results
■ Therapy (respiratory care, physical therapy, etc.)

patient is assigned to a specific Diagnosis Related Group, or **DRG.** There are over 480 DRGs, grouped into about two dozen major diagnostic categories or **MDC**s. Table 2-2 lists the DRGs for MDC 4, Disorders of the Respiratory System.

For each DRG, the Health Care Financing Administration **(HCFA)** prospectively sets a reimbursement rate. Because the amount remains fixed for each admitting diagnosis, hospitals know in advance exactly how much reimbursement they will receive, both for a given admission and for their overall "case mix."

Hospitals that can provide care for less than the fixed rate can keep the difference, thereby realizing a "profit." On the other hand, hospitals whose cost of care exceeds the fixed rate must absorb the cost and thus take a financial loss. By placing hospitals at risk financially, this system provides a powerful incentive for cost-efficiency.

The primary factors determining hospital cost are acuity of care and length of stay (LOS). Since acuity cannot be directly controlled, most hospitals try to achieve cost-efficiency by minimizing length of stay. In addition, prevention of needless admissions (cases that can be handled effectively on an outpatient basis) can also help lower costs.

For the respiratory care department, this reimbursement system means that services must be rendered in the most cost-efficient manner possible. Specifically, respiratory care services must contribute to getting patients well as quickly as possible, thereby decreasing their length of stay. Typically, this practice has increased the intensity of services provided to patients. In addition, there is now greater emphasis on documenting the need for and results of respiratory care interventions (see subsequent discussion).

Respiratory care record. The respiratory care section of the patient's medical record must document: (1) the origin of prescribed treatments, (2) respiratory-related consultations, (3) actual service provided, and (4) evaluation of the results of intervention.

The respiratory care prescription. All respiratory care must be prescribed by a member of the hospital's medical staff. According to **JCAHO** standards, such orders must specify the type, frequency, and duration of treatment. Where applicable, the type and dosage

Table 2-2 Diagnosis related groups for major diagnostic category 4—disorders of the respiratory system

DRG Number	DRG Title
75 (Sur)	Major chest procedures
76 (Sur)	Other respiratory system or procedures with CC *
77 (Sur)	Other respiratory system or procedures without CC
78 (Med)	Pulmonary embolism
79 (Med)	Respiratory infections and inflammation, age >17, with CC
80 (Med)	Respiratory infections and inflammation, age >17 without CC
81 (Med)	Respiratory infections and inflammations, age 0 to 17
82 (Med)	Respiratory neoplasms
83 (Med)	Major chest trauma with CC
84 (Med)	Major chests trauma without CC
85 (Med)	Pleural effusion with CC
86 (Med)	Pleural effusion without CC
87 (Med)	Pulmonary edema and respiratory failure
88 (Med)	Chronic obstructive pulmonary disease
89 (Med)	Simple pneumonia and pleurisy, age >17 with CC
90 (Med)	Simple pneumonia and pleurisy, age >17 without CC
91 (Med)	Simple pneumonia and pleurisy, age 0 to 17
92 (Med)	Interstitial lung disease with CC
93 (Med)	Interstitial lung disease, without CC
94 (Med)	Pneumothorax with CC
95 (Med)	Pneumothorax without CC
96 (Med)	Bronchitis and asthma, age >17 with CC
97 (Med)	Bronchitis and asthma, age >17 without CC
98 (Med)	Bronchitis and asthma, age 0 to 17
99 (Med)	Respiratory signs and symptoms with CC
100 (Med)	Respiratory signs and symptoms without CC
101 (Med)	Other respiratory system diagnoses with CC
102 (Med)	Other respiratory system diagnoses without CC
475 (Med)	Respiratory system diagnosis with ventilator support
483 (Med)	Tracheostomy

* CC is complications or co-morbidity.

of medication, including the desired oxygen concentration, must also be provided.

For purposes of both progress monitoring and quality assurance, the prescription should also specify the goals and objectives of the respiratory care. Ideally, these goals and objectives should derive from a respiratory assessment of the patient, conducted by either the attending physician, medical director or trained RCPs. Further, these goals and objectives should provide the basis for a respiratory care plan, individualized according to patient needs.

Unfortunately, adding goals and objectives to the respiratory care order does not assure that the therapy is needed. To be cost-effective, all therapy must be justified and discontinued when no longer needed. Examples of medical policies governing the use of respiratory care services are provided in the accompanying box.

Many departments have implemented physician order forms to assist physicians in ordering and evaluating patients requiring respiratory care services (Figure 2-3 on page 26).

An alternative and increasingly popular alternative to the traditional prescription is the respiratory care protocol (also called Therapist-Driven Protocol, or **TDP**). Physicians have traditionally written orders for respiratory care services that were specific and allowed no variation by the RCP giving the treatment. Under this arrangement, if the patient's status changed, the ordering physician would be contacted to modify the order.

Recently, protocols have been developed that allow properly trained RCPs to independently initiate and adjust therapy, within guidelines previously established by the medical staff. The key elements required in a medically acceptable respiratory care protocol are listed in the accompanying box. An example of a respiratory care protocol algorithm appears in Figure 2-4 on page 27.

According to the American College of Chest Physicians, respiratory care protocols have the following advantages over traditional prescription-driven therapy:

1. Therapy can be adjusted more frequently in response to changes in patient status;
2. Physicians can still be contacted for major changes, but not minor adjustments, thus reducing nuisance calls;
3. Consistency of therapy can be maintained and nonpulmonary physicians can use appropriate up-to-date methods by simply requesting that protocol therapy be used;
4. RCPs become actively involved in achieving good patient outcomes instead of performing

---

Examples of medical policies governing the use of respiratory care services

1. The objective of the prescribed procedure must be documented
2. The desired outcome of the procedure, specific to the patient's condition, must be documented
3. The indications for therapy must be documented (examples include infiltrate on X-ray, abnormal PFT results, auscultation findings, etc.)
4. Results needed to discontinue or change therapy must be specified
5. Therapy must be reevaluated and reordered at periodic intervals, such as 72 hours

---

Elements of an acceptable respiratory care protocol

- Clearly stated objectives
- Outline of the protocol, including a decision tree or algorithm
- Description of alternative choices at decision and action points
- Description of potential complications and corrections
- Description of end-points and decision-points where the physician must be contacted

Source: American College of Chest Physicians, Respiratory Care Section Steering Committee, Chicago, Illinois, 10/27/92.

---

rigid tasks. This enhanced responsibility attracts and retains better educated and qualified practitioners.

Effective respiratory care protocols must be based on state-of-the-art scientific knowledge (and changed accordingly). Implementation requires strong medical director support, medical staff approval and confidence in the protocols, intensive education of RCPs, and frequent auditing of outcomes. Properly implemented, respiratory care protocols can enhance the quality of patient care by assuring timely, safe, and cost-effective therapy.

Documentation of care. Whether provided separately or incorporated into the general progress notes, there must be ongoing documentation of the respiratory care provided to patients. Such documentation must include the type of therapy provided, the date and time of administration, the effects of the therapy, and any adverse patient reactions. An example of a respiratory care progress note appears in Figure 2-5 on page 28.

Evaluation. In consultation with the respiratory care staff, the physician must provide timely and pertinent evaluation of the outcomes of respiratory care. Such evaluations help determine the need to continue, modify, or end a therapeutic regimen. Moreover, evaluation of the results of respiratory care can be used later in retrospective quality assurance audits.

Departmental records. Each respiratory care service maintains its own records, separate from the legal medical record of the patient. The departmental record system may be maintained either manually or on computer (see Chapter 8).

The departmental record system serves three purposes. First, it provides a portable or "in-the-room" charting system by which RCPs keep a short record for each patient under their care. Second, it is the basis for communicating essential patient information between staff members. Last, it provides the basis for departmental charges for patient services.

In addition to the required entries in the patient's

CHILDREN'S SPECIALIZED HOSPITAL

RESPIRATORY THERAPY ORDER FORM	PATIENT STAMP
ALL PERTINENT AREAS MUST BE COMPLETED BELOW	

Diagnosis _____

Specific Indication for Therapy _____

THERAPY

☐ Continuous Aerosol	☐ Oxygen Therapy	☐ Chest Physical Therapy	☐ Mechanical Ventilation	☐ Special Procedures

THERAPY OBJECTIVES

| ☐ Humidify Airway
☐ Reverse Hypoxemia
☐ Relief of Mucosal
☐ Edema | ☐ Reverse Hypoxemia

_____ Room Air PaO$_2$
Goal | ☐ Achieve Airway Patency

☐ Mobilize Secretions | Mode _____
Rate _____
Peep/Cpap_____
PIP_____
Sigh _____
Tidal Volume_____
Flowrate _____
Inspiratory Time _____
I:E Ratio _____
☐ Continuous
Other:_____ | ☐ Arterial Blood Gas
☐ Capillary Blood Gas
☐ Incentive Spirometer
      Frequency _____
☐ Assess PaO^2 Level
☐ F$_1$O$_2$ / Device Change |

FREQUENCY

| ☐ Continuous

☐ For _____ Hours | ☐ Continuous

☐ For _____ Hours | ☐ QID ☐ TID
☐ BID ☐ QD
☐ Q ___ Hour
☐ While Awake Only | | ☐ Bedside Pulmonary
      Spirometry
☐ Peak Flow
☐ End Tidal CO2
      Frequency _____ hrs. |

SPECIAL INSTRUCTIONS

| GAS MIXTURE
☐ Room Air
☐ Heated
☐ Cool
DEVICE
☐ Aerosol Mask
☐ Trach Collar
☐ "T" Piece
☐ Mist Tent
☐ Oxyhood
☐ Other: | GAS MIXTURE
☐ _____ LPM Oxygen
☐ _____ % Oxygen
☐
DEVICE
☐ Nasal Cannula
☐ Venturi Mask
☐ Simple Mask
☐ Partial Rebreather
☐ Non-rebreather
☐ Other: | Anterior   Posterior
R   L   L   R

Circle Lobe To Be Treated:
1 Rt Upper   6 Lt Upper
2 Rt Middle   7 Lt Lower
3 Rt Lower   8 Rt Upper
4 Lt Upper   9 Rt Lower
5 Lt Lower | ☐ Sputum Culture
☐ Suction
   ☐ Q___ Hours
   ☐ With Treatment

☐ Pulse Oximetry
☐ Keep Sats Greater Than___
☐ Continuous x _____ hours |

MEDICATION

| ☐ Proventil
   _____ mg= _____ ml
☐ Intal
   _____ mg= _____ ml
☐ Normal Saline
   _____ mg= _____ ml
☐ Other
   _____ mg= _____ ml | FREQUENCY

☐ Increase/Decrease
   Q _____ Hour
☐ While Awake Only
☐ Other _____
☐ STAT | OBJECTIVES

☐ Reverse Bronchospasm
☐ Improve Distribution of Ventilation
_____
☐ Aerosol Tx
☐ MDI |

Other: _____
_____
_____
_____
_____

Physician Signature: _____ Date _____ Time _____

Date: _____ Time: _____ Nurses Signature: _____

Date: _____ Time: _____ Therapist Signature: _____

CHILDREN'S SPECIALIZED HOSPITAL   DEPARTMENT OF RESPIRATORY THERAPY   FORM#730-005 REV. 7/92
MEDICAL RECORDS

Fig. 2-3 Examples of respiratory therapy order form (Courtesy Children's Specialized Hospital.)

comprehensive medical record, the RCP enters all treatments or services for a given day on the departmental record card or chart. At the end of the shift, charges for each service rendered are submitted manually to the accounting office or entered into the computer information system.

Accounting records

From the accumulated departmental records and charges, data is obtained for purposes of both patient discharge billing and statistical accounting of the respiratory care service activities.

Statistical accounting of respiratory care service

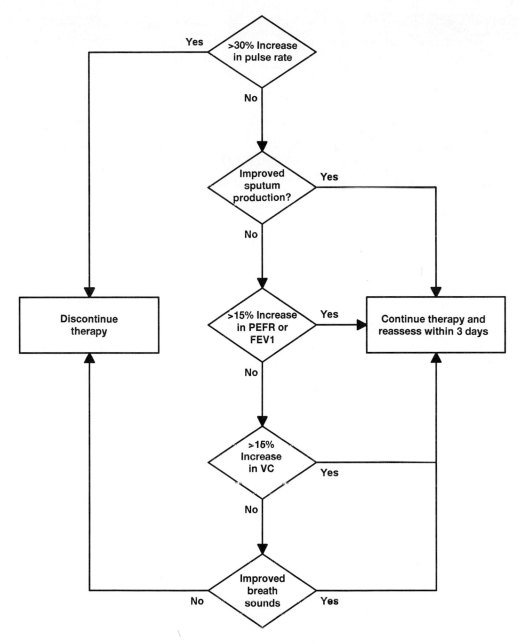

Fig. 2-4 Example of a respiratory care protocol algorithm for aerosol bronchodilator therapy. From Smoker JM: A protocol to assess and administer aerosol bronchodilator therapy, Respir Care 31:780–785, 1986.

activities may involve periodic (daily, weekly, monthly, quarterly, and/or yearly) tabulation of the number and types of patients treated, the number of days patients have received treatment, the number of services, and patient charges according to the type of service provided.

More recently, statistical accounting of respiratory care service activities provides comparative data by admitting DRG. Such comparative data may include respiratory costs as a percentage of total costs for a given DRG, mean length of stay (LOS) as compared to national or regional norms, and even a comparison of

DRG costs and mean LOS to other hospitals. Moreover, new computerized information systems are providing the capability to compare DRG **morbidity** and **mortality** statistics within or among hospitals, and according to the admitting physician or surgeon.

Although such statistical portrayals have limitations, the merger of patient and cost accounting data is becoming a reality for health care facilities in general, and respiratory care services in particular. Rather than perceiving such an orientation as a threat, progressive respiratory care services use this data to improve both cost-efficiency and quality.

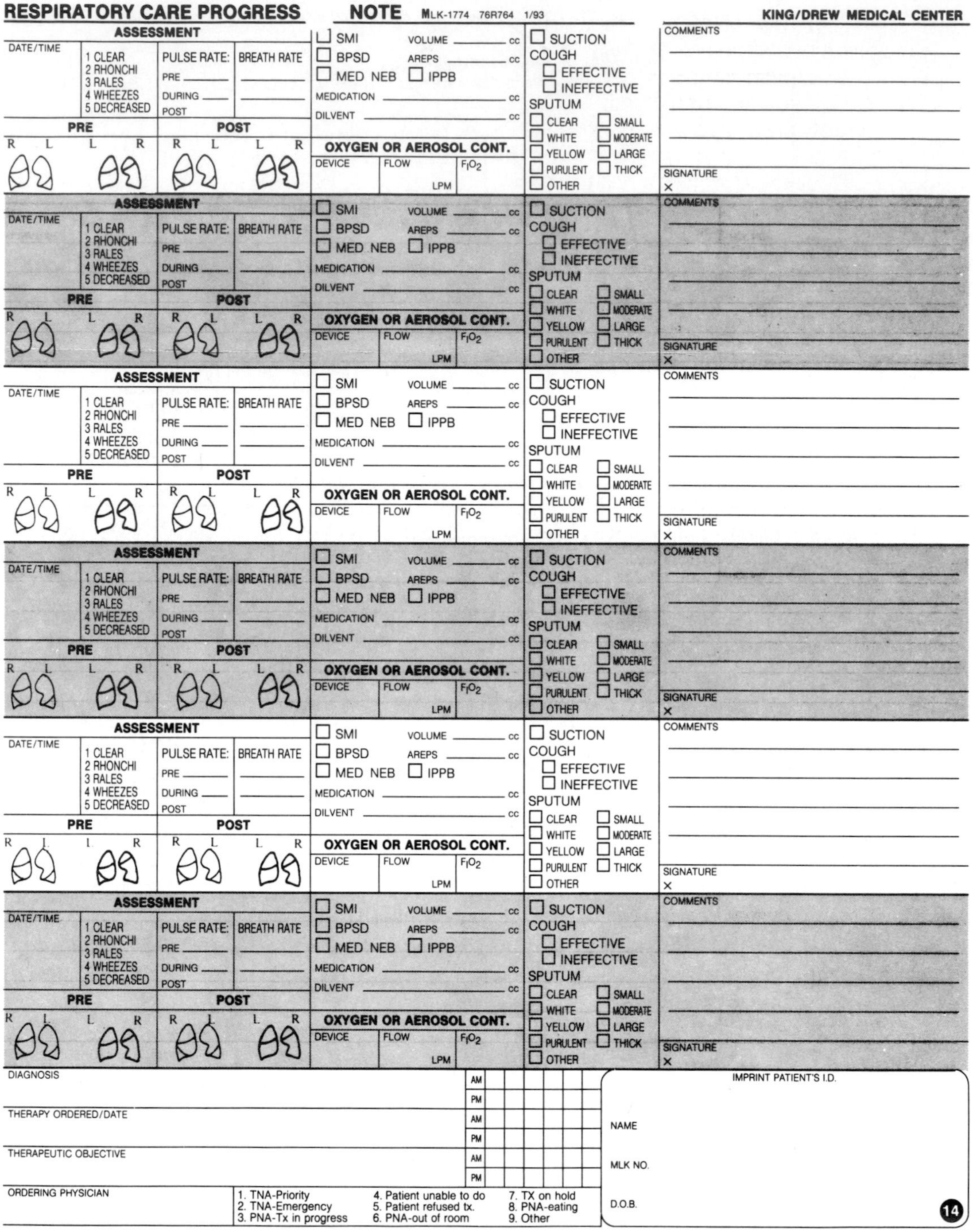

Fig. 2-5 Example of respiratory care progress note form (Courtesy King Drew Medical Center.)

STANDARDS OF CARE AND QUALITY IMPROVEMENT

Standards for respiratory care services

Accreditation standards for hospitals are set by the Joint Commission on Accreditation of Healthcare Organizations (JCAHO). Until recently, JCAHO standards were organized around the structure of a hospital's departments and services. For example, for each hospital service department, like respiratory care, JCAHO established a set of specific standards. Most of these department standards focused on assuring the adequacy of personnel and material resources, and the appropriateness and availability of services.

During the early 1990s, the JCAHO began switching to a more performance or outcome-oriented system. To be fully implemented in 1995, this system will focus on the ability of the total organization to provide high-quality, cost effective and integrated patient care. With full implementation, most department-specific standards will be eliminated. Instead, accreditation will emphasize organization-wide efforts at continuous quality improvement **(CQI)** of patient services, using specific objective indicators. For example, a proposed infection control indicator is the proportion of mechanically ventilated patients who develop pneumonia. Such an indicator clearly cuts across services and departments, thereby requiring a team approach to assure quality.

Quality improvement

Despite increased emphasis on cost containment, quality care remains the first goal of hospitals and respiratory care services. CQI is an ongoing process designed to detected and correct factors hindering the provision of quality and cost-effective health care.

Figure 2-6 provides a basic flowchart of the continuous quality improvement cycle, as recommended by the JCAHO. The accompanying box lists the current JCAHO standards for improving organizational performance.

Organization of a quality improvement program

Table 2-3, page 30 outlines the key responsibilities of various levels of staff needed to implement an organization-wide quality improvement program. Overall authority and responsibility for a hospital's quality improvement program rests with its board of directors. Normally, the board delegates its authority to the medical and administrative staffs, through a

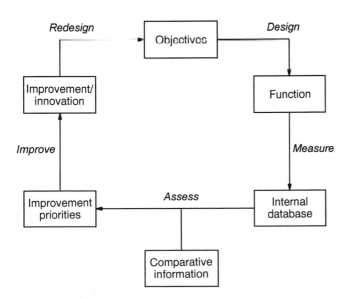

Fig. 2-6 Flowchart for continuous quality improvement as recommended by the Joint Commission on Accreditation of Healthcare Organizations (JCAHO).

JCAHO standards for improving organizational performance

PI.1 The organization has a planned, systematic, organization-wide approach to designing, measuring, assessing, and improving its performance

PI.2 New processes are designed well

PI.3 The organization has a systematic process in place to collect data needed to:
- Design and assess new processes;
- Assess the dimensions of performance relevant to functions, processes, and outcomes;
- Measure the level of performance and stability of important existing processes;
- Identify areas for possible improvement of existing processes; and
- Determine whether changes improved the processes.

PI.4 The organization has a systematic process to assess collected data in order to determine:
- Whether design specifications for new processes were met;
- The level of performance and stability of important existing processes;
- Priorities for possible improvement of existing processes;
- Actions to improve the performances of processes; and
- Whether changes in the processes resulted in improvement.

PI.5 The organization systematically improves its performance by improving existing processes.

Source: Joint Commission on Accreditation of Healthcare Organizations: 1994 accreditation manual for hospitals, Volume I: standards, Oakbrook Terrace, IL, 1993, Joint Commission on Accreditation of Healthcare Organizations.

---

facility-wide CQI committee. This committee develops general policies and objectives for the overall quality improvement effort, and monitors and evaluates implementation across departments. Sources of data that the CQI committee may use are described in the box on page 31.

In the traditionally organized hospital, each service department, in turn, develops a quality improvement program consistent with the institution's general objectives. To carry out these efforts at the department level, a departmental coordinator and committee are desirable.

For the respiratory care service department, quality improvement activities must focus on identifying and resolving problems related to patient care and clinical performance. According to the American Association for Respiratory Care's (AARC) Standards Committee, ultimate authority for the continued development and practice of quality improvement within a respiratory care service must lie with the medical director.

The departmental committee develops and carries its quality improvement plan. According to the

Table 2-3   Quality Improvement Responsibilities

Category of Staff	Responsibilities
Administration/ board of directors	Ensure presence and implementation of a planned systematic process for monitoring, evaluation, and problem solving.
	Analyze and receive reports regarding quality of services at least annually.
	Allocate adequate resources to establish and maintain an organization-wide CQI program.
	Evaluate the organization's performance.
	Undertake education concerning the approaches and methods of quality improvement.
Facility's CQI department or committee	Develop planned systematic process to evaluate organizational activities.
	Receive CQI reports from all departments at least annually, summarize findings, and report to the administration.
	Investigate employee incidents as appropriate.
	Initiate risk management program in response to needs for same.
	Assist in resolving organizational complaints when requested.
	Provide consultative guidance regarding the organization's CQI activities.
	Assist in the development of policies and procedures in response to information provided by CQI reports.
	Tabulate CQI findings received from department reviews and evaluative surveys; summarize results; and provide data and recommendations to senior management and facility personnel annually or as indicated.
	Develop additional aspects of care, criteria, and performance goals for the organization as appropriate.
Department manager	Ensure that the department's CQI plan is developed and implemented, and involves all department personnel.
	Modify the overall evaluative effort to ensure manageability in terms of manpower and resources.
	Develop additional topics, criteria, and performance goals that are relevant to the local setting in conjunction with the medical director.
	Implement elective surveys in accordance with the deparment's policy for same. Respond expediently to issues associated with patient safety, accreditation, government regulations, professional liability, and economics.
	Assign personnel as needed to participate in quality improvement activities. Submit CQI findings to facility CQI committee.
	Schedule staff development activities to discuss CQI findings and initiate corrective plan in response to noted deficiencies.
Patient care department staff	Seek to achieve standards set by the organization.
	Administer procedures in accordance with protocol.
	Identify opportunities for improving service and/or delivery and report same to supervisory staff.
	Assist with the development of action plans to resolve noted deficiencies.
	Initiate corrective actions to resolve deficiencies noted in CQI review.
	Adhere to personnel and documentation standards that are specified in the organization's policies.
	Notify management and/or supervisory staff of aberrations in quality.
	Participate in staff development activities as indicated.
Department's CQI committee	Meet to review the department's services.
	Obtain required quality indicators:
	Reports
	Statistical data
	Logs
	Satisfaction surveys
	Evaluative surveys
	Patient record review summaries
	Analyze data.
	Monitor follow-up activities.
	Report findings in accordance with reporting standards.

AARC's Standards Committee, the goals of a respiratory care quality improvement plan should include at least the following:

1. To provide a method for ongoing monitoring both the quality and appropriateness of respiratory care;

2. To assure that respiratory care methods and procedures are cost-efficient;

3. To assure that respiratory care methods and procedures are effective;

4. To identify, rank, and resolve patient care-related problems;

Sources of data for continuous quality improvement

1. Incident Reports. An incident reporting system must be in place to ensure that potential and experienced injury situations/incidents are automatically and immediately reported. These situations/incidents would include patient-sustained injury from equipment or adverse treatment outcome, a protocol deviation possibly endangering the safety and welfare of a patient, an employee-sustained injury while on the job, and patient service complaints. All incident reports should be formally documented individually and reviewed for proposed problem resolution. These reviews should also be documented in a summary format and reported in the department CQI report.
2. Performance Standards Compliance Evaluations. Mock regulatory audits should be performed periodically to ensure all standards are met. Audit results and areas in need of improvement should be reported to the CQI committee with information regarding current corrective actions in progress.
3. Safety Inspection Surveys. Health care facilities periodically conduct safety inspections to prevent fire and ensure that safe practices are strictly enforced. The findings of these inspections should be reported to the CQI committee, with actions for improvement or correction.
4. Medical Record Reviews. Periodic (usually monthly) chart audits are conducted by department managers to assess compliance with documentation policy and procedures. These chart audits include review of the following:
   a. Physician order completeness
   b. Documentation of therapeutic objectives and desired outcomes
   c. Practitioner documentation completeness
   d. Diagnostic results flowcharts
   e. Ordered procedures and frequency compared to charged procedures
   The complete review of all documentation inspected should be reported to CQI.
5. Elective Surveys. Elective surveys based on high volume, high risk or problem-prone services.
6. Random CQI Audits. Audits are often conducted by CQI committee members of all departments to ensure the CQI plan is ongoing and correctly maintained. Again, report the findings of these audits to the CQI committee.
7. Communication Log Review. It is important to maintain open and documented communication with all staff members regarding patient care services. Communication must be two-way and include policy changes, identified problems with proposed solutions, in-service notification and information, etc. Highlights of communication recorded by both management and staff in the communication log should be reported to the CQI committee.
8. External Quality Reviews/Audits (State and JCAHO Surveys). Any formal inspections should be reported with specific details and findings to the CQI committee. The committee should support and advise the department manager on any revisions or policy changes that should be carried out as a result of said findings. The CQI committee must serve as an advisory committee to each department on an ongoing basis to ensure the best course of action is always taken to improve quality.
9. Financial Review. Recently, many CQI committees are including financial reviews and cost reduction plans as part of their total review. This review mechanism is to ensure that the quality of care is not adversely effected as a result of cost reduction actions.

---

5. To develop, carry out and monitor intervention strategies aimed at problem resolution; and
6. To evaluate the respiratory care quality improvement plan at least annually, and to revise it as necessary.

Quality improvement procedures in respiratory care

As recommended by the AARC Standards Committee, nine key steps are needed to systematically implement a quality improvement plan. As depicted in Figure 2-7, page 32 these steps include: the identification of problem(s), the determination of problem cause(s), the ranking of problems, the development of strategies for problem resolution, the development of appropriate measurement techniques, the implementation of problem resolution strategies, the analysis of intervention results, the reporting of results, and the ongoing evaluation of intervention outcomes.

Successful implementation of the quality improvement plan demands that the respiratory care service develop criteria addressing the therapeutic goals, appropriateness, and means of evaluating the effectiveness of each specific high-utilization and high-risk procedure. The box on page 32 provides an example of such criteria for oxygen therapy.

Problem identification. Using the quality improvement process just described, various data sources, including the patient's medical record, would be used to determine the extent to which oxygen therapy services are being appropriately used.

Normally, an objective problem indicator, such as "90% of all patients receiving oxygen therapy will meet the appropriateness of care criteria" is helpful in problem identification. If the indicator is not being met (e.g., if only 70% of the patients meet the appropriateness of therapy criteria), a problem exists.

Determining causes. Once a problem has been identified, its cause must be determined. For example, the fact that only 70% of the patients receiving oxygen

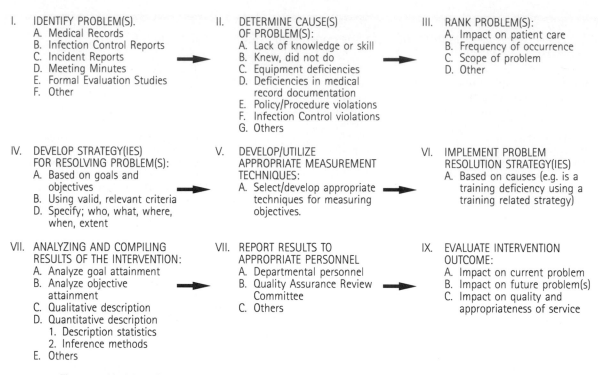

I. IDENTIFY PROBLEM(S).
A. Medical Records
B. Infection Control Reports
C. Incident Reports
D. Meeting Minutes
E. Formal Evaluation Studies
F. Other

II. DETERMINE CAUSE(S) OF PROBLEM(S):
A. Lack of knowledge or skill
B. Knew, did not do
C. Equipment deficiencies
D. Deficiencies in medical record documentation
E. Policy/Procedure violations
F. Infection Control violations
G. Others

III. RANK PROBLEM(S):
A. Impact on patient care
B. Frequency of occurrence
C. Scope of problem
D. Other

IV. DEVELOP STRATEGY(IES) FOR RESOLVING PROBLEM(S):
A. Based on goals and objectives
B. Using valid, relevant criteria
D. Specify; who, what, where, when, extent

V. DEVELOP/UTILIZE APPROPRIATE MEASUREMENT TECHNIQUES:
A. Select/develop appropriate techniques for measuring objectives.

VI. IMPLEMENT PROBLEM RESOLUTION STRATEGY(IES)
A. Based on causes (e.g. is a training deficiency using a training related strategy)

VII. ANALYZING AND COMPILING RESULTS OF THE INTERVENTION:
A. Analyze goal attainment
B. Analyze objective attainment
C. Qualitative description
D. Quantitative description
   1. Description statistics
   2. Inference methods
E. Others

VII. REPORT RESULTS TO APPROPRIATE PERSONNEL
A. Departmental personnel
B. Quality Assurance Review Committee
C. Others

IX. EVALUATE INTERVENTION OUTCOME:
A. Impact on current problem
B. Impact on future problem(s)
C. Impact on quality and appropriateness of service

Fig. 2-7 Model respiratory care quality assurance plan flow chart (Redrawn from Hastings D: The AARC's model quality assurance plan. AARC Times 12(2):25, 1988.)

therapy meet the specified criteria may result from factors such as the ordering physicians' lack of knowledge of the criteria, their failure to follow known criteria, or their failure to discontinue therapy when indicated.

Resolving identified problems. Once the underlying cause is identified, a strategy to resolve the problem must be developed, implemented and evaluated. For example, if the problem with oxygen therapy use is based on the new medical residents' failure to follow the appropriateness of care criteria, proper orientation and/or in-service education may be needed. Once conducted, the impact of the selected strategy on the desired outcome should be assessed. Ideally, evaluation of the outcomes of intervention should be based on the initial problem indicator. For example, we

---

Quality assurance criteria for oxygen therapy*

Therapeutic goals:

1. To prevent or reverse hypoxemia and tissue hypoxia
2. To decrease myocardial work
3. To decrease the work of breathing

Appropriateness of care

1. The patient must be diagnosed as having or being at risk of developing hypoxemia and/or tissue hypoxia; or
2. The patient must be diagnosed as having suffered a myocardial infarction within the last 72 hours; and
3. Oxygen dosing and mode of therapy will follow the criteria specified in the Respiratory Care Service Policy and Procedure Manual.

Evaluation of the effectiveness of therapy

The effectiveness of therapy will be evaluated by comparing the pre-treatment and post-treatment status of the patient according to the following criteria (at least one must apply):

1. Increase in PaO_2 or in arterial saturation; or
2. Reversal or absence of cyanosis; or
3. Decrease in heart rate; or
4. Decrease in blood pressure; or
5. Decrease or absence of cardiac dysrhythmias; or
6. Decrease in respiratory rate; or
7. Increase in level of consciousness; or
8. Decrease in carboxyhemoglobin saturation; or
9. Relief of dyspnea.

*Adapted from Larson, K.: The well-defined quality assurance plan, AARC Times, 12(2): 15–24, 1988.

would want to know whether the in-service education program for the medical residents increased the percentage of patients meeting the appropriateness criteria.

Reporting and ongoing monitoring. Problem identification and resolution activities, including the relative success of intervention strategies, must be documented and reported regularly. Moreover, even successful interventions must be monitored over time to assure that a given problem does not recur. Only in this manner can the respiratory care service ensure that its services are appropriately utilized and effective in meeting patient needs.

CHAPTER SUMMARY

Respiratory care services play a vital role in comprehensive and acute health care. A quality respiratory care department is organized under medical and technical directorship to provide a broad range of services, according to both patient and staff needs. In order to ensure that these services are both efficiently delivered and effective in achieving desired patient outcomes, the service must have appropriate performance standards, adequately trained personnel, and state-of-the-art equipment.

Moreover, the operation of the service must be guided by clear and comprehensive policies and procedures. Last, the respiratory care service must be an active partner in organization-wide efforts to assure optimum and cost-effective care. Advancements in technology notwithstanding, the ability of a respiratory care service to provide quality and cost-effective care rest primarily on the shoulders of a dedicated and committed professional staff.

BIBLIOGRAPHY

American Association for Respiratory Care: Respiratory Care Uniform Reporting Manual, ed 3, Dallas, 1993, American Association for Respiratory Care.

American Association for Respiratory Therapy, Administrative standards for respiratory care services and personnel (official statement), *Respir Care* 28(8):1033–1038, 1983.

American College of Chest Physicians, Respiratory Care Section Steering Committee: Position paper: Respiratory care protocols (Position paper), Chicago, 1992, American College of Chest Physicians.

Bartow SL: Quality assurance: A good management tool for respiratory care services, *AART Times,* 6(12): 26–30, 1982.

Bunch D: Restructuring hospitals for the future, *AARC Times* 16(3):29–36, 1992.

Bunch D: CQI concept leads to successful restructuring at OHSU, *AARC Times* 17(7):54–55, 1993.

Bunch D: Iowa Methodist, experiments with clinical pathways, *AARC Times* 17(7):58, 1993.

Burns R: Quality Assessment Improvement Plan, Primedica, 1993.

Crockett RJ: Quality assurance: Setting up department goals, *AART Times,* 6(12): 20–22, 24–25, 1982.

Durren M: Strategies for quality assurance in the respiratory care department, Mich Soc Respir Therap J 17(1): 3–6, 1983.

Elliott CG: Quality assurance for respiratory care services: a computer-assisted program, *Respir Care* 38(1):54–59, 1993.

Falck S: ECG testing as a function of the respiratory therapy department, *Respir Ther* 13(5):37–8, 42, 44, 1983.

Fink JB, Fink AK: The respiratory therapist as manager, Chicago, 1986, Mosby.

Greenway L, Jeffs M, Turner K: Computerized management of respiratory care. *Respir Care* 38(1):42–53, 1993.

Gulliford D, Sherman J: Respiratory-ECG services department, Memorial Hospital of Union County, Ohio. *Respir Ther* 12(5):133–136, 1982.

Hastings D: The AARC's model quality assurance plan, *AARC Times,* 12(2): 26–26, 28–33, 1988.

Joint Commission on Accreditation of Healthcare Organizations: 1994 accreditation manual for hospitals, Oakbrook Terrace, IL, 1993, Joint Commission on Accreditation of Healthcare Organizations.

Kipp LJ: Practical aspects of quality assurance, *Respir Ther* 13(5):47–50, 1983.

Larson K: The well-defined quality assurance plan, *AARC Times,* 12(2): 15–24, 1988.

Luquire R: St. Luke's Episcopal Hospital practices outcomes management, *AARC Times* 17(7):62–64, 1993.

Mark ML, Sharke KL: Therapy evaluation protocol as a management technique, *Respir Ther* 13(1):67–69, 1983.

McCarthy TP, Yaculak G: Organizing RC services for efficient patient care and cost containment, *AARC Times* 17(12):46–51, 1993.

McLaughlin AJ: Organization and management for respiratory therapists, St. Louis, 1979, Mosby.

Miller WF, et al.: Guidelines for organization and function of hospital respiratory care services: section on respiratory therapy, American College of Chest Physicians, *Chest,* 78:1, 1980.

Monaghan EJ: The UMMS clinical practice ladder, *AARC Times* 17(12):49, 1993.

Rakich JS, Longest BB, O'Donovan T: Managing health care organizations, Philadelphia, 1977, WB Saunders.

Ritz RH: The modern respiratory care department, In: Burton GG, Hodgkin JE, Ward JJ, Eds: Respiratory Care: A Guide to Clinical Practice. 3 ed. Philadelphia: JB Lippincott; 1991.

Sabo J: Reshaping hospitals for the future: hospital restructuring and respiratory care, *AARC Times* 17(7):46–47, 1993.

Sabo J, Milligan S: Clarkson ventures into "new world" of patient-focused care, *AARC Times* 17(7):48–52, 1993.

Scanlan CL: The prospective payment system: What you see is what you get, *Pul Med Tech* 1(5): 19–34, 1984.

Shaffran-Larson K, Eiserman J: Utilization of alternate staff patterns as a cost-effective measure. *Respir Ther* 10(6):121–126, 1980.

Snyder GM: Patient-focused hospitals: an opportunity for respiratory care practitioners, *Respir Care* 37(5):448–454, 1992.

St. Pierre R: A four-day workweek. A retrospective evaluation. *Respir Ther* 13(5):53–4, 1983.

Yanda RL: The need for leadership in hospital respiratory services, *Chest,* 68:81, 1975.

3

Patient Safety, Communication and Recordkeeping

■

Craig L. Scanlan

Robin A. Harvan

CHAPTER LEARNING OBJECTIVES

1. Describe the basic safety considerations involved in patient care, including patient movement and ambulation, and electrical and fire safety.
2. Define the importance of communication as related to patient care and professional performance and job satisfaction.
3. Identify the basic components of communication and factors that affect communication effectiveness.
4. Identify ways to improve your interpersonal communication skills.
5. Identify the key components of a medical record and the RCP's responsibilities in recordkeeping.

Respiratory Care Practitioners (RCPs) share general responsibilities for providing safe and effective patient care with other members of the health care team. These responsibilities include basic patient safety and medical recordkeeping. In addition to performing these technical skills, all health professional must be able to effectively communicate with each other, and with their patients and patients' families. The purpose of this chapter is to provide the foundation skills needed to effectively assume these general aspects of patient care.

SAFETY CONSIDERATIONS

Patient safety must always be the first consideration in respiratory care. Although the RCP does not usually have full control over the patient's environment, efforts must be made to minimize safety hazards and patient risks whenever possible. The key areas of potential risk common to most patients receiving respiratory care are: (1) patient movement and ambulation, (2) electrical hazards, and (3) fire hazards.

Patient movement and ambulation

Basic body mechanics

Posture is the relationship of the body parts to each other both in a resting state and in activity states. Good posture is necessary for psychological, physiological, and safety reasons. Improper posture may affect appearance and place inappropriate stress on certain bones, muscles, and organs. Good body mechanics are the postures patients and practitioners should use in various activities to minimize the likelihood of injury.

Figure 3-1 illustrates the correct and incorrect body mechanics for lifting a heavy object. Figure 3-2 applies this concept to lifting and moving a patient.

Moving the patient in bed

Conscious people assume positions in bed that are the most comfortable for them. For example, patients with acute or chronic respiratory dysfunction often assume a high Fowler position, with arms flexed and thorax leaning forward. This position helps them achieve maximal inhalation with a minimum of effort. In other cases, however, patients may be required to assume certain positions for therapeutic reasons. Good examples of situations requiring special positioning are neurosurgical patients and patients with hip replacements.

Figure 3-3 demonstrates the correct technique for lateral movement of a bedbound patient. Figure 3-4 illustrates the ideal method for moving a conscious patient toward the head of a bed. Last, Figure 3-5 shows the proper technique for assisting a patient to the bedside position for dangling of legs or transfer to a chair.

Ambulation

Ambulation (walking) is required to maintain normal body function. Bed rest, even with appropriate movement exercises, produces many bad effects. Progressive ambulation for a hospitalized patient should

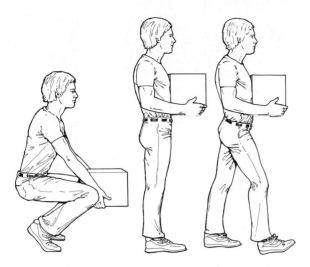

Fig. 3-1 Body mechanics for lifting and carrying objects.

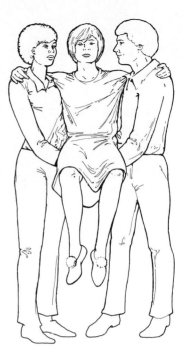

Fig. 3-2 Carrying technique for patient able to sit.

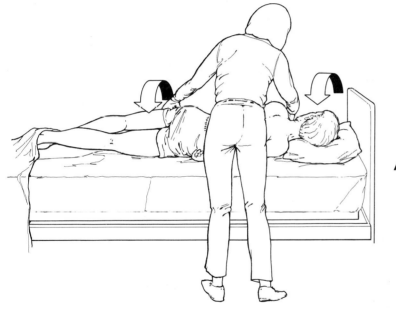

A

Fig. 3-3, A, Method to pull bed patient. **B,** Method to push bed patient.

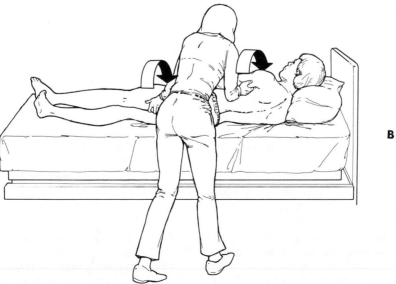

B

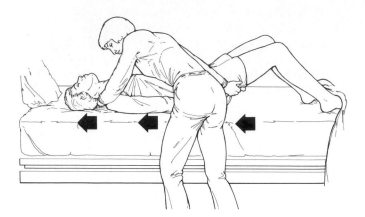

Fig. 3-4 Method to move patient up in bed with patient's assistance.

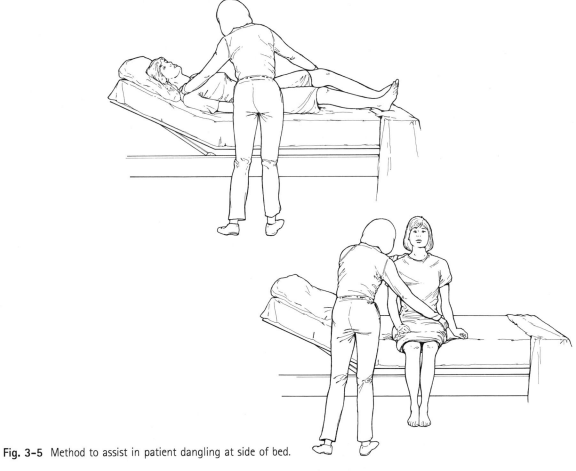

Fig. 3-5 Method to assist in patient dangling at side of bed.

be approached in an orderly and safe fashion by all health team members.

Ambulation is initiated if the patient is physiologically stable and free of severe pain. Thus the patient must be assessed before he or she undertakes ambulation. The most critical factors required for ambulation are stable vital signs and absence of severe pain.

Safe patient movement includes the following steps:

1. Placing the bed in a low position and locking its wheels;
2. Placing all equipment close to the patient to prevent dislodging during ambulation (e.g., **IV** equipment, nasogastric tube, surgical drainage tubes);
3. Moving the patient toward the nearest side of bed;
4. Assisting the patient to sit up in bed (i.e., arm

under nearest shoulder and one under farthest armpit);

5. Placing one hand under the patient's farthest knee and gradually rotating the patient so that the legs are dangling off the bed;

6. Letting the patient remain in this dangling position until dizziness or lightheadedness lessons (encouraging the patient to look forward rather than look at the floor may help);

7. Assisting the patient to a standing position;

8. Encouraging the patient to breathe easily and unhurriedly during this initial change to a standing posture;

9. Walking with the patient using no, minimal, or moderate support (moderate support requires the assistance of *two* practitioners, one on each side of the patient); and

10. Limiting walking to 5 to 10 minutes for the first exercise.

The patient must be monitored during ambulation. The RCP should note the patient's level of consciousness, color, breathing, strength or weakness, and complaints throughout the activity. The RCP should make sure that chairs are present so that emergency seats are available if the patient becomes uncomfortable. Patients must be encouraged to ambulate better until no assistance is required.

Electrical safety

With the production of new electrical equipment in hospitals, the potential for electrical accidents has multiplied.[1,2] These problems have been compounded by the fact that invasive devices such as internal catheters and pacemakers make patients more susceptible to electric shock. Because respiratory care often involves use of electrical devices in or around electrically susceptible patients, RCPs must understand the fundamentals of electrical safety.[3,4]

Physiological effects of electrical current

Current is the primary factor determining the effect of a shock.[5] Voltage and resistance are important only because they determine how much current flows.

The harmful effects of electrical current depend on: (1) the amount of current flowing through the body, (2) the duration for which this current is applied, and (3) the path the current takes through the body.

For example, as long as a person is insulated by normal clothing and shoes and is in a dry environment, a 120 V shock may hardly be felt. However, if the same person was standing without shoes on a wet floor, the same voltage could be fatal. This difference is due to differences in the resistance to current and thus the amount of current that actually flows through the body. In the first case, resistance is high; thus current flow through the body is low. In the second situation, resistance is low, and the current flow is dangerously high.

A shock hazard exists only if the electrical "circuit" through the body is complete. Even when a voltage is applied to an internal conductor, a current will not flow unless there is a second conductor to complete the circuit. Therefore, *two* electrical connections to the body are required for a person to receive a shock. In electrical devices, these connections typically consist of a "hot" wire and a "neutral" wire. The neutral wire completes the circuit by taking the electrical current to a *ground*. A ground is simply a low-resistance pathway to a point of zero voltage, such as the earth (thus the term ground).

Figure 3-6 shows how a circuit can be created for current flow through the body. In this case, a piece of electrical equipment is connected to AC line power by way of a standard three-prong plug. However, unknown to the practitioner, the cord has a broken ground wire. Normally, current leakage from the equipment would flow back to the ground through the ground wire. However, this pathway is not available.

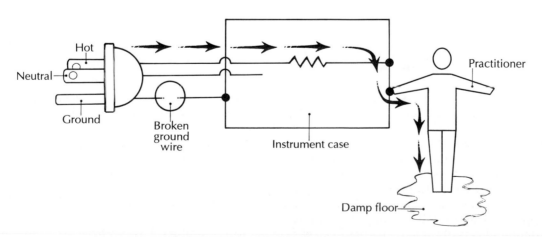

Fig. 3-6 Hazard created by broken ground wire.

■ MINI C LINI ■

3-1

Patient safety

Problem—An RCP is caring for a patient on a mechanical ventilator which requires both electrical and pneumatic power for operation. When the RCP touches the metal frame of the ventilator, a shock is felt. How should the RCP handle the situation based on this observation?

Discussion—All therapeutic instruments used in patient care, including mechanical ventilators, should be connected to grounded outlets (three wire) to prevent the dangerous build-up of voltage which can occur on the metal frames of some electrically powered equipment. Since the ground wire is only a protection device and not part of the main circuit, equipment may continue to operate without the clinician being aware that a problem exists. Since the RCP observed a shock or tingling sensation when touching the metal frame of the ventilator, this may very well represent an improper grounding situation and possible serious electrical current leak. In this situation, the RCP should immediately have the equipment taken out of service and temporarily provide manual ventilation with a resuscitation bag and oxygen until a replacement ventilator is available. It is important for all electrical equipment used in patient care to be routinely checked for appropriate grounding.

Instead, the leakage current finds a path of low resistance through the practitioner to the damp flow (an ideal ground).

Once such a path is established, the direction the electrical current takes through the body will determine the severity of the shock. Normally, the skin offers high resistance to current flow. However, this resistance is strongly affected by moisture. Depending on the amount of moisture present, electrical resistance across the intact body can vary from more than 1,000,000 Ω (for very dry skin) to less than 1,000 Ω (for wet skin).

If dry skin's normally high resistance is bypassed, as in patients with pacemaker wires or saline saline–filled intravascular catheters, current can readily flow into the body, causing damage to vital organs. Even urinary catheters and catheters used to drain fluid from the body can provide a pathway for current flow. The heart is particularly sensitive to electric shock. Experiments with dogs have shown that **ventricular fibrillation** can occur when currents as low as 20μA (20 microamperes or 20 millionths of an **ampere**) are applied directly to the heart. Although potentially lethal, a current this low is not normally noticed.[6]

Thus, according to the current's magnitude and path through the body, we can differentiate between two different types of shock hazards: **macroshock** and **microshock**. A macroshock exists when a relatively high current (usually greater than 1 mA, or one thousandth of an ampere) is applied externally to the skin. A microshock, on the other hand, exists when a small, usually imperceptible current (usually less than 1 mA) is allowed to bypass the skin and follow a direct, low-resistance pathway into the body. Patients susceptible to microshock hazards are termed **electrically sensitive** or **electrically susceptible**.[7] Table 3-1 summarizes the different effects of these two types of electrical shock hazards.

Preventing shock hazards

Most shock hazards are due to inappropriate or inadequate grounding. Shock hazards can thus be eliminated or minimized if you attend to a few basic rules for patient and equipment grounding.

General precautions. General precautions for all patient situations include: (1) never grounding the patient and (2) always ensuring that all patient-related equipment is properly grounded.

Do not ground the patient. The primary purpose of electrical safety measures is to ensure that the patient does not become part of an electrical circuit. If a patient is grounded, he or she can become part of an electrical circuit. In such cases, patient contact with *any* source of electrical voltage will cause current to flow through the body.

Figure 3-7 shows how a microshock to the heart can occur when a patient is electrically grounded. Current flows normally from the line plug to an electrical amplifier and transducer. In this case, however, the equipment line power cord has a broken ground wire. Low-amperage leakage current thus seeks out an alternative low potential ground. In this case, the leakage current finds its ground by flowing through a saline–filled vascular catheter and into the patient's heart. The result is a microshock, with possible ventricular fibrillation and death.

Eliminating the electrical path to ground from the patient would have eliminated the possibility of current flow. Thus ensuring that the patient is isolated from electrical ground is the best way to minimize electrical shock hazards.

Unfortunately, isolating the patient from a ground connection is not always easy. For example, older EKG equipment typically uses the right leg lead as a patient ground. Because many patients on continuous EKG monitors have other electrical apparatus in contact with the body, this is an obvious hazard.

Table 3-1 Effects of Electric Shock

Amperes	Milliamperes (mA)	Microamperes (μA)	Effects
APPLIED TO SKIN (MACROSHOCK)			
6 or more	≥6000	>6,000,000	Sustained myocardial contraction followed by normal rhythm; temporary respiratory paralysis; burns, if small area of contact
0.1 to 2–3	100 to 3000	100,000	Ventricular fibrillation; respiratory center intact
0.050	50	50,000	Pain, fainting, exhaustion, mechanical injury; heart and respiratory function intact
0.016	16	16,000	"Let go" current, muscle contraction
0.001	1	1000	Threshold of perception; tingling
APPLIED TO MYOCARDIUM (MICROSHOCK)			
		100	Ventricular fibrillation

Physiologic effects of AC shocks applied for 1 second to the trunk or directly to the myocardium. Duration of exposure and current pathway are major determinants of human response to electrical shock.

Modern EKG monitors overcome this problem by the use of isolation transformers, which isolate the patient from ground.

In addition to EKG equipment, other patient devices, such as indwelling catheters, may close an electrical circuit by providing a conducting pathway to ground. For this reason, *all* devices connected to a patient should be checked to ensure that the patient is indeed isolated from electrical ground.

Ground electrical equipment near the patient. All electrical equipment—such as lights, electric beds motors, and monitoring or therapeutic instruments used in patient care—should be connected to grounded outlets with three-wire cords. In these cases, the third (ground) wire prevents the dangerous buildup of voltage that can occur on the metal frames of some electrically powered equipment.

Modern electrical devices used in hospitals are designed so that their frames are grounded but their connections to the patient are not. In this manner, all electrical devices in reach of the patient are grounded, but the patient remains isolated from ground. Unfortunately, because the ground wire is simply a protection device and not part of the main circuit, equipment will continue to operate normally even if the ground wire is broken. Therefore, *all* electrical equipment, particularly those devices used with electrically susceptible patients, must be checked for appropriate grounding on a regular basis.

For equipment in use, a faulty ground may be revealed by a tingling sensation that occurs when the metal parts of a piece of equipment are touched. The presence of such tingling indicates improper grounding and the possibility of a serious leakage current. In these cases, the RCP must ensure that the faulty equipment is immediately taken out of service.

Precautions for electrically sensitive patients. Additional precautions should be followed by the RCP when the patient is considered electrically susceptible because of the presence of indwelling catheters or pacemaker wires.

Avoid contact with transcutaneous conductors. The RCP should avoid contacting a bare pacemaker wire or the conducting part of a catheter while simultaneously touching any metal object with the other hand. As shown in Figure 3-8 on page 40, this action can close the circuit between a defective instrument with a low-amperage current leak and a grounded patient. This hazard can be minimized by covering exposed pacemaker wires with a nonconducting material such as plastic or rubber.

Connect all electrical equipment to a common ground. If two pieces of electrical equipment have different grounds, a malfunction in one can produce a voltage difference between the two instruments and thus a flow of current. For this reason, the RCP should make sure that all electrical devices being used with a microshock-sensitive patient are connected to wall

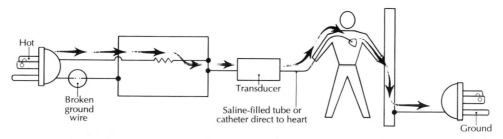

Hot

Broken ground wire

Transducer

Saline-filled tube or catheter direct to heart

Ground

Fig. 3-7 Possible microshock hazard due to patient grounding.

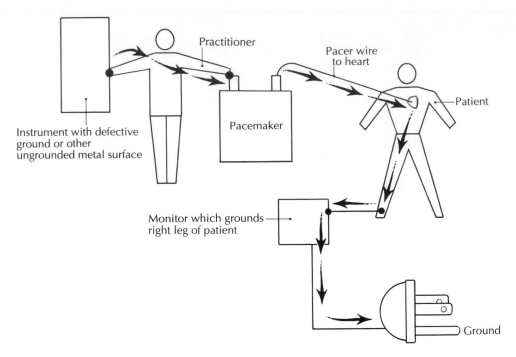

Fig. 3-8 Possible hazard through use of certain cardiac monitors and a pacemaker.

outlets with a *common* low-resistance ground. In most modern hospitals, patient areas have a special electrical panel to which all electrical equipment should be connected. These panels usually provide the safest grounding for equipment and should be used exclusively for connecting equipment to a power source.

Modern electrical equipment has made possible great advances in health care, and the use of sophisticated electronic devices will undoubtedly increase. The benefits of such devices can be maintained without shock hazards if proper attention is paid to the grounding of equipment and the electrical isolation of the patient from hazardous current paths. The RCP can contribute to this effort by maintaining a close watch on the ground wires of equipment, noting frayed wires or other obvious electrical hazards, and strictly following the key precautions just described.

Fire hazards

Three conditions are needed to start a fire: (1) flammable material must be present, (2) oxygen must be present, and (3) the flammable material must be heated to or above its ignition temperature. When all three conditions are present, a fire will start. On the other hand, removing any one of these conditions can prevent a fire from starting or extinguish a fire once it has begun.

With the high oxygen concentrations used in respiratory care, fire is a real and serious hazard. Although oxygen is **nonflammable,** it greatly accelerates the rate of combustion. Burning speed increases with an in-

crease in either the concentrations or partial pressure of oxygen.

The safe use of oxygen thus demands that flammable materials and potential ignition sources be removed from the vicinity of use. Flammable materials include cotton, wool, and polyester fabrics and bed clothing, paper materials, plastics, and certain lotions or salves such as petroleum jelly. The most common potential ignition sources are smoking materials, sparks from electrical equipment, and static electrical discharges.

To minimize the fire hazards associated with oxygen use, the RCP should ensure wherever possible that flammable materials are not used in its presence. This is particularly important whenever oxygen enclosures, such as tents or croupettes, are employed.

In terms of sources of ignition, the RCP must make certain that smoking is not allowed in rooms where oxygen is in use. Also, great care must be taken to avoid electrical equipment capable of generating high-energy sparks, such as exposed switches. Moreover, all appliances that transmit house current should be kept out of oxygen enclosures.

A frequent source of worry is the presence of **static electrical** sparks generated by the friction of movements of the patient in bed or by uniforms of personnel rubbing against bed clothing. For any spark to ignite flammable material, the spark must be able to generate enough heat energy to start the process.

Studies with oxygen concentrations varying from 21% to 100% show that static electrical sparks applied to such fabrics as vinyl plastic canopies, tissue paper, nylon, wool, cotton, muslin, and Dacron-cotton can cause ignition. However, ignition generally occurs only at increased oxygen concentrations and only with a barrage of sparks at a frequency of 60 per minute. Under no circumstances did a single spark produce a fire.

Such studies suggest that, even in the presence of high oxygen concentrations, the overall hazard from static sparks with the materials in common use is very low. In general, solitary static sparks do not have sufficient heat energy to raise common materials to their flashpoints. The minimal risk that may be present can be further reduced by maintaining the relative humidity in oxygen enclosures at 60% or more.

COMMUNICATION

Communication is a dynamic process involving sharing of information, meanings, and rules among people. Communication has five basic components: *sender, message, channel, receiver,* and *feedback* (Figure 3-9).[8,9]

The sender is the individual or group transmitting the message. The message is the idea, information, event, or attitude that is communicated by the sender. Messages may be verbal or nonverbal. Verbal messages are voiced or written down. Examples are discussions with colleagues, letters, and memos. Nonverbal communication is any communication that is not voiced or written. Nonverbal communication includes gesture, facial expression, eye behavior, voice tone, space, and touch.[10]

The channel of communication is the method used to transmit messages. The most common channels are those involving sight and hearing, such as written and oral messages. However, other sensory input, such as touch, may be used with or for visual or **auditory** communication. In addition, communication channels may be formal (memos or letters) or informal (conversation). In organizations, the informal communication channel is often called the "grapevine."

The receiver is the target of the communication. Depending on the message being transmitted, the receiver can be an individual or a group.[8]

The last essential part of communication is **feedback.** Human communication is a two-way process in which the receiver serves an active role. Feedback from receiver to sender allows change of later messages and the interaction as a whole. Because of feedback, both sender and receiver are mutually influenced by communication interactions.[10-13]

Health communication

Health communication is a subset of human communication. Health communication is the cement that binds, coordinates, and integrates human efforts to treat and prevent human suffering due to illness and disease.[14] Health communication takes place in a health care context and involves health **transactions** between and among health care professionals, their patients or clients, and significant others (Figure 3-10 on page 42).

Communication is a key component of health care. After all, health care is a great human undertaking, with social relationships at its core. Considering the differences of the relationships and health-related interactions, communication has a tremendous impact on health care. Communication influences the evaluation and treatment of patients, including their willingness to comply with regimental treatment, their satisfaction with services, and even their emotional well-being. Communication also affects the morale and performance of health care professionals.[11,15]

Communication skills play a key role in the RCP's ability to identify a patient's problems, to evaluate the patient's progress, and to make recommendations for respiratory care. The outcome of treatment may also be affected by communication. Through effective communication, the RCP can help patients cope with hospitalization and obtain maximum benefit from the care they provide. This can improve the patient's emotional well-being and the outcome of therapy.

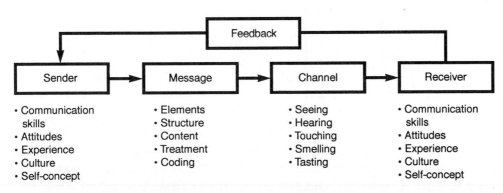

Fig. 3-9 Elements of human communication. See text for details.

■ MINI CLINI ■

3-2

Communication

Problem—A 73 year old male with chronic obstructive lung disease (COPD) is admitted to the emergency department for acute shortness of breath which is not relieved with rest. The patient has been admitted over 8 times during the past year for various respiratory problems. The attending physician feels that this episode may reflect an exacerbation of his COPD process and orders for a RCP to administer an inhaled bronchodilator using a meter dose inhaler (MDI) device are written. When the RCP enters the room and begins to introduce himself to the patient along with the purpose of the visit, the patient becomes quite defensive, stating that he doesn't require any assistance with respiratory treatments and that he should just leave the medication in the room. The RCP has not treated the patient in the past and has to decide how to respond to the patients request.

Discussion—Although this patient exhibited reluctance in allowing the RCP to administer the medication, there was enough verbal and perhaps nonverbal communication (message) expressed by the patient (sender) for the RCP (receiver) to determine a plan of action based on his response. Since human communication is a two-way process, the RCP serves an active role for further messages and interaction. This is a key concept for the RCP to master since it helps in identifying a patient's problems, evaluation of progress, and for recommending further respiratory care. The RCP must recognize that when an individual verbalizes disagreement with an treatment order and exhibits defensive behavior, he/she must attempt to understand what they are saying and not become defensive. For example, the RCP could try to put the patient at ease by demonstrating good eye contact, effective gesturing, and maintaining a safe distance from the patient when talking. Voice tone and facial expressions should match what is actually being said to the patient so as not to confuse the message being delivered. The RCP should seek feedback from the patient to insure that the message was understood as it was intended. In this situation, it may be appropriate for the RCP to just observe the patient self administer the medication so long as he can demonstrate proper technique. Allowing the patient to actively participate in medical care when feasible, may serve to help him maintain a sense of control over his disease process. The RCP benefits by serving as a patient advocate while promoting autonomy.

In terms of morale and job performance, most RCPs work in complex health care organizations. In this setting, the quality of communication among health care professionals has a major impact on one's job satisfaction, performance, and productivity. Indeed, failed communication is the primary source of conflict in complex organizations. Conflict and conflict resolution are discussed in a subsequent section.

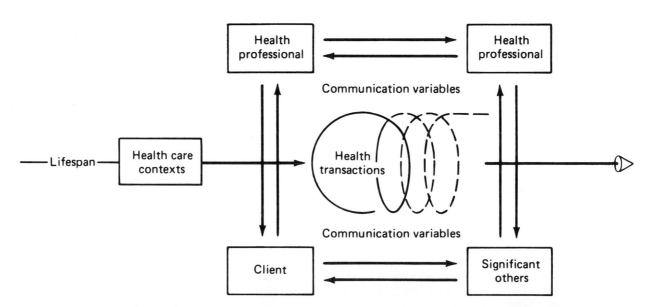

Fig. 3-10 Health communication model. (From Northouse PG and Northouse LL: Health communication: a handbook for health professionals, Englewood Cliffs, NJ, 1985, Prentice-Hall.)

Factors affecting communication

Many factors affect the communication process. Figure 3-11 portrays some of the key factors that affect health communication. The uniquely human or "internal" qualities of sender and receiver—including their prior experiences, attitudes, values, cultural backgrounds, and self-concepts and feelings—play a large role in the communication process. Consider, for example, how a COPD patient's prior difficulties with uncaring RCPs might affect his communication with you. Or what about the interaction between a physician who is committed to extending an elderly patient's life and her family, who value relief of her suffering above all else? And what of an RCP with strong negative feeling against homosexuals being assigned to treat a victim of AIDS who happens to be gay?

Likewise, verbal and nonverbal modes of expression affect health communication, as do the communication skills of sender and receiver. Consider the following interaction between an RCP and a patient:

RCP: Now, Mr. Jones, an SMI is simple: all you have to do is to inspire from your resting expiratory level up to your total lung capacity, then perform a volume hold with your glottis open. This will prevent atelectasis and improve your V/Q ratio. Understand?
Patient: *Nods head up and down.*
RCP: Very good; now let's get started . . .

Generally, the verbal and nonverbal components of a communication should enhance and reinforce each other. For example, the RCP that combines a verbal message in a compassionate tone such as "You're going to be all right now" with the confirming touch of the hand is sending a much stronger message to the anxious patient than that provided by either component alone. On the other hand, consider the same verbal message delivered in a brusque manner while the RCP purposely avoids eye contact with the patient. Which message would you be inclined to believe?

In addition, sensory/emotional and environmental factors can affect health communication. In combination, these factors are often referred to as *noise*.[16] Just as noise interferes with transmission of electronic signals, so too can noise disturb the transmission or receipt of human communication.

Examples of sensory/emotional noise include the severe anxiety of the patient in an acute asthmatic attack and the withdrawal characterizing some terminally ill patients. A literal example of environmental noise would be the effect of a patient moaning in the next bed while you try to communicate with your patient.

Of course, sensory/emotional and environmental factors are not necessarily limited to the patient. An RCP still angry over an earlier encounter with a grumpy doctor could bring this noise to the bedside of the next patient visited. Or what if the RCP's favorite team is on the patient's TV at the same time that he or she is providing treatment?

Last, both the complexity of the message and the channel of communication used affect the out-

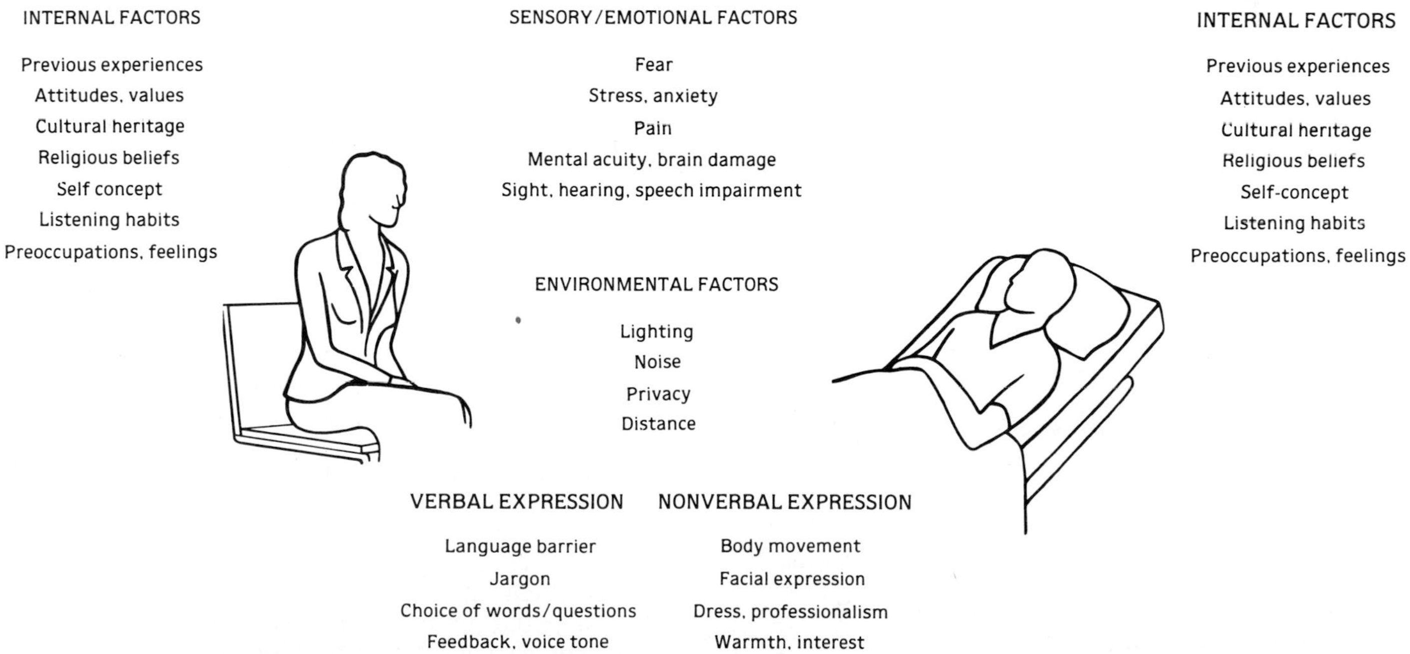

Fig. 3-11 Factors influencing communication. (From Wilkins RL, Sheldon RL, and Krider SJ: Clinical assessment in respiratory care. St. Louis, 1985, Mosby.)

comes of health communication. A communicated message consists of more than just content. A message's elements, structure, treatment, and coding can also affect how it is received and interpreted.[9] Take the simple example of a written patient consent form. The more "legalese" it contains, the less likely it is that the patient will pay attention to its meaning.

In regard to the channel of communication, take the clinical supervisor who was asked by the program faculty to tell the students that their final lab projects were due the next day.[8] The clinical supervisor orally conveyed this message to a student and told her to inform the rest of the class. The student told some of her peers but did not inform everyone. In this case, the failure to use a more formal channel of communication to convey the message (such as a written notice) resulted in failed communication.

Effective health communication

RCPs must be effective communicators. Effective health communication occurs when the intent or purpose of the interaction is achieved. The several key purposes of health communication are summarized in the box below.

To help achieve these purposes when communicating, the RCP must consider the roles involved, the message, the channel, and the appropriate feedback.

Roles

In terms of role, the RCP may be primarily the sender or the receiver. For example, when teaching a patient how to perform a lung function test, the RCP's role of sender is paramount. On the other hand, when interviewing a patient to obtain information, the RCP's role as receiver is most important.

Message and channel

In terms of the message and channel, charting the results of a patient's treatment (to inform other health professionals) requires formality, objectivity, brevity, accuracy, and consistent use of medical **jargon**. Obvi-

ously you would not use this type of message or channel to establish rapport with a patient. Instead, you would use a less formal channel, avoid jargon, and emphasize feelings and feedback, both verbal and nonverbal.

Feedback

The central role played by feedback is evident in all of the listed purposes of health communication. For example, when instructing a patient to perform a lung function test, it is only by judging the patient's understanding and actual performance that the RCP can assess the effectiveness of the teaching effort. Likewise, the feedback received by an RCP while trying to establish rapport with a patient's family indicates the success of that effort and can provide clues as to how to improve the relationship.

Improving communication skills

To enhance their ability to communicate effectively, all health care professionals should focus on improving sending, receiving, and feedback skills. In addition, the RCP must be able to identify and overcome common barriers to effective communication.

The practitioner as sender

There are several ways to improve your effectiveness as a sender of messages. These suggestions may be applied to the clinical setting as follows.[8]

Share information rather than telling. Health professionals often provide information in an authoritative manner by telling colleagues or patients what to do or say. This approach can cause defensiveness and lead to uncooperative behavior. On the other hand, sharing information creates an atmosphere of cooperation and trust.

Seek to relate to people rather than control them. This is of particular significance during communication with patients. Health care professionals often attempt to control patients. Few people like to be controlled. Patients feel much more important if you treat them as an equal partner in the relationship.

Value disagreement as much as agreement. People will often disagree with what you say. When individuals express disagreement, you must make an attempt to understand what they are saying and not become defensive. Be prepared for disagreement, and be open to the input of others.

Eliminate threatening behavior. The first step in effective communication is to put your listeners at ease. If you appear to be a threat to patients or staff, they will resist communication.

Use effective nonverbal communication techniques. The nonverbal communication that you use is just as important as what you say. Nonverbal techniques include good eye contact, effective gesturing, distance between yourself and others when talking, facial ex-

---

Basic purposes of health communication

- *To establish rapport with another individual,* such as a colleague, a patient, or a member of the patient's family
- *To obtain information,* such as during a patient interview
- *To relay pertinent information,* as when charting the results of a patient's treatment
- *To give instructions,* as when teaching a patient how to perform a lung function test
- *To persuade others to take action,* as when attempting to convince a patient to quit smoking

pressions, and voice tone. It is important that your nonverbal communications match what you are actually saying. For instance, if you are trying to gain the rapport of a patient but do not look her in the eye, your communication will not be as effective. Your eye contact and facial expressions help convey what you are trying to say.

The practitioner as receiver/listener

Receiver skills are just as important as sender skills. Messages sent are of no value unless they are received as intended. This requires active listening on the part of the receiver. Learning to listen requires a strong commitment and great effort. Following a few simple principles can help improve your listening skills.[8,17,18]

Work at listening. Listening is often a difficult process. It takes great effort to hear what others are saying. Focus your attention on the speaker and on the message.

Stop talking. Practice silent listening and avoid interrupting the speaker during an interaction. Studies have consistently shown that, with the exception of patient interviews, health professionals consistently dominate communication interactions with patients.[19]

Resist distractions. It is easy to be distracted by surrounding noises and conversations. This is particularly true in a busy environment such as a hospital. When listening, you should try to tune out other distractions and give full attention to the person who is speaking.

Keep your mind open; be objective. Being open-minded is often very difficult. All people have their own opinions that may influence what they hear. Try to be objective in your listening so that you treat everyone fairly.

Hear the speaker out before making an evaluation. Do not just listen to the first few words. This is a common mistake made by listeners. Often, listeners hear the first sentence and tune out the rest, assuming that they know what is being said. It is important to listen to the entire message; otherwise, you may miss important information.

Judge content, not delivery. Many people have difficulty communicating what they are trying to say. When listening to others, you should listen to what they are saying rather than to their style of delivery.

Maintain composure; control emotions. Allowing emotions such as anger or anxiety to distort your understanding or drawing conclusions before a speaker completes their thoughts or arguments is a common error in listening.

Active listening is a key component in health care communication. Many of the messages being sent are vital to patient care. If you do not listen effectively, important information may be lost and the care of your patients jeopardized.[8]

Providing feedback

To enhance communication with others, you need to provide effective *feedback*.[11] Examples of effective feedback mechanisms in oral communication with patients include *attending, paraphrasing, requesting clarification, perception checking,* and *reflecting feelings.*

Attending. Attending involves the use of gestures and posture that communicates one's attentiveness. Attending also involves confirming remarks such as, "I see what you mean."

Paraphrasing. Paraphrasing, or repeating the other's response in one's own words, is a technique useful in confirming that understanding is taking place between the parties involved in the interaction. Overuse of paraphrasing, however, can be irritating.

Requesting clarification. Requesting clarification begins with an admission of misunderstanding on the part of the listener, with the intent being to better understand the message through restating or the use of alternative examples or illustrations. As with paraphrasing, overuse of this technique can hamper effective communication, especially if it is used in a condescending or patronizing manner. Requests for clarification should thus be used only when truly necessary and always be nonjudgmental in nature.

Perception checking. Perception checking involves confirming or disproving the more subtle components of a communication interaction, such as messages that are implied but not stated. As an example, the RCP might sense that a patient is unsure of the need for a treatment. In this case, the RCP might check this perception by saying, "You don't seem to be sure that you need this treatment. Is that correct?" Of course, by verifying or disproving this perception, both the professional and patient will come to understand each other better.

Reflecting feelings. Reflecting feelings involves the use of statements as "verbal mirrors" to better determine the emotions of the other party. Nonjudgmental statements such as, "You seem to be anxious about (this situation)", provide the opportunity for the other party to express and reflect on their emotions and can help them confirm or deny their true feelings.

Minimizing barriers to communication

There are many potential barriers to effective communication. The skillful communicator will try to identify and eliminate or minimize the influence of these barriers in all interactions. By minimizing the influence of these barriers, the RCP can help ensure that the message will be received as intended. Key barriers to effective communication are detailed below:[8]

Use of symbols or words that have different meanings. Words and symbols (including nonverbal communication) can mean different things to different people. These differences in meaning derive from differences in the background or culture between sender and receiver and the context of the communication.

Different value systems. Everyone has their own value system, and many people do not recognize the values held by others. A large difference between the values held by individuals can interfere with communication. For instance, a clinical supervisor may inform her students of the penalties for being late with clinical assignments. If a student does not value timeliness, he or she may not take seriously what is being said.

Different perceptions of the problem. Problems exist in all organizations. Different individuals perceive these problems in different ways. The perceptual differences often cause a lack of understanding among individuals, impairing communication.

Consider the following situation. Dr. Thompson became angry at Carol, the pulmonary function technologist, because a test he ordered was not completed by a certain time. Dr. Thompson needed the results of the test before leaving for a conference. He left angrily, without telling Carol why he had needed the test results early.

Carol did not see the importance of the problem and assumed that Dr. Thompson would eventually cool off. In this case, the individual perceptions of the problem were different, and the problem was not resolved.

Emphasis on status. A hierarchy of positions and power exist in most health care organizations. If superiority is emphasized by those of higher status, communication can be stifled. We have all experienced interactions with professionals who make it clear who is in charge. Emphasis on status can be a barrier to communication not only among health professionals but between health professionals and their patients.

Conflict of interest. Many people are affected by decisions made in health care organizations. If someone is afraid that a decision will take away their advantage or invade their territory they may try to block communication. An example might be a staff member who is unwilling to share expertise with students. This person may feel that a student is invading his or her territory.

Lack of acceptance of differences in points of view, feelings, values, or purposes. Most of us are aware that people have different opinions, feelings, and values. These differences can thwart effective communication. To overcome this barrier, the effective communicator allows others to express their differences. Encouraging individuals to communicate their feelings and points of view is a benefit to all. Most of us think we are always correct. Accepting input from others promotes growth and cooperation.

Feelings of personal insecurity. It is very difficult for people to admit feelings of inadequacy. Those who are insecure will not offer information for fear that they appear ignorant, or they may be defensive when criticized, thus blocking clear communication. Many of us have worked with individuals who are insecure, thereby realizing the difficulty in communicating with them.

In summary, to become an effective communicator, the RCP should first identify the purpose of each communication interaction and his or her role in it. The RCP should also use specific sending, receiving, and feedback skills in each interaction. Last, to ensure that messages are received as intended, the RCP should try to minimize any identified barriers to communication with patients or peers.

Conflict and conflict resolution

Conflict is sharp disagreement or opposition among people's interests, ideas, or values.[8] Because no two people are exactly alike in their backgrounds or attitudes, conflict can be found in every organization.

Health care professionals experience a great deal of conflict in their jobs. Rapid changes occurring in health care have made everyone's jobs more complex and often more stressful.[8] Because conflict is inevitable, all health care professionals must be able to recognize its sources and help resolve or manage its impact on people and on the organization.

Sources of conflict

The first step in conflict management is to identify its potential sources. Four primary sources of conflict in organizations exist: poor communication, structural problems, personal behavior, and role conflict.[8,20]

Poor communication. Poor communication is the primary source of conflict in organizations. The previously discussed barriers to communication are all potential sources of conflict. For example, if a supervisor is not willing to accept different points of view for dealing with a difficult patient, an argument may occur. The importance of good communication cannot be overemphasized.[8]

Structural problems. The structure of the organization itself can increase the likelihood of conflict. Conflict tends to grow as the size of an organization increases. Conflict is also greater in organizations whose employees are given less control over their work and in organizations where certain individuals or groups have excessive power. Structural sources of conflict are the most rigid and are often impossible to control.[8]

Personal behavior. Personal behavior factors are a major source of conflict in organizations. Different personalities, attitudes, and behavioral traits create the possibility of great disagreement among health care professionals and between health care professionals and patients.

Role conflict. *Role conflict* is the experience of

being pulled in several directions by individuals with different expectations of a person's job functions.[8] For example, a clinical supervisor is often expected to function both as a staff member and as a student supervisor. Trying to fill both roles simultaneously can cause stress and create **interpersonal** conflict.

Conflict resolution

Conflict resolution or management is the process by which people control and channel disagreements within an organization. There are five basic strategies for handling conflict: *competing, accommodating, avoiding, collaborating,* and *compromising.*[8,21] Figure 3-12 compares these strategies on the dimensions of cooperativeness and assertiveness.

Competing. Competing is an assertive and uncooperative conflict resolution strategy. Competing is a power–oriented method of resolving conflict. For example, the supervisor who uses rank or other forces to attempt to win is using the competing strategy. This strategy may be useful when an unpopular decision must be made or when one must stand up for his or her rights. However, because it often causes others to clam up, competing should be used cautiously.[8,21]

Accommodating. Accommodating is the opposite of competing; accommodating is unassertive and cooperative. When people accommodate others involved in conflict, they neglect their own needs to meet the needs of the other party. Accommodation is a useful strategy when it is essential to maintain harmony in the environment. Accommodation is also appropriate when an issue is much more important to one party or the other in a dispute.[8,21]

Avoiding. Avoiding is both an unassertive and an uncooperative conflict resolution strategy. In avoiding conflict, one or both parties decide *not* to pursue their concerns. Avoidance may be appropriate if there is no possibility of meeting one's goals. Also, if one or both

of the parties are hostile, avoidance may be a good strategy, at least initially. However, too much avoidance can leave important issues unattended or unresolved.[8,21]

Collaborating. As a conflict resolution strategy, collaborating is the opposite of avoiding. Collaborating is assertive and cooperative. In collaboration, the involved parties try to find mutually satisfying solutions to their conflict. Collaboration usually takes more time than other methods and simply cannot be applied when the involved parties harbor strong negative feelings about each other.[8,21]

Compromising. Compromising is a middle-ground strategy that combines assertiveness and cooperation. Those who compromise give up more than those who compete but less than those who accommodate. Compromise is best used when a quick resolution is needed that both parties can live with. However, because both parties often feel they are losing, compromise should not be used exclusively.[8,21]

Deciding which type of conflict resolution strategy to use requires knowledge of the context, the specific underlying problem(s), and the desires of the involved parties.[22]

RECORDKEEPING

A medical record or *chart* presents a written picture of occurrences and situations pertaining to a patient throughout his or her stay in a health care institution.[23] Medical records are the property of the institution and are strictly confidential. This means that the content of a patient's medical records are not to be read or discussed by anyone except those directly caring for the patient in a hospital or medical care facility.

Because the law requires that a record be kept of the patient's care, a patient's chart is also a legal docu-

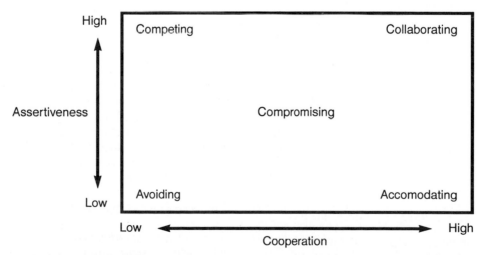

Fig. 3-12 Methods of conflict resolution. (From: Marriner A: Managing conflict—comparing strategies and their use, *Nurs Management* 13(5):29-35, 1982.)

ment. For this reason, charting or record keeping must be done so that it is meaningful for days, months, or years later in case it must be used in court.[23]

Components of a traditional medical record

Each health care facility has its own specification for the medical records it keeps. Although the forms themselves vary between institutions, most acute-care medical records share common sections (see box below).

See Figure 2-5 for an example of a respiratory care progress note form. Note the opportunity for the RCP to provide a brief assessment of breath sounds and vital signs, along with a specification of treatment(s) given and outcome achieved.

Figure 3-13 provides an example of a combined

flow sheet and progress note form for patients undergoing mechanical ventilation. Flow sheets are designed to briefly report data and to decrease time spent in documentation. Note how a single time entry can include dozens of measurements and how review of a sequence of entries can reveal trends in patient status.

Legal aspects of recordkeeping

Legally, documentation of the care given to a patient means that care was given; no documentation means that care was not given. Hospital accreditation agencies critically evaluate the medical records of patients. Again, if the RCP does not document care given (i.e., patient assessment data, interventions, and evaluation of care rendered), the practitioner and the hospital may be accused of patient neglect.

Adequate documentation of care is only valuable in reference to standards and criteria of care. Respiratory care departments, like all departments in health care facilities, must generate their own standards of patient care. For each standard, criteria must be outlined so that the adequacy of patient care can be measured. Documentation must reflect these standards.

Practical aspects of recordkeeping

Record keeping is one of the most significant duties that the RCP performs. Documentation is required for each medication, treatment, or procedure. Accounts of the patient's condition and activities must be charted accurately and in clear terms.[23] Briefness is essential, as is the use of standardized terms (see Chapter 6).

In general, accounts of care and the patient's condition are hand-printed or written. In some institutions, computerized patient information systems also facilitate data entry by selection from menus of choices or direct typing (see Chapter 8). In either case the RCP must document only what is—not one's interpretation or judgment. Assessments of data must be clearly within one's professional domain.[23] When a practitioner cannot interpret the data obtained, he or she should state so in the record and contact another professional for advice or referral. Other general rules for medical record keeping are listed in the box on page 50.[23] In addition to these general rules, each institution has its own additional policies governing medical record keeping.

The Problem-Oriented Medical Record

The *problem-oriented medical record* (POMR) is an alternative documentation format used by some health care institutions. Problem-oriented medical records contain four basic parts: the database, the

---

General sections found in a patient's medical record

- *Admission sheet*—records pertinent patient information (name, address, religion, nearest of kin, etc.), admitting physician, and admission diagnosis
- *History and physical*—records the patient's admitting history and physical examination, as performed by the attending physician or resident
- *Physician's orders*—records the physician's orders and prescriptions
- *Progress sheet*—allows the physician to keep a continuing account of the patient's progress
- *Nurses' notes*—describes the nursing care given to the patient, including the patient's complaints (subjective symptoms), nurses' observations (objective signs), and the patient's response to therapy
- *Medication record*—notes drugs and IV fluids that are given to the patient
- *Vital signs graphic sheet*—records the patient's temperature, pulse, respirations, and blood pressure over time
- *I/O sheet*—records patient's fluid intake (I) and output (O) over time
- *Laboratory sheet*—summarizes the results of laboratory tests
- *Consultation sheet*—for the use of physicians who are called in to examine a patient to make a diagnosis.
- *Surgical or treatment consent*—records the patient's authorization for surgery or treatment
- *Anesthesia and surgical record*—notes key events before, during, and immediately after surgery
- *Specialized therapy records/progress notes*—records specialized treatments or treatment plans and patient progress for various specialized therapeutic services, including respiratory care and physical therapy
- *Specialized flow sheets*—records measurement made over time during specialized procedures such as mechanical ventilation or kidney dialysis

B.S.A. _____

DATE	ARTERIAL LINE						SG DISTAL						FLUSH	ICP	INT.	PROCEDURES		
SHIFT 7 3 11	INSERTION SITE	EXTREMITY TEMPERATURE	EXTREMITY COLOR	DISTAL PULSE	WAVE FORM	CALIBRATION	INSERTION SITE	WAVE FORM	CALIBRATION	TIME C.O. DONE	C.O. L/MIN	C.I. L/MIN/M²	500 ML NS 1000U HEPARIN	WAVE FORM CALIBRATION		TIME	PROCEDURE #	INT.
TIME																		

TIME	MODE	RATE (PER MIN)	TIDAL VOLUME (CC)			PRESSURE (cmH₂O)				MISCELLANEOUS				BLOOD GAS VALUES							INT.	PROCEDURE CODE
	INVERSE I:E ASSIST CONT. IMV SIMV & PS SIMV CPAP	MECHANICAL / SPONTANEOUS	MACHINE DELIVERED	EXHALED MEASURED	SPONTANEOUS	PEAK	EQUAL SYSTEM / PEEP CPAP / SET LIMIT	PS	I:E RATIO	FIO2 (ANALYZED)	FLOW RATE (L/MIN) / INSP. TIME (SEC.)	H₂O LEVEL / ALARM FUNCT.	GAS TEMP.	PH	PCO₂	PO₂	O₂ SAT.	OXIMETER SAT.	B.E.		

PROCEDURE CODE list:
1. INTUBATION
2. EXTUBATION
3. TRACH △
4. HEMO-PROFILE
5. CARDIO-PROFILE
6. A-LINE INITIAL SET UP
7. ARTERIAL CANNULATION
8. A-LINE, TRANS, LINE, FLUSH △
9. SG TRANS, LINE, FLUSH
10. SG TRANS, LINE FLUSH △
11. FEMORAL SHEATH INITIAL SET UP
12. FLUSH △
13. DRESSING △
14. PORT — O2
15. IABP △
16. VENT △
17. VENT TUBING △

PROC. IN MIN. NEEDED
18. VENT TRANSPORT
19. IABP TO SURGERY
20. IABP TRANSPORT
21. CARDIO VERSION
22. CODE 90
23. AIRWAY MAINT.
24. SG INSERTION STANDBY
25. IABP INSERTION

ENDO-TRACH TUBES

LOCATION -

SIZE -   mm

TAPE MARK -   cm

CUFF PRESS-   cmH₂O

OXIMETER ALARM SETTINGS

HIGH-

LOW-

TIME	PROGRESS NOTES

INT.	SIGNATURE	PATIENT STAMP

PAGE #

GP-40952

FLORIDA HOSPITAL
763-1 (288 REV.)   **RESPIRATORY CARE FLOWSHEET**

Fig. 3-13 Respiratory care flowsheet. (Reprinted with permission from the Department of Respiratory Care Services, Florida Hospital Medical Center, Orlando.)

■ MINI CLINI ■

3-3

Recordkeeping

Problem—A patient was given a respiratory treatment by a respiratory care student who then forgot to chart that the therapy was given. The student reasoned that since he did not observe any adverse effects during or immediately following the treatment and furthermore, he knew that the treatment was in fact, given; not documenting the treatment in the medical record this one time would be acceptable. What are the problems associated with this students judgement and subsequent actions?

Discussion—The medical record is a legal document intended to identify types of care given to a patient and to serve as a source of information to the physician, RCP (including the student), and other health care providers in developing an individualized plan of care. It further serves as a tool for evaluating the effectiveness in reaching the goals of therapy. Hospitals and other health care agencies critically evaluate the medical records of patients in order to maintain high quality patient care. Failure to document care rendered, such as a respiratory treatment hinders the process of providing high quality care in several ways. First and foremost, important information to the physician and other caregivers interested in the patients respiratory status will be missing. In this situation, even though the student observed a lack of response by the patient during and immediately following the treatment, a delayed effect could still have taken place. The physician or RCP would in turn, have difficulty in establishing the etiology of a condition change in the patient related to the respiratory treatment. From a legal perspective, patient care not documented may be viewed as care not rendered, thus making the hospital or institution vunerable to charges of patient neglect which would be difficult to defend in a court of law.

problem list, the plan, and the progress notes.[23] The precise forms these records take vary between institutions.

The database contains information of a routine nature about the patient, including a general health history, physical examination results, and the results of diagnostic tests.

In the POMR, a problem is something that interferes with a patient's physical or psychological health or ability to function. From the information provided by the database, the patient's problems are identified and listed. The list of problems is dynamic; new problems are added as they develop, and others are removed as they are resolved.

The POMR progress notes contain the findings, assessment, plans, and orders of the doctors, nurses, and other practitioners involved in the care of the patient. In many institutions, all caregivers chart on the same form, using the *SOAP* format (see box on page 51).

General rules for medical recordkeeping[23]

1. Entries on the patient's chart should be printed or handwritten. After completing the account, sign the chart with one initial and your last name, and your title (CRTT, RRT, LRCP, Resp Care Student; e.g., S. Smith, CRTT). Institutional policy may require student entries to be countersigned by supervisory personnel.
2. Do not use ditto marks.
3. Do not erase. Erasures provide reason for question if the chart is used later in a court of law. If a mistake is made, a single line should be drawn through the mistake and the word "error" printed above it. Then continue your charting in a normal manner.
4. Record after completing each task for the patient, and sign your name correctly after each entry.
5. Be exact in noting the time, effect, and results of all treatments and procedures.
6. Record patient complaints and general behavior. Describe the type, location, onset, and duration of pain. Describe clearly and concisely the character and amount of secretions.
7. Leave no blank lines in the charting. Draw a line through the center of an empty line or part of a line. This prevents charting by someone else in an area signed by you.
8. Use standard abbreviations.
9. Use the present tense. Never use the future tense, as in "Patient to receive treatment after lunch."
10. Spell correctly. If you are not sure about the spelling of a word, use the dictionary at the desk to look it up.

SOAP CHARTING FORMAT

SOAP stands for:

S Subjective information obtained from the patient, his or her relatives, or a similar source;

O objective information based on caregivers' observations of the patient, the physical examination, or diagnostic or laboratory tests;

A assessment, which refers to the analysis of the patient's problem;

P plan of action to be taken to resolve the problem.

Example:

Problem 1: pneumonia
11/21/94

Subjective: "My chest hurts when I take a deep breath."

Objective: Awake, alert, oriented to time, place and person; sitting upright in bed with arms leaning over the bedside stand; pale, dry skin; respirations 26/minute, thoracic in nature, shallow; pulse 98/minute, regular and faint to palpation; blood pressure 112/68, left arm, sitting position; bronchial breath sounds in lower posterior lung fields; occasionally expectorating small volumes of mucopurulent sputum.

Assessment: Pneumonia continues

Plan: Therapeutic—assist with coughing and deep breathing at least every 2 hours; postural drainage and percussion every 4 hours; assist with ambulation as per physician orders and patient tolerance. Diagnostic—continue to monitor lung sounds before each treatment. Education—teach to cough and deep-breathe and evaluate return demonstration.

REFERENCES

1. Bruner J: Hazards of electrical apparatus, *Anesthesiology,* 28:945–957, 1967.
2. *Safe Use of Electricity in Hospitals,* (NFPA 76BM), Boston, National Fire Protection Association.
3. Scanlan CL: *Electrical safety in respiratory therapy, part I,* Dallas, 1978, American Association for Respiratory Therapy.
4. Scanlan CL: *Electrical safety in respiratory therapy, part II,* Dallas, 1978, American Association for Respiratory Therapy.
5. Dalziel CF: Electric shock hazards, *IEEE Spectrum* 9(2):41, 1972.
6. Dalziel CF, Lee WR: *Reevaluation of lethal electrical currents,* IEEE Transactions on Industry and General Applications, 1968.
7. Starmer CF, Whalen RE, McIntosh HD: Hazards of electric shock in cardiology, *Am J Cardiol* 14:537–546, 1964.
8. University of Illinois College of Education: *Clinical supervision skills: communication and conflict management,* Champaign-Urbana, IL, 1985, Illinois State Board of Education.
9. Berlo DK: *The process of communication: an introduction to theory and practice,* New York, 1960, Holt, Reinhart & Winston.
10. Northouse PG, Northouse LL: *Health communication,* Englewood Cliffs, NJ, 1985, Prentice-Hall.
11. Klinzing D, Klinzing D: Communication for allied health professionals, Dubuque, IA, 1985, William C. Brown.
12. Miller GR: *An introduction to speech communication,* ed 2, Indianapolis, 1972, Bob-Merril.
13. Ruffner M, Burgoon M: *Interpersonal communication,* New York, 1981, Holt, Reinhart & Winston.
14. Pettegrew LS, Arntson P, Bush D, Zoppi K, editors: *Explorations in provider and patient interaction,* Louisville, KY, 1982, Humana.
15. DiMatteo MP: A social-psychological analysis of physician-patient rapport: toward a science of the art of medicine, *J Soc Issues* 35:17–31, 1979.
16. Shannon C, Weaver W: *The mathematical theory of communication,* Champaign, IL, 1949, University of Illinois Press.
17. Sanford AC, Hunt GT, Bracey HJ: *Communication behavior in organizations,* Columbus, OH, 1976, Charles E. Merrill.
18. Smith E: Improving listening effectiveness, *Tex Med* 71:98–100, 1975.
19. Bain DJL: Doctor-patient communication in general practice, *Med Ed* 10:125–131, 1976.
20. Robbins SP: *Managing organizational conflict: a nontraditional approach,* Englewood Cliffs, NJ, 1974, Prentice-Hall.
21. Marriner Λ: Managing conflict: comparing strategies and their use. *Nurs Management* 13(5):29–35, 1982.
22. Bray KA: Managing conflict, *Crit Care Nurs,* 3(2):77–78, 1983.
23. Wood LA, Rambo BJ: *Nursing skills for allied health services,* ed 2, Philadelphia, 1977, WB Saunders.

Principles of Infection Control

■

Craig L. Scanlan

Halcyon St. Hill

CHAPTER LEARNING OBJECTIVES

1. Apply the major categories of microorganisms to identify and describe those most pathogenic to man;
2. Describe the three major elements necessary for the spread of infection in general, and respiratory infections in particular;
3. Compare and contrast the various infection control methods used in respiratory care equipment processing;
4. Differentiate among the various infection control techniques used to (a) maintain in-use respiratory care equipment, (b) process reusable respiratory care equipment, and (c) protect fluids and medications;
5. Describe the appropriate use of general barrier methods of infection control;
6. Differentiate among the special categories of patient isolation, including acceptable modifications;
7. Outline the universal infection control precautions currently recommended by the Centers for Disease Control;
8. Describe the key components of a departmental bacteriologic surveillance program.

Between 5% to 10% of all hospitalized patients acquire an infection during their stay. The direct cost of treating these *nosocomial* infections is over a billion dollars per year. The indirect cost is even more staggering, amounting to some 5 to 10 billion dollars per year in lost economic productivity.[1]

Between 10% and 40% of all nosocomial infections are pulmonary. Moreover, among all hospital-acquired infections, those affecting the lungs are most likely to result in death.

Historically, respiratory care equipment and procedures have been identified as a major cause of nosocomial infections.[2-6] Early studies showed that as many as one of every 10 hospital epidemics involved respiratory care equipment.[7] However, as the sophistication of respiratory care procedures have evolved, so too has our understanding of infection control.[8] As a result, infection due to respiratory care equipment has decreased significantly.[9,10]

This progress notwithstanding, respiratory care practitioners (RCPs) must always be on guard to protect their patients against infection. Moreover, health professionals are now giving increased attention to protecting *themselves* against infection, especially those transmitted by blood or body fluids.[1]

Protecting our patients and ourselves against infections requires strict adherence to infection control procedures. Infection control procedures aim to (1) eliminate the sources of infectious agents, (2) create barriers to their transmission, and (3) monitor and evaluate the effectiveness of control.

Infection control is a major and ongoing responsibility of all RCPs. This responsibility requires a general understanding of clinical microbiology, and specific skill in a variety of infection control procedures. The purpose of this chapter is to provide the foundation knowledge and skills needed to fulfill this critical role.

CLINICAL ASPECTS OF MICROBIOLOGY

Microbiology involves the study of microorganisms, including bacteria, viruses, fungi, protozoa, and algae (Figure 4-1). Microbiology is closely related to respiratory care in two ways. First, many respiratory disorders are caused by microorganisms and treated, in part, by antimicrobial drugs. Second, as previously discussed, respiratory care equipment and procedures are a potential cause of nosocomial infections. For these reasons, RCPs must have a sound basic knowledge of microbiology.

All microorganisms, with the possible exception of the algae, are capable of invading a human host and causing disease. An organism capable of causing disease is called a *pathogen.* Using the standard classification scheme, we will highlight the major pathogens and describe their importance in both pulmonary medicine and hospital epidemiology.

Bacteria

Bacteria are the most common cause of nosocomial infections. Bacteria are **procaryotic,** unicellular organisms ranging in size from about 0.5 to 40 μm. Bacteria exist in three basic shapes: cocci (spherical), bacilli (rod-shaped), and spirochetes (helical or spiral).

Two approaches are used to identify and describe bacteria. The first is visual classification by shape, or *morphologic analysis.* The second approach uses more detailed assessment of structural and metabolic features. Usually, both approaches are used together to confirm an organism's identity.

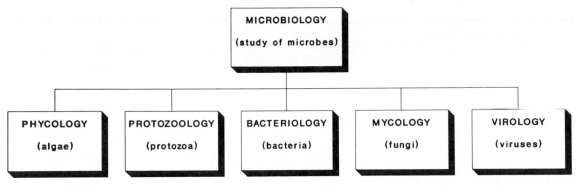

Fig. 4-1 Branches of microbiology.

Staining is used to aid visual identification. The *Gram stain* separates bacteria into those that retain an initial violet stain after alcohol wash (Gram-positive) and those that do not (Gram-negative). The *acid-fast stain* (also called the Ziehl-Neelsen stain) is used to help identify organisms in the genus *Mycobacterium*. *Mycobacterium,* such as the tuberculosis bacillus, are acid-fast because they retain a red carbolfuchsin stain after an acid wash. More complex staining methods may be needed to identify some bacteria.

Metabolic tests are also used. These are based on differences in growth media, metabolic need for oxygen, and enzyme production. For example, based on metabolic need for oxygen, bacteria form three groups: those that require oxygen to live (aerobes), those that don't (anaerobes), and those that can do with or without (**facultative** bacteria).

For example, combining visual classification with staining and metabolic tests, *Staphylococcus aureus* is identified as a Gram positive cocci that appears singly, paired or in irregular clusters, produces the catalase and coagulase enzymes, and is capable of fermenting mannitol.

While staining can be done immediately, metabolic tests require lengthy period of culturing, often as long as 18 to 48 hours. These timelines mean that the treatment of an infection usually begins before the causative organism is identified. Quicker immunologic techniques that detect microbial antigens, like countercurrent immunoelectrophoresis and ELISA, are promising but presently not practical for screening purposes.[11,12]

Table 4-1, page 54 summarizes the major bacterial pathogens. The rest of this section describes these infectious agents, grouped according to their major categories.

Gram-positive cocci

The most common respiratory bacterial pathogens in this category are *Staphylococcus aureus, Streptococcus pyogenes,* and *Streptococcus pneumoniae,* also known as *Diplococcus pneumoniae.*

S. aureus is a aerobe or facultative aerobe that is part of the normal flora of the skin and upper airway. *S. aureus* is a common cause of skin disorders, but can also cause pneumonia and other organ or **systemic** infections, especially among the very old, the very young, and those **debilitated** by disease.

Most streptococci are facultative anaerobes. Lansfield groups A, B, C, D, and G are the most common human pathogens. Group A beta-hemolytic streptococci, or *Streptococcus pyogenes,* causes most human infections, including rheumatic fever, **endocarditis, glomerulonephritis, septicemia,** and scarlet fever. *Streptococcus pneumoniae,* an alpha-hemolytic organism, is the primary cause of community-acquired pneumonia, but is also responsible for acute infectious bronchitis, **peritonitis, meningitis,** and **otitis media.**

Gram-negative cocci

The clinically important Gram-negative cocci are *Neisseria gonorrhoeae* (the gonococcus), *Neisseria meningitidis* (the meningococcus) and *Moraxella catarrhalis.* Both *Neisseria* are facultatively **anaerobic** to **aerobic** diplococci, growing best in 3% to 10% CO_2. *N. gonorrhoeae* causes the sexually transmitted gonorrhea infection. *N. meningitides* causes meningitis, but can also cause septicemia, especially in susceptible hosts.

Moraxella catarrhalis is an aerobic Gram-negative diplococcus that is part of the normal flora of the upper airway.[13] In patients with COPD, alcoholism, and other immunocompromising disorders, *M. catarrhalis* can cause bronchitis and pneumonia.

Gram-negative coccobacilli

Some bacteria fall between the cocci and bacilli in shape. These are called coccobacilli. The coccobacilli most often implicated as human pathogens are Gram-negative, facultative, **nonmotile** organisms capable of capsule formation. The capsule protects these organisms against certain host defense mechanisms, like **phagocytosis.** Thus the encapsulated forms are more virulent than the noncapsulated forms.

Table 4-1   Major pathogenic bacteria

Category	Organisms	Diseases
Gram-positive cocci	Staphylococcus aureus	Skin infections Pneumonia, enteritis
	Streptococcus pyogenes	Pharyngitis, rheumatic fever
	Streptococcus pneumoniae	Pneumonia, meningitis
Gram-negative cocci	Neisseria gonorrhoeae	Gonorrhea
	Neisseria meningitidis	Meningitis
	Moraxella catarrhalis	Bronchitis, pneumonia
Gram-negative coccobacilli	Hemophilus influenzae	Meningitis, pneumonia Epiglottitis
	Bordetella pertussis	Whooping cough
	Brucella	Brucellosis
Gram-positive spore-forming bacilli	Bacillus anthracis	Anthrax
	Bacillus cerus	Endocarditis
	Clostridium tetani	Tetanus
	Clostridium perfringens	Gas gangrene
	Clostridium botulinum	Botulism
Gram-positive nonspore-forming bacilli	Corynebacterium Diphtheriae	diphtheria
Gram-negative bacilli	Escherichia coli	Pneumonia, diarrhea, sepsis
	Klebsiella pneumoniae	Pneumonia, diarrhea, sepsis
	Serratia marcescens	Pneumonia, sepsis
	Shigella dysenteriae	Diarrhea, dysentery
	Salmonella typhi	Diarrhea, sepsis
	Proteus vulgaris	Pneumonia, sepsis
	Pseudomonas aeruginosa	Pneumonia, sepsis
	Bacteroides fragalis	Endocarditis, pneumonia
	Legionella pneumophilia	Legionellosis
Acid-fast bacilli	Mycobacterium tuberculosis	Tuberculosis (classical)
	Mycobacterium kansasii	Atypical tuberculosis
	Mycobacterium avium intracellulare	Atypical tuberculosis
Spirochetes	Treponema pallidum	Syphilis
	Leptospira	Conjunctivitis
	Borrelia	Lyme disease

Hemophilus influenzae is the most important Gram-negative coccobacilli causing respiratory infections. In its encapsulated form, *H. influenzae* is the primary cause of bacterial meningitis in small children. *H. influenzae* also causes pneumonia, bronchitis, epiglottitis and otitis media in children.

The noncapsulated form of *H. influenzae* is part of the normal flora of the upper airway. For this reason, most adult infections with *H. influenzae* occur in hosts with impaired defense mechanisms.[14]

Other Gram-negative coccobacilli of clinical importance are *Bordetella pertussis* and the *Brucella* species. *B. pertussis* causes whooping cough. Whooping cough is a highly communicable disease which, if not treated, can be fatal, especially in infants. Currently, the best treatment is prevention by immunization.

Brucella species are primarily pathogenic to animals, and only secondarily to man. Cattle, pigs, sheep and goats are carriers of the *Brucella* species. In humans, infection with one of these species is called brucellosis, or undulant fever.

Gram-positive bacilli

Gram-positive bacilli are further divided into two major categories: spore-formers and nonspore-formers.

Gram-Positive Spore-Forming Bacilli. Sporulation protects an organism against adverse environmental conditions. In its spore form, a bacterium can stay alive for many years. For example, most nonspore-formers are easily killed by temperatures in excess of 150°F. On the other hand, some spore-former can withstand live steam at 212°F. Spore-forming bacteria also are highly resistant to certain chemical disinfectants that easily kill other bacteria.

Two clinically significant genera of bacilli are spore-formers: the genus *Bacillus* and the genus *Clostridium*. Members of the genus *Bacillus* are mainly aerobic, although some are facultative. *Bacillus anthracis* is the most virulent, causing anthrax in both animals and man. Invasion of the blood or respiratory system with this organism can be fatal. The pulmonary infection is characterized by severe edema and hemorrhaging. Septicemia may also occur. *Bacillus cerus,* is the more common but less virulent pathogen in this genus. This organism can cause endocarditis, pulmonary and wound infections, and food poisoning.

Members of the genus *Clostridium* are **obligate** anaerobes. The three most common pathogens in this genus are *Clostridium tetani* (the cause of tetanus), *Clostridium perfringens,* (one of the causes of gas gangrene), and *Clostridium botulinum* (the cause of botulism).

C. tetani is found mainly in the soil, but may exist in the intestinal tract. The organism enters the body through piercing wounds or abrasions. Toxins produced by the organism cause **tetany** of skeletal muscle. Without treatment, tetanus result in death due to respiratory failure. Tetanus antitoxin is the primary treatment. Mechanical ventilation may be needed for some victims.

C. perfringens also enters the body through deep wounds, causing either an anaerobic **cellulitis** (not severe) or anaerobic **myositis** (gas gangrene). Gas gangrene can cause toxemia and death. Gas gangrene is treated by wound **debridement,** in conjunction with antibiotics. Oxygen under pressure (hyperbaric oxygen) may also help limit further tissue involvement.[15]

C. botulinum causes botulism. Botulism is a noninfectious disease caused by ingesting the potent toxin produced by this organism. The toxin affects the cranial nerves, causing double vision, dizziness, **dyspahgia,** and muscle paralysis, potentially leading to respiratory failure. As with tetanus, botulism is treated with an antitoxin. Antitoxin use has decreased the average mortality rate for botulism from nearly 60% to as low as 12%. Prevention, however, is the first line of defense. Botulism is easily prevented by careful food preparation and preservation.

In their spore phase, spore-forming bacilli are very hard to kill. As discussed later, the ability to kill spores differentiates true sterilization from disinfection.

Gram-Positive Non-Spore Forming Bacilli. *Corynebacterium diphtheriae* is the most important organism in this category. Facultative, nonmotile and **pleomorphic** (many-shaped), *C. diphtheriae* causes diphtheria. Invasion of the upper airway's mucous membranes produces the typical grey-white coating that leads to life-threatening obstruction. The acute disease is treated with diptheria antitoxin, followed by a course of antibiotics. In some cases, an artificial tracheal airway may need to be inserted. Widespread immunization against diphtheria in the US has greatly decreased the incidence of this disease.

Gram-negative enteric bacilli

Gram-negative enteric bacilli (GNBs), also called coliforms bacteria, are found in the digestive tract of all animals, including humans. Most are facultative anaerobes belonging to the family Enterobacteriaceae. Some produce toxins generically called bacteriocins. Among the most important of the enteric bacteria are *Escherichia coli, Klebsiella pneumoniae, Serratia marcescens, Shigella dysenteriae,* and members of the *Proteus* and *Salmonellae* genera. Members of the family Pseudomonadaceae will also be described here. Although not true enterics, the Pseudomonadaceae are often isolated with coliforms and cause similar infections.

E. coli is part of the normal flora of the intestinal tract, and normally not pathogenic. *E. coli* is a common cause of urinary tract infections, and can result in pneumonia, neonatal meningitis, and septicemia in debilitated or **immunosuppressed** patients. *E. coli* can also cause a dysentery-like intestinal infection.

K. pneumoniae is an opportunistic organism that frequently colonizes the upper respiratory tract of hospitalized patients. Lower respiratory tract invasion can cause a severe pneumonia with tissue necrosis. *K. pneumoniae* can also cause **septicemia.**[16]

S. marcescens can often be cultured from "aseptic" solutions used to fill humidifiers and nebulizers, and is also frequently isolated from the hands of hospital workers. Also opportunistic, it commonly causes primary infections in patients with indwelling catheters, and a secondary infection among those being treated for Gram-positive pneumonias.

S. dysenteriae, and members of the *Salmonellae* genera all cause intestinal infection via the ingestion of contaminated food or water. *Salmonella typhi* causes dysentery, **gastroenteritis,** and typhoid fever. Infection with *S. dysenteriae* also causes gastroenteritis and may result in septicemia. *Proteus* infections, on the other hand, are normally spread by direct contact, causing secondary intestinal, urinary, and respiratory tract infections.

Of all the members of the family Pseudomonadaceae, *Pseudomonas aeruginosa* is the most significant. *P. aeruginosa* is a motile, aerobic bacillus commonly found in the soil and water. In the hospital, it can be cultured from sinks, soap trays, drinking water, food, and respiratory care equipment. It is estimated that 10% or more of hospital-acquired infections are due to this organism. *P. aeruginosa* is particularly virulent among burn patients and those receiving immunosuppressive drugs.

Gram-negative anaerobic bacilli

Gram-negative anaerobic bacilli are the most common microorganisms in the human intestinal tract. Members of the genera *Bacteroides* are the most common Gram-negative anaerobes causing hospital infections. *Bacteroides* can cause a wide variety of localized infections, including endocarditis, **osteomylitis,** pneumonia, **empyema,** and urinary tract infections. Systemic *Bacteroides* infections can occur following perforation of abdominal viscera, or after septic abortion. Because this species is very slow-growing, *Bacteroides* infections are often not recognized.

L. pneumophilia is an aerobic Gram-negative bacillus that stains poorly. *Legionella* is treated separately here because it does not grow on common culture media and is very difficult to identify. *Legionella* appears to colonize in water, and has been found in air conditioning units, shower heads, and respiratory care equipment. The infection is acquired mainly by direct inhalation of aerosols carrying the organism and is not very communicable between patients.[17] *L. pneumophilia* causes a high fever, chills, and myalgia, and can progress to a life-threatening pneumonia (refer to Chapter 20).

Acid-fast bacilli (mycobacteria)

Acid-fast bacilli, such as *Mycobacterium tuberculosis,* are non-spore-forming, nonmotile, small aerobic organisms found throughout the environment. In addition to *M. tuberculosis,* other acid-fast bacilli pathogenic to man include *Mycobacterium kansasii, Mycobacterium avium-intracellulare,* and *Mycobacterium leprae.*

M. tuberculosis causes the chronic **granulomatous** infection most often localized to the lung. Pulmonary tuberculosis is classically transmitted by aerosol droplets and droplet nuclei produced by coughing. Although much less common, *M. kansasii* and *M. avium-intracellulare* (MAI) produces similar infections, but are usually spread through contaminated water. As such, they have caused nosocomial infection among patients undergoing invasive procedures like renal dialysis and **extracorporeal** circulation. *M. avium-intracellulare* is also common among patients with AIDS.[18]

Spirochetes

Pathogenic spirochetes belong mainly to the family Spirochaetaceae. These include members of the genera *Treponema, Borrelia,* and *Leptospira. Treponema pallidum* causes the sexually transmitted disease syphilis. Members of the genus *Borrelia* are transmitted by insect vectors. For example, Borrelia burglorferi is transmitted by ticks and causes Lyme disease. *Leptospira* species can cause infection of central nervous system, kidneys, liver, or lungs. Direct contact with infected rats or contaminated water is the most source of infection.

Viruses

Viruses are submicroscopic, noncellular, parasitic particles, composed of a protein shell and a nucleic acid core.[8] Viruses replicate by invading host cells and altering their genetic material. Depending on the virus involved, these infections can be transmitted by essentially all common routes. Viruses are resistant to common antibiotics and can withstand many decontamination procedures. Although some antiviral drug do exist, immunization is currently the best way to control viral infections.

Viruses may be classified according to both their structure and nucleic acid composition. For example, adenoviruses are composed of DNA, have an icosahedron shape and no outer envelope. The influenza virus, on the other hand is composed of RNA strands, is helical in shape, and is enclosed in an envelope.

The major pathogenic viruses are listed in Table 4-2. Influenza viruses are of three major types: A, B, and C. Type B is the most common cause of annual influenza epidemics, for which immunization is the only prevention. Influenza epidemics are a major concern in hospital infection control, especially among debilitated patients, such as those with COPD (see Chapter 20).

The paramyxoviruses include the mumps virus, rubeola (measles), the parainfluenza virus, and the respiratory syncytial virus (**RSV**). The parainfluenza virus causes croup (laryngotracheal bronchitis) in infants, but also can cause bronchiolitis and pneumonia. RSV is the major cause of bronchiolitis in children less than one year old.

The adenoviruses consist of over 30 serologic subgroups and are responsible for a variety of pulmonary-related infections. Although pharyngitis, tracheobronchitis and **conjunctivitis** are most common, fatal pneumonias have been reported in both children and adults infected with some strains of the adenovirus.

The rhinoviruses are small RNA viruses, with over 100 serologic subgroups. The rhinoviruses are respon-

Table 4-2 Viruses that cause disease in man

Virus	Transmission Route	Diseases
INFLUENZA	Respiratory tract	Tracheobronchitis Pneumonia Susceptibility to bacterial pneumonia
PARAMYXOVIRUSES		
Mumps	Respiratory tract	Parotitis Orchitis Pancreatitis Encephalitis
Measles (rubeola)	Respiratory tract	Rash, systemic illness Pneumonia Encephalomyelitis
Parainfluenza	Respiratory tract	Upper respiratory disease Croup, pneumonia
Respiratory syncytial	Respiratory tract	Bronchitis Bronchiolitis Pneumonia
ADENOVIRUSES	Respiratory tract Conjunctivae	Tracheobronchitis Pharyngitis Conjunctivitis
RHINOVIRUSES	Respiratory tract	Rhinitis Pharyngitis
ENTEROVIRUSES		
Coxsackie	Respiratory tract Gut	Systemic infections Meningtitis Tracheobronchitis Myocarditis
Polio	Gut	CNS damage (including anterior horn cells; paralysis)
HERPESVIRUSES		
Herpes simplex	Oral Genital Eye	Blisters → latent infection Keratoconjunctivitis
Varicella Herpes zoster	Respiratory tract	Vesicles → all ectodermal tissues (skin, mouth, respiratory tract)
Cytomegalo- virus	Not known	Usually disseminated disease in newborn and immune deficient
RUBELLA	Respiratory tract	Systemic mild illness, rash, congenitalanomalies in embryo
HEPATITIS	Blood, body fluids	Hepatitis Systemic disease
RABIES	Bites, or saliva on cut	Fatal CNS damage
HIV	Blood, body fluids	AIDS

sible for as much as 40% of all acute respiratory illness, including the common cold.

The enteroviruses include the coxsackie viruses and polio virus. The coxsackie viruses cause a variety of conditions, including meningitis, myocarditis and tracheobronchitis. The polio virus causes poliomyelitis, a neuromuscular disorder that can result in respiratory failure.

The herpesviruses include herpes simplex, varicella-zoster, Epstein-Barr virus and cytomegalovirus. Herpes simplex causes a variety of human infections, including genital and neonatal herpes and pneumonia.[19] Varicella-zoster virus is the cause of chickenpox and shingles (herpes zoster), but can also cause pneumonia. Epstein-Barr virus is associated with infectious mononucleosis.

Hepatitis infections are of four major types: A (HAV), B (HBV), C (HCV), and D (HDV). HAV, or *infectious hepatitis,* is normally transmitted via the fecal-oral route, or can be food or water-borne. Parenteral transmission (via contact with contaminated blood) is rare. Incubation is short (15 to 45 days), onset is acute, and mortality is low.

HBV, or *serum hepatitis* is transmitted mainly through contact with contaminated blood or body fluids. Incubation is long (30 to 120 days), onset is slow, and mortality is as high as 10%. Type B hepatitis may also exist chronically.

HDV is usually present as a coinfection or suprainfection with the HBV. The combined infection is more serious than HBV alone, with mortality as high as 30%. HCV hepatitis is responsible for over 90% of post-transfusion infections. Although less severe than type B, HCV results in a higher rate of chronic infection.

The human immunodeficiency virus **(HIV)** responsible for AIDS impairs the body's immune system by directly attacking the T lymphocytes (refer to Chapter 20). Current knowledge indicates that AIDS can be transmitted by only one of three routes: (1) sexual contact, (2) parenteral exposure via contaminated IV needles, and (3) **transplacental** and/or **intrapartum** perinatal exposure. Transfusion with contaminated blood is also a risk factor. However, mandatory testing of donated blood for HIV antibodies has nearly eliminated transmission via this route.

Given the high rate of exposure of hospital personnel to blood and body fluids, both hepatitis (B and C) and HIV have become the focus of major hospital infection control efforts. Current evidence indicates that the risk of acquiring hepatitis and AIDS through occupational exposure is very low.[20]

In those cases where health care workers have acquired hepatitis or AIDS on the job, neglect of standard infection control procedures has been identified as the primary reason for infection. To help avoid hepatitis B, all health care personnel at high risk should be immununized against this virus.[21] Unfortunately, no human HIV vaccine yet exists. In both cases, however, infection risk can be reduced by safe work practices. More details on these procedures are provided later in this chapter.

Rickettsiae and chlamydiae

Like viruses, Rickettsiae and Chlamydiae require a living cell to replicate. Like bacteria, however, these organisms have a complex structure. Both are very small, generally less than a μm in size. Rickettsiae are transmitted mainly via the vector (insect) route.

Table 4-3 Rickettsial diseases of man

Group	Principal Diseases	Etiologic Agent	Reservoir in Nature	Usual Occurrence
Typhus	Epidemic typhus	*Rickettsia prowazekii*	Man, lice	Worldwide in winter and spring
	Murine typhus	*R. mooseri*	Rats and rat fleas	Worldwide where rats abound
Spotted fever	Rocky Mountain spotted fever	*R. rickettsii*	Ticks	North and South America
	Rickettsial pox	*R. akari*	Mite	New York City Boston
Q fever	Q fever	*R. burneti (Coxiella burnetii)*	Ticks; infected cattle and sheep	Probably worldwide
Trench fever	Trench fever	*R. quintana*	Body lice, man	Europe, Africa North America

Chlamydiae can be transmitted via the airborne route (psittacosis) or via direct contact, including genital.

The common Rickettsial diseases, including their etiologic agent and vectors, are listed in Table 4-3. Ninety percent of all Rickettsial infections in the US are Rocky Mountain spotted fever, caused by *Rickettsia rickettsii.*

Chalamydia pneumoniae, strain TWAR is a common cause of pneumonia among otherwise healthy older children and young adults.[22] Sinusitis, pharyngitis, and bronchitis may also occur. *Chlamydia trachomatis,* the infectious agent in trachoma, is the most common cause of blindness in the world. *C. trachomatis* can also cause a nongonococcal **urethritis,** and newborn conjuntivitis (by contact with the mother's genital tract). *Chlamydia psittaci* causes psittacosis (orinithosis), a highly infectious pneumonia transmitted by contact with parrots, parakeets, pigeons, and other birds.

Mycoplasmas

Mycoplasmas were first identified as causing severe pneumonia in cattle. Due to their extremely small size and ability to pass through bacterial filters, it was initially thought that mycoplasmas were viruses. However, like bacteria, mycoplasmas grow on artificial media.

Mycoplasmas have no rigid cell wall, are pleomorphic, and do not retain the Gram stain. *Mycoplasma pneumoniae* is the key pathogen, which causes primary atypical pneumonia.[23] The infection is spread mainly by contact with respiratory tract secretions.

Identification of the organism is difficult, usually requiring comparative serologic studies.

Fungi

Fungi are found everywhere. Most have a preference for warm, moist environments, such as found in the hospital. As compared to bacteria, fungi are much larger and more complex (**eukaryotic** cell structure). Fungi reproduce either sexually or by spore formation, and include both molds and yeasts. Molds are branching multicellular filaments. Yeasts are unicellular, ranging in size from about 2.5 to 6 μm.[8]

Fungal infections, called *mycoses,* are of two general types: those occurring in otherwise healthy individuals, and those affecting hosts with impaired resistance (opportunistic infections). Common organisms in the first category are *Coccidioides immitis, Histoplasma capsulatum, Blastomyces dermatitidis,* and *Cryptococcus neoformans.*[24] Opportunistic fungi include *Candida albicans* and *Aspergillus fumigatus.*[25] Opportunistic fungal infections are a major problem in hospitals, due to the large number of debilitated and immunosuppressed patients. Table 4-4 summarizes the common mycoses.

Another important organism that is probably a fungi is *Pneumocystis carinii.*[26] *Pneumocystis* causes an opportunistic infection among patients with an abnormal or altered immunologic status, particularly those suffering from the acquired immune deficiency syndrome (AIDS). Infection with *Pneumocystis* causes an acute interstitial pneumonia, with fatality rates of 50% or higher.

Table 4-4   Major fungal infections

Organism	Disease	Comments
Coccidioides immitis	Coccidiodomycosis	Also called San Joaquin fever because of prevalence in southwestern United States; initial illness like influenza; some patients progress to severe systemic infection; transmission via airborne dust
Cryptococcus neoformans	Cryptococcosis	Also known as torulosis; acquired via contact with bird excreta; causes solitary pulmonary nodule in most cases; may progress to fatal meningoencephalitis in some
Histoplasma capsulatum	Histoplasmosis	Acquired via contact with soil containing fecal matter from birds and bats; prevalent in Mississippi valley area; mimics tuberculosis
Blastomyces dermatitidis	Blastomycosis	Acquired via contact with soil contaminated with animal feces; frequently disseminates to skin, bones, GI tract, kidneys, brain
Candida albicans	Candidiasis	Occurs almost exclusively in immunosuppressed patients or those with hematologic malignancies
Aspergillus fumagatus	Aspergillosis	Occurs in three forms: (1) allergic, (2) invasive (common in immunosuppressed patients or those with hematologic malignancies), and (3) "fungus ball" or aspergilloma colonization in pulmonary cavitary lesions; invasive form is the most serious.

Protozoa

Protozoa are single-celled eucaryotic microbes ranging in size from 5 to 60 μm.[8] Protozoal infections are prevalent in many tropical areas of the world, and may also be found under conditions of crowding and poor sanitation. Amebiasis, malaria, and trypanosomiasis are examples of these protozoal infections. Although protozoa do not commonly cause lung infections, they may do so in immunosuppressed patients.[8]

SPREAD OF INFECTION

Three elements must be present for an infection to spread: a source of pathogens, a susceptible host, and a mode of transmission.[27]

Source

The primary source of pathogens in the hospital are either people (patients, personnel, or visitors) or contaminated objects, such as equipment and medications. People may have an acute disease, may be in the incubation period of the disease, or may simply be colonized by pathogens, with no apparent symptoms. People may also serve as their own source of infection, via **endogenous** flora. This latter mechanism is called *autogenous infection.*

Microorganisms differ in their relative **virulence.** Highly virulent organisms need only be present in small numbers to cause an infection. On the other hand, microorganisms that are relatively avirulent must be exist in large numbers to cause infection, or be present in an immunocompromised host.

Most cases of nosocomial pneumonia are due to bacteria.[9] Aerobic Gram-negative bacilli and aerobic Gram-positive cocci each account for about 40% of all reported cases of nosocomial pneumonia.

Host

The mere presence and growth of microorganisms in a host, without tissue invasion, damage, or toxin response is called *colonization.* Whether a host actually develops an infection depends on the virulence of the organism, *and* the host's resistance.

Resistance to infection varies greatly. Some individuals may be immune to certain pathogens or able to resist their colonization. Others exposed to the same organism may become asymptomatic carriers. Still others may develop clinical disease. Persons with diabetes mellitus, **lymphoma,** leukemia, neoplasia, or **uremia** and those treated with certain antimicrobials, corticosteroids, irradiation, or immunosuppressive agents may be particularly susceptible to infection. Age, chronic debilitating disease, shock, coma, traumatic injury, or surgical procedures also increase patient susceptibility to infection.

The high incidence of Gram-negative bacterial pneumonias in the hospital is believed to be the result of factors that promote colonization of the pharynx with these organisms. Colonization dramatically increases in patients with severe underlying illness and predisposes such patients to Gram-negative pneumonias (see accompanying box).[28]

Three-quarters of all nosocomial pneumonias occur in surgical patients, especially those having had chest or abdominal procedures. In these patients, normal swallowing and clearance mechanisms are impaired, allowing bacteria to enter and remain in the lower respiratory tract. Intubation, anesthesia, surgical pain, and use of narcotics and sedatives further impair host defenses.

The risk of pneumonia is not the same for all surgical patients. Patients at highest risk include the elderly, the severely obese, those with COPD or a history of smoking, and those having an artificial airway in place for long periods.[29]

Patients with an artificial tracheal airway are at high risk for nosocomial pneumonia for several reasons. Typically, patients requiring prolonged intubation already have one or more factors predisposing to infection, such as severe COPD. Other risk factors may be increased upper airway colonization with aerobic Gram-negative bacteria. Moreover, since the tube bypasses normal upper airway protective mechanisms, bacteria have easy access to the lower respiratory tract. Last, manipulation of these tubes increases the likelihood of cross-contamination, particularly during suctioning.

Some pneumonias occur primarily in immunocompromised hosts. Immunosuppression may be purposefully induced by drugs, as in patients who receive an organ transplant, or may result from an underlying disease process, such as AIDS. Regardless of cause, immunocompromised hosts are prone to develop opportunistic pneumonias due to unusual bacteria, fungi or viruses.

Conditions associated with colonization of the oropharynx by gram-negative bacilli

Endotracheal intubation
Underlying respiratory disease
Respiratory distress syndrome
Diabetes mellitus
Chronic alcohol abuse
Nasogastric tube
Neutralization of gastric secretions
Hypotension
Coma
Acidosis
Azotemia

Transmission

Pathogens are transmitted via four major routes: contact, vehicle, airborne, and vectorborne. Some pathogens may be transmitted by more than one route. For example, the HIV virus can spread either by direct contact (sexual intercourse) or by indirect contact with a contaminated inanimate object (needles). Examples of the common routes for transmission of selected microorganisms are provided in Table 4-5.[30]

Contact transmission

Contact transmission is the most important and most frequent route for spread of nosocomial infections. Methods of contact transmission include: (1) direct contact, (2) indirect contact, and (3) droplet contact.

Direct contact involves direct physical transfer between a susceptible host and an infected or colonized person. Sexually transmitted diseases such as gonorrhea, syphilis and AIDS are transmitted this way. In the hospital, infection spreads by this route when a colonized or infected worker touches a patient, changes a tracheostomy dressing, or perform other procedures requiring direct contact. This is the common route for many nosocomial *Staphylococcus* and en-

teric bacterial infections. Direct contact can also occur between patients.

Indirect contact involves contact between a susceptible host and a contaminated object. Objects that harbor infectious agents are called *fomites*. Common fomites include clothing, dressings, instruments, and equipment. For example, indirect patient contact with a contaminated nebulizer is a common route for spread of *P. aeruginosa*. Contaminated needles are another common fomite for indirect contact transmission, especially for hepatitis and HIV.

Droplet contact transmission occurs when a pathogen reaches the mucous membranes of a host via an infected person or carrier who is coughing or sneezing. This is considered "contact" transmission rather than airborne, since droplets usually travel no more than three feet. Measles and streptococcal pneumonia are examples of infections transmitted via droplet contact.

Vehicle transmission

Vehicle transmission occurs when a host is exposed to pathogens in contaminated food or water. Salmonellosis and hepatitis A are examples of food-borne infections. Shigellosis and cholera are examples of water-borne infections.

Airborne transmission

Airborne transmission occurs when a pathogen is spread via the air. Airborne spread may occur in the form of aerosol droplets, droplet nuclei or dust particles. Aerosol droplets are liquid particles in the 10 to 100 μm size range. Aerosol droplets can be produced by aerosol generators, or created by coughing and sneezing. Droplet nuclei are the residue of evaporated water droplets. Due to their smaller size (0.5 to 12 μm), droplet nuclei can remain suspended in the air for long periods of time. Dust or dirt particles, usually greater than 50 μm in size, act as minute fomites.

Organisms carried in this manner can be widely dispersed by air currents before being deposited in a susceptible host. Legionellosis (Legionnaire' disease) is probable transmitted via actual aerosol droplets. Tuberculosis is a classical example of an infection transmitted via droplet nuclei. Most fungal infections are transmitted via the airborne route on dust particles.

Vectorborne transmission

Vectorborne transmission occurs when an animal, especially an insect, transfers an infectious agent from one host to another. Vectorborne transmissions such as malaria (mosquito vector) are of major concern in tropical countries. Although vectorborne transmissions are also responsible for many types of infections in United States, they are of little significance in hospital acquired infections.

Table 4-5 Routes of infectious disease transmission

Mode	Type	Examples
Contact	Direct	Hepatitis A Venereal disease HIV Staphylococcus Enteric bacteria
	Indirect	Pseudomonas Enteric bacteria Hepatitis B and C HIV
	Droplet	Measles Streptococcus
Vehicle	Waterborne	Shigellosis Cholera
	Foodborne	Salmonellosis Hepatitis A
Airborne	Aerosols	Legionellosis
	Droplet nuclei	Tuberculosis Diphtheria
	Dust	Histoplasmosis
Vectorborne	Ticks and mites	Rickettsia, Lyme's disease
	Mosquitos	Malaria
	Fleas	Bubonic plague

Spread of infection into the lungs

Spread of infectious agents into the lungs occurs by one or more of three major routes: (1) aspiration of oropharyngeal or gastric secretions, (2) inhalation of aerosol droplets, droplet nuclei or dust particles containing bacteria, and (3) blood-borne **(hematogenous)** spread from a distant site of infection.

Of these three routes, aspiration is believed to cause most cases of bacterial pneumonia.[28] The likelihood of aspiration is greatest in persons with abnormal swallowing mechanisms. These patients usually have one or more of the following risk factors: decreased consciousness, dysphagia, or a nasogastric tube. Patients who have undergone instrumentation of the respiratory or GI tracts are also at high risk for aspiration.

INFECTION CONTROL METHODS

Infection control aims to break the chain of events causing the spread of infection. This can be done by eliminating the source of pathogens, decreasing host susceptibility, and interrupting transmission routes.

Decreasing host susceptibility to infection is the most difficult and least feasible approach. Hospital efforts to achieve this end focus mainly on employee immunization. Depending on the relative risks involved, hospital personnel may be immunized against influenza, hepatitis, **diphtheria,** tetanus and sometimes tuberculosis (BCG vaccine).

With the exception of BCG, these vaccines do not help halt the spread of *bacterial* infections. Moreover, employee immunization programs do not protect patients or visitors. For this reason, we will focus on eliminating the source of infection and interrupting its spread.

Eliminating the source of pathogens

It is impossible to eliminate all pathogens from the hospital. This is exactly why a multifaceted approach to infection control is needed. Nonetheless, standard infection control procedures always include efforts to remove pathogens from the environment.

Infection control procedures designed to remove environmental pathogens fall into two major categories: general sanitation measures, and specialized equipment processing.

If the environment is dirty, all other infection control efforts will be futile. *General sanitation measures* help keep the overall environment clean. General sanitation aims to reduce the number of pathogens to a safe level. This is done via sanitary laundry management, food preparation, and housekeeping. Environmental control of the air (via specialized ventilation systems) and water complement these efforts.

The goal of *specialized equipment processing* is to decontaminate equipment that is linked to infection. Equipment processing involves cleaning and disinfection or sterilization. *Cleaning* is the removal of dirt and organic material from equipment, usually by washing.[31] *Disinfection* is a process which kills the vegetative form of pathogenic organisms.[31] *Sterilization* completely destroys all microbial life.[31] True sterilization kills *both* the vegetative and spore forms of all bacteria, and fungi, yeast and viruses. Disinfection may not kill spore-forming bacteria.

Cleaning

Cleaning is the first step in equipment processing. Cleaning should take place in a designated location that is divided into dirty and clean areas.[8] Cleaning procedures remove infectious materials, particularly organic matter, from equipment that has been in-use.

All equipment should be disassembled and examined for worn parts. Complete disassembly helps assure that as much surface area as possible is exposed to the cleaning agent. Small parts with tiny crevices can be treated in an ultrasonic cleaner.[8] After disassembly, parts should be placed in a clean basin filled with hot water and soap or detergent.

A soap or detergent is needed because water alone cannot penetrate or dissolve substances like fat or grease.[8] Soaps act by lowering surface tension and forming an emulsion with organic matter. Soaps are not bactericidal, but may be combined with a disinfectant.

Like soaps, detergents reduce surface tension, thereby aiding penetration of water into organic matter. Unlike soaps, detergents work in hard water and are weakly bactericidal against Gram-positive bacteria.[8] Unfortunately, detergents are inactivated by contact with proteins, and are not effective against tubercle bacilli and viruses.[8] Some commercial products combine a germicide with a detergent, thus providing the dual action of cleaning and preliminary disinfection.[8]

As an alternative to manual washing, automatic systems similar to kitchen dish washers can be used. These devices go through several cycles to wash, rinse, and pasteurize or chemically disinfect the equipment. Typically, the disinfectant is held in a side tank and pumped into the holding tub when needed. After disinfection, the liquid is pumped back into the holding tank for re-use.[32]

Objects that cannot be immersed, such as electrical equipment, should at least be surfaced disinfected with a 70% alcohol solution or the equivalent. Where possible, these items should undergo subsequent gas sterilization.

After cleaning, equipment should be carefully rinsed and dried. Good rinsing ensures that any soap or detergent residues are removed. Such residues can be irritating to human tissue and can impair subsequent disinfection or sterilization efforts.

Drying is important because residual water dilutes and alters the pH of disinfectant solutions.[8] Also, if equipment is to be gas sterilized, residual water may combine with ethylene oxide gas to form ethylene glycol, which is toxic. Drying is important even if no further disinfection occurs, because a humid environment encourages bacterial growth.[8]

When clean equipment has to be reassembled prior to further processing, care must be taken to avoid recontamination. To avoid recontamination, the processed equipment should be moved to the clean area. Prior to reassembly, the equipment worker should conduct a vigorous hand scrub. Ideally, reassembly should take place in a filtered hood designed for this purpose. Cleaned equipment should never be allowed to sit on open counters for prolonged periods of time.

Although careful cleaning will remove most pathogens from equipment, it cannot totally eliminate the risk of infection. For this reason, most equipment must undergo either disinfection or sterilization.

Disinfection

Disinfection destroys the vegetative form of pathogenic organisms. Disinfection can be achieved by either physical or chemical means. The most common physical method of disinfection is pasteurization. Numerous chemical methods are used to disinfect respiratory care equipment (Table 4-6).

Pasteurization. Pasteurization is an efficient and cost effective method for disinfecting respiratory care equipment.[33,34] Like some sterilization methods, pasteurization uses moist heat to coagulate cell proteins. However, the temperatures used are not high enough to kill bacterial spores (Table 4-6).

The major spore-forming bacterial that are pathogenic to man include *B. anthracis, C. tetani, C. perfringens,* and *C. botulinum.* Anthrax is a rare cause of human infection, especially in the hospital. Although *Clostridia* can produce lethal toxins, these organisms are obligate anaerobes, and thus of little threat in free atmospheric oxygen. Thus, the fact that pasteurization does not kill spores is of minor practical concern in hospital infection control.

The exposure time needed to kill vegetative bacteria by pasteurization depends on the temperature. The *flash* process, (used mainly to disinfect milk), consists of exposing the material to 72° C for a period of 15 seconds. More applicable to respiratory care equipment processing is the *batch* process. In the batch process, equipment is immersed in a water bath

Table 4-6 Capabilities of various disinfecting agents

Disinfectant	Gram-positive Bacteria	Gram-negative Bacteria	Tubercle bacillus	Spores	Viruses*	Fungi
Soaps	0[†]	0	0	0	0	0
Detergents	±	≈	0	0	0	0
Hot water	+	+	+	±	±	?
Quats	+	±	0	0	±	±
Acetic acid	?	+	?	?	?	±
Alcohols	+	+	+	0	±	±
Phenols	+	+	+	±	±	+
Iodophors	+	+	+	≈	±	+
Glutaraldehyde	+	+	+	±	+	+
Hydrogen-peroxide	+	+	+	±	+	+
Sodium Hypochlorite	+	+	+	±	+	+
Peracetic Acid	+	+	+	+	+	+
Chlorine dioxide	l	+	+	+	+	+
Steam (> 100° C)	+	+	+	+	+	+
Ethylene oxide	+	+	+	+	+	+

Adapted from Chatburn RL: Decontamination of respiratory care equipment: what can be done, what should be done, *Respir Care,* 34(2):98–110, 1989.
*Viral activity depends on whether the virus is lipophilic or hydrophilic.
[†]+ = good; ± = fair; ≈ = poor; ? = unknown; 0 = little or none.

heated to 63° C for 30 minutes. These conditions will kill all vegetative bacteria and some viruses, including HIV.[8] Most respiratory care equipment can easily withstand these conditions without damage.

The major problem with pasteurization is not the process itself, but the difficulty in avoiding equipment recontamination following immersion. Special filtered dryers, used with laminar flow assembly hoods and scrupulous aseptic technique, can help minimize recontamination.

Chemical disinfection. Chemical disinfection involves application of chemical solutions to contaminated equipment or surfaces. Depending on their make-up, these agents may kill microorganisms by disrupting their cell membranes, coagulating their proteins, or destroying their enzyme processes.[31,35]

The Centers for Disease Control (**CDC**) recognize three levels of chemical disinfection: low, intermediate and high (Table 4-7).[36] According to this scheme, high-level chemical disinfection is equivalent to sterilization if exposure time is long enough.

Low and intermediate-level disinfection. Low and intermediate-level disinfectants can kill most vegetative bacteria and fungi, but have variable activity against spores and nonlipid viruses. Agents in this category include the alcohols, phenols, halogens, iodophors, quaternary ammonium compounds, and acetic acid.

Alcohols. Alcohols disinfect by **denaturing** cell proteins.[31] Both ethyl and isopropyl alcohol are good disinfectants when combined with water. Ethyl alcohol is best at a 70% concentration, while the optimum concentration for isopropyl alcohol is 90%.[8] Alcohol solutions kill most vegetative bacteria and fungi, including *M. tuberculosis,* but not spores (Table 4-6).[37] Activity against viruses varies, with ethyl alcohol being the better **virucide.**[31] To inactivate the hepatitis virus, the CDC recommends exposure to 70% ethyl alcohol for 15 minutes; 1 minute is sufficient to kill HIV.[38] Alcohols are inactivated by protein and can

damage rubber, plastics, and the shellac mounting of lensed instruments.[31]

Phenolics. Lister first used phenol (carbolic acid) in the 1800s to reduce postoperative infections. A number of synthetic derivatives of phenol (phenolics) have been developed as disinfectants. The two most common are ortho-phenylphenol and ortho-benzyl-para-chlorophenol. These agents have stronger antimicrobial activity than plain phenol.[31] In addition, phenolics retain their activity in the presence of organic matter, and can remain effective on surfaces long after application.[35]

Phenolics kills by injuring the cell wall, inactivating enzymes and denaturing proteins.[31] Simple phenol in a 5% solution is effective against most vegetative forms of bacteria, including, *M. tuberculosis.*[31,35] Phenolics are also fungicidal, but activity against spores and viruses varies (Table 4-6).[31] Unfortunately, phenolics are absorbed easily by porous material, and the residual disinfectant causes tissue irritation.[31] Phenolics are also associated with neonatal hyperbilirubinemia when used in nurseries.[31] For these reasons, phenolics are generally limited to use as surface disinfectants. An exception is an equipment disinfectant formulation that combines a phenolic with glutaraldehyde (discussed under glutaraldehydes).

Halogens. Of the halogens, chlorine and iodine are the only two commonly used as disinfectants. Chlorine is a potent and rapid acting disinfectant. For disinfectant use, chlorine is prepared either as a sodium hypochlorite (bleach) solution or as chlorine dioxide.

Sodium hypochlorite has a broad spectrum of antimicrobial activity, being bactericidal in 10 minutes and fungicidal in 1 hour (see Table 4-6).[31] Most viruses, including HBV and HIV, are inactivated in 10 minutes or less with a 1:100 dilution of bleach. A 1:10 dilution is recommended by the CDC to clean blood spills. Unfortunately, sodium hypochlorite so-

Table 4-7   Levels of disinfection

	Bacteria				Viruses	
Level	Vegetative	Tubercle bacillus	Spores	Fungi	Lipid and medium size	Nonlipid and small
Low	+	−	−	±	+	−
Intermediate	+	+	±₂	+	+	±₃
High	+	+	+₁	+	+	+

NOTES
1—Sporicidal only with extended exposure times.
2—Some intermediate-level disinfectants are sporicidal.
3—Some intermediate-level disinfectants are virucidal.

Adapted from *Am J Infect Control* 14:110–129, 1986.
+ = killing effect under normal conditions
− = little or no killing effect

lutions are unstable and corrosive. In addition, sodium hypochlorite is inactivated by organic matter.[31]

Demand release chloride dioxide is a relatively new disinfectant that may also sterilize with prolonged exposure (see Table 4-6).[31] Unfortunately, chloride dioxide corrodes most metals.

Iodine in alcohol (tincture of iodine) is among the most popular wound and skin bactericidal agents. In addition to being effective against most vegetative bacteria, iodine has fungicidal, sporicdal, and virucidal action. However, high concentrations of iodine cause tissue necrosis, and its staining properties limit its use with many materials.

Iodophors are mixtures of iodine with surface-active organic compounds.[31] The most common iodophor is povidine-iodine (polyvinylpyrrolidone with iodine). Unlike tincture compounds, iodophors are water soluble, nonstaining, and less irritating to tissue. Like iodine, iodophors are bactericidal and virucidal (see Table 4-6). However, iodophors have limited sporicdal activity and can require prolonged contact to kill fungi.[31] Also, proper dilution is critical to ensuring the antimicrobial activity of iodophors.

Quaternary ammonium compounds. Quaternary ammonium compounds, or "quats," are **cationic** detergents containing ammonium ions.[39] Quats are thought to kill bacteria by destroying the plasma membrane and inactivating cellular enzymes.[8]

When compared to most other chemical disinfectants, quats are bland, nontoxic and inexpensive. In addition, when kept free of organic matter, quat solutions retain their activity for up to two weeks. However, the bactericidal activity of quats is selective.[39] Quats are most active against Gram-positive vegetative bacteria. The ability to kill Gram-negative organisms, such as *Pseudomonas aeruginosa,* varies according to the formulation, the concentration, and time of exposure.[40] Sporicidal activity is minimal, and tuberculocidal and virucidal activity is questionable (see Table 4-6).

Perhaps most important of all, quats are neutralized by soaps and anionic detergents, and their activity is reduced by contact with organic material and hard water.[41] Thus it is essential that soap and organic material be removed from equipment before immersion in the disinfectant. Further, dilution of quats with rinse water alters the pH and reduce disinfectant activity. As with any liquid chemical disinfectant, processed equipment must be dried and reassembled carefully to prevent recontamination.

Recently developed third-generation quats remain active in hard water and with anionic detergents.[31] These "triple quats" may be more active against gram-negative bacteria, fungi, and viruses than earlier preparations. However, these new preparations are still considered intermediate-level disinfectants. For these reasons, the use of quats in hospitals is limited. The most common use is for surface disinfection of countertops and devices that cannot be soaked (eg, ventilators).[8] For this purpose, triple quat preparations are available in aerosol spray cans.

Because they are bland, nontoxic and inexpensive, quats have become increasingly popular in the home care setting for equipment disinfection. However, quats do not provide high level disinfection. For this reason, activated glutaraldehyde is recommended as the disinfectant of choice in the home care setting.[42]

Acetic acid. Acetic acid, in the form of white vinegar, has been used as a disinfectant in both the hospital and home.[8] Acetic acid (pH 2.0–3.0) probably kills bacteria by lowering intracellular pH and inactivating enzymes. In general, the bactericidal action of acetic acid is similar to that of quats, with stronger activity against *Pseudomonas aeruginosa.*[43] A 1.25% solution, equivalent to 1 part 5% household vinegar to 3 parts water, appears optimum. Unfortunately, neither the **sporicidal** nor virucidal activity of acetic acid has been documented.[8] For this reason, acetic acid should probably be used only as an emergency alternative to commercial disinfectants in the home care setting.[8]

The addition of an oxygen atom to the acetic acid molecule produces peracetic acid. Alone or in combination with hydrogen peroxide, peracetic acid appears to be a powerful new disinfectant with sterilization capabilities (see Table 4-6).[44]

High-level disinfection. Common high-level chemical disinfectants include glutaraldehyde, hydrogen-peroxide, and peracetic acid.

Glutaraldehydes. Glutaraldehydes are chemically related to formaldehyde, a fumigant and specimen fixative. Glutaraldehydes kill microorganisms by attacking the lipoproteins in bacterial cell membranes and cytoplasm.[8] Under appropriate conditions, glutaraldehydes kill all living material, and can thus be classified as sterilizing agents (see Table 4-6).[31] Two forms of glutaraldehyde are available for use as disinfectants and sterilizing agents: alkaline glutaraldehyde and acid glutaraldehyde.

Alkaline glutaraldehyde (eg, Cidex) is a 2% glutaraldehyde solution buffered by $NaHCO_3$ to a pH between 7.5 and 8.5. Alkaline glutaraldehyde is bactericidal, tuburculocidal, fungicidal, and virucidal at room temperature in ten minutes.[45] Three to 10 hours immersion is required to kill spores (sterilization).[46] With short exposure times, alkaline glutaraldehyde does not harm metals, rubber or plastics, and can be used with fiberoptic endoscopes.[8] Depending on the brand, alkaline glutaraldehyde solutions are reusable for up to 14 to 28 days.[8]

Direct skin contact with alkaline glutaraldehyde can cause dermatitis.[47] To avoid skin reactions, rubber gloves should always be worn when using this disinfectant. In addition, equipment must be thoroughly rinsed before use. Failure to do so can result in inflammatory reactions by patients to invasive devices, such as artificial airways.[48]

Acid glutaraldehyde is available as a ready-to-use 2% solution with a pH between 2.7–3.7. At room temperature, its action is similar to alkaline glutaraldehyde, but requires 20 minutes for high-level disinfection. Warming enhances its activity. At 60° C, the acid formulation is bactericidal, virucidal, and fungicidal in 5 minutes, tuberculocidal in 20 minutes, and sporicidal in 60 minutes.[49] Acid glutaraldehyde is noncorrosive to most materials but should not be used to disinfect plated metal instruments. It does not irritate the eyes or nose, and gloves are not needed when using it. Solutions can be reused for up to 30 days.[49]

The major disadvantage of glutaraldehydes is their effect on mucous membranes and the eyes. Short-term human exposure to glutaraldehyde causes eye, nose and throat irritation. Due to these concerns, the Occupational Safety and Health Administration (OSHA) has set a ceiling limit of 0.2 **ppm** airborne glutaraldehyde exposure.[50]

More recently, glutaraldehyde-phenates (phenolic derivatives combined with glutaraldehyde) have been developed to overcome this problem. Examples include Sporicidin and ColdSpor.[50] At full strength and with proper exposure time (7 to 12 hours), these agents provide true sterilization for up to 30 days use, without the irritating side effects of plain glutaraldehyde.[51] Dilution, however, causes loss of bactericidal activity, especially in the presence of organic matter.[31]

Hydrogen-peroxide-based compounds. Hydrogen peroxide has been used for years as a wound antiseptic. Recently, hydrogen peroxide-based compounds have proved themselves as high-level disinfectants (see Table 4-6). At room temperature, these solutions are bactericidal, fungicidal and virucidal (against influenza and herpes simplex) in 10 minutes.[8] Sterilization (sporicidal action) is achieved in 6 hours at 20° C or in 10 minutes at 50° C.[8] Stabilized hydrogen peroxide combined with peracetic acid is an even more effective sporicide.

Stabilized hydrogen peroxide-based solutions retain effective germicidal activity for up to six weeks. In addition, they require no mixing or activation, do not produce harsh fumes, and are safe for use with rubber, plastic, and stainless steel.[8] They do, however, corrode copper, zinc and brass.[31]

Peracetic acid. Peracetic acid has been recognized for years as a powerful germicide. Until recently, however, its corrosive nature has prevented its use for medical instruments.[52]

Recently, a specially formulated buffered peracetic acid solution with anticorrosives has been developed for this purpose.[53] Early reports indicate that this solution meets or exceed both the EPA and FDA requirements for high-level disinfectants and steriliz-

ing agents (see Table 4-6). When used in a special processor, this peracetic acid solution sterilized medical devices, including endoscopes, in less than 30 min.[53] Mixtures of peracetic acid and hydrogen peroxide with detergents are also being used for one-stage disinfection in settings requiring simultaneous disinfection and washing.[54]

All items subjected to high-level chemical disinfection should be rinsed in sterile water to remove toxic residues and then thoroughly dried. These objects should then be handled aseptically with sterile gloves and towels during the packaging process.[36]

Sterilization

Sterilization can be achieved by either physical or chemical means.[31] Both methods act by denaturing, coagulating, or inactivating essential cell proteins. Table 4-8 compares and contrasts the major methods of sterilization.[55,56]

Physical methods of sterilization. The two most common physical methods used to sterilize equipment are heat and ionizing radiation.

Heat. For most objects, heat is the most practical and efficient means of sterilization.[57,58] In general, the higher the temperature, the shorter the time needed for sterilization. However, different temperatures and time periods are needed to kill various organisms.

Heat sterilization would be simple were it not for spores. The bacterial spore is probably the most resistant form of life known; some will survive boiling water for several hours. Because there is no standard pattern of heat resistance for spores, all heat sterilization methods must be able to kill the most resistant spore forms.

Common methods of heat sterilization include incineration, dry heat, boiling, and moist heat under pressure (autoclaving).

Incineration, or burning, is used for sterilization only when the object has no further use, or is so contaminated as to prohibit its reuse. Although incineration is the surest sterilization method, its use is limited.

Dry heat sterilization is performed in an oven similar to that used in the home. With the exception of incineration, dry heat sterilization requires the highest temperatures of all methods. The most common procedure is to use a temperature of 160° to 180° C for 1 to 2 hours. Dry heat is ideal for most glass and metal objects. However, most equipment used in respiratory care cannot undergo dry heat sterilization.

Boiling water at sea level (100°C) kills all vegetative forms of bacteria and nearly all viruses within 30 minutes.[8] Some spores, however, can withstand boiling for long periods. Thus, boiling water does not assure complete sterilization. Moreover, since water boils at lower temperatures at high altitudes, steriliza-

Table 4-8 Comparison of sterilization methods

Method	Applicable Equipment	Advantages	Disadvantages
Incineration	Disposables; grossly contaminated articles	Surest method; simple	Limited use; may result in air pollution
Dry heat	Laboratory glassware; metal instruments	Inexpensive; simple; nontoxic	Damages heat-sensitive equipment
Boiling	Metals; heat-resistant plastics	Inexpensive; simple	Time consuming; altitude dependent; may damage some equipment
Autoclave	Metal instruments; linens	Inexpensive; fast; nontoxic; prewrapping of items	May damage heat- or moisture-sensitive equipment
Ionizing radiation	Foods; some medical supplies	Fast; effective; prewrapping of items	Expensive; toxic byproducts may be produced
Ethylene oxide	Heat-sensitive items	Effective; prewrapping of items	Time consuming; expensive; toxic residues must be removed by aeration

tion by boiling may be ineffective, particularly with **thermophilic** organisms.

Moist heat, or steam under pressure, is the most efficient sterilization process. Steam under pressure, using an autoclave, quickly coagulates cell proteins. The time needed for sterilization depends on both the temperature and pressure. As the pressure increases, the temperature increases, and time needed for sterilization decreases.

For example, at 15 psig, the temperature of steam is 121° C, and full sterilization can be achieved in 15 minutes. On the other hand, if the pressure is raised to 20 psig, the temperature increases to 126° C, and the sterilization time decreases to 10 minutes. 15 psig at 121° C is the combination most commonly used for autoclave sterilization.[59]

Equipment must be cleaned before autoclaving. The clean equipment is then wrapped in muslin, linen, or paper, which steam easily penetrates.[8] Items must be properly packed in the autoclave to ensure exposure.[60] In addition, the chamber must be free of air and contain only steam.[61] Most autoclaves are equipped with controls which evacuate the air before the steam pressure rises to 15 psig. After sterilization, the packaging material prevents recontamination during subsequent handling and storage.[8] Because so many factors affect steam sterilization, both heat-sensitive and biological indicators should be used to maintain quality control (discussed subsequently).[8]

Steam autoclaving is efficient, quick, cheap, clean and reliable.[8] Unfortunately, most respiratory care equipment is **heat-labile** and can be damaged by the process. For this reason, application of steam heat for respiratory care equipment processing is somewhat limited.

Ionizing radiation. Short wavelength electromagnetic rays are an extremely effective sterilizing agent. Both X-rays and gamma rays can be used to this end, with gamma radiation the most common application.[62] X-rays are produced by electron generators similar to those used in diagnostic radiology. Gamma rays are emitted from radioactive isotopes such as cobalt.

Ionizing radiation kills microorganisms either by destroying cellular nucleic acids or by ionizing intracellular water. Although many commercial products are sterilized in this manner, the required equipment and shielding costs are too expensive for most hospitals. Moreover, in the dose required for sterilization, ionizing radiation can chemically alter some materials, creating toxic by-products.

Ultraviolet (UV) light is another ionizing source used in infection control. UV light is effective in killing most bacteria, but poorly penetrates most common materials. To be effective, UV light must have direct contact with the offending organisms. For this reason, ultraviolet light is not considered a true sterilizing agent. It may, however, be useful in reducing pathogens found in the air of operating rooms, nurseries, communicable-disease wards, and bacteriologic labs.[63]

Chemical methods of sterilization. Chemical methods of sterilization include ethylene oxide gas, and selected liquid solutions.

Ethylene oxide. Ethylene oxide (EtO) is a colorless, toxic gas with an ether-like odor at concentrations above 700 ppm.[64] In concentrations above 3%, EtO is also explosive.[8] To decrease its flammability, EtO is sometimes mixed with Freon or CO_2.

EtO is a potent sterilizing agent. Chemically, EtO

kills microorganisms by alkylation. This action effectively kills all microorganisms. Because EtO exists as a vapor at room temperature, it is readily diffusible and thus effective under ambient conditions. The gas does not damage plastic or rubber materials. Moreover, since EtO penetrates most packaging materials, items to be sterilized can be packaged *before* being placed in the sterilizer. For these reasons, EtO is particularly useful as a sterilant for heat- and moisture-sensitive items which cannot be steam sterilized.

Safe use of EtO requires special attention to materials preparation, cycle parameters, and aeration methods. Personnel operating EtO equipment must be skilled in all aspects of sterilization, including aeration. Further, expert surveillance should be provided to assure safety and quality control.[64]

Preparation of material. Prior to EtO sterilization, items must be disassembled and thoroughly cleaned, with all organic material removed. This assures adequate penetration of the gas.[8] In addition, items must be free from water droplets, which could interfere with sterilization. Water can also combine with EtO to form ethylene glycol (antifreeze), which is irritating to tissues.

Wrapping materials. Materials used to wrap items for EtO sterilization must be gas permeable. Muslin and paper wrapping can be used, but heat-sealed polyethylene pouches are faster and easier to use. Aluminum foil, nylon film, Saran, Mylar, cellophane, polyester, and polyvinylidene film should be avoided because they are not permeable to EtO.[8]

Loading the sterilizer. An EtO sterilizer is loaded in the same manner as a steam autoclave. Space must be provided between items to ensure gas circulation. Overloading may impede sterilization and must be avoided. Manufacturer's loading instructions should always be followed.

Sterilization cycle. Four major factors determine proper EtO sterilization: gas concentration, temperature, humidity and time. In terms of gas concentration, 450 mg/L is the minimum.[65] Since heat enhances EtO activity, most commercial sterilizers offer heated cycles. Humidity is needed to catalyze the reaction between EtO and bacterial proteins.[8] Normally, relative humidity is kept at 30% to 60% by injecting water into the chamber. Depending on the other three factors, exposure time varies from 1-½ to 6 hours. For example, at a relative humidity of 30% to 50% and temperature of 50° to 60° C, EtO sterilization takes 4 hours.[66]

After completion of a cycle, the sterilizer door should be open and personnel should leave the immediate area for at least 15 minutes.[64] Obviously, smoking must not be permitted in the area. Manufacturer's instructions regarding all parameters of the cycle must be followed.

Aeration. Sterilized articles must be aerated to remove residual EtO.[67] Nonporous materials like metal and glass do not absorb EtO and can be used right after sterilization.[67] However, EtO is retained in porous materials following sterilization. This residual EtO is toxic to human tissues, and can cause severe tissue inflammation and other toxic reactions, including hemolysis.[68-71] For this reason, adequate aeration of porous materials, such as plastics or rubber, is essential.[67] All items requiring aeration must be labeled when packaged. After the cycle is complete, these items should be separated from glass or metal equipment, and aerated long enough to insure removal of residual EtO.

Actual aeration time depends on several variables (see accompanying box). Polyvinyl chloride, commonly called PVC, needs the longest aeration time. Other plastics such as polyethylene and polypropylene require less time than PVC. If the composition of an item is in doubt, it should be treated as if it were PVC.

It used to be common to aerate EtO-sterilized articles by simply exposing them to room air. This is now considered an unacceptable hazard.[72] Current evidence indicates that EtO inhalation can cause several acute side effects, including airway inflammation, nausea, diarrhea, headache, dizziness, and convulsions.[73] Chronic exposure may also lead to respiratory infection, anemia, and altered behavior.[74] Additional concerns include possible carcinogenic, mutagenic and **teratogenic effects.**[75]

The current OSHA standard for EtO exposure is 1 ppm for 8-hours, with a recommended maximum short-time exposure of 5 to 10 ppm for a 15-minute period.[76,77] To keep EtO exposure below these limits requires adequate aeration and ventilation, personal and area monitoring, a written compliance program, and employee information and education.[72] The box on page 69 provides guidelines for the safe use of EtO.[64]

Proper aeration and handling of EtO-sterilized items is the key to minimizing patient and worker exposure.[64,67,78] The minimum times recommended for materials that are difficult to aerate are 8 hours at 60° C or 12 hours at 50° C in a mechanical aeration chamber.[79] Of course, these are general guidelines. The manufacturer's instructions always must be consulted to set the required aeration time.[8]

Factors affecting aeration of EtO sterilized equipment

- Composition of the sterilized item
- Configuration and intended use of item
- Aeration temperature
- Air flow during aeration
- Type of sterilizer used
- Time of aeration

Source: Emergency Care Research Institute: Ethylene oxide: hazards and safe use, Tech Respir Therapy 9(12):1–4, 1989.

Guidelines for the safe use of ethylene oxide (EtO)

- EtO irritates the eyes, nose, and throat and causes nausea and disorientation. Report these symptoms immediately.
- EtO is toxic and combustible; know proper handling, use, storage, labeling, spill, and first-aid procedures. Locate fire extinguishers, safety showers, and emergency respiratory equipment.
- After the sterilizer cycle, open the door about 6 inches (or according to the manufacturer's recommendations) and leave the immediate vicinity for at least 15 minutes. [The actual time will depend on your EtO exposure monitoring results.]
- Do not leave materials in a closed sterilizer after the cycle. [The heated environment allows the materials to release EtO more rapidly; high concentrations of EtO build up in the sterilizer and can be released into the room.]
- Transfer sterilized materials to the aerator as quickly as possible with minimal handling. Never leave unaerated materials outside the aerator to contaminate the environment or to be used inadvertently.
- Aerate only in approved sterilizers and aeration chambers. Ambient aeration is unacceptable unless a room is specially designed for this purpose.
- Always wear gloves and a face shield when changing EtO cylinders. Secure tanks to permanent structures and transport on appropriate equipment.
- Store only the minimum number of EtO cartridges or cylinders necessary for sterilizer operation, since 100% EtO is explosive. Store in approved flammable storage areas.
- Include EtO sterilizers/aerators and ventilation systems in a routine preventive maintenance program.
- Monitor EtO levels periodically per OSHA and JCAHO guidelines.

These guidelines are general in nature and are not intended as substitutes for comprehensive, detailed instructions in the safe use of ethylene oxide.

As with steam sterilization, it is necessary to monitor the effectiveness of EtO sterilization with appropriate indicators.[8]

Interrupting routes of transmission

Trying to eliminate the source of infection is not enough; efforts also must be made to stop the spread of pathogens. The two major infection control methods which help prevent the spread of pathogens are equipment handling procedures and barrier and isolation techniques.

Equipment handling procedures

Equipment handling procedures that help prevent the spread of pathogens include (1) maintenance of in-use equipment, (2) processing of reusable equipment, (3) the use of disposables, and (4) fluid and medication precautions.[80]

Maintenance of in-use equipment. In order of importance, in-use respiratory care equipment most likely to spread pathogens includes large reservoir jet nebulizers, ventilator circuits, bag-valve-mask devices (manual resuscitators), and oxygen therapy apparatus. In-use pulmonary function laboratory equipment is a special category.

The principal agent responsible for spreading pathogens is the large reservoir jet nebulizer. This device can become contaminated via non-sterile fluids or air, by handling of its internal components, or by backflow of contaminated condensate (from the delivery tubing) into its reservoir. Once introduced into the reservoir, bacteria can multiply enough within 24 hours to cause infection if nebulized and inhaled.

Several procedures can be used to prevent nebulizers from spreading pathogens (see accompanying box).[80]

In-use ventilator circuits, including their humidifiers and nebulizers, are another potential vehicle for the spread of infection. Prior recommendations were to change and replace these circuits every 24 hours.[80] However, recent research indicates that this is unnecessary.[81-85] Instead, circuits with water humidifiers need be changed only every second or third day (48 to 72 hours). If a heat-moisture exchanger/bacterial filter is used instead of a water humidifier, changing the circuit between patient may be satisfactory.[81,86,87] Regardless of approach, it is critically important that hands be washed after circuit removal.[81]

Methods to prevent nebulizers from spreading pathogens

- Nebulizers should always be filled with sterile distilled water (see fluid and medication precautions).
- Fluid reservoirs should be filled immediately before use. Fluid should not be added to replenish partially filled reservoirs. If fluid is to be added, the remaining old fluid should first be discarded.
- Tubing condensate should be discarded and not allowed to drain back into the reservoir.
- Large volume jet nebulizers, medication nebulizers and their reservoirs should be routinely changed and replaced with equipment that has been sterilized or has undergone high level disinfection every 24 hours.
- Humidifiers or nebulizers that create droplets for purposes of room humidification should *never* be used.

When a ventilator is used to treat multiple patients, as with IPPB, the breathing circuit should be changed between patients and replaced with a sterilized or disinfected one.[80]

Bag-valve-mask devices (BVMs) have long been recognized as a potential vehicle for spread of infection between patients.[88] BVMs are a source for colonizing the airways of intubated patients and the hands of medical personnel.[89] Obviously, nondisposable BVMs should be sterilized between patients (see next section). In addition, the exterior surface and port of in-use BVMs should be cleaned of visible debris and disinfected at least once a day.[89]

Oxygen therapy apparatus pose much less threat than other in-use devices, but should still be treated as vehicles for spreading infection. This is especially true for multiple-use humidifiers, for which the in-use contamination rate is as high as 33%.[90] Prefilled sterile disposable humidifiers, on the other hand, present a negligible infection risk.[90-92] Long-term costs (including personnel) are higher with disposable humidifiers, but only if they are frequently changed.[90] In fact, the use-time of prefilled disposable humidifiers can be safely extended to as long as 6 to 12 days.[91] Based on this knowledge, the accompanying box outlines procedures that can help prevent oxygen therapy apparatus from spreading pathogens.

The role of pulmonary function equipment in the spread of infections has not been established.[94] Nonetheless, all standard CDC procedures governing handwashing, fluids and medications precautions, blood specimen handling, equipment maintenance, patient/ staff protection, and microbiologic surveillance should be followed.[94] In addition, since mouthpieces and spirometer tubing can become contaminated during testing, these components should be changed between patients.[95] Although the likelihood of contaminating the inside of volumetric spirometers is small, low-resistance filters can be used to isolate internal components from the patient. This approach also can help avoid costly disassembly and cleaning.

Processing reusable equipment. Improperly processed reusable equipment is another potential source for pathogens. General guidelines for cleaning, disinfection and sterilization were previously provided. This section provides specific procedures for processing reusable respiratory care equipment.

Several factors must be considered in selecting processing methods for reusable equipment (see accompanying box).[8] First, since the infection potential of equipment varies according to use, devices should be categorized by their infection risk. Medical devices fall into three infection risk categories: critical, semicritical, and noncritical (Table 4-9).[8,36] Once a device's risk category is known, its composition must be matched to the resources available for hospital disinfection and sterilization. In this manner, each reusable device will undergo the most effective and least costly processing approach available (see boxed guidelines for processing reusable equipment on page 71).

Disposable equipment. The use of disposable equipment is a major approach to preventing spread of pathogens in the hospital.[96] Before 1970, only oxygen therapy modalities, suction apparatus and supply items were common disposables in respiratory care. Today, humidifiers, nebulizers, incentive spirometers, ventilator circuits, bag-valve-mask resuscitators, and monitoring transducers are available as disposables.

Although these devices generally function as well as their reusable counterparts, concern has been expressed by clinicians over poor quality control.[97] In any case, disposable devices should be chosen carefully and evaluated before application in the clinical environment.[98] In addition, to assure reliability, evaluation should include physical testing of *multiple* units of each model under consideration.[97]

Initially, the CDC recommended against reuse of disposable equipment.[99] Despite this early recommendation, financial pressures during the 1980s forced many hospitals to begin reusing selected high-cost, high volume disposable items, such as ventilator circuits.[8,96]

Methods to prevent oxygen therapy apparatus from spreading pathogens

- Humidifiers are not needed with flows less than 4 L/min.[93]
- Wherever possible, prefilled sterile disposable humidifiers should be used with oxygen therapy apparatus.
- Reusable oxygen humidifier reservoirs should be emptied and then replenished with sterile distilled water; tap water must be avoided!
- The tubing and oxygen delivery device should be changed between patients; prefilled sterile disposable humidifiers need not be changed between patients, especially in high-use areas (eg, recovery room, ER).
- The use-time of prefilled disposable humidifiers can be safely extended to 6–12 days, or longer (if on stand-by).[91]

Factors to consider in processing reusable equipment[8]

- Infection risk (critical, semicritical, and noncritical)
- Material and equipment configuration
- Available hospital disinfection resources
- Relative cost (both labor and materials)

Table 4-9 Infection risk categories of medical equipment

Category	Description	Examples	Processing
Critical	Devices introduced into the blood-stream or other parts of the body	Surgical devices Cardiac catheters Implants Heart-lung and hemodialysis components	Sterilization
Semicritical	Devices that contact intact mucous membranes	Endoscopes Tracheal tubes Ventilator tubing	High-level disinfection
Noncritical	Devices that touch only intact skin or do not contact patient	Face masks Blood-pressure cuffs Ventilators	Detergent washing Low/intermediate level disinfection

Adapted from Chatburn RL: Decontamination of respiratory care equipment: what can be done, what should be done, *Respir Care* 34(2):98–110, 1989.

Guidelines for processing reusable respiratory care equipment[8,80]

- All reusable respiratory care equipment should undergo low or intermediate-level disinfection as part of the initial cleaning.
- All reusable breathing circuit components (including tubing and exhalation valves, medication nebulizers and their reservoirs, large volume jet nebulizers and their reservoirs, and cascade humidifiers and their reservoirs) should be considered semicritical items.
- Semicritical items should be sterilized between use on patients; heat-stable items should be autoclaved and heat-labile items should undergo EtO sterilization.
- If sterilization is not feasible, semicritical items should undergo high-level disinfection or pasteurization.
- The internal machinery of ventilators and breathing machines need not be routinely sterilized or disinfected between patients.
- Respirometers and other equipment used to monitor multiple patients should not directly touch any part of a ventilator circuit or a patient's mucous membranes. Rather, disposable extension pieces and low-resistance HEPA filters should be used to isolate the device. If the device cannot be isolated from the patient or circuit, it must be sterilized or receive high-level disinfection before use on other patients.
- Once they have been used on one patient, nondisposable resuscitation bags (BVMs) should be sterilized or receive high-level disinfection before use on other patients.

Because no hard evidence has come forward disputing the safety of reusing disposable devices,[8,100] the CDC prohibition was lifted in 1986.[36,85] Instead, the burden of proof has been shifted to individual respiratory care service departments.[8] Clearly, more study in this area is needed because manufacturers rarely, if ever, provide reprocessing information.[8]

Fluids and medications precautions. Fluids and medications represent a major source for spreading infections. The AARC has recommended several procedures to help prevent fluids and medications from becoming vehicles for the spread of infection (see accompanying box).[80] In addition, recent research suggests that hospital tap water should be treated as a contaminated fluid, and never used to clean or rinse-out in-use equipment.[101]

Fluids and medications precautions[80]

- Only sterile fluids should be used to fill nebulizers and humidifiers. These fluids should be dispensed aseptically. Contaminated equipment should not be allowed to enter or touch the fluid while it is being dispensed.
- After a large container (bottle) of fluid intended for use in a nebulizer or humidifier has been opened, unused fluid should be discarded within 24 hours.
- Either single-dose or multi-dose vials can be used for respiratory care. If multi-dose vials are used, they should be stored (refrigerated or at room temperature) according to directions on the label or package insert. Vials should be used no longer than the expiration date given on the label.

Barrier and isolation methods

A major route for the spread of nosocomial infections is by contact with infected persons. Thus, infection control measures that place "barriers" between the source and the host should help disrupt spread of pathogens. General barrier-type precautions include handwashing, and the use of gloves masks and/or gowns. When combined with the separation of infected patients by disease, these techniques are called *isolation protocols.*

General barrier-type precautions. General barrier-type precautions include handwashing, and the use of gloves, masks and/or gowns.[102]

Handwashing. Proper handwashing is the single most important way to prevent the spread of infection.[36] In fact, if handwashing is done properly, glove and gown barrier precautions may have no added benefit in protecting the patient.

RCPs must always wash their hands after any patient contact, even when gloves are used. In addition, personnel should wash their hands after coming into contact with any body excretions, such as feces and urine, or wound, skin or respiratory secretions. Hands should also be washed *before* performing invasive procedures, touching wounds, or touching patients who are at high risk for infection. Hand washing between all patient contacts is particularly critical in intensive care units and newborn nurseries.

When taking care of patients that are infected or colonized with virulent organisms, RCPs should use antiseptics for handwashing, rather than simple soap and water. Antiseptics will inhibit or kill many organisms that may not be completely removed by normal handwashing. Moreover, good antiseptics have a residual effect that continues to suppress microbial growth after handwashing. Such antiseptics should not be used as a substitute for adequate mechanical handwashing.

Gloves. There are three major reasons for using gloves. First, gloves protect health personnel from becoming infected by contacting infected patients. Second, gloves protect patients from acquiring an infection from colonized health personnel. Last, gloves decrease colonization on the hands of health personnel.

Under most conditions, proper attention to handwashing reduces the need for gloves. However, since handwashing practices vary greatly, gloves represent a practical means of preventing transient hand colonization and spread of some infections. Moreover, recent concern over the spread of AIDS and other blood-borne pathogens suggests that gloves should be used for all patient contacts (details on the prevention of AIDS transmission follows).

For these reasons, RCPs should wear gloves whenever excretions, secretions, blood, or body fluids are likely to be contacted. Gloves are especially important wherever the risk of exposure to blood is increased and the infection status of the patient is unknown, such as in the emergency-care settings.

When gloves are indicated, disposable single-use gloves should be worn. Depending on their purpose, either sterile or aseptically clean gloves are chosen. Sterile gloves are required when trying to protect patients from acquiring an infection; clean gloves are all that is needed when the goal is to protect one's self from an infected patient. In either case, gloves should be changed after direct contact with a patient's excretions or secretions, even if in the middle of a treatment or procedure. Used gloves should be discarded into appropriate receptacles.

Masks. Masks help prevent the transmission of infectious agents via the airborne route. Masks protect the wearer from inhaling both large particle aerosols droplets (transmitted by close contact), and the smaller droplet nuclei (true airborne transmission). High efficiency disposable filtration masks called *respirators* are more effective than cotton gauze or paper tissue masks in preventing both aerosol particle and droplet nuclei spread.

If the infection is transmitted by large-particle aerosols, masks need only be used by those close to the patient. If the infection is spread over longer distances by air, masks should be used by all persons entering the room or area.

Masks also can prevent transmission of some infections that are spread by direct contact with mucous membranes. This is because masks discourage personnel from touching their eyes, nose, and mouth until after they have washed their hands and removed the mask.

All masks should fully cover both the nose and the mouth. Because masks become ineffective when moist, they should be discarded after single use. Masks should never be lowered around the neck and reused.

Gowns. Gowns protect clothing from contamination that might occur in patient care activities. Because such soiling occurs infrequently, gowns are not needed for most patient care activities.

Gowns are indicated when clothes are likely to be soiled with contaminated material from a patient in isolation. Even when gross soiling is not foreseen, gowns are indicated for all persons entering the room of patients with highly contagious disorders that cause serious illness, such as varicella (chickenpox) or disseminated zoster. As with gloves and masks, gowns should be worn once only and then discarded. In most situations, aseptically clean, freshly laundered or disposable gowns are satisfactory. Sterile gowns may be needed in some instances, as with extensive burns or wounds.

Isolation precautions. Isolation precautions are designed to prevent the spread of infectious agents among patients, personnel, and visitors.[103]

There are two current approaches to selecting

isolation precautions: disease-specific and categorical. The disease-specific method is based on detailed isolation specifications for *each* disease, as provided by the Centers for Disease Control. The categorical method groups diseases which require similar isolation precautions.

There are seven isolation categories: Strict Isolation, Contact Isolation, Respiratory Isolation, Tuberculosis (AFB) Isolation, Enteric Precautions, Drainage/Secretion Precautions, and Blood/Body Fluid Precautions. The specifications for each category and the diseases and conditions included in the category are discussed below. Table 4-10 provides a summary of these specifications.[103]

Strict isolation. Strict isolation is designed to prevent transmission of highly contagious or virulent infections that may be spread by both air and direct contact. Diseases requiring strict isolation include diphtheria, pneumonic plague, smallpox, and varicella (chickenpox).[103]

Contact isolation. Contact isolation is designed to prevent transmission of highly contagious infections or colonizations that do not need strict isolation. Examples of infections in this category include acute respiratory infections in infants and young children (croup, colds, pharyngitis, bronchitis, viral pneumonias, influenza, and viral bronchiolitis); disseminated Herpes simplex; **pediculosis;** Staphylococcal pneumonia; group A Streptococcal pneumonia; rabies; rubella; scabies; and any major skin, wound, or burn infection that is draining and not covered. Also, contact isolation may be indicated when a patient is infected or colonized with bacteria proven resistant to multiple antibiotics.[103]

Not all the contact isolation precautions listed in Table 4-10 are needed for all diseases. For example, masks and gloves are not generally needed for infants and young children with acute viral respiratory infec- tions, and care of patients infected with resistant bacteria does not normally require masks unless a pneumonia is present. Due to these variations within the contact isolation category, some degree of "over-isolation" may occur.

Respiratory isolation. Respiratory isolation is designed to prevent transmission of infectious diseases via the droplet contact route. Diseases requiring respiratory isolation include: epiglottitis, meningitis, or childhood pneumonia due to *Haemophilus influenzae;* measles; Meningococcal pneumonia; mumps; and pertussis.[103]

Tuberculosis isolation (AFB Isolation). Tuberculosis or AFB isolation is designed for patients with pulmonary tuberculosis who have a positive sputum culture or a chest X-ray that strongly suggests active disease.

In general, infants and young children with pulmonary TB do not require isolation precautions because they rarely cough, and, as compared to adults, their bronchial secretions contain few bacilli. To protect the patient's privacy, this category is visibly posted as "AFB Isolation."[103]

Enteric precautions. Enteric precautions are designed to prevent infections that are transmitted by contact with feces. Examples of diseases requiring enteric precautions include: amebic dysentery; cholera; coxsackievirus disease; encephalitis; gastroenteritis caused by *Escherichia coli,* Salmonellae, or Shigellae; type A viral hepatitis; poliomyelitis; viral meningitis; necrotizing enterocolitis; viral pericarditis or myocarditis; and any enteroviral infection or acute diarrhea suspected of being infectious.[103]

Drainage/secretion precautions. Drainage/secretion precautions are designed to prevent transmission of infections that occur by indirect contact with purulent material or drainage from an infected site. Diseases in this category include Chlamydial infections, gan-

Table 4-10 Specifications for isolation categories

Isolation Category	Private Room?	Wear Mask?	Wear Gloves?	Wear Gown?	Hand-Wash?	Article Handling
Strict	Yes[1]	Yes	Yes	Yes	Yes	Discard or bag and label
Contact	Yes[1]	Yes	Yes[2]	Yes[2]	Yes	Discard or bag and label
Respiratory	Yes[1]	Yes	No	No	Yes	Discard or bag and label
AFB	Yes[1,4]	Yes[3]	No	Yes[2]	Yes	Discard; no bagging
Enteric	No[5]	No	Yes[2]	Yes[2]	Yes	Discard or bag and label
Drainage/secretion	No	No	Yes[2]	Yes[2]	Yes	Discard or bag and label
Blood/body fluids	No[5]	No	Yes[6]	Yes[6]	Yes	Discard or bag and label

NOTES
1—In general, patients with same infection may share a room.
2—Gloves and gowns if touching infective material is likely.
3—Only if the patient is coughing and does not cover mouth.
4—Room should have negative pressure ventilation.
5—Private room is indicated if patient hygiene is poor.
6—Gloves/gowns for touching blood or body fluids.

grene, conjunctivitis, minor infected decubiti ulcers, and minor or limited skin, wound, or burn infections. Infections caused by resistant microorganisms and major skin, wound, or burn infections require contact isolation.[103]

Blood and body fluid precautions. Blood and body fluid precautions are designed to prevent infections that are transmitted by direct or indirect contact with contaminated blood or body fluids. For some diseases included in this category, such as malaria, only blood is infective; for other diseases, such as hepatitis B and AIDS, *both* blood and body fluids may be infective.[103]

Diseases requiring blood and body fluid precautions include the acquired immunodeficiency syndrome (AIDS); hepatitis B, C, and D; yellow fever; Colorado tick fever; leptospirosis, malaria; and primary or secondary syphilis with skin and mucous membrane lesions.

In addition to the barrier methods listed in Table 4-10 for blood and body fluid precautions, care should be taken to avoid needle-stick injuries. Generally, used needles should not be recapped or bent; they should be placed in a prominently labeled, puncture-resistant container designated specifically for such disposal.[104] Blood spills should be cleaned up promptly with a solution of 5.25% sodium hypochlorite diluted 1:10 with water.

Other considerations. Other isolation considerations include: (1) the handling of contaminated articles and equipment, (2) the use of needle and syringes, and (3) the transportation and handling of laboratory specimens.[103]

Contaminated Articles and Equipment. Used articles that have been contaminated should be enclosed in an impervious bag before removal from the room of a patient on isolation precautions. Bagging is intended to prevent accidental exposure of both personnel and the environment to contaminated articles. A single bag is probably adequate if: (1) the bag is strong and impervious and (2) bagging can be accomplished without contaminating the bag's outer surface. Otherwise, a double bagging procedure is needed. Bags used for articles or waste materials that have been contaminated should be clearly labeled or color coded for this purpose.

Use of disposable articles reduces the possibility that equipment will serve as a source of transmission. However, disposable articles must be disposed of safely and adequately. Contaminated disposable equipment should be bagged, labeled, and disposed of in accord with both hospital and applicable local, state or federal regulations.

Reusable patient-care equipment should be returned to the applicable processing area. Contaminated equipment in bags should remain bagged until decontaminated or sterilized.

Needles and Syringes. All personnel should exercise extreme caution when handling used needles and syringes. In order to prevent accidental needle-stick injuries, used needles should not be recapped,* but rather placed in a prominently labeled, puncture-resistant container that is designated solely for this purpose. Needles should never be bent or broken by hand, since this is a common cause of needle-stick injuries. If the patient's blood is infective, disposable syringes and needles are recommended. If reusable syringes are used, they should be treated as contaminated articles, using the precautions described above.

Laboratory Specimens. When gathering laboratory specimens (such as sputum), extreme care should be taken to prevent contamination of the external surface of the container. If the outside of the container is contaminated, it must be disinfected or placed in an impervious bag. In order to minimize the likelihood of leaking during transport, laboratory specimens should always be placed in a sturdy container with a secure lid. When a specimen comes from a patient on isolation precautions, the container normally should be placed in an impervious bag and appropriately labeled *before* removal from the room.

Modifications to standard isolation procedures. Isolation precautions may have to be modified for patients needing intensive care or emergency interventions. Whenever such changes are needed, efforts must be made to ensure minimal risk to both patients and hospital personnel. As a general guideline, modification of any isolation protocol should never compromise adherence to the generic aseptic procedures, particularly conscientious handwashing with antiseptic solutions.

Intensive Care. ICU patients are among those at highest risk for acquiring nosocomial infections. There are several reasons for this increased risk. First, contact between patients and health personnel in an ICU is more frequent than in other settings. Second, ICUs typically cluster patients together in a confined area. Third, ICU patients tend to have impaired host resistance, and are thus more susceptible to infection. Last, ICU patients are more likely to undergo multiple invasive procedures.

The isolation precaution that is most modified in ICUs is the use of a private room. Patients with serious contagious infections should be placed in a private room, even if one is not available in the ICU. When a private room or cubicle in ICU is not feasible, and if airborne transmission of infectious agents is not likely, an isolation area can be defined with physical barriers such as curtains or partitions, or by marking the area with floor tape. In addition, standard instructional cards should be posted to notify personnel and visitors of the applicable isolation precautions.

---

*There are those that argue that *not* recapping needles is also a problem, especially in procedures like arterial puncture. Alternatives recapping methods include a wide-mouth needlecap, a one-handed scoop technique, and a recapping device.[104]

Newborns and Infants. Isolation precautions for newborns and infants often have to be modified due to the lack of private rooms for these patients.

Specifically, grouping infants together is permissible if facilities and procedures assure that all personnel properly wash their hands, and sufficient space (4 to 6 feet) is provided between patients. Enclosed incubators are satisfactory for limited isolation of infants, but should not be considered a primary means of infection control.

In addition to these precautions, grouping of patients with the same infection (cohorting) may be needed. Cohorting is allowed only if the patients can be separated into a single large room with dedicated personnel.

Immunocompromised Patients. Patients with leukemia, cancer, and severe burns, or patients receiving immunosuppressive therapies are highly susceptible to infection. In the past, these patients were placed in "protective isolation." Recent evidence indicates that this approach is no more useful in preventing infection than rigorous handwashing. This is because the most common source of infection in immunocompromised patients is their own (endogenous) flora.

Nonetheless, patients who are immunocompromised should be separated from patients with infectious diseases, preferably in a private room. Under these conditions, careful adherence to routine standards for asepsis are generally all that is needed to minimize the risk of infection.

Burn Patients. Most major burn wounds become infected within 48 to 72 hours after the initial incident. For this reason, care of patients with severe burns must always involve efforts to minimize wound colonization and prevent infection. Although procedures for major burns vary, most burn centers enforce strict contact isolation procedures.[105]

Special considerations with the HIV virus

As indicated earlier, the HIV virus is causing major concern in both the health care community and general population. Regarding its potential for transmission in the hospital, the Centers for Disease Control have issued specific guidelines to minimize risk.[106-109] These guidelines emphasize the use of universal blood and body fluid precautions, and provide special protocols for invasive procedures.

Universal precautions

Since it is impossible to identify all patients infected with the HIV virus or other blood-borne infectious agents, *the CDC recommends that blood and body-fluid precautions should be used for all patients.* This approach is particularly important in emergency-care settings, where the risk of blood exposure is high and the infection status of the patient is usually unknown.

Specific guidelines for universal precautions are provided in the box on page 76. As is evident, these guidelines strengthen normal blood and body fluid precautions. In fact, use of these universal precautions for *all* patients effectively eliminates the blood and body fluid isolation category.

Universal precautions apply to blood, semen, vaginal secretions, body tissues, cerebrospinal fluid, synovial fluid, pleural fluids, peritoneal fluid, pericardial fluid, and amniotic fluid. Other fluids are excluded from universal precautions because studies have failed to implicate them in HIV transmission. These include feces, nasal secretions, sputum, sweat, tears, urine, vomitus, breast milk, and saliva, unless they contain visible blood. However, routine precautions (handwashing, gloves, etc.) to prevent exposure to other diseases transmitted by these fluids should be followed.[111]

Precautions for invasive procedures

All health-care personnel involved in invasive procedures must routinely use appropriate barrier precautions to prevent skin and mucous-membrane contact with blood and other body fluids. Gloves and surgical masks are *required* for all invasive procedures. Protective eyewear and gowns or aprons are recommended for any procedure that could result in the generation of droplets or the splashing of blood or other body fluids. If hands or other skin surfaces become contaminated during an invasive procedure, the gloves should be removed, and the affected area thoroughly washed.

As previously indicated, existing evidence indicates that the risk of acquiring AIDS on the job is extremely small. Simple adherence to these CDC precautions further decreases this risk. Hospital personnel who are careful and meticulous in applying these standards should feel confident in delivering quality care to all their patients.

SURVEILLANCE

Surveillance is an ongoing process designed to ensure that infection control procedures are working. Surveillance generally involves three components: equipment processing quality control, routine sampling of in-use equipment, and microbiological identification. During major outbreaks of nosocomial infections, surveillance will also involve epidemiological investigation.

The policies and procedures governing a hospital surveillance program are normally set by an infection control committee and administered by an infection control nurse or epidemiologist. Depending on institutional policy, surveillance may be centralized or decentralized (to the various service departments). In the latter case, RCPs will work directly with the infection control nurse or epidemiologist in implementing department-level surveillance procedures.

Centers for Disease Control (CDC) Universal Precautions[106-110]

1. All health-care workers should routinely use appropriate barrier precautions to prevent skin and mucous-membrane exposure when contact with blood or other body fluids of any patient is anticipated. Gloves should be worn for touching blood and body fluids, mucous membranes, or non-intact skin of all patients, for handling items or surfaces soiled with blood or body fluids, and for performing venipuncture and other vascular access procedures. Gloves should be changed after contact with each patient. Masks and protective eyewear or face shields should be worn during procedures that are likely to generate droplets of blood or other body fluids to prevent exposure of mucous membranes of the mouth, nose, and eyes. Gowns or aprons should be worn during procedures that are likely to generate splashes of blood or other body fluids.
2. Hands and other skin surfaces should be washed immediately and thoroughly if contaminated with blood or other body fluids. Hands should be washed immediately after gloves are removed.
3. All health-care workers should take precautions to prevent injuries caused by needles, scalpels, and other sharp instruments or devices during procedures; when cleaning used instruments; during disposal of used needles; and when handling sharp instruments after procedures. To prevent needlestick injuries, needles should not be recapped, purposely bent or broken by hand, removed from disposable syringes, or otherwise manipulated by hand. After they are used, disposable syringes and needles, scalpel blades, and other sharp items should be placed in puncture-resistant containers for disposal; the puncture-resistant containers should be located as close as practical to the use area. Large-bore reusable needles should be placed in puncture-resistant containers for transport to the reprocessing area.
4. Although saliva has not been implicated in HIV transmission, to minimize the need for emergency mouth-to-mouth resuscitation, mouthpieces, resuscitation bags, or other ventilation devices should be available for use in areas in which the need for resuscitation is predictable.
5. All blood and body fluid specimens should be placed in a sturdy, leakproof container (such as a ziplock bag) for transport to the laboratory. The lab requisition should be placed outside the container to avoid contamination.
6. Health-care workers who have exudative lesions or weeping dermatitis should refrain from all direct patient care and from handling patient-care equipment until the condition resolves.

Equipment processing quality control

The first step in equipment processing quality control is monitoring and evaluating personnel adherence to policies and procedures. Supplementing this evaluation must be assessment of the *outcomes* of equipment processing, that is determining whether the procedures used actually result in sterile or disinfected equipment. This is accomplished using both specially prepared processing indicators and culture sampling methods.

Processing indicators

As the name implies, processing indicators show whether or not a sterilization or disinfection process worked. There are two types of processing indicators: chemical and biological.

Chemical indicators. Chemical indicators are usually impregnated on packaging tape. These indicators change color when exposed to specific conditions. Autoclave chemical indicators change color after exposure to a given temperature for a sufficient period of time. Likewise, chemical indicators used in EtO processing change color after exposure to a given concentration of the gas.

Chemical indicators provide visual evidence that a package has been through a sterilizing process. Since neither autoclave nor EtO processing changes the appearance of packs or packaging, indicator tape also helps distinguish between processed and unprocessed items.

However, while a chemical indicator tells us that a package has been through a sterilizer cycle, it can not assure either that the process was effective or the item is truly sterile. Only biological indicators can provide these assurances.

Biological indicators. Biological indicators consist of strips of paper impregnated with spores. *Bacillus stearothermophilus* is the primary biological indicator used for autoclave processes, while *Bacillus subtilis* is used for EtO sterilization.

These spore strips are housed in a plastic capsule with a glass ampule that contains a selected growth medium, usually tryptic soy broth (Figure 4-2). To prevent contamination with other organisms, the capsule cap contains a gas-permeable bacterial filter.

The capsule is wrapped in the recommended packaging material and placed in the most inaccessible location in the sterilizer load. After sterilization, the glass ampule is crushed, exposing the spores to the growth medium. The capsule is then incubated according to the manufacturer's instructions. Turbidity or color change in the growth medium after the specified incubation period indicates bacterial growth and failure of the sterilization process.

Unfortunately, the incubation period required to verify sterility of a given processing cycle can range

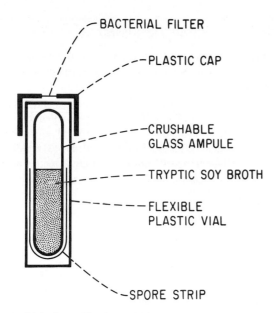

- BACTERIAL FILTER
- PLASTIC CAP
- CRUSHABLE GLASS AMPULE
- TRYPTIC SOY BROTH
- FLEXIBLE PLASTIC VIAL
- SPORE STRIP

Fig. 4-2 Biologic sterilization indicator. The capsule contains a strip impregnated with bacterial spores, pH indicator, and culture medium in a crushable ampule. After removal from the sterilizer the ampule is crushed, releasing the culture medium onto the spore strip. A yellow color after incubation indicates incomplete sterilization. (Redrawn from Boyd and Hoerl: Basic medical mictrobiology, ed 3, Boston 1986, Little, Brown.)

from one to three days. This requires that the processed equipment be held from use until its sterility is assured. Obviously, this "down time" adds to the cost of care by demanding larger inventories of reusable equipment. For this reason, the CDC recommends that sterilizers be checked with biological indicators at least once a week.[8]

In addition, biological indicators should be used when experimenting with new packaging materials, or modifying processing procedures. Any deviation in procedure from that recommended by a sterilizer's manufacturer must be pretested with a biological control.

Culture sampling

Processing indicators are generally used only when assessing sterilization methods using heat, ionizing radiation, and gas. To evaluate other procedures, especially pasteurization and chemical disinfection, bacteriologic samples must be obtained and cultured from processed equipment. When performed correctly, culture sampling determines how much residual bacteria remains on equipment. This provides essential information on the efficacy of the disinfection process.

Unfortunately, contamination during sampling procedures is common, making equipment culture results difficult to interpret. Moreover, if adherence to

disinfection protocols is carefully monitored, regular culture sampling is not needed. Thus, in the absence of a nosocomial epidemic, regularly culturing of *processed* equipment is not warranted.[85,99]

Random sampling and culturing of *stored* items is used to assess packaging adequacy and material shelf life. Culturing also may be a useful tool when assessing a new disinfectant or disinfectant process. Last, sampling of *in-use* equipment is a normal component of bacteriologic surveillance.

Sampling of in-use equipment

In addition to selected sampling of processed equipment, surveillance procedures usually involve random sampling and culturing of in-use equipment. The purpose of sampling in-use equipment is twofold: (1) it helps establish the frequency with which in-use items should be removed from use and reprocessed, and (2) it can help identify the source of nosocomial epidemics *before* they become widespread.

There are three common methods used to sample respiratory care equipment: (1) swab sampling, (2) liquid broths, and (3) aerosol impaction. Each method is designed to aid sample collection from particular equipment or equipment locations.[30] Personnel responsible for sampling of in-use equipment must be trained in these techniques.

Swab sampling

Swab sampling is used to obtain cultures from easily accessible surfaces of respiratory care equipment. As shown in Figure 4-3, a specially-prepared sterile swab is rubbed on the equipment surface at a

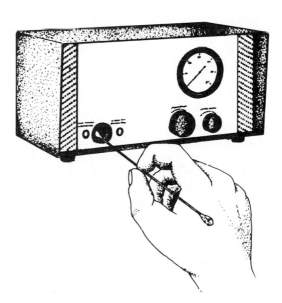

Fig. 4-3 Swab sampling. (From McLaughlin AJ: Manual of infection control in respiratory care, Boston, 1983, Little Brown.)

single location. Each location sampled requires a new swab. Using aseptic technique, the swab is placed either in a tube of sterile liquid broth or used to inoculate a plate of growth media. Information regarding the date, time, equipment source, and location from which the sample was taken must be provided. Samples are then transported to the microbiology laboratory for incubation and identification.

Liquid broths

Swab sampling cannot reach many parts of respiratory care equipment, especially inside tubing. In these situations, sterile liquid broths are used to obtain a sample. Using aseptic technique, the broth is poured into circuitry tubing and "swished" back and forth. Once exposed, the broth is poured into a sterile container for culturing. Labeling protocol is the same as with swab sampling.

Aerosol impaction

Because jet nebulizers are a major source for the spread of infection, it is often necessary to sample the actual particulate output of these devices. Sampling of liquid particle aerosols is done by inertial impaction devices. These range in complexity from a simple funnel with attached culture plate, to sophisticated multichamber devices that segregated aerosol particles according to size. Regardless of the device used, asepsis must be maintained during equipment setup and sample collection. Labeling protocol is the same as with other sample collection methods.

Microbiological identification

The hospital microbiology laboratory fulfills a central role in bacteriologic surveillance. Here, organisms are cultured, isolated and identified according to a variety of specialized procedures.

Although most of its work focuses on diagnostic procedures, the microbiology laboratory works closely with the infection control nurse or epidemiologist in support of the surveillance program. Indeed, regular diagnostic activities often reveal patterns of infection with certain microorganisms that can precede widespread outbreaks. When combined with ongoing surveillance activity, such information can prevent or minimize large scale in-hospital epidemics.

When the surveillance program is decentralized to the departmental level, RCPs may work closely with the microbiology laboratory staff to develop, maintain and evaluate the methods and procedures used to gather and interpret bacteriologic samples.

CHAPTER SUMMARY

Nosocomial infections represent a major problem in health care delivery, causing substantial morbidity and mortality and costing billions of dollars each year.

The incidence of nosocomial infections can be reduced only by strict adherence to infection control procedures. Infection control procedures include techniques designed to (1) eliminate the sources of pathogens, (2) prevent their spread, and (3) monitor and evaluate the effectiveness of control methods. Effective application of infection control procedures is a major and ongoing responsibility of all RCPs.

REFERENCES

1. Hooton TM: Protecting ourselves and our patients from nosocomial infections, *Respir Care,* 34(2):111–115, 1989.
2. Reinarz JA, Pierce AK, Mays BB, Sanford JP: The potential role of inhalation therapy equipment in nosocomial pulmonary infections, *J Clin Invest* 44:831–839, 1965.
3. Mertz JJ, Scharer L, McClement JH: A hospital outbreak of Klebsiella pneumonia from inhalation therapy with contaminated aerosol solution, *Am Rev Respir Dis* 94:454–460, 1966.
4. Sanders CV Jr, Luby JP, Johanson WG Jr, et al.: Serratia marcescens infections from inhalation therapy medications: Nosocomial outbreak, *Ann Intern Med* 73:15–21, 1970.
5. Darin J: Respiratory therapy equipment in the development of nosocomial respiratory tract infections, *Curr Rev Respir Ther* 4:83, 1985.
6. Johanson WG: Infectious complications of respiratory therapy, *Respir Care* 27:445, 1982.
7. Stamm WE: Infections related to medical devices, *Ann Intern Med* 89:764–769, 1978.
8. Chatburn RL: Decontamination of respiratory care equipment: What can be done, what should be done, *Respir Care* 34(2):98–110, 1989.
9. Masferrer R, DuPriest M: Six-year evaluation of decontamination of respiratory therapy equipment, *Respir Care* 22:145–148, 1977.
10. Cross AS, Roup B: Role of respiratory assistance devices in endemic nosocomial pneumonia, *Am J Med* 70:681–685, 1981.
11. Goldstein E, Koo J: Immunologic tests in the diagnosis of pulmonary infection, *Clin Rev Allergy* 8(2–3), 229–252, 1990.
12. Tobin MJ: Diagnosis of pneumonia: techniques and problems, *Clin Chest Med* 8(3):513–527, 1987.
13. Spence TH: Pneumonia, in Civetta JM, Taylor RW, Kirby RR (eds): Critical care, 2nd ed, Philadelphia, JB Lippincott, 1992.
14. Quinones CA, Memon MA, Sarosi GA: Bacteremic *Hemophilus influenzae* pneumonia in the adult, *Semin Respir Infect* 4(1):12–8, 1989.
15. Grim PS, Gottlieb LJ, Boddie A, Batson E: Hyperbaric oxygen therapy, *JAMA* 263(16):2216–2220, 1990.
16. Montgomerie JZ: Epidemiology of Klebsiella and hospital-associated infections, *Rev Infect Dis* 1:736, 1979.
17. Doebbeling BN, Wenzel RP: The epidemiology of *Legionella pneumophila* infections. *Semin Respir Infect* 2(4):206–221, 1987.
18. Horsburgh CR Jr: Mycobacterium avium complex infection in the acquired immunodeficiency syndrome, *N Engl J Med* 324:1332–1338, 1991.
19. Greenberg SB: Viral pneumonia, *Infect Dis Clin North Am* 5(3):603–621, 1991.

20. Bowden FJ, Pollett B, Birrell F, Dax EM: Occupational exposure to the human immunodeficiency virus and other blood-borne pathogens. A six-year prospective study. *Med J Aust* 158(12):810–812, 1993.
21. Centers for Disease Control: Recommendations for protection against viral hepatitis, MMWR 37:178–179, 1985.
22. Grayston JT: *Chlamydia pneumoniae,* strain TWAR, *Chest* 95:664, 1989.
23. Luby JP: Pneumonia caused by *Mycoplasma pneumoniae* infection, *Clin Chest Med* 12(2):237–244, 1991.
24. Sarosi GA: Community-acquired fungal diseases, *Clin Chest Med* 12(2):337–347, 1991.
25. Cairns MR, Durack DT: Fungal pneumonia in the immunocompromised host. *Semin Respir Infect* 1(3):166–85, 1986.
26. Edman JC, Kovacs JA, Masur H, et al.: Ribosomal RNA sequence shows *Pneumocystis carinii* to be a member of the fungi, *Nature* 334:519, 1988.
27. Schaberg DR: How infections spread in the hospital, *Respir Care* 34(2):81–84, 1989.
28. Bjornson HS: Diagnosis and treatment of bacterial pneumonia in the intensive care unit: an overview, *Respir Care* 32(9):773–780, 1987.
29. Garibaldi RA, Britt MR, Coleman ML, et al: Risk factors for postoperative pneumonia, *Am J Med* 70:677–680, 1981.
30. McLaughlin AJ: Manual of infection control in respiratory care, Boston, 1983, Little, Brown and Company.
31. Rutala WA: APIC guideline for selection and use of disinfectants, *Am J Infect Control* 18(2):99–117, 1990.
32. Borick PM, Dondershine FH, Hollis RA: A new automated unit for cleaning and disinfecting anesthesia equipment and other medical instruments, *Dev Ind Microbiol* 12:266–272, 1971.
33. Roberts FJ, Cockcroft WH, Johnson HE: A hot water disinfection method for inhalation therapy equipment, *Can Med Assoc J* 101:30–32, 1969.
34. Nelson EJ, Ryan KJ: A new use for pasteurization: disinfection of inhalation therapy equipment, *Respir Care* 16:97–103. 1971.
35. Favero MS: Chemical disinfection of medical and surgical materials, In: Block SS, ed. Disinfection, sterilization and preservation. 3rd ed. Philadelphia: Lea & Febiger, 1983.
36. Garner JS, Favero MS: CDC guidelines for the prevention and control of nosocomial infections: Guideline for handwashing and hospital environmental control, 1985, *Am J Infect Control* 14:110–129, 1986.
37. Spaulding EH: Chemical disinfection and antisepsis in the hospital, *J Hosp Res* 9:7–31, 1972.
38. Ayliffe GAJ: Hospital disinfection and antibiotic policies, *Chemotherapy* 6:228–233, 1987.
39. Dixon RE, Kaslow RA, Maackel DC, et al.: Aqueous quaternary ammonium antiseptics and disinfectants, *JAMA* 236:2415–2417, 1976.
40. Lee JC, Failkow PJ: Benzalkonium chloride: Source of hospital infection with gram-negative bacteria, *JAMA* 177:708–710, 1961.
41. Frank MJ, Schaffner W: Contaminated aqueous benzalkonium chloride: An unnecessary hospital infection hazard, *JAMA* 236:2418–2419, 1976.
42. American Respiratory Care Foundation: Guidelines for disinfection of respiratory care equipment used in the home, *Respir Care* 33:801–808, 1988.
43. Chatburn RE, Kallstrom TJ, Bajaksouzian MS: A comparison of acetic acid with a quaternary ammonium compound for disinfection of hand-held nebulizers, *Respir Care* 33:179–187, 1988.
44. Alasri A, Valverde M, Roques C, et al.: Sporocidal properties of peracetic acid and hydrogen peroxide, alone and in combination, in comparison with chlorine and formaldehyde for ultrafiltration membrane disinfection, *Can J Microbiol* 39:52–60, 1993.
45. Gorman SP, Scott EM, Russell AD: A review: antimicrobial activity, uses and mechanisms of action of glutaraldehyde, *J Appl Bacteriol* 48:161–190, 1980.
46. Kelsey JC, Mackinnon IH, Maurer IM: Sporicidal activity of hospital disinfectants, *J Clin Pathol* 27:632–638, 1974.
47. Fisher AA: Reactions to glutaraldehyde with particular reference to radiologists and x-ray technicians, *Cutis* 28:113–114, 1981.
48. Belani KG, Priedkalns J: An epidemic of pseudomembranous laryngotracheitis. *Anesthesiology* 47:530–531, 1977.
49. Boucher RM: Cidex and Sonacide compared, *Respir Care* 22:790–799, 1977.
50. Emergency Care Research Institute: Alternatives to glutaraldehyde: coping with OSHA's new ceiling limit, *Technol Respir Therapy* 10(6):1–4, 1989.
51. Miner NA, Ross C: Clinical evaluation of ColdSpor, a glutaraldehyde-phenolic disinfectant, *Respir Care* 36:104–109, 1991.
52. Crow S: Peracetic acid sterilization: a timely development for a busy healthcare industry, *Infect Control Hosp Epidemiol* 13(2):111–3, 1992.
53. Malchesky PS: Peracetic acid and its application to medical instrument sterilization, *Artif Organs* 17(3):147–152, 1993.
54. Melichercikova V: Disinfectant effect of Persteril in combination with detergents, *J Hyg Epidemiol Microbiol Immunol* 33(1):19–28, 1989.
55. Crow S: Sterilization processes. Meeting the demands of today's health care technology, *Nurs Clin North Am* 28(3):687–695, 1993.
56. Dempsey DJ, Thirucote RR: Sterilization of medical devices: a review, *J Biomater Appl* 3(3):454–523, 1989.
57. Schnierson SS: Sterilization by heat, *Int Anesthesiol Clin* 10:67–83, 1972.
58. Ernst RR: Sterilization by heat, In: Block SS. Disinfection, sterilization and preservation. Philadelphia: Lea & Febiger, 1977.
59. Medical Research Council: Sterilization by steam under increased pressure, *Lancet* 1:425–435, 1959.
60. Failon RJ: Factors concerned in the efficient steam sterilization of surgical dressings, *J Clin Pathol* 14:505–511, 1961.
61. Hoyt A, Chancy AL, Caveli K: Studies on steam sterilization and the effects of air in the autoclave, *J Bacteriol* 36:639–652, 1938.
62. Artandi C: Sterilization by ionizing radiation, *Int Anesthesiol Clin* 10(2):123–130, 1972.
63. Riley RL, Nardell EA: Clearing the air. The theory and application of ultraviolet air disinfection, *Am Rev Respir Dis* 139:1286–1294, 1989.
64. Emergency Care Research Institute: Ethylene oxide: hazards and safe use, *Technol Respir Therapy* 9(12):1–4, 1989.
65. American National Standards Institute Sectional Committee Z-79 and ASA Subcommittee on Standardization. Ethylene oxide sterilization of anesthesia apparatus, *Anesthesiology* 33:120, 1970.
66. Edge RS Infection control. In: Barnes TA, Lisbon A, eds: Respiratory care practice. Chicago: Year Book Medical Publishers, 1988.
67. Rendell-Baker L: Ethylene oxide. II. Aeration. *Int Anesthesiol Clin* 10:101–122, 1972.
68. Anderson SR: Ethylene oxide residues in medical materials, *Bull Parenteral Drug Assoc* 27:49–57, 1973.
69. Anderson SR: Ethylene oxide toxicity, *J Lab Clin Med* 77:346–355, 1971.
70. Hirose T, Goldstein R, Bailey CP: Hemolysis of blood due to exposure to different types of plastic tubing and the influence of ethylene oxide sterilization, *J Thorac Cardiovasc Surg* 45:245–251, 1963.
71. O'Leary RK, Guess WL: The toxiogenic potential of medical plastics sterilized with ethylene oxide vapors, *J Biomed Mater Res* 2:297–311, 1968.

72. Haney PE, Raymond BA, Lewis LC: Ethylene oxide. An occupational health hazard for hospital workers, *AORN J* 51(2):480–481, 483, 485–486, 1990.

73. Gross JA, Haas ML, Swift TR: Ethylene oxide neurotoxicity: report of four cases and review of the literature, *Neurology* 29:978–983, 1979.

74. Glaser ZR: Special occupation hazard review with control recommendations for the use of ethylene oxide as a sterilant in medical facilities. US Dept HEW DHEW (NIOSH), Publication No. 77–200, August 1977.

75. US Department of Health and Human Services, DHSS (NIOSH): NIOSH current intelligence bulletin 35: Ethylene oxide. Publication No. 81–130, May 22, 1981.

76. Occupational Safety and Health Administration: Occupational exposure to ethylene oxide—OSHA. Final standard, Fed Regist 49(122):25734–25809 (Jun 22), 1984.

77. Kruger DA: What is 5 ppm? Understanding and complying with the new EO STEL, (short-term exposure limit) regulation, J Healthc Mater Manage Feb-Mar;7(2):34–8, 40–1, 44–5, 1989.

78. Steelman VM: Ethylene oxide. The importance of aeration, *AORN J* 55(3):773–5, 778–9, 782–3, 1992.

79. Association for the Advancement of Medical Instrumentation. Good hospital practice: Ethylene oxide gas-ventilation recommendations and safe use. AAMI DO-VRSU 1981.

80. American Association for Respiratory Therapy, Technical Standards and Safety Committee: Recommendations for respiratory therapy equipment—Processing, handling and surveillance, *Respir Care* 22:928, 1977.

81. Cadwallader HL, Bradley CR, Ayliffe GA: Bacterial contamination and frequency of changing ventilator circuitry, *J Hosp Infect* 5(1):65–72, 1990.

82. Craven DE, Connolly MG Jr, Lichtenberg DA, et al.: Contamination of mechanical ventilators with tubing changes every 24 or 48 hours, *N Engl J Med* 306:1505–1509, 1982.

83. Goularte TA, Manning M, Craven DE: Bacterial colonization in humidifying cascade reservoirs after 24 and 48 hours of continuous mechanical ventilation, *Infect Control* 8:200–203, 1987.

84. Dreyfuss D, Djedaini K, Weber P, et al.: Prospective study of nosocomial pneumonia and of patient and circuit colonization during mechanical ventilation with circuit changes every 48 hours versus no change. *Am Rev Respir Dis* 143 (4 Pt 1):738–743, 1991.

85. Boyce JM, White RL, Spruill EY, et al.: Cost-effective application of the Centers for Disease Control guideline for prevention of nosocomial pneumonia, *Am J Infect Control* Oct;13(5):228–32, 1985.

86. Gallagher J, Strangeways JE, Allt-Graham J: Contamination control in long-term ventilation. A clinical study using a heat- and moisture-exchanging filter, *Anaesthesia* 42(5): 476–481, 1987.

87. Martin C, Perrin G, Gevaudan MJ, et al.: Heat and moisture exchangers and vaporizing humidifiers in the intensive care unit, *Chest* 97:144–149, 1990.

88. Fierer J, Taylor PM, Gezon HM: Pseudomonas aeruginosa epidemic traced to delivery-room resuscitators, *N Engl J Med* 276(18):991–996, 1967.

89. Weber DJ, Wilson MB, Rutala WA, et al.: Manual ventilation bags as a source for bacterial colonization of intubated patients, *Am Rev Respir Dis* 142(4):892–894, 1990.

90. Castel O, Agius G, Grignon B, et al.: Evaluation of closed sterile prefilled humidification, *J Hosp Infect* 17(1):53–59, 1991.

91. Seigel D, Romo B: Extended use of prefilled humidifier reservoirs and the likelihood of contamination, *Respir Care* 35(8):806–810, 1990.

92. Seto WH, Ching TY, Yuen KY, Lam WK: Evaluating the sterility of disposable wall oxygen humidifiers, during and between use on patients, *Infect Control Hosp Epidemiol* 11(11):604–605, 1990.

93. Levine ER: Low-flow oxygen without humidity, *Respir Ther* 16(4):11, 50, 1986.

94. Tablan OC, Williams WW, Martone WJ. Infection control in pulmonary function laboratories. *Infect Control* 1985;6:442–444.

95. Rutala DR, Rutala WA, Weber DJ, et al.: Infection risks associated with spirometry. *Infect Control Hosp Epidemiol* 12(2):89–92, 1991.

96. Greene VW: Reuse of disposable medical devices: historical and current aspects, *Infect Control* 7(10):508–513, 1986.

97. Alvine GF, Rodgers P, Fitzsimmons KM, et al.: Disposable jet nebulizers. How reliable are they? *Chest* 101(2):316–319, 1992.

98. Kissoon N, Nykanen D, Tiffin N, et al.: Evaluation of performance characteristics of disposable bag-valve resuscitators, *Crit Care Med* 19(1):102–107, 1991.

99. Simmons BP, Wong ES: Guide for prevention of nosocomial pneumonia, *Infect Control* 3:327–333, 1982.

100. Institute for Health Policy Analysis, Georgetown University Medical Center: Proceedings of international conference on the re-use of disposable medical devices in the 1980s, March 29–30, 1984. Washington DC: Institute for Health Policy Analysis, 1984.

101. Mastro TD, Fields BS, Breiman RF, et al.: Nosocomial Legionnaires' disease and use of medication nebulizers, *J Infect Dis* 163(3):667–671, 1991.

102. Williams, WW: Guideline for infection control in hospital personnel, *Infect Control* 4(suppl): 326–439, 1983.

103. Garner JS, Simmons BP: Centers for Disease Control guideline for isolation precautions in hospitals (publication no. 83–8314), Atlanta, 1983, Centers for Disease Control.

104. Emergency Care Research Institute: Needlestick injuries, *Technol Respir Care* 11(12):1–5, 1991.

105. American College of Surgeons: Total care for burn patients: a guide to hospital resources, *Bull Am Coll Surg* 62:6–14, 1977.

106. Centers for Disease Control: Acquired immunodeficiency syndrome (AIDS): Precautions for health-care workers and allied professionals, *MMWR* 32:450–451, 1983.

107. Centers for Disease Control: Recommendations for preventing transmission of infection with human T-lymphotropic virus type III/lymphadenopathy-associated virus in the workplace, *MMWR* 34:681–6, 691–5, 1985.

108. Centers for Disease Control: Update: universal precautions for prevention of transmission of human immunodeficiency virus, hepatitis B virus, and other bloodborne pathogens in health-care settings. *MMWR* 37(24):377–382, 387–388, 1988.

109. Centers for Disease Control: Guidelines for prevention of transmission of human immunodeficiency virus and hepatitis B virus to health-care and public-safety workers. *MMWR* 38(Suppl 6):1–37, 1989.

110. Technical Panel on Infections within Hospitals: Management of HIV infection in the hospital, Chicago, American Hospital Association, 1988.

111. Crutcher JM, Lamm SH, Hall TA: Procedures to protect health-care workers from HIV infection: category I (health-care) workers, *Am Ind Hyg Assoc J* 52(2):A100–103, 1991.

5

Ethical and Legal Implications of Practice

■

Raymond Edge

CHAPTER LEARNING OBJECTIVES

1. Define the basic goal of the respiratory care code of ethics.
2. Relate the respiratory care code of ethics to the basic principles of biomedical ethics.
3. Describe the two basic biomedical ethics viewpoints and show how they relate to the dichotomy so often found in ethical decision making.
4. List the major criticisms of duty-oriented and consequence-oriented reasoning.
5. Outline the theoretical position known as virtue ethics.
6. List the major criticisms of the virtue ethics position.
7. Delineate the basic information that must be gathered before a reasoned ethical decision is made.
8. Define the differences between public and private law and relate them to current practice.
9. Describe the nature and elements of a malpractice suit and relate the various torts to current practice.
10. Relate the current practice of respiratory care to professional liability.
11. Describe the nature of unlawful and unethical practice as it relates to the diversification of respiratory care into home care and durable medical equipment.
12. Relate the process of licensing to increased legal responsibility and liability.
13. Explain how the emerging physician/patient relationship, centered on patient independence and responsibility, is shaping the ethical and legal aspects of practice.

Conventional knowledge and technical standards of good practice are generally all that is needed to ensure that respiratory care practitioners (RCPs) fulfill their roles competently. However, special circumstances can arise in which technical standards fail to provide a sufficient basis for our choices and actions. More often than not, these special situations involve ethical issues or the law.

Ethics and law help society maintain order and continuity. Professional ethics guide RCPs in their dealings with others, toward actions designed to bring about a particular result. In the case of respiratory care, the ideal result is restoration of health to the patient. Law, unlike ethics, does not set an ideal but, rather, a minimum standard for social behavior. The force behind law is some enforceable punishment. For ethics, it is censorship by or expulsion from the profession.

ETHICAL DILEMMAS OF PRACTICE

The growth of respiratory care has been closely associated with a rather remarkable series of advances in medical technology and treatment protocols. At the same time, an ever-growing and sophisticated pa-tient population has developed rising expectations. These changes in health care have not only helped create this new specialty, but have also created a new world of ethical and legal dilemmas. In this new world of practice, much of the geography still lies uncharted, yet to be mapped by ethicists and lawyers.

The approaches used to address ethical issues in health care range from the specific to the general. Specific guidance in resolving ethical dilemmas is usually provided by a professional code of ethics. General approaches involve use of ethical theory to help resolve moral decisions.

Codes of ethics

A code of ethics is an essential part of any profession that claims to be self-regulating. In addition to setting forth rules for conduct, a code may try to limit competition, restrict advertisement, or promote a particular image.[1]

The first American medical code of ethics (1847) was as much concerned with separating orthodox practitioners from nontraditionalists ones as it was with regulating behavior. Even modern codes tend to be quite vague as to what is prescribed and what is to be avoided. Indeed, some professions have had to create separate statements just to explain what is meant by the various rules in their codes.

The Code of Ethics established by the American Association for Respiratory Care (AARC) appears here (see accompanying box). This code represents a set of general principles and rules that have been developed to help assure that the health needs of the public are provided in a safe, effective, and caring manner. Codes for different professions might well differ from that governing respiratory care because they may seek different goals.

Ethical codes, then, depend on a group's decision about what is needed to achieve an ideal good, rather than general morality or personal value systems. Personal ethics or morals grow out of an individual's world view and are shaped by the experiences of that person's cultural past. Personal ethics or morals are the social screen by which individuals decide what ought to be, on the basis of social convention and community expectations. Personal ethics provide individuals with general rules of conduct, which tell them which kinds of actions, such as lying and stealing, are inherently wrong.[2]

In a complex world, values help people set priorities and help give life meaning and structure. Ideally, the RCP's professional code always matches his or her personal value system. Unfortunately, many times personal values conflict with what is considered medically and legally acceptable or ethical. In a **pluralistic** society, it would be a remarkable code of ethics that manages to fit each RCP's personal value system all the time.

Another limitation of professional codes of ethics is their narrow focus. Unfortunately, and all too often, codes of ethics represent overly simplistic or prohibitive notions of how to deal with open misbehavior or flagrant abuses of authority over which few would disagree.

The really difficult moral decisions stem from situations in which two or more right choices are incompatible, in which the choices represent different priorities, or in which limited resources exist to achieve a desired end. As the American Hospital Association (AHA) notes, reducing these issues to simple formulations is no easy task. Indeed, the number and complexity of ethical dilemmas have grown dramatically in recent years. Factors contributing to this growth include the increasing sophistication of technology, concerns about the practical limits on financial resources for health care, changes in

---

AARC code of ethics

The principles set forth in this document define the basic ethical and moral standards to which each member of the American Association for Respiratory Care should conform.

1. The respiratory care practitioner shall practice medically acceptable methods of treatment and shall not endeavor to extend his practice beyond his competence and the authority vested in him by the physician.
2. The respiratory care practitioner shall continually strive to increase and improve his knowledge and skill and render to each patient the full measure of his ability. All services shall be provided with respect for the dignity of the patient, unrestricted by considerations of social or economic status, personal attributes, or the nature of health problems.
3. The respiratory care practitioner shall be responsible for the competent and efficient performance of his assigned duties and shall expose incompetence and illegal or unethical conduct of members of the profession.
4. The respiratory care practitioner shall hold in strict confidence all privileged information concerning the patient and refer all inquiries to the physician in charge of the patient's medical care.
5. The respiratory care practitioner shall not accept gratuities for preferential consideration of the patient. He shall not solicit patients for personal gain and shall guard against conflicts of interest.
6. The respiratory care practitioner shall uphold the dignity and honor of the profession and abide by its ethical principles. He should be familiar with existing state and federal laws governing the practice of respiratory therapy and comply with those laws.
7. The respiratory care practitioner shall cooperate with other health care professionals and participate in activities to promote community and national efforts to meet the health needs of the public.

---

society, and growing emphasis on individual independence.[3]

Resolution of these more complex problems requires a more general approach than that provided by a code of ethics. This more general perspective is provided by the broad principles of ethical theory.

Principles of ethical theory

Underlying the codes of ethics of health specialties like respiratory care is a common core of broad ethical principles. Any consideration of ethical principles eventually must address the meaning of such terms as "right" and "good." Obviously, without some benchmark of what is morally right, it is possible to argue in favor of almost any position.

Contemporary ethical principles have evolved from many sources. These include Aristotle and Aquinas' natural law, Judeo-Christian morality, Kant's universal duties, and the values characterizing modern democracy. Although some controversy exists, most ethicists agree that autonomy, veracity, nonmaleficence, beneficence, confidentiality, justice, and role fidelity are the primary guiding principles in moral decision making.

As applied to professional practice, each of these ethical principles consists of two components: a professional duty and a patient right (Figure 5-1). For example, the principle of autonomy obliges health professionals to uphold others' freedom of will and freedom of action. The principle of beneficence obliges us to further the interests of others, either by promoting their good or by actively preventing their harm. The principle of justice obliges us to ensure that others receive what they rightfully deserve or legitimately claim.

Expressed in each duty is a reciprocal patient right. Reciprocal patient rights include the right to autonomous choice, the right not to be harmed, and the right to fair and equitable treatment. From these general principles of rights and obligations one can generate more specific rules, such as those included in a code of ethics.

Autonomy

The principle of autonomy acknowledges patients' personal liberty, and their right to decide their own course and follow through a plan that they freely agree on.

It is from this principle that rules about **informed consent** are derived. To decide freely requires that an individual has adequate information to comprehend the available options. However, true informed consent requires more than just information. Individuals must also be "situated as to exercise free power of choice, without the intervention of any element of

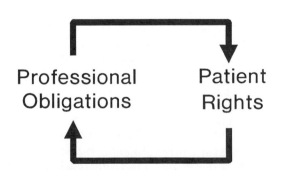

Fig. 5-1 Reciprocal relationship between professional obligations and patient rights.

force, fraud, deceit, duress, overreaching or other ulterior form of constraint or coercion" (The Nuremberg Code, Rule 1).

Autonomy, then, has two basic requirements: *freedom to decide* and *freedom to act without coercion*. Freedom to decide depends on information and comprehension. Freedom to act without coercion depends on the respect for personal autonomy granted by health care professionals and the families involved.

Thus, under the principle of autonomy, an RCP's use of deceit or coercion to get a patient to reverse the decision to refuse a treatment would be considered unethical. Likewise, it would be unethical to threaten a patient unwilling to sign a consent form.

Unfortunately, the principle of autonomy is not regularly followed. There is a tendency among healthcare professionals to assume that they know what is best for the patient. This view, called *paternalism,* has long been a mainstay of health care practice. Take, for example, the following excerpts from the 1848 Medical Code of Ethics:[4]

"Obligations of Patients to their Physicians"

The obedience of a patient to the prescriptions of his physician should be prompt and implicit. He should never permit his own crude opinion as to their fitness to influence his attention to them.

"Duties of Physicians to their Patients"

A physician should not be forward to make gloomy prognostications, because they savor of empiricism, by magnifying the importance of his services in the treatment or cure of disease. But he should not fail, on proper occasions, to give to the friends of the patients timely notice of danger when it really occurs; and even to the patient himself if absolutely necessary.

In the past, medical care was based mainly on good bedside manners and, often, bad science. Patients were made well as much by their faith in the caring and authority of the caregiver as by the opinions and medications prescribed. Today medicine has given up much of its home-based art for the benefits of modern science. The rising expectations of the population, as well as the heavy involvement of the government and third-party payers, has created a new consumerism. Essential in this new consumerism is the expectation that lay people will be given greater responsibility and authority in personal health care decision-making.

Indeed, Robert Veatch, of the Kennedy Institute of Ethics, believes that the old ethic of patient benefit is now outmoded and should be replaced by an ethic of patient responsibility.[5,6] Many authorities feel that the growing conflict between patient autonomy and the paternalism of health care providers is the central crisis in medical relationships today.[7]

To help patients and providers better understand these new expectations, the American Hospital Associ-

---

AHA patient's bill of rights

1. The patient has the right to considerate and respectful care.
2. The patient has the right to obtain from his physician complete current information concerning his diagnosis, treatment, and prognosis in terms the patient can be reasonably expected to understand. When it is not medically advisable to give such information to the patient, the information should be made available to an appropriate person in his behalf. He has the right to know, by name, the physician responsible for coordinating his care.
3. The patient has the right to receive from his physician information necessary to give informed consent prior to the start of any procedure and/or treatment. Except in emergencies, such information for informed consent should include but not necessarily be limited to the specific procedure and/or treatment, the medically significant risks involved, and the probable duration of incapacitation. Where medically significant alternatives for care or treatment exist, or when the patient requests information concerning medical alternatives, the patient has the right to such information. The patient also has the right to know the name of the person responsible for the procedures and/or treatment.
4. The patient has the right to refuse treatment to the extent permitted by law and to be informed of the medical consequences of his action.
5. The patient has the right to every consideration of his privacy concerning his own medical care program. Case discussion, consultation, examination, and treatment are confidential and should be conducted discreetly. Those not directly involved in his care must have the permission of the patient to be present.
6. The patient has the right to expect that all communications and records pertaining to his care should be treated as confidential.

7. The patient has the right to expect that within its capacity a hospital must make reasonable response to the request of a patient for services. The hospital must provide evaluation, service, and/or referral as indicated by the urgency of the case. When medically permissible, a patient may be transferred to another facility only after he has received complete information and explanation concerning the needs for and alternatives to such a transfer. The institution to which the patient is to be transferred must first have accepted the patient for transfer.
8. The patient has the right to obtain information as to any relationship of his hospital to other health care and educational institutions insofar as his care is concerned. The patient has the right to obtain information as to the existence of any professional relationships among individuals, by name, who are treating him.
9. The patient has the right to be advised if the hospital proposes to engage in or perform human experimentation affecting his care or treatment. The patient has the right to refuse to participate in such research projects.
10. The patient has the right to expect reasonable continuity of care. He has the right to know in advance what appointment times and physicians are available and where. The patient has the right to expect that the hospital will provide a mechanism whereby he is informed by his physician or a delegate of the physician of the patient's continuing health care requirements following discharge.
11. The patient has the right to examine and receive an explanation of his bill regardless of source of payment.
12. The patient has the right to know what hospital rules and regulations apply to his conduct as a patient.

---

ation (AHA) has published "The Patients' Bill of Rights" (see box above). This document, although lacking the force of law, provides excellent insight into the emerging patient-provider relationship. A careful reading of this document provides the RCP with a helpful guide in addressing issues in this vital and changing area.

Many states have adopted specific legislation giving patients "the fundamental right to control the decisions relating to their own medical care, including the decision to have life-sustaining procedures withheld or withdrawn in circumstances where such persons are diagnosed as having a terminally and irreversible condition."[8]

Veracity

The principle of veracity is often linked to autonomy, especially in the area of informed consent. In general, veracity binds the health provider and the patient to tell the truth. The nature of the health process is such that both parties involved are best served in an environment of trust and mutual sharing of all information.

Problems with the veracity principle revolve around such issues as *benevolent deception*. In actions of benevolent deception, the truth is withheld from the patient for his or her own good.

When the physician decides to withhold the truth from a conscious, well-oriented adult, the decision

■ MINI CLINI ■

5-1

Ethical and Legal Implications of Practice

Problem—A RCP working at a hospital receives a physician order to administer an aerosolized bronchodilator treatment to a 26 year old female asthmatic patient admitted for suspected pneumonia. Upon entering the room, the patient refuses the treatment, stating that she is having a "bad day" today and doesn't want to be bothered by anyone. The patient is regarded as being competent and fully capable of making health care decisions for herself. How could the RCP handle this situation?

Discussion—The RCP must acknowledge and respect the patient's right to freely decide whether or not to allow the respiratory care treatment. According to the principles of ethical theory and conduct, health care professionals have an obligation to promote patient autonomy by permitting freedom of will and freedom of action. An additional requirement on the part of the practitioner is that coercion or deceit not be used in order to get a patient to reverse their decision to refuse a treatment. Indeed, according to the American Hospital Association Patient's Bill of Rights, the patient has the right to refuse treatment to the extent permitted by law and to be informed of the medical consequences of her action. The RCP could however, talk to the patient and explore what the term "bad day" meant to her. It might be that she is not feeling well due to breathing problems of her asthma condition and worsening symptoms of a possible pneumonia. The RCP has an important role in ensuring that the patient understands what the benefits of the respiratory treatment are as well as the health consequences of refusal. Thus, the patient can make a well-informed decision. By approaching the patient in a professional, nonthreatening manner, she may feel more at ease and be willing to discuss in greater depth why she doesn't want to take the treatment. Not infrequently, patients may initially refuse therapy only to change their mind following communication with the RCP. Should the patient still refuse the treatment following discussion with the RCP, the RCP should remain nonjudgemental, even if he or she disagrees with the patient's decision. Appropriate documentation in the medical record and physician notification should then occur.

affects the interactions between health care providers and the patient, and has a chilling effect on the rapport so necessary for good care. In a poll conducted by the Louis Harris group, 94% of Americans surveyed indicated that they wanted to know everything about their cases, even the dismal facts.[9] Outside of pediatrics and in rare cases where there is evidence that the truth would lead to a harm (such as suicide), the truth, provided in as pleasant a manner as possible, is probably the best policy.[2,10,11]

Nonmaleficence

In the Hippocratic Oath taken by physicians as they enter practice, they swear to "never use treatment to injure or wrong the sick." This principle of nonmaleficence obligates health care providers to avoid harming patients and to actively prevent harm where possible.

In a simpler time this was an easier principle to uphold in practice. Now, many drugs and procedures have undesirable secondary effects. As an example, we might ask whether it is ethical to give a high dose of steroids to an asthmatic patient, knowing the many harmful consequences of these drugs.

One solution to these dilemmas is based on the understanding that many helping action inevitably have both a good and a bad, or *double* effect.[11,12] The key is the first intent. If the first intent is good, then the harmful effect is viewed as an unintended result.

For an action with unintended but harmful results to be considered ethically acceptable, it must meet four basic conditions, as outlined in accompanying box below.[2]

A simple example of the principle of double effect is drawing an arterial blood gas. The intent, to provide diagnostic information to help properly treat the patient, is good. However, this procedure has harmful effects: pain, anxiety, and complications. But the RCP does not desire to or intend to cause pain or complications; these are unintended results. Moreover, the adverse effects are not the means to diagnosis; they are side effects. Last, the good that can occur (and bad that might occur without) outweighs the immediate adverse effects. Accordingly, drawing an arterial blood gas is consistent with the principle of nonmaleficence.

Principle of double effect

An action that helps but may harm a patient may be ethical if:
1. The action itself is good.
2. The doer intends only the good effect.
3. The bad effect is not a means to a good end.
4. A favorable balance exists between the good and bad effects.

Not all people agree with the principle of double effect. According to some, foreseen secondary effects are avoidable and thus become intended if they are not avoided. Even if this critical position holds and the principle of double effect is rejected, it leads us to ask the right question: Under what circumstances can you be said to act morally when some of the foreseeable effects of your actions are harmful?

Beneficence

In simple terms, the principle of beneficence requires that health providers go beyond doing no harm and actively contribute to the health and well-being of their patients. In this dictum lies many quality-of-life issues, for practitioners of medicine today possess the technology to keep some individuals alive well beyond any rational good to themselves. This presents real dilemmas for those who are confronted with the ability to prolong life but not the ability to restore any uniquely human qualities.

In these cases, some interpret the principle of beneficence to mean that they must do everything to promote a patient's life, regardless of how useful the life might be to that individual. Other professionals in the same situation might believe they are allowing the principle to be better served by doing nothing and allowing death to occur without taking heroic measures to prevent it.

In most such cases, patients cannot decide for themselves. Instead, the matter is left to the family, the health care team, ethics committees, or, at times, the legal system. Decision making by others is easier when individuals make their wishes known by way of an advanced directive or "living will" (see box below in left column). In the past, living wills have been ignored by health care practitioners, and their legal weight has been challenged in court. Recently, however, state legislatures have begun to support these documents. Beginning with the 1976 California law, more than 40 states have adopted similar legislation.[9,13,14] In addition, the Patient Self-Determination Act of 1990 requires that all health care agencies receiving federal reimbursement under Medicare/Medicaid legislation provide adult clients with information on advanced directives.[14]

The professions have also been active in addressing the complex issues involved in artificial life support. As an example, the American Medical Association (AMA) recently has provided physicians with a set of broad guidelines on the withholding or withdrawal of life-prolonging medical treatments (see box below).

Example of a living will

To My Family, My Physician, My Lawyer
And All Others Whom It May Concern

Death is as much a reality as birth, growth, maturity, and old age—it is the one certainty of life. If the time comes when I can no longer take part in decisions for my own future, let this statement stand as my expression of my wishes and directions, while I am still of sound mind.

If at such a time the situation should arise in which there is no reasonable expectation of my recovery from extreme physical or mental disability, I direct that I be allowed to die and not be kept alive by medications, artificial means, or "heroic measures." I do, however, ask that medication be mercifully administered to me to alleviate suffering even though this may shorten my remaining life.

This statement is made after careful consideration and is in accordance with my strong convictions and beliefs. I want the wishes and directions here expressed carried out to the extent permitted by law. Insofar as they are not legally enforceable, I hope that those to whom this Will is addressed will regard themselves as morally bound by these provisions.

AMA statement on withholding or withdrawing life-prolonging medical treatment

The social commitment of the physician is to sustain life and relieve suffering. Where the performance of one duty conflicts with the other, the choice of the patient, or his family or legal representative if the patient is incompetent to act in his own behalf, should prevail. In the absence of the patient's choice or an authorized proxy, the physician must act in the best interest of the patient.

For humane reasons, with informed consent, a physician may do what is medically necessary to alleviate severe pain, or cease or omit treatment to permit a terminally ill patient whose death is imminent to die. However, he should not intentionally cause death. In deciding whether the administration of potentially life-prolonging medical treatment is in the best interest of the patient who is incompetent to act on his own behalf, the physician should determine what the possibility is for extending life under humane and comfortable conditions and what are the prior expressed wishes of the patient and attitudes of the family or those who have responsibility for the custody of the patient.

Even if death is not imminent but a patient's coma is beyond doubt irreversible and there are adequate safeguards to confirm the accuracy of the diagnosis and with the concurrence of those who have responsibility for the care of the patient, it is not unethical to discontinue all means of life-prolonging medical treatment.

Life-prolonging medical treatment includes medication and artificially or technologically supplied respiration, nutrition or hydration. In treating a terminally ill or irreversibly comatose patient, the physician should determine whether the benefits of treatment outweigh its burdens. At all times, the dignity of the patient should be maintained.

Confidentiality

The principle of confidentiality is founded in the Hippocratic Oath; it was later reiterated by the World Health Association in 1948. It obliges health care providers to "respect the secrets which are confided. . . . even after the patient has died." As with the other axioms of ethics, confidentiality must often be balanced against other principles, such as beneficence.

A classic confidentiality case involved a young man who had voluntarily visited an outpatient psychiatric unit for evaluation. During his time with the psychologist, he related that he was planning to kill a certain young woman. Although the psychologist briefly had the patient detained, the young man appeared quite normal and demanded to be released. Given the voluntary nature of the man's visit and his otherwise normal behavior, he was released. The psychologist's decision not to hold the patient or to warn the woman was based on confidentiality. The tragedy of this case is that the patient did go on to kill the young woman.

When the parents of the murdered woman learned that the psychologist and security officers had been aware of the threat to their daughter's life but had made no effort to warn her of the potential harm, they sued. The court ruled for the parents, stating that the obligation to the innocent party outweighed the obligation to maintain patient confidentiality.

The main ethical issue surrounding confidentiality is whether more harm is done by occasionally violating its mandate or by always upholding it, regardless of the consequences. This limitation to confidentiality is known as the *Harm Principle*.[15] This principle requires that practitioners refrain from acts or omissions that would forseeably result in harm to others, especially where the others are vulnerable to risk.

For example, this principle would require that confidentiality be maintained for an AIDS patient in matters involving his or her landlord. In this case, confidentiality is justified because the landlord is not particularly vulnerable. However, if the patient were planning to marry, the Harm Principle would require that confidentiality be broken because of the special vulnerability of the spouse.

Confidentiality is usually considered a qualified, rather than an absolute, ethical principle in most health care provider–patient relationships. These qualifications are often written into codes of ethics. For example, the AMA Code of Ethics, Section 9, provides the following guidelines: "A physician may not reveal the confidences entrusted to him in the course of medical attendance or the deficiencies he may observe in the character of patients, unless he is required to do so by law or unless it becomes necessary in order to protect the welfare of the community or a vulnerable individual." Under the requirements of public health and community welfare there is often a legal requirement to report such things as child abuse, poisonings, industrial accidents, communica-

ble diseases, blood transfusion reactions, narcotic use, and injuries caused with knives or guns.[16] Child abuse statutes in many states protect the practitioner from liability even if the report should prove false, as long as the report was made in good faith. Failure to report a case of child abuse by one required to do so can leave that practitioner legally liable for additional injuries that the child may sustain after being returned to the hostile environment.

Unfortunately, breaches of confidentiality are more often due to careless slips of the tongue than to rational decision making. Such social trading in gossip about patients is unprofessional, unethical, and in certain cases, illegal.

As a result of the widespread use of computerized databases, confidential information—once highly protected—is now relatively easy to obtain. Clinical data are available for close scrutiny by the clerical staff, laboratory personnel, and other health care providers. The widespread use of these data systems represents a real threat to patient confidentiality.

Potential violations of the individual's right to privacy in such populations as patients with AIDS pose a special threat because disclosure may result in economic, psychological, or bodily harm to the patient. RCPs would do well to adhere to the dictum found in the Hippocratic Oath: "What I may see or hear in the course of the treatment or even outside of treatment of the patient in regard to the life of men, which on no account one must spread abroad, I will keep to myself, holding such things to be shameful to be spoken about."

Justice

The principle of justice requires that like cases be treated alike and that different cases be treated differently. Under this principle we find such issues as the fair distribution of care.

In an environment of rising expectation in regard to health care, issues of justice are coming to the forefront as policymakers wrestle with questions of how much care can be provided and on what basis. Current population trends indicate that in the year 2000, the number of individuals over 75 will have increased by 30% from the 1980s.

The United States is rapidly approaching a period in history when the number of those who contribute to the financial resources of our health care system will be smaller in number than those who rely on its resources. Nations such as Britain have long found it necessary to set up criteria for rationing certain kinds of care. Under the British health care system, for example, the government will not pay for kidney dialysis for patients over the age of 55.

As U.S. health care reimbursement policies change, our society is beginning to question the level of care citizens can claim or expect.[17] *Distributive justice* deals with the proper allotment of the benefits and burdens in a society, as represented by taxes and subsidies. Questions of justice seem rather straightforward and possible to answer when they are seen as abstract policies, guidelines, or laws designed to allocate scarce resources. It is more difficult to address questions related to care of an individual patient, such as whether we should deny needed care to an individual on the basis of his or her inability to pay.

A second form of justice seen in health care is *compensatory justice.* This form of justice calls for the recovery for damages that were incurred as a result of the action of others. Damage awards in civil cases of medical malpractice or negligence are examples of compensatory justice. Industries that have been found to pollute or produce harmful agents such as asbestos have been sued for damages under this form of justice. Pulmonary function technologists have long been part of the process that determines the amount of loss suffered and degree of impairment caused by industrial agents that cause lung damage.

Role duty

By necessity, modern health care is a team effort. This is because no single individual can be solely responsible for providing all of a patient's health care needs. Today there are more than 100 specialties under the heading of allied health. Along with nursing, these professions provide more than 80% of all patient care. Each of these specialties has its own practice niche, defined by tradition or by licensure law. Practitioners have a duty to understand the limits of their role and to practice with fidelity. As an example, because of differences in role duty, an RCP might be ethically obliged *not* to tell a patient's family how critical the situation is, instead having the attending physician do so.[1]

Ethical viewpoints and decision making

In deciding ethical issues, some practitioners try to adhere to a strict interpretation of one or more ethical principles (such as those just described). Others seek to decide the issue solely on a case-by-case basis, considering only the potential good (or bad) consequences. Still others would appeal to the image of a "good practitioner," asking themselves what a virtuous person would do in a similar circumstance.

These different viewpoints represent the three dominant theories underlying modern ethics.[18-22] The viewpoint that relies on rules and principles is called *formalism* or *duty-oriented reasoning.* The viewpoint in which decisions are based on the assessment of consequences is called *consequentialist-oriented reasoning.* The viewpoint that asks what a virtuous person would do in a similar circumstance is called *virtue ethics.*

Formalism

Formalist thought asserts that certain features of an act itself determine its moral rightness. In this framework, ethical standards of right and wrong are described in terms of rules or principles. These rules function apart from the consequences of a particular act. An act is considered morally justifiable only if it upholds the rules or principles that apply.

The major objection to this duty-oriented approach lies in its potential for inconsistency. Critics of formalist reasoning insist that no principle or rule can be framed that does not have exceptions. Moreover, claim these critics, no principle or rule can be framed that does not conflict with other rules.

The scenario described earlier regarding confidentiality of psychiatric information is a good example of the problems inherent in applying ethical rules without considering the consequences. Basically, this case involved a conflict between the principle of confidentiality and the principle of beneficence. The court decision underscored the fact that principles must admit exceptions, in particular the exception that the principle of confidentiality can not always apply.

Conflicts among competing principles can only be resolved if they are given a "weight," or relative priority. In this way, various alternatives are compared against a set of prioritized rules. As shown in Figure 5-2, if one or more alternatives are consistent with all applicable rules or principles, the decision is easy. On the other hand, if there is a conflict among rules, the decision maker must appeal to the higher level rule to resolve the conflict. As indicated in Figure 5-2, this approach may not always be successful (note the question marks following unsuccessful appeal).

Consequentialism

For the consequentialist, an act is judged to be right or wrong on the basis of its consequences. Each possible act is assessed in terms of the relative amount of good (over evil) that it will bring into being. The most common application of consequentialism judges acts according to the principle of utility. In its simplest form, the principle of utility aims to promote the greatest general good for the greatest number.

As shown in Figure 5-3, this approach requires the practitioner to identify all alternative actions and to each assign a value of "happiness," or the relative amount of good over evil brought into being.[23] In this framework, the ethically correct choice is simple: that which would result in the greatest general good among those involved in the situation.

Critics of this approach claim that it has two fundamental flaws. First, the "calculus" involved in projecting and weighing the amount of good over evil that might occur is not always possible. Second, reliance on the principle of utility to the exclusion of all else can result in actions that are incompatible with

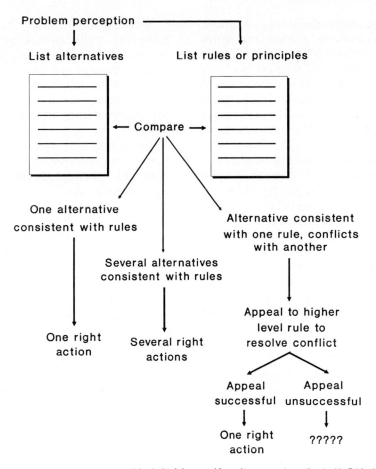

Fig. 5-2 The formalist approach to ethical decision making. (Redrawn from Brody H: Ethical decisions in medicine, ed 2, Boston, 1981, Little, Brown.)

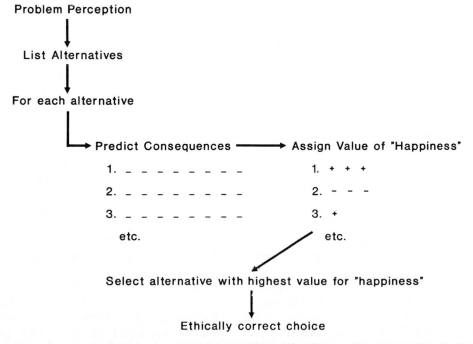

Fig. 5-3 The consequentialist approach to ethical decision making. (Redrawn from Brody H: Ethical decisions in medicine, ed 2, Boston, 1981, Little, Brown.)

ordinary judgments about right and wrong. A classic example of this problem can be seen in the true World War II case of the battle for North Africa. In this scenario, there were two groups of soldiers but only enough antibiotics for one group. One group required the medication for syphilis contracted in the local brothels; the other group needed antibiotics for wounds sustained in battle. Thus the dilemma arose as to who should receive the antibiotics.

Formalist or duty-oriented reasoning would base the decision about who should receive the antibiotics on some concept of justice, such as giving priority to the sickest or to those most in need. However, the actual decision in this case was a consequentialist one, based not on the desire to justly distribute the drug, but rather on the need to obtain a quick victory with as few casualties as possible. Thus the scarce medication was given to those who were "wounded" in the brothels rather than in battle because these soldiers could be restored quickly and returned to the front lines to aid the war effort.

Mixed approaches

Mixed approaches to moral reasoning try to capitalize on the strengths inherent in these two major lines of ethical thought. One approach, called *rule utilitarianism,* is a variation of consequentialism. Under this framework, the question is not which act has the greatest utility, but which rule would promote the greatest good if it were generally followed.

As an example, the rule utilitarian would agree with the formalist that truth-telling is a necessary ethical principle, but for a different reason. To the rule utilitarian, truth-telling is a needed principle not because it has any underlying moral rightness, but because it promotes the greatest good in professional patient relationships. Specifically, if truth-telling were not followed consistently, trusting relationships between patients and health professionals would be impossible.

The rule utilitarian approach is probably the most appealing and useful to health professionals. It is appealing because it addresses both human rights and obligations and the consequences of our actions. Moreover, rule utilitarianism seems best able to account for the modern realities of human experience that so often affect the day-to-day practice of health care.

Virtue ethics

Based in part on the limits of both formalism and consequentialism, a theory of *virtue ethics* has evolved. Virtue ethics is founded not in rules or consequences but in personal attributes of character or virtue. Under this formulation, the first question is not, "How do I act in this situation?" but, rather, "How should I carry out my life, if I am to live well?" or "How would the good RCP act?"

Virtue-oriented theory holds that professions have historical traditions. Thus individuals entering a profession enter not only into a relationship with current practitioners but also with those who have come before. With these traditions come a history of character standards set by those who have previously distinguished themselves in that profession.

According to this perspective, the established practices of a profession can give guidance, without an appeal to either the specific moral principles or consequences of an act.[1,22] Thus, when faced with an ethical dilemma, the professional need only envision what the "good practitioner" would do in a similar circumstance. For instance, it is hard to imagine the good RCP stealing from the patient, charging for services not provided, or smothering a patient with a pillow.

Rapidly changing fields like respiratory care do pose some problems for virtue ethics. What might be considered good ethical conduct at one time might be deemed wrong the next. An example of this change over time is the RCP who is asked not only to disconnect a brain-dead patient from a ventilator but also to remove the feeding tubes and IV lines.

In addition to its difficulty with changing values, virtue ethics provides no specific directions to aid decision making. Moreover, the heavy reliance of virtue ethics on past experience rather than on reason makes creative solutions less likely. Last, practitioners often find themselves in conflicting role situations for which virtue ethics has no answers. A good example is the RCP who practices the virtue of being a good team player but is confronted with the need to "blow the whistle" on a negligent or incompetent team member.[1] Despite these limitations, virtue ethics is probably the way most practitioners make their ethical decisions.

Comprehensive decision-making models

To aid in the process of decision-making in bioethics, several comprehensive models have developed. Figure 5-4 depicts one example of a comprehensive decision-making model that combines the best elements of formalism, consequentialism, and virtue ethics.[23]

As is evident in this approach, the ethical problem is framed in terms of the conditions and who is affected. Initially, an action is chosen on the basis of its predicted consequences. Then the potential consequences of this decision are compared with the human values underlying the problem. The short test of this comparison is a simple restatement of the Golden Rule—that is, "Would I be satisfied to have this action performed on me?" The initial decision is considered ethical if and only if it passes this test of human values.

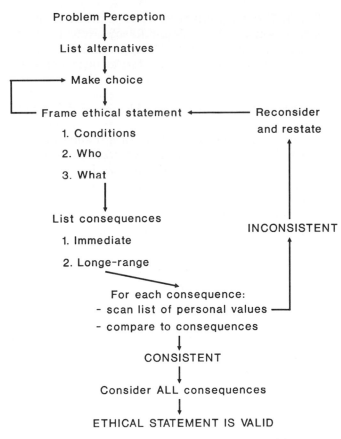

Problem Perception

↓

List alternatives

↓

→ Make choice

↓

Frame ethical statement ← Reconsider and restate

1. Conditions

2. Who

3. What

↓

List consequences

1. Immediate

2. Longe-range

INCONSISTENT

For each consequence:
- scan list of personal values
- compare to consequences

↓

CONSISTENT

↓

Consider ALL consequences

↓

ETHICAL STATEMENT IS VALID

Fig. 5-4 A comprehensive ethical decision-making model. (Redrawn from Brody H: Ethical decisions in medicine, ed 2, Boston, 1981, Little, Brown.)

A somewhat simpler but nonetheless comprehensive model has been proposed by Francoeur.[11] In this framework, ethical decision-making involves eight key steps (see accompanying box).

With or without these models, RCPs are often at a double disadvantage in ethical decision making. This is because RCPs must not only live with their own

---

A comprehensive ethical decision-making model[11]

1. Identify the problem or issue.
2. Identify the individuals involved.
3. Identify the ethical principle or principles that apply.
4. Identify who should make the decision.
5. Identify the role of the practitioner.
6. Consider the alternatives (long-term *and* short-term consequences).
7. Make the decision (including the decision not to act).
8. Follow the decision to observe its consequences.

From Francoeur RT Biomedical ethics: a guide to decision making. New York, 1983, Wiley Medical Publications.

---

decisions but must also support (and act on) the decisions of their physician colleagues. Unless excellent communications exists, misunderstandings can occur. Such misunderstandings may be a key factor in the high job stress, burnout, and attrition in respiratory care.

Classes in ethics, decision making, and communication skills are needed to prepare RCPs for the often confusing and frustrating practice in today's clinics. The specialty requires practitioners who can go beyond simple assertions of their beliefs of rightness or wrongness and provide justifications that are both right and reasoned.

LEGAL ISSUES AFFECTING RESPIRATORY CARE

Unfortunately, there are times when decisions cannot be made in the confines of the medical community and with the help of the patients it serves. These problems often find their way to the courts. The problem of professional liability in the delivery of health care is immense and plays a key role in skyrocketing health care costs.[24]

Practitioners are caught in the middle. On one hand, they are being squeezed by the government to hold down costs by avoiding overuse of technology and therapeutics. On the other hand, they are faced with a level of consumerism that holds them accountable as never before. These dynamics are also causing maldistribution of health care resources. For example, many physicians avoid or limit their participation in high-risk practices such as obstetrics because of the liability risk.

Clearly the costs, losses, frustration, and distraction brought about by the current level of legal intervention in health care practice is a national crisis.

Systems of law

Under our legal system, the law is divided into two broad classes: public and private law. *Public law* deals with the relationships of private parties and the government. *Private law* is concerned with the recognition and enforcement of the rights and duties of private individuals and organizations.

Public law

The two major divisions of public law are *criminal law* and *administrative law*. Criminal law deals with acts or offenses against the welfare or safety of the public. Offenses against criminal law are punishable by fines, imprisonment, or both. In these cases the accuser is the state, and the person prosecuted is the defendant. As shown in Table 5-1, page 92, three types of criminal acts are recognized by the law.[25] RCPs are usually not involved in problems involving criminal

Table 5-1 Types of Criminal Acts Recognized by the Law

Type	Example	Penalty
Infraction	Disorderly conduct; traffic violation	Fines
Misdemeanor	Small theft; perjury; assault (no weapon)	Fine, jail or probation
Felony	Major robberies; assault (weapon); rape; arson	Jail, usually at least 1 year

law, except as mentioned later in our discussion of criminal malpractice.

Administrative law is the second major branch of public law. Administrative law consists of the countless regulations set by governmental agencies. Good examples of administrative law are Medicaid reimbursement regulations and state licensure rules for RCPs.

Violation of administrative law generally results in action to restrict or restrain the activity of the offender. For example, a clinic that is reimbursed under the Medicare/Medicaid programs must follow specific guidelines for record-keeping, allowable charges, and accessibility of records. Failure to comply with these regulations may result in government restriction of that facility from participating in the program. Modern hospitals are inundated by a host of administrative and agency rules that affect almost every aspects of operation. RCPs are obligated to abide by regulations and rules made by such diverse agencies as the Department of Health and Human Services, the Social Security Administration, the Health Care Financing Administration, and the Occupational Safety and Health Administration.

Private law

Private or civil law protects private citizens and organizations from others who might seek to take unfair and unlawful advantage of them. If an individual feels that his or her rights have been compromised, he or she can seek redress in the civil courts. In these cases, the individual bringing the complaint is known as the *plaintiff*, and the individual accused of wrong is the *defendant*. Civil courts decide between the two parties with regard to the degree of wrong and the level of **reparation** required.[25] The category of civil law best related to respiratory care is tort law.[26-28]

Tort law. A *tort* is a civil wrong, other than a breach of contract, committed against an individual or property, for which a court provides a remedy in the form of an action for damages. Causes for the complaints may range from assault and battery to invasion of privacy. The basic functions of torts are to keep the peace between individuals and to substitute a remedy for personal injury instead of vengeance.

There are three basic forms of torts: negligent torts, intentional torts, and torts in which liability is assessed regardless of fault (as in the case of manufacturers of defective products). The basic differences between negligent and intentional torts is the element of *intent*. An intentional tort always involves a willful act that violates another's interest. A negligent tort does not have to involve any action at all. Instead, a negligent tort can consist of an omission of an action.

Professional negligence. In its simplest terms, *negligence* is the failure to perform one's duties competently. Negligence may involve acts of commission or omission. The five basic types of negligence recognized under civil law are described in Table 5-2.[16]

The tort of negligence is concerned with the compensation of an individual for loss or damages arising from the unreasonable behavior of another. The normal standard for the claim is the duty imposed on individuals not to cause risk or harm to others, the standard being what a reasonable and prudent person should have foreseen and avoided. With health care providers, a higher standard than that of the average individual is recognized; health professionals are recognized to owe a special duty to patients and to act with special skill and attention.[29-31]

In negligence cases, the breach of duty often involves the matter of foreseeability. Cases in which the patient falls, is burned, is given the wrong medication, or is harmed by defects in an apparatus often revolve around the health care provider's duty to anticipate the harm.[29,32,33] *Duty* can be defined as an obligation to do a thing, a human action exactly conformable to the law that requires us to obey.[25]

Table 5-2 Types of Negligence[16]

Type	Description
Malfeasance	Execution of an unlawful or improper act
Misfeasance	Improper performance of an act that causes injury
Nonfeasance	Failure to perform and act when there is a duty to do so and under circumstances where a normally prudent individual in a similar circumstance would have done so
Criminal negligence	Willful and reckless disregard for the safety of another
Malpractice	Negligence or carelessness of a professional

■ MINI CLINI ■

5-2

Ethical and Legal Implications of Practice

Problem: A RCP receives an order to set up a venturi mask system on a acutely ill adult patient hospitalized with a newly diagnosed right lower lobe pneumonia and a long standing history of congestive heart failure. The physician order calls for an FIO_2 of .50. The venti-mask system utilizes color coded adapters to indicate both the oxygen percentage and liter flow which must be set on the oxygen flow meter. The RCP sets up the venti-mask using the wrong adapter which is set to deliver an FIO_2 of .24. Over the next 20 minutes, the patient experiences worsening shortness of breath and chest pain with new electrocardiographic changes consistent with evolving acute myocardial infarction. An arterial blood gas is obtained which shows a marked deterioration in arterial oxygenation status. Upon being informed of the patient's blood gas values, the RCP checks the equipment for proper functioning and determines that a serious error was made. If the patient filed a medical malpractice law suit against the hospital and RCP, claim-

ing negligence on the part of the RCP, would there be a valid claim?

Discussion: If the patient makes a claim of medical malpractice, the claim of negligence against a professional, such as a RCP, can fall under three classifications. These include; criminal malpractice, civil malpractice, or ethical malpractice. In its most elementary terms, negligence means failing to perform one's duties competently. RCP's as health care providers, are often held to a higher standard than that of the average person since they are recognized to owe a special duty to patients and to act with special skill and attention. Four conditions must be met in order for the tort of negligence to be a valid

claim. First, the RCP owes a duty to the patient, that is a legal duty to conform with the special standards of the relationship which includes protecting patient interests. Second, the RCP has to demonstrate failure to conform to or depart from the required standards of care. Importantly, the required standard is that care that a reasonably prudent RCP would provide in a similar circumstance. Third, the breach of duty by the RCP must be the direct cause of damage or patient injury. Evidence would typically come from either direct expert testimony or by circumstantial evidence. Last, there must be a claim of direct damage or harm to the patient which could be supported in a court of law by a preponderance of evidence. In this current scenario, it may be argued that the RCP was negligent by incorrectly setting up the oxygen equipment. However, whether or not the resultant patient injury was directly caused by the RCP's error could be vigorously debated by both plaintiff (patient) and defendant (RCP and/or hospital) attorneys.

For the tort of negligence to be a valid claim, four conditions must be met (see box below).[25,27,28]

The legal duty to care is usually inherent in the patient/provider relationship. This requires that the health care provider conform to the special standards of that relationship and protect the interests of the patient.

Breach of duty (dereliction) is established when the practitioner fails to conform to or departs from the required standards of care. The required standard is that care that a reasonably prudent individual would provide in a similar circumstance.

In regard to this *reasonable person standard,* the courts have generally moved from a local perspective to a national one. For example, the **Clinical Practice**

Guidelines being established by the AARC could easily serve as the basis for determining what a reasonably prudent RCP should do in a given situation.

Evidence for a breach of duty also can be established by means of direct expert testimony or circumstantial evidence. In the latter case, the legal principle *res ipsa loquitur* (the thing speaks for itself) may apply. *Res ipsa loquitur* is sometimes invoked to show that the harm would not ordinarily have happened if those in control had used appropriate care.[25] In these cases, negligence is established by inference.

For a claim of *res ipsa loquitur* to be supported, three basic conditions must be met: (1) the harm was such that it would not normally occur without someone's negligence, (2) the action responsible for the injury was under the control of the defendant, and (3) the injury did not result from any contributing negligence or voluntarily assumed risk on the part of the injured party.[25,26,34]

Good examples of *res ipsa loquitur* are a nasopharyngeal airway that becomes displaced and lodges inside a patient's nose or a surgical sponge being left inside a patient after surgery. To protect practitioners from suits arising from cases where the practice was adequate but the results were unsuccessful, limita-

---

The "four ds" of negligence

1. The practitioner owes a **duty** to the patient.
2. The practitioner was **derelict** with that duty.
3. The breach of duty was the **direct** cause of damages.
4. **Damage** or harm came to the patient.

tions to the use of *res ipsa loquitur* have been developed.

For negligence to occur, the breach in duty must also cause actual damage or injury to the individual. The injured party must file the lawsuit within the time frame set by the statute of limitations. The term *injury*, in this sense, may include not only physical harm but also mental anguish and other invasions of the patient's rights and privilege. The claim must be supported by a preponderance of evidence to prevail.

Last, for the tort of negligence to be sustained, the breach of duty must be shown to be the direct or "proximate" cause of the injury. A causal relationship must exist between the negligent action and the resulting damage. The mere failure to provide the appropriate standard of care is insufficient to necessitate payment of damages unless injury occurs as a direct result of the action or omission.

Malpractice. As a form of negligence, *malpractice* can involve professional misconduct, unreasonable lack of skill or fidelity in professional duties, evil practice, or unethical conduct. There are three classifications of malpractice: (1) criminal malpractice, including such crimes as assault and battery or euthanasia (handled in criminal court); (2) civil malpractice, such as negligence, or practice below a reasonable standard (handled in civil court); and (3) ethical malpractice, which includes violations of professional ethics and may result in censure or disciplinary actions by licensure boards.[26,27]

Intentional torts. An intentional tort is a wrong perpetrated by one who intends to break the law. This is in contrast to negligence, in which the professional fails to exercise adequate care in doing what is otherwise permissible. The acts must be intentionally done to produce the harm or done with the belief that the result was likely to follow.

These torts are more serious than the tort of negligence in that the defendant intended to commit the wrong.[27] As a result, punitive, as well as actual, damages may be awarded. Examples of intentional torts are those that involve defamation of character, invasion of privacy, deceit, infliction of mental distress, and assault and battery.[25]

In the hospital, the unwarranted discussion of the patient's condition, diagnosis, or treatment for purposes other than the exchange of information is always deemed suspect in regard to defamation of character. Under the general title of defamation of character are the torts of *libel* and *slander*. Slander is the verbal defamation of an individual by false words by which his or her reputation is damaged. Libel is printed defamation by written words, cartoons, and such representations to cause the individual to be avoided or held in contempt.[25] Libel and slander do not exist unless they are seen or heard by a third person. If the practitioner directed such remarks only to the individual involved, it would not be slanderous.

If, on the other hand, the remark was made in the presence of a third party, it might constitute slander.

Caution in regard to unauthorized disclosure of patient information is especially critical in cases involving such diseases as AIDS, which often carries a high degree of medical and social stigma. Patients have the legal right to expect that all information about their illness will be held in strict confidence. Several states now have civil liability and criminal penalties for the release of confidential HIV test results in which the breach of confidence results in economic, psychological, or bodily harm to the patient.

An *assault* is an intentional act that places another person in fear of immediate bodily harm. Threatening to injure someone is considered an act of assault. *Battery,* on the other hand, represents unprivileged, **nonconsensual** physical contact with another person. In the classic act of assault and battery, one individual threatens and actually injures another.

Although battery is an unusual charge against a clinician, because of the nature of the work, it is one that creates special problems. The major element of battery is physical contact without consent. When a practitioner performs a procedure without the patient's consent, this contact may be considered battery.[35] In most instances, there is an *implied consent,* created when the patient solicits care from the physician. This implied consent allows the performance of ordinary procedures without written consent. In all cases of unusual, difficult, or dangerous procedures, such as surgery, the courts requires written consent. For this reason, to avoid being accused of battery, RCPs should always explain all procedures involving physical contact to their patients before they proceed.

There are two general defenses against intentional torts. The first defense is that there was a lack of intent to harm and that only clinicians who engage in intentional conduct are liable. For example, if a practitioner fainted during a procedure and thereby caused the patient injury, he or she would not be liable because the action was not voluntary. The second defense is that the patient gave consent to the procedure. If the patient consented to the action, knowing the risks involved, the practitioner would not be liable.[36] Thus consent by the patient for both nonroutine and routine procedures should be obtained before care is rendered.

Strict liability. *Strict liability* is a theory in tort law that can be used to impose liability without fault, even in situations where injury occurs under conditions of reasonable care.[25,30] The most common cases of strict liability are those involving the use of dangerous products or techniques. Courts have imposed this principle on medical equipment manufacturers as well as on hospitals. However, strict liability has generally not been extended to professional services.

Breach of contract. *Breach of contract* is a much

rarer malpractice claim than negligence. This claim is based on the theory that when a health care professional renders care, an implicit or explicit professional/patient "contract" is established.[25,27] Essentially, the contract binds the health care professional to place the patient's welfare as the foremost concern, to act only in the patient's behalf, to protect the patient's life, preserve the patient's health, relieve suffering, and protect privacy. When—as a result of the services rendered under this contract—the patient is injured, the patient may claim that the failure of the health care professional to competently perform the service is a breach of the contract.

Like members of all other professions, RCPs are responsible for their actions.[37] When these actions results in the injury of another, the injured party may turn to the courts for redress. If the RCP, while acting for the physician, injures the patient through some negligent act, the patient may sue both the practitioner and the physician.

Civil suits

Civil action can be brought for many reasons, such as to challenge a law or to enjoin an activity. However, as in the case of malpractice suits, most seek monetary damages. The following scenario is an example of a situation that might involve the RCP. In this scenario, the physician means to order 0.5 mL of a bronchodilator for his three-year-old asthmatic patient but inadvertently prescribes 5.0 mL of the drug. As a result of the overdose, given by the RCP, the child dies.

A clearly articulated legal principle in negligence is that the duty owed to the patient is commensurate with the patient's needs. In short, the more vulnerable the patient, the greater the caregiver's duty to protect.[29,31] Under this principle, when the order is not clear or seems inappropriate, clinicians have an obligation to clarify rather than risk harm.

The suit could be brought against the physician for negligence for ordering the overdose, against the nurses and RCP for failing to recognize that the dose was incorrect for the child, and, possibly, against the pharmacist for failing to gain adequate information as to the nature of the patient so that an appropriate dosage could be calculated. The plaintiff would base the secondary charges against the nurses and allied health practitioners on the theory that liability would be incurred by those who missed an opportunity to correct the first wrongdoer's mistake.[13]

Steps in a civil suit

The basic steps of such a civil suit are as follows.[25,26,38]

1. A petition or complaint is filed in the appropriate court for that jurisdiction. The complaint is a statement of the material facts on which the plea for judicial relief is based.

2. A summons is served on the accused by the officer of the court, and the defendants must file their answers with the court responding to each allegation within a specified period of time.
3. Normally at this time the individuals who have received the summons or complaint naming them as a defendant contact their insurers. The insurers assign attorneys to defend the suit; the assigned counsel represents the insured rather than the insurer. In many multiple-defendant cases, each defendant has a separate attorney.
4. After the complaints have been filed with the courts and the defendants notified, there are pretrial activities by both parties to elicit all the facts of a situation. These activities are known as the *discovery phase*. This preliminary fact-finding stage is used by the attorneys to narrow the legal issues and expand the liability and defense theories. During the discovery phase, each party may submit a series of written questions (*interrogatories*) that must be answered under oath. An example of this might be the plaintiff's question of which physicians supervised the practitioner or the defendant's request for a list of all physicians who treated the plaintiff in the last five years.
5. A *deposition*—an oral testimony transcribed as it is given,—is taken in the presence of all attorneys involved in the suit. The deposition serves to establish a record of the events in the case and allows the attorneys to judge the effectiveness of the individuals as witnesses. The defendant should cooperate with and be completely candid with his or her attorney in the deposition. A cardinal rule for the process is that the individual must tell the truth, without embellishment, speculation, or volunteered information. In that the deposition involves material that is more familiar to the clinician than the lawyers involved, the practitioner can approach the questioning with a certain degree of confidence. Before signing the document, the *deponent* is allowed to read the copy of the transcription and make corrections. An individual named as a defendant should prepare for the deposition by reviewing all records of the incident and by discussing the issues with the lawyer. Often a review of other depositions is helpful, in that it familiarizes the individual with the process.

Court appearance

Court appearance is very important, and the clinician who is called upon to testify must appear honest, competent, and sincere. Cross-examination by the plaintiff's attorneys can be very aggressive and abusive or gentle and soft-spoken. Either way, the practitioner should understand that the attorney is working for his or her client. All the material given in deposition applies equally in the courtroom. The practitioner *must* tell the truth. If the initial facts contained in the formal deposition are correct, one need not fear cross-examination in court. Under civil law, the court would then decide the merits of the case and who had committed the wrong and determine the level of restitution to be made.

Medical supervision

RCPs are required by their scope of practice to work under competent medical supervision. This requirement creates not only a professional relationship but a legal one as well. If the RCP is employed by the physician, the physician is liable for his or her actions. The legal framework for this liability is found in the principle *respondeat superior* (let the master answer).[25,26,39]

Under this doctrine, the physician assumes responsibility for the wrongful actions of the RCP as long as such negligence occurred in the course of the employer-employee relationship. For this liability to be incurred, two conditions must be met: (1) The act must be within the scope of employment, and (2) the injury caused must be the result of an act of negligence.

If the RCP acted outside his or her scope of practice, as outlined by licensure laws or by institutional regulations, the court would have to decide whether the physician is still be liable. For instance, if the RCP, while in the patient's room to deliver an aerosol treatment, went beyond the normal scope of practice and adjusted cervical traction, thereby causing injury, it is doubtful that the physician could be held fully responsible. However, under the principle of *respondeat superior,* the hospital, as a corporate entity, could be held responsible for the actions of its employees.[36,39]

Historically, RCPs have not been named individually as defendants in malpractice cases because the law has generally not yet recognized their role as specialized health care providers. Either the hospital or the physician is usually named as the defendant for the acts of the practitioner. RCPs in these cases have been viewed simply as employees, merely carrying out the orders of a superior. However, with the increased application of state licensure regulations governing respiratory care, this relative protection from liability is changing rapidly.

Scope of practice

One measure of professionalism is the extent to which the group is willing to direct its own development and regulate its own activities. This self-direction is carried out mainly through state licensure boards, which attempt to ensure that professionals exhibit minimum levels of competence.

Basis element of a practice act

Some practice acts emphasize one area over another, but most acts address the following elements:

1. Scope of professional practice
2. Requirements and qualifications for licensure
3. Exemptions
4. Grounds for administrative action
5. Creation of examination board and processes
6. Penalties and sanctions for unauthorized practice

Licensure laws and regulations

In licensure legislation there is always a clause specifying a scope of practice (see above box). The scope-of-practice statutes give general guidelines and parameters for the clinician's practice. Deviation from these statutes could be a source of legal problems as the specialty seeks to add new duties. Practitioners must know the limits of their scope of care and seek amendments to the licensure regulations as they expand their practice. Ideally, the original language of a licensure law should be broad enough to account for changes in practice without requiring continual amendment.

Implications for the practitioner

The Jolene Tuma case gives some indication of the problems associated with going beyond the legal scope of practice.[19] In this case Tuma, a nurse, counseled a patient on alternate forms of cancer therapy such as laetrile and nutritional therapies. The state board of licensure sought to revoke her license for unprofessional conduct on the grounds that this form of counseling went well beyond the scope of practice set out in her practice act. Tuma retained her license on the basis that the state nurse practice act did not identify unprofessional conduct clearly enough. She was, however, stopped from performing any further acts of this nature.

Providing emergency care without physician direction

One unique area that allows practice without the direction of a competent physician is that of rendering emergency medical care to injured persons. *Good Samaritan laws* protect citizens from civil or criminal liability for any errors they make while attempting to give emergency aid. Most states have legislated Good Samaritan statutes to encourage individuals to give needed emergency medical assistance. It is necessary for this aid to be given in good faith and free of gross negligence or willful misconduct. However, it is unlikely that the RCP would be protected for giving aid that clearly went beyond the expected skills of the individual or beyond that which could be defined as first aid, such as performing a tracheostomy. Good

Samaritan rules in general apply only to roadside accidents and emergency situations outside the hospital.[26]

INTERACTION OF ETHICS AND THE LAW

A good example of the interaction of ethics and the law in respiratory care is the diversification of the field into home care and durable medical equipment supply. This diversification has led to new relationships between these elements of the health care system and has created real potential for unethical and unlawful activity. For example, if the practitioner accepts some remuneration, such as a finder's fee or percentage of the total lease costs for referring patients to a particular home-care company or equipment service, he or she should be prepared to face charges of unethical and perhaps illegal practice. Statute 42 of U.S. Code 139nn deals directly with the legal component of this problem. According to this code, anyone who knowingly or willfully solicits, receives, offers, or pays directly or indirectly any remuneration in return for Medicare business is guilty of a criminal offense. Violation of this statute carries the potential for prison and or a substantial fine.[40] If the practitioner is aware of others who are engaged in these practices, he should report these activities to the Department of Health and Human Services or the Judicial Committee of the AARC.

To aid the clinician in maintaining an ethical stance on these new issues, the AARC has established a position statement about ethical performance of respiratory home care (see accompanying box).

AARC statement in regard to the ethical performance of respiratory home care

The Code of Ethics of the AARC applies to all respiratory care practices regardless of the environment in which care may be delivered. In general, the following definition of conflict of interest is provided:

Under no circumstances should any respiratory care practitioner engage in any activity which compromises the motive for the provision of any therapy procedures, the advice or counsel given patients and/ or families, or in any manner profit from referral arrangements with home care providers.

Specifically, conflict of interest shall be defined as any act of a respiratory care practitioner during or outside the practitioner's principle employment for which the practitioner receives any form of consideration for:

1. The referral of patients to specific home care providers.
2. The solicitation of others for specific home care provider referrals.
3. Recommendations for ordering of specific therapy procedures and/or equipment.
4. Recommendations for the continuation of unwarranted procedures and/or equipment.
5. The association of any practitioner with any home-care provider, when profit or revenue generation influences the selection, evaluation, or continuation of any home-care procedure and/ or equipment.
6. Individuals who are either employed by, or receive remuneration from, both the health care institutions which may refer patients and by durable medical equipment suppliers who offer respiratory home care must openly disclose this relationship to both parties.
7. Institutionally based RCPs who have significant ownership interest in a durable medical equipment company which provides respiratory home care must openly disclose this relationship to both parties.

Awareness of activities that may be viewed as being a conflict of interest and in violation of the Code of Ethics of the AARC shall be documented and sent to the Judicial Committee of the AARC.

CHAPTER SUMMARY

If ethical reasoning is to be of any value, it must account for the reality of human experience and take its rightful place among the many considerations that compete for our attention. These considerations include: (1) factual premises and beliefs, such as the definition of death; (2) legal concepts, such as tort laws; and (3) externally imposed mandates or expectations, such as hospital accreditation standards.

In many instances, such considerations uphold our underlying moral convictions and strengthen support for a given action. The real challenge to RCPs arises when moral principles dictate one course of action and factual knowledge, legal concepts, or external expectations dictate another.

Respiratory care aspires to professional status. Long ago, Socrates demanded that professionals acknowledge the social context of their activities and that they recognize their obligations toward the segment of society that they profess to serve. As our analysis of ethical reasoning and the law has made clear, only by identifying, justifying, and prioritizing basic principles of human values can the RCP resolve the difficult questions of professional behavior consistently. To the extent that clearly articulated principles guide our choices and actions, all involved will be well served.

REFERENCES

1. Edge R, Groves R: *The ethics of health care: a guide for practice,* Albany, NY, 1994, DelMar.
2. Fowler MD, Ariff JL: *Ethics at the bedside,* Philadelphia, 1987, Lippincott.
3. American Hospital Association: *Values in conflict: resolving ethical issues in hospital care,* Chicago, 1985, American Hospital Association.
4. Katz J: *The silent world of the doctor and patient,* New York 1986, Free Press.
5. Veatch RM: *A theory of medical ethics,* New York, 1981, Basic Books.
6. Veatch RM: Models for ethical medicine in a revolutionary age, *Hastings Center Report,* June 1973.
7. Beauchamp TL, McCullough LB: *Medical ethics,* Englewood Cliffs, NJ, 1984, Prentice-Hall.
8. Cook SE, Anderson CC: The current medical malpractice crisis, *Schumpert Medical Quarterly,* November 1987.
9. Scully TC, Scully C: *Playing God,* New York, 1987, Simon & Schuster.
10. Bok S: *Lying: moral choice in public and private life,* New York, 1978, Vintage Books.
11. Francoeur RT: *Biomedical ethics: a guide to decision making,* New York, 1983, Wiley Medical Publications.
12. Ramsey P, McCormick R, editors: *Doing evil to achieve good,* Chicago, 1978, Loyola University Press.
13. Dennis C: *The power of attorney book,* Berkeley, CA, 1985, Nolo Press.
14. Allen A: Advanced directives provide answers for tough questions, *J Post Anesth Nurs* 7:183-185, 1992.
15. Bok S: *Secrets: on the ethics of concealment,* New York, Vintage Books, 1983.
16. Pozgar, G: *Legal aspects of health care administration,* Gaithersburg, MD, 1990, Aspen Publishers.
17. Evans RE: Health care technology and the inevitability of resource allocation and rationing decisions, *JAMA* 249:2208-2219, 1983.
18. Beauchamp TL, Childress JF: *Principles of biomedical ethics,* ed 3, New York, 1989, Oxford University Press.
19. Purtillo RB, Cassel CK: *Ethical dimensions in the health professions,* Philadelphia, 1981, Saunders.
20. Frankena WK: *Ethics,* ed 2, Englewood Cliffs, NJ, 1973, Prentice-Hall.
21. Ross WD: *The right and the good,* Oxford, 1930, Clarendon Press.
22. MacIntyre A: *After virtue,* Bloomington University of Indiana Press, 1981.
23. Brody H: *Ethical decisions in medicine,* ed 2, Boston, 1981, Little, Brown.
24. Todd JS: The problem of professional liability, *Schumpert Medical Quarterly,* November 1987.
25. Black HC: *Black's law dictionary,* St. Paul, MN, 1983, West Publishing.
26. Hemelt MD, Mackert ME: *Dynamics of law in nursing and health care,* Reston, VA, 1982, Reston Publishing Co.
27. Fiesta J: *The law and liability,* New York, 1983, Wiley Medical Publishers.
28. Murchison I, Nichols TS, Hanson R: *Legal accountability in the nursing process,* St Louis, 1982, Mosby.
29. Cushing M: Who transcribed that order?, *Am J Nurs* 83:1107-1108, October 1986.
30. Gaare R: *Introduction to the legal system of bioethics: biolaw,* Frederick, MD, 1988, University Publications of America.
31. *Wooten* v. *U.S.,* 574. Supp. 200 (1982); affirmed 722 f.2d 743 (1983) (Duty owed patient is commensurate with the patient's needs).
32. *Burks* v. *Christ Hospital,* 19 Ohio St.2d, 249 N.E.2d 829 (Failure to follow procedures results in liability for patient's fall).
33. *Norton* v. *Argonaut Insurance Co.,* 144 So.2d 249 (La. Ct. App, 1962) (Nurse held liable for overdose after failure to clarify confusing medication order).
34. *Ybarra* v. *Spangard,* 25 Cal.2nd 486, 154 p.2d 687 (1944) Supreme Court of CA (Injury held under principle of *res ipsa loquitur*).
35. *Burton* v. *Leftwich,* 123 So.2d 766 (La.Ct.App.1960) (Damages recovered after assault by practitioner).
36. Hogue E: *Nursing and legal liability,* New York, 1985, National Health Publishing.
37. *Morrison* v. *MacNamara,* 407 A.2d 555 (D.C. 1979) (Nonphysician found liable for improper performance of laboratory test).
38. Cushing M: How a civil suit starts, *Am J Nurs* 82:655-656, June 1985.
39. *Bernardi* v. *Community Hospital Association,* 166 Colo. 280, 443 P.2d 708 (1968) Supreme Court of Colo. (Hospital held responsible under principle of *respondeat superior*).
40. Larson K: DME referrals: what's legal and what's not, *AARTimes* 10(8):28-31, 1986.

SUGGESTED READINGS

Blendon RJ: Health policy choices for the 1990s, *Issues in Science and Technology* 2:65, 1986.
Eisendrath SJ, Jonson AR: The living will: help or hindrance?, *JAMA* 249:2054-2058, 1983.
Epstein D: Medicare fraud, abuse, and respiratory therapy, *AARTimes* 9(10):21-26, 1985.
Krekler K: Critical care nursing and moral development, *Crit Care Nurs Q* 10(2), 1987.
Leikin SL: An ethical issue in pediatric cancer care: nondisclosure of a fatal prognosis, *Pediatr Ann* 10:37-41, 44-45, 1981.
Starr P: *The social transformation of American medicine,* New York, 1982, Basic Books.
The President's Commission for the Study of Ethical Problems in Medicine and Biomedical and Behavioral Research, Washington, DC, U.S. Government Printing Office, 1983. (10 reports)

2

Technologic Bases of Respiratory Care

Terms, Symbols, and Units of Measure

■

Craig L. Scanlan

CHAPTER LEARNING OBJECTIVES

1. Apply standard conventions of medical terminology to define and translate common medical terms.
2. Identify the common medical abbreviations used in written communication and medical record-keeping.
3. Identify and apply the primary and secondary symbols used in pulmonary physiology and respiratory care.
4. Apply the concepts of scientific notation and Greek and Latin prefixes to clinical measurement.
5. Define the major units of measure used in the cgs, fps (British) and SI systems and convert a given value between any two systems.

The clinical practice of respiratory care involves extensive observation and communication. Consistency in the use and application of these skills among health professionals requires a common frame of reference. This common frame of reference is embodied in various systems of clinical communication and measurement.

Like any branch of knowledge, medicine has its own language. This language, called *medical terminology,* is a system of word-building that generally follows a few basic rules. Once these rules are mastered, the respiratory care practitioner (RCP) can build and define thousands of new medical terms.

If medical terminology is the language of medicine, abbreviations and symbols are its shorthand. Abbreviations are used mainly in charting and medical record-keeping. Although there are exceptions, abbreviations are not as well standardized as medical terms. Fortunately, the abbreviations and symbols used in respiratory care are an exception. RCPs must be well versed in the use of both general medical abbreviations and those used exclusively in pulmonary medicine.

RCPs also regularly measure, describe, and communicate physical events. These responsibilities require that RCPs master a variety of measurement systems. In the United States, three primary systems of measurement are used in the clinical setting. Until complete standardization occurs in the United States, RCPs must be adept in working with all three systems.

MEDICAL TERMINOLOGY

Like any branch of knowledge, medicine has its own language. This language, medical terminology, provides consistent meanings among diverse groups of health professionals, thus facilitating communication and interaction.

Unlike many languages, medical terminology is a strict system of word-building that follows a few basic rules. Once these rules are learned, the user can build and define thousands of new medical terms. As in all languages, exceptions to these rules exist. However, these exceptions are uncommon, making the language of medicine easy to learn and use.

Most medical terms are Greek or Latin derivatives, representing a blend of root words combined with suffixes and prefixes. Building a medical vocabulary begins with mastering key root, suffix, and prefix terms. Once you master these key terms, you are ready to translate and apply new words by breaking them down into their component parts.

Word roots and combining forms

In medical terminology, a word root represents a "stem" or building block. These roots provide the basis for describing most anatomical terms, medical and surgical procedures, and laboratory tests.

Word roots are seldom used alone. More often than not, a prefix or suffix is added to the word root, or it is combined with another root to form a compound word. For this reason, each word root has a combining form, usually consisting of the word root with an added combining vowel, most often an "o."

Table 6-1 lists several of the most common word roots and their combining forms. The word root appears before the slash, with the combining vowel after the slash. For each root, a definition of its meaning and an example of its use is provided. For example, the root word *cardi* is derived from the Greek word *kardia,* meaning "heart." The combining form of cardi is *cardio.*

Many medical terms are built simply by a combination of root words. These combinations of root words are called compound words. As an example, the

Table 6-1   Selected wood roots and combining forms

Word Root	Meaning	Example	Word Root	Meaning	Example
aden/o	gland	adenopathy	immun/o	safe, protected	immunoglobin
adren/o	adrenal gland	adrenergic	lapar/o	abdomen	laparotomy
angi/o	blood vessel	angioplasty	laryng/o	larynx	laryngoscopy
arteri/o	artery	arterial	later/o	side	lateromedial
atel/o	incomplete	atelectasis	leuk/o	white	leukocyte
brachi/o	arm	brachiocephalic	lob/o	lobe	lobectomy
bronch/o	bronchus	bronchitis	lymph/o	lymph	lymphoma
cardi/o	heart	cardiopulmonary	medi/o	middle	mediosternal
cephal/o	head	cephalad	medull/o	medulla	medullary
cerebr/o	brain	cerebrovascular	my/o	muscle	myopathy
cervic/o	neck	cervical	nas/o	nose	nasopharynx
chondr/o	cartilage	costochondral	nephr/o	kidney	nephrectomy
cost/o	ribs	costochondral	neur/o	nerve	neuropathy
crani/o	skull	craniotomy	or/o	mouth	oral
cutane/o	skin	subcutaneous	oste/o	bone	osteomylitis
cyan/o	blue	cyanosis	ox/o	oxygen	hypoxia
cyst/o	bladder	cystoscopy	oxy/o	oxygen	oxyhemoglobin
cyt/o	cell	cytology	pharyng/o	pharynx	glossopharyngeal
derm/o	skin	dermoid	phleb/o	vein	phlebotomy
dermat/o	skin	dermatotome	phren/o	diaphragm	phrenic
encephal/o	brain	encephalitis	pleur/o	pleura	pleurisy
enter/o	intestines	enteritis	pneum/o	lung, air	pneumotachygraph
epiglott/o	epiglottis	epiglottitis	pneumat/o	lung, air	pneumatocele
crythr/o	red	erythrocyte	poster/o	posterior	posterolateral
esophag/o	esophagus	esophageal	pulm/o	lung	pulmonary
fibr/o	fiber	fibrosis	py/o	pus	pyogenic
gastr/o	stomach	gastritis	rhin/o	nose	rhinoplasty
glomerul/o	glomerulus	glomerulonephritis	thorac/o	thorax	thoracotomy
gloss/o	tongue	glossopharyngeal	thromb/o	clot	thrombolysis
hem/o	blood	hemostasis	thyr/o	thyroid gland	thyroidectomy
hemat/o	blood	hematocrit	trache/o	trachea	tracheostomy
hepat/o	liver	hepatomegaly	vas/o	vessel	vasocontrictor
histo/o	tissue	histocyte	ven/o	vein	venous

combination of *cardi/o* ("heart") with *pulmon/o* (from the Latin *pulmo,* for "lung") yields the compound word *cardiopulmonary,* meaning "heart and lungs," as in "cardiopulmonary resuscitation." Combining *cost/o* ("ribs") with *chondr/o* ("cartilage") gives us the new term *costochondral,* referring to the cartilaginous portion of the ribs.

A few basic rules apply to the use of roots and their combining forms. First, in building a compound word, one should always retain the combining vowel when the second word root begins with a consonant. "Cardiopulmonary" and "costochondral" are good examples. Second, even if the second root begins with a vowel, one usually retains the combining vowel, as in the following example:

Root	Root	Suffix	New Word
gastr/o	enter/o	-itis	gastroenteritis
(stomach)	(intestine)	(inflammation)	

In this example, the two root words *gastr/o* and *enter/o* are combined to form a compound word meaning "stomach *and* intestines." Although enter/o begins with a vowel, the combining "o" of gastr/o is not dropped. The suffix *itis* "inflammation", completes the word-building, giving us the new term *gastroenteritis,* meaning "inflammation of the stomach and intestines."

Suffixes

A suffix is a word element that, when placed at the end of a word, creates a new or modified meaning. Suffixes common in ordinary English include -*less* (doubt*less*), -*y* (dirt*y*), and -*al* (person*al*).

As in standard English, adding a suffix to a medical word changes its meaning. In medical terminology, there are two broad categories of suffixes: (1) suffixes that simply modify the meaning of a noun, verb, or adjective; and (2) combinations of suffixes that actually give new meanings to root words.

Table 6-2 lists some modifying suffixes that simply alter the meaning of nouns, verbs, or adjectives. For example, by adding the suffix *al* to the noun root *neur/o* "nerve", we form the new adjective *neural*, meaning "pertaining to the nerves." Other good examples of the use of the simple modifiers include immun*ize*, hepat*ic*, hypox*ia*, pneuma*tic*, and ven*ous*.

Actual new meanings also can be created with medical suffixes. Table 6-3 lists some combining suffixes that give root words new or extended meanings. For example:

Root	Suffix	New Word	Meaning
atel/o	-ectasis	atelectasis	incomplete expansion
bronch/o	-itis	bronchitis	inflammation of the bronchi
trache/o	-malacia	tracheomalacia	softening of the trachea
cardi/o	-megaly	cardiomegaly	enlargement of the heart
hem/o	-ptysis	hemoptysis	spitting (coughing) of blood

When a root word is combined with a suffix that begins with a vowel, as in "atelectasis" and "bronchitis," the combining vowel is usually dropped. However, the combining vowel is usually retained if the suffix

---

Table 6-2   Selected modifying suffixes

Suffix	Use	Examples
ize, ate	Add to nouns or adjectives to make verbs expressing to use and to act like, to subject to, make into	visual*ize* (able to see)
ist, or, er	Add to verbs to make nouns expressing agent or person concerned or instrument	anesthet*ist* (one who practices the science of anesthesia)
ent	Add to verbs to make adjectives or nouns of agency	recipi*ent* (one who receives)
sia, y, tion	Add to verbs to make nouns expressing action, process, or condition	thera*py* (treatment), inhala*tion* (act of inhaling), anesthe-*sia* (process or condition of not feeling)
ia, ity	Add to adjectives or nouns to make nouns expressing quality or condition	septicem*ia* (poisoning of blood), acid*ity* (condition of excess acid), neuralg*ia* (pain in nerves)
ma, mata, men, mina, ment, ure	Add to verbs to make nouns expressing result of action or object of action	trau*ma* (injury), fora*mina* (openings), liga*ment* (tough fibrous band holding bone or viscera together), fiss*ure* (groove)
ium, olus, olum, culus, culum, cule, cle	Add to nouns to make diminutive nouns	bacter*ium*, alve*olus* (air sac), folli*cle* (little bag)
ible, ile	Add to verbs to make adjectives expressing ability or capacity	contract*ile* ("ability to contract"), flex*ible* ("capable of being bent")
al, c, ic ious, tic	Add to nouns to make adjectives expressing relationship, concern, or pertaining to	neur*al* (referring to nerve), neoplas*tic* (referring to neoplasm), cardi*ac* (referring to the heart)
id	Add to verbs or nouns to make adjectives expressing state or condition	flacc*id* ("state of being weak or lax"), flu*id* ("state of being liquid")
tic	Add to a verb to make an adjective showing relationship	caus*tic* (referring to burn), acous*tic* (referring to sound or hearing)
oid, form	Add to nouns to make adjectives expressing resemblance	polyp*oid* ("resembling a polyp"), plexi*form* ("resembling a plexus"), fusi*form* ("resembling a fusion"), muc*oid* (resembling mucous)
ous	Add to nouns to make adjectives expressing material	ferr*ous* ("composed of iron"), ser*ous* ("composed of serum")

Table 6-3	Selected combining suffixes	
Suffix	**Meaning**	**Example**
algesia	pain	analgesia
algia	pain	myalgia
asthenia	without strength	myasthenia
capnia	carbon dioxide	hypercapnia
cele	swelling	pneumatocele
centesis	puncture	thoracentesis
crine	to secrete	endocrine
ectasis	expansion	atelectasis
ectomy	removal of	pnemonectomy
emia	blood	anemia
esthesia	feeling	anesthesia
genic	origin, cause	carcinogenic
globin	protein	hemoglobin
graph	recording instrument	electrocardiograph
itis	inflammation	bronchitis
lysis	breaking up	hemolysis
malacia	softening	tracheomalacia
megaly	enlargement	hepatomegaly
oma	tumor	adenoma
paresis	partial paralysis	hemiparesis
pathy	disease	neuropathy
penia	decrease	leukocytopenia
phagia	swallowing	dysphagia
phylaxis	protection	anaphylaxis
plasia	growth	dysplasia
plegia	paralysis	hemiplegia
pnea	breathing	dyspnea
ptysis	spitting	hemoptysis
rrhea	discharge	rhinorrhea
sclerosis	hardening	atherosclerosis
scopy	visual exam	laryngoscopy
spasm	involuntary contraction	bronchospasm
stasis	standing still	hemostasis
tomy	cut	tacheotomy
toxic	poison	cytotoxic
trophy	development	hypertrophy
tropin	stimulate	adrenocorticotropin
uria	urine	nocturia

begins with a consonant, as in "tracheomalacia," "cardiomegaly," and "hemoptysis."

Prefixes

A prefix is a word element that, when placed at the beginning of a word, creates a new or modified meaning. Prefixes common in ordinary English include *pre-* (*pre*cooked), *bi-* (*bi*cycle), and *retro-* (*retro*active). As with suffixes, adding a prefix to a medical word changes its meaning. In medical terminology, prefixes most often occur in combination with a word root but may also serve as a combining form.

Table 6-4 provides several of the most common prefixes used in medical terminology. A good example of a prefix in combination with a word root is *anoxia*. Breaking this term down into its component parts demonstrates its derivation.

Prefix	**Root**	**Suffix**	**Meaning**
an- (lack of)	ox/o (oxygen)	-ia (condition)	a condition characterized by the lack of oxygen

On the other hand, a prefix may sometimes serve as the combining form itself, without a root word, as in *dyspnea*.

Prefix	**Root**	**Suffix**	**Meaning**
dys- (difficult)		-pnea (breathing)	difficult breathing

Translating medical terms

After mastering the common root, suffix, and prefix terms, a learner can begin translating and applying new words he or she encounters in reading or hears in discussions or presentations. This is accomplished by systematically breaking the term down into its constituent parts, using the following steps:
1. Identify and define the suffix.
2. Identify and define the prefix.
3. Define the middle part of the word.

Table 6-4	Selected prefixes	
Prefix	**Meaning**	**Examples**
a, an	without, lack of	*a*pnea ("without breath"), *an*oxia ("without oxygen")
ab	away from	*ab*ductor ("leading away")
ad	to, toward	*ad*ductor ("leading toward")
ante	before, forward	*ante*cubital ("before elbow")
anti	against, opposed	*anti*sepsis ("against infection")
auto	self	*auto*immune ("protection against self")
bi	twice, double	*bi*furcation ("two branches")
brady	slow	*brady*pnea ("slow breathing")

continued

Table 6-4 Selected prefixes—*con't.*

Prefix	Meaning	Examples
cata	down, complete	*cata*bolism ("breaking down")
circum	around, about	*circum*flex ("winding about")
contra	against, opposite	*contra*indicated ("not indicated")
crypto	hidden, concealed	*crypto*genic ("unknown origin")
de	away from,	*de*hydrate ("remove water")
dia	through, across	*dia*phragm ("wall across")
diplo	double, twice	*diplo*coccus ("paired grape-shaped bacteria")
dis	reversal, apart from, separation	*dis*infection ("apart from infection")
dys	difficult	*dys*pnea ("difficult breathing")
e, ex	out, away from	*e*viscerate ("take out viscera or bowels")
ec	out from	*ec*topic ("out of place")
ecto	on outer side, situated on	*ecto*derm ("outer skin")
em, en	in	*em*pyema ("pus in")
endo	within	*endo*cardium ("within heart")
epi	upon, on	*epi*dermis ("on skin")
eu	good, normal	*eu*pnea ("normal breathing")
exo	outside, on outer side, outer layer	*exo*genous ("originating outside")
extra	outside	*extra*cellular ("outside cells")
hetero	other	*hetero*geneous ("different")
homo	same	*homo*geneous ("similar")
hyper	over, above	*hyper*trophy ("overgrowth")
hypo	under, below	*hypo*tension ("low blood pressure")
im, in	in, into	*in*filtration ("act of filtering in")
im, in	not	*in*voluntary ("not voluntary")
infra	below	*infra*clavicular ("below clavicle")
inter	between	*inter*pleural ("between the pleura")
intra	within	*intra*vventricular ("within ventricles")
intro	into, within	*intro*version ("turning inward")
mal	bad, abnormal	*mal*absorption ("bad absorption")
meta	beyond, after	*meta*stasis ("beyond original position")
micro	small	*micro*electrode ("small electrode")
neo	new	*neo*natal ("newborn")
oligo	few, scanty	*oligo*uria ("scanty urine")
para	near	*para*thyroid ("near the thyroid")
per	through	*per*cutaneous ("through the skin")
peri	around	*peri*bronchial ("around bronchus")
platy	flat	*platy*pnea ("easy breathing in flat position")
poly	many	*poly*cythemia ("many blood cells")
post	after, behind	*post*operative ("after surgery")
pre	before, in front	*pre*maxillary ("in front of maxilla")
pro	before, in front	*pro*gnosis ("foreknowledge")
pseudo	false	*pseudo*stratified ("falsely layered")
re	back, again, contrary	*re*gurgitation ("backward, flowing contrary to normal")
retro	backward, located behind	*retro*grade ("going backward")
semi	half, partial	*semi*permeable ("partially permeable")
steno	narrow	*steno*sis ("narrowing")
sub	under	*sub*cutaneous ("under skin")
super	above, upper, excessive	*super*numerary ("excessive number")
supra	above, upon	*supra*sternal ("above sternum")
sym, syn	together, with	*syn*apsis ("joining together")
tachy	fast	*tachy*cardia ("fast heart rate")
trans	across, through	*trans*ection ("cut across")
ultra	beyond, in excess	*ultra*sonic ("sound waves beyond hearing")

If an unfamiliar root, prefix, or suffix is encountered, you should write it down and use a medical dictionary to learn its meaning. Then practice with the new term, adding other familiar components to build new words. Don't simply memorize a whole new term. By always applying the building blocks and rules of medical terminology, you can easily understand new terms and avoid rote memorization.

Throughout the rest of this text, key terms are highlighted in bold face. To assist you in defining these terms, a comprehensive glossary is located at the end of the text.

Pronunciation

All good medical dictionaries include pronunciation guides, which provide direction in oral usage of medical terms. However, several basic rules of pronunciation are useful in the early stages of building one's medical vocabulary.

In general, the vowels and consonants of medical terms have ordinary English sounds. Exceptions to this generalization include the following.

- *c* and *g* have a hard sound when they occur before other letters. Examples of this hard sound include *cardiac* (kar'-dē-ak), *cranial* (kra'-nē-al), and *gastric* (gas'-trik).
- *c* and *g* carry the soft sounds of *s* and *j* when they occur before the vowels *e*, *i*, and *y*. Examples of these soft sounds are *cephalic* (sef-al'-ik) and *gynecology* (jīn-e-kol'-ō-jē).
- *ch* is sometimes pronounced as a *k*. Examples of this sound include *cholesterol* (kō-les'-ter-ol) and *chromatograph* (krō-mat'-ō-graf).
- When an *ae* or *oe* is encountered, only the second vowel, the *e* is pronounced. Examples of this dropped vowel sound are *pleurae* (ploor'-ē) and *coelom* (se'-lom).
- When found at the end of a word, *es* is often pronounced as a separate syllable. *Nares* (nar' ēz) is a good example.
- When *i* is used as to form the Latin plural at the end of a word, it is pronounced long. Examples are *bronchi* (brong'-kī) and *fungi* (fun'-jī).
- When *pn* or *ps* occurs at the beginning of a word, the *p* is silent, as in *pneumonectomy* (nū-mō-nek'-to-me) or *psittacosis* (sit-ah-kō'-sis).

ABBREVIATIONS

Whereas medical terminology is the language of medicine, abbreviations are its shorthand. Abbreviations, unlike medical terms, are used exclusively in written communication, especially in charting and medical record-keeping. We will first look at medical abbreviations in general and then analyze those specific to respiratory care and pulmonary physiology.

General medical abbreviations

Many general abbreviations used in medicine, especially those associated with medical prescriptions, are simple shorthand for Latin words. A good example of this type of abbreviation is *b.i.d.,* standing for the Latin *bis in die,* meaning "twice a day." Many other medical abbreviations are **acronyms.** Acronyms are abbreviations formed from the initial letters of a series of words. *COPD* is a good example of an acronym, standing for **c**hronic **o**bstructive **p**ulmonary **d**isease. Usually, all letters in an acronym are capitalized.

Most of the abbreviations used in prescription writing are well standardized. Unfortunately, most other medical abbreviations are not used as consistently. Variations in the use of these nonstandardized abbreviations occur between geographic regions, even among hospitals within a given region. Nonetheless, there exists sufficient agreement on many medical abbreviations to be included here for review. Table 6-5 provides an alphabetical listing of these commonly accepted medical abbreviations, along with their meanings.

Abbreviations used in respiratory care and pulmonary medicine

In the late 1940s, the field of respiratory physiology grew rapidly. With this growth came many scholarly publications and research articles. As in many new fields of study, there was little standardization in the use of the terms and abbreviations. This created substantial confusion and hindered effective communication.

To eliminate confusion and promote uniform communication in the field, researchers and scholars developed a set of standard abbreviations to be used in respiratory physiology and medicine. Over the years, and with the help of the American College of Chest Physicians and the American Thoracic Society, this set of standard abbreviations has undergone several changes and is now well accepted as the basis for written communication in this field.

Four major categories of abbreviations are found in this system: general abbreviations and usages, abbreviations related to the gas phase, abbreviations related to the blood phase, and abbreviations related to the mechanics of breathing.

General abbreviations

The following general abbreviations and usages are recognized:

   P   pressure in general
   V   volume in general
   $\bar{X}$ dash above symbol indicates a mean value (i.e., $\bar{P}$ stands for the "mean or average pressure")

Table 6-5 Common medical abbreviations

Abbreviation	Meaning	Abbreviation	Meaning
ABG	arterial blood gas	FBS	fasting blood sugar
a.c.	before meals	FHR	fetal heart rate
ACTH	adrenocorticotropic hormone	FUO	fever of undetermined origin
ad lib.	as desired	Fx	fracture
ADH	antidiuretic hormone	GI	gastrointestinal
ADL	activities of daily living	Gm, gm	gram
AFB	acid-fast bacillus	grav I, II, etc	pregnancy (gravida) one, two
AIDS	acquired immunodeficiency syndrome	GSW	gunshot wound
Ant.	anterior	Gtt., gtt.	drops
AP	anterior-posterior; anteroposterior	GU	genitourinary
ARDS	adult respiratory distress syndrome	Gyn	gynecology
ASHD	arteriosclerotic heart disease	Hb; Hgb	hemoglobin
AV, A/V, A-V	atriovenous; atrioventricular	HCT, Hct	hematocrit
BE	base excess	Hg	mercury
B.I.D., b.i.d.	twice a day	HGB, Hgb, Hb	hemoglobin
BM	bowel movement	HR	heart rate
BMR	basal metabolic rate	h.s.	at bedtime
BP	blood pressure	Hx	history
bpm	beats per minute	ICF	intracellular fluid
BSA	body surface area	ICU	intensive care unit
BUN	blood urea nitrogen	IM	intramuscular
bx	biopsy	I.V., IV	intravenous
$\bar{c}$	with	kg	kilogram
CA, Ca	cancer	L	liter; left
CAD	coronary artery disease	LAT, lat.	lateral
CAT (scan)	computerized axial tomography	lb	pound
CBC	complete blood count	LLL	left lower lobe (lung)
CC	chief complaint	LUL	left upper lobe (lung)
cc	cubic centimeter	MAP	mean arterial pressure
CHF	congestive heart failure	mcg; μg	microgram
CI	cardiac index	mEq	milliequivalent
cm	centimeter	mg	milligram
CNS	central nervous system	MI	myocardial infarction
CO	cardiac output	mm	millimeter
COPD	chronic obstructive pulmonary disease	MS	multiple sclerosis
CPR	cardiopulmonary resuscitation	NPO	nothing by mouth
CSF	cerebrospinal fluid	OB	obstetrics
CV	cardiovascular	od	once a day
CVA	cerebrovascular accident	OR	operating room
CXR	chest X-ray; chest radiograph	os	mouth
D5W	5% dextrose in water	oz	ounce
d	day (24 hours)	PA; P-A	posteroanterior
/d	per day	paren	parenterally
D/C	discontinue	P.C., p.c.	after meals
diff	white cell differential	P.E.; Px	physical examination
DTR	deep tendon reflex	PEEP	positive end-expiratory pressure
Dx	diagnosis	PFT	pulmonary function test
ECG, EKG	electrocardiogram	PIP	peak inspiratory pressure
ECF	extracellular fluid	PMI	point of maximum impulse
ECMO	extracorporeal membrane oxygenation	PN	percussion note
EEG	electroencephalogram	PND	paroxysmal nocturnal dyspnea
EMG	electromyogram	P.O.	prally
ER	emergency room	p.r.n.	as required
ESR	erythrocyte sedimentation rate	PT	prothrombin time
ET	endotracheal	PTT	partial thromboplastin time
PVC	premature ventricular contraction	SOB	short(ness) of breath

Table 6-5 Common medical abbreviations—*con't.*

Abbreviation	Meaning	Abbreviation	Meaning
Px	pneumothorax; physical exam	Stat.	immediately
q	every	subcu., SC	subcutaneous
q.d.	every day	T	temperature; thoracic
q.h.	every hour	T&A	tonsilectomy and adenoidectomy
Q.I.D., q.i.d.	four times a day	TB	tuberculosis
qm	every morning	T.I.D., t.i.d.	three times a day
qn	every night	top.	topically
R	right; respiration	TPR	temperature, pulse, and respiration
RBC	red blood cell; red blood count	UA	urinalysis
RESP	respiratory (system)	URI	upper respiratory infection
RLL	right lower lobe (lung)	VC	vital capacity
RML	right middle lobe (lung)	VSD	ventricular septal defect
R/O	rule out (differential diagnosis)	WBC	white blood cell; white blood cell count
RUL	right upper lobe (lung)	Wt.	weight
Rx	prescription	x	multiplied by
$\bar{s}$	without	YO	year(s) old

$\dot{X}$ dot above symbol indicates time derivative (i.e., $\dot{V}$ stands for volume per unit time, or flow)

%X percent sign preceding a symbol indicates percentage of the predicted normal value

X/Y% percent sign after a symbol indicates a ratio function with the ratio expressed as a percentage. Both components of the ratio must be designated (e.g., FEV_1/FEV% = 100 × FEV_1/FVC)

f frequency of any event in time (e.g., respiratory frequency: the number of breathing cycles per unit of time)

T time

anat anatomical

max maximum

Gas phase symbols

Gas phase abbreviations are divided into primary symbols and qualifying symbols. Primary symbols include the following:

V gas volume in general. Pressure, temperature, and percent saturation with water vapor must be stated.

F fractional concentration (usually in the dry gas phase)

Primary symbols are normally associated with a qualifying symbol, either a small capital letter or a subscript. Qualifying symbols applicable to the gas phase include the following:

I inspired or inspiratory

E expired or expiratory

A alveolar

T tidal

DS dead space

B barometric

L lung

Thus PB stands for barometric pressure (at a specified altitude), VT is the accepted symbol for tidal volume, $\dot{V}E$ the standard abbreviation for the volume of gas expired per minute, FIO_2 the proper term for the fractional concentration of inspired oxygen, $\dot{V}O_2$ the appropriate symbol for oxygen consumption per minute, TI inspiratory time, and VDSanat stands for the volume of anatomic deadspace.

Regarding the *conditions* of pressure, temperature, and humidity associated with gas phase measurements, the following standard abbreviations apply:

STPD Standard temperature and pressure, dry. These are the conditions of a volume of gas at 0° C, at 760 mm Hg, without water vapor.

BTPS Body temperature (37° C), barometric pressure (at sea level, 760 mm Hg), and saturated with water vapor.

ATPD Ambient temperature, pressure, dry

ATPS Ambient temperature and pressure, saturated with water vapor

By tradition, gas volumes in the lung are measured under BTPS conditions, whereas oxygen and carbon dioxide production per minute are measured at STPD. Methods used for conversion from one condition of pressure, temperature, and humidity to another (e.g., from BTPS to STPD) are discussed in the next chapter.

Blood phase symbols

Blood phase abbreviations also are divided into primary and qualifying symbols. Primary symbols include the following:

Q volume of blood

C concentration in blood phase

S saturation in blood phase

Unlike symbols used to describe the gas phase, qualifying symbols applicable to the blood phase are normally expressed as lowercase letters. Blood phase qualifying symbols include the following:

    a arterial (exact location to be specified)
    v venous (exact location to be specified)
    c capillary (exact location to be specified)
    p pulmonary
    s shunt

These qualifying symbols can also be modified and combined. For example, c' signifies a location at the end of the capillary, whereas $\bar{v}$ indicates average or mixed venous. Combining terms gives even more detail:

    pc′ pulmonary end-capillary
    pa pulmonary arterial

Thus $C\bar{v}O_2$ stands for the concentration of oxygen in the mixed venous blood, SaO_2 represents the saturation of hemoglobin with oxygen in the arterial blood, and $\dot{Q}pc$ is the standard abbreviation for pulmonary capillary blood flow per minute.

Combining the general symbol for pressure, P, with the blood phase qualifying symbols is also very common. For example,

    $P\bar{v}O_2$ Mixed venous pressure of oxygen
    $PaCO_2$ Arterial pressure of carbon dioxide

Mechanics of breathing symbols

Most symbols used to represent pulmonary mechanics are pressure terms. The modifying symbols usually indicate where the pressure is being measured. Modifying symbols used in describing pulmonary mechanics include the following:

    A alveolar (also *alv*)
  ab abdomen
  am ambient
  ao airway opening
  aw airway
    B barometric
  bs body surface
  di diaphragm
  ds downstream
 dyn dynamic
    E expiratory
  el elastic
  es esophageal
  fr frictional
    I inspiratory
    L transpulmonary
 max maximum
  pl pleural
  rc ribcage
  rs respiratory system
  st static
 tm transmural
 us upstream
  W chest wall

Thus Pao stands for pressure at the airway opening (i.e., mouth, nose, tracheal cannula), Pimax indicates maximum inspiratory pressure, Pw is the pressure difference across the chest wall (or transthoracic pressure), and Ppl is the pressure in the pleural space (between visceral and parietal pleura).

Although pressure (P) is the main symbol used in pulmonary mechanics, several others will be used throughout this text. These include:

    C compliance
    E elastance
    G conductance
    R resistance
    W work

Combining these additional main symbols with their modifiers yields several common combinations:

  Cwst static compliance of the chest wall
  Raw airway resistance
  WI,el elastic work during inspiration
  $\dot{W}$di diaphragm work/unit time (power)

SCIENTIFIC NOTATION AND MEASUREMENT PREFIXES

Scientific notation is a simple method for representing very large or very small numbers as powers of 10. This is done by converting the number to an integer between 1 and 10 and then multiplying it by the appropriate power of 10.

To convert a number larger than 10 into scientific notation, one simply moves the decimal to the right of the first integer and multiplies the new number by 10 raised to the power equal to the number of places the decimal was moved. Zeros to the right of the last integer may be dropped. For example:

$$2655 = 2.655 \times 10^3$$
$$54{,}000 = 5.4 \times 10^4$$
$$301{,}010 = 3.0101 \times 10^5$$
$$866.67 = 8.6667 \times 10^2$$

To convert a number smaller than 1 into scientific notation, move the decimal to the right of the first integer but multiply the new number by 10 raised to the *negative* power equal to the number of places the decimal was moved. For example:

$$0.454 = 4.54 \times 10^{-1}$$
$$0.00306 = 3.06 \times 10^{-3}$$
$$0.00000703 = 7.03 \times 10^{-6}$$
$$0.01010 = 1.01 \times 10^{-2}$$

Powers of 10 also are used to define multiples and divisions of both measurement units in decimal-based systems. As depicted in Table 6-6, several prefixes are expressed in Greek, whereas fractional prefixes are expressed in Latin. The following examples of se-

Table 6-6   Standard units prefixes

Prefix	Abbreviation	Power of 10
deka	da	10^1
hecto	h	10^2
kilo	k	10^3
mega	M	10^6
giga	G	10^9
tera	T	10^{12}
deci	d	10^{-1}
centi	c	10^{-2}
milli	m	10^{-3}
micro	μ	10^{-6}
nano	n	10^{-9}
pico	p	10^{-12}
femto	f	10^{-15}
atto	a	10^{-18}

lected linear, volumetric, and mass measures demonstrate the use of these prefixes:

Linear measure	kilometer (km)	$m \times 10^3$
	meter (m)	
	decimeter	$m \times 10^{-1}$
	centimeter (cm)	$m \times 10^{-2}$
	millimeter (mm)	$m \times 10^{-3}$
	micrometer (μm)	$m \times 10^{-6}$
	namometer (nm)	$m \times 10^{-9}$
Volume	liter (L)	
	deciliter (dL)	$L \times 10^{-1}$
	milliliter (mL)	$L \times 10^{-3}$
	microliter (μL)	$L \times 10^{-6}$
	nanoliter (nL)	$L \times 10^{-9}$
Mass	kilogram (kg)	$g \times 10^3$
	gram (g)	
	milligram (mg)	$g \times 10^{-3}$
	microgram (μg)	$g \times 10^{-6}$
	nanogram (ng)	$g \times 10^{-9}$

UNITS OF MEASURE

Measurement is the key to both basic and applied science. Ideally, the same system should be used by scientists and clinicians worldwide to measure, describe, and communicate physical events. Unfortunately, this ideal situation does not exist. Indeed, at least three primary systems of measurement are used in the clinical setting. Were one to add the apothecary and avoirdupois systems used in pharmacy, clinicians would have to master *five* different systems! We will only review three.

Measurement systems

Two different measurement systems were developed separately in Great Britain and continental Europe.

The British system of measure—adopted early on by the United States—is based on the foot (length), pound (mass), and second (time). For this reason, the British system is referred to as the **fps system.** During the French Revolution, a separate system was developed on the Continent. The basic units in this decimal-based system were the centimeter (length), gram (mass), and second (time). This system is referred to as the **cgs system.**

In 1960, worldwide efforts were initiated to adopt a single standard, referred to as *le Système International d'Unites,* or **SI system.** SI units are a simple modification of cgs units. Length is based on the *meter* instead of the centimeter, and mass is based on the *kilogram* instead of the gram. Seconds remain as the time standard, with electric current expressed in amperes, temperature in degrees Kelvin, and chemical amounts of substances in moles. Other SI units of measure are derived from the base units described. For example, the SI unit for force is the *newton* (N), and the unit for work or energy is the *joule* (J). Because of its primary units for length, mass, and time, the SI system is also known as the meter-kilogram-second system, or *mks system.* Table 6-7 compares the major units of measure used in the SI, cgs, and fps systems.

Because both are decimal-based systems, the changeover from the cgs to the SI system is easy. However, given the nondecimal nature of the fps system, "metrification" generally has not fully succeeded in the United States. For this reason, the RCP is still faced with the necessity of working with a variety of units of measure in clinical practice. This skill often requires the clinician to convert units among these various systems.

Table 6-7   The three measurement systems

Quantity	SI	cgs	fps
Length	meter (m)	centimeter (cm)	foot (ft)
Volume	cubic meter (m^3)	cubic centimeter (cm^3 or cc)	cubic foot (ft^3)
Time	second (s)	second (s)	sec (s)
Mass	kilogram (kg)	gram (g)	pound (lb)*
Velocity	m/s	cm/s	ft/s
Acceleration	m/s^2	cm/s^2	ft/s^2
Force	newton (N) ($kg \cdot m/s^2$)	dyne ($gm \cdot cm/s^2$)	pound (lb)
Pressure	pascal (Pa) (N/m^2)	$dyne/cm^3$	lb/ft^2
Work, energy	joule (J) ($N \cdot m$)	erg (dyne $\cdot$ cm)	ft $\cdot$ lb
Power	watt (W) (J/s)	erg/s	ft $\cdot$ lb/s

*The "slug", not the pound, is the true fps unit of mass. A pound is actually a measure of force (mass × acceleration). See text for discussion of mass versus weight versus force.

Unit conversions

To convert measures between these systems, the RCP must know and apply several conversion factors. Table 6-8 provides the most common factors used to convert between cgs, fps and SI units.

To convert from a conventional unit to an alternate

unit, *multiply* the conventional unit by the listed conversion factor. To convert from an alternate unit back to a conventional unit, *divide* the alternate unit by the conversion factor.

For example, the factor to convert inches (fps) to centimeters (cgs) is 2.540. To convert a patient's height of 72 inches to centimeters, simply multiply the old unit by the conversion factor:

$$Old\ unit \times conversion\ factor = New\ unit$$
$$72\ in \times 2.54\ cm/in = 182.88\ cm$$

The following sections discusses common conversions among measures of length, volume, mass, weight, force, pressure, work (and energy), and power used in clinical practice. Although not all factors must be committed to memory, the RCP must be proficient in using selected conversions at the bedside. For this reason, these "must-know" conversion factors are highlighted.

Length

The most common length conversions in clincal practice are between inches and centimeters (Table 6-8). For this reason, RCPs should memorize the following two conversions:

$$inches \times 2.54\ (cm/in) = centimeters$$

$$\frac{centimeters}{2.54} = Inches$$

Volume

The standard unit of volume in each system is based on the cube of its length standard—that is, the cubic meter (m^3), cubic centimeter (cm^3, or *cc*), and cubic foot (ft^3). Related volume measures are the liter (L), deciliter (dL), and milliliter (mL); and the fluid ounce and gallon (U.S.). Table 6-8 compares the common units of volume in the SI, cgs, and fps systems.

The most common volume conversions in clincal practice are between liters and milliliters or deciliters, cubic feet and liters, cubic feet and gallons, and gallons and liters (Table 6-8). For this reason, RCPs should commit to memory the following conversions:

$$milliliters \times 0.001 = Liters$$

$$\frac{Liters}{0.001} = milliliters$$

$$\frac{Liters}{0.1} = deciliters$$

$$cubic\ feet \times 28.32 = liters$$

$$cubic\ feet \times 7.48 = gallons$$

$$gallons \times 3.785 = liters$$

The RCP also will see the cubic centimeter used as a small-volume measure. In clinical practice, 1 cc is equivalent to 1 mL.

Table 6-8   Conversion factors for units commonly used in medicine

Physical quantity	Conventional unit	Alternate unit	Conversion factor*
Length	inch (in)	meter (m)	0.0254
	inch (in)	+centimeter	2.540
	foot (ft)	m	0.3048
Volume	dL (=100 mL)	L	0.10
	ft^3	m^3	0.0283
	ft^3	L	28.32
	ft^3	+gallon (US)	7.48
	gallon (US)	L	3.785
	fluid ounce	+mL	29.57
Force (weight)	pound (lb)	newton (N)	4.448
	dyne	N	0.00001
	kilogram (kg)	N	9.807
	kg	+gm	1000.0
	pound	+kg	0.4536
	ounce	+gm	28.35
Amount of substance	mg/dL	mmol/L	10/molecular weight
	mEq/L	mmol/L	1/valence
	mL of gas (STPD)	mmol	0.04462
Pressure	cm H_2O	kilopascal (kPa)	0.09806
	mm Hg (torr)	kPa	0.1333
	lbs/in² (psi)	kPa	6.895
	psi	+cm H_2O	70.31
	cm H_2O	+torr	0.7355
	standard atmosphere	kPa	101.3
Work, energy	kg · m	joule (J)	9.807
	L · cm H_2O	joule (J)	0.09806
	calorie (cal)	joule (J)	4.185
	BTU	joule (J)	1055.0
Power	kg · m/min	watt (W)	0.1634

*To convert from conventional to alternate unit, multiply conventional unit by factor. To convert from alternate unit back to conventional unit, divide alternate unit by factor.

Examples:
  10 torr = 10 × 0.1333 kPa = 1.333 kPa
  1 L = 1 L/0.10 = 10 dL

+ non SI units
Adapted with permission from Chatburn RL: Measurement, physical quantities and le systeme international d'unites (SI units), *Respir Care* 33(10):861–873, 1988.

Mass and the amount of a substance

Mass represents an absolute quantity of matter. The standard SI unit of mass is the kilogram (kg), with the gram (g) being the cgs mass unit.

True mass is seldom used as a clinical measure. Instead, we measure the force or weight of a substance (see below). The exception involves chemical or solution computation. Here, we need to know the actual quantity of matter available for chemical reactions or combination in a solution. These common clinical measures include milligrams per deciliter (mg/dL), milliequivalents per liter (mEq/L), milliliters of a gas at STPD, and millimoles (mmol).

The most common of these conversions are from mg/dL, mEq/L or mL of a gas at STPD to the standard SI unit, millimoles per liter (mmol/L) (Table 6-8). Although none of these must be memorized, converting from mEq/L to mmol/L is a common and easy enough task. Whenever the valence of the ion is 1 (e.g., Na^+, K^+, HCO_3^-), 1 mEq/L is equivalent to 1 mmol/L. For ions with a valence other than 1 (e.g., Ca^{++}, SO_4^{--}), divide by the valence. Thus 10 mEq/L Ca^{++} equals 5 mmol/L Ca^{++}.

Force

Newton's second law of motion tells us that the acceleration of an object is directly proportional to the force exerted and inversely proportional to its mass:

$$\text{acceleration (a)} = \frac{\text{force (F)}}{\text{mass (m)}}$$

The equation may be rearranged to solve for force (F):

$$\text{Force (F)} = \text{Mass (m)} \times \text{acceleration (a)}$$

Thus force is a measure of mass times acceleration. In the SI system, the unit of force is the *Newton* (N), where $1 N = 1 kg \cdot m/sec^2$. The cgs unit of force is the *dyne* ($1 g \cdot cm/sec^2$), with the fps unit of force being the *pound* (lb).

Weight represents a special case of force, with the acceleration factor due to gravity:

$$\text{force (F)} = \text{mass (m)} \times \text{acceleration (a)}$$
$$\text{weight} = \text{mass (m)} \times \text{acceleration due to gravity}$$

Weight and mass and are the two most commonly confused concepts in physics. Weight, unlike mass, is affected by gravity. Thus the mass of an object always remains the same. However, the weight of the same object changes in different gravitational fields. For example, although your mass on the earth is the same as on the moon, your weight is about two-thirds less on the moon, due to its weaker gravity.

On the earth's surface, the acceleration due to gravity is a constant at any given altitude. For example, at sea level the acceleration due to gravity is 9.807 m/sec^2 (SI). Because acceleration due to gravity is a constant at a given altitude, an object's weight and the mass are directly proportional to each other. For this reason, it is common practice to interchange mass, weight and force units.

The most common force (weight) conversions used in clincal practice are between kilograms and grams, and pounds and kilograms (see Table 6-8). For this reason, RCPs should commit to memory the following conversions:

$$\text{kilogram} \times 1000 = \text{grams}$$
$$\frac{\text{grams}}{1000} = \text{kilograms}$$
$$\text{pounds} \times 0.454 = \text{kilograms}$$
$$\frac{\text{kilograms}}{0.454} = \text{pounds}$$

Pressure

Pressure is a measure of force per unit area, where area is the square of length. Thus the SI unit of pressure is the Newton per square meter (N/m^2), also called the *pascal* (Pa). Because the pascal is such a small unit of pressure, we use the kilopascal (kPa) instead. One kilopascal equals 10^3 pascals. The standard cgs unit of pressure is the dyne per square centimeter (dyne/cm^2). Although the standard fps unit of pressure is the pound per square foot (lb/ft^2), it is more common to express pressure in this system as pounds per square inch (lb/in^2).

With the exception of lb/in^2, few of these pressure units are used in clinical practice. Instead, we commonly measure pressure as the height of a fluid column. Typically we use either centimeters of water (cm H_2O) or millimeters of mercury (mm Hg, or torr).

The most common pressure conversions used in clinical practice are between cm H_2O and mm Hg (torr) (Table 6-8). With the SI system making inroads into scientific publications, the RCP also must know how to convert between these units and kilopascals. Thus RCPs should commit to memory the following conversions:

$$\text{cm } H_2O \times 0.7355 = \text{mm Hg (torr)}$$
$$\frac{\text{mm Hg (torr)}}{0.7355} = \text{cm } H_2O$$
$$\text{cm } H_2O \times 0.098 = \text{kilopascal (kPa)}$$
$$\frac{\text{kilopascal (kPa)}}{0.098} = \text{cm } H_2O$$
$$\text{mm Hg} \times 0.1333 = \text{kilopascal (kPa)}$$
$$\frac{\text{kilopascal (kPa)}}{0.1333} = \text{mm Hg (torr)}$$

More detail on clinical pressure measurements is provided in Chapter 7.

Work and energy

Work is a measure of the force exerted on an object over a given distance. Therefore the SI unit of work is the Newton-meter (N · m), also called the *joule* (J). The cgs unit of work is the *dyne-centimeter* (dynes × cm), or *erg*. Because the erg is such a small unit of work, we often use the *kilogram-meter* (kg · m) instead. The standard fps unit of work is the *foot-pound* (lb · ft).

According to the first law of thermodynamics, an object's total internal energy must equal the work performed on that object plus any heat transferred to it from a hotter substance:

$$\text{internal energy} = \text{work done} + \text{heat energy transferred}$$

According to this formula, we can change the internal energy of an object by: (1) performing work on it or (2) heating it. Thus, in physical terms, heat and work energy are equivalent. For this reason, we could use the same units to measure both work and heat energy —that is, the joule, erg, or foot-pound.

However, heat energy in the cgs and fps systems is not expressed in these units. Instead, the cgs system uses the *calorie* (cal) and the fps system the *British thermal unit,* or BTU. A calorie is defined as the quantity of heat required to raise the temperature of 1 g of water from 14.5° to 15.5° C. A BTU is the amount of heat required to raise the temperature of 1 lb of water 1° F. One BTU equals 252 cal.

As work of breathing measurements become more commonplace at the bedside, RCPs will have to become proficient in converting between work units. The most common conversions are from kilogram-meters or L · cm H_2O to joules. As shown in Table 6-8, 1 kilogram-meter equals approximately 10 J, whereas 1 L · cm H_2O equals about 0.10 J.

Power

Power is a measure of work performed over time. The SI unit of power is the joule per second (J/sec), also called the *watt* (W). The cgs unit of power is the *erg per second* (erg/sec), although kilogram-meters/sec is also used. The standard fps unit of power is the *foot-pound per second* (ft · lb/sec). RCPs currently do not need to memorize power conversions, but they may be required to apply them to clinical measurement.

CHAPTER SUMMARY

As with most health professions, respiratory care involves extensive observation and communication. Accurate and consistent observation and communication among health professionals requires a common frame of reference. This common frame of reference is embodied in various systems of clinical communication and measurement.

Medical terminology provides consistent meanings among all health professionals, thus aiding communication and interaction. Complementing medical terminology is a system of abbreviations, used extensively in charting and medical record–keeping. Unlike most abbreviations, those used in pulmonary medicine are well standardized. Effective clinical interaction demands that RCPs master and consistently apply these terms and symbols.

The purpose of a measurement system is to measure, describe, and communicate physical events. Unfortunately, at least three systems of measurement are used in the clinical setting, namely the Système International d'Unites (SI) system, the centimeter–gram–second (cgs) system, and the British foot-pound–second (fps) system. Until complete standardization on the SI systems occurs in the United States, RCPs must to be skilled in working with all three systems.

BIBLIOGRAPHY

Barclay WR: Medicine, metrication, and SI units, *JAMA* 244: 241–242, 1980.

Chatburn RL: Measurement, physical quantities and le système international d'unites (SI units), *Respir Care* 33(10):861–873, 1988.

Cotes JE: SI units in respiratory medicine, *Am Rev Respir Dis,* 112:753–755, 1975.

Glanze WD, ed.: *Mosby's medical and nursing dictionary,* ed 3, St. Louis, 1986, Mosby.

Gylys BA, Wedding ME: *Medical terminology: a systems approach,* ed 2, Philadelphia, 1988, F.A. Davis

Lough MD, Chatburn RL: *Handbook of respiratory care,* ed 2, St Louis, Mosby, 1990.

McQueen MJ: Conversion to SI units, *JAMA* 256:3001–3002, 1986.

Nave CR, Nave BC: *Physics for the health sciences,* ed 3, Philadelphia, WB Saunders, 1985.

Pappenheimer Committee: Standardization of definitions and symbols in respiratory physiology, *Fed Proc* 9:602, 1950.

Pennycuick CJ: *Conversion factors: SI units and many others,* Chicago: University of Chicago Press, 1988.

Pulmonary terms and symbols: A report of the ACCP-ATS Joint Committee on Pulmonary Nomenclature, *Chest* 67:583, 1975.

Riggs JH: *Respiratory facts,* Philadelphia, FA Davis, 1989.

U.S. Department of Commerce, National Bureau of Standards: *The English and metric systems of measurement,* Special Pub. 304A, revised edition, 1970.

Vawter SM, DeForest RE: The international metric system and medicine, *JAMA* 218:723, 1971.

Young DS: Standardized reporting of laboratory data, *N Engl J Med* 290:368, 1974.

Physical Principles in Respiratory Care

■

Craig L. Scanlan

CHAPTER LEARNING OBJECTIVES

1. Differentiate among the three primary states of matter, with a special emphasis on the physical properties of fluids (liquids and gases).
2. Relate the concepts of heat transfer and change of state to the internal energy of matter and the measurement of temperature.
3. Relate the concept of vaporization to the presence of water vapor in gases and gas mixtures and its quantification as "humidity."
4. Apply the standard laws of gas behavior to explain changes in the temperature, pressure, volume, or mass of an ideal gas.
5. Explain how the behavior of gases deviates from ideal under extremes of pressure and temperature.
6. Relate the key principles of hydrodynamics to the behavior of fluids in motion and their application in respiratory care.

As a field of applied scientific and clinical study, respiratory care has a strong technological base. Much of the technology used in respiratory care is based on the application of basic physical principles. The study of the physical principles governing the world around us is called physics.

Physics is further divided into several branches, including thermodynamics (heat and energy), mechanics, sound, electricity, magnetism, and light. Although all branches of physics have an impact on respiratory care, we will limit our focus to a few key principles involving matter, thermodynamics, mechanics, and electricity.

STATES OF MATTER

There are three primary states of matter: solid, liquid, and gas. Figure 7-1, on page 114 shows the similarities and differences among these three states of matter.

The solid state is characterized by a high degree of internal order, in which the positions of the atoms or molecules are essentially fixed. As depicted in Figure 7-1, *A,* you can think of the atoms of a solid as being held together by springs. In this framework, the atoms are limited to back-and-forth motion about an equilibrium position. The atoms are kept in place by strong mutual attractive forces, called *van der Waals forces.* In solids, these forces are strong enough to ensure that the mass keeps its shape.

Like the atoms or molecules of a solid, those in a liquid state also exhibit strong mutual attractive forces. These cohesive forces among liquid molecules are responsible for such phenomena as surface tension and viscosity (discussed later). However, the attractive forces in liquids do not restrict molecular motion as much as in solids. Instead, liquid molecules are free to move about in relation to each other (Figure 7-1, *B*). This relative freedom of motion explains why liquids take the shape of their containers and can flow from one place to another. However, both liquids and solids are quite dense and cannot be easily compressed.

In a gas, the attractive forces between atoms or molecules are very weak. Lacking restriction to movement, gas molecules exhibit rapid, random motion with frequent collisions (Figure 7-1, *C*). Unlike solids and liquids, gases have no inherent boundaries. Also, they are easily compressed and expanded. However, like liquids, gases are capable of flow. For this reason, both liquids and gases are considered *fluids.*

Internal energy of matter

All matter possesses energy. The energy matter possesses is called *internal energy.* There are two primary forms of internal energy: (1) the energy of position, or *potential energy;* and (2) the energy of motion, or *kinetic energy.*

At ordinary temperatures, the atoms or molecules of solids, liquids, and gases all exhibit constant motion. Thus all matter exhibits some degree of kinetic energy. However, most of the internal energy in solids and liquids is in the form of potential energy. This potential energy is due to the strong forces of attraction between molecules. These intermolecular forces cause rigidity in solids and cohesiveness and viscosity in liquids. In contrast, because these forces of attrac-

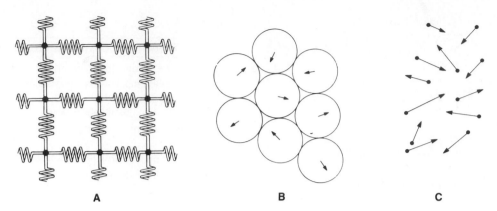

Fig. 7-1 Simplified models of the three states of matter. **A,** Solid. **B,** Liquid. **C,** Gas. (From Nave CR and Nave BC: Physics for the health sciences, ed 3, Philadelphia, 1985, WB Saunders.)

tion are so weak in gases, most of their internal energy is kinetic energy.

Internal energy and temperature

The temperature of a substance and its kinetic energy are closely related. With most of its internal energy spent keeping molecules in motion, the temperature of a gas is directly proportional its kinetic energy. In contrast, the temperatures of solids and liquid represent only part of their total internal energy.

Absolute zero

In concept, there should exist a temperature at which all kinetic activity of matter ceases. This temperature is called *absolute zero*. Although researchers have come close to absolute zero, they have never actually reached it.

Temperature scales

Absolute zero provides a logical zero point on which to build a temperature scale. The SI units for temperature are based on the *Kelvin scale,* with a zero point equal to absolute zero (0° K). Because the Kelvin scale has 100 degrees between the freezing and boiling points of water, it is considered a *centigrade,* or 100-step, temperature scale.

The cgs system for temperature measurement is based on *Celsius* units (° C). Like the Kelvin scale, the Celsius scale has 100 degrees between the freezing and boiling points of water and is thus a centigrade scale. However, the zero point of the Celsius scale is not absolute zero but instead represents the freezing point of water (0° C).

In Celsius units, kinetic molecular activity stops at about −273° C. Therefore 0° K equals −273° C, and 0° C equals 273° K. Conversion between Kelvin and Celsius units is therefore accomplished with the following simple formula:

$$° K = ° C + 273$$

Thus, to convert degrees Celsius to Kelvin, simply add 273. For example:

$$
\begin{aligned}
25° C &= 25 + 273 &&= 298° K \\
37° C &= 37 + 273 &&= 310° K \\
-15° C &= -15 + 273 &&= 258° K
\end{aligned}
$$

And to convert degrees Kelvin to Celsius, simply subtract 273:

$$
\begin{aligned}
310° K &= 310 - 273 = &&37° C \\
373° K &= 373 - 273 = &&100° C \\
0° K &= 0 - 273 = &&-273° C
\end{aligned}
$$

In the fps or British system of measurement, either the *Rankine* or *Fahrenheit* scale is used. The Rankine scale is used frequently in engineering applications but rarely in medical science. The Fahrenheit scale is more common in clinical practice but is used minimally in scientific measurement. Absolute zero on the Fahrenheit scale is equivalent to −460° F.

The following formula is used to convert degrees Fahrenheit to degrees Celsius:

$$° C = 5/9(° F - 32)$$

For example:

$$
\begin{aligned}
° F &= 98.6 \\
° C &= 5/9(98.6 - 32) \\
° C &= 5/9(66.6) \\
° C &= 37
\end{aligned}
$$

Obviously, to convert degrees Celsius back to degrees Fahrenheit, this formula is reversed:

$$° F = (9/5 \times ° C) + 32$$

For example:

$$
\begin{aligned}
° C &= 100 \\
° F &= (9/5 \times 100) + 32 \\
° F &= (180) + 32 \\
° F &= 212
\end{aligned}
$$

Figure 7-2 shows the relationship between the kinetic activity of matter and temperature on all four temperatures scales. For ease of reference, five key points are defined. These include the zero point of each scale (absolute zero for the Kelvin and Rankine scales), the freezing point of water (0° C), body temperature (37° C), and the boiling point of water (100° C).

Heat and the first law of thermodynamics

The **First Law of Thermodynamics,** or the *Law of Conservation of Energy,* states that in any physical process energy is neither created nor destroyed, only transformed in nature. Thus any energy gained by a substance must exactly equal the energy lost by its surroundings. Conversely, if a substance loses energy, this must be offset by a gain in the energy of its surroundings.

In mathematical terms, the First Law of Thermodynamics may be formulated as follows:

$$U = E + W$$

where U is the internal energy of an object, E is the energy transferred to (or taken away from) the object, and W is the external work performed on the object. In this sense, the quantity E is equivalent to heat. Heating is the transfer of internal energy from a high-temperature object to a low-temperature object.

According to this formula, you can increase the internal energy of an object by heating it or by performing work on it. Let's take a close look at the first of these physical phenomenon, the transfer of heat.

Heat transfer

When a temperature difference exists between two objects, the first law of thermodynamics tells us that heat will move from the hotter object to the cooler object until their temperatures are equal. Two objects with the same temperature exist in thermal **equilibrium.**

This transfer of internal energy occurs by way of at least one of three primary mechanisms: (1) conduction, (2) convection, or (3) radiation. Heat transfer also occurs through evaporation and condensation.

Conduction

Conduction is the primary means by which heat transfer occurs in solids. Conduction is the transfer of heat by direct contact between hot and cold molecules. The efficiency of heat transfer by conduction depends on both the number and force of molecular collisions between the adjoining substances.

We quantify the efficiency of heat transfer between objects using a measure called *thermal conductivity.* In cgs units, thermal conductivity is measured as (cal/sec)/(cm² × ° C/cm). As shown in Table 7-1, page 116, solids, particularly metals, have the highest thermal conductivity. This is why metals feel cold to the touch, even when at room temperature. In this case, the high thermal conductivity of the metal quickly draws heat away from the skin, creating a feeling of "cold." In contrast, because their molecules collide less often than do those in solids and liquids, gases are poor heat conductors.

Convection

Convection is the primary means of heat transfer among fluids, both liquids and gases. Convection

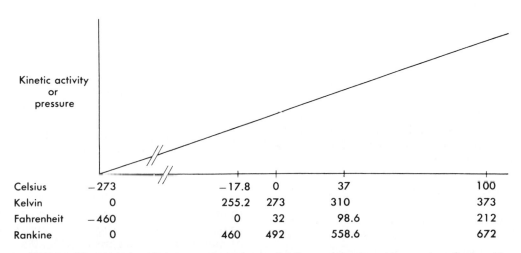

Fig. 7-2 Linear relationship between gas molecular activity, or pressure, and temperature. Comparable readings of the four scales are indicated for five temperature points.

Table 7-1 Thermal conductivities in $(cal/sec)/(cm^2 \times °C/cm)$

Material	Thermal conductivity (k)
Silver	1.01
Copper	0.99
Aluminum	0.50
Iron	0.163
Lead	0.083
Ice	0.005
Glass, ordinary	0.0025
Concrete	0.002
Water at 20° C	0.0014
Asbestos	0.0004
Hydrogen at 0° C	0.0004
Helium at 0° C	0.0003
Snow (dry)	0.00026
Fiberglass	0.00015
Cork board	0.00011
Wool felt	0.0001
Air at 0° C	0.000057

From Nave CR and Nave BC: Physics for the health sciences, ed 3, Philadelphia, 1985, WB Saunders.

involves the mixing of fluid molecules at different temperature states. For example, although air is a poor heat conductor, it can efficiently transfer heat by convection. To do so, we first warm the air in one location and then circulate it to carry the heat elsewhere. This is the principle behind forced-air heating in houses and convection heating in infant incubators. The movements of fluids carrying heat energy are called *convection currents*.

Radiation

The transfer of heat by radiation is very different from both conduction and convection. In these first two methods, energy transfer only occurs by way of direct contact between two substances. Radiant heat transfer occurs without direct physical contact. Indeed, heat transfer by radiation occurs even in a **vacuum,** as when the sun warms the earth.

Thus radiant energy is similar in concept to light. Radiant energy given off by objects at room temperature is mainly in the **infrared** range, invisible to the human eye. On the other hand, objects such as an electrical stove burner or a kerosene heater radiate some of their energy as visible light. In the clinical setting, we commonly use radiant heat energy to keep newborn infants warm.

You calculate the rate at which an object gains or loses heat by radiation with the following formula:

$$\frac{E}{t} = ekA(T_2 - T_1)$$

In this formula, *E/t* is the heat loss or gain per unit time. The symbol *e* stands for the *emissivity* of the object, or its relative effectiveness in radiating heat. The constant *k* is the Stefan-Boltzman constant (based on mass and surface area). *A* is the area of the radiating object, and T_1 and T_2 are the temperatures of the environment and the object, respectively. In simple terms, for an object with a given emissivity, the larger the surface area (relative to mass) and the lower the surrounding temperature, the greater the radiant heat loss per unit time.

Vaporization

Vaporization is the change of state from liquid to gas. Heat energy is needed to cause vaporization. According to the First Law of Thermodynamics, this heat energy must come from the surroundings. In one form of vaporization, called *evaporation,* heat is taken from the air surrounding the liquid, thereby cooling the air. In warm weather or during strenuous exercise, the body takes advantage of this principle of "evaporation cooling" by producing sweat. The liquid sweat evaporates and thus cools the skin.

The opposite of evaporation is *condensation.* During condensation, the gaseous form of a substance changes back into a liquid. Because vaporization takes heat from the air around a liquid (causing cooling), condensation must give heat back to the surroundings (causing warming). The next section expands on the concept of change of state and provides more detail on the processes of vaporization and condensation.

CHANGE OF STATE

All matter can change from solid to liquid to gas. This process is called a *change of state.* As an RCP, you will deal extensively with both liquids and gases. For this reason, you must master the basic processes occurring during phase changes and the key qualities of each state of matter.

Liquid–solid phase changes (melting and freezing)

When heat is applied to a solid body, the kinetic energy of its atoms or molecules increases. This added internal energy increases the intensity of molecular vibrations. If enough heat is added, these vibrations will eventually be great enough to weaken the intermolecular attractive forces. At this point, the molecules will break free of their rigid structure, and the solid will change into a liquid.

Melting

The breakdown of this rigid structure corresponds to *melting.* The temperature at which a solid converts to its liquid form is called its *melting point.* The range of melting points is considerable. For example, water (ice) has a melting point of 0° C, carbon more than 3500° C, and helium less than −272.2° C.

Figure 7-3 depicts the phase change caused by the application of heat (in calories) to water. At the left origin of −50° C, water exists as a solid (ice). As we apply heat energy to the ice, its temperature rises. At its melting point of 0° C, the ice begins to change into liquid water. However, the full change to liquid water requires additional heat energy. Notice this additional heat energy brings about the change of state but does not immediately change the water temperature.

The extra heat needed to bring about the change-over from solid to liquid is called the *latent heat of fusion*. In the cgs system, the latent heat of fusion is defined as the calories required to change 1 g of a solid into a liquid without changing its temperature. The term *latent* means that the heat is used solely to melt the substance, without changing its temperature. To give some idea of the range of energy needed for this change in state, the latent heat of fusion of ice is 80 cal/g, that of calcium chloride is 54 cal/g, and that of oxygen is 3.3 cal/g. Compared with the process of simply heating a solid, this change of phase requires a large amount of internal energy.

Freezing

Freezing is the opposite of melting. Because melting requires large amounts of externally applied energy, you would expect freezing to return energy to the surroundings. This is exactly what occurs. During freezing, heat energy is transferred from a liquid back to the environment, usually by exposure to cold.

As the kinetic energy of the substance decreases, its molecules begin to regain the stable structure of a solid. According to the First Law of Thermodynamics, the energy required to freeze a substance must equal that needed to cause melting. Thus the freezing and melting points of a substance are the same.

Properties of liquids

As was discussed previously, liquids are fluids. Specifically, liquids can flow and take the shapes of their container. Liquids also exert pressure, which varies with depth and density. Variations in liquid pressure within a container produce an upward supporting force, called *buoyancy.*

Although the molecular forces of attraction are weakened when a solid melts, liquid molecules are still attracted to one another. The relative strength of these cohesive forces among molecules help explain other important qualities of liquids such as viscosity, capillary action, and surface tension.

Pressure in liquids

The pressure exerted by a liquid is directly proportional to the depth of the liquid and its density. Mathematically, this relationship is expressed as follows:

$$P_1 = dgh$$

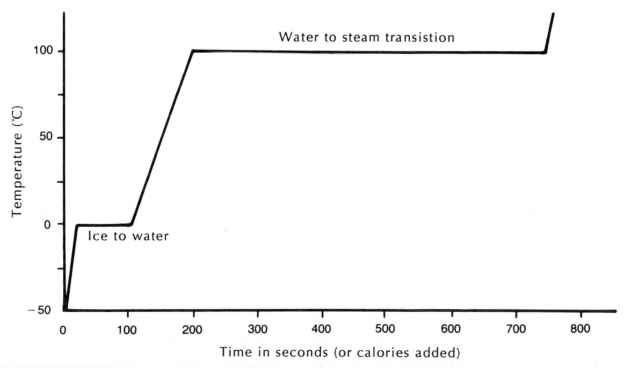

Fig. 7–3 Temperature as a function of time for 1 g of water to which heat is added at the rate of 1 cal/s.
(From Nave CR and Nave BC: Physics for the health sciences, ed 3, Philadelphia, 1985, WB Saunders)

where P_l is the static pressure exerted by the liquid, d is the density of the liquid, g is the acceleration due to gravity, and h is the height of the liquid column.

Density (d) is a measure of a substance's mass per unit. Given the relationship between mass and weight at a given distance from the earth (see Chapter 6), density is usually expressed as weight per unit volume, called *weight density,* or d_w. Because under most clinical conditions $d_w = d \times g$, we replace dg with weight density and simplify the above equation to:

$$P_l = d_w \times h$$

In the cgs system, the weight density of solids and liquids are usually measured in grams per cubic centimeter. The density of gases is usually expressed in grams per liter. As an example, let's compute the pressure at the bottom of a 33.9 foot (1034 cm) high column of water (density = 1 gm/cm^3):

$$
\begin{aligned}
P_l &= d_w \times h \\
&= (1 \text{ gm/cm}^3) \times 1034 \text{ cm} \\
&= 1034 \text{ gm/cm}^2
\end{aligned}
$$

As we shall see, our answer (1034 gm/cm^2) also equals *1 atmosphere* of pressure, or about 14.7 lb/in^2. Of course, this figure does not account for the additional atmospheric pressure (PB) acting on the top of the liquid. The total pressure at the bottom of the column equals the sum of the atmospheric and liquid pressures. In this case, the total pressure would be 2068 gm/cm^2, equal to 29.4 lb/in^2, or 2 atmospheres.

Moreover, the pressure exerted by a liquid depends only on the depth and density of the liquid, and not the shape of the vessel. As shown in Figure 7-4, the pressure exerted by a liquid at a depth (h) is the same, regardless of the container's shape. This is because the pressure in a liquid acts equally in all directions. This concept is known as *Pascal's Principle.*

Buoyancy (Archimedes's principle)

Thousands of years ago, Archimedes showed that an object submersed in water appeared to weigh less that in air. This effect, called *buoyancy,* explains why certain objects float in water.

Liquids exert buoyant force because the pressure below a submerged object always exceeds the pressure above it. This difference in liquid pressure creates an upward or supporting force. If this upward buoyant force is greater than the weight of a submersed object, it will float. Conversely, if the weight of the object exceeds the buoyant force, it will sink.

According to Archimedes's Principle, the buoyant force exerted on an object equals the weight of the fluid displaced by the object. Because the weight of fluid displaced by an object equals its weight density times its volume ($d_w \times V$), the buoyant force ($F_{buoyant}$) may be calculated as follows:

$$F_{buoyant} = d_w \times V$$

Thus, if the weight density of an object is less than water (1 gm/cm^3), it will displace a weight of water greater than its own weight. In this case, the upward buoyant force will exceed the downward force of gravity, and the object will float. Conversely, if an object's weight density exceeds that of water, the downward force of gravity will overcome the upward buoyant force, and the object will sink.

Clinically, Archimedes's Principle is used to measure the *specific gravity* of certain liquids, such as urine. Specific gravity is a variation of the weight density measurement in which we compare the density of a substance to water. It is also possible to measure the specific gravity of a gas. In this case, we use oxygen or hydrogen as the standard instead of water.

In the clinical setting, we measure specific gravity with a device called a *hydrometer.* Figure 7-5 depicts a

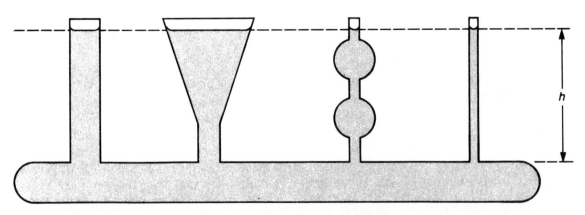

Fig. 7-4 The pressure is dependent only on the height (*h*) and not on the shape of the vessel or the total volume of water. (From Nave CR and Nave BC: Physics for the health sciences, ed 3, Philadelphia, 1985, WB Saunders.)

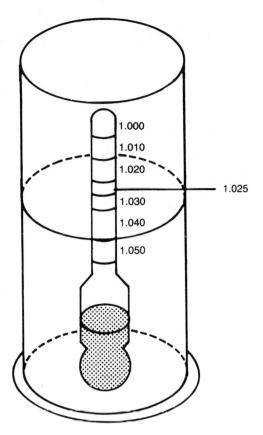

Fig. 7-5 A hydrometer used to measure the specific gravity of a urine specimen. The narrow tubing is calibrated so that the specific gravity 1.025 can be read from the tube. (From Nave CR and Nave BC: Physics for the health sciences, ed 3, Philadelphia, 1985, WB Saunders.)

hydrometer being used to measure the specific gravity of urine. The scale value of 1.025 indicates that this urine sample has a weight density 1.025 times greater than that of water.

Gases also exert buoyant force, although much less than that provided by higher density liquids. For example, buoyancy helps solid particles suspended in

gases. These suspensions, called **aerosols,** play an extremely important role in respiratory care. More detail on the characteristics and use of aerosols is provided in Chapter 25.

Viscosity

Viscosity is the force opposing a fluid's flow. Viscosity in fluids is equivalent to friction in solids.

A fluid's viscosity is directly proportional to the strength of cohesive forces between its molecules. The stronger these cohesive forces, the greater the viscosity of the fluid. The greater a fluid's viscosity, the greater its resistance to deformation and the greater its opposition to flow.

Viscosity is most important when a fluid is moving in discrete cylindrical layers, called *streamlines.* This pattern of motion is termed *laminar flow.* As shown in Figure 7-6, frictional forces between the streamlines and the wall of the tube impede movement of the fluid's outer layers. As we move toward the center of the tube, each layer hinders the motion of the next inner layer less and less. Thus laminar flow consists of **concentric** layers of fluid flowing parallel to the tube wall at velocities that increase toward the center.

The difference in the velocity among these concentric layers is called the *shear rate.* The shear rate is simply a measure of how easily the layers separate. How easily the layers separate depends on two factors: the pressure applied to drive the fluid, called the *shear stress;* and the viscosity of the fluid. Shear rate is directly proportional to shear stress and inversely proportional to viscosity:

$$\text{Shear rate} \propto \frac{\text{Shear stress}}{\text{Viscosity}}$$

Rearranging the equation to solve for viscosity,

$$\text{Viscosity} \propto \frac{\text{Shear stress}}{\text{Shear rate}}$$

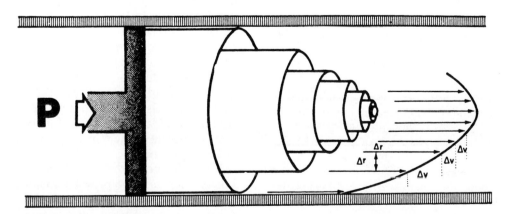

Fig. 7-6 The effects of shear stress or pressure (*P*) on shear rate (velocity gradient) in a newtonian fluid. (Redrawn from Winters WL and Brest AN, editors: The microcirculation, Springfield, Ill, 1969, Charles C Thomas, Publisher.)

The cgs unit for viscosity is the *poise*. A poise equals the force of 1 dyne over an area of 1 cm² for a period of 1 second (dyne · sec/cm²). The viscosity of liquids is measured in centipoises (10^{-2} poises), and that of gases is measured in micropoises (10^{-6} poises). Table 7-2 provides a few examples of these measures. The SI unit for viscosity is the *Pascal-second* (Pa · s), with 1 Pa · s equal to 10 poises.

In **homogeneous** fluids such as water or oil, viscosity varies with changes in temperature. Because an increase in temperature weakens the cohesive forces between fluid molecules, heating a homogeneous fluid lowers its viscosity. Conversely, cooling a fluid increases its viscosity. This is why your car's engine is so hard to start on a cold winter morning. The oil becomes so viscous that it impedes movement of the engine's parts.

Blood, unlike water or oil, is a complex fluid. This is because blood contains not only water (**plasma**) but also particles (cells) in suspension and dissolved substances in solution. For this reason, blood has a viscosity about five times greater than that of water. The greater the viscosity of a fluid, the more energy required to make it flow. Thus the heart performs more work pumping blood than it would pumping water or plasma. The heart must perform even more work when blood viscosity increases, as it does in polycythemia (an increase in red blood cell mass).

Cohesion and adhesion

Cohesive forces represent attraction between like molecules. Attractive forces between unlike molecules are called *adhesive forces.*

You can observe cohesive and adhesive forces at work by placing a liquid in a small-diameter tube. As illustrated in Figure 7-7, the liquid forms a curved surface, or *meniscus*. When the liquid is water, the meniscus that forms is **concave** (Figure 7-7, *A*). This is because water molecules at the surface adhere to the glass more strongly than they cohere to each other. In contrast, a mercury meniscus is **convex** (Figure 7-7, *B*). In this case, the cohesive forces pulling the mercury atoms together exceed the adhesive forces trying to attract the mercury to the glass.

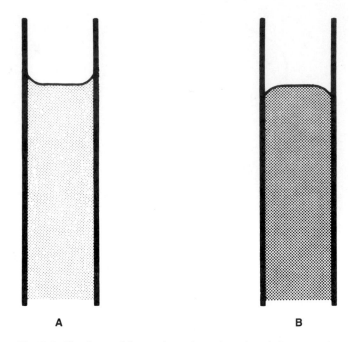

A   **B**

Fig. 7-7 The shape of the meniscus depends on the relative strengths of adhesion and cohesion. **A,** Water; adhesion stronger than cohesion. **B,** Mercury; cohesion stronger than adhesion. (From Nave CR and Nave BC: Physics for the health sciences, ed 3, Philadelphia, 1985, WB Saunders.)

Surface tension

Surface tension is a force exerted by like molecules at a liquid's surface. All liquids display some surface tension. Surface tension occurs at the junction or interface between a liquid and a gas and is best illustrated in a small drop of fluid. As shown in Figure 7-8, molecules inside the drop are subjected to balanced cohesive forces from all directions. However, molecules on the surface are attracted only inwardly. This imbalance in forces at the surface causes the surface film to contract into the smallest possible area, usually a sphere or curve (meniscus). This phenomenon explains why liquid droplets retain a spherical shape, especially when placed in an aerosol suspension (see Chapter 25). Surface tension also permits an insect to walk on the surface of a pond and enables you to float a needle in a glass of water.

Surface tension is measured by determination of the force needed to produce a "tear" in the surface layer of a liquid. Table 7-3 lists the surface tensions of selected liquids in cgs units (dynes/cm). For a given liquid, surface tension varies inversely with temperature. Thus, the higher the temperature, the lower the surface tension.

Like a fist compressing a ball, the force of surface tension increases the pressure inside a drop of liquid. According to the Laplace formula, the pressure within a drop depends on the surface tension of the liquid and the radius of the drop:

$$P = 2 \times \frac{ST}{r}$$

Table 7-2   Examples of viscosity measurements

	Substance	°C	Poises
Liquids	Water	20	1.005×10^{-2}
	Alcohol, ethyl	20	1.2×10^{-2}
	Glycerine	20	1490×10^{-2}
	Oil, castor	10	2420×10^{-2}
Gases	Air	18	182.7×10^{-6}
	Carbon dioxide	20	148×10^{-6}
	Oxygen	19	201.8×10^{-6}
	Helium	20	194.1×10^{-6}

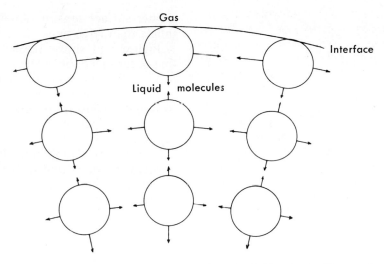

Fig. 7-8 The force of surface tension in a drop of liquid is shown by the action of its fluid molecules. Those molecules within the substance of the drop are mutually attracted to one another (*arrows*) and can move about randomly in a state of balance. Mass attraction can pull the molecules of the outermost layer inward only, creating a centrally directed force, called surface tension, which tends to contract the liquid into a sphere. Pressure within the drop is raised above atmospheric pressure and is expressed by the formula of Laplace, described in text.

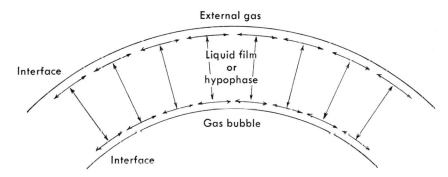

Fig. 7-9 A bubble is a volume of gas enclosed by a thin film of fluid, which has two surfaces. Thus, the forces of surface tension on both surfaces produce a pressure within the bubble twice that in a liquid drop of the same substance and radius.

Table 7-3   Examples of surface tension

Substance	°C	ST in dynes/cm
Water	20	73
Water	37	70
Tissue fluid	37	50
Whole blood	37	58
Plasma	37	73
Ethyl alcohol	20	22
Mercury	17	547

where P is the pressure within the drop, ST is the surface tension, and r is the radius in of the drop.

As an example, to compute the pressure within a 2 mm drop of water at 37° C (surface tension, 70 dynes/cm):

$$P = 2 \times \frac{70}{0.2} = \frac{140}{0.2} = 700 \text{ dynes/cm}^2$$

The same formula applies to gas bubbles that exist within liquids. For example, a 2 mm bubble of oxygen floating upward in a humidifier water reservoir would be subject to the same pressure as the 2 mm droplet described above.

Compared with liquid droplets or gas bubbles, the effect of surface tension on a liquid bubble is somewhat different. As shown in Figure 7-9, a liquid bubble is basically a spherical volume of gas enclosed in a thin fluid film. The thin film contains a finite amount of liquid called the *hypophase*. This hypophase has two surfaces, one exposed to the outside and one enclosing the gas inside. Because a liquid bubble has two gas-fluid interfaces, the surface tensions of the two surfaces act together to compress the gas bubble. Thus the force of surface tension on a gas in a liquid bubble is twice that exerted on a drop of the same size:

$$P = 4 \times \frac{ST}{r}$$

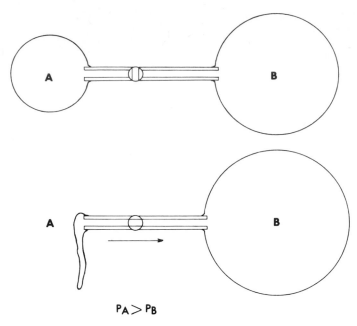

$$P_A > P_B$$

Fig. 7-10 When two bubbles of different sizes, *A* and *B*, but with the same surface tension, are allowed to communicate, the greater pressure in the smaller causes it to empty into the larger.

With the radius in the denominator of both equations, it becomes clear that the smaller the drop or bubble, the greater the pressure due to surface tension. As a result, smaller bubbles (of the same liquid) are under more pressure and are thus more prone to collapse than larger bubbles. Indeed, as shown in Figure 7-10, if a large and small bubble communicate with each other, the smaller bubble will always empty into the larger one. Conversely, because of their greater surface tension, small bubbles are harder to inflate than large ones.

Figure 7-11 shows the actual changes in pressure that occur in a bubble when we alter its size or surface tension. When the size of the bubble increases from A to B, the pressure drops, as predicted by the LaPlace formula. In contrast, bubble C shows how the pressure can remain unchanged as long as we lower the surface tension.

Because the alveoli in the lungs resemble clumps of bubbles, it follows that surface tension plays a key role in the mechanics of ventilation (see Chapter 11). Moreover, changes in alveolar surface tension are responsible for certain abnormal conditions, such as respiratory distress syndrome of the newborn. The role of surface tension in disease is addressed in Chapters 29 and 35.

Capillary action

Capillary action is a phenomenon in which a liquid in a small tube tends to move upward, against the force of gravity. Capillary action involves both adhesive and surface tension forces. As shown in Figure 7-12, *A*, the adhesion of water molecules to the walls of a thin tube causes an upward force on the liquid's edges and produces a concave meniscus.

Because surface tension acts to maintain the smallest possible liquid-gas interface, instead of just the edges of the liquid moving up, the whole surface is pulled upward. The force with which this occurs depends on how much liquid is in contact with the tube surface. Because a small capillary tube creates a more concave meniscus and thus a greater area of contact, liquid will rise higher in tubes with smaller cross-sectional areas (Figure 7-12, *B*).

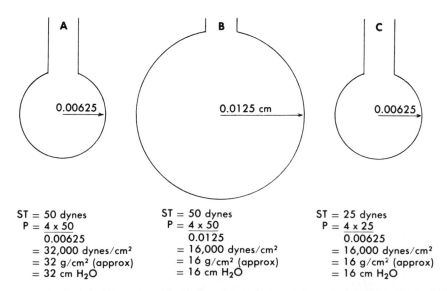

	A	B	C
	0.00625	0.0125 cm	0.00625
ST	= 50 dynes	= 50 dynes	= 25 dynes
P	$= \dfrac{4 \times 50}{0.00625}$	$= \dfrac{4 \times 50}{0.0125}$	$= \dfrac{4 \times 25}{0.00625}$
	= 32,000 dynes/cm²	= 16,000 dynes/cm²	= 16,000 dynes/cm²
	= 32 g/cm² (approx)	= 16 g/cm² (approx)	= 16 g/cm² (approx)
	= 32 cm H₂O	= 16 cm H₂O	= 16 cm H₂O

Fig. 7-11 The internal pressure of a single bubble varies with the size of the bubble and the surface tension of its liquid film. An increase in radius from **A** to **B** drops the pressure, but **C** shows that the same pressure drop can accompany a reduction in surface tension without changing bubble size.

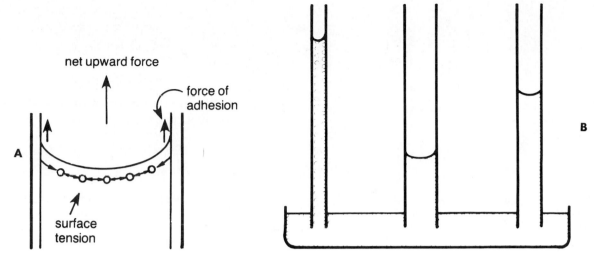

Fig. 7-12 The basis of capillary action. **A,** Adhesion and surface tension contribute to capillarity. **B,** The liquid rises highest in the smallest tube. (From Nave CR and Nave BC: Physics for the health sciences, ed 3, Philadelphia, 1985, WB Saunders.)

The principle of capillary action is the basis for "capillary-stick" blood samples. The absorbent wicks used in some gas humidifiers are also an application of this principle, as are certain types of surgical dressings.

Liquid–vapor phase changes

Returning to Figure 7-3, page 117, only after ice completely melts does additional heat raise the temperature of the newly formed liquid. As the temperature of the water reaches 100° C, a new change of state begins, from liquid to vapor. This change of state is called *vaporization*. There are two different forms of vaporization: *boiling* and *evaporation*.

Boiling

Boiling occurs at the boiling point. The boiling point of a liquid is defined as the temperature at which its vapor pressure equals the pressure exerted by the surrounding atmosphere. When a liquid boils, its molecules must have enough kinetic energy to force themselves into the atmosphere, against its opposing pressure. Because the weight of the atmosphere retards the escape of vapor molecules, the greater the atmospheric pressure, the greater the boiling point. Conversely, when atmospheric pressure is low, liquid molecules escape more easily and boiling occurs at lower temperatures. This is why changes in cooking times are needed at higher altitudes.

Although we associate boiling with high temperatures, the boiling points of most liquefied gases are very low. For example, at normal atmospheric pressure, oxygen boils at −183° C.

Just as energy is needed to liquefy a solid, energy is also required to vaporize a liquid. The energy required to vaporize a liquid is called the *latent heat of vaporization*. In cgs units, the latent heat of vaporization is the number of calories required to vaporize 1 g of a liquid at its normal boiling point.

As previously described, melting weakens the attractive forces between molecules but does not eliminate them. On the other hand, to vaporize a substance we must completely abolish these forces. In doing so, we convert essentially all the substance's internal energy into the kinetic energy of motion. For this reason, vaporization requires substantially more energy than does melting. As shown in Figure 7-3, page 117, nearly seven times as much energy is needed to convert water to steam (540 cal/gm) as is required to change ice to water. For comparison, see Table 7-4 for the latent heats of fusion and vaporization of some other common substances.

Table 7-4   Normal melting and boiling points and latent heats of fusion and vaporization of some common substances

Substance	Melting point (° C)	Heat of fusion (cal/g)	Boiling point (° C)*	Heat of vaporization (cal/g)
Water	0	80	100	540
Ammonia	75	108	−33	327
Ethyl alcohol	−114	26	78	204
Nitrogen	−210	6.2	−196	48
Oxygen	−219	3.3	−183	51
Lead	327	5.9	1620	208
Mercury	−39	2.7	357	68

*At standard atmospheric pressure of 760 mm Hg.

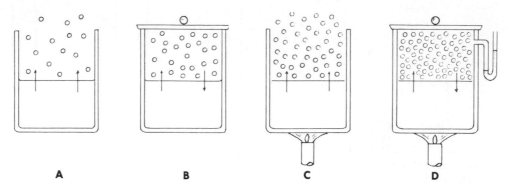

Fig. 7-13 The factors influencing vaporization of water are shown in these four sketches. **A,** The kinetic activity of molecules at the surface carries the molecules into the surrounding air, and evaporation gradually reduces the reservoir. **B,** If the container is covered, vaporization does not stop, but a state of equilibrium is reached when the air trapped in the container becomes saturated. At this point, water molecules leave and return to the reservoir in equal numbers. **C,** If the open container is heated, the increased molecular activity speeds the rate of vaporization. **D,** When the container is both covered and heated, more vapor will crowd into the trapped air, raising the vapor pressure as indicated by the attached manometer.

Evaporation, vapor pressure, and humidity

Boiling is only one means of vaporization. A liquid can change into a gas without being heated to its boiling point. The vaporization of a liquid occurring below its boiling point is called evaporation. Water is a good example (Figure 7-13).

Below its boiling point, water enters the atmosphere by evaporation. As in the gas phase, the molecules of liquid water are in constant motion. Although less intense than in the gaseous state, this kinetic energy allows some molecules near the surface to escape into the surrounding air as water vapor (Figure 7-13, A).

Once converted to its vapor form, water assumes the characteristics of a gas. To distinguish it from visible particulate water, such as mist or fog, this invisible gaseous form of water is often called *molecular water.* Molecular water obeys the same physical principles as other gases and therefore exerts a pressure, called *water vapor pressure.*

Of course, evaporation requires heat. The heat required for evaporation is taken from the air immediately next to the water surface, thus cooling the air. This is the principle of evaporation cooling, previously described.

If we place a cover over water container, water vapor molecules will continue to enter the trapped air until it can hold no more (Figure 7-13, B). At this point, the air over the water becomes *saturated* with water vapor. However, vaporization does not stop once saturation occurs. Instead, a state of equilibrium develops. In this equilibrium state, for every molecule escaping into the air another returns to the water reservoir.

Influence of temperature. No other factor influences evaporation more than temperature. Temperature affects evaporation in two ways. First, the warmer the air, the more vapor it holds. Specifically, the capacity of air to hold water vapor increases with temperature. Thus, when warm air comes into contact with a water surface, evaporation will occur at a faster rate than it would with cold air.

Second, if we heat the liquid water, we increase its kinetic energy and thus help more molecules escape from the water surface (Figure 7-13, C). Last, if we cover the container of heated water, the air will again become saturated (Figure 7-13, D). However, compared with air in the unheated state, (Figure 7-13, B), the heated saturated air now contains more vapor molecules and thus exerts a higher vapor pressure. Therefore the water content and the degree of saturation of air or any gas are a function of temperature.

The quantitative relationship between water vapor pressure and temperature appears in Figure 7-14. The *left* vertical axis of the graph plots water vapor pressure in both mm Hg and kPa (*kiloPascals*). Temperatures between 0° and 70° C are plotted on the horizontal x-axis. The intersection of any two axis points represents the water vapor pressure of air at that temperature. As is clear, the saturated water vapor pressure (indicated by the bold black dots) increases with increasing temperature. Table 7-5 lists the actual water vapor pressures in saturated air in the clinical range of temperatures (20° to 37° C).

Water vapor pressure is a measure of the kinetic activity of water molecules in air. If we want to know the actual amount of water vapor in a gas, we must measure its *water vapor content.* The actual amount or weight of water present in a volume of gas is called the *absolute humidity.*

Absolute humidity is expressed in grams of water vapor per cubic meter (gm/m³) or milligrams per liter (mg/L). You can measure the absolute humidity in air by physically removing the water vapor with an absorbing agent and then weighing the extracted water. Alternatively, you can compute absolute hu-

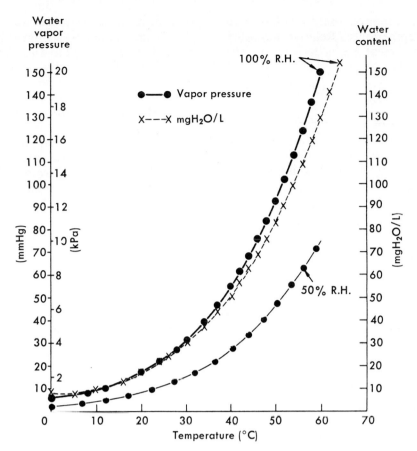

Fig. 7-14 Water vapor pressure (PH₂O) and absolute humidity (H₂O mg/L) curves for gas that is fully saturated (RH = 100%) and gas that is half saturated (RH = 50%). (From Sykes MK, McNicol MW, and Campbell EJM: Respiratory failure, ed 2, Oxford, England, 1976, Blackwell Scientific Publications.)

Table 7-5   Water vapor pressures and contents at selected temperatures

Temp (°C)	Vapor pressure (mm Hg)	Water vapor content (mg/L)	ATPS to BTPS correction factor*
20	17.50	17.30	1.102
21	18.62	18.35	1.096
22	19.80	19.42	1.091
23	21.10	20.58	1.085
24	22.40	21.78	1.080
25	23.80	23.04	1.075
26	25.20	24.36	1.068
27	26.70	25.75	1.063
28	28.30	27.22	1.057
29	30.00	28.75	1.051
30	31.80	30.35	1.045
31	33.70	32.01	1.039
32	35.70	33.76	1.032
33	37.70	35.61	1.026
34	39.90	37.57	1.020
35	42.20	39.60	1.014
36	44.60	41.70	1.007
37	47.00	43.80	1.000

*Correction factors based on 760 mm Hg pressure.

midity with meteorologic data according to the techniques of the U.S. Weather Bureau.

Values for absolute humidity of saturated air at various temperatures are plotted against the right vertical axis of Figure 7-14, using "x" hash marks. The middle column of Table 7-5 provides specific numeric values of absolute humidity for saturated air between 20° and 37° C.

A gas need not be fully saturated with water vapor. If a gas is only half-saturated with water vapor, its water vapor pressure and absolute humidity are only half that in the fully saturated state. As an example, air saturated with water vapor at 37° C and 760 mm Hg has a water vapor pressure of 47 mm Hg and an absolute humidity of 43.8 mg/L (Table 7-5). However, if the same volume of air was only 50% saturated with water vapor, its water vapor pressure would be 0.50 × 47, or 23.5 mm Hg, and its absolute humidity would be 0.50 × 43.8, or 21.9 mg/L.

When gas is less than fully saturated with water vapor, it is useful to express its water vapor content in relative terms. For this purpose, we apply a third measure of water vapor content, called *relative humidity*. The relative humidity of a gas is defined as the ratio of its actual water vapor content to its saturated capacity at a given temperature. Relative humidity (*RH*) is expressed as a percent and is derived with the following simple formula:

$$\%RH = \frac{\text{Content (absolute humidity)}}{\text{Saturated capacity}} \times 100$$

For example, at a room temperature of 20° C, saturated air has the *capacity* to hold about 17.3 mg/L water vapor (Table 7-5, page 125). If the absolute humidity is 12 mg/L, then the relative humidity is calculated as

$$\%RH = \frac{\text{Content (absolute humidity)}}{\text{Saturated capacity}} \times 100$$

$$\%RH = \frac{12}{17.3} \times 100$$

$$\%RH = 69\%$$

In reality, one need not measure the actual content of water vapor to derive the relative humidity. Simple instruments called *hygrometers* allow direct measurement of relative humidity without extraction and weighing of the water content of air samples.

When the water vapor content of a volume of gas equals its capacity, the relative humidity is 100% (fully saturated). Even slight cooling of a saturated gas will cause *condensation*. Condensation is the reverse of vaporization. During condensation, the gaseous form of a substance changes back to a liquid. Condensation occurs on whatever surface is available, such as on the sides of a container, on the walls of tubing, or on liquid or solid particles suspended in the gas.

The concept of latent heat of vaporization tell us that heat must be given up during condensation. When water condenses, this heat is given up to the air immediately next to the water surface, thereby warming the air. This is exactly the opposite of the principle of evaporation cooling previously described.

Take the example of air with a relative humidity of 90%. Should the temperature fall, air's capacity to hold water vapor will decrease. While its capacity decreases, its content remains the same, causing the relative humidity to increase. Eventually, a temperature will be reached at which the falling water vapor capacity equals the content. At this point the air is fully saturated with water vapor, and the relative humidity is 100%.

Because relative humidity never exceeds 100%, any further drop in temperature causes condensation. The temperature at which condensation begins is called the *dew point*. The greater the relative humidity of a gas, the higher its dew point. As a saturated gas is cooled below its dew point, more and more water vapor condenses out of the gas phase into liquid water droplets.

Figure 7-15 provides a useful analogy of the relationship between water vapor content, capacity, and relative humidity. The various-sized cups represent the capacity of a gas to hold water vapor. The bigger the cup, the greater its holding capacity. The water in the cups represents the actual water vapor content. Thus a cup that is half-full is at 50% capacity, or 50% relative humidity. A full cup represents the saturated state, equivalent to 100% relative humidity.

Figure 7-15, *A* shows what happens when a saturated gas is heated. When we heat a gas we raise its

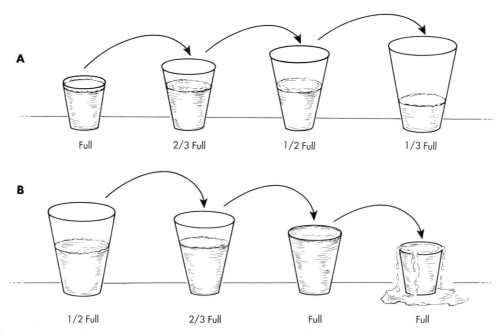

Fig. 7-15 Relative humidity analogy. **A** shows effect of increasing capacity without changing content, as when heating a saturated gas. **B** shows effect of decreasing capacity, as with cooling a gas (see text for details).

capacity to hold water vapor, but we do not change its content. This is equivalent to pouring the contents of the full cup at the left into larger and larger cups. The amount of water doesn't change, but as the cups get bigger and bigger, they become less full. We started with a full cup (100% relative humidity) but end up with one only one-third full (33% relative humidity).

Of course, a decrease in capacity would have the opposite effect. In Figure 7-15, *B,* we start with a large cup that is half full (50% relative humidity). We decrease the capacity by pouring our water into smaller and smaller cups (equivalent to decreasing the temperature). Eventually, the amount of water is enough to fill a smaller cup (100% relative humidity). What if we try to pour the water from this full cup into an even smaller cup? Because the smaller cup has less capacity, the excess content will have to spill over. This spillover is equivalent to the condensation of water that occurs when a saturated gas is cooled below its dew point. But note that although the excess moisture has been removed from the air by condensation, the smaller cup is still full (100% relative humidity).

The best clinical example of these processes is the hygroscopic condenser humidifier, or artificial nose (Figure 7-16). These devices consist of layers of water-absorbent material encased in plastic. When a patient exhales into an artificial nose, the warm saturated expired gases cool, causing condensation on the absorbent surfaces. As this condensation occurs, heat is generated in the device. When next the patient inhales from the device, the inspired gases are warmed, and the previously condensed water now evaporates, aiding in humidification of the airway. Chapter 25 provides more detail on humidification devices, including the artificial nose.

In clinical practice, we use a third measure of humidity called *percent body humidity* (%BH). The %BH of a gas is the ratio of its actual water vapor content to the water vapor capacity in saturated gas at body temperature (37° C). %BH is thus the same as relative humidity, except that the capacity (or denominator) is fixed at 43.8 mg/L.

$$\%BH = \frac{\text{Content (absolute humidity)}}{\text{Capacity at 37° C}} \times 100$$

or

$$\%BH = \frac{\text{Content (absolute humidity)}}{43.8 \text{ mg/L}} \times 100$$

For example, saturated air at a room temperature of 20° C contains about 17.3 mg/L water vapor, whereas saturated air at body temperature contains 43.8 mg/L. In this case, the room air could be said to provide about 40% (17.3/43.8 × 100) of the body's humidity.

Influence of pressure. Although high temperatures increase the rate of vaporization, high pressures hinder this process. Remember, water molecules trying to escape from a liquid surface must push their way out against the opposing air molecules. If the surrounding air pressure increases, there will be more opposing air molecules, and the rate of vaporization will decrease. Conversely, a decrease in atmospheric pressure will increase the rate of vaporization.

Influence of surface area. Logically, the greater the surface area available for evaporation, the easier it will be for liquid molecules to escape into the surrounding gas. For this reason, the rate of evaporation is directly proportional to the available surface area. You can easily prove this by comparing how quickly equal volumes of water evaporate under dry conditions from a flat plate versus a tall, narrow glass.

Properties of gases

As fluids, gases share many properties with liquids. Specifically, gases exert pressure, are capable of flow, and exhibit the property of viscosity. However, unlike liquids, gases are readily compressed and expanded and fill the spaces available to them by diffusion.

Kinetic activity of gases

Because the intermolecular forces of attraction in a gas are so weak, most of its internal energy is kinetic energy. Kinetic theory tells us that gas molecules travel about randomly at very high speed and with frequent collisions. For example, hydrogen molecules travel more than a mile a second. During that short time, more than a billion collisions will occur between the gas molecules and the surface of their container! The velocity of gas particles is directly proportional to temperature. As the temperature rises, the kinetic

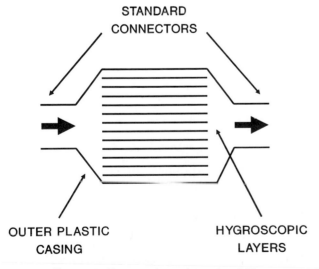

Fig. 7-16 Hygroscopic condenser humidifier.

STANDARD
CONNECTORS

OUTER PLASTIC
CASING

HYGROSCOPIC
LAYERS

activity of a gas increases, molecular collisions increase, and the pressure rises. Conversely, when the temperature drops, molecular activity declines, particle velocity and collision frequency drop, and pressure falls.

It is actually possible to see this intense kinetic activity at work. To do so, simply view a suspension of smoke particles under a microscope. Under low magnification, the smoke particles can be seen moving about in a rapid and erratic manner. This phenomenon, called *brownian movement,* is produced by the kinetic activity of the gas molecules randomly striking the larger smoke particles.

Molar volume and gas density

One of the major principles governing chemistry is *Avogadro's Law.* This law states that the 1 g atomic weight of any substance contains exactly the same number of atoms, molecules, or ions. This number— 6.023×10^{23} —is referred to as *Avogadro's number.* In SI units, this quantity of matter is known as a *mole.*

Molar volume. As applied to gases, Avogadro's Law states that equal volumes of gases under the same conditions contain the same number of molecules. Conversely, at a constant temperature and pressure, equal numbers of molecules of all gases occupy the same volume. The volume occupied by one mole of gas is termed the *molar volume.*

At STPD, the ideal molar volume of any gas is 22.4 L. In reality, variations in intermolecular behavior among different gases result in small deviations from this ideal. As indicated in Table 7-6, the molar volumes of most gases of clinical importance are very close to the predicted value of 22.4 L. The one exception is carbon dioxide, with a molar volume of about 22.3 L. We will use these values later to calculate gas densities and convert dissolved gas volumes into moles per liter.

Table 7-6 Molar volume of selected gases under standard conditions

Gas	Symbol	Molar volume (L)
"Ideal gas"		22.414
Ammonia	NH_3	22.094
Carbon dioxide	CO_2	22.262
Carbon monoxide	CO	22.402
Chlorine	Cl_2	22.063
Helium	He	22.426
Hydrogen	H_2	22.430
Hydrogen chloride	HCl	22.248
Nitrogen	N_2	22.402
Oxygen	O_2	22.393
Sulfur dioxide	SO_2	21.888

Modified from Pimental GC, editor: Chemistry, an experimental science, San Francisco, 1963, WH Freeman.

Density. Density is the ratio of a body's mass to its volume. A dense substance is characterized by heavy (high atomic weight) particles packed closely together. Uranium is a good example of a dense substance. Conversely, a low-density substance has a low concentration of light atomic particles per unit volume. Hydrogen gas is a good example of a low-density substance.

In clinical practice, we substitute weight for mass and thus actually measure weight density (weight per unit volume). Abbreviated as d_w, the weight densities of solids and liquids are most often measured in cgs units of grams per cubic centimeter. For gases, the most common unit is grams per liter.

Because weight density equals weight divided by volume, you can easily compute the density of any gas at STPD by dividing its molecular weight by the universal molar volume of 22.4 L (22.3 for CO_2). Examples of simple gas density calculations are shown in Table 7-7.

You can also calculate the density of a gas mixture if you know the percentage of each gas in the mixture. For example, to calculate the density of air at STPD, we first must know the proportion of gases constituting this mixture:

Gas	Percent	Fraction
Oxygen	21%	0.21
Nitrogen	79%	0.79

Using the gram molecular weights of these gases (Table 7-7), we set up a proportionality as follows:

$$\text{Density of mixture } (d_w) = \frac{(F_1 \times gmw_1) + (F_2 \times gmw_2) + \text{etc.}}{22.4}$$

where F_1 equals the fractional concentration of gas number 1, gmw_1 equals the gram molecular weight of gas number 1, F_2 equals the fractional concentration of gas number 2, gmw_2 equals the gram molecular weight of gas number 2, and so on, according to the number of gases in the mixture.

We thus compute the weight density of air as follows:

$$d_w \text{ air} = \frac{(FN_2 \times gmwN_2) + (FO_2 \times gmwO_2)}{22.4}$$

$$d_w \text{ air} = \frac{(0.79 \times 28) + (0.21 \times 32)}{22.4}$$

$$d_w \text{ air} = 1.29 \text{ g/L}$$

Gaseous diffusion

Diffusion is the physical process whereby molecules move from an area of high concentration to an area of lower concentration. Kinetic energy is the driving force behind diffusion. For this reason, diffusion is most rapid among gases. However, diffusion also occurs in liquids and can even take place in solids.

Among gases, rates of diffusion are defined by

Table 7-7   Examples of gas densities (D) under standard conditions

$$D\ O_2 = \frac{gmw}{22.4} = \frac{32}{22.4} = 1.43\ g/L \qquad D\ He = \frac{gmw}{22.4} = \frac{4}{22.4} = 0.1785\ g/L$$

$$D\ N_2 = \frac{gmw}{22.4} = \frac{28}{22.4} = 1.25\ g/L \qquad D\ CO_2 = \frac{gmw}{22.3} = \frac{44}{22.3} = 1.973\ g/L$$

Graham's Law. According to Graham's Law, lighter gases diffuse rapidly, whereas heavy gases diffuse more slowly. Mathematically, the rate of diffusion of a gas (*D*) is inversely proportional to the square root of its gram molecular weight:

$$D \approx \frac{1}{\sqrt{gmw}}$$

Because diffusion is based on kinetic activity, anything that increases the activity of molecules will increase their rate of diffusion. Thus heating and mechanical agitation speed the diffusion of both gases and liquids.

Gas pressure

All gases exert pressure, whether they are free in the atmosphere, enclosed in a container, or dissolved in a liquid such as blood. In physiology, the pressure exerted by a gas in a liquid is commonly referred to as its *tension.*

The pressure or tension of a gas depends mainly on its kinetic activity. In addition, gravity affects gas pressure. Although the kinetic activity of gas molecules is random, the pressure exerted by a gas is always higher near the earth's surface. This is because gravity increases gas density, thereby increasing the frequency of molecular collisions.

As we learned in Chapter 6, pressure equals force per unit area. The SI unit of pressure is the N/m², or pascal (Pa). In CGS units, pressure is measured in dynes/cm². In the British system, the most common unit for pressure measurement is pounds per square inch (lb/in²), sometimes abbreviated as *psi.* Also in common use are pressure units based on the *height* of liquid columns, because such columns are often used for pressure measurements. This is the method used most often in measurements of atmospheric pressure.

Measurement of atmospheric pressure. Many miles of atmospheric gases rest on the earth, exerting force on its surface. We call this force *atmospheric pressure.*

We measure atmospheric pressure with a *barometer.* A barometer consists of an **evacuated** glass tube about one meter long. This tube is closed at the top end, with its lower, open end immersed in a reservoir of mercury (Figure 7-17). The pressure of the atmosphere on the mercury reservoir forces the mercury up the vacuum tube a distance equivalent to the force exerted.

In this manner, the height of the mercury column represents the downward force of atmospheric pressure. The actual height is measured in inches (fps system) or millimeters (cgs system). Thus we report barometer pressure with readings such as 30.4 inches of mercury (Hg) or 772 mm Hg. This means that the atmospheric pressure is great enough to hold up a column of mercury 30.4 inches or 772 mm high.

Alternatively, you may see the term *torr* used in pressure readings. Torr is short for Torricelli, the 17th century inventor of the mercury barometer. At sea level, 1 torr equals 1 mm Hg. Thus a pressure reading of 772 torr is the same as 772 mm Hg.

Of course, the height of a column of mercury is not a true measure of pressure. Height is a linear measure, whereas pressure represents force per unit area. We already know that the pressure exerted by a liquid is

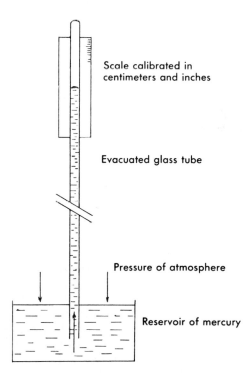

Fig. 7-17 The major components of a mercury barometer include a mercury reservoir, into which is inverted the open end of an evacuated glass tube, and a scale, by which the height of the mercury column can be read in inches and centimeters above the surface of the reservoir. The atmospheric pressure, acting on the surface of the mercury reservoir, is balanced by the weight of the column of mercury in the tube.

directly proportional to the depth of the liquid times its density. Thus, to compute the actual pressure exerted by the liquid (and thus the atmosphere), we need to know both the height of the column and the density of the liquid:

$$\text{pressure (P) in g/cm}^2 = \text{height in cm} \times \text{density in g/cm}^3$$
$$P = \text{cm} \times \text{g/cm}^3$$
$$P = \text{g/cm}^2$$

or

$$\text{pressure (P) in lb/in}^2 = \text{height in inches} \times \text{density in lb/in}^3$$
$$P = \text{inches} \times \text{lb/in}^3$$
$$P = \text{lb/in}^2$$

At sea level the average atmospheric pressure will support a column of mercury 76 cm (760 mm) or 29.9 inches high. If we also know that mercury has a density of 13.6 g/cm^3 (0.491 lb/in^3), then we can calculate the atmospheric pressure (P$_B$) by the formulas just given:

$$P \text{ in g/cm}^2 = 76 \times 13.6 = 1034 \text{ g/cm}^2$$
$$P \text{ in lb/in}^2 = 29.9 \times 0.491 = 14.7 \text{ lb/in}^2$$

Standard measures in the cgs and fps systems, equivalent to *one atmosphere of pressure* (1 atm), are 1034 g/cm^2 and 14.7 lb/in^2. Of course, the column heights of 29.9 inches or 760 mm Hg, though not really pressure measurements, are also *equivalent* to 1 atm of pressure. This equivalence (based on fluid column height) simplifies pressure measuring and recording and is the basis for most clinical measurements.

Like any solid material, a barometer housing reacts to temperature changes by expanding and contracting. Even more important, the mercury column barometer behaves like a large thermometer. Therefore, when you read a mercury barometer, you see the effects of both pressure and temperature. For accuracy you must correct your reading for changes caused by temperature.

The U.S. Weather Bureau provides factors for correcting barometric readings at any given temperature (Appendix 1). The pertinent value in the table is subtracted from the observed reading. For example, at 30° C you would correct an observed barometric reading of 750 mm Hg for temperature by subtracting 3.66 from 750 for a corrected reading of 746.34 (usually rounded off to 746.3 or just 746). For P$_B$ values between those listed in the table, simple linear interpolation is used.

Clinical pressure measurements. Mercury is the most common fluid used in pressure measurements, both in barometers and at the bedside. Because of its high density (13.6 g/cm^3), mercury assumes a height

that is easy and convenient to read for most pressures in the clinical range.

Water is also used as a fluid in pressure measurements, but only for relatively low pressures. Of course, we could construct a water barometer to measure atmospheric pressure. However, at 1 atm, water, which is 13.6 times lighter than mercury, would rise to a height of 33.9 feet or about as high as a two-story building!

Mercury and water columns are still used in clinical practice, especially in measuring vascular pressures. However, these traditional tools are rapidly being replaced by analog devices that measure pressure indirectly. Still, the accuracy of these newer analog devices depends on measures made with traditional columns of fluid. Indeed, most analog pressure gauges must still be calibrated against a mercury or water column before being used.

The simplest analog pressure gauge is the aneroid barometer, common in homes. An aneroid barometer consists of a sealed evacuated metal box with a flexible, spring-supported top that responds to external changes in pressure (Figure 7-18). This motion is magnified by levers to activate a geared pointer, which

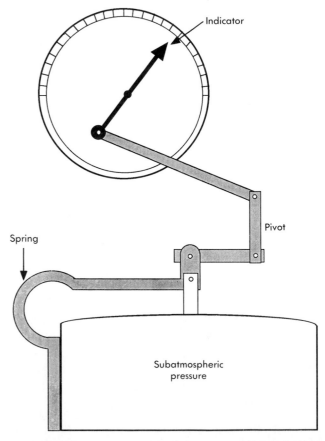

Fig. 7-18 Aneroid barometer opposes pliable strength of evacuated metal box with gas pressure. As gas pressure increases, box is forced to contract. Spring is pulled down, causing lever to pivot and move indicator to higher value on scale.

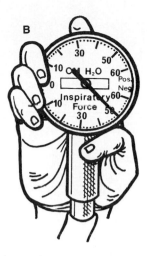

Fig. 7-19 An inspiratory force measurement. The gauge is attached to the patient's airway. **B.** The negative pressure detection, measured here as −50 cm of water, is the patient's maximum inspiratory force. (From Pilbeam SP: Mechanical ventilation: physiological and clinical applications, ed 1, St Louis, 1986, Multimedia Publishing.)

provides a scale reading *analogous* to pressure (thus the term *analog gauge*).

This same concept underlies the simple mechanical manometers used to measure blood or airway pressure at the bedside (Figure 7-19). However, rather than having the pressure act on the outside of the sealed chamber, we connect the inside to the pressure source. In this manner, the flexible chamber wall expands and contracts with increases or decreases in pressure.

Taking this principle one step further, we can use expansion and contraction of a flexible diaphragm to electronically measure pressure. In this device, called a strain-gauge pressure transducer, pressure changes cause expansion and contraction of a flexible metal diaphragm to which are attached electrical wires (Figure 7-20). The physical strain caused by expansion and contraction of the diaphragm changes the amount of electrical flow through the wires. This change in electrical flow is therefore analogous to pressure changes and can easily be measured (see subsequent section on electrical principles). Figure 7-21 shows a strain-gauge pressure transducer and pressure monitor being calibrated against a mercury fluid column (sphygmomanometer).

Millimeters of mercury (mm Hg) and centimeters of water (cm H_2O) are still the most common pressure units used in clinical practice. But neither is a standard SI unit. Because many clinicians encourage use of SI units for all physiologic measures, you must also be familiar with a third unit of pressure, the pascal (Pa).

In the SI system, 1 Pa equals 1 N/m^2. Because this is a very small quantity of pressure, we tend to express our pressure measurements in kilopascals (kPa). One kilopascal is roughly equal to 10 cm H_2O.

Figure 7-22, on page 132 is an alignment nomogram designed to help you convert one pressure unit to another. To use the nomogram, find the pressure being converted and place a ruler across the vertical scale at the point selected. Then read the equivalent pressure from the parallel scale corresponding to the

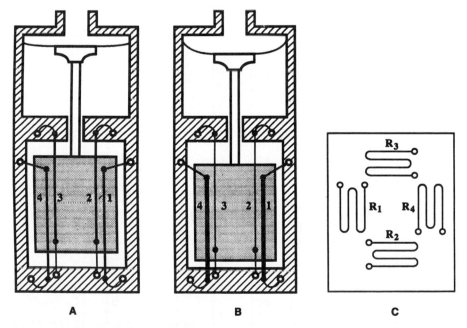

Fig. 7-20 Resistive strain gauge pressure transducer. Elements 1, 2, 3, and 4 are resistive wires. **A,** no pressure is applied. **B,** Pressure is applied to the transducer—the movement of the diaphragm is greatly exaggerated to illustrate the operating principle. **C,** Layout of resistors on a semiconductor "chip" for a modern disposable pressure transducer.

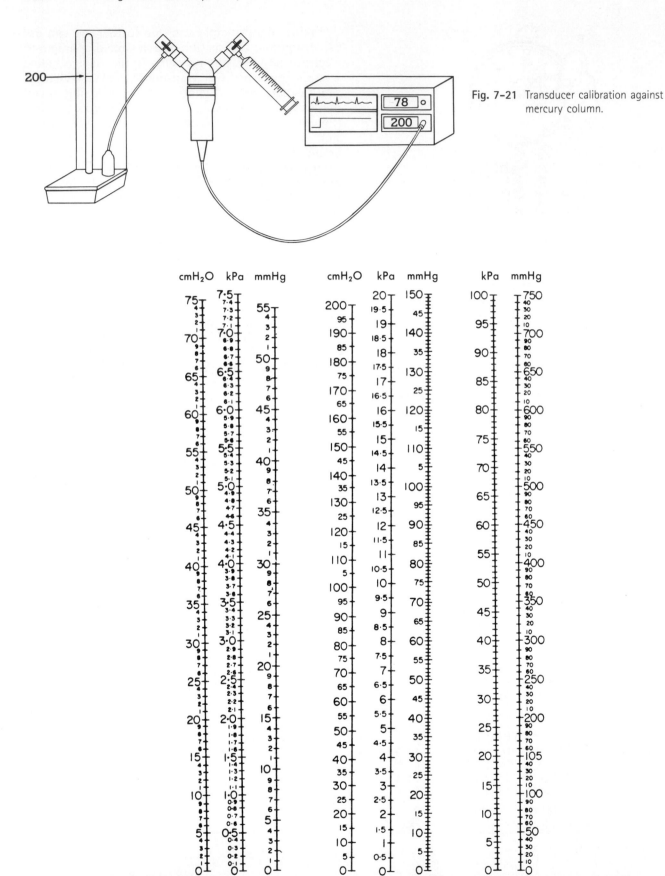

Fig. 7-21 Transducer calibration against mercury column.

Fig. 7-22 Chart for converting the more traditional units of pressure of cm H₂O and mm Hg to SI units: kPa. (From Sykes MK, McNichol MW, and Campbell EJM: Respiratory failure, ed 2, London, 1976, Blackwell Scientific Publications.)

units desired. Alternatively, the following table of conversions factors may be used:

cm H$_2$O	kPa	mm Hg
10.197	1	7.501
1.359	0.133	1
1	0.098	0.736

Partial pressures (Dalton's law)

Many gases exist together as mixtures. Air is a good example of a gas mixture, consisting mainly of oxygen and nitrogen. Like a solitary gas, a gas mixture exerts pressure. The pressure exerted by a mixture of gases must equal the sum of the kinetic activity of all the component gases. The pressure exerted by a single gas in a mixture is called the *partial pressure.*

Dalton's Law describes the relationship among the partial pressures and the total pressure in a gas mixture. According to this law, the total pressure of a gas mixture must equal the sum of the partial pressures of the component gases. Moreover, the partial pressure exerted by a component gas will always be proportional to its percentage in the mixture.

Thus a gas that represents 25% of a mixture would exert 25% of the total pressure. For purposes of computation and consistency, we always express the percentage of a gas in a mixture as a decimal and use the term *fractional concentration.* A gas that represents 25% of a mixture thus has a fractional concentration of 0.25.

As an example, air consists of about 21% O$_2$ and 79% N$_2$. To compute the partial pressure of each component gas, you simply multiply it fractional concentration times the total pressure. Assuming a normal atmospheric pressure of 760 mm Hg, you compute the individual partial pressures as follows:

Partial pressure = Fractional concentration × total pressure

$$PO_2 = 0.21 \times 760 = 160 \text{ mm Hg}$$
$$PN_2 = 0.79 \times 760 = \underline{600 \text{ mm Hg}}$$
$$760 \text{ mm Hg}$$

As predicted by Dalton's Law, the sum of the partial pressures equals the total pressure of the gas mixture.

What if the total (barometric) pressure were to change? In addition to minor fluctuations due to weather, barometric pressure changes are mainly a function of altitude. Focusing solely on oxygen, we know that is fractional concentration, or FIO_2, remains constant at about 0.21. At a PB of 760 mm Hg, the PO_2 is equal to 0.21 × 760, or 160 mm Hg. At 25,000 feet, the FIO_2 of air is still 0.21. However, the PB is only 282 mm Hg and the resulting PO_2 is 0.21 × 282, or 59 mm Hg, just over a third of that available at sea level! Because the PO_2 (not its percent) determines its physiologic activity, high altitudes can impair oxygen uptake by the lungs. This explains why mountain climbers must sometimes use extra oxygen on high mountains. By increasing the concentration of O2 above 0.21, we can raise its partial pressure and assure adequate uptake by the lungs. For a practical application of this principle, see the accompanying MiniClini 7-1.

Now this PIO_2 (about the same as at sea level) is sufficient to keep the passengers alive until the crew can bring the plane to a safe altitude.

In contrast, high atmospheric pressures increase the PIO_2 in an air mixture. Pressures significantly higher than atmospheric pressure are called *hyperbaric* pressures. Hyperbaric pressures commonly occur only in underwater diving and in special hyperbaric chambers.

For example, at a depth of 66 feet under the sea, water exerts a pressure of 3 atm, or 2280 mm Hg (3 × 760). At this depth, the oxygen in an air mixture breathed by a diver exerts a PO_2 of 0.21 × 2280 or about 479 mm Hg. This is nearly three times the partial pressure of oxygen at sea level!

The same conditions can be created on dry land in a hyperbaric chamber. In the armed forces and in industry, hyperbaric chambers are used for controlled

---

■ MINI **C**LINI ■

7-1

Why are Oxygen Masks Needed on Airplanes?

$$PIO_2 = 0.21 \times 226 = 47 \text{ mm Hg}$$

Problem: People who have traveled by air are familiar with the safety instructions given by the crew before flight. Part of these instructions describe how to use the oxygen masks. When and why are these masks needed?

Discussion: At a typical cruising altitude of 30,000 feet, the PB outside the airplane cabin is about 226 mm Hg. Thus the PIO_2 would be calculated as follows:

Should the cabin depressurize, travelers inside would be exposed to this low PIO_2. At this PIO_2, most people become unconscious within seconds and will eventually die of lack of oxygen (anoxia).

To overcome this problem, emergency oxygen masks are available when the cabin depressurizes. Assuming a tight fit, these masks probably provide about 70% oxygen, or an FIO_2 of 0.70. Wearing the mask, your PIO_2 would now be:

$$PIO_2 = 0.70 \times 226 = 158 \text{ mm Hg}$$

depressurization of deep sea divers and to treat certain types of diving accidents. Clinically, hyperbaric chambers and oxygen are used together to treat a variety of conditions, including carbon monoxide poisoning and gangrene. Chapter 26 provides more details on this use of high pressure oxygen.

Solubility of gases in liquids

Gases can dissolve in liquids. Carbonated water and soda pop are good examples of a gas (CO_2) dissolved in a liquid (water).

Henry's Law predicts exactly how much of a given gas will dissolve in a liquid. According to this law, for a given temperature, the volume of a gas that dissolves in a liquid equals its solubility coefficient times its partial pressure:

$$V_{dissolved\ gas} = \alpha \times P_{gas}$$

where α is the solubility coefficient of the gas in the given liquid and P_{gas} is the partial pressure of the gas above the liquid.

Each gas has a different *solubility coefficient* for each different liquid. This coefficient is the volume of gas that dissolves in 1 mL of a given liquid at standard pressure and specified temperature. For example, at 37° C and 760 mm Hg pressure the solubility coefficient of oxygen in plasma is 0.023 mL/mL. Under the same conditions, 0.510 mL of CO_2 will dissolve in 1 mL of plasma.

As you can see, temperature plays a crucial role in determining gas solubility in liquids. High temperatures decrease the amount of gas that dissolves in a liquid, whereas low temperatures have the opposite effect. This is why an open can of soda pop may still fizz if left in the refrigerator but quickly goes flat when left out at room temperature.

This effect is due to the changes in kinetic activity that occur with changes in temperatures. As the temperature of a liquid rises, the kinetic activity of its dissolved gas molecules also increases. This increased kinetic activity increases the escaping tendency of these molecules and thus their partial pressure. With an increased rate of molecular escape, the amount of gas left in solution decreases rapidly. For a practical application of this principle, see MiniClini 7-2 on page 135.

Solid–vapor phase changes (sublimation)

To complete our discussion of change of state, we must take a brief look at the transition from solid to vapor. Just like liquids, some solids can vaporize. Moreover, solids can exert vapor pressure. The strong odor of mothballs (napthalene) proves that vapor can and does escape from some solids.

The direct transition from a solid to a gas is called *sublimation*. As with all change of states, sublimation requires energy. The energy required during sublimation is called the *heat of sublimation*. The heat of sublimation equals the sum of the heats of fusion and vaporization.

Sublimation resembles boiling because it occurs when the vapor pressure of the solid equals that of the opposing **ambient** pressure. Also like boiling, increasing or decreasing the surrounding pressure alters the temperature at which sublimation occurs. High pressures impede sublimation, whereas low pressures aid the transition from solid to gas.

Solid CO_2, or dry ice, is a good example. If you cool CO_2 to −57° C under high pressure (5.1 atm), it will freeze. If you then expose this solid CO_2 to normal atmospheric pressure, the drop in pressure to 1 atm causes the solid state to sublime directly into vapor, leaving no trace of moisture.

GAS BEHAVIOR UNDER CHANGING CONDITIONS

Because of the relatively great distances between their molecules, gases are easily compressed and expanded. When pressure is applied to a gas, the molecules are pushed closer together. On the other hand, if a container holding a gas enlarges, the gas expands to accommodate the new volume, and its molecules spread further apart.

Figure 7-23 illustrates the concepts of gas compression and expansion, and the corresponding temperatures and pressure changes. As compression brings the molecules closer together, the frequency of collisions increases, and both temperature and pressure rise (Figure 7-23, *B*). Conversely, the expansion of a gas decreases the rate of molecular collisions, producing a drop in temperature and pressure (Figure 7-23, *C*).

The relationships among the pressure, temperature, mass and volume of gases are expressed in the gas laws. These laws allow us to explain and predict the behavior of gases under a variety of conditions. Underlying all these laws are three basic assumptions: (1) that no energy is lost during collisions between gas molecules, (2) that the volume actually occupied by these molecules is negligible, and (3) that no forces of mutual attraction exist between these molecules.

These three assumptions describe an "ideal gas." As we shall see, no gas is truly ideal. Gas behavior often fails to conform to these assumptions, especially at the extremes of pressure and temperature. However, under normal conditions most gases behave as if they were ideal.

Constant temperature processes (Boyle's law)

During the 1600s, Robert Boyle, a British physicist and chemist, observed that if the temperature and

■ M I N I **C** L I N I ■

7-2

Blood Gases vs. Patient Temperature

Problem: We frequently need to sample and measure the partial pressures of oxygen and carbon dioxide in patients' arterial blood. These samples are called **arterial blood gases,** or *ABGs.*

Typically, ABG samples are measured in analyzers kept at a normal body temperature of 37° C. But not all patients have normal body temperatures. Many will be feverish (*hyperpyrexia*); some will have low body temperatures (*hypothermia*). What effect does this have on our measurements?

Discussion: The direct relationship between temperature and partial pressure causes higher arterial PO_2 and PCO_2 readings at higher temper-

atures. At 37° C, the normal adult arterial PO_2 is about 100 mm Hg. However, at 47° C the PO_2 would be nearly twice as high. A smaller increase from 37° C to 39° C increases the arterial PO_2 less markedly, from 100 to about 110 mm Hg. Likewise, an increase in temperature raises the arterial PCO_2. Arterial PCO_2

values increase approximately 5% per degree Celsius. Thus an increase in temperature from 37° C to 39° C increases the PCO_2 by about 10%, from 40 to 44 mm Hg. Of course, the reverse is also true. Decreases in temperature decrease the arterial partial pressures of oxygen and carbon dioxide. Nomograms are available to help compute these corrections; however, the nomograms only correct for the relationship between temperature and pressure. They do not take into account metabolic and cardiovascular changes that accompany a change in a patient's temperature. For this reason, the use of corrected PO_2 and PCO_2 readings remains controversial.

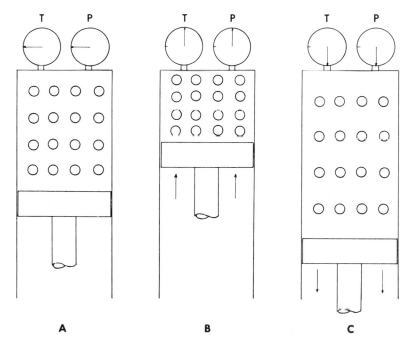

Fig. 7-23 A mass of gas in the resting state exerts a given pressure at a given temperature, in cylinder **A.** In **B,** as the piston compresses the gas, the molecules are crowded closer together, and the increased energy of molecular collisions is reflected in a rise of both temperature and pressure. Conversely, retraction of the piston in **C** allows the gas to expand, and temperature and pressure drop as molecular interaction decreases.

mass of a gas remained constant, its volume varied inversely with its pressure. Expressed as a formula,

$$PV = k$$

where P is the pressure of the gas, V its volume, and k a constant of proportionality.

According to Boyle's Law, if you keep the temperature of a given mass of a gas constant, increasing its pressure will decrease its volume. Conversely, decreasing its pressure will increase its volume.

To calculate the change in volume that occurs when a gas is subject to a change in pressure, you simply set up an equality between the conditions of pressure and volume *before* (condition 1) and *after* (condition 2) the change, as follows:

$$P_1V_1 = P_2V_2$$

To solve for a new volume (V_2), simply rearrange the equation above:

$$V_2 = V_1 \times \frac{P_1}{P_2}$$

As an example, suppose you have a 2 L of a gas (V_1) existing at 1 atm, or 760 mm Hg of pressure (P_1). What would be the new volume of the gas (V_2) if you were to *increase* its pressure to 1520 mm Hg (P_2)? Using the above equation,

$$V_2 = V_1 \times P_1/P_2$$
$$V_2 = 2\ L \times 760\ mm\ Hg/1520\ mm\ Hg$$
$$V_2 = 2\ L \times 0.5$$
$$V_2 = 1\ L$$

Thus, by doubling the pressure on the gas, you halve its original volume.

Boyle's Law describes gas behavior under conditions of constant temperature. Processes of gas compression or expansion in which the temperature remains constant are called *isothermal* processes. The First Law of Thermodynamics dictates that to keep the temperature constant during such processes, heat must be added (during expansion) or taken away (during compression) to maintain the energy equilibrium.

During isothermal expansion in which no external work is performed, the temperature of a gas should not change. For example, when a gas is allowed to escape from a high-pressure cylinder into the atmosphere, there should be no temperature change. However, this is not the case. In fact, the rapid expansion of a gas causes substantial cooling. This phenomenon of expansion cooling is called the *Joule-Thompson Effect*.

Cooling occurs during the rapid expansion of a gas because the forces of mutual attraction (van der Waals

forces) between molecules must be broken. Because the energy needed to break these forces must come from the gas itself, the temperature of the gas must decrease. Depending on the pressure drop that occurs, this decrease in temperature can be large enough to actually liquefy the gas. This is the primary method used to liquefy air for the production of oxygen, as described in Chapter 24.

Whereas isothermal processes keep the temperature constant by adding or removing heat, *adiabatic* processes have no such restrictions. During adiabatic compression or expansion, heat energy is neither added to nor taken away from the gas. Under these conditions, the gas' heat energy will vary according to changes in its pressure or volume.

For example, adiabatic compression of a gas can cause a rapid increase in its temperature. A diesel engine uses this principle to ignite the fuel mixture without a spark. Adiabatic compression can also occur in medical gas delivery systems when a gas undergoes rapid compression within a fixed container. The increase in temperature caused by this rapid compression can cause ignition of any **combustible** material in the system. It is for this reason that RCPs must take care to clear any combustible matter from high-pressure gas delivery systems before pressurization.

Constant pressure processes (Charles' law)

About a century after Boyle's discovery, the Frenchman Jacques Charles observed that if the pressure and mass of a gas were kept constant, its volume varied directly with changes in its *absolute* temperature. Expressed as a formula:

$$\frac{V}{T} = k$$

where T is the temperature of the gas (in degrees Kelvin), V its volume, and k a constant of proportionality. According to this law, if a given mass of a gas is kept at a constant pressure, an increase in its absolute temperature causes an increase in its volume. Conversely, decreasing the temperature of the gas will decrease its volume.

To calculate the change in volume that occurs when a gas is subject to a change in temperature, you establish another simple equality:

$$\frac{V_1}{T_1} = \frac{V_2}{T_2}$$

To solve for a new volume (V_2), simply rearrange the equation above:

$$V_2 = V_1 \times \frac{T_2}{T_1}$$

As an example, suppose you have a 8 L of a gas (V_1) existing at 0° C, or 273° K (T_1). To compute the new volume of the gas (V_2) after decreasing its temperature to 200° K (−73° C), you simply apply the equation above:

$$V_2 = V_1 \times T_2/T_1$$
$$V_2 = 8 \text{ L} \times 200° \text{ K}/273° \text{ K}$$
$$V_2 = 8 \text{ L} \times 0.73$$
$$V_2 = 5.84 \text{ L}$$

Constant volume processes (Gay-Lussac's law)

As a corollary to Boyle's and Charles' laws, the Frenchman Joseph Louis Gay-Lussac observed that if the volume and mass of a gas remained fixed, the pressure exerted by the gas varied directly with its absolute temperature. Expressed as a formula,

$$\frac{P}{T} = k$$

where T is the temperature of the gas (in degrees Kelvin), P its pressure, and k a constant of proportionality. According to this law, if a given mass of a gas is kept at a constant volume, an increase in its absolute temperature will cause its pressure to rise. Conversely, decreasing the temperature of the gas will decrease its pressure.

To calculate the change in pressure that occurs when a gas is subject to a change in temperature, you set up another simple equality:

$$\frac{P_1}{T_1} = \frac{P_2}{T_2}$$

To solve for a new pressure (P_2), simply rearrange the equation above:

$$P_2 = P_1 \times \frac{T_2}{T_1}$$

As an example, suppose you have a volume of gas in a fixed-size cylinder at 2200 lb/in² (P_1), at a room temperature of 20° C or 293° K (T_1). To compute the new pressure of the gas (P_2) if the temperature were to increase to 323° K, or 50° C (T_2), you simply apply the equation above:

$$P_2 = P_1 \times T_2/T_1$$
$$P_2 = 2200 \text{ lb/in}^2 \times 323° \text{ K}/293° \text{ K}$$
$$P_2 = 2200 \text{ lb/in}^2 \times 1.102$$
$$P_2 = 2425 \text{ lb/in}^2$$

Combined gas law

Seldom is the pressure, volume, or temperature of a gas actually constant. For this reason, it is useful to treat all these properties (including mass) as variables and combine them into a single equation. This single equation is called the *combined gas law*. Expressed as a formula,

$$PV = nRT$$

where P is the pressure of the gas, V its volume, n its mass, T its temperature, and R a combined constant of proportionality, often called the *gas constant*.

In clinical practice, we are interested mainly in how changes in pressure, volume, and temperature affect each other. Because the gas constant does not change, it need not be included in your calculations. Moreover, because the total mass of a gas will not be affected, you can eliminate it from your computations. You then set up a simple equality between the three main variables: pressure, volume, and temperature:

$$\frac{P_1 V_1}{T_1} = \frac{P_2 V_2}{T_2}$$

This equation represents the working form of the combined gas law under conditions of constant mass. By rearranging this equation, you can determine the combined effect of changes in any two variables on the third. For example, to solve for V_2 under conditions of changing temperature and pressure, you rearrange the equation as follows:

$$V_2 = \frac{V_1 \times P_1 \times T_2}{P_2 \times T_1}$$

Thus, to calculate the new volume (V_2) of 3 L of gas existing at 273° K (T_1) and 760 mm Hg (P_1) when heated to 300° K (T_2) and subject to 1520 mm Hg (P_1) pressure:

$$V_2 = \frac{V_1 \times P_1 \times T_2}{P_2 \times T_1}$$
$$V_2 = \frac{3 \text{ L} \times 760 \text{ mm Hg} \times 300° \text{ K}}{1520 \text{ mm Hg} \times 273° \text{ K}}$$
$$V_2 = 1.65 \text{ L}$$

Correcting for water vapor

In clinical practice, most gas calculations involve gases saturated with water vapor. Like any gas, water vapor occupies space. For this reason, removal of water vapor from a gas mixture shrinks the total volume. Conversely, the addition of water vapor increases the total volume.

Therefore, whenever we need to know what volume a saturated gas would occupy if dry, we must subtract that amount due to water vapor. Thus the dry volume of a gas at a constant pressure and temperature is always smaller than its saturated volume. The opposite is also true. Correcting from the dry state to the saturated state always yields a larger gas volume.

In addition to its effect on the volume of a gas mixture, water vapor also affects the partial pressure of gases in a gas mixture. Water vapor pressure is not affected by the other gases with which it mixes, depending only on the temperature and relative humidity. For this reason, the addition of water vapor to a gas mixture always lowers the partial pressures of the other gases present.

Corrected pressure computations

To compute the new or corrected partial pressure of a gas after the addition of water vapor, apply the following formula:

$$P_C = F_{gas}(P_T - P_{H_2O})$$

where *PC* is the corrected gas pressure, F_{gas} the fractional concentration of the gas in the gas mixture, *PT* the total gas pressure of the mixture, and P_{H_2O} the water vapor pressure at the given temperature, as listed in Table 7-5. If only a single gas is present, then F_{gas} equals 1, and the formula can be simplified:

$$P_C = (P_T - P_{H_2O})$$

For example, in the presence of saturated gas, you would have to modify Boyle's Law as follows:

$$V_2 = V_1 \times \frac{(P_1 - P_{H_2O} \text{ at } T_1)}{(P_2 - P_{H_2O} \text{ at } T_2)}$$

Correction factors

Instead of doing repetitive calculations, you can use correction factors. In gas volume conversions, the three most common computations are: (1) correction from ATPS to BTPS, (2) correction from ATPS to STPD, and (3) correction from STPD to BTPS.

Factors to correct volumes from ATPS to BTPS. The values in the third column of Table 7-5, when multiplied by V_1, will convert a gas volume from ATPS to BTPS. Because these factors are based on a PB of 760 mm Hg, they provide only a close estimate of the corrected gas volume at other pressures. However, this discrepancy will usually be of little clinical significance at sea level.

For example, to convert a saturated gas volume

of 3 L at an atmospheric pressure of 760 mm Hg and a room temperature of 20° C to its equivalent saturated volume at 37° C, you simply find the appropriate factor, in this case 1.102. Then multiply the original volume (at ATPS) by the conversion factor:

$$V_{BTPS} = V_{ATPS} \times \text{conversion factor}$$
$$V_{BTPS} = 3.0 \text{ L} \times 1.102$$
$$V_{BTPS} = 3.306 \text{ L}$$

Factors to correct volumes from ATPS to STPD. Appendix 2 provides the factors needed to convert a gas volume from ATPS to STPD. Because these factors already incorporate a temperature correction for your barometric readings, you should use the *uncorrected* barometric value to obtain the appropriate factor.

For example, to correct a saturated gas volume of 2 L at an observed PB of 770 mm Hg and a room temperature of 20° C to its equivalent dry gas volume at 760 mm Hg and 0° C (STPD), you simply find the appropriate factor, in this case 0.919. Then multiply the original volume (at ATPS) by the conversion factor:

$$V_{STPD} = V_{ATPS} \times \text{conversion factor}$$
$$V_{STPD} = 2.0 \text{ L} \times 0.919$$
$$V_{STPD} = 1.838 \text{ L}$$

Factors to correct volumes from STPD to BTPS. Factors for this conversion appear in Appendix 3. In this conversion, ambient pressure is the only variable.

For example, to convert a dry gas volume of 4 L at a standard pressure of 760 mm Hg to its equivalent saturated volume at 37° C and a PB of 740 mm Hg, you again use the table to identify the appropriate factor, in this case 1.245. Then multiply the original volume (at STPD) by the conversion factor:

$$V_{BTPS} = V_{STPD} \times \text{conversion factor}$$
$$V_{BTPS} = 4.0 \text{ L} \times 1.245$$
$$V_{BTPS} = 4.98 \text{ L}$$

Properties of gases at extremes of temperature and pressure

Up to this point, we have only looked at how gases behave in the ideal state. Now we will consider variations from the ideal, in which gases undergo extreme changes in temperatures and pressure. Only under such circumstances do gases begin to deviate substantially from ideal behavior.

As previously discussed, the weak attractive forces between gas molecules oppose their kinetic activity. Both temperature and pressure affect these forces. For example, at high temperatures, the increased kinetic activity of gas molecules far overshadows these relatively weak forces, rendering them relatively unimportant. At very low temperatures, however, the decrease in kinetic activity increases the effect of these forces. Likewise, very low pressures permit gas molecules to move freely about with little mutual attraction. In contrast, high pressures crowd molecules together, increasing the influence of the van der Waals forces.

In addition to the mutual attractive forces they share, the actual space occupied by the molecules can influence gas behavior. At low pressure, the total mass of matter in a gas is a negligible fraction of the total volume. However, at very high pressures molecular density become important, altering the expected relationship between pressure and volume.

Critical temperature and pressure

For every liquid there is a temperature above which the kinetic activity of its molecules is so great that the attractive forces cannot keep them in a liquid state. This temperature is called the *critical temperature.*

Because no amount of pressure can keep the molecules in a liquid state above this temperature, the critical temperature is the highest temperature at which a substance can exist in liquid form. The pressure needed to maintain equilibrium between the liquid and gas phases of a substance at this critical temperature is called the *critical pressure.* Together, the critical temperature and pressure represent the *critical point* of a substance.

For example, the critical temperature of water is 374° C. At this temperature, a pressure of 218 atm is needed to maintain equilibrium between water's liquid and gaseous forms. Beyond 374° C, no pressure can return water vapor to its liquid form.

Compared with liquids, gases tend to have much lower critical points. Table 7-8 lists the critical points of three common therapeutic gases: oxygen, helium, and carbon dioxide. Note that the critical temperatures of all the gases except carbon dioxide are well below room temperature.

Heretofore, we have used the terms *gas* and *vapor* more or less interchangeably. Now that you understand the concept of critical temperature, you can better distinguish between these terms. A true gas is a substance with a critical temperature so low that at

Table 7-8   Critical points of three gases

	°C	°F	atm
Helium	−267.9	−450.2	2.3
Oxygen	−118.8	−181.1	49.7
Carbon dioxide	31.1	87.9	73

room temperature and pressure it simply cannot exist as a liquid. In contrast, a vapor is the gaseous state of a substance coexisting with its liquid or solid state.

Thus oxygen is a true gas because it has no solid or liquid phase under ambient conditions. Water exists as both liquid and gas at room temperature and pressure. Under these conditions, the gaseous phase of water is properly referred to as a *vapor*. Appendix 4 lists the critical temperatures of several gaseous and vaporous substances.

Understanding the concept of critical temperature and pressure also helps explain some practical aspects of gas liquefaction. To change a gas into a liquid, you must cool the gas below its critical temperature and then compress it. Of course, it is possible to liquefy a gas by means of cooling alone, dropping its temperature below its boiling point. But under no circumstances can you liquefy a gas by pressure alone if its temperature is above its critical point. The further below its critical temperature a gas is cooled, the less pressure is needed to liquefy it.

According to these principles, any gas with a critical temperature above ambient can be liquefied by pressure alone. For example, the critical temperature of CO_2 (31° C) is slightly above normal room temperature. At a room temperature of 21.5° C, you can liquefy CO_2 by simply applying about 60 atm of pressure. To convert the liquid CO_2 back to its gaseous state, you simply lower its pressure.

Like CO_2, any gas with a critical temperature above ambient can be kept in the liquid state at room temperature. However, such liquids still need to be stored under pressure, usually in strong storage cylinders. Along with CO_2, the **anesthetic** gases cyclopropane and nitrous oxide are commercially supplied as tanked liquids. Table 7-9 compares their critical points with the approximate pressures at which they are kept at room temperature to maintain their liquid state. Oxygen presents a more complicated problem.

Table 7-9   Pressures needed to maintain liquid state of gases at room temperature

Gas	Critical temperature		Critical pressure		Approximate pressure in commercial cylinder at room temperature	
	°C	°F	atm	psi	atm	psi
Cyclopropane	125	257	54.2	797	5.4	79
Nitrous oxide	36.5	97.7	71.8	1054	50.6	745
Carbon dioxide	31.1	87.9	73.0	1071	57.0	838

Because of the widespread medical and industrial use of oxygen, moving and storage are made easier when it is stored in the liquid state. However, compared with the three gases discussed earlier, oxygen has a low critical temperature, $-118.8°$ C ($-181.1°$ F). This tells us that no pressure can keep oxygen as a liquid above that temperature.

In the manufacture of oxygen, large quantities of filtered air are compressed to very high pressures, up to 200 atm. Once compressed, the air is subjected to a rapid drop in pressure. This large pressure drop expands the gas, and according to the Joule-Thompson Effect, rapidly lowers its temperature. In this manner the oxygen in the air mixture is taken below its boiling point of $-183°$ C ($-297°$ F), and it liquefies.

Once removed from air and liquefied, the oxygen can be kept in an insulated container. As long as its temperature does not exceed its boiling point, the oxygen will remain liquid at atmospheric pressure. Should higher temperatures be needed, higher pressures must be used. If at any time the liquid oxygen is allowed to exceed its critical temperature of $-118.8°$ C, it will convert immediately back to a gas.

FLUID DYNAMICS

So far, we have limited our look at the physical principles of liquids and gases to static, or nonmov-ing, conditions. However, both liquids and gases exhibit the dynamic characteristic of *flow*. Unlike the random process of diffusion, flow represents the bulk movement of a substance through space.

The branch of physics involved in the study of fluids in motion is called *hydrodynamics*. Because much of the equipment used in respiratory care is based on hydrodynamic concepts, careful analysis of its underlying principles is essential to further study.

Pressures in flowing fluids

As we have seen, in a static liquid the pressure depends solely on the depth and density of the fluid. In contrast, the pressure exerted by a flowing liquid is dictated by the nature of the flow itself.

As depicted in Figure 7-24, *A,* the pressure exerted by a static fluid is the same at all points along a horizontal tube, depending only on the height of the liquid column. However, when the fluid flows out through the bottom tube, the pressure drops continuously all along the tube length (Figure 7-24, *B*).

Careful analysis also shows that the relative pressure drops between each of the equally spaced vertical tubes are the same. That is, the drops in pressure along each successive unit length in a flowing fluid are equal.

This progressive drop in pressure during flow re-

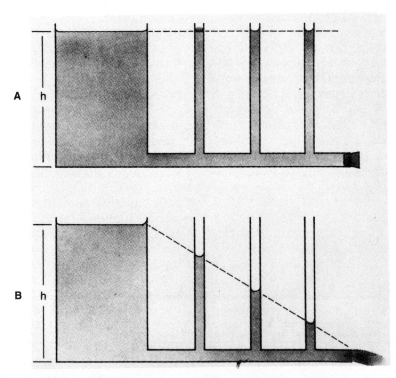

Fig. 7-24 A, The pressure is the same at all points along the horizontal tube when there is no flow. **B,** A uniform pressure drop occurs when there is smooth flow through a uniform tube. (From Nave CR and Nave BC: Physics for the health sciences, ed 3, Philadelphia, 1985, WB Saunders.)

flects a cumulative loss of energy, as predicted by the *Second Law of Thermodynamics*. In simple terms, this law states that in any mechanical process, there will always be a decrease in the total energy available to do work.

This decrease in available work energy is due mainly to frictional resistance against flow. Frictional resistance exists both within the fluid itself (viscosity) and between the fluid and the tube wall. In general, the greater the viscosity of the fluid and the smaller the cross-sectional area of the tube, the greater will be the drop in pressure along the tube.

For any given tube length, this *resistance* to flow equals the difference in pressure between the two points along the tube, divided by the actual flow. Expressed as a formula,

$$R = \frac{P_1 - P_2}{\dot{V}}$$

where R is the total resistance to fluid flow, P_1 the pressure at the upstream point (point 1), P_2 the pressure at the downstream point (point 2), and $\dot{V}$ the flow (volume/time).

The pressure difference due to flow also varies according to the nature of the flow itself. There are three primary patterns of flow through tubes.

Patterns of flow

The three primary patterns of fluid flow through tubes are laminar, turbulent, and tracheobronchial or transitional (Figure 7-25).

Laminar flow

As described earlier in our discussion on viscosity, during laminar flow a fluid moves in discrete cylindrical layers or streamlines. Under conditions of laminar flow through a smooth tube of fixed size, the difference in pressure required to produce a given flow is defined by *Poiseuille's Law:*

$$\triangle P = \frac{n8l\dot{V}}{\Pi r^4}$$

where $\triangle P$ is the driving pressure gradient, n the viscosity of the fluid, l the tube length, $\dot{V}$ the fluid flow, r the tube radius, and Π and 8 constants.

According to this formula, the pressure difference needed for laminar flow through a tube is directly proportional to the viscosity of the fluid, the length of the tube, and the rate of flow. In contrast, this pressure difference varies inversely with the fourth power of the tube radius.

In practical terms, when a fluid flows through a tube in a laminar pattern, higher driving pressures will be needed whenever the fluid viscosity, tube length, or flow increases. Likewise, you can predict that higher driving pressures will be required if the radius of the tube decreases.

Turbulent flow

Under certain conditions, the nature of fluid flow through a tube changes significantly. The orderly pattern of concentric layers is lost. Molecular movement becomes chaotic, with the formation of irregular eddy currents. This pattern is called turbulent flow.

When flow becomes turbulent, Poiseuille's Law no longer applies. Instead, the driving pressure required to move a volume of fluid through a tube is defined by the following equation:

$$\triangle P = \frac{fl\dot{V}^2}{4\Pi^2 r^5}$$

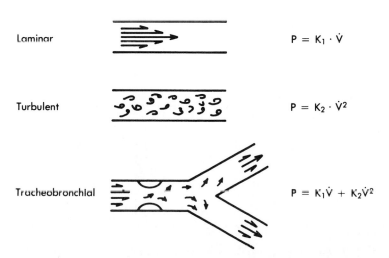

Laminar		$P = K_1 \cdot \dot{V}$
Turbulent		$P = K_2 \cdot \dot{V}^2$
Tracheobronchial		$P = K_1\dot{V} + K_2\dot{V}^2$

Fig. 7-25 The three patterns of flow: laminar, turbulent, and tracheobronchial. (From Moser KM and Spragg RG: Respiratory emergencies, ed 2, St Louis, 1982, Mosby.)

where $\triangle P$ is the driving pressure gradient; f a friction factor that incorporates fluid density, fluid viscosity, and the roughness of the tube wall; l the tube length; $\dot{V}$ the fluid flow; and r the tube radius.

The major difference between this formula and Poiseuille's Law is the relationship between driving pressure and flow. In Poiseuille's Law, the driving pressure is linearly proportional to the flow. In contrast, when flow is turbulent the driving pressure is proportional to the *square* of the flow.

Transitional flow

A mixture of laminar and turbulent flow is termed transitional or tracheobronchial flow. Under these conditions, the pressure-flow relationship depends on the relative influence of the laminar and turbulent components. When flow is mainly laminar, the driving pressure varies linearly with the flow. In contrast, when flow is mainly turbulent, the driving pressure will vary the square of the flow. Moreover, if laminar flow is dominant, pressure and flow changes will be affected mainly by the fluid's viscosity. On the other hand, if flow is mainly turbulent, pressure and flow changes will be affected most by the fluid's density.

Flow, velocity, and cross–sectional area

As we have seen, flow is measured as the bulk movement of a volume of fluid per unit of time. Clinically, the most common units of flow are liters/minute or liters per second. In contrast, velocity is a measure of linear distance traveled by the fluid per unit of time. Centimeters per second is a common velocity unit used in pulmonary physiology.

Although fluid flow and velocity are different measures, the two concepts are closely related. The key factor relating velocity to flow is the cross-sectional area available for flow. Figure 7-26 demonstrates this relationship.

At the beginning of the tube, fluid is moving at a constant rate of 5 L/min (the volumetric flow rate). At point A, the cross-sectional area is 5.08 cm^2, and the velocity of the fluid is calculated as 16.4 cm/sec. As the fluid approaches point B, the cross-sectional area is halved to 2.54 cm^2. At this point, the velocity of the fluid doubles to 32.8 cm/sec. Finally, as we move toward point C, the tube divides into eight smaller conduits. Although each of these tubes by itself is smaller than its "parent," together they result in a 10-fold increase in the total cross-sectional area available for flow, compared with point B. Here the velocity of the fluid decreases proportionately, from 32.8 to 3.28 cm/sec.

On the basis of these observations, we may state that the velocity of a fluid moving through a tube at a constant flow varies inversely with the available cross-sectional area. Mathematically, this relationship is expressed as follows:

$$(A_1 \times v_1) + (A_2 \times v_2) + (A_n \times v_n) = k$$

where A is the cross-sectional area of the tube; v the velocity of the fluid; $1, 2,$ and n different points in the conduit; and k a constant value.

This relationship between fluid velocity and cross-sectional area is called *Law of Continuity.* Although the principle holds true only for the flow of incompressible liquids, the qualitative features are similar for gas flow. This principle also underlies the application of nozzles or jets in fluid streams. Nozzles and jets are simply narrow passages in a tube designed to increase the velocity of the fluid flowing through

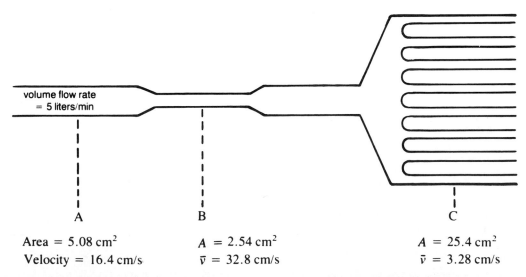

Area = 5.08 cm^2	A = 2.54 cm^2	A = 25.4 cm^2
Velocity = 16.4 cm/s	$\bar{v}$ = 32.8 cm/s	$\bar{v}$ = 3.28 cm/s

Fig. 7-26 The flow rate is maintained at a constant value by varying the velocity of the fluid. (From Nave CR and Nave BC: Physics for the health sciences, ed 3, Philadelphia, 1985, WB Saunders.)

them. A garden-hose nozzle is a good example of this principle in action. Clinically, jets are used in many types of respiratory care equipment, including pneumatic nebulizers (see Chapter 25) and gas entrainment or mixing devices (Chapter 26).

The Bernoulli effect

As we have seen, when a fluid flows through a tube of uniform diameter, the pressure drops progressively over the length of the tube. This pressure drop is illustrated by the first three water columns in Figure 7-27. However, when the fluid passes through a **constriction** in the tube, the pressure drop is much greater. This large pressure drop is evident in the fourth water column in Figure 7-27.

The eighteenth-century scientist Daniel Bernoulli was the first to carefully study this effect, which now bears his name. On the basis of his analysis, Bernoulli formulated a theorem to explain the interaction of variables causing this pressure drop. Central to his theorem is the concept that a moving fluid has three types of energy: potential energy, kinetic energy, and pressure energy.

The potential energy of a moving fluid is based on its position. If any section of the flow tube is elevated above the horizontal plane, gravity will impart potential energy on the fluid. The potential energy of a moving fluid is thus equivalent to the static pressure exerted by a liquid column. In a level tube, this static pressure (and thus potential energy) remains constant and is disregarded.

Kinetic energy is the amount of work performed by matter in motion. The kinetic energy of a moving fluid is directly proportional to both its velocity and density. The greater the velocity and density (mass) of a fluid, the greater its kinetic energy. If density is constant, kinetic energy varies directly with velocity only.

Whereas potential and kinetic energy are well understood concepts, the principle of pressure energy is unique to fluid flow. The pressure energy of a fluid is the radial or outward force exerted by the moving fluid. This radial force is measured as the *lateral pressure* exerted by the fluid.

According to the First Law of Thermodynamics, the total energy at any given point in a fluid stream must be the same everywhere throughout the tube. If potential energy is held constant, then the sum of the kinetic and pressure energies at any given point in a fluid stream must equal their sum at any other point.

Of course, velocity is the kinetic energy of a fluid, and lateral force its pressure energy. Because their sum must always be equal, the velocity and lateral pressure in a fluid stream must be inversely related. In other words, if additional energy is expended to increase velocity, then the amount of energy available to exert pressure must decrease. As velocity increases, lateral pressure decreases. Conversely, as velocity decreases, lateral pressure increases.

Figure 7-28 demonstrates this relationship. Fluid

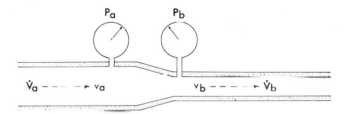

Fig. 7-28 The Bernoulli effect demonstrates that the *pressure* exerted by a steady flow of gas or liquid in a conducting tube varies *inversely* as the *velocity* of the fluid. With an abrupt narrowing of the passage since the volume of fluid per unit of time leaving ($\dot{V}_b$) must equal the time-volume entering the tube ($\dot{V}_a$), the linear motion of the fluid per unit of time (velocity, v) must increase as it traverses the structure ($v_b > v_a$). Thus there is a pressure drop distal to the restriction ($P_b < P_a$).

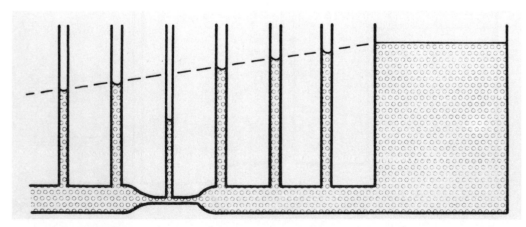

Fig. 7-27 The Bernoulli effect. (From Nave CR and Nave BC: *Physics for the health sciences,* ed 3, Philadelphia, 1985, WB Saunders.)

is flowing through a tube at point ⓐ with a certain velocity (v_a) and a lateral pressure (P_a). As dictated by the Law of Continuity, as the fluid moves through the constriction its velocity increases. Thus at point ⓑ (after the constriction), the fluid's velocity (v_b) is greater than that at point ⓐ. According to the Bernoulli theorem, the higher velocity at point ⓑ should result in a lower lateral pressure at that point (P_b). Thus, as a fluid flows through a restriction, its velocity increases and its lateral pressure decreases.

Fluid entrainment

According to the Bernoulli theorem, as a fluid flows through a restriction its velocity increases and its lateral pressure decreases. If the restriction is small enough, the resulting large increase in velocity will actually drop the lateral pressure below atmospheric pressure. Pressure that is less than atmospheric is termed *negative pressure.*

As shown in Figure 7-29, if we place an open tube distal to such a constriction, the negative pressure will literally pull another fluid into the tube of flow. The use of the Bernoulli effect to draw a second fluid into a stream of flow is called *entrainment.*

In this example, the entrained fluid is air. This use is common in the home, where aerator attachments on faucets mix air into the water stream. In the laboratory setting, the negative pressure produced at a constriction in a water faucet can also be used as a source of negative pressure. This application is called the *water aspirator.*

Of course, any fluid (liquid or gas) may provide the primary flow source, and any fluid can be entrained into the stream of flow. In respiratory care, the most common application of the Bernoulli effect is the *air injector.* An air injector is a device designed to increase the total flow in a gas stream. In this case, a pressurized gas, usually oxygen, serves as the primary flow source. This pressurized gas passes through a nozzle or jet, beyond which is an air entrainment port. The negative pressure created at the jet **orifice** entrains air into the primary gas stream, thereby increasing the total flow output of the system.

As depicted in Figures 7-30 and 7-31, the amount of air entrained depends on the diameter of the jet orifice and on the size of the air entrainment ports. For a fixed jet size, the larger the entrainment ports, the greater the volume of air entrained and the higher the total flow (Figure 7-30). With entrainment ports that are fixed in size, the volume of entrained air can still be altered by changing the diameter of the jet (Figure 7-31). A large jet results in a lower gas velocity and less entrainment, whereas a small jet boosts velocity, entrained volume, and total flow.

The Venturi tube

A modification of the Bernoulli principle, called the Venturi tube, was developed some 200 years ago by Giovanni Venturi. As illustrated in Figure 7-32, a Venturi tube includes a dilation just distal to the tube jet. Venturi proved that if the angle of dilation is kept at less than 15 degrees, the original fluid pressure can be almost completely restored.

This smooth tapering helps prevent turbulence and allows much of the kinetic energy generated at the jet to be transformed back into pressure energy. With restoration of the pressure energy to prerestriction levels, the pressure gradient needed to maintain flow is also restored, thereby permitting more entrainment. Moreover, the Venturi design helps keep the

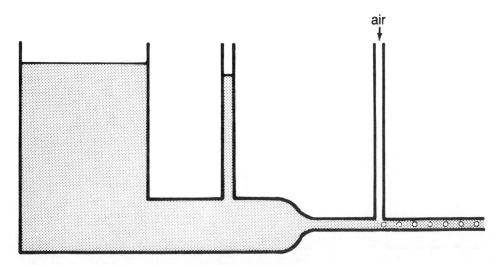

Fig. 7-29 The entrainment of gas into a liquid by means of the Bernoulli effect. (From Nave CR and Nave BC: Physics for the health sciences, ed 3, Philadelphia, 1985, WB Saunders.)

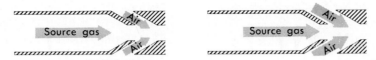

Fig. 7-30 Same orifice size in jet provides (1) same forward velocity, (2) same lateral subatmospheric pressure, and therefore (3) same pressure gradient (atmospheric to subatmospheric) for air entrainment. Entrainment-port size on right is larger; therefore more air will be entrained at set pressure gradient. (From McPherson SP: Respiratory therapy equipment, ed 4, St Louis, 1989, Mosby.)

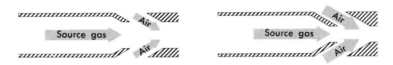

Fig. 7-31 Smaller restriction (right) causes greater increase in forward velocity of gas, resulting in lower lateral pressure and larger quantity of air entrained through ports. (From McPherson SP: Respiratory therapy equipment, ed 4, St Louis, 1989, Mosby.)

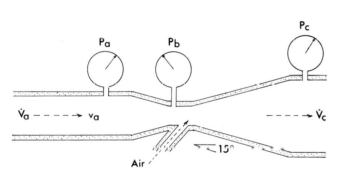

Fig. 7-32 The venturi principle states that the pressure drop distal to a restriction can be closely restored to the prerestriction pressure if there is a dilation of the passage immediately distal to the stenosis, with an angle of divergence not exceeding 15 degrees. Thus P_c approximately equals P_a. The venturi is a widely used device to entrain a second gas to mix with the main-flow gas. The subambient pressure distal to the restriction draws in the second gas just past the restriction, and the increased outflow ($\dot{V}_c > \dot{V}_a$) is accommodated by the widened distal passage.

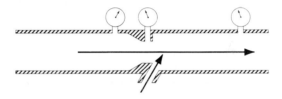

Fig. 7-33 Pitot tube. By retaining high forward velocity and forward pressure after air entertainment, molecules of mixture composed of source gas and entrained air hit the sides less frequently. Ideally they exert low lateral pressure similar to that at the restriction (jet) so that forward pressure is maximum.

Fluidics and the Coanda effect

Fluidics is a branch of engineering in which hydrodynamic principles are used in flow circuits for purposes such as switching, pressure and flow sensing; and amplification. Because such devices use only the driving force of the fluid in precisely designed flow circuits, no moving parts are required. Without moving parts to fail or wear out, fluidic devices are very dependable and require little maintenance.

The primary physical principle underlying most fluidic circuitry is a phenomenon called *wall attachment,* or the *Coanda effect.* One observes this effect mainly when a fluid flows through a small orifice with properly contoured downstream surfaces.

We know from the Bernoulli theorem that negative pressure distal to a fluid jet causes entrainment of surrounding fluid, such as air, into the primary flow stream (Figure 7-34, *A,* on page 146). If a carefully contoured curved wall is added to one side of the orifice, as shown in Figure 7-34, *B,* the confinement of the wall causes the pressure near the wall to become more negative relative to atmospheric. Thus the atmospheric pressure on the other side of gas stream

percentage of entrained fluid constant, even when the total flow varies.

When used as an entrainment device, the Venturi tube has one major drawback. Any buildup of downstream pressure (Figure 7-32) causes a large decrease in fluid entrainment. This problem is partly overcome with an alternate design, called the Pitot tube (Figure 7-33). Instead of being used to restore pressure, the Pitot tube is designed to restore fluid velocity. Thus the volume of fluid entrainment in the Pitot tube is less affected by downstream pressure than in the Venturi tube.

We will apply all these principles in subsequent chapters while discussing certain respiratory care equipment.

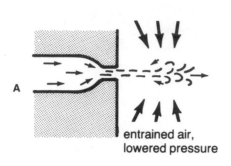 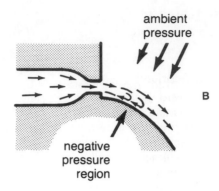

Fig. 7-34 The Coanda wall effect. **A,** Entrainment into the driving airstream. **B,** Wall attachment initiated by negative pressure near wall. (From Nave CR and Nave BC: Physics for the health sciences, ed 3, Philadelphia, 1985, WB Saunders)

pushes the stream against the wall, where it remains locked until interrupted by some counterforce. Using this principle, Coanda demonstrated that a fluid stream could be deflected through a full 180-degree turn by means of careful extension of the wall contour.

As applied in respiratory care equipment, fluidic switches, pressure- and flow-sensing devices, and flow amplifiers are often combined into an integrated fluidic logic circuit, which functions much like an electronic circuit board. This fluidic logic circuit can provide overall control of most equipment function without electrical power. Chapter 31 provides details on the application of fluidic circuits in ventilatory support equipment.

ELECTRICITY

Years ago, most respiratory care equipment was pneumatically controlled, and common bedside monitoring devices used simple mechanical principles. This is no longer true. Today, most therapeutic and diagnostic equipment is electrically powered and controlled. Electrically and computer-controlled ventilators, physiologic monitoring electrodes, pressure and flow transducers, cathode-ray tube displays, strip-chart and X-Y recorders are all commonplace at the bedside.

Safe and effective use of this equipment requires a basic understanding of the principles of electrical circuitry. This knowledge is applied in Chapter 3 (electrical safety) and again in Chapters 17 and 18 (monitoring and pulmonary function testing equipment).

Basic electrical circuitry

Electricity is the flow of electrons from one place to another. Electrons flow through substances called *conductors*. The wires found in your home and in biomedical equipment are good examples of electrical

conductors. The electrical conductivity of substances varies greatly. Most metals are good electrical conductors, as are salt solutions (such as body water). Other substances—such as plastic, rubber, and glass—are very poor conductors of electricity.

For electrons to flow through a conductor, there must be an energy source, such as a generator or battery. This energy source pumps electrons through the conductor. All electrical energy sources have two poles, one negatively charged and one positively charged. The negative pole, or *cathode,* has an excess of stored electrons. The positive pole, or *anode,* has a relative shortage of electrons. Being negatively charged, electrons always flow away from the negative pole toward the positive pole. In combination, an electrical energy source that causes electron flow through a conductor from its negative to positive pole constitutes an *electrical circuit* (Figure 7-35). Electrical circuits can perform work, such as producing heat or creating light. In addition, we can use the principles of electrical circuitry to measure biophysical signals (such as blood pressure) or control complex machines.

Ohm's law

There are three basic physical parameters governing electrical circuitry: *voltage, current,* and *resistance.*

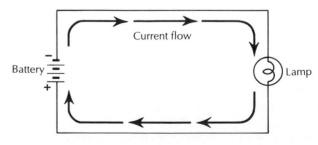

Fig. 7-35 Basic components of an electrical circuit.

As indicated in Table 7-10, these three parameters are analogous to the driving pressure, flow, and resistance in fluid circuits.

Voltage (electromotive force)

Voltage, like fluid pressure, pushes electrons through a circuit. This driving force may be supplied by a battery, as is the case in portable instruments. However, most electronic equipment is designed to operate from line voltage available at a wall outlet. The voltage available at wall outlets is produced at a remote location by a power company's electrical generators.

The unit used to measure this electromotive force is the *volt* (V). We use an instrument called a *potentiometer* to measure voltage. Automobile batteries, for example, produce an electrical pressure or potential of 12 V. Nine-volt batteries are commonly used in portable equipment, whereas flashlight cells (used in laryngoscopes) produce 1.5 V. Wall outlets in the United States provide about 110 V. Low voltage is specified in mV (10^{-3} V) or μV (10^{-6} V); high voltage is specified in KV (10^{3} V) or mV (10^{6} V).

Current

Current is the flow of electrons through a circuit; it is analogous to fluid flow through a tube. The unit used to measure current is the ampere (A). Currents much smaller than one ampere are recorded in mA (10^{-3} A), or μA (10^{-6} A). As previously discussed, current flow produces heat. In some cases, such as a humidifier heating element, this heat is desirable. In most electronic instruments, however, heat is an undesirable by-product of current flow. For this reason, some means of cooling must be provided to prevent circuit components from overheating. Ventilation ducts in equipment cabinets and internal cooling fans are common means of preventing over-

heating of electronic instruments. Of course, covering equipment vent openings can cause overheating and damage to the electronic components and increases the risk of fire. One must therefore always be careful not to obstruct the ventilation ducts of electronic equipment.

Resistance

Electrical resistance, like resistance in fluid circuits, represents opposition to flow. In electrical circuits, resistance opposes the flow of electrons or current. The unit used to measure electrical resistance is the ohm (Ω).

Resistance is a property of conductors. A good conductor of electricity has very low resistance to current flow. As previously mentioned, most metals and salt solutions are good electrical conductors. This means they offer low resistance to current flow. Copper has very low electrical resistance and is therefore an excellent conductor. This is why most electrical wires are made of copper. Silver and gold, although more expensive, are even better conductors of electricity. This is why these precious metals are often used in circuit components and as measuring electrodes.

Conversely, substances such as plastic, rubber, and glass are poor electrical conductors because they have high resistance to current flow (sometimes millions of ohms). Such materials are used for insulation around wires and on other electrical components.

Resistance is sometimes purposefully included in electric circuits to limit or direct current flow, or to reduce voltage. Electrical components designed for this purpose are called *resistors*.

The relationship among the three basic physical parameters of voltage, current, and resistance is described by *Ohm's Law:*

$$\text{electromotive force} = \text{current} \times \text{resistance}$$

You can rearrange the equation to solve for resistance:

$$\text{resistance} = \frac{\text{electromotive force}}{\text{current}}$$

Careful inspection of this revised equation reveals a direct and simple analogy to fluid dynamics. You will remember that the resistance to fluid flow in a tube equals the difference in pressure between the two points along the tube, divided by the actual flow of fluid:

$$R = \frac{P_1 - P_2}{\dot{V}}$$

The same concept applies to electrical circuits, as expressed in Ohm's Law. Resistance to the flow of

Table 7-10

Parameter	Unit	Description	Fluid analogy
Voltage	Volt (V)	Force pushing electrons through a circuit; also called *electromotive force* or *difference in potential*	Pressure difference across a tube; driving pressure
Current	Ampere (A)	Flow of electrons through a conductor	Flow of fluid; volume/unit time
Resistance	Ohm (Ω)	Opposition to flow of electrons; opposition to current	Resistance to flow; opposition to movement of fluid

electrons equal the difference in pressure across the electrical circuit (electromotive force or voltage) divided by the actual flow (current). In measurable terms:

$$\text{ohms} = \frac{\text{voltage}}{\text{amperes}}$$

One can easily perform numeric computations with this formula. For our purposes, however, your understanding of the relationships among these three parameters is more important.

According to Ohm's Law, voltage and current are directly related; the higher the voltage (all else being equal), the higher the current. For example, connecting an electronic device to a 220 V outlet will cause higher current flow through its circuits than will using a regular 110 V source. Indeed, such a high current might either damage the equipment or create excess heat and thus be a fire hazard. For prevention of such accidents, two safety features exist. First, a 220 V outlet has a plug configuration different than that of a 110 V outlet, making it nearly impossible to make the connection. Second, were the connection actually made, all biomedical electronic devices have built-in current limiters. Consisting of fuses or circuit-breakers, these devices prevent excessive current by literally breaking the circuit connections. To restore the circuit connection, you must replace the fuse or reset the circuit breaker.

On the other hand, Ohm's Law tells us that current and resistance are inversely related. With voltage constant, the higher the resistance, the lower the current. Of course, the opposite is also true: The lower the resistance, the higher the current.

The strain-gauge pressure transducer previously discussed (Figure 7-20, page 131) is a good example of this relationship. In one common design, a constant low voltage is passed through the transducer's wires. As pressure changes flex the diaphragm, strain is placed on the transducer's wires, altering their resistance to current flow. According to Ohm's Law, if the voltage is kept constant and the resistance changes, the current will change in the opposite direction:

$$\text{voltage (constant)} = \text{current}(\downarrow) \times \text{resistance}(\uparrow)$$

In this manner, the changes in current represent the effect of pressure on the flexible diaphragm. We observe these changes in current either as the needle displacement on a gauge or as a digital readout on a numeric display panel.

These basic relationships underlie the principles of electrical safety discussed in Chapter 3 and the design of biomedical measuring instruments described in Chapter 17.

CHAPTER SUMMARY

Much of the technology involved in respiratory care is based on simple physical principles. Although all areas of physics have their impact on respiratory care, the properties of matter, thermodynamics, mechanics, and electricity are fundamental areas of knowledge for the practitioner.

With regard to the properties of matter, we recognize three primary states: solid, liquid, and gas. The solid state has a high degree of internal order, in which the positions of the molecules are more or less fixed by strong mutual attractive forces. When these forces are weakened by melting, the resulting liquid can flow; they tend to take the shape of their containers. Liquids also exert pressure and buoyant force, and they exhibit the properties of viscosity, capillary action, and surface tension.

In the gas phase, the attractive forces between molecules are negligible. Lacking restriction to movement, these molecules exhibit rapid, random motion, characterized by frequent collisions. Thus, unlike a solid or a liquid, a gas has no inherent boundary and is readily compressed and expanded. However, like liquids, gases are capable of flow. For this reason, both liquids and gases are considered fluids.

In both solids and liquids, most of the internal energy of the matter is potential energy. On the other hand, because the forces of attraction among gas molecules are negligible, essentially all the internal energy of a gas is kinetic energy. With most of its internal energy expended in maintainance of molecular motion, the temperature of a gas is a direct measure of its average kinetic energy.

The First Law of Thermodynamics tells us that heat moves from objects of high temperature to objects of low temperature until equilibrium is reached. This transfer of internal energy occurs by way of at least one of three primary mechanisms: (1) conduction, (2) convection, and (3) radiation. Heat transfer may also occur during evaporation.

Heat transfer provides the basis for matter's change of state. The additional heat energy needed to effect the changeover from solid to liquid is referred to as the latent heat of fusion. The heat energy required to vaporize a liquid into a gas is the latent heat of vaporization. There are two forms of vaporization: boiling and evaporation. In boiling, liquid molecules must be given enough kinetic energy to force them into the surrounding atmosphere, against its opposing pressure. In evaporation, random surges in kinetic energy allow some liquid molecules to escape into the surrounding air.

The relationships among the pressure, temperature, mass, and volume of gases are expressed in the gas laws. These laws allow us to explain and quantitatively predict the behavior of gases under a variety of conditions. Underlying all these laws are three basic assumptions: (1) that collisions between molecules are perfectly elastic, (2) that the volume occupied by the gas molecules is negligible, and (3) that no forces of mutual attraction exist between the molecules. These three assumptions describe an ideal gas. Variations in the behavior of gases from this ideal do occur, especially at the extremes of pressure and temperature. However, under normal conditions, most gas behavior is consistent with the conception of an ideal gas.

In contrast to a static liquid, in which the pressure depends solely on the depth and density of the fluid, the pressure exerted by a flowing liquid varies according to the characteristics of the flow itself. The three main patterns of fluid flow through tubes are laminar, turbulent, and transitional. Under conditions of laminar flow through a tube, the difference in pressure required to produce a given flow is defined by Poiseuille's Law.

The velocity of a fluid flowing through a tube at a constant rate of flow varies inversely with the available cross-sectional area. Moreover, as a fluid flows through a stricture its velocity increases and its lateral pressure decreases. If a tube is narrowed sufficiently, the large increase in fluid velocity will result in a negative lateral fluid pressure relative to atmospheric, which allows additional fluids to be entrained. Design variations on this principle allow restoration of downstream pressures, as in the Venturi tube, or direction of the fluid stream along a wall, as in the Coanda effect.

Similar in concept to fluids, the flow of electricity in circuits is described by a few basic parameters and relationships. The three basic parameters governing electrical circuitry are voltage, current, and resistance. These parameters are directly analogous to driving pressure, flow, and resistance in fluid circuits. The interelationships among voltage, current, and resistance are described by Ohm's Law. Ohm's Law has broad application for practitioners, especially in the understanding of the safe and effective use of biomedical instrumentation.

REFERENCES

1. Barker JA, Henderson D: The fluid phases of matter, *Scientific American,* Nov 1981.
2. Chatburn RL: Measurement, physical quantities and le système international d'unites (SI units), *Respir Care* 33:861–873, 1988.
3. Epstein II: *Basic physics in anesthesiology,* Chicago, 1976, Year Book.
4. Flitter HH: *An introduction to physics in nursing,* ed 7, St. Louis, 1976, Mosby.
5. Green JF: *Mechanical concepts in cardiovascular and pulmonary physiology,* Philadelphia, 1977, Lea & Febeger.
6. Hill DW: *Physics applied to anesthesia,* London, 1976, Butterworth.
7. Kacmarek RM: Chemical and physical background. In: Pierson DJ, Kacmarek RM, editors: *Foundations of respiratory care,* New York, 1992, Churchill Livingstone.
8. Kimball WR: Fluid mechanics. In: Kacmarek RM, Hess D, Stoller JK, editors: *Monitoring in respiratory care,* St. Louis, 1993, Mosby–Year Book.
9. List RJ, editor: *Smithsonian meteorological tables,* Washington, DC, 1958, Smithsonian Institute.
10. Nave CR, Nave BC: *Physics for the health sciences,* ed 3, Philadelphia, 1985, W.B. Saunders.
11. Parbrook GD: *Basic physics and measurement in anesthesia,* ed 2, Baltimore, 1986, Appleton-Lange.
12. Quagliano JV: *Chemistry,* Englewood Cliffs, NJ, 1964, Prentice-Hall.
13. Rau JL: An evaluation of fluidic control in ventilators. *Respir Ther,* 6:29–32, 1976.
14. Richardson IW: *Physics for biology and medicine,* New York, 1972, John Wiley & Sons.
15. Smith RK: Respiratory care applications for fluidics, *Respir Ther* 3:29, 1973.
16. Weast RC, editor: *Handbook of chemistry and physics,* ed 69, Cleveland, 1988, Chemical Rubber Co.
17. Whitaker S: *Introduction to fluid mechanics,* Englewood Cliffs, NJ, 1968, Prentice-Hall.
18. Williams AL, et al: *Introduction to chemistry,* Reading, MA, 1973, Addison-Wesley.

Computer Applications in Respiratory Care

■

Craig L. Scanlan

Gregg L. Ruppel

CHAPTER LEARNING OBJECTIVES

1. Identify the primary components of a small computer system;
2. Define and describe hardware and software;
3. List at least two uses of computers in department management in respiratory care;
4. Describe at least one implementation of a computer in the delivery of respiratory care;
5. Describe three applications of computers in the diagnosis of respiratory disease.

Computers have supported clinical respiratory care for many years. Much of the equipment used by the respiratory care practitioner is microprocessor controlled. This equipment includes ventilators, bedside monitors, and laboratory instruments. Computers are used for storing patient data and medical records. Most departmental and hospital management functions are performed by the computer. Computer-assisted bedside monitoring is commonplace. Computer technology assists clinicians in interpreting data, reaching diagnoses, and planning patient care. Closed-loop computer systems to control certain aspects of patient management, including mechanical ventilation, have been described.

The involvement of respiratory care practitioners with computer technology has increased dramatically in the past decade. In order to function in the modern health care setting, practitioners should understand the strengths and limitations of computerized systems.

DEVELOPMENT OF COMPUTERS

The earliest modern computers were developed by the armed services during World War II. These huge devices consisted of thousands of vacuum tubes. Unlike modern computers, programming consisted of supplying instructions and data on paper tape. These systems typified early computer architecture. Each had five key components: (1) a *central control unit* designed to "orchestrate" overall operations; (2) an *arithmetic logic unit* (**ALU**), capable of arithmetic and logical functions; (3) an *input mechanism* to let the user provide both data and instructions to the computer; (4) a *memory* to store these data and instructions; and (5) an *output mechanism* to provide the results of data analysis for the user. This scheme is still widely applied.

During the 1950s and 1960s several important advances in computer technology occurred. Transistors replaced vacuum tubes as the logic element of the computer. Magnetic memory was developed. The earliest forms of modern programming languages (**FORTRAN, COBOL, BASIC**) were developed. These languages allowed a single instruction to execute a series of machine commands. The most important development was the **integrated circuit (IC)**. An IC is a small silicon-base semiconductor chip, upon which thousands of miniaturized transistors can be placed. Early ICs lowered the cost and increased the dependability of computer circuitry by a factor of 10. Modern ICs may have over a million transistor components. This provides a thousandfold improvement in both cost and computational power over their early counterparts.

During the late 1960s and early 1970s semiconductors also became the primary mode for storing data and instructions for use by the computer (**primary memory**). Enhancements in **mass storage** technology (secondary memory) also occurred with IBM's development of the magnetic disk. **Software** developments were equally important. Up until this time, a computer could only attend to a single task or serve a single user. The development of *operating systems* changed this limited approach by allowing the computer's time to be divided into extremely small "slices." Computers with this new capability could switch rapidly between separate tasks, appearing to do two or more things simultaneously. This capability to "juggle" activities rapidly by using separate time allocations is called *multitasking*. Multitasking also allows a single computer to serve more than one user concurrently, a concept called **timesharing.**

The last 20 years has been characterized by continued miniaturization of components. Such components combine many diverse functions into a single computer chip. This has been accomplished through a concept called *very large scale integration* (VLSI). VLSI allows several components to be combined on a single chip. There has also been an increase in the computational abilities of *microprocessors*. These developments made possible the modern personal computer (PC), which relies heavily on VLSI technology. It also allowed the use of microprocessors in many instruments commonly used in respiratory care. Software developments during this era include sophisticated data base management systems and programming languages, such as **PASCAL, FORTH,** and **C.**

In the current era of computer technology refinements in IC technology are likely as are alternatives to classic computer architecture. Such alternatives include parallel processing and reduced instruction set computers (RISCs). Both of these developments are designed to challenge the computational "speed limits" of conventional computer designs. Also typical of current computer technology are advances in software, including computer-aided software engineering (CASE) applications, natural language processors, and expert systems.

HOW COMPUTERS WORK

Respiratory care practitioners who use computers for diagnostic or therapeutic purpose should have a basic understanding of both hardware and software. This section provides an overview of computer equipment and programs.

Hardware

Modern computers consist of five key hardware components: a central control unit, an arithmetic logic unit (ALU), input devices, memory to store data and instructions, and output devices (Figure 8-1).

Central processing unit

The central control unit and arithmetic logic unit are combined to form the **central processing unit** (CPU). Microprocessors, such as those found in personal computers, are single CPU chips. The CPU contains a decoder that translates a sequence of instructions. These instructions form a **program.** The arithmetic logic unit (ALU) performs basic arithmetic (i.e., addition, subtraction). It also performs logical operations, such as comparisons (i.e., greater than, less than). The CPU also has a number of registers used to store and transfer data. Some microprocessors are designed for specialized functions. These devices are sometimes called *coprocessors*. Coprocessors are often used to perform floating-point decimal arithmetic (math coprocessor). Other processors perform tasks such as high-resolution video display. The most sophisticated CPU designs include coprocessor functions in the main chip.

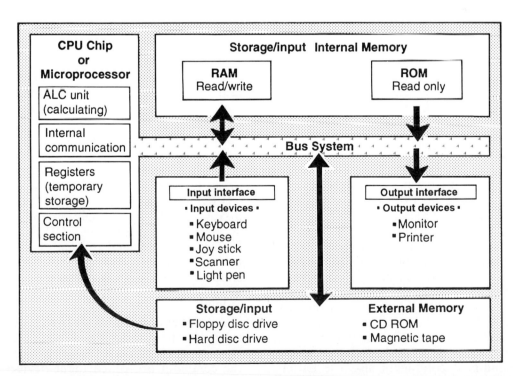

Fig. 8-1 Components of a computer system. (Copyright 1993 by Microscoft Corporation. Reproduced with permission.)

Memory

Memory is the electronic "space" where the computer stores data or instructions. Information is stored in the form of **binary** digits, or **bits,** symbolized as either a 0 or a 1. Eight bits combine to form a **byte.** One byte may be used to represent a character, such as the letter A. A single byte can also be used to represent a computer instruction. The largest decimal number that can be represented by a byte is 256. To work with large numbers, current computers use registers that handle 32 or 64 bits at one time.

The byte is still used to describe the basic unit of memory. One **kilobyte** (Kb) equals 1024 bytes. A **megabyte** (Mb) equals 1024 Kb, approximately a million bytes. Small amounts of memory are usually described in kilobytes (Kb), while large memory volumes are described in megabytes (Mb). Desktop computers, such as those used for pulmonary function systems, are equipped with 4 Mb of memory or more. Dedicated microprocessors, such as those in pulse oximeters, often use smaller amounts of memory to match a specific task.

Computers have two general types of memory: primary and secondary. Primary memory is immediately available to the CPU, usually in the form of memory chips. Secondary memory is external to the CPU. Mass storage devices such as disk drives are considered secondary memory.

Primary memory. Primary memory consists of two types: ROM and RAM. **Read only memory** (ROM), contains preprogrammed instructions that allow the CPU to function. The ROM in a desktop computer contains the basic instructions necessary to get the computer up and operating once it is powered on. Also in ROM is much of the operating system that handles **input** and **output.** Instructions in ROM are permanently stored within the physical structure of one or more semiconductor chips. These instructions remain in ROM regardless of the power status of the computer. ROM instructions can only be "read" by the CPU and cannot normally be altered by the user.

Random access memory (RAM), consists of semiconductor chips that store binary data or instructions for use by the CPU. Unlike ROM, RAM is normally empty unless data or instructions are entered into it. "Loading" a program causes the CPU to store the program's instructions and associated data into RAM for subsequent use. The data stored in RAM is maintained electronically. Loss of electrical power causes all data stored in the computer's RAM to be lost. For this reason, RAM is also referred to as "volatile" memory.

Most desktop computers include at least one battery powered RAM chip. This chip stores important information about the computer's configuration (i.e., amount of memory, type of disk drive). Portable, laptop, and hand-held computers also use battery power to maintain data and programs when disconnected from conventional power. In these devices nickel-cadmium (NiCad) or other rechargeable batteries provide power not only to maintain memory but to operate the entire computer.

Secondary memory. To avoid keeping all data and instructions in RAM, computers use secondary memory or mass storage. Data is stored externally, usually on magnetic tapes or disks. Optical storage methods are also used to provide secondary memory (see later discussion).

The *storage capacity* of tape or disk media varies according to the density of the magnetized material on its surface. **Floppy disks** have relatively low storage capacities per unit area (i.e., 1 to 3 Mb per disk). For example, a typical 3.5 inch floppy disk is capable of storing about 1.44 Mb of data (1,440,000 bytes). This equals 700 double-spaced pages of typewritten information. Floppy disks may be used to transfer small amounts of information from one system to another. Most software for desktop computers is supplied on floppy disks. Because of their slow access time, floppy disks are not used in CPU operations in which time is critical.

Hard disks have greater storage ability, with sizes ranging from a few hundred megabytes to more than a gigabyte (1024 Mb). Hard disks allow fast access by the CPU. This permits the hard disk to be used to save and retrieve program instructions. Access time is an important factor in large multiuser systems, when the CPU is performing multiple tasks for multiple users.

Tape systems are typically used for large-volume data storage when rapid access is not critical. High-capacity tape drives are often used to **backup** data stored on hard drives. Data backup is required in case the hard disk itself should fail. The backup tape can be used to restore the data or programs after repair or replacement of the hard drive.

Optical disks, similar to audio compact disks, are also used for mass storage. Optical disk capacity varies from about 300 Mb to 900 Mb, depending on the recording method. The most common type of optical disk is the WORM—*write once read many.* These disks are used for archiving (storing) data such as medical records or electrocardiograms. WORM drives both read and write to the optical media. The **CD-ROM** player simply reads a prerecorded optical disk. CD-ROM disks supply large volumes of data for access by desktop computers. CD-ROM disks are used for large medical **databases** and references. A magneto-optical drive is available that allows data to be stored (written to disk) and later erased.

Input and output devices

A number of methods are used for supplying information to the computer and receiving results from it. Devices used to instruct, program, or supply data to the computer are called input devices. Devices the computer uses to communicate the results of computations or data searches are called output devices.

Input devices. Input data may consist of a program of instructions or the words, numbers, or graphic information needed by the program to complete its task. Common input devices include the **keyboard** and the **mouse,** or a similar pointing device. Other input methods are **optical scanners,** digitizing pads, and **analog-to-digital converters.** Some sophisticated systems include pen-based input and voice recognition.

Keyboard. The most common way for a user to enter data into a computer is through a keyboard (Figure 8-2). A typical computer keyboard consists of four major components: (1) a typewriterlike section of **alphanumeric** keys, (2) a numeric keypad, (3) special purpose **function keys,** and (4) cursor control keys.

The typewriter-like section of the keyboard is used to input individual letters or strings of characters that form words. The numeric keypad allows data entry much like a calculator. The cursor controls, usually arrow keys, allow the user to point to options on the screen. This simplifies making choices from menus. Some keyboards combine the numeric keypad and cursor controls, with a toggle key used to select between functions.

Function keys (i.e., F1, F2, and so on) are usually defined by the application program being used. For example, pressing F1 in a word processing program may save the document to a disk file. Alternatively, F1 in a statistical application may be used to calculate the mean of a group of numbers. Function keys may also be used as *soft keys*. **Soft keys** change their function within an application. This method is often used with medical instruments that include a keyboard. The function of a soft key is displayed on the screen and changes with each choice made by the user (Figure 8-3, on page 154). This allows an entire **menu** of options to be accessible with a limited number of function keys.

Mouse. Pointing devices, such as the mouse or trackball, allow very rapid access to options displayed on the screen. Rather than typing a keyboard command or using cursor keys, the user simply points to an item displayed on the computer screen. Selection is made by clicking one or more buttons on the mouse. Pointing devices are particularly useful in graphic-based applications or **operating systems.** In such applications, data or programs can be represented by *icons.* For example, the icon for a text **file** can be clicked on, then "dragged" to the icon for a **word processor.** Dropping the text icon on the word processor icon causes the word processor program to start using the text file. The mouse does require a hard surface. This makes it impractical for many medical applications (i.e., bedside monitors).

Touch screens. The computer screen is normally considered an output device. It may be used for user input by adapting it to respond to touch. The simplest type of touch screen is made up of a grid of sensing lines that determine the location of the touch by matching vertical and horizontal contacts. Another type, commonly used in medical applications, employs infrared light-emitting diodes (LEDs). These LEDs and sensors create an invisible infrared grid in front of the computer screen. The user's finger interrupts the infrared beam when pointing to an option

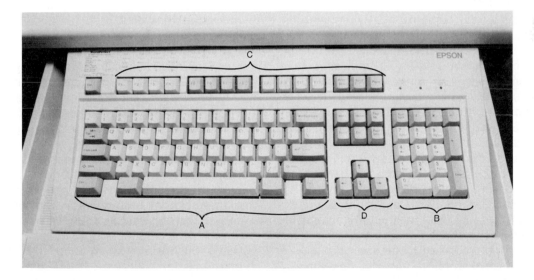

Fig. 8-2 Computer keyboard. *A,* Alphanumeric keys for data entry, arranged similar to a standard typewriter keyboard. *B,* Numeric keypad for rapid entry of numbers. On some systems the numeric keypad is also used for cursor control by toggling back and forth. An LED lights to indicate whether the keypad is set to number entry or cursor movement. *C,* Function keys F1 through F12, arranged at the top of the keyboard. On some systems the function keys are located to the left of the standard keys; some systems have function keys in both positions. *D,* Cursor control keys (arrow keys) for navigating through menus or screen choices. This key board has cursor control keys in addition to those available on the numeric keypad.

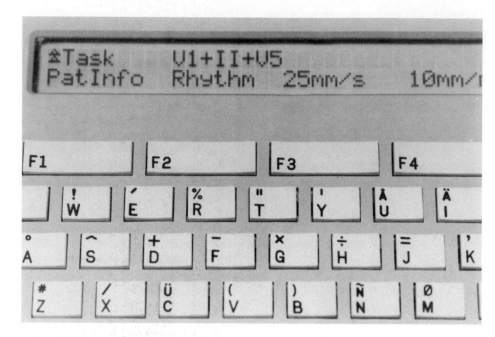

Fig. 8-3 Soft keys, so named because their functions are controlled by the application software. The data entry keyboard of a computerized electrocardiograph is shown. Function keys F1–F4 are related to the menu choices displayed directly above them on the LCD display. Pressing one of these soft keys brings up a different menu, reassigning the function of each key. The use of function keys and soft keys allows the user to quickly navigate through a series of choices, without having to remember specific commands. (Courtesy St. Louis University Health Sciences Center.)

on the screen. Touch screens are often used in "dirty" environments such as critical care units or laboratory settings. Touch screens can completely replace the conventional keyboard in many instances. They are limited because the users must hold their hands in midair, and this is very tiring over extended periods. Touch screens do not offer high resolution.

Analog-to-digital converters. **Analog** information is data which correspond to or is analogous to a physical measurement. A mercury thermometer is an example of a simple analog measurement device. The height of the mercury column is a physical representation of temperature. Analog information is usually provided electronically as a change in either voltage or current. A good example of electronically acquired analog data is data obtained from a flow-volume tracing made during a pulmonary function test. An electronic pneumotachometer is used to measure expiratory flow. The signal from the pneumotachometer is either a voltage or a current change over time. This analog signal can be recorded by an appropriate X-Y recorder. The signal cannot, however, be directly analyzed by a computer.

Analog signals must be converted to digital format. This is accomplished by using a special input device called an analog–to–digital converter, (ADC). An analog-to-digital converter transforms the changing analog input (such as voltage) into a series of pulses by sampling the signal at known intervals. The converter assigns a value to each segment (interval) of the analog

signal (Figure 8-4). By sampling at a rapid rate (i.e., thousands of times per second), the digital value can closely approximate the analog signal. After the analog signal has been converted to digital form, the computer can manipulate the data. Analog-to-digital conversion is widely used in medical applications. Electrocardiographs, pulse oximeters, gas analyzers, hemodynamic monitors, spirometers, and most laboratory instruments produce analog signals. Interfacing these devices to a computer requires an ADC.

Serial communications. Many medical instruments contain their own microprocessors. In order to allow one instrument to communicate with an external computer, a serial port is needed. The serial **port** is a communication device that is standardized between computers. It allows the transfer of digital data, by an appropriate cable, between two computers. Serial communications require specialized **application software,** so that the sending and receiving computers can transfer data. Suppliers of medical equipment often specify the format which their instrument uses to communicate.

Miscellaneous input devices. Other devices used occasionally in medical applications include optical scanners, bar code readers, and pen-based systems.

Optical scanners. Optical scanners translate a printed image into digital form for computer input. The simplest scanners look for a mark on a form in a particular location. A graphics scanner is an input device that converts a graphic image, such as an

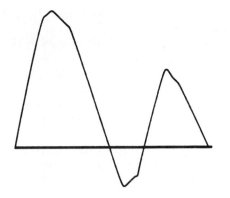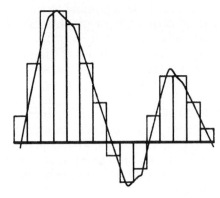

Fig. 8-4 Analog-to-digital conversion. The analog signal (left) may be a voltage, current, or physical movement, usually supplied by a transducer. The analog-to-digital converter (ADC) "samples" the signal at a high frequency (right) and assigns a digital value proportional to the analog signal. The greater the sampling frequency, the more accurately a particular portion of the signal can be represented. The number of bits the converter uses to represent the signal also affects the sensitivity of the measurement. Many medical applications use "12-bit" ADC devices. A 12-bit converter can represent a signal using 4096 different values ($2^{12} = 4096$).

anatomic drawing or X-ray, into a digitalized format. Typically, a scanned graphic image is converted into thousands of binary picture elements, called **pixels.** Each pixel represents a light dot that can be turned on or off on the screen display. Some scanners can input typed or written words using optical character recognition (OCR) software.

Bar code readers. Bar code readers are widely used in hospitals. Any item that can have a bar code attached can be scanned with a bar code reader. This includes patient supplies, pharmaceuticals, and laboratory specimens. Bar codes for patient specimens are widely used in automated laboratory systems to prevent mislabeling.

Pen-based systems. Pen-based systems use penlike devices to input data into a computer. Pen-based computing is a relatively new field, but the number of applications is increasing. Pen-based systems allow the user to enter data either on a computer "form" or on a blank screen. The main problem with pen-based input is the limited ability of the computer to decipher the user's handwriting.

Output devices. Common output devices include the computer **monitor** or screen, a variety of **printers,** and plotters. Output data may also consist of digital or analog signals designed to activate or control specialized equipment.

Computer monitor. The computer monitor is the most common output device. Results of computations are usually displayed on a monitor screen. The output may include alphanumeric and graphic information. Most computer monitors are simple cathode ray tubes (CRTs). New display technologies, such as liquid crystal (LCDs) and gas plasma, provide alternatives to the CRT. The resolution available with modern display devices approaches photographic quality. Many medical devices use a computer display to represent both analog signals and computer graphics. For exam-

ple, a pressure waveform may be accompanied by hemodynamic calculations.

Printers. The printer is the primary means for converting computer output into *hard copy.* **Hard copy** represents words, numbers, and/or graphic information that is transferred to paper. Several types of printers are used in medical applications. These include: (1) dot-matrix, (2) thermal, (3) ink-jet, and (4) laser printers.

Dot-matrix printers use a print head made up of pins arranged in one or more columns. As the print head moves across the paper, the pins fire to form the dot pattern of the individual characters or graphic image. Dot-matrix printers can produce a **printout** (printed output) very rapidly and are capable of graphics reproduction. Newer dot-matrix printers use a print head with a larger number of pins (usually 24) to produce near-letter-quality type. By using color ribbons and controlling print head movement, color images can be created. Four-color ribbons are common. Color dot-matrix images are useful for certain graphic images such as those used in pulmonary function and exercise tests.

Thermal printers are widely used for medical applications because they are small, lightweight, and quiet. Many instruments include thermal printers that can reproduce alphanumeric or graphic images. Thermal printers require special paper that may be costly.

Ink-jet printers form images by ejecting a small jet of ink from a special print head. The ink-jet sprays small dots to form letters. Ink-jet printers are small and quiet. Modern ink-jet printers rival laser printers for print quality. In addition, ink-jet technology can be used to produce multicolored images. This is particularly useful in some diagnostic areas in which hard copy color images must be produced.

Laser printers use electrophotographic technology to print a full page of characters or graphics at one time. A small laser beam is used to neutralize the surface of a positively charged drum, creating a reverse image. The drum is then coated with a positively charged toner. When negatively charged paper contacts the drum, toner is attracted to it, forming the desired image. The image is fused to the paper by a combination of heat and pressure. Laser printers can produce images with resolutions of 600 dots per inch (dpi). The laser printer is a relatively fast output device, capable of printing 6 to 50 pages per minute. Although laser printers produce the highest-quality output, they are large and expensive. A single laser printer can be shared by multiple users to control operating expenses.

Plotters. A plotter is a specialized X-Y recorder used as an output device for a computer. Plotters are used to produce complex graphic images. A plotter translates digital computer output into the motion of a drawing pen on paper. Special codes sent to the plotter can cause it to switch pens; this ability allows for different line thicknesses and colors.

Output control signals. Output data may also consist of digital or analog signals designed to activate or control specialized equipment. In respiratory care, a microprocessor-based ventilator can take an input signal, such as flow, convert it to volume, and send an output signal that tells the exhalation valve to open when the desired volume is achieved.

Software

Software instructs the computer what to do, and how to do it. A complete set of such instructions is called a **program.** Individuals who develop computer software are called programmers. A respiratory care practitioner does not need to be a programmer to use a computer, although understanding the basic concepts of computer programming and the types of software is useful.

Computer programs

Most computer programs are based on algorithms. An **algorithm** is a clearly defined, step-by-step procedure for solving a specific problem (Figure 8-5). The algorithm is written like a flow chart to describe the decision making process the computer will use to solve a problem. From the algorithm, a sequence of instructions or commands is developed. The program tells the computer exactly what operations to carry out.

Most programs are written as a series of subroutines or functions. Each routine can be used as often as needed. One subroutine supplies data, input by the user or by an interfaced instrument. The input data can be changed so that the program can solve similar problems over and over.

Three basic concepts underlie conventional computer algorithms:
1. *Simple Sequence:* Each step in the algorithm is performed in sequence, one after another.
2. *Conditional Branching:* Depending on the value of a given conditional statement, the program will either branch to other portions of the algorithm or continue in the programmed sequence, but not both.
3. *Looping:* An operation or sequence of operations is done over and over again until some condition is satisfied.

Types of software

Software, or computer programs, may be best thought of as existing at various levels. The "lowest" level of computer instruction occurs within the microprocessor itself. This level consists of binary coded instructions (i.e., 1s and 0s) called **machine language.** Early computers required programs written directly in machine language. Higher-level computer languages are now used to program computers.

Programming languages. The lowest level of programming is referred to as *assembly language.* Assembly language uses very basic instructions specific to the microprocessor being used. Assembly language routines are often programmed into ROM. This is particularly common in computerized instruments that perform monitoring functions.

The next level of computer software is high-level programming languages. **High-level languages** consists of English-like instructions that describe the task they perform. Each high-level instruction translates into many machine language statements. High-level programming languages include BASIC, FORTRAN, COBOL, PASCAL, LISP, FORTH, and C. These programming languages do not depend directly on the design of the microprocessor. This means that programs written in high-level languages can often be used on many different computers.

Application generators. An application generator is halfway between a programming language and an application program. An application generator is used to develop a set of instructions so the computer can perform a specific task. The instructions are created by the application generator, rather than by a programmer. The technique of using an application generator to assist in software design is often referred to as *computer-aided software engineering* (CASE). Application generators allow nonprogrammers to develop programs to solve specific problems.

Many types of application programs have programming features built in. Such applications include data base programs, word processors, and spreadsheets. The built-in programming often takes the form of recorded *macros.* A **macro** is a set of instructions that can be repeated as often as needed. For example, a spreadsheet program may be used to produce a

Algorithm   **Pseudocode**

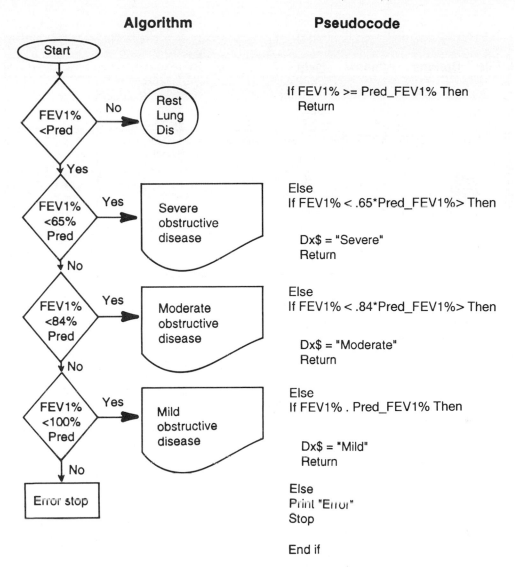

```
If FEV1% >= Pred_FEV1% Then
  Return




Else
If FEV1% < .65*Pred_FEV1%> Then


  Dx$ = "Severe"
  Return



Else
If FEV1% < .84*Pred_FEV1%> Then


  Dx$ = "Moderate"
  Return



Else
If FEV1% . Pred_FEV1% Then


  Dx$ = "Mild"
  Return

Else
Print "Error"
Stop


End if
```

Fig. 8-5 Program algorithm and pseudocode for a portion of a program to interpret a pulmonary function study. **Left** The algorithm or flow chart is the starting point for constructing the program. In this example the $FEV_1\%$ (FEV_1/FVC × 100) is compared to the patient's predicted value (Pred) to determine the extent of obstruction present. **Right** Pseudocode showing the computer commands that would be used by a high level language, such as BASIC, PASCAL, or C. The code uses the "If . . . Then . . . Else" construct to evaluate the $FEV_1\%$ according to the algorithm. $FEV_1\%$ and $PredFEV_1\%$ are variables, representing their respective values determined from the pulmonary function study. Dx$ is a "string" variable that holds a text string that will be used to produce the output statements. See Fig. 8-19 for an example report. (From Ellis JR, Perera SP, Levin DC: A computer program for calculation and interpretation of pulmonary function studies. Chest, 68:209–13, 1975.)

monthly department report (see Figure 8-7). Formatting and printing the report may require many keystrokes. These keystrokes can be stored in a "macro" so that the entire sequence can be repeated by simply using the macro.

Other built-in programming features include *user defined configurations.* Applications that are configurable by the user allow a general program to be customized to fit a specific need. This is usually accomplished by allowing the user to describe the way the application is to be used and then store the responses in a configuration file. The configuration file is then read each time the application is started.

Application programs

An application program is a set of preprogrammed instructions that allow a computer to perform a specific function. Common functions provided by application programs include word processing, data base management, and statistical computation. Such applications can be used in any area, including health care. Applications specific to respiratory care include programs to perform monitoring functions, programs to operate laboratory equipment, and programs to control therapeutic interventions.

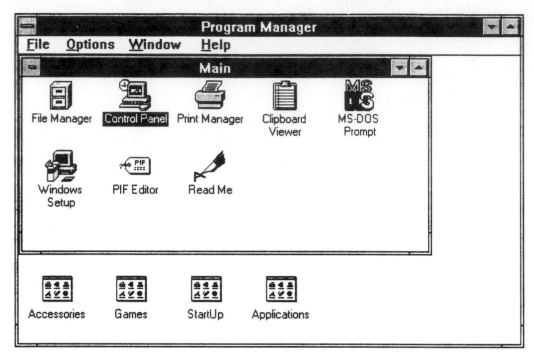

Fig. 8-6 A graphics-based user interface (Windows[1]). Programs are grouped together according to their function (Main, Accessories, Startup, etc.). A program group is selected by clicking on its icon with a mouse or cursor. The icon then becomes a window from which program icons can be selected. The box title "Main" in this display contains the program icons for several system programs (File Manager, Control Panel, etc.) A graphical user interface such as this makes it easy for users to learn program operation, since program functions are similar across a range of different applications.

---

[1]Windows is a registered trademark of Microsoft, Inc.

Operating systems

An **operating system** oversees the basic functions of the computer. A typical operating system (OS) provides six key functions, which are necessary to use other application programs:

- Command and program execution
- Input and output **(I/O)** control
- Memory management
- File management
- Multitasking
- Applications interface

The command and program execution function determines both the sequence and the time certain functions will be executed by the CPU. I/O control directs the operations of both input and output devices, such as the keyboard and screen. The memory management component controls the use of and access to the computer's primary and secondary memory systems. File management includes copying, moving, editing, and deleting program and data files. Multitasking, if provided, allows the computer to divide CPU time among many different tasks, as previously described. The applications interface allows application programs to use the other functions effectively, providing a "platform" for controlling other programs.

Two basic forms of operating systems are widely used: command-driven and graphics-based. A command-driven operating system uses English-like commands such as "COPY" (to copy a file) or "EXEC" (to execute a program). Commands may be grouped together to perform a series of operating system tasks in sequence. A series of operating system commands designed to function in sequence is called a **batch file.** For example, a batch file can direct the computer to: (1) list a directory of files, (2) sort the files by date of creation, and (3) send the sorted list of files to an output device, such as a printer.

The most common command-driven operating systems used in **microcomputers** and **minicomputers** are MS-DOS, OS/2, and Unix. MS-DOS (i.e., Microsoft Disk Operating System) is a single-user operating system that gained popularity with the introduction of the IBM Personal Computer in 1982. OS/2 is a second-generation microcomputer operating system for IBM PCs and compatibles that gives the single user multitasking capabilities and an optional graphics-oriented user interface. Unix was originally developed by AT&T as a multitasking, multiuser operating system. Unix, in many different variations, is used extensively in engineering and scientific workstation applications.

Graphics-based operating systems employ *icons* as the basis for user interface. The icons represent programs, functions, or groups of programs (Figure 8-6). By pointing to an icon, the user can instruct the

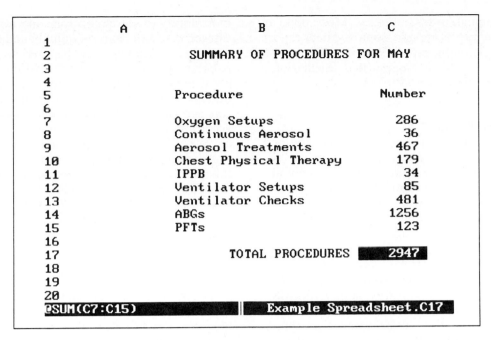

	A	B	C
1			
2		SUMMARY OF PROCEDURES FOR MAY	
3			
4			
5		Procedure	Number
6			
7		Oxygen Setups	286
8		Continuous Aerosol	36
9		Aerosol Treatments	467
10		Chest Physical Therapy	179
11		IPPB	34
12		Ventilator Setups	85
13		Ventilator Checks	481
14		ABGs	1256
15		PFTs	123
16			
17		TOTAL PROCEDURES	2947
18			
19			
20			
@SUM(C7:C15)		Example Spreadsheet.C17	

Fig. 8-7 A spreadsheet for manipulation of numeric data. A blank sheet is set up as a series of columns (A, B, C in this example) and rows (1–20). The intersection of each column and row forms a *cell*, which is referenced by its address. Cells may contain labels (text), numbers, or mathematical formulas. In this sheet cell B7 contains the label "Oxygen Setups", while C7 contains the associated number of procedures "286". Cell C17 contains the formula "@SUM(C7:C15)". This formula adds the numbers in column C from row 7 to row 15, and displays the total on the worksheet. Spreadsheets can be used to record and analyze almost any type of numeric data, including quality control statistics, and physiologic measurements.

computer to perform a specific task. With this type of operating system, the user can have the computer start an application by pointing to it with a mouse or light pen. The graphical operating system gained popularity with the introduction of the Apple MacIntosh personal computers. Graphics-based operating systems are easier for new users to master. By standardizing the way applications appear, once a user learns a particular function, he or she can use that function repeatedly in other applications. Windows-based operating systems also make transfer or sharing of data (objects) between applications easier.

Word processing

Application programs that deal primarily with text and documents are commonly referred to as word processors. Word processors may operate on **mainframes,** minicomputers, or desktop computers (PCs). These application programs have the ability to create, edit, store, and retrieve text files called documents. Multipurpose word processing software generally includes a variety of editing functions, including margin control, justification, search and replacement of text strings, block copy and move operations, and spell checking.

Word processing programs are particularly useful in creating or maintaining documents that must be updated periodically. Such documents include policy and procedure manuals, monthly reports, and depart-

ment forms. By maintaining such documents in word processor format, modifications and enhancements can be made easily. Word processors can also be used to generate reports of tests or procedures. Some respiratory care application programs have text editing capacity built in. These may be more limited in scope, being used for specific purposes such as adding comments to a formatted report.

Spreadsheets

One type of application that is widely used to perform numeric analysis is the spreadsheet. A spreadsheet is divided into rows and columns. The intersection of one row and column represents a cell; the row and column represents the "address" of the cell on the sheet. Each cell may contain either a number, a formula, or a text label. By referencing other cells, a formula in a cell can perform one of many standard mathematical operations on the data. For example, the formula in a cell may reference a range of cells to be added (Figure 8-7). The cell containing the formula displays the result of the calculation. Once a formula is set up, it can be replicated so that similar functions occur across a range of columns or rows. This makes the spreadsheet an ideal tool for presenting reports that contain tables.

Complex spreadsheets can look up data from another source, perform statistical operations, and provide "what-if" modeling of numeric data to predict the effect of changing assumptions. Most popular spreadsheet programs include sophisticated report formatting and graphing capabilities. This allows the user not only to perform complicated calculations, but to display the data in multiple formats.

Database programs

Large volumes of data can usually be grouped into categories. For example, a patient's name, admitting date, diagnosis, and attending physician are all categories of information. By applying such categories to many observations, large volumes of text and numeric data can be organized, stored, retrieved, and manipulated according to specific information needs.

Organizing text and numeric data in such a way that it can be easily stored, retrieved, and manipulated is called a *database management system* (DBMS). A database management system consists of two related components: an underlying program of computer instructions that provide the storage, retrieval, and manipulation functions, and one or more databases.

A database is simply a collection of records. A record represents data that describe a single person, object, or event (Figure 8-8). Each piece of information within a record is called a field. In the previous example, each patient would represent a record in the database; the name, admission date, diagnosis, and physician would be fields.

The power of a database management system lies in its ability to search for, sort, and report on specific categories of information quickly and accurately. For example, a database can be used to report on the respiratory care procedures for patients admitted in a given period. The database management system can quickly search for patients who received respiratory care services. The list of patients can then be sorted according to diagnosis, age, admitting physician, or any other field in the database records.

Advanced database management systems simplify this process by allowing the user to retrieve data by using English-like commands. This approach is called **structured query language** (SQL). A related technique is called *query by example* (QBE). Both methods are designed to make data retrieval and reporting easier. Some database management systems also provide for extensive manipulation of numeric data within their fields.

The most sophisticated database systems are called *relational databases*. Relational databases allow the user to work with more than one database at a time. This capacity allows one to relate or link data in one file with relevant data in another file (Figure 8-9). Relational databases offer great flexibility since similar types of data can be grouped into separate databases. The individual databases are "linked" by one or more key fields, such as the patient's name or ID. Fields from any linked databases can be combined when organizing a report. Once established, these linkages not only minimize the need to reenter data, but decrease the likelihood of input error.

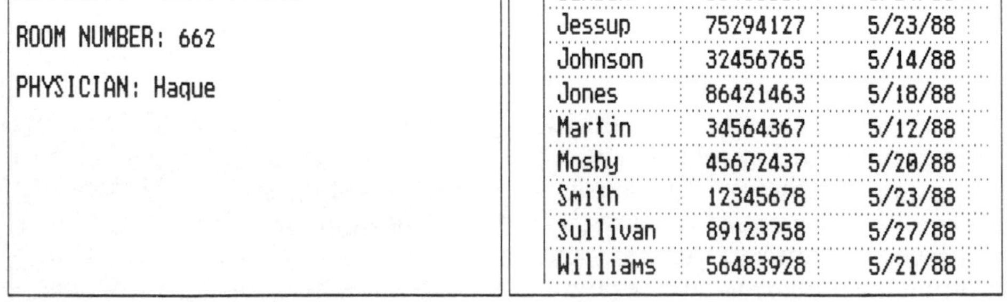

Fig. 8-8 A simple patient database displayed on a computer screen. The right half of the display shows a list of *records* in the database; each row represents a record. Each record is divided into *fields,* shown here as columns. By scrolling to a particular record with the cursor, the detailed contents of the record can be viewed. The left half of the display shows a single patient record with the field names (i.e., LAST NAME, ID NUMBER, etc.) and the field contents displayed. A simple database such as this can be used to store, retrieve, sort, and report large amounts of categorical data.

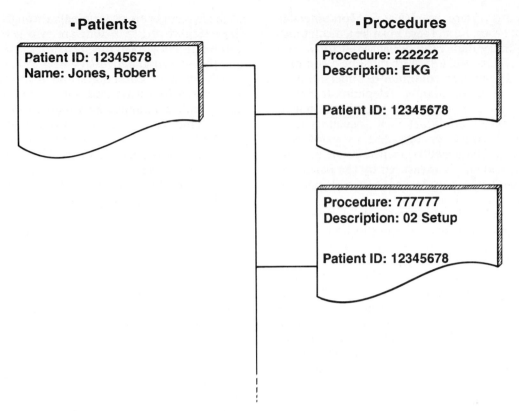

Fig. 8-9 A relational database management system. To handle large volumes of data over a wide range of topics, relational databases are often used. In a relational database, smaller databases (also called tables) are established. Each table contains a different aspect of related data. In a hospital system, one table might contain patient data, while another contains a list of procedures performed. The data tables are "linked" by having one or more common fields. In the diagram both the Patient database and the Procedures database contain a Patient ID field. Using these types of links data from the two databases can be combined to generate a report. For example, all procedures for a specific patient can be identified, or all patients that received a specific procedure can be determined using the same databases.

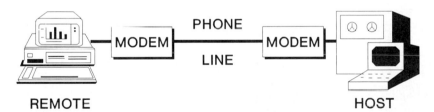

Fig. 8-10 Data communications using standard telephone connections. A microcomputer or simple terminal (REMOTE) access a mainframe or similar large system (HOST) by means of modems. The modem converts a digital signal into an acoustic one that can be transmitted via standard telephone lines. Special communication software is needed to encode/decode the modem signals, and to control the data transfer process. Modem speed is very important since it determines the cost of data transfer via telephone.

Data communication

The process of sharing data among computers is called data communication. There are two primary types of communication systems: host-remote systems and networks.

Host-remote telecommunication

The simplest example of data communication using computers is the linkage between a mainframe computer, called the **host,** and a terminal or micro-computer, called the **remote.** This link is often made by using standard voice telephone lines (Figure 8-10). The purpose of this type of linkage is usually to transfer data stored on one system to the other. When data is sent from the host to the remote microcomputer, the process is called *downloading.* For example, a respiratory therapist might need to download literature references on a specific pulmonary disease from a host computer that maintains a medical reference data base. The reverse process, terminal-to-host transfer, is called *uploading.*

Two components are necessary for computers to "talk" to each other. First, there must be a mechanism to transmit binary data rapidly back and forth over the telephone lines. Second, there must be a common language that allows each computer to understand the other's actions and commands. Telephone transmission is based on analog acoustic signals. A **modem** (i.e., modulator-demodulator) is a special type of analog-to-digital converter designed to work with acoustic signals. The speed of transmission of computer data via modem is measured by the **baud rate.** The fastest modems can transmit a full page of characters in just a few seconds.

Common communication protocols ensure effective communication between the two systems. These protocols provide a means for the computers to exchange status signals. Status signals allow the computers to notify each other when data has been sent, when it is ready to be accepted, or when it has been accepted. Most communication protocols also provide an error correction mechanism. Automatic error correction helps identify errors that occur during data transmission. If an error is detected, the error correction mechanism attempts to retransmit the data until accuracy is verified.

Computer networks

A computer **network** is a system that connects one or more computers or **terminals** through transmission lines (Figure 8-11). There are two general types of computer networks: the *local area network* (LAN), and the *wide area network* (WAN). A LAN is usually a small group of computers and terminals linked by specialized hardware and software. LANs are often set up within a particular work area, such as an office or building. A wide area network is an extension of the LAN concept in which computers communicate across long distances, such as between cities or between continents.

Computer networks differ from simple host-remote systems in two ways. First, a computer network allows all linked computers to communicate with each other. Messages or data from any one computer can readily be sent to all other computers on the network. Second, most networks use high-speed communication lines designed solely for data transmission. Compared to standard telephone lines, special coaxial cables can provide a hundredfold increase in the rate of data transmission. Fiberoptic cables can transmit data a million times faster than standard telephone lines.

COMPUTER APPLICATIONS IN RESPIRATORY CARE

Computers have been used in respiratory care for more than 20 years. The early use of computers

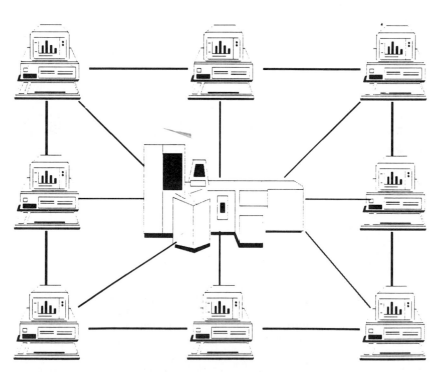

Fig. 8–11 A computer network. Illustrated is a series of microcomputers connected to each other and to a mainframe, a common network configuration in the health care setting. Many hospital information systems utilize a mainframe for maintenance of the primary patient databases. Microcomputers (PCs) are then used as "smart" terminals. Data can be downloaded from the mainframe for use in application programs such as spreadsheets. The microcomputers can also communicate with each other using one of several local area network (LAN) protocols.

coincided with the introduction of hospitalwide financial and patient information management systems. At about the same time, the computer began to be used to increase the speed and accuracy of diagnostic and monitoring devices. Computers are particularly useful in conjunction with bedside monitors or laboratory instruments. They are being used to help clinicians to interpret data, reach diagnoses, and provide patient care.

Information management

Hospitalwide information systems

The first use of computers in the hospital setting was limited to business applications. Hospitals developed and incorporated computerized patient billing systems to replace manual bookkeeping methods. Direct involvement of clinicians with the computer system was minimal.

The next logical step was to incorporate clinical data as components of the hospital information system. This was accomplished after patient discharge. Selected elements of patient data, such as the admitting diagnosis and discharge status, were incorporated into the data base. Such information was used primarily for reimbursement reporting. In the late 1970s,

advances in technology resulted in the creation of interactive patient information management systems. These systems incorporate a large mainframe data base with a remote terminal network. The remote terminals provide simultaneous access to relevant patient data by hospital staff and clinicians.

Patient information management systems allow access to commonly needed data elements, such as admitting diagnosis, attending physician, or physician orders. More sophisticated patient information management systems replace some or all of the manual medical record keeping functions. For example, a sophisticated patient information system can not only provide physician order entry but allows users to enter progress notes, chart data such as vital signs, and maintain a cumulative record of diagnostic test results. To minimize user training and aid in data input, such systems are often *menu-driven*. This format allows the user to select common treatment options or data needs. When it is combined with specialized input devices, such as bar code readers, the clinician can enter information into the record very quickly. Locating terminals in most hospital departments give easy access to patient records (Figure 8-12).

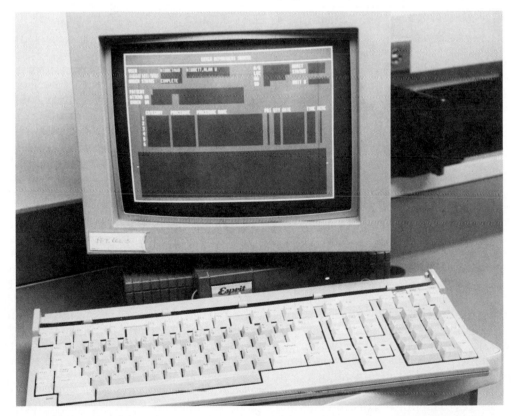

Fig. 8-12 A standard terminal. This terminal consists of a simple video display along with a keyboard. The terminal is linked directly to the hospital mainframe, and can access patient data via several application modules. This type of terminal is relatively inexpensive and can be located in any area of the hospital that requires access to the hospital information system. A microcomputer running terminal emulation software can be used in a similar fashion. (Courtesy St. Louis University Health Sciences Center.)

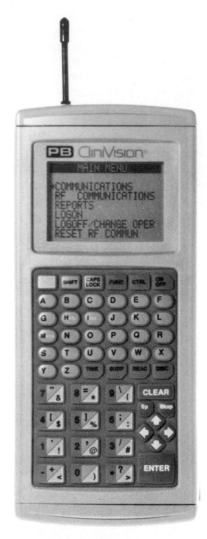

Fig. 8-13 Portable hand-held computer. The hand-held computer provides an alphanumeric keyboard along with a liquid crystal display (LCD). The computer is taken to the point-of-care, where patient data, charting, and records can be entered and stored. Data can be "uploaded" from appropriately equipped devices, such as microprocessor controlled ventilators. Information stored in the hand-held system can be transferred (downloaded) either to another computer (workstation) or directly to a printer. This type of bedside data collection is becoming increasingly common in fields such as nursing and respiratory care. (Courtesy of Puritan-Bennet Corporation, Carlsbad CA)

Modern hospital information systems integrate a number of functions. These functions include admission, discharge, and transfer of patients within the hospital. Other functions involve laboratory information management, nursing care documentation, and resource scheduling. Many hospital information systems support interfaces to laboratory instruments and other diagnostic equipment. Since many instruments use microcomputers, software and hardware capacity for communicating with the hospital mainframe is essential. Management of very busy departments such as pharmacy, radiology, and respiratory care often requires dedicated modules within the hospital information system.

Departmental management

Many respiratory care departments use computer-based management systems. As noted, hospital information systems often provide specialized departmental modules to streamline department functions. In the absence of a hospitalwide patient information system, departmental computing may be used to track physician orders, record patient treatments, and create billing/procedure summaries. Where a hospitalwide patient information system is used, departmental computing may focus on personnel management and material resources. Departmental computing may be used to facilitate scheduling of staff, monitor productivity, maintain inventory, and keep track of equipment maintenance schedules.

Two methods are commonly used to track physician orders and record patient treatments. In the first method, respiratory care practitioners enter relevant data into a department computer after completing their rounds. This process may be time consuming. It requires both transcription of treatment notes and their transfer into the computer. When there is a limited number of computers or terminals, access by a large staff may be problematic.

Instead of manually recording notes on the hospital wards, practitioners can use hand-held computers for "remote" data entry (Figure 8-13). Selected patient information, new orders, treatment times, and even ventilator settings can be logged directly into the hand-held unit. This information can be downloaded into a central workstation or off-loaded to a printer. Software operating on the central station combines each therapist's report with that downloaded by other practitioners. This allows all data for a given shift to be compiled. Automation of day-to-day procedures enhances standardization of care and assures accuracy in charting and billing.

In addition to dedicated respiratory care management systems, many general purpose software packages can be used to improve department management. Spreadsheets are readily adapted to report everything from department statistics to actual diagnostic test results. Word processing can be used for procedure manuals, reports, correspondence, and intradepartment communications. Statistics and financial packages designed for small businesses often lend themselves to improved departmental record keeping and management.

Selecting and implementing computer tools for department management should include all levels of practitioners. Front-line therapists most often understand the demands placed on them both to provide high-quality care and to document that care adequately. The problems of a poorly organized department are seldom remedied by converting to a computer-

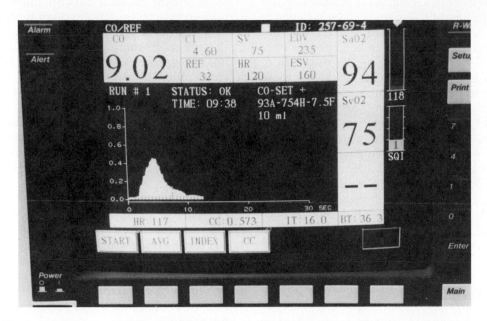

Fig. 8-14 Computer-aided bedside hemodynamic monitor. The main display of a computerized monitor used with a pulmonary artery catheter. The catheter provides pulmonary artery pressures, thermodilution cardiac output, and measurement of mixed-venous saturation. An additional pulse oximeter provides arterial saturation. The computer allows multiple parameters to be calculated using the various measurements as inputs. In addition, the user can enter data such as blood gases to calculate a wide range of cardiopulmonary variables. Displayed here is a graph of a thermodilution cardiac output injection along with the calculated values. Note soft keys along the bottom for selecting options. (Courtesy St. Louis University Health Sciences Center)

based system. Careful planning, by care givers as well as managers, is needed to implement an automated system effectively. Well-defined objectives should be the starting point for setting up either a hospitalwide or a departmental information management system.

Clinical applications

Use of the computer to measure and/or interpret clinical data is a natural extension of its capabilities. Simple algorithms are satisfactory for data acquisition, retrieval, and computation. Computer-based interpretation and diagnosis necessarily employs concepts of **artificial intelligence** (AI). The most common interpretive applications used in respiratory care focus on pulmonary function, blood gas analysis, and hemodynamic data.

Computer-aided monitoring

Perhaps the most common application of computers encountered in respiratory care is their use in bedside monitoring equipment.

Ventilation monitors. Simple electronic integrators and timers have long been used to process analog signals. These devices compute tidal volumes, airway and vascular pressures, as well as breathing and heart rates. The use of microprocessors with appropriate ROM-based software to store, display, and interpret these signals has become commonplace in the past 20 years. For example, the analog-to-digital conversion of a tidal volume signal from a ventilator can be combined with breathing rate, measured electronically, to compute minute ventilation. Combination of flow and airway pressure signals permit monitoring of airway resistance, and static and dynamic compliance. Most contemporary mechanical ventilators use one or more microprocessors. Not only is the ventilator controlled by microprocessor, but flows, pressures, and gas fractions are all monitored by computer.

Hemodynamic monitors. Dedicated microprocessors are also used in bedside monitoring of hemodynamic data. The indwelling reflective oximeter is a good example of such an instrument. The reflective oximeter measures mixed venous oxygen saturation in vivo. This information is combined with thermodilution cardiac output measurements to derive several hemodynamic parameters (Figure 8-14). Typical of many computerized bedside monitors, this instrument combines data acquired "on-line" with external parameters entered by the user. Function keys and softkeys (see Input Devices, this chapter) are used extensively to simplify data entry, display selection, and printing of results.

Electrocardiographic monitoring. Monitoring of electrocardiographic (ECG) signals is often computer assisted. The amplified ECG signal can be sampled at an appropriate rate by an analog-to-digital converter. The resulting digital signal can then be stored for later review (Figure 8-15). By comparing the stored ECG complexes with known arrhythmia patterns, cardiac function can be monitored and interpreted. In addition to monitoring, computers can be used to store 12-lead electrocardiograms. Digital storage allows interpretation of rate, rhythm, and axis, along with signs of hypertrophy or infarction. Another advantage of digital ECG storage is that individual tracings can be managed in a data base (Figure 8-16). Data base storage permits comparisons of electrocardiographic changes over time. Digital storage also lends itself to easy access to ECG data. ECGs can be displayed on remote computers or terminals, or even transferred by facsimile (FAX).

Laboratory information systems

Because of the large volumes of data produced, most clinical laboratories employ computers to reduce data, store it, and report results. Blood gas laboratories are often interfaced to either a hospitalwide system or a dedicated laboratory computer. Laboratory systems may be categorized as one of three types: (1) as a module in a larger hospital mainframe-based system, (2) as a stand-alone minicomputer lab system, or (3) as a desktop computer interfaced to one or more instruments.

Blood gas analyzers, like many other instruments, may be designed with serial communications capabilities. This allows the analyzer to be interfaced to any of the three categories of systems described. Many manufacturers supply both software and hardware (i.e., a microcomputer) so that patient results can be stored by computer. Some blood gas analyzers include disk drives or other computer components, so that an external microcomputer is not necessary. Vendors of hospital and laboratory information systems typically provide interface hardware and software that can be adapted to a wide range of analyzers (Figure 8-17, page 168).

Laboratory information systems have many advantages over manual methods. Patient data can be stored and retrieved systematically. Reports can be generated in multiple formats to meet specific needs. Serial reports can be generated to track a patient's progress. Billing information and department reports can be maintained with greater accuracy than is possible with most manual systems. Quality assurance data, such as daily quality controls or proficiency test results, can be stored as well.

One disadvantage of automated instrumentation is the large volume of data that must be maintained. A year's worth of blood gas results can quickly fill several hundred megabytes of disk space. In addition, some means of data backup must be provided. A backup system usually involves both an **archive** copy of stored data and a manual system to report results in the event of computer downtime. Tape backup or optical storage is often used if a large database of results must be maintained.

Pulmonary function testing

Most pulmonary function test systems are computerized. Three levels of automation are commonplace. These are dedicated microprocessors, desktop computer interfaced systems, and mainframe interfaced systems.

Most portable (i.e., bedside) pulmonary function devices use a dedicated microprocessor. The pulmonary function software itself is coded into ROM. Data storage may be during power-on only, or limited data may be stored in battery-powered RAM. Many portable systems can "dump" stored data to an external printer or to a desktop computer. These systems often include a miniature keypad equipped with softkeys or function key.

The majority of laboratory pulmonary function systems now use desktop computers. A typical system includes an IBM-compatible PC with high-resolution graphics display interfaced to a spirometer, gas analyzers, and associated equipment (Figure 8-18, page 169). The pulmonary function software is loaded from disk. Patient data is stored on hard disk, with floppy disk or tape used for backup. Some systems support a data base format for data storage. Color dot-matrix printers are commonly used to print both reports and spirograms or flow-volume loops. Laser printers can also be used for high-resolution graphic images, but not in color.

A number of flow-based systems (i.e., using a flow-sensing spirometer rather than a volume-based spirometer) are interfaced with portable or laptop microcomputers. This combination permits use of sophisticated pulmonary function software in a system that is compact and portable. Some flow sensors contain all interface electronics in the flow sensor head itself. A serial port and the pulmonary function software loaded into the computer are all that is required to use the laptop as a pulmonary function testing system.

Some hospitals decide to interface a pulmonary function system with the hospital information system, or with a large laboratory system. This arrangement requires significant expertise in not only interfacing but programming. More commonly, PC-based pulmonary function systems are networked in a LAN. This allows reports and graphics to be accessed from multiple workstations. Cardiopulmonary exercise and metabolic measurement systems are two other types of equipment that use desktop computers in the pulmonary function laboratory.

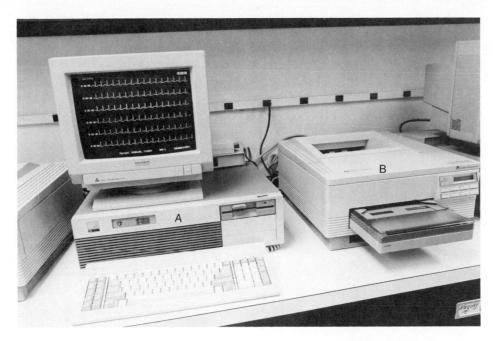

Fig. 8-15 Computerized ECG monitoring. *A* Personal computer equipped with an analog-to-digital converter and special diagnostic software. This type of system can store ECG tracings from multiple patients. The tracings can be retrieved as needed for display or review. *B* A laser printer is used to permanently record the ECG. Because of its high resolution, the laser printer can accurately reproduce data signals such as ECG or pressure waveforms. Similar computerized systems can be used to store other physiologic signals such as pulse oximetry data. (Courtesy St. Louis University Health Sciences Center.)

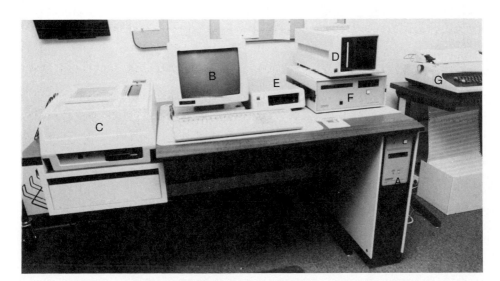

Fig. 8-16 Computer-based ECG system. *A* Minicomputer with large hard disk, *B* standard terminal for editing or retrieving stored records, *C* digital writer for reproducing ECGs, *D* optical storage device (WORM) for archiving ECG records, *E* tape backup system, *F* diskette reader for transferring ECG tracings from computerized electrocardiographs, and *G* system printer for reports. Hundreds of thousands of ECG records can be stored and retrieved via a database system. (Courtesy St. Louis University Health Sciences Center.)

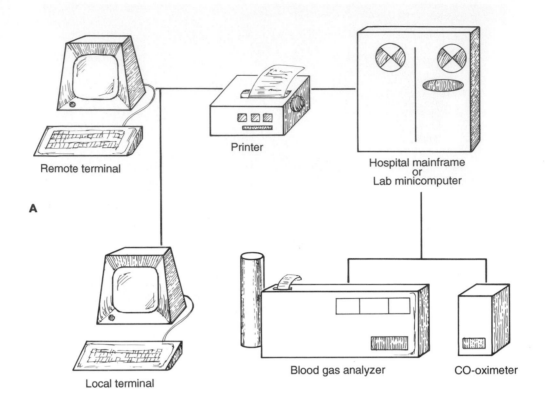

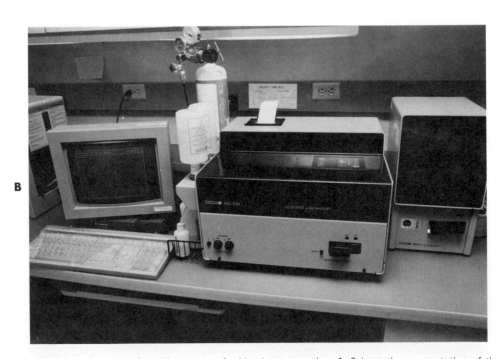

Fig. 8-17 Laboratory information system for blood gas reporting. **A,** Schematic representation of the components of a laboratory information system in which a blood gas analyzer and CO-oximeter are interfaced. The blood gas devices communicate with the hospital or laboratory computer through standard serial ports. The system then makes the data available to all terminals and printers. **B,** An automated blood gas system using the type of interface described. The blood gas analyzer and CO-oximeter are linked to the hospital mainframe, which echoes results back to the local terminal. (Courtesy St. Louis University Health Sciences Center.)

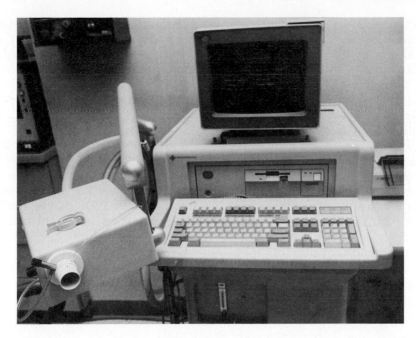

Fig. 8-18 Computer-based pulmonary function system. A typical pulmonary function system interfaced to a microcomputer. Signals from a flow sensor and various gas analyzers are digitized and processed by the computer. Spirograms and related tracings are displayed directly on the computer screen, and can be printed if necessary. Patient data is stored as hard disk files. Interfacing to standard desktop computers permits various components (memory, disk drives, printers, etc.) to be upgraded as necessary. (Courtesy St. Louis University Health Sciences Center.)

Mechanical ventilation

As noted previously, mechanical ventilators are one of several devices that use microprocessors for monitoring and control. Systems designed for monitoring and control can assess complex data and either suggest appropriate actions (**open-loop systems**) or take such actions automatically (**closed-loop systems**). The systems already described are open-loop computer systems. They provide clinical data or advice, but defer to the user to take appropriate actions. Closed-loop computerized control systems use input data provided by one or more sensors. The data from the sensors are the basis for predefined actions; there is no need for user input. A predetermined result is achieved by monitoring one or more responses continuously and making adjustments to achieve the desired end.

An example of a closed-loop control system used in respiratory care is the servo-controlled heated humidifier. The therapist sets a desired gas temperature. On the basis of input from an electronic temperature sensor, the controller increases or decreases the power output to the heating element. This feedback maintains the desired gas temperature. This type of closed-loop control can be accomplished without a microprocessor, by using a simple electromechanical relay. By incorporating a microprocessor circuit with software stored in ROM, the humidifier becomes an "intelligent" system. This provides additional functions such as default temperature control in the event of sensor failure or recognition of operational problems (i.e., automated troubleshooting).

Closed-loop computer control is not limited to simple devices such as a ventilator humidifier. Microprocessor-controlled oxygen delivery systems have been implemented in neonates. A microcomputer receives input from a standard pulse oximeter and then controls a mechanical blender to maintain a prescribed SaO_2. This system requires a real-time multitasking operating system to allow control, data display, alarm monitoring, and user input. The key to implementation of such a closed-loop control system are the software algorithms that interpret the input data. Closed-loop systems must include carefully defined criteria for rejecting bad input.

The next logical step in the management of patients who require mechanical ventilation is closed-loop control of the ventilator itself. The clinical application of closed-loop ventilator control actually preceded the advent of digital computers in medicine. A closed-loop ventilator designed to provide appropriate minute ventilation and gas concentrations in patients who were undergoing general anesthesia was first reported in 1957. In 1973 a ventilator was linked to a computer for purposes of ventilator control. This closed-loop system was applied successfully in animal anesthesia experiments to regulate minute ventilation and anesthetic gases.

Closed-loop computer control of ventilation has been limited by the accuracy of the devices available to provide input. Infrared CO_2 analyzers and pulse oximeters frequently lack the sensitivity to allow even sophisticated control algorithms to be useful. This is due to the fact that expired CO_2 and SaO_2 by pulse oximeter are indirect measures of gas exchange parameters. Recent refinements of indwelling blood gas electrodes (i.e., optodes) may provide the necessary level of sensitivity to allow computer control of ventilator settings.

Similar approaches have been used (in animal models) to optimize positive end-expiratory pressure (PEEP) levels. In these experiments, input to the computer comes from invasive measures of pulmonary pressures and calculations of lung mechanics.

One application of closed-loop ventilatory control has reached the bedside—mandatory minute ventilation (MMV). MMV does not employ expired or arterial gas analysis as a basic input for adjusting ventilatory parameters. Instead, expired minute ventilation itself is used as input to the microprocessor. This approach has significant limitations and may require substantial refinements before clinicians can confidently use it.

Computer-assisted interpretation and diagnosis

Use of computers to interpret clinical data and diagnose patient conditions represents a natural extension of their unique capabilities. Simple algorithms are satisfactory for data acquisition, retrieval, and computation. Computer-based interpretation and diagnosis must necessarily employ **artificial intelligence** (AI) software. Computerized AI applications in respiratory care focus on interpretation of pulmonary function studies, blood gas analysis, hemodynamic assessment, and diagnosis of patient conditions.

```
                      St. Louis University Hospital
                       Pulmonary Function Laboratory
       PT: Smith, Mary
       AGE: 47      SEX: F        RM#: 809-1      HT: 65.5 in    WT: 150.0 lb
       DATE: 01/05/94                             PHYSICIAN: Jones

            ----- Predicted Values Have Been Race Corrected -----
                          Pre-Drug*                       Post-Drug*    ALBUTEROL
       Spirometry         Actual   %Pred     Predicted     Actual  %Pred  %Change
```

Spirometry		Actual	%Pred	Predicted	Actual	%Pred	%Change
FVC	(L)	2.96	97	3.02	3.03	100	2
FEV1	(L)	1.87	80	2.31	1.98	85	5
FEV1/FVC	(%)	63	82	76	65	85	3
FEF25-75%	(L/S)	1.00	32	3.07	1.10	35	10
FEFmax	(L/S)	6.29	100	6.28	5.79	92	-7
FEF25%	(L/S)	2.78	48	5.74	2.88	50	3
FEF50%	(L/S)	1.16	26	4.40	1.31	29	13
FEF75%	(L/S)	0.38	17	2.12	0.37	17	-3
FEF50/FIF50	(%)	27			25		-9
MVV	(L/MIN)	84.79	82	103.00	94.66	91	11

Lung Volumes		Actual	%Pred	Predicted
TLC	(L)	4.32	93	4.59
FRC	(L)	2.06	82	2.51
RV	(L)	1.46	92	1.57
VC	(L)	2.86	94	3.02
IC	(L)	2.26	108	2.08
ERV	(L)	0.60	63	0.94
RV/TLC	(%)	34	98	34

Diffusion	Actual	%Pred	Predicted
Dsb ml/min/mmHg	11.66	56	20.82
VA(sb) (L)	4.34	80	5.40

```
_____ Computerized Interpretation _____

Moderate obstructive disease
Lung volumes within normal limits
Moderate decrease in Dsb
No change after bronchodilator
_____ End of Computerized Interpretation _____
```

Fig. 8-19 Pulmonary function report with computer assisted interpretation. Pulmonary function data is stored in a relational database. The interpreter program then accesses the database and analyzes the data according to a set of algorithms (see also Figure 8-5). The software then adds computer generated statements to the tabular report. Computer assisted diagnostic statements should always be clearly identified.

Pulmonary function test interpretation

A number of interpretation algorithms are currently used to aid in interpretation of results of pulmonary function studies. These algorithms examine data obtained from standard pulmonary function studies, including spirometry, lung volume, diffusing capacity, and bronchodilator response (Figure 8-19). In most instances, the patient's measured values are compared with reference values based on age, height, sex, and race. By applying statistical standards of normality or abnormality, generalized statements about the patient data can be derived. Computer-assisted interpretation of pulmonary function focuses on pattern recognition. Obstructive and restrictive lung diseases display characteristic changes in lung volumes and flows. The computer can classify these patterns just as a trained observer would.

Diagnosis of specific diseases cannot be made by simple pattern recognition. Diagnosis requires input of additional clinical data. Expert systems that allow clinical findings to be assessed along with results of standard pulmonary function studies are now available. Computer-assisted interpretation is ideal for screening purposes. Subjects who may require more sophisticated testing can be identified. Because of the variability of "normal" pulmonary function parameters in healthy subjects, and because of the effect of patient effort on test results, computer-assisted interpretation should be reviewed by a qualified interpreter.

Arterial blood gas interpretation

Interpretation of arterial blood gas test results by both physicians and respiratory care practitioners may be unreliable. Since blood gas interpretation employs a fixed set of rules, expert system software (AI) has been developed and applied in this area (Figure 8-20).

Blood gas values, including the patient's temperature and FIO_2, are input by the user. Standard algorithms are used to derive the PaO_2, A-a gradient, hemoglobin saturation, HCO_3^- and $[H^+]$. Using a knowledge base of known rules, both acid-base status and oxygenation status are interpreted. Some interpretive systems allow the user to compare results with expected acid-base responses to specific conditions, such as chronic hypercapnia. The results of computer-assisted analyses are highly consistent with the interpretations provided by experts. All computer-assisted interpretations should be reviewed by a qualified clinician, preferably before therapeutic intervention.

Hemodynamic assessment

The number and complexity of hemodynamic measurements make their interpretation difficult. Hemodynamic assessment represents an ideal area for applying clinical expert systems.

Pertinent data are input by the user (Figure 8-21, *A,* on page 172). Using this information, the expert system produces a standard hemodynamic profile for the patient. With the derived data, the system consults a knowledge base consisting of 80 production rules.

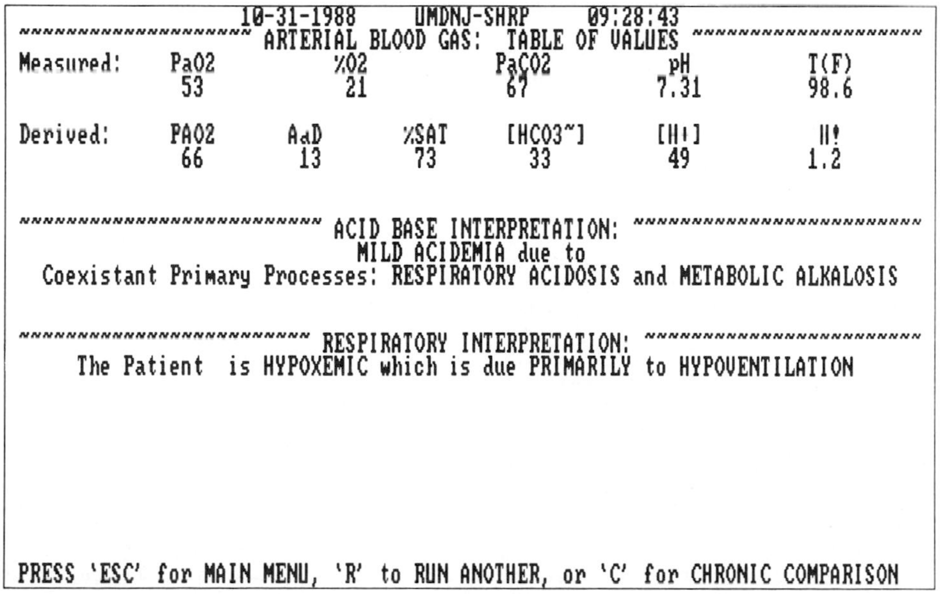

```
            10-31-1988      UMDNJ-SHRP     09:28:43
~~~~~~~~~~~~~~~~~~~~~~~ ARTERIAL BLOOD GAS:  TABLE OF VALUES ~~~~~~~~~~~~~~~~~~~~
Measured:    PaO2           %O2             PaCO2          pH          T(F)
             53             21              67             7.31        98.6

Derived:    PAO2    AaD     %SAT    [HCO3~]     [H]        H!
            66      13      73      33          49         1.2


~~~~~~~~~~~~~~~~~~~~~~~~~~~~~~ ACID BASE INTERPRETATION: ~~~~~~~~~~~~~~~~~~~~~~~~~~
                           MILD ACIDEMIA due to
      Coexistant Primary Processes: RESPIRATORY ACIDOSIS and METABOLIC ALKALOSIS


~~~~~~~~~~~~~~~~~~~~~~~~~~ RESPIRATORY INTERPRETATION: ~~~~~~~~~~~~~~~~~~~~~~~~~~~~
       The Patient  is HYPOXEMIC which is due PRIMARILY to HYPOVENTILATION




PRESS 'ESC' for MAIN MENU, 'R' to RUN ANOTHER, or 'C' for CHRONIC COMPARISON
```

Fig. 8-20 Summary interpretation of expert system analysis of arterial blood gas data. (From Wears RL and Kamen DR: Blood gas consultant. 1984.)

**EXAMPLE OF INTERACTION WITH
A HEMODYNAMIC MONITORING
EXPERT SYSTEM**

What is the patient's first name?
→Mary
What is the patient's last name?
→Smith
What is Mary Smith's patient number?
→123456789
There is no record of Mary Smith, #123456789, on file.
  Do you wish to establish a file for this patient (Y/N)?
→Y
What is Mary Smith's height (in inches)?
→65
What is Mary Smith's weight (in pounds)?
→160
What is Mary Smith's heart rate (in beats/min)?
→90
What is Mary Smith's cardiac output (in L/min)?
→3.0
What is Mary Smith's CVP or right atrial pressure (in
  mm Hg)?
→−1
What is Mary Smith's mean pulmonary artery pressure
  (in mm Hg)?
→10
What is Mary Smith's mean pulmonary wedge pressure
  (in mm Hg)?
→5
What is Mary Smith's mean arterial pressure (in mm
  Hg)?
→50
Which of the following clinical signs does Mary Smith
  exhibit?
(check all that apply):

postural hypotension	altered sensorium
skin pallor*	cool skin*
oliguria	concentrated urine*
weak pulse*	flat neck veins*

A

If all premises that fit a specific conclusion are true, the system provides a definitive hemodynamic interpretation (Figure 8-21, *B*). If the system cannot make a definitive assessment, the clinician is alerted. The expert system may provide suggestions to help refine the diagnosis.

Other applications of computer-assisted interpretation

Expert systems may be used in other applications of interest to the respiratory care practitioner. These include general diagnostic systems, computer-assisted interpretation of electrocardiograms, and cardiopulmonary fitness profiles.

Expert systems designed to support general clinical diagnosis have a broad scope. They must deal with a large number of clinical disorders by examining extensive lists of clinical signs and symptoms. Patient data is used to predict plausible hypotheses, similar to differential diagnoses. The preliminary hypotheses are then used to predict other clinical manifestations that must be confirmed or used to alter the original hypotheses. The output of these general diagnostic systems is usually a ranked list, with the most likely diagnoses listed in order of probability.

Computer-assisted ECG interpretation uses an extensive set of rules applied to numerous measurements taken from standard 12-lead ECG signals. In most systems, the rule-based software is encoded in a

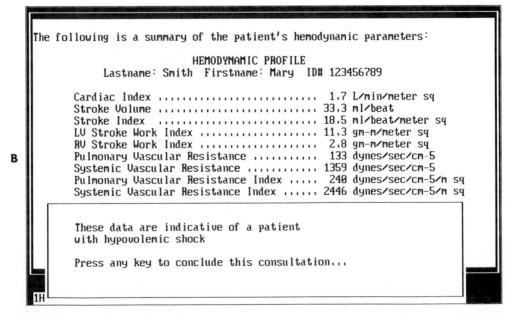

B

```
The following is a summary of the patient's hemodynamic parameters:

                    HEMODYNAMIC PROFILE
        Lastname: Smith  Firstname: Mary  ID# 123456789

        Cardiac Index ..........................    1.7 L/min/meter sq
        Stroke Volume ..........................   33.3 ml/beat
        Stroke Index  ..........................   18.5 ml/beat/meter sq
        LV Stroke Work Index ...................   11.3 gm-m/meter sq
        RV Stroke Work Index ...................    2.8 gm-m/meter sq
        Pulmonary Vascular Resistance ..........    133 dynes/sec/cm-5
        Systemic Vascular Resistance ..........   1359 dynes/sec/cm-5
        Pulmonary Vascular Resistance Index .....   240 dynes/sec/cm-5/m sq
        Systemic Vascular Resistance Index ......  2446 dynes/sec/cm-5/m sq


        These data are indicative of a patient
        with hypovolemic shock

        Press any key to conclude this consultation...
```

Fig. 8-21 Expert system for hemodynamic assessment. **A,** Script of the input required for hemodynamic assessment as entered by the practitioner. **B,** Output of the consultation with the expert system. Calculated data is presented along with diagnostic statements reflecting the expert system's interpretation of the data.

ROM chip inside the electrocardiograph instrument. After digitizing and storing appropriate samples of all 12 ECG leads, the software applies its rules. The output consist of the standard ECG measurements (i.e., rate, intervals, axis) and a list of interpretive statements. The interpretation is stored as a series of acronyms, which can be edited as necessary by the user.

Cardiopulmonary data, derived from an exercise test, can be used to assess the level of fitness of an individual. An expert system can examine variables stored during an exercise test. These variables include oxygen consumption, ventilation, heart rate, and blood pressure responses. By comparing the observed patterns to those known to occur in various diseases or conditions, the system can suggest which factors might limit the subject's ability to perform exercise. Such systems can also suggest the frequency and intensity of training appropriate for rehabilitation or conditioning.

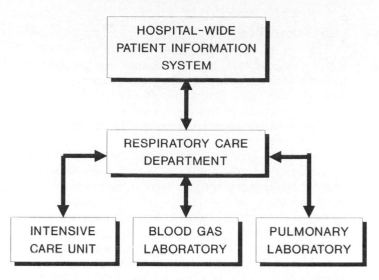

Fig. 8-22 Schema of an integrated clinical information system, combining clinical areas with the Respiratory Care Department and the hospital information system.

Integrated approaches

The clinical use of computers may actually make patient care more difficult. Large volumes of patient data made available by computers can be overwhelming. Data from multiple sources is seldom integrated into a unified package. The hospital information system (HIS) maintains one type of information, a departmental database may focus on another aspect of relevant data, and a computer-based intensive care unit (ICU) system may emphasize different clinical information.

Since certain elements of this diverse information may be pertinent to providing high-quality care to the patient, some hospitals are beginning to develop integrated approaches to acquisition, storage, and retrieval of relevant clinical data. For example, a respiratory care department's computer may be linked to both the hospital information system and selected clinical patient management systems (Figure 8-22). These might include blood gas and pulmonary function laboratories and the ICU monitoring system. By using such a framework, both general patient information and pertinent clinical data can be integrated. The patient record can be continuously updated across all systems. This gives clinicians full access to the information needed to plan, provide, and evaluate patient care.

Such systems are beginning to appear. Many HIS vendors offer subsystems that allow specialization on a departmental level. For example, results of pulmonary function studies or blood gas analyses can be uploaded into a patient care database. Because of the lack of standards for communicating text and data between small computers and mainframes, total systems integration is not yet a reality.

Nontechnical issues related to computers

Several concerns become apparent as computers are used for storing patient information and automating data reduction. These concerns include confidentiality and technical skills.

Confidentiality

Computer storage of patient records raises several concerns in regard to sensitive data. Most hospital information systems regulate access to patient data by means of passwords. Individuals using the system must "log on" by using a **password** that identifies them and determines their level of access. Comprehensive algorithms are available to manage various levels of access. The greatest concern is how to apply these algorithms so that appropriate personnel can view or edit patient data.

Implementing a password system requires policies that define who may access patient demographic, clinical, and billing information. These policies should define not only levels of access but the way data is to be handled. This may include regulations for printing of patient information versus simple screen viewing. Most systems provide utilities for auditing which users performed specific functions. The use of such audit functions can help ensure observance of hospital policies.

Hospital information systems generally provide capabilities for "blacking out" selected patient information. Departmental computer systems or PC-based equipment may not offer the same capability. In these cases, it is important that policies be established to regulate how patient data are to be handled.

Technical skills

The use of computers interfaced to spirometers, blood gas analyzers, and ventilators can promote a false sense of complacency. This complacency occurs when the user has an incomplete understanding of the technical aspects of the instrument-computer interface. This phenomenon has been termed the "black box mentality."

Many tasks previously performed by a technologist or therapist are now managed by computer. Calculations and measurement that were done manually are now executed by the computer. This promotes a tendency to teach individuals to use the computerized instrument without a detailed understanding of the process involved. In effect, the computer allows an individual with minimal understanding of a technical procedure (such as blood gas analysis) to perform the task. Serious problems can arise when a computerized system malfunctions, and the user fails to detect an irregularity. Users of computerized instruments (monitors, ventilators) need a greater understanding of the technical process than someone using a similar instrument in the manual mode. Computer-based equipment requires that the user be knowledgeable not only about the specific device, but about the computer itself and how it is interfaced.

CHAPTER SUMMARY

The computer is a versatile tool. Computers can perform complex mathematical and logical operations quickly and accurately. They can store, retrieve, translate, and sort multiple types of data. They can monitor external events and control external devices. Modern computer technology involves both hardware and software. There are five key components in most computer systems: (1) a CPU, (2) an arithmetic logic unit, (3) input devices, (4) memory to store data and instructions, and (5) output devices. Software represents how the user instructs the computer what to do and how to do it. A set of instructions is called a program.

Programs can be divided into groups according to the specific functions they allow the computer to perform. Operating system programs are essential to the computer's ability to perform tasks such as data storage and retrieval and memory management. Application programs are run under the control of the operating system to accomplish specific tasks. These tasks include text processing, manipulation of numeric data, data base management, artificial intelligence, and monitoring or control of external devices.

Computers have been used in respiratory care for over 20 years. The first application of computers dealt with hospital-based financial and patient information systems. Computers have also been involved in areas such as pulmonary function testing, where calculation and display of numerical data were important. The introduction of microprocessors revolutionized monitoring and therapeutic devices such as ventilators. Now, most monitors and ventilators incorporate one or more microprocessor-controlled components. Computers themselves are being used to assist clinicians in interpreting data, reaching diagnoses, and automating certain aspects of patient care.

Patient care in general and respiratory care in particular are at the same time human and humane endeavors. The computer can assist the health care provider in almost every area. In many instances, it is indispensable. The computer cannot replace the practitioner. As a clinical tool, the computer can perform those tasks that are repetitive and time consuming. Its use should allow the respiratory care practitioner to devote more time to direct patient care. To do this requires not only understanding of therapeutic and diagnostic protocols, but skill in using the computer to improve patient care.

BIBLIOGRAPHY

Andrews RD, Gardner RM: Portable computers used for respiratory care charting, *Int J Clin Monit Comput* 5:45–52, 1988.

Aquino MM: A respiratory profile from a hand-held computer, *Heart Lung,* 14:88–90 1985.

Baldwin J: Continuous breath-by-breath monitoring greatly enhances patient care capabilities: incorporating the pneumotach and real time computer based system, *Crit Care Nurse* 3(3):33–35, 1983.

Bhutani VK et al: Adaptive control of inspired oxygen delivery to the neonate, *Pediatr Pulmonol* 14:110–117, 1992.

Caceres CA: Computer-assisted ECG: an overview of computerized analysis, *Consultant* 24:237–239, 242–243, 247–248, 1984.

Chatburn RL: Computation of cardiorespiratory variables with a programmable calculator, *Respir Care* 28:447–451, 1983.

Clemmer TP, Gardner RM: Medical informatics in the intensive care unit: state of the art, *Int J Clin Monit Comput,* 8:237–250, 1991–1992.

Coon RR, Zuperky EJ, Kampine JP: Systemic arterial blood pH servocontrol of mechanical ventilation, *Anesthesiology* 49:201–204, 1978.

Crapo RO et al: Automation of pulmonary function equipment: user beware! Chest 90:1–2, 1986 (editorial).

Demers RR: Some potential pitfalls associated with the use of computers and microprocessors, *Respir Care* 27:842–845, 1982.

East TD: Microcomputer data acquisition and control, *Int J Clin Monit Comput* 3:225–238, 1986.

East TD, Andriano KP, Pace NL: Computer-controlled optimization of positive end-expiratory pressure, *Crit Care Med* 14:792–797, 1986.

Ellis JR, Perera SP, Levin DC: A computer program for calculation and interpretation of pulmonary function studies, *Chest* 68:209–213, 1975.

Gardner RM, Elliott CG, Greenway L: The computer for charting and monitoring. In Kacmarek RM, Hess D, Stoller JK, editors: *Monitoring in Respiratory Care,* St. Louis, 1993, Mosby.

Gardner RM et al: Computer guidelines for pulmonary laboratories, *Am Rev Respir Dis* 134:628–629, 1986.

Gardner RM et al: Computerized decision-making in the pulmonary function laboratory, *Respir Care,* 27:799–808, 1982.

Henderson S et al: Performance of computerized protocols for the management of arterial oxygenation in an intensive care unit, *Int J Clin Monit Comput* 8:271–280, 1991–1992.

Hess D, Eitel D: A portable and inexpensive computer system to interpret arterial blood gases, *Respir Care* 31:792–795, 1986.

Klar R, Zaiss A: Medical expert systems: design and applications in pulmonary medicine, *Lung* 168(suppl):1201–1209, 1990.

Korst RJ et al: Validation of respiratory mechanics software in microprocessor-controlled ventilators, *Crit Care Med* 20:1152–1156, 1992.

Kunz JC et al: *A physiologic rule-based system for interpreting pulmonary function test results.* Report HPP-78-19. Stanford, Calif, 1979, Stanford University, Computer Science Department, Heuristic Programming Project.

Lampotang S: Microprocessor controlled ventilation systems and concepts. In Kirby RR, Banner MJ, Downs JB, editors: *Clinical Application of Ventilatory Support.* New York, 1990, Churchill Livingstone.

Levine R, Drang DE, Edelson B: A comprehensive guide to AI and expert systems, New York, McGraw-Hill, 1986.

Maxwell C, Silage DA: Hand-held computers in pulmonary medicine, *Respir Care* 28:35–36, 1983.

McPeck M: Fifth annual international symposium on computers in critical care and pulmonary medicine, *Respir Care* 29:384–394, 1984.

Meehan PA: Hemodynamic assessment using the automated physiologic profile, *Crit Care Nurse* 6(1):29–46, 1986.

Miller PL, Blumenfrucht SJ, Rose JR: Computer technology: state of the art and future trends, *J Am Coll Cardiol* 9:204–214, 1987.

Mishelevich DJ et al.: Respiratory therapy as a component of an integrated hospital information system: the Parkland on-line information system, *Respir Care* 27:846–854, 1982.

Morozoff PE, Evans RW: Closed-loop control of SaO2 in the neonate, *Biomed Instrum Technol* 26:117–123, 1992.

Nelson SB et al: Performance evaluation of contemporary spirometers, Chest 97:288–297, 1990.

Ohlson KB, Westenskow DR, Jordan WS: A microprocessor based feedback controller for mechanical ventilation, *Ann Biomed Eng* 10:35–48, 1982.

Schwartz WB, Patil RS, Szolovits P: Artificial intelligence in medicine: where do we stand? *N Engl J Med* 316:685–688, 1987.

Sittig DF et al: Clinical evaluation of computer based respiratory care algorithms, *Int J Clin Monit Comput* 7:177–185, 1990.

Thompson JD: Computerized control of mechanical ventilation: closing the loop, *Respir Care* 32:440–444, 1987.

Westenskow DR: Fundamentals of feedback control applied to microcomputer instrumentation design, *Int J Clin Monit Comput* 3:239–244, 1986.

Worthley JA, Disalvo PS: *Managing Computers in Health Care,* ed 2, Ann Arbor, Mich, 1989, Health Administration Press.

3

Applied Anatomy and Physiology

9

Functional Anatomy of the Respiratory System

■

Gregg L. Ruppel

John Tesoriero

1. Identify and describe the gross structures of the thorax and their functions;
2. Characterize the actions of the primary and accessory muscles of ventilation during various levels of activity;
3. Describe the origin and action of the somatic and autonomic pathways innervating the lung and thoracic musculature;
4. Compare and contrast the pulmonary and bronchial circulations;
5. Describe the major structures of the upper respiratory tract and list their functions;
6. Describe the structure of the lower respiratory tract as a system for conducting gas;
7. Identify the pulmonary segments and differences between the right and left lungs;
8. Describe the differences in structure and function of the large airways and small airways;
9. Identify the components of the respiratory zones of the lung.

The respiratory system is made up of cells, tissues, and organs. It sustains the body under both normal and stressful conditions. Working with the cardiovascular system, the respiratory system functions primarily to exchange oxygen and carbon dioxide between the atmosphere and the cells of the body.

The process of respiration involves specialized structures that perform complex functions. The respiratory system must protect itself against inhaled contaminants. It must condition inspired gas, moving it in and out of the lungs with a minimum of work. The respiratory system must expose gases to blood to assure rapid and efficient exchange. It must respond and adapt to changing conditions within the body. Respiratory care is founded on the appreciation and understanding of the anatomic and physiologic relationships in health and disease.

The development of the respiratory system is detailed in Chapter 35 (Neonatal and Pediatric Respiratory Care). This chapter focuses on the adult respiratory system.

THE THORAX

Overview

The thorax is formed by the rib cage, the thoracic vertebrae, and the sternum. It contains the esophagus, trachea, lungs, heart, and great vessels (Figure 9-1). The thorax has a wide base, bounded by the diaphragm below and a narrow opening at the top. The opening, called the operculum, is bounded by the first ribs and the upper portion of the sternum.

The thorax may be viewed as consisting of three "compartments." These are the mediastinum and the left and right pleural cavities. These spaces are actually filled by the major organs just described. The centrally located mediastinum contains the trachea, esophagus, heart, and great vessels of the circulatory system. The left and right pleural cavities contain the lungs.

The "cage" around these thoracic compartments serves two purposes. First, its bony structures protect the vital organs inside. Second, the thoracic bones and muscles interact to vary its volume. This action generates the pressure differences necessary to cause gas flow into and out of the lungs.

Gross Structure and Function

The mediastinum

The mediastinum is the central compartment of the chest. It divides the thorax vertically and separates the left and right pleural cavities. The mediastinum is bounded laterally by the parietal pleura along the **medial** aspects of both lungs. It is bounded anteriorly by the sternum, posteriorly by the thoracic vertebrae, inferiorly by the diaphragm, and superiorly by the thoracic inlet.

The mediastinum is divided into three subcompartments.[1] The anterior compartment lies between the sternum and **pericardium.** It contains the thymus gland and the anterior mediastinal lymph nodes. The middle compartment contains the pericardium and heart. It also contains the great vessels, phrenic and upper portions of the vagus nerves, the trachea and mainstem bronchi, and their associated lymph nodes. The posterior compartment lies between the pericardium and the vertebral column. It contains the tho-

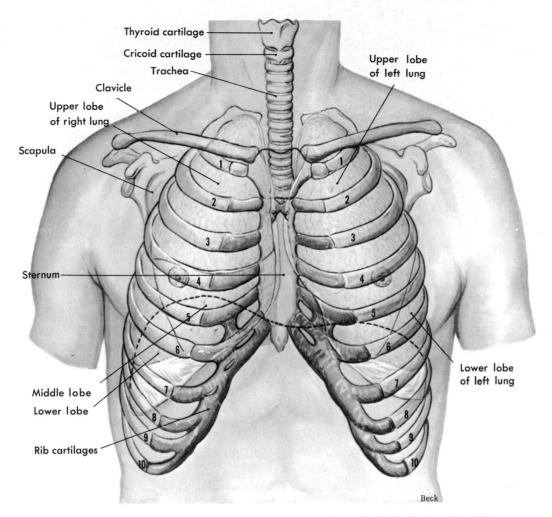

Thyroid cartilage

Cricoid cartilage

Trachea

Upper lobe
of left lung

Clavicle

Upper lobe
of right lung

Scapula

Sternum

Lower lobe
of left lung

Middle lobe

Lower lobe

Rib cartilages

Beck

Fig. 9-1 Projection of the lungs and trachea in relation to the rib cage and clavicles. Dotted line indicates location of the dome-shaped diaphragm at the end of expiration and before inspiration. Note that apex of each lung projects above the clavicle. Ribs 11 and 12 are not visible in this view. (From Anthony CP and Thibodeau GA: Textbook of anatomy and physiology, ed 12, St Louis, 1987, Mosby.)

racic aorta, esophagus, and thoracic duct. The sympathetic chains and lower portions of the vagus nerve, as well as the posterior mediastinal lymph nodes, are in the posterior mediastinum.

The lungs and pleura

The lungs are paired cone-shaped organs. They lie in the pleural cavities, separated by the mediastinum. Although the adult lungs weigh about 800 grams, their volume consists of nearly 90% air and only 10% tissue. The heart and mediastinum protrude to the left, forming a cavity called the *cardiac notch*. As a result, the left lung is somewhat narrower than the right. The liver elevates the right hemidiaphragm, making the right lung shorter than the left.

The lungs extend from the diaphragm to a point approximately 1 to 2 cm above the clavicles. The tops of the lungs are called the *apices*. The lung surfaces lying against the ribs form the curved costal margins. The medial surfaces of the lungs are adjacent to the mediastinum. The mediastinal surface contains a vertical opening called the *hilum*. The major airways, blood vessels, lymphatics, and nerves enter and exit through the hilum. This grouping of pathways, bound together by connective tissue, is often referred to as the *lung root*. The apices, hilum, and lung root are often referenced in the interpretation of chest radiographs (see Chapter 19).

Each lung is divided into smaller anatomic units called *lobes* (Figure 9-1). The lobes are separated by one or more *fissures*. The right lung has upper, middle, and lower lobes. The upper and middle lobes of the right lung are separated by a horizontal fissure. Its middle and lower lobes are set apart by an oblique fissure. The left lung has only an upper and a lower lobe, separated by a single oblique fissure. The lobes are divided into *segments* according to the branches of the tracheobronchial tree. The bronchopulmonary segments are subdivided into *secondary lobules*. These are the smallest gross anatomic units of lung tissue set apart by true connective tissue septa (Figure 9-2, on page 180). Secondary lobules contain clusters of three

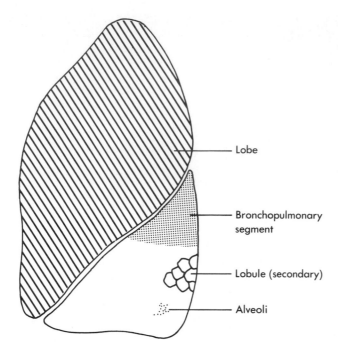

Fig. 9-2 Diagram of units of lung. Alveoli are actually microscopic in size.

to five terminal bronchioles. These lobules can be observed from the external and cut surface of the lung (Figure 9-3). Secondary lobules are polygonal in shape, from 1 to 2.5 cm on a side.[2] Localized infection, hemorrhage, and aspiration are initially contained by the boundaries between these lobules.

The surface of the lungs and the inside of the chest walls are covered by a thin layer of **mesothelium** called the *pleura.* Pleural tissue also covers portions of the interlobular fissures, the diaphragm, and the lateral portions of the mediastinum. That portion covering the lungs is called the *visceral pleura.* The visceral pleura extends onto the hilar bronchi and vessels, and into the major fissures. The deeper portions of the visceral pleura contain elastic and fibrous tissue, as well as small venules and lymphatics. The interlobular septa are continuous with this layer. The veins and lymphatics course along these septa, starting as fine-caliber vessels in the visceral pleura.

The pleura covering the inner surface of the chest wall and the mediastinum is called the *parietal pleura* (Figure 9-4). Portions of the parietal pleura are named according to the structures that they contact. The costal pleura lines the inner surface of the rib cage. The mediastinal pleura covers the mediastinum. The diaphragmatic pleura covers the diaphragm. The acute angle where the costal pleura joins the diaphragmatic pleura is known as the *costophrenic angle.* This area contains no lung tissue and is clearly visible on normal chest radiographs. Excess fluids in the pleural space have a tendency to pool here in an upright subject. This causes the angle to appear blunted or flattened on the chest radiograph (see Chapter 19). The upper dome of the parietal pleura extends above the first rib and encloses the thoracic inlet. At the lung root, the parietal pleura becomes continuous with the visceral pleura as it passes onto the surface of the lung. Although the two portions of the pleura are

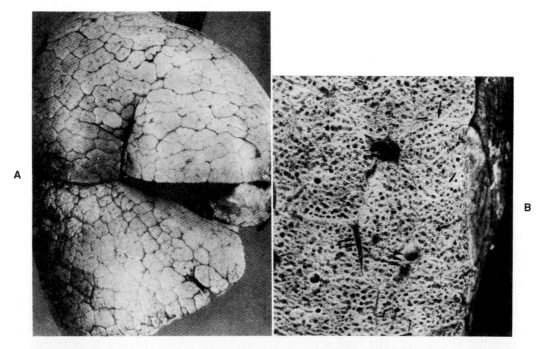

Fig. 9-3 Outer surface (**A**) and cut surface (**B**) of lung. **B,** One arrow marks an interlobular septum, two arrows mark small veins in these septa, and three arrows point to a pulmonary artery and bronchiole near center of secondary lobule. (From Heitzman ER: The lung: radiologic-pathologic correlations, St Louis, 1973, Mosby.)

■ M I N I **C** L I N I ■

9-1

Penetrating Chest Injury

Normally, the parietal and visceral pleura are in physical contact with one another, separated only by a thin liquid film of fluid. This liquid film allows these two pleural membranes to slide over one another with very little friction. At the same time, the film provides a cohesive force that resists separation of the membranes, much as a film of water between two glass microscope slides makes pulling the slides apart almost impossible. Thus, when the respiratory muscles move the rib cage outward in an inspiratory effort, the lung is literally pulled with it by the cohesive forces between the parietal and visceral pleural membranes. The elastic recoil forces of the lung resist this outward movement.

Problem: A person suffers a traumatic penetrating wound to the chest such that the chest wall and parietal pleural membrane are punctured, leaving the visceral pleura intact. What are the consequences of this injury to the lungs and chest wall?

Answer: The lungs would collapse, sucking atmospheric air into the chest, separating the parietal and visceral pleura. The chest wall would simultaneously expand. (Air in the pleural space is called pneumothorax.)

Analysis: The natural elastic recoil of the lung normally creates a subatmospheric intrapleural pressure. In the intact chest, the lung is expanded beyond its resting shape and the chest wall is pulled inward beyond its resting shape. Both structures tend to recoil in opposite directions but each is held in position by the other's equal and oppositely directed recoil force. If the pleural cavity communicates with the atmosphere, as it would in the previous problem, air would rush into the pleural space down its pressure gradient. Elastic recoil of the lungs would be unopposed, collapsing the lung and pulling more air into the chest. The thorax, unopposed, would recoil outward. Treatment of this condition would involve inserting a tube into the chest cavity and applying vacuum to reexpand the lung.

---

described by different names, they form one continuous lining.

Between the visceral and parietal pleura is the *pleural cavity.* This "cavity" is really a potential space, occupied by a thin layer of serous fluid. This fluid forms a thin film of uniform thickness that couples the visceral and parietal pleural surfaces. The fluid allows the pleura to slip easily over one another.[3] It also permits chest wall forces to be transmitted to the lungs. If air, blood, or other fluids are introduced into this space, the two pleural surfaces can separate. If this happens, the parietal pleura remains fixed against the inner wall of the thorax, while the lung and the visceral pleura are displaced away from the chest wall.

The lung itself has elastic properties. This elasticity is due to surface tension forces in the alveoli and to tissue forces. The presence of **elastin** fibers in the alveolar walls, around the small airways, and in pulmonary capillaries produces elastic recoil. **Collagen** fibers probably contribute little to the elastic

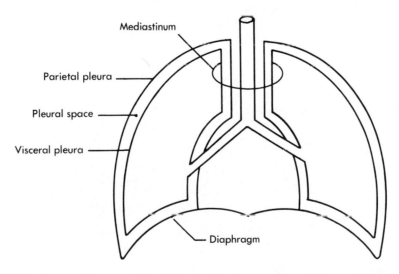

Fig. 9-4 This diagram shows overall relationship of chest organs, cavities, and investments. The mediastinum occupies space between lungs. Each lung sits within its chest cavity. This cavity is lined by parietal pleura, which covers chest cage, diaphragm, and lateral mediastinum, and by visceral pleura, which covers lungs.

properties of the lungs, acting primarily to limit expansion at high lung volumes.[4] Because of its elasticity, the lung always tends to recoil to a lower volume. When a lung is removed from the chest cavity, it quickly collapses to a smaller size. The same occurs when air or fluid is introduced into the pleural space. This tendency of the lung to contract permits development of subatmospheric intrapleural pressure (see Chapter 11). It is possible for individual lobes of the lung to collapse. The most common cause of a lobar collapse is obstruction of its bronchus.

Bones of the thoracic cage

Thoracic bones include the thoracic vertebrae, the sternum, and the ribs and costal cartilages (Figure 9-5). These bony structures provide support and protection to the thoracic viscera. They serve as points of origin and insertion for the respiratory muscles.

Vertebrae

The 12 thoracic vertebrae share a common structure with the entire vertebral column. Each vertebrum has a *body* with **pedicles, laminae, spinous** and **transverse processes.** Thoracic vertebrae differ from their **cervical** and **lumbar** counterparts. The bodies and transverse processes of the thoracic vertebrae have *facets* that serve as points of articulation for the head of each rib. The orientation of these facets provides for the rotation and elevation that characterize rib movement.

Sternum

The sternum is a dagger-shaped bony structure in the median line at the front of the chest. It serves as the point of attachment for the costal cartilages and numerous muscles. It also provides protection for the underlying organs. The adult sternum averages 18 cm in length. It consists of three portions: the upper triangular *manubrium;* the long, narrow *body;* and the pointed lower *xiphoid process.*

The manubrium articulates with the first and second ribs and the clavicle. Between the clavicles, the upper surface of the manubrium forms an easily identified depression called the *suprasternal notch.* The manubrium is a point of attachment for portions of the pectoralis major muscle. It also serves as the sternal origin of the sternomastoid muscle. Between the levels of the fourth and fifth thoracic vertebrae, the manubrium articulates with the body of the sternum and second costal cartilages (second ribs). A slightly oblique angle called the *angle of Louis* is formed. The angle of Louis is an important external landmark. It marks the point at which the trachea divides into left and right mainstem bronchi. It also marks the upper margin of the heart. In the adult, the body of the sternum (corpus sterni) is a single bone, articulating with the second through seventh ribs via the costal cartilages.

The xiphoid process is a **cartilaginous** structure. It is located at approximately the level of the 10th thoracic vertebra. The xiphoid process is the smallest portion of the sternum and its shape varies. It articu-

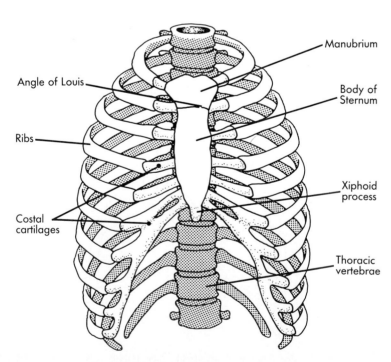

Fig. 9-5 Chest cage. Ribs arch around from vertebral column joining sternum through cartilaginous extensions.

lates with the seventh rib pair. The xiphoid process serves as an attachment point for portions of the diaphragm and abdominal muscles.

Ribs

Corresponding to the twelve thoracic vertebrae are twelve pairs of ribs. The first seven pairs are the vertebrosternal ribs. They connect directly to the sternum via the costal cartilages (see Figure 9-5). The 8th through 10th pairs are the vertebrochondral ribs. These ribs connect to the ribs above and indirectly to the sternum through the costal cartilages. This **cartilage** is soft and moderately flexible during childhood and adolescence. As the individual ages the cartilages become calcified. The rib cage then becomes less flexible. The 11th and 12th rib pairs have no connection to the other rib pairs or sternum. These ribs are often referred to as "floating ribs." The floating ribs terminate in cartilaginous free ends in the wall of the abdomen.

Each rib consists of a *head,* a *neck,* and a body or *shaft* (Figures 9-6 and 9-8, on page 184). Except for ribs 10–12, the rounded head has two *facets* for articulation with corresponding facets on the thoracic vertebrae. The flattened neck is about 2.5 cm long and extends outward from the head. The neck provides an attachment point for the costotransverse ligaments. On the posterior surface of the neck is a *tubercle,* most prominent in the upper ribs. The tubercle articulates with the transverse process of the lower of the two vertebrae to which the head of the rib is connected. The rib shaft is thin and curved, with numerous ridges and grooves. The ridges serve as points of origin or attachment for muscles. The *costal groove* on the underside of each rib (Figures 9-6 and 9-7, on page 184) contains an intercostal artery, vein, and nerve. To prevent damage to these structures, placement of needles or tubes into the intercostal space must always be done *above* the rib.

Rib movements

The first rib moves slightly, raising and lowering the sternum. Its small motion increases the **anteroposterior** (AP) diameter of the chest. This action is not used during quiet breathing. It becomes important under conditions that require increased ventilation, such as exercise.

The six vertebrosternal ribs play an important role in ventilation. These ribs move simultaneously about two axes (Figure 9-8). As they rotate about the axes of their necks, their sternal ends rise and fall. This movement increases the AP thoracic diameter. This action is described as "pump handle" motion. At the same time these ribs move about the long axes from their angles to the sternum. This motion causes the middle segments of the ribs to move up and down. This "bucket handle" motion produces increases and decreases in the transverse diameter of the chest. The

compound action of these ribs changes both the AP and transverse diameters smoothly and evenly.

The vertebrochondral ribs rotate in a pattern similar to that of the vertebrosternal group. Elevation of the anterior ends of these ribs, however, produces a backward movement of the lower sternum. This reduces the thoracic AP diameter (Figure 9-9, page 185). As with the vertebrosternal ribs, outward rotation of the middle portions of the ribs increases the transverse diameter of the thorax. Ribs 11–12 do not participate in changing the contour of the chest but act as muscular insertion points.

Muscle action

Various muscles of the thorax and abdomen contribute to the movement of gas into and out of the lungs. These muscles may be divided into the *primary* and the *accessory* muscles of ventilation. The diaphragm and intercostal muscles are the primary muscles of ventilation. They are active during both quiet breathing and exercise. The accessory muscles of ventilation assist the diaphragm and intercostals under conditions of increased ventilatory demand. The scalenes, sternomastoids, pectoralis major, and abdominals are the predominant accessory muscles. Other abdominal and chest wall muscles may also function as accessory muscles.

Diaphragm

This large transverse muscle arises from the lumbar vertebrae, the costal margin, and the xiphoid process. Its fibers converge into a broad connective sheet called the *central tendon.* The diaphragm is configured like a dome. It divides the chest from the abdomen. The central tendon combines with the **pericardium** to divide the dome into two "leaves." These leaves are referred to as the *right* and *left hemidiaphragms.* Because the liver is located immediately below it, the right hemidiaphragm is about 1 cm higher than the left at the end of a quiet breath. Movements of the hemidiaphragms are synchronous in healthy subjects. However, innervation by separate phrenic nerves allows each hemidiaphragm to function independently. Many clinical situations arise in which one or both hemidiaphragms move asynchronously.

The diaphragm accounts for about 75% of the change in thoracic volume during quiet inspiration. During tidal breathing, the diaphragm moves approximately 1.5 cm. Each centimeter of vertical movement results in approximately 350 mL of volume change. At high levels of ventilation the diaphragm may move 6 to 10 cm. The ability of the diaphragm to change thoracic volume is altered in the presence of obstructive or restrictive lung disease (see Chapter 11, Ventilation).

During quiet breathing, the excursions of both

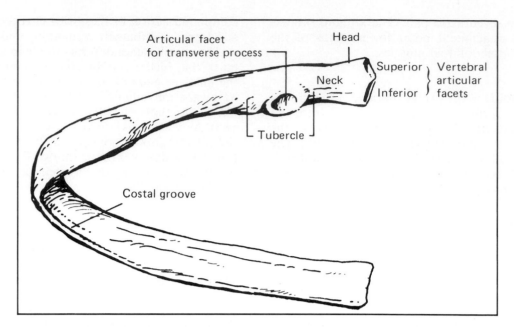

Fig. 9-6 A typical middle rib, from the left side of the body, viewed posteriorly (from the back). The head end (and tubercle) articulate with the vertebral column, while the shaft articulates with the sternum. (From Martin DE and Youtsey JW: Respiratory anatomy and physiology, St Louis, 1988, Mosby.)

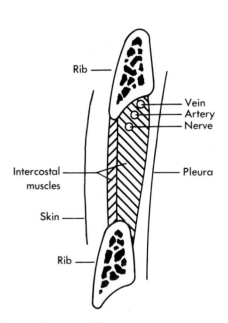

Fig. 9-7 Intercostal muscles fill spaces between ribs. An intercostal artery, veins, and nerve run in groove just beneath lower edge of each rib.

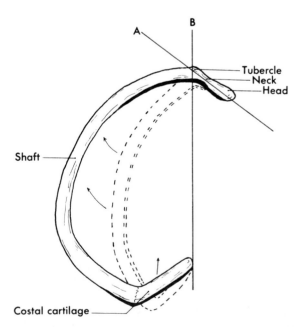

Fig. 9-8 The two axes about which the vertebrosternal ribs rotate during ventilation are indicated by lines *A* and *B*. The former passes through the length of the rib head and neck; the latter follows an AP direction from the tip of the costal cartilage to the tubercle. The rib undergoes a compound movement from its starting position (*dotted outline*), the shaft swinging upward and laterally about axis *B,* and the anterior end moving upward about axis *A.*

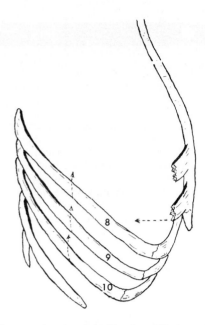

Fig. 9-9 The vertebrochondral ribs, *8* to *10,* have laterosuperior movement, but elevation of their anterior ends retracts the lower end of the sternum, shortening the AP diameter of the thorax in that plane.

leaves of the diaphragm are about equal. With a deep inspiration the right diaphragm may descend more than the left. Total diaphragmatic movement is approximately the same in the erect and supine positions. In a head-down, 45-degree supine tilt, however, the resting level of the diaphragm rises about 6 cm. This causes a reduction of the functional residual capacity (FRC) and the expiratory reserve volume (ERV). When a subject lies in a lateral position, the lower hemidiaphragm tends to rise into the chest.[5]

The mechanical action of the diaphragm is twofold. First, contraction draws the central tendon down. This flattens the diaphragm, increasing the thoracic volume and lowering intrathoracic pressure. As the diaphragm descends, intra-abdominal pressure increases. The muscles of the abdominal wall relax, allowing the upper abdomen to balloon outward. Splinting or rigidity of the abdominal wall interferes with diaphragmatic descent during inspiration. The second mechanical action of the diaphragm is achieved through contraction of its costal fibers. This raises and everts the lateral costal margins (Figure 9-10, *A*). Increasing abdominal pressure during inspiration acts as a fulcrum. Continued contraction of the diaphragmatic fibers pulls up and outward on the costal margin.

This dual action of the diaphragm may be disturbed by various pulmonary diseases. For example, in advanced emphysema air is trapped in the lungs. The diaphragm is displaced to an abnormally low and flat position. When this happens, there is less vertical excursion during inspiration. Contraction of the costal fibers often pulls the lower chest boundary *inward*. This results in *narrowing* rather than expansion of the lateral dimensions of the thorax (Figure 9-10, *B*).

Although the diaphragm is the principal ventilatory muscle, it is not essential for survival. Adequate ventilation is possible even if the diaphragm is paralyzed. If either or both of the diaphragm leaves are paralyzed, the affected component(s) stays in the resting position. During deep inspiration, the paralyzed diaphragm rises as other ventilatory muscles reduce the intrathoracic pressure. During quiet breathing the paralyzed diaphragm may remain immobile or may move in either direction. The pressure above and below a paralyzed diaphragm tends to make it rise during inspiration. The outward movement of the lower ribs tends to stretch and flatten it. The final course is the result of these two forces.

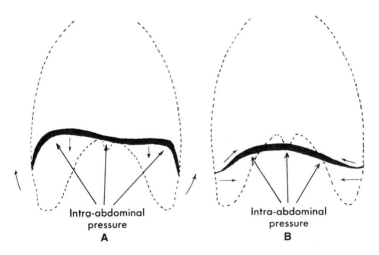

Fig. 9-10, A, as the normal diaphragm contracts, it descends, gradually building up pressure in the abdomen until the intraabdominal pressure acts as a fulcrum against which continued contraction everts the costal margin, enlarging the thorax further. **B,** Contraction of the diaphram, which is abnormally low at the start of inspiration, can only pull in the costal margin, reducing the lower thoracic diameters.

■ M I N I C L I N I ■

9-2

Hyperinflated Lungs, Enlarged Thorax, and Flattened Diaphragms in Emphysema

Emphysema is a disease characterized by the destruction of elastic lung tissue. The emphysematous lung has less elastic recoil force than the normal lung.

Problem: Why do people with severe emphysema have enlarged, overinflated lungs; flattened diaphragms; and a thorax that appears to be overexpanded, even at the end of a normal quiet exhalation?

Answer: Emphysema destroys elastic fibers in the lung. This causes it to lose some of its natural tendency to recoil. As the disease worsens, the inward recoil force of the lung becomes less than the normal outward recoil force of the chest wall; these two oppositely directed recoil forces are no longer equal in magnitude. The balance between these two recoil forces is broken. The stronger outward recoil force of the chest wall overcomes the weak inward recoil force of the lung, pulling the lung outward to a new enlarged volume. When the lung becomes stretched enough, its inward recoil force increases until once again it counterbalances the outward recoil of the chest wall. The results are an expanded chest wall and an overinflated lung, even at the end of a normal quiet exhalation. The diaphragm is flattened for similar reasons. Its normal upward, domed position is due to the elastic pull of a normally recoiling lung. In emphysema, loss of elastic lung recoil allows the diaphragm to move downward and assume a more flattened position, even at the end of a normal exhalation. This flattened position limits the extent to which the diaphragm can descend during an inspiration, thus causing the inspiratory capacity to be abnormally small. The volume in the lung at the end of a normal exhalation is, on the other hand, abnormally large. The emphysema patient appears to be in a continual inspiratory position.

The diaphragm does not actively participate in exhalation. It returns to its resting position during the passive recoil of the thorax. During forced exhalation or against resistance the diaphragm acts as a passive piston. It expels gas from the lung as it is pushed upward by increased pressure in the abdomen. The abdominal pressure increase is generated by contracting abdominal muscles. The diaphragm performs important functions other than ventilation. It aids in generating high intraabdominal pressures by remaining fixed while the abdominal muscles contract. The diaphragm facilitates vomiting, coughing and sneezing, defecation, and parturition.

Intercostal muscles

The intercostal muscles consist of two sets of fibers located between each rib pair (Figures 9-7 and 9-11). The *external intercostal* muscles arise from the inferior edge of each rib from the rib tubercle to its costochondral junction. The fibers pass inferiorly and anteriorly to insert into the superior edge of the rib below. These muscles are thicker posteriorly than anteriorly and are thicker than the internal intercostals.

The *internal intercostal* muscles are located beneath the external intercostals. They arise from the inferior edge of each rib from the anterior end of the intercostal space to the rib angles. The fibers pass inferiorly and posteriorly to insert into the superior edge of the rib below. This muscle group is divided into two functional parts: (1) an interosseous portion located between the sloping parts of the ribs and (2) an intercartilaginous portion located where the costal cartilages slope superiorly and anteriorly.

Considerable controversy exists regarding the function of the intercostal muscles. **Electromyographic** studies indicate that the external intercostals and the intercartilaginous portion of the internal intercostals are active during breathing. Contraction of these muscles during inspiration elevates the ribs, increasing thoracic volume. This action occurs primarily near the resting expiratory level. At high lung volumes the intercostals actually lower the ribs.[6] The absence of this function is documented during paralysis. These muscles probably serve to stabilize the chest wall and prevent intercostal bulging or retraction during large intrathoracic pressure changes. Myographic studies also reveal intercostal activity continuing from quiet inspiration into early exhalation. This expiratory activity may help to retard high airflows and facilitate less turbulent exhalation. At flows greater than 50 L/min or during maximum voluntary exhalation, the intercostals of the lower spaces also contract toward the end of exhalation. This action presumably stabilizes the chest in the presence of powerful abdominal contraction.

Scalene muscles

The anterior, medial, and posterior scalene muscles are considered as a functional unit (Figure 9-11). The scalenes are primarily skeletal muscles of the neck. They also function as accessory muscles of ventilation and play an important role in breathing. The scalenes arise from the transverse processes of the

■ MINI CLINI ■

9-3

Significance of Intercostal Retractions

Intercostal retractions are inward movements of the tissues between the ribs of the chest wall during inspiration. This causes the ribs to stand out prominently during inspiratory efforts.

Problem: Why may a patient who is experiencing respiratory difficulty because of severe airway obstruction or noncompliant "stiff" lungs exhibit inspiratory intercostal retractions?

Answer: The intrathoracic space (i.e., space between the lungs and chest wall) normally exhibits a subatmospheric pressure. This is caused by the tendency of the lung to recoil inward while the chest wall tends to recoil outward. The magnitude of this subatmospheric pressure increases with inspiration; that is, during inspiration, ventilatory muscles enlarge the chest wall and the diaphragm descends, thus enlarging the intrathoracic volume and decreasing its pressure (Boyle's law). During normal quiet breathing with open, unobstructed airways, the drop in intrathoracic pressure during inspiration is relatively small. However, if the airways are severely obstructed (e.g., foreign body aspiration, asthmatic bronchoconstriction) much greater muscular effort is required to inhale because of the high resistance to airflow. This greater muscular effort translates into a much greater drop in intrathoracic pressure as the thorax enlarges and tries to pull air through obstructed airways. The drop in intrathoracic pressure pulls or "sucks" the soft tissues between the ribs inward, causing intercostal retractions. Abnormally "stiff" noncompliant lungs (e.g., pneumonia, atelectasis, fibrotic lung diseases) may cause intercostal retractions for similar reasons. In this case, the lungs have an abnormally high recoil force that resists inflation. Again, greater inspiratory muscular efforts generate greater than normal subatmospheric pressure in the intrathoracic space, and intercostal retractions occur, signaling greatly increased work of breathing.

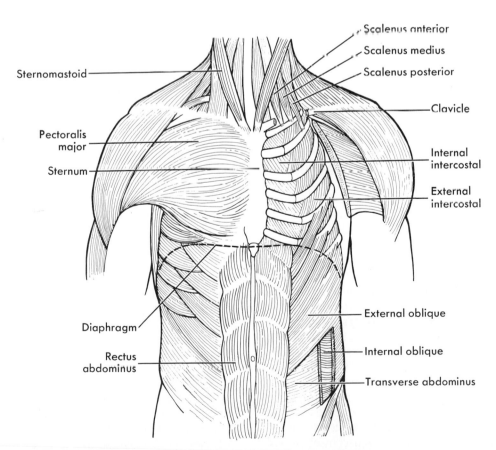

Fig. 9-11 The muscles of ventilation. (See text for description.)

lower five cervical vertebrae. The anterior and medial scalenes insert into the upper surface of the first rib. The posterior scalene inserts at the upper surface of the second rib. The scalenes elevate and fix the first and second ribs. Their most important function is to assist in inspiration when the diaphragm and intercostal muscles cannot meet ventilatory demands. Such instances may occur in healthy subjects during exercise or in patients who have pulmonary disease. In healthy subjects inspiratory efforts against a closed glottis or obstructed airway activate the scalenes. When intraavleolar pressure reaches -10 cm H_2O, scalenes are active in all subjects. The scalene muscles are inactive during expiratory efforts until intraalveolar pressure reaches $+40$ cm H_2O. The function of the scalene muscles during expiration is considered to be fixation of the ribs as the abdominal muscles contract. This action may prevent herniation at the apices of the lung during coughing.

Sternomastoid muscles

The sternomastoids are another important accessory muscle group (see Figure 9-11). The sternomastoids help to rotate the head and support it. They arise bilaterally by two heads. One head is from the manubrium of the sternum and the other on the medial end of the clavicle. The heads fuse into a single muscle that courses superiorly and slightly posteriorly. It inserts into the mastoid process and occipital bone of the skull. This muscle is prominent on either side of the neck. It is especially noticeable with rotary movements of the head.

When functioning to mobilize the head, the sternomastoids pull from their sternoclavicular origin. This rotates the head to the opposite side and turns it slightly upward. When the head and neck are held fixed by other skeletal muscles, the sternomastoids act as ventilatory muscles. They pull from their skull insertions and elevate the first rib and the sternum. This motion increases the AP diameter of the chest. In all subjects the sternomastoids contract when intraalveolar pressures reach -10 cm H_2O. These muscles exhibit no action during exhalation. The sternomastoids are activated at high lung volumes or with high ventilatory demands, such as during exercise.[7]

In chronic obstructive pulmonary disease (COPD) the sternomastoids become active during inspiration. The thorax becomes enlarged and air trapping flattens the diaphragm. The diaphragm fails to function effectively, as discussed previously. The sternomastoids contract and pull up on the sternum. The ribs rotate about their neck axes but not about the rib angle–sternal junction axes. This produces an up and down motion with little side expansion. In extreme cases AP expansion of the thorax may cause the lower ribs to draw in, partially negating the increase in chest volume.

Pectoralis major muscle

A third important accessory muscle of ventilation is the pectoralis major. The pectoralis is a powerful bilateral anterior chest muscle whose primary function is pulling the upper arms into the body in a hugging motion (see Figure 9-11). It arises from the medial half of the clavicle, the anterior surface of the sternum, the first six costal cartilages, and a fibrous sheath enclosing muscles of the abdominal wall. The muscle fibers converge into a thick tendon that inserts into the upper part of the humerus. The pectoralis major forms the anterior fold of the **axilla**. In muscular subjects its outlines are plainly visible beneath the skin.

When used as an accessory muscle of ventilation, the pectoralis pulls in a direction opposite to that of its primary function. If the arms and shoulders are fixed, the pectoralis can use its insertion as an origin. Fixing the arms and shoulders can be accomplished by leaning on the elbows or firmly grasping a wide object. The pectoralis can then pull on the anterior chest. This motion lifts the ribs and sternum, increasing AP diameter of the thorax. Patients who have COPD often lean on their elbows or support their arms for maximum use of the pectoralis. In advanced COPD most of the air moved may result from the action of this accessory muscle. It aids inspiration only, taking no part in exhalation.

Abdominal muscles

Several muscles make up the abdominal wall, providing support for the abdominal contents (see Figure 9-11). Four abdominal muscle groups play an indirect but important role in ventilation. These include the external and internal obliques, the transverse abdominal, and the rectus abdominis groups.

The *external oblique* muscle arises from the lower eight ribs. Its posterior fibers insert into the iliac crest. The remaining fibers course obliquely down and forward. They insert into a fibrous sheath (**aponeurosis**) with their counterparts from the other side. The *internal oblique* arises from the iliac crest and the inguinal ligament. Its posterior fibers pass upward to insert onto the last three ribs. The remainder slope upward and forward to a fibrous aponeurosis.

The *transverse abdominus* arises from the costal cartilages of the lower ribs, iliac crest, and lateral part of the inguinal ligament. It courses horizontally forward to an aponeurosis. The *rectus abdominus* arises from the pubic bones. It passes upward in a sheath and inserts into costal cartilages five through seven.

The abdominal muscles function mainly in expiration. Their action is twofold. Contraction of the rectus abdomini decreases the distance from the xiphoid to the pubis. Contraction of the external oblique decreases the transverse diameter of the rib cage. Both actions normally result in a decrease in rib cage diameter, and hence deflate the lungs. Paradoxically, increasing intraabdominal pressure causes an inflationary force on the lower rib cage. These muscles are normally inactive during quiet breathing. They become active when the elastic recoil of the thorax cannot provide the needed expiratory flow. Such conditions occur when expiratory flows reach or exceed 40 L/min, significant resistance impedes exhalation, or gas is forcibly exhaled below the resting expiratory level. Contraction of the abdominals increases intraabdominal pressure, driving the diaphragm upward.

The abdominals can also contribute to inspiration by contracting during end exhalation. This tends to reduce end-expiratory lung volume, so the chest wall stores elastic energy that assists in the next inspiratory effort.[8] Increasing intraabdominal pressure increases the length of the diaphragm as well as its radius of curvature. Both of these effects result in greater transdiaphragmatic pressure for a given contractile tension. With any increase in ventilatory demand, patients with COPD significantly increase their use of the abdominal muscles. Loss of effective use of these accessory muscles places patients with airway obstruction at a disadvantage.

The abdominal muscles are also used for voluntary maneuvers such as forceful expiration. Forced expiration is employed in various pulmonary function tests (see Chapter 18). Such maneuvers are performed in measuring the forced vital capacity (FVC), forced expiratory flow (FEF), and maximal expiratory pressure (MEP). High intraabdominal pressures are transmitted to the lungs to generate maximal transpulmonary pressures. This results in maximal expiratory airflow, measured to assess the status of the airways. Subjects with weak or dysfunctional abdominal muscles are often unable to generate normal maximal expiratory flows.

Actions of the primary and secondary muscles of ventilation are summarized in Table 9-1.

INNERVATION OF THE LUNG AND THORACIC MUSCULATURE

The lung is innervated by both the autonomic and somatic nervous systems. The autonomic system provides both motor and sensory pathways to the lung. The somatic system provides only motor innervation to the respiratory muscles.[9]

Somatic innervation

Somatic innervation of the respiratory system consists of efferent motor stimulation of the diaphragm and intercostals (Figure 9-12, on page 190).

The diaphragm is innervated by paired *phrenic nerves.* The phrenic nerves originate as branches of spinal nerves C3-C5 in the cervical **plexuses.** They

Table 9-1   Summary of respiratory muscle action

Level	Inspiration	Expiration
Quiet ventilation	Diaphragm in all subjects Intercostals in most subjects Scalenes in some subjects	Some persistence of inspiratory muscle contraction in expiration
Modest increase in ventilation (<50 L/min)	Diaphragm in all subjects Intercostals in most subjects Scalenes in some subjects	Some persistence of inspiratory muscle contraction in expiration
Moderate increase in ventilation (50–100 L/min)	Diaphragm in all subjects Intercostals in most subjects Scalenes in most subjects Sternomastoid action toward end inspiration	Some persistence of inspiratory muscle contraction Abdominal and intercostals at end expiration
Significant increase in ventilation (>100 L/min)	All inspiratory accessories active	Abdominals active throughout inspiration

enter the chest in front of the subclavian arteries, lateral to the carotid arteries. The phrenic nerves run down each side of the mediastinum anterior to the hilar structures. The left phrenic nerve travels a longer course than the right. It extends around the heart. Injury to the phrenic nerves may result in paralysis of the diaphragm. Such injuries include neck trauma and chest wounds.

The intercostal muscles receive their motor innervation via the *intercostal nerves.* The intercostal nerves (T2-T11) leave the vertebral column from the intervertebral **foramina** between adjacent vertebrae. Unlike other spinal nerves, the intercostals do not form plexuses. They are distributed directly to the structures they innervate. The ventral rami of the intercostal nerves provide motor innervation to the intercostal muscles. The dorsal rami innervate the muscles and skin of the back.

Autonomic innervation

Autonomic innervation is via branches of the paired *vagus nerves* and the upper four or five thoracic sympathetic ganglia.[10] Both contribute fibers to the anterior and posterior pulmonary plexuses at the roots of the lung (Figure 9-12).

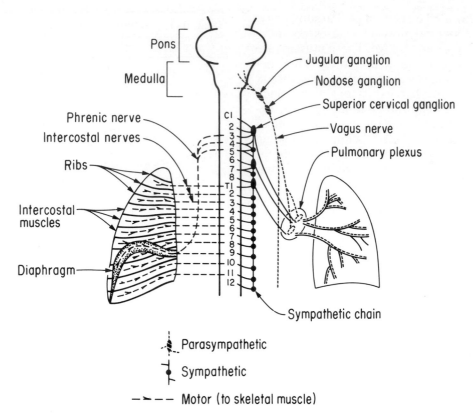

Fig. 9-12 Schema of the autonomic innervation (motor and sensory) of the lung and the somatic (motor) nerve supply to the intercostal muscles and diaphragm. (Redrawn from Murray JF: The normal lung, ed 2, Philadelphia, 1986, WB Saunders.)

Efferent pathways

On entry into the chest, each vagus nerve sends off a branch that curves back up to the larynx. These branches are the *recurrent laryngeal nerves.* The left recurrent laryngeal nerve leaves the vagus at the level of the aortic arch. It loops around the arch and follows the trachea upward through the mediastinum to the larynx. The right recurrent laryngeal nerve originates at the level of the subclavian artery. It loops deep toward that vessel, then **cephalad** toward the larynx.

Each vagus nerve also gives off a branch called the *superior laryngeal nerve.* The external branch of this nerve supplies the cricothyroid muscle. The internal branch provides sensory fibers to the larynx. The recurrent laryngeal nerves provide the primary motor innervation to the larynx. Depending on which branches are involved, damage to the laryngeal nerves can cause unilateral or bilateral paralysis of the vocal cords. This may result in hoarseness, loss of voice, and an ineffective cough. The most common causes of laryngeal nerve damage are trauma and thoracic or mediastinal tumors.

Entering at the hilum, autonomic nerve fibers subdivide with the airways. The largest branches accompany the bronchi. The smallest nerve fibers parallel the pulmonary veins.[11] Both sympathetic and parasympathetic efferents innervate the smooth mus-

cle and glands of the airways. Anatomic and physiologic evidence indicates that the parasympathetic system predominates.[4] Autonomic motor fibers from both systems combine to influence the caliber of the conducting airways. Both systems affect the volume of the terminal respiratory units, the activity of the bronchial glands, and the diameter of the pulmonary blood vessels.[12]

Afferent pathways

Most afferent nerve fibers from the lung to the central nervous system are vagal in origin. Important sensory paths are associated with well-defined receptor sites in both the airways and lung parenchyma. Three of these vagal sensory sites are the *bronchopulmonary stretch receptors,* the *irritant receptors,* and the *J receptors.* Additional receptors are located outside the lung. The muscle **proprioceptors** and the peripheral **chemoreceptors** are involved in the control of ventilation (see Chapter 14, Acid Base Balance and Regulation of Ventilation).

Characteristics of the pulmonary vagal receptors are summarized in Table 9-2.[4] Pulmonary stretch receptors are located in the smooth muscle of the bronchi and bronchioles. They progressively discharge during lung inflation up to the end of inspiration. This *inflation reflex* was thought to adjust the

Table 9-2   Characteristics of the three pulmonary vagal sensory reflexes

Receptor	Location	Fiber type	Stimulus	Responses
Pulmonary stretch, slowly adapting	Associated with smooth muscle of intrapulmonary airways	Medullated	Lung inflation Increased transpulmonary pressure	Hering-Breuer inflation reflex Bronchodilatation
Irritant, rapidly adapting	Epithelium of (mainly) extrapulmonary airways	Medullated	Irritants Mechanical stimulation Anaphylaxis Pneumothorax Hyperpnea Pulmonary congestion	Bronchoconstriction Hyperpnea Expiratory constriction of the larynx Cough
Type J	Alveolar wall	Nonmedullated	Increased interstitial volume (congestion) Chemical injury Microembolism	Rapid shallow breathing Severe expiratory constriction of larynx Hypotension, **bradycardia** Spinal reflex inhibition

depth of inspiration. Recent animal studies indicate that these receptors influence the duration of the expiratory pause between breaths.[13] The inflation reflex is probably very weak or absent during quiet breathing in healthy adults. There appears to be a strong inflation reflex only in newborn infants.[4,12]

A special reflex thought to be associated with the stretch receptors is *Head's paradoxical reflex*. This reflex stimulates a deeper breath rather than inhibiting further inspiration. It may be the basis for occasional deep breaths. Deep breaths or sighs occur with normal breathing, presumably preventing alveolar collapse. Head's reflex may also be responsible for gasping in newborn infants as they progressively inflate their lungs.[12,14]

Irritant receptors or mechanoreceptors are located in the subepithelial tissues of the larger airways.[15] They are found mainly in the posterior wall of the trachea and at the bifurcations of the larger bronchi. These receptors respond to a variety of mechanical, chemical, and physiologic stimuli. The stimuli include physical manipulation or irritation, inhalation of noxious gases, histamine-induced **bronchoconstriction,** asphyxia, and microembolization of the pulmonary arteries.[10-12]

Stimulation of the irritant receptors can result in bronchoconstriction, **hyperpnea,** glottic closure, and cough. Stimulation of these receptors can also cause a reflex slowing of the heart rate **(bradycardia).** This response is referred to as the *vagovagal reflex.* It may occur during tracheobronchial **aspiration, intubation,** or **bronchoscopy.** These procedures may cause significant mechanical irritation of the airway. The vagovagal reflex can be blunted by applying local anesthetics.

J receptors are named because they are found primarily in "juxtaposition" to the pulmonary capillaries. The primary role of the J receptors is their response to increases in pulmonary capillary pres-sures.[10-12] When capillary pressure increases, as in congestive heart failure, stimulation of the J receptors results in rapid, shallow breathing. J receptor stimulation can also cause bradycardia, **hypotension,** and expiratory narrowing of the glottis. Stimulation of these receptors may contribute to the sensation of **dyspnea** that accompanies pulmonary **edema,** pulmonary **embolism,** and pneumonia.[4]

VASCULAR SUPPLY

The vascular supply of the lungs is composed of the pulmonary and bronchial circulations. The pulmonary circulation carries mixed venous blood from the tissues through the lungs to restore its oxygen content and remove carbon dioxide. The bronchial circulation provides arterial blood to the lungs to meet their metabolic requirements. Also involved in fluid transport from the lungs is a network of lymphatics. The lymphatic system removes fluid from the lung parenchyma and pleural space and returns it to the systemic circulation.

Pulmonary circulation

The pulmonary circulation originates on the right side of the heart. Poorly oxygenated mixed venous blood is delivered to the lungs through the pulmonary artery. The main pulmonary artery exits from the heart and passes superiorly (Figure 9-13, on page 192). The pulmonary artery divides into right and left pulmonary arteries just below the point of tracheal division (the carina). The pulmonary arteries accompany the right and left mainstem bronchi. This symmetry continues through all the divisions into the distal air spaces. The pulmonary arteries are always adjacent to the bronchi and bronchioles. Pulmonary arterioles extend to the terminal lung units. The arterioles

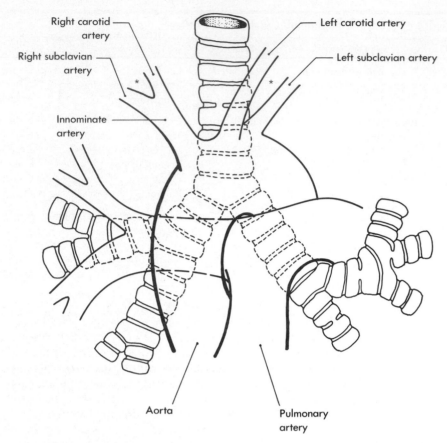

Right carotid artery

Right subclavian artery

Innominate artery

Left carotid artery

Left subclavian artery

Aorta

Pulmonary artery

Fig. 9-13 Diagram of relationship between main pulmonary artery and aorta, with their main branches, as they leave right and left ventricles of heart. Trachea is in background. The aorta arches over main pulmonary artery, which divides into right and left branches that enter the lungs. The aorta supplies oxygenated blood to remainder of body. The asterisk (*) on each side indicates the course of phrenic and vagus nerves as they enter thorax.

subdivide into a bed of alveolar capillaries. The alveolar capillaries provide a large surface area to exchange oxygen and carbon dioxide with the alveoli.[16,17] Arterialized blood leaves the alveoli via the pulmonary venules. The venules combine into larger veins. Four to five major pulmonary veins drain the arterialized blood into the left atrium of the heart, then into the systemic circulation.

Pressures in the normal pulmonary circulation average about one sixth of that in the systemic circulation.[16-18] Even though the entire cardiac output passes through both systems, the pulmonary circulation offers much less resistance. The pulmonary circulation, including the right ventricle, is a low-pressure, low-resistance system. These low pressures are essential in maintaining fluid balance at the alveolar-capillary interface. Increased pressure in the pulmonary circulation, as occurs in congestive heart failure, can disrupt fluid balance. Rising back-pressure from the left side of the heart can cause fluid leaks into the **interstitial** spaces and alveoli, impairing gas exchange.

Since the pulmonary circulation is a low-pressure system, blood flow is highly dependent on gravity. In the upright lung, hydrostatic pressure in the pulmonary circulation decreases about 1 cm H_2O for each 1

cm distance from the base to the apex.[17] Blood flow is very low at the apex of the lung in resting subjects. Perfusion increases linearly down the lung in proportion to the hydrostatic pressure. The lung bases receive nearly *20 times* as much blood flow as the apices.[17] Gravity-related effects also occur in recumbent positions, but are less pronounced. Hydrostatic pressure differences always cause the dependent portions of the lungs to receive the greatest proportion of blood flow. The distribution of pulmonary blood flow is closely related to pulmonary gas exchange (see Chapter 12, Gas Exchange and Transport).

Bronchial circulation

Mixed venous blood in the pulmonary arteries lacks sufficient oxygen for the metabolic needs of the lung. A separate arterial supply called the bronchial circulation also accompanies the bronchi.[19] The metabolic needs of the lung are comparatively low, and much of the lung parenchyma is oxygenated by direct contact with inspired gas. Because of this, blood flow through the bronchial circulation is only 1% to 2% of the total cardiac output.

Bronchial arteries vary in number and origin.[20] A

single right artery arises from an upper intercostal, right subclavian, or internal mammary artery. Two bronchial arteries supply the left lung. They branch directly from the upper thoracic aorta. Bronchial arteries follow their respective bronchi. Two or three branches accompany each subdivision of the conducting airway. The bronchial arterial circulation terminates in a plexus of capillaries that anastomose with the alveolar capillary bed.

Return flow of the bronchial circulation to the right side of the heart takes one of two courses (Figure 9-14). From 25% to 33% of bronchial venous blood returns to the heart through true *bronchial veins.* These veins empty into the azygos, hemizygos, or intercostal veins. The remaining bronchial venous flow courses through "bronchopulmonary veins." These veins originate from the bronchial capillaries and empty into the pulmonary veins. Direct vascular connections between the bronchial and pulmonary arteries may also exist. These *bronchopulmonary arterial anastomoses* represent a third path for return to the heart.

The bronchial and pulmonary circulations share an important compensatory relationship.[4] Decreased perfusing pressure in the pulmonary arterial circulation tends to cause an increase in bronchial artery blood flow to the affected area. This minimizes the danger of pulmonary infarction, such as that which occurs with **embolization.** Similarly, loss of bronchial circulation can be partially offset by increases in pulmonary arterial perfusion. This may occur after lung transplantation. When such compensatory pathways are blocked, tissue necrosis of the affected area often results.

Lymphatics

The lymphatic system consists of a network of lymphatic vessels, lymph nodes, and the tonsils, thymus gland, and spleen. Its primary function is to clear fluid from the interstitial spaces. The lymphatic system also plays an important role in the body's immune system. It removes bacteria, foreign material, and cell debris from the lymph fluid. It also produces lymphocytes and plasma cells to aid in defense. Both roles are essential for maintaining normal function of the respiratory system.

The pulmonary lymphatic system consists of superficial and deep vessels.[21] The superficial (pleural) network drains the lung surface and pleura. The deep (peribronchovascular) network drains the lung parenchyma. Both originate as dead-end lymphatic capillaries in their respective regions. Deep lymph vessels are closely associated with the terminal lung units.

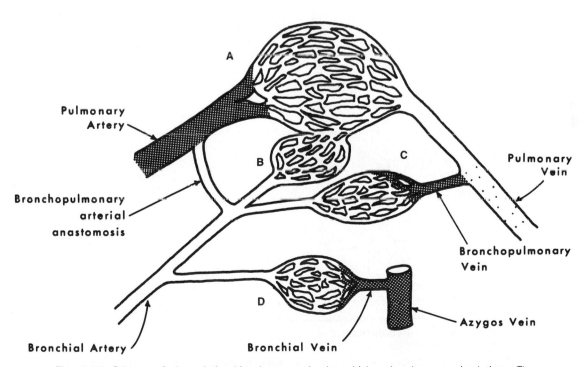

Fig. 9-14 Schema of the relationships between the bronchial and pulmonary circulations. The pulmonary artery supplies the pulmonary capillary network, **A.** The bronchial artery supplies capillary networks **B, C,** and **D.** Network **B** represents the bronchial capillary supply to bronchioles that anastomoses with pulmonary capillaries and drains through pulmonary veins. Network **C** represents the bronchial capillary supply to most bronchi; these vessels form bronchopulmonary veins that empty into pulmonary veins. Network **D** represents the bronchial capillary supply to lobar and segmental bronchi; these vessels form true bronchial veins that drain into the azygos, hemiazygos, or intercostal veins. (From Murray JF: The normal lung, ed 2, Philadelphia, WB Saunders.)

They do not, however, extend to the level of the alveolar-capillary membrane. The lymphatic system works with phagocytic cells in the alveoli to provide defense against foreign material able to penetrate to the alveolar level.[22]

Lymph fluid returns to the circulatory system through lymphatic channels that course toward the hilum. These channels join in the pleura. They travel toward the hilum in the septa accompanying veins, and in the bronchopulmonary artery complexes (Figures 9-15 and 9-16). Lymph flow is directed

through one or more lymph nodes clustered about each hilum. From there lymph travels through the mediastinum. It rejoins the general circulation via either the right lymphatic or the thoracic duct.

Lymphatic channels are usually not visible on chest radiographs. They may be detected if they are distended or thickened by disease (see Chapter 19). Kerley "A" lines on chest films represent distension and thickening of lymph vessels accompanying the pulmonary veins and arteries. Kerley "B" lines are the radiologic manifestation of distended lymph vessels

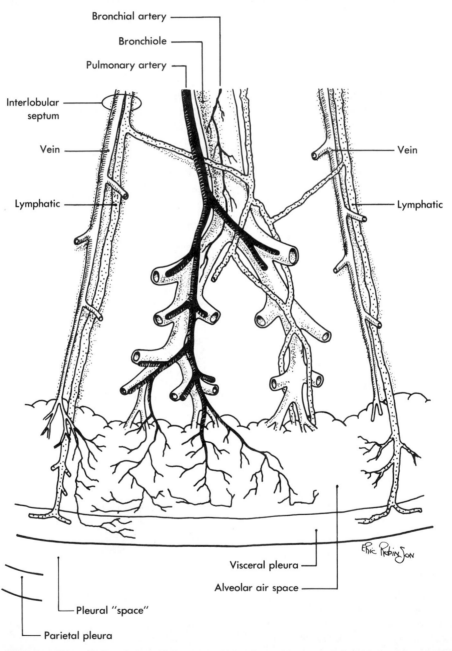

Fig. 9-15 Diagram of distal pulmonary arteries, bronchioles, and air spaces with their associated bronchial arteries. Pulmonary veins lie in fibrous tissue septa between these paired pulmonary arteries and airways. Note that lymphatic channels travel with both sets of structures.

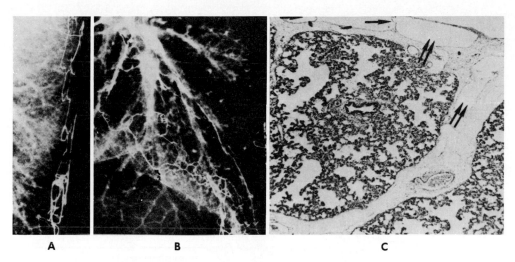

Fig. 9–16 Radiographs of lymphatic channels following their injection with contrast material. The pleural lymphatics are seen in profile in **A.** One lymphatic channel marked with an arrow in **B** is following a pulmonary vein. Tissue section, **C,** shows pleural lymphatics marked with one arrow, and septal lymphatics marked with two arrows. (From Heitzman ER: The lung: radiologic-pathologic correlations, St. Louis, 1973, Mosby.)

in the interlobular septa.[23] Pulmonary edema and pleural **effusion** become evident on chest radiographs when the lymphatic system is unable to remove excess fluid in the lung.

ANATOMY OF THE RESPIRATORY TRACT

The respiratory tract is divided into an upper and a lower portion. The upper tract includes the oral and nasal cavities, the pharynx, and the larynx. The upper respiratory tract warms, humidifies, and filters inspired gas. The lower respiratory tract begins at the inferior border of the larynx at the cricoid cartilage. It extends through the airway divisions to the alveoli. The lower respiratory tract is devoted almost entirely to conduction and exchange of gas.

Upper respiratory tract

The upper respiratory tract consists of the nasal and oral cavities, the pharynx, and the larynx (Figure 9-17, on page 196). It performs four important respiratory functions. The nose, pharynx, and larynx *conduct respiratory gases* to and from the lungs. These structures serve as frontline *defense mechanisms* for the lungs.[24] The nasal passages also *humidify inspired air* and *exchange heat* for the respiratory system and body as a whole.

The nose

Adults normally breathe through the nose. Conditions such as nasal polyps or mucosal edema sometimes prohibit nasal breathing. High ventilatory flows, as occur during strenuous exercise, may cause mouth breathing. This is due to the higher resistance to flow through the nasal passages when compared to the mouth. This resistance to flow is caused by the structures of the nose that heat, humidify, and filter inspired gas.

The external nose is formed by the frontal process of the maxilla, two nasal bones, cartilage, and fatty connective tissue (Figure 9-17). There are two flexible, flared entryways called *alae.* The alae, or wings, enclose a space on each side called the *vestibule.* The vestibules are lined by squamous **epithelium.** They have large hairs that act as a gross filter. Posterior to the vestibules are the openings to the internal nose, the *anterior nares.* These openings have the smallest cross-sectional area in the adult respiratory tract.[25]

The internal nasal passages begin at this point. They are separated in the midline by a *septum.* The septum is formed anteriorly by cartilage. The vomer bone and the perpendicular plate of the ethmoid bone make up the posterior septum. The nasal septum frequently deviates to one side or the other. Three bony shelves extend from the lateral wall and project into the nasal cavity. They are formed by projections of the superior, middle, and inferior conchae. These *turbinates* divide the nasal cavities into superior, middle, and inferior passages, or meati. The olfactory receptors lie above the superior turbinates on each side.

The turbinates are lined by highly vascularized tissue. This lining consists of pseudostratified, ciliated columnar epithelium. The epithelium is interspersed with mucus-secreting goblet cells. These structures provide a large surface area for heat and water exchange. Both inspired and expired gases are conditioned.

The nose warms inspired air close to body temperature (37°C). It saturates inspired gas with water vapor when it reaches the nasopharynx.[25,26] During expira-

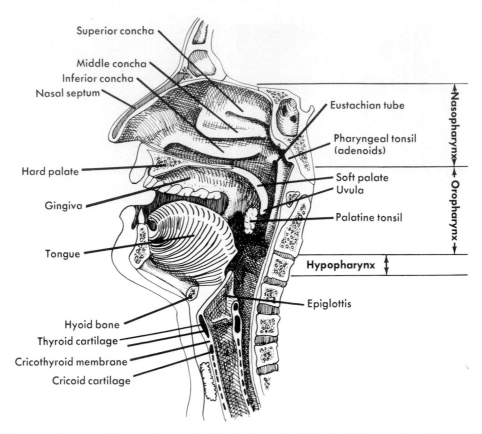

Fig. 9-17   Structures of upper airway and oral cavity. Larynx is the landmark for separation of upper and lower airway. (From Ellis PD and Billings DM: Cardiopulmonary resuscitation: procedures for basic and advanced life support, St Louis, 1980, Mosby.)

tion, water vapor condenses in the nose. This retains heat and moisture for the next inhalation. The nasal mucosa functions unimpaired even in very dry environmental conditions.[25] Bypassing the nose can severely compromise the respiratory system's ability to warm and humidify inspired gas. This occurs with **endotracheal** intubation or **tracheostomy.**

The defense function of the nose involves several mechanisms. Large hairs in the vestibule provide gross filtration. Filtration is augmented by pattern of airflow through the nasal cavity. Inspired gas is accelerated to a high velocity through the anterior nares. It then changes direction sharply as it enters the internal nasal cavity. This flow pattern causes particles larger than a few μm to impact on the nasal mucosa. These particles are cleared by ciliary action or nose blowing.

Beyond the external nares the cross-sectional area increases. This results in a decrease in the velocity of the inspired gas. Gas flow is *turbulent* because of the narrow convolutions of the passages. Low velocity and turbulence combine to ensure that remaining particles are removed. Filtration is based on impaction, sedimentation, and diffusion.

Surface fluids originate from the goblet cells and submucosal glands. This fluid lining has mild antibacterial properties. Mucosal fluids also remove water-soluble irritant gases such as sulfur dioxide. Ciliary activity transports surface fluids *backward.* Surface fluids move into the nasopharynx at a rate of about 6 mm/min. Foreign matter is then cleared by swallowing. These defense mechanisms ensure that inspired air is free of inanimate or bacterial contamination, and of common air pollutants.

Paranasal sinuses

The paranasal sinuses are symmetrically paired spaces adjacent to the nasal cavity. Most of the sinuses open into the nasal cavity between the turbinates (Figure 9-18, *A*). The paranasal sinuses consist of the frontal, maxillary, ethmoid, and posterior sphenoid sinuses (Figures 9-18, *A* and *B*). All are named for the bones in which they occur. The purposes of the sinuses are unclear. The sinuses may provide temperature insulation, strengthen the skull without additional weight, or enhance voice resonance.[14] Problems can develop when drainage of the paranasal sinuses becomes impaired. Chronic sinus infections are a source of contaminated materials that may be aspirated into the lower respiratory tract.

Oral cavity

The oral cavity serves multiple purposes. It is involved in digestion, as well as in speech and respira-

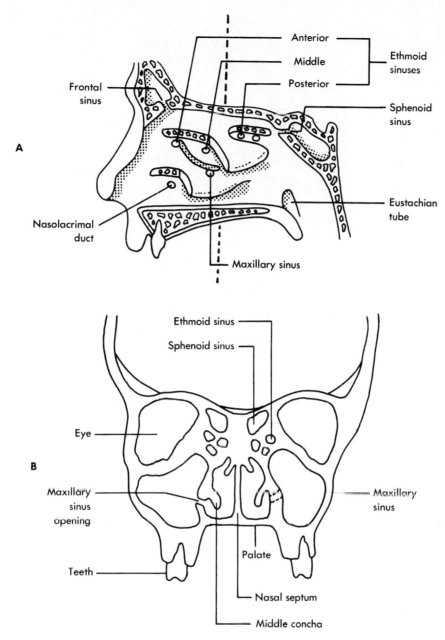

Fig. 9-18 The nasal sinuses are named for bones in which they occur. **A,** In lateral view (as in Fig. 3-2) but with conchae cut away. Note entrances into nasal cavity of various sinuses and their location within these cavities. **B,** Frontal view of face taken at level of dotted line in **A.** Note position of maxillary sinuses in each cheekbone. Sphenoid sinuses are behind ethmoid sinuses, although they appear to be at same level in this frontal view.

tion. The oral cavity is considered an accessory respiratory passage. Mouth breathing, in adults, is used mainly during speech and strenuous exercise. It also is used when the nose is obstructed by upper respiratory tract infections or foreign materials.

The *palate* separates the nasal cavity from the oral cavity (Figure 9-19, on page 198). The anterior two thirds has a bony skeleton and is called the hard palate. The posterior third does not have such support and is called the soft palate. The uvula extends from the midline of the soft palate at the back of the mouth (Figure 9-19). The uvula and the surrounding walls

control flow in eating, drinking, sneezing, coughing, and vomiting.

The lips, teeth, tongue, and jaw muscles protect the mouth from injury or intrusion. The tongue is involved in mechanical digestion, taste, and phonation. The posterior surface of the tongue is supplied with many sensory nerve endings. These nerves produce a vagal gag reflex when stimulated. This is a protective reflex. It must be considered when passing tubes or instruments through the mouth in conscious or semiconscious patients. The *lingual tonsils* are located at the base of the tongue.

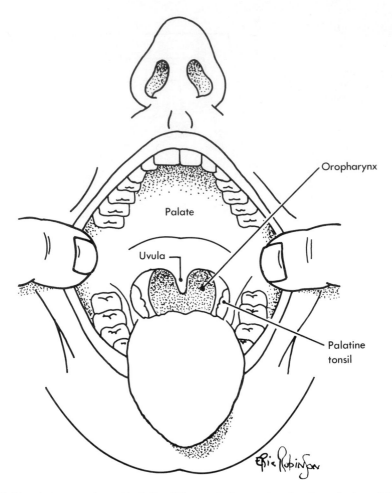

Fig. 9-19 View into opened mouth. Soft midline uvula is seen hanging from fleshy palatine pillars. Pharynx is seen at back of mouth.

The mucosal surfaces of the oral cavity also provide humidification and warming of inspired air. These surfaces are much less efficient than those provided by the nose. Saliva is produced by major and minor salivary glands. Saliva functions primarily as a wetting and digestive agent for food. It provides some humidification of inspired gas.

The oral cavity ends at a double web on each side called the palatine folds (Figure 9-19). The palatine tonsils sit between these folds on each side. These tonsils are vascularized lymphoidal tissues. The palatine tonsils appear to play an immunologic role, especially in childhood.

The protective reflexes of the mouth, pharynx, and larynx during swallowing protect the lower respiratory tract. These protective functions can be severely compromised during anesthesia or unconsciousness. Poor oral hygiene may expose the lower respiratory tract to pathogenic bacteria, increasing the risk of infection.

Pharynx

Posterior to the nasal cavities and mouth is the pharynx. The pharynx extends to the point where the airway and the digestive tract separate. It is divided into three sections: the nasopharynx, the oropharynx, and the hypopharynx (see Figure 9-17). The entire pharynx is lined with stratified squamous epithelium.

The *nasopharynx* lies behind the nasal cavities. The muscles of the palate occlude the nasopharynx during swallowing and coughing. The *Eustachian* tubes open into the lateral nasopharynx. These tubes connect the nasopharynx with each middle ear, and with the mastoid sinuses. The *adenoid tonsils* are located on the posterior wall of the nasopharynx. These tonsils are also called the adenoids. The palatine, lingual, and adenoid tonsils make up Waldeyer's ring. This ring of lymphoid tissue protects the entrances to the respiratory and gastrointestinal tracts.

In back of the oral cavity is the *oropharynx*. It extends from the uvula to the epiglottis and base of the tongue. Nasotracheal and nasogastric tubes must turn inferiorly at the nasopharynx in order to reach the trachea, lungs, or stomach.

The inferior portion of the pharynx between the epiglottis and the larynx is the *hypopharynx*. This short segment extends into the neck. Immediately below it the digestive and respiratory tracts separate.

The hypopharynx changes its shape dramatically during swallowing and speech.

The positions of the oral cavity, pharynx, and larynx are critical to the **patency** of the upper airway. Their relative positions are important in unconscious patients. In upright subjects, the head and neck form a 90-degree angle with the axis of the pharynx and larynx (Figure 9-20, *B*). With loss of consciousness, the head droops downward and decreases the angle (Figure 9-20, *A*). This positional change can partially or completely obstruct the upper airway. Extension of the head and lower jaw alleviates this obstruction (Figure 9-20, *C*). Extension of the head moves the tongue away from the rear of the pharynx. This technique is used to maintain the airway in unconscious patients. It also facilitates placement of artificial airways.

Larynx

The larynx is a complex structure located immediately below the pharynx. The larynx "hangs" from the hyoid bone at the base of the tongue. It can be palpated (felt) at the thyroid cartilage or Adam's apple. The larynx consists of nine cartilages, and numerous muscles and ligaments (Figure 9-21, on page 200). These structures combine to protect the lower airway during breathing and swallowing.[27] Its major function is sound production.

The *epiglottis* is a flat cartilage that extends from the base of the tongue backward and upward (Figures 9-17 and 9-21). It is attached by ligaments to the hyoid bone anteriorly. Its pointed stalk attaches to the thyroid cartilage below. The epiglottis is 2 to 4 cm long and 2 to 3 cm wide. Its thickness averages only 2 to 5 mm. This structure is not easily visualized in

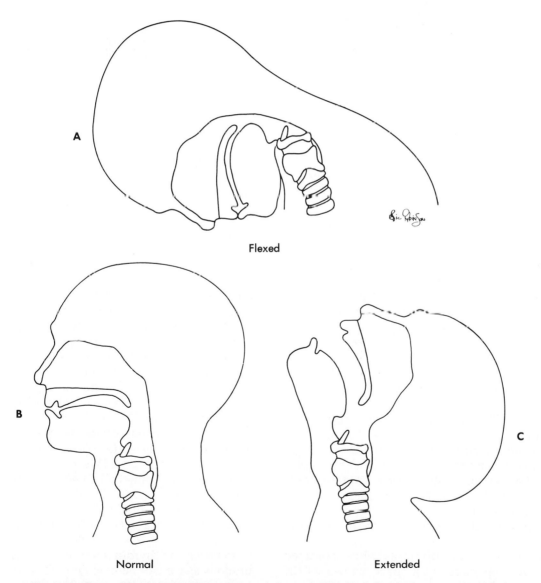

A   Flexed

B   Normal

C   Extended

Fig. 9-20 The position of head affects patency of airway. **A,** With head flexed, airway may be kinked, making breathing or intubation difficult. **B,** Normal upright relationship of head and neck to chest. **C,** Extension of head straightens airway, making breathing, clearance of material, or intubation easier.

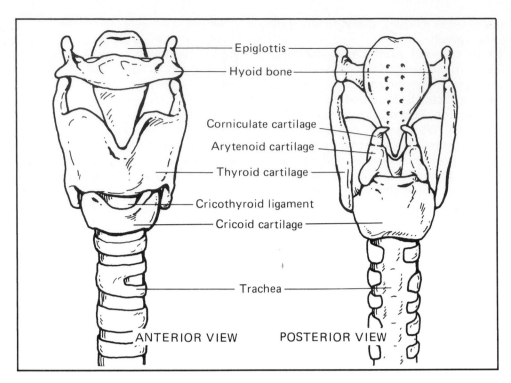

Fig. 9-21 Anterior and posterior views of the laryngeal cartilages and trachea. (From Martin DE and Youtsey JW: Respiratory anatomy and physiology, St Louis, 1988, Mosby.)

adults. It can be seen in small children and crying babies because of its higher position. The position of the larynx in infants partially explains why they are obligatory nose breathers.

The epiglottis does not close off the airway during swallowing. It is pushed down and back by the tongue and rising larynx. This motion simply diverts food into the esophagus.[27] Surgical removal of the epiglottis does not impair swallowing.

The inlet to the larynx lies below and behind the base of the tongue. Figure 9-22 shows the larynx inlet as it appears when viewed with a **laryngoscope**. The base of the tongue is attached to the epiglottis by three folds. These folds form a space between the tongue and the epiglottis called the *vallecula*. The vallecula is a key landmark in oral intubation.

Above the true vocal cords are the *false vocal cords*. These vestibular folds can act together with the true cords to close off the lower airway. This action is essential for an effective cough. Patients who have artificial airways cannot produce an effective cough. The artificial airway prevents the true and false cords from sealing the airway. The false cords can also completely obscure the view of the true cords. This may occur during reflex contraction of the laryngeal muscles.

The true vocal cords appear as white bordered veils. They are separated by a space known as the *glottis*. The vocal cords are composed of muscle, ligament, and submucosal soft tissue. They have a mucous membrane covering. The space below this mucous membrane readily accumulates fluid. Since the lymphatic drainage to this area is sparse, swelling caused by the fluid resolves slowly.

The vocal cords project from the paired *arytenoid cartilages*. They insert on the posterior surface of the thyroid cartilage. The distance between the vocal cords changes with **adduction** or **abduction** of the arytenoids. These movements of the arytenoids alter the tension on the vocal cords, producing phonation.

Sound is produced by vibration of the cords in the air stream. By varying cord tension, the pitch of the sound made changes. Varying the volumes of air passing the cords varies the sound intensity. The cords may flutter during normal breathing. They are drawn apart during inspiration by active muscular contraction. They relax toward the midline during expiration (Figure 9-23).

The lower border of the larynx is formed by a cartilaginous ring called the *cricoid cartilage* (see Figure 9-21). The cricoid cartilage is the only rigid structure that completely encircles the airway. Its inner diameter sets the limit for the size of endotracheal tubes passed through the larynx. In infants the cricoid ring represents the narrowest portion of the airway.

Between the thyroid and cricoid cartilages a membranous space can be palpated. This space is the *cricothyroid ligament* (Figure 9-21). Emergency opening of the airway, called a **cricothyrotomy**, is performed

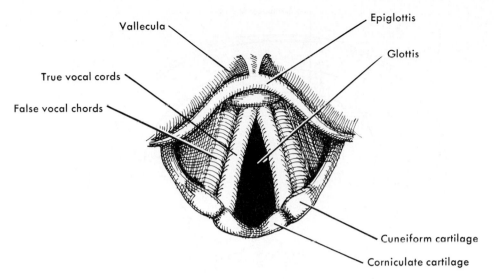

Fig. 9-22 Interior of larynx. (From Ellis PD and Billings DM: Cardiopulmonary resuscitation: procedures for basic and advanced life support, St Louis, 1980, Mosby.)

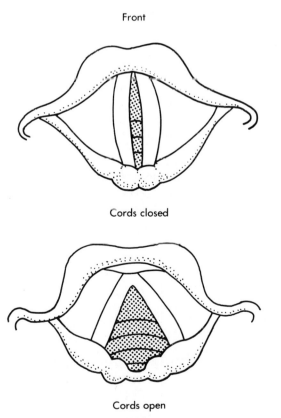

Fig. 9-23 View into larynx from back of mouth to the front. Vocal cords vary in tension, length, and relationship to one another. Note open inspiratory position versus expiratory or resting closed position. Inside of trachea with its cartilaginous rings is seen through opening between vocal cords.

through this ligament. Catheters for removal of secretions, supply of supplementary oxygen, or ventilation can be inserted through the cricothyroid ligament. Because of the proximity of the laryngeal nerves and vocal cords, extreme caution must be used in these procedures. True surgical tracheostomy is usually placed 1 to 3 cm below the cricoid cartilage.

Lower respiratory tract

The lower respiratory tract begins at the inferior border of the cricoid cartilage. The lower respiratory tract serves two primary functions. It conducts the respiratory gases and allows gas exchange with the blood. Movement of gas is accomplished by a system of airway branchings. These branches lead to an enormous surface where blood and gas contact each other.

Trachea

The trachea marks the beginning of the conducting system, often called the tracheobronchial tree. The trachea is a tubular structure that begins at the cricoid cartilage. It proceeds through the neck into the mediastinum. The trachea extends to the articulation between the manubrium and body of the sternum (angle of Louis). At this point it divides into the two mainstem bronchi.

The adult trachea averages 2.0 to 2.5 cm in diameter. It ranges from 10 to 12 cm long. The trachea's support comes from 16 to 20 *C-shaped* cartilaginous rings. Each tracheal cartilage is 4 to 5 mm high. These rings cannot be felt easily except in very thin individuals. Posteriorly, a thin muscle, the *trachealis,* extends between the ends of the cartilages (Figure 9-24, on page 202). This structure of muscle and cartilage provides support yet allows variation in diameter.

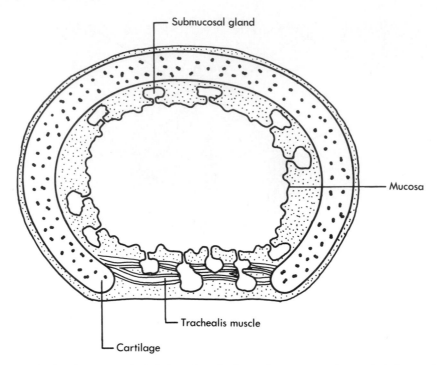

Fig. 9-24 Trachea is composed of **C**-shaped cartilaginous rings connected posteriorly by membrane covering thin trachealis muscle. This arrangement allows variation in tracheal caliber. Note mucosal and submucosal glands lining airway.

The portion of the trachea within the thorax is particularly affected by pressure differences across its walls. The most dramatic compression occurs during coughing.[27]

The trachea can be seen on a chest radiograph as an air-filled structure (Figure 9-25). On the usual negative X-ray film, the trachea as well as other air spaces appear dark. Soft tissues appear gray and bones appear white (see Chapter 19).

The trachea is almost midline in the neck. In the superior mediastinum it deviates slightly to the right. This allows room for the aorta to pass by on its left side (see Figure 9-13). At the point of tracheal bifurcation, there is a sharp dividing cartilage. This cartilage, the *carina,* helps divide flow to the right or left side. The right mainstem bronchus angles off at 20 to 30 degrees from the midline. The left mainstem bronchus deflects more sharply at 45 to 55 degrees (Figure 9-26). Objects aspirated in upright subjects have a tendency to follow the straighter course into the right mainstem bronchus. In supine subjects **aspiration** goes into the dependent lung units.

Airway divisions and segmental anatomy.

Each mainstem bronchus divides into branches that supply the lung lobes. The right mainstem bronchus gives rise to the upper lobe bronchus. It then divides into the middle and lower lobe bronchi. The left mainstem bronchus divides into a left upper and a lower lobe bronchi. The left lung lacks a middle lobe. A division of the left upper lobe, the *lingula,* corre-

sponds to the right middle lobe. Its bronchus arises from the left upper lobe bronchus.

The lobes are divided into uniform anatomic units called *bronchopulmonary segments.* There are normally 10 segments in the right lung and 8 segments in the left (Table 9-3 and Figure 9-27, on page 204). Detailed knowledge of segmental anatomy is very useful in physical assessment of the thorax. Under-

Table 9-3   Bronchopulmonary segments*

Segment	Number	Segment	Number
RIGHT UPPER LOBE		**LEFT UPPER LOBE**	
Apical	1	Upper division	
Posterior	2	Apical-posterior	1 and 2[†]
Anterior	3	Anterior	3
RIGHT MIDDLE LOBE		Lower division (lingula)	
Lateral	4	Superior lingula	4
Medial	5	Inferior lingula	5
RIGHT LOWER LOBE		**LEFT LOWER LOBE**	
Superior	6	Superior	6
Medial basal	7	Anteromedial	7 and 8[†]
Anterior basal	8	Lateral basal	9
Lateral basal	9	Posterior basal	10
Posterior basal	10		

The subdivisions of the lung and bronchial tree are fairly constant. Slight variations between the right and left sides are noted by combined names and numbers.

[†]*Editor's note:* Some authors feel that the left lung should be numbered such that there are eight segments, where the apical-posterior is numbered 1 and anteromedial is numbered 6.

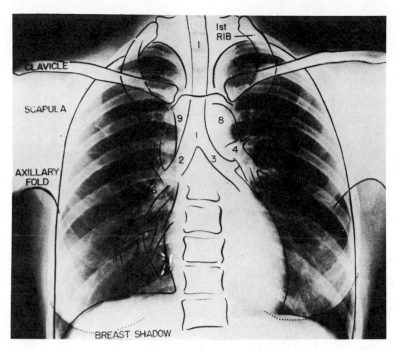

Fig. 9-25 Roentgenogram of mediastinum and lungs. Air-containing structures such as trachea and lungs are dark on this negative. The mediastinum is the central structure between lungs. Note air-filled trachea within this structure (*1*). Hilus of each lung is its connection with the mediastinum. It contains mainstem and first division airways (*2* and *3*) as well as the major pulmonary blood vessels (*4, 5, 6,* and *7*). (From Fraser RG and Paré JA: Structure and function of the lung with emphasis on roentgenology, Philadelphia, 1971, WB Saunders.)

standing the orientation of each segment is necessary for those providing chest physical therapy (see Chapter 28).

The segmental patterns of the right and left lungs are similar, except as noted in Table 9-3 and Figure 9-27. A standardized naming system is widely used in North America.[28] This system helps to show which segments on the left correspond to those on the right.

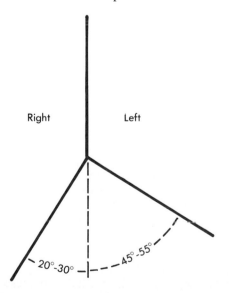

Fig. 9-26 Course of trachea and right and left main stem bronchi. Notice that right mainstem bronchus continues on straighter course from midline than left mainstem bronchus.

Since the right middle lobe and the lingula differ slightly, their names describe their segmental relationships. Some lobes of the left lung are combined to form single segments (Table 9-3).

The bronchi continue to divide into smaller, but more numerous airways.[29] Each branch gives rise to two lower "generations" (Table 9-4). Lobar bronchi divide into segmental bronchi. Segmental bronchi divide into subsegmental bronchi. These divisions continue until airways called the *bronchioles* arise. Bronchioles begin from 5 to 14 generations below the segmental bronchi. They are 1 to 2 mm in diameter and are referred to as the *small airways*. Bronchioles are the smallest "conducting" airways of the lower respiratory tract. Bronchioles differ from the larger airways in that they lack cartilage in their walls.

With further divisions, the number of airways increases tremendously. The cross-sectional area of the conducting system increases exponentially (Table 9-4). At the level of the terminal bronchioles, the cross-sectional area is about 20 times greater than at the trachea. Gas flow in the airways conforms to the laws of fluid physics. The increase in cross-sectional area results in a *decreased* velocity of gas flow during inspiration. When inspired gas reaches the alveoli, its average velocity is about the same as the rate of diffusion.[30] Low velocity in the small airways and alveoli is useful for two reasons. First, it allows *laminar flow* to develop. Laminar airflow minimizes resistance in the small airways. This decreases the

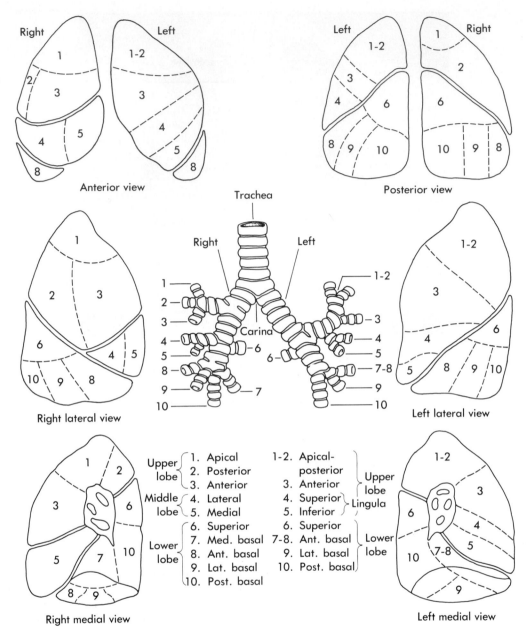

Right · Left

1-2

Anterior view

Left · Right

Posterior view

Trachea

Right · Left

Carina

Right lateral view

Left lateral view

Upper lobe {	1. Apical	1-2. Apical-posterior } Upper lobe
	2. Posterior	
	3. Anterior	3. Anterior
Middle lobe {	4. Lateral	4. Superior } Lingula
	5. Medial	5. Inferior
Lower lobe {	6. Superior	6. Superior
	7. Med. basal	7-8. Ant. basal } Lower lobe
	8. Ant. basal	9. Lat. basal
	9. Lat. basal	10. Post. basal
	10. Post. basal	

Right medial view

Left medial view

Fig. 9-27 Bronchopulmonary segments diagrammed. Again note similarities, with minor variations, between right and left lungs. (See editor's note for Table 6-5.)

work associated with inspiration. Second, low gas velocity facilitates rapid mixing of gases. This provides a stable environment for gas exchange.[31]

Tissues of the conducting airways

The walls of the conducting airways of the lungs share a similar gross structure. They vary considerably, however, in the number and type of cellular elements (Figure 9-28, page 206). All conducting airways have three major tissue layers. These layers are the *mucosa,* the *submucosa,* and a connective tissue envelope called the *adventitia.*[32]

The *mucosa* is composed of an epithelial lining and a layer of connective tissue known as the lamina propia Between these is a basement membrane. The primary cell type of the mucosa in the larger airways is *pseudostratified, ciliated columnar epithelium.* Between these ciliated cells are mucus-secreting *goblet cells.* Basal cells are also found on the basement membrane beneath these primary cell types. Basal cells are thought to differentiate into ciliated and goblet cells. This occurs in the normal growth process and in mucosal repair.[33]

The ciliated cells of the mucosa are essential in clearing and defending the respiratory tract. Each ciliated cell has about 200 cilia. This results in an estimated 1 to 2 billion cilia per square centimeter of mucosa.[32] Each cilia is about 6 to 7 μm long. These

Table 9-4   Bronchial and bronchiolar divisions

Structure	Trachea	Segmental bronchus	Terminal bronchiole	Number	Diameter of individual structures	Total cross-sectional area	
Trachea	0			1	2.5 cm	5.0 cm^2	
Main bronchi	1			2	11–19 mm	3.2 cm^2	
Lobar	2–3			5	4.5–13.5 mm	2.7 cm^2	
Segmental	3–6	0		19	4.5–65. mm	3.2 cm^2	Cartilaginous
Subsegmental	4–7	1		38	3–6 mm	6.6 cm^2	conducting
Bronchi		2–6		Varies	Varies	Varies	structures
Terminal bronchi		3–7		1000	1.0 mm	7.9 cm^2	
Bronchioles		5–14		Varies	Varies	Varies	
Terminal bronchioles		6–15	0	35000	0.65 mm	116 cm^2	
Respiratory bronchioles			1–8	Varies	Varies	Varies	
Terminal respiratory bronchioles			2–9	630000	0.45 mm	1000 cm^2	No cartilage in walls
Alveolar ducts/sacs			4–12	4 × 10^6	0.40 mm	1.71 m^2	
Alveoli				300 × 10^6	0.25–0.30 mm	70 m^2	

cilia "beat" in a rhythmic manner about 20 "strokes" per second. This sequential motion of the cilia is called a *metachronal wave* (Figure 9-29, page 206). The metachronal wave length is about 20 μm. Each wave propels surface material in a specific direction. In the nose this "ciliary escalator" propels material back to the pharynx. From the bronchioles up to the larynx it moves material toward the pharynx. In healthy lungs inhaled particles are removed within 24 hours.[34]

The effectiveness of ciliary action depends on the fluid layer above the mucosal epithelium.[35] Particulates are carried on a mucous blanket atop the cilia. The cilia beat in a less viscous *sol* layer (see Figure 9-29). Drying of the respiratory mucosa inhibits ciliary action. Excessive mucus production can also alter ciliary clearance. Certain drugs may affect ciliary activity. Atropine slows the rate of movement of the mucous blanket. This may be due to atropine's drying effect on the production of secretions. Drugs that stimulate the parasympathetic nervous system can increase ciliary activity.

Beneath the lamina propria of the mucosa is the submucosa (Figure 9-28). The submucosa of large airways contains *bronchial glands*. It also contains a capillary network, smooth muscle, and elastic tissue. The bronchial glands vary in size up to a millimeter in length. They connect to the bronchial surface by long, narrow ducts. These glands are the major source of respiratory tract secretions in healthy lungs. The number of these glands increases significantly in diseases such as chronic bronchitis. *Mast cells* are also found in the submucosa. Mast cells can release a potent vasoactive substance called histamine. Histamine causes vasodilatation and bronchoconstriction, acting directly on smooth muscle. This type of reaction is characteristic in diseases such as asthma.

The smooth muscle of the airways varies in location and structure. In the large airways, such as the trachea, smooth muscle is bundled in sheets. In smaller airways, smooth muscle forms a helical pattern. Muscle fibers crisscross and spiral around the airway walls. This placement causes a reduction in diameter and shortening of the airway during muscle contraction. This pattern of smooth muscle continues into the terminal lung units, even to the alveolar ducts.

Between the submucosa and adventitia of the large airways are incomplete rings or plates of cartilage (Figure 9-28). This cartilage provides structural support for the larger airways. The small airways depend on transmural pressure gradients and the "traction" of surrounding elastic tissue to remain open. During forced expiration, pressures across the wall of the small airways exceed the supporting forces of the elastic tissues. As a result, the small airways can collapse. The cartilage in the larger airways prevents their collapse during such maneuvers.

The adventitia is a sheath of connective tissue that surrounds the airways. It is interspersed with bronchial arteries, veins, nerves, lymph vessels, and adipose tissue.

The cells making up the respiratory mucosa change as they progress into the smaller airways (Figure 9-30, page 207). As the thickness of the walls of the airways decreases, bronchial glands become fewer in number. At the bronchiolar level, the number of ciliated cells

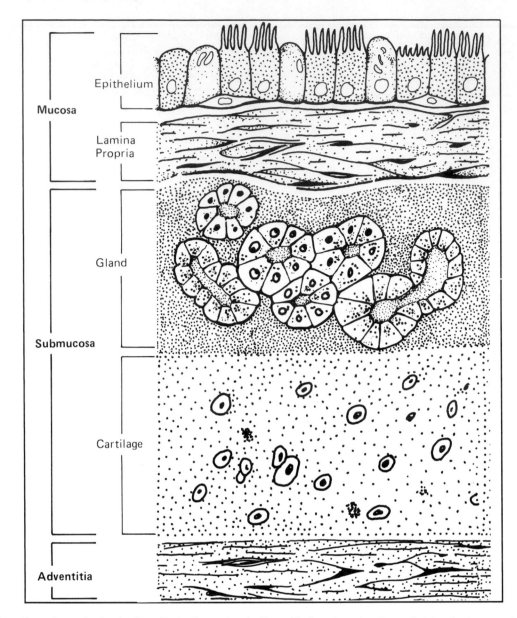

Mucosa
- Epithelium
- Lamina Propria

Submucosa
- Gland
- Cartilage

Adventitia

Fig. 9-28 Various tissue layers in the trachea, illustrating not only the epithelium but also the underlying lamina propria of the mucosa. Submucosal glands below this, whose ducts reach the tracheal lumen, allow secretory contribution to the mucus layer. Incomplete cartilaginous rings ensure a noncollapsible tube for airflow. (From Martin DE and Youtsey JW: Respiratory anatomy and physiology, St Louis, 1988, Mosby.)

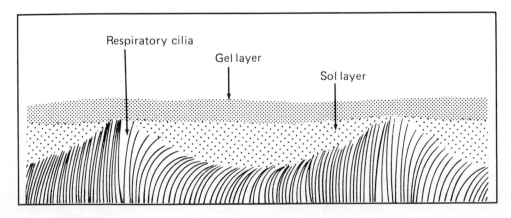

Respiratory cilia

Gel layer

Sol layer

Fig. 9-29 Respiratory cilia are bathed in the sol portion of the mucus layer above them. Their power strokes allow mucus movement by contacting the viscous gel layer, always in the same direction. (From Martin DE and Youtsey JW: Respiratory anatomy and physiology, St Louis, 1988, Mosby.)

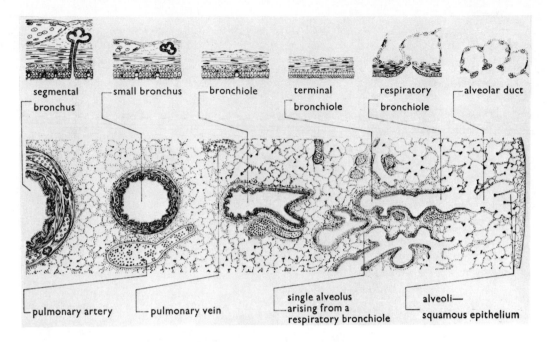

Fig. 9-30 Histologic diagram of airways from segmental bronchus to alveolus. (From Freeman WH and Bracegirdle B: An atlas of histology, London, 1966, Heinemann Educational Books Ltd.)

decreases. Simple columnar and **cuboidal** epithelial cells begin to predominate. These cells are interspersed with goblet cells. Nonciliated Clara cells are also found at the bronchiolar level. These cells are believed to have secretory functions.

Transitional and respiratory zones

The terminal bronchioles begin about 17 generations beyond the trachea. All of the airways above the terminal bronchioles simply condition and/or conduct gases. Further subdivisions below the terminal bronchioles are unique passageways called *respiratory bronchioles* (Figures 9-31 and 9-32, on page 208).

Respiratory bronchioles have a dual function. Like conducting airways, they move gas forward. Alveolar pouches on their surfaces also allow gas exchange. The respiratory bronchioles constitute the *transitional zone* in the lung. They lie between zones dedicated purely to conduction and purely to gas exchange.

The primary function of the lung, gas exchange, takes place in the *terminal respiratory unit*.[4] Terminal respiratory units begin at about the 17th division of bronchi. They consist of all structures distal to a terminal bronchiole (Figure 9-31). Terminal respiratory units have two to five orders of respiratory bronchi-

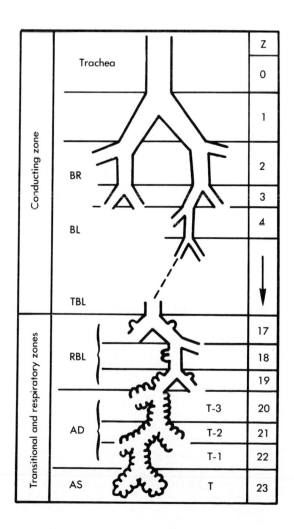

Fig. 9-31 The airways that only conduct gases back and forth are designated the conducting zone of lung. These include approximately the first 17 divisions of the tracheobronchial tree. The unit where gas exchange occurs, from respiratory bronchiole to alveolar space, is called the respiratory zone. *BR* = bronchus, *BL* = bronchiole, *TBL* = terminal bronchiole, *RBL* = respiratory bronchiole, *AD* = alveolar duct, *AS* = alveolar space, *Z* = order of airway division. (From Weibel ER: Morphometry of the human lung, Heidelberg, 1963, Springer-Verlag.)

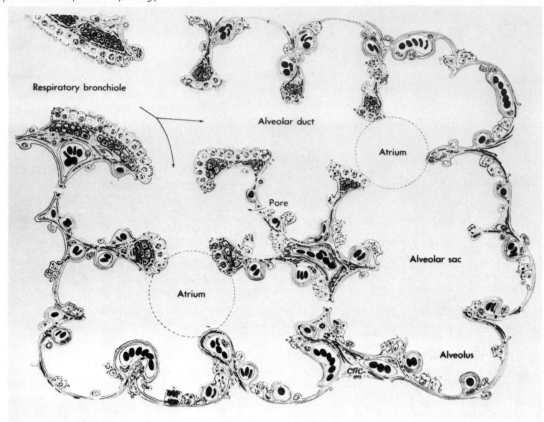

Fig. 9-32 Diagram of microscopic view of terminal airways. These units compose the respiratory zone of lung. (From Sorokin SP: The respiratory system. In Greep RO and Weiss L, editors: Histology, New York, 1973, McGraw-Hill. Used with permission of McGraw-Hill.)

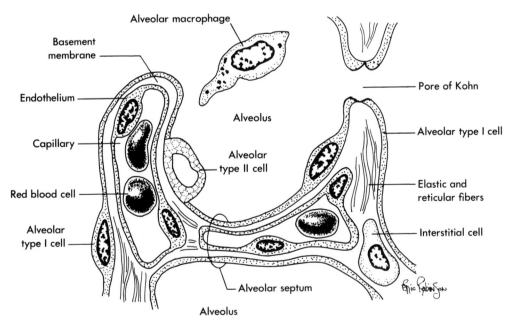

Fig. 9-33 Very high-power view of alveolus. Alveolar walls or septae are occupied mainly by capillaries. Basement membrane of capillary is fused with that of alveolar lining. Interstitium contains a few interstitial fibers, composed mostly of reticular support fibers, elastic fibers, and one interstitial cell. An incomplete portion of alveolar septum called a pore of Kohn is shown (see also Figure 6-5). Type I lining cells are very flat. Small distance between blood and air makes gas exchange remarkably efficient. Type II cells are much less numerous than type I cells. Type II cells are source of surfactant. The alveolar macrophages are mobile phagocytic cells that migrate into alveoli from the bloodstream.

oles. These are followed by a similar number of generations of *alveolar ducts.* Alveolar ducts are only as long as they are wide. They terminate in clusters of 10 to 16 alveoli.

The *alveolus* is the final anatomic unit in the respiratory system. It is the primary site of gas exchange. The adult lungs have approximately 300 million alveoli. The surface area for gas exchange ranges from 40 to 100 m^2, averaging 70 m^2. By comparison, the lung has 35 times more area than the skin in the average adult. The architecture of the alveolar region is essentially a pocket of air (Figure 9-33). It is surrounded by a thin membrane containing an extensive capillary network.

Scanning electron microscopy of the alveolar region provides a detailed view of its various structures (Figure 9-34, on page 210). The two principal cells found in the alveolus are type I, *squamous pneumocytes,* and type II, *granular pneumocytes* (see Figure 9-33). Type I cells are the very thin, flat cells that line the alveoli. Openings between type I cells provide communication between adjacent alveoli. These openings are called the *pores of Kohn.* Type II cells are cuboidal. They are also called septal cells and are more numerous than type I cells. Because of their shape they occupy less than 5% of the alveolar surface. These cells are thought to be the source of the surface-active substance called *pulmonary surfactant.*[36] Type II cells proliferate in cases of injury. They may also give rise to new type I cells. A third cell type is also found in the alveolar region. The *alveolar macrophage* is a phagocytic cell that clears bacteria and other material invading the alveoli.[37] Unlike type I and II cells, alveolar macrophages do not originate in the lung. They differentiate from stem cell precursors in the bone marrow. Alveolar macrophages are transported to the lung by the circulatory system.[4]

The tissue between alveolar air and capillary blood is the *alveolar septum* or *alveolar-capillary membrane.* Each septum contains a dense capillary network (Figure 9-35, *A*, on page 211). The short length and multiple branches of the capillaries around the alveolus present a sheetlike surface for gas exchange. This network is structured so that 100 to 300 mL of capillary blood capillaries is spread over 70 m^2 of surface. For example, each square meter of alveolar surface would be covered by just a teaspoon of blood.

In addition to the large surface area for gas exchange, the distance between alveolar gas and blood is small. The alveolar-capillary membrane ranges from 0.35 to 2.5 μm, separating capillary blood from alveolar air (Figure 9-35, *B*). Only very thin tissue and fluid layers ($\approx$ 1 μm) must be crossed for gas exchange to occur (Figure 9-35, *C*).

These short distances are essential for efficient gas exchange. Transfer of O_2 and CO_2 in the lung depends on diffusion gradients across this membrane. The red blood cell spends less than 1 second in transit through the pulmonary capillaries. Gas exchange is so efficient in the healthy lung that it is complete before the blood reaches the end of the capillary. At rest in upright subjects, the top one third of the lung receives little blood flow. During exercise these **unperfused** capillaries are "recruited" for gas exchange. These normal reserves become important in disease states.

Intercommunicating channels

Gas exchange lung units are not "dead-end" passages. Several forms of intercommunicating channels exist throughout the lung. Such channels may be found at the alveolar level, between bronchioles and alveoli, and among bronchioles.[38]

The pores of Kohn (Figures 9-33 and 9-34) range from 5 to 15 μm in diameter, varying their size during breathing. They allow collateral air movement between adjacent alveoli. These pores may explain why a lobule beyond an obstructed bronchiole remains partially inflated. Alveolar pores are not present during early postnatal phases of lung development. They increase in size and number throughout life, by an unknown mechanism. The number of alveolar pores increases in some diseases that affect the lung parenchyma.

A second type of intercommunicating channel between terminal bronchioles are the *canals of Lambert.* These openings are approximately 30 μm in size. They appear to remain open even when bronchiolar smooth muscle contracts. The canals of Lambert provide for gas movement between primary lobules.

A third larger pathway for collateral ventilation may also exist. *Intersegmental respiratory bronchioles* have been demonstrated in normal human lungs. These channels are found in airways with diameters of 80 to 150 μm, especially in the lower lobes.[39] Such channels may represent a major source for collateral gas exchange. Intercommunicating channels probably facilitate even distribution of ventilation during breathing. They may also contribute to the lung's ability to respond to structural damage accompanying certain lung diseases.

OTHER FUNCTIONS OF THE LUNG

In addition to gas exchange, the lungs perform other functions related to **homeostasis.** These functions involve both anatomic and metabolic roles.

The pulmonary circulation serves as a *blood reservoir* for the left ventricle. This reservoir maintains stable left ventricular volumes despite small changes in cardiac output. The pulmonary blood volume (about 600 mL) is sufficient to maintain normal left ventricle filling for several cardiac cycles. This is important if filling of the right side of the heart is decreased or interrupted.

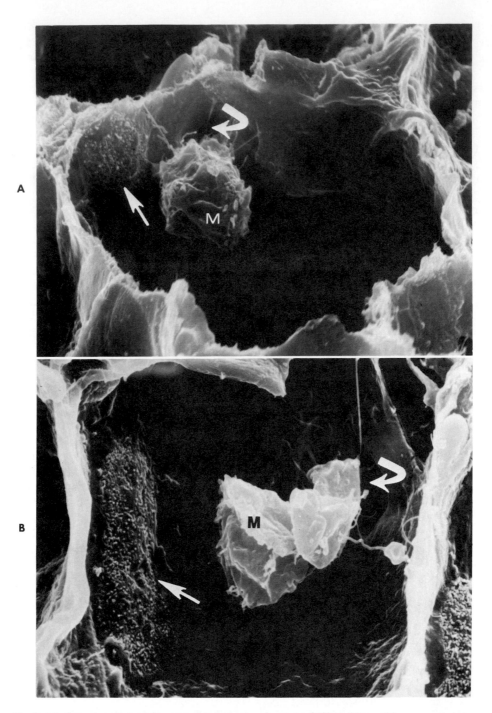

Fig. 9-34 Scanning electron micrographs of alveolar air spaces. **A,** Note thin partitions or septa between adjacent alveoli. The thin platelike type I cells compose most of these. Type II cells have projections off their surfaces that appear dotted or hairy (*straight arrow*). Alveolar macrophage (*M*) is seen at back partially covering pore of Kohn (*upper curved arrow*). **B,** Similar view with two or three macrophages passing through pore of Kohn. (Grateful appreciation is given to Mr. Mike Wagner, of San Diego, Calif, for use of the electron micrographs.)

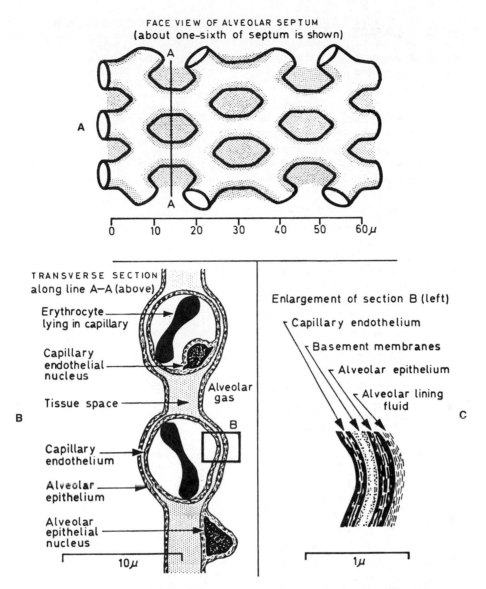

FACE VIEW OF ALVEOLAR SEPTUM
(about one-sixth of septum is shown)

A

0   10   20   30   40   50   60μ

TRANSVERSE SECTION
along line A—A (above)

Erythrocyte
lying in capillary

Capillary
endothelial
nucleus

Tissue space

Alveolar
gas

B

B

Capillary
endothelium

Alveolar
epithelium

Alveolar
epithelial
nucleus

10μ

Enlargement of section B (left)

Capillary endothelium

Basement membranes

Alveolar epithelium

Alveolar lining
fluid

C

1μ

Fig. 9-35 A, Face view of an alveolar septum (of which about one sixth is shown). The capillary network is dense, with the spaces between the capillaries being rather less than the diameter of the capillaries. **B,** Section (*A-A*) through two capillaries, demonstrating the very thin membrane through which gas exchange takes place. **C,** Enlargement of **B.** (From Nunn JF: Applied respiratory physiology, ed 2, London, 1977, Butterworth.)

The pulmonary circulation is also a *filter* for the systemic circulation. It traps particles before they enter the systemic circulation. This protects capillary beds where blockages could be life-threatening. Such areas include the coronary and cerebral circulations. Harmful particles that are filtered include fibrin and blood clots, fat cells, platelet aggregates, and debris found in stored blood or intravenous (IV) fluids.

The lungs play an active role in metabolism. They are responsible for synthesis, activation, inactivation, and detoxification of many bioactive substances. Heparin, histamine, bradykinin, serotonin, and certain prostaglandins are stored or synthesized in the lung. The lung releases these substances in response to physiologic or immunologic challenges. Angiotensin is converted to its active form by the lung. Adenosine triphosphate (ATP) and norepinephrine are partially removed from the blood and inactivated by the lungs.

CHAPTER SUMMARY

The respiratory system fulfills its primary purpose of gas exchange by integrating its form and functions. The thorax houses and protects the lungs. It is also the mechanical bellows that makes ventilation possible. Motor and sensory neurons innervate the muscles of ventilation. They provide feedback mechanisms for responding to changing conditions. Dual circulatory systems sustain the lung and provide a capillary network for gas exchange. The upper respiratory tract heats and humidifies inspired air. It also protects the lungs against foreign substances. The lower respiratory tract conducts respired gases from the atmosphere to the respiratory zones of the lung. It too participates in clearance and defense. Finally, the respiratory lung units provide a large surface that facilitates external respiration.

In healthy persons, these structures perform efficiently throughout life. The reserve capacities of the respiratory system provide the ability to respond to changing physiologic needs. Alterations in structure or function can compromise this ability, threatening survival. The basis of respiratory care is to maintain the structure or restore normal function.

REFERENCES

1. Fraser RG, Paré JA: *Structure and function of the lung with emphasis on roentgenology,* Philadelphia, 1971, WB Saunders.
2. von Hayek H: *The human lung,* New York, 1960, Hafner.
3. Lai-Fook SJ: Mechanics of the pleural space: fundamental concepts. *Lung* (165(5):249, 1987.
4. Murray JF: *The normal lung: the basis for diagnosis and treatment of pulmonary disease,* ed 2, Philadelphia, 1986, WB Saunders.
5. Wade OL, Gilson JC: The effect of posture on diaphragmatic movement and vital capacity in normal subjects, *Thorax* 6:103, 1951.
6. DeTroyer A et al: Mechanics of intercostal space and actions of external and internal intercostal muscles, *J Clin Invest* 75(3):850, 1985.
7. Celli BR: Clinical and physiologic evaluation of respiratory muscle function, *Clin Chest Med* 10(2):199, 1989.
8. Mier A et al: Action of the abdominal muscles on the ribcage in humans. *J Appl Physiol* 58:1438, 1985.
9. Richardson JB: Nerve supply to the lung, *Am Rev Respir Dis* 119:785, 1979.
10. Barnes PJ: Neural control of human airways in health and disease, *Am Rev Respir Dis* 134(6):1289, 1986.
11. Spencer H and Leof D: The innervation of the human lung, *J Anat* 98:599, 1964.
12. Coleridge HM, Coleridge JCG: *Reflexes evoked from the tracheobronchial tree and lungs.* In Fishman AF et al, editors: *Handbook of physiology, sect 3, The respiratory system, vol II, Control of breathing,* Bethesda, Md, 1986, American Physiological Society.
13. Fishman NH, Phillipson EA, Nadel JA: Effect of differential vagal cold blockade on breathing patterns in conscious dogs, *J Appl Physiol* 34:754, 1973.
14. Crofton J, Douglas A: *Respiratory diseases,* ed 3, Oxford, England, 1981, Blackwell Scientific Publications.
15. Karlsson JA, Sant'Ambrogio G, Widdicombe JG: Afferent neural pathways in cough and reflex bronchoconstriction, *J Appl Physiol* 65:1007, 1988.
16. Harris P, Heath D: *The human pulmonary circulation,* Edinburgh, 1962, E and S Livingstone.
17. Green JF: The pulmonary circulation. In Zelis R, editor: *The peripheral circulation,* New York, 1975, Grune & Stratton.
18. Milnor WR: *Pulmonary hemodynamics.* In Bergel DH, editor: *Cardiovascular fluid dynamics,* vol 2, New York, 1972, Academic Press.
19. Daly I, Hebb CO: *Pulmonary and bronchial vascular systems,* Baltimore, 1967, Williams & Wilkins.
20. Charan NB: The bronchial circulatory system: structure, function and importance, *Respir Care* 29:1226, 1984.
21. Nagaishi C: *Functional anatomy and histology of the lung,* Baltimore, 1972, University Park Press.
22. Lauweryns JM, Baert JH: Alveolar clearance and the role of the pulmonary lymphatics. *Am Rev Respir Dis* 115:625, 1977.
23. Heitzman ER: *The lung: radiologic-pathologic correlations,* St. Louis, 1973, Mosby.
24. Johanson WG: Lung defense mechanisms, *Basics Respir Disease,* 6(2):7, 1977.
25. Proctor DF: The upper airways. Part I. Nasal physiology and defense of the lung. *Am Rev Respir Dis* 115:97, 1977.
26. Lough mL, Boat T, Doershuk CF: The nose, *Respir Care* 20:286, 1975.
27. Proctor DF: The upper airways. Part II. The larynx and trachea. *Am Rev Respir Dis* 115:315, 1977.
28. Boyden EA: *Segmental anatomy of the lungs,* New York, 1955, McGraw-Hill.
29. Weibel ER: *Morphometry of the human lung,* New York, 1962, Academic Press.
30. Foster RE, et al: *The lung: Physiologic basis of pulmonary function tests,* ed 3, St Louis, 1986, Mosby.
31. Engel LA: Gas mixing within the acinus of the lung, *J Appl Physiol* 54(3):609, 1983.
32. Rhodin JAG: Ultrastructure and function of the human tracheal mucosa, *Am Rev Respir Dis* 93 (suppl 1): 1966.
33. Breeze RG, Wheeldon EB: The cells of the pulmonary airways, *Am Rev Respir Dis* 116:705, 1977.
34. Pavia D et al: General review of tracheobronchial clearance, *Eur J Respir Dis* 153 (suppl):123, 1987.
35. Widdicombe JG: Control of secretions of tracheobronchial mucus, *Br Med Bull* 34:57, 1978.
36. Clements JA et al: Pulmonary surface tension and alveolar stability, *J Appl Physiol* 16:444, 1972.
37. Fels AO, Cohn ZA: The alveolar macrophage, *J Appl Physiol* 60(2):353, 1986.
38. Menkes HA, Traysman RJ: Collateral ventilation, *Am Rev Respir Dis* 116:287, 1977.
39. Anderson JB, Jespersen W: Demonstration of intersegmental respiratory bronchioles in normal human lungs, *Eur J Respir Dis* 61(6):337, 1980.

The Cardiovascular System

■

Craig L. Scanlan
Norman Schussler

CHAPTER LEARNING OBJECTIVES

1. Relate the gross anatomy and microanatomy of the heart and vascular system to their functions;
2. Differentiate among the key properties of cardiac tissue;
3. Delineate the various factors responsible for local and central control of the heart and vascular system;
4. Describe how the cardiovascular system coordinates its functions under normal and abnormal conditions;
5. Explain the normal mechanisms responsible for conduction of electrical impulses and their graphic representation on ECG;
6. Relate the mechanical and electrical events that occur during a normal cardiac cycle.

The cardiovascular system provides the vital link between external gas exchange at the lung and internal respiration at the tissues. It transports needed oxygen and nutrients to the trillions of body cells and removes their metabolic waste, including carbon dioxide. By distributing the blood and body fluids throughout the body, the cardiovascular system maintains what Claude Bernard long ago called "le milieu interieur," or balanced internal environment.[1]

The heart and vascular system must work closely together to ensure that each body region receives adequate blood flow according to its individual need. In addition, the cardiovascular system must have enough reserve capacity to respond to both normal stress, as occurs during exercise, as well as abnormal conditions, such as blood loss.

Respiratory care practitioners (RCPs) must understand that the cardiovascular and respiratory systems share structural and functional relationships. Clinical disorders in one system are often closely related to dysfunction in the other. Terms such as *shock lung, cor pulmonale,* and *pulmonary vascular hypertension* remind us that in clinical practice the boundaries that separate the two systems are meaningless. More often than not, RCPs must deal with not just the patient's lungs, heart, or vasculature, but with a single, integrated cardiopulmonary system. This chapter provides the necessary foundations to apply this integrated perspective in clinical practice.

FUNCTIONAL ANATOMY

The Heart

Gross anatomy of the heart

The heart is a hollow, muscular organ about the size of a fist. It is positioned **obliquely** in the middle compartment of the mediastinum of the chest, just behind the sternum (Figure 10-1, page 214). About two thirds of the heart lies to the left of the sternum's midline. The heart's pointed apex is formed by the tip of the left ventricle and lies just above the diaphragm at the level of the fifth intercostal space. The base of the heart is formed by the atria. It projects to the right and lies just below the second rib. Surface grooves called *sulci* mark the boundaries of the heart chambers. The coronary sulcus lies between the atria and the ventricles, while the anterior and posterior longitudinal sulci mark the boundaries between the ventricles themselves.

The heart is enclosed in a loose, membranous sac called the parietal *pericardium.* The outer fibrous layer consists of tough connective tissue. The inner serous layer is thinner and more delicate, being continuous with a similar visceral layer (the visceral pericardium) on the outer surface of the heart and great vessels. Pericardial fluid separates these two layers. This fluid helps minimize friction as the heart contracts and expands within the pericardium. "Inflammation of the pericardium results in a clinical condition called *pericarditis."*

The heart wall consists of three layers: the outer visceral layer (epicardium), the middle myocardium, and the inner endocardium. The endocardium is a thin layer of tissue continuous with the inner layer of blood vessels. The myocardium composes the bulk of the heart and consists of bands of involuntary striated muscle fibers. It is the contraction of these muscle fibers that creates the pumplike action needed to move blood throughout the body.

Four rings of dense connective tissue, or *annuli fibrosi,* form a fibrous "skeleton" for the heart. This

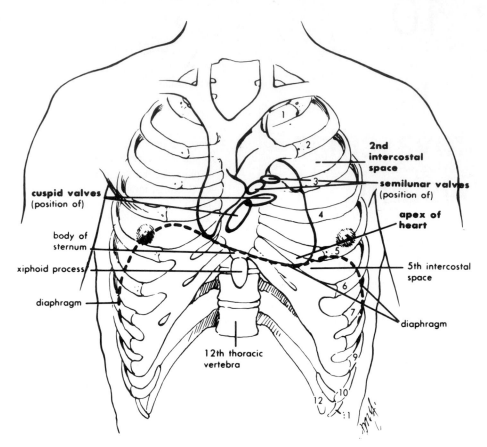

Fig. 10-1 Anterior view of the thorax showing the position of the heart in relationship to the ribs, sternum, diaphragm, and the position of the heart valves. (From Crouch JE: Functional human anatomy, ed 4, Philadelphia, 1985, Lea & Febiger.)

AV ring (Figure 10-2), provides support for the heart's four interior chambers and valves (Figure 10-3). The two atrial chambers are thin-walled "cups" of myocardial tissue separated by an interatrial septum. On the right side of the interatrial septum is an oval depression called the *fossa ovalis.* The fossa ovalis is the remnant of the fetal foramen ovale. Each atrium also has an appendage, or auricle, the function of which is unknown.

The two lower chambers, or ventricles, make up the bulk of the heart's muscle mass and provide the major force for circulating the blood. The mass of the left ventricle is about two thirds greater than that of the right and appears spherical in shape when viewed in anteroposterior (AP) cross section. The right ventricle is thin-walled and oblong in shape, forming a pocket-like attachment to the left ventricle. Because of this relationship, contraction of the left ventricle actually pulls in the right ventricular wall, aiding its contraction (Figure 10-4). The effect, called *left ventricular aid,* explains why some forms of right ventricular failure have a less harmful effect than would otherwise be expected.[2]

The right and left ventricles are separated by a muscle wall called the *interventricular septum* (Figure

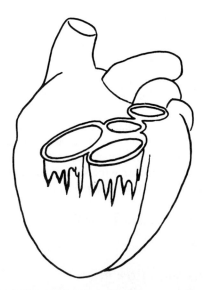

Fig. 10-2 Four rings that form anulus fibrosus with cusps hanging curtain-like from edges. (From McLaughlin AJ Jr: Essentials of physiology for advanced respiratory therapy, St Louis, 1977, Mosby.)

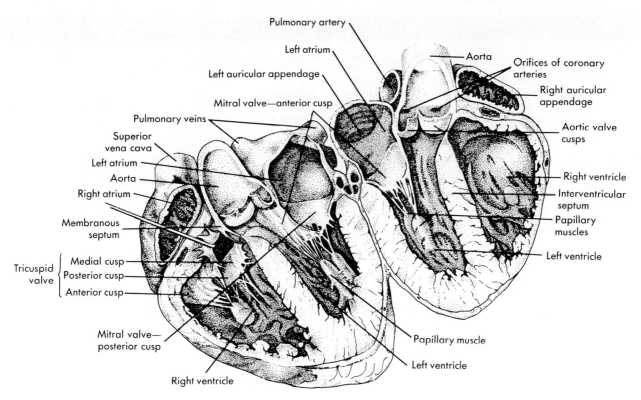

Fig. 10-3 Drawing of a heart split perpendicular to the interventricular septum to illustrate the anatomic relationships of the leaflets of the AV and aortic valves. (From Berne RM and Levy MN: Cardiovascular physiology, ed 5, St Louis, 1986, Mosby.)

10-3). Ventricular muscle fibers are arranged in an overlapping spiral fashion, much like the wrappings of a turban. Contraction of these fibers results in a wringing action that helps eject blood from the ventricles.

The valves of the heart are flaps of fibrous tissue firmly anchored to the annuli fibrosi (Figure 10-2). Those located between the atria and ventricles are called atrioventricular (AV) valves (Figure 10-5, page 216). The valve between the right atrium and ventricle is called the *tricupid valve*. The valve between the left atrium and ventricle is called the bicuspid, or *mitral valve*. The AV valves close during systole, thereby preventing backflow of blood into the atria. This provides a critical period of **isovolemic** contraction during which chamber pressures quickly rise without blood being ejected.

The free ends of the AV valves are anchored to papillary muscles of the endocardium via *chordae tendenae* (Figure 10-3). During systole, papillary muscle contraction prevents the AV valves from swinging upward into the atria. Damage to either the chordae tendenae or the papillary muscles can impair function of the AV valves. Common valve problems include regurgitation and stenosis. *Regurgitation* is the backflow of blood through an incompetent or damaged valve. **Stenosis** is a pathologic narrowing or constriction of a valve outlet, which causes increased pressure

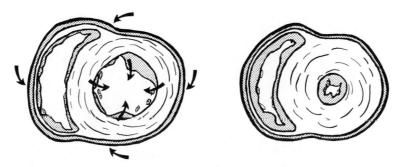

Fig. 10-4 Cross section of ventricles showing changes in size of left and right ventricles during contraction. (Adapted from Guyton AC: Textbook of medical physiology, ed 4, Philadelphia, 1971, WB Saunders Co. From McLaughlin AJ Jr: Essentials of physiology for advanced respiratory therapy, St Louis, 1977, Mosby.)

■ MINI CLINI ■

10-1

The mitral valve separates the left atrium and ventricle. A stenotic mitral valve is one that is narrowed and offers high resistance to the blood flowing through it into the ventricle. Pulmonary edema is a condition in which fluid collects in the spaces between alveolar and capillary walls, known as the interstitial space.

Problem: Why does a patient with mitral stenosis have poor oxygenation of the blood and increased work of breathing?

Discussion: Blood flows from the lungs to the left atrium, where it encounters high resistance through a narrowed, stenotic valve. This causes

Mitral Stenosis, Poor Oxygenation, and Increased Work of Breathing

high pressure to build in the left atrium. Pressure in the pulmonary veins, and eventually, the pulmonary capillaries also increases. This high pressure within the capillaries engorges them and forces fluid components of the blood plasma out of

the vessels into the interstitial space, creating pulmonary edema. This collection of fluid interferes with oxygen diffusion from the lung into the blood. Engorged capillaries surrounding the alveoli create a stiff "web" around each alveolus that makes expanding the lungs difficult. Some areas of the lung expand more easily than other areas. This causes inhaled air to be preferentially directed into these compliant regions while "stiffer" noncompliant regions are underventilated. The underventilated regions do not properly oxygenate the blood perfusing them. Thus, mitral stenosis, a cardiac problem, has significant pulmonary consequences.

in the affected chamber. In either condition, cardiac performance is affected. For example, in mitral stenosis, high pressures in the left atrium back up into the pulmonary circulation. This can cause pulmonary edema.

A separate set of *semilunar valves* separate the ventricles from their arterial outflow tracts (Figure 10-5). Consisting of three half-moon-shaped cusps attached to the arterial wall, these valves prevent backflow of blood into the ventricles during diastole. The pulmonary valve is at the outflow tract of the right ventricle. During systole, blood flows through

the open pulmonary valve from the right ventricle into the pulmonary artery. The aortic valve is located at the outflow tract of the left ventricle. During systole, blood flows through the open aortic valve from the left ventricle into the aorta. As with the AV valves, the semilunar valves can leak (regurgitation) or become obstructed (stenosis).

Like the lung, the heart has its own circulatory system, called the *coronary circulation*. Unlike the lung, however, the heart has a very high metabolic rate. As a result of its high metabolism, the heart requires more blood flow per gram of tissue weight

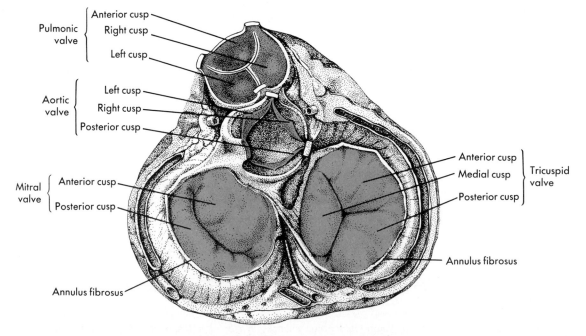

Fig. 10-5 Four cardiac valves as viewed from the base of the heart. Note how the leaflets overlap in the closed valves. (From Berne RM and Levy MN: Cardiovascular physiology, ed 5, St Louis, 1986, Mosby.)

■ MINI CLINI ■

10-2

Heart Rate and Coronary Perfusion

Problem: Why might a very high heart rate decrease blood flow through the coronary arteries?

Discussion: Blood flow through the coronary arteries occurs only during ventricular diastole. During systole, the myocardium contracts with such force that coronary artery pressures actually rise above aortic pressures. Thus, myocardial perfusion occurs only during diastole. As heart rate increases, both systolic and diastolic times must necessarily decrease. As diastolic time decreases, less and less time is available for coronary artery perfusion until finally coronary blood flow can be significantly reduced. This is critically important in the individual who already has compromised coronary circulation caused by arteriosclerotic heart disease. Not only is coronary artery perfusion compromised with severe tachycardia; decreased ventricular filling time causes decreased stroke volume and decreased cardiac output.

---

than any other organ except the kidney.[3] To meet these needs, the coronary circulation provides an extensive network of branches to all myocardial tissue (Figure 10-6, page 218).

Two main coronary arteries, a left and a right, arise from the root of the aorta. Because of their position, the coronary arteries get the maximum pulse of pressure generated by contraction of the left ventricle. Although there can be major individual differences in the branching of the coronary circulation, the basic layout is similar in all humans.

The left coronary artery divides into two branches between the pulmonary artery and the tip of the left atrial appendage. An *anterior descending branch* courses down the anterior sulcus to the apex of the heart. A *circumflex branch* moves along the coronary sulcus toward the back and around the left atrial appendage. The circumflex branch further divides into smaller arteries which feed the back side of the left ventricle. In combination, the left coronary artery normally supplies most of the left ventricle, the left atrium, the anterior two thirds of the interventricular septum, the lower half of the interatrial septum, and part of the right atrium.

The right coronary artery also begins at the aorta, where it proceeds diagonally to the right across the coronary sulcus. As it moves across the front surface of the right ventricle, it divides into many small branches. The right coronary artery ends in its *posterior descending branch,* which descends within the posterior interventricular sulcus (Figure 10-6). In about one of five people, this posterior descending branch arises from the terminal branch of the left circumflex coronary artery.[4] In these cases, the person is said to have a predominant left coronary artery system.

Together, the branches of the right coronary artery supply the anterior and posterior portions of the right ventricular myocardium, the right atrium, the sinus node, the posterior third of the interventricular septum, and a portion of the base of the right ventricle.

The coronary veins closely parallel the arteries (Figure 10-6). The great cardiac vein follows the anterior descending artery in the anterior interventricular sulcus. The small cardiac vein accompanies the right coronary artery in the coronary sulcus. The left posterior coronary vein follows a branch of the circumflex artery, and the middle cardiac vein parallels the posterior descending artery. These veins gather together into a large vessel called the coronary sinus, which passes left to right across the back of the heart. The coronary sinus empties into the right atrium between the opening of the inferior vena cava and the tricuspid valve.

In addition to these major routes for return blood flow, some coronary venous blood flows back into the heart through the *thebesian* veins. The thebesian veins empty directly into all heart chambers. Thus any blood coming from the thebesian veins that enters the left atrium or ventricle will mix with arterial blood coming from the lungs. Whenever venous blood mixes with arterial blood, the overall oxygen content falls. Because the thebesian veins bypass or **shunt** around the pulmonary circulation, this phenomenon is called an "anatomic shunt." When combined with a similar bypass in the bronchial circulation (see Chapter 9), these normal anatomic shunts total about 2% to 3% of the total cardiac output.

Properties of the heart muscle

The heart's performance as a pump depends on its ability to initiate and conduct electrical impulses and to synchronously contract its muscle fibers quickly and efficiently. These actions are possible only because myocardial tissues possess four key properties: excitability, inherent rhythmicity, conductivity, and contractility.[5,6]

The myocardial property of *excitability* is the same as that exhibited by other muscles and tissues. Excitability is the ability of cells to respond to electrical, chemical, or mechanical stimulation. In the clinical setting, factors such as electrolyte imbalances and certain drugs can increased myocardial excitability.

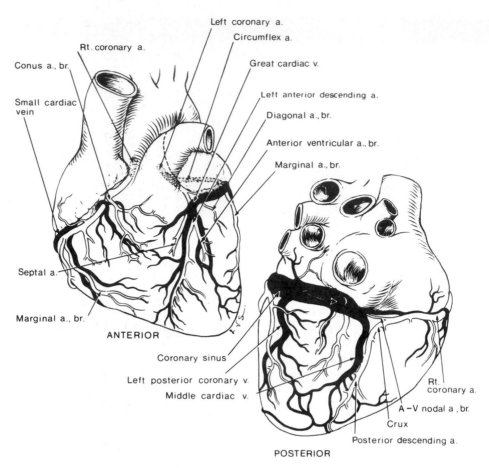

Left coronary a.
Circumflex a.
Rt. coronary a.
Great cardiac v.
Conus a., br.
Left anterior descending a.
Small cardiac vein
Diagonal a., br.
Anterior ventricular a., br.
Marginal a., br.
Septal a.
Marginal a., br.
ANTERIOR
Coronary sinus
Left posterior coronary v.
Middle cardiac v.
Rt. coronary a.
A–V nodal a., br.
Crux
Posterior descending a.
POSTERIOR

Fig. 10-6 Arteries and veins of the heart. Veins are black; arteries are clear-colored. Major vessels are described in the text. Note how the major cardiac veins parallel the coronary arteries. The direction of flow of blood in the coronary sinus is indicated by the arrow, whose tip is at the site of the coronary sinus ostium. (From Sanderson RG: The cardiac patient: a comprehensive approach, ed 2, Philadelphia, 1983, WB Saunders.)

As a result, abnormalities in electrical conduction can occur.

The unique ability of the cardiac muscle to initiate a spontaneous electrical impulse is called *inherent rhythmicity,* or automaticity. Although such impulses can arise from any cardiac tissue, this ability is highly developed in specialized areas called pacemaker, or nodal tissues. The sinoatrial (SA) node and the atrioventricular (AV) node are good examples of specialized heart tissues that are designed to initiate electrical impulses. The origin of an electrical impulse from other than a normal pacemaker is considered abnormal and represents one of the many causes of what are called cardiac arrhythmias.

Conductivity is the ability of myocardial tissue to spread or radiate electrical impulses. This property is similar to that of smooth muscle, in that it allows the myocardium to contract without direct neural innervation (as required by skeletal muscle). The rate with which electrical impulses spread throughout the myocardium is extremely variable.[2] In the nodal areas, impulses move as slowly as 5 cm/sec. In contrast, the Purkinje fibers conduct impulses at 300 to 400 cm/sec. These differences in conduction velocity are needed to assure synchronous contraction of the cardiac chambers. Abnormal conductivity can affect the timing of chamber contractions and thus decrease cardiac efficiency.

Contractility in response to an electrical impulse is the primary function of the myocardium. Unlike those of other muscle tissues, however, cardiac contractions cannot be sustained or tetanized. This is because myocardial tissue exhibits a prolonged period of inexcitability after contraction.[2] This period during which the myocardium cannot be stimulated is called the *refractory period.*

Microanatomy

To understand how cardiac muscle contracts requires knowledge of the heart's microanatomy. Under the microscope, myocardium tissue is seen to consist of an arrangement of striated, cylindrically shaped muscle fibers averaging 10 to 15 μm wide, and 30 to 60 μm long. Individual fibers are enclosed in a membrane called the *sarcolemma,* surrounded by a rich capillary network (Figure 10-7). Cardiac fibers are separated by irregular transverse thickenings of the sarcolemma called *intercalated discs.* These discs pro-

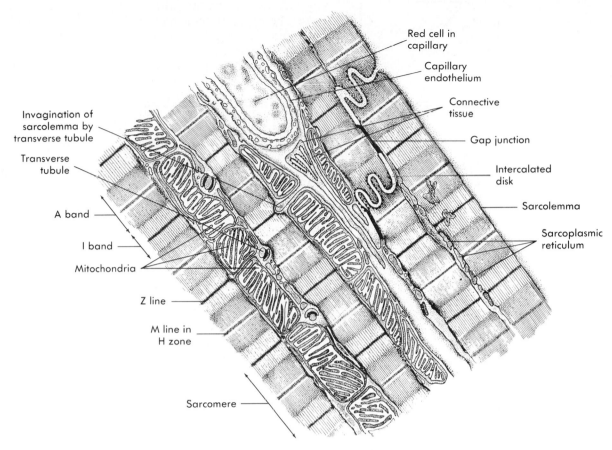

Fig. 10-7 Diagram of an electron micrograph of cardiac muscle showing large numbers of mitochondria and the intercalated disks with nexi (gap junctions), transverse tubules, and longitudinal tubules. (From Berne RM and Levy MN: Cardiovascular physiology, ed 5, St. Louis, 1986, Mosby.)

vide structural support and aid in electrical conduction between fibers.[7]

Each muscle fiber consists of many smaller units called *myofibrils.* Myofibrils contain repeated structures about 1.5 to 2.5 μm in size called *sarcomeres.* Within the sarcomeres are contractile protein filaments responsible for shortening the myocardium during systole.[7,8] These proteins are of two types: the thick filaments are composed mainly of myosin, and thin filaments consist mostly of actin.

According to the sliding filament theory, myocardial cells contract when actin and myosin combine to form reversible bridges between these thick and thin filaments. These cross bridges cause filaments to slide over one another, shortening the sarcomere and thus muscle fibers as a whole.

In principle, the tension developed during myocardial contraction is directly proportional to the number of cross bridges between the actin and myosin filaments. In turn, the number of cross bridges is directly proportional to the sarcomere's length. This principle underlies Starling's law of the heart, also known as the *Frank-Starling principle.* According to this principle, the more a cardiac fiber is stretched, the greater will be the tension it generates when contracted.

The Frank-Starling principle is depicted in Figure 10-8, page 220. Note that this relationship holds true only up to a sarcomere length of 2.2 μm. Beyond this point, the actin and myosin filaments become partially disengaged, and fewer cross bridges can be formed. With fewer cross bridges, the overall tension developed during contraction is less. This relationship is of major importance, and will be explored later in discussion of the heart as a pump.

The Vascular System

Figure 10-9, page 220 represents the basic plan of blood flow to and from the heart. Venous, or deoxygenated blood from the head and upper extremities enters the right atrium from the superior vena cava, while blood from the lower body enters from the inferior vena cava. From the right atrium, blood flows through the tricuspid valve into the right ventricle. The right ventricle pumps blood through the pulmonary valve, into the pulmonary arteries, and on to the lungs. Oxygenated blood returns to the left atrium through the pulmonary veins. The left atrium pumps

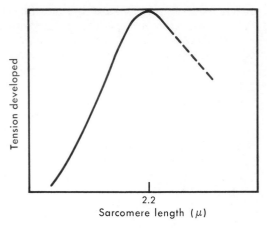

Fig. 10-8 The ultrastructural basis for the Frank-Starling curve, showing that peak tension development occurs at a sarcomere length of 2.2 μm; whether a downslope of the curve after peak tension exists is not known. (From Schroeder JS and Daily EK: Techniques in bedside hemodynamic monitoring, St Louis, 1976, Mosby.)

blood through the mitral valve into the left ventricle. The blood is then pumped through the aortic valve and into the aorta. From the aorta, the blood flows out to the tissues of the upper and lower body. From the capillary network of the various body tissues, venous blood returns to the vena cava.

Although a single organ, the heart functions as two separate pumps. The right side of the heart provides the pressures needed to drive blood through the low-resistance, low-pressure pulmonary circulation. The left side of the heart generates enough pressure to propel blood through the higher-pressure systemic circulation.

Components of the systemic vasculature

Because the pulmonary circulation has already been described in Chapter 9, the emphasis here will be on the systemic vasculature. The systemic vasculature consists of three major components: the arterial system, the capillary system, and the venous system. Although all three components are responsible for circulating blood to and from the tissues and lungs, these various vessels are more than just passive conduits. In fact, they regulate not only the amount of

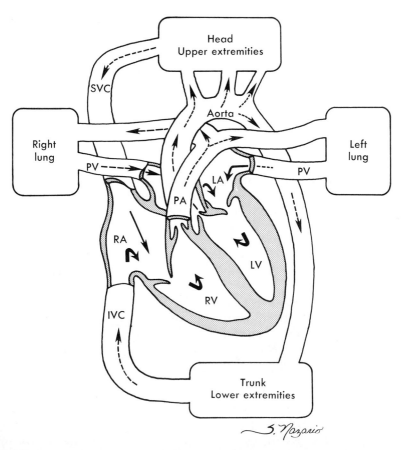

Fig. 10-9 Schematic of plan of circulation. *RA*, right atrium; *RV*, right ventricle; *LA*, left atrium; *LV*, left ventricle; *IVC*, inferior vena cava; *SVC*, superior vena cava; *PA*, pulmonary artery; *PV*, pulmonary vein.

blood flow per minute (cardiac output), but also its bodily distribution.[2] To achieve this function, each component has a unique structure and serves a somewhat different role in the circulatory system as a whole.[9]

The arterial system consists of large, highly elastic, and low-resistance arteries and small, muscular, variable-resistance **arterioles.** With their high elasticity, the large arteries help transmit and maintain the head of pressure generated by the heart. Together, the large arteries are called *conductance vessels.*[5,9]

Just as faucets control the flow of water into a sink, the smaller arterioles control blood flow into the capillaries. Arterioles provide this control by varying their flow resistance. For this reason, arterioles are often referred to as *resistance vessels.*[5,9]

The vast capillary system, or microcirculation, maintains a constant environment for the body's cells and tissues via the transport and exchange of nutrients and waste products. It is for this reason that the capillaries are commonly referred to as *exchange vessels.*[5,9]

Figure 10-10 shows the basic structure of a typical capillary network.[10] Blood flows into the network via an arteriole (A) and out through a **venule** (V). A direct communication between these vessels is called an arteriovenous **anastomosis** (AVA). When open, AVAs allows arterial blood to shunt around the capillary bed and flow directly into the venules. Downstream from the AVA, the arteriole divides into terminal arterioles (TAs), which further branch into thoroughfare channels (TCs) and true capillaries (Cs). Capillaries have smooth muscle rings at their proximal ends, called precapillary sphincters. Contraction of these sphincters decreases blood flow in that area, while relaxation increases perfusion. In combination, these various channels, sphincters, and bypasses allow precise control over the direction and amount of blood flow to a given area of tissue.

The venous system consists of small, expandable venules and veins and larger, more elastic veins. Besides conducting blood back to the heart, these vessels act as a reservoir for the circulatory system. At any given time, the veins and venules hold about three

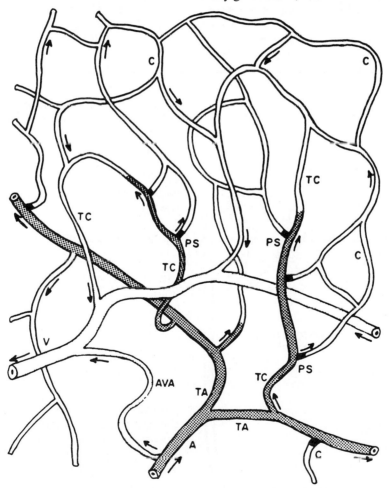

Fig. 10-10 Components of a microcirculatory network.*C,* Capillary; *TC,* thoroughfare channel; *V,* venule; *PS,* precapillary sphincter; *AVA,* arteriolovenous **anastomosis;** *A,* arteriole; *TA,* terminal arteriole. (From Zweifach BW: The microcirculation of the blood, January 1959, pp. 54–60. Copyright © 1959 by Scientific American. All rights reserved.)

quarters of the body's total blood volume. Moreover, the volume held in this reservoir can be quickly changed simply by altering the tone of these vessels. By quickly changing its holding capacity, the venous system can match the volume of circulating blood to that needed to maintain adequate perfusion. Accordingly, the components of the venous system, especially the small, expandable venules and veins, are termed *capacitance vessels.*

As the part of the circulation with the lowest pressures, the venous system must overcome gravity to return blood to the heart. As shown in Figure 10-11, four mechanisms combine to aid venous return to the heart: (1) **sympathetic** venous tone, (2) skeletal muscle pumping or "milking" (combined with venous one-way valves), (3) cardiac suction, and (4) thoracic pressure differences caused by respiratory movements.

This last mechanism is often called the "thoracic pump." As an aid to venous return, the thoracic pump is particularly important to RCPs. This is because artificial ventilation with positive pressure reverses normal thoracic pressure gradients. Positive pressure ventilation thus impedes, rather than assists venous return. Fortunately, as long as blood volume, cardiac function, and **vasomotor** tone are adequate, positive pressure ventilation has a minimal effect on venous return. If this were not the case, positive pressure ventilatory support would be impossible.

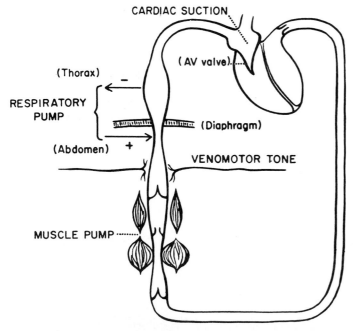

Fig. 10-11 Mechanisms that assist venous flow from the extremities. See text for details. (From Richardson DR: Basic circulatory physiology, Boston, 1976, Little, Brown.)

Vascular resistance

Like the movement of any fluid through tubes, blood flow through the vascular system is opposed by frictional forces. The sum of all frictional forces opposing blood flow through the systemic circulation is called the *systemic vascular resistance.*

In terms of the concept of resistance developed in Chapter 7, systemic peripheral resistance must equal the difference in pressure between the beginning and the end of the circuit, divided by the flow. The beginning pressure for the systemic circulation is the mean aortic pressure; ending pressure equals right atrial pressure. Flow for the system as a whole equals the cardiac output. Thus, systemic vascular resistance (SVR) can be calculated by the following formula[11]:

$$SVR = \frac{\text{mean aortic pressure} - \text{right atrial pressure}}{\text{cardiac output}}$$

Given a normal mean aortic pressure of 90 mm Hg, a mean right atrial pressure of about 4 mm Hg, and a normal cardiac output of 5 L/min, the normal systemic vascular resistance is computed as follows:

$$SVR = \frac{90 \text{ mm Hg} - 4 \text{ mm Hg}}{5 \text{ L/min}}$$
$$= 17.2 \text{ mm Hg/L/min}$$

The same concepts can be used to compute flow resistance in the pulmonary circulation. Beginning pressure for the pulmonary circulation is the mean pulmonary artery pressure; ending pressure equals left atrial pressure. Flow for the pulmonary circulation is the same as for the systemic system, which equals the cardiac output. Thus pulmonary vascular resistance (PVR) can be calculated by using the following formula:

$$PVR = \frac{\text{mean pulmonary artery pressure} - \text{left atrial pressure}}{\text{cardiac output}}$$

Given a normal mean pulmonary artery pressure of about 16 mm Hg and a normal mean left atrial pressure of 8 mm Hg, the normal pulmonary vascular resistance is computed as follows:

$$PVR = \frac{16 \text{ mm Hg} - 8 \text{ mm Hg}}{5 \text{ L/min}}$$
$$= 1.6 \text{ mm Hg/L/min}$$

On the basis of these computations, we can conclude that resistance to blood flow in the pulmonary circulation is much less than in the systemic circulation. Indeed, the pulmonary vasculature is characterized as a low-pressure, low-resistance circulation.[11]

Determinants of blood pressure

Just as adequate pressure is needed to move water throughout your house or apartment building, so too must the cardiovascular system maintain sufficient pressure to propel blood throughout the body. In fact, the cardiovascular system's first priority is to keep perfusion pressures normal, even under changing conditions.[2]

By rearranging our equation for computing vascular resistance (and dropping the normally small atrial pressure), we see that the average blood pressure in the circulation is directly related to both cardiac output and flow resistance:

mean arterial pressure = cardiac output × vascular resistance

With a constant rate and force of cardiac contractions, cardiac output is about equal to the circulating blood volume. Under similar conditions, vascular resistance varies inversely with the size of the blood vessels, that is, the capacity of the vascular system. All else being constant, mean arterial pressure is directly related to the volume of blood in the vascular system, and inversely related to its capacity[2]:

$$\text{mean arterial pressure} = \frac{\text{volume}}{\text{capacity}}$$

On the basis of this relationship, we see that mean arterial pressure can be regulated by: (1) changing the volume of circulating blood, (2) changing the capacity of the vascular system, or (3) changing both. Volume changes can reflect absolute changes in total blood volume, such as those in shock or blood transfusion. Alternatively, "relative" volume changes can occur when cardiac output rises or falls. Changes in system capacity occur mainly via changes in blood vessels' smooth muscle tone, particularly in the expandable venules and veins.

To maintain adequate perfusion pressures under changing conditions, the cardiovascular system balances these two factors. In exercise, for example, the circulating blood volume undergoes a relative increase. Blood pressure, however, remains near normal. This is because the skeletal muscle vascular beds dilate, causing a large increase in system capacity. On the other hand, when blood loss occurs, as with hemorrhage, system capacity is decreased by constricting the venous vessels. Perfusing pressures can thus be kept near normal until the volume loss overwhelms the system.

Of course, regulation of blood flow and pressure is much more complex than indicated in these simplified equations and examples. Cardiovascular control is accomplished via a complex array of integrated functions, to which we now turn.

CONTROL OF THE CARDIOVASCULAR SYSTEM

The cardiovascular system is responsible for transporting metabolites to and from the tissues under a variety of conditions and demands. As such, it must act in a highly coordinated fashion. This coordination is achieved by integrating the functions of the heart and vascular system. The goal is to maintain adequate perfusion to all tissues according to their needs.

Contrary to common thinking, the heart plays a secondary role in regulating blood flow. The cardiovascular system regulates blood flow mainly by altering the capacity of the vasculature and the volume of blood it holds. In essence, the vascular system tells the heart how much blood it needs, rather than the heart's dictating what volume the vascular system will receive.[2]

These integrated functions involve both local and central control mechanisms. Local or *intrinsic* mechanisms operate independently, without central nervous control. Intrinsic control alters perfusion under normal conditions to meet metabolic needs. Central or *extrinsic* control involves both the central nervous system (CNS) and circulating **humoral** agents. Extrinsic control mechanisms are responsible mainly for maintaining a basal level of vascular tone. However, central control mechanisms will take over when the competing needs of local vascular beds must be coordinated.

A useful analogy is Richardson's comparison of the cardiovascular system to a factory.[2] As long as the supply of raw materials equals the production rate in all the manufacturing areas, materials keep flowing smoothly. However, should production rates begin to vary among areas, the "head office" will have to intervene and alter materials flow to restore a coordinated function. Otherwise raw materials will needlessly build up or the productivity of dependent areas will drop.

With keeping this analogy in mind, we will first explore vascular regulatory mechanisms; this discussion is followed by an analysis of factors controlling cardiac output. Finally, we will combine these perspectives to demonstrate the full integration of the cardiovascular system under both normal and abnormal conditions.

Regulation of peripheral vasculature

A basal level of vascular muscle tone is normally maintained throughout the vascular system at all times.[2,3,5,7] Basal muscle tone must be present to allow for effective regulation. If blood vessels remained in a completely relaxed state, further dilatation would be impossible, and local increases in perfusion could not occur.

Local vascular tone is maintained by the smooth muscle of the precapillary sphincters of the microcirculation and can function independent of neural control. Central control of vasomotor tone involves either direct CNS innervation or circulation hormones. Central control mainly affects the high-resistance arterioles and capacitance veins.

Local control

Local regulation of tissue blood flow probably involves at least two related mechanisms: myogenic and metabolic control. *Myogenic control* involves the relationship between vascular smooth muscle tone and perfusing pressure. Increased perfusing pressures increase vascular muscle tone, while decreased pressures decrease vascular tone. Myogenic control ensures relatively constant flows to capillary beds despite changes in perfusion pressures.[12]

Metabolic control involves the relationship between vascular smooth muscle tone and the level of local cellular metabolites. High amounts of carbon dioxide or lactic acid, low pH levels, and low partial pressures of oxygen all cause relaxation of the smooth muscle, thereby increasing flow to the affected area. Metabolic control thus provides tissue flow according to metabolic needs.[13]

As shown in Figure 10-12, these local regulatory mechanisms probably work together.[14] However, their influence varies in different organ systems. The brain is most sensitive to changes in the local metabolite levels, particularly CO_2 and pH. The heart, on the other hand, shows a strong response to both muscular and metabolic factors.

Central control

Central control of blood flow is achieved mainly via the autonomic nervous system, particularly its sympathetic division.[15] As with local regulation, the level of central control varies among organs and tissues. The brain is minimally regulated by this mechanism.[16] However, skeletal muscle and skin are regulated mainly by central control.

Smooth muscle contraction and increased flow resistance are due mainly to **adrenergic** stimulation and the release of norepinephrine.[17,18] Smooth muscle relaxation and vessel dilatation occur via stimulation of either **cholinergic** or specialized adrenergic beta receptors. Whereas the contractile response is distributed throughout the entire vascular system, dilatation response appears to be limited to the precapillary vessels.

Regulation of cardiac output

Like the vascular system, the heart is regulated by both intrinsic and extrinsic factors. These mechanisms act together with vascular control to ensure that the heart's output matches the varying needs of the tissues.[19]

The total amount of blood pumped by the heart per minute is called the *cardiac output*. Cardiac output is simply the product of the heart rate times the volume ejected by the left ventricle on each contraction, or *stroke volume:*

$$\text{cardiac output} = \text{heart rate} \times \text{stroke volume}$$

Substituting a normal rate (70 contractions per minute) and stroke volume (75 mL or 0.075 L per contraction):

$$\text{cardiac output} = 70 \text{ beats/min} \times 0.075 \text{ L/beat}$$
$$= 5.25 \text{ L/min}$$

we can calculate a normal resting cardiac output of about 5 L/min. Of course, this is a hypothetical average; actual cardiac output varies considerably in both health and disease.

Whether in health or disease, a change in cardiac output must involve a change in stroke volume, a change in rate, or both (Figure 10-13). Stroke volume is affected mainly by intrinsic control of three factors: preload, afterload, and contractility. Rate is affected primarily by extrinsic or central control mechanisms.

Changes in stroke volume

Stroke volume is the volume of blood ejected by the left ventricle during each contraction or systole. The heart does not eject all the blood it contains during systole. Instead, a small volume, called the end-systolic volume (ESV), remains behind in the ventricles. During the resting phase or diastole, the ventricles fill back up, to a volume called the end-diastolic volume (EDV).

Stroke volume thus equals the difference between the end-diastolic volume and the end-systolic volume:

$$\text{stroke volume} = EDV - ESV$$

In a normal man at rest, the EDV ranges between 110 and 130 mL.[20] Given a normal stroke volume of about

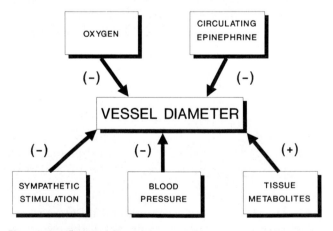

Fig. 10-12 Factors influencing vessel diameter in the microcirculation; (+) indicates dilation, (−) indicates constriction. Note that a variety of constrictor influences of circulating blood or neurogenic origin are balanced by dilatory influences related to local tissue metabolism. (Redrawn from Richardson DR: Basic circulatory physiology, Boston, 1976, Little, Brown.)

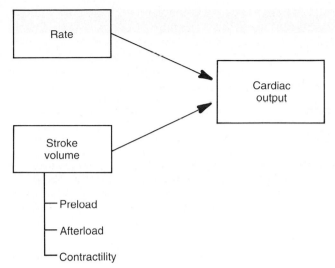

Fig. 10-13 Factors determining cardiac output (see text for details).

75 mL (see earlier discussion), we can compute a normal **ejection fraction (EF)**, or proportion of the EDV ejected on each stroke, as follows:

$$EF = \frac{SV}{EDV}$$
$$= \frac{75}{110}$$
$$= .68 \text{ or } 68\%$$

Thus, on each contraction, the normal heart ejects about two thirds of its stored volume. Decreases in ejection fraction are normally associated with a weakened myocardium and decreased contractility.

As shown in Figure 10-14, an increase in stroke volume can occur only if either the EDV increases or the ESV decreases. On the other hand, a decrease in stroke volume occurs when either the EDV decreases or the ESV increases.

The heart's ability to change stroke volume solely according to the EDV is an intrinsic regulatory mechanism based upon the Frank-Starling principle.[19] Since the EDV corresponds to the initial stretch or tension placed on the ventricle, the greater the EDV (up to a point), the greater will be the tension developed on contraction, and vice versa. The concept is similar to stretching a rubber band: the greater the stretch (up to a point), the greater the contractile force.

In clinical practice, this initial ventricular stretch is called *preload,* while the tension of contraction is equivalent to stroke volume. Figure 10-15 applies the Frank-Starling principle to ventricular function as a whole by plotting ventricular stretch against stroke volume. Ventricular stretch is directly proportional to EDV. EDV, in turn, is directly related to the pressure difference across the ventricle wall. Thus, preload can be measured indirectly as the ventricular end-diastolic pressure.[5]

The second major factor affecting stroke volume is the force against which the heart must pump. This is called *afterload.* In clinical practice, left ventricular afterload equals the systemic vascular resistance. In other words, the greater the resistance to blood flow, the greater the afterload.

With all else constant, the greater the afterload on the ventricles, the harder it is for them to eject their volume. Thus, for a given EDV, an increase in afterload causes the volume remaining in the ventricle after systole (the ESV) to increase. Of course, if the EDV remains constant while the ESV increases, the stroke volume (EDV − ESV) will decrease (Figure 10-14). Normally, however, the heart muscle responds to increased afterload by altering its contractility.

Contractility represents the amount of systolic force exerted by the heart muscle at a given preload.[2] At a given preload (EDV), an increase in contractility results in a higher ejection fraction, a lower ESV, and thus a higher stroke volume. Conversely, a decrease in

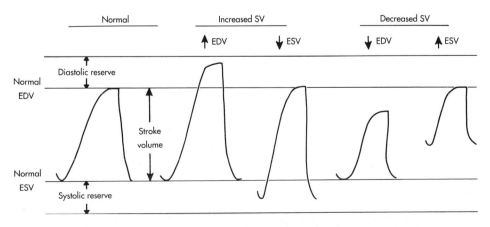

Fig. 10-14 Relationship between stroke volume (SV), end-diastolic volume (EDV) and end-systolic volume (ESV).

■ M I N I C L I N I ■

10-3

Afterload is the force against which the heart works to eject its stroke volume. Afterload can be thought of as outflow resistance. It is apparent that as afterload increases, the stroke volume ejected by the ventricle decreases, assuming that the heart's contractility (force with which the heart contracts) remains constant.

Problem: During exercise, the healthy person's blood pressure rises considerably, indicating that the afterload has increased. And yet the healthy heart's stroke volume and cardiac output do not decrease. Why is this so?

Discussion: When afterload increas-

The Effect of Increased Afterload on Cardiac Output in the Normal Heart

es, the first ventricular contraction that experiences the increased afterload does produce a smaller stroke volume. This in turn causes more

blood to be left in the ventricle at the end of systole (i.e., the end systolic volume [ESV] is increased). During the subsequent diastole, blood rushes in from the atria to fill the ventricle, and because of the higher than normal ESV, the ventricle becomes more distended and stretched than before. The healthy heart muscle responds to increased stretch in a way described by the Frank-Starling principle: that is, the heart now contracts with greater force than before, ejecting a greater stroke volume. By increasing contractility in this fashion, stroke volume and cardiac output are not compromised by increased afterload in the healthy heart.

contractility results in a lower ejection fraction, higher ESV, and decreased stroke volume.

Changes in contractility affect the slope of the ventricular function curve (Figures 10-15 and 10-16). Greater stroke volumes for a given preload (increased slope) indicate a state of increased contractility, often referred to as *positive inotropism*. The opposite is also true: lesser stroke volumes for a given preload indicate decreased contractility, referred to as *negative inotropism*.

Although cardiac contractility is affected mainly by local mechanisms, neural control, circulating hormo-

nal factors, and certain drugs also can exert an influence.[20,21]

Whether local or central in origin, all these factors influence the reactivity of contractile proteins, mainly by affecting calcium metabolism in the sarcomere. In general, neural or drug-mediated sympathetic stimulation has a positive inotropic effect. Conversely, **parasympathetic** stimulation exerts a negative inotropic effect.[21] Profound hypoxia and acidosis impair myocardial metabolism and decrease cardiac contractility.

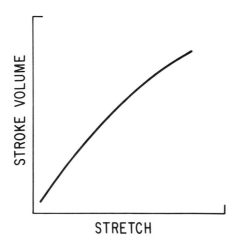

Fig. 10-15 The Frank-Starling relationship—stroke volume as a function of ventricular end diastolic stretch. An increase in the stretch of the ventricles immediately before contraction (end diastole) results in an increase in stroke volume. Note that ventricular end diastolic stretch is synonymous with the concept of preload. (From Green JF: Fundamental cardiovascular and pulmonary physiology, ed 2, Philadelphia, 1987, Lea & Febiger.)

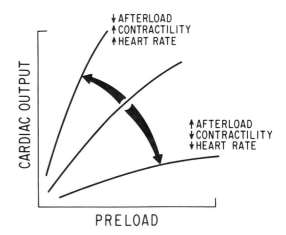

Fig. 10-16 Effects of preload, afterload, contractility, and heart rate on cardiac output function curve. (From Green JF: Fundamental cardiovascular and pulmonary physiology, ed 2, Philadelphia, 1987, Lea & Febiger.)

Changes in rate

The last factor influencing cardiac output is heart rate. Unlike the factors controlling stroke volume, those affecting rate are mainly of central origin, that is, neural or hormonal.[20,21]

All else being equal, cardiac output rises and falls with like changes in heart rate. Because of the normal rapid filling and emptying of the heart chambers, this relationship is maintained up to about 180 beats per minute. At higher rates, there is not enough time for the ventricles to fill completely. This causes a drop in EDV, a decrease in stroke volume, and a fall in cardiac output.[22]

The combined effects of preload, afterload, contractility, and heart rate on cardiac performance are graphically portrayed in Figure 10-16. The middle ventricular function curve represents the normal state. The upper, steeper curve represents a hypereffective heart. In the hypereffective heart, a given preload results in a greater than normal cardiac output. Factors contributing to this state include decreased afterload, increased contractility, and increased heart rate. The bottom curve has less slope than normal, indicating a hypoeffective heart. Factors contributing to this state include increased afterload, decreased contractility, and decreased rate.[5]

Coordination of functions

Cardiovascular control is achieved by integrating local and central regulatory mechanisms that affect both the heart and the vasculature. The underlying goal is to ensure that all tissues receive enough blood flow to meet their metabolic needs. Under normal resting conditions, this goal is achieved mainly via local regulation of the heart and vasculature.[2,5] Where there are increased or abnormal demands, such as during exercise or massive bleeding, central mechanisms take over primary control.

Central control of cardiovascular function occurs via interaction between the brainstem and selected peripheral receptors. The brainstem constantly receives data from these receptors about the pressure, volume, and chemical status of the blood. The brainstem also receives input from higher brain centers, such as the hypothalamus and cerebral cortex. These inputs are integrated with those coming from the heart and blood vessels to maintain adequate blood flow and pressure under all but the most abnormal conditions.[15,21]

The cardiovascular centers

Figure 10-17 provides a simplified diagram of the cardiovascular centers and their various interconnections. Excitatory and depressor interactions are depicted by plus (+) and minus (−) signs, respectively.

These "centers" are actually diffuse areas of neural tissue located in the reticular formations of the **medul-**

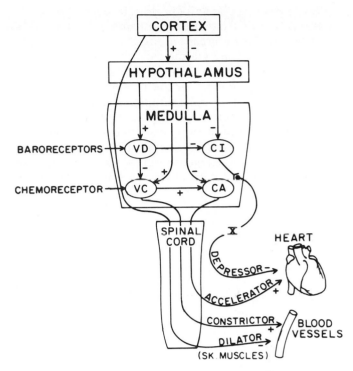

Fig. 10-17 Schematic summarizing major known neural pathways involved in central regulation of cardiovascular function. This design is oversimplified to illustrate the major relationships between excitatory (+) and depressor (−) fibers. *VD*, Vasodepressor area; *VC*, vasoconstrictor area; *CA*, cardioaccelerator area; *CI*, cardioinhibitory area. (From Green JF: *Fundamental cardiovascular and pulmonary physiology*, ed 2, Philadelphia, 1987, Lea & Febiger.)

la. Stimulation of the vasoconstrictor area, labeled VC, increases output to adrenergic receptors in the vascular smooth muscle, causing **vasoconstriction** and increased vascular resistance. A vasodepressor area, labeled VD, probably works mainly by inhibiting the vasoconstrictor center.

Closely associated with the vasoconstrictor center is a cardioaccelerator area, labeled CA. Stimulation of this center increases heart rate by increasing sympathetic discharge to the heart's SA and AV nodes. A cardioinhibitory area, labeled CI, plays the opposite role. Stimulation of this center decreases heart rate by increasing vagal (parasympathetic) stimulation to the heart.

The vascular and cardiac centers also interact among themselves. For example, stimulation of the vasoconstrictor area tends to excite the cardioaccelerator center, causing a rise in both blood pressure and heart rate. Conversely, excitation of the vasodepressor area inhibits both the vasoconstrictor and cardioinhibitory areas. This causes **vasodilatation** and an increase in heart rate.

Higher brain centers also influence the cardiovascular system, both directly and through the medulla. Signals coming from the cerebral cortex in response to exercise, pain, or anxiety pass directly via cholinergic fibers to the vascular smooth muscle, causing vasodilatation. Signals from the hypothalamus, particularly its heat regulating areas, indirectly affect heart rate and vasomotor tone via the cardiovascular centers.

The cardiovascular centers are also affected by local chemical changes in the surrounding blood or cerebral spinal fluid. For example, decreased levels of carbon dioxide tend to inhibit the medullary centers. General inhibition of these centers causes a decrease in vascular tone and thus a fall in blood pressure. A local decrease in oxygen tension has the opposite effect. Mild hypoxia in this area tends to increase sympathetic discharge rates. This tends to elevate both heart rate and blood pressure. Severe hypoxia has a depressant effect.

Peripheral receptors

In addition to high-level and local input, the cardiovascular centers receive signals from peripheral receptors (Figure 10-17). There are two types of peripheral cardiovascular receptors: baroreceptors and chemoreceptors. *Baroreceptors* respond to pressure changes.[23] *Chemoreceptors* respond to changes in blood chemistry.[24]

Baroreceptors. The cardiovascular system has two different sets of baroreceptors. The first set is located in the aortic arch and carotid sinuses. These receptors monitor arterial pressures generated by the left ventricle. The second set is located in the walls of the atria and the large thoracic and pulmonary veins. These low-pressure sensors respond mainly to changes in vascular volumes. Baroreceptor output is directly proportional to the stretch on the vessel wall. The greater the blood pressure, the greater the stretch, and the higher the rate of neural discharge to the cardiovascular centers in the medulla.

Together with the cardiovascular centers, these receptors form a negative feedback loop (Figure 10-18). A negative feedback system is designed to stabilize a controlled variable, in this case blood pressure. In a negative feedback loop, stimulation of a receptor causes an *opposite* response by the effector. In the case of the arterial receptors, a rise in blood pressure

increases aortic and carotid and receptor stretch, thus discharge rate. This increased discharge rate causes an *opposite* response by the medullary centers, that is, a *depressor* response. Venomotor tone decreases, blood vessels dilate, and heart rate and contractility both decrease. Decreased blood pressure (decreased baroreceptor output) will have the opposite effect, causing vessel constriction and increased heart rate and contractility.

While the high-pressure arterial receptors provide minute-to-minute control of blood pressure, the low-pressure sensors are responsible for long-term regulation of plasma volume.[2] The low-pressure atrial/venous baroreceptors regulate plasma volume mainly via their effects on: (1) renal sympathetic nerve activity; (2) release of antidiuretic hormone (ADH; vasopressin); (3) release of atrial natriuretic factor (ANF); and (4) the renin-angiotensin-aldosterone (RAA) system.[20]

Figure 10-19 outlines the major pathways for plasma volume control. As indicated, an increase in blood volume stimulates the atrial/venous baroreceptors. This causes a decrease in ADH and aldosterone levels, and an increase in ANF level. ADH and aldosterone cause sodium and water retention, while ANF is a potent diuretic. Thus decreases in ADH and aldosterone, and increases in ANF all promote sodium and water excretion. Combined with a CNS-mediated rise in renal filtration, these humoral mechanisms decrease the overall plasma volume. A decrease in blood volume would have the opposite effect, that is, sodium and water retention and an increase in plasma volume.

Chemoreceptors. Chemoreceptors are small, highly vascularized tissues located near the high-pressure sensors in the aortic arch and carotid sinus. Whereas baroreceptors respond to pressure changes, chemoreceptors are sensitive to changes in blood chemistry.[24] They are strongly stimulated by decreased oxygen tensions, although low pH or high levels of carbon dioxide can also increase their discharge rate. The major cardiovascular effects of chemoreceptor stimulation are vasoconstriction and increased heart rate.

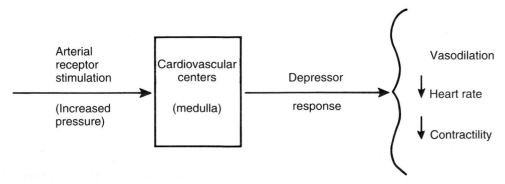

Fig. 10-18 Schematic representation of hemodynamic control via a negative feedback loop. See text for details.

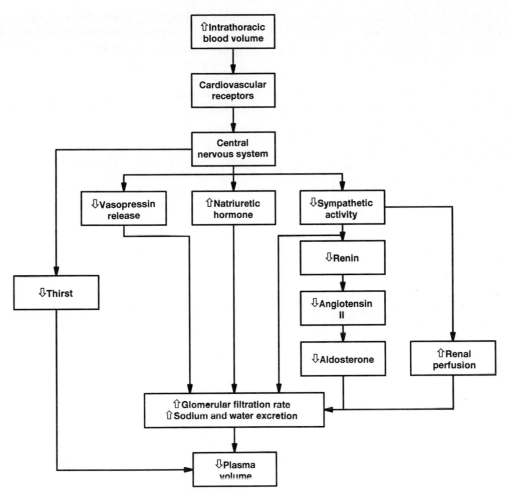

Fig. 10-19 Major pathways for plasma volume control. See text for details. (Adapted from Smith JJ, Kampine JP: Circulatory physiology—the essentials, ed 3, Baltimore, 1990, Williams & Wilkins.)

Since these changes occur only when the cardiopulmonary system is overtaxed, the chemoreceptors probably have little influence under normal conditions.[22] Their influence on respiration, however, is clinically important. For this reason, the peripheral chemoreceptors are discussed in detail in Chapter 14.

Response to changes in overall volume

The coordinated response of the cardiovascular system is best demonstrated under abnormal conditions. Among the most common clinical conditions in which all key regulatory mechanisms come into play is the large blood loss that occurs with hemorrhage. Figure 10-20, page 230 portrays changes in these key factors during progressive blood loss in an animal model.[2]

With 10% blood loss, the immediate drop in the central venous pressure causes a 50% decrease in the discharge rate of the low-pressure (atrial) baroreceptors; there is little change in the activity of the high-pressure (arterial) receptors. The initial response, mediated through the medullary centers, is an increase in sympathetic discharge to the sinus node. This causes a progressive rise in heart rate. At the same time, plasma levels of ADH (vasopressin) begin to rise. These two initial changes are sufficient to maintain normal arterial blood pressure.

As the blood loss becomes more severe (20%), atrial receptor activity decreases further. This increases the intensity of sympathetic discharge from the cardiovascular centers. Plasma ADH and heart rate continue to climb, as does peripheral vasculature tone. An increase in vascular tone occurs mainly through constriction of the capacitance vessels in the venous system, thereby slowing the drop in central venous pressure.

Not until blood loss approaches 30% does the arterial pressure start to drop. At this point, arterial receptor activity begins to decrease, resulting in a marked rise in systemic vascular tone. Despite the magnitude of blood loss, central venous pressure levels off. As long as no further hemorrhage occurs, blood pressure, and therefore tissue perfusion, can be maintained at adequate levels.

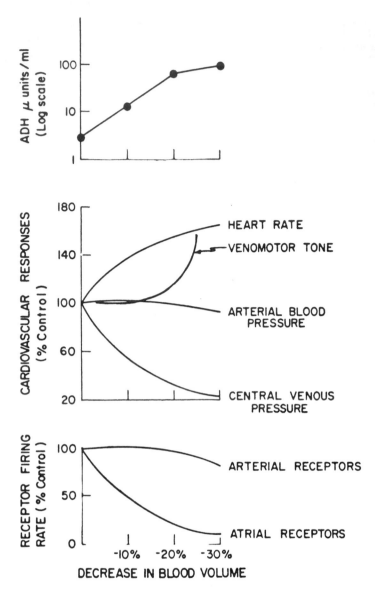

Fig. 10-20 Plasma levels of antidiuretic hormone (*ADH*), cardiovascular responses, and receptor firing rates in response to graded hemorrhage in the dog. See text for details. (From Richardson DR: Basic circulatory physiology, Boston, 1976, Little, Brown & Co. Venomotor tone data are those of WJ Sears as cited in Gauer OH, Henry JP, and Behn C: The regulation of extracellular fluid volume, Annu Rev Physiol 32:547–595, 1970. All other data are from Henry JP et al: The role of afferents from the low-pressure system in the release of antidiuretic hormone during nonhypotensive hemorrhage, Can J Physiol Pharmacol 46:287–295, 1968.)

Should blood loss continue, central control mechanisms begin to take over. Massive vasoconstriction occurs in the resistance vessels, shunting blood away from skeletal muscle in order to maintain blood flow to the brain and heart.[5,22] Rising levels of local metabolites in these areas—especially CO_2 and other acids—override central control and cause further vessel dilatation and increased blood flow.[16,25] Unfortunately, as these metabolites build up, and as the tissues

become hypoxic, cardiac function becomes impaired and vasodilatation occurs throughout the body. This signals the onset of a state of irreversible shock, after which death ensues.[22,26]

ELECTROPHYSIOLOGY OF THE HEART

Although loss of blood pressure caused by hemorrhage is a common occurrence, RCPs will observe many other causes of cardiovascular failure. Among the most frequent of these problems are abnormalities in the heart's electrical conduction, called arrhythmias. Arrhythmias can severely impair cardiac function and thus compromise blood flow and tissue perfusion. To understand arrhythmias, one must first develop a sound understanding of normal cardiac electrophysiology.

Electrical potentials and depolarization

As with other muscles, myocardial contraction occurs as the result of electrical events. These electrical events involve the buildup, discharge, and conduction of tiny electrical currents occurring within individual muscle fibers.[27]

As shown in Figure 10-21 in the resting state there exists a difference in concentration between potassium and sodium across the fiber cell membrane. This difference in ion concentration creates a difference in charge between the inside and the outside of the cell. The difference in charge or electrical potential is called the *resting potential*. This resting potential averages −90 mV in ventricular tissue.

This resting potential can be altered by electrical stimulation. The resulting *action potential* (Figure 10-21) is due to a change in membrane permeability for sodium ions, which rapidly diffuse into the cell and reverse its charge. This process is called *depolarization*. During the plateau phase of depolarization (Phase 2), calcium ions move into the cell through what are called slow channels. Once inside the cell, these calcium ions help activate the actual contractile process.

During most of depolarization (Phases 1–3), the muscle fiber cannot respond to additional stimulation. This is called the *refractory period*. As compared to fibers of other types of muscle, cardiac fibers have a much longer refractory period. In fact, since the refractory period of cardiac fibers exceeds the peak of contraction, heart tissue cannot normally go into a tetanic or sustained contraction.[2]

After depolarization and contraction, the myocardium must be returned to its initial resting potential, a process called *repolarization*. During repolarization, the influx of sodium ions slows, while membrane permeability for potassium increases (Phases 3–4 in Figure 7-21). As repolarization is completed, active

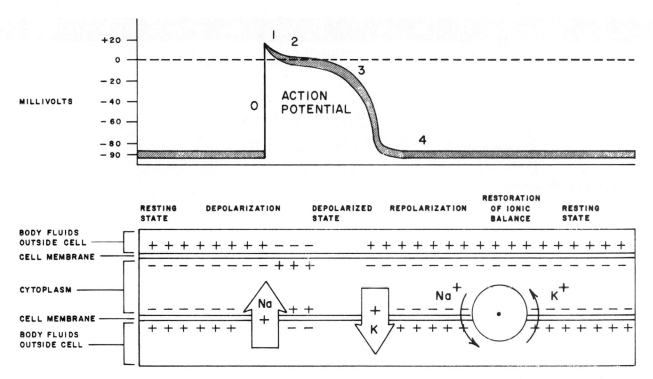

Fig. 10-21 Process of depolarization and repolarization. *Above:* The action potential of a single myocardial cell. Phase 0 is the rapid depolarization of the cell from a negative charge to a slightly positive charge. Phases 1, 2, and 3 represent repolarization; during this time the cell is refractory to a second depolarization. Phases 1 and 2 are periods of absolute refractoriness; during phase 3 the cell is relatively refractory. Phase 4 is the resting phase; repolarization is complete and the cell can be depolarized by another impulse. *Below:* The ionic shifts that occur with depolarization and repolarization. Sodium ions rapidly enter the cell with depolarization; as the cell repolarizes, potassium ions leave the cell, restoring the net negative electrical charge. Ionic balance is then restored by a sodium potassium exchange across the cell membrane. (From Sanderson RG: The cardiac patient: a comprehensive approach, ed 2, Philadelphia, 1983, WB Saunders. After Netter FH: The CIBA collection of medical illustrations, Heart, vol 5, Ciba, 1969.)

sodium-potassium exchange occurs across the cell membrane. This reestablishes the prior ionic balance and fully restores the resting potential.

The action potential for pacemaker tissue is slightly different. As seen in Figure 10-22, the resting potential of pacemaker tissue "decays" over time. This is due to a slow but steady influx of sodium ions.

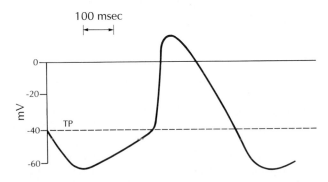

Fig. 10-22 The normal decay in resting potential of pacemaker tissue over time. When a threshold potential of about 40mV is reached, spontaneous depolarization occurs. This provides pacemaker tissue with its unique property of automaticity.

Eventually, the potential difference reaches about −40 mV, called the *threshold potential.* Once the threshold potential is reached, spontaneous depolarization occurs. Of course, the spontaneous depolarization of pacemaker tissue is the basis for the heart's property of inherent rhythmicity or automaticity.

The rate of decay in pacemaker resting potential determines its rate of depolarization, and thus the rate of impulse formation in the tissue as a whole. As discussed earlier, all myocardial tissue has the potential to originate such impulses. These "dormant" pacemakers, called *ectopic foci,* only take command if: (1) their excitability is increased, (2) the sinoatrial (SA) node is depressed, or (3) conducting pathways are blocked.[5,27]

Anatomy of the conducting system

Under normal resting conditions, the adult heart contracts rhythmically 60 to 100 times per minute. Effective function demands that the electrical and mechanical events of each cycle be highly synchronized. Synchronization is made possible by a special-

■ MINI CLINI ■

10-4

Heart Rate and the Administration of Bronchodilator Drugs

You are giving a bronchodilator aerosolized drug to a patient, and you notice a significant increase in heart rate. Would you expect increased heart rate to be a common side effect of drugs that cause bronchodilatation?

Discussion: The discharge rate of the sinus node and thus the heart rate is increased by sympathetic nervous stimulation and decreased by parasympathetic nervous stimulation.

The airways of the lung are dilated by sympathetic nervous stimulation and constricted by parasympathetic stim-

ulation. Drugs that cause bronchodilatation either mimic sympathetic stimulation (sympathomimetic) or block parasympathetic stimulation (parasympatholytic). Both of these drug actions also cause heart rate to increase, as noted. Parasympatholytic drugs bring about effects similar to sympathetic stimulation because by inhibiting parasympathetic activity, they allow sympathetic impulses to predominate, ultimately causing a sympatheticlike response.

---

ized system of tissues that conduct electrical impulses through the myocardium. These specialized tissues include the sinoatrial (SA) node, the atrioventricular (AV) node, the atrioventricular bundles, and the bundle branches and Purkinje fibers (Figure 20-23).[27,28]

Sinoatrial node

The SA node is a small tissue nodule located in the right atrium just anterior to the opening of the superior vena cava. Because it has the fastest rate of spontaneous depolarization, the SA node is the dominant pacemaker in the normal heart. Impulses initiated by the SA node radiate outward and travel at speeds of 80 to 100 cm/sec throughout the atria. Special interatrial pathways help direct these impulses through the atria, causing the chambers to contract in a coordinated fashion.

The SA node discharge rate can be increased or decreased by both neural and humoral control. Factors that increase SA node discharge rate are said to exert a positive chronotropic effect; those that slow impulse formation have a negative chronotropic effect.

In terms of neural control, sympathetic stimulation increases the SA node discharge rate, and parasympathetic (vagal) stimulation has the opposite effect.[21] In fact, strong parasympathetic stimulation caused by certain vagal reflexes can actually block SA output altogether. This can result in sinoatrial arrest, an abrupt and potentially lethal cessation of the cardiac cycle.

Circulating humoral agents and drugs also affect SA node discharge rate. For example, adrenergic drugs like the **catecholamine** isoproterenol increase SA node discharge rate. A similar effect occurs with administration of a cholinergic blocking agent such as atropine. Conversely, an adrenergic blocking agent such as propranolol and cholinergic drugs such as

edrophonium bromide decrease the rate of SA node impulse formation.

Atrioventricular node

The atria and ventricles are separated by a fibrous skeleton of nonconductive connective tissue. Thus depolarization cannot proceed directly between them. Instead, the depolarization wave is routed through a specialized relay station called the AV node. Similar in structure to the sinus node, the AV node is located in the right atrium just above the tricuspid valve and near the orifice of the coronary sinus.

The primary role of the AV node is to delay, then relay the SA nodal impulse onto the ventricles. The delay at the AV node is due to its slow conduction velocity (about 5 cm/sec). This delay ensures that the atria have sufficient time to empty before ventricular contraction. It also prevents too high a rate of atrial impulses from being transmitted to the ventricles. In addition the AV node also functions as a backup pacemaker. Should the SA node fail, the AV node can take over as the heart's pacemaker. However, because of its slower rate of spontaneous depolarization, the AV node provides only about 40 to 60 impulses per minute.

Atrioventricular bundle (bundle of His)

The bundle of His is a well-defined array of conducting tissue that begins at the AV node and runs horizontally forward to the upper part of the interventricular septum. SA impulses received by the AV node are transmitted through the bundle and on to the ventricles. Because it is the only link between the atria and ventricles, damage to the bundle of His can have serious consequences. Specifically, impulses coming from the SA and AV nodes can be blocked at this point. AV block is a cardiac condition commonly encountered in clinical medicine.

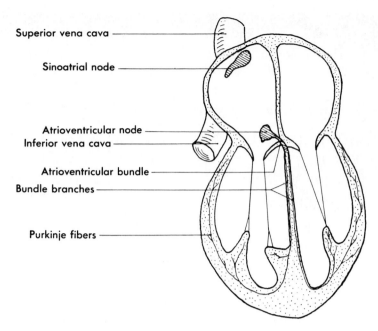

Superior vena cava

Sinoatrial node

Atrioventricular node
Inferior vena cava

Atrioventricular bundle
Bundle branches

Purkinje fibers

Fig. 10-23 Conduction system of the heart. (See text for description.)

Bundle branches/Purkinje fibers

The AV bundle terminates on the upper part of the interventricular septum. At this point it divides into two bundle branches, right and left, each going into its respective ventricle. The bundles pass down the septum, giving off branches to the papillary muscles and septal wall. They then continue into the ventricles, where they divide into many fine filaments. This network of conducting filaments, called the Purkinje fibers, extends into the depths of the ventricular muscle.

Conduction velocity in the bundle branches and Purkinje system is extremely fast, as high as 5000 mm/sec. This high speed of impulse transmission causes a nearly simultaneous depolarization of all ventricular fibers. This rapid depolarization helps assure uniform ventricular contraction.

Electrocardiography

Electrocardiography (ECG) is the measurement of the electrical events of the cardiac cycle. It is used clinically both to monitor heart rhythms and to help diagnose cardiac arrhythmias.[27] Our approach here is to emphasize the basic concepts of normal electrocardiography. This knowledge will be applied later to develop skills in recognizing cardiac arrhythmias (see Chapter 23).

The basic principles of electrocardiography are simple.[2] Since the heart is located in a large conducting medium (tissues and electrolyte fluids), its electrical activity generates current flow throughout the body. We can detect this current flow by placing electrodes on the body's surface.

Obviously, the strength of the heart's activity varies from point to point on the body surface. By placing *two* electrodes at different locations, we can measure the actual difference in potential, or voltage changes, caused by the heart's electrical activity. If we record these voltages over time, we obtain a graphic representation of the electrical events of the cardiac cycle. This is called the electrocardiogram (ECG).

Although electrodes can be placed anywhere on the body, in clinical practice electrode (or lead) positions are highly standardized. The simplest of these positions are the three bipolar leads, which together form Einthoven's triangle (Figure 10-24, page 234). Classically, this configuration requires placement of electrodes on both arms and the left leg. For monitoring purposes, the arm leads are usually placed to either side of the upper thorax (just below the clavicles), while the left leg electrode is usually moved to below the left nipple.

Limb leads are set up so that a wave of depolarization progressing toward a positive electrode creates a positive or upward deflection on the ECG. Conversely, a wave of repolarization should cause a negative deflection.

As shown in Figure 10-24, the net direction or *axis* of cardiac depolarization (the large arrow) is from atria down to the ventricles, that is, from upper left to lower right. Thus lead II, between the right arm (−) and the left leg (+), should record a positive deflection during depolarization. Moreover, the amount of electricity produced by various portions of the heart is directly related to the mass of depolarizing tissue. Because of their large mass, ventricular depolarization should thus produce the greatest voltage changes.

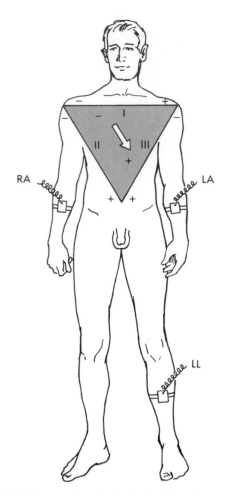

Fig. 10-24 Einthoven triangle, illustrating the galvanometer connections for standard limb leads I, II, and III. (From Berne RM and Levy MN: Cardiovascular physiology, ed 5, St. Louis, 1986, Mosby.)

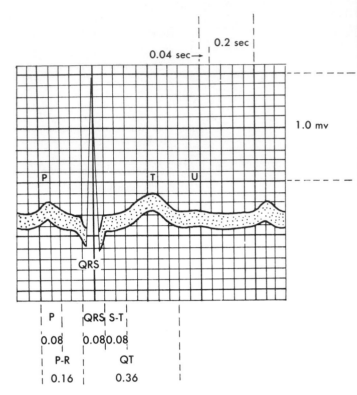

Fig. 10-25 A normal electrocardiographic pattern. (See text for description.)

Figure 10-25 shows a segment of a typical lead II ECG recording. The bold vertical lines represent time intervals of 0.2 second, subdivided into five small 0.04 boxes. Bold horizontal lines are 1 cm apart, measuring an amplitude of 0.5 **millivolt** (mV). Each smaller horizontal box equals 0.1 mV.

The major electrical events of the cardiac cycle appear as distinctive waveforms. The small positive P wave represents atrial depolarization, and the large positive QRS complex shows ventricular depolarization. Because atrial repolarization occurs during ventricular activity, it is masked by the large QRS complex. Ventricular repolarization follows, producing a T wave. The T wave is sometimes followed by a small U deflection, probably caused by ventricular after potentials.

Time intervals between these waves are used to indicate certain conduction events. The P-R interval equals the time taken by the SA impulse to go through the AV node and reach the ventricles. The length of the QRS complex equals the duration of ventricular depolarization. The S-T segment represents the acti-

vated state of the ventricles immediately after depolarization. During this period, the ventricles are refractory to additional electrical stimulation. Last, the Q-T segment is the time interval needed for complete electrical excitation and recovery of the ventricles. This is often referred to as "electrical systole," as opposed to mechanical systole.

Comprehensive examination of an ECG rhythm strip proceeds through four basic steps. First, you determine the regularity of the rhythm. This is done by measuring the distance between consecutive sets of R waves (Figure 10-26). If the distance for each set is the same (± 0.1 second), the rhythm is considered regular. Otherwise, the rhythm is judged irregular.

Next, you compute the heart rate. There are two methods to determine heart rate. If the rhythm is regular, you can simply count the number of large (0.2 second) boxes between two R waves:

Distance	Rate
1 box	300/min
2 boxes	150/min
3 boxes	100/min
4 boxes	75/min
5 boxes	60/min
6 boxes	50/min

This method cannot be used if the rhythm is irregular. Instead, you must count the number of R-R intervals over a longer time span, usually at least 6 seconds (3 second markings on most ECG paper makes this

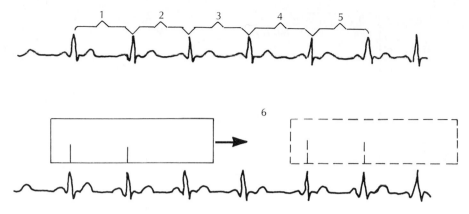

Fig. 10-26 To determine regularity of heartbeat, measure the distance between consecutive R waves (*1* through *5*) using calipers. If calipers are unavailable, mark the distance of one set of consecutive R waves and compare it to consecutive sets (*6*).

easy). For example, if you count 9 complete R-R intervals over 6 seconds, the rate is about 90/min.

After assessing the rhythm and rate, you next determine whether P waves are present or not. If they are present, you note their shape and measure the P-R interval. Last, you inspect the QRS complex and measure its duration.

Within the range of normal cardiac rates (60 to 100/min), the regular occurrence of the P, QRS, and T waveforms according to preestablished intervals indicates a *normal sinus rhythm.*[27,28] Any variations in the occurrence, duration, or pattern of these waveforms is called an arrhythmia. Arrhythmia recognition is addressed in Chapter 23.

EVENTS OF THE CARDIAC CYCLE

Up to this point, we have focused on the heart's electrical and mechanical activities as if they were separate events. In fact, these events are interdependent. Given the critical role of RCPs in dealing with cardiovascular problems, an in-depth knowledge of how these events relate is essential.

Figure 10-27 portrays the events of the cardiac cycle. At the very top is a time axis scaled in tenths of a second. Pressure events in the left heart and the aorta appear next, with timing bars for ventricular systole and diastole and heart sounds immediately below. Right and pulmonary artery pressure curves appear next, followed by flow measurements in the aorta and pulmonary artery. At the bottom of Figure 10-27, page 236 is the standard ECG.

Going from left to right, we will start at the P wave of the ECG, equivalent to late diastole. Before this point, the ventricles have been passively filling with blood through the open AV valves. The P wave signals atrial depolarization. Within 0.1 second, the atria contract, causing a slight rise in both atrial and ventricular pressures (the "a" waves). This atrial

contraction helps preload the ventricles, increasing their volume by as much as 25%.[20]

Toward the end of diastole, the electrical impulses from the atria reach the AV node and bundle branches. This initiates ventricular depolarization (the QRS complex). Within a few hundredths of a second after depolarization, the ventricles begin to contract. As soon as ventricular pressures exceed those in the atria, the AV valves close. Closure of the mitral valve occurs first (indicated by the vertical line marked MC), followed immediately by tricuspid closure (vertical line TC). Closure of the AV valves marks the end of ventricular diastole. This event produces the first heart sound on the **phonocardiogram.**

Immediately after AV valve closure, the ventricles become closed chambers. During this short *isovolemic phase* of contraction (marked by the diagonal hatching on the timing bars), ventricular pressures rise very rapidly. Upward bulging of the AV valves during this phase causes a slight upswing in atrial pressure graphs, called the "c" wave.

Within 0.05 second, ventricular pressures rise to exceed those in the aorta and pulmonary artery. This opens the semilunar valves, as indicated by the vertical AO and PO markers.

Toward the end of systole, as repolarization starts (indicated by the T wave), the ventricles begin to relax. As a result, ventricular pressures drop rapidly. When arterial pressures exceed those in the relaxing ventricles, the semilunar valves close, a point marked by the vertical AC and PC markers. Closure of the semilunar valves generates the second heart sound.

Rather than immediately dropping off, aortic and pulmonary pressures rise again after semilunar valve closure. This *dichrotic notch* is caused by the elastic recoil of the arteries. This recoil provides an extra "push" that helps maintain the head of pressure created by the ventricles.

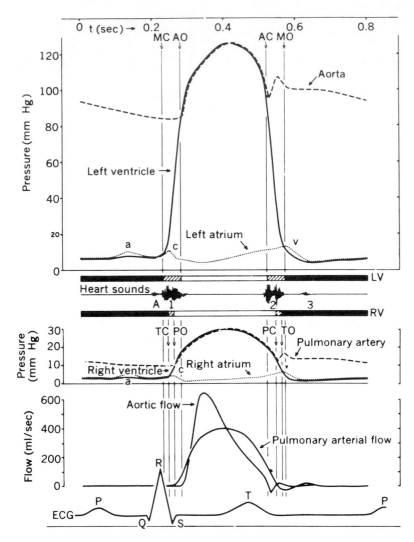

Fig. 10-27 Schematic of the hemodynamic events that occur during the cardiac cycle. *From the top downward:* pressure in the aorta, left ventricle, and left atrium; duration of left ventricular diastole (heavy shading), isovolumic periods (diagonal lines), and systole; pressure in the pulmonary artery, right ventricle, and right atrium; blood flow in the aorta and pulmonary artery; and electrocardiogram. Aortic valve opening and closure are indicated by AO and AC, respectively; MO and MC for the mitral valve; PO and PC for the pulmonic valve; and TO and TC for the tricuspid valve. (From Milnor WR: The heart as a pump. In Mountcastle VB, editor: Medical physiology, ed 14, vol 2, St Louis, 1980, Mosby.)

As the ventricles continue to relax, their pressures drop below those in the atria. This reopens the AV valves (indicated by the vertical MO and TO lines). As soon as the AV valves open, the blood collected in the atria rushes to fill the ventricles, causing a rapid drop in atrial pressures (the "v" wave). Thereafter, ventricular filling slows as the heart prepares for a new cycle.

Knowledge of these normal events helps one understand many of the diagnostic and monitoring procedures used for patients with cardiopulmonary disorders. Among the most common of these are: (1) the measurement of central venous pressure (CVP) (Figure 10-28), (2) balloon-directed pulmonary artery catheterization (Figure 10-29), and (3) direct arterial pressure monitoring.

Despite the "widening" effect of its fast time scale, Figure 10-27 provides a useful point of reference for each of these procedures. Normal CVP pressures correspond to those shown in the right atrium, including the characteristic a-c-v wave. An indwelling pulmonary artery catheter produces a waveform similar to that shown in Figure 10-27 for the pulmonary artery. Last, arterial pressure measurements look much like the aortic waveform, although this pattern changes with increased distance from the heart (Figure 10-30).

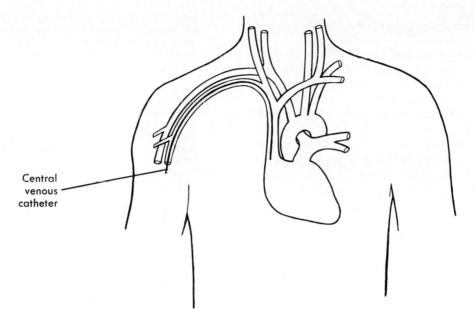

Fig. 10-28 Placement of central venous catheter.

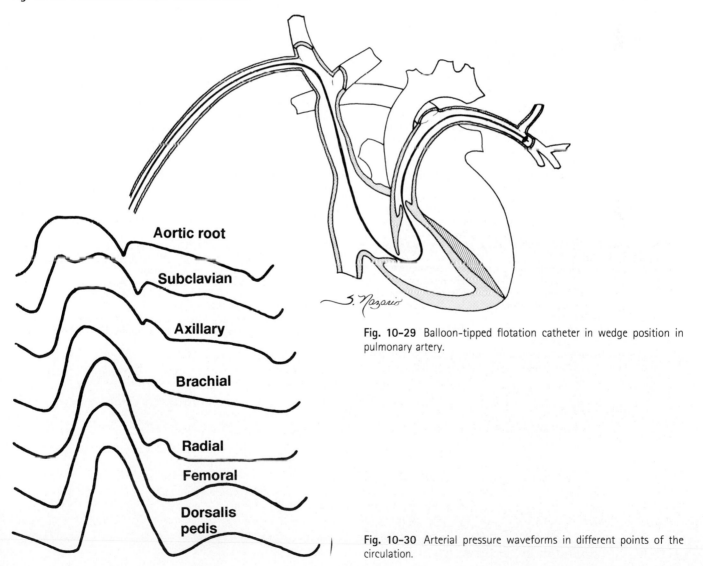

Fig. 10-29 Balloon-tipped flotation catheter in wedge position in pulmonary artery.

Aortic root

Subclavian

Axillary

Brachial

Radial

Femoral

Dorsalis pedis

Fig. 10-30 Arterial pressure waveforms in different points of the circulation.

CHAPTER SUMMARY

The cardiovascular system consists of a highly efficient pump, the heart, and a complex vascular network. These structures work together to maintain **homeostasis** by continually distributing and regulating blood flow throughout the body.

Specialized mechanical and electrical properties of cardiac tissue, combined with internal and external control mechanisms, provide the basis for coordinated cardiac function. Like the heart, the vascular system is regulated by both local and central control mechanisms. Rather than passively receiving blood from the heart, the vascular network assumes an active role in the control and distribution of blood flow.

Normally these two components work together in a coordinated fashion to ensure that all body tissues receive sufficient blood to meet their metabolic needs. Under conditions of increased demand, or when one component falters, special compensatory mechanisms are called on to maintain stable conditions. Failure of these mechanisms often requires the intervention of RCPs to help restore and maintain normal function.

REFERENCES

1. Bernard C: *Lecons sur les phenomenes de la vie communes aux animaux et aux vegetaux,* Paris, 1879, B. Bailliere et Fils.
2. Richardson DR: *Basic circulatory physiology,* Boston, 1976, Little, Brown.
3. Detweiler DK: *Circulation.* In Brobeck JR, editors: *Best and Taylor's physiologic basis of medical practice,* ed 9, Baltimore, 1973, Williams & Wilkins.
4. Sanderson RG: *The cardiac patient: a comprehensive approach,* Philadelphia, 1972, WB Saunders.
5. Green JF: *Fundamental cardiovascular and pulmonary physiology,* ed 2, Philadelphia, 1987, Lea & Febiger.
6. Brady AJ: *Mechanical properties of cardiac fibers.* In Berne SR, Sperelakis N, Geiger SR, editors: *Handbook of physiology, Sect 2, The cardiovascular system, Vol I, The heart,* Bethesda, Md, 1979, American Physiological Society.
7. Berne RM, Levy MN: *Cardiovascular physiology,* ed 4, St Louis, 1981, Mosby.
8. Tortora GJ, Anagnostakos NP: *Principle of anatomy and physiology,* ed 4, New York, 1984, Harper and Row.
9. Mellander S, Johansson B: Control of resistance, exchange, and capacitance functions in the peripheral circulation, *Pharmacol Rev* 20:117, 1968.
10. Wiedeman MP: *Microcirculation,* Stroudsburg, Pa, 1974, Dowdon, Hutchingson & Ross.
11. Green JF: *Mechanical concepts in cardiovascular and pulmonary physiology,* Philadelphia, 1977, Lea & Febiger.
12. Johnson PC: *The myogenic response.* In Bohr DF, Somlyo AP, Sparks HV, editors: *Handbook of physiology, Sect 2, The cardiovascular system, Vol II, Vascular smooth muscle,* Bethesda, Md, 1980, American Physiological Society.
13. Sparks HV Jr: *Effect of local metabolic factors on vascular smooth muscle.* In Bohr DF, Somlyo AP, Sparks HV, editors: *Handbook of physiology, Sect 2, The cardiovascular system, Vol II, Vascular smooth muscle,* Bethesda, Md, 1980, American Physiological Society.
14. Johnson PL: *The microcirculation and local and humoral control of the circulation.* In Guyton AC, Jones CE, editors: *Cardiovascular physiology,* Baltimore, 1974, University Park Press.
15. Korner PI: *Central nervous control of autonomic cardiovascular function.* In Berne SR, Sperelakis N, Geiger SR, editors: *Handbook of physiology, Sect. 2, The cardiovascular system, Vol. I, The heart,* Bethesda, 1979, American Physiological Society.
16. Scheinberg P: *The cerebral circulation.* In Zelis R, editor: *The peripheral circulation,* New York, 1975, Grune & Stratton.
17. Bevan JA, Bevan RD, Duckles SP: *Adrenergic regulation of smooth muscle.* In Bohr DF, Somlyo AP, Sparks HV, editors: *Handbook of physiology, Sect 2, The cardiovascular system, Vol II, Vascular smooth muscle,* Bethesda, Md, 1980, American Physiological Society.
18. Rothe CF: Reflex control of veins and vascular capacitance, *Physiol Rev* 63:1281. 1983.
19. Guyton AC, Jones CE, Coleman TC: *Circulatory physiology: cardiac output and its regulation,* Philadelphia, 1973, WB Saunders.
20. Smith JJ, Kampine JP: *Circulatory physiology: the essentials,* ed 3, Baltimore, 1990, Williams & Wilkins.
21. Levy MN, Martin PJ: *Neural control of the heart.* In Berne SR, Sperelakis N, Geiger SR, editors: *Handbook of physiology, Sect 2, The cardiovascular system, Vol I, The heart,* Bethesda, Md, 1979, American Physiological Society.
22. Rushmer RF: *Structure and function of the cardiovascular system,* ed 2, Philadelphia, 1976, WB Saunders.
23. Downing SE: *Baroreceptor regulation of the heart.* In Berne SR, Sperelakis N, Geiger SR, editor: *Handbook of physiology, Sect 2, The cardiovascular system, Vol I, The heart,* Bethesda, Md, 1979, American Physiological Society.
24. Coleridge JCG, Coleridge HM: *Chemoreflex regulation of the heart.* In Berne SR, Sperelakis N, Geiger SR, editors: *Handbook of physiology, Sect 2, The cardiovascular system, Vol I, The heart,* Bethesda, Md, 1979, American Physiological Society.
25. Mark AL, Abboud FM: *Myocardial blood flow: neuro-humoral determinants.* In Zelis R, editor: *The peripheral circulation,* New York, 1975, Grune & Stratton.
26. Bordicks KJ: *Patterns of shock,* New York, 1965, Macmillan.
27. Goldberger AL, Goldberger E: *Clinical electrocardiography,* ed 2, St Louis, 1981, Mosby.
28. Phillips RE, Feeney MK: *The cardiac rhythms: a systematic approach to interpretation.* Philadelphia, 1973, WB Saunders.

11

Ventilation

■

Craig L. Scanlan
Gregg L. Ruppel

CHAPTER LEARNING OBJECTIVES

1. Describe the events of a normal breathing cycle in terms of changes in pressure, flow, and volume;
2. Apply definitions to describe various lung volumes and capacities;
3. Compare and contrast the elastic and frictional forces opposing inflation of the lung;
4. Explain factors contributing to expiratory flow limitation in health and disease;
5. Differentiate between the mechanical and metabolic work (oxygen cost) of ventilation and describe their significance in health and disease;
6. Relate the mechanical properties of the lung to regional and local differences in the distribution of ventilation;
7. Define efficiency and effectiveness of ventilation as related to alveolar ventilation and CO_2 removal.

The primary function of the lung is to supply the body with oxygen and to remove carbon dioxide. To do both of these, the lung must be adequately ventilated. Ventilation may be defined simply as the process of moving air in and out of the lungs. This distinguishes it from respiration, which involves complex chemical and physiologic events at the cell level.

In health, ventilation is regulated to meet body needs under a wide variety of circumstances. In disease, however, this process can be disrupted. The result may be inadequate ventilation or excessive work of breathing. Respiratory care often restores adequate and efficient ventilation in such circumstances. Respiratory care modalities reduce the work of breathing and even provide artificial ventilation if necessary. Providing effective respiratory care demands understanding of the normal ventilatory processes as well as abnormalities that affect ventilation.

MECHANICS OF VENTILATION

Normal ventilation is a cyclic activity consisting of two components. The inward flow of air is called *inspiration,* and the outward flow is called *expiration.* During each cycle, a volume of gas moves in and out of the respiratory tract. This volume, measured during either inspiration or expiration, is called the *tidal volume* or V_T. The normal V_T satisfies resting metabolic needs. There must be sufficient reserves to meet increased ventilatory demands, as occur during exercise.

Lung volumes and capacities

Four lung volumes make up the *total lung capacity* (TLC).[1] These include the tidal volume (already described), the inspiratory reserve volume, the expiratory reserve volume, and the residual volume. The *end-expiratory level* marks the end of quiet tidal volume breath. The *end-inspiratory level* denotes the end of a quiet inspiration (Figure 11-1, on page 240).

The *inspiratory reserve volume* (IRV) is the maximum volume of air that can be inhaled after a normal quiet inspiration. The *expiratory reserve volume* (ERV) is the volume that can be exhaled from the end-expiratory level. These reserve volumes allow the tidal volume to increase as necessary. The *residual volume* (RV) is the volume of gas remaining in the lungs after a maximal exhalation. The RV remains in the lungs despite maximal expiratory effort. As the lungs empty, the airways decrease in size. Near residual volume the airways begin to close. When all the airways have closed (after a maximal exhalation) some gas remains in the lungs. The residual volume stabilizes the lung, facilitating expansion on subsequent breaths.

A lung capacity consists of two or more lung volumes. Four lung capacities have been defined. These are *total lung capacity* (TLC), *function residual capacity* (FRC), *inspiratory capacity* (IC), and *vital capacity* (VC) (see Figure 11-1).

TLC is the sum of the four lung volumes (i.e., RV + ERV + V_T + IRV). TLC is defined as the total volume of gas in the lungs after a maximum inspiration. In healthy adults, the TLC ranges from approximately 5 to 8 L.

The FRC is the sum of the residual volume and the expiratory reserve volume (RV + ERV). The FRC is defined as the volume of gas left in the lungs at the end of a quiet breath. This resting expiratory level is maintained by the opposing forces of the chest wall and lungs.

The VC is the sum of the inspiratory reserve volume, the tidal volume, and the expiratory reserve volume (IRV + V_T + ERV). The VC is defined as the

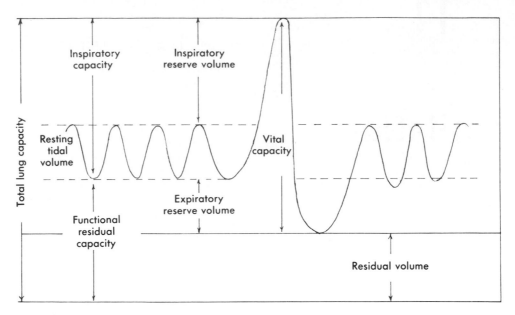

Fig. 11-1 Lung capacities and volumes. Volumetric divisions of the total gas capacity of the lungs. A capacity consists of two or more volumes. (See text for description.)

largest volume of air that can be moved in or out of the lungs. The VC makes up approximately 80% of the TLC in healthy young adults.

The IC is the sum of the tidal volume and inspiratory reserve volume (VT + IRV). The IC represents the volume of air that can be inhaled from the resting end-expiratory level (i.e., FRC).

Chapter 18, Basic Pulmonary Function Testing, reviews lung volumes and capacities in more detail, describing their measurement and use in clinical diagnosis.

Pressure differences during breathing

Lung volumes change in response to pressure gradients created by thoracic expansion and contraction.[2] Figure 11-2 shows the key pressures and gradients involved in ventilation. These pressures are usually measured in centimeters of water (cm H_2O), but are sometimes expressed in millimeters of mercury (mm Hg). Respiratory pressures are often expressed *relative* to atmospheric pressure. A respiratory pressure of "0" is equivalent to 1 atmosphere (i.e., 1034 cm H_2O or 760 mm Hg). A "positive" pressure is considered one that is greater than atmospheric. Although not correct, the term "negative" pressure is sometimes used to describe subatmospheric pressures.

Mouth pressure, that is, at the airway opening, is abbreviated by the term P_{ao}. Unless positive pressure is applied to the airway, P_{ao} is always zero. Pressure at the body surface (P_{bs}), equal to atmospheric pressure, is also usually zero. Alveolar pressure (P_{alv}), often referred to as **intrapulmonary** pressure, varies throughout the breathing cycle. Pleural pressure (P_{pl}) is usually negative (i.e., subatmospheric) during quiet breathing. P_{pl} also varies during the breathing cycle.

The difference between two pressures is called a *pressure gradient*. Three important pressure gradients are involved in ventilation. These are the transrespiratory, the transpulmonary, and the transthoracic pressure gradients.[3]

The transrespiratory pressure gradient (P_{rs}) represents the difference in pressure between the atmosphere (body surface) and the alveoli:

$$P_{rs} = P_{alv} - P_{bs}$$

In a spontaneously breathing subject, the pressure at the body surface and at the airway opening both equal atmospheric pressure. Substituting P_{ao} for P_{bs}:

$$P_{rs} = P_{alv} - P_{ao}$$

The transrespiratory pressure gradient causes gas to flow into and out of the alveoli during breathing.[2]

The transpulmonary pressure gradient, or P_L, equals the pressure difference between the alveoli and the pleural space:

$$P_L = P_{alv} - P_{pl}$$

P_L is the pressure difference that maintains alveolar inflation. Changes in P_L during breathing result in corresponding changes in alveolar volume.[4]

The transthoracic pressure gradient, or Pw, represents the difference in pressure between the pleural space and the body surface:

$$Pw = P_{pl} - P_{bs}$$

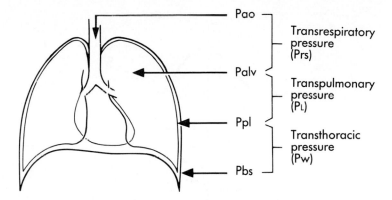

Fig. 11-2 Pressures involved in ventilation. Pao = pressure at the airway opening (mouth pressure); Palv = pressure in the alveoli (intrapulmonary pressure); Ppl = pressure in the pleural space (intrapleural pressure); Pbs = pressure at the body surface. Transrespiratory pressure gradient (Prs = Palv − Pao) is responsible for gas flow into and out of lungs. Transpulmonary pressure gradient (PL = Palv − Ppl) is responsible for degree of alveolar inflation. Transthoracic pressure gradient (Pdw = Ppl − Pbs) is difference in pressure across chest wall, or total pressure necessary to expand or contract lungs and chest wall together. (From Martin L: Pulmonary physiology in clinical practice: the essentials for patient care and evaluation, St Louis, 1987, Mosby.)

Pw is the pressure across the chest wall. It represents the total pressure necessary to expand or contract the lungs and chest wall together.[3]

During a normal breathing cycle, the glottis remains open.[2] Since P_{bs} and P_{ao} remain at zero throughout the cycle, only changes in P_{alv} and P_{pl} are of interest. Before the beginning of inspiration, pleural pressure is about −5 cm H_2O and alveolar pressure is 0 cm H_2O (Figure 11-3, page 242). The transpulmonary pressure gradient (PL) is about −5 cm H_2O in the resting state. This pressure gradient maintains the lung at its resting volume, the FRC. The alveolar pressure and the airway opening pressure are both zero. The transrespiratory pressure gradient is zero, and no gas moves into or out of the respiratory tract.

As inspiration begins, muscular effort expands the thorax. Thoracic expansion increases the transthoracic pressure gradient by causing a *decrease* in pleural pressure. As the pleural pressure drops, the transpulmonary pressure gradient widens, causing the alveoli to expand. As the alveoli expand, their pressures fall below the pressure at the airway opening. This *negative* transrespiratory pressure gradient causes air to move from the airway opening to the alveoli, increasing their volume.

Intrapleural pressure continues to decrease until the end of inspiration. Alveolar pressure reaches equilibrium with the atmosphere. Alveolar filling slows, and inspiratory flow decreases to zero. At this point, called *end-inspiration,* alveolar pressure has returned to zero. At end-inspiration, the transpulmonary pressure gradient reaches its maximum value of about −10 cm H_2O. This point also corresponds to peak inflation volume.

As expiration begins, the thorax recoils, and pleural pressure starts to rise. As pleural pressure rises, the transpulmonary pressure gradient narrows, and alveoli begin to deflate. As the alveoli become smaller, alveolar pressure exceeds that at the airway opening. This *positive* transrespiratory pressure gradient causes air to move from alveoli toward the airway opening. When alveolar pressure has fallen back to atmospheric pressure, flow ceases and a new cycle begins.

These events occur during normal tidal volume excursions. Similar pressure changes accompany deeper inspiration and expiration. The magnitude of the pressure changes is greater with deeper breathing. During a forced expiration, pleural pressure may actually rise *above* atmospheric pressure.

Forces opposing inflation of the lung

In order to generate the pressures necessary to cause gas flow into the lungs, the lungs must be distended. This distension requires that several opposing forces be overcome. Normal expiration is passive, using the energy stored during inspiration.[5] The forces opposing lung inflation may be grouped into two categories: *elastic* forces and *frictional* forces.[6] Elastic forces represent *static* opposition to expansion of the lungs and thorax. Frictional forces represent *dynamic* opposition to gas flow and tissues movement during breathing.

Elastic opposition to ventilation

Elastic and **collagen** fibers are found in the lung parenchyma. These tissues give the lung the property of *elasticity.* Elasticity is the physical tendency of an object to resist stretching.[7] When stretched, an elastic body tends to return to its original shape.

Hooke's law. Elastic behavior is defined by Hooke's law. The tension developed when an elastic structure is stretched is proportional to the degree of deformation produced.[5] An example of Hooke's law is a simple spring (Figure 11-4, page 242). When tension on a spring is increased, the spring lengthens in a linear

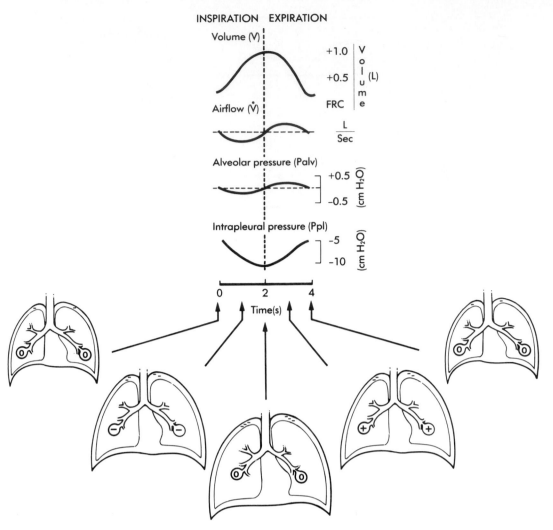

Fig. 11–3 Changes in pressure, volume, and flow during a single breath. (From Martin L: Pulmonary physiology in clinical practice: the essentials for patient care and evaluation, St Louis, 1987, Mosby.)

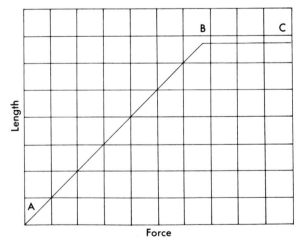

Fig. 11–4 Graphic demonstration of compliance of a simple spring (increase in length/increase in force). With increasing force, the spring lengthens in a linear manner, from *A* to *B*, but at the point of maximum stretch, further force produces no additional increase in length, *B* to *C*.

manner. The ability of the spring to stretch, however, is limited. Once the point of maximum stretch is reached, further tension produces little or no increase in length. Additional tension may actually break the spring.

In terms of the lung, inflation is equivalent to stretching. Inflation is opposed by elastic forces. To increase lung volume, pressure must be applied. The property of elastance may be demonstrated by subjecting a lung that has been removed from the body to different pressures and measuring the changes in volume (Figure 11-5). To simulate the pressures during breathing, the lung is placed in an airtight jar. The force to inflate the lung is provided by a pump that varies the pressure around the lung inside the jar. This action mimics thoracic expansion and contraction. The amount of stretch (i.e., inflation) is measured as

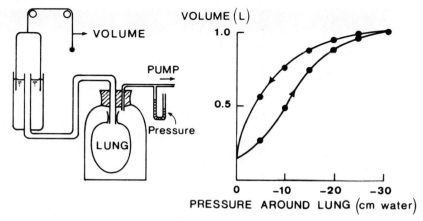

Fig.11–5 Measurement of the pressure-volume curve of an excised lung. The lung is held at each pressure for a few seconds while its volume is measured. The curve is nonlinear and flattens at high expanding pressures. Note that the inflation and deflation curves are not the same; this difference is called *hysteresis*. (From West JB: Respiratory physiology: the essentials, ed 3, Baltimore, 1985, Williams & Wilkins.)

volume by a **spirometer.** Changes in volume for a given pressure are plotted on a graph.

During inspiration greater and greater negative pressures are required to stretch the lung to a larger volume. As the lung is stretched to its maximum, the inflation "curve" becomes flat. This flattening indicates *increasing* opposition to expansion.

As with a spring under tension, deflation occurs passively as pressure in the jar rises back toward atmospheric. Deflation of the lung does not follow the inflation curve exactly. During deflation the lung volume at any given pressure is slightly greater than during inflation. This difference between the inflation and deflation curves is called *hysteresis.*[8] Hysteresis of the curves indicates that factors other than simple elastic tissue forces are present.

Surface tension forces. Part of the hysteresis exhibited by the lung is due to surface tension forces in the alveoli.[9] Von Neergaard demonstrated the role of surface tension forces in the lung in 1929.[10] He compared pressure-volume curves of lungs filled with saline solution with those of lungs filled with air (Figure 11-6). He observed that less pressure was needed to inflate a saline solution–filled lung to a given volume. Only when he filled the lung with air did it exhibit hysteresis.

These observations indicated that a gas-fluid **interface** in the air-filled lung changed its inflation-deflation characteristics. This interface is not present in the fluid-filled lung. The gas-fluid interface *increases* the elastic recoil of the lung, making it harder to inflate. It also changes lung elasticity depending on the lung's volume.

A lung filled with air is harder to inflate than a saline solution–filled lung because of surface tension at the gas-fluid interface in the alveoli. The lung contains millions of alveoli. Each alveolus is lined with a thin film of fluid. This gas-fluid interface causes

surface tension forces so that alveoli resemble "bubbles." According to LaPlace's law (see Chapter 7), surface tension forces contract the alveoli, compressing the gas inside them.

The elasticity of the lung is due to tissue elasticity and surface tension forces in the alveoli. Alveolar surface tension forces partially explain the hysteresis of the lung's pressure-volume curves. During inflation, additional pressure is needed to expand alveoli collapsed by surface tension forces. During deflation from maximum lung volume, most alveoli are open. Less pressure is required to maintain a given volume.

The inflation and deflation pressures of the lung are less than predicted by LaPlace's law.[8] The instability expected in a lung made up of 300 million bubbles of different sizes does not occur. The surface tension forces in the lung appear lower than expected at a simple gas-water interface. If surface tension forces in the lung were not lower than expected, small alveoli would become highly unstable. Deflation would result

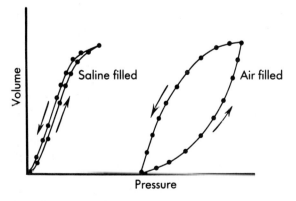

Fig.11–6 Static pressure-volume curves of saline-filled and air-filled excised lungs, demonstrating the effects of elastic forces (left) and elastic plus surface tension forces (right) on static compliance of the lung. (From Slonim NB and Hamilton LH: Respiratory physiology, ed 5, St Louis, 1987, Mosby.)

Surfactant Replacement Therapy and Lung Mechanics

Problem: If an infant is born prematurely, the lungs may be underdeveloped and fail to synthesize adequate amounts of pulmonary surfactant. How does this condition affect lung mechanics, and what effect will surfactant replacement therapy have on lung compliance and the work of breathing?

Discussion: The liquid molecules that line each alveolus attract one another. This intramolecular attraction creates a force, called surface tension, that tends to shrink alveolar size and cause collapse. Pulmonary surfactant molecules have very weak intramolecular attractive forces. When surfactant molecules are mixed with other liquid molecules that have higher intramolecular attraction, the surfactant molecules are pushed to the surface of the liquid, where they become the air-liquid interface. Because of the weak intramolecular attraction between these surfactant molecules at the surface, the liquid lining of the alveoli exhibits much less surface tension than it would in the absence of pulmonary surfactant. The infant with premature lungs lacking surfactant has abnormally high intraalveolar surface tension; this produces a collapsing force that increases lung recoil and reduces lung compliance. Greater muscular effort is required to overcome this increased recoil during inspiration, and work of breathing is increased. The infant may eventually fatigue and develop ventilatory failure. Instillation of surfactant into the lungs reduces surface tension down toward its normal level. This increases lung compliance, reduces lung recoil force, and reduces the muscular work required to inflate the lung.

---

in massive alveolar collapse. Each inflation would require extraordinary pressures to reopen collapsed alveoli.[11]

Surface tension in the lung is lowered by a substance called *pulmonary surfactant.* Alveolar type II cells probably produce pulmonary surfactant. This surfactant consists mainly of a **phospholipid,** dipalmitoyl lecithin, synthesized from fatty acids.[9] A physiologic saline solution has a surface tension of about 70 dynes/cm. Lung extract, however, displays an average surface tension of 25 dynes/cm.[8] This reduction in surface tension permits alveoli to be inflated easily. Surfactant decreases the pressure (i.e., work) necessary to achieve a given lung volume.[12]

Unlike typical surface-active agents, pulmonary surfactant varies surface tension according to its area.[8] Its ability to lower surface tension decreases as surface area increases. Conversely, when surface area decreases, the ability of pulmonary surfactant to lower surface tension increases.

This unique property of pulmonary surfactant is critical in stabilizing alveoli. In alveoli with small surface areas, pulmonary surfactant exerts its maximum effect. It dramatically lowers their surface tension, increasing their stability. Surface tension in larger alveoli is less affected. This variable action equalizes deflation pressures, preventing small alveoli from collapsing into large ones.[11-13]

The half-life of pulmonary surfactant is a few hours. If replacement is impaired, alveolar collapse (i.e., atelectasis) rapidly develops.[14] Without pulmonary surfactant, inflating partially collapsed alveoli requires high pressures. This makes inspiration very difficult. The work of breathing may be insurmounta-ble in diseases that affect pulmonary surfactant. The best clinical example of the effects of surfactant deficiency is newborn *respiratory distress syndrome* (see Chapter 35).

Surfactant therapy is being used with encouraging results in studies involving infants and adults with acute lung injury.[15] Naturally occurring as well as synthetic surfactants have been used. These agents, when instilled in the lungs, improve alveolar stability and decrease the work of breathing (see Chapter 35).

Lung compliance. Tissue elastic forces and surface tension impede inflation of the lung. *Compliance* measures the opposition of the lung to inflation. Elastance is the property of resisting deformation. Compliance represents the ease with which a body stretches, or its **distensibility.** Compliance is the reciprocal of elastance:

$$\text{Compliance} = \frac{1}{\text{Elastance}}$$

Compliance of the lung (C_L) is defined as the volume change per unit of pressure change. It is measured in liters per centimeter of water:

$$C_L = \frac{\Delta V \text{ (liters)}}{\Delta P \text{ (cm } H_2O)}$$

The volume in this equation is measured simply as the inspired volume at a known inflation pressure. The inflation pressure is the difference between the alveolar and pleural pressure, the transpulmonary pressure gradient.[1] Normal compliance of the adult lung averages 0.2 L/cm H_2O.[2]

Compliance is usually measured under *static* conditions (i.e., no airflow). When there is no airflow, alveolar pressure equals zero. Under static conditions the transpulmonary pressure gradient equals intrapleural pressure. Lung compliance (C_L) then equals:

$$C_L = \frac{\Delta V \text{ (liters)}}{\Delta P_{pl} \text{ (cm H}_2\text{O)}}$$

In spontaneously breathing subjects, measurement of compliance requires placement of a balloon in the esophagus.[1] The balloon is connected to a sensitive pressure transducer. The subject then holds his or her breath at different lung volumes. Intrapleural pressure is measured by the esophageal balloon at each volume. A graph of change in lung volume versus change in intrapleural pressure (Figure 11-7, *A*) is the compliance curve of the lung.

Figure 11-7, *B*, compares a normal compliance curve to those observed in emphysema and pulmonary fibrosis. The curve of the subject with emphysema is steeper. This slope represents a large change in volume for a given pressure change (i.e., increased compliance). Increased compliance results from loss of elastic fibers that occurs in emphysema. There is an increase in **distensibility** of the lungs. The compliance curve of the patient with fibrosis is flatter than the normal curve. This indicates a smaller change in volume for any given pressure change (i.e., decreased compliance). Interstitial fibrosis is characterized by an increase in connective tissue. As a result, the lungs become stiffer.

Chest wall compliance. Inflation and deflation of the lung occur with changes in the dimensions of the chest wall. The relationship between the lungs and chest wall can be illustrated when they are separated (Figure 11-8, page 246). The lungs and chest wall separate when the "seal" between them is broken. This occurs during surgical procedures such as **thoracotomy.**

In the intact thorax, the lungs and chest wall recoil to the resting level, or FRC (Figure 11-8, *A*). When the chest wall is opened, the pleural space is exposed to atmospheric pressure. The transpulmonary pressure gradient is lost, since pleural pressure equals atmospheric. The lungs collapse to a smaller volume, called the *minimal air volume.* The chest wall expands outward to its unopposed resting position (Figure 11-8, *B*). The normal resting volume of the intact thorax (i.e., the FRC) is about 40% of the TLC. When the normal lung–chest wall relationship is disrupted, the lung collapses to a volume less than the RV. The thorax expands to a volume larger than the FRC.

The chest wall, like the lung, has elastic properties. The elastic properties of the chest wall are due to its bones and muscles, as described in Chapter 9. Unlike the lungs, which only collapse, the chest wall may recoil either inward or outward. The direction in which the chest wall moves depends on the volume of lung inflation.

The lung–chest wall system may be compared to a bowed flat spring (i.e., the chest wall) tied to a stretched coiled spring (i.e., the lungs). The bowed flat spring tends to expand while the coiled spring tends to contract (Figure 11-9, page 246). Expansion or contraction of the coiled spring represents an increase or decrease, respectively, in lung volume. At the resting level, the forces of the chest wall and lungs balance. The tendency of the chest wall to expand is offset by the contractile force of the lungs. This balance of forces determines the resting lung volume, or FRC. The opposing forces between the chest wall and lungs are partially responsible for the subatmospheric pressure in the intrapleural "space."

Inhalation occurs when the balance between the lungs and chest wall is shifted. Energy from the

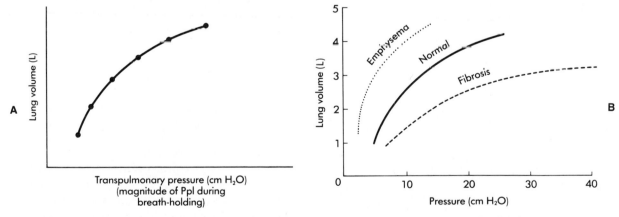

Fig. 11-7 A, Compliance measurement. After swallowing an esophageal tube, the patient inhales to a specified lung volume and holds his breath with the glottis open, assuring an alveolar pressure of zero. The amount of air inhaled (change in volume) divided by the change in esophageal pressure (read from a pressure meter) is the compliance at that point. Measurements are recorded at several different lung volumes, generating a compliance curve. **B,** Compliance curves. Normal lung compliance is approximately 0.2 L/cm H_2O. Compliance is high in emphysema and low in pulmonary fibrosis. (From Martin L: *Pulmonary physiology in clinical practice: the essentials for patient care and evaluation,* St Louis, 1987, Mosby.)

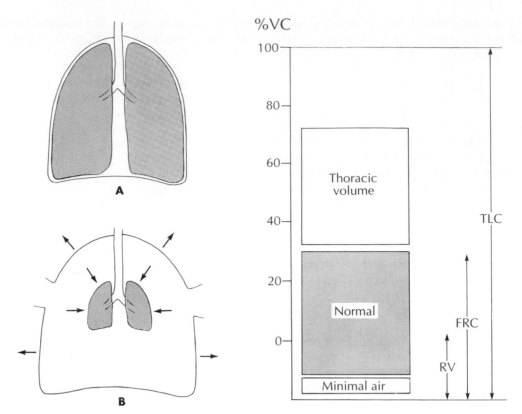

Fig. 11-8 The relationship between the lungs and chest wall. In the intact thorax **(A)**, opposing forces between the lungs and chest wall establish the resting level, or FRC (A). The resting volume of the intact thorax is about 40% of the TLC. When the chest wall is opened **(B)**, the pleural space is exposed to atmospheric pressure, which causes the transpulmonary pressure gradient to drop to zero. With no transpulmonary pressure gradient to keep them inflated, the lungs collapse to a smaller volume, called the minimal air volume. At the same time, the chest wall expands outward to its unopposed resting position (about 70% of the TLC).

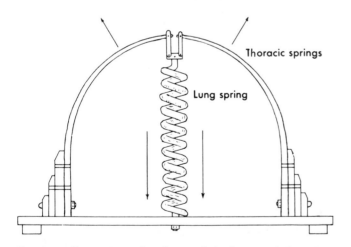

Fig. 11-9 The counteracting forces of the lungs and thorax are schematically represented by two sets of springs. In the resting position, the bowed flat *thoracic springs* are shown as held under bent tension by the coiled *lung spring*, itself partially stretched by the action. *Arrows* indicate the direction each spring tends to move to reach its own position of rest. From the lung-thorax resting position, the thorax can expand or contract, depending on the action of the ventilatory muscles. These muscles can assist the *thoracic springs* to overcome the restraint of the *lung spring*, or they can compress the *thoracic springs* and assist the recoil of the *lung spring*.

respiratory muscles overcomes the contractile force of the lungs.[5] Early in the breath, the tendency of the chest wall to expand facilitates lung expansion. When lung volume nears 70% of the vital capacity, the chest wall reaches its natural resting level. Above this volume, it resists further expansion. Inspiratory muscle effort must overcome the recoil of both the lungs and the chest wall to reach total lung capacity.

During exhalation, potential energy "stored" in the stretched lung (and chest wall at high volumes) causes passive deflation. Exhalation below the resting level (i.e., FRC) requires muscular effort to overcome the tendency of the chest wall to expand. This energy is provided by the expiratory muscles (see Chapter 9).

Compliance of the chest wall, like lung compliance, is a measure of distensibility. The compliance of the normal chest wall approximates that of the lungs (i.e., 0.2 L/cm H_2O). Obesity, **kyphoscoliosis,** and **ankylosing spondylitis** can reduce chest wall compliance and limit lung expansion.

Total compliance. The total compliance of the respiratory system equals lung compliance (C_L) plus the compliance of the thorax (C_T). The lung and chest wall work in parallel as described previously. Total compliance of the lung-thorax system (CLT) may be calculated as follows:

$$1/C_{LT} = 1/C_L + 1/C_T$$

As with resistors in a parallel circuit, the CLT is *less* than either individual component.

Lung-thorax compliance (CLT) is difficult to measure. A relaxed or anesthetized subject may be placed in a body respirator (Figure 11-10). Negative pressure applied to the surface of the body produces ventilation. By measuring pressures and volumes as the subject is ventilated, the CLT can be calculated. The CLT of healthy subjects measured this way is about 0.1 L/cm H_2O. CLT can also be measured in a subject intubated with a cuffed **endotracheal** tube. The lungs are inflated to various levels by positive pressures. By measuring the resulting volume changes, compliance data can be obtained. This method is often employed in patients who are receiving mechanical ventilation (see Chapter 33). CLT of healthy subjects measured by this method is also about 0.1 L/cm H_2O. The total compliance of the respiratory system can be altered by disorders affecting compliance of the lungs, chest wall, or both.

Frictional (nonelastic) opposition to ventilation

Frictional forces also oppose ventilation. Frictional opposition is unrelated to the elastic properties of the lungs and thorax. It occurs only when the system is in motion. Frictional opposition to ventilation has two components: tissue viscous resistance and airway resistance.[16]

Tissue viscous resistance. Tissue viscous resistance is the **impedance** to motion caused by displacement of tissues during ventilation.[16] The tissues displaced include the lungs, rib cage, diaphragm, and abdominal organs. The energy to displace these structures is comparable to the impedance caused by friction in any dynamic system. Tissue resistance accounts for

about 20% of the total resistance to lung inflation. Obesity, fibrosis, and **ascites** can alter tissue viscous resistance, increasing the total impedance to ventilation.[5]

Airway resistance. Gas movement through the airways also causes frictional resistance. Impedance to ventilation by the movement of gas through the airways is called *airway resistance*. Airway resistance accounts for about 80% of the frictional resistance to ventilation.

Airway resistance (Raw) is the ratio of driving pressure responsible for gas movement to the flow of the gas:

$$Raw = \frac{\Delta P}{\dot{V}}$$

Driving pressure (ΔP) is the pressure difference between the alveoli and the airway opening (i.e., transrespiratory pressure gradient, or [$P_{alv} - P_{ao}$]). Substituting for ΔP:

$$Raw = \frac{P_{alv} - P_{ao}}{\dot{V}}$$

The driving pressure is measured in centimeters of water (cm H_2O) and the flow in liters per second (L/sec). The units for airway resistance are centimeters of water per liter per second (cm H_2O/L/sec). Airway resistance in healthy adults ranges from 0.5 to 2.5 cm H_2O/L/sec.[2]

Measurement. Airway resistance is usually measured in a pulmonary function laboratory.[1] Flow is measured with a **pneumotachometer.** Alveolar pressures are determined in a body **plethysmograph,** an airtight box in which the subject sits. Pressure changes in the plethysmograph reflect alveolar pressures. By measuring flow and alveolar pressure, airway resistance can be calculated (see Chapter 18).

Factors Affecting Airway Resistance. Two airflow patterns characterize gas movement in the respiratory tract. These are laminar flow and turbulent flow.[17] A third pattern, called tracheobronchial flow, is a combination of laminar and turbulent flow (Figure 11-11, page 248).

In *laminar flow,* gas moves in discrete layers or streamlines. In an airway, movement of the layer closest to the wall is less than at the center of the tube. This is due to friction between the streamlines and the wall. Gas flowing in a laminar pattern consists of concentric layers parallel to the tube wall. Flows increase toward the center of the tube.[18]

Poiseuille's law defines laminar flow through a smooth, unbranched tube of fixed dimension. The pressure required to move a volume of gas through a tube is:

$$\Delta P = \frac{\eta 8 l \dot{V}}{\pi r^4}$$

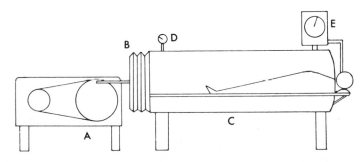

Fig. 11-10 This is a schematic representation of a subject in a body respirator. The motor, *A,* operates bellows, *B,* to create a rhythmic subatmospheric pressure in the cylindrical respirator, *C,* which is recorded by gauge, *D.* As the subject is ventilated by negative pressure applied to his or her body, exhaled air is collected and measured in a meter, *E.* Volume change of the lung-thorax per unit of pressure applied can be determined.

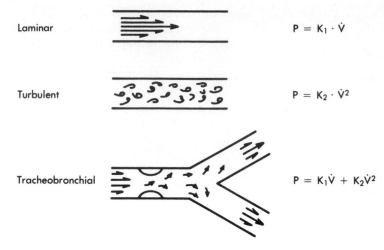

Fig. 11-11 The three patterns of flow: laminar, turbulent, and tracheobronchial. (From Moser KM and Spragg RG: Respiratory emergencies, ed 2, St Louis, 1982, Mosby.)

where

ΔP = driving pressure (dynes/cm^2)
η = viscosity of the gas
l = tube length (cm)
$\dot{V}$ = gas flow (mL/sec)
r = tube radius (cm)

π and 8 are constants.[19]

By eliminating those factors that remain constant (i.e., viscosity, length, known constants), this equation can be rewritten:

$$\Delta P \approx \frac{\dot{V}}{r^4}$$

Rearranging to solve for $\dot{V}$:

$$\dot{V} \approx \Delta P r^4$$

This equation has great significance when applied to clinical situations involving the airways:

1. For gas flow to remain constant, delivery pressure must vary *inversely* with the fourth power of the airway's radius. Reducing the radius of a tube by half requires a 16-fold pressure increase to maintain a constant flow. To maintain ventilation in the presence of narrowing airways, large increases in driving pressure may be needed.

2. If gas delivery pressure ventilating the lung remains constant, gas flow will vary *directly* with the fourth power of the airway's radius. Reducing the airway radius by half will decrease flow 16-fold at a constant pressure. Small changes in bronchial caliber can markedly change gas flow through an airway.

Under certain conditions, gas flow through a tube changes significantly. The orderly pattern of concentric layers is no longer maintained. Gas molecules form irregular eddy currents. This pattern is called *turbulent flow.*[19] Transition from laminar to turbulent

flow depends on several factors.[18] These factors include gas density (d), viscosity (n), linear velocity (v), and tube radius (r). They may be combined mathematically to determine *Reynold's number* (NR):

$$N_R = \frac{v \times d \times 2r}{\eta}$$

Reynold's number is dimensionless. In a smooth-bore tube, laminar flow changes to turbulent flow when Reynold's number exceeds 2000. If the tube wall is irregular, turbulent flow may occur at lower values of N_R.[12] Turbulence (increasing N_R) is increased by:

- increased linear velocity of gas
- increased gas density
- decreased gas viscosity
- increased tube radius

When flow becomes turbulent, Poiseuille's law no longer applies. The pressure required to generate flow is defined by the following equation[12]:

$$\Delta P = \frac{fl\dot{V}^2}{4\pi^2 r^5}$$

where

ΔP = driving pressure
f = friction factor (including gas density, viscosity, and tube wall roughness)
l = tube length
$\dot{V}$ = gas flow
r = tube radius

In Poiseuille's law, driving pressure is directly proportional to flow. Under conditions of turbulent flow, driving pressure is proportional to the *square* of flow ($\dot{V}^2$). To double flow under laminar conditions, the driving pressure must double (Table 11-1). To double the flow under turbulent conditions, the driving pressure must be increased fourfold.

Transitional or tracheobronchial flow describes the

Table 11-1 Comparison of driving pressures, laminar versus turbulent flow

Flow (V̇)	Driving Pressures (ΔP)	
	Laminar	Turbulent
1	1	1
2	2	4
4	4	16
8	8	64
16	16	256

Nondimensional units demonstrating proportionate effect.

Table 11-2 Distribution of airway resistance (ΔP)

Location	Reynold's Number	ΔP cm H₂O
Mouth	2986	0.170
Trachea	3513	0.220
Primary bronchi	2930	0.125
Bronchiole	47	0.016
Terminal bronchiole	3	0.008
	Total	1.089

mixture of laminar and turbulent flows found in the normal respiratory tract. The equations relating ΔP and ΔV under laminar and turbulent conditions can be combined. The resulting equation (Rohrer's equation[18]) approximates the total driving pressure necessary to move gas through the respiratory tract:

$$\Delta P = (K_1 \times \dot{V}) + (K_2 \times \dot{V}^2)$$

This driving pressure represents the sum of the factors associated with laminar and turbulent flow. The magnitude of K_1 and K_2 expresses the relative contributions of each flow pattern to overall airway resistance. When flow is mainly laminar, driving pressure varies linearly with the flow. When flow is mainly turbulent, driving pressure varies exponentially with the flow. If all other conditions (i.e., pressure, flow, tube size) are equal, laminar flow depends on gas viscosity, while turbulent flow depends on gas density.

Distribution of airway resistance. Approximately 90% of the resistance to gas flow occurs in the nose, mouth, and large airways. Only about 10% of the total resistance to flow is attributable to airways less than 2 mm in diameter.[20] This appears to contradict the fact that resistance is inversely related to the radius of the conducting tube.

Branching of the tracheobronchial tree increases the cross-sectional area with each airway generation (Figure 11-12). As gas moves toward the alveoli, the combined "radius" of the conducting system increases exponentially. According to the laws of fluid dynamics, this increase in cross-sectional area causes a decrease in gas velocity. The decrease in gas velocity promotes a laminar flow pattern (i.e., lower NR).

Reynold's numbers are highest in the mouth, trachea, and primary bronchi (Table 11-2). Gas velocity is high, and flow is turbulent. At the level of the terminal bronchioles the cross-sectional area increases more than 30-fold. Gas velocity is very low here. As indicated by a Reynold's number of 3, flow is laminar. The driving pressure at this level is about 0.008 cm H₂O. This is less than 1% of the total driving pressure for the system.

The diameter of the airways is not constant. During inspiration, the stretch of surrounding lung tissue and widening transpulmonary pressure gradient increase the diameter of the airways. The higher the lung volume, the more these factors influence airway caliber (Figure 11-13, page 250). This increase in airway diameter with increasing lung volume decreases airway resistance.[1] As lung volume decreases toward residual volume, airway diameters also decrease. Airway resistance rises dramatically at low lung volumes.

Mechanics of exhalation

Airway caliber is determined by several factors. These factors include anatomic support provided to the airways and pressure differences across their walls. Anatomic support comes from cartilage in the wall of

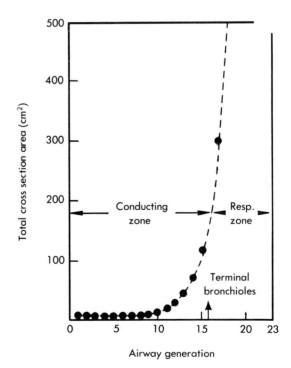

Fig. 11-12 Since no gas exchange takes place in the conducting zone, this region is called the anatomic dead space (see Chapter 9). The gas exchange surface increases markedly at the level of the terminal bronchiole. (From West J: Respiratory physiology—the essentials, Baltimore, 1974, Williams & Wilkins.)

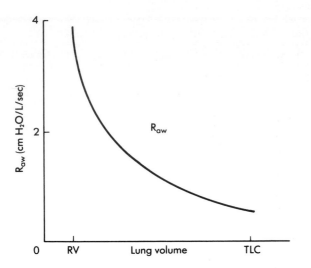

Fig. 11-13 Change in airways resistance (Raw) with change in lung volume. See text for discussion. (From Martin L: Pulmonary physiology in clinical practice: the essentials for patient care and evaluation, St Louis, 1987, Mosby.)

the airway and the "traction" provided by surrounding tissues. The larger airways of the lung depend mainly on **cartilaginous** support. Because smaller airways lack cartilage, they depend on support provided by surrounding lung parenchyma.[21]

The airways are also supported by the pressure difference across their walls. This transpulmonary pressure gradient helps stabilize the airways, particularly the small ones. The difference between the pleural pressure and pressure inside the airway is called the *transmural pressure gradient*.

During quiet breathing pleural pressure is normally negative (subatmospheric). Airway pressure varies minimally about zero. The transmural pressure gradient during normal quiet breathing is negative. It ranges between -5 cm H_2O and -10 cm H_2O. This negative transmural pressure gradient helps maintain the caliber of the small airways.

During a forced exhalation, contraction of expiratory muscles can increase pleural pressure above atmospheric. This reverses the transmural pressure gradient, making it positive. If the positive transmural pressure gradient exceeds the supporting force provided by the lung parenchyma, the small airways may collapse.

Forceful contraction of the expiratory muscles causes pressure across the thorax to rise. This increases pleural pressure from its normal negative value to above atmospheric (Figure 11-14). Alveolar pressure during forced exhalation equals the sum of pleural pressure and that of the elastic forces of alveolar contraction.[2]

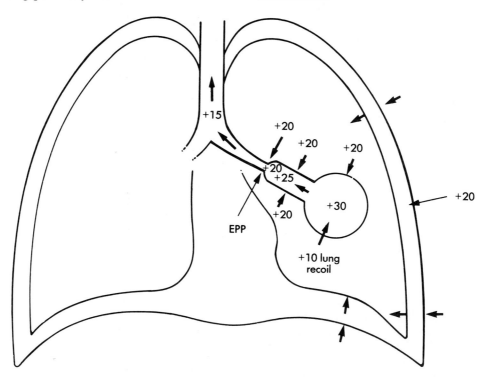

Fig. 11-14 Generation of equal pressure point (EPP) in normal lungs: pleural pressure (Ppl) 20 cm H_2O. This figure shows generation of the EPP when Ppl is 20 cm H_2O during forced exhalation. Alveolar pressure is the sum of Ppl (20 cm H_2O) plus lung elastic recoil pressure (10 cm H_2O), or 30 cm H_2O. Airway pressure falls continually from the alveolus to the mouth. At the EPP, pressure within the airway equals Ppl. Further toward the mouth, airway pressure falls below Ppl, resulting in a narrowed airway and limitation of airflow. (From Martin L: Pulmonary physiology in clinical practice: the essentials for patient care and evaluation, St Louis, 1987, Mosby.)

The "upstream" pressure drops as gas flows from the alveoli toward the mouth. Moving "downstream" (i.e., toward the mouth), transmural pressure continually drops. At some point along the airway, the pressure inside equals the pressure outside in the pleural space. This point is referred to as the *equal pressure point* (EPP). Downstream of this point, pleural pressure exceeds the airway pressure. The resulting positive transmural pressure gradient causes airway compression and can lead to actual collapse.[6]

Airway compression increases expiratory airway resistance and limits flow. At the EPP, greater expiratory effort only increases pleural pressure, further restricting flow.[22] *Dynamic compression* is responsible for the characteristic flow patterns observed in forced expiratory tests of pulmonary function (see Chapter 18).

In healthy subjects, dynamic compression occurs only at lung volumes well below the resting expiratory level. Additional anatomic support is provided by the surrounding lung parenchyma. This tissue support opposes the collapsing force created by negative transmural pressure gradients.

In pulmonary emphysema, the elastic tissue responsible for supporting the small airways is de-stroyed. Destruction of elastic tissue has two outcomes. It increases the compliance of the lung, decreasing its elastic recoil. It also obliterates the anatomic structures responsible for small airway support.[21]

These two factors have a significant effect on exhalation in subjects who have emphysema. If the emphysema patient makes an expiratory effort comparable to that of a healthy subject, pleural pressure rises to +20 cm H_2O. As a result of decreased elastic recoil of the emphysematous lung (P_{recoil} = +5 cm H_2O), alveolar pressure is only +25 cm H_2O (Figure 11-15). The small airways are also more prone to collapse. The EPP occurs farther upstream (toward the alveoli) than in a healthy lung. Airway collapse occurs earlier in exhalation. It also begins at higher volumes than in healthy subjects. As a result air is trapped in the lung.

Air trapping often complicates chronic bronchopulmonary disease. One consequence of air trapping is a gradual elevation of the end-expiratory lung volume. This produces an increase in both the functional residual capacity and the residual volume (Figure 11-16, page 252). Over time, the thorax increases in size, especially its anterior-posterior diameter. The resulting physical abnormality is called a "barrel chest."

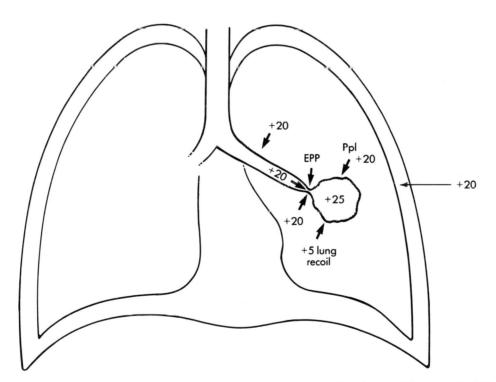

Fig.11–15 EPP in emphysematous lungs. Despite maximal expiratory effort from total lung capacity, Ppl is 20 cm H_2O, but lung elastic recoil pressure is only 5 cm H_2O (compare with Fig. 8–13). As a result, airway driving pressure in the emphysematous lungs is only 25 cm H_2O. Airway driving pressure dissipates further down the airway and equals the Ppl (EPP) at a point earlier than it is reached in healthy lungs. As a result, the airways narrow or collapse at a larger lung volume than is normal. In patients with emphysema, airway collapse is contributed to by the weakened bronchial walls. (From Martin L: Pulmonary physiology in clinical practice: the essentials for patient care and evaluation, St Louis, 1987, Mosby.)

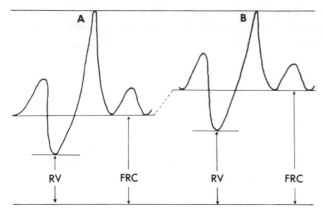

Fig. 11-16 Sketch **A** shows the resting level before, and **B** after, the effect of long-standing airway resistance and/or loss of lung elasticity, as the expansile thoracic springs dominate the pulmonary. Both functional residual capacity and residual volume enlarge. As disease progresses, loss of pulmonary flexibility decreases the expiratory reserve volume, further enlarging the residual volume, and continuing distention may depress the diaphragm to expand the total lung capacity.

WORK OF BREATHING

The work of breathing is done by the respiratory muscles.[23] This work requires energy to overcome the elastic and frictional forces opposing inflation. Assessment of *mechanical work* involves measurement of the physical parameters of force and distance. Assessment of *metabolic work* involves measurement of the oxygen cost of breathing.

During normal breathing, the work of exhaling is recovered from potential energy "stored" in the expanded lung and thorax. Forced exhalation requires additional work by the expiratory muscles. The actual work of forced expiration depends on the mechanical properties of the lungs and thorax, as previously described.

Mechanical work of breathing

Work done on an object is the product of the force exerted on the object, times the distance it is moved. Work may be measured either in dyne-centimeters (dyne-cm) (CGS) or joules (J) (SI):

$$\text{Work} = \text{force} \times \text{distance}$$

Pressure equals force per unit area (distance^2). Volume is the cube of length (distance^3). The product of pressure (P) and volume (V) has the same dimension as work:

$$P \times V = \text{force/area} \times \text{volume}$$
$$P \times V = \text{force/distance}^2 \times \text{distance}^3$$

or

$$P \times V = \text{force/distance}^2 \times (\text{distance}^2 \times \text{distance})$$

Cancelling out distance^2 in both numerator and denominator yields:

$$P \times V = \text{Force} \times \text{distance}$$

The mechanical work of breathing can be calculated as the product of the pressure across the respiratory system and the resulting change in volume:[24]

$$\text{Work of breathing} = \Delta P \times \Delta V$$

The mechanical work of breathing cannot be easily measured during spontaneous breathing. This is due to the fact that the respiratory muscles contribute to the resistance offered by the chest wall. Total mechanical work can be measured during artificial ventilation, if the respiratory muscles are completely at rest. Change in lung volume may be related to the pressure difference between the airway opening and the body surface.[23]

Work of breathing is calculated by integration of the pressure and volume. This is equivalent to determining the area under a volume-pressure curve of the lung (Figure 11-17). Change in pressure is plotted on the x-axis. Change in volume is plotted on the y-axis. The product of pressure and volume represents an area on the graph. The larger this area, the greater the amount of work.

If the lung is inflated slowly, with airflow interrupted to plot volume and pressure changes, a straight line is obtained (Figure 11-17, dashed line A–B). Because conditions during these measurements are static, the straight line represents the change in volume for a given change in pressure, caused solely by the elastic

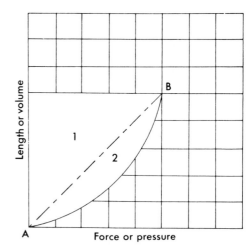

Fig. 11-17 Point *A* is the resting level, and *B* is end-inspiration. *Dashed A-B* represents the pressure-volume relationship of pure elastic resistance, and *curved A-B* the "drag" added by nonelastic friction. At *B*, where airflow momentarily ceases, nonelastic resistance is inactive because it is dependent on movement. The curved line thus disappears, leaving only the elastic resistance of stretch. Areas *1* and *2* represent the work of overcoming elastic nonelastic resistance, respectively.

properties of the lung. The slope of the line is the compliance of the lung. The work done overcoming purely elastic forces opposing inflation is represented by the triangular area 1 in Figure 11-17. If the lung pressure and volume changes are measured during dynamic inflation, the linear relationship no longer holds true. Instead, a curvilinear relationship is obtained between end-expiration and end-inspiration (Figure 11-17, solid line A–B). This curve represents the additional resistance produced by the friction of tissue and gas movement. Most of this resistance is airway resistance. At points of zero flow (Figure 11-17, A and B), resistance is nonexistent, and the curve rejoins the static compliance line. The work done to overcome these frictional forces is represented by the loop labeled as area 2 in Figure 11-17.

The total mechanical work for one breath is the sum of the work overcoming both the elastic and frictional forces opposing inflation. This is represented as the sum of areas 1 and 2 in Figure 11-17. In healthy adults about two thirds of the work of breathing can be attributed to elastic forces opposing ventilation. The remaining third is due to frictional resistance to gas and tissue movement.

In diseased states, the work of breathing can dramatically increase (Figure 11-18). The areas of the volume-pressure curves in both obstruction and restriction are greater than those of healthy subjects. The reasons for these increases in the mechanical work are quite different. In patients who have restrictive lung disease, the area of the volume-pressure curve is greater because the slope of the static component (i.e., compliance) is less than normal. The area of the volume-pressure curve in patients with obstructive lung diseases is increased because the portion associated with frictional resistance is markedly widened. The leftward "bulge" of the loop indicates positive pleural pressure during expiration (Figure 11-18, C).

In healthy subjects the mechanical work of breathing depends on the pattern of ventilation. Large tidal volumes increase the elastic component of work. High breathing rates (flows) increase frictional work. When changing from quiet breathing to exercise ventilation, healthy subjects automatically adjust their tidal volumes and breathing frequencies to minimize the work of breathing.

Similar adjustments occur in subjects who have lung disease (Figure 11-19, page 254).[13] Individuals with disorders characterized by increased elastic work of breathing, such as pulmonary fibrosis, assume a rapid, shallow breathing pattern. This pattern minimizes the mechanical work of ventilating the lungs. Patients who have airway obstruction assume a ventilatory pattern that reduces the frictional work of breathing. Breathing slowly and deeply minimizes tissue and airway resistance.

Increased work of breathing can be complicated by *respiratory muscle weakness*.[25] Respiratory muscle weakness may result from electrolyte imbalance, **acidemia,** shock, or **sepsis.** When increased work of breathing combines with respiratory muscle weakness, inspiratory muscle fatigue can occur. Tidal volumes decrease and respiratory rates increase with muscle fatigue. Gas exchange is compromised by ventilation/perfusion imbalances and increased deadspace (see Efficiency and Effectiveness of Ventilation, this chapter).

Treatment of acute respiratory muscle failure involves resting the muscles. This is usually accomplished by mechanical support of ventilation and removal of the cause of the weakness (i.e., infection, metabolic disorder). Treating chronic respiratory muscle weakness is slightly different. Muscles are rebuilt through nutritional replacement and specific training exercises (see Chapter 37).

Metabolic work of breathing

In order to perform work, the respiratory muscles consume oxygen. The rate of oxygen consumption by the respiratory muscles reflects their energy requirements. It also provides an indirect measure of the work of breathing.[26]

The oxygen cost of breathing is assessed by measuring the total body oxygen consumption at rest and at increased levels of ventilation.[23] If no other factors increase oxygen consumption, the additional O_2 uptake is due to respiratory muscle metabolism. The O_2 cost of breathing in healthy subjects averages 0.5 to 1.0 mL of O_2 for each liter of increased ventilation. This represents less than 5% of total body oxygen consumption.[23] At high levels of ventilation (i.e., greater than about 120 L/min), the oxygen cost of breathing increases tremendously.

The oxygen consumption of the respiratory muscles correlates with the inspiratory pressures generated by the diaphragm.[27] The transdiaphragmatic pressure is measured by a technique like that for intrapleural pressure (see Lung Compliance, this chapter). In addition to a balloon in the esophagus, a

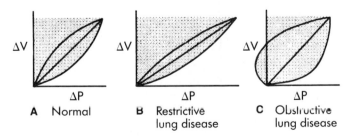

Fig. 11-18 Analysis of the work of breathing (shaded areas) for **A,** a healthy subject; **B,** a patient with restrictive ventilatory impairment; and **C,** a patient with chronic diffuse obstructive bronchopulmonary disease. (From Slonim NB and Hamilton LH: Respiratory physiology, ed 5, St Louis, 1987, Mosby.)

■ M I N I C L I N I ■

11-2

Optimal Breathing Pattern in Obstructive Airway Diseases

You have a patient with advanced emphysema, which means this patient's lungs have lost elastic tissue and have reduced elastic recoil (i.e., the lung compliance is abnormally high). This also means there is a lack of elastic fibers available to apply "radial traction" around the outside circumference of small airways, and thus small, noncartilaginous airways are prone to collapse. When your patient exhales (especially during forced exhalation) airway resistance is abnormally high because the small airways prematurely narrow or collapse as a result of an adverse pressure gradient. That is, the equal pressure point phenomenon occurs and distal to this point, extraluminal pressure exceeds intraluminal pressure. (See the Mechanics of Exhalation section in the text.) This situation greatly increases the work of breathing. How would you instruct this patient to breathe to minimize work of breathing?

Discussion: This patient's increased work of breathing arises from high **frictional** resistance during exhalation. (Work required to overcome **elastic** resistance is actually less than normal because lung compliance is high.) To minimize the work required to overcome frictional resistance, airflow should be slow in order to reduce turbulence and increase the laminar flow characteristics of the gas stream. To keep airways patent and prevent their premature closure, exhaling against resistance may be helpful; this would increase pressure in the airways throughout the expiratory phase and counteract the collapsing effect of extraluminal pressure surrounding the airways. Therefore, you should instruct your patient to breathe slowly and deeply, and to exhale slowly through pursed lips to create expiratory resistance. This should reduce the frictional work of breathing.

second balloon is placed in the stomach. The pressure difference between the two balloons represents pressure across the diaphragm. The greater the pressure required to overcome inspiratory resistance, the higher the O_2 consumption of the respiratory muscles.

The pressure generated by the diaphragm (Pdi) is often expressed in relation to the maximal pressure obtainable (Pdimax). The ratio of Pdi/Pdimax represents the pressure required to maintain ventilation, compared with maximal capacity. It is also possible to determine the time the muscles spend in inspiration (Ti). Ti is expressed in relation to the total breath time (Ttot). These two ratios can be combined as the *tension-time index* (TTdi).

$$TTdi = \frac{Pdi}{Pdimax} \times \frac{Ti}{Ttot}$$

A TTdi above 0.15 is indicative of a potentially fatiguing pattern of ventilation.[28] Fatigue can develop

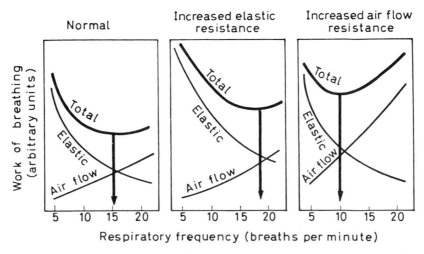

Fig. 11-19 Work done against airflow and elastic resistance together equal total work. Under normal circumstances, the total work of breathing is at a minimum at about 15 breaths per minute (left). For the same minute volume, but with increased elastic resistance (low compliance), minimum work is performed at higher frequencies (middle). However, with increased air flow resistance (right), minimum work occurs at lower rates of breathing. (From Nunn JF: Applied respiratory physiology, ed 2, London, 1977, Butterworth.)

as a result of increased elastic work (i.e., Pdi/Pdimax increases). Fatigue can also develop when inspiratory resistance increases the length of time needed to breath in (Ti/Ttot).

In certain diseases the O_2 cost of breathing increases dramatically with increasing ventilation (Figure 11-20). As ventilation increases, the oxygen consumption of the emphysema patient's respiratory muscles increases at a much faster rate than a normal subject's. This abnormally high oxygen cost of breathing is one factor that limits exercise in such patients.

THE DISTRIBUTION OF VENTILATION

Ventilation is not distributed evenly in the healthy lung. Regional as well as local factors account for this unevenness in the distribution of ventilation.[29] Uneven ventilation helps explain why the lung is less than perfect for gas exchange (see Chapter 12). In disease, the distribution of ventilation can worsen dramatically. The resulting deficiencies in gas exchange can be life-threatening. The maldistribution of ventilation in disease represents a primary cause of impaired oxygen and carbon dioxide exchange (see Chapter 15).

Regional Factors

Two factors affect regional distribution of gas in the healthy lung: (1) relative differences in thoracic expansion and (2) regional transpulmonary pressure gradients.[30] These factors combine to direct more ventilation to the bases and periphery of the lungs than to the apices and central zones.

Differences in thoracic expansion

The configuration of thoracic bony structures and the action of the respiratory muscles cause proportionately greater expansion at the lung bases than at the apices. Expansion of the lower chest is about 50% greater than that of the upper chest.[2] The action of the diaphragm preferentially inflates the lower lobes of the lung.

Transpulmonary pressure gradients

The transpulmonary pressure gradient is not equal throughout all portions of the thorax. It varies substantially, both from outside to inside, and from top to bottom.

At a given level of alveolar inflation, the transpulmonary pressure gradient is directly related to the pleural pressure. Pleural pressure represents the pressure on the outer surface (i.e., periphery) of the lung. Its effect lessens toward more centrally located alveoli. Changes in the transpulmonary pressure gradient are greatest in peripheral alveoli. The changes are less in alveoli in the central zones.[2] Peripheral alveoli expand proportionately more than their more central counterparts.

Top-to-bottom differences in pleural pressure have an even greater effect on distribution of ventilation, especially in the upright lung.[8] Pleural pressure increases about 0.25 cm H_2O/cm distance from the lung apex to its base. This increase in pressure is due to the weight of the lung and the effect of gravity. Pleural pressure at the apex is approximately -10 cm H_2O. At the base pleural pressure is only about -2.5 cm H_2O.[7] Because of these differences, the transpulmonary

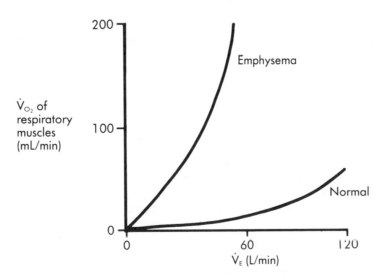

Fig. 11-20 Relationship of oxygen cost of breathing to expiratory minute volume for a healthy subject and for a patient with bronchitis-emphysema syndrome. (From Slonim NB and Hamilton LH: Respiratory physiology, ed 5, St Louis, 1987, Mosby. After Campbell EJM, Westlake EK, and Cherniack RM: J *Appl Physiol* 11:303, 1957.)

pressure gradient at the top of the upright lung is greater than at the bottom. Alveoli at the apices have a higher volume than those at the bases.

In spite of their higher volume, alveoli at the apices expand less during inspiration than those at the bases. Apical alveoli "sit" on the upper portion of the pressure-volume curve (Figure 11-21). This part of the curve is relatively flat. Each unit of pressure changes causes only a small change in volume. Alveoli at the lung bases are positioned on the middle portion of the pressure-volume curve. That part of the curve is relatively steep. For each unit of pressure change there is a larger change in volume.

For a given transpulmonary pressure gradient, alveoli at the bases expand more than those at the apices. The bases of the upright lung receive about four times as much ventilation as the apices.[7]

These gravity-dependent differences are also observed in recumbent subjects. The magnitude of the differences is less than in the upright lung. Ventilation is greatest in the dependent zones of the lung. In recumbent subjects, the posterior regions are dependent. Lying on the side causes more ventilation to go to whichever lung is lower.

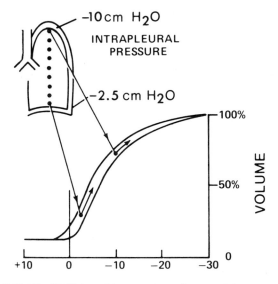

Fig. 11-21 Causes of regional differences in ventilation down the lung. Due to the weight of the lung and the influence of gravity, the intrapleural pressure at the apex is more negative than at the base. Thus alveoli at the apex are maintained at a higher *resting* inflation volume than those at the base. However, alveoli at the apex reside on the higher portion of the pressure-volume curve, whereas those at the base are positioned on the lower, *steeper* portion. Thus, for an equal change in intrapleural pressure, alveoli at the base expand more on inspiration than those at the apex. (From West JB: Respiratory physiology: the essentials, ed 3, Baltimore, 1985, Williams & Wilkins.)

Local Factors

Alveolar filling and emptying are also affected by "local" factors. Individual respiratory units and their associated airways may differ from each other. These local factors contribute to uneven ventilation in healthy lungs. Their influence on gas distribution is particularly important in disease.

Each respiratory unit has an elastic element, the alveolus, and a resistive element, the airway. Change in alveolar volume and the time required for the change to occur depend on the compliance and resistance of each respiratory unit.[8]

In terms of compliance, the more distensible the unit, the greater the volume change will be (at a given transpulmonary pressure). Lung units with high compliance have less elastic recoil than normal. These units fill and empty more slowly than normal units. Lung units with low compliance (i.e., high elastic recoil) increase their volume less. They also fill and empty faster than normal.

Airway resistance also affects emptying and filling. Airway caliber influences how much driving pressure reaches distal lung units. In healthy airways the pressure drop between the airway opening and the alveolus is minimal. Most of the driving pressure is available for alveolar inflation. If there is airway obstruction, high resistance to gas flow can occur. The pressure drop across the obstruction may be substantial. Less driving pressure is available for alveolar inflation. As a result there is less alveolar volume change.

Time constants

Compliance and resistance determine local rates of alveolar filling and emptying. The relationship between the compliance and resistance of a lung unit can be measured. This property of each lung unit is called its *time constant*. The time constant is simply the product of each unit's compliance and resistance:

$$\text{Time Constant} = C \times R$$

where:

$$C = \text{compliance (L/cm H}_2\text{O)}$$
$$R = \text{resistance (cm H}_2\text{O/L/sec)}$$

The pressure and volume units (i.e., cm H_2O and L, respectively) cancel out. The time constant is expressed in units of seconds.

A lung unit will have a long time constant when its resistance or compliance (or both) is high. Units with long time constants take longer to fill and to empty than units with normal compliance and resistance (Figure 11-22).

Lung units have a short time constant when either resistance or compliance (or both) is low. Lung units

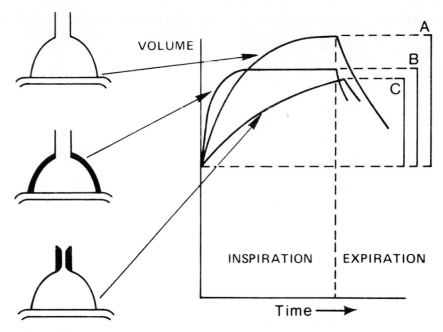

Fig. 11-22 Effect of changes in resistance and compliance on filling and emptying of lung units inflated with equal pressures. Lung unit A has normal resistance and compliance, and fills and empties at a normal rate (normal time constant). Lung unit B has normal resistance but low compliance, fills and empties faster than normal (low time constant), but at a lower volume. Lung unit C has normal compliance but high resistance. It fills and empties slower than normal (high time constant), but also at a lower volume. (From West JB: Respiratory physiology: the essentials, ed 3, Baltimore, 1985, Williams & Wilkins.)

with short time constants fill and empty more rapidly than those with normal compliance and resistance.

Time constants affect local distribution of ventilation in the lung. When the time available for inflation is fixed, units with long time constants fill less and empty more slowly than normal units. Units with short time constants also fill less than normal, as a result of low compliance. These units also fill and empty quickly. The ventilation going to lung units with either long or short time constants is less than that received by units with normal compliance and resistance.

Frequency dependence of compliance

Variations in time constants can affect ventilation throughout the lung. Abnormal ventilation is characteristic of obstruction in the small airways. This type of obstruction occurs in emphysema. The time constants of many lung units are increased. These long time constants are due mainly to increased resistance to flow in the small airways. Loss of normal tissue elastic recoil also contributes to slowed filling and emptying.

At increased breathing rates, units with long time constants fill less and empty more slowly than units with normal compliance and resistance. More and more inspired gas goes to lung units with relatively normal time constants. When more inspired volume goes to a smaller number of lung units, higher trans-

pulmonary pressures must be generated to maintain alveolar ventilation. Compliance of the lung will appears to decrease as breathing frequency increases.

This phenomenon is called *frequency dependence of compliance*. Compliance measured during breathing is not static, as described previously (see Mechanical Work of Breathing, this chapter). It includes pressure changes created by resistance to airflow. The term *dynamic compliance* is used to assess pressure-volume relationships during breathing. If dynamic compliance decreases as the respiratory rate increases, some lung units must have abnormal time constants.

Distribution of ventilation is influenced by breathing frequency in patients with abnormal time constants. Any stimulus to increase ventilation, such as exercise, may redistribute inspired gas. Mismatching of ventilation and perfusion can result in hypoxemia, severely limiting the individual's ability to perform daily activities (see Chapters 15 and 37).

EFFICIENCY AND EFFECTIVENESS OF VENTILATION

Ventilation moves respired gases into and out of the lungs. To be effective, the process must meet body needs for O_2 uptake and CO_2 removal. To be efficient, ventilation should require little O_2 and produce the minimum amount of CO_2.

Efficiency of ventilation

Even in healthy lungs, ventilation is not entirely efficient. A substantial volume of inspired gas is "wasted" with each breath. Wasted ventilation does not participate in gas exchange.

Ventilation is wasted because the lungs are a dead-end circuit. Gases must move in and out through the same pathway. Some of the gas must occupy space in the airways leading to the exchange area. This volume does not participate in gas exchange. For each breath, the gas left in the conducting tubes is wasted.

Minute ventilation

To determine how much ventilation is wasted, total ventilation must be measured. Ventilation is usually assessed in liters per minute. The total volume moving in or out of the lungs per minute is called *minute ventilation.* Expired volume is commonly measured. Minute ventilation is symbolized as $\dot{V}_E$. $\dot{V}_E$ is calculated as the product of frequency of breathing (*f*) times the expired tidal volume:

$$\dot{V}_E = f \times V_T$$

For example, for a healthy adult breathing at a rate of 12 breaths/minute and a V_T of 500 mL:

$$\dot{V}_E = 12 \times 500 \text{ mL}$$
$$= 6000 \text{ mL/min, or } 6.0 \text{ L/min}$$

Minute ventilation depends on the size of the subject and his or her metabolic rate. $\dot{V}_E$ values range from about 5 to 10 L/min in a resting subject.

Deadspace ventilation

Not all of the $\dot{V}_E$ participates in gas exchange. Some of this volume occupies space in the conducting zones of the lung. The conducting zones do not participate in gas exchange. The volume occupying this space is wasted. Wasted ventilation is referred to as *deadspace.*

Anatomic deadspace

The volume of the conducting airways is called the anatomic deadspace, or $V_{DS_{anat}}$. $V_{DS_{anat}}$ averages about 1 mL per pound of body weight. For a subject who weighs 150 pounds, $V_{DS_{anat}}$ is about 150 mL.

$V_{DS_{anat}}$ does not participate in gas exchange because it is *rebreathed.* During exhalation of a 500 mL tidal breath, the first 150 mL of gas comes from the anatomic deadspace. The remaining 350 mL is alveolar gas. At the end of exhalation, the airways contain 150 mL of alveolar gas. During the next inhalation, this 150 mL volume is rebreathed. Only about 350 mL of "fresh" gas reaches the alveoli per breath.

Alveolar ventilation

The volume of fresh gas reaching the alveoli per breath is called the *alveolar ventilation,* symbolized as V_A. V_A may be calculated by subtracting the anatomic deadspace ($V_{DS_{anat}}$) from the tidal volume (V_T):

$$V_A = V_T - V_{DS_{anat}}$$

or, substituting average normal values:

$$V_A = 500 \text{ mL} - 150 \text{ mL}$$
$$= 350 \text{ mL}$$

Instead of calculating V_A for a single breath, it is usually expressed per unit of time (i.e., per minute). *Alveolar minute ventilation,* abbreviated as $\dot{V}_A$, is the product of breathing rate (f) and alveolar ventilation per breath (V_A):

$$\dot{V}_A - f \times V_A$$

Since $V_A = V_T - V_{DS_{anat}}$, this equation may be rewritten as:

$$\dot{V}_A = f \times (V_T - V_{DS_{anat}})$$

For example, in a healthy adult with a V_T of 500 mL and a $V_{DS_{anat}}$ of 150 mL:

$$\dot{V}_A = 12 \times (500 \text{ mL} - 150 \text{ mL})$$
$$= 12 \times 350 \text{ mL}$$
$$= 4200 \text{ mL}$$

The anatomic deadspace ventilation per minute in normal subjects may also be calculated as the difference between $\dot{V}_E$ and $\dot{V}_A$. Using the values given:

$$\dot{V}_{DS_{anat}} = \dot{V}_E - \dot{V}_A$$
$$= 6000 \text{ mL} - 4200 \text{ mL}$$
$$= 1800 \text{ mL/min}$$

Approximately one third of the minute ventilation in healthy resting subjects is wasted as anatomic deadspace.

Alveolar deadspace

The preceeding calculations assume that all fresh gas reaching the alveoli participates in gas exchange. In healthy subjects this assumption is usually true. In certain disease states, some alveoli may be ventilated but not participate in gas exchange. These alveoli are ventilated but not perfused with mixed venous blood. Without perfusion, gas exchange cannot occur. Any gas that ventilates unperfused alveoli is also wasted (i.e., deadspace).

The volume of gas ventilating unperfused alveoli is called *alveolar deadspace,* or $V_{DS_{alv}}$. Significant amounts of $V_{DS_{alv}}$ are pathologic. $V_{DS_{alv}}$ is usually related to defects in the pulmonary circulation. A clinical example of such a defect is a pulmonary **embolism.** A pulmonary embolus blocks a portion of the pulmonary circulation. This obstructs perfusion to ventilated alveoli, creating alveolar deadspace. Alveolar deadspace occurs in addition to the anatomic deadspace.

Physiologic deadspace

The sum of anatomic and alveolar deadspace is called *physiologic deadspace* ($V_{DS_{phy}}$):

$$V_{DS_{phy}} = V_{DS_{anat}} + V_{DS_{alv}}$$

The total volume of wasted ventilation, or physiologic deadspace, equals the sum of the conducting airways and the alveoli that are ventilated but not perfused (Figure 11-23).

Physiologic deadspace includes both the normal and abnormal components of wasted ventilation. $V_{DS_{phy}}$ is the preferred clinical measure of ventilation efficiency. Alveolar ventilation is more accurately assessed by using $V_{DS_{phy}}$:

$$\dot{V}_A = f \times (V_T - V_{DS_{phy}})$$

or

$$\dot{V}_A = \dot{V}_E - \dot{V}_{DS_{phy}}$$

Physiologic deadspace is measured clinically by using a modified form of the Bohr equation:

$$V_{DS_{phy}} = \left[V_T \times \left(\frac{PaCO_2 - P\overline{E}CO_2}{PaCO_2} \right) \right] - V_{DS_{mec}}$$

where

$V_{DS_{phy}}$ = physiologic deadspace
V_T = tidal volume (averaged)
$PaCO_2$ = partial pressure of CO_2 in the arterial blood
$P\overline{E}CO_2$ = partial pressure of CO_2 in the mixed expired air
$V_{DS_{mec}}$ = mechanical deadspace (of the collection device)

A sample of the subject's exhaled air is collected over several minutes. This is done by using a nonrebreathing valve and gas collection bag. The bag must be large enough to hold several minutes of ventilation (i.e., 10 to 100 liters). The volume exhaled by the subject can be measured by a **respirometer** (see Chapter 37). The respiratory rate is measured by counting the number of breaths per minute. The mechanical deadspace of the collection apparatus should be measured. Larger volumes of mixed expired air usually improve the accuracy of the calculation.

During the expired gas collection, an arterial blood sample is drawn. The value for $PaCO_2$ is obtained from blood gas analysis. The $P\overline{E}CO_2$ may be measured by using either the blood gas analyzer or a separate CO_2 analyzer. These values are entered into the modified Bohr equation. For example, a subject has an arterial PCO_2 of 40 mm Hg, a mixed expired PCO_2 of 20 mm Hg, and a tidal volume of 500 mL. If the mechanical deadspace is 100 mL, then by the previous equation:

$$\begin{aligned} V_{DS_{phys}} &= \left[500 \times \left(\frac{40 - 20}{40} \right) \right] - 100 \\ &= [500 \times 0.50] - 100 \\ &= 250 - 100 \\ &= 150 \text{ mL} \end{aligned}$$

Deadspace/tidal volume ratio

In clinical practice $V_{DS_{phy}}$ is often expressed as a ratio to the tidal volume. This ratio, or V_{DS}/V_T, provides an index of the wasted ventilation (i.e., anatomic and alveolar deadspace) per breath. The V_{DS}/V_T ratio represents the *efficiency* of ventilation. Using the data from the previous example, the V_{DS}/V_T ratio is:

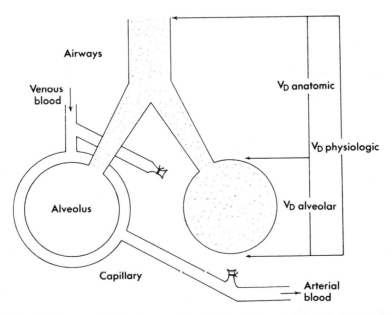

Fig. 11-23 The three types of dead space are shown in this sketch, which schematically represents two alveoli, their supporting airways, and capillaries. One alveolus is normally perfused and ventilated; but the capillary to the other is shown as if it were tied off and removed, so that the alveolus is freely ventilated but not perfused. The relationships of the dead spaces are indicated, as defined in the text.

$$\frac{V_{DS_{phy}}}{V_T} = \frac{150 \text{ mL}}{500 \text{ mL}}$$
$$= 0.30$$

In this example the physiologic deadspace is approximately one third of the tidal volume. The V_{DS}/V_T ratio varies in healthy subjects, with a normal range of 0.2 to 0.4.

Clinical significance

Table 11-3 lists the effect of changes in various parameters on alveolar ventilation. In healthy subjects, alveolar ventilation depends on the rate of breathing and V_T. High rates and low tidal volumes result in a high proportion of wasted ventilation per minute (i.e., low alveolar ventilation). The most efficient breathing pattern is slow, deep breathing.

In pulmonary disease, an increased $V_{DS_{phy}}$ causes a decrease in alveolar ventilation, unless compensation occurs. An increased breathing rate by itself worsens the problem. Effective compensation for increased $V_{DS_{phy}}$ requires an increased tidal volume. Elevating V_T increases the elastic work of breathing. This increases oxygen consumption by the respiratory muscles. In some patients these increased demands cannot be met. In such cases, alveolar ventilation may not be adequate to meet body needs.

Effectiveness of ventilation

Ventilation is effective when it removes CO_2 at a rate that maintains a normal pH. Under resting metabolic conditions, the body produces about 200 mL of CO_2 per minute. Carbon dioxide production must be matched by sufficient alveolar ventilation per minute to ensure **homeostasis.**

The balance between CO_2 production and $\dot{V}_A$ determines the PCO_2 in the lungs and in arterial blood. This balance also helps determine the pH of arterial blood. The partial pressure of CO_2 in the alveoli and blood is directly proportional to its production ($\dot{V}CO_2$). PCO_2 is inversely proportional to its rate of removal by alveolar ventilation ($\dot{V}_A$):

$$PCO_2 \cong \frac{\dot{V}CO_2}{\dot{V}_A}$$

Alveolar and arterial partial pressures of CO_2 are normally in equilibrium at about 40 mm Hg. If alveolar ventilation falls, $\dot{V}CO_2$ will exceed its rate of removal. The $PaCO_2$ will rise above its normal value of 40 mm Hg, and arterial pH will fall. Ventilation that does not meet metabolic needs (i.e., maintain a normal pH) is termed *hypoventilation.* Hypoventilation is indicated by the presence of an elevated $PaCO_2$ and a pH below the normal range (i.e., 7.35 to 7.45).

If alveolar ventilation increases, the $\dot{V}CO_2$ will be less than its rate of removal. $PaCO_2$ will fall below its normal value of 40 mm Hg, and pH will rise. Ventilation in excess of metabolic needs is termed *hyperventilation.* Hyperventilation is indicated by a lower than normal $PaCO_2$ and a pH above the normal range.

Hyperventilation is sometimes confused with the increased ventilation that occurs in response to increased metabolism. A good example is the changes observed during low or moderate levels of exercise. Ventilation rises in proportion to the increased $\dot{V}CO_2$ from exercise. The $PaCO_2$ remains in the normal range of 35 to 45 mm Hg, and pH remains near 7.40. The increase in ventilation that occurs with increased metabolic rates is termed *hyperpnea.*

Effectiveness of ventilation is determined by partial pressure of CO_2 and the resulting pH, specifically in arterial blood. Ventilation is effective when the $PaCO_2$ is maintained at a level that keeps the pH within normal limits.

Ineffective ventilation occurs when CO_2 production and alveolar ventilation are out of balance. Hypoventilation is ineffective because CO_2 removal is inadequate to meet metabolic needs. Hyperventilation is

---

Table 11-3 Changes in alveolar ventilation (mL) associated with changes in rate, volume, and physiologic deadspace

	Rate of breathing	Tidal volume	Minute ventilation	Physiologic deadspace	Alveolar ventilation
Normal	12	500	6000	150	4200
High rate, low volume	24	250	6000	150	2400
Low rate, high volume	6	1000	6000	150	5100
Increased deadspace	12	500	6000	300	2400
Compensation for increased deadspace	12	650	7800	300	4200

MINI CLINI
11-3

Minute Ventilation, Deadspace Ventilation, Alveolar Ventilation, and PaCO₂

Problem: A patient breathing at a rate of 12 breaths per minute has a tidal volume of 600 mL and an estimated anatomic deadspace of 150 mL. This ventilatory pattern produces an arterial carbon dioxide tension ($PaCO_2$) of 40 mm Hg. Several hours pass and your assessment of the patient reveals a breath rate of 24/min, but the minute ventilation ($\dot{V}_E$) has remained the same as before. You now measure the $PaCO_2$ and find that it has risen to 60 mm Hg. Explain how the $PaCO_2$ increased even though $\dot{V}_E$ remained constant.

Explanation:
The initial $\dot{V}_E$ and $\dot{V}_A$ were as follows:

$$\dot{V}_E = 600 \times 12 = 7200 \text{ mL/min}$$
$$\dot{V}_A = (600 - 150) \times 12$$
$$= 5400 \text{ mL/min}$$

This $\dot{V}_A$ of 5400 mL/min was respon-sible for maintaining the $PaCO_2 = 40$ mm Hg.

When respiratory rate increased to 24 breaths/min and $\dot{V}_E$ remained at 7200 mL/min, tidal volume (V_T) must have decreased:

$$7200 = V_T \times 24$$
$$V_T = 7200/24 = 300 \text{ mL}$$

However, anatomic deadspace re-mained at 150 mL. Alveolar ventila-tion subsequently decreased:

$$\dot{V}_A = (300 - 150) \times 24$$
$$= 3600 \text{ mL/min}$$

This reduced $\dot{V}_A$ (from 5400 mL/min to 3600 mL/min) explains the in-crease in $PaCO_2$ from 40 mm Hg to 60 mm Hg. This patient, although tachypneic, is hypoventilating.

---

ineffective because excessive energy is expended need-lessly. There is no direct or consistent correlation between measures of ventilation (i.e., $\dot{V}_E$, V_T, f) and effectiveness of ventilation. Hypoventilation or hyper-ventilation must be determined by arterial blood gas analysis (see Chapters 12 and 14).

Ventilation is considered effective when CO_2 removal meets the body's needs. CO_2 production must be matched by sufficient alveolar ventilation per minute to maintain a normal pH. The desired result is maintenance of a normal pH by adjusting the PCO_2 with maximum efficiency and minimum work.

CHAPTER SUMMARY

Ventilation is the movement of air into and out of the lungs. This process is accomplished by the action of the respiratory muscles on the thorax. Their action creates pressure gradients necessary to overcome the elastic and frictional forces opposing lung and thoracic expansion.

In overcoming the forces opposing inflation, work is performed by the respiratory muscles. During normal breathing, the work of expiration is recovered from potential energy "stored" during expansion of the lungs and thorax. Forced exhalation requires that additional work be performed by the expiratory muscles. How much work is involved in breathing depends on the mechanical properties of the lungs and thorax.

The mechanical properties of the lungs and thorax also affect the distribution of ventilation. Regional and local factors make the lung a less than perfect organ for gas exchange. In disease, the distribution of ventilation can dramatically worsen, causing signif-icant gas exchange abnormalities.

The process of ventilation should be both efficient and effective in removing CO_2. Even the normal lung wastes a portion of ventilation on each breath. Changes in the pattern of breathing also affect the efficiency of ventilation. Pulmonary disease can increase the volume of wasted ventilation. This makes it difficult for the lung to remove CO_2 effectively.

REFERENCES

1. Fishman AP: *Assessment of pulmonary function,* New York, 1980, McGraw-Hill.
2. Martin L: *Pulmonary physiology in clinical practice: the es-sentials for patient care and evaluation,* St. Louis, 1987, Mosby.
3. Report of the ACCP-ATS Joint Committee on Pulmonary Nomenclature, *Chest* 67:583, 1975.
4. Tisi GM: *Pulmonary physiology in clinical medicine,* ed 2, Baltimore, 1984, Williams & Wilkins.
5. Peters RM: *The mechanical basis of respiration,* Boston, 1969, Little, Brown.
6. Green JF: *Mechanical concepts in cardiovascular and pulmo-nary physiology,* Philadelphia, 1977, Lea & Febiger.
7. Green JF: *Fundamental cardiovascular and pulmonary physi-ology,* ed 2, Philadelphia, 1987, Lea & Febiger.
8. West JB: *Respiratory physiology: the essentials,* ed 4, Balti-more, 1991, Williams & Wilkins.
9. Murray JF: *The normal lung,* ed 2, Philadelphia, 1986, WB Saunders.
10. Von Neergaard K: Neue auffassungen uber einen grundbegriff der atemmechanik: Die retraktionkraft der lunge, abhangig von der oberflachenspannung in der alveolen, *Z Gesamte Exp Med* 66:373, 1929.
11. Clements JA et al: Pulmonary surface tension and alveolar stability, *J Appl Physiol* 16:444, 1972.
12. Jacquez JA: *Respiratory physiology,* New York, 1979, Mc-Graw-Hill.
13. Cherniack RM, Cherniack L: Respiration in health and dis-ease, ed 3, Philadelphia, 1983, WB Saunders.
14. Wright JR, Hawgood S: Pulmonary surfactant metabolism, *Clin Chest Med,* 10(1):83, 1989.

15. Lachmann B: *Surfactant replacement in acute respiratory failure: animal studies and first clinical trials.* In B Lachmann, editor: *Surfactant replacement therapy,* New York, 1987, Springer.

16. Foster RE et al: *The lung: physiologic basis of pulmonary function tests,* ed 3, St Louis, 1986, Mosby.

17. Olson DE, Dart GA, Filley GF: Pressure drop and fluid flow regime of air inspired into the human lungs, *J Appl Physiol* 28:482–484, 1970.

18. Slonim NB, Hamilton LH: *Respiratory physiology,* ed 5, St Louis, 1985, Mosby.

19. Whitaker S: *Introduction to fluid mechanics,* Englewood Cliffs, NJ, 1968, Prentice-Hall.

20. Ferris BG Jr, Mead J, Opie LH: Partitioning of respiratory flow resistance in man, *J Appl Physiol* 19:653–658, 1964.

21. Nunn JF: *Applied respiratory physiology,* ed 2, London, 1977, Butterworth.

22. Robinson DR, Chaudhary BA, Speir WS: Expiratory flow limitation in large and small airways, *Arch Intern Med* 144:1457, 1984.

23. Altose MD: *Pulmonary mechanics.* In Fishman AP, editor: *Assessment of pulmonary function,* New York, 1980, McGraw-Hill.

24. Otis AB: The work of breathing, *Physiol Rev* 34:449–458, 1954.

25. Rochester DF: Respiratory muscles and ventilatory failure: 1993 perspective. *Am J Med Sci* 305:394–402, 1993.

26. Cournand A et al: The oxygen cost of breathing, *Trans Assoc Am Physician* 67:162–173, 1954.

27. Field S, Sanci S, Grassino A: Respiratory muscle oxygen consumption estimated by the diaphragm pressure-time index. *J Appl Physiol* 57:44–51, 1984.

28. Celli BR: Clinical and physiologic evaluation of respiratory muscle function, *Clin Chest Med* 10(2):199–214, 1989.

29. Macklem PT: Relation between lung mechanics and ventilation distribution, *Physiologist,* 16:580–588, 1973.

30. Milic-Emili J et al: Regional distribution of inspired gas in the lung, *J Appl Physiol* 21:749–759, 1966.

12

Gas Exchange and Transport

■

G. Woodard Gross
Craig L. Scanlan

CHAPTER LEARNING OBJECTIVES

1. Delineate the normal gradients in oxygen and carbon dioxide partial pressure between the atmosphere and tissues.
2. Explain, using mathematical formulas, the determinants of alveolar oxygen and carbon dioxide partial pressures.
3. Apply pertinent physical laws to describe the factors affecting diffusion at the alveolar-capillary membrane.
4. Describe the normal relationship between ventilation and perfusion in the healthy lung and its impact on local gas tensions in various lung zones.
5. Differentiate between how oxygen and carbon dioxide are transported in the blood and describe the factors affecting their movement to and from the tissues.

Ventilation is only one component of human respiration. In addition to simply moving in and out of the lungs, gases must be efficiently distributed to the alveoli, exchanged with the pulmonary circulation, and transported to and from the tissues.

Normally, these processes of gas exchange and transport occur in a well-integrated manner under a wide variety of circumstances. In disease states, however, one or more of these critical processes may become impaired. Impaired gas exchange or transport can cause physiologic imbalances that can alter function or even threaten survival. At such times, respiratory care intervention may be the only way to maintain or restore a level of function consistent with life.

DIFFUSION

Whole-body diffusion gradients

Although enhanced by various mechanisms, the actual movement of gases between lungs and the tissues depends mainly on diffusion. Proper diffusion between lungs and tissues requires partial pressure gradients of sufficient size and direction throughout the body.

These normal diffusion gradients for both oxygen and carbon dioxide are shown in Figure 12-1. For oxygen, there is a stepwise downward "cascade" of partial pressures from the normal atmospheric P_{IO_2} of 159 torr to a low point of 40 torr or less at the systemic capillaries. The intracellular PO_2, estimated to be 5 torr or less, provides the final gradient necessary for movement of oxygen into the cell.[1]

Likewise, a partial pressures gradient exists for carbon dioxide. In this case, however, the direction of

the gradient is reversed. The partial pressure of carbon dioxide is highest in the cells (estimated at 60 torr) and lowest in room air (<1 torr). This reverse cascade governs carbon dioxide movement from the tissues to the lungs and—with the aid of ventilation—out to the atmosphere.

Determinants of alveolar gas tensions

Diffusion in the lung requires pressure gradients for both oxygen and carbon dioxide between alveoli and pulmonary capillaries. Pulmonary capillary gas pressures depend mainly on the rate of cellular metabolism in relation to blood flow; thus they are beyond the direct control of the clinician. Alveolar oxygen and carbon dioxide tensions, however, can be controlled by the clinician. For this reason, RCPs must know what determines partial pressures in both the normal and abnormal lung.

Alveolar carbon dioxide tensions

The alveolar partial pressure of carbon dioxide, or $PACO_2$, varies directly with the body's production of carbon dioxide ($\dot{V}CO_2$) and inversely with alveolar ventilation ($\dot{V}A$).[2] Using a constant of 0.863 to convert $\dot{V}CO_2$ from STPD to BTPS, these relationships can be expressed in the following formula:

$$PACO_2 = \frac{\dot{V}CO_2 \times 0.863}{\dot{V}A}$$

Given a normal VCO_2 of 200 mL/minute and a normal alveolar ventilation of 4.2 L/minute, applica-

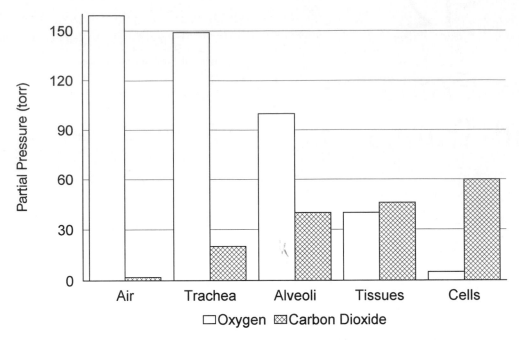

Fig. 12-1 Normal diffusion gradients for oxygen and carbon dioxide. Note downward cascade for oxygen from air to cells, with a reverse gradient for carbon dioxide.

tion of this formula yields a P_ACO_2 of about 40 torr:

$$PACO_2 = \frac{200 \times 0.863}{4.2}$$
$$= 40 \text{ torr}$$

The P_ACO_2 will increase above this level if: (1) carbon dioxide production increases, (2) alveolar ventilation decreases, or (3) both conditions coexist.[3] Likewise, a decrease in P_ACO_2 below this normal level will occur if carbon dioxide production decreases or alveolar ventilation increases. Normally, complex respiratory control mechanisms maintain the P_ACO_2 within a range of 35 to 45 torr under a wide variety of conditions (see Chapter 14).

Alveolar oxygen tensions

Unlike carbon dioxide, oxygen makes up a substantial portion of the inspired air. The alveolar partial pressure of oxygen, or P_AO_2, is thus determined, mainly by its partial pressure in the inspired gas. Under Dalton's Law (see Chapter 7), the partial pressure of inspired oxygen must equal its fractional concentration (FIO_2) times the total barometric pressure (PB):

$$PIO_2 = FIO_2 \times PB$$

At sea level ($PB = 760$ torr), PIO_2 is calculated as:

$$PIO_2 = 0.2095 \times 760 \text{ torr} = 159 \text{ torr}$$

Correcting for water vapor pressure. As humidification occurs in the nose and upper airways, inspired oxygen molecules are effectively "displaced" by water vapor. The resulting oxygen partial pressure is thus lowered by an amount equal to the water vapor pressure (PH_2O) at BTPS (see Figure 12-1). At BTPS, the water vapor pressure is 47 torr. Thus, to correct for the addition of water vapor, we use the following formula to compute the partial pressure of inspired oxygen:

$$PO_2 \text{ (tracheal)} = FIO_2 \times (PB - PH_2O)$$

or

$$PO_2 \text{ (tracheal)} = FIO_2 \times (PB - 47 \text{ torr})$$

Placing normal values at sea level in these equations, we calculate a tracheal PO_2 of about 149 mm Hg:

$$PO_2 \text{ (tracheal)} = 0.2095 \times (760 \text{ torr} - 47 \text{ torr})$$
$$= 149 \text{ torr}$$

Accounting for carbon dioxide. As oxygen moves into the gas exchange areas of the lung, it is further diluted by carbon dioxide. However, we cannot simply subtract the P_ACO_2, as we did for water vapor. Instead, we must correct for the difference between oxygen and carbon dioxide movement into and out of the alveoli. The amount of CO_2 moving into the alveoli per minute is abbreviated as $\dot{V}CO_2$. The amount of oxygen leaving the alveoli per min is abbreviated as $\dot{V}O_2$.[4] The ratio of the two, $\dot{V}CO_2/\dot{V}O_2$, is called the **respiratory exchange ratio** (*R*).* R averages 0.8 throughout the lung, indicating a slightly greater rate of oxygen uptake than CO_2 excretion.

For any given R, the partial pressure of CO_2 in alveolar gas is linearly related to the alveolar partial pressure of oxygen. Thus we must also correct the P_ACO_2 for the amount of oxygen in the inspired air, or F_IO_2.

You correct the P_ACO_2 for both for the respiratory exchange ratio (R) and the F_IO_2 as follows:

$$\text{Corrected } P_ACO_2 = \frac{P_ACO_2}{R} \times [1 + F_IO_2(R - 1)]$$

Alveolar air equation. Applying this corrected P_ACO_2 to the calculation of the alveolar partial pressure of oxygen, we derive the classical form of the alveolar air equation:[3]

$$P_AO_2 = F_IO_2(P_B - PH_2O) - \frac{P_ACO_2}{R}[1 + F_IO_2(R - 1)]$$

In clinical practice we usually drop the F_IO_2 correction for alveolar carbon dioxide. Because the arterial

---

*Not to be confused with the respiratory quotient (RQ), or whole-body rate of CO_2 production to oxygen consumption, the respiratory exchange ratio varies throughout the lung. For the lung as a whole, R is normally equal to 0.8.

PCO_2 nearly equals the alveolar level of this gas, we also substitute the P_ACO_2 for the P_ACO_2. On the basis of these two changes, we derive a clinical estimation form of the alveolar air equation:

$$P_AO_2 = F_IO_2(P_B - PH_2O) - \frac{P_ACO_2}{R}$$

As an example, if the F_IO_2 is 0.21, the P_B 760 torr, the PH_2O 47 torr, the P_ACO_2 40 torr, and R 0.8, we can estimate the normal alveolar partial pressure of oxygen as follows:

$$P_AO_2 = 0.21(760 \text{ torr} - 47 \text{ torr}) - \frac{40 \text{ torr}}{0.8}$$
$$= 149 \text{ torr} - 50 \text{ torr}$$
$$\approx 100 \text{ torr}$$

In clinical practice, if a patient is breathing 60% or more oxygen ($F_IO_2 \geq 0.60$), the correction for R can be dropped. This yields the following simplified form of the alveolar air equation:[3]

$$P_AO_2 = F_IO_2(P_B - PH_2O) - P_ACO_2$$

See the accompanying MiniClini for some common clinical applications of the alveolar air equation.

■ MINI CLINI ■

12-1

The alveolar-arterial PO₂ difference P(A−a)O₂ and the a/A ratio

Not all oxygen from the alveoli gets into the blood. The many reasons why blood oxygen levels fall short of those in the alveoli are discussed later in this chapter. For now, let's look at how we can actually compute the efficiency of oxygen transfer from alveoli to blood.

Two common bedside computations are used to compute the efficiency of oxygen transfer in the lungs. The first is the *difference* between the alveolar and arterial PO_2, called the **gradient** and abbreviated as $P(A-a)O_2$. Normally this difference is small, only 5 to 10 torr while breathing air and no more than 65 torr when breathing 100% oxygen.

The second common bedside computation is the *ratio* of arterial to alveolar PO_2, called the **a/A ratio**. You should think of the a/A ratio as the proportion of oxygen getting from alveoli to blood. Normally this proportion is at least 90% (a ratio of 0.9).

Problem: Compute and interpret the $P(A-a)O_2$ and a/A ratio for a 45-year-old patient breathing 70% oxygen at sea level with the following blood gases: PaO_2, 50 torr; $PaCO_2$, 50 torr.

Discussion: First, the computations:
1. Compute the P_AO_2:
$P_AO_2 = F_IO_2(P_B - PH_2O) - PaCO_2$
(patient breathing more than 60% oxygen)
$P_AO_2 = 0.70(760 - 47) - 50$
$P_AO_2 = 449.10$

2. Compute the $P(A-a)O_2$:
$P(A-a)O_2 = P_AO_2 - PaO_2$
$P(A-a)O_2 = 449 - 50$
$P(A-a)O_2 \approx 400$ torr

3. Compute the a/A:
$a/A = PaO_2/P_AO_2$
$a/A = 50/400$
$a/A = 0.13$

Both the $P(A-a)O_2$ and a/A are abnormal. Compared with a normal of 65 torr or less, the $P(A-a)O_2$ of 400 torr is very high. This indicates a large difference between the alveolar and arterial PO_2 values—that is, inefficient oxygen transfer. Likewise, the a/A ratio of 0.13 indicates that only about 13% of the oxygen in the alveoli is getting into the blood.

Conclusion: Even though she is receiving a high F_IO_2 (0.70), this patient has a severe problem getting oxygen into her blood.

Changes in alveolar gas partial tensions

Other than carbon dioxide, oxygen, and water vapor, alveoli normally contain nitrogen. Because nitrogen is inert, it takes no part in gas exchange. However, nitrogen does occupy space and exerts a partial pressure. According to Dalton's Law (see Chapter 7), the partial pressure of alveolar nitrogen must equal the pressure it would exert if it alone was present. Thus to compute the partial pressure of alveolar nitrogen, you must subtract the pressures exerted by all the other alveolar gases:

$$P_{A}N_2 = P_B - (P_{A}O_2 + P_{A}CO_2 + P_{H_2}O)$$
$$P_{A}N_2 = 760 \text{ torr} - (100 \text{ torr} + 40 \text{ torr} + 47 \text{ torr})$$
$$P_{A}N_2 = 760 \text{ torr} - (187 \text{ torr})$$
$$P_{A}N_2 = 573 \text{ torr}$$

Because both water vapor tension and $P_{A}N_2$ remain constant, the only partial pressures that change in the alveolus are those of oxygen and carbon dioxide. On the basis of the alveolar air equation shown above and assuming a constant $F_{I}O_2$ of 0.21, the $P_{A}O_2$ should vary *inversely* with the $P_{A}CO_2$.

Of course, the $P_{A}CO_2$ itself is inversely related to the level of alveolar ventilation. Thus we would expect increases in $\dot{V}_A$ to simultaneously decrease $P_{A}CO_2$ and increase $P_{A}O_2$. Decreases in $\dot{V}_A$ should have the opposite effect. As indicated in Figure 12-2, this is precisely what occurs. With constant carbon dioxide production, a decrease in $\dot{V}_A$ causes a proportional increase in $P_{A}CO_2$; this rise in $P_{A}CO_2$ causes a equivalent fall in $P_{A}O_2$. Likewise, an increase in $\dot{V}_A$ causes a drop in $P_{A}CO_2$ and a resultant rise in $P_{A}O_2$.[5]

The size of this change is governed by the limited ability of the lungs to decrease the $P_{A}CO_2$. Regulatory mechanisms and the high workload that occurs with increased alveolar ventilation prevent decreases in $P_{A}CO_2$ much below 15 to 20 torr.[3] Thus, whenever a patient is breathing room air at sea level, you should not expect to see a $P_{A}O_2$ any higher than 120 to 130 torr. PO_2 values above 120 to 130 torr indicate that the patient is breathing supplemental oxygen.

Because the total combined partial pressures of oxygen and carbon dioxide in room air is about 140

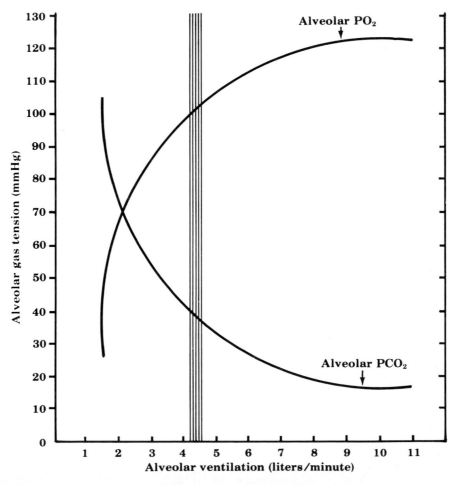

Fig. 12-2 The effect of alveolar ventilation on alveolar gases. (From Pilbeam SP: Mechanical ventilation: physiological and clinical applications, Denver, 1986, Multi-Media Publishing.)

■ MINI CLINI ■

12-2

Assessing Arterial Gas Partial Pressures

Problem: You are given the following arterial blood gas report for a patient just admitted to the emergency room:

PaO$_2$ 170 torr
PaCO$_2$ 23 torr

Without additional data, what conclusions can you draw about this patient?

Discussion: In room air, the total pressure exerted by oxygen and carbon dioxide in the alveoli (and blood) should be about 140 torr. In this case, the total is 170 (PaO$_2$) + 23 (PaCO$_2$), or 193 torr. Whenever this total significantly exceeds 140 *and* the PaO$_2$ is above 120 to 130 torr, you can be sure that the patient is breathing supplemental oxygen.

torr, you can estimate the impact of a change in PaCO$_2$ on PaO$_2$ with the following rule of thumb:

$$PaO_2 = 140 \text{ torr} - PaCO_2$$

Of course, this rule of thumb assumes that the respiratory exchange ratio remains stable at 0.8. In reality, even in the normal lung, the respiratory exchange ratio varies greatly. These variations are due to imbalances in the amount of ventilation and perfusion throughout the normal lung.[6] However, before discussing this important relationship, we must first analyze how respiratory gases are exchanged between the alveoli and the blood and the blood and the tissues.

See the accompanying MiniClini for some common clinical applications of these principles.

Mechanism of diffusion

Not too long ago, physiologists thought that pulmonary gas exchange was an active process of secretion and **absorption**. Today, we know that the movement of gases throughout the body depends on the relatively simple physical process of diffusion.

Barriers to diffusion

As described in Chapter 7, *diffusion* is the process whereby gas molecules move from an area of high partial pressure to an area of low partial pressure. As all motion requires some driving force, so diffusion depends on a pressure gradient. The two gases with which we are concerned, oxygen and carbon dioxide, not only must diffuse from one area to another but also must move through formidable barriers.

The barrier to gaseous diffusion in the lung is the *alveolar-capillary membrane*. At the cellular level, gases must traverse a similar barrier between the tissue capillary and cell wall. Thus, for gases to pass throughout the body, pressure gradients must be sufficient to overcome these diffusion barriers. Of primary concern to the RCP is the process of diffusion at the site of external respiration—that is, the alveolar-capillary membrane.

Figure 12-3 shows how this process occurs. For CO$_2$ or O$_2$ to move between alveolus and blood, four "layers" must be penetrated. In sequence for oxygen movement into the blood, these layers are the pulmonary surfactant, the alveolar epithelial membrane, the interstitial fluid space, and the capillary endothelial membrane.[7] Moreover, for CO$_2$ or O$_2$ to pass in and out of the red blood cell, they also must traverse the **erythrocyte** cell membrane.

Fick's law of diffusion

The bulk movement of a gas through a biological membrane ($\dot{V}_{gas}$) is described by *Fick's Law of Diffusion.*[8]

$$\dot{V}_{gas} = \frac{A \times D}{T} (P_1 - P_2)$$

In this formula, *A* is the cross-sectional area available for diffusion, and *D* is the diffusion coefficient of the gas. *T* is the thickness of the membrane, and $P_1 - P_2$ is the partial pressure gradient across the membrane.

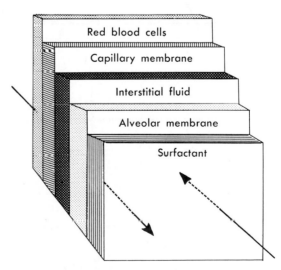

Fig. 12-3 The five barriers through which O$_2$ and CO$_2$ pass at the alveolocapillary membrane. (From McLaughlin AJ Jr: Essentials of physiology for advanced respiratory therapy, St Louis, 1977, Mosby.)

According to Fick's Law, the volume of a gas diffusing across a biological membrane per unit time will be greatest when the area, gas diffusion constant, and partial pressure gradient are all large; and the distance across the membrane is small. Conversely, a small area, low gas diffusion constant, small partial pressure gradient, or large diffusing distance can, alone or in combination, impede diffusion.

Given that the cross-sectional area and distance across the alveolar-capillary membrane is relatively constant in the normal lung, we will focus mainly on the actual partial pressure gradients and the relative ease with which oxygen and carbon dioxide diffuse in and out of the alveoli.

Pulmonary diffusion gradients

For gas exchange to occur between alveolus and pulmonary capillary, a difference in partial pressures $(P_1 - P_2)$ must exist. Figure 12-4 shows the size and direction of these gradients for oxygen and carbon dioxide.

As previously described, the partial pressures of oxygen and carbon dioxide in the ideal alveolus are determined mainly by the FIO_2 and level of alveolar ventilation relative to CO_2 production. Although these pressures vary somewhat with the breathing cycle, the alveolar PO_2 averages 100 torr, whereas the mean PCO_2 is about 40 torr.

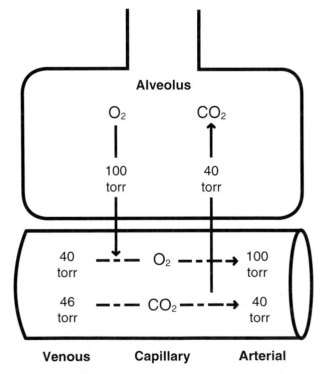

Fig. 12-4 Ventilation maintains the mean alveolar gas pressures for O_2 and CO_2. As blood enters the venous end of the capillary it gives up CO_2 and loads O_2 until these two gases are in equilibrium with alveolar pressures. At this point the blood is "arterialized."

Mixed venous blood returning to the lungs has a lower partial pressure of oxygen (40 torr) than alveolar gas. Thus the pressure gradient for movement of O_2 is about 60 torr (100 torr − 40 torr) and favors diffusion from alveolus into the blood. Conversely, venous blood returning to the lungs has a higher partial pressure of oxygen (46 torr) than alveolar gas. Thus the pressure gradient for CO_2 is smaller than that for oxygen but opposite in its direction. This favors diffusion of CO_2 from the blood into the alveolus.

Oxygen therefore diffuses from the alveolus into the pulmonary blood. As blood flows past the alveolus, it takes up oxygen, leaving the capillary with a PO_2 nearly equal to the alveolar value of 100 torr. At the same time, carbon dioxide diffuses in the opposite direction until the capillary blood PCO_2 **equilibrates** with the alveolar PCO_2. This "arterialized" blood thus leaves the capillary with a PCO_2 of about 40 torr.

Diffusion coefficients

Like the partial pressure gradient, the amount of a gas diffusing across a biological membrane is directly proportional to its diffusion coefficient. The diffusion coefficient is defined as the amount of gas (in milliliters per minute) that will diffuse a distance of 1 μm over a square-centimeter area with a pressure gradient of 760 torr.[9]

Because gas movement through the alveolar-capillary membrane is essentially diffusion through a liquid barrier, the diffusion coefficient must take into account both the density of the gas and its solubility in the liquid. *Graham's Law* states that the diffusion coefficient of a gas (D) is inversely proportional to the square root of its density (or gram molecular weight):

$$D \propto \frac{1}{\sqrt{gmw}}$$

The solubility coefficient is defined as the volume of a gas that can dissolve in 1 mL of a given liquid at standard pressure (760 torr) and specified temperature. The higher a gas' solubility coefficient, the faster it will diffuse through a liquid.

Combining these two concepts, the diffusion coefficient for gas movement across the alveolar-capillary membrane must be directly proportional to the solubility coefficient of the gas, and inversely proportional to the square root of its gram molecular weight:

$$D \propto \frac{Solubility\ coefficient}{\sqrt{gmw}}$$

Given that the solubility coefficient of oxygen in plasma at 37° C is 0.023 mL/760 torr and that for carbon dioxide is 0.510 mL/760 torr, we may compare the relative ease with which each diffuses across the alveolar-capillary membrane:

$$D_{O_2} \approx \frac{0.023}{\sqrt{32}} \approx 0.004$$

$$D_{CO_2} \approx \frac{0.510}{\sqrt{44}} \approx 0.077$$

$$\frac{D_{CO_2}}{D_{O_2}} \approx \frac{0.077}{0.004} \approx \frac{19}{1}$$

Thus carbon dioxide diffuses about 20 times faster across the alveolar-capillary membrane than oxygen, mainly because of its higher solubility in plasma. In the normal lung, this difference explains why a much smaller pressure gradient (6 torr) is required to move CO_2 across the alveolar-capillary membrane than is needed to move like amounts of oxygen (60 torr). Moreover, this difference in diffusibility explains why disorders that impair the lung's diffusion capacity mainly affect oxygen, with little effect on carbon dioxide.[10] That such disorders can and do impede the movement of oxygen from alveolus into the pulmonary capillary circulation is due entirely to the lower diffusion coefficient of oxygen.

Time limits to diffusion

For blood to leave the pulmonary capillary adequately oxygenated, it must spend enough time in contact with the alveolus to allow equilibration. Because of the higher diffusion coefficient of carbon dioxide, its movement across the alveolar-capillary membrane is seldom affected by time. However, the time available for oxygen diffusion from the alveolus into the pulmonary circulation can be critical. Should inadequate time be available for diffusion, blood leaving the lungs may not be fully oxygenated.

The diffusion time in the lung depends on the rate of pulmonary blood flow. As depicted in Figure 12-5, blood normally takes about 0.75 seconds to pass through the pulmonary capillary.[5] This time is more than enough to ensure complete diffusion of oxygen across the alveolar-capillary membrane.[11]

Should blood flow increase, as during heavy exercise, time spent in the pulmonary capillary can decrease by as much as two thirds, down to about 0.25 seconds.[11] Even this short a time frame is adequate to ensure that equilibration takes place, as long as no other factors impair diffusion.[12]

However, when disorders that impede diffusion occur together with conditions that increase cardiac output, rapid blood flow through the pulmonary circulation can further impair the lung's ability to provide adequate oxygenation.[5] Fever and **septic shock** are good examples of clinical conditions that limit the time available for diffusion by increasing blood flow through the lung.

Measuring diffusing capacity

In clinical practice, knowledge of the lung's diffusing capacity can be helpful in evaluating certain disease states. The diffusing capacity of the lung (D_L) is defined as the value, in milliliters per minute, of a specific gas that diffuses across the alveolar-capillary membrane into the blood, for each millimeter mercury difference in the pressure gradient.[13-14]

Although oxygen can be used to measure the diffusion capacity of the lung, it is more common to use low concentrations (0.1% to 0.3%) of carbon monoxide. Carbon monoxide is preferred over oxygen because its higher affinity for hemoglobin keeps its capillary partial pressure extremely low. This minimizes the effect of variations in blood flow on the measurement.[4]

The normal value for the diffusing capacity of the lung (D_LCO), as measured with the single-breath carbon monoxide test, is about 27 mL/min/torr.[5] Because oxygen's diffusion coefficient is about 1.23 times greater than that of carbon monoxide, you can convert the value obtained with carbon monoxide to that for oxygen by multiplying the D_LCO by this factor. Details on the theory underlying the measurement of diffusing capacity and the clinical implications of abnormal test results are provided in Chapter 18.

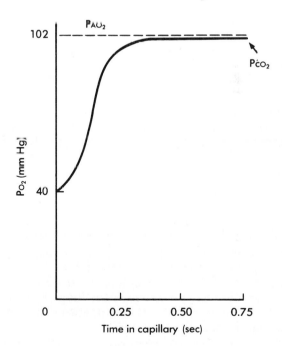

Fig. 12-5 Alveolar-capillary PO_2 gradient. Normal transit time for a red blood cell in the pulmonary capillary is approximately 0.75 sec. Blood PO_2 reaches near equilibrium with alveolar PO_2 (PA_{O_2}) well before the end of capillary transit time. (From Martin L: Pulmonary physiology in clinical practice: the essentials for patient care and evaluation, St Louis, 1987, Mosby.)

Systemic diffusion gradients

So far we have focused only on gas pressure gradients at the alveolar-capillary membrane. For a complete picture of diffusion, we must include the equally important gradients at the tissue level.

The partial pressure gradients in the tissues are the opposite of those in the lung. As the metabolism of the cell depletes its oxygen, the intracellular PO_2 drops below that of the blood entering the tissue capillary. Oxygen thus diffuses from the tissue capillary blood ($PO_2 = 100$ torr) to the cells ($PO_2 < 40$ torr). Simultaneously, carbon dioxide diffuses from the cells ($PCO_2 > 46$ torr) into the capillary blood ($PCO_2 = 40$ torr). After equilibration, blood leaves the tissue capillaries as venous blood. Venous blood gas tensions roughly equal those at the tissue level, that is, a PO_2 of about 40 torr, and a PCO_2 of about 46 torr.

Just as arterial blood reflects the gas exchange occurring in the lung, venous blood reflects events in tissues. For this reason, assessment of gas exchange at the tissue level, especially tissue oxygenation, requires measurement of venous blood parameters. The collection and use of venous blood in the assessment of tissue oxygenation is discussed further in Chapters 17 and 33.

VARIATIONS FROM IDEAL GAS EXCHANGE

Up to this point, we have focused almost entirely on the gas partial pressures in a "perfect" alveolus—that is, one with ideal ventilation and blood flow. In reality, the normal lung is an imperfect organ of gas exchange. Clinically, this becomes clear when we measure the arterial partial pressures of oxygen in normal subjects.

In theory, if all the blood leaving the lung were to pass through "ideal" alveoli with a $P_{A}O_2$ of 100 torr, then partial pressure of oxygen in the arterial blood would equal that in the alveoli, 100 torr. In reality, the PaO_2 of normal subjects breathing air at sea level is always about 5 to 10 torr less than the calculated $P_{A}O_2$ (see MiniClini 12-1).[5]

Two factors account for this normal difference: (1) anatomic shunts in the pulmonary circulation, and (2) regional differences in ventilation and blood flow throughout the lung.[4,6] In addition to these normal factors, pathologic processes in the lung can increase this difference even more. These abnormal factors are described in detail in Chapter 15.

Anatomic shunts

An anatomic shunt is a direct connection between the venous and arterial sides of the circulation. A right-to-left anatomic shunt occurs when venous blood flow bypasses the pulmonary circulation, thereby never contacting the areas of gas exchange. This venous blood then enters the arterial circulation without picking up oxygen or removing excess carbon dioxide. This "dilutes" the oxygen content and raises the amount of carbon dioxide in the arterial blood. Two such anatomic shunts exist in the normal human: the bronchial venous drainage and the thebesian venous drainage.

As discussed in Chapter 9, as much as two thirds of the return flow of the bronchial circulation (venous blood) empties into the pulmonary veins (arterialized blood). Although the flow through this anatomic shunt is small, it does decrease the oxygen content of arterial blood. The thebesian veins drain a portion of the coronary circulation and empty into both sides of the heart. Those that flow into the left side mix venous blood with arterial, thereby furthering lowering the oxygen content of the arterial blood.

In combination, these normal anatomic shunts account for some 70% to 80% of the difference between the observed and expected levels of arterial oxygenation in normal subjects. The remaining 20% to 30% is due to normal inequalities in ventilation and perfusion in the lung.

Regional inequalities in ventilation and perfusion

The normal respiratory exchange ratio of 0.8 assumes that both ventilation and perfusion in the lung are in perfect balance. Perfect balance would require that every liter of alveolar ventilation ($\dot{V}_A$) be matched by a liter of pulmonary capillary blood flow ($\dot{Q}c$).

Any variation from this perfect balance should alter gas tensions in the affected alveoli. If pulmonary blood flow remains constant and $\dot{V}_A$ increases, we would expect the alveolar PCO_2 to fall and the alveolar PO_2 to rise. On the other hand, a decrease in $\dot{V}_A$ should result in a higher alveolar PCO_2 and a lower alveolar PO_2.[6]

Changing blood flow will also disrupt the ideal balance in alveolar gas partial pressures. If alveolar ventilation remains constant but $\dot{Q}c$ increases, carbon dioxide coming from the tissues will be delivered to the alveolus faster than it can be removed. This will cause the alveolar PCO_2 to rise. Conversely, as blood flow increases, oxygen will be taken up by the capillaries faster than it can be restored by ventilation. This will cause a fall in alveolar PO_2. Should pulmonary capillary blood flow decrease, alveolar gas tensions would change in the opposite direction.

The ventilation-perfusion ratio

Changes in $\dot{V}_A$ and $\dot{Q}c$ are expressed as a ratio, called the ventilation-perfusion ratio (V/Q). An ideal ratio of 1.0 indicates that ventilation and perfusion in the pulmonary exchange units are in perfect balance. A high V/Q indicates that ventilation is greater than normal, perfusion is less than normal, or both. In the presence of a high V/Q, the alveolar PO_2 is always increased above normal, whereas the PCO_2 is always lower than normal.[16]

On the other hand, a low V/Q indicates that ventilation is less than normal, perfusion is greater than normal, or both. In the presence of a low V/Q, the alveolar PO_2 is always below normal, whereas the PCO_2 is always above normal.[16] These relationships are summarized below:

V/Q	PAO_2	$PACO_2$
High	↑	↓
Low	↓	↑

Effect of alterations in the V/Q

Obviously, these changes in ventilation and perfusion affect the respiratory exchange ratio. Figure 12-6 graphs the effect of V/Q changes on the respiratory exchange ratio (R), plotting all possible values of alveolar PO_2 and PCO_2.[6]

Note that when ventilation and perfusion are in perfect balance (V/Q = 1.0), the respiratory exchange ratio equals 0.8. At this point, the alveolar PO_2 and PCO_2 values equal the ideal values of 100 and 40 torr, respectively.

As the V/Q rises above 1.0 (following the curve to the right), the ratio of carbon dioxide excretion to oxygen uptake (R) also increases. The result is a higher alveolar PO_2 and a lower alveolar PCO_2. At the extreme right of the graph, perfusion is zero, and the V/Q is infinitely large. An infinitely large V/Q indicates the presence of ventilation without blood flow. With no blood flow to unload CO_2 or take up oxygen,

the makeup of gases in an area with an infinitely large V/Q will be like that of inspired air (PO_2 = 150 torr; PCO_2 = 0 torr). Exchange units with an infinite V/Q ratio represent alveolar deadspace, as defined in Chapter 11. The normal lung has little or no alveolar deadspace.

As the V/Q drops below 1.0 (following the curve to the left), the ratio of carbon dioxide excretion to oxygen uptake (R) decreases. The result is a lower alveolar PO_2 and a higher alveolar PCO_2. At the extreme left of the graph, ventilation is nil, resulting in a V/Q ratio of 0. At this point, there is perfusion but no ventilation. With no ventilation to remove CO_2 and restore fresh oxygen, the makeup of gases in an area with a V/Q of 0 would be like that of mixed venous blood (PO_2 = 40 torr; PCO_2 = 46 torr).

Because exchange units with V/Q values of 0 provide no gas exchange, blood passing through them cannot pick up oxygen or unload carbon dioxide. In these areas, venous blood arrives and leaves unchanged. When it later mixes with the arterial circulation, such blood has the same effect as that coming from a right-to-left anatomic shunt. To distinguish such areas from true anatomic shunts, we call exchange units with V/Q values of 0 called "alveolar shunts." Although small anatomic shunts are normal, alveolar shunts always indicate a disease process.

Although alveolar deadspace and shunts do not exist in the normal lung, V/Q values do vary substantially from the ideal. Reasons for this variation, and its impact on gas exchange, are the focus of the next section.

Causes of regional differences in V/Q

Regional variations in V/Q in the normal lung are due mainly to gravity and thus are most evident in the

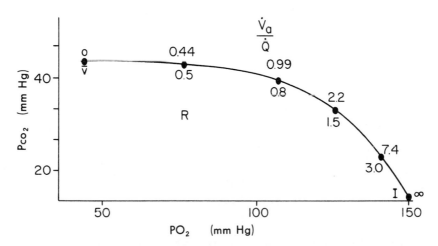

Fig. 12-6 A curve may be drawn that joins the points (representing the values of PO_2 and PCO_2) that are determined by given values for the respiratory exchange ratio (R), the ventilation/perfusion ratio (VA/Q), the composition of mixed venous blood (v̄), and inspired air (I). (From Cherniack RM and Cherniack L: Respiration in health and disease, ed 3, Philadelphia, 1983, WB Saunders.)

upright posture. Although gravity affects the distribution of both blood flow and ventilation in the lung, it has a greater impact on perfusion than on ventilation.

Perfusion. Because the pulmonary circulation is a low-pressure system, blood flow in the upright lung varies considerably from top to bottom. As described in Chapter 9, **hydrostatic** pressures in the pulmonary circulation decrease about 1 cm H_2O for every centimeters of distance from the lung base to its apex.[8] Toward the apex of the lung, perfusion is minimal (low $\dot{Q}c$). As one moves down the lung, perfusion increases linearly in proportion to the hydrostatic pressure, such that the lung bases receive nearly 20 times as much blood flow as the apices.[8]

Ventilation. Regional differences in ventilation throughout the lung also occur, but are less drastic than those for perfusion. Like perfusion, ventilation also increases from lung apex to base. These regional differences in ventilation are due to gravity's effect on pleural pressures (see Chapter 11).

Pleural pressures decrease by about 0.25 cm H_2O for each cm distance from the lung base to its apex, such that apical pleural pressures (about -10 cm H_2O) are about 7.5 cm H_2O less than pleural pressures at the lung bases.[8] Because of these differences in pleural pressures, the transpulmonary pressure gradient at the top of the lung is greater than at the bottom. Alveoli at the apices are thus kept at a higher resting volume than those at the bases. However, because they are positioned on the steeper portion of the lung's pressure-volume curve, alveoli at the bases expand more than alveoli at the apex during inspiration (refer to Chapter 11). Thus about four times as much ventilation goes to the bases of the upright lung than to its apices.

Figure 12-7 summarizes the relationship between ventilation and perfusion in the normal upright lung. As you can see, both blood flow and ventilation decrease from bottom to top, but blood flow decreases proportionately more than ventilation.[6] At the bottom of the lung, blood flow is greater than ventilation, resulting in a low V/Q. As we work our way up the lung, blood flow decreases more than ventilation, such that toward the middle, the two are about equal (V/Q = 1.0). As we progress up toward the apices, ventilation begins to exceed blood flow, resulting in increasing V/Q values.

Of course, these regional differences in V/Q alter the respiratory exchange ratio, thereby affecting the partial pressures of oxygen and carbon dioxide in the alveoli.[6] Indeed, at the top of the upright lung, the V/Q ratio is about 3.3, R is about 2.0, the alveolar PO_2 averages 132 torr, and the alveolar PCO_2 is maintained at about 28 torr. On the other hand, at the lung bases, where the V/Q ratio is about 0.6, R is about 0.66, the alveolar PO_2 averages 89 torr, and the alveolar PCO_2 is maintained at about 42 torr.

These deviations from the ideal balance help explain why gas exchange within the lung is not perfect. Were all blood to pass through ideal exchange units, arterial partial pressures of oxygen and carbon dioxide would equal those in a perfectly ventilated and

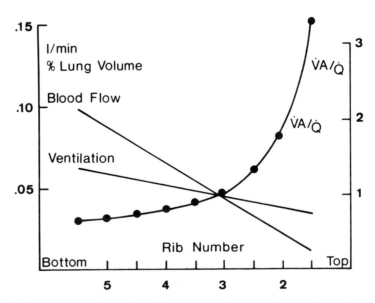

Fig. 12-7 Distribution of ventilation, blood flow, and ventilation-perfusion ratio up the normal upright lung. Straight lines have been drawn through the ventilation and blood flow data. Because blood flow falls more rapidly than ventilation with distance up the lung, the ventilation-perfusion ratio rises, slowly at first, then rapidly. (From West JB: Ventilation/bloodflow and gas exchange, Oxford, 1970, Blackwell Scientific Publishers.)

perfused alveolus. However, most blood flows through exchange units at the bases of the lung. Here blood flow exceeds ventilation (low V/Q), and PO_2 values are lower and PCO_2 values are higher than those in a perfect exchange unit. After leaving the lung, this relatively large volume of blood combines with the smaller volume coming from the apices. The result is a mixture with less oxygen and more carbon dioxide than would come from an idea gas exchange unit.[4]

In reality, V/Q inequalities always have a greater impact on the exchange of oxygen than on carbon dioxide.[3] To understand this complex phenomenon (discussed in detail in Chapter 15), we must first analyze the differences in how these two respiratory gases are transported in the blood.

OXYGEN TRANSPORT

Oxygen is carried in the blood in two different states.[17,18] A small amount of oxygen always exists in simple physical solution, dissolved in the plasma and erythrocyte intracellular fluid. However, the vast majority of oxygen is carried in reversible chemical combination with hemoglobin inside the red blood cell.

Physically dissolved oxygen

As oxygen diffuses into the blood, it immediately dissolves in the plasma and erythrocyte intracellular fluid. According to Henry's Law, the amount of oxygen that dissolves will be directly proportional to its solubility coefficient and inversely proportional to the temperature. Assuming a constant body temperature of 37° C, 0.023 mL of oxygen will dissolve in each mL of plasma at a PO_2 of 760 torr.[17]

In clinical practice, we measure and record dissolved blood gases in milliliters of gas per deciliter (100 mL) of plasma, or mL/dL. Because 0.023 mL O_2/mL equals 2.3 mL O_2/100 mL, 2.3 mL/dL of oxygen are carried in physical solution at a pressure of 760 torr PO_2. By dividing 2.3 by 760, we derive a constant equal to the milliliters of oxygen that dissolve in each deciliter of blood for each torr PO_2:

$$\text{mL/dL } O_2/\text{torr } PO_2 = 2.3/760 = 0.003$$

Thus you can compute the volume of dissolved oxygen for any PO_2 by simply multiplying this factor times the partial pressure of oxygen in the blood:

$$\text{Dissolved oxygen (mL/dL)} = PO_2 \times 0.003$$

Figure 12-8 depicts this equation. As you can see, the relationship between partial pressure and dissolve oxygen is direct and linear. For example, in normal arterial blood with its PaO_2 of about 100 torr, there is about 0.3 mL/dL dissolved oxygen. However, if a normal subject breathes pure oxygen, the arterial PO_2 increases to about 670 torr. In this case, the dissolved

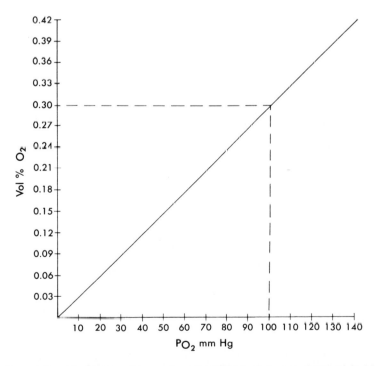

Fig. 12-8 The relationship between the number of milliliters of oxygen dissolved in blood and its consequent partial pressure is linear. Each 0.003 mL of oxygen dissolved in 100 mL of blood (vol% of O_2) exerts a pressure of 1 torr. The *dashed line* emphasizes the fact that arterial blood, with an average PO_2 of 100 torr, has 0.3 mL of oxygen dissolved in each 100 mL.

oxygen would increase to about 2.0 mL/dL. The blood of a subject breathing pure oxygen in a **hyperbaric** chamber at 3 atm pressure (2280 torr) would carry nearly 6.5 mL/dL dissolved oxygen in the plasma. This amount is itself enough to supply most tissue needs!

However, this high PO_2 is not normally available to the lung. Moreover, even if it were, PO_2 values this high quickly cause direct damage to the lungs and nervous system. Instead of relying solely on dissolved oxygen for transport, the body has developed a unique and efficient chemical means for carrying this essential gas.

Chemically combined oxygen

The nature of hemoglobin

Most oxygen in the body is carried chemically combined with hemoglobin (Hb) in the erythrocytes. Hb is a **conjugated protein,** consisting of four linked **polypeptide** chains (the globin portion), each of which is combined with a **porphyrin** complex called heme. The four polypeptide chains of Hb are coiled together into a ball-like structure, the shape of which determines its affinity for oxygen.[1]

As shown in Figure 12-9, each heme complex contains a centrally located ferrous iron ion (Fe^{++}). When hemoglobin is not carrying oxygen, this ion has four unpaired electrons.[17,18] In this deoxygenated state, the molecule exhibits the characteristics of a weak acid and is referred to as reduced reduced hemoglobin (Hb^-). As such, Hb^- serves as an important blood **buffer** for hydrogen ions, a factor critically important in CO_2 transport (addressed subsequently).

Oxygen molecules bind to hemoglobin by way of the ferrous iron ion, one for each protein chain. With complete oxygen binding, all electrons become paired, and the Hb^- is converted to its oxygenated state (HbO_2, or *oxyhemoglobin*).

Oxygen-carrying capacity of hemoglobin

Knowing that each Hb^- molecule can combine with four molecules of O_2, you can compute the total oxygen carried by each gram of Hb. With a molecular weight of about 66,700, 1 mol of hemoglobin weighs 66,700 g. This weight of hemoglobin can combine with 4 mol of oxygen. Because 1 mol of oxygen at STPD is equivalent to 22.4 L or 22,400 mL (Avogadro's Law), 66,700 g of Hb can chemically combine with $4 \times 22,400$ mL oxygen. To compute the amount of oxygen carried by 1 g of hemoglobin, simply divide

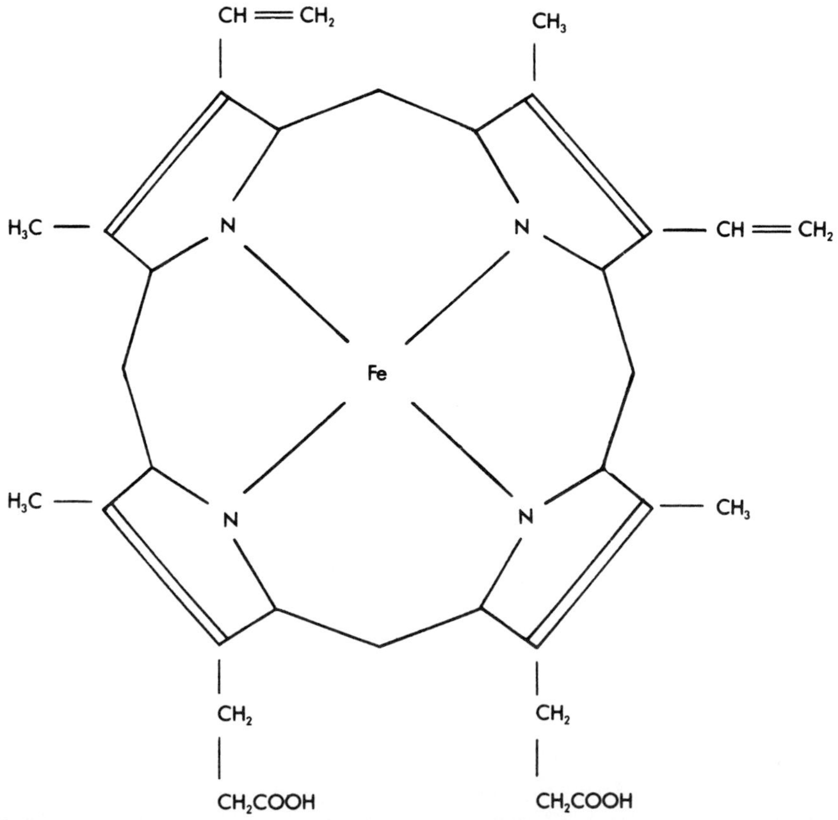

Fig. 12-9 Structure of heme. (From Lane EE and Walker JF: Clinical arterial blood gas analysis, St Louis, 1987, Mosby.)

the volume equivalent of 4 mol of oxygen by the gram molecular weight of Hb:

$$\frac{4 \times 22,400 \text{ mL/mol}}{66,700 \text{ gm/mol}} = 1.34 \text{ mL/gm*}$$

Thus each gram of Hb can carry about 1.34 mL of oxygen. Given an average Hb content in whole blood of 15 g/100 mL (15 g/dL), you can compute the oxygen-carrying capacity of the blood due to chemical combination with Hb:

$$1.34 \text{ mL/g} \times 15 \text{ g/100 mL} = 20.1 \text{ mL/100 mL} = 20.1 \text{ mL/dL}$$

Compared with the blood's limited ability to carry disolved oxygen (0.3 mL/dL), the addition of hemoglobin increases the oxygen-carrying capacity nearly 70-fold! How much of the oxygen-carrying capacity of Hb is actually used depends on its saturation.

Hb saturation

Saturation is a measure of the proportion of available hemoglobin that is actually carrying oxygen. Specifically, you compute saturation as the ratio of HbO_2 (content) to total Hb (capacity).[17] Hb saturation (SaO_2) is always expressed as a percentage of this ratio of content to capacity and calculated according to the following formula:

$$SaO_2 = \frac{[HbO_2]}{[Hb^-] + [HbO_2]} \times 100$$

where $[HbO_2]$ equals the amount of HbO_2 (the content), and $[Hb^-] + [HbO_2]$ is the total Hb available to carry oxygen, both reduced and oxygenated (the capacity).

For example, were there a total of 15 g/dL Hb in the blood ($Hb^- + HbO_2$), of which 7.5 g was HbO_2, SaO_2 would be calculated as:

$$SaO_2 = \frac{7.5}{15} \times 100 = 50\%$$

In this example, the Hb is said to be *50% saturated.* This means that only half the available Hb is actually carrying oxygen, with the remainder being reduced or unoxygenated. In actual clinical practice, we directly measure both SaO_2 and total Hb content ($[Hb^-] + [HbO_2]$) and thereby derive the $[HbO_2]$.

The HbO_2 dissociation curve

The degree of Hb saturation is determined by its affinity for oxygen at various partial pressures. The relationship between Hb saturation and PO_2 is described by the HbO_2 dissociation curve.[19]

Unlike dissolved O_2, hemoglobin saturation is not linearly related to PO_2. Instead, this relationship forms an S-shaped curve (Figure 12-10, on page 276). The relatively flat upper part of this curve represents the normal operating range for arterial blood. Because the slope is minimal in this area, minor changes in PaO_2—resulting from disease or environmental abnormalities—have little effect on Hb saturation, indicating a strong affinity of Hb for oxygen. For instance, with a normal arterial PO_2 of 100 torr, Hb is about 97% saturated with oxygen. Were some abnormality to reduce the PaO_2 to 65 torr, the hemoglobin would still be about 90% saturated with oxygen.

However, below a PO_2 of 60 torr, the curve steepens dramatically. Here, in the normal operating range of the tissues, even a small drop in PO_2 causes a large drop in Hb saturation, indicating a lessening affinity for oxygen. This normal change in the affinity of Hb for oxygen helps assure release of large amounts of oxygen in the systemic capillaries in response to relatively small decreases in tissue PO_2.

Total oxygen content of the blood

The total amount of oxygen in a given volume of blood, or total oxygen content, must equal the sum of that in physical solution and that chemically combined with hemoglobin. Total oxygen content is abbreviated as CxO_2, with the x referencing the type of blood being measured. Typically, x will be replaced with either an *a*, indicating arterial blood, or a *v*, indicating venous blood (see Chapter 6).

To calculate total oxygen contents, you must know three values: PO_2, the total hemoglobin content (g/dL), and SaO_2. Given these values, you proceed in three steps. First, calculate the dissolved oxygen. Then calculate the oxygen chemically combined with Hb. Last, add these two quantities to derive the total (dissolved + chemically combined).

For example, assume that you obtain a sample of arterial blood with a PO_2 of 100 torr containing 15 g/dL of Hb that is 97% saturated with oxygen. As a first step, you calculate the amount of dissolved oxygen by multiplying the PaO_2 by 0.003:

$$\text{Dissolved } O_2 = PO_2 \times 0.003$$
$$\text{Dissolved } O_2 = 100 \times 0.003 = 0.30 \text{ mL/dL}$$

To calculate the amount of oxygen chemically combined with Hb, you multiply the hemoglobin content (15 g/dL) times its carrying capacity (1.34 mL/gm) by the saturation of hemoglobin with oxygen (derived from the oxyhemoglobin dissociation curve):

$$\text{Chemically combined } O_2 = \text{Hb (g/dL)} \times 1.34 \text{ mL/g} \times SaO_2$$
$$\text{Chemically combined } O_2 = 15 \text{ g/dL} \times 1.34 \text{ mL/g} \times 97\%$$
$$= 19.50 \text{ mL/dL}$$

---

*The figure 1.34 mL/gm is based on STPD conditions. Theoretically, at BTPS the carrying capacity of Hb is higher, about 1.39 mL/gm. However, the STPD value of 1.34 is most widely used and therefore retained for this section.

■ MINI CLINI ■

12-3

Relating Hemoglobin Saturation and PaO$_2$

Problem: Pulse **oximeters** are simple bedside devices that measure Hb saturation by way of a noninvasive probe that is taped to the finger or forehead. Although oximeters measure percent Hb saturation, we still tend to quantify blood oxygenation according to arterial PO$_2$. Is there a simple way to relate these two measures (without carrying around an oxyhemoglobin dissociation curve)?

Discussion: First, although extremely useful, pulse oximeters are not very accurate ($\pm4\%$) and only measure normal hemoglobin saturation. For this reason, their use should be limited to following trends or warning of significant changes in hemoglobin saturation with oxygen.

Even so, you will often need to estimate arterial PO$_2$ from oximeter readings. The following simple rule of thumb should help. We call it the **40–50–60/70–80–90 rule.** Assuming normal pH, PCO$_2$ and normal Hb,

saturations of 70%, 80% and 90% are roughly equivalent to PO$_2$ values of 40, 50, and 60 torr, respectively:

Hemoglobin saturation	Approximate arterial PO$_2$
70%	40 torr
80%	50 torr
90%	60 torr

Thus a patient with a pulse oximeter reading of 90% has a PaO$_2$ of about 60 torr. Should saturation drop to 80%, PaO$_2$ will fall to about 50 torr. Note that this rule of thumb only works in the middle range of PO$_2$ values (where the curve is most linear); do not apply it with saturations above 90%. For example, a saturation of 100% may represent a PaO$_2$ of 200 torr.

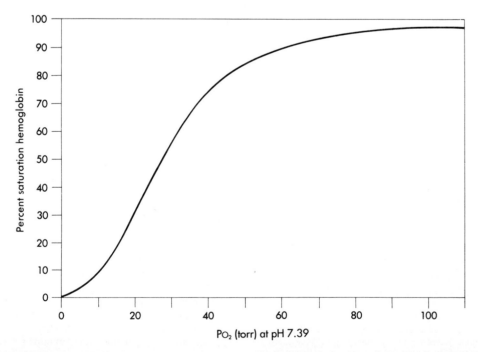

Fig. 12–10 The oxygen dissociation curve plots the relation between hemoglobin saturation (y-axis) and plasma PO$_2$ (x-axis). (From Lane EE and Walker JF: Clinical arterial blood gas analysis, St Louis, 1987, Mosby.)

Last, you add the dissolved oxygen to that carried by hemoglobin. This yields the total arterial oxygen content, or CaO_2:

$$CaO_2 = \text{Dissolved } O_2 + \text{chemically combined } O_2$$
$$= 0.30 \text{ mL/dL} + 19.50 \text{ mL/dL}$$
$$= 19.80 \text{ mL/dL}$$

For a clinical application of these computations, see the accompanying MiniCini on the effect of **anemia** on oxygen content.

Of course, you also can also calculate the oxygen content of blood returning from the tissues after it unloads its oxygen. By comparing the difference in oxygen content between the point of oxygen loading (the lungs) and the point of oxygen unloading (the tissues), you can gain important insight into the overall mechanism of oxygen transport.

Normal loading and unloading of oxygen (arterial-venous differences)

In Figure 12-11, the oxyhemoglobin dissociation curve is labeled to show the effects of oxygen loading unloading, relative to changes in saturation and oxygen content of arterial and venous blood. Point Ⓐ represents normal values for arterial blood, with point Ⓥ indicating normal venous parameters.

Blood leaving the lungs (point Ⓐ) has a PO_2 of about 100 torr. At this PO_2, the hemoglobin is about 97% saturated with oxygen. When arterial

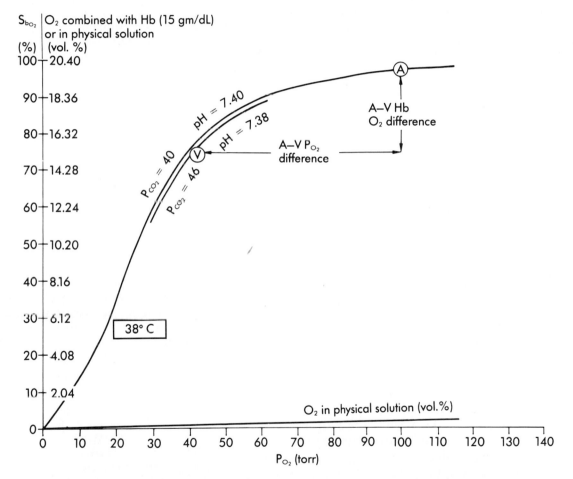

Fig. 12-11 The oxyhemoglobin dissociation curve, showing the basic relationship of blood O_2 transport. Its shape has great physiologic importance. The full curve above applies to the arterial blood of healthy man at rest, whereas the small section to its right applies to venous blood. Point A represents normal values for arterial blood, and point V, for venous blood. Changes in CO_2 pressure, pH, or temperature displace the oxyhemoglobin dissociation curve to the right or left. A physiologic shift from the venous to the arterial curve takes place as blood flows through the pulmonary capillaries, losing CO_2 and increasing in pH. The reverse shift occurs as blood flows through the systemic capillaries. Note that this effect, termed the Bohr shift, facilitates O_2 uptake in the lungs and O_2 dumping in the tissues. Note also the relatively small amount of O_2 carried by the blood in physical solution in the physiologic range of O_2 pressure. (From Slonim NB and Hamilton LH, ed 5, St Louis, 1987, Mosby.)

■ M I N I **C** L I N I ■

12-4

Effect of Anemia on Oxygen Content

In its most common form, anemia is a clinical disorder in which the number of red blood cells is decreased. Because the red blood cells carry hemoglobin, anemia decreases the amount of this oxygen-carrying protein.

Problem: What effect will anemia that causes a progressive drop in hemoglobin from (a) 15 to (b) 12 to (c) 8 to (d) 4 g/dL have on the amount of oxygen carried in a patient's blood? Assume that the PO_2 and saturation stay normal—100 torr and 97% respectively.

Discussion: First, the computations:
1. Calculate dissolved oxygen (the same for all four):

Dissolved O_2 = 100 × 0.003 = 0.30 mL/dL

2. Compute chemically combined oxygen

Chemically combined O_2 = Hb (g/dL) × 1.34 mL/gm × SaO_2

a. 15 g/dL × 1.34 mL/gm × 97% = 19.50 mL/dL
b. 12 g/dL × 1.34 mL/gm × 97% = 15.60 mL/dL
c. 8 g/dL × 1.34 mL/gm × 97% = 10.40 mL/dL

d. 4 g/dL × 1.34 mL/gm × 97% = 5.20 mL/dL

3. Compute total oxygen contents:

CaO_2 = Dissolved O_2 + chemically combined O_2

a. 0.30 + 19.50 = 19.80 mL/dL
b. 0.30 + 15.60 = 15.90 mL/dL
c. 0.30 + 10.40 = 10.70 mL/dL
d. 0.30 + 5.20 = 5.50 mL/dL

Loss of hemoglobin decreases the amount of oxygen carried in a patient's blood, even though the PO_2 and saturation remain normal. For example, with a hemoglobin concentration of 4 g/dL, the amount of oxygen carried in a patient's blood is only about one-fourth the normal concentration normal (5.50 vs. 19.80 mL/dL).

---

blood perfuses body tissues, its PO_2 and saturation drop to the venous levels of about 40 torr and 73%, respectively (point Ⓥ).

To assess the actual change in blood oxygen content between the points of oxygen loading and unloading, we must know the amount of Hb in the blood. Using a normal Hb content of 15 g/dL, and knowing the hemoglobin saturation at each possible PO_2, we can calculate total oxygen contents at any PO_2 in the manner previously described. The y axis of Figure 12-11 provides this information for us, in SaO_2 increments of 10%. Table 12-1 summarizes the difference between the oxygen content of these normal arterial and venous points.

As indicated in Table 12-1, the difference between the arterial and venous oxygen contents is normally about 5 mL/dL. This is the arterial-venous oxygen contents difference, abbreviated as $C(a-v)O_2$. $C(a-v)O_2$ is the amount of oxygen given up by every 100 mL of blood on each pass through the tissues. Obviously, this value reflects the mean of the body as a whole, with different organ systems extracting more or less oxygen according to need.

Fick equation

The $C(a-v)O_2$ indicates oxygen extraction in proportion to blood flow. If you combine this measure with total body oxygen consumption, you can calculate cardiac output. The basis for this calculation is the classic *Fick Equation:*

$$\dot{Q}T = \frac{\dot{V}O_2}{C(a-\overline{v})O_2 \times 10}$$

In this equation, $\dot{Q}T$ is cardiac output in liters per minute, $\dot{V}O_2$ is total body oxygen consumption in milliliters per minute, and $C(a-\overline{v})O_2$ is the arterial-venous oxygen contents difference in milliliters per deciliter. The factor of 10 converts milliliters per deciliter to milliliters per liter. Given a normal $\dot{V}O_2$ of 250 mL/min and a normal $C(a-\overline{v})O_2$ of 5 mL/dL, you calculate a normal cardiac output as:

$$\dot{Q}T = \frac{250 \text{ mL/min}}{5 \text{ mL/dL} \times 10}$$
$$\dot{Q}T = \frac{250 \text{ mL/min}}{50 \text{ mL/L}}$$
$$\dot{Q}T = 5.0 \text{ L/min}$$

Significance of the $C(a-\overline{v})O_2$

According to the Fick Equation, if the oxygen consumption remains constant, a decrease in cardiac output will cause an increase in the $C(a-\overline{v})O_2$. Conversely, should cardiac output rise and oxygen consumption remain constant, the $C(a-\overline{v})O_2$ will fall proportionally. Although the Fick method of calculating cardiac output has been replaced by other tech-

---

Table 12-1 Oxygen content of arterial and venous blood

	Arterial O_2 (mL/dL)	Venous O_2 (mL/dL)
Combined O_2 (1.34 × 15 × Sat)	19.5	14.7
Dissolved O_2 (Po_2 × 0.003)	0.3	0.1
Total O_2 content	19.8	14.8

niques, the principle relating $C(a-\overline{v})O_2$ to perfusion is used to monitor tissue oxygenation at the bedside.[20] More details on these methods are provided in Chapter 33.

Factors affecting oxygen loading and unloading

Many factors besides the shape of the HbO_2 curve affect oxygen loading and unloading. Among those most important in clinical practice are: (1) the hydrogen ion concentration of the blood (pH), (2) the body temperature, and (3) the concentration of certain organic phosphates in the erythrocyte. Also affecting oxygen loading and unloading are variations in the chemical structure of Hb. Last, chemical combinations of Hb with substances other than oxygen, such as carbon monoxide, can also affect oxygen loading and unloading.[21]

pH

The clinical significance of blood pH changes are discussed in detail in Chapter 14. At this point, all we need to understand is that the affinity of Hb for oxygen is significantly affected by blood pH changes.

Bohr effect. The impact of changes in blood pH on the affinity of Hb for oxygen is called the *Bohr effect*. As shown in Figure 12-12, the Bohr effect describes changes in the actual position of the HbO_2 dissociation curve. A low pH (acidity) shifts the curve to the right, whereas a high pH (alkalinity) shifts it to the left.[22] This alteration in position of the curve is caused

by pH-induced changes in the shape of the Hb molecule. Changes in the molecule's shape alter the accessibility of the heme complex for oxygen binding.[1]

As blood pH drops and the curve shifts to the right, the Hb saturation for a given PO_2 falls. A lower saturation for a given PO_2 indicates decreased Hb affinity for oxygen. Conversely, as blood pH rises and the curve shifts to the left, the Hb saturation for a given PO_2 rises, indicating that the affinity of Hb for oxygen has increased.

Physiologic significance. Even in the narrow range of pH changes between arterial and venous blood, the Bohr effect has physiologic importance. As shown in Figure 12-13, on page 280, blood pH varies about 0.03 unit between the normal venous and arterial points. As blood becomes venous, its carbon dioxide content rises, causing the pH to drop from 7.40 to about 7.37. As a result, the HbO_2 curve shifts to the right, lowering the affinity of Hb for oxygen. With this lowered affinity for oxygen, Hb more readily gives up its oxygen, thus aiding its unloading at the tissues.

Conversely, when venous blood returns to the lungs, the pH rises back to 7.40. This increase shifts the HbO_2 curve back to the left, thereby increasing the affinity of Hb for oxygen and enhancing its uptake from the alveoli. The Bohr effect thus aids both pulmonary uptake and tissue delivery of oxygen.[16]

Effect of Wide Fluctuations in pH. According to the Bohr effect, even when there is no change in PO_2 changes in blood pH can substantially modify blood's oxygen-carrying capacity. Figure 12-13 shows the impact that wide fluctuations in pH can have on the

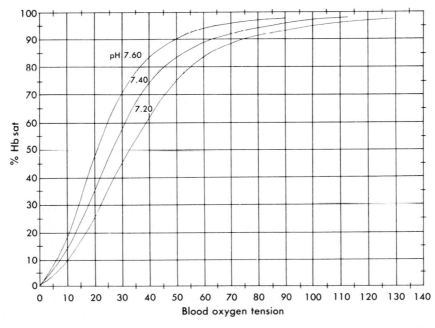

Fig. 12–12 Oxygen dissociation curve of blood at 37°C, showing variations at three pH levels. For a given oxygen tension, the higher the blood pH, the more the hemoglobin holds onto its oxygen, maintaining a higher saturation.

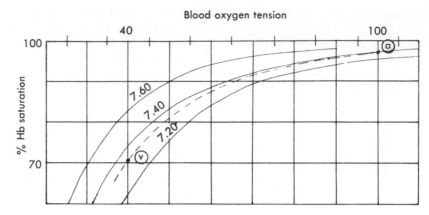

Fig. 12-13 Bohr effect. The *dashed line* indicates the physiologic shift in oxygen dissociation curve as changing blood carbon dioxide content alters blood pH between arterial, ⓐ, and venous, ⓥ, points.

blood's oxygen-carrying capacity. As an example, with a PaO$_2$ of 50 torr, there is a difference of about 15% in Hb saturation between the pH values of 7.20 and 7.60.

Because the blood can maintain higher oxygen saturations when alkalotic, one might presume that **alkalosis** is a desirable state. Comparison of the pH 7.60 and pH 7.20 dissociation curves (Figure 12-13) demonstrates that this premise is false.

Assuming a Hb concentration of 15 g/dL and complete oxygen equilibration at arterial and venous PO$_2$ values of 100 torr and 40 torr, respectively, we read oxygen saturations of 98% for arterial blood and 84% for venous blood on the pH 7.60 curve. Likewise, we read saturations of 94% and 62% on the pH 7.20 curve. You can now compare the C(a−v)O$_2$ between the arterial and venous points for each abnormal pH value and compare them with the normal C(a−v)O$_2$, as outlined in Table 12-2.

Although there is less than 1 mL/dL difference between the two abnormal pH blood samples at the arterial point, after tissue perfusion the C(a−v)O$_2$ of the blood with the low pH is more than double that of the blood with a pH of 7.60. This indicates that Hb in alkaline blood (high pH) holds its oxygen more strongly, making it less available to tissues than that normally provided.

This does not mean that a low blood pH is beneficial. Under conditions of **acidosis** (low pH), Hb does more readily releases oxygen to the tissues. However, the damaging effects of acidosis more than outweigh any benefits gained by increased oxygen unloading. Only by keeping the pH in the normal range and maintaining normal arterial oxygen saturations can adequate loading and unloading of oxygen from Hb be assured.[23]

Body temperature

Variations in body temperature also affect the position of the HbO$_2$ dissociation curve. As shown in Figure 12-14, a drop in body temperature shifts the curve to the left, resulting in a higher Hb saturation for a given PO$_2$ and thus a greater affinity of Hb for oxygen. Conversely, as body temperature rises, the curve shifts to the right and the affinity of Hb for oxygen decreases.

Like the Bohr effect, changes in Hb affinity for oxygen due to temperature enhance normal oxygen uptake and delivery.[16] At the tissues, temperature changes are directly related to metabolic rate, such that areas of high metabolic activity have higher temperatures. In areas such as exercising muscle, higher temperatures decrease Hb affinity for oxygen, thereby enhancing its release to the tissues. In clinical practice, this same phenomenon occurs bodywide under conditions of **hyperpyrexia.** Conversely, in **hypothermia,** the oxygen demands of the tissues are greatly reduced, and Hb need not give up as much of its oxygen.

Because temperature does influence Hb saturation, and because patients' temperatures may vary substantially over time, it is customary to measure oxygen tension at a standard temperature of 37° C. If needed, both tension and saturation can be corrected to the patient's actual temperature by means of tabulated factors or nomograms.

Table 12-2 Arterial-venous oxygen difference at three pH levels

| | Total O$_2$ (mL/dL) | | a−v (mL/dL) |
	Arterial	Venous	O$_2$
pH 7.60	20.0	17.0	3.0
pH 7.40	19.8	14.8	5.0
pH 7.20	19.2	12.6	6.6

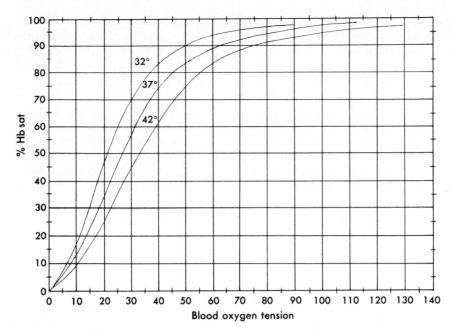

Fig. 12-14 Oxygen dissociation curve of blood at a pH of 7.40, showing variations at three temperatures. For a given oxygen tension, the lower the temperature, the more the hemoglobin holds onto its oxygen, maintaining a higher saturation.

Organic phosphates

Organic phosphates play vital roles in many cellular biochemical reactions and are essential to the transfer of energy on which cell function depends. In the past few years, attention has been directed to the involvement of phosphates in respiration. The two most significant organic phosphates involved in respiration are 2,3-diphosphoglycerate (2,3 DPG) and adenosine triphosphate (ATP). In the interest of brevity and because of its relatively greater importance, we describe DPG as the prototype.[24,25]

At 0.85 mol/mol of Hb, 2,3 DPG is the most abundant phosphate in the erythrocyte.[21] 2,3 DPG is synthesized during glucose metabolism and can form a loose chemical bound with the globin chains of the unsaturated Hb molecule. In combination with Hb, 2,3 DPG stabilizes the molecule in its unsaturated state, thereby reducing its affinity for oxygen.[26] Indeed, without the existence of 2,3 DPG, Hb affinity for oxygen would be so great that normal oxygen unloading would be impossible. The ability of 2,3 DPG to decrease Hb affinity for oxygen is in direct proportion to its concentration in the erythrocyte. Therefore increased concentrations of 2,3 DPG shift the HbO_2 dissociation curve to the right, promoting oxygen unloading at the tissues. Conversely, a decrease in 2,3 DPG concentration shifts the curve to the left, increasing Hb affinity for oxygen and impairing its capacity to unload oxygen.[27]

Changes in the intracellular level of 2,3 DPG occur during the events of normal gas exchange in the erythrocyte and in response to certain chronic conditions. These factors and their clinical significance are outlined below.

Changes in pH. Intracellular 2,3 DPG concentrations vary directly with changes in pH. Thus, although an increase in blood pH immediately shifts the HbO_2 curve to the left (the Bohr effect), the primary pH change increases intracellular 2,3 DPG. This increase in 2,3 DPG in turn causes a compensatory shift back toward the original position. Conversely, a drop in pH immediately shifts the HbO_2 curve to the right; however, because of decreasing levels of 2,3 DPG, the curve will tend to move back toward its normal position. The time required for these changes is on the order of several hours.[26,28]

Hypoxemia. Hypoxemia increases intracellular 2,3 DPG concentrations.[29] This change shifts the HbO_2 curve to the right, increasing the availability of oxygen to the tissues. This response is seen in normal individuals exposed to low barometric pressure for sustained periods (living at high altitude)[30] and among those with diseases causing chronic hypoxemia. Among the disorders causing chronic hypoxemia, none is more common than chronic obstructive pulmonary disease (COPD).

Anemia. Intracellular 2,3 DPG levels increase when the whole-blood concentration of Hb falls (**anemia**).[31] Like the response to chronic hypoxemia, this change is an adaptation that can help compensate for up to half the oxygen deficit caused by the loss of erythrocytes. Unlike the response to chronic hypoxemia, the increased 2,3 DPG levels observed with anemia can occur within minutes.[31] Moreover, this rapid response may account for the common observation that hypoxic symptoms are not always present in patients with severe anemia.

Banked blood. Stored or banked blood exhibits a substantial decrease in 2,3 DPG levels over time; after 1 wk of storage, the concentration of this organic phosphate is about a third of the normal value.[26] This change shifts the HbO_2 curve to the left, thereby decreasing the availability of oxygen to the tissues. Large **transfusions** of banked blood more than a few days old can severely impair oxygen delivery, even in the presence of a normal PO_2. Furthermore, banked blood may have undesirable levels of carboxyhemoglobin (above 1.5%). This is especially noteworthy in cardiac or pulmonary disease patients who receive multiple transfusions.[32]

Abnormal hemoglobins

Abnormal variants in the structure of the hemoglobin molecule can also affect oxygen loading and unloading. Normal adult hemoglobin is abbreviated *HbA*. Abnormal Hb varieties are given different letter designations, often according to the geographic locale where they were identified. Thus *HbR* is the abbreviation for hemoglobin Rainier and *HbK* shorthand for hemoglobin Kansas. Each of the abnormal forms varies according to the composition of the **amino acids** in the polypeptide chains of the globin portion of the molecule. More than 120 abnormal Hbs have been identified.[33,34] Even in normal individuals, anywhere from 15% to 40% of the circulating Hb may have a structure different from that of normal HbA.[21,35]

Abnormal molecular structures. Variations in the composition of hemoglobin's amino acids alter its shape, thereby increasing or decreasing the accessibility of the heme portion to oxygen. Changes in the accessibility of the heme complex result in greater or lesser affinity for oxygen and are manifested by a shift in the oxyhemoglobin curve. HbC (Chesapeake), HbR (Rainier), and HbY (Yakima) all exhibit varying degrees of increased affinity for oxygen; HbY causes a clinically significant shift to the left. HbK, on the other hand, has a lesser affinity for oxygen than HbA, causing a dramatic shift of the HbO_2 curve to the right.[36]

Despite significant differences in the oxygen affinity exhibited by the abnormal Hbs, individuals with large percentages of these variants have near-normal arterial-venous oxygen contents differences [$C(a-\bar{v})O_2$], indicating adequate O_2 delivery to the tissues. Compensation probably occurs through changes in cardiac output, erythrocyte production or both.

Sickle-cell anemia also represents a condition caused by an abnormal Hb variant. Genetically determined, sickle-cell anemia is caused by a single different amino acid on two of the four chains of the globin moiety, producing HbS. HbS has less affinity for oxygen than does HbA. From a clinical standpoint this is less important than the changes that occur in HbS solubility. Deoxygenated HbS is less soluble than oxygenated HbS or HbA. In its deoxygenated form, HbS can actually crystallize inside the erythrocyte, causing the characteristic deformation in the shape of the cell. This increases the fragility of the erythrocyte and raises the possibility of **thrombus** formation.[4]

Oxidized hemoglobin (methemoglobin). Normally, the iron ion of the heme complex exists in the ferrous state (Fe^{++}). If oxidized, the ferrous iron loses an electron, changing to the ferric state (Fe^{+++}). This abnormal form of hemoglobin, called *methemoglobin* (metHb), cannot bind with oxygen and is thus useless in oxygen transport.

Oxidation of Hb to metHb produces a condition called *methemoglobinemia*. Because methemoglobin cannot carry oxygen, methemoglobinemia is similar to other forms of anemia. The most common cause of methemoglobinemia is **nitrite** poisoning. However, many oxidizing agents, including aniline, paraaminosalicylic acid, and phenylhydrazine, can have similar effects.[21] **Congenital** methemoglobinemias, though rare, also exist. These may be associated with a specific **enzyme** deficiency, either acquired or inherited.

In large quantities, metHb gives the blood a characteristic brownish color. This produces a slate-gray skin coloration that may be confused with cyanosis.[1] However, the actual presence of metHb can only be confirmed on **spectrophotometry**. Treatment of methemoglobinemias due to poisoning by oxidants involves removing the offending chemical and restoring the hemoglobin to its ferrous state. Normally, this is done by giving the patient a reducing agent such as methylene blue or ascorbic acid.

Fetal Hb. During fetal life and for up to one year after birth, the blood has a high proportion of an Hb variant called *fetal hemoglobin* (HbF). HbF has a greater affinity for oxygen than does adult Hb, as manifested by a leftward shift of the HbO_2 curve.[37] Given the low PO_2 values available to the fetus at the **placenta,** this leftward shift aids the loading of oxygen at the site of maternal-fetal gas exchange. Because of the relatively low pH of the fetal environment, oxygen unloading at the cell level is not greatly affected. After birth, however, this enhanced oxygen affinity is less advantageous; fetal hemoglobin is gradually replaced over the first year of life with HbA. However, HbF production in adults can be stimulated by anemia.[26]

Carboxyhemoglobin. The affinity of hemoglobin for carbon monoxide is about 200 to 300 times greater than that for oxygen. Thus even extremely low concentrations of carbon monoxide quickly displace oxygen from the hemoglobin molecule, forming HbCO, or *carboxyhemoglobin.* A carbon monoxide partial pressure of as low as 0.12 torr can result in as much as 50% saturation of hemoglobin with carbon monoxide.[20] Because HbCO cannot carry oxygen, each gram of Hb saturated with carbon monoxide represents a loss in carrying capacity. For example, 50% saturation of hemoglobin with carbon monoxide has the same effect as an anemia with an Hb content of 7.5 mL/dL. Moreover, the combination of carbon monoxide with hemoglobin shifts the HbO_2 curve to the left, further impeding oxygen delivery to the tissues.[38,39] The treatment for carbon monoxide poisoning involves giving the patient as high a partial pressure of oxygen as possible, sometimes via a hyperbaric chamber.[40]

Measurement of hemoglobin affinity for oxygen

We quantify variations in the affinity of Hb using a measure called the P_{50}. The P_{50} is the partial pressure of oxygen at which the Hb is 50% saturated, standardized to a pH of 7.40. A normal P_{50} is about 26.6 torr. Conditions that cause a decrease in Hb affinity for oxygen (a shift of the HbO_2 curve to the right) increase the P_{50} above normal. Conditions associated with a increase in affinity (a shift of the HbO_2 curve to the

left) decrease the P_{50} below normal. For example, with 15 gm/dL Hb, a 4 torr increase in P_{50} results in about 1 to 2 mL/dL more oxygen being unloaded at the tissues than when the P_{50} is normal.[41] Figure 12-15 shows the effect of changes in P_{50} and summarizes how the major factors previously discussed affect Hb affinity for oxygen.

CARBON DIOXIDE TRANSPORTATION

Figure 12-16, on page 284 portrays the physical and chemical events of gas exchange at the systemic capillaries. At the level of the pulmonary capillaries, all events occur in the opposite direction. Although our primary focus here is with carbon dioxide transport, Figure 12-16 also includes the basic elements of oxygen exchange. Oxygen exchange is included here not only for completeness; as you will see, the exchange and transport of these two gases are closely related.

Transport mechanisms

Forty-five to 55 mL/dL of carbon dioxide is normally carried in the blood, in three forms: (1) dissolved in

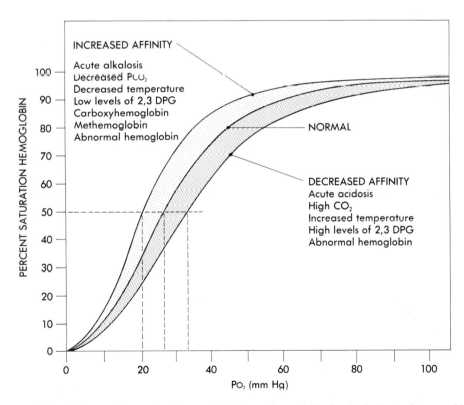

Fig. 12-15 Conditions associated with altered affinity of hemoglobin for O_2. P_{50} is the Pao_2 at which hemoglobin is 50% saturated, normally 26.6 torr. A lower than normal P_{50} represents increased affinity of hemoglobin for O_2; a high P_{50} is seen with decreased affinity. Note that variation from the normal is associated with decreased (low P_{50}) or increased (high P_{50}) availability of O_2 to tissues *(dotted lines)*. The shaded area shows the entire oxyhemoglobin dissociation curve under the same circumstances. (From Lane EE and Walker JF: Clinical arterial blood gas analysis, St Louis, 1987, Mosby.)

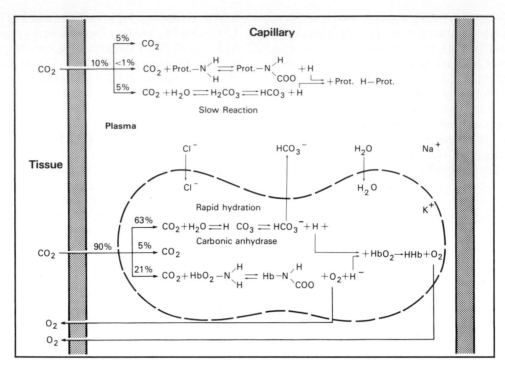

Fig. 12-16 Summary diagram of the various fates of CO_2 as it diffuses from cells and interstitial space into the peripheral capillaries prior to its transport toward the venous circulation. (From Martin DE and Youtsey JW: Respiratory anatomy and physiology, St Louis, 1988, Mosby.)

physical solution, (2) chemically combined with protein, and (3) ionized as bicarbonate.[14]

Dissolved carbon dioxide

As with oxygen, carbon dioxide produced by the tissues dissolves in the plasma and erythrocytes' intracellular fluid. Unlike oxygen, however, dissolved carbon dioxide plays an important role in transport, accounting for about 10% of the total released at the lungs. This is due to carbon dioxide's higher solubility coefficient and thus the greater amount transported in physical solution.

Still, most of the carbon dioxide that goes into physical solution does not remain in that state. Instead, it chemically combines with other elements in the blood, including protein and water.

Chemically combined with protein

Molecular carbon dioxide has the capacity to chemically combine with free amino groups (*NH₂*) of protein molecules (*Prot*), forming a carbamino compound:

$$Prot-NH_2 + CO_2 \rightleftarrows Prot-NHCOO^- + H^+$$

About 1% of the carbon dioxide leaving the tissues combines with plasma proteins to form these carbamino compounds.[10] This fraction of the carbon dioxide in the blood is relatively insignificant.

A larger fraction of the CO_2 combines with erythro-

cyte Hb to forms a carbamino compound called *carbamino-Hb*.[14] As indicated in the equation above, this reaction produces H^+ ions. These H^+ ions are buffered by the reduced hemoglobin (Hb^-), made available by the concurrent release of oxygen.

The availability of additional sites for H^+ buffering increases the affinity of Hb for CO_2. Moreover, because reduced Hb is a weaker acid than HbO_2, pH changes associated with the release of the H^+ ions in the formation of carbamino-Hb are minimized. Although the carbamino-Hb constitutes only about 5% of the total carbon dioxide transported, it accounts for nearly 30% of that released at the lungs.[42]

Ionized as bicarbonate

Of the carbon dioxide that dissolves in plasma, a small portion (about 5%) chemically combines with water in a process called *hydrolysis*. Hydrolysis of carbon dioxide initially forms carbonic acid, which quickly ionizes into hydrogen and bicarbonate ions:[5]

$$CO_2 + H_2O \rightleftarrows H_2CO_3 \rightleftarrows HCO_3^- + H^+$$

The H^+ ions produced in this reaction are buffered by the plasma proteins, in much the same way as hemoglobin buffers H^+ in the red blood cell. However, the rate of this plasma hydrolysis reaction is extremely slow, producing minimal amounts of H^+ and HCO_3^-.

Most carbon dioxide (about two thirds, or 63%) undergoes hydrolysis inside the erythrocyte. This reaction is greatly enhanced by an enzyme catalyst called **carbonic anhydrase** (CA). The resulting H^+ ions are buffered by the imidazole group ($R\text{-}NHCOO^-$) of the reduced Hb molecule. Again, the concurrent conversion of HbO_2 to reduced Hb helps buffer H^+ ions, thereby enhancing the loading of carbon dioxide as carbamino-Hb.

As the hydrolysis of carbon dioxide continues, HCO_3^- ions begin to accumulate in the erythrocyte. To maintain a concentration equilibrium across the cell membrane, some of these anions diffuse outward into the plasma. Because the erythrocyte is not freely permeable by cations, electrolytic equilibrium must be maintained by way of an inward migration of anions. This is achieved by the shifting of chloride ions (Cl^-) from the plasma into the erythrocyte, a process called the *chloride shift,* or the *Hamburger phenomenon.*

Carbon dioxide dissociation curve

Like oxygen, carbon dioxide has a dissociation curve. The relationship between blood PCO_2 and carbon dioxide content is depicted in Figure 12-17, on page 286.

The first point to note is the effect of Hb saturation on this curve. We already know that carbon dioxide levels, through their influence on pH, modify the oxygen dissociation curve (Bohr effect). As shown in Figure 12-17, we see that Hb saturation with oxygen also affects the position of the carbon dioxide dissociation curve. The influence of oxyhemoglobin saturation on carbon dioxide dissociation is called the *Haldane effect.* As previously explained, this phenomenon is due to changes in the affinity of hemoglobin for CO_2 that occur as a result of its buffering of H^+ ions.

Figure 12-17, *A* shows the carbon dioxide dissociation curves for three levels of blood oxygen saturation. The first two are physiologic values; the third extreme value is provided for contrast. Figure 12-17, *B* "zooms in" on selected segments of these curves in the physiologic range of PCO_2. Note first the arterial point (ⓐ) lying on the curve representing an SaO_2 of 97.5%. At this point, the PCO_2 is 40 torr, and the carbon dioxide content is about of 48 mL/dL. In contrast, the venous point (ⓥ) falls on the curve representing an SaO_2 of about 70%. At this point, the

PCO_2 is 46 torr, and the carbon dioxide content is about 53 mL/dL. Because oxygen saturation changes from arterial to venous blood, the true physiologic carbon dioxide dissociation curve must lie somewhere between these two points. This physiologic curve is represented as the dashed line in Figure 12-17, *B*.

At point ⓐ, the high SaO_2 decreases the blood's capacity to hold carbon dioxide, thus helping unload this gas at the lungs. At point ⓥ, the lower SvO_2 increases blood's capacity for CO_2, thus aiding tissue uptake.

Table 12-3 compares and contrasts the total carbon dioxide content of both arterial and venous blood according to its major components. Here, "combined CO_2" is equivalent to that portion ionized as bicarbonate, whereas "dissolved CO_2," is that portion in simple physical solution in the plasma and erythrocyte water. Note that the amounts of CO_2 are expressed in both gaseous volume equivalents (milliliters per deciliter) and as millimoles per liter. This latter measure of the chemical combining power of CO_2 in solutions is critical in understanding the role of this gas in acid-base balance.

Relationship of CO_2 to acid–base balance

Of utmost importance in acid-base homeostasis is the relationship between the CO_2 carried as bicarbonate (a salt) and that transported as carbonic acid (a weak acid). Together, this salt and its weak acid form the primary buffer system of the body. This buffer system helps minimize the effect of changes in hydrogen ion concentrations on the blood's pH.

Because we cannot directly measure H_2CO_3, we must estimate its concentration. We know that the amount of carbonic acid in the plasma is directly proportional to the amount of CO_2 in solution. Thus we can use the amount of dissolved CO_2 to estimate the H_2CO_3 concentration. As indicated in Table 12-3, the ratio of combined CO_2 (24 mmol/L) to that physically dissolved in the arterial blood (1.2 mmol/L) is maintained at a remarkably constant ratio of 20:1. Maintenance of this ratio ensures a normal blood pH. Any deviation from this ratio will cause an abnormal pH. These important concepts will be pursued in depth in the next chapter.

Table 12-3   Carbon dioxide content of arterial and venous blood plasma

	Arterial		Venous	
	mL/dL	mmol/L	mL/dL	mmol/L
Combined CO_2	46.1	24.0	50.4	26.3
Dissolved CO_2	2.3	1.2	2.7	1.4
Total CO_2	48.4	25.2	53.1	27.7
PCO_2	40 torr		46 torr	

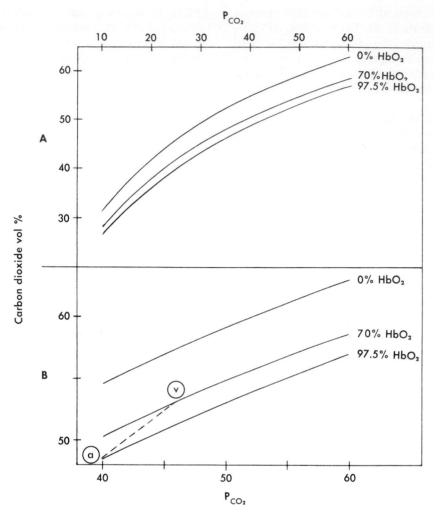

Fig. 12-17 Haldane effect and carbon dioxide dissociation curves. **A,** The relationship between carbon dioxide content and tension at three levels of hemoglobin saturation. **B,** Close-up of the curves between PCO_2 of 40 torr and 60 torr (see text for details). (Modified from Comroe JH Jr et al: The lung, ed 2, St Louis, 1962, Mosby.)

CHAPTER SUMMARY

The movement of gases between lungs and the tissues depends mainly on diffusion. Normal pressure gradients at the alveolar-capillary membrane ensure rapid movement of oxygen and carbon dioxide between the alveoli and pulmonary circulation. However, anatomic shunts and regional differences in ventilation and perfusion make the lung a less than perfect organ of gas exchange.

The loading and unloading of oxygen and carbon dioxide in the lung and tissues is further enhanced by specialized blood gas transport mechanisms. These mechanisms mutually aid each other, such that oxygen uptake and delivery assists in the excretion and removal of carbon dioxide. Moreover, carbon dioxide transport plays a critical role in acid-base homeostasis.

Normally, these processes are well integrated and maintained in a constant state of balance. However, abnormalities in structure or function can alter this balance and potentially disrupt normal gas exchange and transport between the atmosphere and tissue. Under such conditions, restoration of normal gas exchange and transport is a primary goal of respiratory care.

REFERENCES

1. Nunn JF: *Applied respiratory physiology,* ed 2, Kent, UK, 1977, Butterworth.
2. Tisi GM: *Pulmonary physiology in clinical medicine,* ed 2, Baltimore, 1984, Williams & Wilkins.
3. Martin L: *Pulmonary physiology in clinical practice: the essentials for patient care and evaluation,* St. Louis, 1987, Mosby.
4. West JB: *Respiratory physiology: the essentials,* ed 4, Baltimore, 1990, Williams & Wilkins.
5. Foster RE, Dubois AB, Briscoe WA, Fisher AB: *The lung: physiologic basis of pulmonary function tests,* ed 3, St. Louis 1986, Mosby.
6. West JB: Ventilation-perfusion relationships, *Am Rev Resp Dis* 116:919, 1977.
7. Divertie MB, Brown AL Jr: The fine structure of the normal alveolocapillary membrane, *JAMA* 187:938, 1964.
8. Green JF: *Fundamental cardiovascular and pulmonary physiology,* ed 2, Philadelphia, 1987, Lea & Febiger.
9. Weast RC, ed: *Handbook of chemistry and physics,* ed 69, Cleveland, 1988, Chemical Rubber Co.
10. Comroe JH: *Physiology of respiration,* ed 2, St Louis, 1974, Mosby.
11. Roughton FJW: The average time spent by the blood in the human lung capillary, and its relation to the rates of carbon monoxide uptake and elimination in man, *Am J Physiol* 143:621, 1945.
12. Wagner PD, West JB. Effects of diffusion impairment on O_2 and CO_2 time courses in pulmonary capillaries. *J Appl Physiol* 33:62-71, 1972.
13. Ogilvie C. The single-breath carbon monoxide transfer test 25 years on: a reappraisal, *Thorax* 38:5-9, 1983.
14. American Thoracic Society: Single breath carbon monoxide diffusing capacity (transfer factor): recommendations for a standard technique, *Am Rev Respir Dis* 136:1299-307, 1987.
15. Harris EA, et al.: The normal alveolar-arterial oxygen tension gradient in man, *Clin Sci Mol Med,* 46:89, 1974.
16. Murray JF: *The normal lung,* ed 2, Philadelphia, 1986, WB Saunders.
17. Roughton FW: Transport of oxygen and carbon dioxide. In *Handbook of physiology,* Washington, DC, 1964, American Physiological Association.
18. Kacmarek RM: Oxygen carriage, transport and utilization. In: Pierson DJ, Kacmarek RM, eds: *Foundations of respiratory care,* New York, 1992, Churchill-Livingstone.
19. Wagner PD. The oxyhemoglobin dissociation curve and pulmonary gas exchange. *Semin Hematol* 11(4)405-21, 1974.
20. Dantzker DR, Guiterrez G. The assessment of tissue oxygenation. *Respir Care* 1985; 30(6):456-462.
21. Lane EE, Walker JF: *Clinical arterial blood gas analysis,* St. Louis, 1987, Mosby.
22. Astrup P: Red-cell pH and oxygen affinity of hemoglobin, *N Engl J Med* 283:202, 1970.
23. Bryan-Brown CW, Baek SM, Makabali G, Shoemaker WC. Consumable oxygen availability of oxygen in relation to oxy-hemoglobin dissociation, *Crit Care Med* 1973;1(1):17-21.
24. Benesch R, Benesch RE: Intracellular organic phosphates as regulators of oxygen release by haemoglobin, *Nature* 221:618, 1969.
25. Klocke RA: Oxygen transport and 2,3-diphosphoglycerate (DPG), *Chest* 62 (suppl):79s, 1972.
26. Slonim NB, Hamilton LH: *Respiratory physiology,* ed 5, St. Louis, 1985, Mosby.
27. Thomas HM III, Lefrak SS, Irwin RS, Fritts HW Jr, Caldwell PR. The oxyhemoglobin dissociation curve in health and disease: role of 2,3-diphosphoglycerate, *Am J Med* 57(3):331-348, 1974.
28. Agusti AG, Rodriguez-Roisin R, Roca J, Aguilar JL, Agusti-Vidal A. Oxyhemoglobin affinity in patients with chronic obstructive pulmonary disease and acute respiratory failure: role of mechanical ventilation, *Crit Care Med* 14(7):610-613, 1986.
29. Oski FA, et al.: Red-cell 2,3-diphosphoglycerate levels in subjects with chronic hypoxemia, *N Engl J Med* 280:1165, 1969.
30. Cymerman A, Maher JT, Cruz JC, Reeves JT, Denniston JC, Grover RF. Increased 2,3-diphosphoglycerate during normocapnic hypobaric hypoxia, *Aviat Space Environ Med* 47(10):1069-1072, 1976.
31. Torrance J, et al.: Intraerythrocyte adaptation to anemia, *N Engl J Med* 283:165, 1970.
32. Aronow WS, O'Donohue WJ Jr, Freygang J, Sketch DE: Carboxyhemoglobin levels in banked blood, *Chest* 85(5):694-695, 1984.
33. Wells RM, Brennan SO. The detection and importance of functionally abnormal haemoglobins, *N Z Med J* 105(940):329-330, 1992.
34. Jones RT, Shih TB. Hemoglobin variants with altered oxygen affinity, *Hemoglobin* 4(3-4)243-261, 1980.
35. Nagel RL, Bookchin RM: Human hemoglobin mutants with abnormal oxygen binding, *Semin Hematol* 11:385, 1974.
36. Parer JT: Oxygen transport in human subjects with hemoglobin variants having altered oxygen affinity, *Resp Physiol* 9:43, 1970.
37. Gregory IC: The oxygen and carbon dioxide capacities of fetal and adult hemoglobin, *J Physiol* 236:625, 1974.
38. Dolan MC. Carbon monoxide poisoning, *Can Med Assoc J* 133(5)392-399, 1985.
39. Winter PM. Miller JN. Carbon monoxide poisoning, *JAMA* 236(13):1502, 1976.
40. Norkool DM, Kirkpatrick JN: Treatment of acute carbon monoxide poisoning with hyperbaric oxygen: a review of 115 cases, *Ann Emerg Med* 14:1168, 1985.
41. Miller MF: *Laboratory evaluation of pulmonary function,* Philadelphia, 1987, JB Lippincott.
42. Kacmarek RM: Carbon dioxide production, carriage and transport. In: Pierson DJ, Kacmarek RM, eds: *Foundations of respiratory care,* New York, 1992, Churchill-Livingstone.

Solutions, Body Fluids, and Electrolytes

■

Gregg L. Ruppel

Craig L. Scanlan

In health, body water and various substances are carefully regulated to maintain an environment in which biochemical processes continue. Imbalances in the amount or concentration of chemicals in the body occur in many diseases. The nature and importance of body fluids and electrolytes requires an understanding of physiologic chemistry.

SOLUTIONS

Definition of a solution

The body is a watery medium. In this medium, chemical substances and particles exist in solution or suspension. These substances and particles combine with water in three ways: as *colloids, suspensions,* or *solutions.*

Colloids (sometimes called *dispersions* or *gels*) consist of large molecules that attract and hold water molecules. These molecules become uniformly distributed throughout the dispersion. That is, they tend not to settle. Intracellular protoplasm is a common example of a colloid.

Suspensions comprise large particles that float in a liquid. Suspensions do not behave like the solvent and solute found in a true solution. Red blood cells in plasma are an example of a suspension. Dispersion of suspended particles depends on physical agitation. When the suspension is allowed to stand, particles settle.

A solution is a stable mixture of two substances. One substance is evenly dispersed throughout the other. The substance that dissolves is called the *solute.* The medium in which it dissolves is the *solvent.*

The ease with which a solute dissolve in a solvent is its *solubility.* Four primary factors influence solubility:

1. Nature of the solute. The ease with which substances go into solution in a given solvent is a physical characteristic of matter and varies widely.
2. Nature of the solvent. Solvents vary widely in their ability to dissolve substances.
3. Temperature. Solubility of most solids increases with temperature. The solubility of gases, however, varies *inversely* with temperature.
4. Pressure. Solubility of gases in liquids varies *directly* with pressure.

The effects of temperature and pressure on solubility of gases is important. Oxygen and carbon dioxide transport can change markedly with changes in body temperature or the pressure to which the body is exposed (see Chapter 12).

Concentration of solutions

A solution is described as *dilute* if the amount of solute is relatively small in proportion to solvent (Figure 13-1, *A*). A *saturated* solution has the maximum amount of solute that can be held in a given volume of a solvent at a constant temperature. An excess of solute must be present. In such a mixture the dissolved solute is in equilibrium with undissolved solute. Saturated solutions are prepared by the addition of excess solute to the solvent. The excess solute remains in contact with the solution (Figure 13-1, *B*). This excess solute is not completely inert. Solute particles precipitate into the solid state at the same rate that other particles go into solution. This

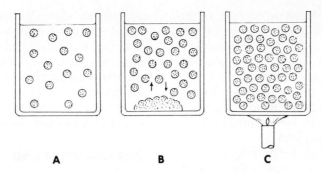

Fig. 13–1 In the dilute solution, **A,** the solute particles are relatively few in number, whereas in the saturated solution, **B,** the solvent contains all the solute it can hold in the presence of an excess of solute. Heating the solution, **C,** dissolves more solute particles, which may remain in solution if gently cooled, creating a state of supersaturation.

state of equilibrium characterizes a saturated solution.

A solution is said to be *supersaturated* when it contains more solute than a saturated solution at the same temperature and pressure. If a saturated solution is heated, the solute equilibrium is upset. More solute goes into solution. If undissolved solute is filtered and the solution cooled gently, there will be an excess of dissolved solute (Figure 13-1, *C*). Additional particles may remain in solution, even after cooling to the original temperature. Supersaturated solutions are unstable. The excess solute may be precipitated out of solution by physical stimuli such as shaking or vibrating. Precipitation may occur if more solute is added to the supersaturated solution.

Osmotic pressure of solutions

Most of the solutions of physiologic importance in the body are dilute. Solutes in dilute solution demonstrate many of the properties of gases. This behavior results from the relatively large distances between the molecules in dilute solutions. The most important physiologic characteristic of solutions is their ability to exert pressure.

Osmotic pressure is the force produced by solvent particles under certain conditions. A membrane that permits molecules passage of solvent, but not solute, is called a *semipermeable membrane*. If such a membrane divides a solution into two compartments, molecules of solvent can pass through it from one side to the other (Figure 13-2, *A*). The number of molecules passing (or diffusing) in one direction must equal the number passing in the opposite direction. An equal ratio of solute to solvent particles (which determines the concentration of the solution) is maintained on both sides of the membrane.

If a solution is placed on one side of the semipermeable membrane and pure solvent on the other, solvent molecules will move through the membrane into the solution. The force driving solvent molecules through the membrane is osmotic pressure. You can

measure osmotic pressure by connecting the expanding column of the solution to a manometer (Figure 13-2, *B* and *C*). This pressure tries to distribute solvent molecules so that the same ratio of solute to solvent exists on both sides of the membrane.

Osmotic pressure can also be visualized as an attractive force of solute particles in a concentrated

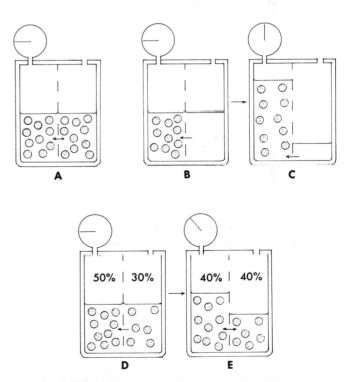

Fig. 13–2 Osmotic pressure is illustrated by the solutions in the above five containers. The containers are divided into two compartments by semipermeable membranes that permit the passage through them of solvent molecules but not solute (*dotted circles*). The numbers of solute particles represent relative concentrations of the solutions; since they are fixed in number and are confined by the membranes, volume changes are a function of the diffusible solvent, movements of which are indicated by the arrows through the membranes. The arrows between containers **B** and **C** and **D** and **E** indicate progressive sequences of osmotic pressure. (See text for further description.)

solution. If a 50% solution is placed on one side of the membrane and a 30% solution on the other, solvent molecules will move from the dilute to the concentrated side (Figure 13-2, *D* and *E*). The greater number of solute particles in the concentrated solution attracts solvent molecules from the dilute solution until equilibrium occurs. An equilibrium condition exists when the ratios of solute to solvent in both compartments are equal (40% in the example given).

Osmotic pressure depends on the number of particles in solution. A 2% solution has twice the osmotic pressure of a 1% solution. For a given amount of solute, osmotic pressure is inversely proportional to the volume of solvent. Osmotic pressure varies directly with temperature, increasing 1/273 for each 1° C.

Most cell walls are semipermeable membranes. Through osmotic pressure, water is distributed throughout the body within physiologic ranges. *Tonicity* is the degree of osmotic pressure exerted by a solution. Average body cellular fluid has the tonicity of a 0.9% solution of NaCl (i.e., physiologic saline). Other solutions with similar tonicity are called *isotonic.* Those with greater tonicity are *hypertonic,* and those with less *hypotonic.* Some cells possess selective permeability. These cells allow passage not only of water but of specific solutes. Through this mechanism, nutrients and physiologic solutions are distributed throughout the body.

There are three basic types of physiologic solutions. Depending on the solute, solutions are *ionic,* (electrovalent), *polar covalent,* or *nonpolar covalent* (Table 13-1). In ionic and polar covalent solutions, some of the solute ionizes into separate particles known as *ions.* A solution in which this dissociation occurs is termed an electrolyte solution (Figure 13-3). If an electrode is placed in such a solution, positive ions migrate to the negative electrode. These ions are called *cations.* Negative ions migrate to the positive electrode and are called *anions.* In nonpolar covalent solutions, molecules of solute remain intact. They do not carry electrical charges. They are referred to as nonelectrolytes. All three types of solutions coexist in the body. These solutions also serve as the media in which colloids and simple suspensions are dispersed.

Quantifying solute content and activity

There are two ways to quantify the amount of solute in a solution: (1) by actual weight (grams or milligrams) and (2) by chemical combining power. The weight of a solute is relatively easy to measure and specify. It does not, however, indicate chemical combining power. For example, the sodium ion (Na^+) has a gram ionic weight of 23. The bicarbonate ion (HCO_3^-) has a gram ionic weight of 61. Because the gram atomic weight of every substance has 6.023×10^{23} particles, these ions have the same chemical combining power in solution. The number of chemically reactive units is more meaningful than their weight.

Equivalent weights

In medicine it is customary to refer to physiological substances in terms of chemical combining power. The measure commonly used is *equivalent weight.* Equivalent weights are amounts of substances that have equal chemical combining power. For example, if chemical A reacts with chemical B, one equivalent weight of A will react with exactly one equivalent weight of B. No excess reactants of A or B will remain.

Two magnitudes of equivalent weights are used to calculate chemical combining power: the gram equivalent weight (gEq), and the milligram equivalent

Table 13-1 Types of physiologic solutions

Type	Characteristics	Physiologic example
Ionic (electrovalent)	Ionic compounds dissolved from crystalline form, usually in water (hydration); form strong electrolytes with conductivity dependent on concentration of ions.	Saline solution (0.9% NaCl)
Polar covalent	Molecular compounds dissolved in water or other solvents to produce ions (ionization). Electrolytes may be weak or strong, depending on degree of ionization. Solutions polarize and are good conductors.	Hydrochloric acid (HCl) (strong electrolyte) Acetic acid (CH_3COOH) (weak electrolyte)
Nonpolar covalent	Molecular compounds dissolved into electrically neutral solutions (i.e., do not polarize). Solutions are not good conductors; nonelectrolytes.	Glucose ($C_6H_{12}O_6$)

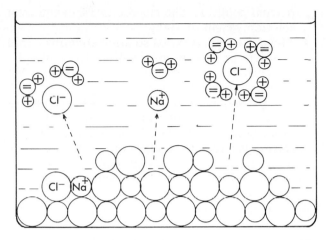

Fig. 13-3 Sodium chloride is shown as a crystalline mass of ions being dissociated by the attraction of water **dipoles**. (See text for a more detailed description.)

weight, or milliequivalent (mEq). One milliequivalent is 1/1000 of a gEq.

Gram equivalent weight values A gEq of a substance is calculated as its gram atomic (i.e., formula) weight divided by its **valence**. The valence sign is disregarded. Therefore:

$$gEq = \frac{gram\ atomic\ (formula)\ weight}{valence}$$

For example, the gEq of sodium (Na^+), with a valence of +1, equals its gram atomic weight of 23 g. The gEq of calcium (Ca^{++}) is its atomic weight divided by 2, or 20 g. The gEq of ferric iron (Fe^{+++}) is its atomic weight divided by 3, or about 18.6 g.

For radicals such as sulfate (SO_4^{--}), the formula for sulfuric acid (H_2SO_4) shows that one sulfate group combines with two atoms of hydrogen. Half (0.5) a mol of sulfate is equivalent to 1 mol of hydrogen atoms. The gEq of SO_4^{--} is half its gram formula weight, or 48 g. If an element has more than one valence, the valence must be specified or be apparent from the observed chemical combining properties.

Gram equivalent weight of an acid. The gEq of an acid is the weight of the acid (in grams) that contains 1 mol of replaceable hydrogen. You can calculate the gram equivalent weight of an acid by dividing its gram formula weight by the number of atoms of hydrogen atoms in its formula.

For example, in the reaction

$$HCl + Na^+ \rightarrow NaCl + H^+$$

the single H^+ of hydrochloric acid (HCl) is replaced by Na^+. One mol of HCl has 1 mol of replaceable hydrogen. By definition, the gEq of HCl must be the same as its gram formula weight, or 36.5 g. The two H^+ of sulfuric acid (H_2SO_4) are both considered re-

placeable. Therefore 1 mol of sulfuric acid contains 2 mol of replaceable hydrogen. The gram equivalent weight of H_2SO_4 is therefore half its gram formula weight, or 49 g.

Those acids in which H^+ are not completely replaceable are exceptions to the above rule. In some acids H^+ replacement varies according to specific reactions. Carbonic acid (H_2CO_3) and phosphoric acid (H_3PO_4) are good examples of such exceptions. Their equivalent weights are determined by the conditions of their chemical reactions.

For example, H_2CO_3 has two hydrogen atoms. In physiologic reactions, only one is considered replaceable:

$$H_2CO_3 + Na^+ \rightarrow NaHCO_3 + H^+$$

Only one hydrogen is released; the other remains bound. One mole of carbonic acid contains only 1 mol of replaceable hydrogen. The gram equivalent weight of carbonic acid is the same as its gram formula weight, or 62 g.

Gram equivalent weight of a base. The equivalent weight of a base is its weight (grams) containing 1 mol of replaceable hydroxyl (OH^-) ions. Like acids, the gEq of bases is calculated by dividing gram formula weight by the number of OH groups in its formula.

Conversion of gram weight to equivalent weight. To determine the number of gram equivalent weights in a substance, the gram weight is divided by its calculated equivalent weight. For example, 58.5 g of NaCl divided by its gram equivalent weight of 58.5 g equals 1 gEq; 29.25 g of NaCl divided by 58.5 g equals 0.5 gEq.

Milligram equivalent weights. The concentrations of most chemicals in the body are very small. The term *milligram equivalent weight,* or mEq, is preferred. A milliequivalent is simply 0.001 gEq:

$$mEq = \frac{gEq}{1000}$$

For example, the normal concentration of potassium (K^+) in the plasma ranges between 0.0035 and 0.005 gEq/L. These values may be converted to milliequivalents by multiplying by a factor of 1000. The normal concentration of K^+ in the plasma ranges between 3.5 and 5.0 mEq/L.

Solute content by weight

The measurement of most electrolytes is based on actual weight rather than on milliequivalents. This weight is expressed as mg/100 mL of blood or body fluid. The units for this method are abbreviated as mg% or mg/dL (i.e., milligrams per **deciliter**). This text uses the modern designation, mg/dL.

Values in mg/dL may be converted into their corresponding equivalent weights and reported as mEq/L. Conversion between mEq/L and mg/dL may be performed as follows:

$$mEq = mg \text{ weight/equivalent weight} \quad (1)$$
$$mEq/L = mg/dL \times 10/\text{equivalent weight}$$

$$mg = mEq \times \text{equivalent weight} \quad (2)$$
$$mg/dL = mEq/L \times \text{equivalent weight}/10$$

For example, to convert a serum value of 322 mg/dL of Na^+ to mEq/L:

$$mEq/L = mg/dL \times 10/\text{equivalent weight}$$
$$= 322 \times 10/23$$
$$= 140 \text{ mEq/L}$$

In clinical practice, electrolyte replacement is common. The electrolyte content of intravenous solutions is usually stated in milligrams per deciliter or in mEq per liter. Lactated Ringer's solution is one such infusion used for electrolyte replacement (Table 13-2).

Calculating solute content

In addition to gEq, mEq, and mg/dL, several other methods of calculating solute content exist. These common chemical standards are used to compute solute content and dilution of solutions.

Quantitative classification of solutions

There are six methods by which the amount of solute in a solution may be quantified:

1. **Ratio solution.** The relationship of the solute to the solvent is expressed as a proportion (i.e., 1:100). Ratio solutions are used frequently in describing concentrations of pharmaceuticals.
2. **Weight per volume solution.** The W/V solution is commonly used for solids dissolved in liquids. This method is sometimes erroneously referred to as a "percent solution." It is defined as weight of solute per volume of solution. W/V solutions are commonly expressed as grams of solute per 100 mL of solution. For example, 5 g of glucose dissolved in 100 mL of solution is properly called a 5% solution according to the weight-per-volume scheme. In contrast, a liquid dissolved in a liquid is measured as volumes of solute to volumes of solution.
3. **Percent solution.** A percent solution is weight of solute per weight of solution. Five grams of glucose dissolved in 95 g of water is a true

percent solution. The glucose is 5% of the total solution weight of 100 g.

4. **Molal solution.** A molal solution contains 1 mol of solute per kilogram of solvent (or 1 mmol/g solvent). The concentration of a molal solution is independent of temperature.
5. **Molar solution.** A molar solution has 1 mol of solute per liter of solution (or 1 mmol/mL solution). Solute is measured into a container, and solvent is added to produce the solution volume desired. Equal volumes of molar solutions of equal molarity contain the same number or fractions of solute mols.
6. **Normal solution.** A normal solution has 1 gEq solute/L solution (or 1 mEq/mL solution). For all monovalent solutes, normal and molar solutions are the same. The equivalent weights of their solutes equal their gram formula weights. Equal volumes of solutions of the same normality contain chemically equivalent amounts of their solutes. If the solutes react chemically with one another, then equal volumes of the solutions will react completely. Neither substance will remain in excess. Normal solutions are often used as standards in the analytic process of **titration** to determine the concentrations of other solutions.

Dilution calculations

Dilute solutions are made from a stock preparation. Dilution problems often involve medications. Dilution calculations are based on the weight per unit volume percent principle.

Diluting a solution increases its volume without changing the amount of solute it contains. This reduces the concentration of the solution. The amount of solute after dilution is the same as in the original volume. The amount of solute in a solution can be expressed as volume times concentration. For example, 50 mL of a 10% solution (i.e., 10 g/dL) contains 50×0.1, or 5 g. In dilution of a solution, initial volume (V_1) times initial concentration (C_1) equals final volume times final concentration. This can be expressed as:

$$V_1C_1 = V_2C_2$$

When three of the variables are known, the fourth can be calculated.

1. Given 10 mL of a 2% (0.02) solution, dilute to a concentration of 0.5% (0.005).
   This requires finding the new volume (V_2):

$$V_1C_1 = V_2C_2$$

rearranging:

$$V_2 = V_1C_1/C_2$$
$$V_2 = 10 \text{ mL} \times 0.02/0.005$$
$$V_2 = 40 \text{ mL}$$

Table 13-2   Concentrations of ingredients in lactated Ringer's solution

	mg/dL		Approximate mEq/L
NaCl	600	Na	130
NaC$_3$H$_5$O$_3$ (sodium lactate)	310	Cl	109
KCl	30	C$_3$H$_5$O$_3$	28
CaCl$_2$	20	K	4
		Ca	3

2. Fifty milliliters of water is added to 150 mL of a 3% (0.03) solution; calculate the new concentration.

This requires finding the new concentration (C_2):

$$V_1C_1 = V_2C_2$$

rearranging:

$$C_2 = V_1C_1/V_2$$
$$C_2 = 150 \text{ mL} \times 0.03/(50 + 150 \text{ mL})$$
$$C_2 = 0.0225 \text{ or } 2.25\%$$

3. Given 50 mL of a 0.33N solution, dilute it to a 0.1N concentration. Here, concentration is given as normality, but it can be used similar to a percent. The new volume (V_2) must be calculated.

$$V_1C_1 = V_2C_2$$

rearranging:

$$V_2 = V_1C_1/C_2$$
$$V_2 = 50 \text{ mL} \times 0.33/0.1$$
$$V_2 = 165 \text{ mL}$$

ELECTROLYTIC ACTIVITY AND ACID-BASE BALANCE

Acid-base balance depends on the concentration and activity of electrolytic solutes in the body. Clinical application of acid-base *homeostasis* is covered in detail in Chapter 14.

Characteristics of acids, bases and salts

Acids

An *acid* is a compound that yields hydrogen ions when placed in aqueous solution. Such substances consist of hydrogen atoms covalently bonded to a negative valence nonmetal or radical. An example of such a compound is hydrochloric acid (HCl). A newer definition of an acid is that of Brönsted-Lowry. In this scheme, an acid is any compound that is a proton donor. Many substances other than traditional acids can be included. For example, the ammonium ion (NH_4^+) qualifies as an acid because it donates a proton (H^+) in the following reaction:

$$NH_4Cl + NaOH \rightarrow NH_3 + NaCl + HOH$$

In this reaction, the sodium and chloride ions are not involved in the proton transfer. The equation can be rewritten ionically to demonstrate the acidity of the ammonium ion:

$$NH_4^+ + OH^- \rightarrow NH_3 + HOH$$

The ammonium ion donates a hydrogen ion (proton) to the reaction. The H^+ combines with the hydroxide ion (OH^-). This converts the former into ammonia gas and the latter into water.

Acids with single ionizable hydrogen. Simple compounds such as HCl ionize into one cation and anion each:

$$HCl \rightarrow H^+ + Cl^-$$

Acids with multiple ionizable hydrogens. The H^+ ions in an acid may become available in stages. The degree of ionization increases as an electrolyte solution becomes more dilute. Concentrated sulfuric acid ionizes only one of its two hydrogen atoms per molecule:

$$H_2SO_4 \rightarrow H^+ + HSO_4^-$$

With further dilution, second-stage ionization occurs:

$$H_2SO_4 \rightarrow H^+ + H^+ + SO_4^{--}$$

Bases

A *base* is a compound that yields hydroxyl ions (OH^-) when placed into aqueous solution. A base is also considered as a substance capable of inactivating acids. These compounds, called *hydroxides,* consist of a metal ionically bound to a hydroxide ion or ions. The hydroxide may also be bound to an ammonium cation (NH_4^+). A good example of this type of base is sodium hydroxide (NaOH).

The Brönsted-Lowry definition of a base is any compound that accepts a proton. This includes substances other than hydroxides. Nonhydroxide bases include ammonia, carbonates, and certain proteins.

Hydroxide bases. In aqueous solution, the following are typical dissociations of hydroxide bases:

$$Na^+OH^- \rightarrow Na^+ + OH^-$$
$$K^+OH^- \rightarrow K^+ + OH^-$$
$$Ca^{++}(OH^-)_2 \rightarrow Ca^{++} + 2(OH^-)$$

Inactivation of an acid is part of the definition of a base. This is accomplished by OH^- reaction with H^+, forming water:

$$NaOH + HCl \rightarrow NaCl + HOH$$

Nonhydroxide bases. Ammonia and carbonates are good examples of *nonhydroxide bases.* Proteins, with their amino groups, can also serve as nonhydroxide bases.

Ammonia. Ammonia qualifies as a base because it reacts with water to yield OH^-:

$$NH_3 + HOH \rightarrow NH_4^+ + OH^-$$

and neutralizes H^+ directly:

$$NH_3 + H^+ \rightarrow NH_4^+$$

In both instances NH_3 accepts a proton to become NH_4^+. Ammonia plays an important role in renal excretion of acid (see Chapter 14).

Carbonates. The carbonate ion, CO_3^{--}, can react with water to produce OH^-. First:

$$Na_2CO_3 \rightleftharpoons 2Na^+ + CO_3^{--}$$

then

$$CO_3^{--} + HOH \rightleftharpoons HCO_3^- + OH^-$$

In this reaction, the carbonate ion accepts a proton from water, becoming the bicarbonate ion. It simultaneously produces a hydroxide ion. The carbonate ion can also directly react with H^+ to inactivate it:

$$CO_3^{--} + H^+ \rightleftharpoons HCO_3^-$$

Protein bases. Proteins are composed of amino acids bound together by peptide linkages. Physiologic reactions in the body occur in a mildly alkaline environment. This allows proteins to act as anionic proton receptors, or bases. Cell and blood proteins acting as bases are symbolized as *prot*⁻.

The imidazole group of the amino acid histidine serves as a primary proton acceptor on protein molecules (Figure 13-4). Imidazole groups produce the buffering effect of hemoglobin. Each hemoglobin molecule contains 38 histidine residues. The oxygen carrying component (heme group) of hemoglobin is attached to a histidine residue. Hemoglobin's ability to accept H^+ ions depends on the oxygenation state of the molecule. Deoxygenated (reduced) hemoglobin is a stronger base (i.e., better proton acceptor) than oxygenated hemoglobin. This difference partially accounts for the ability of reduced hemoglobin to buffer more acid than oxygenated hemoglobin (see Chapter 14). Plasma proteins also act as buffers. Their buffering power is less than that of hemoglobin because they contain less histidine.

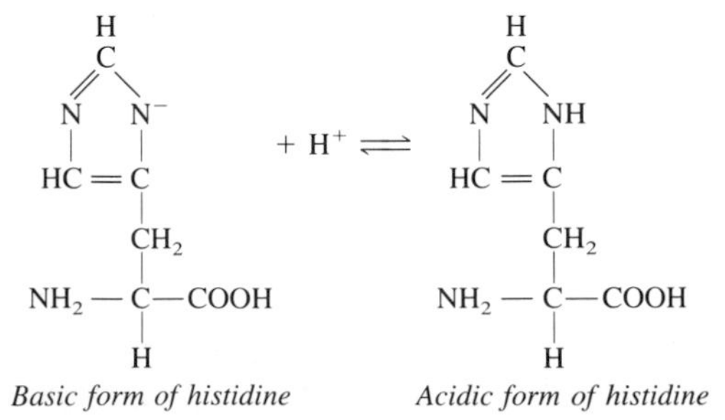

Basic form of histidine   *Acidic form of histidine*

Fig. 13-4 Histidine portion of protein molecule serving as a proton acceptor (base).

Designation of acidity and alkalinity

Pure water can be used as a reference point for determining acidity or alkalinity. The concentration of both H^+ and OH^- in pure water is 10^{-7} mmol/L. Any solution that has a greater H^+ concentration or lower OH^- concentration than water acts as an acid. A solution that has a lower H^+ concentration or greater OH^- concentration than water is alkaline or basic.

The H^+ concentration $[H^+]$ of pure water has been adopted as the standard by which to compare reactions of other solutions. Electrochemical techniques are used to measure the $[H^+]$ of unknown solutions. Acidity or alkalinity is determined by variation of the $[H^+]$ above or below 1×10^{-7}. For example, a solution with an $[H^+]$ of 89.2×10^{-4} has a higher $[H^+]$ than water and is therefore acidic. A solution with a $[H^+]$ of 3.6×10^{-8} has fewer hydrogen ions than water and is alkaline.

There are two related techniques for recording acidity or alkalinity of solutions using the $[H^+]$ of water as a neutral: (1) the $[H^+]$ in nanomoles per liter and (2) the logarithmic pH scale.

Nanomolar concentrations

Acidity and alkalinity of solutions may be reported using the molar concentration of hydrogen ions compared with that of water. The $[H^+]$ of water is 1×10^{-7} mol/L, or 0.0000001 (one ten millionth of a mole). The prefix for billionths is *nano*. The $[H^+]$ of water can be designated as 100 nanomoles per liter (100 nmol/L). A solution that has a $[H^+]$ of 100 nmol/L is neutral. One with greater than 100 nmol/L is acidic; one with less than 100 nmol/L, alkaline.

This system is limited because of the wide range of possible $[H^+]$. The system is applicable in clinical medicine because the physiologic range of $[H^+]$ is narrow. $[H^+]$ in healthy subjects is usually between 30 and 50 nmol/L.

pH scale

pH is the negative logarithm of the $[H^+]$ used as a positive number. It is derived by converting the value for $[H^+]$ to a negative exponent of 10 and calculating its logarithm. For example, the $[H^+]$ of water is 1×10^{-7} mol/L. Because the negative logarithm of 1×10^{-7} is -7, the pH of water is 7. Similarly:

$$\begin{aligned}
[H^+] &= 4.0 \times 10^{-8} \text{ mol/L} \\
pH &= -\log(4.0 \times 10^{-8}) \\
&= -\log 4.0 + -\log 10^{-8} \\
&= -\log 4.0 + \log 10^8 \\
&= -0.602 + 8 \\
&= 7.40
\end{aligned}$$

With this scheme, any solution with a pH of 7 is neutral, corresponding to the $[H^+]$ of pure water. For pH values below 7, the $[H^+]$ increases logarithmically, becoming more acid. As the pH value increases above 7, the $[H^+]$ decreases logarithmically, becoming more alkaline. A pH of 7 is equivalent to an $[H^+]$ of 100 nmol. A pH of 8 is equivalent to an $[H^+]$ concentration of 10 nmol. A change of 1 pH unit is equivalent to a 10-fold change in $[H^+]$ (Figure 13-5).

BODY FLUIDS AND ELECTROLYTES

Body fluids

Water is the major component of the body. It constitutes 45% to 80% of an individual's body weight. The percentage of total body water depends on an individual's weight, sex, and age. Leanness is associated with a higher body water content. Obese subjects have a lower percent of body water (as much as 30% less).

The total body water of the average man is approximately 60% of his body weight. That of the average woman is about 50%. The lower percentage in women correlates with a larger volume of subcutaneous fat tissue. The percentage of weight attributable to water in infants and children is substantially greater than that in adults. In the newborn, water comprises 80% of the total weight (Table 13-3). There is a rapid decline in the proportion of body water to body weight during the first six months of life. This proportion then remains constant until puberty. At puberty differences begin to occur between males and females. As age increases, there is a steady decrease in total body water content.

Distribution

Total body water is divided into two major compartments: (1) the *intracellular water* (within the cells) and (2) the *extracellular water* (outside the cells). Intracellular water represents about two thirds of total body water. The remaining third of body water is extracellular. Extracellular water is further divided into two subcompartments: (1) *intravascular water* and (2) *interstitial water*. Intravascular water makes up about 5% of the body weight. Interstitial water is water in the tissues between cells. It makes up about 15% of the body weight.

Composition

The compositions of solutes in intracellular and extracellular fluids differ markedly. Sodium, chloride,

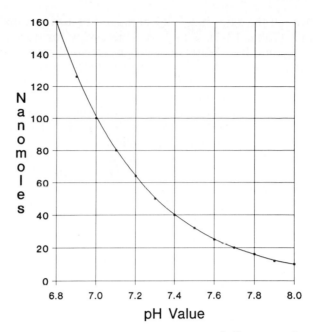

Fig. 13-5 Relationship between pH and nmol $[H^+]$ concentrations.

and bicarbonate are predominantly extracellular electrolytes. Potassium, magnesium, phosphate, sulfate, and protein constitute the main intracellular electrolytes. Intravascular and **interstitial** fluid have similar electrolyte compositions. Plasma, however, contains substantially more protein than does interstitial fluid. Proteins, chiefly albumin, account for the high colloid osmotic pressure of plasma. Osmotic pressure is an important determinant of fluid distribution between vascular and interstitial compartments.

Regulation

Movement of certain ions and proteins between body compartments is restricted. Water, however, diffuses freely. Control of total body water occurs through regulation of water intake (i.e., thirst), and water excretion (i.e., urine production, insensible loss, and stool water). The kidneys are mainly responsible for this regulation. If water intake is low, the kidneys reduce urine volume. This can raise urine solute concentration to four times that in the plasma. If water intake is high, the kidneys can excrete large volumes of dilute urine.

The kidneys maintain the volume and composition of body fluids. This is done by way of two related mechanisms. First, filtration and reabsorption of sodium adjusts urinary sodium excretion to match changes in dietary intake. Second, water excretion is regulated by secretion of antidiuretic hormone (ADH or vasopressin). These mechanisms allow the kidneys to maintain the volume and concentration of body fluid despite variations in salt and water intake. Analysis of the composition and volume of the urine often provides diagnostic clues in disorders of body fluid volume.

Water losses. Water may be lost from the body

Table 13-3   Distribution of body fluids

Body water	Adult male (% body wt)	Adult female (% body wt)	Infant (% body wt)
Total body water	60 ± 15	50 ± 15	80
Intracellular	45	40	50
Extracellular	15–20	15–20	30
Interstitial	11–15	11–15	24
Intravascular	4.5	4.5	5

through the skin, lungs, kidneys, and gastrointestinal tract (Table 13-4). This loss is necessary for normal body function. Water loss can be divided into that which is *insensible,* such as the vaporization of water from the skin and lungs, and *sensible* losses from urine and gastrointestinal tract.

Insensible loss accounts for about 900 mL/day. Of that volume, 500 to 700 mL is lost through skin vaporization in the body's regulation of temperature. About 200 mL is lost in the expired air from the lungs.

Sensible losses are approximately 1200 mL/day. The kidneys require 30 mL of water to excrete 1 g nitrogen. The average adult produces 15 g of nitrogenous waste in 24 hours. The minimum urine output required to excrete this waste is about 450 mL/day. The average urine output in the healthy adult is 1000 to 1200 mL/day. Daily stool contains approximately 200 mL of water.

Other fluid losses from the body are called *additive losses.* They are not essential for body function. Such losses may occur in vomiting, diarrhea, or suctioning from the intestines. Fever, in conjunction with sweating, can also cause additive losses. For each degree of temperature above 99° F that persists for 24 hours, an additional 1000 mL of fluid will be required. Perspiration contains dilute concentrations of NaCl. The healthy adult may excrete 10 to 70 mEq of NaCl/L perspiration.

The gastrointestinal tract manufactures some 8 to 10 L of fluid per day. More than 98% of this volume is reclaimed in the large intestine. In patients who are vomiting or have diarrhea, water losses through the gastrointestinal tract can be considerable. Individuals with open wounds can also lose large quantities of water (in both plasma and lymph).

Other causes of abnormal fluid loss include certain renal and respiratory disorders. Patients with renal disease may have to excrete larger quantities of urine to get rid of extra nitrogenous wastes. Patients with

increased ventilation also have increased water losses as a result of increased evaporation from the respiratory tract. Patients with artificial airways whose inspired air is not adequately humidified are particularly prone to evaporative water loss. The artificial airway bypasses the normal heat and water exchange processes of the nose. The lower airway must make up the difference between the low humidity content of inspired air and the saturated conditions in the lung. This difference, called the *humidity deficit,* can result in large evaporative water losses. A patient with a tracheostomy may lose an additional 700 mL/day if humidification is inadequate. Water loss can be minimized by providing adequate humidification to the inspired air (see Chapter 25).

Infants have a greater amount of body water, particularly in the extracellular compartment. Water loss in infants may be twice that of adults. Infants have a proportionately greater body surface area, making basal heat production twice as high as an adult's. Higher metabolic rates in infants necessitate greater urinary excretion. Infants turn over approximately half of their extracellular fluid volume daily. Adults turn over about one seventh. Fluid loss or lack of intake depletes the infant of water much more rapidly.

Water replacement. Water is replenished in two major ways: by ingestion and by metabolism (Table 13-4).

Ingestion. Water is replaced mainly by ingestion, through the consumption of liquids. Meat and vegetables also contain as much as 60% to 90% water. The average adult drinks 1500 to 2000 mL of water/day. Another 500 to 600 mL of water is ingested from solid food.

Metabolism. Water also is gained from oxidation of fats, carbohydrates, and proteins in the body. The destruction of cells also releases some water. During total starvation, 2000 mL of water is produced daily by the metabolism of 1 kg fat. Recovery after surgery is similar to starvation. During this period, approximately 0.5 kg of protein and a similar amount of fat is metabolized. This yields about 1 L/water day.

Transport between compartments. Homeostasis depends on the total quantity of body fluids. It also depends on transport of fluids between different body compartments.

The first stage of this process is exchange of fluids between the systemic capillaries and interstitial fluid. Transport proceeds by passive diffusion. The capillary wall is permeable to crystalline electrolytes, so that equilibrium between the two extracellular compartments occurs quickly. Plasma, except for its large protein molecules, can also move through capillary walls into the tissue spaces.

This movement of fluid and solutes from capillary blood to interstitial spaces is enhanced by the difference in *hydrostatic pressure* between compartments. This hydrostatic pressure difference depends on blood

Table 13-4 Daily water exchange

	Average daily volume	Maximum daily volume
Water Losses		
Insensible		
Skin	700 mL	1500 mL
Lung	200 mL	
Sensible		
Urine	1000–1200 mL	2000+ mL/hr
Intestinal	200 mL	8000 mL
Sweat	0 mL	2000+ mL/hr
Water Gain		
Ingestion		
Fluids	1500–2000 mL	1500 mL/hr
Solids	500–600 mL	1500 mL/hr
Body metabolism	250 mL	1000 mL

pressure, blood volume, and the distance of the capillary from the heart (relative to gravity).

Opposing hydrostatic pressure is osmotic pressure between the interstitial and intravascular compartments. This osmotic pressure difference is mainly a function of proteins in colloidal suspension in the plasma. Proteins such as albumin are too large to be filtered through the pores of the capillary. Instead, these proteins remain in the intravascular compartment. They draw water and small solute molecules back into the capillaries.

For example, mean arterial blood pressure may be assumed to be 100 mm Hg (Figure 13-6). As a result, capillary blood pressure is about 30 mm Hg at the arterial end and about 20 mm Hg at the venous end. The colloidal osmotic pressure of the intravascular fluid remains constant at about 25 mm Hg. Hydrostatic pressure along the capillary continually decreases. By the time blood reaches the venous end, hydrostatic pressure is less than the osmotic pressure. On the venous side, colloidal osmotic pressure overcomes hydrostatic forces. Water returns into the vascular compartment.

The outflow of water and electrolytes from the capillary on the arterial end is not completely balanced by the return on the venous end. Slightly more diffuses out than is reabsorbed. This slight outward excess is balanced by fluid return through the lymphatic circulation.

Return of tissue fluid by way of lymphatic channels also depends on pressure differences. The pressure in the interstitial space is determined by the volume of interstitial fluid and its electrolyte content. Interstitial fluid moves from a region of greater pressure (i.e., interstitial space) to a region of lower pressure (i.e., lymphatic channels). This "lymph" moves into larger lymphatics, where the pressure is continuously decreasing. Ultimately it returns to the innominate vein in the chest. The return of lymph to the central circulation is enhanced by skeletal muscle activity.

These relationships may be expressed in the *Starling equilibrium equation*:

$$Q_f = K_1 (P_{ch} - P_{ih}) - K_2 (P_{co} - P_{io})$$

where Q_f is bulk flow of fluid between intravascular and interstitial compartments, P_{ch} is capillary hydrostatic pressure, P_{ih} is interstitial fluid hydrostatic pressure, P_{co} is capillary osmotic pressure, P_{io} is interstitial osmotic pressure, K_1 is capillary permeability coefficient for fluids and electrolytes, and K_2 is capillary permeability coefficient for proteins. Three good

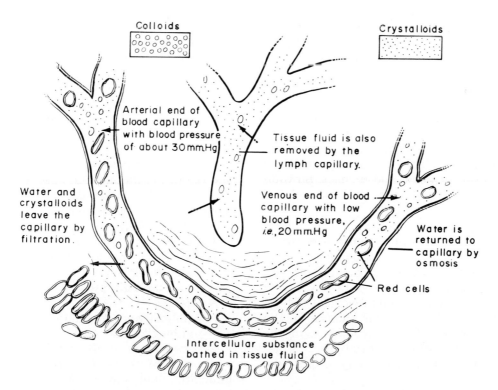

Fig. 13-6 Tissue fluid is formed by a process of filtration at the arterial end of the blood capillary, where blood pressure exceeds colloidal osmotic pressure. The fluid is absorbed by the blood capillaries and lymphatic vessels. It will return to the venous end of the capillary when colloidal osmotic pressure exceeds blood pressure. Fluid is absorbed into the lymphatic capillary when interstitial fluid pressure is greater than pressure within the lymphatic capillary. Normally, little colloid escapes from the blood capillary. Colloid that does escape is returned to the blood circulation by the lymphatic vessels. (From Burke SR: The composition and function of body fluids, ed 3, St Louis, 1980, Mosby.)

examples of the forces in this equation are fluid return from gravity dependent areas of the body, fluid exchange in the lung, and tissue edema.

Because of hydrostatic effects, capillary pressure in the feet can be as high as 100 mm Hg when a person standing. Reabsorption of tissue fluid can be accomplished even though hydrostatic pressure greatly exceeds colloidal osmotic pressure. Three factors favor reabsorption under these circumstances. First, high intravascular hydrostatic pressure is somewhat balanced by a proportionally greater interstitial pressure. Second, "pumping" action of skeletal muscles surrounding leg veins lowers venous pressures. Third, lymph flow back to the thorax is enhanced by a similar mechanism. This facilitates clearance of excess interstitial fluid.

The lung presents a somewhat different problem. In systemic tissues, a constant exchange of interstitial fluid is essential. In the lungs the alveolar region must be kept relatively "dry." Otherwise, interstitial fluid in the alveolar-capillary spaces would impede diffusion of gas. Colloidal osmotic pressure in the pulmonary circulation is the same as that in the systemic circulation. For minimum filtration of fluids in the alveolar-capillary region, the hydrostatic pressure difference must be kept low. The pulmonary circulation is in fact a low-pressure system. The mean pressures are about one-sixth of those in the systemic circulation. Colloid osmotic pressure tends to draw fluid back into the pulmonary circulation. This pressure exceeds hydrostatic forces across the length of the capillary. As a result, the alveoli are relatively free of excess interstitial water.

If hydrostatic pressure increases in the pulmonary circulation, this balance can be upset. This causes fluid movement into the alveolar-capillary interstitium. Excess fluid in the interstitial space is called *edema.* In the lungs, edema caused by increased hydrostatic pressure is often due to back pressure from a failing left ventricle (i.e., congestive heart failure).

Edema can be caused by other factors. The Starling equilibrium equation shows that edema also can be caused by decrease in colloid osmotic pressure or an increase in capillary permeability. For example, if a person loses albumin from the blood, the balance of forces is upset, favoring increased movement of fluid into the interstitium. Likewise, an increase in the capillary permeability results in more fluid leaving the capillaries. Increased capillary permeability is a major factor in certain types of acute lung injuries (see Chapter 29).

Unequal concentrations of potassium, chloride, and phosphate are maintained across cell walls without appreciable hydrostatic pressure differences between compartments. Some molecules are transported across membranes in the direction opposite to that expected from simple diffusion. Such transport re-quires that energy be supplied to the molecules by the membrane. These molecules are moved against the normal osmotic gradient. This process, termed *active transport,* can be accomplished only by membranes that have an energy source.

Electrolytes

Electrolytes in the various body fluids are not passive solutes. These substances are essential to life. They serve to maintain the internal environment while making key chemical and physiologic events possible. There are seven major electrolytes: sodium, chloride, bicarbonate, potassium, calcium, magnesium, and phosphorus (phosphate).

Sodium

Regulation of the sodium concentration in plasma and urine is related to regulation of total body water. Fifty percent of the total body stores of sodium are extracellular. The remainder is found in bone (40%) and in the cells (10%). The normal serum concentration of sodium ranges from 136 to 145 mEq/L. In the cells, the sodium concentration is much lower, averaging only 4.5 mEq/L.

The average adult ingests and excretes about 100 mEq of sodium every 24 hours. Children require about half this amount. Infants typically exchange 20 mEq of sodium/day. Most sodium is reabsorbed through the kidney. About 80% of the body's sodium is reclaimed passively in the proximal tubules. The remainder is actively reabsorbed in the distal tubules. Sodium reabsorption in the kidneys is governed mainly by the level of the hormone **aldosterone.** Aldosterone is secreted by the adrenal cortex. Na^+ reabsorption in the distal tubules of the kidney occurs in exchange for other cations. Sodium balance is involved in acid-base **homeostasis** (i.e., H^+ exchange) and the regulation of potassium (K^+).

Abnormal losses of sodium (*hyponatremia*) may be due to one of the following:
- gastrointestinal losses
- excessive sweat or fever
- prolonged use of certain diuretics (e.g., **acetazolamide**)
- **Addison's disease**
- **ascites**
- congestive heart failure
- kidney failure

Serum sodium levels may be seriously decreased when sodium shifts from the intravascular to the interstitial fluid compartment, as occurs with serious burns. Clinical symptoms of hyponatremia include weakness, **lassitude,** apathy, and headache. In the presence of a decrease in intravascular volume, orthostatic hypotension and tachycardia may also be present.

Hypernatremia is usually associated with an excess

accumulation of body water. Intrinsic factors causing hypernatremia are increased aldosterone production or a decrease in its inactivation. Steroids administration can also cause hypernatremia.

Chloride

Chloride is the most prominent anion in the body. Two thirds of the body's stores of chloride are extracellular. The remainder is in solution in the cells. Intracellular chloride is present in significant amounts in red and white blood cells. It is also present in cells that have external excretory functions, such as the gastrointestinal mucosa.

Normal serum levels of chloride (Cl^-) range between 98 and 106 mEq/L. The concentration of chloride in the extracellular compartment is inversely proportional to that of the other major anion, bicarbonate (HCO_3^-). [Cl^-] is regulated by the kidney in much the same manner as Na^+ (80% reabsorbed in the proximal tubules, 20% in the distal tubules). Chloride is usually excreted with potassium in the form of KCl. Thus inbalances in one of these electrolytes usually affects both. Replacement therapy usually includes both K^+ and Cl^-. The stomach and the small bowel also affect the balance of Cl^-. Sweat also contains hypotonic quantities of chloride.

The most common cause of low serum Cl^- *(hypochloremia)* is gastrointestinal loss. Hypochloremia is also caused by diuretics, such as furosemide (Lasix) and ethacrynic acid. Loss of Cl^- is equivalent to a gain in HCO_3^- (a base). Hypochloremia is usually associated with metabolic alkalosis (see Chapter 14). Hypochloremia may cause muscle spasm and, in severe cases, coma. Hyperchloremia can occur in dehydration, metabolic acidosis, and respiratory alkalosis, and with the administration of excessive amounts of K^+ and NaCl.

Bicarbonate

Next to chloride, bicarbonate (HCO_3^-) is the most important body fluid anion. It plays a key role in acid-base **homeostasis.** It is the strong base in the bicarbonate/carbonic acid buffer pair (Chapter 14). HCO_3^- is the primary means for transport of CO_2 from the body through the lungs.

Bicarbonate stores are evenly divided between intracellular and extracellular compartments. Normal serum HCO_3^- levels range from 22 to 26 mEq/L. The ratio of HCO_3^- to carbonic acid in healthy subjects is maintained close to a 20:1 ratio. This results in a pH of close to 7.40.

More than 80% of the blood HCO_3^- is reabsorbed in the proximal tubules of the kidney. The remainder is reclaimed in the distal tubules. A reciprocal relationship exists between Cl^- and HCO_3^- concentrations. Bicarbonate retention is associated with chloride excretion, and vice versa (see Chapter 14).

Potassium

Potassium (K^+) is the main cation of the intracellular compartment. Most (98%) of the body's K^+ is found in cells. Active transport of K^+ into cells occurs through an ionic pump mechanism. An electrical differential across the cell membrane also facilitates K^+ movement into the cell. For each three K^+ ions that enter a cell, two Na^+ ions and one H^+ ion must leave. This transfer maintains electrical neutrality in the cell.

The difference in K^+ distribution is evident when comparing concentrations between fluid compartments. The intracellular K^+ concentration is approximately 150 mEq/L. Serum K^+ concentration normally ranges between only 3.5 and 5.0 mEq/L. Serum K^+ is only an indirect indicator of the total body potassium. Analysis of serum potassium is usually combined with assessment of both its intake and excretion.

The average adult excretes 40 to 75 mEq of potassium in the urine per 24 hours. An additional 10 mEq is excreted in the stool. Average dietary intake of potassium is 50 to 85 mEq/day. Patients undergoing surgery or with trauma or disease have greater K^+ losses. Consequently, they need K^+ replacement, averaging 100 to 120 mEq/day.

Serum K^+ concentration is determined primarily by the pH of extracellular fluid and the size of the intracellular K^+ pool. In extracellular acidosis, excess H^+ ions are exchanged for intracellular K^+. Movement of K^+ from intracellular to extracellular spaces may produce dangerous levels of hyperkalemia. Alkalosis has the opposite effect. When pH rises, K^+ moves into cells. In the absence of acid-base disturbances, serum K^+ reflects total body potassium. With excessive loss of K^+ from the gastrointestinal tract, serum K^+ falls. A 10% loss of total body K^+ drops serum K^+ level about 1 mEq/L.

Renal excretion of K^+ is controlled by aldosterone levels. Aldosterone inhibits the enzyme responsible for K^+ transport in distal renal tubular cells of the kidney. Metabolic acidosis also inhibits the transport system. Na^+ and H^+ ions enter cells at the expense of increased K^+ excretion. Alkalosis has the reverse effect. It stimulates cellular retention of potassium. Kidney failure results in potassium retention and hyperkalemia.

Hypokalemia due to excessive renal excretion may follow administration of diuretics or adrenal steroids. It is also associated with certain renal tubular disorders. Hypokalemia is commonly associated with vomiting, diarrhea, malnutrition, and trauma (i.e., crush injury, burns). Severe trauma releases large quantities of K^+ into extracellular fluid. Unlike many electrolytes, K^+ is not conserved by the kidney. Despite body depletion, the loss of K^+ can continue.

Hypokalemia disturbs cellular function in a number of organ systems. Affected organs include the gastrointestinal, neuromuscular, renal, and cardiovascular systems. Muscle weakness and paralysis are common. Abnormal electrocardiograms are found in about 50% of cases of hypokalemia. These findings include depressed S-T segments, prolonged Q-T and P-R intervals, and supraventricular arrhythmias (see Chapter 23). **Extrasystoles,** circulatory failure, and cardiac arrest can also develop with diminished K⁺ stores. Hypokalemia may also lead to decreased motility of the gastrointestinal tract.

Management of hypokalemia involves replacement of K⁺ losses and treatment of the underlying disorder. To manage the associated Cl⁻ deficit, K⁺ is given with Cl⁻. Caution is required in the administration of intravenous K⁺. Cardiac muscle is very sensitive to extracellular concentrations of this electrolyte.

Excess K⁺ *(hyperkalemia)* is most common in renal insufficiency. Patients with chronic renal disease do not adequately excrete potassium. Other causes of hyperkalemia include hemorrhage or tissue necrosis. The clinical manifestations of excess K⁺ are similar to those of hypokalemia. The effect on the cardiac muscle is even greater. Hyperkalemia is often diagnosed on the basis of serum K⁺ levels and electrocardiogram changes. With severe K⁺ intoxication, irregular ventricular rhythms and even cardiac arrest may develop. Drug-induced hyperkalemia has become increasingly common. It is usually caused by nonsteroid antiinflammatory drugs, angiotensin converting enzyme inhibitors, cyclosporine, and K⁺-sparing diuretics.

The primary treatment of hyperkalemia is restriction of K⁺ intake. The processes that precipitated the hyperkalemia must also be controlled. Temporary measures for reducing serum K⁺ levels include administration of insulin, calcium gluconate, sodium salts, or large volumes of hypertonic glucose. Cation exchange resins may be given orally or rectally. If these measures fail, **peritoneal** or renal **dialysis** can aid in K⁺ removal.

Calcium

Calcium is an important mediator of neuromuscular function and cellular enzyme processes. The usual dietary intake of calcium is 1 to 3 g/day. Most Ca⁺⁺ is excreted unabsorbed in the feces. Urinary excretion of Ca⁺⁺ averages 150 mg/day. Most of the body's calcium is contained in the bones.

The normal serum calcium concentration is 9.0 to 10.5 mg/L, or 4.5 to 5.25 mEq/L. This concentration is maintained by humoral factors such as vitamin D, parathyroid hormone, calcitonin, and thyrocalcitonin. Calcium in blood is present in three forms: ionized, protein-bound, and complex. The proportion of calcium in each form is affected by blood pH, concentration of plasma proteins, and presence of calcium-combining anions (i.e., HCO_3^- and HPO_4^{--}). About half of the serum calcium is nonionized and bound to plasma albumin. Five percent is in the form of a calcium anion complex. The remaining 45%

is ionized Ca⁺⁺. Ionized calcium is physiologically active in processes such as enzyme activity, blood clotting, neuromuscular irritability, and bone calcification. Acidemia increases, and alkalemia decreases, the concentration of ionized Ca⁺⁺ in the serum.

Hypocalcemia occurs in **hypoparathyroidism,** severe **pancreatitis,** kidney failure, and severe trauma. Clinical manifestations of hypocalcemia are mainly neuromuscular. They include hyperactive tendon reflexes, muscular twitching and spasm, abdominal cramps, and, rarely, convulsions. Hypocalcemia is reflected in the electrocardiogram by a prolonged Q-T interval (see Chapter 10). Treatment consists of correcting the underlying cause and replacing Ca⁺⁺, either orally or intravenously.

Hypercalcemia most frequently is caused by **hyperthyroidism,** hyperparathyroidism, cancer with **metastases** to the bones, ectopic production of parathyroid hormone, vitamin D or A intoxication, **sarcoidosis,** milk-alkali syndrome, or prolonged immobilization. Hypercalcemia is also a rare complication of thiazide diuretic administration. The symptoms of hypercalcemia are fatigue, depression, muscle weakness, anorexia, nausea, vomiting, and constipation. With severe hypercalcemia, stupor and coma may occur.

Treatment of acute hypercalcemia is an emergency. Death may quickly occur if serum Ca⁺⁺ rises above 17 mg/L (8.5 mEq/L). In such cases there is usually an associated deficit of extracellular fluid. Volume replacement will lower the serum calcium by dilution. Steroids and **chelating agents** (such as EDTA) are sometimes helpful in lowering serum calcium.

Magnesium

Magnesium is an important electrolyte for muscle function. It is also related to neural conduction, particularly in the cardiac conduction system.

Normal values for serum Mg⁺⁺ range from 1.3 to 2.1 mEq/L in healthy adults. Serum levels of magnesium may remain normal even if total body stores are depleted up to 20%. Fatty acids and excess phosphates impair magnesium uptake. At least 65 to 70% of magnesium is in a diffusible state. Approximately 35% of serum magnesium is bound to proteins.

Decreased serum Mg⁺⁺ levels are associated with inadequate intake or impaired absorption of magnesium. This may be due to malabsorption syndromes or a diet low in proteins and calories. Pancreatitis, hypoparathyroidism, and alcoholism are often accompanied by increased Mg⁺⁺ requirements or inadequate replacement. Low levels of Mg⁺⁺ are also found in hypercalcemia, hyperaldosteronism, and inappropriate secretion of antidiuretic hormone. Symptoms of deficiency usually do not occur until the serum level is less than 1.0 mEq/L. Severe depletion causes muscle weakness (including respiratory muscles), irritability, tetany and electrocardiogram changes. Delirium and convulsions may follow. Decreased serum magnesium may cause cardiac arrhythmias. Mg^{++} deficiency may also play a role in the development of congestive heart failure.

Hypomagnesemia may accompany the use of certain drugs. Pentamidine, used to treat *Pneumocystis carinii* pneumonia, is one such preparation. Cyclosporine, an antirejection drug used in organ transplantation, may also cause decreased serum Mg^{++}. Low serum magnesium is common in digitalis intoxication.

Increased serum levels of magnesium accompany dehydration and renal insufficiency. Tissue trauma, hypothyroidism, and lupus erythematosus may precipitate increased Mg^{++}. In rare cases, uncontrolled diabetes mellitus may cause hypermagnesemia. Increased magnesium levels potentiate the cardiac effects of hyperkalemia. At levels from 5.0 to 10 mEq/L, the cardiac conduction system is retarded. Magnesium levels of 15 mEq/L may cause respiratory paralysis. Above levels of 25.0 mEq/L, hypermagnesemia results in cardiac arrest.

Phosphorus

About 80% of body phosphorus is contained in the bones and teeth. Ten percent is combined with proteins, carbohydrates, and lipids in muscle tissue and blood. The remainder is incorporated into a variety of complex organic compounds. Organic phosphate (HPO_4^{--}) is the main anion in cells. Inorganic phosphate plays a primary role in cellular energy metabolism, being the source from which ATP is synthesized. In acid-base **homeostasis,** phosphate is the main urinary buffer for titratable acid excretion (see Chapter 14).

Serum phosphate level (1.2 to 2.3 mEq/L) is only an approximate indicator of total body phosphorus. Serum phosphate levels are influenced by several factors, including the serum calcium concentration and the pH of blood.

Hyperphosphatemia (i.e., high serum phosphorus) is associated with endocrine disorders, such as hypoparathyroidism and **acromegaly.** Phosphorus excesses may also occur in chronic renal insufficiency and acute kidney failure. Tissue destruction may also cause hyperphosphatemia, especially in the presence of renal insufficiency. High serum phosphorus is also associated with hypocalcemia. Treatment is directed at the underlying disorder. Dialysis can be used to reduce a sharply increased serum phosphate.

Hypophosphatemia (i.e., low serum phosphorus) may be due to a diminished supply, as in starvation. It also occurs with poor absorption, as when the small bowel is bypassed. Increased loss of phosphorus may occur in hyperparathyroidism, hyperthyroidism, certain renal tubular defects, and uncontrolled diabetes mellitus. Hypophosphatemia is also associated with hypercalcemia and respiratory alkalosis. Low serum phosphate has been implicated in diaphragmatic weakness during respiratory failure. Treatment involves either intravenous administration of a potassium phosphate buffer mixture, or oral phosphate salts.

CHAPTER SUMMARY

The body is a water-based organism in which chemical substances and particles exist in solution or suspension. A major characteristic of solutions involves the action of osmotic pressure. Body cell walls are semipermeable membranes, and osmotic pressure maintains the distribution of water in physiologic ranges.

The electrolytes in the body fluids are essential. They serve a variety of important roles in maintaining the internal environment and making possible key chemical and physiologic events.

There are two primary ways to quantify the concentration of electrolytes in a solution: (1) by actual weight (grams or milligrams) and (2) by chemical combining power. The weight of a solute does not necessarily give us an indication of its chemical combining power. It is customary in medicine to measure electrolyte concentrations in the body in terms of chemical combining power. This is done using either gram equivalent weights (gEq) or milliequivalents (mEq). There are several other ways to classify solute content. These standards are useful for calculating solute contents and dilution of solutions.

Physiologically active compounds of the body are mostly weak electrolytic covalent substances. In aqueous solution only a proportion of the molecules of these substances ionize, with the remainder persisting intact. At a given temperature and concentration, equilibrium is maintained between the ions and the unionized molecules. This equilibrium is quantified by the ionization constant (K).

Electrochemical techniques are used to measure the hydrogen ion concentration of unknown solutions. The degree of acidity or alkalinity is determined by variation of $[H^+]$ above or below 1×10^{-7} mol/L. There are two related techniques for recording acidity and alkalinity of solutions. Both use H^+ concentration of water as the neutral standard: (1) the actual measured molar concentration of hydrogen ions, in nanomoles per liter; and (2) the logarithmic pH scale.

Water is the major component of the body. It makes up between 45% and 80% of an individual's body weight. Percentage of total body water depends on an individual's weight, sex, and age. Total body water is divided into intracellular and extracellular water. Extracellular water is further divided into intravascular and interstitial water.

The composition of solutes in the intracellular and extracellular fluid compartments differ markedly. The predominantly extracellular electrolytes are sodium, chloride, and bicarbonate. Potassium, magnesium, phosphate, sulfate, and protein (prot$^-$) are the main intracellular electrolytes. Intravascular water and interstitial fluid have similar electrolyte compositions. Plasma contains substantially more protein than interstitial fluid. The plasma proteins account for the high colloid osmotic pressure of plasma. Colloid osmotic pressure determines distribution of fluid between vascular and interstitial compartments.

Control of total body water occurs through regulation of water intake and water excretion. The kidneys maintain the volume and composition of body fluids constant by two related mechanisms: (1) filtration and reabsorption of sodium, and (2) regulation of water excretion in response to changes in secretion of antidiuretic hormone (ADH).

Certain electrolytes are essential to **homeostasis**. These include sodium, chloride, bicarbonate, potassium, calcium, magnesium, and phosphorus. Increased or decreased concentrations of any of these can result in disease and sometimes death. Patient care often involves monitoring, replacement, or drug therapy for electrolyte imbalances.

Bibliography

Burgess A: *The nurse's guide to fluid and electrolyte balance,* ed 2, 1979, New York, McGraw-Hill.

Burke SR: *The composition and function of body fluids,* 1976, St. Louis, Mosby.

Carrol HJ, Oh MS: *Water, electrolyte, and acid-base metabolism,* Philadelphia, 1978, JB Lippincott.

Chenevey B: *Overview of fluids and electrolytes, Nurs Clin North Am.* 22: 749–759, 1987.

Gettes LS: Electrolyte abnormalities underlying lethal and ventricular arrhythmias. *Circulation,* 85(suppl):I70–I76, 1992.

Humes HD: *Pathophysiology of electrolyte and renal disorders,* New York, 1985, Churchill-Livingstone.

Keyes JL: *Fluid electrolyte and acid-base regulation: physiology and pathophysiology,* New York, 1985, Jones and Bartlett.

Kruck F: *Endocrine regulation of electrolyte balance,* New York, 1986, Springer-Verlag.

Masiak MJ: *Fluids and electrolytes through the life cycle,* New York, 1985, Appleton and Lange.

Maxwell MH, Kleeman CR, eds: *Clinical disorders of fluid and electrolyte metabolism,* ed 3, New York, 1980, McGraw-Hill.

Metheny NM: *Fluid and electrolyte balance: Nursing considerations,* ed 3, Philadelphia, 1987, JB Lippincott.

Mishoe SC: A review of the physiology, measurement, and clinical significance of colloid osmotic pressure, *Respir Care,* 28:1129–1142, 1983.

Pestana C: *Fluids and electrolytes in the surgical patient,* ed. 3, Baltimore, 1985, Williams & Wilkins.

Puschett JB: *Disorders of fluid and electrolyte balance: diagnosis and management,* New York, 1985, Churchill-Livingstone.

Reed GM: *Regulation of fluid and electrolyte balance: a programmed instruction in clinical physiology,* ed. 2, Philadelphia, 1977, WB Saunders.

Rose BD: *Clinical physiology of acid-base and electrolyte disorders,* New York, 1977, McGraw-Hill.

Stroot VR, Lee CAB, Barrett CA: *Fluids and electrolytes: a practical approach,* ed. 3, Philadelphia, 1984, FA Davis.

Tietz NW, editor: *Clinical guide to laboratory tests,* ed 2, Philadelphia, 1990, WB Saunders.

Webster PO: Electrolyte balance in heart failure and the role for magnesium ions. *Am J Cardiol* 70:44s-49s, 1992.

Williams ME: Endocrine crises: hyperkalemia. *Crit Care Clin,* 7:155–174, 1991.

York K: The lung and fluid-electrolyte and acid-base imbalances, *Nurs Clin North Am* 22:805–814, 1987.

CHAPTER

14

Acid-Base Balance and the Regulation of Respiration

Will Beachey
Craig L. Scanlan

CHAPTER LEARNING OBJECTIVES

1. Compare and contrast the role of the body buffer systems, lungs and kidneys in normal acid-base **homeostasis;**
2. Describe buffering capacity with respect to a buffer's pK and its function as an open or closed buffer system;
3. Apply the concept of ionization constant to the calculation of the pH of the bicarbonate buffer system (the Henderson-Hasselbalch equation);
4. Employ the parameters of the Henderson-Hasselbalch equation to differentiate among the four primary (uncompensated) and four secondary (compensated) states of acid-base imbalance;
5. Compare the four primary states of acid-base imbalance according to underlying causes, and mechanisms of compensation and correction;
6. Explain the interrelationships between renal regulation of electrolytes (sodium, potassium, chloride) and acid-base states;
7. Interrelate the various physiologic processes responsible for regulating ventilation;
8. Describe the responses of the neural and chemical control mechanisms under abnormal conditions, including selected acid-base disorders.

A central component of body **homeostasis** is the maintenance of a narrow range of pH in the blood. Although this range differs among tissues and organ systems, deviations in the hydrogen ion concentration of 25% or more (a pH > 7.5 or < 7.3) can alter intracellular enzyme activity and increase the irritability of nerve and muscle tissue, especially that of the heart.[1] Survival is unlikely when the pH of body fluids drops below 7.0 or exceeds 7.8.

Normal metabolic processes of the body produce more than 24,000 mmol/L of acid/day.[2] Therefore mechanisms must exist to (1) prevent this acid load from causing wide fluctuations in pH and (2) remove or excrete this by-product of metabolism. Physiologic buffering systems assist in preventing wide fluctuations of pH in the body fluids. Excretion of body acids is accomplished by both the kidneys and lungs.

The respiratory system plays a vital role in both the buffering and the excretion components of acid-base **homeostasis.** The primary mechanisms involved in the regulation of breathing cause acid excretion to equal acid production through minute to minute changes in ventilation. Disorders of the respiratory system, including alterations in neural control mechanisms, can disrupt this delicate balance, thereby altering normal acid-base homeostasis.

For this reason, RCPs must be able to assess the patient's acid-base balance and the respiratory system's influence on pH **homeostasis.** This critical ability requires in-depth knowledge of normal and abnormal acid-base chemistry and its relationship to the neural control of breathing.

ACID-BASE CHEMISTRY

Maintaining normal acid-base balance is one of the body's more important functions, and one in which respiration plays a major role. The body's goal in acid-base **homeostasis** is to maintain a balance between acid production and acid excretion while preventing large changes in the pH of its internal environment.

Normal aerobic metabolism of carbohydrates and fats results in the production of carbon dioxide. In solution, CO_2 forms the weak carbonic acid, which dissociates into H^+ and HCO_3^- (see Figure 14-1, page 304). Because this acid exists in equilibrium with gaseous carbon dioxide, it is called a **volatile acid**—that is, an acid that can be excreted in its gaseous form through ventilation of the lungs. About 24,000 mmol of CO_2 are eliminated from the body daily by way of normal ventilation.[2]

Nonvolatile or **fixed acids** are also produced continuously, mainly from the catabolism of proteins (Figure 14-1). Examples of fixed acids regularly produced by the body include sulfuric acid (H_2SO_4) and phosphoric acid (H_2PO_4). Other acids, such as lactic acid, can be produced by the incomplete oxidative metabolism of carbohydrates and fats. Unlike carbonic acid, these fixed acids are not in equilibrium with nor do they originate from a gaseous component.

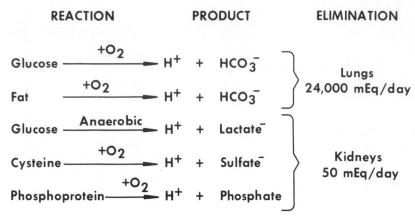

Fig. 14-1 Condensed chemical reactions show the products of several important metabolic pathways and the routes by which H^+ is eliminated. (From Murray JF: The normal lung, ed 2, Philadelphia, 1986, WB Saunders.)

They are therefore not eliminated by the lungs. Compared with the daily production of CO_2, the amount of fixed acid produced by the body is small, averaging approximately 1 mEq acid/kg of body weight, or about 50 to 70 mmol/day.[2] The kidney is responsible for removal of the body's fixed acid load.

If mechanisms to buffer and excrete both volatile and fixed acids did not exist, normal acid production would continuously increase the hydrogen ion concentration of body fluids and eventually cause cell death. The following discussions address the mechanisms whereby buffer systems, in concert with ventilation, maintain acid-base homeostasis.

Body buffer systems

A **buffer system** represents a physiologic mechanism designed to counteract the effects of adding acid or base (alkali) to body fluids, thereby limiting large changes in hydrogen ion concentration and preventing wide swings in pH.[3]

A buffer may be simply defined as a solution that has the ability to resist changes in pH when either an acid or a base is added to it. This solution may be called a *buffer system* or a *buffer pair* because it contains both acid and base components. The acid component is the hydrogen ion formed from the dissociation of a weak acid in solution. The simultaneously formed base component is the anion portion of the acid molecule, also known as the **conjugate base** of the acid. A typical example of a buffer system is a solution of carbonic acid, which dissociates slightly as shown in this reaction:

$$H_2CO_3 \rightleftharpoons H^+ + HCO_3^-$$

The bicarbonate ion is the conjugate base of carbonic acid.

Blood contains two general categories of buffer systems: the bicarbonate system and the nonbicarbonate system. The bicarbonate buffer system consists of the weak acid, carbonic acid (H_2CO_3), and its conjugate base, bicarbonate (HCO_3^-). In the blood, the bicarbonate ion is generally associated with the sodium cation to form sodium bicarbonate ($NaHCO_3$). The nonbicarbonate buffer system consists mainly of phosphates and proteins, including Hb.[4]

The total quantity of all blood buffers capable of binding hydrogen ions is called the **total buffer base,** abbreviated as *BB*. Normal buffer base (NBB) ranges from 48 to 52 mEq/L.[5]

The approximate contribution of the various blood buffers to the normal buffer base is summarized in Table 14-1. The bicarbonate buffer system, both within and outside the erythrocyte, is the most important of all blood buffer mechanisms, for reasons explained later.

The chemical actions of the two primary buffer systems are shown in simplified equations in Figure 14-2. For simplicity, the conjugate base component

Table 14-1 Approximate contribution of blood buffers to total buffering capacity

Buffer category	Percent buffering in whole blood
BICARBONATE	**Percent (%)**
Plasma bicarbonate	35
Erythrocyte bicarbonate	18
Total Bicarbonate	53
NONBICARBONATE	
Hemoglobin	35
Plasma proteins	7
Organic phosphate	3
Inorganic phosphate	2
Total Nonbicarbonate	47

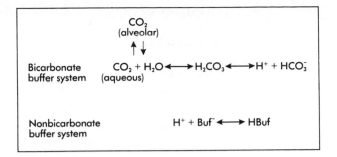

Fig. 14-2 Bicarbonate and nonbicarbonate buffer system. The two systems are in equilibrium with each other. (From Martin L: Pulmonary physiology in clinical practice: the essentials for patient care and evaluation, St Louis, 1987, Mosby.)

of the nonbicarbonate buffer system is represented as *Buf,* with *HBuf* the weak acid and *Buf⁻* the conjugate base of the buffer pair.

Although Figure 14-2 portrays these two systems separately, in reality they exist in equilibrium with each other. For this reason, measuring the components of *either* the bicarbonate or nonbicarbonate buffer system provides an accurate overall picture of acid-base relationships in the blood.[1]

Normally, the bicarbonate buffer system is the focus for acid-base analysis. Not only is it the major contributor to the blood's buffering capacity, it is the easiest component to measure. As shown in Figure 14-2, the bicarbonate buffer system is an **open buffer system,** meaning that its acid component (carbonic acid) is in contact with its gaseous component (CO_2) and can thus be readily excreted through the lungs in large quantities. Carbonic acid is therefore called a **volatile** acid. In its gaseous form (CO_2), the volatile acid of the bicarbonate buffer system, is highly diffusible across cell membranes. As a result, the chemical actions of this buffer system occur quickly within the body's cells.[1] For these reasons, our focus on blood buffers will emphasize the bicarbonate buffer system, addressing the role of the nonbicarbonate system as necessary.

Buffer action

If a strong acid is added to a buffer pair, the chemical reaction will yield a weak acid and a neutral salt. Conversely, if a strong base is added to a buffer pair, the result will be a weakly alkaline salt and water.

Thus, if hydrogen chloride, a strong acid, is added to the carbonic acid/sodium bicarbonate buffer system, the bicarbonate ion reacts with the added hydrogen ions to form more of the weak carbonic acid molecules:

$$HCl + H_2CO_3/NaHCO_3 \rightarrow H_2CO_3 + NaCl$$

Thus the strong acidity of hydrogen chloride is con-

verted to the relatively weak acidity of carbonic acid, thereby preventing a large drop in pH.

Similarly, if sodium hydroxide, a strong base, is added to this buffer system, it will react with the carbonic acid molecule to form a weak base, $NaHCO_3$, and water:

$$NaOH + H_2CO_3/NaHCO_3 \rightarrow NaHCO_3 + HOH$$

The strong alkalinity of sodium hydroxide is thus "buffered" into the relatively weak alkalinity of sodium bicarbonate. Eventually the buffer will be used up, but in the meantime the [H⁺] of the reaction, and thus the pH, will change gradually rather than abruptly.

Calculating the pH of a buffer solution

In a true buffer pair, the weak acid component is only slightly dissociated such that most of the acid exists as undissociated acid molecules. The conjugate base, created by the slight dissociation of the acid, exists in its ionic, or dissociated, form. The ratio between the concentrations of weak acid molecules and base ions determines the hydrogen ion concentration [H⁺] of the buffer solution. The [H⁺] of any buffer pair can be calculated if the concentration of its components and the ionization constant of the acid are known.

For example, the chemical dissociation of carbonic acid in solution occurs in this manner:

$$H_2CO_3 \rightleftharpoons H^+ + HCO_3 \quad \text{(only slight dissociation)}$$

As described in Chapter 13, the ionization constant for H_2CO_3 (K_{ac}) would be the product of the concentrations of H⁺ and HCO_3^- divided by the concentration of H_2CO_3:

$$K_{ac} = \frac{[H^+][HCO_3^-]}{[H_2CO_3]}$$

Solving this equation for [H⁺] yields this equation:

$$[H^+] = K_{ac}\frac{[H_2CO_3]}{[HCO_3^-]}$$

This equation states that the concentration of hydrogen ions in a bicarbonate buffer system is equal to the ionization constant of carbonic acid multiplied by the ratio of carbonic acid concentration to bicarbonate ion concentration. (All concentrations are expressed in terms of moles per liter.) This equation applies to buffer systems in general.[3-6] A generic equation for calculating the hydrogen ion concentration of any buffer system is:

$$[H^+] = K_{ac} \times \frac{acid}{base}$$

pH and the Henderson–Hasselbalch equation

Compared with other electrolytes in the blood, hydrogen ions are present in minute quantities. Table 14-2 compares the plasma ion concentrations of the major cations found in the plasma.[1] The concentration of hydrogen ions is several hundred thousand times less than that of the other major electrolytes. Despite their comparatively low concentration, hydrogen ions exert profound effects on body chemistry.

As explained in Chapter 13, hydrogen ion concentration can be expressed in terms of moles per liter. In the plasma, this concentration is so small that it is expressed in billionths of a mole per liter (nanomoles per liter). Normal plasma hydrogen ion concentration is 40 billionths of a mole per liter (or 40 nmol/L). It is more commonplace to express hydrogen ion concentration in terms of pH—that is the negative log of the hydrogen ion concentration. This yields a positive number (see Chapter 13). The normal plasma hydrogen ion concentration of 40 nmol/L is equivalent to a pH of 7.40.

The **Henderson-Hasselbalch equation** allows you to calculate the pH of the plasma's bicarbonate buffer system:

$$pH = 6.1 + \log \frac{[HCO_3^-]}{[PCO_2 \times 0.03]}$$

Calculation of this pH is important because it is equal to blood pH. The blood does not contain just one buffer system, but many different systems, all of which are in equilibrium with the same $[H^+]$. Therefore, in blood plasma, which has a uniform distribution of several buffer systems, detailed knowledge of one buffer's characteristics (e.g., its pH) permits you to know the pH of the entire plasma solution. The *isohydric principle* explains the fact that all buffer pairs in a well-mixed solution are in equilibrium, with the same pH.[7]

The Henderson-Hasselbalch equation is specific for calculating the pH of the blood's bicarbonate buffer system. As explained above, this pH is the same as the blood's pH. The Henderson-Hasselbalch equation is derived from the ionization constant for carbonic acid (the acid component of the bicarbonate buffer system):

Table 14-2 Plasma ion concentrations

Ion*	nmol/L	mEq/L
H⁺	40	4×10^{-5}
K⁺	4,000,000	4
Ca⁺⁺	2,500,000	5
Mg⁺⁺	1,000,000	2
Na⁺	140,000,000	140

*K⁺, potassium ion; Ca⁺⁺, calcium ion; Mg⁺⁺, magnesium ion; Na⁺, sodium ion.
From Martin L: Pulmonary physiology in clinical practice: the essentials for patient care and evaluation, St Louis, 1987, Mosby.

$$H_2CO_3 \rightleftharpoons H^+ + HCO_3^-$$

The ionization constant is:

$$\frac{[H^+] \times [HCO_3^-]}{[H_2CO_3]} = K_{ac}$$

We know that pH is a logarithmic expression of $[H^+]$. To express $[H^+]$ in terms of pH, we find the log (to the base 10) of both sides of the equation:

$$\text{Log } ([H^+] \times [HCO_3^-])/[H_2CO_3] = \log K_{ac}$$

which is equivalent to:

$$\text{Log } [H^+] + \log ([HCO_3^-]/[H_2CO_3]) = \log K_{ac}$$

Transposing:

$$\text{Log } [H^+] = \log K_{ac} - \log ([HCO_3^-]/[H_2CO_3])$$

We know that $pH = -\log [H^+]$; therefore we multiply both sides of the equation by -1:

$$-\log [H^+] = -\log K_{ac} + \log ([HCO_3^-]/[H_2CO_3])$$

The negative logarithm of the ionization constant, K_{ac}, is the definition of **pK,** which is the pH of the buffer system when H_2CO_3 is exactly 50% dissociated.[7] We can now substitute pH and pK for the negative logarithms of $[H^+]$ and K_{ac}, respectively, and the equation becomes:

$$pH = pK + \log \frac{[HCO_3^-]}{[H_2CO_3]}$$

The Henderson-Hasselbalch equation substitutes dissolved CO_2 for H_2CO_3. This is possible because, dissolved carbon dioxide is responsible for and directly proportional to blood carbonic acid concentration:[5]

$$CO_2 + H_2O \rightleftharpoons H_2CO_3 \rightleftharpoons H^+ + HCO_3^-$$

Carbonic acid is a rare, transitory intermediate compound between CO_2 and H^+, and CO_2 itself is treated as though it were the acid instead of H_2CO_3.[8] Dissolved CO_2 is a more clinically useful quantity than carbonic acid because physiologically it is about 500 times more abundant than H_2CO_3,[8] and it is much easier to determine in the laboratory than H_2CO_3.

The partial pressure of the blood's carbon dioxide, routinely measured with a blood gas analyzer, can be used to compute the dissolved carbon dioxide in millimoles per liter. This is done by multiplying the PCO_2 by a conversion factor of 0.03. Derivation of this factor is provided in the box on page 307.

The final Henderson-Hasselbalch equation then becomes:

$$pH = pK' + \log \frac{[HCO_3^-]}{[PCO_2 \times 0.03]}$$

> ### Derivation of the conversion factor for dissolved carbon dioxide
>
> (1) 1 mol CO_2 = 22,300 mL at 760 torr pressure
> (2) 1 mmol CO_2 = 22.3 mL
> (3) Sol coefficient of CO_2 at 760 torr = 0.51 mL CO_2/mL plasma
> (4) Thus mL CO_2/mL plasma at any PCO_2 = PCO_2 × 0.51/760
> (5) Thus mL CO_2/L plasma = PCO_2 × 0.51 × 1000/760
> (6) Thus mmol CO_2/L plasma = PCO_2 × 0.51 × (1000/760)/22.3
> = PCO_2 × 0.03009

When dissolved CO_2 (i.e., PCO_2 × 0.03) is treated as the acid of the bicarbonate buffer system and is substituted for H_2CO_3 in the Henderson-Hasselbalch equation, the pK, now termed *pK'*, has a value of 6.1. This is a different pK then would be used if H_2CO_3 were left in the denominator of the above equation that is, it is incorrect to use the pK' of 6.1 with the ratio of $[HCO_3^-]/[H_2CO_3]$.[8] As applied in clinical practice then, the Henderson-Hasselbalch equation takes this form:

$$pH = 6.1 + \log \frac{[HCO_3^-]}{[PCO_2 \times 0.03]}$$

Buffer strength

A buffer solution's strength is determined by measuring the quantity of hydrogen ions that must be added to or taken away from the solution to change the pH by one unit.[9] A buffer's strength will vary,

however, depending on the pH of the solution before hydrogen ions are added or subtracted. In other words, a buffer solution has a unique pH range in which it is most effective in resisting pH changes. A titration curve for the bicarbonate buffer system, $[HCO_3^-]/PCO_2$, illustrates this point (see Figure 14-3). Traditionally, this buffer system is symbolized by the ratio between the concentrations of bicarbonate ion and carbonic acid $[HCO_3^-/H_2CO_3]$. Dissolved CO_2, which is equal to PCO_2 × 0.03, is substituted for H_2CO_3 in Figure 14-3 because this substitution also occurs in the Henderson-Hasselbalch equation.

As stated in the previous section, the value 6.1 is specific for the HCO_3^-/PCO_2 buffer system. Although the Henderson-Hasselbalch equation is often written with the term H_2CO_3 in the denominator, the correct form must use $(PCO_2 \times 0.03)$ when 6.1 is used.[8]

Figure 14-3 shows how pH changes when hydrogen ions are added to or subtracted from the buffer solution. The upper left of the graph shows the theoretical situation in which the concentration of dissolved CO_2 is 0% and that of HCO_3^- is 100%. At this point, the quantity of H^+ required to effect a pH change of one unit (i.e., from 7.90 to 6.90) is relatively small, as denoted by the dotted zone. Progressively greater amounts of H^+ are required to change the pH by one unit as more and more acid is added to the solution. When the system contains exactly 50% dissolved CO_2 and 50% HCO_3^-, its buffering power is maximal. Note the comparatively large amount of H^+ (compare the hatched zone with the dotted zone) required to change the pH by one unit (from 6.50 to 5.50). The system's pH at this maximal buffering point (point A) is known as the **pK,** which in this case is 6.10. A given buffer is most effective in resisting pH changes when the system's pH is equal to its pK.

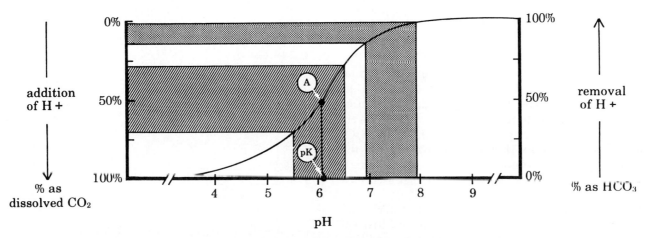

Fig. 14-3 Titration curve for the (HCO_3^-)/(dissolved CO_2) buffer system. (From Beachey WD: Physiologic Buffering Systems: Bicarbonate and Non-Bicarbonate Buffers. *Current Reviews in Respiratory Therapy,* Miami, Lesson 12, Vol 8, 1986, Current Reviews in Respiratory Therapy.)

Physiological importance of the bicarbonate buffer system

The HCO_3^-/CO_2 system would not appear to be an effective buffer in humans considering the fact that the system's pK is 6.10, which is well out of even the pathological range for human blood. Why, then, is it considered one of the most important buffers in the blood? The answer lies in the fact that HCO_3^-/CO_2 is an open buffer system and is an extremely effective way to transport CO_2 from the tissues to the lungs.[4] Therefore it is the most effective buffer against fixed, nonvolatile acids in the body. This fact is best understood if you comprehend the difference in function between open and closed buffer systems.

An open buffer system is one in which a reactant or product of an acid-base reaction is continually removed. In the body, the bicarbonate buffer system is an open one.[4] Pulmonary ventilation provides the mechanism for continuous CO_2 removal, as shown in this reaction:

$$HCO_3^- + H^+ \rightarrow H_2CO_3 \rightarrow H_2O + CO_2 \text{ (exhaled as gas)}$$

Carbonic acid, a volatile acid, is thus removed by way of ventilation. Continuous removal of carbon dioxide prevents equilibrium from being reached; therefore buffering activity occurs as long as ventilation continues. In fact, this buffering activity can continue until virtually all HCO_3^- is used up in binding H^+ ions.[4]

In a closed buffer system, all components of acid-base reactions remain in the system. Products accumulate and reach equilibrium with reactants, and chemical activity ceases (i.e., no further buffering activity can take place). Unlike the open system, not all buffer anions are available for binding of H^+ ions. Examples of closed buffer systems in the body are nonbicarbonate buffers (e.g., plasma proteins, Hb, and phosphates).[4]

To illustrate the effectiveness of the open bicarbonate buffer system, it is helpful to visualize what would occur if the system were a closed one, as depicted in Figure 14-4.

Initially, the buffer solution has HCO_3^- and dissolved CO_2 concentrations equal to those of normal plasma, and pH is 7.40 (Figure 14-4, A). When 12 mmol of a strong acid, HCl, is added, 12 mmol of HCO_3^- is converted to 12 mmol CO_2, which lowers HCO_3^- from 24 mmol to 12 mmol and raises CO_2 from 1.2 to 13.2 mmol (Figure 14-4, B). Because the CO_2 thus produced cannot escape from the system, it increases the denominator of the Henderson-Hasselbalch equation and decreases the pH to 6.06.

However, in the body, the HCO_3^-/CO_2 system is an open one. This system is much more effective in resisting the pH change brought about by addition of 12 mmol HCl (Figure 14-5). A gas with a PCO_2 of 40 torr is bubbled through the HCO_3^-/CO_2 buffer

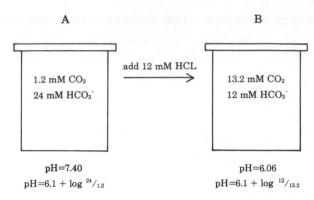

Fig. 14-4 Bicarbonate buffer activity in a closed system. (From Beachey WD: Physiologic Buffering Systems: Bicarbonate and Non-Bicarbonate Buffers. *Current Reviews in Respiratory Therapy*, Miami, Lesson 12, Vol 8, 1986, Current Reviews in Respiratory Therapy.)

solution in Figure 14-5, A to simulate the effects of normal ventilation. Figure 14-5, A represents normal plasma values for HCO_3^-, PCO_2 and pH. As in Figure 14-4, adding 12 mmol HCl converts an equal amount of HCO_3^- to 12 mmol CO_2. Again, HCO_3^- decreases from 24 to 12 mmol, (Figure 14-5, B) but the newly generated 12 mmol CO_2 escapes to the atmosphere. Thus the amount of dissolved CO_2 remains constant (it is 1.2 mmol in both A and B of Figure 14-5), which means the denominator of the Henderson-Hasselbalch equation remains constant. The pH can fall no lower than 7.07 (Figure 14-5, B) because dissolved CO_2 cannot build up in the solution. For this reason, the bicarbonate buffer system is very effective in buffering fixed acids if lung ventilation is normal, even though its pK is well outside the normal physiological range.

Roles of the bicarbonate and nonbicarbonate buffer systems

Bicarbonate buffer system

The bicarbonate buffer system is effective only in buffering fixed (noncarbonic) acid. An increased load

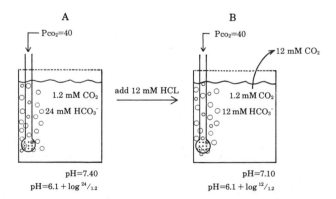

Fig. 14-5 Bicarbonate buffer activity in an open system. (From Beachey WD: Physiologic Buffering Systems: Bicarbonate and Non-Bicarbonate Buffers. *Current Reviews in Respiratory Therapy*, Miami, Lesson 12, Vol 8, 1986, Current Reviews in Respiratory Therapy.)

of fixed acid in the body (e.g., lactic acid) reacts with HCO_3^- of the bicarbonate buffer system, which causes this reaction to occur:

$$H^+ + HCO_3^- \rightarrow H_2CO_3 \rightarrow H_2O + CO_2 \text{ (exhaled as gas)}$$
↑
Fixed acid

The CO_2 produced is eliminated in exhaled gas through the process of alveolar ventilation. Large quantities of acid can be buffered in this fashion. The bicarbonate stores are reduced during this activity, but tissue metabolism provides a continual source of CO_2, which is the source of HCO_3^-:

$$CO_2 + H_2O \rightarrow H^+ + HCO_3^-$$
↑
Tissue metabolism

The bicarbonate buffer system is, of course, ineffective in buffering carbonic acid.[7] Carbonic acid accumulates in the blood only when the PCO_2 of the blood increases. Increased PCO_2 is caused only by hypoventilation, which excretes CO_2 at a rate slower than that at which the body's tissues produce it. This state of affairs drives the CO_2-H_2O reaction to the right. This produces carbonic acid which dissociates into hydrogen and bicarbonate ions:

$$CO_2 + H_2O \rightarrow H^+ + HCO_3^-$$
↑
Hypoventilation

Because inadequate CO_2 elimination forces this reaction to be driven to the right (which will continue to be the case as long as a state of inadequate CO_2 removal exists), the hydrogen ions cannot be buffered by bicarbonate ions and thus must be buffered by other mechanisms.

Nonbicarbonate buffer system

The *nonbicarbonate buffer system* includes plasma proteins, Hb, and phosphates. These buffers may be collectively designated by the symbol *Buf⁻*. Of these, Hb is the most important because it is the most abundant (see Table 14-1). These buffers are the only effective buffers for carbonic acid, but their activity is not restricted to this acid alone. The nonbicarbonate buffers can buffer the H^+ ions produced by any acid, fixed or volatile. These buffers operate as a closed system, and as noted earlier, not all of this kind of buffer is available, because the buffering reaction eventually reaches equilibrium and ceases. In contrast, in the bicarbonate buffer system, virtually all of the HCO_3^- is available for buffering activity. That is, all HCO_3^- can theoretically be used up in binding of H^+ ions because the bicarbonate buffer is an open system. This is illustrated by the following reactions, which show both open and closed systems functioning in a common fluid compartment (plasma):

(Eliminated by (HCO_3^-
ventilation)   stores)
↑   ↓
Open system: $CO_2 + H_2O \leftarrow H^+ + HCO_3^-$
↑
Added fixed acid
↓
Closed system: $H\text{ Buf} \rightleftharpoons H^+ + \text{Buf}^-$
↑
(Buf⁻ stores)

Most of the added H^+ is buffered by HCO_3^- because ventilation frees the reaction to go to the left.[4] Smaller amounts of H^+ react with Buf⁻ of the closed system because equilibrium is approached (denoted by the double arrow) and the reaction slows down. Note that at equilibrium, Buf⁻ still exists in solution, but is unavailable for further combination with H^+.

Although all HCO_3^- is theoretically available for buffering H^+, it is never totally depleted in reality. When metabolically produced CO_2 reacts with H_2O in the erythrocyte to form H^+ and HCO_3^-, hemoglobin buffers the hydrogen ion and causes bicarbonate to be continuously generated. At the same time, ventilation serves as an escape mechanism for CO_2; these two events operate simultaneously to provide a continuous removal mechanism for hydrogen ions as shown in this reaction:

Fixed acid
H^+ ventilation
+   ↑
$CO_2 + H_2O \rightarrow H^+ + HCO_3^- \rightarrow H_2CO_3 \rightarrow H_2O + CO_2 \text{ (gas)}$
↑   ↓
Tissue CO_2 Buffered by
production   Hb

Measurement and computation

Of the three variables in the Henderson-Hasselbalch equation, any one can be calculated if the other two are known. In actual cardiopulmonary practice, modern blood gas analyzers allow concurrent measurement of the pH, PCO_2, and PO_2 on the same blood sample.[10] Assuming that an arterial blood sample has a normal pH of 7.40 and a normal $PaCO_2$ of 40 torr, the Henderson-Hasselbalch equation would allow computation of the blood bicarbonate value as follows:

$$\text{pH} = 6.1 + \log [HCO_3^-] / [PCO_2 \times 0.03]$$
$$7.40 = 6.1 + \log [HCO_3^-] / [40 \times 0.03]$$
$$7.40 = 6.1 + \log [HCO_3^-] / [1.2 \text{ mmol/L}]$$

Rearranging to solve for HCO_3^- yields the normal value for bicarbonate in the arterial blood (expressed in mEq/L):

$$[HCO_3^-] = 1.2 \times [\text{antilog } (7.40 - 6.1)]$$
$$= 1.2 \times [\text{antilog } (1.3)]$$
$$= 1.2 \times 20$$
$$= 24 \text{ mEq/L}$$

Just as the HCO_3^- can be derived if we know the pH and PCO_2, so too can we calculate the pH or PCO_2 if the other values are known. The various forms of the Henderson-Hasselbalch equation necessary to derive any one unknown value are provided in the box below.

Although an RCP equipped with a scientific hand calculator can quickly derive unknowns from this equation, in clinical practice such manipulations generally are unnecessary. Modern blood gas analyzers automate these computations, quickly deriving the HCO_3^- value from the measured pH and PCO_2.

On the other hand, the Henderson-Hasselbalch equation is useful for checking the internal consistency of pH, PCO_2, and HCO_3^- in a blood gas report; in this way, transcription errors and incompatible blood gas values can be detected. Also, it may be clinically useful to compute the effect that a change in one component of the Henderson-Hasselbalch equation will have on another component in the equation. For example, one may wish to know how a given change in $PaCO_2$ may affect the pH. A clinical example would be the mechanically ventilated patient in whom we wish to maintain an acceptable arterial blood pH. We know from Chapters 11 and 12 that the patient's $PaCO_2$ depends on the patient's alveolar ventilation. We can manipulate alveolar ventilation by manipulating the patient's minute ventilation (i.e. tidal volume and ventilatory frequency). Therefore, by changing the patient's minute ventilation by way of the mechanical ventilator we can change the $PaCO_2$ and, according to the Henderson-Hasselbalch equation, the arterial pH.

For example, let us assume that we are ventilating a patient with a tidal volume of 800 mL at a frequency of 10 breaths/min. for a minute ventilation of 8 L/min. Let us further assume that the $PaCO_2$ is 55 torr, the pH is 7.30, and the bicarbonate is 26 mEq/L,

and that we wish to maintain a pH of 7.35. How much would we need to change the $PaCO_2$ to achieve this desired pH, and what kind of change in the patient's tidal volume would this require?

First, we would calculate the $PaCO_2$ required to achieve a pH of 7.35 (according to the boxed information above) using our known values:

$$PaCO_2 = \frac{26 \text{ mEq/L}}{0.03 \times \text{antilog} (7.35 - 6.1)}$$

$$PaCO_2 = 26/0.53$$

$$PaCO_2 = 49 \text{ torr}$$

Next, we must calculate the minute ventilation required to produce a $PaCO_2$ of 49 torr. We know from Chapter 11 that minute ventilation is inversely proportional to $PaCO_2$; therefore, we can state:

$$(\dot{V}_E)_1 \times (PaCO_2)_1 = (\dot{V}_E)_2 \times (PaCO_2)_2$$

where *1* and *2* represent current and future values, respectively. We now solve for $(\dot{V}_E)_2$ using our hypothetical patient:

$$(8 \text{ L/min}) \times 55 \text{ torr} = (\dot{V}_E)_2 \times 49 \text{ torr}$$

$$(8 \times 55)/49 = (V_E)_2$$

$$8.99 \text{ L/minute} = (V_E)_2$$

If we increase our patient's minute ventilation from 8 L/min to approximately 9 L/min, we will achieve a $PaCO_3$ of 49 torr and a pH of approximately 7.35. Now we simply divide our new minute ventilation of 9 L/min by the respiratory frequency to calculate the new tidal volume required:

$$9 \text{ L/minute}/10 = 900 \text{ mL}$$

A tidal volume of 900 mL at a rate of 10 breaths/minute should produce an arterial pH of 7.35 in our hypothetical patient.

Computations involving the Henderson-Hasselbalch equation may also be accomplished with a variety of acid-base alignment **nomograms**.[5] The nomogram shown in Figure 14-6 page 308 is useful for this purpose and can also aid the user in understanding the relationships among the variables involved in acid-base *homeostasis*.[1] The *nomogram* plots PCO_2 on the x-axis. pH and $[H^+]$ (in nanomoles per liter) are plotted on the y-axes. HCO_3^- isopleths fan out from the lower left. If you plot the two known values and draw intersecting lines, you can easily derive the third unknown.

ACID EXCRETION

The body's buffer systems represent the first line of defense against the accumulation of hydrogen ions. However, if mechanisms for continuous excretion of acid by-products of metabolism did not exist, body

---

Forms of Henderson-Hasselbach equation used to compute an unknown value

To calculate the pH if the PCO_2 and HCO_3^- are known:

$$pH = 6.1 + \log [[HCO_3^-]/(PCO_2 \times 0.03)) \qquad (1)$$

To calculate the PCO_2 if the pH and HCO_3^- are known:

$$PCO_2 = [HCO_3^-]/(0.03 \times \text{antilog}[pH - 6.1]) \qquad (2)$$

To calculate the HCO_3^- if the pH and PCO_2 are known:

$$[HCO_3^-] = (0.03 \times PCO_2) \times \text{antilog} (pH - 6.1) \qquad (3)$$

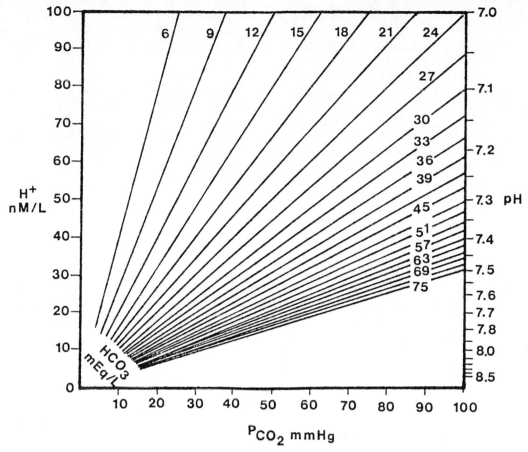

Fig. 14-6 Graphic solution of the Henderson-Hasselbalch equation. (From Martin L: Pulmonary physiology in clinical practice: the essentials for patient care and evaluation, St Louis, 1987, Mosby.)

buffers would be quickly exhausted, and the pH of body fluids would rapidly drop to lethal levels.

Acid excretion is shared in a complementary fashion by the lungs and kidneys. The lungs can excrete only volatile acid (CO_2) but are capable of quickly removing vast quantities of this by-product of metabolism. However, as discussed above, H^+ which originates from fixed acid is very effectively converted to volatile acid (CO_2) by the bicarbonate buffer system, which in concert with the lungs, rapidly removes large quantities of fixed acid from the blood. The kidneys also function to remove fixed acids, but do so at a relatively slow pace.[11] In health, the acid excretion mechanisms of these two organ systems remain in delicate balance. In disease, compromise or failure of one system can be partially offset by a compensatory response of the other. Failure of both systems obviously will result in rapid acid accumulation and, without correction, death of the organism.

The lungs

The lungs are responsible for the excretion of the volatile acid H_2CO_3 in the form of CO_2. Because CO_2 is the end product of normal aerobic metabolism, the amount of H_2CO_3 formed from the reaction between CO_2 and H_2O is more than 500 times that of all other acids combined.[2] In addition to this normal pathway, H_2CO_3 also is produced by the reaction of fixed acids with the bicarbonate buffer system, as mentioned above. H_2CO_3 generated by way of both pathways is eliminated as CO_2 through the lungs. About 24,000 mmol of CO_2 is removed from the body daily through normal ventilation.

In reality, excretion of CO_2 does not by itself remove hydrogen ions; instead, the chemical reaction that releases CO_2 from H_2CO_3 binds active hydrogen ions into the harmless water molecule:

$$H^+ + HCO_3^- \rightarrow H_2CO_3 \rightarrow H_2O + CO_2$$

As described in Chapter 11, CO_2 excretion is directly proportional to the level of alveolar ventilation. Normally, the level of CO_2 in both the lungs and blood is maintained in a very narrow range by sensitive and rapidly responding neural control mechanisms. These neural control mechanisms maintain near constant levels of CO_2 by carefully monitoring changes in hydrogen ion concentration, thereby constantly altering CO_2 excretion to match its production. More detail on these regulatory mechanisms is provided in the last section of this chapter.

Renal regulation of hydrogen ion concentration

Nonvolatile or fixed acids are not, by definition, in equilibrium with a gas that the lungs can exhale. Such acids can be eliminated in solution form by the kidneys. The process by which the kidneys eliminate fixed acids is called *acidification of the urine.*[11]

The kidneys influence the blood hydrogen ion concentration by excreting either acidic or basic urine.[12] To understand how the kidneys determine whether to excrete acidic or basic urine, one must understand some fundamental facts about kidney function. First, however, it is important to define basic terms. **Excretion** refers to the elimination of substances from the body through the urine. **Secretion** refers to the process whereby renal tubule cells actively transport substances across the cell membrane into the fluid in the tubular lumen. **Reabsorption** is the active or passive movement of substances in the tubule lumen back into the tubule cell and then into the blood of the peritubular capillaries.

The glomerulus is the component of the renal nephron responsible for filtering the blood. Hydrostatic blood pressure in the glomerular capillaries forces water, electrolytes and other nonprotein substances through the semipermeable glomerular membrane. This resulting **filtrate** passes out of the glomerulus and is greatly modified in both volume and composition as it flows through the proximal tubules, loop of Henle, distal tubules, and collecting ducts. In the renal pelvis, the modified filtrate is called **urine,** which is then excreted.

At the glomerulus, bicarbonate ions in the blood pass through the glomerular membrane to become part of the tubular filtrate. This process removes base from the blood. But at the same time, the tubular epithelium actively secretes hydrogen ions into the tubular lumen to join the filtrate. This process of secretion removes acid from the blood. Under normal conditions, the rate of hydrogen ion secretion is almost the same as the rate of bicarbonate ion filtration into the glomerular filtrate.[12] This means that these two ions, one an acid and the other a base, are normally **titrated** against each other such that they neutralize one another and create carbon dioxide and water.

The secretion of hydrogen ions begins with the diffusion of carbon dioxide from the blood (extracellular fluid) into the tubule cell (see Figure 14-7). Aided by the enzyme, carbonic anhydrase, carbon dioxide reacts with water to form carbonic acid, which breaks down into bicarbonate and hydrogen ions. The hydrogen ion is actively secreted by the tubule cell into the filtrate by a mechanism termed *countertransport,* which involves the simultaneous diffusion of a sodium ion from the filtrate into the tubule cell.[12] That is, Na^+ first combines with a carrier protein in the luminal border of the tubule cell membrane. At the

same time, H^+ in the tubule cell combines with the opposite end of the same carrier molecule. Na^+ moves into the cell down its concentration gradient which, because of its linkage with the H^+ by way of the carrier protein, provides the energy to secrete H^+ into the tubule filtrate (Figure 14-7).[12]

The rate of hydrogen ion secretion is increased as the concentration of hydrogen ion in the extracellular fluid (blood plasma) rises; likewise, the rate of hydrogen ion secretion is decreased as blood plasma hydrogen ion concentration decreases. Therefore any factor that increases $PaCO_2$ (e.g., hypoventilation) increases H^+ secretion and any factor which decreases $PaCO_2$ (e.g., hyperventilation) decreases H^+ secretion.

The bicarbonate ion that was formed in the tubule cell from the reaction between carbon dioxide and water (Figure 14-7) diffuses back into the blood plasma because the luminal side of the tubule cell is relatively impermeable to bicarbonate ion.[12] Therefore both bicarbonate ion and sodium ion are reabsorbed whenever a hydrogen ion is secreted into the tubular filtrate.

Reabsorption of HCO_3^-

Because bicarbonate is freely filtered out of the blood by the glomerulus, blood bicarbonate would be quickly depleted and lost in the urine unless it were actively reabsorbed into the blood. Because the renal tubule lumen is relatively impermeable to bicarbonate ion, reabsorption of this ion occurs in an indirect fashion, as shown in Figure 14-7. The bicarbonate ions in the filtrate react with the hydrogen ions secreted by the tubular cells. The resulting carbonic acid breaks down into CO_2 and water. Because CO_2 is extremely diffusible through biological membranes, it diffuses instantly into the tubule cell. Here the CO_2 rapidly reacts with water in the presence of carbonic

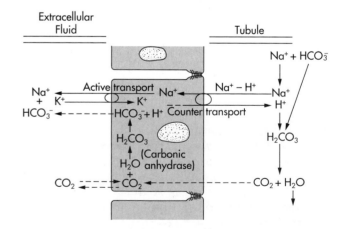

Fig. 14-7 Chemical reactions for (1) secondary active secretion of hydrogen ions into the tubule, (2) sodium ion reabsorption in exchange for the hydrogen ions secreted, and (3) combination of hydrogen ions with bicarbonate ions in the tubules to form carbon dioxide and water. (From Guyton, AC: Basic human physiology, ed 8, Philadelphia, WB Saunders, 1991.)

anhydrase to form HCO_3^- and H^+, and the HCO_3^- diffuses back into the blood. Thus HCO_3^- in the tubular filtrate is "reabsorbed" into the blood, although it is not the same HCO_3^- ion which existed in the tubular fluid. If sufficient H^+ is secreted by the tubule cells, all HCO_3^- in the tubular fluid is reabsorbed in this manner.

Renal elimination of acid and base

The titration of bicarbonate ions against secreted hydrogen ions in the tubular filtrate is not always complete. For example, the number of H^+ ions secreted by the tubule cells when blood CO_2 is increased is greater than the number of HCO_3^- ions present in the filtrate. This is true because when blood CO_2 is high, as is the case in a state of hypoventilation, the ratio of dissolved CO_2 to HCO_3^- increases which causes tubular H^+ secretion to exceed HCO_3^- filtration at the glomerulus. The excess H^+ combines with other buffer anions present in the filtrate (to be explained later) and is excreted in the urine. The net effect of secreting excess H^+ (due to high blood CO_2 in this example) is to reabsorb all of the HCO_3^- in the filtrate and to increase the quantity of HCO_3^- in the blood.[12] According to the Henderson-Hasselbalch equation, this increased reabsorption of the HCO_3^- component of the bicarbonate buffer system would shift the blood pH in the alkaline direction, thereby correcting acidic blood.

On the other hand, if blood CO_2 is low, as would be the case in a state of hyperventilation, the ratio of bicarbonate ions to dissolved CO_2 molecules increases. Again, titration of HCO_3^- against H^+ is incomplete (i.e. there are more bicarbonate ions in the filtrate than there are hydrogen ions available). Because HCO_3^- cannot be reabsorbed without first reacting with H^+ (as explained earlier), the remaining excess HCO_3^- is excreted in the urine, carrying with it some other positive ion such as Na^+ or K^+. The net effect of reduced secretion of H^+ is an increased quantity of HCO_3^- lost in the urine. The Henderson-Hasselbalch equation reveals that because the bicarbonate portion of the bicarbonate buffer system is decreasing, the blood pH is shifted back in an acid direction, thereby correcting alkaline blood. These renal responses to high and low blood PCO_2 just described are the basis for the kidney's **compensation** for respiratory abnormalities, as discussed in later sections.

Excess hydrogen ion excretion and the role of urinary buffers

Only a small amount of H^+ can be carried in the free form by the tubular filtrate into the urine because when the tubular pH drops to 4.5, H^+ secretion ceases.[12] Hydrogen ion secretion by the tubule cell is "gradient limited" so that as filtrate $[H^+]$ builds up, secretion slows until it stops at a filtrate pH of 4.5. Therefore, if no buffers existed in the filtrate with which excess H^+ could combine, the H^+-secreting

mechanism could not function to any great extent. Buffers in the tubular fluid, then, are essential for the secretion and elimination of excess hydrogen ions in acidotic states. After bicarbonate, the two most important urinary buffers in this regard are the phosphate and ammonia buffers.

Phosphate buffers

The phosphate buffer system consists of both HPO_4^{--} and $H_2PO_4^-$. These buffers are fairly concentrated in the tubular fluid because of the relative impermeability of the tubular membrane to them and because of the loss of water from tubular fluid. Thus the phosphate buffer, although weak in the blood, is much more powerful in the tubular fluid.[12] Moreover, the pK of the phosphate buffer system is 6.8, within the range of tubular filtrate when blood is acidotic; therefore in the tubules, the phosphate buffer system functions in its most effective range.[12] Figure 14-8 shows that for each H^+ secreted by the tubule cell (which then combines with HPO_4^{--}), a bicarbonate ion is formed in the tubule cell and transported into the blood. Thus when the blood is acidic and the tubule cell secretes more hydrogen ions than there are bicarbonate ions available in the tubular fluid, the urinary phosphate buffer helps to further correct the acidic state of the blood.

Ammonia buffer system

Figure 14-9, page 314, illustrates the function of the renal ammonia buffer system. The tubule cells continually synthesize and secrete ammonia (NH_3), which diffuses into the tubular fluid down a concentration gradient where it combines with any excess H^+ remaining in the filtrate. This forms ammonium cations (NH_4^+) which are excreted into the urine with chloride anions. Whenever an ammonium ion is formed, the concentration of NH_3 in the tubular fluid decreases which causes more NH_3 to diffuse out of the tubule

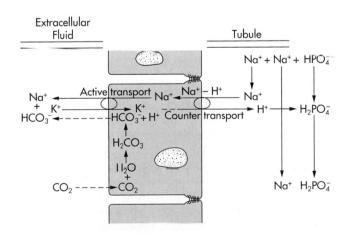

Fig. 14-8 Chemical reactions in the tubules involving hydrogen ions, sodium ions, and the phosphate buffer system. (From Guyton, AC: Basic human physiology, ed 8, Philadelphia, WB Saunders, 1991.)

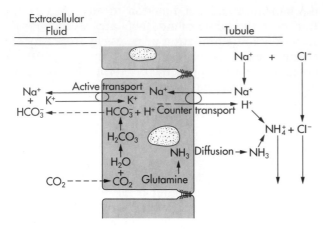

Fig. 14–9 Secretion of ammonia by the tubular epithelial cells and reaction of the ammonia with hydrogen ions in the tubules. (From Guyton AC: Basic human physiology, ed 8, Philadelphia, 1991, WB Saunders.)

cell. Thus the rate of NH_3 secretion by the tubule cell is controlled by the quantity of excess H^+ present in the tubular fluid. In chronic acidotic states in which tubular fluid has a high excess of H^+ for long periods of time, ammonia secretion greatly increases and may increase as much as 10-fold.[12]

Most negative ions in the tubular fluid are chloride ions; if H^+ were to combine with Cl^-, the tubular fluid pH would fall rapidly because hydrochloric acid is a very strong acid. By first combining with ammonia, the hydrogen ion is carried as an ammonium ion, which then combines with the chloride ion. Because NH_4Cl is only weakly acidic, tubular fluid pH does not decrease significantly, and H^+ secretion by the tubule cell is not hampered. Figure 14-9 shows that when H^+ is secreted by the tubule cell to combine with NH_3, an HCO_3^- ion diffuses from the tubule cell back into the blood. The net effect of the ammonia buffer system activity is cause more bicarbonate to be reabsorbed into the blood, counteracting the acidic state of the blood. It is important to note that while a chloride ion is excreted in the urine in combination with an ammonium ion, a bicarbonate ion is gained by the blood.

Bicarbonate and chloride ion relationships

As stated in the preceding sections, in acidotic states, the kidneys conserve (reabsorb) bicarbonate ions while in alkalotic states, the kidneys remove (excrete) bicarbonate ions. Thus the kidneys cause bicarbonate ions to fluctuate between high and low concentrations as the major means of correcting the pH in the blood. This fluctuation in plasma bicarbonate ion concentration requires the removal of some other anion from the plasma, or the addition of some other anion to the plasma, depending on whether bicarbonate ion increases or decreases. This anion, which decreases and increases reciprocally with the bicarbonate anion, is chloride, the most abundant

anion in the blood plasma. The ammonia buffer system is an example of a mechanism whereby this reciprocation occurs. As noted above, in an acidotic state when the ammonia buffer system is active, hydrogen ion combines with NH_3 to form NH_4^+, and a chloride ion is excreted with the NH_4^+ into the urine; simultaneously, a bicarbonate ion is gained by the blood (Figure 14-9). On the other hand, in alkalotic states the ammonia system is inoperative, and excess bicarbonate is excreted into the urine instead of chloride. This means that an additional amount of Cl^- is reabsorbed into the blood, the amount of reabsorption being equal to the quantity of HCO_3^- that was excreted into the urine.

ACID–BASE IMBALANCES

In health, the combined activity of the body buffer systems, the lungs and the kidneys assure that acid-base **homeostasis** is maintained under a wide variety of conditions. However, should *any* of these three components fail, this balance can be disrupted.

Normal acid–base balance

Normally, the renal mechanisms maintain an arterial blood bicarbonate concentration of 24 mEq/L, while the lungs excrete carbon dioxide to maintain a constant blood PCO_2 level of 40 torr.[3-6] On the basis of these normal values, we may compute a normal pH of 7.40:

$$pH = 6.1 + \log [HCO_3/(PCO_2 \times 0.03)]$$
$$pH = 6.1 + \log [24/1.2]$$
$$pH = 6.1 + \log [20]$$
$$pH = 7.4$$

Because the pK is constant at 6.1, it is important to note that pH is determined by the *ratio* of the concentrations of buffer to weak acid, *not* their absolute values. Therefore, as long as the ratio of HCO_3 buffer to weak acid (H_2CO_3) is 20:1, the pH will be normal (i.e., 7.40).

Abnormal pH values

In health, the body maintains the arterial blood pH in a narrow normal range of 7.35 to 7.45. However, variations from this normal range can and do occur. When the blood pH is higher than normal (above 7.45), a state of **alkalemia** exists. When the blood pH is lower than normal (below 7.35), a state of **acidemia** exists.[14] Acidemia and alkalemia refer specifically to blood states, whereas the terms **acidosis** and **alkalosis** are more general and refer to abnormal hydrogen ion concentrations in the body. Unfortunately, knowledge of the pH alone provides little useful information regarding the *process* underlying an abnormal value. Indeed, as will be demonstrated, an abnormal acid-base state can exist with a normal pH.

Primary acid–base abnormalities

To analyze the processes underlying acid-base imbalances, we need to return to the Henderson-Hasselbalch equation. Beyond providing the basis for computing the parameters of acid-base balance, the Henderson-Hasselbalch equation can assist us in understanding the interrelationships that occur between the various components of acid-base balance, particularly those underlying abnormal acid-base states.

As we now know, the HCO_3^- component of the Henderson-Hasselbalch equation relates primarily to renal buffering and excretion of the body's fixed acid load. Likewise, the dissolved CO_2 component of the equation relates primarily to the excretion of the volatile acid load by the lungs. Based on this understanding, we can rewrite the equation to reflect in concept these critical components of acid-base balance:

$$pH \propto \frac{\text{Fixed acid buffering } (HCO_3^-) \text{ by kidneys}}{\text{Volatile acid regulation } (CO_2) \text{ by lungs}}$$

According to this conceptual formula, the pH will increase if either the buffer capacity increases (kidneys), or the volatile acid (CO_2) decreases (lungs). On the other hand, if either the buffer capacity decreases, or CO_2 increases, the pH will fall.

Thus alkalemia (pH > 7.45) can be caused either by an increase in buffer base (as indicated by an increase in $[HCO_3]$) or by a decrease in CO_2. Likewise, acidemia (pH < 7.35) can be caused either by a decrease in buffer base (as indicated by a decrease in $[HCO_3]$) or by an increase in CO_2. Because *two* primary causes can be associated with an abnormally high pH, and *two* primary causes can be associated with an abnormally low pH, *four* primary abnormal acid-base processes exist (Table 14-3).

Respiratory processes

Because changes in CO_2 are mainly a function of ventilation, imbalances resulting solely from ventilation abnormalities are considered respiratory in origin. Respiratory processes resulting in acidemia are termed *respiratory acidosis*. Respiratory acidosis occurs whenever the denominator of the Henderson-Hasselbalch equation (CO_2) increases ($\rightarrow$ = normal or no change; $\uparrow$ = increased; $\downarrow$ = decreased):

$$\downarrow pH \propto \frac{\rightarrow HCO_3^-}{\uparrow PaCO_2} \text{ (respiratory acidosis)}$$

Respiratory processes resulting in alkalemia are termed *respiratory alkalosis*. Respiratory alkalosis occurs whenever the denominator of the Henderson-Hasselbalch equation (CO_2) falls:

$$\uparrow pH \propto \frac{\rightarrow HCO_3^-}{\downarrow PaCO_2} \text{ (respiratory alkalosis)}$$

Metabolic processes

On the other hand, changes in HCO_3^- are primarily caused by variations in the kidney's response to the fixed acid load, that is these changes are "metabolic" or nonrespiratory in origin. The term *metabolic* is arbitrarily, and by convention, the term used to designate all nonrespiratory processes that affect acid-base status of the blood.[12] Nonrespiratory processes resulting in acidemia are termed *metabolic acidosis*. Metabolic acidosis occurs whenever the numerator of the equation (HCO_3^-) falls:

$$\downarrow pH \propto \frac{\downarrow HCO_3^-}{\rightarrow PaCO_2} \text{ (metabolic acidosis)}$$

Nonrespiratory processes resulting in alkalemia are termed *metabolic alkalosis*. Metabolic alkalosis occurs whenever the numerator of the equation (HCO_3^-) rises.

$$\uparrow pH \propto \frac{\uparrow HCO_3^-}{\rightarrow PaCO_2} \text{ (metabolic alkalosis)}$$

Restoring a normal pH

The goal of acid-base homeostasis is maintenance of a normal pH. The body restores an abnormal pH through a mechanism called compensation. Therapeutic intervention by health care personnel aimed at restoring a normal pH is termed **correction.**

Compensation

Because the pH is proportionate to the ratio of bicarbonate ion concentration (controlled by the kidneys) to dissolved carbon dioxide (controlled by the lungs), a primary failure of one organ system can be compensated for by the other. In compensation, the system not primarily affected assumes responsibility for returning the pH to normal.[15] Compensation represents a normal response of the body to a failure in one component of the acid-base regulatory mechanism.

For example, if the $PaCO_2$ rises to 60 torr because of hypoventilation (respiratory acidosis), the pH would fall to approximately 7.22:

$$pH = 6.1 + \log [24/(60 \times 0.03)]$$
$$pH = 6.1 + \log [13.3]$$
$$pH = 7.22$$

Table 14-3   Primary acid-base disturbances

pH Change	Main Abnormality	Designation
Alkalemia (pH>7.45)	Decreased PCO_2	Respiratory alkalosis
	Increased HCO_3	Metabolic (nonrespiratory) alkalosis
Acidemia ph<7.35	Increased PCO_2	Respiratory acidosis
	Decreased HCO_3	Metabolic (nonrespiratory) acidosis

With an increase of the amount of HCO_3^- buffer in the numerator of the equation to 36 mEq/L (by way of increased renal reabsorption of bicarbonate), the original normal ratio of buffer to acid (20:1) is restored and the pH is returned to 7.40:

$$pH = 6.1 + \log [36/(60 \times 0.03)]$$
$$pH = 6.1 + \log [36/1.8]$$
$$pH = 6.1 + \log [20]$$
$$pH = 7.40$$

Likewise, if a metabolic or nonrespiratory process alters HCO_3^- concentrations above or below normal, the lungs would respond by increasing or decreasing their excretion of CO_2 (through hyperventilation or hypoventilation) in an attempt to restore the normal ratio of base to acid and thereby return the pH toward normal.

The foregoing examples are somewhat oversimplified in that a change in blood CO_2 does affect the HCO_3^- concentration slightly. This is due to the *hydrolysis effect*[16]:

$$CO_2 + H_2O \rightarrow H_2CO_3 \rightarrow H^+ + HCO_3^-$$

As more CO_2 dissolves in the plasma, the reaction is driven to the right, and more HCO_3^- ions are formed.

Table 14-4 summarizes the four primary acid-base disorders and the compensatory responses that normally characterize the body's efforts to restore pH values back toward normal.[1] Large arrows indicate the direction of the changes caused by the primary disturbance; small arrows indicate the nature of the compensatory response. The mechanisms whereby the compensatory retention or elimination of bicarbonate by the kidney occur have been explained in previous sections of this chapter.

Obviously, compensatory responses require that the unaffected system is functioning normally. Otherwise, compensation will either not occur or, if it occurs, will not be effective. The speed with which compensation occurs varies substantially according to the organ system responsible. More details on these compensatory processes, including their clinical applications, are provided in the following sections.

Correction

In compensation for an acid-base abnormality, the system not primarily affected assumes responsibility for returning the pH to normal. On the other hand, therapeutic correction of an acid-base abnormality aims to restore the pH toward normal by treating the abnormal component. For example, correction of the acute respiratory acidosis in the above example would require that the $PaCO_2$ be lowered to its normal value of 40 torr. You could accomplish this by using a mechanical ventilator to increase alveolar ventilation to match CO_2 production, thereby restoring the pH back toward its normal value of 7.40.

In general, actions designed to correct acid-base abnormalities must focus on removing the underlying cause of the disturbance. However, correction of compensated acid-base abnormalities must be done slowly and with extreme care. Otherwise, correction could cause rapid and potentially harmful fluctuations in pH. For example, in the above case in which the HCO_3^- rose to 36 mEq/L to compensate for the high $PaCO_2$ of 60, if the high $PaCO_2$ is rapidly corrected to a normal 40 torr, a severe swing to alkalosis occurs because the kidneys require hours to days to bring HCO_3^- back to normal limits.[12]

CLINICAL ACID-BASE STATES

To effectively manage acid-base imbalances one must accurately identify the patient's underlying acid-base status. Although RCPs are mainly involved in implementing treatment plans designed to correct respiratory acid-base abnormalities, the metabolic component must be taken into account. Certain metabolic acid-base abnormalities (both primary and compensatory) result from disorders of the cardiopulmonary system. For this reason, the skilled RCP must be able to distinguish between the clinical manifestations and potential underlying causes of *all* types of acid-base disturbances.

Graphic interpretation

Given the complexity of clinical acid-base chemistry, it is sometimes helpful to visualize various acid-base states with a graphic "map." Figure 14-10 illustrates such a map. The map portrays various acid-base states as overlays on the nomogram previously used to graphically solve the Henderson-Hasselbalch equation. The areas of acid-base abnormalities surrounding a central normal axis are plotted as 95% confidence bands, based on the clinical and statistical

Table 14-4 Primary event and compensatory response for acid-base disorders

Acid-base disorder	Primary event	Compensatory response
Metabolic acidosis	$\downarrow pH = \dfrac{\downarrow HCO_3^-}{PaCO_2}$	$\downarrow pH = \dfrac{\downarrow HCO_3^-}{\downarrow PaCO_2}$
Metabolic alkalosis	$\uparrow pH = \dfrac{\uparrow HCO_3^-}{PaCO_2}$	$\uparrow pH = \dfrac{\uparrow HCO_3^-}{\uparrow PaCO_2}$
Respiratory acidosis	$\downarrow pH = \dfrac{HCO_3^-}{\uparrow PaCO_2}$	$\downarrow pH = \dfrac{\uparrow HCO_3^-}{\uparrow PaCO_2}$
Respiratory alkalosis	$\uparrow pH = \dfrac{HCO_3^-}{\downarrow PaCO_2}$	$\uparrow pH = \dfrac{\downarrow HCO_3^-}{\downarrow PaCO_2}$

From Martin L: Pulmonary physiology in clinical practice: the essentials for patient care and evaluation, St Louis, 1987, Mosby.

analysis of a large number of patients. Intersects outside the mapped area indicate mixed acid-base problems.

Although they are no substitute for sound knowledge of acid-base chemistry or clinical understanding, maps such as these are particularly useful as learning aids. For this reason, we will make frequent reference to Figure 14-10 as we further explore the major categories of acid-base imbalances.

Systematic clinical assessment

In analyzing an acid-base problem, it is helpful to approach the data with a series of systematic steps.[17,18] Consistently applying the same systematic approach to all acid-base disturbances helps avoid the tendency to jump to conclusions and ensures that all relevant information is applied to solve the problem at hand. We will apply the following approach in the interpretation of selected examples of acid-base imbalances in arterial blood.

Step 1: categorize the pH

If pH is greater than 7.45, a state of alkalosis exists; if pH is less than 7.35, a state of acidosis exists. The next steps will help us determine whether the acid-base abnormality is of respiratory or nonrespiratory origin.

Step 2: determine the respiratory involvement

Assessing the respiratory involvement entails inspecting the $PaCO_2$; this is logical because the lungs control the level of carbon dioxide in the arterial blood. (The normal range for $PaCO_2$ is 35 to 45 torr.) The $PaCO_2$ must be evaluated in light of the arterial pH. That is, if the pH is abnormal, we then ask ourselves: would this observed $PaCO_2$, by itself, cause this pH abnormality? For example, suppose that the pH is below 7.35 (denoting acidosis) and the $PaCO_2$ is above 45 torr. According to the Henderson-Hasselbalch equation, a high $PaCO_2$ would indeed cause a low pH (i.e., acidosis). Therefore we know that the respiratory system is at least in part, if not entirely, responsible for the acidosis. On the other hand, if pH is less than 7.35 and the $PaCO_2$ is in the normal range, then we know that the acidosis must be of nonrespiratory (metabolic) origin.

Step 3: determine the metabolic involvement

Assessing the metabolic involvement requires that we inspect the plasma $[HCO_3^-]$; this is logical because $[HCO_3^-]$ is controlled by nonrespiratory factors. (The normal plasma $[HCO_3^-]$ of arterial blood is 22 to 26 mEq/L.) Again, we must evaluate the $[HCO_3^-]$ in light of the arterial pH. That is, if the pH is abnormal, we ask ourselves: would this observed $[HCO_3^-]$, by itself,

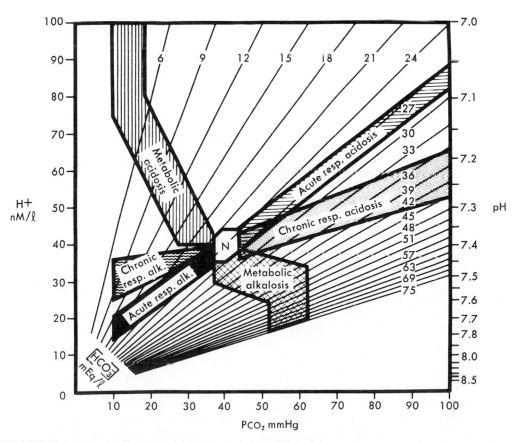

Fig. 14-10 Acid-base map. (See text for description.) (Reprinted from Goldberg M et al: *JAMA* 223:1973. Copyright 1973, American Medical Association.)

cause this pH abnormality? For example, suppose that the pH is less than 7.35 (denoting acidosis) and the $[HCO_3^-]$ is below 22 mEq/L. Indeed, according to the Henderson-Hasselbalch equation, the low $[HCO_3^-]$ is consistent with acidosis. Thus we know that nonrespiratory factors are in part, if not entirely, responsible for the acidosis. If $[HCO_3^-]$ were in the normal range in the presence of this acidosis, then we would know that the acidosis must be of respiratory origin.

Step 4: assess for compensation

Once the acid-base disorder is identified as respiratory or metabolic, we must look for the degree of compensation that may or may not be occurring. We know that the system not primarily responsible for the acid-base abnormality must assume the responsibility for returning the pH to the normal range. This compensation may be complete (pH is brought into the normal range) or partial (pH is still out of the normal range but is in the process of moving toward the normal range). In pure respiratory acidosis (high $PaCO_2$, normal $[HCO_3^-]$, and low pH) we would expect an eventual compensatory increase in plasma $[HCO_3^-]$ that would work to restore the pH to normal. Similarly, we expect respiratory alkalosis to elicit an eventual compensatory decrease in plasma $[HCO_3^-]$. A pure metabolic acidosis (low $[HCO_3^-]$, normal $PaCO_2$, and low pH) should elicit a compensatory decrease in $PaCO_2$, and a pure metabolic alkalosis (high $[HCO_3^-]$, normal $PaCO_2$, and high pH) should cause a compensatory increase in $PaCO_2$. All compensatory responses work to restore the pH to the normal range (7.35 to 7.45).

In cases where compensation has occurred, if the pH is on the acid side of 7.40 (7.35 to 7.39), the acid-base component that would cause acidosis (either increased $PaCO_2$ or decreased plasma HCO_3^-) is generally the main cause of the original acid-base imbalance. If compensation is present but pH is on the alkaline side of 7.40 (7.41 to 7.45), the component that would cause an alkalosis (either decreased $PaCO_2$ or increased HCO_3^-) is generally the primary cause of the original acid-base disturbance.

The term *complete compensation* refers to any case in which the compensatory response returns the pH to the normal range (7.35 to 7.45). The term *partial compensation* refers to cases in which the expected compensatory response, as described above, has begun but has had insufficient time to return the pH to the normal range.

For example, suppose a patient has partially compensated respiratory acidosis; this would be characterized by a high $PaCO_2$, a pH less than 7.35, and a plasma $[HCO_3^-]$ greater than 26 mEq/L. The compensatory response (increased HCO_3^-) is not yet sufficient to return the pH to the normal range, although the expected compensatory activity has clearly begun. In contrast, completely compensated respiratory acido-

sis is illustrated by the same patient several hours later, when the kidneys have had enough time to retain sufficient plasma HCO_3^- to bring the pH into the normal range. This completely compensated respiratory acidosis would be characterized by the same originally observed high $PaCO_2$, a pH that is now in the 7.35 to 7.39 range, and a plasma $[HCO_3^-]$ that is greater than it was before complete compensation took place. The reason that the pH is on the acid side of 7.40 (7.35 to 7.39) is that the primary disturbance (high $PaCO_2$) created an acidotic environment; moreover, the body generally does not overcompensate for acid-base disturbances.

Respiratory acidosis

Respiratory acidosis is a primary physiologic process that causes an increase in the arterial PCO_2 called **hypercapnia**.[1,18] Respiratory acidosis lowers the pH of the blood because of a gain in carbonic acid. An acute increase in PCO_2 of 20 torr will lower the pH by about 0.12. Table 14-5 illustrates acute $PaCO_2$- pH relationships. These acute relationships between $PaCO_2$ and pH assume normal and constant metabolic factors (i.e., a normal and constant HCO_3^-). Under these conditions, any change in pH must be caused by a change in respiratory status. Thus an expected pH for a given change in $PaCO_2$ can be precisely predicted.[16] The extent to which the expected pH differs from the actual measured pH reflects the degree of nonrespiratory or metabolic influence on pH. For example, if the actual measured pH is considerably more acidic than the calculated expected pH, then metabolic processes must exist that tend to cause acidosis. Likewise, if measured pH exceeds expected pH, metabolic factors exist that tend to cause alkalosis. From Table 14-5, expected pH formulas can be derived:[16]

In hypocapnia:
$$\text{Expected pH} = 7.4 + (40 \text{ torr} - PaCO_2)\ 0.01$$

In hypercapnia:
$$\text{Expected pH} = 7.4 - (PaCO_2 - 40 \text{ torr})\ 0.006$$

A different pH change factor is used for hypocapnia than for hypercapnia because of the logarithmic nature of the $PaCO_2 - $ pH relationship.[16]

Table 14-5 Acute $PaCO_2$-pH relationship

$PaCO_2$ change	pH change
Decrease	*Increase*
1 torr	0.01
10 torr	0.10
Increase	**Decrease**
1 torr	0.006
10 torr	0.06

From Malley WJ: Clinical blood gases, Philadelphia, 1990, WB Saunders. Used by permission.

Causes

Hypercapnia (respiratory acidosis) is caused by hypoventilation (i.e., alveolar ventilation that does not eliminate CO_2 as fast as the metabolic processes of the body produce it). The result is an increase in PCO_2 of arterial blood, which represents a gain in volatile acid (H_2CO_3). One can conceive of different ways in which hypercapnia may occur. For example, a patient may have an absolute decrease in alveolar ventilation because of a depressed central nervous system or due to neuromuscular weakness. Or an infection and fever may increase metabolic rate and CO_2 production, thus placing an increased demand on the lungs for CO_2 excretion, which a debilitated patient may not be able to accommodate. This would cause the $PaCO_2$ to rise even though measured alveolar ventilation may appear normal. The common feature of all causes of respiratory acidosis is increased $PaCO_2$. The boxed material summarizes common causes of respiratory acidosis in both normal and abnormal lungs.[10,13,17]

As indicated on the acid-base map (see Figure 14-10), if the process causing the disturbance is acute in onset, the patient with respiratory acidosis will exhibit increased arterial PCO_2, decreased arterial pH, and a normal or slightly elevated serum HCO_3^-. The slight elevation of HCO_3^- is not a sign of metabolic involvement or kidney compensation; rather, it is simply due to the hydrolysis effect. A clinical example of acute respiratory acidosis, including analysis, is provided as Mini Clini 14-1, page 320.

Common causes of respiratory acidosis

With normal lungs

Central nervous system depression
    Anesthesia
    Sedative drugs
    Narcotic analgesics
Neuromuscular disease
    Poliomyelitis
    Myasthenia gravis
    Guillain-Barre syndrome
Trauma
    Spinal cord
    Brain
    Chest wall
Severe restrictive disorders
    Obesity (Pickwickian syndrome)
    Kyphoscoliosis

With abnormal lungs

Chronic obstructive pulmonary disease
Acute airway obstruction (late phases)

Compensation

The kidney begins to compensate for respiratory acidosis as soon as carbon dioxide starts to accumulate. It does so by increasing reabsorption of bicarbonate to keep pace with the rising levels of dissolved carbon dioxide.[2]

The kidney reabsorbs bicarbonate when respiratory acidosis is present by increased H^+ secretion, which reacts with tubular fluid HCO_3^-, as explained in detail in previous sections. When HCO_3^- is reclaimed from the tubular fluid and added to the blood, a chloride ion (Cl^-) is secreted from the blood into the tubular fluid. This causes plasma Cl^- to decrease as plasma HCO_3^- increases.[12]

If the onset of respiratory acidosis is acute, renal compensation may not be able to keep up with the rising level of carbon dioxide on a minute-by-minute basis, and the compensatory bicarbonate reabsorption and hydrogen ion secretion may not reach maximum efficiency for 3 or 4 days. However, the clinician will usually start to see evidence of a response within 24 hours.

On the other hand, if the respiratory acidosis develops slowly, as is often seen in the course of chronic pulmonary disease, the compensatory process may have sufficient time to keep pace with the increase in $PaCO_2$. In such instances, pH levels may be kept stable at or near the low end of the normal range. This is often referred to as "chronic" respiratory acidosis (Mini Clini 14-2, page 321). The high bicarbonate level that accompanies the high $PaCO_2$ is a revealing sign that the high $PaCO_2$ has been present for a considerable period of time. In such cases, the underlying process is still present; renal compensation simply masks the effect of respiratory acidosis by preventing a serious drop in pH. Examination of arterial blood still reveals an elevated PCO_2, the hallmark of respiratory acidosis. However, as demonstrated in the example (Mini Clini 14-2), the HCO_3^- is elevated above normal.[19] One would also find that serum Cl^- is decreased and that the pH of the urine is below normal.

The absolute upper limit of the kidney's ability to compensate for respiratory acidosis is unknown. One study concluded that renal compensation was rarely complete for a $PaCO_2$ greater than 70 torr.[20] Other clinical case reports have demonstrated compensation for, and good tolerance of, arterial PCO_2 as high as 90 torr.[21]

Hydrolysis effect

Differentiation between acute and chronic respiratory acidosis is complicated by the fact that plasma HCO_3^- concentrations are affected by factors other than kidney function. As indicated earlier, increased levels of dissolved CO_2 increase H_2CO_3 concentrations by way of the hydrolysis effect. According to the

■ MINI CLINI ■

14-1

Case Study

The patient is a 35-year-old woman admitted to the emergency room with a diagnosis of heroin overdose. Her breathing is shallow and slow. Arterial blood gas analysis reveals the following:

pH   7.30
PaCO$_2$ 55 torr
HCO$_3$ 27 mEq/L

■ **Step 1** *categorize the pH*
The pH is below normal, indicating the presence of acidemia.

■ **Step 2** *determine respiratory involvement*
The PCO$_2$ is elevated above nor-

Acute (uncompensated) respiratory acidosis

mal, consistent with a low pH, indicating hypoventilation as a contributing factor for acidemia (respiratory acidosis).

■ **Step 3** *determine the metabolic involvement*

The HCO$_3^-$ is elevated slightly above normal; however, this is in the expected range for acute respiratory acidosis (1 mEq for each 10 torr increase in PCO$_2$).

■ **Step 4** *assess for compensation*
As explained in step 3, the HCO$_3^-$ is within the expected range for acute respiratory acidosis; therefore there is no evidence of metabolic compensation.

Conclusion: *acute (uncompensated) respiratory acidosis*

---

principles of mass action, the resulting dissociation of carbonic acid into its ionic components is enhanced, thereby increasing the levels of HCO$_3^-$:

$$CO_2 + H_2O \rightarrow H_2CO_3 \rightarrow H^+ + HCO_3^-$$

This reaction occurs mainly in the red blood cells because of the presence of carbonic anhydrase, an enzyme that greatly increases the speed of the reaction. Thus H$^+$ and HCO$_3^-$ are rapidly produced; H$^+$ is immediately buffered by the hemoglobin molecule, which results in the continual generation of HCO$_3^-$. The HCO$_3^-$ then diffuses down its concentration gradient out of the red blood cell and into the plasma. The amount of plasma HCO$_3^-$ increase is almost exactly equal to the amount of carbonic acid buffered by the blood's major nonbicarbonate buffer, hemoglobin. Figure 14-11, page 322, illustrates the hydrolysis effect. Normal status is represented by a PaCO$_2$ of 40 torr, a pH of 7.40, and a plasma HCO$_3^-$ of 24 mEq/L. An acute rise in PaCO$_2$ from 40 to 80 torr proceeds from point A, moving to the left up the normal blood buffer line (*line BAC*) to point D, where the buffer line intersects the PaCO$_2$ (80 torr isopleth). Point D indicates a HCO$_3^-$ of about 28.5 mEq/L and a pH of about 7.18.

As a rule of thumb, acute respiratory acidosis can be expected to raise the HCO$_3^-$ by about 1 mEq/L for each 10 torr increase in PCO$_2$. On the other hand, if renal compensation is occurring—as in chronic respiratory acidosis—the plasma HCO$_3^-$ can be expected to increase by about 4 mEq/L for each 10 torr rise in PCO$_2$ (see Figure 14-10).[17]

Standard bicarbonate

To eliminate the influence of the hydrolysis effect, some laboratories report an additional value called the **standard bicarbonate.** The standard bicarbonate is defined as the plasma concentration of HCO$_3^-$ (mEq/L) obtained from a blood sample that has been equilibrated (at body temperature) with a PCO$_2$ of 40 torr. In concept, measuring the HCO$_3^-$ when the PaCO$_2$ of the blood sample is 40 torr eliminates the effect of dissolved CO$_2$ on HCO$_3^-$ levels. This HCO$_3^-$ measurement should then allow one to assess strictly the metabolic component of acid-base balance, unhampered by the influence of CO$_2$ on HCO$_3^-$. However the process of standardizing the bicarbonate under in vitro laboratory conditions creates an artificial situation that is not present in the patient's body, or in vivo conditions. That is, the blood in the patient's vascular system is separated from the extravascular fluid (fluid outside of the vessels) by a thin capillary endothelial membrane, readily permeable to nonprotein ions such as HCO$_3^-$. When a patient hypoventilates and the blood PaCO$_2$ rises, the plasma HCO$_3^-$ rises also in accordance with the hydrolysis effect. This increased plasma HCO$_3^-$ equilibrates with extravascular HCO$_3^-$ because of the capillary membrane's permeability to HCO$_3^-$. If the patient were now to hyperventilate such that PaCO$_2$ was once again 40 torr, the hydrolysis reaction between CO$_2$ and H$_2$O would be reversed, and plasma HCO$_3^-$ would decrease. The HCO$_3^-$ that earlier diffused into extravascular fluid when the PaCO$_2$ rose would now diffuse back into the plasma to maintain equilibrium between plasma and extravascular fluid.

■ MINI CLINI ■

14-2

Chronic (compensated) respiratory acidosis

Case Study

The patient is a 73-year-old man being treated on an outpatient basis for pulmonary emphysema, diagnosed some 7 years ago. His breathing is labored at rest, with marked use of accessory muscles. Arterial blood gas analysis reveals the following:

pH 7.36
$PaCO_2$ 64 torr
HCO_3^- 35 mEq/L

■ **Step 1** *categorize the pH*
The pH is on the acid side of the normal range but normal.

■ **Step 2** *determine the respiratory involvement*
The PCO_2 is above normal, indicating hypoventilation as a contributing factor to the low-normal pH (respiratory acidosis).

■ **Step 3** *determine the metabolic involvement*
The HCO_3^- is substantially elevated above normal. This would, by itself, cause alkalemia. But because pH is on the acid side of normal, primary metabolic alkalosis is ruled out. Compensation for the respiratory acidosis has occurred.

■ **Step 4** *assess for compensation*
The HCO_3^- is about 8 to 10 mEq above normal; this is consistent with a compensatory response by the kidneys (about 5 mEq/L for each 10 torr increase in PCO_2). In addition, the expected pH for a $PaCO_2$ of 64 torr would be $7.40-(64-40 torr) 0.006$, or 7.26. Because the actual pH is 7.36, metabolic compensation (retention of HCO_3^-) must have occurred.

Conclusion: *chronic (compensated) respiratory acidosis*

In the laboratory blood sample, however, when blood of the hypercapnic patient is lowered artificially to a PCO_2 of 40 torr, again, plasma HCO_3^- falls, but the extravascular HCO_3^- that would have diffused back into the plasma in vivo is obviously unavailable to the sample's plasma. Therefore the standard bicarbonate, measured in vitro, yields a falsely low HCO_3^- compared with what the HCO_3 would be in actual in vivo conditions.[16]

Base excess

Base excess (*BE*) is defined as the difference between the normal buffer base (*NBB*) and the actual buffer base (*BB*) in a whole blood sample, expressed in mEq/L:[22]

$$BE - NBB - BB$$

More precisely, the BE is obtained by equilibrating a blood sample in the laboratory to a PCO_2 of 40 mm Hg (at 37 ∝ C) and observing the number of milliequivalents of acid or base needed to titrate 1 L of blood to a pH of 7.40.[4]

A normal BE is ± 2 mEq/L. A positive BE (greater than +2 mEq/L) indicates a gain of base *or* loss of acid from nonrespiratory causes. A negative BE (< −2 mEq/L) or *base deficit* indicates a shortage of base or excess of acid from non respiratory causes.[5,22]

Base excess is derived by graphic solution of a nomogram developed by Siggaard-Andersen.[5] Derivation of BE requires prior measurement of the blood pH, $PaCO_2$, and hemoglobin concentration.

The BE suffers from the same limitation as the standard bicarbonate in that it is an in vitro rather than an in vivo measurement. That is, in hypercapnia, the buffer base that diffused into the extravascular fluid in vivo cannot be recovered during laboratory in vitro titrations.

The reliance on BE to quantitate metabolic acid-base abnormalities can be misleading to the casual observer. In acute (uncompensated) respiratory acidosis, BE would generally be in the normal range, indicating correctly that the disturbance is purely respiratory in origin. However, when renal compensation has occurred for chronic hypercapnia, the BE measurement is elevated above the normal range because of the compensatory increase in plasma HCO_3^-.

To illustrate, consider Mini Clini 14-2 on chronic respiratory acidosis. If this patient's blood is equilibrated in vitro to a $PaCO_2$ of 40 torr, HCO_3^- will fall by 2 or 3 mEq/L (to 32 to 33 mEq/L) and pH will rise well above 7.45. Thus this patient's BE will be well above normal. The high BE may lead one to erroneously conclude that this patient has primary metabolic alkalosis, which is, of course, not the case. The high BE in this case merely points out that compensation has occurred for the respiratory acidosis and does not mean that the patient has primary metabolic alkalosis.

Expected pH relationships

The concept of an expected pH derived from the acute relationships between $PaCO_2$ and pH was discussed briefly at the beginning of this section on respiratory acidosis. This method of determining metabolic involvement has been termed *indirect metabolic assessment*.[16] It is predicated on the idea that

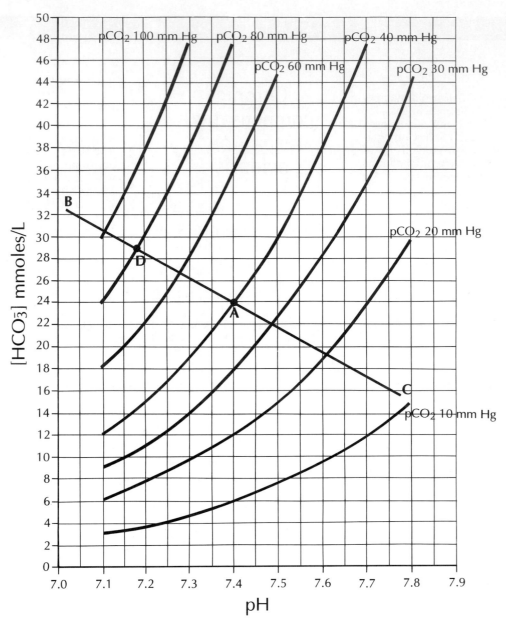

Fig. 14-11 pH-HCO$_3^-$ diagram of blood under *in vitro* tonometer conditions. (From: Masoro & Siegel: Acid-Base Regulation: Its Physiology and Pathophysiology, Philadelphia, 1971, WB Saunders.)

any change in pH must be caused by either metabolic or respiratory factors (i.e., if pH changes, and it is not of respiratory origin, it must be of metabolic origin). One can calculate the pH expected from PaCO$_2$ (respiratory) changes alone when HCO$_3^-$ (the metabolic factor) is held constant at normal values. Under conditions of a constant, normal HCO$_3^-$, any change in pH must be due to a change in respiratory status.

Suppose, for example, that a patient experienced an arterial pH change. The expected pH for the measured PaCO$_2$ can then be calculated and compared with the actual measured pH of the patient. If the two pH values are equal, then metabolic status must be normal, because in the expected pH calculation any change in pH must be due to a change in respiratory status. However, if these two pH values are not equal, then nonrespiratory or metabolic changes must have occurred. Very small differences between actual measured and calculated expected pH values do not denote metabolic involvement. If the measured pH falls within a value of ±0.03 range of the expected pH, metabolic influences on pH are not present; that is, an actual pH more than 0.03 pH units greater than expected pH denotes metabolic alkalosis, whereas an actual pH more than 0.03 pH units less than expected pH denotes metabolic acidosis.[16]

Despite the efforts of many researchers to arrive at

an ideal index of metabolic involvement in acid-base disturbances, plasma bicarbonate, and base excess continue to be the most commonly reported indexes in this regard.[16] If the clinician understands the limitations and physiologic determinants of these indexes, metabolic status can be accurately assessed.

Correction

As previously described, correction of an acid-base abnormality aims to restore the pH toward normal by treatment of the component primarily responsible for the acid-base imbalance. In acute or uncompensated respiratory acidosis, this may be accomplished by increasing alveolar ventilation and thereby lowering the $PaCO_2$. This usually implies some intervention by the therapist aimed at improving ventilation. In chronic or compensated respiratory acidosis, the pH has already been adjusted toward normal by renal retention of HCO_3^-, and "corrective" action aimed at restoring a normal $PaCO_2$ is neither indicated nor desirable. In this case, a rapid increase in alveolar ventilation, induced by a mechanical ventilator, for example, would quickly raise the pH above normal, further complicating the acid-base imbalance.[10]

Respiratory alkalosis

Respiratory alkalosis is a primary physiologic process that causes a decrease in the arterial PCO_2 called hypocapnia.[1] Respiratory alkalosis raises the pH of the blood. An acute drop in PCO_2 of 10 mm Hg will raise the pH by about 0.10 units.

Causes

As with respiratory acidosis, the processes underlying respiratory alkalosis may occur in patients with normal lungs or those with pulmonary disease.[2] In either case, alveolar ventilation and CO_2 excretion exceeds the rate of the body's CO_2 production. This lowers arterial blood PCO_2, which is the fundamental definition of hyperventilation. As indicated in the boxed material, respiratory alkalosis in patients with normal lungs is generally attributable to disorders causing stimulation of the central nervous system. On the other hand, respiratory alkalosis in patients with cardiopulmonary disorders is most likely due to one of two factors: arterial hypoxemia or direct stimulation of certain parasympathetic receptors located in the lung **parenchyma**. Both mechanisms will be described later in this chapter.

A third cause of respiratory alkalosis in patients receiving respiratory care is *iatrogenically induced hyperventilation*. An iatrogenic condition is a problem or complication resulting from treatment. Iatrogenically induced hyperventilation is most commonly associated with the application of mechanical ventilators. Overzealous artificial ventilation can quickly

Common causes of respiratory alkalosis
With normal lungs
Anxiety
Fever
Stimulant drugs
Central nervous system lesions
Pain
Sepsis
Hypobarism (high altitude)
With abnormal lungs
Hypoxemia-causing conditions
Acute asthma
Pneumonia
Stimulation of vagal lung receptors
Pulmonary edema
Pulmonary vascular disease
Either
Iatrogenic hyperventilation

result in acute respiratory alkalosis. A transient respiratory alkalosis may also occur during the assay on arterial blood gas as a result of patient anxiety or pain. Such results can easily be misinterpreted unless the clinician who obtains the sample records information about the patient's ventilatory status on the blood gas report.

Clinical manifestations

An early indicator of acute respiratory alkalosis is paresthesia, a sensation of numbness or tingling in the extremities. Later, neural reflexes become hyperactive, and true tetanic contractions can occur. Because a rapid decrease in PCO_2 produces marked contraction of cerebral arterioles, respiratory alkalosis can also impair cerebral circulation.[23] Depending on its severity, this reduction in blood flow to the brain can cause symptoms ranging from speech difficulty to muscular paralysis. Hypocapnia and the resulting alkalosis also predisposes the patient to serious disturbances in myocardial conductivity, resulting in potentially life-threatening cardiac arrhythmias.[1] Mini Clini 14-3, page 324, provides a clinical example of acute respiratory alkalosis, including the acid-base analysis.

Compensation

Compensation for respiratory alkalosis is accomplished by an increased renal excretion of bicarbonate. This occurs because the low arterial PCO_2 reduces the number of hydrogen ions secreted by the renal tubule cell; because of the reduced H^+ in the filtrate, HCO_3^- in the filtrate cannot react with H^+ and be

■ MINI CLINI ■

14-3

Case Study

A distraught 77-year-old man experiencing anxiety of apparent psychosomatic origin is brought into the hospital by his wife. The patient exhibits rapid and deep breathing, has slurred speech, and complains about tingling in the extremities. Arterial blood gas analysis reveals the following:

pH	7.57
$PaCO_2$	23 torr
HCO_3^-	21 mEq/L

■ **Step 1** *categorize the pH*

The pH is substantially higher than normal, indicating the presence of an alkalemia.

Acute (uncompensated) respiratory alkalosis

■ **Step 2** *determine the respiratory involvement*

The PCO_2 is well below normal, which is consistent with the high pH, indicating hyperventilation as a contributing factor in the alkalemia (respiratory alkalosis).

■ **Step 3** *determine the metabolic involvement*

The HCO_3^- is slightly lower than normal; however, this is within the expected range for acute respiratory alkalosis (hydrolysis effect).

■ **Step 4** *assess for compensation*

The drop in HCO_3^- is within the expected range for acute respiratory alkalosis (1 mEq for each 5 torr decline in PCO_2).

Conclusion: *acute uncompensated respiratory alkalosis*

---

reabsorbed into the blood. Therefore HCO_3^- is excreted in the urine, accompanied by some positive ion such as Na^+ and K^+. Because most Na^+ is usually reabsorbed, more than normal amounts of K^+ are secreted by the kidney to accompany HCO_3^- as it is lost in the urine. This condition predisposes to the development of hypokalemia.

While HCO_3^- is excreted in the urine, Cl^- is reabsorbed along with Na^+. The overall result of these events is the lowering of the blood bicarbonate level, bringing the acid-base ratio back toward 20:1 and reducing the pH back toward normal (Mini Clini 14-4 on page 325).

As with respiratory acidosis, the expected change in plasma HCO_3^- with respiratory alkalosis depends on the magnitude and the longevity of the problem. One should keep in mind that in acute respiratory alkalosis the HCO_3^- is expected to drop by about one 1 mEq/L for each 5 torr decline in PCO_2 because of the hydrolysis effect; patients with chronic or compensated respiratory alkalosis exhibit about 5 mEq/L decrease in HCO_3^- for every 10 torr decrement in PCO_2.[17]

Correction

As with respiratory acidosis, the therapeutic correction of respiratory alkalosis aims to restore the pH back toward normal. Normally this is accomplished indirectly by eliminating or treating the stimulus that caused the increased alveolar ventilation. For example, in Mini Clini 14-4 on page 325, oxygen therapy would presumably raise the PaO_2 and eliminate the stimulus for hyperventilation, thus allowing the $PaCO_2$ to rise and the pH to return toward the middle of the normal range. Another example would be the iatrogenically induced respiratory alkalosis caused by a mechanical ventilator. In this case respiratory alkalosis could be directly corrected by decreasing the ventilator's rate and tidal volume.

Metabolic (nonrespiratory) acidosis

Metabolic or nonrespiratory acidosis is a primary physiologic process that causes a decrease in the plasma bicarbonate, a condition called *hypobasemia*.[1,14] Metabolic acidosis lowers the pH of the blood.

Causes

Metabolic or nonrespiratory acidosis is caused by either a gain in fixed (nonvolatile) acids or an excessive loss of buffer base.[2] The boxed material delineates the common clinical disorders associated with each of these two major categories of metabolic acidosis. Regardless of underlying cause, the hallmark of metabolic acidosis is a reduction in the buffering capacity of the blood, as manifested by a low HCO_3^- and a large negative BE or, more accurately, a base deficit.

Although the end result of all types of metabolic acidosis is the same (a decreased HCO_3^- or negative BE), the effective clinical management of this acid-base disorder relies on accurately identifying the underlying cause. In most cases, a careful history and related clinical assessment will allow the clinician to

■ MINI CLINI ■

14-4

Case Study

A 27-year-old man is admitted to the hospital with a persistent case of bacterial pneumonia that has not responded to six days of ambulatory care with antimicrobials. He exhibits mild cyanosis and labored breathing. Arterial blood gas analysis (breathing room air) reveals the following:

pH 7.44
$PaCO_2$ 26 torr
HCO_3^- 17 mEq/L
PaO_2 53 torr

- **Step 1** *categorize the pH*
  The pH is on the alkalotic side of the normal range but normal.

- **Step 2** *determine the respiratory involvement*
  The PCO_2 is well below normal,

Compensated (chronic) respiratory alkalosis

indicating hyperventilation as a contributing factor to the high-normal pH. (respiratory alkalosis)

- **Step 3** *determine the metabolic involvement*
  The HCO_3^- is substantially lower than normal; but because the pH is on the alkalotic side of

normal, primary metabolic acidosis is ruled out. Compensation for the respiratory alkalosis has occurred.

- **Step 4** *assess for compensation*
  The HCO_3^- is about 7 mEq below normal; this is consistent with a compensatory response by the kidneys (about 5 mEq/L for each 10 torr drop in PCO_2). In addition, the *expected* pH for a $PaCO_2$ of 26 torr would be 7.40 + (40−26 torr) 0.01, or 7.54. Because actual pH is 7.44, metabolic compensation (excretion of HCO_3^-) must have occurred.

Conclusion: *compensated (chronic) respiratory alkalosis*

Common causes of metabolic (nonrespiratory) acidosis

Loss of base (normal anion gap)
Direct loss of bicarbonate

Diarrhea
Pancreatic fistula
Carbonic anhydrase inhibition
Chloride retention
Renal tubular acidosis
Chloride administration
NH_4Cl
Parenteral nutrition (arginine/lysine)

Gain of acid (increased anion gap)
Metabolically produced

Diabetic ketoacidosis
Alcoholic ketoacidosis
Lactic acidosis
Renal insufficiency (phosphate, sulfate retention)
Starvation

Drug- or chemical-induced

Salicylate intoxication
Carbenicillin therapy
Methanol (formic acid)
Ethylene glycol (oxalic acid)
Paraldehyde (acetic acid)

distinguish between metabolic acidosis due to a gain in fixed acids and that caused by an excessive loss of base. However, in some situations, this difference is not so clear.

Differentiating among the various types of metabolic acidosis often requires further analysis of the plasma electrolytes. In metabolic disorders, acid-base balance depends in part on the balance between the plasma cations and anions.[15] The cations comprise sodium, calcium, potassium, and magnesium; the anions include bicarbonate, protein, (serum protein and hemoglobin), phosphate, chloride, sulfate, and organic acids. As shown in Figure 14-12, page 326, the sum of the anions must equal the sum of the cations, which is consistent with the *law of electroneutrality*.[16] This law states that the total positive charges must equal the total negative charges in a volume of fluid.

Anion gap

In clinical practice, the only electrolytes commonly measured are Na^+, K^+, Cl^-, and HCO_3^-. This leads to the so-called anion gap, which in reality does not exist, but simply reflects the fact that the routinely measured cations (Na^+ and K^+) outnumber the routinely measured anions (Cl^- and HCO_3^-). The relative balance between measured cations and anions

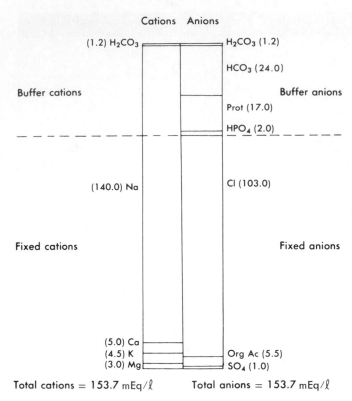

Cations Anions

(1.2) H$_2$CO$_3$ — H$_2$CO$_3$ (1.2)

HCO$_3$ (24.0)

Buffer cations — Buffer anions

Prot (17.0)

HPO$_4$ (2.0)

(140.0) Na — Cl (103.0)

Fixed cations — Fixed anions

(5.0) Ca
(4.5) K — Org Ac (5.5)
(3.0) Mg — SO$_4$ (1.0)

Total cations = 153.7 mEq/ℓ   Total anions = 153.7 mEq/ℓ

Fig. 14-12 Balance between fixed and buffer electrolytes of plasma.

is therefore determined by calculating the difference between the total of the two primary anions (Cl$^-$ and HCO$_3^-$) and the two primary cations (Na$^+$ and K$^+$). This computation is called the **anion gap**[1]:

$$\text{Anion gap} = (Na^+ + K^+) - (Cl^- + HCO_3^-)$$

Usually, K$^+$ is ignored in the computation. Therefore the normal anion gap range is about 8 to 16 mEq/L.[1] An anion gap greater than 16 mEq/L is usually caused by metabolic acidosis, specifically those types of metabolic acidosis associated with accumulation of unusual fixed acids in the body. These acids combine with plasma HCO$_3^-$, which lowers the concentration of HCO$_3^-$ in the blood, leading to an increased anion gap. That is, the anions from the dissociated fixed acids are *unmeasured* anions. Such unmeasured anions include those of lactic acid, ketones (B-hydroxybutyric acid and acetoacetic acid), salicylic acid, formic acid, and oxalic acid. Lactic acid and ketones are metabolically produced, whereas salicylic acid, formic acid, and oxalic acid represent ingested anions. Metabolic acidosis caused by renal insufficiency also causes an increased anion gap because of the retention of phosphate and sulfate anions, both of which are usually unmeasured.

On the other hand, not all types of metabolic acidosis increase the anion gap. Specifically, conditions in which the acidosis is caused by a loss of

HCO$_3^-$ (as opposed to a gain of acid) generally will not increase the anion gap (see boxed material). In these situations, bicarbonate loss and chloride retention offset each other, keeping the anion gap in normal limits. This inverse relationship between bicarbonate and chloride anions is best understood in light of the law of electroneutrality. If electroneutrality is to be maintained, a loss of bicarbonate (when cation concentration is constant) means that the kidney must reabsorb more chloride anions. This causes hyperchloremia.

Because of the characteristic elevation of serum chloride, nonrespiratory acidosis with a normal anion gap is called *hyperchloremic metabolic acidosis.* Hyperchloremic metabolic acidosis may be caused by any condition in which HCO$_3^-$ is lost or Cl$^-$ is gained. Among the most common causes of bicarbonate loss are diarrhea, pancreatic fistula, and renal tubular acidosis. Chloride ingestion may also cause hyperchloremic metabolic acidosis. Ammonium chloride (NH$_4$Cl) ingestion is a primary cause of hyperchloremic metabolic acidosis, as are amino acid–chloride formulas used in parenteral nutrition (hyperalimentation).

Compensation

Compensation for metabolic acidosis occurs by way of an increase in the excretion of volatile acid (H$_2$CO$_3$) in the form of CO$_2$ by the lungs (i.e., hyperventilation). In this manner, the ratio of bicarbonate to H$_2$CO$_3$ is raised back toward a normal ratio of 20:1, restoring the pH to its normal range). Mini Clini 14-5 provides an example of compensated metabolic acidosis.

Because the response of the normal respiratory system to metabolic acidosis is rapid, uncompensated metabolic acidosis is rare.[17] Therefore one expects the PCO$_2$ of a patient with metabolic acidosis to be below normal. Indeed, if a metabolic acidosis is confirmed and the PCO$_2$ is normal or high, a ventilatory disorder must coexist. Mini Clini 14-6 is an example of partially compensated metabolic acidosis, a more common clinical entity.

Correction

As with the other acid-base abnormalities, therapeutic correction of metabolic acidosis aims to restore the pH to normal. Normally this is accomplished by treatment of the underlying process causing the gain of acid or loss of base. However, because respiratory compensation normally accompanies metabolic acidosis, the pH may already be adjusted toward normal. Corrective action in these situations may not be indicated. An obvious corrective action would be to infuse sodium bicarbonate intravenously to combat metabolic acidosis. However, rapid correction of metabolic acidosis by sodium bicarbonate infusion is generally not indicated if respiratory compensation is

■ MINI CLINI ■

14-5

Compensated Metabolic Acidosis

Case Study

A 38-year-old man has suffered for weeks from severe diarrhea without medical attention. Arterial blood gas analysis reveals the following:

pH   7.36
$PaCO_2$ 24 torr
HCO_3^- 13 mEq/L
BE   −11 mEq/L

■ **Step 1** *categorize the pH*
The pH is on the acid side of the normal range, but normal never the less.

■ **Step 2** *determine the respiratory involvement*
The PCO_2 is below normal, indicating hyperventilation. This by

itself would cause alkalosis. However, because the pH is on the acid side of normal, the presence of primary respiratory alkalosis is ruled out. The low PCO_2 is likely a compensatory response to a primary metabolic problem (possible metabolic acidosis).

■ **Step 3** *determine the metabolic involvement*

The HCO_3^- level is substantially lower than normal, consistent with a low pH; given that pH is on the acid side of normal, this low HCO_3^- signals a possible metabolic acidosis. This is confirmed by the large base deficit (−11 mEq/L).

■ **Step 4** *assess for compensation*
The hyperventilation previously described must represent a compensatory response to primary metabolic acidosis. The pH is in the normal range.

Conclusion: *compensated metabolic acidosis*

---

in progress. In such cases the pH may swing rapidly above normal, further complicating the acid-base imbalance. Sodium bicarbonate administration is generally indicated when the arterial pH is less than 7.20 because a pH at this level is usually considered more dangerous than the complication of the thera-

py.[16] A fairly common cause of metabolic acidosis is the accumulation of lactic acid due to anaerobic metabolism, which accompanies the severe tissue hypoxia of cardiac arrest (loss of tissue perfusion). Because sodium bicarbonate therapy has not been shown to improve survival in cardiac arrest, its role in

---

■ MINI CLINI ■

14-6

Partially Compensated Metabolic Acidosis

Case Study

A 42-year-old woman enters the emergency room in a diabetic coma. She exhibits gasping, deep respirations. Arterial blood gases reveal the following:

pH   7.22
$PaCO_2$ 20 torr
HCO_3^- 8 mEq/L
BE   −16 mEq/L

■ **Step 1** *categorize the pH*
The pH is below the normal range, indicating the presence of acidemia.

■ **Step 2** *determine the respiratory involvement*
The PCO_2 is below normal, indicating severe hyperventilation. This by itself would cause alkalo-

sis, but the presence of acidemia rules out primary respiratory alkalosis. The low $PaCO_2$ is probably a compensatory response to primary metabolic acidosis, although this response is insufficient to restore pH to the normal range.

■ **Step 3** *determine the metabolic involvement*

The HCO_3^- is severely reduced, consistent with the low pH. This low HCO_3^- in the presence of low pH and a low $PaCO_2$ (which would cause a high pH) signals primary metabolic acidosis. This is confirmed by the large base deficit.

■ **Step 4** *assess for compensation*
The severe hyperventilation represents a compensatory response to the primary metabolic acidosis, although compensation is far from complete. Nevertheless, the pH would be lower still if $PaCO_2$ were normal.

Conclusion: *partly compensated metabolic acidosis*

cardiopulmonary resuscitation has been seriously questioned, and its initial use in cardiopulmonary resuscitation has greatly declined.[16]

Metabolic (nonrespiratory) alkalosis

Metabolic or nonrespiratory alkalosis is a primary physiologic process that causes an increase in the plasma bicarbonate, a condition called **hyperbasemia**.[1,14] Metabolic alkalosis raises the pH of the blood.

Causes

Metabolic or nonrespiratory alkalosis is associated with a loss of fixed (nonvolatile) acids or an excessive gain of blood buffer base.[24] The boxed material lists the common clinical disorders associated with each of these two major categories of metabolic alkalosis. Regardless of underlying cause, the hallmark of metabolic alkalosis is an increase in the buffering capacity of the blood, as manifested by an elevated HCO_3^- and a positive base excess. Mini Clini 14-7, on page 329, is an example of metabolic alkalosis.

Metabolic alkalosis due to ingestion or administration of excessive HCO_3^- is a relatively rare occurrence. This is because the normal kidney can rapidly excrete excessive loads of HCO_3^-. More commonly, metabolic alkalosis is caused by gastric loss of fixed acid, as with severe vomiting or nasogastric suctioning, or by low plasma Cl^- (hypochloremia) and augmented renal excretion of H^+ and K^+.

To understand how hypochloremia and augmented renal excretion of H^+ and K^+ can cause metabolic alkalosis, it is important to understand how the kidney regulates sodium; sodium regulation is intimately related to acid-base balance. About 26,000 mEq of Na^+ passes through the glomerular membrane into the filtrate daily; yet daily intake of Na^+ averages only 150 mEq.[12] Therefore the main role of the renal tubules in sodium regulation is to reabsorb sodium, not to excrete it. Otherwise the body would rapidly be depleted of sodium.

Renal excretion of H^+ and K^+ in hypochloremia

When sodium, a positive ion, is removed from the tubular filtrate (i.e., reabsorbed), the law of electroneutrality dictates that: (1) it must be accompanied by a negative ion from the filtrate or (2) a different positive ion must be secreted into the filtrate by the tubule cell when sodium leaves. Sodium is reabsorbed through two different mechanisms: (1) primary active transport of sodium, in which sodium is accompanied by the chloride anion and (2) secondary active secretion of hydrogen and potassium into the tubular lumen in exchange for sodium. In primary active transport, sodium is actively pumped out of the tubule cell into the extracellular fluid (and ultimately, the blood) using energy derived from breakdown of ATP in the cell membrane.[12] Potassium is simultaneously transported into the cell from the blood by way of the same mechanism, but more sodium ions are pumped out than potassium ions pumped in. This process keeps intracellular $[Na^+]$ very low and creates an intracellular electronegativity. Because $[Na^+]$ is very high in the filtrate, it rapidly diffuses from the tubular lumen into the cell as a result of its concentration gradient and the electronegative attractive forces in the cell.[12] To maintain electrical neutrality within the tubule, Cl^- passively diffuses into the cell with Na^+ (Figure 14-13).

Reabsorption of Na^+ through secondary active secretion of H^+ and K^+ is a somewhat more complex process (Figures 14-14 and 14-15). In the case of

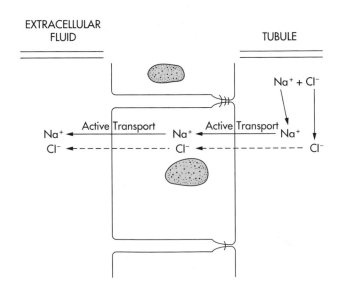

Fig. 14-13 Sodium reabsorption via primary active transport. Sodium is actively transported from the tubule cell to the extracellular fluid and then to the blood. Sodium then diffuses from the tubular lumen into the cell down concentration and electrical gradients. Chloride passively accompanies sodium to maintain electroneutrality. (From Malley WJ: Clinical blood gases, Philadelphia, 1990, WB Saunders.)

Common causes of metabolic (nonrespiratory) alkalosis

Increase in base

Administration/ingestion of HCO_3
Hypochloremia
Diuretic therapy
Contraction of blood volume

Loss of fixed acid

Severe vomiting
Nasogastric suction
Hypokalemia
Potassium deficiency
Corticosteroids

■ MINI **C**LINI ■

14-7

Case Study

A 83-year-old woman with heart disease has been taking a powerful diuretic to remove excess edematous fluid from her legs and help keep her free of pulmonary edema. Her blood gases and serum electrolytes reveal the following:

pH	7.58
PaCO$_2$	48 torr
HCO$_3^-$	44 mEq/L
BE	+19 mEq/L
Serum K$^+$	2.5 mEq/L
Serum Cl$^-$	95 mEq/L

■ **Step 1** *categorize the pH*
The pH is substantially above normal, indicating the presence of alkalemia.

■ **Step 2** *determine the respiratory involvement*

Metabolic Alkalosis

The PCO$_2$ is slightly above normal, indicating mild hypoventilation. However, because alkalemia is present, the existence of primary respiratory acidosis is ruled out. The elevated PCO$_2$ may be a compensatory response to a primary metabolic problem (possible metabolic alkalosis).

■ **Step 3** *determine the metabolic involvement*
The HCO$_3^-$ is substantially high-

er than normal; given the high pH, this elevated HCO$_3^-$ signals a metabolic alkalosis. This is confirmed by the large base excess (+19 mEq/L). Further, the low serum K$^+$ and Cl$^-$ values indicate hypokalemic/hypochloremic metabolic alkalosis.

■ **Step 4** *assess for compensation*
Although there is a slight elevation in the PCO$_2$, compensation for metabolic alkalosis is minimal. This lack of compensation is consistent with the presence of hypokalemic metabolic alkalosis.

Conclusion: *uncompensated metabolic alkalosis*

---

hydrogen ion secretion, the process proceeds in this manner: first, H$^+$ is generated in the tubule cell by the reaction between CO$_2$ and H$_2$O in the presence of carbonic anhydrase, as explained earlier. The H$^+$ in the tubule cell and the Na$^+$ in the filtrate then simultaneously combine with opposite ends of a protein carrier molecule in the luminal border of the cell membrane. In the countertransport process described earlier, sodium moves down its concentration gradient into the tubule cell, which provides the energy for

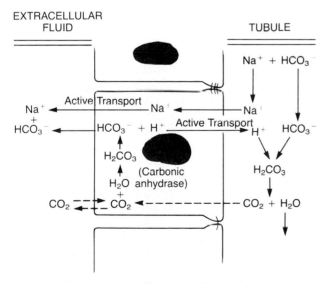

Fig. 14-14 Sodium reabsorption via secondary active secretion of hydrogen ion. Hydrogen ions, available through the hydrolysis reaction, are secreted into the filtrate in exchange for sodium. The sodium is then transported from the renal cell to the extracellular fluid and ultimately to the plasma. Bicarbonate, also available from the hydrolysis reaction, accompanies sodium into the extracellular fluid to maintain electroneutrality. (From Malley WJ: Clinical blood gases, Philadelphia, 1990, WB Saunders.)

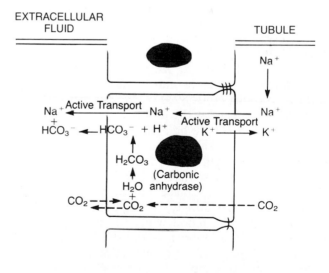

Fig. 14-15 Sodium reabsorption via secondary active transport of potassium ion. Potassium ions are secreted into the filtrated in exchange for sodium. The sodium is then transported from the renal cell to the extracellular fluid and ultimately to the plasma. Bicarbonate accompanies sodium into the extracellular fluid to maintain electroneutrality. (From Malley WJ: Clinical blood gases, Philadelphia, 1990, WB Saunders.)

moving the hydrogen ion in the opposite direction into the filtrate. In the primary active transport mechanism described above, chloride ion passively accompanied Na^+ into the tubule cell. In the countertransport process, the bicarbonate anion, generated by the reaction between CO_2 and H_2O in the tubule cell, accompanies sodium's transport out of the cell into the blood.[16] This same countertransport mechanism can involve potassium ions rather than hydrogen ions.

About 80% of total Na^+ reabsorption occurs by way of the primary active transport process, which involves the passive reabsorption of Cl^- with Na^+.[16] The remaining 20% occurs by way of the active secretion of H^+ and K^+ in exchange for Na^+, as described above. When an H^+ or K^+ ion is secreted to reabsorb Na^+, an HCO_3^- ion rather than a Cl^- ion accompanies Na^+ into the blood, as shown in Figures 14-14 and 14-15. Therefore any condition that increases the demand for Na^+ reabsorption through H^+ and K^+ secretion mechanisms, such as a shortage of Cl^- ion (caused, for example, by diuretic therapy) causes more HCO_3^- to be added to the blood, which in turn causes metabolic alkalosis. This helps explain the reciprocal relationship between plasma Cl^- and HCO_3^- concentrations and also why hypochloremia would cause alkalosis.[4]

Hypochloremic metabolic alkalosis is sometimes a complication of therapies used in chronic obstructive pulmonary disease. Low-salt diets, diuretics, and steroid therapy help bring this condition about. Nasogastric suction also depletes the body of Cl^-. Moreover, in chronic destructive pulmonary disease (COPD) with chronic CO_2 retention and compensating HCO_3^- retention, increased Cl^- is lost in the urine because the increased H^+ secreted by the tubules causes increased NH_3 synthesis by the kidney and, subsequently, excretion of NH_4Cl. Regardless of the cause, hypochloremia tends to cause metabolic alkalosis and, also, hypokalemia. This is true because low Cl^- in the filtrate increases the demand for both H^+ and K^+ secretion for Na^+ to be reabsorbed.

The metabolic alkalosis caused by hypochloremia can only be alleviated by bicarbonate diuresis, which cannot occur as long as inadequate Cl^- is available to take the HCO_3^- ion's place in the process of Na^+ reabsorption.[7] Interestingly, in this case all HCO_3^- is reabsorbed into the blood while the urine becomes acidified; thus the blood is alkalotic, but an acidic urine is produced. The corrective action in this case is to infuse NaCl to supply Cl^- for reabsorption with Na^+ so that HCO_3^- diuresis can occur.[4,7]

Causes of hypokalemia and hypochloremia, both of which cause metabolic alkalosis, include gastric or intravenous infusion of nutrition with inadequate K^+ content; severe diarrhea resulting because the lower bowel is rich in K^+; nasogastric suction, which depletes both K^+ and Cl^-; and diuretics such as ethacrynic acid, furosemide, thiazides, and mercurials.[7] In addition, corticosteroid administration and clinical entities such as Cushing's syndrome and aldosteronism cause increased loss of these ions.[11]

Potassium and acid–base states

It is important to remember that the kidney's main task in sodium regulation is to reabsorb it; in fact, about 99% of the sodium in the filtrate is reabsorbed.[12] The body will reabsorb sodium even at the expense of imbalances in other electrolytes. For example, in a state of alkalosis, sodium will be reabsorbed through the countertransport mechanism involving potassium ion secretion rather than hydrogen ion secretion, because of the relative shortage of hydrogen ions. This leads to selective loss of potassium, and is a major reason why *alkalosis tends to cause hypokalemia.* Furthermore, in an alkalotic state, more bicarbonate anions enter the filtrate at the glomerulus than normal; at the same time, fewer hydrogen ions are secreted by the tubule. Because they have few hydrogen ions with which to react, bicarbonate anions are lost in the urine, but they must be accompanied by a positive ion. Because hydrogen ion is scarce and sodium ion reabsorption is a priority, potassium ion secretion increases to accompany urinary bicarbonate anions; this promotes hypokalemia.

Similarly, a state of hypokalemia would cause the kidney tubules to secrete inappropriately large amounts of hydrogen ion so that sodium can be reabsorbed by way of the countertransport mechanism. (For example, hypokalemia may be induced by certain diuretics.) Thus hypokalemia would lead to alkalosis. This alkalosis is compounded in coexisting hypokalemia and extracellular volume depletion.[7] Frequently, during diuretic therapy, both extracellular volume depletion and hypokalemia are induced. This produces a profound stimulus for renal sodium reabsorption. This aggressive sodium reabsorption, coupled with hypokalemia, further exaggerates the increased tubular cell secretion of hydrogen ions into the filtrate. This occurs because buffer anions in the filtrate are not diffusible through tubular membranes, and the kidney is confronted with the need to excrete an equivalent amount of cation (Na^+, H^+, or K^+). Avid reabsorption of sodium makes this ion unavailable, and the hypokalemia means that potassium ion is scarce. Therefore the tubules increase hydrogen ion secretion to meet the demand for cation excretion, and metabolic alkalosis is further exacerbated.

The relationship between extracellular (plasma) potassium levels and plasma pH (e.g., alkalosis and hypokalemia) has a further explanation at the cellular level in the blood.[4] Plasma hypokalemia causes intracellular potassium to diffuse out of the cell down its concentration gradient. The resulting intracellular electronegativity causes a net movement of Na^+ and H^+ into the cell. Thus plasma H^+ is depleted, causing alkalosis. In alkalosis, intracellular H^+ diffuses out of the cell down its concentration gradient, causing a net movement of K^+ and Na^+ into the cell. Thus plasma K^+ is depleted, causing hypokalemia.

As would be expected, in an acidotic plasma H^+ diffuses into the cell and K^+ diffuses out of the cell to maintain electrical neutrality. Thus acidemia creates hyperkalemia. Similarly, if hyperkalemia exists (e.g., as may occur with KCl infusion), K^+ diffuses into the cell and H^+ diffuses out, causing acidemia. The effect of plasma pH on plasma potassium levels is illustrated in Figure 14-16.

Because of the intracellular-extracellular shifts in K^+ that accompany pH changes, plasma $[K^+]$ must be interpreted carefully. For example, $[K^+]$ may be elevated in acidemia, but total K^+ stores may actually be depleted. If K^+ is *normal* in acidemia, then intracellular K^+ stores must be below normal. Similarly, low plasma $[K^+]$ in alkalemia may not indicate severe depletion of K^+ stores. Generally, K^+ should be administered slowly, with a goal of a $[K^+]$ in the low normal range.[16]

Compensation for metabolic alkalosis

The expected compensatory response to metabolic alkalosis is CO_2 retention by way of hypoventilation.[25] Traditionally, it has been thought that this response may not be observed in hypokalemic metabolic alkalosis. The failure to compensate in this case has been explained in part by the cation exchange that occurs across cellular membranes in this condition.[2] As explained earlier, when serum K^+ decreases, K^+ ions

diffuse out of the cells in exchange for H^+ ions. This increase in intracellular hydrogen ion concentration, especially in the respiratory chemoreceptive centers, has been thought to offset the influence of the extracellular alkalosis, thereby maintaining a normal stimulus to breathe. However, more recent evidence does not support this theory.[26]

Hypoventilation and carbon dioxide retention do occur to compensate for metabolic alkalosis, although it has been commonly assumed that the stimulatory effect of hypoxemia, which accompanies hypoventilation, would greatly limit the degree of hypoventilation. More recent evidence shows that marked hypoventilation occurs in severe metabolic alkalosis even when the PaO_2 is as low as 55 torr.[26] It is thought that the metabolic alkalosis itself may blunt the hypoxic chemoreceptor response, thus allowing hypoventilation to occur even in the face of significant hypoxemia.[26] The reason why significant CO_2 retention is often not seen in metabolic alkalosis may be that this condition is commonly associated with other factors that may cause hyperventilation, such as anxiety, pain, infection, fever, and pulmonary edema.

Correction

Correction of metabolic alkalosis aims to restore normal fluid volume and electrolyte concentrations, especially potassium and chloride levels. As stated earlier, inadequate fluid volume, especially if coupled with hypochloremia, causes excessive secretion and loss of hydrogen and potassium ions. Thus, in treatment of this type of alkalosis, it is important to supply adequate fluids containing chloride ion. If hypokalemia is a primary factor, KCl is the preferred corrective agent. Metabolic alkalosis due to excess corticosteroids is often resistant to chloride therapy, as a result of the kidney's inability to retain this electrolyte.

Mixed and combined acid-base states

It is obvious that combinations of acid-base disorders may occur in the same patient.[27,28] A combined disturbance is one in which both respiratory and metabolic disturbances exist and the two promote the same acid-base disturbance. For example, consider the arterial blood gas results below:

pH   7.62
$PaCO_2$ 32 torr
HCO_3^- 29 mEq/L

The pH shows alkalemia, consistent with both the low $PaCO_2$ and the elevated HCO_3^-. This is interpreted as a combined alkalosis and indicates that the patient has two primary acid-base problems (i.e., respiratory and metabolic alkalosis combined). A combined disturbance, by definition, cannot have compensation.

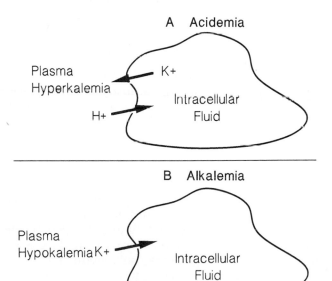

A   Acidemia

Plasma Hyperkalemia

K^+

H^+

Intracellular Fluid

B   Alkalemia

Plasma Hypokalemia K^+

Intracellular Fluid

H^+

Fig. 14-16 pH and plasma potassium. **A,** Plasma acidemia tends to cause hyperkalemia as hydrogen ions form the plasma exchange with potassium ions from the intracellular fluid. **B,** Plasma alkalemia tends to cause plasma hypokalemia as potassium ions from the plasma move into the intracellular fluid in exchange for hydrogen ions. (From Malley WJ: Clinical blood gases, Philadelphia, 1990, WB Saunders.)

A mixed acid-base disturbance is defined as one in which two primary acid-base disturbances which have opposite effects on pH coexist.[16] This may give the appearance of simple compensation because pH may coincidentally be in the normal range. A useful tool in distinguishing between simple compensation and a mixed acid-base disturbance is the acid-base map in Figure 14-10. The labeled areas denote with 95% confidence the ranges of pH, $PaCO_2$, and HCO_3^- that are expected if simple compensation exists.[16] If a patient's arterial blood gas values define a point outside of the 95% confidence bands, the disturbance is most likely a mixed disturbance. The point is defined by the intersection of two straight, perpendicular lines that pass through the measured $PaCO_2$ and arterial pH.

REGULATION OF RESPIRATION

For the lungs to effectively exchange respired gases and participate in acid-base **homeostasis,** a regulatory mechanism must exist. Exactly how these diverse and sometimes conflicting roles are integrated is an ongoing subject of inquiry.

Contemporary studies of the regulation of respiration have made it clear that the control mechanisms underlying this process are exceedingly complex.[29,30] Even today, our knowledge in this area is incomplete and often speculative. Our focus will be to apply what is currently known in this area to the clinical practice of respiratory care.

Rhythmicity of breathing

Among the facts best known about the regulation of breathing is that the rhythmic cycle of inspiration and expiration is mainly mediated by way of the central nervous system.[31] We know that this cycle originates in the brainstem, mainly from neurons located in the medulla.[32,33]

Medullary respiratory "centers"

By use of microelectrodes, clusters of neurons having activity patterns linked with inspiration and expiration have been identified (Figure 14-17).[34,35] A dorsal respiratory group of neurons is located on either side of the medulla, in the nucleus of the tractus solitarius (NTS). These dorsal neurons appear to be the main source of inspiratory activity, probably through direct efferent innervation of the phrenic nerves. Moreover, the dorsal respiratory group appears to receive *afferent* impulses through the vagal and glossopharyngeal cranial nerves. These nerves are responsible for transmitting sensory impulses from the lungs, airways, and peripheral chemoreceptors to the brainstem.

A ventral respiratory group of neurons is located in the ventrolateral portion of the medulla, in the region of the nucleus ambiguous (NA) and nucleus retroambigualis (NRA). Some of these neurons cause inspiration while others cause expiration. However, the ventral respiratory group of neurons is most important for strong expiratory signals to the abdominal muscles during active expiration.[12] Unlike the dorsal neurons, the ventral respiratory group receives no afferent input. These neurons are almost completely inactive during normal quiet breathing, which indicates that normal breathing at rest is caused only by the repetitive inspiratory signals from the dorsal respiratory group, and that expiration occurs because of passive elastic recoil of the lungs and chest wall.[12]

Until recently, it was thought that these dorsal and ventral groups served, respectively, as inspiratory and expiratory "centers." It was believed that the cyclic pattern of inspiration and expiration was simply a result of self-excitation and mutual inhibition between these groups. Recent evidence suggests that this explanation may be an oversimplification.[36-39]

The basic oscillatory rhythm of respiration originates in the dorsal respiratory neurons, and there is no evidence to support any involvement of the ventral neurons.[12] The cause of these repetitive dorsal neuronal signals remains unknown.

The dorsal signal transmitted to the inspiratory muscles is characterized as a "ramp" signal, as opposed to an instantaneous, abrupt burst. The signal is initially very weak, gradually strengthening in a ramp fashion for about 2 seconds, then abruptly ceasing for about 3 seconds.[12] This cycle is continually repeated. Because of the ramplike signal, inspiration proceeds gradually rather than in an abrupt gasp. This inspiratory signal can be controlled through adjustment of the rate of increase, or steepness, of the ramp, or by limiting the point at which the ramp signal abruptly ceases. The latter is the usual method for controlling respiratory rate in quiet breathing, whereas the former predominates during exercise.[12] For unknown reasons, limiting the duration of inspiration also shortens expiratory time, resulting in an increased respiratory rate.

Pons

If the brainstem is transected above the medulla, spontaneous respiration continues, although in a more irregular pattern. This finding has led to the conclusion that the pons is not involved in the genesis of rhythmic breathing but may only modify the activity of the lower medullary centers. Recent evidence suggests that the neurons of the pons, unlike their medullary counterparts, have no periodic activity.[8]

As shown in Figure 14-17, two localized collections of neurons in the pons have been shown to influence the medullary respiratory centers: the *apneustic center* (located at the level of the area vestibularis), and the *pneumotaxic center* (located in the region of the nucleus parabrachealis medialis, or NPBM). The pri-

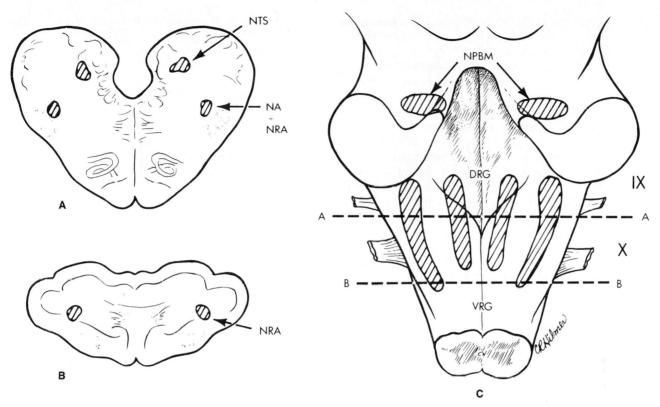

Fig. 14-17 Diagram of central respiratory centers in the midbrain. **A,** Transverse section of the medulla oblongata slightly rostral to the obex at the level indicated by the dashed line *AA* in **C. B,** Transverse section of the medulla slightly caudal to the obex at the level indicated by the dashed line *BB* in **C. C,** Dorsal view of the medulla and pons, showing the location of central respiratory neuron groups: *NTS,* nucleus solitarius; *NA,* nucleus ambiguus; *NRA,* nucleus retroambigualis; *NPBM,* nucleus parabrachialis medialis; *DRG,* dorsal respiratory group; *VRG,* ventral respiratory group; *IX,* ninth cranial (glossopharyngeal) nerve; and *X,* tenth cranial (vagus) nerve. (From Slonim NB and Hamilton LH: Respiratory physiology, ed 5, St Louis, 1987, Mosby.)

mary function of the pneumotaxic center is to control the "switch-off" point of the inspiratory ramp, thus controlling the inspiratory time. This has a secondary effect of controlling respiratory rate, as explained above, such that strong pneumotaxic signals can increase respiratory rate up to 30 to 40 breaths/minute.[12]

The function of the apneustic center is not clearly understood. If the vagus nerve to the medulla is blocked and the neural connection between the apneustic center and pneumotaxic center is also blocked, then the apneustic center stimulates the dorsal inspiratory neurons to prevent the switch-off of the inspiratory ramp signal. Otherwise, the apneustic center's function cannot be demonstrated.[12] In this explanation, the "off switch" is activated by pneumotaxic stimulation or vagal afferent input. This theory helps explain the inspiratory spasms (apneustic breathing) that occur with suppression of the pneumotaxic center or blockage of vagal afferent input to the brainstem. However, the exact details on how the pontine and medullary centers interact or modify the basic cyclical rhythm are still being sought.[36-39]

Gamma-efferent feedback system

Impulses generated by the brainstem respiratory centers are delivered over efferent pathway to the respiratory muscles, causing their contraction. How *much* these muscles contract, however, is determined by a separate regulatory mechanism common to all skeletal muscle. This system is called the *gamma-efferent feedback system.*

The gamma-efferent feedback system represents a reflex arc that automatically adjusts muscle contractions to accommodate varying loads. As depicted in Figure 14-18, page 334, impulses arising from the brainstem centers travel over efferent nerves to both the alpha and gamma fibers. As both fibers contract, stretch receptors in the spindle of the gamma fibers send impulses *back* to the spinal cord over gamma-afferent pathways, in proportion to the change in spindle tension. In turn, the reflex impulses arising from the stretch receptors are transmitted to the alpha fibers over alpha-efferent pathways.

As long as muscle contraction is unopposed, both the alpha and gamma fibers will shorten to the same degree, and increases in spindle tension will be mini-

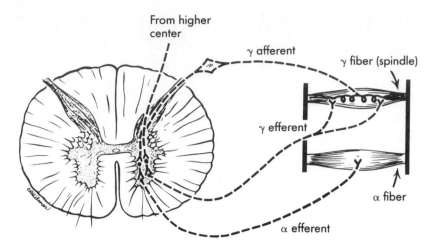

Fig. 14–18 The extravagal gamma-efferent system is a feedback system that modifies the breathing pattern. (From Slonim NB and Hamilton LH: Respiratory physiology, ed 5, St Louis, 1987, Mosby.)

mal. However, if the shortening of the muscle fibers meet resistance, for example, if pulmonary compliance is decreased, the tension in the stretch receptors of the spindle will increase. An increase in the tension on the spindle fiber stimulates the ventral horn motorneurons of the cord through the gamma-afferent fibers, and by way of the alpha-efferent portion of the arc, causes further contraction of the main muscle (alpha) fibers.

An increase in tension on the respiratory muscle spindle fibers will occur whenever the transpulmonary pressure gradient must be increased, as with an increase in airway resistance or a decrease in lung or thoracic compliance (refer to Chapter 11). These conditions impose an increased load on the respiratory muscles, to which the gamma-efferent system responds by increasing their strength of contraction. In this manner, muscle contractions are automatically adjusted to accommodate the varying loads associated with changes in the mechanical properties of the lungs and thorax.

Sustained increases in gamma-afferent activity occur when the effort required to contract the muscle exceeds the actual shortening, as would be the case with a decrease in compliance. Current theory suggests that such conditions affect the brainstem centers by causing early cessation of inspiration.[8] This theory explains, in part, the increased frequency of breathing associated with conditions that lower lung or thoracic compliance.

Influence of higher centers

Stimulation of selected neurons in the mesencephalon (midbrain) and diencephalon (hypothalamus and thalamus) can augment tidal volume, respiratory rate or both.[2] These responses may simply represent a general increase in the "arousal" reaction of the reticular activating system.

Modification of the basic respiratory rhythm more commonly occurs by way of the cerebral cortex.[8] Good examples of the modifying influence of the cerebral cortex are the variations in breathing pattern that occur with breath-holding, voluntary hyperventilation, isometric muscular efforts, singing, crying, and swallowing. However, the ability of the cerebral cortex to override the basic cyclic pattern established by the medullary centers is limited. This limitation is due to the strong influence of other factors on the regulation of breathing, particularly the chemical constituency of the blood and cerebral spinal fluid.

Chemical regulation of respiration

It has long been known that the normal rhythmic pattern of breathing is modified by a variety of chemical stimuli, particularly hypercapnia, acidemia, and hypoxia. Research conducted over the past 75 years has demonstrated that the major factor responsible for changes in ventilation is neural input to the medullary centers through specialized structures called **chemoreceptors**.[40-42] A chemoreceptor is a group of nerve cells that senses and responds to changes in the chemical composition of its fluid environment.

There are two sets of chemoreceptors: the central or medullary chemoreceptors and the peripheral chemoreceptors. The central chemoreceptors lie on the ventrolateral surfaces of the medulla in proximity to the exit of the ninth and tenth cranial nerves. The peripheral chemoreceptors are located in the bifurcations of both carotid arteries and the arch of the aorta, but far more chemoreceptors are located in the carotid structures.[12] Afferent neurons from the carotid bodies ascend as part of the carotid nerve to join the glossopharyngeal nerve. The afferent nerve fibers from the aortic bodies enter the vagal nerve pathways, usually along with the recurrent laryngeal nerves.

Both the central and peripheral chemoreceptors send impulses to the medullary center, and although there are similarities in their functions there are also significant differences. These differences are most pronounced in regard to their relative response to CO_2 and O_2.

Response to carbon dioxide

Carbon dioxide exerts the main chemical influence on breathing. High inspired partial pressure of carbon dioxide has a direct stimulating effect on ventilation (Figure 14-19). Ventilation increases gradually as inspired CO_2 concentrations rise to 8% to 10%. Concentrations in the 10% to 20% range cause a proportionately greater increase in ventilation. However, at concentrations in the 20% range, CO_2 exerts a depressant effect on both ventilation and the central nervous system as a whole, not unlike an anesthetic gas.

Early experiments demonstrated that this effect was due in part to changes in the chemical environment of the brainstem. Perfusion of the ventricles of the brain with fluid containing a high PCO_2 and a low pH stimulated breathing. On the other hand, perfusion with fluid containing a low PCO_2 and a high pH depressed respiration. These findings pointed to the existence of a central chemoreceptive area.

Central Chemoreceptors. The central chemoreceptors are mainly stimulated by hydrogen ions rather than by the CO_2 molecule. However, they are exquisitely sensitive to CO_2 in an indirect fashion. These specialized cells are not in direct contact with the blood. Instead, they are exposed to the circulating cerebrospinal fluid (CSF), which is separated from the blood by a semipermeable membrane referred to as the *blood-brain barrier.*

The blood-brain barrier is relatively impermeable by hydrogen and bicarbonate ions, but is freely permeable by molecular carbon dioxide. Elevations in

blood CO_2 therefore cause rapid diffusion of this gas into the CSF, where it dissociates into H^+ and HCO_3^-, lowering the CSF pH. These H^+ ions so generated in the CSF, and not the high CO_2, have a potent stimulatory effect on the central chemoreceptors. Thus increased levels of CO_2 in the blood increase ventilation indirectly by altering the pH of the CSF, thereby stimulating the central chemoreceptors. The central chemoreceptors, in turn, signal the medullary centers to increase ventilation.

Because of the impermeability of the blood-CSF barrier to hydrogen ions, changes in blood hydrogen ion concentration have much less effect on the central chemoreceptors than do changes in blood carbon dioxide. When blood PCO_2 rises, CSF PCO_2 rises immediately, forming hydrogen ions in the CSF as it reacts with water. However, when blood hydrogen ion concentration increases, these ions cannot cross the blood-CSF barrier in great enough numbers to be as effective as CO_2 in stimulating the chemoreceptors. The response to metabolic acidosis, then, is not as rapid as the response to increases in $PaCO_2$.

The stimulatory effect of $PaCO_2$ on the central chemoreceptors gradually declines after 1 to 2 days because of the renal compensatory response to high $PaCO_2$ (i.e., retention of blood bicarbonate and the return of pH toward normal). That is, blood bicarbonate eventually slowly diffuses through the blood-brain barrier to reduce the hydrogen ion concentration of the fluid that bathes the chemoreceptors.

Changes in blood oxygen concentration have no direct effect on central chemoreceptors. Compared with blood CO_2, blood O_2 is much more poorly regulated by the neural control system; however, there is less need for precise control of oxygen because nearly normal amounts of oxygen are delivered to the tissues for a PaO_2 that changes from 60 torr to 1000 torr. This is because of the nature of the oxygen-hemoglobin equilibrium curve, which reveals that hemoglobin is 90% saturated with oxygen at a PO_2 of 60 torr. Therefore adequate oxygen delivery can occur even when ventilation is less than half of normal. This is not true for CO_2 because blood PCO_2 changes linearly and inversely with ventilation. Therefore carbon dioxide, not oxygen, is the major controller of ventilation.

Peripheral chemoreceptors. Early research demonstrated that when blood high in CO_2 or low in O_2 perfused the left ventricle and first part of the aorta, stimulation of breathing occurred. However, such stimulation was observed only when the vagus nerves were intact. Later investigations showed a similar effect with the carotid arteries. These findings pointed to the existence of peripheral chemoreceptors.

As compared to the central chemoreceptors, the carotid and aortic bodies are not very sensitive to CO_2 changes.[12,41] In general, the $PaCO_2$ must rise to 20 to 30 torr above normal before a significant increase in

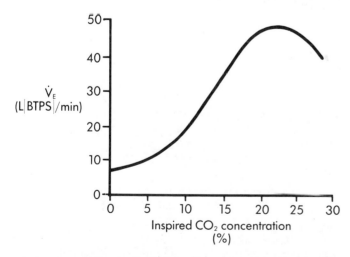

Fig. 14-19 Ventilatory response to CO_2 concentration in inspired gas. (From Slonim NB and Hamilton LH: Respiratory physiology, ed 5, St Louis, 1987, Mosby.)

ventilation occurs. For this reason, it is estimated that less than a third of the response to hypercapnia in normal subjects is due to the activity of the peripheral chemoreceptors. For practical purposes, then, CO_2 effects on peripheral chemoreceptors need not be considered.

The peripheral chemoreceptors are also responsive to changes in H^+. This response occurs even in the presence of normal or low pressures of CO_2, as might be observed in metabolic acidosis. However, the response to changes in blood pH is less sensitive than that to CO_2. The pH must change by 0.05 to 0.1 units before a ventilatory response is observed.

Although the peripheral chemoreceptors are stimulated by hypercapnia and acidemia, their primary role appears to be in response to hypoxia.

Response to oxygen lack

Ventilation is not stimulated significantly until inspired concentrations of oxygen fall to 12% or less—equivalent to an arterial PO_2 between 50 and 60 torr. Indeed, in normal individuals living at sea level, the hypoxic stimulus to breathing, which is mediated through the peripheral chemoreceptors, is not considered part of the regular mechanism controlling respiration.[8] The carotid bodies' rate of nerve impulse transmission does not increase significantly until PaO_2 falls below 60 torr. As PaO_2 falls from 60 torr to 30 torr, the rate of nerve impulses greatly increases.[12] Interestingly, this corresponds to the PaO_2 range in which arterial hemoglobin saturation with oxygen falls most rapidly.

In contrast to hypercapnia, which acts both centrally and peripherally, hypoxia appears to stimulate breathing solely through the peripheral chemoreceptors. In fact, if the peripheral chemoreceptors are removed, arterial hypoxemia actually suppresses ventilation, presumably by depression of the medullary centers.

The peripheral chemoreceptors respond to decreased partial pressures of oxygen rather than to an actual decrease in the oxygen content of the blood. This sensitivity to PaO_2 is explained, in part, by the extraordinarily high blood flow they receive in comparison to their metabolic rates.[41] the blood flow through the carotid bodies each minute is twenty times greater than the weight of the bodies themselves.[12] Thus the fraction of oxygen extracted from the blood by these bodies is extremely low. Because the arterial-venous oxygen content difference $(C(a - v)O_2)$ of the peripheral chemoreceptors is so small, most of their oxygen need are met by the small amount of dissolved O_2 in the plasma. Therefore, a decrease in PO_2 or blood flow will stimulate the peripheral chemoreceptors, causing increased ventilation.

The sensitivity of the peripheral chemoreceptors to PaO_2, as opposed to CaO_2, explains why conditions in

which the arterial oxygen contents is low but the oxygen partial pressure is normal do not stimulate breathing. Such conditions include anemia and carbon monoxide poisoning. Although a decrease in PaO_2 below 60 torr excites peripheral chemoreceptors and increases ventilation, this effect is attenuated by the fact that as ventilation increases, $PaCO_2$ decreases. This decrease in $PaCO_2$ raises blood pH, and both of these factors suppress the central chemoreceptors. That is, the increase in ventilation and subsequent decrease in blood hydrogen ion concentration tends to limit the stimulatory effect of hypoxemia on ventilation.[12]

On the other hand, in some conditions such as emphysema and advanced chronic bronchitis, the presence of ventilation-perfusion imbalances and deranged pulmonary mechanics may interfere with gas exchange to the extent that $PaCO_2$ cannot be lowered significantly regardless of patient effort and total minute ventilation. In such cases, there is no opposing hypocapneic effect to suppress the stimulatory effect of hypoxemia on ventilation, and hypoxemia drives ventilation quite strongly.

Interactions

Hypercapnia and hypoxemia together have an additive effect on ventilation.[36] As shown in Figure 14-20, in the presence of hypoxemia, the ventilatory response to hypercapnia occurs earlier and is greater than when the PO_2 is normal. Likewise, in the presence of hypercapnia the ventilatory response to hypoxemia is augmented. In clinical practice, these

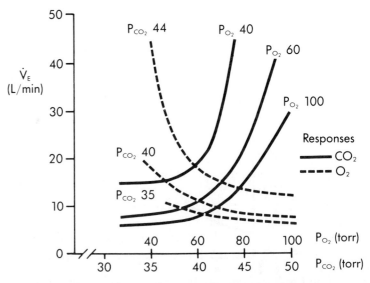

Fig. 14-20 Set of curves illustrating the ventilatory response to hypercapnia and hypoxia. The curves were constructed from published data. The solid lines represent the ventilatory response to PCO_2 at constant PO_2. The broken lines represent the response to PO_2 at constant PCO_2. (From Slonim NB and Hamilton LH: Respiratory physiology, ed 5, St Louis, 1987, Mosby.)

interactions help explain the differential impact of and response to hypercapnia and hypoxemia in patients with respiratory insufficiency and failure.

Reflex control of respiration

In addition to input provided by the chemoreceptors, the respiratory centers of the brainstem constantly receives and processes other sensory information. This information arises from a variety of mechanical sensors called **proprioceptors.** Impulses from these proprioceptors travels over afferent pathways of the vagus nerve to the medullary respiratory centers, where they are integrated with other input to vary the breathing pattern.

Proprioceptive mechanisms thus provide the third major regulatory influence on respiration, termed reflex control.[43,44] The major reflex control mechanisms include the Hering-Breuer inflation reflex, Head's paradoxic reflex, the deflation reflex, airway irritant reflexes, a vascular congestive reflex, and the baroreceptor reflex to changes in systemic perfusion pressures.

Inflation reflex (Hering–Breuer reflex)

The Hering-Breuer inflation reflex originates in specialized stretch receptors located mainly in the bronchi and bronchioles. As the lung inflates, these stretch receptors discharge progressively move nerve impulses. Because such impulses continue as long intratracheal pressure remains high, the stretch receptors responsible for the Hering-Breuer reflex are called "slowly adapting" receptors. These impulses travel through the vagus nerve to the dorsal respiratory group of neurons where they switch off the inspiratory ramp signal, stopping further inspiration.[8] The Hering-Breuer reflex in adult humans is only activated at large tidal volumes (1.5 L or greater) and is apparently not an important control mechanism in quiet normal breathing.[12] The only evidence of a strong inflation reflex in human beings is among newborn infants.[2]

Head's paradoxic reflex

When the afferent pathways for the Hering-Breuer reflex are blocked by cooling of the vagus nerve, inflation of the lung causes an additional inspiratory effort. This response, called Head's paradoxic reflex, is also initiated through sensory stimulation of pulmonary stretch receptors. However, compared with those receptors responsible for the Hering-Breuer reflex, the stretch receptors involved in Head's reflex are stimulated mainly by rapid volume changes. Hence these receptors are referred to as "rapidly adapting."

Head's reflex may be the basis for the occasional deep breath or sigh that punctuates normal breathing, thereby preventing alveolar collapse or microatele-

ctasis. It may also be responsible for maintaining high tidal volumes during exercise and the successive gasping exhibited by newborn infants as they progressively inflate their lungs at birth.[8]

Deflation reflex

Injury to the lung or chest wall that causes deflation results in an increased force and frequency of inspiratory effort. This response, which is distinct from the Hering-Breuer reflex, is referred to as the deflation reflex. Like Head's reflex, the deflation reflex is initiated through sensory stimulation of rapidly adapting stretch receptors located primarily in the bronchi and bronchioles. The deflation reflex may help explain the hyperpnea that is frequently observed with chest compression and pneumothorax. Because the deflation reflex is observed mainly in response to injury and not during the normal process of breathing, it is sometimes referred to as a **nociceptive** reflex.[2]

Irritation reflexes

Irritant receptors are located in the subepithelial tissues of the larger airways, mainly in the posterior wall of the trachea and at the bifurcations of the larger bronchi. Not active during normal breathing, these receptors respond to a variety of mechanical, chemical and physiological stimuli, including physical manipulation or irritation, inhalation of noxious gases, histamine-induced bronchoconstriction, asphyxia, and microembolization of the pulmonary arteries. Stimulation of the irritant receptors can result in bronchoconstriction, hyperpnea, reflex closure of the glottis, and cough. These responses are readily observed at the bedside during procedures such as tracheobronchial intubation or bronchoscopy and can be reduced by the application of local anesthetics.

Alveolar J receptors

Pulmonary embolism, pulmonary edema, and congestive heart failure all can evoke a rapid, shallow breathing pattern. That such a pattern is abolished by vagotomy demonstrates its reflex origin.

The source of this reflex response is thought to be the "J" receptors, which are sensory nerve ending located in alveolar walls in **juxtaposition** to pulmonary capillaries. These receptors respond to irritant chemicals—as well as to engorged capillaries, such as may occur in congestive heart failure. Besides causing rapid, shallow breathing, stimulation of the J receptors can result in **bradycardia,** hypotension, and expiratory narrowing of the glottis. J-receptor stimulation also may contribute to the sensation of dyspnea accompanying pulmonary vascular congestion.[2]

Baroreceptor reflexes

It has long been observed that a decrease in arterial blood pressure results in hyperventilation and an increase in arterial blood pressure causes hypoventilation.[8] This reflex is mediated mainly by the aortic and carotid baroreceptors, described in Chapter 10.

The hyperventilation that occurs with decreased perfusion pressures does slightly increase arterial oxygen content, thereby providing a very small increment in oxygen delivery. Of perhaps more importance is the potential increase in venous return that would result from such a breathing pattern. However, these effects are minimal, and the actual role of the baroreceptor reflex in the regulation of respiration remains unknown.

Ventilatory response to exercise

Because arterial pH, PCO_2 and PO_2 all remain almost exactly normal even during strenuous exercise, control of ventilation during exercise has been a subject of much interest. Ventilation, oxygen consumption, and carbon dioxide production all increase greatly; however, there seems to be no chemical basis for the increase in ventilation, especially the abrupt and immediate increase at the onset of exercise. The hyperpnea of exercise is not understood, but two effects seem to predominate[12]: (1) the higher centers of the brain may transmit collateral impulses to the respiratory centers as it transmits signals to contracting skeletal muscle, and (2) excitation of proprioceptors in moving limb joints stimulate the respiratory centers. Even passive joint movements are known to increase ventilation.

Integrated responses

Figure 14-21 provides an integrated perspective on the interaction among the three major mechanisms involved in the regulation of respiration. The basic rhythmicity of the breathing pattern is established by the medullary and pontine centers. The response of the respiratory muscles to varying mechanical loads is adjusted by way of the gamma-efferent feedback system. Modification to the basic breathing pattern occurs by way of input from local and peripheral chemoreceptors in the aortic and carotid bodies and from proprioceptors located in the lung parenchyma. Last, input from higher brain centers provides voluntary control when necessary. In combination, these control mechanisms normally assure that ventilation is efficient, that gas exchange is adequate, and that acid-base homeostasis is maintained.

When faced with abnormal circumstances, these control mechanisms must adjust their activity to maintain as near a normal level of body function as possible. As with any deviation from normal, such adjustments represent compromise. Good examples of adjustments made by the regulatory mechanisms are those that occur in chronic hypoxemia, chronic hypercapnia, and metabolic acidosis.

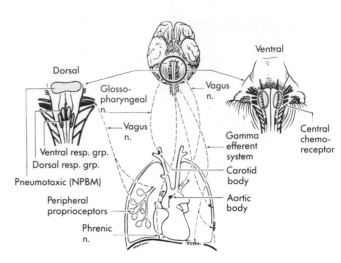

Fig. 14-21 The system that regulates pulmonary ventilation and generates the breathing pattern. (From Slonim NB and Hamilton LH: *Respiratory physiology*, ed 5, St Louis, 1987, Mosby.)

Chronic hypoxemia

An initial reduction in arterial PO_2 to 60 torr or less is immediately detected by the peripheral chemoreceptors, causing an immediate increase in ventilation. The resulting hyperventilation lowers blood CO_2 levels, causing diffusion of this gas out of the CSF. As CO_2 leaves the CSF, brain pH rises, causing suppression of ventilation. This secondary action slightly offsets the initial hypoxic stimulus, resulting in a lower level of hyperventilation than would otherwise occur, as discussed earlier.

Beyond the acute phase, continued low arterial PO_2 levels provoke a series of compensatory responses designed to improve oxygen delivery and restore a normal pH.

Within a few hours, active transport of HCO_3^- out of the CSF begins, causing decrease of CSF pH back toward normal. As the pH of the CSF is restored toward normal, the early secondary suppression to ventilation is removed, and a new balance (with greater hyperventilation) is established. That is, the hypoxia-induced hyperventilation is no longer opposed by suppressive CSF alkalosis.

In essence, chronic hypoxemia causes the medullary chemoreceptors to be "reset" to maintain a lower-than-normal PCO_2. Under such circumstances, should the hypoxic stimulus be removed, ventilation will gradually decrease. Then, as the PCO_2 rises over time, CSF HCO_3^- will rise, and ventilation will eventually be restored to normal.

Chronic hypercapnia

An acute increase in arterial PCO_2 causes an immediate increase in ventilation by way of stimulation of both the peripheral and central chemoreceptors. If hypercapnia persists, the kidneys begin to preferentially retain bicarbonate and excrete fixed acids restoring blood pH back toward normal even though the $PaCO_2$ remains high. Eventually, the high blood bicarbonate level caused by renal compensation diffuses across the blood-brain barrier into the CSF, bringing its pH back to normal also. The $PaCO_2$ remains high, but pH—and thus hydrogen ion—stimulus of the central chemoreceptors, is now normal. In this manner, the central chemoreceptors are reset to operate normally at a high PCO_2. This means the high $PaCO_2$ is no longer a stimulus to ventilation.

However, as long as one is breathing room air, the increase in $PaCO_2$ causes a reciprocal fall in the PaO_2. When this fall in PaO_2 is of sufficient magnitude (< 60-70 torr), the peripheral chemoreceptors are again stimulated, this time by the arterial hypoxemia. Therefore, in spite of the loss of central sensitivity to CO_2, ventilation is maintained by way of a hypoxic stimulus.

If the main drive to breathing is arterial hypoxemia, oxygen administration could eliminate this hypoxic stimulus and result in depression of ventilation, increased hypercapnia, and even death. The potential for this oxygen-induced hypoventilation is the reason for the use of controlled low-concentration oxygen therapy in patients with chronic hypercapnia.

Chronic (compensated) metabolic acidosis

An increase in fixed acid in the blood lowers its pH, quickly causing stimulation of the peripheral chemoreceptors and hyperventilation. The lowered blood PCO_2 causes a similar decrease in the CSF PCO_2, thereby raising its pH. This CSF alkalosis causes a secondary central inhibition to ventilation that partially blunts the initial peripheral stimulation.

As with chronic hypoxia, should the hyperventilation persist, active transport of HCO_3^- out of the CSF begins, causing a lowering of its pH back toward normal. As the pH of the CSF is restored toward normal, the early secondary suppression to ventilation is removed, and a new balance (with greater hyperventilation) is established. The central chemoreceptors are reset to this lower level of CO_2 and become more sensitive to increases in the CSF level of this gas.

If the metabolic acidosis is now rapidly corrected, hyperventilation will persist initially, and the patient will swing from compensated metabolic acidosis to acute respiratory alkalosis. Events such as these explain the persistent hyperventilation that is observed with rapid correction of compensated metabolic acidosis, as in the treatment of renal tubular acidosis by dialysis or diabetic ketoacidosis by insulin.[2]

CHAPTER SUMMARY

Metabolic processes of the body produce more than 24,000 mmol of acid/day. Normal acid–base homeostasis involves minimizing the pH changes caused by this acid load and excreting these by-products of metabolism. Buffer systems are the first line of defense against wide fluctuations in pH of the body fluids. Excretion of body acids is accomplished by both the kidneys and lungs.

Imbalances in acid–base homeostasis can arise from abnormal respiratory or metabolic function, from ingestion of chemicals or drugs, or as a result of treatment. The lungs represent the respiratory component of acid–base regulation and act within minutes to rapidly control the level of volatile acid (carbon dioxide) in the blood. The kidneys control the nonrespiratory, or metabolic, component of acid–base balance and act within hours or days to gradually excrete or retain bicarbonate and fixed acids. The control of fluid volume and electrolytes—such as sodium, potassium, and chloride—by the kidneys is an integral part of maintaining acid–base balance. The body minimizes the impact of respiratory or metabolic acid–base disturbances by causing the system not affected to compensate for the abnormality in the other. Correcting an acid–base imbalance involves treating the system primarily affected and restoring it to normal function.

The respiratory system plays a vital role in acid–base regulation because it controls ventilation and, thus, carbon dioxide levels in the blood. This control is mediated through neurological structures, both central and peripheral, which are sensitive to blood carbon dioxide, pH, and oxygen levels. Mechanical stretch receptors and neural reflexes modify this control of ventilation. Control of carbon dioxide is intimately connected to maintenance acid–base balance. It is critically important that RCPs understand the role of ventilation in controlling acid–base balance, and especially ventilation's interaction with kidney function in the process of compensation and restoration of pH homeostasis.

REFERENCES

1. Martin L: *Pulmonary physiology in clinical practice: the essentials for patient care and evaluation,* St. Louis, 1987, Mosby.
2. Murray JF: *The normal lung,* ed 2, Philadelphia, 1986, WB Saunders.
3. Winters RW, Knud E, Dell RB: *Acid-base physiology in medicine,* Copenhagen, 1967, The London Co.
4. Filley G: *Acid-base and blood gas regulation,* Philadelphia, 1971, Lea & Febiger.
5. Siggaard-Andersen O: *The acid-base status of the blood,* ed 4, Baltimore, 1974, Williams & Wilkins.
6. Jones NL: *Blood gases and acid-base physiology,* New York, 1980, Decker.
7. Masoro EJ, Siegel PD: *Acid-base regulation: physiology and pathophysiology.* Philadelphia, 1971, WB Saunders.
8. Slonim NB, Hamilton LH: *Respiratory physiology,* ed. 5, St. Louis, 1987, Mosby.
9. Comroe JH: *Physiology of respiration,* ed 2, Chicago, 1974, Mosby.

10. Shapiro BA, Harrison RA, Walton JR: *Clinical application of blood gases,* ed 3, Chicago, 1982, Mosby.
11. Narins RG: Acid-base metabolism. In: Gonick HC, ed: *Current nephrology,* vol 1, Boston, 1977, Houghton-Mifflin.
12. Guyton AC: *Textbook of medical physiology,* ed. 8, Philadelphia, 1991, WB Saunders.
13. Lane EE, Walker JF: *Clinical arterial blood gas analysis,* St. Louis, 1987, Mosby.
14. ACCP-ATS Joint Committee on Pulmonary Nomenclature: Pulmonary terms and symbols, *Chest* 67:583, 1975.
15. Rose BD: *Clinical physiology of acid-base and electrolyte disorders,* New York, 1977, McGraw-Hill.
16. Malley WJ: *Clinical blood gases: application and noninvasive alternatives,* Philadelphia 1990, WB Saunders.
17. Wilkins RL: Interpretation of blood gases. In: Wilkins RL, Sheldon RL, Krider SJ, eds. *Clinical assessment in respiratory care,* St. Louis, 1985, Mosby.
18. Flenley DC: Blood-gas and acid-base interpretation, *Basics RD,* 10:1, September 1981.
19. Robin ED: Abnormalities of acid-base regulation in chronic pulmonary disease, with special reference to hypercapnia and extracellular alkalosis, *N Engl J Med* 268:917, 1963.
20. Refsum HE: Acid-base disturbances in chronic pulmonary disease, *Ann N Y Acad Sci* 133:142, 1966.
21. Petty TL, Neff TA: Renal function in respiratory failure, *JAMA* 217:82, 1971.
22. Collier CR, Hackney JD, Mohler JD: Use of extracellular base excess in diagnosis of acid base disorders: a conceptual approach, *Chest,* 61:65, 1972.
23. Nunn JF: *Applied respiratory physiology,* ed 2., Kent, UK, 1977, Butterworth.
24. Selden DW, Rector FC Jr.: The generation and maintenance of metabolic alkalosis, *Kidney Int,* 1:306, 1972.
25. Goldring RM: Respiratory adjustments to chronic metabolic alkalosis in man, *J Clin Invest,* 47:188, 1968.
26. Jovaheri S, Kazemi H: Metabolic alkalosis and hypoventilation in humans, *Am Rev Respir Dis* 136:1011–1016, 1987.
27. McCurdy DK: Mixed metabolic and respiratory acid-base disturbances: diagnosis and treatment, *Chest* 62:355, 1972.
28. Narins RG, Emmett M: Simple and mixed acid-base disorders: a practical approach, *Medicine* 59:161, 1980.
29. Mitchell RA, and Berger AJ: Neural regulation of respiration. *Am Rev Respir Dis* 111:206, 1975.
30. Berger AJ, Mitchell RA, Severinghaus JW.: Regulation of respiration, *N Eng J Med* 297, 1977.
31. Euler CV: Brain stem mechanisms for the generation and control of breathing pattern. In: Fishman AF, et al editors: *Handbook of physiology,* Bethesda, MD, 1986, American Physiological Society.
32. Bradley GW: Control of breathing pattern. In: Widdicombe JG, ed, *International review of physiology,* vol 14, Baltimore, University Park Press, 185–217, 1974.
33. Cohen MI: Central determinants of respiratory rhythm. *Annu Rev Physiol* 43: 91–104, 1981.
34. Kalia MP: Anatomical organization of central respiratory neurons. *Annu Rev Physiol* 43:105–120, 1981.
35. Long SE, Duffin J: The medullary respiratory neurons: a review. *Can J Physiol Pharmacol* 62:161–182, 1984.
36. Feldman JL: Interactions between brainstem respiratory neurons. *Fed Proc* 40:2384–2388, 1981.
37. Wang SC, Ngai SH: Respiration coordinating mechanisms of the brain stem: a few controversial points, *Ann NY Acad Sci* 109:550, 1963.
38. Merrill EG: Where are the real respiratory neurons? *Fed Proc* 40:2389–2394, 1974.
39. Richter DW, Ballantyne D, Remmers JH: How is the respiratory rhythm generated? A model. *News Physiol Sci,* 1:109–112, 1986.
40. Sorenson SC: The chemical control of ventilation, *Acta Physiol Scand* 361 (suppl):1–72, 1971.
41. Torrance RW: Arterial chemoreceptors. In: Widdicombe JG, ed, *International review of physiology,* vol 2 Baltimore, University Park Press, 1974.
42. Fitzgerald RS, Lahiri S: reflex response to chemoreceptor activity. In: Fishman AF, et al, editors, *Handbook of physiology,* Bethesda, MD, 1986, American Physiological Society.
43. Coleridge HM, Coleridge JCG: Reflexes evoked from the tracheobronchial tree an lungs. In: Fishman AF et al, editors, *Handbook of physiology,* Bethesda, MD, 1986, American Physiological Society.
44. Widdicombe JG: Reflex control of breathing. In: Widdicombe JG, editor: *International review of physiology,* Baltimore, 1974, University Park Press.

4

Assessment
of
Respiratory
Disorders

Patterns of Cardiopulmonary Dysfunction*

■

Craig L. Scanlan

Cardiopulmonary dysfunction exists when the lungs, heart, or vascular system fails to function adequately or efficiently. In general terms, this means that O_2 or CO_2 exchange is impaired, or that the energy cost needed to exchange these gases is prohibitive.

On the basis of this general definition, most clinical disorders can be grouped into one or more major patterns. These patterns include hypoxia, ventilation-perfusion (V/Q) imbalances, airway obstruction/hyperinflation, and pulmonary restriction.

Only by understanding these major patterns of abnormality can the respiratory care practitioner (RCP) effectively participate as a member of the patient care team.

GENERAL CONCEPTS

Cardiopulmonary dysfunction exists when either O_2 or CO_2 exchange is impaired, or when the energy cost needed to exchange these metabolites is prohibitive.

Impaired oxygen delivery

As discussed in Chapter 12, O_2 delivery (DO_2) to the tissues is a function of arterial O_2 content (CaO_2) times cardiac output ($\dot{Q}T$)[1]:

$$DO_2 = CaO_2 \times \dot{Q}T$$

When O_2 delivery falls short of cellular needs, a condition of *hypoxia* exists. According to the preceding equation, hypoxia occurs if: (1) the arterial blood O_2 content is decreased, (2) cardiac output or perfusion is decreased, or (3) both conditions exist.

---

*The section on ventilation-perfusion imbalances has been adapted with permission from Martin L: *Pulmonary physiology in clinical practice: the essentials for patient care and evaluation,* St. Louis, 1987, Mosby.

A decrease in arterial blood O_2 content is called *hypoxemia.*[2] Hypoxemia can result from a decrease in PaO_2, a decrease in available hemoglobin, or hemoglobin saturation abnormalities. Alone or in combination, these factors decrease the amount of O_2 available to the tissues. Thus, without compensation by the cardiovascular system, hypoxemia can cause tissue hypoxia.

Tissue hypoxia can occur even when the arterial blood O_2 content is normal.[3] In this case, poor perfusion is the cause. Decreased perfusion may be localized to a tissue region (ischemia) or occur throughout the body (shock). Whether decreased perfusion causes tissue hypoxia depends on how poor the blood flow is, how long the blood flow is reduced, and the metabolic rate of the affected tissues.

Impaired carbon dioxide removal

As presented in Chapter 11, impaired CO_2 removal by the lung causes hypercapnia and respiratory acidosis. Alveolar CO_2 levels are governed by the relationship between production and excretion of this metabolic waste product, as follows:

$$PaCO_2 = \frac{\dot{V}CO_2 \times 0.863}{\dot{V}A}$$

Given this relationship, any disorder that lowers alveolar ventilation ($\dot{V}A$) relative to metabolic need will impair CO_2 removal.

A decrease in alveolar ventilation in relation to metabolic need may occur when: (1) the minute ventilation ($\dot{V}E$) is inadequate, (2) the deadspace ventilation per minute ($\dot{V}D$) is increased, or (3) both an inadequate $\dot{V}E$ and an increased $\dot{V}D$ coexist.[4]

Clinically, an inadequate minute ventilation is usually caused by decreased tidal volumes. Decreased tidal volumes occur in restrictive conditions, such as respiratory center depression, neuromuscular disorders, or impeded thoracic expansion (refer to the subsequent section on pulmonary restriction). An increase in deadspace ventilation is due to either: (1) rapid, shallow breathing (an increase in *anatomic* deadspace per minute) or (2) the presence of areas of the lung with abnormally high V/Q ratios (an increase in *physiologic* deadspace per minute).[5]

Regardless of cause, when alveolar ventilation decreases relative to metabolic need, the $PaCO_2$ rises (hypercapnia). Since hypercapnia normally increases ventilatory drive, an abnormally high $PaCO_2$ indicates that other problems exist. Specifically, a high $PaCO_2$ means that either: (1) the patient is not responding normally to the elevated $PaCO_2$; (2) the patient is responding normally, but the signal is not getting through to the respiratory muscles; or (3) despite normal neural responses, the respiratory pump (lungs and chest bellows) cannot provide adequate ventilation, as a result of restrictive disease or muscular fatigue.[5]

Prohibitive energy costs

The lungs and the heart normally meet the metabolic needs of the tissues over a wide range of physiologic demands. During exercise, for example, a healthy individual can maintain a fivefold increase in minute ventilation and a tripling of cardiac output.

However, even in healthy individuals, there is an upper limit to the work that the respiratory and cardiovascular systems can do. At a point determined, in part, by the individual's overall physical conditioning, lactic acidosis and muscle fatigue combine to limit further activity.

Of course, this limit is much lower for patients with either respiratory or cardiovascular disease. In respiratory disease, the major factors limiting an increase in workload are an inadequate ventilatory reserve and dyspnea. Moreover, unlike healthy individuals, those with respiratory disease often undergo an *increase* in PCO_2 at higher work levels, which can lead to respiratory failure.

In patients with cardiovascular disease, it is an inability to increase cardiac output that limits workload. This may be due to inadequate stroke volume or heart rate, although inadequate stroke volume is the more common factor. Regardless of cause, these limitations lead to an early increase in lactic acid production (caused by anaerobic metabolism) and hyperventilation. Sustained increases in workload may cause cardiac failure.

Thus, if the workload needed to maintain normal exchange of O_2 and CO_2 exceeds the ability of the lungs or heart, the body may opt to conserve energy and accept an abnormal state. Thus, hypoventilation and hypercapnia may have to be "accepted" in order to prevent respiratory muscle fatigue. Likewise, a decreased cardiac output may have to be "accepted" in lieu of risking acute cardiac failure.

In summary, the three major physiologic disturbances underlying all forms of cardiopulmonary dysfunction are: (1) impaired O_2 delivery, (2) impaired CO_2 removal, and (3) energy costs in excess of those which the respiratory and cardiovascular systems can maintain.

Associated with these major physiologic disturbances are a large number of discrete clinical disorders. In general, these numerous disorders may be grouped into one or more major pathophysiologic patterns. These major patterns include hypoxia, ventilation-perfusion imbalances, airway obstruction and pulmonary hyperinflation, and pulmonary restriction.

HYPOXIA

Hypoxia exists when O_2 delivery to the tissues is inadequate to meet their metabolic needs. In this section we explore the major causes of hypoxia, its physiologic effects, and clinical signs and symptoms. This discussion is followed by a brief discussion on the treatment of hypoxia.

Causes of hypoxia

As previously discussed, hypoxia usually is due to either a decrease in the O_2 content of arterial blood (hypoxemia) or a decrease in perfusion.[3] Both these conditions decrease O_2 delivery to the tissues. A third major category of hypoxia, called *dysoxia,* can occur even when O_2 delivery to the tissues is normal. Dysoxia is an abnormal metabolic state in which the tissues are unable to utilize the O_2 made available to them.[6] The major causes of hypoxia and their primary indicators are summarized in Table 15-1, page 344.

Hypoxemia

Hypoxemia is a condition of reduced arterial blood O_2 content. Hypoxemia occurs when either the PaO_2 or hemoglobin is low, or when hemoglobin saturation abnormalities are present. Alone or in combination, these factors lower the amount of O_2 carried to the tissues. Without compensation by the cardiovascular system, hypoxemia can cause tissue hypoxia.

Decreased PaO_2. A decreased PaO_2 may be due to a low ambient PO_2, hypoventilation, impaired diffusion, right-to-left shunting, or ventilation-perfusion (V/Q) imbalances.

Low ambient PO_2. Breathing gases with a low O_2 concentration at sea level or breathing air at pressures less than atmospheric lowers the alveolar O_2 tension, thereby decreasing the PaO_2. A common example of

Table 15-1 Causes of Hypoxia

Cause	Primary indicator	Mechanism	Example
HYPOXEMIA			
Low $P_{I}O_2$	Low PaO_2	Reduced P_B	Altitude
	Low PaO_2		
Hypoventilation	Low PaO_2	Decreased $\dot{V}_A$	Drug overdose
	High PCO_2		
Diffusion defect	Low PaO_2	Barrier at A-C membrane	Interstitial lung disease
	High $P_{(A\text{-}a)}O_2$ on air; resolves with O_2		
Anatomic shunt	Low PaO_2	Blood flow between right and left sides of circulation	Congenital heart disease
	High $P_{(A\text{-}a)}O_2$ on air; does not resolve with O_2		
$\dot{V}/\dot{Q}$ imbalance			
Low $\dot{V}/\dot{Q}$	Low PaO_2	Decreased $\dot{V}_A$ relative to perfusion	Chronic obstructive lung disease; aging
	High $P_{(A\text{-}a)}O_2$ on air; resolves with O_2		
Physiologic shunt	Low PaO_2	Perfusion without ventilation	Atelectasis
	High $P_{(A\text{-}a)}O_2$ on air; does not resolve with O_2		
HB deficiency			
Absolute	Low Hb content	Loss of Hb	Hemorrhage
	Reduced CaO_2		
Relative	Abnormal SaO_2	Abnormal Hb	Carboxyhemoglobin
	Reduced CaO_2		
REDUCED BLOOD FLOW	Increased $C(a\text{-}\bar{v})O_2$	Decreased perfusion	Shock; ischemia
	Decreased $C\bar{v}O_2$		
DYSOXIA	Normal CaO_2	Disruption of cellular enzymes	Cyanide poisoning; septic shock
	Increased $C\bar{v}O_2$		

A-C, alveolar-capillary; *Hb,* hemoglobin.

this problem occurs during travel to high altitudes, where the visitor often suffers the ill effects of hypoxia for several days. This condition is called acute mountain sickness.[7] The compensatory response of the body to this form of chronic hypoxia is described later in this chapter.

Hypoventilation. Assuming a constant FiO_2, the alveolar PO_2 varies *inversely* with the alveolar PCO_2 (refer to Chapter 11). Thus, a rise in the alveolar PCO_2 (hypoventilation) is always accompanied by a proportionate fall in alveolar PO_2.

Impaired alveolar-capillary diffusion. Even when the alveolar PO_2 is normal, disorders of the alveolar-capillary membrane may limit diffusion of O_2 into the pulmonary capillary blood, thereby lowering the PaO_2. Examples include pulmonary fibrosis and interstitial edema. However, a pure diffusion limitation is a relatively uncommon cause of hypoxemia at rest. Diffusion limitations generally occur only when the blood flow through the pulmonary circulation is increased, as during exercise (refer to Chapter 11).

Anatomic shunts. A shunt is a bypass. An anatomic shunt connects the arterial and venous circulations, bypassing the lungs. Small anatomic shunts occur in

normal individuals. These include the bronchial circulation (see Chapter 9) and the thebesian vessels of the heart (see Chapter 10). Abnormal anatomic shunts may be due to congenital cardiac defects, disease, or trauma. Congenital heart disease is the most common cause of anatomic shunting.

There are two types of anatomic shunts: right-to-left and left-to-right. In a right-to-left shunt, blood flows from the venous to the arterial side of the circulation. Under these conditions, poorly oxygenated venous blood mixes with well oxygenated arterial blood. This lowers both the O_2 content and the PO_2 of the arterial blood.

In a left-to-right shunt, blood flows from the arterial to the venous side of the circulation. A left-to-right shunt has little direct effect on the arterial O_2 content. However, because flow through a left-to-right shunt is wasted (like a leak), the heart may have to increase its output to satisfy tissue demands. For this reason, large left-to-right shunts can increase the heart's workload and lead to cardiac failure.

Ventilation-perfusion (V/Q) imbalances. As described in Chapter 11, even the normal lung has a small V/Q imbalance. In conjunction with normal anatomic shunts, this normal V/Q imbalance helps explain why the arterial PO_2 is always slightly less than the alveolar PO_2.

When a low PO_2 is observed, the RCP must also take into account the normal decrease in arterial O_2 tensions that occurs with aging. As shown in Figure 15-1, breathing air at sea level, the "normal" $P(A-a)O_2$ increases in a near-linear fashion with increasing age. This results in a gradual decline in the PaO_2 over time. One may estimate the expected PaO_2 in older adults by using the following formula[8]:

$$\text{Expected } PaO_2 = 100.1 - (0.323 \times \text{age in years})$$

This progressive increase in $P(A-a)O_2$ over time is due to the normal loss of elastic recoil pressure in the aging lung. This loss of elastic recoil changes the V/Q distribution and results in a mildly progressive hypoxemia.

However, when blood perfuses areas of the lung with poor ventilation, or perfusion greatly exceeds ventilation, a marked reduction in the PaO_2 can occur. The most obvious example of this type of V/Q imbalance is the *physiologic shunt*. A physiologic shunt exists when pulmonary blood perfuses unventilated alveoli (V/Q = 0). The result is similar to that previously described for a right-to-left anatomic shunt. That is, venous blood mixes with arterial blood, lowering both CaO_2 and PaO_2.

Of course, less extreme V/Q ratios can and do occur. Indeed, low V/Q ratios (between 1 and 0) are a more common cause of hypoxemia than are true physiologic shunts. Because of the importance of this problem, its principles and consequences are discussed in detail later in this chapter.

Hemoglobin deficiencies. In and of itself, a normal PaO_2 does not guarantee adequate arterial O_2 content or delivery. For the arterial O_2 content to be adequate, there must also be enough normal hemoglobin in the blood. If the blood hemoglobin is low—even when the PaO_2 is normal—hypoxia can occur.[9]

Hemoglobin deficiencies, or anemias, can be either absolute or relative. An absolute hemoglobin deficiency occurs when the hemoglobin concentration is lower than normal. Relative hemoglobin deficiencies are due to either the displacement of O_2 from normal hemoglobin or the presence of abnormal hemoglobin variants.

Absolute hemoglobin deficiencies. A low blood hemoglobin concentration may be due to either a loss of red blood cells, as with hemorrhage, or inadequate **erythropoiesis.** Regardless of cause, a low hemoglobin can seriously impair the O_2-carrying capacity of the blood, even in the presence of a normal supply (PaO_2) and adequate diffusion.

Figure 15-2, page 346, plots the relationship between arterial oxygen content and PaO_2 as a function of hemoglobin concentration. As can be seen, progres-

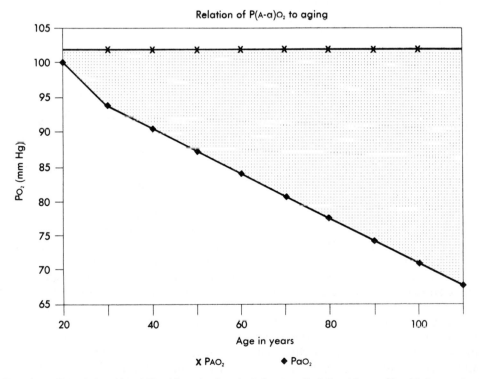

Relation of P(A-a)O₂ to aging

X PaO₂   ◆ PaO₂

Fig. 15-1 The relationship of $P(A-a)O_2$ and aging. As PaO_2 naturally falls with age, $P(A-a)O_2$ increases at the rate of approximately 3 torr each decade beyond 20 years. (From Lane EE and Walker JF: Clinical arterial blood gas analysis, St Louis, 1987, Mosby.)

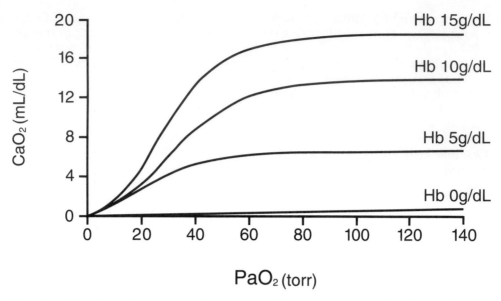

Fig. 15-2 The relationship between CaO$_2$ and arterial PO$_2$ as a function of blood hemoglobin (Hb) concentration. Progressive decreases in Hb cause large drops in CaO$_2$. (From Pierson DJ: Normal and abnormal oxygenation: physiology and clincial syndromes, *Respir Care* 38(6):587-599, 1993.)

sive falls in blood hemoglobin content cause large drops in arterial oxygen content (CaO$_2$). In fact, a 33% decrease in hemoglobin content (from 15 to 10 g/dL) reduces the CaO$_2$ as much as would a drop in PaO$_2$ from 100 to 40 torr.

Relative hemoglobin deficiencies. Not only must there be enough hemoglobin, but it must be capable of normal O$_2$ transport. As described in Chapter 12, both **carboxyhemoglobinemia** and **methemoglobinemia** can cause abnormal O$_2$ transport, as can abnormal hemoglobin variants.

In carboxyhemoglobinemia and methemoglobinemia, each gram of affected hemoglobin is comparable to the loss of a gram of normal hemoglobin. Abnormal hemoglobins have variable effects on O$_2$ transport. Those causing left shifts in the dissociation curve impede O$_2$ unloading and thus are most likely to cause hypoxia. HbC (Chesapeake), HbR (Rainier), and HbY (Yakima) all shift the curve to the left; HbY impairs O$_2$ unloading most.

Reduction in blood flow (shock or ischemia)

Because O$_2$ delivery depends on *both* arterial O$_2$ content and cardiac output, hypoxia can still occur when the CaO$_2$ is normal if blood flow is reduced. There are two types of reduced blood flow: (1) circulatory failure (shock) and (2) local reduction in perfusion (ischemia).

Circulatory failure (shock). In circulatory failure, tissue O$_2$ deprivation is widespread. Although the body tries to compensate for O$_2$ lack by directing blood flow to vital organs, this response is limited. Thus prolonged shock ultimately causes irreversible damage to the central nervous system and eventual cardiovascular collapse. Details on the causes, clinical

manifestations, and body's response to shock are provided in Chapter 20.

Local reductions in perfusion (ischemia). Even when whole body perfusion is adequate, local reductions in blood flow can cause localized hypoxia. Ischemia can result in anaerobic metabolism, metabolic acidosis, and eventual death of the affected tissue. **Myocardial infarction** and stroke (cerebrovascular accident) are good examples of ischemic conditions that can cause hypoxia and tissue death.

Dysoxia. Dysoxia is a form of hypoxia in which the cellular use of O$_2$ is abnormally decreased. The best example of dysoxia is cyanide poisoning. Cyanide disrupts the intracellular **cytochrome oxidase system,** thereby preventing cellular use of O$_2$.

Dysoxia may also occur when tissue oxygen consumption becomes dependent on oxygen delivery. Figure 15-3 plots tissue oxygen consumption ($\dot{V}O_2$) against oxygen delivery (DO$_2$) in both the normal and the pathologic state.

Normally, the tissues extract as much oxygen as they need from what is delivered, and oxygen consumption equals oxygen demand (the flat portion of the solid line).[3] However, if delivery falls, conditions begin to change (Figure 15-3, solid line). At a level called the *point of critical delivery* tissue extraction reaches a maximum. Further decreases in delivery then result in an oxygen "debt." An oxygen debt occurs when oxygen demand exceeds oxygen consumption. Under conditions of oxygen debt, oxygen consumption becomes dependent on oxygen delivery (the sloped line). This, in turn, leads to lactic acid accumulation and metabolic acidosis.

In pathologic conditions such as septic shock and adult respiratory distress syndrome, or ARDS

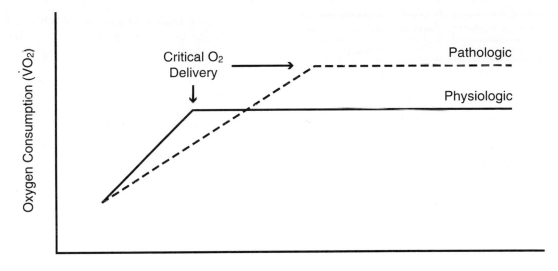

Fig. 15-3 Physiologic versus pathologic O_2 consumption-delivery relationship. Note that critical O_2 delivery occurs at higher O_2 delivery in pathologic state. The slope of the pathologic consumption curve below the critical delivery point reflects the decrease in O_2 extraction ratio that exists in these situations. (From Pasquale MD, Cipolle MD, Cerra FB: Oxygen transport: does increasing supply improve outcome? *Respir Care* 38(7):800-825, 1993.)

(Figure 15-3, dotted line), this critical point may occur at levels of oxygen delivery considered normal. In addition, the slope of the curve below the point of critical delivery may be less than normal, indicating a decreased extraction ratio ($\dot{V}O_2/DO_2$).[10] In combination, these findings indicate that oxygen demands are not being met, and that a defect exists in the cellular mechanisms regulating oxygen uptake.[11,12]

Physiologic effects

Mild hypoxia produces only minor effects. Hyperventilation is an early response in normal people, and subtle changes in intellectual performance and visual acuity may be seen. However, more severe hypoxia can have serious physiologic consequences.[13] The accompanying box lists some of the most serious effects of hypoxia.[14]

Clinical manifestations

Hypoxia results in a variety of signs and symptoms. The clinical findings seen with hypoxia depend on both its severity and its duration.[13] Table 15-2, page 348, compares and contrasts the major clinical findings associated with moderate and severe hypoxia. Two of these clinical findings, cyanosis and clubbing, warrant detailed discussion.

Cyanosis is one of the most commonly cited signs of severe hypoxia. Cyanosis is a blue or blue-gray coloration of skin, mucous membranes, and nailbeds that can occur in both acute and chronic hypoxia. This dis-

---

Harmful physiologic effects of hypoxia

- Pulmonary vasoconstriction resulting in pulmonary vascular hypertension
- Increased cardiovascular workload (produced by a compensatory increase in cardiac output)
- Deleterious effects on myocardial function, especially in the presence of preexisting coronary artery disease
- Impaired renal function, with a tendency to retain sodium and water
- Altered central nervous system (CNS) function, ranging from restlessness and disorientation to convulsions and permanent brain damage
- Anaerobic metabolism, lactic acid accumulation, and metabolic acidosis.

---

tinct coloration is due to abnormally high amounts of reduced hemoglobin (Hb^-) in the capillaries.

There are two types of cyanosis: central and peripheral. Central cyanosis is best observed in the capillary beds of the lips or **buccal** membranes. Central cyanosis occurs when the arterial hemoglobin saturation is low. Peripheral cyanosis, on the other hand, is due to excessive Hb^- in the venous blood. High venous levels of Hb^- occur when the tissues extract more O_2 from the blood than normal. This commonly occurs with poor perfusion or blood **stasis.**

Normally, capillary blood contains about 2.5 g/dL reduced Hb^-.[15] Most observers first recognize cyanosis

Table 15-2 Clinical Manifestations of Hypoxia

	Mild to moderate	Severe
Respiratory findings	Tachypnea	Tachypnea
	Dyspnea	Dyspnea
	Paleness	Cyanosis
Cardiovascular findings	Tachycardia	Tachycardia, eventual
	Mild hypertension	**bradycardia,** arrhythmias
	Peripheral vasoconstriction	Hypertension and eventual hypotention
Neurologic findings	Restlessness	Somnolence
	Disorientation	Confusion
	Headaches	Blurred vision
	Lassitude	Tunnel vision
		Loss of coordination
		Impaired judgment
		Slow reaction time
		Manic-depressive activity
		Coma
Other		Clubbing

From Pilbeam SP: Mechanical ventilation. Denver, 1986, Multi-Media Publishing.

when the capillary Hb⁻ exceeds 5 to 6 g/dL.[16] For central cyanosis, this is equivalent to a SaO_2 of 75% or less.[17] An SaO_2 of 75% corresponds to a PaO_2 of about 40 torr. Thus, we would expect central cyanosis to be evident whenever the arterial PO_2 drops below this level. In peripheral cyanosis, the SaO_2 need not be reduced.

The intensity of cyanosis increases with the hemoglobin content. For this reason, patients with a high hemoglobin content (polycythemia) can be cyanotic yet still have adequate arterial oxygen content. Conversely, patients with low hemoglobin content (anemia) can be severely hypoxic before cyanosis ever appears. Moreover, not all hypoxic states produce cyanosis. For example, both carboxyhemoglobinemia and cyanide poisoning can cause lethal hypoxia, but neither results in cyanosis.

Last, evaluation of the presence and degree of cyanosis depends on the perception of the examiner and is modified by such factors as the ambient lighting, the color of the skin, and the presence of abnormal blood pigments, such as methemoglobin or **sulfhemoglobin.** For these reasons, cyanosis must be considered an unreliable indicator of hypoxemia and hypoxia.[18] Cyanosis is a physical sign to be noted, but not awaited.[16]

Clubbing is one form of a more generalized process that affects bones and joints called hypertrophic osteoarthropathy.[19] Osteoarthropathy is a chronic inflammatory process which thickens the **periosteum.** Joints may also be affected with swelling and inflammation. In a well-developed case, pain and disabling

limitations to motion may occur. Clubbing may occur early in the development of hypertrophic osteoarthropathy, or it may not be associated with long bone changes.

To the observer, clubbing is seen as a bulbous swelling of the terminal phalanges of the fingers and toes. All diameters are affected, giving them a "drumstick" appearance. Although soft tissue swelling may be considerable, pain is seldom a symptom of clubbing.

A key feature of clubbing is the contour of the nail, which becomes rounded both longitudinally and transversely. Although such curvature may be seen in normal individuals, the distortion of the nail in clubbing is marked by the loss of the angle between the junction of the skin and the nail (cuticular angle).

Figure 15-4 compares a normal flat nail, a normal curved nail, and nails having early and late clubbing. As can be seen, both normal nails exhibit a cuticular angle less than 180 degrees. However, this angle increases in the fingers with clubbing. Also seen in the early stages of clubbing is a "floating" nail base. This sponginess under nail allows it to be moved up and down with compression. As the clubbing progresses, the degree of nail curvature gradually increases.

Despite its high incidence, the specific cause of clubbing remains unknown. We do know that patients with clubbing have enlarged capillaries and increased blood flow through the affected areas.[20] In adults, about 75% to 85% of all clubbing is associated with respiratory disease, such as lung tumors, bronchiectasis, or pulmonary **fibrosis.** Of patients with clubbing 10% to 15% have a cardiac disease, such as a congenital right-to-left shunt or chronic bacterial **endocarditis.** Patients with liver or gastrointestinal disorders make up an additional 10% of those with clubbing; the remaining 5% occur in miscellaneous conditions. In children, clubbing is predominantly associated with cystic fibrosis, **bronchiectasis, empyema,** and congenital heart disease.

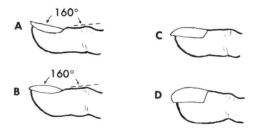

Fig. 15-4 Clubbing is characterized by marked curvature of the nail, a loss of the cuticular angle (an increase in the angle the surface of the nail makes with the terminal phalanx above the normal of 160 degrees) and a bulbous soft tissue swelling of the terminal phalanx. **A** and **B** show the contours of normal straight and curved nails; **C** and **D** represent increasing degrees of clubbing.

Acute hypoxia

Acute hypoxia is caused by a rapid reduction in available O_2. Common causes include asphyxia, airway obstruction, pulmonary edema, pneumonia, abrupt cardiorespiratory failure, and acute hemorrhage. Regardless of cause, tachypnea and dyspnea are common, as is hyperventilation. However, some patients with acute hypoxia cannot increase their alveolar ventilation. For these patients, tachypnea may result in hypoventilation, which will worsen the hypoxia.

Acute hypoxia produces a mental state like alcoholic intoxication.[21] Although mental stimulation may occur early on, disorientation usually follows. Headache is a frequent complaint. As the hypoxia worsens, confusion and **somnolence** occur. Eventually, motor coordination is lost and judgment becomes impaired. Finally, loss of consciousness and coma occur.[13]

The most critical target organ of hypoxia is the central nervous system.[13] With few exceptions, survival after acute hypoxia depends on its effect on the brain. Among the early responses of the brain to hypoxia are vasodilatation and increased cerebral blood flow. However, because nerve tissue is very vulnerable to O_2 lack, a few minutes of severe hypoxia may produce irreversible cell damage. Comas of days' or weeks' duration are not uncommon, and the half-living vegetative existence of the not-quite-dead brain may be the most tragic consequence of hypoxia.

As previously described, other organs are also affected by hypoxia. Hypoxia strains the heart indirectly by causing tachycardia and pulmonary vasoconstriction. Hypoxia may also act directly on the myocardial fibers, causing a decrease in contractility, cardiac arrhythmias or actual tissue death. Likewise, hypoxia interferes directly with the function of the renal tubular cells, impairing the kidney's ability to maintain normal electrolyte and water balance.

In general, the lower limit for brain survival is a PaO_2 between 20 and 22 torr.[13] However, the depth of hypoxia that the body can tolerate varies greatly. Modifying factors include exposure time, circulatory function, metabolic rate, and the speed with which therapy begins. Some patients have recovered from hypoxic incidents in which the arterial PO_2 was as low as 9 torr. Moreover, some individuals have survived total asphyxia (as during cold water immersion) for periods in excess of 30 minutes. In these later cases, survival has been attributed to the low metabolic rate caused by severe **hypothermia.**

Chronic hypoxia

If hypoxia develops slowly, the body has time to compensate for its effects. Diseases most likely to cause chronic hypoxia include **parenchymal** lung disorders (both destructive and fibrotic), chronic airway obstruction, congenital or acquired heart disease, and chronic anemia.

Much of our knowledge of chronic hypoxia has been learned by studying people born at or acclimated to high altitudes. Many of these people live normal and active lives with PO_2s as low as those in severely hypoxemic patients at sea level. Obviously, altitude dwellers must have adjusted to their "hypoxic" environment.

Although many of the details concerning adaptation to altitude are still under study, a few pertinent facts are known. First, all altitude dwellers hyperventilate, thereby raising the alveolar PO_2. This partially offsets the lower ambient PO_2. The respiratory alkalosis caused by the hyperventilation is compensated for by increased renal excretion of HCO_3. Thus normal blood and cerebral spinal fluid pH is maintained.

Altitude dwellers also increase O_2 delivery to their tissues. Enhanced O_2 delivery is achieved by increasing both hemoglobin content and tissue vascularity. More hemoglobin is available as a result of a larger red cell mass. Hypoxemia increases secretion of erythropoietin, a hormone which stimulates the bone marrow to produce more red blood cells. This increase in circulating erythrocyte volume is called *secondary polycythemia.*

Last, most high-altitude dwellers have pulmonary arterial hypertension, caused by hypoxic pulmonary vasoconstriction. This pulmonary hypertension causes electrocardiographic (ECG) changes characteristic of right ventricular hypertrophy, such as right axis deviation.[22]

The patient with chronic hypoxia is in a situation much like that of the altitude dweller. Of course, the important difference is the presence of some underlying abnormality.

For these patients, chronic hypoxia often causes persistent mental and physical fatigue. Mental responses may become sluggish and acuity diminished. These patients frequently complain of an inability to perform even the simplest physical task without difficulty. As a rule, however, chronic hypoxia itself is not the primary cause of their disability; rather the underlying disease limits activity. For example, in patients with certain forms of chronic lung disease, it is the physical effort or work needed to maintain adequate O_2 and CO_2 levels that is the real cause of disability, and not the hypoxia itself.

As among altitude dwellers, secondary polycythemia is common. In some patients, secondary polycythemia is readily detected by a simple blood hematocrit determination. Normally the hematocrit is 45% or less. In secondary polycythemia, it may rise above 55%. The hemoglobin content is also elevated from 15 g/dL to perhaps 20 g/dL. In addition, the red blood cell count often exceeds the normal of about 5 million/mm³.

However, these simple measures do not always indicate a secondary polycythemia. This is particularly true for patients who have an associated increase in plasma volume.[23] If both the cell mass and plasma volume increase together, the hematocrit, hemoglobin content, and red blood cell count may all be within normal limits. More definitive tests, such as those which actually measure the circulating red cell mass, may be the only way to uncover the polycythemia.

However, enough patients show elevated hematocrit or hemoglobin to warrant a few remarks about the significance of such findings. When the hematocrit rises above 55%, the viscosity of the blood increases significantly. As the viscosity of the blood rises, cardiac work increases and blood flow slows. When blood flow is sluggish, the likelihood of intravascular thromboses increases.[24] Of course, these harmful effects offset any advantages gained by increasing the blood's O_2 carrying capacity.[25]

As previously described, the patient with secondary polycythemia is usually cyanotic. Patients often complain of headache, fullness in the head, nasal stuffiness, lethargy, difficulty in taking a deep breath, and **epistaxis** (nosebleed). The small vessels of the **sclera** (the white of the eye) may be seen as grossly congested as a result of increased blood volume. Finally, the increased volume and viscosity of blood increase cardiac workload, especially that on the right ventricle. Together with hypoxic pulmonary arterial hypertension, this increased workload can cause *cor pulmonale,* or right-sided heart disease, secondary to pulmonary disease (see Chapter 20).

Laboratory assessment of hypoxia

The laboratory assessment of hypoxia involves the sampling, calculation, and measurement of various blood parameters. Parameters most commonly used are PaO_2 (or SaO_2), $P(A-a)O_2$, CaO_2, and $C\bar{v}O_2$ (O_2 content of the mixed venous blood). As indicated in Table 15-3, by combining these indicators, it is possible to identify the primary physiologic cause of the hypoxia.

Except for hemoglobin deficiencies, all causes of hypoxemia cause a reduced PaO_2. However, only when hypoxemia is due to a diffusion defect, right-to-left shunting, or V/Q imbalance is the $P(A-a)O_2$ increased when breathing room air. Giving supplemental oxygen decreases the $P(A-a)O_2$ if the problem is a low V/Q or a diffusion defect. However, raising the FIO_2 causes the $P(A-a)O_2$ to widen when the problem is a right-to-left shunt.

With hypoxemia in general, as long as the cardiovascular system compensates for the low arterial O_2 content by increasing cardiac output, the mixed venous O_2 content ($C\bar{v}O_2$) remains normal and tissue hypoxia does not occur. On the other hand, if the cardiovascular system cannot compensate, or if the hypoxemia is severe, the $C\bar{v}O_2$ may drop, indicating tissue hypoxia.

In terms of uncomplicated hemoglobin deficiencies, the PaO_2 is often normal, as is the $P(A-a)O_2$. In combination, these factors indicate normal pulmonary exchange of O_2. However, the measured CaO_2 is always decreased.

As with hemoglobin deficiencies, when hypoxia is due to reduced blood flow, the PaO_2 and $P(A-a)O_2$ may be normal. Moreover, the arterial O_2 content may also be normal. The major laboratory finding signaling hypoxia caused by reduced blood flow is a low $C\bar{v}O_2$.

Table 15-3   Assessment of Hypoxia

Cause	PaO₂	P(A-a)O₂ Air	P(A-a)O₂ O₂	CaO₂	C̄vO₂
HYPOXEMIA					
Low PIO_2	↓↓	N	N	↓↓	N*
Hypoventilation	↓↓	N	N	↓↓	N*
Diffusion defect	↓↓	↑↑	N	↓↓	N*
Anatomic shunt	↓↓↓	↑↑↑	↑↑↑↑	↓↓	N*
$\dot{V}/\dot{Q}$ imbalance					
Low $\dot{V}/\dot{Q}$	↓↓	↑↑	↑	↓↓	N*
Physiologic shunt	↓↓↓	↑↑↑	↑↑↑↑	↓↓	N*
HB deficiency					
Absolute	N or ↓↓	N	N	↓↓	↓↓
Relative	N or ↓↓	N	N	↓↓	↓↓
REDUCED BLOOD FLOW	N	N	N	N	↓↓
DYSOXIA	N	N	N	N	↑↑

*Venous oxygen content will remain normal only if cardiac output increases to compensate.
N, Normal; ↓, decreased; ↑, increased.

Like hypoxia produced by reduced blood flow, the PaO_2, $P(A-a)O_2$, and CaO_2 may all be normal in dysoxia. However, since this is a condition in which tissue O_2 extraction is abnormally low, the $C\bar{v}O_2$ may be *higher* than normal, and oxygen consumption may become dependent on oxygen supply.[26]

Thus, with some important exceptions, the "best" laboratory indicator of the presence or absence of tissue hypoxia is the $C\bar{v}O_2$. Unfortunately, the $C\bar{v}O_2$ can only be obtained via invasive sampling of blood from the distal port of a pulmonary artery catheter. More detail on the clinical assessment of oxygenation is provided in Chapters 17 and 33.

Treatment

In patients with hypoxia, the primary goal is to provide the cells sufficient O_2 to meet their needs. Generally, this requires that: (1) normal arterial O_2 content be restored, (2) adequate tissue perfusion be assured, and (3) toxic levels of oxygen be prevented (refer to Chapter 26). Since oxygen therapy is supportive only, concurrent efforts must be made to correct the underlying problem causing the hypoxia.

When hypoxemia is caused by a low alveolar PO_2, diffusion defect, or moderately low V/Q ratio, normal arterial oxygenation can be achieved by simple oxygen therapy techniques, generally with FIO_2 less than 0.50. Details on the indications, methods, and hazards of simple oxygen therapy are provided in Chapter 26.

When hypoxemia is caused by extremely low V/Q ratios or shunting, even 100% O_2 may not be sufficient to achieve a satisfactory arterial O_2 content. Instead, special methods of ventilatory support designed to open collapsed alveoli, such as CPAP or positive pressure ventilation with positive end-expiratory pressure (PEEP), may be necessary. These methods are described in detail in Chapter 30.

When secondary polycythemia complicates chronic hypoxia, phlebotomy may be useful. Withdrawal of 300 mL venous blood every 3 to 4 days can lower the hematocrit and reduce blood viscosity. The clinical results are often very rewarding, with improvement in exercise tolerance,[27] decreases in both mean pulmonary artery pressure and total pulmonary resistance,[28] and better cerebral blood flow.[29]

VENTILATION–PERFUSION IMBALANCES

As previously discussed, ventilation-perfusion (V/Q) imbalances are the most common cause of hypoxemia. V/Q imbalances are the primary cause of hypoxemia in virtually all parenchymal lung diseases, such as asthma, bronchitis, emphysema, pneumonia, and pulmonary embolism. As we shall see, V/Q imbalances also are a common cause of impaired CO_2 removal in many clinical situations.

Definition

A V/Q imbalance is an abnormal deviation in the distribution of ventilation to perfusion in the lung. Normally, most lung units receive equivalent amounts of ventilation and blood flow, for example, 1 L of air for each 1 L of blood. Such units are "balanced," with a V/Q ratio of about 1.0. When a respiratory unit has more ventilation than blood flow, its ratio is greater than 1.0; if blood flow exceeds ventilation, the ratio is less than 1.0.

In reality, even the normal lung has some V/Q mismatch (refer to Chapter 12). Because of the effects of gravity, some lung units are overventilated and some are overperfused. In the upright lung, both ventilation and perfusion increase toward the bottom of the lung (Figure 15-5). However, because perfusion increases more than ventilation, the V/Q ratio changes from more than 3 at the top of the lung to less than 1 at the bottom. This slight mismatch in the normal lung explains why the arterial PO_2 is always slightly less than the alveolar PO_2.

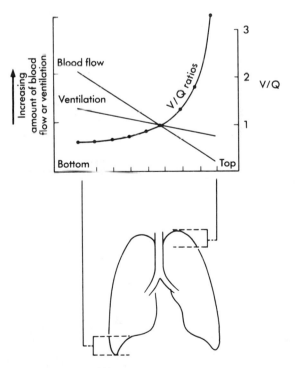

Fig. 15-5 Changes in V̇/Q̇ ratios in the upright lung. At the top of the lung, ventilation is greater than perfusion, resulting in high V̇/Q̇ ratios. From the top to the bottom of the lung, there is a progressive increase in both ventilation and perfusion. Since blood flow increases more than ventilation, the V̇/Q̇ ratios decrease and are lowest at the bottom of the lung. (From Martin L: Pulmonary physiology in clinical practice: the essentials for patient care and evaluation, St. Louis, 1987, Mosby.)

Distribution of V/Q ratios in disease

In disease states, the range of V/Q imbalances becomes much greater than normal. Figure 15-6 shows the possible range of V/Q ratios. As shown in the top two units, when ventilation is greater than perfusion (a *high* V/Q), there is wasted ventilation or *alveolar deadspace.* Conversely, when ventilation is less than perfusion, the V/Q ratio is *low* (bottom two lung units). In this case, blood passing through the lungs is exposed to less O_2 than normal and thus returns to the circulation with an abnormally low O_2 content. When this poorly oxygenated blood mixes with arterial blood, the arterial O_2 content is reduced.

In lung disease, V/Q imbalances usually cause both excess wasted ventilation and poor oxygenation. Since a V/Q imbalance impairs O_2 exchange, the PaO_2 is reduced. V/Q imbalances also hinder CO_2 exchange. However, the effect on CO_2 exchange is usually less than that on oxygenation. Reasons for this difference are discussed later in this section.

Shunts and venous admixture

In the lungs, a shunt exists whenever venous blood bypasses ventilated alveoli and mixes with freshly oxygenated or arterialized blood. This right-to-left shunting lowers the O_2 content of the blood leaving the lungs, a condition called *venous admixture.*

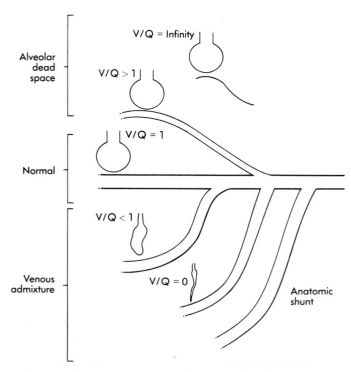

Fig. 15-6 The range of V̇/Q̇ ratios. See text for discussion. (From Martin, L: Pulmonary physiology in clinical practice: the essentials for patient care and evaluation, St. Louis, 1987, Mosby.)

Venous admixture can occur in one of three situations, only two of which are true shunts:

1. A right-to-left *anatomic shunt* occurs when blood bypasses the lungs through an anatomic channel, such as normally exists in the thebesian and bronchial circulations. Abnormal right-to-left anatomic shunts are seen in some forms of congenital heart disease and can develop in certain chronic lung diseases, such as bronchiectasis.

2. A right-to-left *physiologic shunt* occurs when blood perfuses unventilated alveoli (V/Q = 0). In this case, there is no abnormal connection between the venous and arterial circulations; rather, venous blood entering the lung follows its normal course but returns to the arterial circulation unchanged. Physiologic shunting is seen in conditions such as pulmonary edema, pneumonia, and atelectasis.

3. A *low V/Q ratio* ($1 \geq V/Q \geq 0$) occurs when an area of the lung is poorly ventilated in relation to its perfusion. In this case, the blood is exposed to some ventilation, but not enough to achieve full oxygenation. Low V/Q ratios account for most cases of hypoxemia seen clinically.

Whether of physiologic or anatomic origin, a right-to-left shunt has an equivalent effect on oxygenation. In both cases, some unoxygenated blood bypasses the alveoli and mixes with oxygenated blood. Although both types of shunts cause venous admixture, they differ in one important respect from low V/Q ratios. Since shunted blood contacts no air, increasing the inspired oxygen concentration does not significantly improve oxygenation. In contrast, because blood in low V/Q units is in contact with some air, supplemental O_2 can improve blood oxygenation.

In the past, a trial of 100% O_2 was commonly used to distinguish between hypoxemia caused by a low V/Q and that by a right-to-left shunt. It is now known that breathing 100% O_2 can cause shunting by promoting the collapse of alveoli with low V/Q ratios (see Chapter 26). Because of this potential hazard, the 100% O_2 trial has been replaced by a simple incremental FIO_2 test. For example, if the PaO_2 rises significantly when a patient's FIO_2 is increased from 30% to 60%, the main problem is a low V/Q. If the PaO_2 does not rise significantly, a right-to-left shunt exists.

Effect of V/Q imbalances on oxygenation and CO_2 removal

Oxygenation

It has been stated that V/Q imbalances are the most common cause of hypoxemia. The mechanism of this type of hypoxemia can now be examined more closely. Figure 15-7 shows the normal oxyhemoglobin dissociation curve, with content (instead of satura-

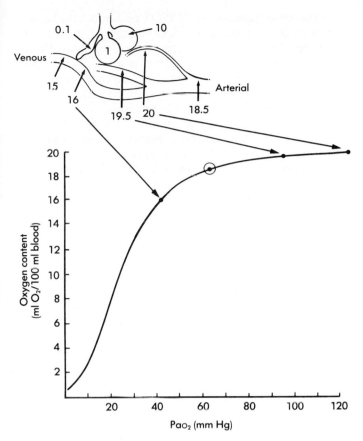

Fig. 15-7 Oxygen dissociation curve: Pa_{O_2} versus oxygen content. Oxygen content from alveolar-capillary units with $\dot{V}/\dot{Q}$ ratios of 0.1, 1, and 10 are, respectively, 16, 19.5 and 20.0 ml O_2/dL blood. Lines are drawn for each content to its point on the dissociation curve. The average oxygen content, 18.5 ml O_2/dL, is represented by a circle on the dissociation curve. Note that the arterial oxygen content after all the blood is mixed (18.5 ml O_2/dL) is lower than the oxygen content from the normal unit (19.5 ml O_2/dL) (From Martin L: Pulmonary physiology in clinical practice: the essentials for patient care and evaluation, St. Louis, 1987, Mosby.)

tion) plotted on the y-axis. Note that the curve is nearly flat in the physiologic range of PaO_2 (above 70 torr) but falls steeply below 60 torr. Points representing the O_2 content of three separate lung units are also shown. These units have V/Q ratios of 0.1, 1.0, and 10.0.

Blood leaving the normal unit (V/Q = 1.0) has a normal O_2 content (19.5 ml/dL). Blood leaving the unit with poor ventilation (V/Q = 0.1) has a low O_2 content (16.0 ml/dL). Blood leaving the overventilated unit (V/Q = 10.0) has an O_2 content just slightly higher than normal (20.0 ml/dL). When the blood from all three units mixes together, the result is an O_2 content below normal (18.5 ml/dL). Thus, the decrease in oxygenation caused by the poorly ventilated unit is *not* compensated for by the high V/Q unit.

The fact is that when blood from areas of high V/Q is mixed with blood perfusing low V/Q areas, the resulting PO_2 is always lower than the average of the

two. This is because the final PaO_2 is determined *not* by an average of PO_2s from various lung units, but by an average of their O_2 contents.

Since hemoglobin is almost fully saturated when the PO_2 is 100 torr (refer to Figure 15-7), raising the PO_2 above this level does little to increase the blood O_2 content. Thus, as compared to normal units (V/Q about 1.0), lung units with high V/Q ratios cannot significantly raise the blood O_2 content. Although the final O_2 content still represents an average, the resulting PaO_2 is lower than would be predicted by averaging the PO_2 values from each pulmonary capillary.

The expected decrease in PaO_2 and the increase in venous admixture resulting from progressive V/Q imbalances are shown in Figure 15-8. As can be seen, as the V/Q imbalance worsens, the venous admixture increases. This increasing venous admixture is accompanied by a steady decline in the PaO_2.

Carbon dioxide removal. As shown in Figure 15-8, V/Q imbalances also impair CO_2 removal.[30] As a V/Q imbalance worsens, physiologic deadspace increases. In concept, this increase in deadspace should cause a progressive rise in $PaCO_2$. However, this expected increase in $PaCO_2$ does not always occur. Indeed, many patients who are hypoxemic as a result of a V/Q

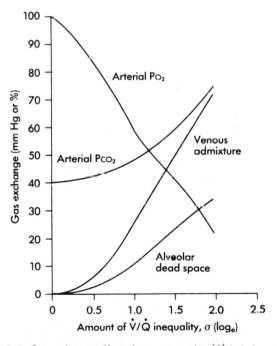

Fig. 15-8 Gas exchange effects from progressive $\dot{V}/\dot{Q}$ imbalance. $\dot{V}/\dot{Q}$ inequality and overall gas exchange in computer model of the lung. For this model, oxygen uptake and carbon dioxide output were kept constant. As the amount of $\dot{V}/\dot{Q}$ inequality increases (represented by a log scale on the abscissa), PaO_2 decreases and $PaCO_2$ increases; this occurs because $\dot{V}/\dot{Q}$ inequality causes increases in both venous admixture and alveolar dead space. (From Martin L: Pulmonary physiology in clinical practice: the essentials for patient care and evaluation, St. Louis, 1987, Mosby)

imbalance have a low or normal $PaCO_2$. This common clinical finding suggests that V/Q imbalances have a greater effect on oxygenation than on CO_2 removal.

Careful inspection of the O_2 and CO_2 dissociation curves supports this concept and helps explain why it is true. Figure 15-9 shows the O_2 and CO_2 dissociation curves plotted on the same scale. The upper CO_2 curve is nearly linear in the physiologic range. The lower O_2 curve is almost flat in the physiologic range. Point *a* on each curve is the normal arterial point for both content and partial pressure. To the right of the graph are two lung units, one with a low V/Q, the other with a high V/Q. The blood O_2 and CO_2 contents from each unit are plotted on the curves.

The final CO_2 content, arrived at by averaging the high and low V/Q points, is shown as point *a* on the CO_2 curve. Note that this is the same as the normal arterial point for CO_2.

The final O_2 content, also arrived at by averaging the high and low V/Q points, is shown as point *x* on the O_2 curve. While the averaged value for CO_2 was normal, that resulting from averaging the O_2 content of the high and low V/Q units is well below normal (point *a* on the O_2 curve).

Thus the effect of low V/Q units is to lower the PO_2 and raise the PCO_2. The effect of high V/Q units is the opposite: that is, to raise the PO_2 and lower the PCO_2. However, the shape of the dissociation curves dictates that a high V/Q unit can reverse the high PCO_2 but not the low PO_2. Thus any increase in PCO_2 from low V/Q units can be corrected by a reduction in PCO_2 from high V/Q units. However, these same high V/Q units cannot compensate for the reduced O_2 content, because the O_2 curve is nearly flat when the PO_2 is above normal.

Of course, patients with V/Q imbalances still must compensate for the high PCO_2 coming from underventilated units. To compensate for these high PCO_2 values, one must increase the minute ventilation (Figure 15-10). Patients who can increase their minute ventilation thus tend to have either a normal or a low $PaCO_2$, combined with hypoxemia.

On the other hand, patients with a V/Q imbalance who cannot increase their minute ventilation are hypercapnic. Generally, this only occurs when the V/Q imbalance is severe and chronic. The most common clinical example is severe chronic obstructive pulmonary disease (COPD) in which the V/Q imbalance causes a large increase in alveolar deadspace. Such a patient must sustain an above-normal minute ventilation just to maintain a normal $PaCO_2$. If the energy costs required to sustain a high minute ventilation are prohibitive, the patient will opt for less work and hence an elevated $PaCO_2$.

AIRWAY OBSTRUCTION AND HYPERINFLATION

Airway obstruction is a common cause of cardiopulmonary disease.[31] Obstruction can occur in the upper or lower airways. Some obstruction is temporary and reversible, while other forms are chronic in nature. Chronic lower airway obstruction is often associated with pulmonary hyperinflation.

Causes of airway obstruction

The primary causes of airway obstruction are mucosal edema, bronchial spasm, increased secretions, and bronchiolar collapse (Figure 15-11). Less common

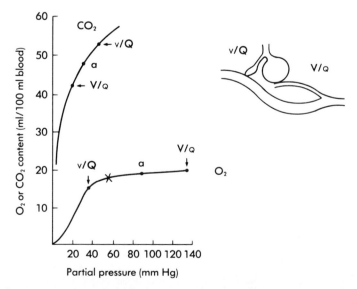

Fig. 15-9 V̇/Q̇ imbalance and the dissociation curves for carbon dioxide and oxygen. v/Q represents low V̇/Q̇ units, and V/Q represents high V̇/Q̇ units. See text for discussion. (From Martin L: *Pulmonary physiology in clinical practice: the essentials for patient care and evaluation*, St. Louis, 1987, Mosby.)

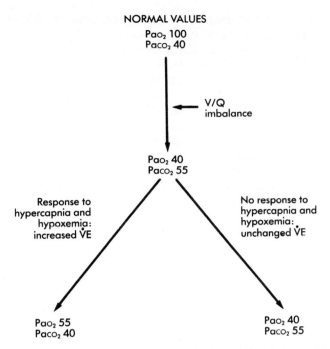

NORMAL VALUES
PaO₂ 100
PaCO₂ 40

← V/Q imbalance

PaO₂ 40
PaCO₂ 55

Response to hypercapnia and hypoxemia: increased V̇E

No response to hypercapnia and hypoxemia: unchanged V̇E

PaO₂ 55
PaCO₂ 40

PaO₂ 40
PaCO₂ 55

Fig. 15-10 Changes in PaO_2 and $PaCO_2$ from V̇/Q̇ imbalance. All values are torr. See text for discussion. (From Martin L: Pulmonary physiology in clinical practice: the essentials for patient care and evaluation, St. Louis, 1987, Mosby.)

Common causes of airway obstruction by locale

Upper airway obstruction
- Rhinitis/pharyngitis
- Diphtheria
- Croup
- Epiglottitis
- Obstructive sleep apnea
- Laryngeal paralysis
- Tracheal stenosis
- Tracheal malacia
- Foreign body
- Tetanus

Lower airway obstruction
- Emphysema
- Chronic bronchitis
- Asthma
- Cystic fibrosis
- Bronchiectasis
- Bronchiolitis
- Bronchial compression (tumor, lymph nodes)
- Endobronchial tumors
- Foreign body
- Mucus plugging

causes of airway obstruction include fibrosis, foreign body aspiration, external compression, and loss of muscle tone. The accompanying box lists the most common diseases that cause airway obstruction according to locale.

Mucosal edema

Edema exists when the interstitial fluid volume is excessive. The major causes of respiratory tract edema are listed in the box on page 356. These mechanisms all cause body water to shift from the plasma to the intercellular space, with resulting swelling of the affected area.

Edema may be either localized or widespread. The most common example of respiratory tract edema is the nasal swelling and inflammation caused by the common cold (rhinitis). This same response can be visualized in the other locales. For example, croup is a localized infection which produces edema and obstruction of the larynx and trachea in children. Likewise, edema and airway narrowing caused by infection can occur in the small bronchi and bronchioles of children, a condition called *bronchiolitis*.

In acute edema, the respiratory mucosa becomes spongy and waterlogged. There is usually an accompanying vascular congestion, which adds to the swelling.

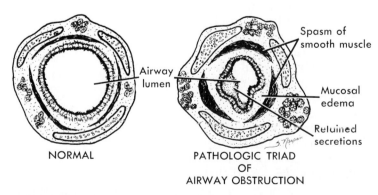

NORMAL

PATHOLOGIC TRIAD
OF
AIRWAY OBSTRUCTION

Airway lumen

Spasm of smooth muscle

Mucosal edema

Retained secretions

Fig. 15-11 Cross-sections of airways comparing normal with obstruction caused by pathologic triad. Note narrowed airway lumen (opening) in obstructed airway.

Major causes of respiratory tract edema

- Mechanical irritation or trauma to the respiratory mucosa, as from instrumentation, the presence of a foreign body, or the inhalation of caustic liquids or irritant fumes
- Infection, bacterial or viral, in which the reaction represents a body defense against the invading organisms
- Allergy to inhaled liquids or particulate matter, exemplified by allergic (**atopic**) bronchial asthma

---

If of short duration, the edema may resolve quickly when the underlying cause is removed. However, if the edema is long lasting or recurs frequently (as with chronic infection), it may become *indurated*. Indurated tissue is permanently thickened and has a firm, rather than soft consistency. Besides causing obstruction, such changes markedly impair mucociliary clearance.

Bronchospasm

A spasm is an involuntary and excessive muscle contraction. Muscle cramps are a good example. Bronchospasm represents an excessive contraction of the bronchial smooth muscle. Whether localized or widespread, bronchospasm can seriously reduce airway caliber. Any reduction in airway caliber obstructs airflow.

In general, the causes of bronchospasm are the same as those of edema. Also as with edema, chronically recurring bronchial spasms can result in a permanent histologic change, bronchial muscle *hypertrophy*. Asthma is a good example of airway obstruction caused by inflammation and bronchospasm.

Increased secretions

Either the volume or the viscosity of bronchial secretions can increase. Infection and inflammation are the most common causes of increased respiratory tract secretions. The common cold, with its abundance of nasal secretions, is again a familiar example. More serious obstructive disorders in which an increased volume or viscosity of secretions plays a role include chronic bronchitis, cystic fibrosis, and bronchiectasis.

Respiratory tract secretions (or sputum) are produced by the goblet cells and mucous glands of the bronchial mucosa. Normal secretions consist mainly of water, mucopolysaccharides, proteins, and electrolytes. Respiratory tract secretions may also contain cellular elements, including leukocytes, epithelial cells, and macrophages.

During inflammation and infection, the respiratory tract increases its production of secretions. In addi-

tion, the makeup of the secretions changes. Typically, there is an increase in granulocytic cells, as well as peroxidases and nucleic acids (released from disintegrating cells). Plasma fluid and proteins, including fibrinogen, may also appear, having escaped from peribronchial capillaries.[32] Blood or blood elements may also be seen, especially if bleeding is a component of the process.

Distinguishing between normal and abnormal secretions depends on the relative concentrations of these components. For clinical purposes, we can differentiate among four major types of sputum (Table 15-4). Each type is associated with one or more respiratory disorders.[33]

Mucoid secretions are clear or white in color. Generally mucoid secretions are produced in response to inflammation. Mucoid secretions are seen commonly during acute asthmatic attacks and in uncomplicated chronic bronchitis.

Purulent secretions are dark yellow or green and are seen mainly in bacterial infections. Purulent secretions contain a large amount of cellular debris, dead bacteria, nucleic acids, and peroxidases. When left to settle, purulent secretions tend to separate into three layers: a white upper mucoid layer, a middle watery layer, and a bottom layer of cellular debris. Purulent secretions tend to be very viscous as a result of the presence of long chain nucleic acids. If anaerobic bacteria are causing the infection, purulent secretions often have a disagreeable, or **fetid**, odor. Purulent secretions are seen in aspiration pneumonia, lung abscess, and bronchiectasis.

Mucopurulent secretions are a mix of mucoid and purulent secretions. Mucopurulent secretions tend to be light to medium yellow and less viscous than purulent secretions. They probably represent either the early or the late (resolution) stage of an infectious process. Mucopurulent secretions are common in

---

Table 15-4 Disease states associated with abnormal gross appearance of the sputum

Type of Sputum	Condition
Mucoid	Asthma
Purulent	Aspiration pneumonia Bronchiectasis (fetid) Lung Abscess (fetid)
Mucopurulent	Chronic bronchitis Cystic fibrosis Pneumonia (blood-streaked)
Bloody	Tuberculosis Lung cancer Pulmonary infarction Pulmonary edema (frothy, pink)

Adapted from MacIntyre NR: Respiratory monitoring without machinery, *Respir Care* 35(6):546–553, 1990.

acute and chronic bronchitis, cystic fibrosis, and pneumonia. Mucopurulent secretions in pneumonia are often blood-streaked.

Bloody secretions may be red to brown in color, depending on their "freshness." Bloody secretions must be distinguished from expectoration of whole blood, or *hemoptysis*. Bloody secretions are tinged with blood but still include mucoid and watery components. Bloody secretions may occur in tuberculosis, lung cancer, and pulmonary infarction. Frothy, blood-streaked secretions are sometimes seen in pulmonary edema. In this case, the blood gives the secretions a pinkish tone.

As the volume and viscosity of respiratory tract secretions increase, the normal mucociliary clearance mechanism becomes less effective. Moreover, high-viscosity respiratory tract secretions cannot be as easily cleared by coughing. In combination, these factors can lead to retained secretions, mucus plugging, and atelectasis.

Bronchiolar collapse

Bronchiolar collapse is an important form of small airway obstruction that can lead to significant **disability.** Conditions predisposing to bronchiolar collapse include emphysema, bronchiectasis, and cystic fibrosis. By far, emphysema is the most common cause.

As discussed in Chapter 11, the caliber of small airways is determined by two factors: (1) the support of surrounding lung tissue and (2) the transmural pressure gradient. In conditions such as pulmonary emphysema, the elastic tissue that normally supports the small airways is destroyed. This loss of elastic tissue has two major impacts. First, it increases the compliance of the lung, thus decreasing its elastic recoil. Second, it abolishes the major structural factor responsible for keeping the small airways open during exhalation.[34]

Because of a loss of elastic recoil, rising pleural pressure during exhalation causes less increase in alveolar pressure than normal. Rising pleural pressure also compresses the unsupported bronchioles more than normal. In combination, these factors cause the equal pressure point (EPP) to "move" farther upstream than in the healthy lung. Airway collapse thus occurs earlier *and* at higher volumes than in the normal subject. The result is premature air trapping.

To prevent air trapping, many patients with bronchiolar collapse learn to breathe through "pursed lips." In this maneuver, the patient slightly purses the lips while exhaling, deliberately prolonging exhalation and trying to maintain an even flow of air. This moderate obstruction at the mouth increases proximal airway pressure. The increase in airway pressure moves the EPP farther downstream toward the larger airways with cartilaginous support, thereby preventing premature small airway closure.[4] Pursed-lip breathing also helps increase the efficiency of ventilation, probably by slowing the respiratory rate and increasing the tidal volume.[35]

Hyperinflation

Hyperinflation is a condition in which the resting lung volume is abnormally high. Pulmonary hyperinflation is the natural consequence of airway obstruction and air trapping. Hyperinflation may occur acutely (as in asthma) or chronically (as in emphysema). Typically, hyperinflation causes an increase in both the functional residual capacity (FRC) and the residual volume (RV). In addition, the inspiratory capacity (IC) is often reduced and the diaphragm assumes an abnormally low and flat position. If chronic, hyperinflation causes a progressive increase in the size of the thorax, especially its anteroposterior (AP) diameter. The resulting physical abnormality is called "barrel chest." Barrel chest is a common clinical finding in emphysema.

Whether acute or chronic, hyperinflation has several harmful effects. It can compress pulmonary capillaries and thus increase deadspace ventilation and pulmonary vascular resistance. In addition, air trapping can prevent alveolar pressures from returning to zero during exhalation. This "auto-PEEP" effect tends to increase the work of breathing. Last, the abnormally low and flat position of the diaphragm impairs its ability to contract effectively.

Clinical manifestations

As a result of high flow resistance, airway obstruction greatly increases the work of breathing. Resistance to breathing may be more pronounced in one phase or the other of ventilation. For example, laryngeal obstruction in croup increases inspiratory resistance. This may require a strong inspiratory effort, resulting in noticeable intercostal and substernal **retractions** during inspiration. Moreover, the flow of air past the obstruction may produce a harsh sound known as *stridor* (see Chapter 16).

The most common cause of obstruction, however, is COPD. In COPD, exhalation is impeded. In COPD patients, normal passive exhalation cannot overcome the high expiratory flow resistance and exhalation often requires strenuous muscular effort. The work needed to overcome the high resistance may be so great as to cause muscle fatigue. As described in Chapter 29, muscle fatigue may lead to hypercapnia, respiratory acidosis, and respiratory failure.

Whether inspiratory or expiratory, all obstructive disorders are characterized by reduced airflow. The extent of airflow reduction can be measured in the pulmonary function laboratory (refer to Chapter 18). If the problem is mainly expiratory flow obstruction, expiration time is usually prolonged beyond that of inhalation, and often contraction of the upper abdomen is evident during the latter part of exhalation. If bronchospasm is extensive or mobile secretions are present, characteristic breath sounds can be heard during exhalation by either auscultation or the unaided ear. These breath sounds may include early inspiratory crackles, rhonchi, and wheezes. More detail on the physical signs and symptoms of obstructive lung disease is provided in Chapter 16.

Treatment

The general strategy for treating obstructive lung disorders depends on the underlying abnormality. For example, therapy in reversible disorders such as asthma aims to restore normal function by reducing inflammation and bronchospasm with drugs. On the other hand, when the disorder involves permanent damage, as in emphysema, therapy is mainly supportive and directed at relief of the symptoms and prevention of complications. More detail on the treatment of obstructive lung disorders is provided in Chapter 20. The various modes of respiratory care applicable to patients with obstructive lung disease are reviewed in detail in the Basic Therapeutics section of the text (Section VI). Last, rehabilitative activities designed to help COPD patients cope with their disorder are covered in Chapter 37.

PULMONARY RESTRICTION

Pulmonary restriction is a general term referring to a large variety of disorders that share a common feature: that is, a *reduction in lung volume*.[36]

Causes

As listed in Table 15-5, there are six major categories of restrictive lung disease: skeletal/thoracic, neuromuscular, pleural, interstitial, alveolar, and abdominal.

Skeletal/thoracic causes

Some thoracic causes of restriction are due to structural changes in the muscles or bones; others are caused by reduced chest compliance. *Kyphoscoliosis* is a good example of a restrictive disorder caused by structural changes. It is characterized by an abnormal curvature of the spine that twists the thoracic cage and compresses the lung.

Ankylosing spondylitis is a restrictive disorder in which the primary problem is reduced compliance of the chest cage. In ankylosing spondylitis the vertebral bodies and the **costrovertebral** joints become fused, causing a dramatic decrease in thoracic wall compliance.

Table 15–5 Categories of Restrictive Pulmonary Disorders

Category	Examples
Skeletal-thoracic	Kyphoscoliosis
	Ankylosing spondylitis
CNS-neuromuscular	Cord transection
	Amyotrophic lateral sclerosis
	Guillain-Barré syndrome
	Myasthenia gravis
Pleural	Pleurisy
	Effusion-empyema
	Pneumothorax
	Hemothorax
Interstitial	Recurrent infections
	Pneumoconiosis
Alveolar	Pneumonia
	Pulmonary edema
Abdominal	Splinting
	Distention
	Ascites

Neuromuscular causes

Processes that interfere with nerve transmission or respiratory muscle function can also cause pulmonary restriction. Included in this category are abnormalities of the spinal cord, peripheral nerves, neuromuscular junctions, and respiratory muscles. Common to all these problems is an inability to generate normal respiratory pressures.

Pleural disorders

Pleural disorders cause restriction by one of two mechanisms. Restriction may be caused by a pathologic disorder of the pleural membranes, such as pleurisy. Alternatively, a lesion may restrict lung expansion by occupying pleural space. Pleural effusion, empyema, pneumothorax, and hemothorax are examples of space-occupying lesions.

Interstitial disorders

Interstitial pulmonary disease processes involve chronic inflammatory or fibrotic changes. Chronic inflammatory processes, such as recurrent respiratory infections, often accompany conditions such as COPD, tuberculosis, and bronchiectasis. Conditions caused by inhalation of inorganic dusts, or pneumoconioses, are the most common cause of fibrotic changes in the lung tissue.

Alveolar disorders

Alveolar restrictive processes involve changes in the area of the terminal respiratory unit, including the pulmonary capillary circulation. Pneumonia, an acute infectious process leading to alveolar consolidation, is a good example. Vascular congestion, such as occurs in cardiogenic pulmonary edema, can also result in restriction. In this case, increased fluid in the pulmonary interstitial spaces and in the alveoli causes a reduction in lung compliance.

Abdominal causes

Abdominal conditions can restrict free movement of the diaphragm. Among the most common abdominal conditions restricting lung expansion are splinting, distension, and fluid accumulation.

Abdominal splinting is a rigid contraction of the abdominal wall musculature. Splinting is usually an involuntary reaction to pain from abdominal disorders, including surgery. Abdominal distension occurs when gas or air accumulates in the stomach or intestinal tract. An abnormal increase in abdominal fluid, referred to as **ascites,** is usually due to liver disease, heart failure, or peritoneal irritation.

Effect of Restriction on Ventilation

All restrictive disorders lower lung volumes. In particular, restriction reduces the vital capacity (VC); in severe instances the VC may not be much greater than the tidal volume. In this case, as in distension, there may be little or no inspiratory reserve volume to accommodate increased ventilatory demands.

In neuromuscular disorders, the FRC may be close to normal. However, as a result of inspiratory muscle weakness, total lung capacity decreases. On the other hand, expiratory muscle weakness causes an increase in the residual volume. As with restrictive disorders in general, both vital capacity and the maximum inspiratory pressure (negative inspiratory force) are decreased.

Only the interstitial and alveolar forms of restrictive disease actually decrease lung compliance. A decrease in lung compliance, in turn, can impair the distribution of ventilation and increase the work of breathing.

Treatment

The goal in treating restrictive disorders is to remove the underlying cause. For example, if the problem is accumulation of pleural fluid, removal by **thoracentesis** should help alleviate the restriction. Likewise, if a structural defect of the thorax is restricting ventilation, surgical intervention can sometimes help. Unfortunately, in many restrictive conditions, such as the pneumoconioses, there is no specific treatment available to correct the primary problem. In these cases, treatment is mainly supportive, with the goal of minimizing symptoms and preventing further complications.

CHAPTER SUMMARY

Cardiopulmonary dysfunction exists when the lungs, heart, or vascular systems fail to fulfill their functions adequately. One or more of three primary physiologic abnormalities underlie all cardiopulmonary dysfunction. Either O_2 delivery to or CO_2 removal from the tissues is impaired, or the energy cost needed to exchange these gases is excessive.

If O_2 delivery is inadequate to meet tissue metabolic needs, hypoxia is present. Hypoxia may be due to either a decrease in blood O_2 content (hypoxemia) or a decrease in blood flow. A third major category of hypoxia, called dysoxia, occurs when the cells cannot properly use the O_2 delivered to them.

Impaired CO_2 removal is always associated with a decrease in alveolar ventilation relative to metabolic need. Clinically, this causes a rise in $PaCO_2$, or hypercapnia. Hypercapnia occurs when minute ventilation is inadequate or deadspace ventilation increases.

Airway obstruction and restriction may affect both O_2 and CO_2 exchange, usually by altering the lung's normal V/Q balance. In addition, each of these major patterns of dysfunction can increase the work of breathing, thereby increasing the energy cost needed to exchange O_2 and CO_2.

An understanding of these major pathophysiologic patterns, including their causes, clinical manifestations, and general treatment approaches, provides the foundation for quality respiratory care.

REFERENCES

1. Dantzker DR: Oxygen transport and utilization, *Respir Care* 33(10):874–880, 1988.
2. Hudson LD, Pierson DJ: Hypoxemia. In Pierson DJ, Kacmarek RM, editors: *Foundations of respiratory care,* New York, 1992, Churchill Livingston.
3. Pierson DJ: Normal and abnormal oxygenation: physiology and clinical syndromes, *Respir Care* 38(6):587–599, 1993.
4. Martin L.: *Pulmonary physiology in clinical practice: the essentials for patient care and evaluation,* St Louis, 1987, Mosby.
5. West JB: Causes of carbon dioxide retention in lung disease, *N Engl J Med* 284:1232, 1971.
6. Robins ED: Dysoxia: abnormal tissue oxygen utilization, *Arch Intern Med,* 137:905, 1977.
7. Sutton JR, Jones N, Houston C, editors: *Hypoxia: man at altitude,* New York, 1982, Thieme-Stratton.
8. Sorbini CA et al: Arterial oxygen tension in relation to age in healthy subjects, *Respiration* 25:3, 1968.
9. Hudson LD, Pierson DJ: Inadequate blood oxygen content. In Pierson DJ, Kacmarek RM, editors; *Foundations of respiratory care,* New York, 1992, Churchill Livingston.
10. Dantzker DR, Gutierrez G: The assessment of tissue oxygenation, *Respir Care* 30(6):456–461, 1985.
11. Phang PT, Russell JA: When does VO_2 depend on DO_2? *Respir Care* 38(6):618–626, 1993.
12. Pasquale MD, Cipolle MD, Cerra FB: Oxygen transport: does increasing supply improve outcome? *Respir Care* 38(7):800–825, 1993.
13. Higgins TL, Yared J: Clinical effects of hypoxemia and tissue hypoxia, *Respir Care* 38(6):603–615, 1993.
14. Burrows B, Knudson RJ, Kettrl LJ: *Respiratory insufficiency,* St Louis, 1975, Mosby.

15. Cherniack RM, Cherniack L, Naimark A: *Respiration in health and disease,* ed 2, Philadelphia, 1972, WB Saunders.

16. Nicholson D: Cyanosis: five grams of history, *Respir Care* 32:113–114, 1987.

17. Med WE et al: Cyanosis as a guide to arterial oxygen saturation, *Thorax* 14:247–250, 1959.

18. Hudson LD: Evaluation of the patient in acute respiratory failure, *Respir Care* 28:542–550, 1983.

19. Shulman LE: Hypertrophic osteoarthropathy, *Bull Rheum Dis* 7:135, 1957.

20. Field AS, Gray FD: The width of the nail fold capillary stream in clubbing, *Dis Chest* 41:631, 1962.

21. Barcroft J: Anoxemia, *Lancet* 2:485, 1920.

22. Slonim NB, Hamilton LH: *Respiratory physiology,* ed 5, St Louis, 1985, Mosby.

23. Shaw DB, Simpson T: Polycythemia in emphysema, *Q J Med* 30:135, 1961.

24. Comroe JH, Jr: *Physiology of respiration,* ed 2, St Louis, 1974, Mosby.

25. Filley GF: *Pulmonary insufficiency and respiratory failure,* Philadelphia, 1967, Lea & Febiger.

26. Mohsenifar Z et al: Relationship between O_2 delivery and O_2 consumption in the adult respiratory distress syndrome, *Chest* 83:267, 1983.

27. Chetty KG et al: Exercise performance of polycythemic chronic obstructive pulmonary disease patients: Effect of phlebotomies, *Chest* 98(5):1073–1077, 1990.

28. Weisse AB et al: Hemodynamic effects of staged hematocrit reduction in patients with stable cor pulmonale and severely elevated hematocrit levels, *Am J Med* 58(1):92–98, 1975.

29. York EL et al: Effects of secondary polycythemia on cerebral blood flow in chronic obstructive pulmonary disease, *Am Rev Respir Dis* 121(5):813–818, 1980.

30. West JB: *Ventilation/blood flow and gas exchange,* ed. 4, Oxford, 1980, Blackwell Scientific.

31. Johnson NT, Pierson DJ: Disorders producing airflow obstruction. In Pierson DJ, Kacmarek RM, editors: *Foundations of respiratory care.* New York, 1992, Churchill Livingston.

32. Tappan V, Zalar V: Pathophysiology of bronchial mucus, *Ann NY Acad Sci* 106:722, 1963.

33. MacIntyre NR: Respiratory monitoring without machinery, *Respir Care* 35(6):546–553, 1990.

34. Nunn JF: *Applied respiratory physiology,* ed 2, London, 1977, Butterworth.

35. Mueller RE, Petty TL, Filley GF: Ventilation and arterial blood gas changes induced by pursed lip breathing, *J Appl Physiol* 28:784, 1970.

36. Johnson NT, Pierson DJ: Restrictive disorders. In Pierson DJ, Kacmarek RM, editors: *Foundations of respiratory care,* New York: 1992, Churchill Livingston.

16

Bedside Assessment of the Patient*

■

Robert L. Wilkins

CHAPTER LEARNING OBJECTIVES

1. Outline the steps normally taken in a comprehensive bed-side assessment of the adult patient;
2. Identify the purposes for and methods used to conduct patient interviews;
3. Outline the contents of a comprehensive medical history;
4. Interpret the findings obtained during examination of the patient with cardiopulmonary disease;
5. Apply specific anatomic and general pathophysiologic knowledge in the systematic examination of the head, neck, thorax, lungs, precordium, abdomen, and extremities;
6. Understand and use the terminology associated with examination of the patient.

Progress in the science of respiratory care has placed increasing demands on respiratory care practitioners (RCPs) to develop sophisticated assessment skills. The integration of assessment with treatment is a necessary outcome of the growing complexity of roles and functions assumed by RCPs. No longer is it acceptable to initiate or alter therapy without careful consideration of the underlying disorder and its clinical manifestations. Decisions regarding when to begin, change, or end therapy must be based on tangible clinical evidence. Although the physician has primary responsibility for these decisions, RCPs must participate in the clinical decision-making process. In order to fulfill this role effectively, the RCP must assume responsibility for gathering and interpreting relevant bedside patient data.

Two key sources of patient data are the history and physical examination. Data initially gathered by interview and physical examination help identify the need for subsequent diagnostic tests. Once a diagnosis is made, these assessment procedures also help clinicians select the best treatment approaches. And once a treatment regimen begins, these procedures are again used to monitor patient progress toward predefined goals.

B edside assessment is the process of interviewing and examining the patient for the signs and symptoms of disease. It is also a cost-effective way of obtaining pertinent information about the patient's health status.

The patient initially is assessed to help identify the correct diagnosis. Once a tentative diagnosis is reached, subsequent physical examinations help monitor the patient's course and evaluate treatment results. Each examination should be conducted with a specific purpose and be tailored to the individual patient's history. With experience, the respiratory care practi-

tioner (RCP) learns which of the techniques described here to use in any given situation. Examinations should be performed in a quiet, well-lighted room. In conducting their assessment, RCPs should avoid exposing the patient to any unnecessary discomfort.

During a physical exam, the RCP must infringe on the intimate space of the patient (0 to 18 inches). This should be done only with permission, and only after rapport has been established with the patient. The only exception to this rule is when the patient needs emergency care.

The skills described here are not difficult to learn; however, mastery requires practice. The beginner first should practice the skills on healthy individuals. This helps improve technique and provides an understanding of normal variations. To detect abnormalities, one must first comprehend normal body functions for comparison.

This chapter emphasizes the techniques used in assessing patients with respiratory disease. Because respiratory disorders may affect other body systems, examination of the entire patient is important. For this reason, the basic techniques used to examine other key body systems are reviewed. Content is presented in the typical order in which the initial assessment is performed (see the box on page 362).

PATIENT INTERVIEWING AND HISTORY TAKING

Because it provides the patient's perspective, interviewing furnishes unique information. It serves three related purposes: it sets the climate for all interpersonal interaction between the RCP and patient; it is the most common method used to obtain patients' medical history; and ongoing bedside interviewing is needed to help monitor changes in patients' symp-

---

*Adapted from Wilkins RL, Sheldon RL, and Krider SJ, eds: *Clinical assessment in respiratory care,* ed. 2, St. Louis, 1990, Mosby.

Typical format for recording the physical examination

Initial impression

Age, height, weight, and general appearance

Vital signs

Pulse rate, respiratory rate, temperature, and blood pressure

Heent (head, ears, eyes, nose, and throat)

Inspection findings

Neck

Inspection and palpation findings

Thorax

Lungs—inspection, palpation, percussion, and auscultation

Heart—inspection, palpation, and auscultation findings

Abdomen

Inspection, palpation, percussion, and auscultation findings

Extremities

Inspection and palpation findings

toms and their response to therapy. For these reasons, interviewing is a crucial aspect of general patient assessment.

Principle of interviewing

Interviewing is a component of therapeutic communication (see Chapter 3), which occurs within a complex context. As depicted in Figure 16-1, this context includes sensory and emotional factors, environmental factors, verbal and nonverbal components of the communication process, and the values, beliefs, feelings, habits, and preoccupations of both the professional and the patient.

Whether used briefly to assess a therapy session or obtain a lengthy history, the ideal interview is one in which the patient feels secure and free to talk about important personal matters.[1] Although developing interviewing skills takes time and experience, beginners can get a head start on effective patient interaction by following several basic guidelines (see the box on page 363).

Given good initial preparation and setting of the right climate, the RCP should structure the interview according to the following general procedures:

1. Determine the subjective information needed to plan specific respiratory care interventions;

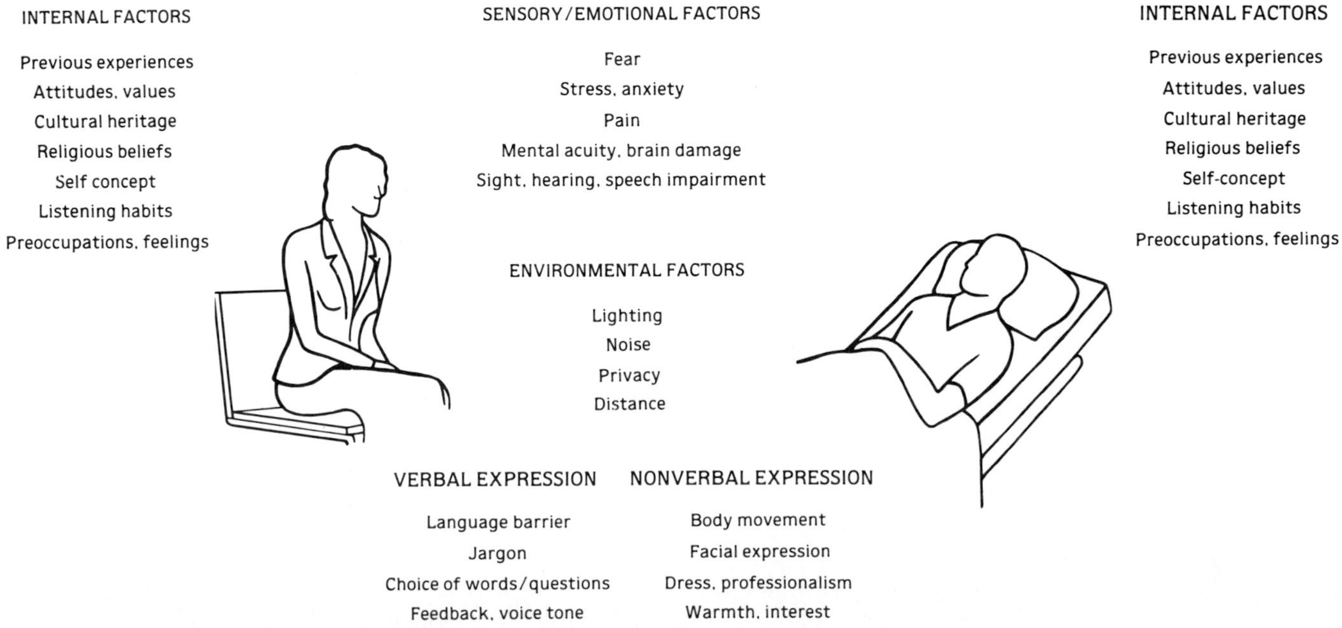

INTERNAL FACTORS

Previous experiences
Attitudes, values
Cultural heritage
Religious beliefs
Self concept
Listening habits
Preoccupations, feelings

SENSORY/EMOTIONAL FACTORS

Fear
Stress, anxiety
Pain
Mental acuity, brain damage
Sight, hearing, speech impairment

ENVIRONMENTAL FACTORS

Lighting
Noise
Privacy
Distance

INTERNAL FACTORS

Previous experiences
Attitudes, values
Cultural heritage
Religious beliefs
Self-concept
Listening habits
Preoccupations, feelings

VERBAL EXPRESSION

Language barrier
Jargon
Choice of words/questions
Feedback, voice tone

NONVERBAL EXPRESSION

Body movement
Facial expression
Dress, professionalism
Warmth, interest

Fig. 16-1 Factors influencing communication. (From Wilkins RL, Sheldon RL, and Krider SJ: Clinical assessment in respiratory care, St. Louis, 1985, Mosby.)

Guidelines for effective patient interviewing[1]

1. *Project a sense of undivided interest in the patient:*
- Provide for privacy and don't permit interruptions;
- Review records and prepare materials before entering the room;
- Listen and observe carefully; be attentive and respond to the patient's priorities, concerns, feelings, and comfort.

2. *Establish your professional role during the introduction:*
- Dress and groom professionally;
- Enter with a smile and unhurried manner;
- Make immediate eye contact;
- If the patient is well enough, introduce yourself with a firm handshake;
- State your role and the purpose of your visit, and define the patient's involvement in the interaction;
- Address adult patients by title—Mr., Mrs., or Ms.—and their last name. Use of these formal terms of address alerts the patient to the importance of the interaction.

3. *Show your respect for the patient's beliefs, attitudes, and rights:*
- Be sure the patient is appropriately covered;
- Position yourself so that eye contact is comfortable for the patient (ideally patients should be sitting up with their eye level at or slightly above yours);
- Avoid standing at the foot of the bed or with your hand on the door (this may send the nonverbal message that you do not have time for the patient);
- Ask the patient's permission before moving any personal items or making adjustments in the room;
- Remember that the patient's dialogue with you and the medical record are confidential;
- Be honest. Never guess at an answer or information you do not know. Do not provide information beyond your scope of practice. Providing new information to the patient is the privilege and responsibility of the attending physician;
- Make no moral judgments about the patient. Set your values for patient care according to the patient's values, beliefs, and priorities;
- Expect the patient to have an emotional response to illness and the health care environment;
- Listen, then clarify and teach, but never argue;
- Adjust the time, length, and content of the interview to your patient's needs.

4. *Employ a relaxed, conversational style:*
- Use questions and statements that communicate empathy;
- Encourage the patient to express his or her concerns;
- Expect and accept some periods of silence;
- Close even the shortest interview by asking whether there is anything else the patient needs or wants to discuss;
- Tell the patient when you will return.

2. Prepare an interview schedule with specific questions needed to obtain the information required;
3. Prepare a general opening question for the interview schedule; the information obtained may guide or focus the remainder of the interview;
4. Guide the patient carefully in the questioning process; use open-ended, closed, direct, indirect, and neutral questions to maintain focus while allowing digression (see box on types of questions used in interviews below);
5. Guide the patient through the interview using the following interpersonal communication techniques:

Facilitation—techniques that encourage the patient to respond. Examples include nonverbal behavior such as maintaining eye contact, leaning toward the patient, nodding the head; and verbal communication such as "please go on," "go on," or "explain that to me again."

Clarification—techniques that seek clearer information from the patient. Examples include questions such as "I don't understand what you

Types of questions used in patient interviews[1]

1. *Open-ended questions* encourage patients to describe events and priorities as they see them and thereby help bring out concerns and attitudes and promote understanding. Questions such as "What brought you to the hospital?" or "What happened next?" encourage conversational flow and rapport while giving patients enough direction to know where to start;
2. *Closed questions* such as "When did your cough start?" or "How long did the pain last?" focus on specific information and provide clarification;
3. *Direct questions* can be either open-ended or closed and always end in a question mark. Though they are used to obtain specific information, a series of direct questions or frequent use of the question "Why?" can be intimidating;
4. *Indirect questions* are less threatening because they sound like statements: "I gather your doctor told you to take the treatments every 4 hours." Inquiries of this type also work well to confront discrepancies in the patient's statements: "If I understood you correctly, it is harder for you to breathe now than it was before your treatment;"
5. *Neutral questions* and statements are preferred for all interactions with the patient. "What happened next?" and "Tell me more about . . ." are neutral open-ended questions. A neutral closed question may give a patient a choice of responses while focusing on the type of information desired: "Would you say there was a teaspoon, a tablespoon, or a half cup?" By contrast, leading questions such as "You didn't cough up blood, did you?" should be avoided because they imply an answer.

have just said; please explain that to me again" and statements or questions that help the RCP understand an initially vague or unclear patient response.

Reflection—restating to the patient that which he or she has just said. For example, the RCP might respond to a patient's complaint of orthopnea with the following questions: "So your shortness of breath goes away when you sit up? Do other positions help ease your breathing?" Reflection often leads to more detail from the patient. It may also "buy" the RCP time to develop or alter strategy.

Empathy—verbal or nonverbal communication that informs the patient that the RCP understands the emotions being expressed. Examples of verbal expressions indicating an empathetic response include statements such as "Yes, I understand your concern" or "I can see why you are so upset." Empathetic responses like these help secure a therapeutic relationship. Such responses do not necessarily imply that the RCP agrees with the patient's emotions; they simply communicate that the expression of such feelings is acceptable.

Interpretation—verbal expressions that help the RCP draw inferences from the patient's verbal and nonverbal responses. For example, "You seem to be anxious about (this situation)" provides the opportunity for the patient to express his or her emotions and can help the RCP validate the patient's true feelings.

6. When exploring the patient's symptoms, use probing questions to elaborate on the onset, characteristics, and course of each subjective complaint. Recognize that a patient's evaluation of a symptom is related to individual factors, such as pain tolerance and perception.

The medical history*

The medical history provides an organized picture of the patient's past and present health problems, including why the patient is seeking health care. By itself, a good history often provides enough information to make a diagnosis. More commonly, the history guides the rest of the assessment process, including physical examination and radiographic and laboratory studies.

Traditionally, history taking was performed only by physicians. Today, however, histories are taken by many health professionals, including nurses, physician's assistants, physical therapists, dietitians, and RCPs. Although nurses and physician's assistants may take complete histories, RCPs tend to emphasize the respiratory or cardiopulmonary component. However, pulmonary assessment cannot be limited to the chest; a comprehensive evaluation of the patient's entire health status is essential. The accompanying box provides a typical content outline for a comprehensive medical history.[1]

All histories describe the patient's current health or illness. Chief complaint (**CC**) and history of present illness (**HPI**) are the most commonly used headings. Since it is this information that most concerns the patient, the interview and recording of the history usually begin here.

After the chief complaint and history of present illness, the interviewer solicits the patient's past medical history, to include major illnesses, hospitalizations, allergies, drugs, and health-related habits. This information gives the RCP a basic understanding of the patient's previous experiences with illness and health care.

The family and social/environmental history focuses on potential genetic or occupational links to disease and the patient's current life situation. A detailed occupational history is particularly important in assessing for pulmonary disorders, since there are so many occupationally related lung diseases.

Assessment of the current life situation should include the impact of culture, attitudes, relationships, and finances on health. Knowing patients' cultural backgrounds, educational levels, and patterns of health-related behavior gives insight into their ability to comprehend their current health status and their willingness or ability to participate in care. This background information also can give clues as to possible psychosocial implications of disease.

The review of symptoms is designed to uncover problem areas the patient forgot to mention or omitted. This information is classically obtained in a head-to-toe review of all body systems. For each body system, the interviewer obtains past and present information on pertinent symptoms, as experienced by the patient. For example, during review of the respiratory system, questioning would determine the presence or history of cough, hemoptysis, sputum production, chest pain, shortness of breath, fever, and so on (see the preceding box, Outline of a Complete Health History).

When exploring the patient's symptoms, the RCP should use probing questions to elaborate on the onset, characteristics, and course of each subjective complaint. The accompanying box outlines the approach taken when analyzing a symptom. As previously discussed, a patient's subjective evaluation of a symptom is related to individual factors, such as pain tolerance and perception. Thus, one should evaluate the intensity or severity of a current symptom in terms of its observable interference with the patient's ability to function.

*Excerpted from Krider SJ: Interviewing and the respiratory history, in Wilkins RL, Sheldon RL, Krider SJ, eds: *Clinical assessment in respiratory care,* ed. 2, St. Louis, 1990, Mosby.

Outline of a complete health history

1. Demographic data (obtained from admission data): Name, address, age, birth date, place of birth, race, nationality, marital status, religion, occupation, source of referral;

2. Date and source of history, estimate of reliability of historian;

3. Brief description of patient's condition at time of history or patient profile;

4. Chief complaint: reason for seeking health care;

5. History of present illness (chronological description of each symptom):
   - Onset: time, type, source, setting
   - Frequency and duration
   - Location and radiation
   - Severity (quantity)
   - Quality (character)
   - Aggravating/alleviating factors
   - Associated manifestations

6. Past medical history:
   - Childhood diseases and development
   - Hospitalizations, surgeries, injuries, accidents, major illnesses
   - Allergies
   - Drugs and medications
   - Immunizations
   - Habits
   - General health and sources of previous health care

7. Family history:
   - Familial disease history
   - Family history
   - Marital history
   - Family relationships

8. Social and environmental history:
   - Education
   - Military experience
   - Occupational history
   - Religious and social activities
   - Living arrangements
   - Hobbies and recreation
   - Satisfaction/stress with life situation, finances, relationships
   - Recent travel or other event that might impact health

9. Review of systems (respiratory system as an example):
   - Cough
   - Hemoptysis
   - Sputum (amount and consistency)
   - Chest pain
   - Shortness of breath
   - Hoarseness/voice changes
   - Dizziness/fainting
   - Fever/chills
   - Peripheral edema

10. Signature

Analysis of a symptom

I. Onset
- When (year, date, time)
- Onset (i.e., gradual or sudden)?
- Precipitating events (injury, exertion, etc.)
- Predisposing factors (age, infection, pregnancy, environment, drugs or other therapeutic agents or treatments, etc.)

II. Characteristics
- Quality
- Consistency
- Duration
- Quantity
- Location
- Radiation
- Intensity
- Aggravating factors
- Relieving factors
- Associated symptoms

III. Course
- Timing (e.g., acute, chronic, daily, periodic)
- Therapy (prescribed or nonprescribed)—effective or otherwise?

INITIAL ASSESSMENT

If the RCP was not involved in acquiring the initial history (see previous section), the medical record should be reviewed first. This gives the RCP insight into the patient's current symptoms and the physical examination findings to expect. Chart review also helps identify the areas of the examination to emphasize.

The RCP should briefly introduce herself or himself to the patient when entering the patient's room. The introduction is followed by a brief interview. The purpose of this interview is to identify what, if any, changes, have occurred in the patient's symptoms. Questions should be worded in a neutral fashion to prevent leading the patient to a desired answer. For example, asking "How is your breathing today?" is more likely to provide an accurate response than asking "Is your breathing better today?"

If the RCP notes any major changes in the patient's symptoms, a more thorough probe is needed. The RCP may need to contact the patient's nurse or physician when a major change in the patient's condition has occurred. Different therapy may be needed. Failing to take the time for this brief interview may result in administration of inappropriate therapy.

In order to ask the right questions, the RCP must be familiar with the common symptoms associated with cardiopulmonary disease. Dyspnea on exertion, cough, sputum production, chest pain, and hemoptysis (spitting up blood-tinged sputum) are symptoms often seen in the patient with cardiopulmonary disease. The interview is generally followed by an initial assessment consisting of observational impressions and the measurement of vital signs.

Initial impressions

One's initial impressions are based on observation of the patient's general appearance, level of consciousness and alertness, and presence of obvious signs of respiratory distress. Initial impressions are usually gathered while conducting the interview.

Overall appearance

The first few seconds of a patient encounter usually help reveal both the acuity and the severity of the problem at hand. These initial impressions should determine the course of subsequent assessment. If, for example, the patient's general appearance indicates an acute problem, the rest of the examination can be postponed until the patient's condition is stabilized. On the other hand, if the initial impressions indicate that the condition is stable and the patient is not in immediate danger, a complete assessment can be conducted.

Several indicators are important in assessing the patient's overall appearance. These include the general look of the body as a whole and the patient's facial expression, level of anxiety or distress, positioning, and personal hygiene.

In observing the body as a whole, the RCP should note any prominent findings. Does the patient appear well nourished or emaciated? Weakness and emaciation (**cachexia**) are signs of general ill health and malnutrition. Is the patient sweating? Diaphoresis can indicate fever, increased metabolism, or acute anxiety.

The general facial expression may help reveal pain or anxiety. Facial expression also can help in evaluating alertness, mood, general character, and mental capacity. More specific facial signs (discussed later) can also indicate respiratory distress. Simple observation of the patient's anxiety level can help reveal how severe the problem is and whether cooperation can be expected. The patient's position may also be useful in assessing the problem's severity and the patient's response to it. Last, personal hygiene indicators can help determine both the duration and the impact of the illness on the patient's daily activities.

Level of consciousness and alertness

After observing the patient's overall appearance, the RCP should quickly assess the patient's level of consciousness and alertness.

Evaluation of the patient's alertness is a simple but important task. If the patient appears conscious, the RCP determines the patient's orientation to time, place, and person. This is often called evaluating the

sensorium. The alert patient, who is well-oriented as to time, place, and person, is said to be "oriented × 3," and sensorium is considered normal.

If, however, the patient is not alert, the RCP should try to determine the level of consciousness. The simple rating scale in the accompanying box allows the RCP to describe the patient's level of consciousness objectively using common clinical terms.

Depressed consciousness may occur with poor cerebral blood flow or when poorly oxygenated blood perfuses the brain. As cerebral oxygenation falls, the patient first become restless, confused, and disoriented. If tissue hypoxia worsens, patients may become comatose. Abnormal consciousness also may occur in chronic degenerative brain disorders, as a side effect of certain medications, and in drug overdose cases.

Signs of respiratory distress

While assessing the patient's overall appearance, the RCP also should be looking for any obvious signs of respiratory distress. Distress often is evident in the

---

Levels of consciousness

Confused
- Exhibits slight decrease of consciousness
- Is slow in mental responses
- Has decreased or dulled perception
- Is incoherent in thought

Delirious
- Confused
- Easily agitated
- Irritable
- Exhibits hallucinations

Lethargic
- Sleepy
- Arouses easily
- Responds appropriately when aroused

Obtunded
- Awakens only with difficulty
- Responds appropriately when aroused

Stuporous
- Does not completely awaken
- Has decreased mental and physical activity
- Exhibits response to pain and deep tendon reflexes
- Is slow to respond to verbal stimuli

Comatose
- Is unconscious
- Does not respond to stimuli
- Does not exhibit voluntary movement
- Exhibits possible signs of upper motor neuron dysfunction (Babinski reflex present and hyperreflexia)
- Loss of reflexes with deep or prolonged coma

patient's position (sitting forward), facial expression (fear), rate of breathing (fast), and speech patterns (interrupted). More detail on the physical signs of respiratory distress are provided in subsequent sections.

VITAL SIGNS

Vital signs are the most frequently used clinical measurements. The four basic vital signs are body temperature, pulse rate, respiratory rate, and blood pressure.

The vital signs provide important diagnostic information and may reveal the first clue of adverse reactions to treatment. In addition, improvement in a patient's vital signs is strong evidence that a given treatment is having a positive effect. For example, a decrease in the patient's breathing and heart rate toward normal after oxygen therapy suggests a beneficial effect.

Body temperature

The average normal body temperature for adults is about 98.6° F (37° C),* with daily variations of about 1° F (0.5° C). Temperature usually is lowest in the early morning and highest in the late afternoon. Metabolic functions occur optimally when the body temperature is normal.

Body temperature is kept normal by balancing heat production with heat loss. Were the body not able to discharge the heat generated by metabolism, temperature would rise about 2° F per hour. The hypothalamus plays an important role in regulating heat loss and can initiate peripheral vasodilatation and sweating (diaphoresis) to dissipate body heat. The respiratory system also helps remove excess heat via ventilation. When the inspired gas is heated to near body temperature, as with heated aerosols, generators, or humidifiers, this mechanism is not functional.

An elevated body temperature (hyperthermia or hyperpyrexia) can result from disease or from normal activities such as exercise. Temperature elevation caused by disease is called *fever,* and the patient is said to be *febrile.* Fever often occurs as a result of infection.

Fever increases the body's metabolic rate, thereby increasing both oxygen consumption and carbon dioxide production. For every 1° C rise in temperature, oxygen consumption and carbon dioxide production increase by about 10%. To maintain homeostasis, this increase in metabolism must be matched by an increase in both circulation and ventilation. This is why febrile patients often have increased heart and breath-

ing rates. However, not all patients can tolerate increased circulation and ventilation. For patients with cardiac or pulmonary disease, this increased demand may overtax the cardiopulmonary system.

A body temperature below normal is called *hypothermia.* Hypothermia can occur when severe head injuries damage the hypothalamus. However, the most common cause of hypothermia is prolonged exposure to cold. When the body temperature is low, the hypothalamus initiates shivering (to generate heat) and vasoconstriction (to conserve heat).

Because hypothermia reduces oxygen consumption and carbon dioxide production, patients with hypothermia may exhibit slow and shallow breathing and reduced pulse rate. Mechanical ventilators in the control mode may need significant adjustments in the depth and rate of delivered tidal volumes as the body temperature of the patient varies above and below normal.

Body temperature is most often measured at one of three sites: the mouth, axilla, or rectum. Rectal temperatures are closest to actual body core temperature. The oral site is the most acceptable for the alert, adult patient but cannot be used with infants, comatose patients, or orally intubated patients. For accuracy, if a patient ingests hot or cold liquid or has been smoking, one should wait 10 to 15 minutes before taking an oral temperature. The **axillary** site is acceptable for infants or small children who do not tolerate rectal thermometers.

The oral temperature is not affected by simple oxygen administration via nasal **cannula** or mask.[3] For this reason, it is *not* necessary to remove the oxygen or use the rectal site when patients are receiving simple oxygen therapy.

However, the oral temperature may not be a valid measurement in patients breathing heated or cooled aerosol via face masks.[4] There is a tendency for oral temperatures to be falsely high in patients receiving heated aerosols. The opposite is true for cool aerosol inhalation. In these cases, when absolute accuracy is essential, the rectal site should be used.

Pulse rate

The peripheral pulse should be evaluated for rate, rhythm, and strength. The normal adult pulse rate is 60 to 100/min and is regular in rhythm. A pulse exceeding 100/min is termed *tachycardia.* Common causes of tachycardia are exercise, fear, anxiety, low blood pressure, anemia, fever, reduced arterial blood oxygen levels, and certain medications. A pulse rate below 60/min is termed *bradycardia.* This is less common but can occur with hypothermia, as a side effect of medications, or with certain cardiac arrhythmias.

The amount of oxygen delivered to the tissues depends on the heart's ability to pump oxygenated

---

*These long-held normal values have recently been challenged. Mackowiak et al. recently found a mean oral temperature of 36.8°C (98.2°F) among normal adults.[2]

blood. The amount of blood pumped through the circulation per minute (cardiac output) is a function of heart rate and stroke volume. When arterial oxygen content falls below normal, usually as a result of lung disease, the heart tries to maintain adequate oxygen delivery by increasing cardiac output. Cardiac output is increased mainly by increasing the rate.

The radial artery is the most common site used to evaluate the pulse. The RCP's second and third finger pads are used in assessment of the radial pulse (Figure 16-2). Ideally, the pulse rate should be counted for 1 minute. If the patient's wrist is held too far above the level of the heart, the pulse may be difficult to obtain. Key pulse characteristics that should be noted and documented are described in the accompanying box.

In terms of amplitude changes, spontaneous ventilation can influence pulse strength. A notable decrease in pulse strength during inhalation is called *pulsus paradoxus,* or paradoxical pulse. Pulsus paradoxus is common in patients with obstructive pulmonary disease, especially those suffering an acute asthma attack. Pulsus paradoxus may also signal a mechanical restriction on the heart's pumping action, as can occur with **constrictive pericarditis** or **cardiac tamponade.** Paradoxical pulse is best assessed by actual blood pressure measurement.

Pulsus alterans is an alternating succession of strong and weak pulses. Pulsus alterans suggests left-sided heart failure and usually is not related to respiratory disease.

The pulse may also be assessed by using the carotid, brachial, femoral, temporal, popliteal, posterior tibial, and dorsalis pedis. The more centrally located pulses (such as carotid and femoral) should be used when the blood pressure is abnormally low. If the carotid site is used, great care must be taken to avoid

---

Key characteristics of the pulse

Rate—is it normal, high, or low?
Rhythm—is it regular, consistently irregular, or irregularly irregular?
Amplitude (strength)—are there any changes in the amplitude of the pulse in relation to respiration? Are there changes in amplitude from one beat to another?
Other abnormalities—are there palpable vibrations (**thrills** or **bruits**)?

---

the carotid sinus area. Pressure on the carotid sinus area can evoke a strong parasympathetic response and cause bradycardia or even asystole.

Respiratory rate

The normal resting adult rate of breathing is 12 to 20/min. *Tachypnea* is an abnormally high respiratory rate. Rapid respiratory rates are associated with exercise, fever, arterial hypoxemia, metabolic acidosis, anxiety, and pain. A slow respiratory rate is called *bradypnea.* Although uncommon, bradypnea may occur in patients who have head injuries or hypothermia, as a side effect of certain medications such as narcotics, and in patients with drug overdose. Along with rate, the pattern of breathing (discussed later) should be assessed.

The respiratory rate is counted by watching the abdomen or chest wall move in and out. With practice, even the subtle breathing movements of the normal individual at rest can be identified easily. In some cases, the RCP may need to place a hand on the patient's abdomen to confirm the breathing rate.

Ideally, the patient should be unaware that the respiratory rate is being counted. One successful method to do so is to count the respiratory rate immediately after evaluating the pulse, while keeping the fingers on the artery.

Blood pressure

The arterial blood pressure is the force exerted against the wall of the arteries as the blood moves through them. Arterial systolic blood pressure is the peak force exerted during contraction of the left ventricle. Diastolic pressure is the force remaining after relaxation. *Pulse pressure* is the difference between the systolic and diastolic pressures. A normal pulse pressure is 35 to 40 mm Hg. When the pulse pressure is less than 30 mm Hg, the peripheral pulse is difficult to detect.

Blood pressure is determined by the force of left ventricular contraction, the systemic vascular resistance, and the blood volume (refer to Chapter 10). Normal systolic pressure ranges from 95 to 140 mm Hg, with an average of 120 mm Hg. Normal diastolic pressure ranges from 60 to 90 mm Hg, with an average

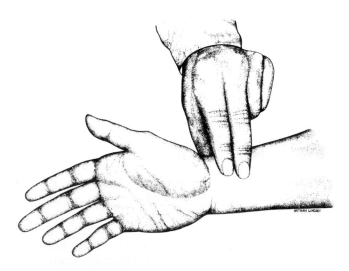

Fig. 16-2 Technique for assessment of radial pulse. (From Wilkins RL, Sheldon RL, and Krider SJ: Clinical assessment in respiratory care, St Louis, 1985, Mosby.)

of 80 mm Hg. The blood pressure is recorded by listing systolic over diastolic, for example, 120/80 mm Hg.

A blood pressure persistently above 140/90 mm Hg is termed *hypertension.* Hypertension is usually caused by high systemic vascular resistance. An increased force of ventricular contraction is a less common cause. Severe hypertension can result in central nervous system abnormalities (such as headaches, blurred vision, and confusion), uremia, congestive heart failure, or cerebral hemorrhage leading to stroke.

Hypotension is defined as a blood pressure less than 95/60 mm Hg. The most common causes are peripheral vasodilatation, left ventricular failure, or low blood volume. With hypotension, vital body organs may receive inadequate blood flow. Without adequate circulation, O_2 delivery to the tissues can be impaired, and tissue hypoxia may occur. For this reason prolonged hypotension must be prevented.

When normal individuals sit or stand up, their blood pressure changes very little. However, similar postural changes may produce an abrupt fall in the blood pressure among **hypovolemic** patients. This condition is called *postural hypotension.* Postural hypotension can be confirmed by measuring the blood pressure in both the supine and sitting positions.

Rapid drops in arterial blood pressure caused by postural hypotension can reduce cerebral blood flow and lead to *syncope,* or fainting. Postural hypotension is generally treated by administration of fluid or vasoactive drugs. Untreated or nonresponsive postural hypotension must always be taken into account when moving or ambulating a patient.

The auscultatory method is the most common technique for measuring arterial blood pressure. This method employs a blood pressure cuff **(sphygmomanometer)** and a stethoscope (Figure 16-3). When the cuff is applied to the upper arm and pressurized to exceed systolic blood pressure, brachial blood flow stops. As the cuff pressure is released slowly to a point just below systolic pressure, blood flows intermittently passes the obstruction. Partial obstruction of the blood flow creates turbulence and vibrations called *Korotkoff sounds.* Korotkoff sounds can be heard over the brachial artery distal to the obstruction with the aid of a stethoscope.

To measure the blood pressure, a deflated cuff is wrapped snugly around the upper arm with the lower edge of the cuff 1 in above the **antecubital fossa.** The brachial pulse is palpated, and the cuff is inflated about 30 mm Hg above the point at which the pulse stops. The bell of a stethoscope is placed over the artery. Then the cuff is deflated at a rate

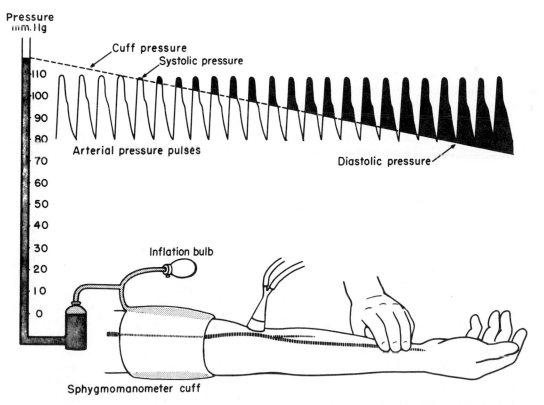

Fig. 16-3 Auscultatory method for measuring arterial blood pressure, using a sphygmomanometer and a stethoscope. (From Rushmer RR: Structure and functions of the cardiovascular system, ed 2, Philadelphia, 1976, WB Saunders.)

of 2 to 3 mm Hg per second while observing the manometer.

The systolic blood pressure is recorded as the point at which the first Korotkoff sounds are heard. The point at which the sounds become muffled is the diastolic pressure. This muffling is the final change in the Korotkoff sounds just before they disappear. At this point, cuff pressure equals diastolic pressure, and turbulence ceases. When muffling and disappearance of the sounds occur at a wide interval, all three pressures are recorded (120/80/60).

The RCP must be careful and perform the procedure rapidly, since the pressurized cuff impairs circulation to the forearm and hand. Since cuff pressures are only estimates of pressure based on blood flowing through an artery, anything that alters flow in the artery may result in erroneous blood pressure measurements. Common mistakes that result in erroneously high pressure measurements are summarized in the accompanying box.

A falsely low reading may occur if the cuff is too wide; however, this produces errors of 3 to 5 mm Hg rather than the 40 mm Hg error often obtained when using too narrow a cuff.

False diastolic readings can occur if pressure is maintained on the artery so that laminar flow is not reestablished. Since turbulent flow can be heard, muffling and/or disappearance of sound may not occur. Causes include applying the cuff too tightly and pressing the stethoscope too tightly over the artery.

Static electricity, ventilators, extraneous room sounds, and presence of an *auscultatory gap* may also cause erroneous cuff measurements. An auscultatory gap is a 20 to 40 mm Hg drop with no sound between the first systolic sound and the continuous pulse sound. Inflating the cuff until the palpated radial pulse can no longer be felt prevents missing the "opening snap." When an auscultatory gap is heard, both the opening snap pressure and the pressure at which continuous pulses are heard should be recorded (160/140/80).

The systolic blood pressure usually decreases slightly with normal inhalation. A drop in systolic pressure of more than 6 to 8 mm Hg during a resting inhalation is, however, abnormal. This condition, previously described, is termed paradoxical pulse.

Paradoxical pulse is due to the intrathoracic pressure swings created by the respiratory muscles during breathing. Negative intrathoracic pressure during inspiration aids venous return to the right ventricle (RV) but impedes arterial outflow from the left ventricle (LV). In addition, increased venous return increases RV pressures, thus constricting LV filling. This reduces LV stroke volume and decreases systolic blood pressure during inhalation.

Although simple palpation may signal its presence, paradoxical pulse can only be quantified by auscultatory measurement. To do so, the cuff is normally inflated until the pulse ceases. Then the cuff is slowly deflated until sounds are heard on exhalation only (point 1). Last, cuff pressure is reduced again until sounds are heard throughout respiration (point 2). The difference between point 1 and 2 indicates the degree of paradoxical pulse.

EXAMINATION OF THE HEAD AND NECK

Head

Besides expression (previously discussed), the face should be inspected for abnormal signs indicating respiratory problems. The most common facial signs are nasal flaring, cyanosis, and pursed-lip breathing. Nasal flaring occurs when the external nares flare outward during inhalation. This occurs especially in neonates with respiratory distress and indicates an increase in the work of breathing.

When respiratory disease reduces arterial oxygen content, cyanosis may be detected, especially around the lips and oral mucosa. Cyanosis may be difficult to detect, especially in a poorly lighted room. Although cyanosis suggests inadequate oxygenation, further investigation is indicated. The absence of cyanosis, however, does not necessarily assure good oxygenation. This is because a sufficient hemoglobin concentration must exist before cyanosis can be identified (Chapter 15).

Patients with chronic obstructive pulmonary disease (COPD) may use pursed-lip breathing during exhalation. Although this is often taught to patients, many develop this technique on their own. Breathing through pursed lips during exhalation creates resistance to flow. This increased resistance causes development of a slight back pressure in the small airways during exhalation, which prevents their premature collapse.

Mistakes causing erroneously high blood pressure measurements

1. Too narrow a cuff. (Cuff and bladder width should be at least the diameter of the arm.)
2. Cuff applied too tightly.
3. Cuff applied too loosely. (When the loose bladder is inflated, the edges rise so the portion pressing on the artery has a tourniquet effect.)
4. Excessive pressure placed in the cuff during measurement.
5. Inflation pressure held in the cuff.
6. Incomplete deflation of cuff between measurements.

Neck

Inspection and palpation of the neck help determine the position of the trachea and the jugular venous pressure (JVP). Normally, when the patient faces forward, the trachea is located in the middle of the neck. The midline of the neck can be identified by palpating the suprasternal notch. The midline of the trachea should be directly below the center of the suprasternal notch.

The trachea can shift away from the midline in certain thoracic disorders. In general, the trachea shifts *toward* an area of collapsed lung. Conversely, the trachea shifts *away* from areas with increased air, fluid, or tissue (such as **pneumothorax,** pleural effusion, or lung tumor). Abnormalities in the lung bases may not shift the trachea unless the defect is large.

JVP is estimated by examining the height of the blood column in the jugular veins. JVP reflects the volume and pressure of venous blood in the right side of the heart. Both the internal and external jugular veins can be assessed, although the internal is more reliable. Individuals with obese necks may not have visible neck veins, even when they are distended.

When lying in a supine position, a normal individual has neck veins that are full. When the head of the bed is elevated gradually to a 45-degree angle, the level of the blood column descends to a point no more than a few centimeters above the clavicle. With elevated venous pressure, the neck veins may be distended as high as the angle of the jaw, even when the patient is sitting upright.

The degree of venous distension is estimated by measuring the distance the veins are distended above the sternal angle. The sternal angle has been chosen since its distance above the right atrium remains nearly constant (about 5 cm) in all positions. With the head of the bed raised 45 degrees, venous distension greater than 3 to 4 cm above the sternal angle is abnormal (Figure 16-4).

Precise measurement of the jugular pressure (in centimeters) is difficult and probably exceeds the accuracy needed for most observers. A simple grading scale of normal, increased, and markedly increased is acceptable.

Jugular pressure may vary with breathing. Typically, the blood column descends toward the thorax during inhalation and rises back up with exhalation. For this reason, JVP should always be estimated at the end of exhalation.

The most common cause of jugular venous distension is failure of the right side of the heart. Right-sided heart failure may occur secondary to left-sided heart failure or chronic hypoxemia. Hypoxemia causes pulmonary vasoconstriction, which increases flow resistance through the pulmonary vasculature. Increased pulmonary vascular resistance increases right

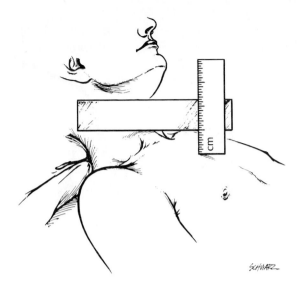

Fig. 16-4 Estimation of jugular venous pressure. (From Malasanos L et al: Health assessment, ed 4, St Louis, 1990, Mosby.)

ventricular workload. Persistent lung disease with hypoxemia may result in right-sided heart failure and jugular venous distension. Jugular venous distension also may occur with **hypervolemia,** and when the venous return to the right atrium is obstructed by mediastinal tumors.

EXAMINATION OF THE THORAX AND LUNGS

Lung topography

To perform an accurate physical assessment of the thorax and lungs, the RCP must first identify key landmarks. Topographic or surface landmarks on the chest help one identify the location of underlying structures or abnormalities. In addition, imaginary lines are used to describe the location of anatomic structures within the chest and abnormal physical examination findings.

Imaginary lines

On the anterior chest, the midsternal line divides the chest into equal halves. The left and right midclavicular lines parallel the midsternal line and are drawn through the midpoints of the left and right clavicles, respectively (Figure 16-5, page 372).

The midaxillary line divides the lateral chest into equal halves. The anterior axillary line parallels the midaxillary line and is situated along the **anterolateral** chest. The posterior axillary line is also parallel to the midaxillary line and is located in the **posterolateral** chest (Figure 16-6, page 372).

Three imaginary vertical lines are described on the posterior chest. The midspinal line divides the posterior chest into two equal halves. The left and right

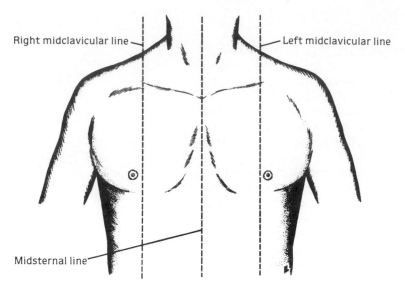

Fig. 16-5 Imaginary lines on anterior chest wall.

midscapular lines parallel the midspinal line and pass through the inferior angles of the scapulae in the relaxed upright individual (Figure 16-7).

Thoracic cage landmarks

The *suprasternal notch* is situated on the anterior chest at the top of the manubrium. It can be located by palpation of the depression at the base of the neck. Directly below this notch is the *sternal angle,* or angle of Louis. The sternal angle is identified by palpating down from the suprasternal notch until the ridge between the manubrium and body of the sternum is felt. Here, the second rib joins the sternum (Figure 16-8). Using this as a reference point, rib identification on the anterior chest is now easy. Usually it is easier to count the ribs slightly to the side of the sternum, rather than along its lateral border.

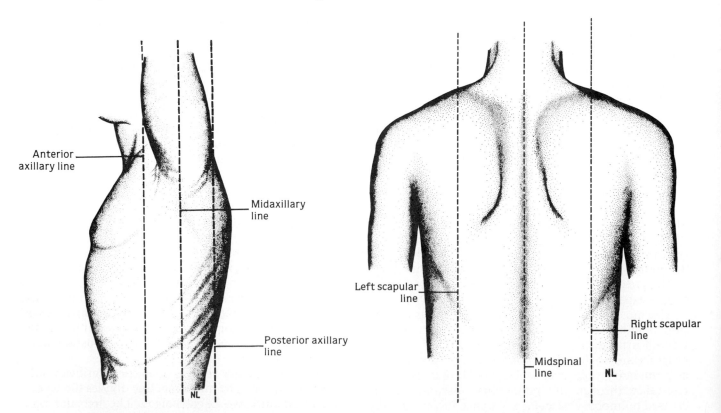

Fig. 16-6 Imaginary lines on lateral chest wall.

Fig. 16-7 Imaginary lines on posterior chest wall.

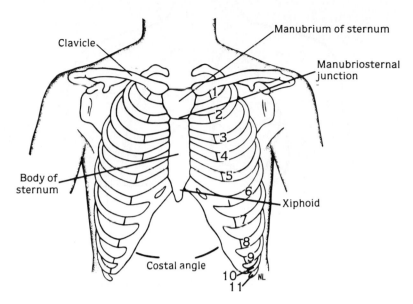

Fig. 16-8 Thoracic cage landmarks on anterior chest.

On the posterior chest, the spinous processes of the vertebrae are useful landmarks (Figure 16-9). The spinous process of the seventh cervical vertebra (C7) usually can be identified by asking the patient to flex his or her head and neck forward and slightly down. At the base of the neck the most prominent spinous process that can be seen and palpated is C7. The spinous process just below C7 is that of the first thoracic vertebra (T1).

The scapular borders also can be useful landmarks on the posterior chest. With the patient's arm raised above the head, the inferior border of the scapula nearly overlies the oblique fissure that separates the upper from the lower lobes on the posterior chest (see the following discussion).

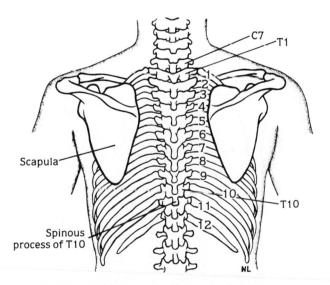

Fig. 16-9 Thoracic cage landmarks on posterior chest.

Lung fissures

Fissures separate the lobes of the lungs. Both lungs have an oblique fissure that begins on the anterior chest at about the sixth rib at the midclavicular line. This fissure extends laterally and upward until it crosses the fifth rib on the lateral chest in the midaxillary line and continues on the posterior chest to approximately T3 (Figures 16-10 and 16-11, page 374).

The right lung also has a horizontal fissure that separates the right upper lobe and middle lobes. The horizontal fissure extends from the fourth rib at the sternal border around to the fifth rib at the midaxillary line. The left lung rarely has a horizontal fissure.

Tracheal bifurcation

On the anterior chest, the carina is located beneath the angle of Louis, and on the posterior chest at about T4 (Figure 16-12, page 375).

Diaphragm

The diaphragm is a dome-shaped muscle that lies between the thoracic and abdominal cavities and moves up and down during breathing. At the end of a normal tidal expiration, the right dome of the diaphragm is located level with T9 posteriorly and the fifth rib anteriorly. On the left side, the diaphragm normally comes to rest at end-expiration at T10 posteriorly and the sixth rib anteriorly. The right hemidiaphragm is usually a little higher than the left hemidiaphragm because of the position of the liver.

Lung borders

On the anterior chest, the lungs extend 2 to 4 cm above the medial third of the clavicles. At end-expiration, the anterior lower lung borders extend to about the sixth rib at the midclavicular line, and to the

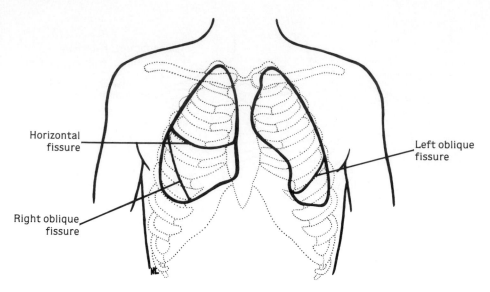

Fig. 16-10 Topographic position of lung fissures on anterior chest.

eighth rib on the lateral chest wall. On the posterior chest, the superior border extends to T1, while the inferior border rises and falls with breathing between T9 and T12 (Figure 16-12).

Techniques of examination

Inspection

The chest is visually inspected to assess the thoracic configuration and the pattern and effort of breathing. For adequate inspection the room must be well lighted and the patient should be sitting upright. When the patient is too ill to sit up, the RCP should carefully roll the patient to one side in order to examine the posterior chest. Male patients should be stripped to the waist. Female patients should be given some type of drape to prevent embarrassing exposure of the breasts.

Thoracic configuration. The normal adult thorax has an anteroposterior (AP) diameter less than the transverse diameter. The AP diameter normally increases gradually with age but may prematurely increase in patients with certain types of chronic obstructive lung disease. This abnormal increase in AP diameter is called *barrel chest*. When the AP diameter increases, the normal 45-degree angle of articulation between the ribs and spine is lost, becoming essentially horizontal (Figure 16-13).

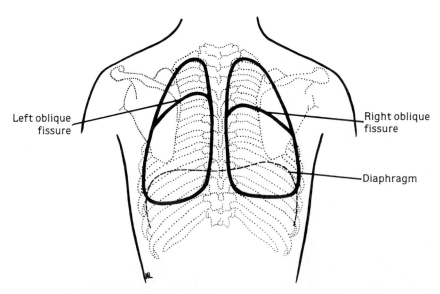

Fig. 16-11 Topographic position of lung fissures on posterior chest.

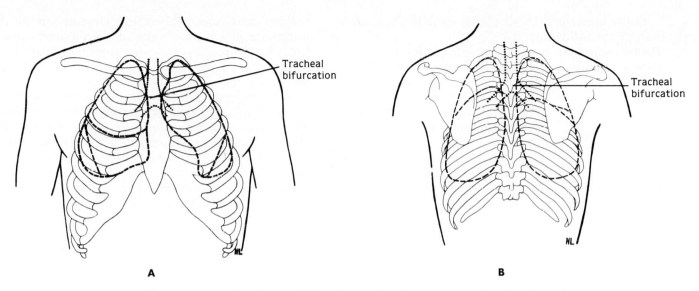

Fig. 16-12 Topographic position of tracheal bifurcation and lung borders on anterior chest, **A,** and posterior chest, **B.**

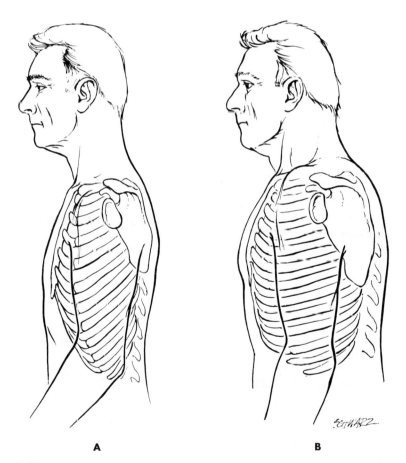

Fig. 16-13 A, Patient with normal thoracic configuration. **B,** Patient with increased anteroposterior diameter. Note contrasts in angle of slope of ribs and development of accessory muscles. (From Malasanos L et al: Health assessment, ed 4, St Louis, 1990, Mosby.)

Other abnormalities of the thoracic configuration include the following:

Pectus carinatum sternal protrusion anteriorly

Pectus excavatum depression of part or all of the sternum, which can produce a restrictive lung defect

Kyphosis spinal deformity in which the spine has an abnormal anteroposterior curvature

Scoliosis spinal deformity in which the spine has a lateral curvature

Kyphoscoliosis combination of kyphosis and scoliosis; may produce a severe restrictive lung defect as a result of poor lung expansion

Breathing pattern and effort. At rest, the normal adult has a consistent rate and rhythm of breathing. Breathing effort is minimal on inhalation and passive on exhalation. Men typically breathe with the diaphragm, causing the stomach to move slightly outward during inhalation. Women tend to use a combination of intercostal muscles and the diaphragm, producing more chest wall movement than men. Table 16-1 describes some of the common abnormal patterns of breathing.

Any respiratory abnormalities that increase the work of breathing may cause the accessory muscles of ventilation to become active, even at rest. This is common in acute and chronic diffuse airway obstruction, acute upper airway obstruction, and disorders that reduce lung compliance. An increased work of breathing can also result in *retractions.* Retractions are indrawings of the skin overlying the chest wall during inspiration. This occurs when the ventilatory muscles contract forcefully enough to cause a large drop in the intrathoracic pressure. Retractions may be seen between the ribs, above the clavicles, or below the rib cage. These are called "intercostal," "supraclavicular," or "subcostal" retractions, respectively.

The patient's breathing pattern often provides reliable clues as to the underlying problem. A significant reduction in lung volume, as occurs with atelectasis, usually results in rapid, shallow breathing. In general, the greater the loss of lung volume, the higher will be the patient's respiratory rate.[5] Obstruction of the intrathoracic airways results in a prolonged exhalation time. This alters the normal ratio of inspiratory to expiratory time from about 1:2 or 1:3 to 1:4 or more. Upper airway obstruction (outside the thorax) usually results in a prolonged inspiratory time.

The diaphragm may be nonfunctional in patients with spinal injuries or neuromuscular disease and severely limited in patients with COPD. When this occurs, the accessory muscles of ventilation may also become active.

In patients with emphysema, the lungs lose their elastic recoil and become hyperinflated. Over time, the diaphragm assumes a low, flat position. Because of the lack of normal curvature, greater pressure differences (thus greater patient effort) are needed to move this muscle. In addition, contraction of a flat diaphragm tends to draw in the lateral costal margins, instead of expanding them (Hoover's sign).

The accessory muscles then must assist ventilation by raising the anterior chest in an effort to increase thoracic volume ("clavicular lift"). In fact, the severity of lung disease is directly related to the magnitude of activity of these accessory muscles.[6]

In some patients with COPD, the diaphragm is overworked and underfed. As a result, the diaphragm is prone to severe fatigue. Diaphragm fatigue usually results in a distinctive breathing pattern. The fatigued diaphragm is flaccid and is drawn upward into the thoracic cavity with each inspiratory effort of the accessory muscles. This is recognized by inward movement of the anterior abdominal wall during inspiration efforts, a sign called abdominal paradox.[7,8]

Palpation

Palpation is the art of touching the chest wall to evaluate underlying structure and function. It is used in selected patients to confirm or rule out suspected problems suggested by the history and initial examination findings. Palpation is performed to: (1) evaluate vocal fremitus, (2) estimate thoracic expansion, and (3) assess the skin and subcutaneous tissues of the chest.

Table 16-1 Abnormal breathing patterns

Pattern	Characteristics	Causes
Apnea	No breathing	Cardiac arrest
Biot's	Irregular breathing with long periods of apnea	Increased intracranial pressure
Cheyne-Stokes	Irregular type of breathing; breaths increase and decrease in depth and rate with periods of apnea	Diseases of central nervous system Congestive heart failure
Kussmaul's	Deep and fast	Metabolic acidosis
Apneustic	Prolonged inhalation	Brain damage
Paradoxic	Portion or all of chest wall moves in with inhalation and out with exhalation	Chest trauma, diaphragm paralysis, muscle fatigue
Asthmatic	Prolonged exhalation	Obstruction to airflow out of lungs

Vocal fremitus. The term *vocal fremitus* refers to the vibrations created by the vocal cords during speech. These vibrations are transmitted down the tracheobronchial tree and through the alveoli to the chest wall. When these vibrations are felt on the chest wall, it is called *tactile fremitus*.

To assess for tactile fremitus, the patient is asked to repeat the words "ninety-nine" while the RCP systematically palpates the thorax. As shown in Figure 16-14, the RCP can use the **palmar** aspect of the fingers or the **ulnar** aspect of the hand. If one hand is used, it should be moved from one side of the chest to

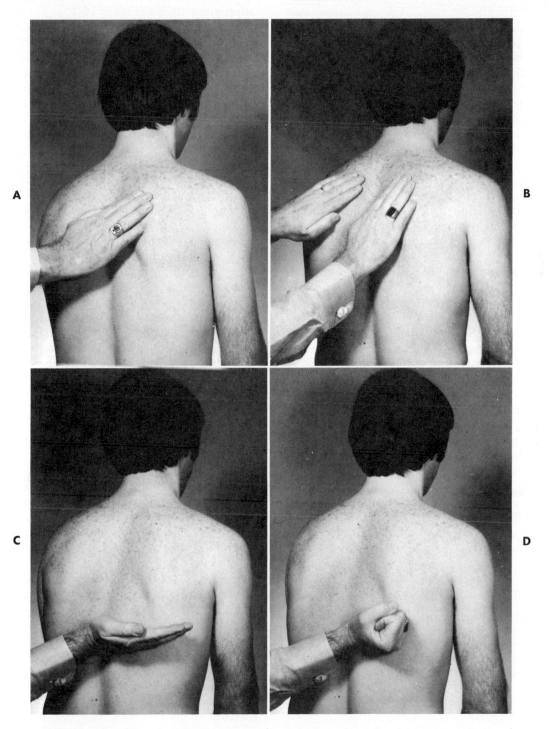

Fig. 16-14 Palpation for assessment of vocal fremitus. **A,** Use of palmar surface of fingertips. **B,** Simultaneous application of fingertips of both hands. **C,** Use of ulnar aspect of hand. **D,** Use of ulnar aspect of closed fist. (From Prior JA, Silberstein JS, and Stang JM: Physical diagnosis: the history and examination of the patient, ed 6, St Louis, 1982, Mosby.)

the corresponding area on the other side. The anterior, lateral, and posterior chest wall should be evaluated.

The vibrations of tactile fremitus may be increased, decreased, or absent. Increased fremitus is due to the transmission of the vibration through a more solid medium. The normal lung structure is a combination of solid and air-filled tissue. Any condition that increases the density of the lung, such as the consolidation that occurs in pneumonia, increases the intensity of fremitus. However, if an area of consolidation is not in communication with an open airway, speech cannot be transmitted to that area, and fremitus will be absent or decreased.

Tactile fremitus is reduced most often in patients who are obese or overly muscular. Also, when the pleural space lining the lung becomes filled with air (pneumothorax) or fluid (pleural effusion), fremitus is significantly reduced or absent.

In patients with emphysema, the lungs become hyperinflated. This reduces the density of lung tissue. Because density is low, speech vibrations transmit poorly through the lung, resulting in a bilateral reduction in fremitus. This reduction in tactile fremitus is more difficult to detect than the unilateral increase in fremitus associated with lobar consolidation. The causes of abnormal tactile fremitus are summarized in the accompanying box.

The passage of air through airways containing thick secretions may produce palpable vibrations referred to as *rhonchial fremitus*. Rhonchial fremitus often is identified during inhalation and exhalation and may clear if the patient produces an effective cough. It frequently is associated with a coarse, low-pitched sound that can be heard without a stethoscope.

Thoracic expansion. The normal chest wall expands symmetrically during deep inhalation. This expansion can be evaluated on the anterior and posterior chest.

To evaluate it anteriorly, the RCP places his or her hands over the anterolateral chest, with the thumbs extended along the costal margin toward the xiphoid. On the posterior chest, the hands are positioned over the posterolateral chest with the thumbs meeting at approximately T8 (Figure 16-15). The patient is then instructed to exhale slowly and completely. When the patient has exhaled maximally, the RCP gently secures his or her fingertips against the sides of the patient's chest and extends the thumbs toward the midline until the tip of each thumb meets at the midline. The patient then is instructed to take a full, deep breath. The RCP should make note of the distance each thumb moves from the midline. Normally, each thumb moves an equal distance of about 3 to 5 cm.

Diseases that affect expansion of both lungs cause a bilateral reduction in chest expansion. This is seen commonly in neuromuscular disorders and COPD. Unilateral reduction in chest expansion occurs with respiratory diseases that reduce the expansion of one lung or a major part of one lung. This can occur with lobar consolidation, atelectasis, pleural effusion, or pneumothorax.

Skin and subcutaneous tissues. The chest wall can be palpated to determine the general temperature and condition of the skin. When air leaks from the lung into subcutaneous tissues, fine bubbles produce a crackling sound and sensation when palpated. This condition is referred to as *subcutaneous emphysema.* The sensation produced on palpation is called *crepitus.*

Percussion of the chest

Percussion is the art of tapping on a surface in an effort to evaluate the underlying structure. Percussion of the chest wall produces a sound and a palpable vibration useful in evaluating underlying lung tissue. The vibration created by percussion penetrates the lung to a depth of 5 to 7 cm below the chest wall.

The technique most often used in percussion of the chest wall is termed *mediate* or *indirect percussion.* The RCP places the middle finger of the left hand (if the RCP is right-handed) firmly against the chest wall parallel to the ribs, with the palm and other fingers held off the chest. The tip of the middle finger on the right hand or the lateral aspect of the right thumb strikes the finger against the chest near the base of the terminal phalanx with a quick, sharp blow. Movement of the hand striking the chest should be generated at the wrist, not the elbow or shoulder (Figure 16-16).

The percussion note is clearest if the RCP remembers to keep the finger on the chest firmly against the chest wall and to strike this finger and immediately withdraw. The two fingers should be in contact only

---

Causes of abnormal tactile fremitus

Increased

Pneumonia
Lung tumor or mass
Atelectasis
Pulmonary fibrosis

Decreased
Unilateral

    Bronchial obstruction with mucus plug or foreign object
      Pneumothorax
      Pleural effusion

Diffuse

    Chronic obstructive lung disease
    Muscular or obese chest wall

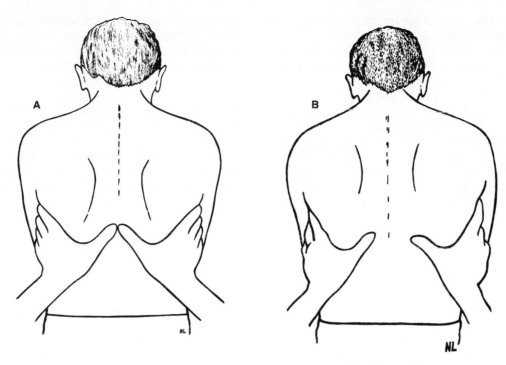

Fig. 16-15 Estimation of thoracic expansion. **A,** Exhalation. **B,** Maximal inhalation.

for an instant. As one gains experience in percussion, the feel of the vibration becomes as important as the sound in evaluating lung structures.

Percussion over lung fields. Percussion of the lung fields should be done systematically, consecutively testing comparable areas on both sides of the chest. Percussion over the bony structures and breasts of the female is not of value and should be avoided. Asking patients to raise their arms above their shoulders will help move the scapulae laterally and minimize their

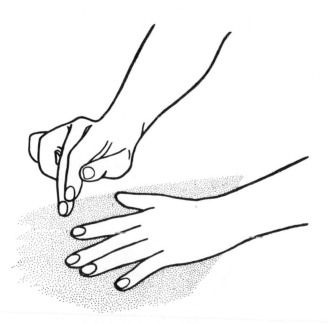

Fig. 16-16 Technique for indirect chest percussion.

interference with percussion on the posterior chest wall.

The sounds generated during percussion of the chest are evaluated for intensity (loudness) and pitch. Percussion over normal lung fields produces a sound moderately low in pitch that can be heard easily. This sound is best described as normal resonance. When the percussion note is louder and lower in pitch than normal, resonance is said to be increased. Percussion may produce a sound with characteristics just the opposite of resonance, referred to as dull or flat. This sound is high pitched, short in duration, and not loud.

Clinical implications. By itself, percussion of the chest is of little value in making a diagnosis. However, when considered along with other findings, it can provide essential information.

Any abnormality that increases lung tissue density, such as pneumonic consolidation, tumor, or atelectasis, results in a loss of resonance and a dull percussion note over the affected area. Percussion over pleural spaces filled with fluid, such as blood or water, also produces a dull or flat percussion note.

An increase in resonance is detected in patients with hyperinflated lungs. Hyperinflation can result from acute bronchial obstruction (asthma) or chronic obstructive disease such as emphysema. The percussion note also can increase in resonance when the pleural space contains large amounts of air (pneumothorax).

Unilateral problems are easier to detect than bilateral ones because the normal side provides an immediate comparison. The dullness heard from percussion over consolidation is a distinct sound that is easier to detect than the subtle increase in resonance heard with hyperinflation or pneumothorax.

Percussion of the chest has limitations that are often clinically important. Abnormalities that are small or deep below the surface are not likely to be detected during percussion of the chest. This may explain why many RCPs do not routinely use chest percussion to evaluate lung resonance.[9]

Diaphragmatic excursion. The range of diaphragm movement can be estimated by percussion. This is best done on the posterior chest wall (Figure 16-17). To estimate diaphragm movement, the patient first is asked to take a deep, full inspiration and hold it. The RCP then determines the lowest margin of resonance by percussing downward in small increments over the lower lung field until a definite change in percussion note is detected. The patient then is instructed to exhale maximally, holding this position while the percussion procedure is repeated. The RCP should work rapidly to prevent the patient from becoming short of breath. The normal diaphragm excursion during a deep breath is about 5 to 7 cm. The range of diaphragm movement is less than normal in certain neuromuscular diseases and in severe pulmonary hyperinflation.

The exact range of movement and position of the diaphragm is difficult to determine by percussion.[10] This is due to the fact that the diaphragm is a dome-shaped muscle with the center of the dome 15 cm beneath the surface of the posterior chest. Percussion can only approximate the position and degree of movement.

Auscultation of the lungs

Auscultation is the process of listening for bodily sounds. Auscultation over the thorax is performed to identify normal or abnormal lung sounds. It is used by RCPs to assess the patient condition and the effects of therapy.[11] A stethoscope is used during auscultation to enhance sound transmission. Whenever auscultation is performed, the room must be as quiet as possible.

Stethoscope. A stethoscope has four basic parts: a bell, a diaphragm, tubing, and earpieces (Figure 16-18). The bell detects a broad spectrum of sounds. It is particularly good for listening to low-pitched sounds, such as those produced by the heart. It also can be used to auscultate the lungs in certain situations, as when emaciation causes rib protrusion that restricts placement of the diaphragm flat against the chest. The bell piece should be pressed lightly against the chest when trying to hear low-frequency sounds. If the bell is pressed too firmly, the patient's skin will be stretched under the bell and may act as a diaphragm, filtering out many low-frequency sounds.

The diaphragm piece is preferred for auscultation of the lungs, since most lung sounds are of high frequency. It also is useful in listening to high-frequency heart sounds. The diaphragm piece should be pressed firmly against the chest so that external sounds are not heard.

The ideal tubing should be thick enough to exclude external noises and about 25 to 35 cm (11 to 16 in) long. Longer tubing may impair sound transmission, and shorter tubing makes it hard to reach the patient's chest.

The stethoscope should be examined regularly for cracks in the diaphragm, wax or dirt in the earpieces, and other defects that may interfere with the transmission of sound. It should be wiped clean with alcohol on a regular basis to prevent a buildup of microorganisms.

Technique. When possible, the patient should be sitting upright in a relaxed position. The patient should be instructed to breathe a little more deeply than normal through an open mouth. Inhalation should be active, with exhalation passive. The bell or

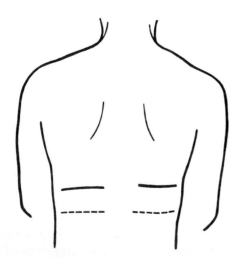

Fig. 16-17 Assessment of diaphragmatic excursion by percussion. Horizontal lines indicate position of diaphragm at maximal inhalation and exhalation.

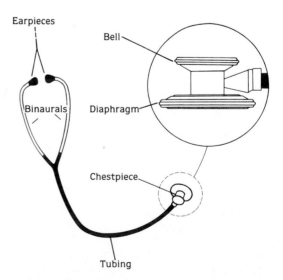

Fig. 16-18 Acoustic stethoscope.

diaphragm must be placed directly against the chest wall, since clothing may alter lung sounds or produce distortion. The tubing should not rub against any objects, since this may produce extraneous sounds.

Auscultation of the lungs should be systematic, including all lobes on the anterior, lateral, and posterior chest. The RCP should begin at the base, compare side with side, and work toward the lung apexes. It is important to begin at the bases because certain abnormal sounds (described later) that occur only here may be altered by several deep breaths. At least one full ventilatory cycle should be evaluated at each stethoscope position. Common errors to avoid during auscultation are summarized in the accompanying box.

The RCP should carefully listen for and distinguish among the four key features of breath sounds. First, the pitch (vibration frequency) should be identified. Second, the amplitude or intensity (loudness) is noted. Third, any distinctive characteristics are listened for. Fourth, the duration of the sound's inspiratory and expiration components is compared. The acoustic characteristics of breath sounds can be illustrated in breath sound diagrams (Figure 16-19). The features of the normal breath sounds are described in Table 16-2. Examiners must be familiar with normal breath sounds before they can expect to identify the subtle changes that may signify respiratory disease.

Terminology. In normal individuals the sounds heard over the trachea have a loud, tubular quality. These are referred to as a *bronchial* or *tracheal* breath sounds. Bronchial breath sounds are high-pitched sounds with an expiratory component equal to or slightly longer than the inspiratory component.

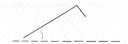

Fig. 16-19 Diagrammatic representation of normal breath sound. Upstroke represents, inhalation, and downstroke represents exhalation; length of upstroke represents duration; thickness of stroke represents intensity; angle between upstroke and horizontal line represents pitch.

A slight variation in bronchial breath sounds is heard around the upper half of the sternum on the anterior chest and between the scapula on the posterior chest. These sounds are not as loud as bronchial breath sounds, are slightly lower in pitch, and have equal inspiratory and expiratory components. They are referred to as *bronchovesicular breath sounds.*

When auscultating over the lung **parenchyma** of a normal individual, soft, muffled sounds are heard. These normal sounds, referred to as *vesicular sounds,* are lower in pitch and intensity (loudness) than bronchial breath sounds. Vesicular sounds are heard primarily during inhalation, with only a minimal exhalation component (Table 16-2 on page 382).

Respiratory disease may alter the intensity of normal breath sounds heard over the lung fields. A slight variation in intensity is difficult to detect even for experienced clinicians. Breath sounds are described as *diminished* when the intensity decreases, and *absent* in extreme cases. They are described as *harsh* when the intensity increases. When the expiratory component of harsh breath sounds equals the inspiratory component, they are considered *bronchial* in nature.

Abnormal sounds or vibrations produced by the movement of air in the lungs are termed *adventitious* sounds. Most adventitious lung sounds can be classified as either continuous or discontinuous. Continuous lung sounds are defined as having a duration longer than 25 milliseconds. (This definition is derived from recording and spectral analysis of lung sounds. Examiners are not expected to time the lung sounds.) Discontinuous lung sounds are intermittent, crackling, or bubbling sounds of short duration, usually less than 20 milliseconds.[12]

Until recently, clinicians used many different terms to describe abnormal breath sounds.[13] Fortunately, the American Thoracic Society and the American College of Chest Physicians formed a committee to help standardize these terms. First published in 1975, their work suggested that the term *rales* be used for discontinuous (intermittent) abnormal sounds and the term *rhonchi* for continuous sounds.[14]

The committee published updated reports in 1977 and 1981. At that time, they recommended that *crackles* replace *rales* as the term for discontinuous sounds.[15,16] Although use of the term *rales* has declined since 1981, it remains a popular term among many clinicians.[17-19]

The updates also suggested that high-pitched con-

Common errors and current methods for auscultation

Errors

- Listening to breath sounds through the patient's gown
- Allowing tubing to rub against bed rails or patient's gown
- Attempting to auscultate in a noisy room
- Interpreting chest hair sounds as adventitious lung sounds
- Auscultating only the "convenient" areas

Correct technique

- Placing bell or diaphragm directly against the chest wall
- Keeping tubing free from contact with any objects during auscultation
- Turning television or radio off
- Wetting chest hair before auscultation if thick
- Asking alert patient to sit up; rolling comatose patient onto side to auscultate posterior lobes

Table 16-2 Characteristics of normal breath sounds

Breath sound	Pitch	Intensity	Location	Diagram of sound
Vesicular or normal breath sounds	Low	Soft	Peripheral lung areas	
Bronchovesicular	Moderate	Moderate	Around upper part of sternum, between scapulae	
Bronchial	High	Loud	Over trachea	

tinuous lung sounds be described as *wheezes* and that *rhonchi* be used specifically for low-pitched, continuous sounds. To be consistent with these recommendations, this text will use the term *crackles* to indicate discontinuous lung sounds; *wheezes* for high-pitched, continuous lung sounds; and *rhonchi* for low-pitched, continuous lung sounds.

Another continuous abnormal sound heard primarily over the larynx and trachea during inhalation is *stridor*. Stridor is a loud, high-pitched sound that sometimes can be heard without a stethoscope. Most common in infants and small children, stridor is a sign of upper (**supraglottic**) airway obstruction.

The reader should be aware that other texts may use different terms to describe abnormal lung sounds. Table 16-3 provides a list of alternative terms that are often used by others.

When the RCP identifies abnormal lung sounds, their location and specific features should be noted. Abnormal lung sounds may be high or low pitched, loud or faint, scanty or profuse, and inspiratory or expiratory (or both). The timing during the respiratory cycle should be noted also (for example, late inspiratory). The RCP must pay close attention to these features because they help determine the functional status of the lungs. This is further discussed in the following sections.

Table 16-3 Recommended* terminology for lung sounds versus alternative terminology

Recommended term	Classification	Alternative terms
Crackles	Discontinuous	Rales
		Crepitations
Wheezes	High-pitched, continuous	Sibilant rales
		Musical rales
		Sibilant rhonchi
Rhonchi	Low-pitched, continuous	Sonorous rales
		Low-pitched wheeze

*According to the Ad Hoc Pulmonary Nomenclature Committee of ATS/ACCP.

Mechanisms and significance of lung sounds. The exact mechanisms that produce normal and abnormal lung sounds are not fully known. However, there is enough agreement among investigators to allow a general description. This knowledge should give RCPs a better understanding of the lung sounds frequently heard through a stethoscope.

Normal breath sounds. Lung sounds heard over the chest of the normal individual are generated primarily by turbulent flow in the larger airways.[20,21] Turbulent flow creates audible vibrations in the airways, producing sounds that are transmitted through the lung and the chest wall. As the sound travels to the lung periphery and the chest wall, it is altered by the filtering properties of normal lung tissue. Normal lung tissue acts as a low-pass filter, which means it preferentially passes low-frequency sounds. This filtering effect is evident when one listens over the periphery of the lung while a subject speaks. The muffled voice sounds are difficult to understand because of low-pass filtering.

This filtering explains the characteristic differences between bronchial breath sounds heard directly over larger airways and vesicular sounds heard over the lung periphery. Normal vesicular lung sounds essentially are filtered bronchial breath sounds.

Abnormal breath sounds. Bronchial breath sounds are considered abnormal when heard over peripheral lung regions. They may replace the normal vesicular sound when lung tissue increases in density, as in atelectasis and pneumonia. When the normal air-filled lung tissue becomes consolidated, the filtering effect is lost, and similar sounds are heard over large upper airways and the consolidated lung.[22]

Diminished breath sounds. Diminished breath sounds occur when the sound intensity at the site of generation (larger airways) is reduced, or when the sound transmission through the lung or chest wall is decreased. Sound intensity is reduced with shallow or slow breathing patterns. Obstructed airways and hyperinflated lung tissue inhibit normal transmission of sounds through the lungs. Air or fluid in the pleural space and obesity reduce sounds transmission through the chest wall.

In patients with chronic airflow obstruction, normal breath sound intensity often is reduced markedly throughout all lung fields. This is the result of poor sound transmission through hyperinflated lung tissue, as occurs with emphysema. Shallow breathing patterns also contribute to decreased breath sounds in patients with COPD.

In fact, research studies indicate that a definite, diffuse reduction in breath sounds is strong evidence that obstructive pulmonary disease is present (as indicated by decreased expiratory flow rates).[23-25] Normal breath sound intensity heard throughout the lung nearly excludes the possibility of COPD. Mild reductions in breath sound intensity are less predictive.

Wheezes and rhonchi. Wheezes and some rhonchi represent vibrations caused when air flows at high velocity through a narrowed or compressed airway.[20,22] Airway diameter can be reduced by bronchospasm, mucosal edema, and foreign objects. The pitch of a wheeze is directly related to the degree of narrowing, but independent of airway length. The greater the narrowing, the higher the pitch. Low-pitched continuous sounds (rhonchi) often are associated with the presence of excessive secretions in the airways. A sputum flap vibrating in the airstream may produce rhonchi that clear after the patient coughs.

The significance of expiratory wheezing during unforced breathing has been studied, and several useful conclusions have been reached. Patients with chronic airflow obstruction who do not wheeze are not likely to show improvement in expiratory flows (measured by spirometry) after bronchodilator treatment. Patients with chronic airflow obstruction who do wheeze are more likely to show improvement after bronchodilator administration. When unforced expiratory wheezing is intense, spirometry consistently demonstrates moderate to severe airway obstruction. Less intense wheezing is associated with a wide range of obstructive defects.[26] Wheezing occurring during *forced* expiration is of little or no predictive value.[26]

It is also useful to monitor the pitch and duration of wheezing.[27] Improved expiratory flow is associated with a drop in the pitch and length of the wheezing. For example, if wheezing is present during both inspiration and expiration before treatment, but occurs only late in exhalation after therapy, the degree of airway obstruction has decreased.[23]

Wheezing may be monophonic (single note) or polyphonic (multiple notes). A single monophonic wheeze indicates that a single airway is partially obstructed. Monophonic wheezing may be heard during inhalation and exhalation or only during exhalation. Polyphonic wheezing suggests that many airways are obstructed, as with asthma, and is heard only during exhalation.

Crackles. Crackles can occur when airflow causes movement of excessive secretions or fluid in the airways. In this situation, crackles are usually coarse and heard during inspiration and expiration. These crackles often clear when the patient coughs and may be associated with rhonchial fremitus.

Crackles also may be heard in patients without excess secretions. These crackles occur when collapsed airways pop open during inspiration.[20,28-31] Airway collapse or closure can occur in peripheral bronchioles or in larger, more proximal bronchi.

Larger, more proximal bronchi may close during expiration when there is an abnormal increase in bronchial compliance or the retractile pressures around the bronchi are low. In this situation crackles usually occur early in the inspiratory phase and are referred to as *early inspiratory crackles* (Figure 16-20). Early inspiratory crackles are usually scanty (few in number) but may be loud or faint. They often are transmitted to the mouth and are not silenced by a cough or change in position. They most often occur in patients with COPD (chronic bronchitis, emphysema, and asthma) and usually indicate a severe airway obstruction.[25]

Peripheral alveoli and airways may close during exhalation when the surrounding intrathoracic pressure increases. Crackles produced by the sudden opening of peripheral airways usually occur late in the inspiratory phase and are referred to as *late-inspiratory crackles*. They are more common in the dependent lung regions, where the peripheral airways are most prone to collapse during exhalation. They often are identified in several consecutive respiratory cycles, producing a recurrent rhythm. They may clear with changes in posture, or if the patient performs several deep inspirations. Coughing or maximal exhalation by the patient may cause late inspiratory crackles to reappear. Late-inspiratory crackles are most common in patients with respiratory disorders that reduce lung volume. These disorders include atelectasis, pneumonia, pulmonary edema, and fibrosis (Table 16-4 on page 384).[29]

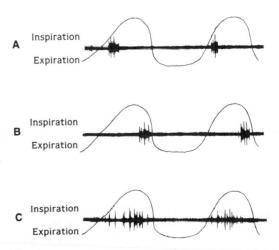

Fig. 16-20 Timing of inspiratory crackles. **A,** Early inspiratory crackles. **B,** Late inspiratory crackles. **C,** Paninspiratory crackles.

Table 16-4   Application of adventitious lung sounds

Lung sounds	Possible mechanism	Characteristics	Causes
Wheezes	Rapid airflow through obstructed airways caused by bronchospasm, mucosal edema	High-pitched; most often occur during exhalation	Asthma, congestive heart failure, bronchitis
Stridor	Rapid airflow through obstructed airway caused by inflammation	High-pitched; often occurs during inhalation	Croup, **epiglottitis,** postextubation
Crackles			
Inspiratory and expiratory	Excess airway secretions moving with airflow	Coarse and often clear with cough	Bronchitis, respiratory infections
Early inspiratory	Sudden opening of proximal bronchi	Scanty, transmitted to mouth; not affected by cough	Bronchitis, emphysema, asthma
Late inspiratory	Sudden opening of peripheral airways	Diffuse, fine; occur initially in the dependent regions	Atelectasis, pneumonia, pulmonary edema, fibrosis

Although inspiratory crackles are considered abnormal, they can occur in normal individuals in certain situations.[32-33] Fine inspiratory crackles can be identified in normal subjects during inhalation from low lung volumes (after maximal exhalation). In addition, an end-expiratory cough may cause late inspiratory crackles that were not present after a normal expiration to appear. Since crackles can be elicited from normal subjects during inspiration from low lung volumes, they are not necessarily abnormal lung sounds. Perhaps fine, late inspiratory crackles should be considered abnormal only when they occur during inhalation from a resting lung volume.

Pleural friction rub. A pleural friction rub is a creaking or grating type of sound that occurs when the pleural surfaces become inflamed and the roughened edges rub together during breathing, as in pleurisy. It may be heard only during inhalation but often is identified during both phases of breathing. Pleural friction rubs often sound similar to coarse crackles but are not affected by coughing. The intensity of pleural rubs may increase with deep breathing.

Voice sounds. If chest inspection, palpation, percussion, or auscultation suggests any abnormality, vocal resonance is assessed. Vocal resonance is produced by the same mechanism as vocal fremitus, described earlier. Vibrations created by the vocal cords during speech travel down the airways and through the peripheral lung units to the chest wall. The patient is instructed to repeat the words "one, two, three" or "ninety-nine" while the RCP listens with a stethoscope over the chest wall, comparing side to side. The normal, air-filled lung tissue filters the voice sounds, producing a significant reduction in intensity and clarity. Pathologic abnormalities in lung tissue alter the transmission of voice sounds, causing either increased or decreased vocal resonance.

Bronchophony. An increase in intensity and clarity of vocal resonance produced by enhanced transmission of vocal vibrations is called *bronchophony*. Bronchophony indicates increased lung tissue density, as occurs in the consolidation phase of pneumonia. Bronchophony is easier to detect when it is unilateral. It often accompanies bronchial breath sounds, a dull percussion note, and increased vocal fremitus.

Vocal resonance is reduced when the transmission of voice sounds through the lung or chest wall is impeded. Hyperinflation, pneumothorax, bronchial obstruction, and pleural effusion all impede transmission of voice sounds and decrease vocal resonance. Decreased vocal resonance usually occurs together with reduced breath sounds and decreased tactile fremitus.

Egophony. When the spoken voice increases in intensity and its character takes on a nasal or bleating quality, it is referred to as *egophony*. Egophony may be identified over areas of the chest where bronchophony is present. The exact reason for this change in voice-sound character is unknown. It is identified most easily when the patient says "e-e-e." If egophony is present, the "e-e-e" will be heard over the peripheral chest wall with the stethoscope as a "a-a-a." Egophony usually is identified only over an area of compressed lung above a pleural effusion.

Whispering pectoriloquy. Whispering pectoriloquy may be a helpful physical finding, especially in patients with small or patchy areas of lung consolidation. The patient is instructed to whisper the words "one, two, three" while the RCP listens over the lung periphery with a stethoscope, comparing side with side. Whispering creates high-frequency vibrations that are filtered out selectively by normal lung tissue and normally heard as muffled, low-pitched sounds. However, when consolidation is present, the lung loses its selective transmission quality, and the characteristic high-pitched sounds are transmitted to the chest wall with clarity.

EXAMINATION OF THE PRECORDIUM

Chronic diseases of the lungs are often associated with other body system abnormalities. Recognition of these other abnormalities can help identify both the respiratory disorder present and its severity. Because of the close working relationship between the heart and lungs, the heart is especially at risk in developing problems secondary to lung disease.

The techniques for physical examination of the chest wall overlying the heart, or *precordium,* include inspection, palpation, and auscultation. Percussion is of little value. Most clinicians examine the precordium at the same time they assess the lungs.

Review of heart topography

The heart lies between the lungs within the mediastinum. The upper portion of the heart, consisting of the atria, is referred to as the *base.* The base lies directly beneath the upper-middle portion of the body of the sternum. The lower portion of the heart, which consists of the ventricles, is called the *apex.* The apex points downward and to the left, extending to a point near the midclavicular line. It usually lies directly beneath the lower left portion of the corpus sterni and near the costal cartilage of the fifth rib (Figure 16-21).

Inspection and palpation

Inspection and palpation of the precordium help identify normal or abnormal pulsations. Pulsations on the precordium are affected by the strength of ventricular contraction, the thickness of the chest wall, and the quality of the tissue through which the vibrations must travel. An apical impulse is produced by the thrust of the contracting left ventricle. This impulse travels through the chest wall to produce a visible bulging during systole. This bulging is called the *point of maximal impulse* (PMI). In normal individuals, the PMI can be felt and visualized near the left midclavicular line in the fifth intercostal space.

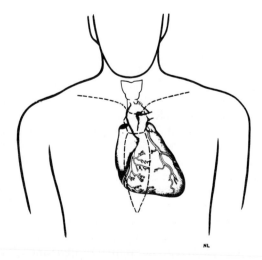

NL

Fig. 16-21 Topographic position of heart.

Right ventricular hypertrophy, a common manifestation of chronic lung disease, often produces a systolic thrust that is felt and possibly visualized near the lower left sternal border. The palmar aspect of the RCP's right hand is placed over the lower left sternal border for identification. Right ventricular hypertrophy may be the result of chronic hypoxemia, pulmonary valve disease, or pulmonary hypertension.

In patients with chronic pulmonary hyperinflation (emphysema), the PMI may be difficult to locate. As a result of the increase in anteroposterior (AP) diameter and the changes in lung tissue, systolic vibrations are not well transmitted to the chest's surface.

The PMI may shift to the left or right, following deviations in the position of the mediastinum. Pneumothorax or lobar collapse can cause a shift in the mediastinum. Typically, the PMI shifts toward lobar collapse, but away from a pneumothorax. The PMI in patients with emphysema and low flat diaphragms may be located in the **epigastric** area.

The second left intercostal space near the sternal border is referred to as the *pulmonic area* and is palpated in an effort to identify accentuated pulmonary valve closure. Strong vibrations may be felt in this area with pulmonary hypertension or valvular abnormalities (Figure 16-22, page 386).

Auscultation of heart sounds

Normal heart sounds are created by the closure of the heart valves (see Chapter 10). The first heart sound (S1) is produced by closure of the mitral and tricuspid valves (AV) during contraction of the ventricles. When systole ends, the ventricles relax and the semilunar valves (pulmonic and aortic) close, creating the second heart sound (S2). As a result of the higher pressures in the left heart, mitral valve closure is louder and contributes more to S1 than closure of the tricuspid valve. For the same reason closure of the aortic valve usually is more significant in producing S2. If the AV or semilunar valves do not close together, a split heart sound is heard. A slight splitting of S2 is normal and occurs in association with breathing. The normal splitting of S2 is increased during inhalation because of the decrease in intrathoracic pressure, which improves venous return to the right side of the heart and further delays pulmonic valve closure.

A third heart sound (S3) may be identified during diastole. S3 is thought to be produced by rapid ventricular filling immediately after systole. The rapid distension of the ventricles causes the walls of the ventricles to vibrate and produce a sound of low intensity and pitch. It is best heard over the apex. In young, healthy children an S3 is considered normal and called a physiologic S3. Otherwise, an S3 is abnormal. For example, in an older patient with a history of heart disease, an S3 may signify **myocardial infarction.**

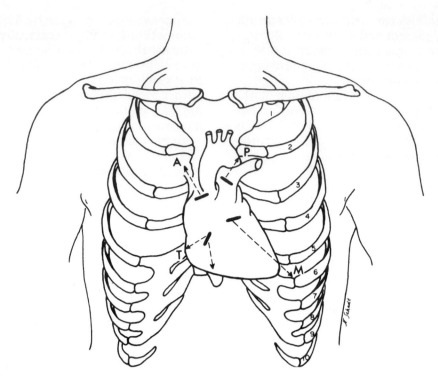

Fig. 16-22 Anatomic and auscultatory valve area. Location of anatomic valve sites is respresented by solid bars. Arrows designate transmission of valve sounds to their respective auscultatory valve areas. *M,* Mitral valve; *T,* tricuspid valve; *A,* aortic valve; *P,* pulmonic valve. (From Prior JA, Silberstein JS, and Stang JM: Physical diagnosis: the history and examination of the patient, ed 6, St Louis, 1982, Mosby.)

A fourth heart sound (S4) is produced by mechanisms similar to those of S3. It may occur in normal individuals or be considered a sign of heart disease. S4 is different from S3 only in its timing during the cardiac cycle. S4 occurs later, just before S1, whereas S3 occurs just after S2.

During auscultation of the heart, alterations in the loudness of either S1 or S2 may be present. Reduced intensity of heart sounds may be due to cardiac or extracardiac abnormalities. Extracardiac factors include alteration in the tissue between the heart and the surface of the chest. Pulmonary hyperinflation, pleural effusion, pneumothorax, and obesity make identification of both S1 and S2 difficult. S1 and S2 intensity also decreases when the force of ventricular contraction is poor, as in heart failure, or when valvular abnormalities exist.

Pulmonary hypertension produces an increased intensity of S2. This "P2" sound is due to more forceful closure of the pulmonic valve. A lack of S2 splitting with inhalation also may be the result of pulmonary hypertension. An increased P2 is identified best over the pulmonic area of the chest.

Cardiac murmurs are identified whenever the heart valves are incompetent or stenotic. Murmurs usually are classified as either systolic or diastolic. Systolic murmurs are produced by an incompetent AV valve or a stenotic semilunar valve. An incompetent AV valve allows a backflow of blood into the atrium, usually producing a high-pitched "whooshing" noise simultaneously with S1. A stenotic semilunar valve produces a similar sound created by an obstruction of blood flow out of the ventricle during systole.

Diastolic murmurs are created by an incompetent semilunar valve or a stenotic AV valve. An incompetent semilunar valve allows a back flow of blood into the ventricle simultaneously with or immediately after S2. A stenotic AV valve obstructs blood flow from the atrium into the ventricles during diastole and creates a turbulent murmur.

A murmur also may be created by rapid blood flow across normal valves. In summary, murmurs are created by: (1) a back flow of blood through an incompetent valve, (2) a forward flow through a stenotic valve, and (3) a rapid flow through a normal valve.

Heart sounds are usually auscultated together with lung sounds. The bell and diaphragm pieces of the stethoscope are used. The heart sounds may be easier to identify by requesting that the patient lean forward or lie on the left side, since this anatomically moves the heart closer to the chest wall. When the peripheral pulses are difficult to identify, auscultation over the precordium may provide an easier method of identifying the heart rate. In addition, RCPs must sometimes compare the rate as heard over the precordium (the apical rate) to the palpated peripheral pulse. Normally, these two rates are the same. However, there are times when the apical rate is higher than the peripheral pulse. This sign, called a *pulse deficit,* is common in atrial fibrillation. Because atrial fibrillation causes an irregular rhythm, some ventricular contractions are too weak to be felt at peripheral locations.

EXAMINATION OF THE ABDOMEN

An in-depth discussion of examining the abdomen is beyond the scope of this text; however, a review of the findings associated with respiratory diseases is presented.

The abdomen should be inspected and palpated for evidence of distension and tenderness. Abdominal distension and pain impair diaphragm movement and contribute to respiratory insufficiency or failure; they also may inhibit the patient from coughing and deep breathing. The ability to deep breathe and cough is extremely important in preventing postoperative respiratory complications.

Typically, the right upper quadrant of the abdomen is palpated and percussed to estimate the size of the liver (Figure 16-23). Among its many causes, an enlarged liver may be seen in patients with chronic right-sided heart failure occurring secondary to

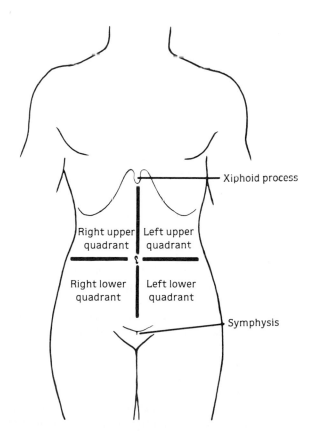

Fig. 16-23 Division of abdomen into quadrants. (From Prior JA, Silberstein JS, and Stang JM: Physical diagnosis: the history and examination of the patient, ed 6, St Louis, 1982, Mosby.)

chronic respiratory disease. In such cases, venous return to the heart is reduced, and engorgement of major veins and organs may occur. The hepatic vein that empties into the inferior vena cava may become engorged in this situation, and the liver increases in size. This is called *hepatomegaly.*

To identify hepatomegaly, the superior and inferior borders of the liver are identified by percussion. Normally, the liver spans about 10 cm at the midclavicular line. If it extends more than 10 cm, it is considered enlarged.

EXAMINATION OF THE EXTREMITIES

Respiratory disease may cause several abnormalities of the extremities. These include digital clubbing, cyanosis, and pedal edema. Each is discussed briefly.

Clubbing

Clubbing of the digits is a significant manifestation of cardiopulmonary disease (refer to Chapter 15). The mechanism responsible for clubbing is not known. It is identified most commonly in patients with bronchogenic carcinoma, COPD, and chronic cardiovascular disease.

Clubbing is a painless enlargement of the terminal phalanges of the fingers and toes that develops over years. As the process advances, the angle of the fingernail to the nail base increases and the base of the nail feels "spongy." The profile view of the digits allows easier recognition of clubbing (Figure 16-24, page 388).

Cyanosis

The digits also should be examined for the presence or absence of cyanosis. Because of the transparency of the fingernails and skin, cyanosis can be detected easily here.

Cyanosis becomes visible to most observers when the amount of reduced hemoglobin in the capillary blood exceeds 5 to 6 g/dL.[34] This may be due to a reduction in either arterial or venous oxygen content or both. When the arterial hemoglobin saturation drops to 75% or less (equivalent to a PO_2 of 40 torr or less),[35] cyanosis is seen by most observers in the mucous membranes of the lips and mouth, as well as the fingers. This type of cyanosis is called *central cyanosis.*

In peripheral cyanosis, the SaO_2 need not be reduced. Peripheral cyanosis is due mainly to poor blood flow, especially in the extremities. When capillary blood flow is poor, the tissues extract more oxygen, lowering the venous O_2 content and raising the amount of reduced hemoglobin. This also results in cyanosis, although the cause differs from that of the central type. Moreover, peripheral cyanosis tends to

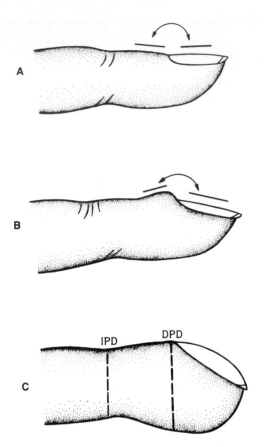

Fig. 16-24 A, Normal digit configuration. **B,** Mild digital clubbing with increased hyponychial angle. **C,** Severe digital clubbing; depth of finger at base of nail (*DPD*) is greater than depth of interpharyngeal joint (*IPD*) with clubbing.

be localized to the extremities; central cyanosis can appear in any visible capillary bed. When observed together with coolness of the extremities, peripheral cyanosis is a sign of circulatory failure. Central cyanosis, on the other hand, indicates arterial hypoxemia caused by a problem in gas exchange at the lung.

The intensity of cyanosis increases with the hemoglobin content. For this reason, patients with a high hemoglobin content (polycythemia) can be cyanotic yet still have adequate arterial oxygen content. Conversely, patients with low hemoglobin content (anemia) can be severely hypoxic before cyanosis ever appears. Additionally, not all hypoxic states produce cyanosis (refer to Chapter 15). Thus cyanosis is a physical sign to be noted, but not awaited.[34]

Pedal edema

Some patients with chronic respiratory disease have pedal edema. Since hypoxemia produces pulmonary vasoconstriction, the right ventricle must work harder than normal whenever significant hypoxemia exists. This chronic increase in right ventricular workload can result in right ventricular hypertrophy and poor venous return to the heart. When return flow to the

right heart is reduced, the peripheral veins engorge. This causes fluid to build up in **dependent** tissues, especially the ankles. This physical sign is called *pedal edema.*

The ankles most often are affected, since they are in a gravity dependent position throughout most of the day. The edematous tissues "pit" or indent when pressed firmly with a finger. The height at which pitting edema occurs can indicate the severity of right-sided heart failure. For example, pitting edema above the knee signifies a more significant problem that edema around the ankles only.

Capillary refill

Capillary refill can be assessed by pressing firmly for a brief period on the fingernail and noting the speed at which the blood flow returns. When cardiac output is reduced and digital perfusion is poor, capillary refill is slow, taking several seconds to complete. In normal individuals with good cardiac output and digital perfusion, capillary refill time is less than 3 seconds.

Peripheral skin temperature

When the heart fails to circulate enough blood, compensatory vasoconstriction in the extremities helps shunt blood to the vital organs (see Chapter 10). This reduction in peripheral perfusion causes the extremities to become cool. Palpation of the patient's feet and hands may provide general information about perfusion. Cool extremities usually indicate poor perfusion.

Actual extremity temperature can be measured and compared to room temperature. The extremity should be at least 2° C warmer than room temperature (unless room temperature is equal to or greater than body temperature). When there is less than a 2° C difference, perfusion is reduced; 0.5° C differences indicate that the patient has serious perfusion problems.

CHAPTER SUMMARY

The history and physical examination are inexpensive and quick methods to help identify important clinical abnormalities of the cardiopulmonary system. The initial evaluation of the patient with acute disease, needing rapid assessment and treatment, should identify the adequacy of tissue oxygenation and pulmonary function with regard to ventilation and oxygenation.

By themselves, the history and physical examination cannot always confirm a specific diagnosis, but they can suggest certain pathologic abnormalities of the lungs. When the physical findings are considered along with the history and the other diagnostic procedures, a more specific diagnosis can be supported. Table 16-5 summarizes the characteristic findings associated with some of the more common pulmonary disorders.

Table 16-5 Physical signs of abnormal pulmonary pathology

Abnormality	Initial impression	Inspection	Palpation	Percussion	Auscultation	Possible causes
Acute airways obstruction	Appears acutely ill	Use of accessory muscles	Reduced expansion	Increased resonance	Expiratory wheezing	Asthma, bronchitis
Chronic airways obstruction	Appears chronically ill	Increased antero-posterior diameter, use of accessory muscles	Reduced expansion	Increased resonance	Diffuse reduction in breath sounds; early inspiratory crackles	Chronic bronchitis, emphysema
Consolidation	May appear acutely ill	Inspiratory lag	Increased fremitus	Dull note	Bronchial breath sounds; crackles	Pneumonia, tumor
Pneumothorax	May appear acutely ill	Unilateral expansion	Decreased fremitus	Increased resonance	Absent breath sounds	Rib fracture, open wound
Pleural effusion	May appear acutely ill	Unilateral expansion	Absent fremitus	Dull note	Absent breath sounds	Congestive heart failure
Local bronchial obstruction	Appears acutely ill	Unilateral expansion	Absent fremitus	Dull note	Absent breath sounds	Mucous plug
Diffuse interstitial fibrosis	Often normal	Rapid shallow breathing	Often normal; increased fremitus	Slight decrease in resonance	Late inspiratory crackles	Chronic exposure to inorganic dust
Acute upper airway obstruction	Appears acutely ill	Labored breathing	Often normal	Often normal	Inspiratory or expiratory stridor or both	Epiglottitis, croup, foreign body aspiration

REFERENCES

1. Krider SJ: Interviewing and the respiratory history. In Wilkins RL, Sheldon RL, Krider SJ, editors: *Clinical assessment in respiratory care,* ed 2, St Louis, 1990, Mosby.
2. Mackowiak PA, Wasserman SS, Levine MM: A critical appraisal of 98.6 degrees F, the upper limit of the normal body temperature, and other legacies of Carl Reinhold August Wunderlich, *JAMA* 268(12):1578-1580, 1992.
3. Hasler ME, Cohen JA: The effect of oxygen administration on oral temperature assessment, *Nurs Res* 31:265, 1982.
4. Lim-Levy F: The effect of oxygen inhalation on oral temperature, *Nurs Res* 31:151, 1982.
5. Gravelyn TR, Weg JG: Respiratory rate as an indicator of acute respiratory dysfunction, *JAMA* 244:1123, 1980.
6. Anderson CL, Chankar PS, Scott JH: Physiological significance of sternomastoid muscle contraction in chronic obstructive pulmonary disease, *Respir Care* 25:937, 1980.
7. Cohen CA et al: Clinical manifestations of inspiratory muscle fatigue, *Am J Med* 73:308, 1982.
8. Mier-Jedrzejowicz A et al: Assessment of diaphragm weakness, *Am Rev Respir Dis* 137:877, 1988.
9. Wilkins RL, Olfert M, Specht L: Chest percussion for resonance is not routinely used by respiratory care practitioners, *Respir Care* 38:1218, 1993 (abstract).
10. Williams TJ, Ahmand D, Morgan WK: A clinical and roentgenographic correlation of diaphragmatic movement, *Arch Intern Med* 141:878, 1981.
11. Wilkins RL, Olfert M, Specht L: Survey of respiratory care practitioners for the perceived value of chest auscultation, *Respir Care* 38:1218, 1993 (abstract).
12. Murphy RLH, Holford E, Knowler W: Visual lung sound characterization by time-expanded waveform analysis, *N Engl J Med* 296:968, 1977.
13. Andrews JL, Badger TL: Lung sounds through the ages, *JAMA* 241:2625, 1979.
14. Report of the ACCP-ATS Joint Committee on Pulmonary Nomenclature, *Chest* 67:583, 1975.
15. Report of the ATS-ACCP Ad Hoc Subcommittee on Pulmonary Nomenclature, *ATS News* 35, 1977.
16. Report of the ATS-ACCP Ad Hoc Subcommittee on Pulmonary Nomenclature, *ATS News* 28, 1981.
17. Wilkins RL, Dexter JR, Smith JR: Survey of adventitious should terminology in case reports, *Chest* 85:523, 1984.
18. Wilkins RL et al: Lung sound nomenclature survey, *Chest* 98:886-889, 1990.
19. Wilkins RL, Dexter JR: Comparing RCPs to physicians for the description of lung sounds: are we accurate and can we communicate: *Respir Care* 35:969-976, 1990.
20. Forgacs P: The functional basis of pulmonary sounds, *Chest* 73:399, 1978.
21. Murphy RLH, Holford SK: Lung sounds, *Basics RD,* 8:1980.
22. Donnerberg RL et al: Sounds transfer function of the congested canine lung, *Br J Dis Chest* 74:23, 1980.
23. Bohadana AB, Peslin R, Uffholtz H: Breath sounds in the clinical assessment of airflow obstruction, *Thorax* 33:345, 1978.
24. Pardee NE et al: Combinations of four physical signs as indicators of ventilator abnormality in obstructive pulmonary syndromes, *Chest* 77:354, 1980.
25. Pardee NE, Martin CJ, Morgan EH: A test of the practical value of estimating breath sound intensity, *Chest* 70:341, 1976.
26. Marini JJ et al: The significance of wheezing in chronic airflow obstruction, *Am Rev Respir Dis* 120:1069, 1979.
27. Baughman RP, Loudon RG: Quantification of wheezing in acute asthma, *Chest* 86:718, 1984.
28. Forgacs P: Crackles and wheezes, *Lancet* 2:203, 1967.
29. Nath AR, Capel LH: Inspiratory crackles, early and late, *Thorax* 29:223, 1974.
30. Nath AR, Capel LH: Inspiratory crackles and mechanical events of breathing, *Thorax* 29:695, 1974.
31. Forgacs P: Lung sounds, *Br J Dis Chest* 63:1, 1969.
32. Thacker RE, Kraman SS: The prevalence of auscultatory crackles in subjects without lung disease, *Chest* 81:672, 1982.
33. Workum P et al: The prevalence and character of crackles (rales) in young women without significant lung disease, *Am Rev Respir Dis* 126:921, 1982.
34. Nicholson D: Cyanosis: five grams of history, *Respir Care* 32:113-114, 1987.
35. Med WE et al: Cyanosis as a guide to arterial oxygen saturation, *Thorax* 14:247-250, 1959.

BIBLIOGRAPHY

Bowers AC, Thompson JM: *Clinical manual of health assessment,* ed 4, St Louis, 1992, Mosby.

Cherniack RM, Cherniack L, Naimark A: *Respiration in health and disease,* ed 3, Philadelphia, 1983, WB Saunders.

Forgacs P: *Lung sounds,* London, 1978, Bailliere Tindall.

Judge RD, Zuidema GD: *Methods of clinical examination,* ed 4, Boston, 1982, Little, Brown.

Malasanos L et al: *Health assessment,* ed 4, St Louis, 1990, Mosby.

Prior JA, Silberstein JS: *Physical diagnosis the history and examination of the patient,* ed 6, St Louis, 1982, Mosby.

Seidel HM et al: *Mosby's guide to physical examination,* ed 2, St Louis, 1991, Mosby.

Wilkins RL, Sheldon RL, Krider SJ: *Clinical assessment in respiratory care,* ed 2, St Louis, 1990, Mosby.

Wilkins RL, Hodgkin JE, Lopez B: *Lung sounds: a practical guide,* St Louis, 1988, Mosby.

Analysis of Gas Exchange

■

Theron Van Hooser

CHAPTER LEARNING OBJECTIVES

1. Describe how and why the analysis of arterial blood is the "standard" for gas exchange analysis;
2. Differentiate between laboratory and point of care (POC) invasive blood gas analysis, including three sources of samples (e.g., capillary, percutaneous, and arterial line);
3. Describe the concepts used in point of care gas exchange analysis, including bedside and in vivo systems;
4. Differentiate transcutaneous gas exchange analysis systems from invasive ones;
5. Differentiate expired gas systems from other approaches and describe how these methods can be used to determine gas exchange analysis.

Gas exchange is the movement of gases into and out of the body tissue cells. This exchange is a critical, sometimes delicate balance of pressures, events, and chemical reactions monitored and controlled by several check points. In Chapter 12 of this text the exchange of gas through the various layers of the alveolar/capillary membrane and the transport of those gases to and from the tissues are presented. Gas exchange can be thought of as a system with a loading dock (the lungs), a conveyance mechanism (the cardiovascular system), and an unloading dock (tissue cells). Normally this system is very efficient and provides our bodies with the correct amount of oxygen and removes the wastes (carbon dioxide) quickly in a businesslike manner. In Chapter 15, the various patterns of cardiopulmonary dysfunction and disturbances are explained. These disturbances of normal function can happen quickly and silently. Gas exchange difficulties have significant effects on all normal body function systems and can even cause them to fail completely.

Because the respiratory care practitioner (RCP) is responsible for therapies and interventions that treat and sometimes correct these dysfunctions, a basic understanding of how this gas exchange is analyzed and monitored is important. This chapter explains most of the methods of analysis of gas exchange. Chapter 33 addresses other aspects of monitoring the information provided by the analysis of these systems. The reader is advised to review Chapters 12 and 15 before reading this chapter.

INVASIVE ANALYSIS

For centuries, it was known that the arteries carry oxygenated blood from the heart and lungs to the cells of the body. Early physicians knew that if the amount of oxygen in arterial blood could be determined, then valuable information about how the heart and lungs were working could be gained. Arterial blood gas analysis was the logical place to start in the analysis of gas exchange.

In 1954, Leland Clark developed a blood gas electrode, which initiated a new method of gas exchange analysis.[1] It analyzed the dissolved oxygen in the blood. Three years later John Severinghaus[2] improved a carbon dioxide electrode originally described by Stow[3] and his colleagues. As a result Clark and Severinghaus are considered to be two of the founders of a common tool used millions of times each day, blood gas analysis. The assessment of oxygen and carbon dioxide with modern versions of the Clark and Severinghaus electrodes is so important in the management of the critically ill that it is hard to imagine practicing respiratory care without them. Arterial blood gases (ABGs) were among the first laboratory tests to measure the function of gas exchange and the oxygen delivery system directly and accurately. They have been, and continue to be, the "gold standard" of gas exchange analysis.

ABG analysis is not without problems. A major disadvantage is that it requires **invasive** sampling of arterial blood. A needle must be placed into the artery and a sample withdrawn. This one drawback to ABGs is significant enough that many other systems and noninvasive strategies have been developed, with varying degrees of success. There have been many recent advances in the noninvasive analysis of gas exchange and ABGs. Some of these systems are discussed later in this chapter.

Laboratory evaluations account for about 25% of total critical care costs. ABGs are the most frequently ordered laboratory test in the critical care patient area.[4] Invasive sampling procedures are still the mainstay of modern gas analysis and ABGs remain foremost in most intensive care units (ICUs).

ARTERIAL SAMPLING

Arterial puncture

Acquisition of an arterial blood sample for analysis is an invasive procedure in which a needle penetrates the protective barrier of the skin and directly enters the bloodstream. Therefore, there are problems and precautions associated with the procedure. RCPs are well advised to pay particular attention to all of the steps of this procedure. Invasive procedures are associated with an increased potential for complications, such as infection and trauma. Invasive procedures entail increased discomfort and pain for the patient and are usually more costly than noninvasive methods. Poorly sampled arterial blood can yield erroneous information, necessitating repeat testing or causing errors in patient care planning.

Arterial blood sampling is more difficult and has greater risk than venous sampling. Clot formation, bleeding, vessel spasm, and cross-contamination all are more serious when they occur in an artery rather than a vein. In spite of this, arterial puncture is performed simply, easily, and safely by RCPs, laboratory technologists, nurses, and others millions of times each day.

Puncture site selection

The best artery to select for arterial puncture should be large and superficial (close to the skin) and an easy target. The artery should not lie near veins or nerves, to prevent accidental venous puncture or significant pain. Collateral circulation should be present. Adjacent arteries that can maintain perfusion to the distal limb if an obstruction occurs in the punctured artery should be assessed (Figure 17-1).

The three most common sites for arterial puncture are the radial, brachial, and femoral arteries. Although other sites can be used, these three are usually chosen because of accessibility, comfort, and safety.

The radial and temporal sites are often chosen in the infant. The umbilical arteries are patent during the first 24 to 48 hours after birth. Although the umbilical arteries are the ideal site for sampling in the newborn, they constrict rapidly if they are not kept open by catheterization.

Radial artery

Of all ABG samples 99% are taken from the radial artery, which is the vessel of choice in the adult. Lying on the thumb side of the forearm, it is very accessible because it is superficial and easy to feel. The radial nerve and vein are not close to the artery and collateral circulation is normally good. The radial artery pulsations are easy to feel approximately 1 in from the wrist where the artery passes over the radius. The radial nerve is avoided at this location because it lies below the bone. Radial artery puncture may be painful if the puncture is deep and if the periosteum is pierced.

Before an arterial puncture in the radial artery is performed, the RCP must determine the presence of adequate collateral circulation. Collateral circulation

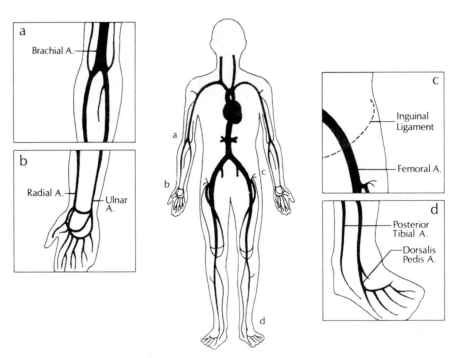

Fig. 17-1 Schematic of collateral circulation. **a,** deep brachial, superior, and inferior ulnar collateral arteries usually provide sufficient flow to the radial and ulnar arteries if the brachial artery is obstructed. **b,** the palmar arches usually provide adequate flow to the hand and fingers when either the ulnar or radial arteries are obstructed. **c,** the deep femoral artery is the only collateral source of flow to the lower extremity—it usually originates well below the level of the inguinal ligament; thus, obstruction to flow in the femoral artery above this point leaves the lower extremity without arterial blood flow. **d,** the arterial arches that provide blood flow to the foot and toes are usually supplied by both the dorsalis pedis and the posterior tibial arteries.

to the hand is via the ulnar artery. Normally, the ulnar artery is able to provide adequate perfusion to the hand if the radial becomes occluded or damaged. In 3% to 5% of the population, ulnar perfusion is either nonexistent or minimal. If adequate collateral circulation is absent, radial artery puncture is not recommended.

Allen test

The most common technique used to determine the adequacy of ulnar circulation is the modified Allen test.[5] The modification of the original test is commonly used to evaluate the adequacy of ulnar circulation. Ulnar circulation can also be assessed with a Doppler ultrasonic flow indicator.

To perform a modified Allen test, ask the patient to extend the arm. The RCP should locate and occlude both the radial and ulnar arteries tightly. Ask the patient to make a tight fist with the hand; then release the ulnar artery and watch the blanched skin in the palm of the hand fill with blood and regain color. The time of the fill should be mentally noted. Next, ask the patient to make a fist again; this time, release the radial artery and mentally compare the time and quality of blood flow into the skin of the palm again. If the radial fills faster, this is normal. If when the ulnar is released, the palm does not flush or flushes extremely slowly, another site should be selected.

Brachial artery

The brachial artery is usually the second choice when the radial arteries are unsuitable. The brachial artery is the major artery of the lower arm. It divides into the radial and ulnar branches just below the elbow. This artery is large and can be palpated a short distance above the bend of the elbow on the internal surface of the arm where it passes over the humerus.

To locate the artery, extend the arm completely, and rotate the wrist outward until the strongest pulse is obtained just above the elbow crease. If this artery is chosen, caution should be exercised to prevent puncture of the median nerve, which will cause intense pain. Venous puncture may also occur accidentally because of the presence of important large veins in this area.

Femoral artery

The femoral artery may be felt just below the **inguinal** ligament. The patient should be lying flat and supine with the knee slightly bent and the foot rotated slightly outward. The femoral artery is the least desirable of the three puncture sites. It has a large diameter and is therefore an easy target. The artery is deeper than it appears to be. Because it is approximately the size of the patient's little finger, the pulse is usually strong and bounding. Therefore, it appears to be nearer the skin than it actually is. A 1.5 inch needle is recommended. Complications of a femoral puncture can be serious. Large quantities of blood may seep from this vessel and may be undetected for a time because the tissues of the leg may be able to absorb large quantities of blood. In addition, **atherosclerotic** plaques are common in this area. These plaques may dislodge, leading to distal occlusion. The femoral artery has almost no collateral circulation; therefore, puncture should be reserved for emergencies. In extreme hypotension this may be the only choice.

Normal ABG ranges

The various parameters shown in Table 17-1 are reported for most blood gas laboratory tests.[6] The values of these parameters are referred to collectively as arterial blood gases (ABGs). High and low normal ranges for adults are also shown. Normal ranges mean that 95% of the normal population have values that fall within this range. Normal values are determined by each laboratory; they are based on the population it serves. Normal values are established by measurements made on normal individuals. The average value is calculated as well as the dispersion, or "spread," of values. The statistical term for "spread" is *standard deviation.* In a normal population, 68% of individuals have ABG values that fall within 1 standard deviation and 95% within 2 standard deviations; 99.73% of measurements fall within 3 standard deviations. One should note that the values in Table 17-1 are those at sea level; PaO_2 and SaO_2 'normals' are lower for populations living at high altitude.

Normal laboratory ranges are 2 standard deviations from the mean because these values represent the majority of the population. It is important to understand that 5% of the normal population has values that fall outside the normal range.

Units of measurement

Units of measurement are involved in the every usage of ABGs. Respiratory care practitioners, however, sometimes use terms loosely even when they are not. For example, although PO_2 is different from PaO_2, the terms are used interchangeably. A review of the units is wise to ensure accurate and concise interpretation of the information given by the ABG report.

The PaO_2 and $PaCO_2$ are measured in millimeters of mercury (mm Hg). "Torr" is sometimes used in place of mm Hg. These two units are identical and can be used interchangeably. (Torricelli was an Italian

Table 17-1   Normal blood gas values

	pH	$PaCO_2$	HCO_3	BE	Hb	PaO_2	SaO_2
High	7.45	45	26	+2	18	100	97
Low	7.35	35	22	−2	12	80	93

From Pagana KD, Pagana TJ: Mosby's diagnostic and laboratory test reference, St Louis, 1992, Mosby.

physicist who studied the measurement of gases in solution.)

The International System of Units (SI) has attempted to standardize the reporting of all scientific data. The recommended SI unit for pressure is the pascal (Pa). Because this unit is too small for clinical use, the kilopascal (kPa) is used for measurement of blood gases. The conversion factor from millimeters of mercury (mm Hg) to kilopascals (kPa) is 0.133. A normal PaO_2 of 80 to 100 mm Hg is thus equivalent to 10.6 to 13.3 kPa. A normal $PaCO_2$ of 35 to 45 mm Hg is thus equivalent to 4.6 to 6 kPa. The decimal has made general usage awkward and most laboratories continue to use mm Hg or torr.

The pH value is a numerical scale. SaO_2 is measured as a percentage. The [HCO3] and [BE] are usually reported in milliequivalents per liter (mEq/L), which is equal to millimoles per liter (mmol/L) in ions with an equivalent charge such as $HCO3^-$ and Na^+. The mmol/L unit is also used by some laboratories.

Complications

A serious, although uncommon complication of arterial puncture is *thrombosis*. Thrombosis is the formation of an abnormal clot within the vessel with a reduction of blood flow. Hemorrhage is also a possibility, particularly for patients who are receiving anticoagulant therapy or have coagulation problems. The leakage of blood into the tissues, known as *hematoma,* is not unusual. Elderly individuals may lack sufficient elastic tissue to seal the puncture site and are therefore more prone to hematoma.

Pain or anxiety may cause arteriospasm reflex. Other complications include infection and peripheral nerve damage. Occasionally, vascular and vagal (vasovagal) responses happen. These responses cause precordial distress, anxiety, feeling of impending doom, nausea, and respiratory difficulty. Even with all of these possibilities, the overall incidence of complication with arterial puncture is low. Arterial puncture is a safe, simple procedure that can be done by qualified RCPs and other health care personnel.[7-9]

Materials

The availability of disposable "blood gas kits" proliferated greatly in the 1980s. Lists of materials needed to perform an arterial puncture vary because hospitals and other employers select particular brands or kits on the basis of price and utilization standards. The following review of why particular components are included emphasizes the importance of each item to be used.

Syringe

Although the debate over glass versus plastic syringes seemed to be settled years ago,[10,11] glass is still preferred by many clinicians given the choice. The low friction between the syringe barrel and plunger offered by a glass syringe has been closely matched by most modern ABG kit syringes.

Unwanted air bubbles are more difficult to remove from a plastic syringe. Either way, the syringe must be capable of filling from the arterial pressure alone, since force from manual aspiration can introduce error, slippage and possible injury to the artery.

Anticoagulant

Even microclots can affect the function of modern blood gas analyzers. Sample size needed for actual exposure to the electrodes has decreased dramatically over the years: 1,000 units/mL of liquid sodium heparin has been the standard for years.[12,13] Because of the sample size and electrode function, lithium heparin is now used in most kits. Dry heparin (lyophilized) is common and has largely replaced the "fill the deadspace of the needle, and squirt out the rest" method of heparin volume measurement.

Needles

Short bevel 20 or 22 gauge needles with a clear hub (in order to visualize flash when entering the artery) has become the standard. Lengths vary from 5/8 to 1-1/2 inches. Longer needles are needed for both brachial and femoral sites. Some kits provide both short and long needles. Children and infants are sampled with a 25 gauge needle.

Needle cap or plug

It was once commonplace to remove the needle with the hands, replace with a cap, insert it into a rubber plug, or even bend it in half. However, Centers for Disease Control (CDC) recommendations for prevention of exposure to blood prohibit touching or recapping needles, to reduce inadvertent sticks. Various kits have various methods to plug or otherwise prevent sample exposure to air. These safeguard methods are designed for the protection of the practitioner *and should not, under any circumstances, be ignored* (see Chapter 4).

Procedure preparation

Before any arterial puncture, the clinician should be aware of several items. The box below provides a list of items to review before arterial puncture. It is mandatory for any respiratory care practitioner who prepares a patient for ABG analysis to have at least three cognitive abilities: the ability to review and understand the patient's medical record, the ability to perform and interpret assessment skills, and a functional understanding of the institution's infection control policies and procedures. Medical history, current status, and current anticoagulant and other drug therapy can be determined from the progress notes and other portions of the medical record.

Prearterial puncture checklist

Patient's primary diagnosis
Current status
Respiratory care (oxygen therapy, mechanical ventilation)
Anticoagulant therapy status
Bleeding disorder history
Vital signs and clinical inspection of patient
Appropriate infection control procedures

Documenting current status. Many times the individual who interprets and applies information from the blood gas report is not the same individual who gathered the sample. It is important that all pertinent information regarding the patient's status at the time of the sample be recorded. Correct decisions and therapy changes can only be made if conditions at the time of sampling are known. At least 10 points should be recorded to establish current status:

1. Time and date of sample
2. Patient name and identity number
3. Site at which sample was drawn
4. Name or initials of individual obtaining sample
5. Patient position at time of sample
6. Patient activity at time of sample
7. Type of oxygen therapy and flow or FIO_2
8. Mechanical ventilation data
   a. Pressures (peak and end-expiratory pressure [PEEP])
   b. Tidal volume
   c. SpO_2 (pulse oximeter reading)
   d. $PETO_2$ (end tidal carbon dioxide)
   e. Transcutaneous monitor readings
9. Vital signs (spontaneous respiratory rate, pulse, and temperature)
10. Results of Allen test (radial puncture)

Although not all these items are appropriate to record in all situations, bedside assessment of the respiratory status, inspired oxygen, respiratory rate, and ventilatory parameters is extremely important. All of these factors should be noted appropriately in the medical record, paperwork, or computer. These items are even more critical when the clinician drawing the sample will not be making the interpretation, even when computerized interpretations are used. If the RCP does not record all these factors, delay or misinterpretation may result. This is especially true if another individual is interpreting the test result.

Infection control[14]

Functional knowledge of infection control policies means that the individual performing the invasive puncture knows how and why to protect both himself or herself and the patient. Because of the types of serious infections which may be transmitted by body fluids, especially blood, universal precautions guidelines should be strictly followed. The RCP should know whether the patient has an infectious disease that may be transmitted by contact with blood. Currently acquired immunodeficiency syndrome (AIDS) is the most commonly thought of disease when infection control is mentioned. AIDS, caused by the human immunodeficiency virus (HIV), can be contracted by contact with the body secretions of an infected individual. The greatest amount of the virus is contained in blood, semen, and vaginal secretions. It may be transmitted percutaneously through the skin and mucous membranes or through cuts, open wounds, or needle punctures. The risk that RCPs may acquire the disease is directly related to the potential for percutaneous exposure or mucous membrane contact with contaminated body secretions. That risk is indirectly related to how well the RCP understands and follows published universal precautions during the sampling and analysis of ABGs. These risks mean that any blood sample from any patient should be treated with full precautions, as if it were known to be contaminated.

Although our attention is on AIDS, there are other serious infectious that should be guarded against, including types A and B viral hepatitis, syphilis, and **septicemia.** Universal precautions require diligent hand washing and use of gloves during arterial blood gas sampling. The CDC recommends the use of masks and protective eyewear to prevent contact with mucous membranes during any procedure likely to generate droplets of blood. Gloves should always be worn when acquiring an ABG sample, keeping in mind that they are an adjunct to, but not a substitute for, hand washing.

To aid the RCP, the American Association for Respiratory Care has published a Clinical Practice Guideline for blood gas analysis.[15]

Radial puncture technique

Steady state. Using an ABG analysis result to determine the ongoing state of gas exchange is similar to using an instant camera to capture a single picture of all the children on a school bus on the way to school. In order to snap a single picture with everyone in it, the photographer must wait until all children have entered the bus and taken their seats and no children are getting on or off the bus. In other words, the bus is in a steady state. Likewise, the RCP must determine that the patient (bus) is in a steady state before obtaining the ABG specimen (snapping the picture). The sample should be drawn only after all changes have been made and the patient's condition has become stable.

Blood gas information often is the major criterion on which therapeutic decisions regarding mechanical ventilation, oxygenation, and acid-base disturbances are made. "Wait 20 minutes and get a blood gas sample" is probably the most common verbal order given in the ICU. It is of utmost importance that this information be able to provide an accurate reflection of the patient's current status. Anytime a patient's status changes or therapy is modified a period of adjustment is necessary to allow the effects of the changes to be reflected in the blood gases. Once the cardiopulmonary system has adapted to the new setting or change and the patient has reached a new "steady state," the blood will accurately reflect the results of that change. ABG samples should always be drawn only when the patient is in a steady state. The actual time required to reach a steady state varies with the patient's pulmonary status. Patients without pulmonary disease achieve a steady state much sooner than those with abnormal lungs. Three to ten minutes is probably long enough for these patients.[16] Patients with chronic airway obstruction may require up to 24 minutes.[17] In actual clinical practice, a 20 to 30 minute waiting period before ABG analysis is usual.[18] A spontaneously breathing patient should be at rest for at least 5 minutes before ABG is sampled. Alterations in therapy also affect steady-state conditions. These fluctuations can happen if the patient temporarily removes the oxygen therapy device. If the patient is not in a steady-state condition, a repeat puncture with related pain, risks, and cost is usually needed. Even worse, incorrect therapy may be prescribed. Thus, before arterial puncture the patient must be carefully assessed to ensure steady-state conditions.

The RCP should be aware that the pain and anxiety of arterial puncture cause changes in ventilation that affect results. The patient should be approached calmly, and the sample should be obtained as quickly as possible. Use of a local anesthetic at the sample site is recommended by some.[13] Some authors feel that the pain and anxiety that result from an arterial puncture may cause hyperventilation and alteration of blood gas values, although this has not been clearly demonstrated.[19] Other studies do not advocate the use of local anesthesia. Some authors believe that the additional cost, time, discomfort, and potential for complications are not justified.[12,20,21]

If local anesthetic is used, 0.5% lidocaine is infiltrated with a 25-gauge or 26-gauge hypodermic needle under the skin and into the tissues surrounding the artery. Sometimes this can be more painful than the arterial puncture itself, but some patients prefer it. Usually the patient is then relatively calm.

The patient should be seated or lying down. The wrist should be extended to approximately 30 degrees by placing a rolled towel below the wrist, taking care not to overextend the wrist.[21] A definite pulse should be palpated by gently pressing the index and middle fingers over the artery. A puncture should not be performed if a palpable pulse cannot be felt. After location of the pulse, the site should be cleansed with 70% isopropyl alcohol or an alcohol or Betadine solution.

The radial artery should again be palpated with one hand while holding the heparinized syringe much like a pencil or dart with the opposite hand. While holding the fingers over the palpable pulse, the needle is then inserted opposite the blood flow at 45-degree angle (or less) with the bevel turned upward.[9,12,13] Because rapid insertion may force the needle completely through the artery, slow insertion is preferred. If the needle is advanced too far, an acceptable technique is to withdraw it slowly until blood flashes in the hub of the needle. Redirection of the syringe may be done if the initial attempt fails to result in entry to the artery, if the tip of the needle is left under the skin. Redirection should not be done while the needle lies deep within the tissue.

After a 3-mL to 4-mL sample of blood has been obtained, the needle is withdrawn and sterile gauze is placed immediately over the puncture site. Digital pressure should normally be applied to the site for a minimum period of 5 minutes.[9,13,20,22] Femoral punctures should be held for 7 to 10 minutes because the pressure is appreciably higher in this large artery. A few minutes after the pressure is released, the site should be inspected for bleeding.

If any bleeding is present, pressure should be continued until bleeding ceases. Pressure bandages and ice packs are sometimes but rarely necessary to stop bleeding. If the patient is on anticoagulant therapy, 10 to 20 minutes of direct pressure may be necessary. Pressure dressings are not a substitute for direct pressure but should be considered an additional safeguard. The pressure of a palpable pulse beyond the puncture site should be determined.[9] Steps to prevent an accidental venous sample include using a clear hub needle and watching for the flash, allowing the syringe plunger to advance from arterial pressure, and carefully palpating the site. If a venous sample is suspected, the RCP should draw a venous sample for comparison.

Arterial line sampling

An additional source of blood samples that will give the RCP information about gas exchange can be obtained from arterial lines that are used to monitor blood pressure. Indwelling arterial lines are common in many ICUs (Figure 17-2). A three-way **stopcock** allows direct sampling of arterial blood, without the risks of a puncture. The same infection risks to the RCP are present, and the same precautions must be taken.

The three ports on a three-way stopcock are the patient port, a sample port, and a flush port that leads to a pressurized heparin solution. The lever on the top of the stopcock can be rotated, and the port to which the handle is pointed is "off" with the other two ports being open.

In the normal resting position for the stopcock on the arterial line, the handle is pointed to the sample port. The pressurized heparin solution is forced slowly and continuously through the system. This slow heparin flush keeps the arterial catheter free and open while not impairing the body's ability to form clots.

Two syringes are needed to obtain a sample from an arterial line. An empty syringe is attached to the sample port. The stopcock is positioned so that blood flows into the syringe, and the flush port is closed. Fluid and blood from inside the arterial line are then aspirated. The volume of fluid withdrawn should be at least 5 mL. When this is completed, the stopcock will

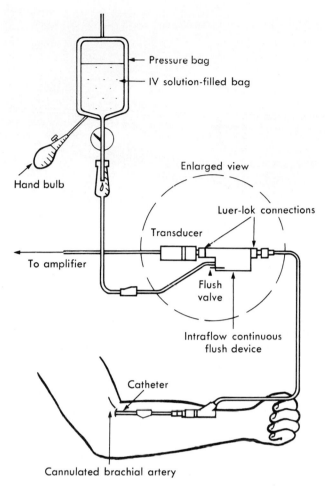

Fig. 17-2 Percutaneous arterial catherter, showing angle and sampling port. (From Schroeder JS and Daily EK: Techniques in bedside hemodynamic monitoring, St Louis, 1976, Mosby.)

have fresh unheparinized blood in the catheter up to the stopcock.

The handle is then repositioned so that all ports are obstructed. The syringe used to clear the sampling line should be discarded properly in a biohazard container. A new heparinized sample syringe is then attached to the sample port. The stopcock is again turned to allow blood to enter the sample syringe; 2 to 4 mL is allowed to enter the syringe from the patient's blood. The stopcock is then returned to the off position.

It is important to flush the line and stopcock at this point. Most arterial line systems have a plunger or button to push to activate the flush, and heparin solution is flushed through the system. This action forces a small amount of blood trapped in the line to return to the patient. The sample port on the stopcock should also be flushed at this point to prevent blood from clotting in the lumen of the port. A clear (undamped) arterial waveform should be present when the flushing procedure has been completed (Figure 17-3).

Capillary sampling

Capillary sampling is used in many neonatal intensive care units as a way to evaluate gas exchange and yet avoid the risks of arterial sampling, which are greater in neonates. Pulse oximetry has reduced the need for capillary blood samples to evaluate oxygenation. It is, however, common enough to warrant a brief review of the theory and principles of this technique.

Arterialization of the capillary beds can be achieved by warming the skin and thereby increasing the flow of blood through the capillary. With warming, blood gas values in the capillary beds approach arterial values. When peripheral perfusion in the patient is normal, arterialized capillary pH and PCO_2 values correlate well with $PaCO_2$ and arterial pH; PaO_2 values below 60 torr correlate well with capillary PO_2s.

Warming of the capillary beds can be accomplished with warm compresses, a water bath, a heat lamp, or commercially available hot packs. The most popular site is the heel. The earlobe or the tip of a finger (or toe) may also be used. The capillary bed should be heated carefully to prevent burns. The skin should be cleaned with an antiseptic solution such as alcohol. A puncture no more than 2.5 mm deep should then be made on the lateral aspects of the plantar surface. The first drop of blood should be wiped away, and the sample should freely flow until the sample tube is completely full. The tube should be filled by capillary action from the middle of the drop of blood. Most labs require a 0.75 to 1.0 mL sample. Squeezing of the heel or capillary bed to increase flow should be avoided because it may alter the values, especially the pH.

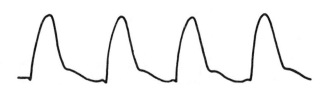

Fig. 17-3 Normal undamped arterial pressure waveform. (From Andreoli KG et al: Comprehensive Cardiac Care, ed 6, St Louis, 1987, Mosby.)

After the tube is full, one end of the capillary tube should be sealed with clay. A small metal wire is placed into the lumen of the capillary tube at this point. A magnet is then moved along the outside of the capillary tube in a forward and backward fashion to mix the blood with the heparin inside the capillary tube. The sample should then be analyzed as soon as possible.

Point of care testing

Because ABG testing involves removing a sample from a patient and taking it to another, sometimes remote location for analysis, there is a built-in time delay. This delay adds to the probability of inaccuracies. Blood that has just been removed from the body is still living tissue, with metabolism and gas exchange that can affect the ABG analysis. Although placement of samples on ice reduces errors due to metabolism, the chance for human error still exists. A simple and logical solution to this type of error is to analyze the blood in the ICU at the bedside. Point of care (POC) testing systems are available for glucose monitoring,[23] and ABG determinations. Some systems now available can measure blood gases, electrolytes, and hematocrit from very small amounts (0.5 mL) of blood,[24] and in as little as 90 seconds. POC is an attractive technology that allows rapid results and gives a "real-time" aspect to the decision. One drawback, however, is that accuracy, quality control, and precision are compromised in exchange for rapid response time. One study[25] found higher agreement between actual and POC PO_2 values at lower ranges than at higher ones. This suggests that this type of technology may not be accurate enough for critically ill patients with high FIO_2 requirements. In addition, manufacturers of these systems advertise their simplicity and ease of operation. In the present health care fiscal climate, this means that it is likely that these systems may be used by untrained or unskilled individuals who are not necessarily able to determine malfunctions or inaccuracies or to make sound clinical judgments. This in turn may make the results less precise than conventional laboratory tests.

Although rapid access to gas exchange (ABG) information is the motivation for the use of these systems, quality control and lack of proficiency issues need to be addressed. Cost effectiveness also must be well established before POC blood gas testing takes the place of the standard ABG sampling in modern critical care. Like other types of technology, POC blood gas analysis will probably achieve a future role in the ICU, once the limitations and pitfalls are determined and defined by research. Figure 17-4 shows the StatPal II (PPG Industries, Biomedial Systems Division). Table 17-2 shows the specifications for this system.

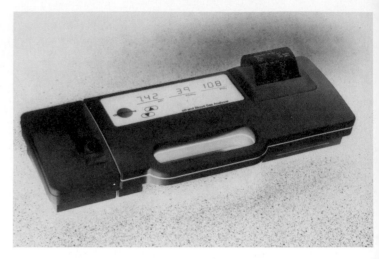

Fig. 17-4 StatPal II on site arterial blood gas analyzer.

In vivo systems

In terms of the gas exchange system example given at the beginning of this chapter (loading dock, conveyance, and unloading dock), **in vivo** systems monitor gas exchange by monitoring the delivery part of the system.

The rapid access to blood gas information gained with POC ABG testing is taken one dimension further with in vivo technology. In vivo technology places the electrode or analyzing device *inside* the patient and displays real-time information on gas exchange. Both POC and laboratory blood gas evaluations are limited because they do not provide us real-time information. Although POC is closer to real time than laboratory ABG analysis, it still gives an "after the fact" picture of what is happening to the gas exchange. Obviously, real-time information is more useful in the evaluation and management of patients. In terms of the school bus analogy, if the laboratory ABG provides an instant snapshot, then in vivo technology is a video camera. Waiting for steady state to occur is no longer necessary. In vivo systems allow the RCP actually to watch the effects of the changes made to the ventilator or oxygen therapy and, in some cases, "fine-tune" it.

Indwelling electrodes. Early research centered around development of in vivo systems in which the

Table 17-2 Specification for StatPal II

Methodology	Microelectrodes
Chamber volume	0.2 mL
Analysis time	60 sec
Dimensions	11.5 in wide by 5.5 in deep by 2.5 in high
Patient temperature correction	25.0° C to 40.0° C
Parameters	pH 6.8–7.8
	PO_2 0–600 torr
	PCO_2 1–99 torr

standard blood gas analyzer electrodes were miniaturized. Kontron Inc. has developed a probe that can be used to monitor *in vivo* PaO_2 continuously. This probe contains a miniature version of the Clark electrode, and the entire probe is small enough to be placed inside a radial artery.

Miniaturized Clark electrodes provide a continuous measure of PaO_2,[26] but numerous problems associated with their use have limited their popularity.[27] Generally, these electrodes have been abandoned because of significant disadvantages and problems. These miniature electrodes must be temperature compensated. Both the amount of oxygen dissolved and the current generated in the electrode itself are sensitive to temperature. Corrections in temperature may be made manually by entering the patient's temperature. Drift in temperature of only a few tenths of a degree can cause system error. The electrode itself consumes oxygen, and the electrode is **thrombogenic.** The electrochemical oxygen probe membrane is susceptible to protein deposits or platelet adhesions. Not only can these deposits be released into the bloodstream, but their existence on the membrane itself causes inaccuracy of the electrode.[28]

Indwelling optodes. An *optode* is a sensor that operates on optical detection and quantification rather than electrochemical properties.[29] Current-generation in vivo systems use optodes, and several manufacturers have FDA approval to market systems.[30] Figure 17-5 shows the PB3300 Intra-Arterial Blood Gas analysis system.

The fluorescence-based optode, located at the tip of a flexible fiber optic strand, is capable of measuring PO_2, PCO_2, and pH.[31-33] *Fluorescence* is the physical capacity of certain molecules to absorb light and then rapidly reemit it at a longer wavelength. Very small amounts of fluorescent material or dye can be measured by determining the amount of emitted light.

Certain dyes decrease output of fluorescence in the presence of oxygen. The decrease is proportionate to the amount of oxygen present. Because oxygen "quenches" or dampens the amount of fluorescence, PO_2 can be determined accurately via fluorescence measurement.

Measurement of pH is accomplished by analyzing the fluorescence of certain weak acids at specific light wavelengths. The degree of dissociation of the acid can be determined on the basis of these measurements. The amount of hydrogen ions (pH) present are determined by the amount of dissociation.

Like the Severinghaus electrode, the fluorescent CO_2 detector has a membrane that is permeable to CO_2. After the CO_2 crosses over the membrane, it functions much as the fluorescent pH sensor does. $PaCO_2$ is determined indirectly through the measured change in pH.[29] Figure 17-6 on page 400 shows a schematic of the Puritan Bennett 3300 optode catheter.

One major advantage of this technology is the

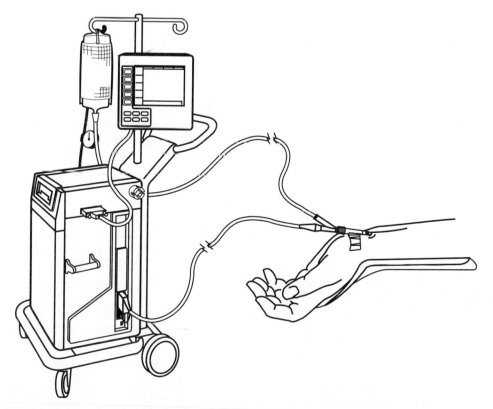

Fig. 17-5 Puritan Bennett 3300 indwelling blood gas in-vivo system.

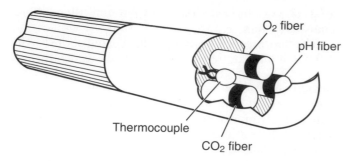

Fig. 17-6 Diagram of the Puritan Bennett optode showing the O_2, CO_2, pH and thermocouple fibers.

ability to collect data over hours and present it in a "trend" format with events marked. Alarm parameters can also be set. The computerization of these data then allows the practitioner to look only at highlights, in much the same way as a coach looks at highlight films of a sporting event. Calculated data can also be presented in a printed report.

Although the technology has been recently improved and refined and several monitoring systems are on the market, only a few clinical studies have been published.[34-37] The accuracy, especially with oxygen, does not approach the gold standard (laboratory ABG). Some authors feel that in vivo blood gas systems may provide information that has "clinically useful accuracy" as opposed to "laboratory accuracy."[30]

Because the technology now exists to monitor blood gases continuously in clinical practice, it does not follow that its use is justified or affordable. These systems are expensive. In addition, care must be taken with the risk of thrombosis or infection. Other unanswered questions about the life span of the optodes in the average ICU, quality control, continuing accuracy, and their role in closed logic ventilator systems remain unanswered. Nevertheless, continuous in vivo measurement of blood gases may be lifesaving in certain rapidly changing clinical situations. With properly designed research to answer these questions, the future holds great promise for in vivo blood gas systems.

NONINVASIVE ANALYSIS OF GAS EXCHANGE

Like in vivo blood gas analysis, noninvasive methods of gas exchange also provide "clinically useful" information that is not "laboratory accurate." In addition, changes in insurance and governmental reimbursement policies have added pressure to use more cost-effective methods. Another factor that has focused attention on noninvasive methods is the need to reduce the hazard of accidental infection inherent in invasive procedures. Added to these factors, the advantage of "real-time" data gives noninvasive

procedures a major role in management of the patient.

Noninvasive analysis of gas exchange can be divided into two categories: transcutaneous and expired gas.

Transcutaneous gas monitoring

Thus far we have seen gas exchange monitored in the blood (ABG) while on the conveyance system (in vivo). These monitors look at gas exchange at the unloading dock (transcutaneous) or tissue level.

In order to monitor the gas exchange, at the unloading dock, transcutaneous monitoring is the technology of choice. Two key ideas must be kept in mind about this technology: (1) all gases diffuse through the skin, and (2) gas diffusion varies with the perfusion of blood beneath the skin.

Through the skin (transcutaneous) monitoring of oxygen and CO_2 started in the neonatal intensive care units of the 1970s,[38] although the technology of transcutaneous gas measurement was first described in 1851 (Table 17-3). This technology is used less in adult intensive care units because age and cardiac output have profound effects on transcutaneous oxygen measurements, and the ratio or correlation between skin oxygen and arterial oxygen is not consistent. Table 17-4 shows how this ratio varies with age and cardiac output.[39]

This discrepancy has generally given adult transcutaneous monitoring systems a poor reputation for accuracy. Carbon dioxide is a little better, perhaps because CO_2 is more diffusible. Several studies[40] have found that $PaCO_2$ changes of 5 mm Hg or more can be monitored or "trended" by the transcutaneous CO_2 monitor.

Technology

Virtually all transcutaneous monitoring systems now incorporate oxygen and carbon dioxide elec-

Table 17-3 History of transcutaneous gas measurements

Date	Individual	Accomplishment
1851	Von Gerlach	Determined that gas diffuses through skin, and this varies with perfusion
1951	Baumgardner	Measured oxygen diffusion
1954	Clark	Developed oxygen electrode
1957	Rooth	Adapted Clark electrode for bloodless determinations
1969	Huch	Reported use of P_{O_2} electrodes
1973	Huch	Reported use of P_{CO_2} electrodes

From Kacmareck RM, Hess D, Stoller J: *Monitoring in respiratory care,* St Louis, 1993, Mosby.

Table 17-4 Ratios correlating $PtcO_2$ with PaO_2

	$PtcO_2/PaO_2$ Ratio
AGE GROUP	
Premature neonates	1.14
Neonates	1.0
Children	0.84
Adults	0.79
Older adults	0.68
CARDIAC OUTPUT	
Stable	0.79
Moderate shock	0.48
Severe shock	0.12

From Tobin MJ: Respiratory Monitoring, *JAMA* 264:244–251, 1990.

trodes combined in the same skin probe. The schematic in Figure 17-7 shows the combined electrodes. This probe is stuck to the skin with a special glue or tape. The probe heats the skin beneath it in order to increase the perfusion. Heat dilates the capillary beds and increases the blood flow to the skin. In neonates, this heating balances the oxygen consumption of the skin itself and leads to a 1:1 ratio between $PtcO_2$ and PaO_2. As the patient becomes older, this relationship decreases (see Table 17-4). Periodic skin site care and location change along with calibration are necessary to keep the information accurate and consistent. These probes must be maintained by a method similar to that used for electrodes on a blood gas analysis system. Membrane procedures must be followed, and application to the skin must be correct to prevent room air from entering the electrode. Temperatures must be meticulously monitored to prevent damage to the skin, yet maintain perfusion and keep the electrode functioning properly. Minimal staff training and education recommended by the American Academy

of Pediatrics[41] should include knowledge of maintenance, quality control, application, accuracy, response limitations, response characteristics, physiologic principles, and underlying technique.

Clinical application

Gas exchange over a given period can be determined by monitoring transcutaneous gases, but the limitations and factors affecting the technology must be taken into account before making clinical decisions (see accompanying box). Many times clinicians do not appreciate the fact that transcutaneous O_2 and CO_2 are not the same as arterial O_2 and CO_2. Several factors are involved. Koff and Hess[40] list these factors as follows:

Electrode
Calibration
Membrane condition
Contact solution
Probe placement
Temperature
Patient
Skin thickness
Perfusion
Blood pressure
Vasodilator
Age
Acidotic conditions

Hess and Kacmarek[30] provide a list of limitations of $PtcO^2$ monitoring; these limitations are related to oxygen (see box).

These considerations make the future use of this technology questionable for all but a specific subgroup of patients. The fact that it is noninvasive keeps it a possibility and appealing as a cost saver when compared to invasive methods. The use of these monitors for peripheral vascular diseases, watching for trends in oxygenation and ventilation, has perhaps the best

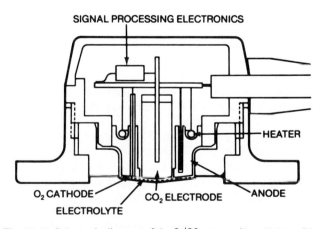

SIGNAL PROCESSING ELECTRONICS

O_2 CATHODE CO_2 ELECTRODE ANODE

ELECTROLYTE

HEATER

Fig. 17-7 Schematic diagram of the O_2/CO_2 sensor. (From Mahutte CK et al: Evaluation of a single transcutaneous PO2-PCO2 sensor in adult patients. Crit Care Med 1984; 12:1063–1066. © by Williams and Wilkins. Used by permission.)

Limitations of $PtcO_2$ monitoring

Frequent calibration is required.

Frequent change of electrode position is required.

Equilibration time is relatively long after electrode placement.

Insufficient electrode temperature that may adversely effect performance.

Performance that may be suboptimal over poorly perfused areas.

$PtcO_2$ tends to underestimate PaO_2.

Compromised hemodynamic status causes underestimation of PaO_2.

Heated electrode may cause skin to blister.

$PtcO_2$ may underestimate PaO_2 during hyperoxemia.

Frequent membrane/electrolyte changes and electrode maintenance are necessary.

Performance is more reliable in neonates than adults.

potential for future application. Even in the neonatal ICU it has largely been replaced by the pulse oximeter.

Pulse oximetry

In another attempt to view the amount of oxygen delivered to the tissues, the pulse oximeter is now used extensively. In terms of the earlier analogy, the pulse oximeter checks the amount of oxygen on each boxcar (the red blood cell) being transported by the conveyance system (the cardiovascular system) as it enters the unloading dock (the capillaries) of the finger, toe, or earlobe.

The pulse oximeter has become the most common tool used in modern ICU to determine the gas exchange status of oxygen. Since its introduction in the mid-1970s, the pulse oximeter has quickly become an indispensable modality. There are at least 35 different companies engaged in the manufacture of pulse oximeter, with sales exceeding the $200 million mark in 1989.[42] No other device in medical history has so quickly and widely become the standard of patient care in the operating room, critical care area, exercise physiology lab, and outpatient clinics as the pulse oximeter. What was only "Star Trek" technology in the 1970s has become the standard for noninvasive monitoring for oxygenation in less than two decades.

Ironically, little scientific evaluation of the impact of pulse oximetry on outcomes has been done to date. Pulse oximetry has become an integral part of virtually all critical care monitoring protocols; it is used in emergency rooms and prehospital care systems through out the world. Information is provided through a small hand-held device incorporated into a mechanical ventilator system or through expensive, sophisticated bedside monitoring systems that allow complete computerization of the data and parameters. The information can be combined with other monitoring data to give more meaningful information to the clinician.

Technology. The two physical principles of spectro-*photometry* and *photoplethysmography* have allowed the development of this device. Spectrophotometry is the technique of measuring the amount of light absorbed by a substance (in this case, hemoglobin): the more substance, the more light absorbed. Photoplethysmography uses light to measure arterial pressure waveforms generated by the pulse in the capillaries (in this case, pulse rate and strength). Instruments based on these principles, combined with high-intensity **light emitting diodes** (LEDs), are the basic components of all pulse oximeters. These three elements are combined in the finger probe (Figure 17-8).

Limitations. Although this technology is well entrenched in the standard of care, it has problems and limitations. The accuracy of these devices depends on several empirical assumptions. Since these instruments are not routinely calibrated, they employ "fac-

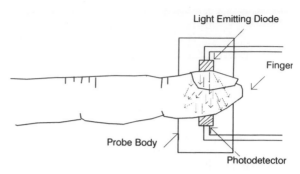

Fig. 17-8 Pulse oximeter finger probe.

tory calibration" based on findings of studies of normal healthy volunteers with normal oxygen/hemoglobin association. When actual arterial saturations are above 80%, the saturation reported by the oximeter, or SpO_2, may be ±5%, according to some factory specifications. Therefore, a patient with an actual SaO_2 of 90% may have a pulse oximeter reading as low as 85% to as high as 95%. If the patient has a normal dissociation curve, the actual PaO_2 may be as low as 55 torr. Upper limit is unpredictable. If there are other irregularities present, such as abnormal hemoglobin, abnormal skin pigments, fingernail polish or other interfering factors, the actual PaO_2 may be anywhere on the scale. This is not very sound information for changing FIO_2 settings or prescription oxygen.

Anyone using this device should be aware of these and other limitations. Some of the most common clinical problems to watch for are the following:

1. *Motion of extremity:* Motion of the finger can lead to false pulse rates and poor quality waveform artifact. Earlobe, toe, or external nares can be used as a substitute.

2. *Light dilution:* Sunlight or high-intensity light from surgical lamps or other appliances may interfere with the ability of the probe to detect the correct wavelength. Direct sunlight can cause the reading to be high.

3. *Abnormal hemoglobin:* The pulse oximeter cannot distinguish between oxyhemoglobin and carboxyhemoglobin and thus can overestimate actual saturation. Methemoglobin may cause interference with the light absorption, producing a false high reading.

4. *Dyes, fingernail polish, and abnormal skin pigments:* Radiologic procedures that use vascular dyes (blue or green) can affect readings. Fingernail polish and extremely dark skin pigment can cause a shunt of the light away from the photodetector.

5. *Anemia:* Pulse oximeter error is extremely likely during open heart surgery, renal dialysis, and other states in which the number of red blood cells may not be normal in a given sample. The

pulse oximeter may be inaccurate in patients with severe anemia (Hb<8g/dL).

6. *Low perfusion states:* The pulse oximeter cannot determine saturation when the pulse signal is weak or missing. Hypovolemia, hypotension, vasoconstriction, and hypothermia may cause a low pulse signal and therefore low saturation readings.

Clinical application. Although Severinghaus and Kelleher[40] called the pulse oximeter a "desaturation meter," it is no better than the "disconnect" and other alarms found on any modern ventilator. Hess and Kacmarek[28] found no clinically important desaturation events that were not otherwise detected and do not recommend the use of this instrument for mechanically ventilated patients. It is difficult to find indications for the use of the pulse oximeter on mechanically ventilated patients with properly functioning ventilators and alarm protocols. Pulse oximeters have a notoriously high failure rate caused by probe disconnections. In addition, false-positive alarms are likely to have a desensitizing effect on the staff.

Use of the pulse oximeter is indicated during interventions in which precipitous desaturations may occur, such as bronchoscopy and transtracheal procedures. Pulse oximeters can be helpful in various stress producing therapeutics, such as **bronchoalveolar lavage,** even though to date there are no published studies on the morbidity or mortality rates associated with their use or nonuse. To assist clinician in the proper application of this technology, the American Association for Respiratory Care has published a Clinical Practice Guideline for the use of Pulse Oximetry.[43]

Capnography: end tidal carbon dioxide (PetCO₂)

Yet another way to look at the gas transport system is to check the amount of carbon dioxide exhaled by the patient. Theoretically, observation of the exhaled tidal gas from the patient's lungs (referred to as end-tidal) and knowledge of what has been inhaled allow the clinician to judge the overall system. *Capnography* is the term for this technology. The partial pressure of carbon dioxide in the end-tidal gas (PetCO₂) is the parameter measured. The ability to measure the patient's exhaled CO₂ has existed for a long time.[44] It has only recently become common in critical care units and emergency rooms. Anesthesiologists used capnography in the operating room for many years before it was used in the critical care area. In fact, the use of capnography during surgery has become the "standard of practice" to ensure that endotracheal **intubation** has occurred correctly and to monitor the respiratory system during anesthesia. Many anesthesiologists prefer to continue to follow their patients with this type of monitor during the postoperative period. In recent years, capnography

technology has improved the equipment greatly. These two influences have caused this type of noninvasive monitoring to be increasingly utilized.

Terms. *Capnometry* is the measurement of carbon dioxide in the patient's breath. A *capnometer* is a device that displays a digital number that indicates the partial pressure of the carbon dioxide. Because the amount of CO₂ varies during the exhaled part of the breath, most capnometers also display a graphic waveform of the CO₂ during the entire respiratory cycle. This waveform is referred to as the *capnograph.* Knowing the number alone is of little value to the respiratory care practitioner, whereas the capnograph waveform can give useful information about the source and nature of each breath. A printed waveform is referred to as the capnogram by some authors.[44] Figure 17-9 shows a normal capnograph waveform.

Technology. Mass spectrometry can be used to measure inspired and expired gases and anesthetic agents. Mass spectrometers are bulky and expensive to operate; they must be frequently maintained and serviced. Although a few hospitals have them at the bedside, use of the infrared capnometer is more common. Carbon dioxide gas has the ability to absorb infrared light; virtually all bedside capnometers use this principle to measure the exhaled CO₂. The patient's exhaled gas must be placed into a sample chamber through which an infrared light source is directed. The amount of light at the end of the sample chamber is analyzed and then compared to the amount going through an adjacent reference chamber. The PCO₂ can then be determined (Figure 17-10, page 404).

Gas sampling. Two types of devices are used to collect the sample. Both can be found on capnometers in the ICU. The mainstream type of sampler places the sample chamber between the endotracheal tube and the ventilator circuit (Figure 17-11, page 404). The side stream has a sample tube connected to a negative pressure pump and actually pumps a small sample of the patient's exhaled gas away from the circuit and into the sample chamber located within

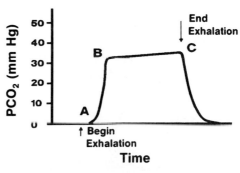

Fig. 17-9 The normal capnogram, showing **A** as anatomic dead-space, **B,** the beginning of the alveolar plateau, and **C** as the end of the alveolar plateau.

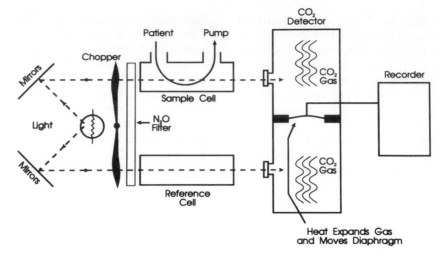

Fig. 17-10 Schematic representation of a double beam capnometer.

the device (Figure 17-12). Both types have advantages and disadvantages over the other. Table 17-5 is a comparison of both types.

Clinical application. If the $P_{ET}CO_2$ were always the same as the $PaCO_2$, then in all probability the capnometer would have replaced the ABG long ago, and the capnograph would be the standard for noninvasive monitoring of $PaCO_2$. In healthy subjects, with normal lungs, $P_{ET}CO_2$ is 1 to 5 torr less than the $PaCO_2$.[39] Capnography is useful in the management of many patients, especially those with a stable cardiovascular system. Once the patient's hemodynamics become unstable, capnography can be used to alert the RCP that pulmonary blood flow has changed. Capnography is useful in resuscitation to monitor the quantity of cardiac output through the pulmonary system, as

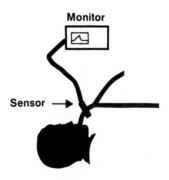

Fig. 17-11 Schematic illustration of mainstream capnograph, with the sensor placed directly at the airway. (From Hess D: Capnometry and capnography: Technical aspects, physiologic aspects, and clinical applications. Respir Care 1990; 35:557–576. Used by permission.)

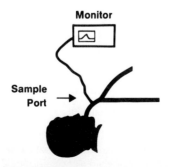

Fig. 17-12 Schematic of a sidestream capnograph.

Table 17-5 Advantages and disadvantages of mainstream and sidestream capnographs

MAINSTREAM CAPNOGRAPH

Advantages:	*Disadvantages:*
Sensor at patient airway	Secretions and humidity blocks
Fast response	sensor window
(crisp waveform)	Sensor requires heating to prevent
Short lag time	condensation
(real-time readings)	Requires frequent calibration
No sample flow to	Bulky sensor at patient airway
reduce tidal volume	Does not measure N_2O
	Difficult to use with nonintubated
	patients
	Reusable adapters requires
	cleaning and sterilization

SIDESTREAM CAPNOGRAPH

Advantages:	*Disadvantages:*
No bulky sensors or	Secretions block sample tubing
heaters at airway	Water trap required to remove
Ability to measure N_2O	water from the sample
Disposable sample line	Frequent calibration required
Ability to use with	Slow response to CO_2 changes
nonintubated patients	Lag time between CO_2 change and
	measurement
	Sample flow may decrease tidal
	volume

From Kacmareck RM, Hess D, Stoller J: *Monitoring in respiratory care,* St Louis, 1993, Mosby.

indicated in several studies.[45-47] Hyperventilation is sometimes used to induce cerebral vasoconstriction in head injuries; capnography is useful in that application. Although the authors found that it had limitations, as in cases of large deadspace and sudden hypercapnia, capnography was used to monitor patients during weaning from mechanical ventilation.[48] Because there is no carbon dioxide produced in the stomach, $P_{ET}CO_2$ monitoring devices are useful in determining whether endotracheal **intubation** has been successful. There are small disposable CO_2 detectors on the market that can be used by prehospital personnel to assess endotracheal tube placement.

$P_{ET}CO_2$ is not $PaCO_2$. $P_{ET}CO_2$ is not $PaCO_2$. Graybeal and coworkers found that 31.3% of the changes in $P_{ET}CO_2$ did not predict changes in $PaCO_2$.[49] In another study, Hess and his colleagues found that 43% of the $P_{ET}CO_2$ changes did not correctly indicate the change in $PaCO_2$.[50] Therein lies the difficulty with the use of capnography; those who use it must understand that the physiologic and technologic limitations of the comparisons of the two values can cause misleading or false conclusions about the patient.

In several clinical situations the capnometer can not be depended on to reflect $PaCO_2$ accurately. Patients with uneven distribution of ventilation have a capnograph waveform in which $P_{ET}CO_2$ never becomes stable but continues to rise throughout the entire expiratory cycle. In addition, patients with deadspace to tidal volume inequities (such as pulmonary embolism) have inaccurate capnographic results. Table 17-6 summarizes the clinical conditions associated with changes in $P_{ET}CO_2$.

Table 17-6 Conditions associated with changes in $P_{ET}CO_2$.*

INCREASES IN $P_{ET}CO_2$
Sudden

Sudden increase in cardiac output
Sudden release of a tourniquet
Injection of sodium bicarbonate

Gradual

Hypoventilation
Increase in carbon dioxide production

DECREASES IN $P_{ET}CO_2$
Sudden

Sudden hyperventilation
Sudden decrease in cardiac output
Massive pulmonary embolism
Air embolism
Disconnection of the ventilator
Obstruction of the endotracheal tube
Leakage in the circuit

Gradual

Hyperventilation
Decrease in oxygen consumption
Decreased pulmonary perfusion

ABSENT $P_{ET}CO_2$

Esophageal **intubation**

*$P_{ET}CO_2$ indicates end tidal carbon dioxide tension.

CHAPTER SUMMARY

Arterial blood gas analysis remains the gold standard for the evaluation of gas exchange, especially for mechanically ventilated patients. Any respiratory care practitioner who wishes to prepare for the future should be well schooled and skilled in the collection, analysis, interpretation, and troubleshooting of arterial blood gas analysis techniques and results. Although point of care and in vivo systems are on the horizon, their costs, limitations, and complexity have prevented them from totally replacing the ABG. They are yet to be proved economical alternatives. In addition, noninvasive monitoring techniques have not yet become the standard: transcutaneous techniques are still too inaccurate, especially in the adult population, and the pulse oximeter, although a giant in the noninvasive arena, still has the largely unrecognized possibility of being 4% to 5% inaccurate. Most serious practitioners do not rely on the pulse oximeter for accurate titration of exact oxygen needs. Capnography has limitations and pitfalls that make it an unlikely to supersede current methods.

All of these technologies are appropriate in some applications and can represent real-time and money savings when used properly. Noninvasive monitoring techniques are useful in assessing "trend" information to predict clinical course. When used properly they constitute an excellent monitor to alert the RCP of sudden or precipitous changes in the gas exchange system. However, they still have not replaced precise and accurate knowledge of a well-trained practitioner exercising good clinical judgment based on information from an accurately calibrated blood gas analyzer.

REFERENCES

1. Clark LC: Measurement of oxygen tension: a historical perspective, *Crit Care Med* 9:690–692, 1981.
2. Severinghaus JW, Bradley AG: Electrodes for blood PO2 and PCO2 determination, *J Appl Physiol* 13:515–520, 1958.
3. Stow RW, Baer RF, Randall B: Rapid measurement of the tension of carbon dioxide in blood, *Arch Phys Med Rehabil* 38:646–650, 1957.
4. Hess D, Kacmarek RM: Techniques and devices for monitoring oxygenation, *Respir Care* 38:646–671, 1993.
5. Allen EV: Thromboangitis obliterans: methods of diagnosis of chronic occlusive arterial lesions distal to the wrist with illustrative cases, *Am J Med Sci* 178:237–244, 1929.
6. Pagana KD, Pagana TJ: Mosby's diagnostic and laboratory test reference, St Louis, Mosby, 1992.
7. Petty TL, Bigelow B, Levine BE: The simplicity and safety of arterial puncture, *JAMA* 195:181–182, 1966.
8. Sackner MA, Avery WG, Sokolowski J: Arterial puncture by nurses, *Chest* 59:97–98, 1971.
9. Felkner D: A protocol for teaching and maintaining arterial puncture skills among respiratory therapists, *Respir Care* 18:700–705, 1973.
10. Winkler JB et al: Influence of syringe material on arterial blood gas measurements, *Chest* 66:518–521, 1974.
11. Scott PV, Horton JN, Mapelson WW: Leakage of oxygen from blood and water samples stored in plastic and glass syringes, *Br Med J* 3:512–516, 1971.
12. American Lung Association of Pennsylvania PTS: *Clinical pulmonary function testing manual of uniform lab procedures,* Harrisburg, Pa, 1981, ALA/PTS.
13. Shapiro BA et al: *Clinical application of blood gases,* ed 4, St Louis, 1989, Mosby.
14. Center for Disease Control: Update: universal precautions for the transmission of human immuno deficiency virus, hepatitis B and other blood borne pathogens in health care settings, *MMWR* 37:377–388, 1988.
15. American Association for Respiratory Care: AARC clinical practice guideline: In-vitro pH and blood gas analysis and hemoximetry, *Respir Care* 38:505–510, 1993.
16. Howe LP et al: Return of arterial PO2 values to baseline after supplemental oxygen in patients with cardiac disease, *Chest* 67:256–258, 1975.
17. Sherter CB et al: Prolonged rate of decay of arterial PO2 following oxygen breathing in chronic airways obstruction, *Chest* 67:259–261, 1975.
18. Woolf CI: Arterial blood gas levels after oxygen therapy, *Chest* 69:808–809, 1976 (letter).
19. Morgan E et al: The effect of arterial puncture on steady state blood gas tensions, *Am Rev Respir Dis* 11:152, 1979 (abstract).
20. Petty TL: *Practical pulmonary function tests,* Philadelphia, 1975, Lea & Febiger.
21. Guenter CA, Welch MH: *Pulmonary medicine,* ed 2, Philadelphia, 1982, JB Lippincott.
22. Burton GC, Hodgkin JE, editors: *Respiratory care,* ed 3, Philadelphia, 1992, JB Lippincott.
23. Belsy R et al: Managing bedside glucose testing in the hospital, *JAMA* 258:1634–1638, 1987.
24. Chernow B: The bedside laboratory: a critical step forward in ICU care, *Chest* 97:183s–184s, 1990.
25. Bashein G, Greydanus WK, Kenny MA: Evaluation of a blood gas and chemistry monitor for use during surgery, *Anesthesiology* 70:123–127, 1989.
26. Barker SJ, Tremper KK: Intra-arterial oxygen tension monitoring, *Int Anesth Clin* 25:199–208, 1987.
27. Tobin MJ: *Essentials of critical care medicine,* New York, 1989, Churchill Livingstone.
28. Malley WJ: Clinical blood gases: *applications and noninvasive alternatives,* Philadelphia, 1990, WB Saunders.
29. Opitz N, Lubbers DW: Theory and development of fluorescence based optical sensors: oxygen optodes, *Int Anesth Clin* 25:177–197, 1987.
30. Hess D, Kacmareck RM: Techniques and devices for monitoring oxygenation, *Respir Care* 38:646–671, 1993.
31. Barker SJ, Tremper KK: Intra-arterial oxygen tension monitoring, *Int Anesth Clin* 25:199–208, 1987.
32. Green GE, Hassell KT, Mahutte CK: Comparison of arterial blood gas with continuous intra-arterial and transcutaneous PO2 sensor in adult critically ill patients, *Crit Care Med* 15:491–494, 1987.
33. Shapiro BA et al: Preliminary evaluation of an intra-arterial blood gas system in dogs and humans, *Crit Care Med* 17:455–460, 1989.
34. Mahutte CK et al: Progress in the development of a flourescent intravascular blood gas system in man, *J Clin Monit* 6:147–157, 1990.
35. Shapiro BA et al: Preliminary evaluation of an intra-arterial blood gas system in dogs and humans, *Crit Care Med* 17:455–460, 1989.
36. Miller WW et al: Performance of an in vivo, continuous blood-gas monitor with disposable probe, *Clin Chem* 33:1538–1542, 1987.
37. Barker SJ et al: Continuous fiberoptic arterial oxygen tension measurement in dogs, *J Clin Monit* 3:48–52, 1987.
38. Huch A, Huch R, Lubbers DW: Transcutaneous measurement of blood PO2: methods and applications in perinatal medicine, *J Perinat Med* 1:183–186, 1973.
39. Tobin MJ: Respiratory monitoring, *JAMA* 264:244–251, 1990.
40. Kacmareck RM, Hess D, Stoller J: *Monitoring in respiratory care,* Chapter 11, St Louis, 1993, Mosby.
41. Avery GB et al: American Academy of Pediatrics Task Force on Transcutaneous Oxygen Monitors: report of consensus meeting, *Pediatrics* 83:122–126, 1989.
42. Severinghaus JW, Kelleher JF: Recent developments in pulse oximetry, *Anesthesiology* 76:1018–1038, 1992.
43. American Association for Respiratory Care: Clinical practice guideline: pulse oximetry, *Respir Care* 36(12): 1406–1409, 1991.
44. Hess D: An overview of noninvasive monitoring in respiratory care: present, past, and future. *Respir Care* 35:482–499, 1990.
45. Gudipati C, Weil MH, Bisera J: Expired carbon dioxide: a noninvasive monitor of cardiopulmonary resuscitation, *Circulation* 77:234–239, 1988.
46. Kalenda Z: The capnogram as a guide to the efficacy of cardiac massage, *Resuscitation* 6:259–263, 1978.
47. Saunders AB et al: Expired CO2 as a prognostic indicator of successful resuscitation from cardiac arrest, *Ann Emerg Med* 14:948–952, 1985.
48. Healey CJ et al: Comparison of noninvasive measurements of carbon dioxide tension during withdrawal of mechanical ventilation, *Crit Care Med* 16:701–705, 1988.
49. Graybeal JM, Russel GB: Capmometry in the surgical ICU: an analysis of the arterial-to-end-tidal carbon dioxide difference, *Respir Care* 38:923–928, 1993.
50. Hess D et al: An evaluation of the usefulness of end-tidal PCO2 to aid weaning from mechanical ventilation following cardiac surgery, *Respir Care* 36:837–843, 1991.

18

Basic Pulmonary Function Measurements

■

F. Herbert Douce

CHAPTER LEARNING OBJECTIVES

1. Define lung volumes, capacities, flowrates, and diffusing capacity of the lung;
2. Describe the general purposes and identify specific uses for pulmonary function testing as a component of respiratory care;
3. Delineate the standards for volume and flow measuring devices used in pulmonary function testing;
4. Describe the methods commonly employed in the measurement of lung volumes, capacities, mechanics, and diffusing capacity;
5. Apply pulmonary function data to distinguish between the major patterns of pulmonary disease and evaluate the effectiveness of respiratory care.

The primary function of the lungs is gas exchange. As mixed venous blood passes through the lungs, the lungs add oxygen and remove excess carbon dioxide before the blood returns to the heart. Normal gas exchange results in normal arterial blood gases. The ability of the lungs to perform gas exchange depends upon several factors. The diaphragm and thoracic muscles must be capable of expanding the thorax and lungs to produce a subatmospheric pressure; the airways must be unobstructed to allow gas to flow into the lungs; the cardiovascular system must circulate blood through the lungs; and oxygen and carbon dioxide must be able to diffuse through the alveolar capillary membrane.

Pulmonary function tests can provide valuable information about these important components of gas exchange. A variety of measurements are available to aid in the diagnosis and assessment of pulmonary diseases and to evaluate the effectiveness of respiratory care. For the respiratory care practitioner (RCP), knowledge of these tests and an ability to interpret the measurements are essential for planning and implementing effective patient care.

DEFINITIONS

Lung volumes and capacities

There are four lung volumes and four lung capacities.[1] A lung capacity consists of two or more lung volumes. The lung volumes are tidal volume, inspiratory reserve volume, expiratory reserve volume, and residual volume. The four lung capacities are total lung capacity, inspiratory capacity, functional residual capacity, and the vital capacity. These volumes and capacities are shown in Figure 18-1, page 408.

Total lung capacity (TLC) is the maximum volume of gas in the lungs at the end of a maximum inhalation. The total lung capacity equals the sum of all four lung volumes (TLC = IRV + V_T + ERV + RV), the sum of the vital capacity and the residual volume (TLC = VC + RV), or the sum of the functional residual capacity and the inspiratory capacity (TLC = FRC + IC).

Inspiratory capacity (IC) is the maximum amount of gas that can be inhaled after a normal, effortless exhalation (also known as resting expiratory level). The inspiratory capacity is the sum of the tidal volume and the inspiratory reserve volume (IC = V_T + IRV).

Functional residual capacity (FRC) is the amount of gas left in the lungs after a normal effortless exhalation at the resting expiratory level. The functional residual capacity equals the sum of the expiratory reserve volume and the residual volume (FRC = ERV + RV).

Vital capacity (VC) is the maximum amount of gas that can be exhaled after a maximum inhalation (or the maximum amount of gas that can be inhaled following a maximum exhalation). The vital capacity equals the sum of the inspiratory reserve volume, the tidal volume, and the expiratory reserve volume (VC = IRV + V_T + ERV).

Inspiratory reserve volume (IRV) is the maximum volume of air that can be inhaled after the tidal volume is inhaled.

Tidal volume (V_T or sometimes TV) is the volume of air that is inhaled or exhaled from the lungs during effortless breathing.

Expiratory reserve volume (ERV) is the amount of gas that can be exhaled from the lungs after a normal quiet exhalation.

Residual volume (RV) is the volume of gas remaining in the lungs after a complete maximal exhalation.

Pulmonary mechanics - spirometry

The tests of pulmonary mechanics include measurements of forced expiratory volumes, forced inspiratory flowrates, forced expiratory flowrates, and the

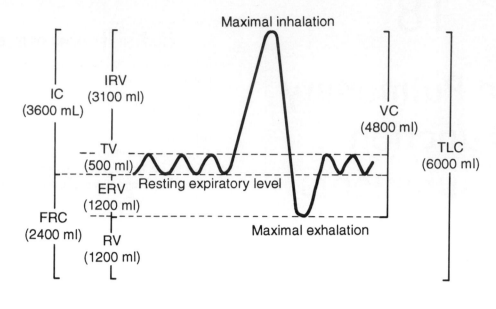

Fig. 18-1 Lung volumes and capacities. Volumes listed are average normals for an adult male.

maximum voluntary ventilation. Many measurements are made while the subject is performing the forced vital capacity maneuver which is shown in Figure 18-2.

The forced vital capacity (FVC) is the maximum volume of gas that the subject can exhale as forcefully and as quickly as possible.

The forced expiratory volume, half second (FEV$_{0.5}$) is the maximum volume of gas that the patient can exhale during the first half second of a forced vital capacity maneuver.

The forced expiratory volume, 1 second (FEV$_1$) is the maximum volume of gas that the patient can

exhale during the first second of the forced vital capacity maneuver.

The forced expiratory volume, 3 seconds (FEV$_3$) is the maximum volume of gas that the patient can exhale during the first 3 seconds of the forced vital capacity maneuver.

The forced expiratory volume in 1 second ratio (%FEV$_1$/FVC) is the percent of the measured forced vital capacity that can be exhaled in 1 second.

The peak expiratory flowrate (PEFR) is the maximum, greatest expiratory flowrate in L/sec.

The forced expiratory flow between 200 mL and 1200 mL (FEF$_{200-1200}$) is a measure of the average

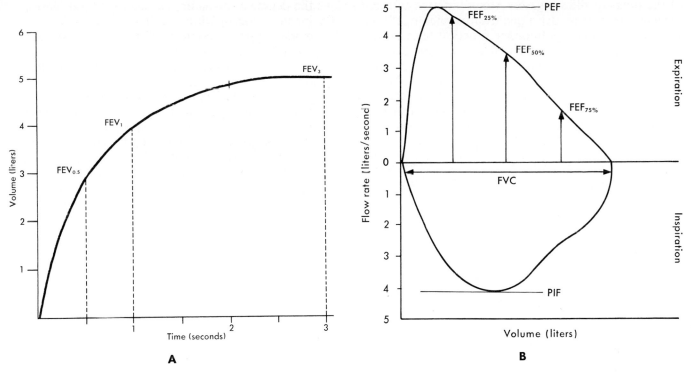

Fig. 18-2 Forced vital capacity, forced expiratory volumes, and flowrates. **A** shows the forced vital capacity on a volume-time graph. **B** shows the forced vital capacity on a flow-volume graph.

expiratory flow during the early phase of exhalation. Specifically, it is a measure of the flowrate for the 1000 mL of expired gas immediately following the first 200 mL of expired gas. This measurement was called the maximum expiratory flow rate (MEFR).

The forced expiratory flow between 25% and 75% of the forced vital capacity ($FEF_{25\%-75\%}$) is a measure of the average expiratory flow during the middle half of the forced vital capacity.

The forced expiratory flow between 75% and 85% of the forced vital capacity ($FEF_{75\%-85\%}$) is a measure of the average expiratory flow during the end of the forced vital capacity.

The forced expiratory flow at 25% ($FEF_{25\%}$ or $\dot{V}max_{25}$) is the maximum expiratory flow after 25% of the forced vital capacity has been exhaled.

The forced expiratory flow at 50% ($FEF_{50\%}$ or $\dot{V}max_{50}$) is the maximum expiratory flow after 50% of the forced vital capacity has been exhaled.

The forced expiratory flow at 75% ($FEF_{75\%}$ or $\dot{V}max_{75}$) is the maximum expiratory flow after 75% of the forced vital capacity has been exhaled.

The forced inspiratory flow at 50% ($FIF_{50\%}$) of the vital capacity is the maximum inspiratory flow after 50% of the forced vital capacity has been inspired.

The maximum voluntary ventilation (MVV) is the maximum volume of air in liters per minute that a subject can breathe during a 12 to 15 second period. The MVV was called the maximum breathing capacity (MBC). Because some laboratories use a 12 second test and others use a 15 second test, the test results are standardized to liters per minute (L/min).

Diffusion

The third major category of pulmonary function testing is measuring the ability of the lungs to transfer gases across the alveolar-capillary membrane. The diffusing capacity of the lung (D_L) is the number of milliliters of gas that transfer from the lungs to the pulmonary blood per minute for each torr partial pressure difference between the alveoli and pulmonary capillary blood.

The diffusing capacity of the lung to alveolar volume ratio (D_LCO/V_A) is an index of the diffusing capacity for each liter of lung volume and an index of the functional alveolar surface area available for diffusion.

GENERAL PRINCIPLES IN PULMONARY FUNCTION TESTING

A complete evaluation of the respiratory system includes the patient history, a physical examination, a chest X-ray, arterial blood gas analysis, and tests of pulmonary function. Basic tests of pulmonary function measure several lung volumes and capacities, flowrates of gases through the airways, and the ability of the lungs to diffuse gases. A combination of these measurements provides a quantitative picture of lung function. Although pulmonary function tests do not diagnose specific pulmonary diseases, these tests do identify the presence and the degree of pulmonary impairments and the type of pulmonary disease. Some basic tests of pulmonary function can be performed at the bedside and some tests also may provide useful information on the effectiveness of therapy.

Purposes of pulmonary function testing

These diagnostic and therapeutic roles of pulmonary function testing cause clinicians to ask some general questions about respiratory patients. These questions are posed in Table 18-1. In general, the purpose of pulmonary function testing is to identify and quantify pulmonary impairments.[2] The specific purposes of assessing pulmonary function include the following:

1. *To quantify changes in the degree of pulmonary function and impairment.* Pulmonary disease may progress or regress, and pulmonary function tests help quantify disease progress or the reversibility of the disease.[3]
2. *Epidemiological surveillance for pulmonary disease.* Screening programs may detect pulmonary abnormalities caused by disease or environmental factors in general populations, occupational settings, smokers, or other high-risk groups. By measuring the pulmonary function of the normal population, researchers also have measured normal pulmonary function.[4,5,6,7]
3. *Assessment of post-operative pulmonary risk.* Pre-operative testing can identify those patients who may have an increased risk of pulmonary complications after surgery.[8] Sometimes the risk for complications can be reduced by pre-operative respiratory care.
4. *To aid in the determination of pulmonary disability.*[9] Pulmonary function tests also can determine the degree of **disability** caused by lung diseases, including occupational diseases such as coal workers pneumoconiosis. Some federal entitlement programs and insurance policies rely on pulmonary function tests to confirm claims for financial compensation.
5. *To evaluate and quantify therapeutic effectiveness.*[10] Pulmonary function tests may be helpful in selecting or modifying a specific therapeutic technique, such as identifying the most effective bronchodilator medication or a rehabilitation exercise protocol. Clinicians and researchers use pulmonary function tests to objectively measure changes in pulmonary function as a result of treatment.

Organization of pulmonary function testing

In most modern pulmonary function laboratories, there are three components to basic pulmonary function measurements; lung volumes and capacities, pulmonary mechanics, and the diffusing capacity of the lung. For each component, there are a variety of techniques and different types of equipment that make the measurements. When the purpose of the testing is to identify the presence and the degree of pulmonary impairments and the type of pulmonary disease, patients usually require all three components of testing. When the purpose of the testing is more limited, such as assessment of post-operative pulmonary risk or to evaluate and quantify therapeutic effectiveness, the scope of measurements also is limited.

A common regimen of pulmonary function testing in the laboratory is to evaluate the effectiveness of bronchodilator therapy. Pulmonary mechanics, especially the FEV_1, are measured as a baseline. Then a bronchodilator is given by inhalation of a diluted aerosol or by metered dose inhaler. Measurements of pulmonary mechanics are repeated, and the percent change is calculated according to the equation:

$$\% \text{ change} = \frac{[(\text{Post-test } FEV_1 - \text{Pretest } FEV_1)]}{\text{Pretest } FEV_1} \times 100$$

An increase in expiratory flow greater than 15% indicates beneficial effects of the medication.

Some pulmonary function laboratories also perform specialized tests of pulmonary function. These specialized tests may include exercise testing, bronchial provocation testing, low density spirometry, and respiratory quotients. Many pulmonary function laboratories also perform arterial blood gas analysis. These specialized tests are less common and not discussed in this chapter. Arterial blood gas analysis is discussed in Chapter 17.

Table 18-1 Basic questions for clinical pulmonary function testing

Diagnostic	Therapeutic
1. Is lung disease present?	1. Is the disease reversible?
2. What type of lung **impairment** is present?	2. What treatments are most effective?
3. What is the degree of lung impairment?	3. To what degree is the disease reversible?
4. Is there more than one type of lung impairment present?	4. Is rehabilitation feasible?
5. Can multiple lung diseases be separated?	5. Can rehabilitation be objectively evaluated?

Equipment for pulmonary function testing

Measuring volumes and flow for pulmonary function testing can be accomplished by a wide variety of instruments and principles of measurement. These instruments are commonly divided into two broad categories: devices that measure gas volumes and devices that measure gas flows. There are three types of volume measuring devices: water-sealed spirometers, bellows spirometers, and dry rolling seal spirometers. There are five general principles for measuring gas flows: **pneumotachometers,** thermistors, turbinometers, and sonic devices. Peak flow meters comprise the fifth group of devices. All flow measuring devices are sometimes called pneumotachometers. Many practitioners reserve the term pneumotachometer for devices that utilize the principle of measurement of the original gas flow measuring device designed by Fleisch.[11,12]

Regardless of the general type of device and the specific principle of measurement, there are several characteristics that are common to all volume and flow measuring devices. Every measuring instrument has the characteristics of capacity, accuracy, error, precision, linearity, and output.[13,14,15]

The *capacity* of an instrument refers to the range or limits of how much it can measure. The *accuracy* of a measuring instrument is how well it measures a known reference value. For volume measurements, standard reference values are provided by a graduated 3.0 liter calibration syringe.[16,17] No measuring instrument is perfect, and there is usually an arithmetic difference between reference values and measured values; this difference is called the error. Accuracy and error are opposite terms; the greater the accuracy, the smaller the error. Accuracy and error are commonly expressed as a percent accuracy or percent error. The sum of the percent accuracy and percent error always equals 100%.

To determine percent accuracy and percent error several reference values are measured and the mean of the measured values is computed and compared to the reference values according to the equations:

$$\% \text{ accuracy} = \frac{\text{mean measured value}}{\text{reference value}} \times 100$$

or

$$\% \text{ error} = \frac{\text{mean measured value} - \text{reference value}}{\text{reference value}} \times 100$$

Precision is synonymous with reproducability and is a measure of the *reliability* of measurements. The standard deviation of the mean measured reference value is the statistic that indicates the precision of an instrument. *Linearity* refers to the accuracy of the instrument over its entire range of measurement or its capacity. Some devices may accurately measure large volumes or high flowrates, but may be less accurate when measuring small volumes or low flowrates. To determine linearity, accuracy and precision are calculated at different points over the range or capacity of the device.

Output includes the specific measurements made or computed by the instrument. Some volume and flow measuring devices measure the FVC and forced expiratory volume in one second (FEV_1). Others may calculate a variety of forced expiratory flowrates (FEF) while some measure tidal volume and minute ventilation. Diagnostic spirometers usually measure and calculate VC, FVC, FEV_1, peak expiratory flowrate (PEFR), and forced expiratory flowrates (FEF). Some measure and calculate maximum voluntary ventilation (MVV). Some of these instruments may be a component of a laboratory system to provide the volume or flow measuring capability for other diagnostic tests of pulmonary function; for example, they are used with gas analyzers to measure functional residual capacity (FRC) and total lung capacity (TLC), or the inspiratory VC during the single breath diffusing capacity (DLCOsb). Whether a **spirometer** is used in a diagnostic laboratory, a physician's office, or at the bedside in the intensive care unit, there are national performance standards for volume and flow measuring devices.

In 1978, the American Thoracic Society (ATS) adopted standards for diagnostic spirometers. These standards were updated in 1987 and have been adopted by other medical organizations and government agencies (Table 18-2, page 412.)[16,10] Some spirometers have been independently evaluated against the ATS Standards or in comparison to instruments that meet those standards.[19,20-25] According to the ATS Standards, when measuring a slow vital capacity, the spirometer should be able to measure for up to 30 seconds, and for the FVC the time capacity should be at least 15 seconds. When measuring the vital capacity and FEV, a volume measuring spirometer should have a capacity of at least 7 liters and should measure volumes with less than 3% error or within 50 milliliters of a reference value, whichever is greater. These standards, even the 7-liter standard for capacity, also apply to children.[26] A diagnostic spirometer that measures flow should be at least 95% accurate (or within 0.2 L/sec, whichever is greater) over the entire 0 to 12 L/sec range of gas flow. A summary of the standards is provided in Table 18-2.

The spirometer standards also require spirometers to have a thermometer or produce BTPS-corrected values, and that a graphic recording be produced of sufficient size for diagnostic testing, validation, and hand measurements. For the diagnostic function, the scale of the volume axis must be $\geq$ 5 mm/L and the scale for the time axis must be $\geq$ 10 mm/sec. For validation and hand measurement functions, the scale of the volume axis must be $\geq$ 10 mm/L and the scale

Table 18-2 1987 American Thoracic Society spirometer performance standards

Test	Volume Range and Accuracy	Flow Range	Time	Back Pressure	Test Signal
VC	7 L ± 3 % or 50 mL*	0–12 L/sec	30 sec	—	3 L syringe
FVC	same as VC	0–12 L/sec	15 sec	—	24 wave forms
FEV$_1$	same as VC	0–12 L/sec	t	< 1.5 cm H$_2$O/L/sec	24 wave forms
FEF$_{25-75\%}$	7 L ± 5 % or ± 0.2 L/sec*	0–12 L/sec	15	same as FEV$_1$	24 wave forms
Flow	12 L/sec ± 5% or ± 0.2 L/sec*	0–12 L/sec	15	same as FEV$_1$	Manufacturer proof
MVV	250 L/min V$_T$ = 2 L, ± 5%	0–12 L/sec ± 5%	12-15	< ±10 cm H$_2$O at 2 L, 120 bpm	Sine wave pump

* Whichever is greater.

for the time axis must be 20 mm/sec. Most manufactures have designed their spirometers to meet or exceed the validation and hand measurement standards. For quality control, the standards include verifying volume accuracy with a 3 liter calibration syringe daily or every 4 hours, if the spirometer is in continuous use. Volume accuracy should be verified quarterly over the entire volume range, and the recorder speed should be checked with a stopwatch quarterly.[16]

Infection control

Pulmonary function testing is safe, but a possibility of cross-contamination exists, either from the patient or from the technologist. Although Universal Precautions do not apply to saliva or mucus unless they contain blood, other potentially hazardous organisms may be present in these fluids, and the use of proper barriers and hand washing is important. Pulmonary function technologists performing procedures on patients with potentially infectious airborne diseases should wear a personal respirator or a close-fitting surgical mask, especially if the testing itself induces coughing. The mouthpiece, tubing, and any parts of the spirometer that come into contact with any subject should be disposed, sterilized, or disinfected between subjects. It is unnecessary to routinely clean the interior surface of the spirometer between subjects.[27-30]

PRINCIPLES OF MEASUREMENT

Lung volumes and capacities

The lung volumes that can be measured directly with a spirometer include tidal volume, inspiratory capacity, inspiratory reserve volume, expiratory reserve volume, and vital capacity. Since the residual volume cannot be exhaled, the residual volume, functional residual capacity, and the total lung capacity must be measured using indirect methods.

The volume of gas measured by a spirometer is often measured at a temperature less than body temperature. The spirometer temperature is related to its design and the environmental temperature. Some instruments are heated to body temperature, while others include an electronic or alcohol thermometer so a temperature correction can be applied. According to Charles's gas law, if pressure remains constant, a volume of gas is indirectly related to its temperature. Volumes measured by spirometers are at ambient temperature, pressure, saturated (ATPS) conditions, and must be adjusted for the temperature difference between the spirometer and the subject's body temperature (BTPS). To make this adjustment, multiply the volume by the ATPS to BTPS correction factor.[31] All lung volumes and capacities are converted to BTPS conditions. There can be a 5% to 10% difference between volumes measured at ATPS versus BTPS conditions.[32]

The tidal volume (V$_T$) is measured directly from a spirogram (Figure 18-1). For the purposes of assuring test **validity** and standardization, the subject should be in a sitting position and wearing a nose clip. It sometimes takes the subject 2 to 3 minutes to become accustomed to the nose clip and mouthpiece. The subject breathes through a tight-fitting mouthpiece until a normal, rhythmic breathing pattern is established. Since the tidal volume will vary normally from breath to breath, an average tidal volume is a more reliable measurement. In the laboratory, sometimes an average tidal volume is measured during 3 minutes of quiet breathing while the spirometer records volumes and graphs volume and time. At the bedside, an average tidal volume usually is measured over 1 minute; the subject breathes normally into a spirometer that stores in a memory each volume exhaled for one minute and computes an average. An alternate approach is to measure the total volume of air exhaled for 1 minute (VE) and then divide by the breathing frequency (f) counted during the same period. The following formula can be used to calculate the tidal volume: $V_T = V_E \div f$.

The inspiratory capacity (IC) is also measured directly from a spirogram. The patient is asked to inhale maximally at the end of a normal effortless exhalation. To assure validity, a consistent resting expiratory level should be obvious on the spirogram before inhaling. To assure reliability, the IC should be measured at least twice, and the two largest measurements should agree within 5%. Since the definition of inspiratory capacity is the maximum volume inhaled, the largest measurement is the subject's IC.

The expiratory reserve volume (ERV) is measured directly from the spirogram. The patient is asked to breathe normally for a few breaths and then exhale maximally. The expiratory reserve volume is that volume of air exhaled between the resting expiratory level and the maximum exhalation level on the spirogram. To assure validity, a consistent resting expiratory level should be obvious on the spirogram before exhaling maximally. To assure reliability, the ERV should be measured at least twice and the two largest measurements should agree within 5%. Since the definition of expiratory reserve volume is the maximum volume exhaled, the largest measurement is the subject's ERV.

The vital capacity (VC) is the most frequently measured lung volume. There are several methods of measuring the vital capacity. When the volume of the vital capacity is most important, the VC can be measured during inspiration or during a slow prolonged expiration. To measure the vital capacity during inspiration, the subject exhales maximally and then inhales as deeply as possible. The volume of the maximal inspiration is the inspiratory vital capacity. To measure the VC during expiration, the subject inhales maximally and then exhales maximally taking all the time necessary to exhale completely. The exhaled volume is the slow VC. An alternative method is to measure the inspiratory capacity and the expiratory reserve volume and add these volumes together; but this method should be reserved only for subjects who cannot otherwise execute the vital capacity. The VC also is measured when it is exhaled forcefully and as rapidly as possible. This technique is called the forced vital capacity (FVC), and it is used to assess pulmonary mechanics, which is the subject of the next section of this chapter.

Since the residual volume cannot be exhaled, neither it nor the, functional residual capacity, or total lung capacity can be measured directly with a spirometer. There are three indirect techniques to measure these lung volumes: helium dilution, nitrogen washout, and body **plethysmography.** The helium dilution and nitrogen washout techniques will measure whatever gas is in the lungs at the beginning of the test, if the gas is in communication with unobstructed airways. The body plethysmographic technique will measure all the gas in the thorax at the resting expiratory volume. Since the plethysmographic technique measures *all* gas in the thorax, including gas that is trapped distal to obstructed airways or gas in the pleural space, the lung volume measured by this technique is called the thoracic gas volume (TGV). In normal individuals, the thoracic gas volume is identical to the FRC measured by both the helium dilution and nitrogen washout techniques. When the FRC is measured the residual volume can be calculated as the difference between the FRC and the ERV. The total lung capacity also can be calculated by adding the residual volume to the vital capacity.

The helium dilution technique for measuring lung volumes uses a closed, **rebreathing** circuit (Figure 18-3).[33,34] This technique is based upon the assump-

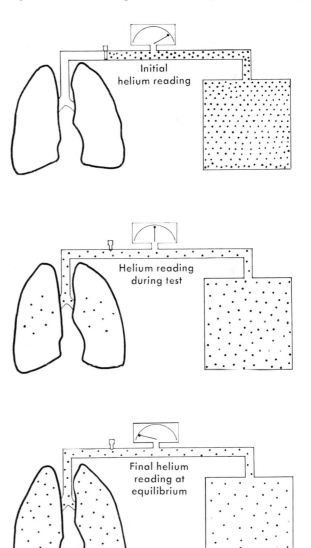

Fig. 18-3 Helium dilution method for measuring the functional residual capacity, the residual volume, and the total lung capacity.

tions that a known volume and concentration of helium in air begin in the closed spirometer, that the subject has no helium in the lungs, and that an equilibration of helium can occur between the spirometer and the lungs. To perform the helium dilution procedure, a measurable volume of helium is added into the spirometer circuit, and the initial concentration of helium (F_iHe) is measured. To measure the FRC following a normal exhalation, a valve is turned to connect the subject to the breathing circuit. The resting expiratory level of the FRC is a common point to begin the test. Starting the test at RV requires maximal expiratory effort by the patient and is not considered a reliable starting point. Although starting the test at the TLC level requires a maximal inspiration, TLC may be a reliable alternate beginning point. The lung volume at the time the subject is connected to the helium is the lung volume measured.

The subject is connected to the helium-air mixture, and the concentration of helium is diluted slowly by the subject's lung volume. Wearing nose clips, the patient breathes normally in the closed circuit. Exhaled carbon dioxide is absorbed with soda lime, and oxygen is titrated at a rate equal to the subject's oxygen consumption. A constant volume is maintained to assure accurate helium concentration measurements. The subject rebreathes the gas in the system until an equilibrium of helium concentration is established. In normal subjects and those with a small functional residual capacity, equilibration occurs in 2 to 5 minutes. In patients with obstructive lung disease **equilibration** may take up to 20 minutes because of slow gas mixing in the lungs. The helium dilution time or the duration of the test is a gross index of the distribution of ventilation.

To calculate the FRC using the helium dilution technique, several measurements must be made. These include the volume of helium added (vol He) to the closed spirometer, the initial helium concentration (F_iHe), the final helium concentration (F_fHe) after equilibrium is established, and the spirometer

temperature. The functional residual capacity can be calculated with the equation:[32]

$$FRC = (He\ Vol \div F_iHe) \times [(F_iHe - F_fHe) \div F_fHe]$$

Applying Charles' law, the calculated FRC must be adjusted for the temperature difference between the spirometer and the subject's body temperature. This is the ATPS to BTPS correction. Although helium is an inert gas with a negligible solubility in plasma, another correction is sometimes applied. A small amount of helium is thought to diffuse across the alveolar capillary membrane and be lost in the measurement of final helium concentration. To account for the loss, 30 mL of BTPS-corrected volume is subtracted for each minute of helium breathing, up to 200 mL for a seven minute test.[35] Once these corrections are made, the residual volume can be calculated by subtracting the expiratory reserve volume from the FRC according to the equation:

$$RV = FRC - ERV$$

The nitrogen washout technique uses a non-rebreathing or open circuit (Figure 18-4).[36] The technique is based upon the assumptions that the nitrogen concentration in the lungs is 78% and in equilibrium with the atmosphere, that the subject inhales 100% oxygen, and that the oxygen replaces all of the nitrogen in the lungs. Similar to the helium dilution technique, the subject is connected to the system at either the resting expiratory level or the TLC. The lung volume at the time the subject begins 100% oxygen breathing and when exhaled gas is measured will be the lung volume measured. The subject's exhaled gas is monitored, and its volume and nitrogen percentage measured.

In general, there are two types of circuits used to measure lung volumes with this technique. In one type of circuit, all of the exhaled gases are collected in a large container where the measurements of volume and concentration of nitrogen are made. In the second

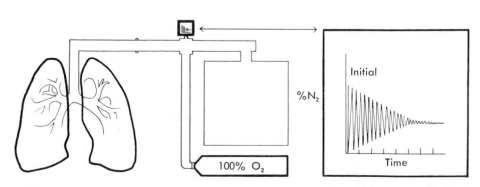

Fig. 18-4 Nitrogen washout method for measuring the functional residual capacity, the residual volume, and the total lung capacity.

type of circuit, the volume and concentration of each exhaled breath are measured separately and stored in a memory; the sum of the volumes and the weighted average of the nitrogen concentration is calculated by a computer.

Wearing nose clips, the patient breathes 100% oxygen until nearly all of the nitrogen has been washed out of the lungs, leaving less than 2.5% nitrogen in the lungs. When the peak exhaled concentration of nitrogen is less than 2.5%, the subject exhales completely and the fractional concentration of alveolar nitrogen (FAN_2) is noted. Similar to the helium technique, the time it takes to wash out the nitrogen is approximately 2 to 5 minutes in normal subjects and longer in those with obstructive disease. Some laboratories take precautions with subjects who have chronic obstructive pulmonary disease and chronic respiratory acidosis, since the subject breathes 100% oxygen. The test must occur in a leakproof circuit, since the presence of any air would alter the measured nitrogen percentages.

To calculate the FRC or TLC by the nitrogen washout technique, several measurements must be made. These include the total volume of gas exhaled during the test (VE), the fractional concentration of nitrogen in the total exhaled gas volume (FEN_2), the fractional concentration of nitrogen in the alveoli at the end of the test (FAN_2), and spirometer temperature. The functional residual capacity (or total lung capacity, if the test began at TLC) can be calculated with the equation.

$$FRC = (\dot{V}E \times FEN_2) \div (0.78 - FAN_2).$$

The calculated FRC (or TLC) must be adjusted for the temperature difference between the spirometer and the subject's body temperature using the BTPS correction factor. During the test, some nitrogen from the plasma and body tissues may have been excreted and exhaled with lung nitrogen, and a correction is needed. The volume of tissue nitrogen excreted (V_{tis} in mL) is directly related to the time (t in minutes) of the test and weight (W in kilograms) of the subject. A correction for this extra nitrogen should be made according to the formula

$$V_{tis} (mL) = (0.1209\sqrt{t} - 0.0665) \times (W/70)$$

V_{tis} (mL) is subtracted from the BTPS-corrected lung volume. The residual volume is the difference between the expiratory reserve volume and the functional residual capacity.

The validity of the helium dilution and nitrogen washout techniques can be assured by measuring known volumes accurately, such as a 3 liter syringe, while recognizing this method would not include oxygen consumption and oxygen **titration** for the helium method nor tissue nitrogen excretion for the nitrogen method. The reliability of these techniques can be established by repeated measurements which agree within 5%.

The whole-body plethysmography technique applies Boyle's Law and uses volume and pressure changes to determine lung volume.[37] The plethysmograph consists of a sealed chamber in which the subject sits (Figure 18-5 on page 416). Pressure **transducers** (electronic manometers) measure pressure at the airway and in the chamber. An electronically controlled shutter allows the airway to be occluded periodically, thereby measuring airway pressure changes under conditions of no airflow. According to Boyle's law ($V \times P = k$), volume changes in the thorax create volume changes in the chamber, which in turn are reflected by pressure changes in the chamber.

When conducting the measurement of thoracic gas volume (TGV), the subject sits in the chamber, breathes normally through the mouthpiece, then holds his cheeks, and pants.[38] During the panting, the technologist closes the airway shutter and measures the airway pressure changes (ΔP) and the chamber volume changes (ΔV). As applied to whole-body plethysmography,

$$TGV = PB \times (\Delta V \div \Delta P)$$

where PB is the barometric pressure in cm H_2O.

Because the body plethysmographic method of measuring FRC actually measures the total amount of gas in the thorax (TGV), the value obtained for some subjects may be somewhat larger than those resulting from either the helium dilution or nitrogen washout techniques. Such a difference would occur whenever there is gas in the thorax that is not in communication with patent airways, as might be the case in pneumothorax, pneumomediastinum, or emphysema. The residual volume is the difference between the thoracic gas volume and the expiratory reserve volume, and the total lung capacity is the sum of the residual volume and vital capacity, or the sum of the thoracic gas volume and the inspiratory capacity.

Pulmonary mechanics – spirometry

Measuring pulmonary mechanics is assessing the ability of the lungs to move large volumes of air quickly to identify airway obstruction. Some measurements are aimed at large intrathoracic airways, some are aimed at small airways, and some assess obstruction throughout the lungs. Most flows are measured by a spirometer or pneumo-tachometer while the subject is performing the forced vital capacity maneuver. Although performing the forced vital capacity is a safe procedure, some adverse reactions have occurred. These include pneumothorax,[39] syncope, chest pain, symptoms of paroxysmal coughing, and bronchospasm associated with exercise-induced asthma.[40]

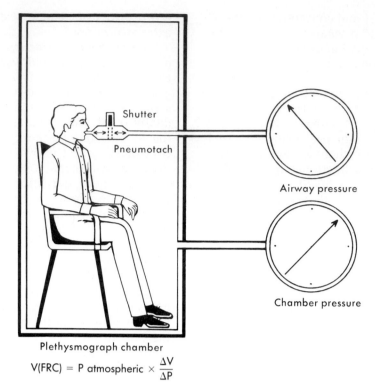

Shutter

Pneumotach

Airway pressure

Chamber pressure

Plethysmograph chamber

$$V(FRC) = P \text{ atmospheric} \times \frac{\Delta V}{\Delta P}$$

Fig. 18-5 Body plethysmography method for measuring lung volumes, V is the change in gas volume in the lungs, as sensed by the chamber pressure manometer. P is the change in pressure produced by the respiratory efforts of breathing against the shutter, as sensed by the airway pressure manometer.

The forced vital capacity (FVC) is the most commonly performed test of pulmonary mechanics. There are few contraindications to performing spirometry, and these are not considered absolute. These contraindications include hemoptysis of unknown origin, untreated pneumothorax, and unstable cardiovascular status which include thoracic, abdominal, or cerebral aneurysms.[10,35] Subjects who have recently had cataracts removed may be at risk due to an increase in cerebral pressure. Performing the FVC on subjects who are acutely ill or who have recently smoked a cigarette may hinder test validity.

National professional standards for performing the FVC, for assuring validity and reliability of the measurements, and for the accuracy and precision of the measuring equipment have been adopted by the American Thoracic Society, the American Association for Respiratory Care, and other professional and government agencies.[10,13,41-43] The FVC may be measured on a spirometer that measures volumes or one that measures flows, one that presents a graph of volume and time or flow and volume, one that is mechanical or electronic, and one that has a calculator or computer. Sometimes the forced expiratory vital capacity is followed by a forced inspiratory vital capacity to produce a complete loop of forced breathing.

The FVC is an effort-dependent maneuver that requires careful subject instruction, understanding, coordination, and cooperation. Spirometry standards for FVC specify that subjects must be instructed in the FVC maneuver and that the appropriate technique be demonstrated.[16] According to the standards, nose clips are encouraged, but not required. In one study, the measurements of FVC and FEV_1 were not significantly affected by the use of nose clips.[44] Subjects may be tested in the sitting or standing position. It is recommended that the position be consistent for repeat testing of the same subject. For adults, the FVC in the standing position is significantly greater than in the sitting position.[45] For children, the earlier ATS recommendation indicated VC is greater in the standing than in the sitting position.[17] Forced vital capacities should be converted to body temperature conditions and reported as liters, BTPS.

To assure validity, each subject must perform a minimum of 3 acceptable FVC maneuvers. To assure reliability, the largest FVC and second largest FVC from the acceptable trials should not vary by more than 5% (expressed as a percentage of the largest observed FVC regardless of the trial on which it occurred) or 0.100 L, whichever is greater. The forced exhalation of an acceptable FVC trial begins abruptly and without hesitation. A satisfactory start of expiration is characterized by an **extrapolated** volume less than 5% of FVC or 0.100 L, whichever is greater (Figure 18-6). An acceptable FVC trial also is smooth, continuous, and complete. While performing a FVC

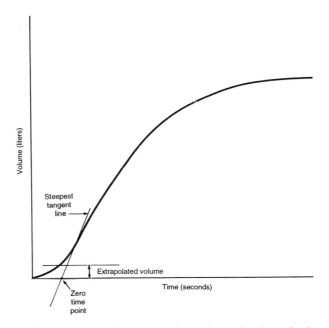

Fig. 18-6 Extrapolated volume and zero time point determination

maneuver, a cough, an inspiration, a **Valsalva** maneuver, a leak, or an obstructed mouthpiece would disqualify the trial. The FVC must be completely exhaled, or an exhalation time of at least 6 seconds must occur (longer times are frequently needed for subjects with airway obstruction). An end-expiratory plateau must be obvious in the volume-time curve resulting in less than 40 mL exhaled for at least 2 seconds of exhalation. Consistent with its definition, the largest acceptable FVC (BTPS) measured of the set of three acceptable trials is the subjects's FVC.

During forced vital capacity testing several other measurements are also made. The FEV_1 is a measurement of the volume exhaled in the first second of the FVC (see Figure 18-2, A). To assure validity of the FEV_1, the measurement must originate from a valid FVC trial. The first second of forced exhalation begins at the "zero time point" (Figure 18-6). The volume exhaled before the "zero time point" is called the extrapolated volume. No more than 5% of the vital capacity can allowed to be exhaled before the "zero time point." To assure reliability of the FEV_1, the largest FEV_1 and second largest FEV_1 from the acceptable trials should not vary by more than 5% (expressed as a percentage of the largest observed FEV_1 regardless of the trial on which it occurred) or 0.100 L, whichever is greater. Consistent with its definition, the largest FEV_1 (BTPS) measured is the subjects's FEV_1. Sometimes the largest FEV_1 comes from a different trial than the largest FVC.

The $\%FEV_1/FVC$, also called the FEV_1/FVC ratio, is calculated by dividing the subject's largest FEV_1 by the subject's largest FVC and converting to a percentage (by multiplying by 100). The two values do not necessarily have to come from the same trial.

All other measurements which originate from the FVC, such as PEFR, $FEF_{200-1200}$, $FEF_{25\%-75\%}$, $FEF_{75\%-85\%}$, and/or the instantaneous expiratory flowrates ($\dot{V}max$ or FEF) should be obtained from the single "best test" or "best curve." The best test curve is defined as the trial that meets the acceptability criteria and gives the largest sum of FVC plus FEV_1. The validity and reliability of these other measurements are based upon their origin from a valid and reliable FVC.

The $FEF_{200-1200}$ and $FEF_{25\%-75\%}$ represent average flowrates that occur during specific intervals of the forced vital capacity. Both measurements can be made on a volume-time spirogram as the slope of a line connecting the two points in their subscripts. For the $FEF_{200-1200}$, the 200 mL point and the 1200 mL point are identified. A straight line is drawn connecting these points, and the line is extended to intersect two vertical time lines one second apart on the graph (Figure 18-7, page 418). The volume of air measured between the two time lines is the $FEF_{200-1200}$ in liters per second. The volume measured must be corrected to BTPS.

The $FEF_{25\%-75\%}$ is a measure of the flow during the middle portion of the forced vital capacity, or the time necessary to exhale the middle 50%. For the $FEF_{25\%-75\%}$, the vital capacity of the "best curve" is multiplied by 25% and 75%, and the points are identified on the tracing. A straight line is drawn connecting these points, and the line is extended to intersect two vertical time lines one second apart on the graph. The volume of air measured between the two time lines is the $FEF_{25\%-75\%}$ in liters per second. The volume measured must be corrected to BTPS (Figure 18-8, page 418).

The peak expiratory flowrate (PEFR) is difficult to identify on a volume-time graph of the FVC. The peak flow is the slope of the **tangent** to the steepest portion of the forced vital capacity curve.[46] The PEFR is easy to identify on a flow-volume graph as the highest point on the graph (refer to Figure 18-2, B). The PEFR is sometimes measured independently of the forced vital capacity (FVC) with a peak flow meter. These devices are designed to only indicate the greatest expiratory flowrate. The validity of PEFR is based upon a preceding inspiration to total lung capacity (TLC) and a maximum effort. The FVC principles of assuring reliability should apply to measurements of PEFR. The two largest repeated measurements should agree within 5%.

In addition to PEFR, the other instantaneous flowrates such as $FEF_{25\%}$, $FEF_{50\%}$, $FEF_{75\%}$, during a forced vital capacity are graphed on a flow-volume curve. When the FVC is followed by a forced inspiratory vital capacity, a flow-volume loop is produced (see Figure 18-2, B). On the flow-volume loop, the maximum inspiratory flowrate at 50% ($FIF_{50\%}$) of the vital capacity can be measured and compared to the $FEF_{50\%}$.

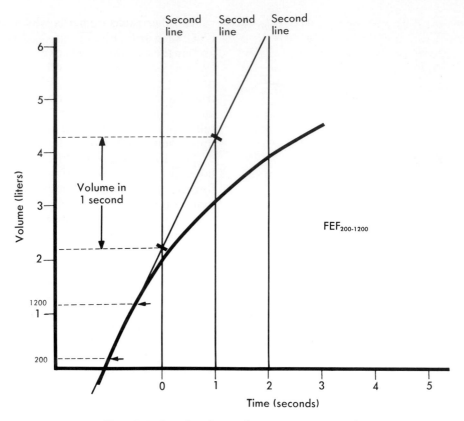

Fig. 18-7 Forced expiratory flowrate 200 to 1200 mL.

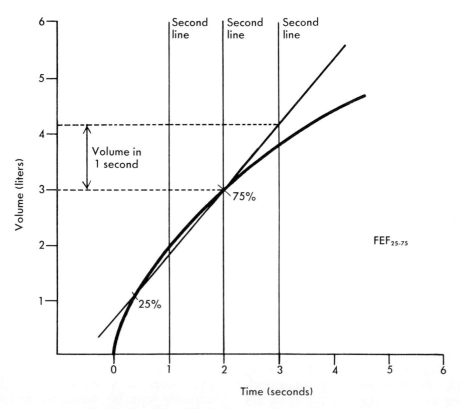

Fig. 18-8 Forced expiratory flowrate 25% to 75% of the FVC.

Another measurement of pulmonary mechanics is the maximum voluntary ventilation (MVV). The maximum voluntary ventilation is another effort dependent test for which the subject is asked to breathe as deeply and as rapidly as possible for at least 12 seconds. The MVV is a test which includes subject cooperation and effort, the ability of the diaphragm and thoracic muscles to expand the thorax and lungs, and airway obstruction.

The subject usually stands with a chair behind him or her and nose clips in place. After a demonstration of the expected breathing pattern, the subject should be instructed to breathe as rapidly and as deeply as possible for 12 or 15 seconds. The subject's breathing is measured on a spirogram (Figure 18-9) or electronically for the specific number of seconds (t), and the volume (V) breathed during the MVV is converted to liters per minute. As with all volumes measured on a spirometer, the recorded values should be in BTPS conditions. The use of an accumulator on many spirometers simplifies the measurement of the volume of gas moved in the specific time period. The accumulator adds all inspiratory volumes using a gear reduction. Once corrected for the gear reduction, the accumulator provides an easy way to measure the volume of gas moved (Figure 18-9) according to the following equation:

$$MVV = V \times VF \times BTPS \times (60 \div t)$$

For example:

Volume (V) breathed in 12 sec: 1.2 L
Gear reduction factor (f) = 25
Spirometer temperature 24° C (BTPS = 1.08)
Correction factor for time 60 ÷ 12 = 5

$$MVV = 1.2 \times 25 \times 1.08 \times 5 = 162 \text{ L/min}$$

Diffusion

The diffusing capacity of the lung or DLCO is sometimes called the transfer factor. DLCO expressed in mL/min/torr under standard temperature and pressure and dry conditions (STPD). The gas normally used to measure the diffusing capacity of the lung is carbon monoxide (CO), according to the equation:

$$D_{L}CO = V_{E}(F_{I}CO - F_{E}CO) \div (P_{A}CO - P_{C}CO)$$

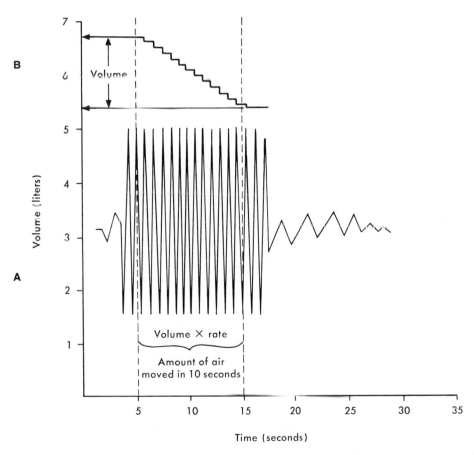

Fig. 18-9 Maximum voluntary ventilation tracing. **A,** Actual ventilations recorded during a 10-second period. **B,** Accumulator recording (addition of inspiratory volume) measured during the 10 seconds. Accumulator volume times correction factor (eg, 25 for Collins spirometer) equals actual volume.

Carbon monoxide is used as the transfer gas because carbon monoxide is similar to oxygen in important ways. Carbon monoxide and oxygen have similar molecular weights and **solubility coefficients.** Similar to oxygen, carbon monoxide also chemically combines with hemoglobin. Carbon monoxide has a very high affinity for hemoglobin and diffuses rapidly into the pulmonary blood. Carbon monoxide has an affinity for hemoglobin nearly 210 times greater than oxygen, and the high affinity keeps the pulmonary capillary partial pressure (PcCO) of carbon monoxide near zero. As a result, the diffusion of carbon monoxide across the alveolar capillary membrane is membrane-limited and not limited as much by the partial pressure gradient. Performing the diffusing capacity on subjects who have recently smoked a cigarette or have been exposed to environmental carbon monoxide may hinder test validity.

There are several techniques and variations of techniques for measuring the diffusing capacity of the lungs. The two most common methods are single breath and steady state techniques. These techniques have several important advantages and differences such as the concentrations of carbon monoxide and the duration of exposure. The single breath technique requires some patient cooperation and breatholding; the steady state technique utilizes a normal breathing pattern. Both techniques assume that the subject has a normal hematocrit and does not have an abnormal level of carboxyhemoglobin. The hematocrit should be measured for all subjects of the diffusing capacity,[47] and the test should be delayed for subjects who have been recently exposed to smoke or excessive auto emissions, unless determining the acute effects of exposure is the purpose of the test.[48]

For the steady state technique (DLCOss), subjects breathe a gas mixture 0.1% to 0.2% CO in air for several minutes until the exhaled concentrations of carbon monoxide become stable. The volume (VE) and concentration of carbon monoxide in the exhaled gases (FeCO) are measured. The volume of carbon monoxide transferred per minute across the alveolar capillary membrane is the minute ventilation multiplied by the difference between inspired and mean expired concentrations of carbon monoxide according to the equation:

$$\text{mL CO} = V_E \times (F_ICO - F_ECO)$$

The partial pressure of carbon monoxide in the pulmonary capillary plasma (PcCO) is assumed to be zero. There are several variations of the steady state technique to determine the alveolar partial pressure of carbon monoxide (PACO); collecting an end-tidal sample is one. The end-tidal sampler collects a small volume of gas at the end of the tidal volume exhalation to represent alveolar gas. The partial pressure of carbon monoxide in the end-tidal sample can be calculated according to the equation:

$$P_ACO = F_{ET}CO \times (P_B - 47)$$

where P_B is the barometric pressure in torr and 47 is the water vapor pressure in torr at body temperature.

The diffusing capacity of the lung for carbon monoxide using the single breath method (DLCOsb) is the most common measurement technique because it is quick. The entire test can be performed in just slightly longer than 10 seconds. The subject inspires a vital capacity of a gas mixture containing 0.3% CO and 10% He in air, maintains breathholding for 10 seconds, and then exhales rapidly at least 1 liter. After a present volume is exhaled, a sample of alveolar gas is collected and analyzed for expired carbon monoxide (F_ECO_t) and helium (F_EHe). The breatholding period (t) begins when inspiration of the gas mixture begins, and the period ends when the alveolar sample is collected; this period should not exceed 11 seconds.[49] To regulate the breathholding period, some measuring systems close the mouthpiece with a timed shutter. The suitable breathing pattern does require some patient cooperation and coordination; some patients benefit from a timer as a visual aid.[50]

The single breath method (DLCOsb) is based upon the diffusion decay curve described by Forster (Figure 18-10).[51] When a bolus of gas is inhaled, the rate of gas diffusion declines logarithmically. The diffusing capacity of the lung is a function of lung volume (V_A), the duration ($60 \div t$) that the test gas is in contact with the lung, and the concentration of test gas in the lung (F_ACO_0) according to the equation:

$$D_LCO = [60(V_A) \div t(P_B - 47)] \times \ln (F_ACO_0 \div F_ACO_t)$$

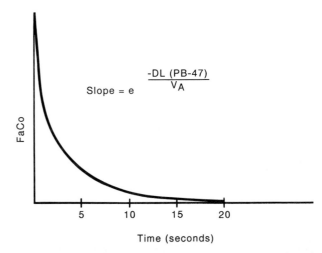

Fig. 18-10 The concentration of alveolar carbon monoxide following a single breath to total lung capacity.

The alveolar volume (VA) must be converted from ATPS conditions to STPD conditions.[52]

Helium is in the gas mixture as a tracer gas for the dilution of the inspired carbon monoxide concentration by the residual volume and to measure the effective total lung capacity by a single breath helium dilution. The inspired carbon monoxide concentration of 0.03% is not the concentration of carbon monoxide received by the lungs because the inspired volume is diluted by the residual volume of the subject. The dilution of carbon monoxide is reflected by the dilution of helium, and the FACO$_0$ can be calculated according to the equation:

$$FACO_0 = FICO (FEHe \div FIHe)$$

The FACO$_0$ is the concentration of carbon monoxide in the lung at "zero time" before any diffusion occurs. The single breath technique distributes the gas mixture through unobstructed airways to an alveolar volume that is also called the effective total lung capacity. The effective total lung capacity (VA) can be calculated according to the equation:

$$VA = VC \times (FIHe \div FEHe)$$

The effective total lung capacity is necessary to calculate the DLCOSB, and it is used in the DLCOSB/VA ratio.

INTERPRETATION OF TEST RESULTS

Pathophysiologic considerations

Pulmonary function testing provides the basis for classifying pulmonary diseases into two major categories, obstructive and restrictive. Figure 18-11 compares normal lungs with the pathophysiologic aspects of obstructive lung diseases and restrictive lung diseases. Sometimes these two types of lung diseases

Table 18-3 Comparisons between obstructive and restrictive types of pulmonary diseases

Characteristic	Obstructive	Restrictive
Anatomy affected	Airways	Non-airways
Breathing phase difficulty	Expiration	Inspiration
Pathophysiology	Increased airway resistance	Decreased lung/thoracic compliance
Useful measurements	Flows	Volumes

occur together. Obstructive and restrictive types of lung diseases are different in several important ways. These comparisons are summarized in Table 18-3. Obstructive diseases affect the airways; restrictive diseases affect the alveoli, the thoracic cage, or the ventilatory muscles. The primary pathophysiology in obstructive disease is an increase in airway resistance; in restrictive disease the primary problem is a reduced lung or thoracic compliance. With obstructive disease, patients have more difficulty exhaling; patients with restrictive disease have difficulty inhaling. Measuring the flow of gases, such as the FEV$_1$ or PEFR, is useful in detecting obstructive disease, and measuring lung volumes, such as the total lung capacity, is useful in detecting restrictive diseases.

The primary problem in obstructive pulmonary disease is an increased airway resistance. Airway resistance is the difference in pressure between the ends of the airways divided by the flowrate of gas moving through the airway, according to the formula, Raw = ΔP $\div$ V. There is an inverse relationship between airway resistance (Raw) and flowrates (V). If the pressure difference is constant, a reduced flowrate indicates an increase in airway resistance. Since the

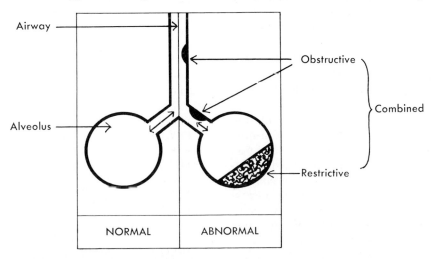

Fig. 18-11 Pathophysiologic aspects of lung disease.

radius of the airways normally lessens slightly during expiration, flowrates are usually measured during expiration. By rearranging the symbols in Poiseuille's law, airway resistance is inversely related to the radius of the airways according to formula, $Raw = \Delta P \div V = n81 \div \pi r^4$. When airway radius (r) decreases, resistance (Raw) increases and flowrates ($\dot{V}$) decrease. Airway radius can be reduced by excessive contraction of the bronchial and bronchiolar muscles (bronchospasm), excessive secretions in the airways, swelling of the airway mucosa, airway tumors, collapse of the bronchioles, and other causes. By measuring flowrates, pulmonary function tests measure indirectly the size of the airways, airway resistance, and the presence of obstructive disease.

The primary problem in restrictive lung disease is a reduced lung compliance, thoracic compliance, or both lung and thoracic compliances. Compliance is the volume of gas inspired for the amount of inspiratory effort; effort is measured as the amount of pressure created in the lung or in the pleural space when the inspiratory muscles contract. Compliance is calculated according to the formula, $C = \Delta V \div \Delta P$. There is a direct relationship between compliance (C) and volume (V). If the pressure difference is constant, a reduced inspiratory volume indicates a reduction in compliance. A reduced lung compliance is usually the result of alveolar inflammation, pulmonary **fibrosis,** or neoplasms in the alveoli; a reduced thoracic compliance may be the result of thoracic wall abnormalities such as kyphoscoliosis. Neuromuscular diseases also can result in reduced lung volumes and restrictive–type pulmonary impairments, mainly by affecting the function of the inspiratory muscles. In these circumstances, lung and thoracic compliance may be normal, but the patient is simply unable to generate enough subatmospheric pressure to take a full, deep breath.

Some obstructive diseases and some restrictive diseases also may affect the ability of the lung to diffuse gases. In some diseases there is damage to the alveolar capillary membrane or less alveolar surface area accessible for diffusion. Measuring the diffusing capacity of the lung can identify the destruction of alveolar tissue or the loss of functioning alveolar surface area.

For each measurement of pulmonary function there is a normal value and a range of normal limits. The severity of pulmonary impairment is based upon a comparison of each subject's measurement compared to the predicted normal value for the subject. There are several methods to compare to the normal value. A common method of comparison is to compute a percentage of the predicted normal value according to the equation:

$$\% \text{ Predicted} = \frac{\text{Measured Value}}{\text{Predicted Normal Value}} \times 100$$

Table 18-4 Severity of pulmonary impairments based upon % of the predicted normal value or standard deviations of the mean predicted normal value

Degree of Impairment	% Predicted	Standard Deviations Below Mean
Normal	80–120%	< 1 SD
Mild	65–79%	1–2 SD
Moderate	50–64%	2–3 SD
Severe	35–49%	> 3 SD
Very Severe	< 35%	

Determining if the subject's value is within one or two standard deviation of the predicted normal value is an alternate method used in some laboratories. The % Predicted or the number of standard deviations from the predicted normal value can be used to quantify severity of impairment. Typical degrees of severity are in Table 18-4.

Lung volumes and capacities

Some lung volumes provide valuable diagnostic information. For example, the total lung capacity is always reduced in restrictive lung disease, unless obstruction and restriction occur together. Then the TLC may be a less sensitive measure of the restrictive impairment.[53] Other volumes and capacities may remain normal with obstructive or restrictive disease. The pattern of lung volume changes also is important. Table 18-5 summarizes lung volume and capacity

Table 18-5 Pulmonary function changes that may occur in advanced obstructive and restrictive lung diseases

Measurement	Normal *	Obstructive	Restrictive
V_T	500 mL	N or ↑	N or ↓
IC	3600 mL	N or ↓	↓
ERV	1200 mL	N or ↓	↓
RV	1200 mL	↑	↓
IC	3600 mL	N or ↓	↓
FRC	2400 mL	↑	↓
TLC	6000 mL	N or ↑	↓
FVC	4800 mL	↓	↓
FEV_1	4200 mL	↓	N or ↓
FEV_1/FVC	> 70%	↓	N or ↑
$FEF_{200-1200}$	8.5 L/sec	↓	N
$FEF_{25\%-75\%}$	4.5 L/sec	↓	N
PEFR	9.5 L/sec	↓	N
$FEF_{25\%}$	9.0 L/sec	↓	N
$FEF_{50\%}$	6.5 L/sec	↓	N
$FEF_{75\%}$	3.5 L/sec	↓	N
MVV	160 L/min	↓	N or ↓
$DLCO_{SB}$	40 mL/min/torr	N or ↓	N or ↓
$DLCO_{SB}/V_A$	6.6 mL/min/torr/L	N or ↓	N or ↓

* "Normal" values are for 70 kg adult male.

changes that may occur in obstructive and restrictive lung diseases.

The normal tidal volume is approximately 500 mL to 700 mL for the average healthy adult. In the normal population, there is great variation of tidal volumes and measurements beyond the normal range are not indicative of a disease process. Normal tidal volumes are often observed in both restrictive and obstructive lung diseases. Therefore, the tidal volume alone is not a valid indicator of the type of lung disease.

The normal inspiratory capacity is approximately 3600 mL with a significant variation in the normal population. The inspiratory capacity may be normal or reduced in restrictive and obstructive lung diseases. A reduction of inspiratory capacity occurs in restrictive lung diseases because the subject's inhaled volume is reduced, and there is a reduction in total lung capacity. In mild obstructive lung diseases, the inspiratory capacity is usually normal. In moderate and severe obstructive disease the inspiratory capacity can be reduced because the resting expiratory level of the functional residual capacity has increased due to **hyperinflation** of the lungs. An increase in inspiratory capacity may occur when the subject is below the resting expiratory level when the measurement is performed; athletes and wind musicians may also have increased inspiratory capacities. Therapists utilize the measurement of inspiratory capacity in clinical protocols to decide between methods of hyperinflation therapy. During intermittent positive pressure breathing and sustained maximal inspirations (SMI) patients inhale the inspiratory capacity.

The Inspiratory reserve volume (IRV) is not commonly measured. Similar to the tidal volume and the inspiratory capacity, the inspiratory reserve volume can be normal in both restrictive and obstructive diseases and is not a very useful diagnostic measurement. The normal value for the inspiratory reserve volume is 3.10 L.

The normal expiratory reserve volume is approximately 1.20 L and represents around 20% to 25% of the vital capacity. It can be either normal or reduced in obstructive and restrictive lung diseases. The expiratory reserve volume is subtracted from the functional residual capacity in order to calculate the residual volume.

The normal value of the vital capacity is 4.80 L and represents approximately 80% of the total lung capacity. Normal values for vital capacity can vary significantly depending on age, gender, height, and ethnicity. A reduction of vital capacity occurs in restrictive lung diseases because the subject's inhaled volume is reduced and there is a reduction in total lung capacity. In mild obstructive lung diseases, the slow vital capacity is usually normal if the subject exhales leisurely and has had enough time to exhale completely, or if the vital capacity is measured during inspiration.

Measurements made from the forced vital capacity provide valuable data for pulmonary mechanics.

The residual volume, functional residual capacity, and total lung capacity are the most important measurements of lung volumes. Age, height, gender, ethnicity, and sometimes weight or body surface area correlate with normal values for these lung volumes.[54] Table 18-6 provides common regression equations to predict the lung volumes for individuals of specific height (in centimeters), age (in years), gender, and body surface area (BSA in square meters).[34] There is a positive correlation between lung volumes and height, and there is a negative correlation between lung volumes and age for subjects older than 20 years. Male values are larger than female values when height and age are equal.

The typical normal total lung capacity is 6.00 L. The normal residual volume is approximately 1.20 L and represents about 20% of the total lung capacity. The functional residual capacity is approximately 2.40 L which represents approximately 40% of the total lung capacity. The residual volume and functional residual capacity are usually enlarged in acute and chronic obstructive lung diseases due to hyperinflation and air trapping (See Figure 18-12 and Mini-Clini 18-1 on page 424). In chronic obstructive pulmonary disease, the total lung capacity may also be enlarged. The total lung capacity is always reduced in restrictive lung diseases due to a loss of lung volume; the residual volume and functional residual capacity are often reduced proportionately. Certain acute disorders, such as pulmonary edema, atelectasis, and consolidation also will cause a reduction of total lung capacity and functional residual capacity.

Pulmonary mechanics – spirometry

The normal values for the spirometric measurements of pulmonary mechanics are based on height, age, gender, and ethnicity. Table 18-7, page 425, provides common regression equations to predict normal values for the measurements of pulmonary mechanics for individuals of specific height (in centi-

Table 18-6 Examples of regression equations for predicted normal lung volumes and capacities in adults

Lung volumes	Regression equations	References
FRC (L)	♂ 0.081(Hcm) − 1.792(BSA) −7.11	53
	♀ 0.0421(Hcm) − 0.00449(A) −3.825	53
RV (L)	♂ 0.027(Hcm) + 0.017(A) − 3.447	53
	♀ 0.032(Hcm) + 0.009(A) − 3.90	53
TLC (L)	♂ 0.094(Hcm) − 0.015(A) 9.167	53
	♀ 0.079(Hcm) + 0.008(A) −7.49	53
VC (L)	♂ 0.0844(Hcm) − 0.0298(A) − 8.7818	45
	♀ 0.0427(Hcm) − 0.0174(A) − 2.9001	45

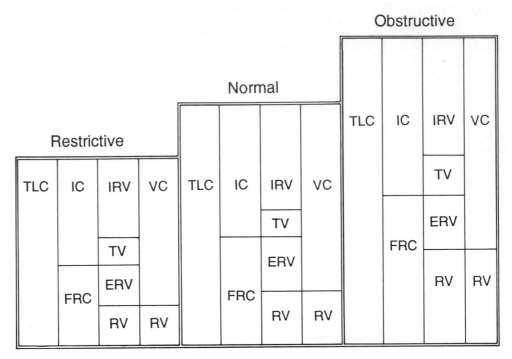

Fig. 18-12 Changes in lung volumes and capacities with pulmonary disease.

meters), age (in years), and gender.[45,55,56] There is a positive correlation between measurements of pulmonary mechanics and height, and there is a negative correlation between measurements of pulmonary mechanics and age for subjects older than 20 years. Male values are larger than female values when height and age are equal. The populations that were studied to determine the normal values of pulmonary mechanics were predominately caucasian. To account for ethnic differences of non-caucasians, the predicted normal caucasian values commonly are reduced by 12% to 15% when applied to non-caucasians. Figure 18-13 presents the **nomogram** produced by Morris in 1971 for predicting spirometric values of males and females. For subjects of each gender, a line connecting the points of age and height is extended to identify the predicted normal values of forced vital capacity, FEV_1, $FEF_{200-1200}$, and $FEF_{25\%-75\%}$.

A typical normal forced vital capacity is 4.80 L. A reduced forced vital capacity (FVC) may occur with

---

■ MINI **C**LINI ■

18-1

Why are Functional Residual Capacity (FRC) and Residual Volume (RV) Increased in Emphysema?

In the advanced stages of chronic obstructive pulmonary disease (COPD) such as pulmonary emphysema, the FRC and the RV are increased; also the vital capacity is often decreased. Why is this so?

Discussion: Emphysema is characterized by a destruction of elastic tissue in the lung which causes low lung recoil force. The size of the FRC is determined by the equilibrium between the oppositely directed recoil forces of the lung and chest wall. The FRC marks the relaxation point or resting level of the lung-thorax system, i.e. ventilatory muscles are in a relaxed state. When lung recoil forces decrease, as in emphysema, chest wall recoil forces predominate and the chest wall expands outward, pulling the lung with it. As the lung stretches to a larger volume, its recoil force increases, and eventually an equilibrium is reestablished between the lung and chest wall. This new equilibrium occurs at an increased lung volume, and thus FRC is increased. This increase is technically due to an increase in RV (FRC = RV + ERV). Because VC = TLC − FRC, an increased FRC decreases the vital capacity. Another reason for the decrease in VC is that expiratory resistance is high in obstructive disease. Small airways narrow and may collapse, trapping gas in the lung, thus increasing FRC and decreasing VC.

Table 18–7 Examples of regression equations for predicted normal pulmonary mechanics in adults

Parameters	Regression equations	References	Parameters	Regression equations	References
FVC (L)	♂ $(0.0580 \times \text{Ht})-(0.025 \times \text{A})-4.24$ ♀ $(0.0453 \times \text{Ht})-(0.024 \times \text{A})-2.852$	55	PEFR	♂ $(0.0567 \times \text{Ht})-(0.024 \times \text{A})+0.225$ ♀ $(0.0354 \times \text{Ht})-(0.018 \times \text{A})+1.130$	54
FEV_1 (L)	♂ $(0.052 \times \text{Ht})-(0.027 \times \text{A})-4.203$ ♀ $(0.027 \times \text{Ht})-(0.021 \times \text{A})-0.794$	45	$\text{FEF}_{25\%}$	♂ $(0.088 \times \text{Ht})-(0.035 \times \text{A})-5.618$ ♀ $(0.043 \times \text{Ht})-(0.025 \times \text{A})-0.132$	45
$\%\text{FEV}_1/\text{FVC}$	♂ $103.64-(0.087 \times \text{Ht})-(0.140 \times \text{A})$ ♀ $107.38-(0.111 \times \text{Ht})-(0.109 \times \text{A})$	45	$\text{FEF}_{50\%}$	♂ $(0.069 \times \text{Ht})-(0.015 \times \text{A})-5.4$ ♀ $(0.035 \times \text{Ht})-(0.013 \times \text{A})-0.444$	45
FEF_{2-1200}	♂ $(0.0429 \times \text{Ht})-(0.047 \times \text{A})+2.010$ ♀ $(0.0570 \times \text{Ht})-(0.036 \times \text{A})-2.532$	55	$\text{FEF}_{75\%}$	♂ $(0.044 \times \text{Ht})-(0.012 \times \text{A})-4.143$ ♀ $3.042-(0.014 \times \text{A})$	45
$\text{FEF}_{25\%-75\%}$	♂ $(0.0185 \times \text{Ht})-(0.045 \times \text{A})+2.513$ ♀ $(0.0236 \times \text{Ht})-(0.030 \times \text{A})+0.551$	55	MVV	♂ $(1.19 \times \text{Ht})-(0.816 \times \text{A})-37.9$ ♀ $(0.84 \times \text{Ht})-(0.685 \times \text{A})-4.87$	55
$\text{FEF}_{75\%-85\%}$	♂ $(0.0051 \times \text{Ht})-(0.023 \times \text{A})+1.21$ ♀ $(0.0098 \times \text{Ht})-(0.021 \times \text{A})+0.321$	55			

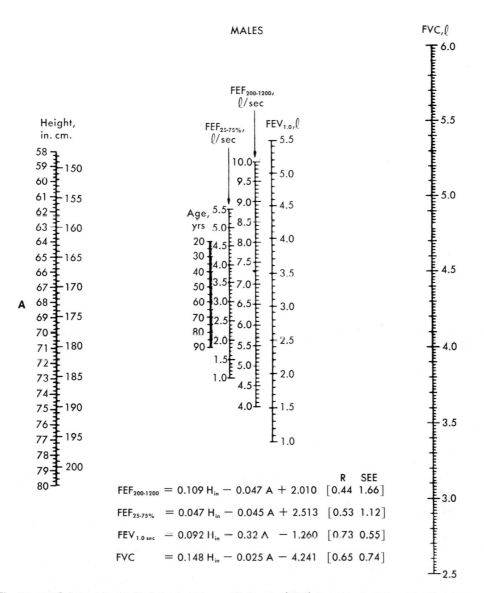

MALES

$$\text{FEF}_{200-1200} = 0.109\, H_{in} - 0.047\, A + 2.010 \quad [0.44 \quad 1.66]$$

$$\text{FEF}_{25-75\%} = 0.047\, H_{in} - 0.045\, A + 2.513 \quad [0.53 \quad 1.12]$$

$$\text{FEV}_{1.0\,sec} = 0.092\, H_{in} - 0.32\, A - 1.260 \quad [0.73 \quad 0.55]$$

$$\text{FVC} = 0.148\, H_{in} - 0.025\, A - 4.241 \quad [0.65 \quad 0.74]$$

Fig. 18–13 Spirometric standards for **A,** males and **B,** females (BTPS). (From Morris JF, Koski WA, and Johnson LC: *Am Rev Resp Dis* 103(1):57, 1971.)

continued

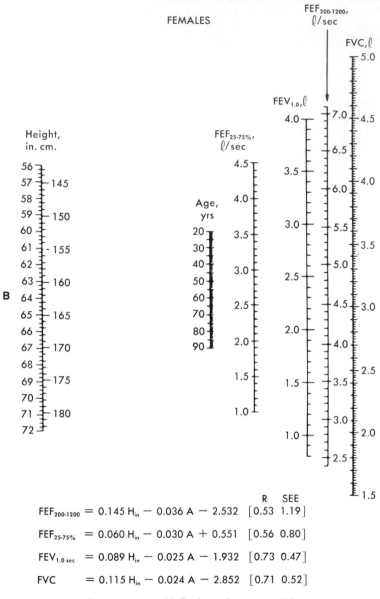

FEMALES

$$FEF_{200\text{-}1200} = 0.145\,H_{in} - 0.036\,A - 2.532 \quad [0.53 \quad 1.19]$$

$$FEF_{25\text{-}75\%} = 0.060\,H_{in} - 0.030\,A + 0.551 \quad [0.56 \quad 0.80]$$

$$FEV_{1.0\,sec} = 0.089\,H_{in} - 0.025\,A - 1.932 \quad [0.73 \quad 0.47]$$

$$FVC = 0.115\,H_{in} - 0.024\,A - 2.852 \quad [0.71 \quad 0.52]$$

Fig. 18-13 *cont'd* For legend see page 425.

obstructive or restrictive impairments. Figure 18-14 demonstrates forced vital capacities from volume-time spirometer tracings for the normal, obstructive, and restrictive conditions. The forced vital capacities in both the obstructed and restricted curves are shown as reduced volumes compared to the normal. The primary difference between the curve in the restricted subject compared to the obstructed subject is the slope of the tracing; obstructive diseases produce flattened slopes.

Figure 18-15 on page 428 displays the forced vital capacities from flow-volume tracings for the obstructive, and restrictive conditions. The shapes of these tracings are different; obstructive diseases produce lower peaks and lower flowrates at all lung volumes. Sometimes forced inspiratory flowrates are useful for identifying extrathoracic airway obstructions. In moderate and severe obstructive lung diseases, the forced vital capacity will be reduced if weakened bronchioles collapse and trap air in the lungs creating an increase in residual volume. Some laboratories compare the volumes of the slow vital capacity and the forced vital capacity to identify air trapping. A reduction of vital capacity occurs in restrictive lung diseases because the subject's inhaled volume is reduced.

The forced expiratory volume, half second ($FEV_{0.5}$) is an indicator of subject effort during the initial phase of the forced vital capacity maneuver. With good effort, a subject should exhale at least 50% of their vital capacity in the initial half second.

Although the units for the forced expiratory volume, 1 second (FEV_1) are volume, the FEV_1 is considered a flowrate. A typical normal FEV_1 is 4.20 L. The

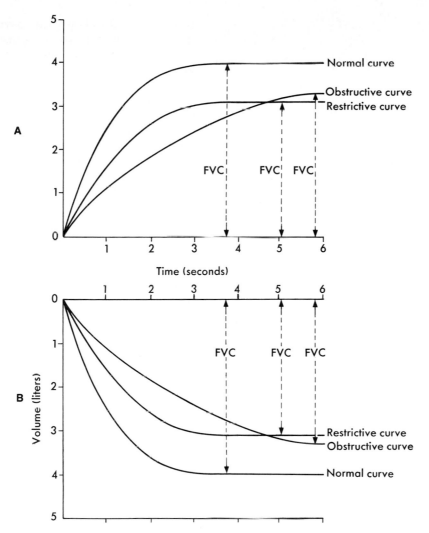

Fig. 18-14 Forced vital capacity curves comparing normal, obstructive, and restrictive disorders. **A** shows curves as they appear on commonly available spirometers with tracings beginning at the bottom left corner. **B** shows same curves as they appear on some spirometers that begin tracings at upper left corner.

FEV_1 may be reduced with obstructive or restrictive impairments. For subjects with airway obstruction, the FEV_1 measures the general severity of airway obstruction. For subjects with restrictive impairment, the FEV_1 may be reduced when the subject's vital capacity is smaller than the predicted FEV_1.

The forced expiratory volume in 1 second ratio (%FEV_1/FVC) separates subjects with airway obstruction from those with normal pulmonary function and from those with restrictive impairment (MiniClini 18-2, page 428). The predicted normal %FEV_1/FVC can be determined by dividing the predicted normal FEV_1 by the predicted normal FVC. In general, individuals without airway obstruction will be able to exhale at least 70% of their vital capacities in the first second, and individuals with airway obstruction will exhale less than 70% of their vital capacities in the first second.

To interpret other flowrates a generalization may be helpful. Gas exhaled during the early portion of the forced vital capacity reflects the resistance in the larger airways, and gas exhaled during the later portion of the forced vital capacity reflects the resistance in the smaller airways. As exhalation of the FVC proceeds, flow decreases, and the airways reflected in the measurements get smaller. Any flow measured in the first half of the forced vital capacity reflects on the bronchi; any flow measured beyond 50% of the vital capacity reflects on the bronchioles.

The PEFR, $FEF_{200-1200}$, $FEF_{25\%}$ occur near the onset of the FVC. Typical normal values are similar; PEFR is 9.5 L/sec; $FEF_{200-1200}$ is 8.5 L/sec; $FEF_{25\%}$ is 9.0 L/sec. A reduced PEFR, $FEF_{200-1200}$, or $FEF_{25\%}$ may occur due to large airway obstruction, as well as lack of sufficient effort to inhale maximally and exhale forcibly. The $FEF_{25\%-75\%}$ and $FEF_{50\%}$ occur in the middle of the FVC. Because the $FEF_{25\%-75\%}$ is an average of half the vital capacity and $FEF_{50\%}$ is an instantaneous flow, these

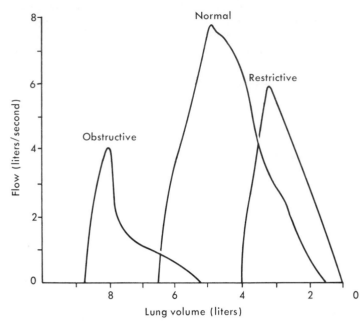

Fig. 18-15 Maximum expiratory flow volume curve example comparing normal with obstructive and restrictive disorders. Displayed as flows at actual lung volumes.

Sometimes subjects who are **asymptomatic** for cough, sputum production, or dyspnea may have reduced flow in the small airways. A singular reduction in small airway flow may indicate nothing at all or may be an early indicator of obstruction.

The shape of the flow-volume loop and the $FEF_{50\%}/FIF_{50\%}$ ratio provide additional information about upper airway obstruction. Compared to the normal flow-volume loop, a fixed upper airway obstruction produces a curve that appears box-shaped (Figure 18-16), both expiratory and inspiratory flows are decreased and limited by the solid obstruction; the $FEF_{50\%}/FIF_{50\%}$ ratio remains normal. Variable upper airway obstructions produce two different shapes depending upon the site of the obstruction. Since the intra-airway pressure during a forced inspiration is less than atmospheric outside the thorax, a variable **extrathoracic** upper airway obstruction limits inspiratory flow, and the $FEF_{50\%}/FIF_{50\%}$ ratio is greater than 1.0. Because the intra-airway pressure during a forced inspiration is greater than atmospheric inside the thorax, a variable intrathoracic upper airway obstruction limits expiratory flow, and the $FEF_{50\%}/FIF_{50\%}$ ratio is less than 1.0.

Similar to other spirometric measurements of pulmonary mechanics, normal values of the maximum voluntary ventilation are based on sex, age, and height. The maximum voluntary ventilation is reduced in patients with moderate and severe airway obstruction. A measured value less than 75% of the predicted is significant. The normal for males is about 160 to 180 L/min; it is slightly lower in females. In

typical normal values are less similar; $FEF_{25\%-75\%}$ is 4.5 L/sec; $FEF_{50\%}$ is 6.5 L/sec. A reduced $FEF_{25\%-75\%}$ or $FEF_{50\%}$ may occur due to small airway obstruction, as well as lack of effort to sustain a maximal exhalation. The $FEF_{75\%}$ and $FEF_{75\%-85\%}$ occur late in the FVC and reflect on the smallest airways. Typical values are 3.5 L/sec for $FEF_{75\%}$ and 1.5 L/sec for $FEF_{75\%-85\%}$.

■ MINI CLINI ■

18-2

Decreased FVC and FEV₁: Obstruction or Restrictive?

Both obstructive and restrictive diseases may exhibit decreased forced vital capacities (FVC) and one-second forced expired volumes (FEV_1). How can one differentiate the two kinds of patterns?

Discussion: FVC and FEV_1 are reduced in both obstructive and restrictive diseases for different reasons. Restrictive disease is associated with low FVC and FEV_1 because total lung volume is low; that is, lung expansion is difficult. Obstructive disease, on the other hand, is associated with a low FVC largely because of high expiratory resistance and air trapping during a forced exhalation; total lung volume is normal or possibly increased. Another reason for low FVC in obstructive disease may be low lung recoil force that causes

an increased FRC. FEV_1 is low in obstructive disease, because of high expiratory resistance which decreases expiratory flow rates.

The key to differentiating obstructive from restrictive patterns when FVC and FEV_1 are known is to compare FEV_1 with FVC. The question is what percentage of the FVC can the individual forcefully exhale in one

second? With normal airways, this value (FEV_1/FVC) should be at least 70%. For example:

Patient A	Patient B
FVC 2.0L	FCV 3.5L
(60% of predicted)	(65% of predicted)
FEV_1 1.56 L	FEV_1 1.57L
(58% of predicted)	(29% of predicted)
FEV_1/FVC 78%	FEV_1/FVC 45%

Patient A has a restrictive impairment with no airway obstruction; patient B has an obstructive impairment as indicated by the low FEV_1/FVC ratio. To determine if patient B also has a restrictive impairment, a TLC determination is required. Normal or high TLC indicates absence of restriction.

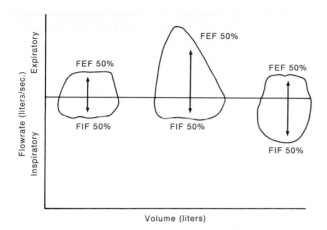

Fig. 18-16 Flow-volume loops of fixed upper airway obstruction, extrathoracic upper airway obstruction, variable intrathoracic upper airway obstruction.

Table 18-8 Examples of regression equations for predicting normal pulmonary diffusing capacities in adults

Parameters	Regression Equations	References
$D_L CO_{SS}$	♂ (0.073 H) − (0.279 A) + 18.167	59
	♀ (0.069 H) − (0.252 A) + 15.863	
$D_L CO_{SB}$	♂ (0.416 H) − (0.219 A) − 26.34	60
	♀ (0.256 H) − (0.144 A) − 8.36	
$D_L CO_{SB}/V_A$	♂ 6.61 − (0.034 A)*	60
	♀ 7.34 − (0.032 A)*	

*Hemoglobin corrected according to Dinikara[62]

restrictive lung disease the maximum voluntary ventilation value may be normal or only slightly reduced. Respiratory muscle strength is a primary determinant of MVV in patients with interstitial lung disease, and an important determinant in patients with chronic obstructive disease.[57] Undernourished patients also may have a reduced MVV.[58]

Diffusion

Because the two techniques use different concentrations of carbon monoxide, different exposure periods, and different breathing patterns, there are different normal values for each technique. For the steady state technique, a typical normal value for an adult is 25 mL/min/torr.[59] For the single breath technique, a typical normal value is 40 mL/min/torr.[60] Table 18-8 provides common regression equations to predict the diffusing capacity for individuals of specific height (in centimeters), age (in years), and gender for the $D_L CO_{SS}$ and the $D_L CO_{SB}$.

The diffusing capacity ($D_L CO$) may be reduced in subjects with obstructive or restrictive lung diseases. With destruction of alveoli in pulmonary emphysema, with small lung volumes, and with fibrosis of alveoli in asbestosis, the diffusing capacity may be less than normal (see MiniClini 18-3). Pulmonary embolism also may decrease the diffusing capacity.[61] Diffusion also can be influenced by hematologic factors, such as hemoglobin type and concentration, the presence of carboxyhemoglobin, and the volume of pulmonary blood flow. A common reason that the diffusing capacity ($D_L CO_{SB}$) may vary from the normal is due to an hematocrit which is not normal. The

■ M I N I **C** L I N I ■

18-3

Diffusion Capacity in Chronic Obstructive Pulmonary Disease

A patient presents with pulmonary function spirometry typical of chronic obstructive pulmonary disease (COPD). All flows are significantly reduced, as are FEV_1, and FEV_1/FVC. Functional residual capacity (FRC) is increased, and total lung capacity is 110% of normal. The diffusion capacity for carbon monoxide ($D_L CO$) is only 45% of predicted. Two major disease entities in the COPD category are pulmonary emphysema and chronic bronchitis. Which of these two entities most closely fits the pulmonary function data?

Discussion: Pulmonary emphysema primarily involves alveolar structures, and is characterized by destruction of alveolar architecture and elastic fibers. Chronic bronchitis involves mostly airways, rather than alveoli, and is characterized by chronic inflammation of the mucosa, hypertrophy of mucous glands, and hypersecreation of abnormal mucous. Both of these pathologies cause an obstructive pattern, although the mechanisms of obstruction are different. In emphysema, the mechanism involves dynamic compression and narrowing of the airways induced by pressure gradients during exhalation (refer to Chapter 11, Mechanics of Exhalation). In chronic bronchitis, the mechanism involves mucosal edema, airway secretions, and possibly bronchospasm, all of which narrow the airways. Because emphysema involves destruction of alveolar-capillary membranes, it deceases gas exchange surface area. Chronic bronchitis does not involve alveoli, therefore does not change surface area for gas exchange. For these reasons, a decreased diffusion capacity is associated with emphysema rather than chronic bronchitis. The test for diffusion capacity is a useful way to find out the extent to which emphysema may be present in a patient with COPD.

diffusing capacity measurement should be corrected for subjects with abnormal hematocrit according to the equation, Corrected DLCOSB = Measured DLCOSB ÷ 0.06965 (Hb).[62] The diffusing capacity may be useful in identifying which subjects with obstructive impairment are likely to desaturate during exercise and who may benefit from oxygen therapy.[63] The DLCO may be increased in subjects with **polycythemia,** congestive heart failure, and who are exercising. Factors that can alter the DLCO above or below the normal value are summarized in Table 18-9.

The DL/VA ratio differentiates between diffusion abnormalities caused by having a small effective total lung capacity compared to diffusion abnormalities caused by alveolar-capillary membrane pathologies. Subjects whose only problem is small lungs will have a decreased DLCO, but their DL/VA ratio will be normal. Subjects with pulmonary emphysema or fibrosis will have a decreased DLCO and DL/VA ratio.

Interpretation of the pulmonary function report

Starting with the %FEV₁/FVC ratio, Figure 18-17 presents an algorithm for systematically assessing a basic report of pulmonary function testing. If the %FEV₁/FVC ratio is > 75% and if the % predicted normal TLC is < 80%, the subject has a restrictive impairment, according to this algorithm. The severity of the restriction is based upon the % predicted or the

Table 18-9   Effect of various factors on the diffusing capacity of the lung

Factor	Effect
Anemia	↓
Polycythemia	↑
Exercise	↑
Carboxyhemoglobin	↓
Diffuse pulmonary fibrosis	↓
Pulmonary emphysema	↓
Pulmonary embolism	↓

number of standard deviations from the mean predicted TLC according to Table 18-4.[64,65,66] If the %FEV₁/FVC ratio is < 75%, the subject may have an obstructive impairment; the severity of the obstruction is based upon the % predicted normal FEV₁. If the % predicted normal DLCO is less than 80%, the subject may have a diffusion impairment, and if the DLCO/VA ratio is also less the 80% of the predicted normal value, the cause of the diffusion impairment is within the lung. The algorithm also can help identify subjects with reversible airway obstruction, small airways disease, hyperinflation, and air trapping.

Most modern pulmonary function laboratories use computers for data acquisition and reduction. Computer-assisted testing can enhance the effective-

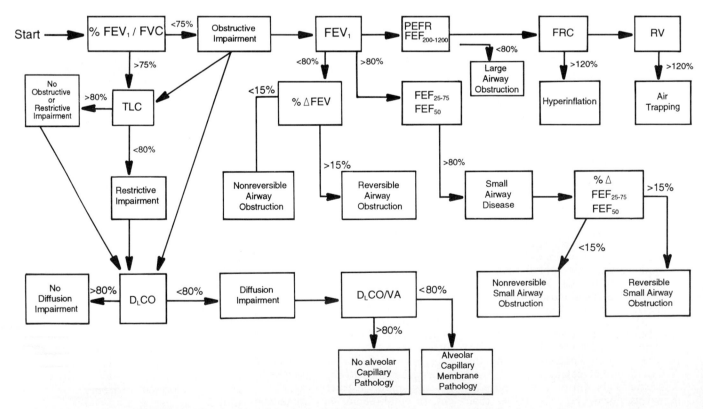

Fig. 18-17 An algorithm for systematically assessing basic pulmonary function test results.

ness of spirometry by increasing accuracy, increasing subject acceptance, and decreasing the time necessary to complete the test and its interpretation.[67] Although ATS spirometry criteria are often applied by a computer, computer analysis should not replace human analysis.[68] Algorithms (Figure 18-17) also can be programmed for computer-assisted interpretations of the pulmonary function report. Computer graphics can enhance subject performance.[69,70]

CHAPTER SUMMARY

Pulmonary function testing provides valuable information on the components of gas exchange in health and disease. The measurements of lung function can aid in the diagnosis of disease and in the assessment of the need for and effectiveness of respiratory therapeutics.

Respiratory care practitioners can use the results of pulmonary function testing to plan and evaluate the care they provide to patients. Only in this manner can objective decisions be made regarding the status of the patient, the selection of appropriate therapy, and the evaluation of therapeutic outcomes.

REFERENCES

1. Pulmonary terms and symbols: A report of the ACCP-ATS Joint Committee on Pulmonary Nomenclature. *Chest* 67:583, 1975.
2. Zibrak JD, O'Donnell CR, Marton K.: Indications for pulmonary function testing. *Ann Intern Med* 112:793-794, 1990.
3. American Thoracic Society: Evaluation of impairment/disability secondary to respiratory disorders. *Am Rev Respir Dis* 133:1205-1209, 1986.
4. Hankinson JL.: Pulmonary function testing in the screening of workers: guidelines for instrumentation, performance, and interpretation. *J Occup Med* 28:1081-1082, 1986.
5. Schmidt CD, Dickman ML, Gardner RM, Brough FK.: Spirometric standards for healthy elderly men and women. *Am Rev Respir Dis* 108:933-939, 1973.
6. Ferris BG Jr, Speizer FE, Bishop Y, Prang G, Weener J.: Spirometry for an epidemiologic study: Deriving optimum summary statistics for each subject. *Bull Eur* Physiopathol Respir 14:146-166, 1978.
7. Ferris BG.: Epidemiology standardization project: Recommended standardized procedures for pulmonary function testing. *Am Rev Respir Dis* 11 8:(Part 2), 1978.
8. Hodgkin JE: Preoperative Assessment of Respiratory Function. *Respir Care* 29:496-503, 1984.
9. Renzetti AD Jr, Bleecker ER, Epler GR, Jones RN, Kanner RE, Repsher LH: Evaluation of impairment/disability secondary to respiratory disorders. *Am Rev Respir Dis* 133:1205-1209, 1986.
10. American Association for Respiratory Care Clinical Practice Guideline: Spirometry. *Respir Care* 36:1414-1417, 1991.
11. Fleisch A: Pneumotachograph: Apparatus for recording respiratory flow. *Arch Ges Physiol* 209:713-722, 1925.
12. Sullivan WJ, Peters GM, Enright PL: Pneumotachographs: Theory and clinical application. *Respir Care* 29:736-749, 1984.
13. Shigeoka JW: Calibration and quality control of spirometer systems. *Respir Care* 28:747-753, 1983.
14. Norton A: Accuracy in pulmonary measurements. *Respir Care* 24:131-137, 1979.
15. Clausen JL, Tisi GM, Moser KM: Methods of evaluation of accuracy of spirometers and pneumotachographs (abstract). *Med Instrum* 8:117, 1974.
16. ATS Statement: Standardization of spirometry 1987 update. *Am Rev Respir* 136:1285-1298, 1987. Reprinted in *Respir Care* 32:1039-1060, 1987.
17. ATS Statement: Quality assurance in pulmonary function laboratories. *Am Rev Respir Dis* 134:625-7, 1986.
18. Gardner RM (chairman): ATS Statement I, Snowbird Workshop on Standardization of Spirometry. *Am Rev Respir Dis* 119:831-838, 1978.
19. Gardner RM, Hankinson JL, West RF: Evaluating commercially available spirometers. *Am Rev Respir Dis* 121:73-82, 1980.
20. Eichenhorn MS, Beauchamp RK, Harper PA, Ward JC: An assessment of three portable peak flow meters. *Chest* 82:306-309, 1982.
21. Hess D, Kacer K, Beener C: An Evaluation of the Accuracy of the Ohmeda 5410 Spirometer. *Respir Care* 33:21-26, 1988.
22. Hess D, Lehman E, Troup J, Smoker J.: An evaluation of the PK Morgan spirometer. *Respir Care* 31:786-791, 1986.
23. Hess D, Chieppor P, Johnson K: An evaluation of the Respiradyne II spirometer. *Respir Care* 32:1123-1130, 1987.
24. Shanks DE, Morris JF.: Clinical comparison of two electronic spirometers with a water-sealed spirometer. *Chest* 69:461-466, 1976.
25. Glindmeyer HW 111, Anderson ST, Diem JF, Weill H: A comparison of the Jones and Stead-Wells spirometers. *Chest* 73:596-8, 1978.
26. Dickman ML, Schmidt CD, Gardner RM: Spirometric standards for normal children and adolescents (ages 8 years through 18 years). *Am Rev Respir Dis* 104:680-687, 1971.
27. Garner JS, Favero MS: CDC guidelines for the prevention and control of nosocomial infections: guideline for hand washing and hospital environmental control. *Am J Infect Control* 14:110-129, 1986.
28. Tablan OC, Williams WW, Martone WJ: Infection control in pulmonary function laboratories. *Infect Control* 6:442-444, 1985.
29. Rutala DR, Rutala WA, Weber DR: Infection risks associated with spirometry. *Infection Control Hospital Epidemiol* 12:89-92, 1991.
30. Centers for Disease Control: Guidelines for preventing the transmission of tuberculosis in health care settings, with special focus on HIV-related issues. *MMWR* 39:1-29, 1990.
31. Hankinson JL, Viola JO: Dynamic BTPS correction factors for spirometric data. *J Appl Physiol* Respirat Environ Exercise Physiol 44:1354-5, 1983.
32. Pincock AC, Miller MR: The effect of temperature on recording spirograms. *Am Rev Respir Dis* 128:894-898, 1983.
33. Hathirat S, Renzetti AD, Mitchell M: Measurement of the total lung capacity by helium dilution in a constant volume system. *Am Rev Respir Dis* 102:760-768, 1970.
34. Meneely GR, Ball CT, Kory RC, et al: A simplified closed circuit helium dilution method for the determination of the residual volume of the lungs. *Am J Med* 28:824-829, 1960.
35. Birath G, Swenson EW: A correction factor for helium absorption in lung volume determinations. *Scand J Clin Lab Invest* 8:155-163, 1956.
36. Boren HG, Kory RC, Snyder JC.: The veterans administration-army cooperative study of pulmonary function II: The lung volume and its subdivisions in normal men. *Am J Med* 41:96-114, 1966.
37. Dubois AB, Botelho SV, Bedel GN, et al: A rapid plethysmographic method for measuring thoracic gas volume: a comparison with a nitrogen washout method for measuring FRC in normal subjects. *J Clin Invest* 35:322-326, 1956.
38. Habib MP, Engel LA: Influence of the panting technique on the plethysmographic measurement of thoracic gas volume. *Am Rev Respir Dis* 117:265-71, 1978.

39. Varkey B, Kory RC: Mediastinal and subcutaneous emphysema following pulmonary function tests. *Am Rev Respir Dis* 108:1393–1396, 1973.

40. Stanescu DC, Teculescu DB: Exercise and cough induced asthma. *Respiration* 27:273–277, 1970.

41. Taussig LM, Chernick V, Wood R, Farrell P, Mellins RC: Conference Committee. Standardization of lung function testing in children. *J Pediatr* 97:668–678, 1980.

42. Zamel N, Altose MD, Speir WA Jr: ACCP Scientific Section Recommendations. Statement of spirometry: A report of the section on respiratory pathophysiology. *Chest* 83:547–550, 1983.

43. Pulmonary Function Standards for Cotton Dust: 29 Code of Federal Regulations; 1910.1043 Cotton Dust, Appendix D. Occupational Safety and Health Administration 808–832, 1980.

44. Verrall AB, Julian JA, Muir DC, Haines AT: Use of nose clips in pulmonary function tests. *J Occup Med* 31:29–31, 1989.

45. Townsend MC: Spirometric forced expiratory volumes measured in the standing versus the sitting posture. *Am Rev Respir Dis* 130:123–124, 1984.

46. Knudson RJ, Slatin RC, Lebowitz MD, Burrows B: The maximal expiratory flow volume curve. *Am Rev Respir Dis* 113:587–600, 1976.

47. Knudson RJ, Kaltenborn WT, Knudson DE, Burrows B: The single-breath carbon monoxide diffusing capacity. Reference equations derived from a healthy nonsmoking population and effects of hematocrit. *Am Rev Respir Dis* 135:805–11, 1987.

48. Knudson RJ, Kaltenborn WT, Burrows B: The effects of cigarette smoking and smoking cessation on the carbon monoxide diffusing capacity of the lung in asymptomatic subjects. *Am Rev Respir Dis* 140:645–51, 1989.

49. Chinn DJ, Harkawat R, Cotes JE: Standardization of single-breath transfer factor (TLCO); derivation of breathholding time. *Eur Respir J* 5:492–6, 1992.

50. ATS Statement: Single breath carbon monoxide diffusing capacity (transfer factor) Recommendations for a standard technique. *Am Rev Respir Dis* 136:1299–1307, 1987.

51. Forster RE, Fowler WS, Bates DV, Van Lingen B: The absorption of carbon monoxide by the lungs during breathholding. *J Clin Invest* 33:1135–1139, 1954.

52. Ogilvie CM, Forster RE, Blakemore WS, Morton JW: A standardized breath holding technique for the clinical measurement of the diffusing capacity of the lung for carbon monoxide. *J Clin Invest* 36:1–17, 1957.

53. Barnhart S, Hudson LD, Mason SE, Pierson DJ, Rosenstock L: Total lung capacity. An insensitive measure of impairment in patients with asbestosis and chronic obstructive pulmonary disease? *Chest* 93:299–302, 1988.

54. Goldman HI, Becklake MR: Respiratory function tests: normal values at median altitudes and the prediction of normal values. *Am Rev TB Pulm Dis* 79:457–467, 1959.

55. Cherniack RM, Raber MB: Normal standards for ventilatory function using an automated wedge spirometer. *Am Rev Respir Dis* 106:38–46, 1972.

56. Morris JF, Koski A, Johnson LC: Spirometric standards for healthy nonsmoking adults. *Am Rev Respir Dis* 116:209–213, 1971.

57. Aldrich TK, Arora NS, Rochester DF: The influence of airway obstruction and respiratory muscle strength on maximal voluntary ventilation in lung disease. *Am Rev Respir Dis* 126:195–9, 1982.

58. Arora NS, Rochester DF: Respiratory muscle strength and maximal voluntary ventilation in undernourished patients. *Am Rev Respir Dis* 126:5–8, 1982.

59. Bates DV, Macklem PT, Christie RV: *Respiratory Function in Disease.* Philadelphia 1971, W B Saunders.

60. Crapo RO, Morris AM: Standardized single breath normal values for carbon monoxide diffusing capacity. *Am Rev Respir Dis* 123:185–189, 1981.

61. Wimalaratna HS, Farrell J, Lee HY: Measurement of diffusing capacity in pulmonary embolism. *Respir Med* 83:481–5, 1989.

62. Dinakara P, Blumenthal WS, Johnston RF, et al: The effect of anemia on pulmonary diffusing capacity with derivation of a correction equation. *Am Rev Respir Dis* 102:965–969, 1970.

63. Owens GR, Rogers RM, Pennock BE, Levin D: The diffusing capacity as a predictor of arterial oxygen desaturation during exercise in patients with chronic obstructive pulmonary disease. *N Engl J Med* 310:1218–21, 1984.

64. Clausen JL: Prediction of normal values in pulmonary function testing. *Clin Chest Med* 10:135–43, 1989.

65. Crapo RO, Morris AH, Gardner RM: Reference spirometric values using techniques and equipment that meet ATS recommendations. *Am Rev Respir Dis* 123:659–64, 1981.

66. ATS Statement: Lung function testing: selection of reference values and interpretative strategies. *Am Rev Respir Dis* 144:1202–18, 1991.

67. Gardner RM, Clausen JL, Cotton DJ, Crapo RO, Epler GR, Hankinson JL, Johnson RL Jr: Computer guidelines for pulmonary laboratories. *Am Rev Respir Dis* 134:628–629, 1986.

68. Glindmeyer HW, Jones RN, Barkman HW, Weill H: Spirometry: quantitative test criteria and test acceptability. *Am Rev Respir Dis* 136:449–52, 1987.

69. Larson JK: Computer-assisted spirometry. *Respir Care* 27:839–41, 1982.

70. Paliotta JJ: The role of the digital computer in the pulmonary function laboratory. *Respir Care* 27:816–20, 1982.

19

Systematic Analysis of the Chest X-ray

■

Richard L. Sheldon

CHAPTER LEARNING OBJECTIVES

1. Describe the technical basis by which an X-ray image is produced;
2. Differentiate among the standard positions used for chest radiographs;
3. Describe the effect of tissue density on X-ray penetration and image projection;
4. Define the key characteristics of a normal chest radiograph;
5. Ascertain the presence of selected abnormalities on a chest radiograph, and their clinical significance;
6. Understand some of the uses of CT and HRCT for the diagnosing of chest disease.

Chest radiologists develop techniques and accumulate experience over their entire lifetime in order to accurately identify abnormal findings on a chest X-ray. Therefore, this chapter cannot make the reader an expert radiologist, but it is worthwhile for the respiratory care practitioner to recognize some of the basic areas of normality and abnormality. All the normal and abnormal chest findings cannot be covered in one brief chapter, so it is our intent to introduce a systematic approach to reading the chest radiograph film. This systematic approach can be used by practitioners as a framework on which to build and refine their understanding of this important diagnostic tool.

FUNDAMENTALS OF RADIOGRAPHY

Conventional chest radiography

X-rays are electromagnetic waves that radiate from a tube through which an electrical current has been passed. The tube is made of a cathode which is attached to a low-voltage electron source called a transformer. The end of the cathode wire is inside the vacuum-sealed tube, and as the electrons flow through the wire they are boiled off, accelerated across a short gap, and strike a positively charged tungsten plate called the anode. The electrons coming off the cathode wire filament are focused so they hit a very small area on the anode. This area is called the target (Figure 19-1, page 434).

On striking the target, physical changes occur, which result in the emission of X-rays. These X-rays are emitted in all directions, but because of the construction of the tube, only a few X-rays are allowed to escape through the window and are actually used. The rest are absorbed harmlessly into the wall of the X-ray machine.

X-rays are not reflected back like light rays but penetrate matter, and their ability to penetrate matter is dependent on the density of the matter. Very dense objects like bone will absorb (not allow penetration) more X-rays than air-filled objects like lung tissue. The four main objects shown in the chest radiograph film are bone, air, soft tissue, and fat.

If a sheet of film is placed on the side of the patient opposite to where the X-ray tube is located, the x-rays passing through the patient will be absorbed by some objects and cast a shadow on the film. X-rays that pass through the low-density objects (air-filled), strike the film full force and turn it black. X-rays that strike bone are partially absorbed, and less darkening of the corresponding area on the X-ray film is seen. This area is relatively unchanged and is seen as white on the film.

The standard chest radiograph film is taken in two directions. First, with the patient standing upright with his or her back to the X-ray tube, the chest is pressed against a metal cassette containing the film and the arms are positioned out of the way. The X-ray beam leaves the tube and first strikes the patient's back (posterior), moves through the chest, exits through the front (anterior), and then strikes the film. Since the beam moves posterior to anterior this is called a **P-A view.** The patient is then turned sideways, and a **lateral** or side view is obtained. Thus two films are routinely taken, a P-A and lateral.

Other views are sometimes obtained when special problems are identified. If the patient is in an intensive care unit and cannot be moved, the film is placed in the bed behind the patient's back, and the X-ray tube positioned in front. Since the X-rays are moving anterior to posterior, this is called an **A-P portable.** Obliques are done, left and right lateral decubitus, with the patient lying on the right or left side in order

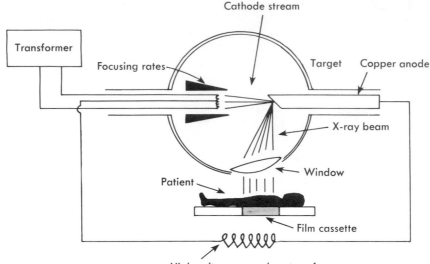

Fig. 19-1 The electrical current is generated by the transformer, passes through the focusing plates, and arrives at the cathode. The electrons are "boiled off" making a cathode stream. They then strike the anode target and are transformed into "X-rays." The X-rays leave the sealed vacuum X-ray tube through a window; strike and pass through the patient, and cast a shadow on the film cassette, making an "X-ray picture."

to see if free fluid (pleural effusion or blood) is present in the chest. Also, an *apical* **lordotic** is sometimes requested in order to look at the right middle lobe or the top (apical region) of the lung.

If an area of the lung consolidates because of pneumonia, tumor, obstruction, or collapse, it will show as a white patch on the film. Cavities will look like black holes. Diffuse patterns (interstitial markings) will be a fine, lace-like pattern in the lung tissue.

Some densities that appear on the film are normal, such as the heart and the lymph nodes. When they become abnormal they change shape, and by developing a clear understanding of what normal looks like one can make an accurate diagnosis of the disease process by how the shape of the structure is altered.

One of the most important jobs the X-ray technician has is to make sure the patient is not rotated or turned. A very slight amount of rotation will so distort normal structures that they will start to appear falsely abnormal.

Newer imaging modalities

Over the last 20 years, computerized tomography (CT) and magnetic resonance imaging (MRI) have been applied to provide more detailed images than available via conventional chest radiography. CT uses a highly columnated X-ray beam and a computer to interpretate the density data to form an image. MRI uses a strong magnetic field to which tuned radio waves are pulsed. Certain electrons are caused to occilate in their orbits giving off weak radio waves which are received by tuned antennae and sent to a computer which turns the signals received from tissue into images.

Computed tomography (CT) of the chest

With improvements in technology and increasing clinical experience, the indications for thoracic computed tomography (CT) have expanded. CT is based on two (2) basic attributes. First, CT of the chest is able to visualize the superimposed structures seen on plain chest radiography in *cross section*. This cross-sectional anatomy obtained provides a very useful dimension to conventional radiology. CT can clarify confusing patterns that may represent pathology. A second important feature of CT is its ability to detect subtle differences in density (as little as 0.5% change in density, compared to about 10% for conventional X-rays). A much higher contrast is seen with CT when settings are properly adjusted, thus enhancing the detectability of lesions.

High resolution tomography (HRCT) of the lung was first described in 1982. It is defined as 1mm–2mm thick CT slices reconstructed with pixel sizes in the range of 200 to 300 microns whereas plain CT imaging is usually done with a slice thickness of

10mm contiguously through the chest. HRCT greatly reduces the superimposition of structures because the slice is so thin. This permits optimal evaluation of lung detail.

Some focal lung lesions have been made easier to diagnose because of the better lung detail seen with HRCT. For example, differentiation of pulmonary nodules (benign versus malignant), **bronchiectasis,** artiovenous malformation, rounded atelectasis, and some of the **pneumoconioses** are generally more easily to diagnosed on HRCT. Although many of the HRCT patterns of disease are nonspecific, our knowledge of HRCT's ability to detect lung pathology continues to expand as more research is done in this area.

Bronchiectasis is a common disease of the airways in which HRCT is the examination of choice. Bronchography has been made obsolete by the introduction of HRCT. HRCT is as accurate as bronchography, is less expensive, and is non-invasive.

HRCT of pulmonary emphysema clearly and beautifully delineates bullae and blebs. This can be helpful to the thoracic surgeon when planning excisional surgery (Figure 19-2, *A, B,* page 436).

Pulmonary emphysema, asthma and cystic lung disease are now being evaluated by a CT protocol called QCT or quantitative CT. This is a research technique for measuring average pixel values within the lungs. It has been found to be a sensitive way to diagnosing emphysema and asthma. Whether it will be practical and cost-effective remains to be seen.

Carcinoma of the lung is the most common form of cancer in men and women. The majority of lung cancer patients will have advanced disease at the time their tumor is discovered. The stage of the cancer directly relates to the surgical resectability. The technical possibility of removing all malignant tissue with one surgical procedure is the only chance of a cure.

CT has been found to be a cost-effective way in help stage lung cancer. The resectability of a lesion prior to surgical intervention is best evaluated by CT, thus saving the patient from unnecessary surgery. CT can recognize cancer invading the pleura, the chest wall, the mediastinum, the mediastinal lymph nodes, and distant **metastases** to the liver and adrenal glands.

Magnetic resonance imaging

Magnetic Resonance Imaging (MRI) of the chest offers unique advantages and disadvantages. Imaging without the use of ionizing radiation is definitely an advantage. The high cost of MRI is a definite limitation to its use. MRI is a problem-solving tool in cases where CT is inconclusive. MRI has the advantage of delineating blood vessels from adjacent lymph nodes and or tumors more easily than CT and can be very valuable in assessing cancer invasion of the chest wall and mediastinum (Figure 19-3 *A, B,* page 437). Thus

MRI is useful in staging patients who have carcinoma of the lung. MRI will allow for detection of even minimal enlargement of the hilar lymph nodes due to the spread of the primary cancer to these nodes. Local spread of cancer to the chest wall can be detected earlier with MRI than using routine chest radiographs or with CT. MRI is the method of choice for imaging thoracic aneurysms, congenital **anomalies** of the aorta, and major thoracic vessels.

SYSTEMATIC INTERPRETATION OF THE CHEST X–RAY

Now we take a step-by-step approach to chest radiograph films, thus forcing the practitioner to concentrate on certain areas of the film rather than letting his or her eye scan it in a random manner. Many of the findings on chest X-ray films are subtle and require the ability to collect many pieces of information that may suggest where the abnormality can be found. Even though the practitioner may be unable to identify what the abnormality is, attention can be directed to the fact that something is wrong with the film and more expert help can be sought in delineating the precise nature of this problem.

We introduce here a systematic approach using the alphabet to make the practitioner concentrate on specific areas of the film as suggested by the subsequent letters of the alphabet. This will make for a thorough inspection of the film.

A. Airways (Figures 19-4, 19-6)

Is the trachea midline? Do the vertebral spines go right through the middle of the tracheal air column? If not, the film has been rotated or the trachea may have been deviated to one side or the other because of fibrosis drawing it to one side, loss of volume in one lung drawing it to one side, or hyperinflation on one side forcing it to the opposite side.

Is the trachea the same width as the vertebral column? If not, **tracheobronchomegaly,** also known as Mounier-Kuhn syndrome, may be present. This is a very rare disorder. Is the trachea buckling to the side opposite the aortic arch? This is a very common, normal finding. Are the larger bronchi, especially just distal to the main carina or at the openings to the lobes, tapering? This may suggest the presence of a bronchogenic carcinoma invading carinal lymph nodes, which in turn are compressing the main bronchi.

B. Bones (Figures 19-4, 19-7 and 19-17)

The ribs should be equal distance apart. If the space between the ribs is narrowed on one side more than on

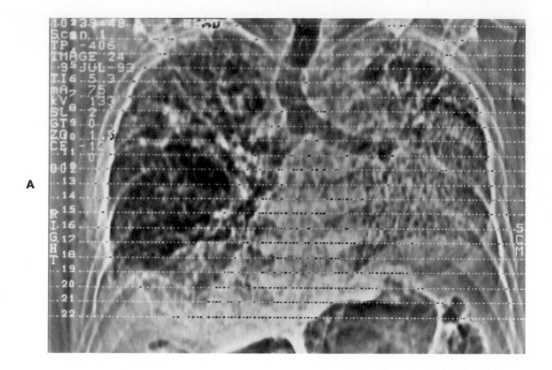

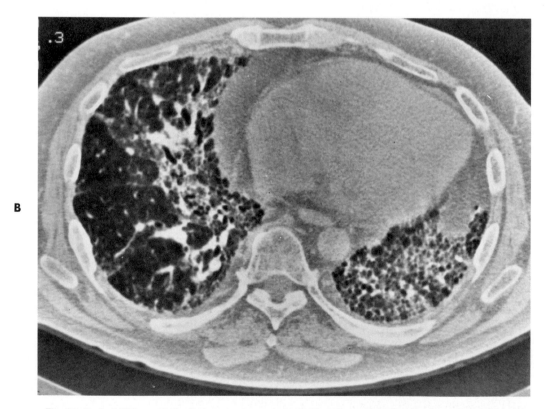

Fig. 19-2 **A,** A CT "scout" film is done to show where the "cuts" are taken. The film is not intended to be detailed. There is however, enough detail to show considerable fibrosis and bullae formation. The example below is cut 15. **B,** This photo shows the detail on the size and exact location of the large bullae in the right chest. Also seen are septae between bullae. Of equal importance is the detail of the severe fibrosis in both lungs. The heart is seen as the large "blob" in the upper right of the picture. This is the correct position for the heart—in the left anterior side of the chest.

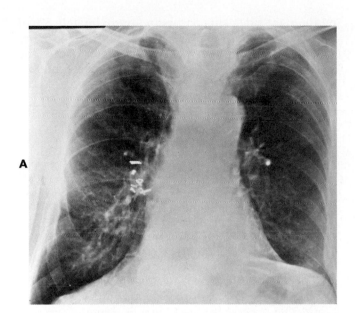
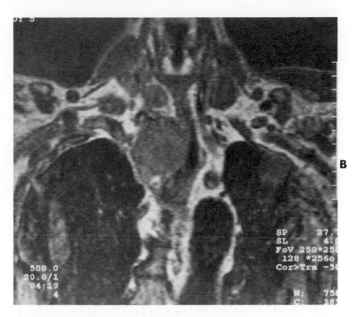

Fig. 19-3 A, This P-A film shows only a mid tracheal deviation to the left to suggest the nearby carcinoma. **B,** The MRI scan for the same patient clearly shows a large carcinoma invading pleura and medialstinal structures.

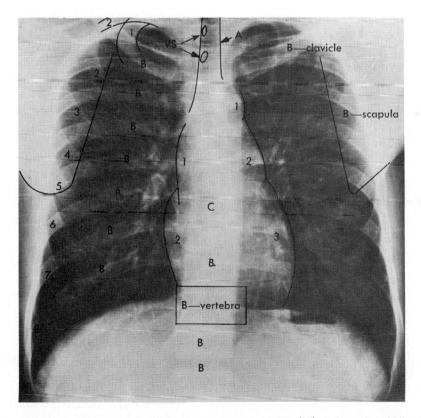

Fig. 19-4 *A,* Airways. Do the vertebral spinous processes seen end on (*VS*) go down the middle of the air column? In this case they do not. This patient is rotated slightly. *B,* Bones. Ribs numbered 1 through 8 on the right side where they swing anteriorly. Clavicles, scapula, and vertebrae are in the *B* category also. *C,* Cor. Cardiac shadow: (*right side*) *1,* superior vena cava, *2,* right atrium; (*left side*) *1,* aortic arch, *2,* pulmonary artery segment, *3,* left ventricle.

the other, this may suggest loss of muscle tone such as in a patient who has a paralysis involving that side of chest. Notching of the ribs can be a significant finding that should be carefully examined. Notching of the superior aspect of the first rib bilaterally is suggestive of **scleroderma** or rheumatoid arthritis (Figure 19-17). Inferior notching of the third through the ninth ribs suggests **coarctation (narrowing) of the aorta. Tetralogy of Fallot** may cause inferior rib notching on the left side only. The ribs can be inspected for cough fractures, which may be seen on the sixth through the ninth rib, usually the seventh in the posterior axillary line. Rib anomalies such as bifid ribs can be seen. These usually have no clinical significance. **Pectus carinatum** (pigeon breast) is associated with congenital atrial and ventricular septal defects or asthma from early childhood. The spine should also be inspected for such things as **kyphoscoliosis,** which, if severe enough, will result in loss of pulmonary volume and subsequently hypoventilation. Demineralization of the bones (washed out bones on the X-ray film) may be seen with steroid therapy, aging, renal disease, or other metabolic diseases.

C. Cor (Figures 19-4, 19-9, 19-11, 19-14, and 19-17)

The right heart border is composed of two bulges that should always be seen. If they are obliterated, it may represent **pectus excavatum,** as suggested in the previous section. The bulges will be blurred or absent in the presence of right middle lobe collapse, pneumothorax, or pneumonia involving the portion of the lung that comes in contact with the heart (Figure 19-11, page 443). Loss of superior bulge may be seen with an abnormal aortic arch. The left heart border is composed of three bulges, the most superior being the aorta, followed by the main pulmonary artery segment, and then the most inferior of the three, the left ventricle. Pneumonias located next to these bulges will obliterate the edges of the bulge. This can be helpful in identifying the presence of pneumonia. There are multiple congenital cardiac lesions that will be present as abnormal cardiac shapes, but they will not be dealt with in this chapter.

If the width of the heart is greater than one-half the distance across the lungs at the level of the diaphragms on the P-A projection, the cardiothoracic (C/T) ratio is increased, and the heart is considered enlarged, usually from congestive heart failure (Figure 19-9, page 442). Other heart problems can also cause the heart to enlarge.

D. Diaphragm (Figures 19-5, 19-10, 19-13, and 19-17)

The right diaphragm is usually about one-half a rib interspace higher than the left. *Scalloping* can appear

on the right side. This occurs in approximately 5% of all cases and is of no clinical significance (Figure 19-5). One diaphragm may be elevated above the normal limits, in which case the following should be thought of: thoracic tumor with resultant paralysis of the phrenic nerve (Figure 19-10, page 443); or old surgery to the chest, which will result in fibrosis, scarring of the pleura, and subsequent entrapment of the diaphragm and elevation. **Subphrenic** abscess will usually result in the posterior portion of the right diaphragm being elevated. This can best be identified from a lateral view. Some rare causes of hemidiaphragm elevation include trauma (Erb's paralysis), stroke, tumor or infection in the neck or cervical spine, pneumonia, and radiation therapy.

An interesting anomaly of the diaphragm is the accessory diaphragm, usually on the right and associated with scimitar syndrome, a congenital cardiac defect composed of both heart and lung malformations. The accessory diaphragm is usually oriented upward and backward to the posterior wall and has a lower lobe between it and the true diaphragm.

E. Esophagus (Figure 19-6)

The esophagus will be located behind the trachea. An air fluid level would suggest certain diseases such as **achalasia** or stricture.

F. Fissures (Figures 19-7, 19-8, 19-10, and 19-11)

The fissure lines divide the lung into various lobes. The two long (major) fissures or the oblique fissures (one each for the right and left lungs) are best seen on the lateral view X-ray film. The inferior end of these fissures never runs into the anterior chest wall but ends in the diaphragm. Sometimes it is important to know which fissure is for the right lung and which is for the left. They usually run with the sixth rib, and on the lateral view the right fissure ends in the higher of the two diaphragms. The left fissure can be identified as the one that ends in the diaphragm that has a stomach bubble under it. If the stomach bubble is not well seen, this may cause some confusion. The heart will usually obliterate the anterior part of the left diaphragm.

The short fissure, also called the minor or horizontal fissure, is seen on the right. It is absent in approximately 20% of normal chest radiograph films. Approximately one half of the normal films show a short fissure, and it is rarely seen projecting all the way across the right lung (Figures 19-7 and 19-8, page 440).

The azygos lobe (Figure 19-13, page 445) is visible in about four tenths of 1% of normal chests. This fissure is very distinctive in its appearance. It is almost always seen on the right, but left azygos lobes

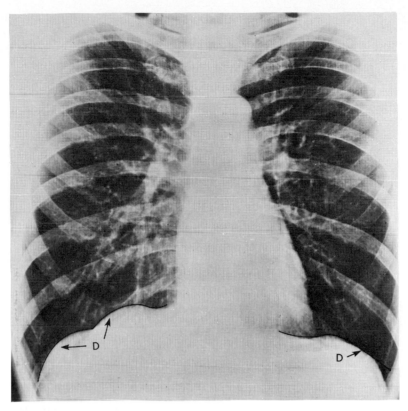

Fig. 19-5 *D*, Diaphragm. This example shows scalloping on the right, with the right side higher than the left. This is normal.

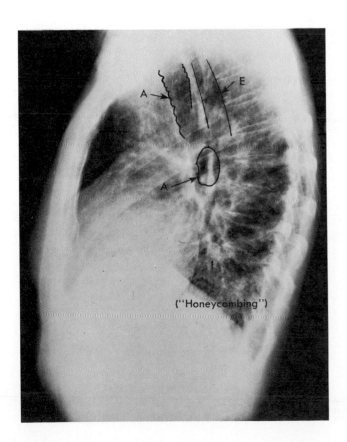

("Honeycombing")

caused by an accessory hemiazygos vein have been identified. The azygos lobe is evidence of a pleural reflection from the azygos vein, which has descended during the embryologic period into its proper resting position, bringing with it a piece of pleura that remains radiographically evident. It looks like an upside-down comma.

There is also a superior accessory lobe, which is found in about 5% of the normal films and is seen below the horizontal fissure on the right. It separates the superior segment of the right lower lobe from the rest of the lobe. Inferior accessory lobes also occur in about 5% of normal films, and it separates the medial basilar segment of the right lower lobe from the rest of the right lower lobe. It therefore runs obliquely from the right heart border. A left minor fissure occurs rarely and represents a separate minor fissure.

Fig. 19-6 *A*, Airway. This is the lateral view of the trachea and the right and left main stem bronchi. *E*, Esophagus. Its proper position is behind the trachea. The vertical lines seen in this area are the scapulae on end. *I*, Interstitial markings are increased with a big esophagus. The increased markings are due in this case to scleroderma. Note the "honeycombed" appearance of the lung markings.

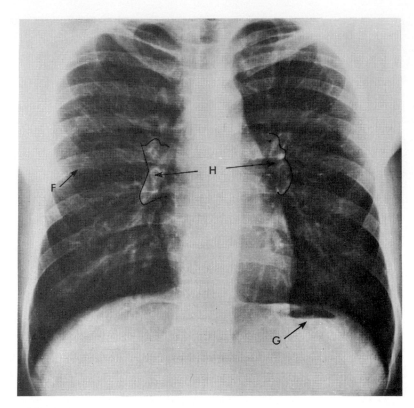

Fig. 19-7 *F,* The horizontal fissure line or "short" fissure is shown on the right. *G,* Gastric bubble. Note the thickness of the left diaphragm above it. This is normal. *H,* Hila. The left hilum is higher than the right. This is the proper relationship.

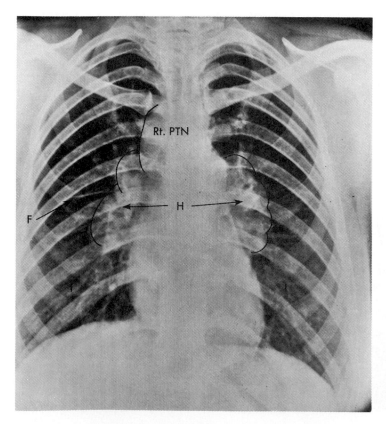

Fig. 19-8 *F,* Another example of a short fissure line. This horizontal fissure is a little thickened. *H,* Enlarged hila bilaterally and right paratracheal nodes (*Rt. PTN*) consistent with sarcoid. *I,* Note the diffuse, multidirectional lines in the lower portion of the lung. These lines are interstitial markings, and they are increased, consistent with interstitial disease. Sarcoidosis causes interstitial infiltrates and is the cause for the finding of hilar node enlargement and interstitial infiltrate in this patient.

G. Gastric bubble (Figure 19-7)

It is important to make sure that the gastric bubble, if present, is seen on the left. If it is found on the right, mislabeling of the chest radiograph film should be suspected, or the patient may have **situs inversus.** If the gastric bubble is absent, the possibility of **achalasia** should be considered. A bubble behind the heart could indicate the presence of a **hiatal hernia.** The top of the gastric bubble should be no more than 2 cm from the top of the dome of the diaphragm.

H. Hila (Figures 19-7 and 19-8)

The displacement of this part of the chest anatomy constitutes the most important indirect sign of collapse of part of the lung. Ninety-seven percent of left hila are higher than right hila. The right is never higher than the left. The left should not be over 3 cm higher than the right. If any of these rules are violated, then the hilum is out of its proper position. This results from either hyperinflation of the lung on one side of the hilum pushing it in the opposite direction, or collapse of an area of lung, which would pull the hilum in the direction of the collapse. Enlargement of the hilar area is also an important finding. The hilar area can enlarge because of spreading cancer, infection somewhere in the lung, immunologic diseases, or sarcoid, to name a few. Enlarging left hila are hard to see. It is not as difficult to observe right hilar enlargement.

I. Interstitium (Figures 19-8, 19-10, 19-11, and 19-17)

Interstitial **infiltrates** are separated classically into alveolar and interstitial patterns. If there is an interstitial infiltrate, its presence can be confirmed by looking at the anterior air space, the area behind the sternum and in front of the heart. This is best seen on the lateral film. If an interstitial infiltrate is seen in the lateral view in the anterior air space, this is good evidence that in fact the patient does have a true interstitial infiltrate. Breast shadows overlying the lower portions of the lung will accentuate normal lung findings, and the practitioner should not be trapped into thinking that there is an abnormal interstitial pattern in female patients.

The alveolar pattern is caused by filling of the alveolus with water or near water density material such as pus, blood, or edema fluid. In the case of near drowning or congestive heart failure, the alveolar space fills up with water. With **Goodpasture's Syndrome** or idiopathic **pulmonary hemosiderosis,** these spaces fill up with blood. In the case of **pulmonary alveolar proteinosis,** these spaces fill up with a protein like material. In the case of disquamative interstitial pneumonitis, these spaces fill up with cells. Some-

times this differential diagnosis can be narrowed if one has an idea of the type of material that the patient is coughing up.

J. Junction lines

Junction lines are vertical lines in the mediastinum seen only on the P-A projection. They include the right paraspinal line, left paraspinal line, right para-aortic line, left paraaortic line, posterior junctional line, anterior junctional line, right paratracheal line, and left paracardial line. These lines may be difficult to find, but if they are outlined or seen to bulge, this suggests a mass lesion displacing them.

K. Kerley's lines (Figure 19-9)

The Kerley B line is 1 mm thick and approximately 1 cm to 2 cm long and is found in the periphery of the lung, usually on the right at the base. The B line is a short, straight, horizontal line originating from the pleural surface. This usually is evidence of congestive heart failure. Kerley A lines are 1 mm thick and 2 mm to 4 cm long within the lung midway between the hila and pleura, oriented in many directions. The actual length of the Kerley C lines is controversial, but they have been reported to be associated with engorgement of the pleural lymphatics. These lines look like an interstitial infiltrate, mentioned previously under Interstitium. They have been called "everywhere lines."

L. Lobes (Figure 19-10)

Collapse of a lobe is the result of obstruction of a bronchus either from an intrinsic mass, narrowing from tuberculosis, traumatic fracture of the bronchus, extrinsic pressure from the lymph nodes or cardiac enlargement, or mucous plugging. There are certain tumors that have been known to metastasize to the large bronchi and result in collapse. These include tumors from kidneys, breasts, and skin.

Cardiac enlargement as a result of certain diseased states has been reported to be associated with obstruction, especially in the newborn infant. The left lower lobe bronchus can be compressed by a very large left atrium or left pulmonary artery.

Right middle lobe syndrome is a distinct clinical entity resulting from collapse of the right middle lobe. It is sometimes seen in persons with asthma and other allergic disorders. The signs of collapse of a lobe include displaced fissure lines, loss of aeration, elevation of the diaphragm on the involved side, deviation of the trachea to the involved side, shifting of the heart to the right, narrowing of the trachea to the right, narrowing of the rib cage, compensatory overaeration, or hilar displacement.

It is helpful to know where each lobe goes when it collapses and how to find it. The right upper lobe is

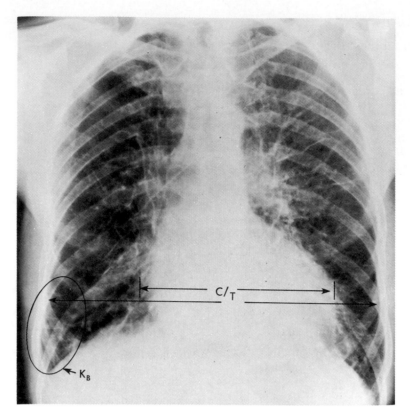

Fig. 19–9 K_B, Kerley B lines seen in their most common position. Note that the cardiothoracic ratio, which normally should be one half, is increased. This chest film is an excellent example of cardiogenic pulmonary edema.

demonstrated by the horizontal fissure swinging up (Figure 19-10) and with complete collapse swinging up to the right paratracheal mediastinum (Figure 19-11). This is best seen on a P-A view. The left upper lobe moves anteriorly, and on P-A projection there is no sharp border to delineate the collapse. It is therefore best to see this form of collapse on a lateral film. The aortic knob can be obliterated.

The right middle lobe is seen best with a lateral or an apical lordotic view. On P-A projection the right heart border is obliterated when the right middle lobe collapses.

With collapse of the lingula, the left heart border is lost or blurred on the P-A projection, with displacement of the lower half of the left major fissure as seen on the lateral view. This displacement is usually forward. The collapse of the right lower lobe results in downward posterior and medial displacement of the lung toward the spine. The right heart border is usually seen well. This collapse is best seen on P-A projections. The left lower lobe has the same direction of collapse as with the right lower lobe. The left heart border is seen well, but the "ivory heart" sign, as described by Dr. B. Felson, may be seen. This constitutes loss of lung markings seen through the heart and results in a pure white heart shadow with no lung markings seen through it. This is best seen on the P-A projection.

M. Mediastinum (Figure 19-12)

The mediastinum is the part of the chest that is found between both lungs. It contains the heart, the great vessels, several very important nerves such as the vagus nerve and phrenic nerve, hilar nodes, and other soft tissue such as fat pads. It is classically described as having an anterior compartment, middle compartment, and posterior compartment. Several organs come to rest in each of these compartments, and enlargements or mass lesions found in these compartments give a clue as to the diagnosis of the disease entity.

Sometimes air gets into the mediastinum, which is called a **pneumomediastinum.** It can best be seen on the lateral view, but the subtle findings of a small line around the heart in the P-A view can be a tip-off that a pneumomediastinum has occurred.

N. Nodules (Figure 19-12)

Nodules can be of two types: **benign,** not indicating a serious clinical problem, or malignant, which is a

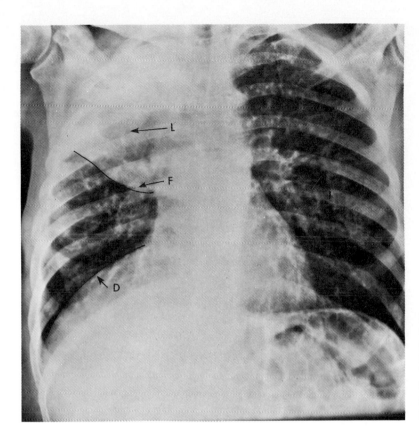

Fig. 19-10 *D,* The diaphragm is markedly elevated. Is the right phrenic nerve paralyzed? *F,* Fissure line. This horizontal fissure drifted up and is bulging. *L,* Lobe. This right upper lobe was full of tumor, which had blocked the bronchus. This resulted in collapse of the lobe. Forceful growth against the fissure line make it bulge, and growth of the tumor into the phrenic nerve caused paralysis of the right diaphragm. *I,* Interstitial marking. Another example of interstitial lines.

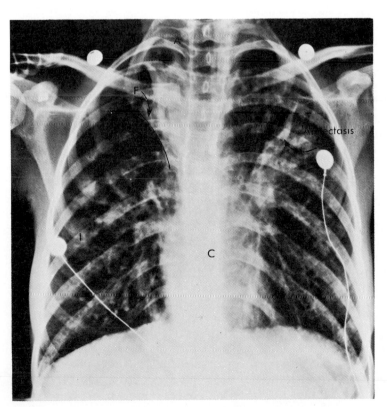

Fig. 19-11 *A,* Because of right upper lobe collapse the trachea is shifted to the right of the vertebral spines. *C,* The cardiac border on the left has been lost because of collapse of the lung on the left and because of several areas of atelectasis. *F,* The horizontal fissure line has been moved up and medially to the right. *I,* Interstitial markings are well seen. Several areas on the right upper-to-mid lung fields appear to be an alveolar infiltrate.

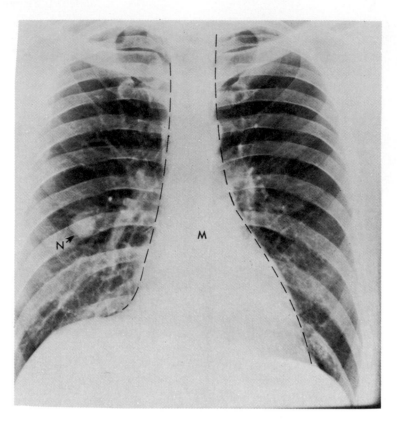

Fig. 19-12 *M*, Mediastinum is outlined with broken lines. *N*, Nodule with an area of calcium deposited in it—small white dot within the nodule at the 3- to 4-o'clock position. This means the nodule is benign; in this case it is a coccidiodomycosis scar.

much more serious diagnosis and prognosis. Nodules that are less than 1 cm are usually benign. Regardless of its size, a lesion that has calcium in it is most likely benign. If the nodule is 1 cm to 6 cm, it may well be malignant. Nodules in the 1 cm to 6 cm size are described as solitary **coin lesions** if they have clear areas of normal lung surrounding them.

Whether or not a nodule is growing can be determined by review of old films, if available. Malignancy is more likely if the lesion is enlarging. However, nonmalignant lesions can slowly enlarge, such as progressive massive **fibrosis** from silicosis.

Sometimes nodules can cavitate so that they have hollow centers. This occurs with squamous cell carcinomas. It also occurs with tuberculosis, **coccidiomycosis,** and **Wegner's granulomatosis.** Sometimes these cavities will become the home of a colony of fungus. The fungus will form itself into a ball and actually be able to roll around inside the cavity. This should suggest a method to diagnose fungous balls. If the patient is made to lie on his or her side, and a lateral decubitus film shows the density inside the cavity moving to a more dependent position because of gravity, the diagnosis of fungus ball is confirmed. If possible, comparison should be made with old films to determine if the fungus ball is growing.

O. Overaeration

A finding of overaeration on a chest radiograph film can be extremely subtle. The film should be checked for an area indicating more air in a part of the lung exceeding the aeration on the matching part of the opposite lung. This will be viewed as a much darker area on the film since air does not stop X-rays. Usually this will not have any distinct borders, so it will be a diffuse area of overaeration. It can be either an obstructed or non-obstructed area of the lung. Non-obstructed areas of overaeration usually suggest emphysematous blebs or bullae. Emphysema will be present with overaeration.

The obstruction form of overaeration is usually secondary to an inhaled foreign body or tumor. Another cause of overaeration is a **pneumatocele,** an area of lung destruction following a staphylococcal pneumonia. It usually has a distinct border caused by a very thin wisp of tissue of overaeration in a tension pneumothorax. This occurs when rupture of the lung forces air into the pleural space, causing the lung to collapse. This will be present with overaeration throughout the entire side of the involved lung.

P. Pleura (Figures 19-13 and 19-14)

The practitioner should run his or her eye all around the lung looking for thickening of the pleura, mass lesions, loss of markings in the lung sitting right next to the pleura, or blunting of the costophrenic (CP) angle. The CP angle is at the very bottom of the lung where the diaphragm and chest wall meet. If there is any blunting of the sharp angle formed by the diaphragm and lateral portion of the chest wall, this suggests the presence of fluid, called **pleural effusion.**

The thickening of the pleura at the apex of the lung field is caused by old tuberculosis in about half of the patients. There is no cause found for the thickening in the other half.

Very rare phrenic tumors called **mesotheliomas** are usually located along the lateral edge of the lung field. It should be determined whether the mass seen on the lung-pleural junction is actually arising from pleural tissue or whether it is arising from the lung itself. This will make a difference in treatment and clinical course depending on whether this lesion comes from the lung or from the pleura. There are two good rules of thumb for this. Pleural-based lesions tend to form an obtuse angle with the chest wall. In contrast, a tumor originating from the lung forms an acute angle. Another important differentiation is that if the vertical dimension of the lesion is greater than the horizontal dimension, then the lesion is pleural based. If the opposite is true (Figures 19-13 and 19-14), then the lesion is based in the lung.

If a pneumothorax occurs (Figure 19-14), the pleural edges will become visible by looking through and between the ribs to see where the lung markings have pulled away from the chest wall. A thin line will be present just parallel to the chest wall. This can be easily missed if not carefully looked for. Pleural effusions have some specific findings on chest X-ray films. One that has been mentioned is blunting of the CP angle (Figure 19-13). However, one form of pleural effusion is called the subpulmonic effusion. This type of effusion will spare the CP angle because the fluid is tucked under the lung and is not free to migrate down to the most dependent corner that makes up the CP angle. If this does occur, the diaphragm will tend to be flattened and go straight out laterally toward the chest wall, almost reaching it, then sharply drop off into the CP angle.

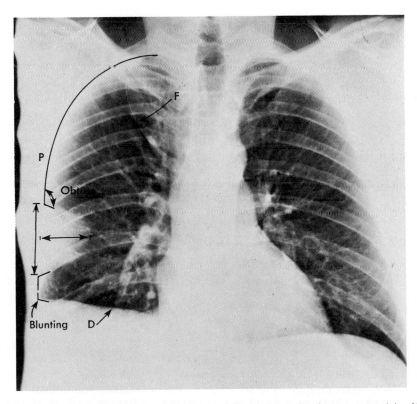

Fig. 19–13   *D*, Right diaphragm abnormally shaped. *F*, Fissured line showing an azygos lobe. Note the typical white, almost almond shape at the end of this fissure line. This is where the azygos vein came to rest. This is a normal, but uncommon, finding. *P*, Pleura with a typical pleural-based lesion showing an obtuse angle with the chest wall and vertical dimensions greater than horizontal. If it were reversed (acute angle with the chest wall and horizontal dimensions greater than vertical), then the lesion would be originating from lung tissue.

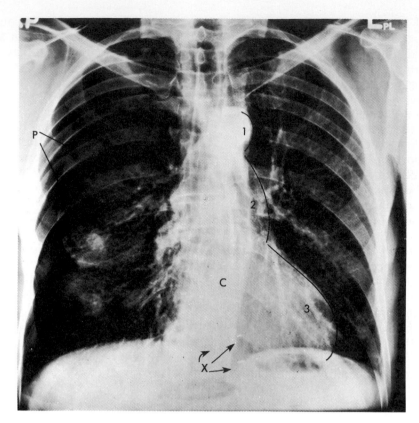

Fig. 19-14 *C,* Cardiac shadow shows the three bulges on the left, and bulge *1* and *2* are absent on the right. *P,* Pleural surface is displaced away from the chest wall, in this case because of a large pneumothorax. With the lung collapsing away from the chest wall, the right heart border has been obliterated. *X,* "X-tra" densities: surgical clips used to stop bleeding during surgery.

Q. "Quickly examine name plate"

Since there does not seem to be a good Q relationship during examination of the radiograph, this would be an excellent time for the practitioner to quickly look at the name plate on the film and make sure that this film belongs to the patient with whom the practitioner is concerned.

R. Respiration

Respiration has effects on the chest film. The lung makes obvious shifts with inspiration and expiration. A great deal can be determined about the nerve supply to the diaphragm via the phrenic nerve by the sniff test, a form of rapid respiration. In addition, the heart size has been described as changing with respiration. Whether this actually happens is under some debate.

If the chest radiograph film has been taken properly, and inspiration has been deep enough, the diaphragm will have descended to the bottom of the sixth rib anteriorly or the tenth rib posteriorly. Anything less than that will misrepresent some of the markings that are used to evaluate the film. Inspiration or expiration films are taken to accentuate and clearly define the presence of a small pneumothorax.

S. Segments (Figure 19-15)

It is sometimes important to find out which segment is involved with an infiltrative process. This requires understanding of the anatomy of the segments and which structures sit next to them. The silhouette sign as described by Dr. B. Felson[1] has been a very helpful technique used for identifying segments that are involved. The **silhouette sign** depends on the fact that an infiltrate will obscure the demarcating line of the structure it sits next to. We show some examples of this as we go through this section.

There are ten segments on the right and eight on the left. Figure 19-15 demonstrates where each of these areas can be found.

T. Thoracic calcifications (Figures 19-16 and 19-18)

Areas of calcification within the lung are frequent and represent benign lesions the majority of the time. However, there are a few that need to be identified and discussed. *Eggshell* calcifications have been described to occur in the hilar lymph nodes in patients who have silcosis, **sarcoidosis,** and other granulomatous diseases. Calcifications of the pulmonary artery,

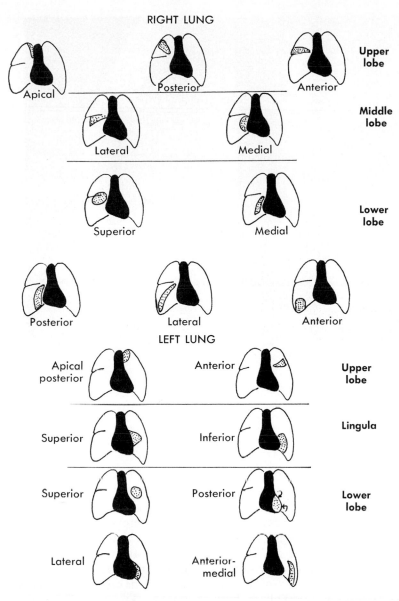

RIGHT LUNG

Apical   Posterior   Anterior   **Upper lobe**

Lateral   Medial   **Middle lobe**

Superior   Medial   **Lower lobe**

Posterior   Lateral   Anterior

LEFT LUNG

Apical posterior   Anterior   **Upper lobe**

Superior   Inferior   **Lingula**

Superior   Posterior   **Lower lobe**

Lateral   Anterior-medial

Fig. 19–15 The *dotted areas* show the approximate location of infiltrates should they occur in segments of the lung. Ten areas are shown for the right lung corresponding to the ten segments in the right, and eight areas are shown for the eight segments of the left lung.

much like the calcification seen in the aorta, can imply severe pulmonary hypertension. The most common cause of calcifications seen in the lung are healed infections caused by **histoplasmosis,** coccidiomycosis, or tuberculosis. Also described are calcifications seen in patients who have had chickenpox, pneumonia, and paragonimiasis, a parasitic worm that will take up residence in the lung. Paragonimiasis is more commonly seen in patients who live in Asia.

The pneumoconioses, that is, silicosis, **asbestosis,** etc., are present with calcifications not only within the lung and the hilar lymph nodes as noted above, but also with calcifications of the pleura.

A very rare, but interesting, lung disease has been called alveolar microlithiasis, a familial disease that presents with calcium phosphate deposits in the lung. With this disease the lung appears like a snowstorm because of the myriads of calcifications within the alveolar sacs and ducts. An interesting pleural sign has been described in this disease. It is called the "negative" pleural sign. It is a dark line running all the way around the outer border of both lungs. Lung tissue has been whited out because of the calcium phosphate deposits. The pleura, which does not absorb any of the calcium, appears as a very thin dark line around the lung making the chest radiograph film look as though it were a negative from a photograph.

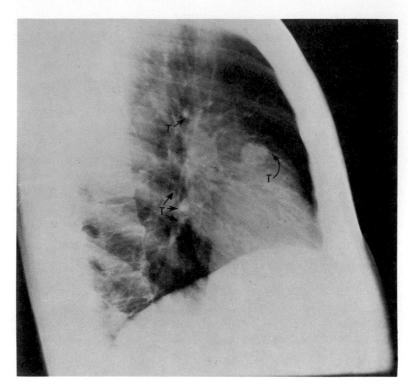

Fig. 19-16 *T*, Thoracic calcifications here represent old scars secondary to histoplasmosis.

U. Under perfusion

Under perfusion involves a loss of blood vessels in a portion of the lung. When this occurs in association with pulmonary embolism it is known as *Westermark's sign*. This is a very subtle finding and sometimes very difficult to spot. It is the loss of vessel markings past where a pulmonary embolism has impacted. This same finding can be associated with the malpositioning of a Swan-Ganz catheter so that the catheter itself becomes an embolic device and blocks the flow of blood from the tip on out.

Another important disease is MacLeod and Swyer-James syndrome. This is associated with loss of small peripheral vessels. There is no overinflation, and a normal to small hilum is associated with the syndrome. It is secondary to acute bronchopneumonia in infancy and may look like unilateral pulmonary agenesis.

V. Volume (Figure 19-17)

In evaluating the lung volume it is important to know that the right lung represents 55% of the total of both lungs and therefore should appear larger than the left lung. A problem is suggested in a lung that disrupts this relationship.

W. Women's breast shadows (Figure 19-18)

The difference in women's and men's anatomy must be taken into account in reading chest radiograph film. Women's breast shadows overlie the lower lung fields and will accentuate the lung markings behind them. This creates an impression of increased interstitial markings—a false impression. Absence of a breast shadow will make the chest film appear to be "overaerated" on the side where the breast is absent. It is a sign that the patient has undergone surgery to remove a breast, usually secondary to cancer.

Also, the nipples will appear as small coin lesions on chest X-ray films of women. Special techniques are used such as X-ray dense markers attached to the patient's nipples. The film is then retaken, and the film with the nipple markers is compared with the previous X-ray film to see if these "coin lesions" correspond to the are in question.

X. "X-tra" densities (Figure 19-14)

"X-tra" densities, such as bullets, other foreign bodies within the chest wall, and radio-opaque dyes, can sometimes be seen. In Figure 19-14 on page 446, surgical clips used in a previous surgery to obtain control of bleeding can be observed.

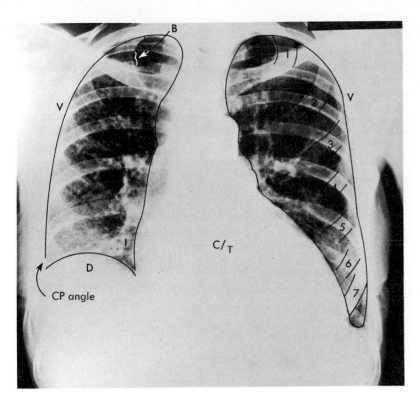

Fig. 19-17 *B*, Bone. The ribs on the left side are down by seven ribs anteriorly, so this is a good inspiration as far as the left side is concerned. The right side does not show as good an inspiration. Note the notching on the first rib on the right. *I*, Interstitial marking at both lung bases in this female patient show more "honeycombing." *V*, Volume. The right lung should be larger than the left. In this case the opposite is true and is therefore abnormal. *D*, Diaphragm. Why is the right diaphragm too high and the CP angle laterally is obscured? This is probably because of a pleural effusion. The *C/T* ratio is increased. The heart is therefore too large.

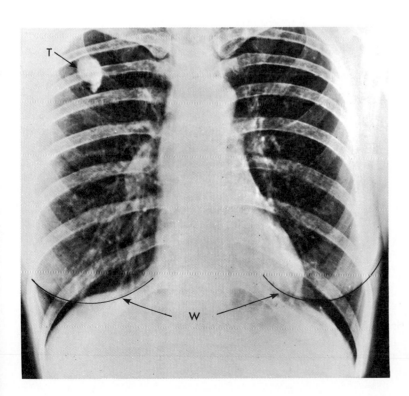

Fig. 19-18 *T*, Thoracic calcifications on this example are a result of old tuberculosis. *W*, Women's breast shadows. Note how the breast shadows accentuate the underlying tissue, making it appear as though there is an interstitial disease process present. As the lung tissue moves out beyond the breast shadow the increased interstitial pattern disappears.

CHAPTER SUMMARY

Chest radiography represents an important tool in the diagnosis and management of disorders of the pulmonary and cardiovascular systems. Under the guidance of a trained radiologist, the interpretation of the chest X-ray provides information essential in the identification and monitoring of disease processes. The respiratory care practitioner can and should understand the application of this key diagnostic tool and its appropriate use in the provision of comprehensive respiratory care.

REFERENCE

1. Felson, B: *Chest roentgenology,* Philadelphia, 1973, WB Saunders.
2. Nadich, DP, Zeritowin, EA, Speelman, SS: *Computed Tomography and Magnetic Resonance of the Thorax,* ed 2: New York, 1991, Raven Press.
3. Freundlich, IM, Bragg, D: *A Radiologic Approach to Diseases of the Chest,* 1992, Williams & Wilkins.

BIBLIOGRAPHY

Felson, B, Weinstein, AS, Spitz, HB: *Principles of chest roentgenology: a programmed text,* Philadelphia, 1965, WB Saunders.

Fraser, RG, Pare, JAP: *Diagnosis of diseases of the chest,* ed 3, Philadelphia, vols. I to IV, 1989, WB Saunders.

Lillington, GA: In Burton, GG, Gee, GN, Hodgkin, JE, editors: *Respiratory care,* Philadelphia, JB Lippincott, 1977.

Lillington, GA, Jamplis, RW: *A diagnostic approach to chest diseases,* ed 2, Baltimore, 1976, Williams & Wilkins.

Synopsis of Cardiopulmonary Disease

■

Craig L. Scanlan

Gregg L. Ruppel

Alaa El-Gendy

CHAPTER LEARNING OBJECTIVES

1. Describe the major respiratory infectious disorders including their causes, clinical signs and symptoms, and treatment;
2. Describe the immune mechanisms and their relationship to both respiratory hypersensitivity reactions and decreased host defenses (with an emphasis on AIDS);
3. Identify the major components of obstructive sleep apnea;
4. Compare and contrast the disorders associated with chronic airways obstruction, including asthma, chronic bronchitis, emphysema, bronchiectasis, and cystic fibrosis;
5. Describe the major pneumoconioses and diseases associated with noxious fumes and chemicals;
6. Describe common pulmonary neoplasms;
7. Identify the causes and symptoms of skeletal and thoracic disorders;
8. List at least three neuromuscular conditions commonly present with respiratory complications;
9. Define the causes of pleurisy, pleural effusions, and pneumothoraces;
10. Differentiate between the causes, signs and symptoms of left versus right heart failure;
11. List at least three types of shock;
12. Describe the major postoperative respiratory complications and the therapies used to treat them.

Respiratory care involves treating patients with a wide variety of cardiopulmonary disorders. This broad scope of care requires understanding of the causes, clinical features, and management approaches for a large number of diseases. This chapter provides a review of the major disease categories that confront the respiratory care practitioner (RCP). Included are the causes, clinical manifestations, and current treatment approaches used for most common adult disorders.

PULMONARY INFECTIONS

Infection is the most common cause of respiratory disease. The most common respiratory infection is pneumonia. Pneumonia is an inflammatory process of the lung tissue.

Pneumonia remains a major medical problem. Over a million cases occur each year in the United States. In the elderly, pneumonia and influenza together are the leading infections that cause death.

Pneumonia also strikes between 12% to 23% of all hospitalized critically ill patients. In addition, 50% to 60% of patients with **ARDS** develop some form of pneumonia. Pneumonia has the highest mortality rate of all hospital-acquired infections, ranging from 20% to 50%.

Pneumonias were once classified as either community or hospital-acquired. This traditional division is no longer so clear-cut. Medical care is more complex, and as patients live longer, unusual infections are becoming more common, both inside and outside the hospital. For example, the AIDS epidemic has dramatically increased the incidence of formerly rare pneumonias, such as those caused by cytomegalovirus (CMV), *Mycobacterium avium-intracellulare* (MAI) and *Pneumocystis carinii.*

Rather than trying to identify where a pneumonia was acquired, today it is more useful to identify the type of host and nature of the organism. The host may be either normal (having normal defense mechanisms) or abnormal (lacking in one or more host defenses). The organism may be usual (a common cause of infection) or unusual/uncommon. Using this classification results in four major categories of pneumonia (Table 20-1, page 452).

Normal hosts

Usual organisms

About 95% of normal adults in whom pneumonia develops in the usual community setting are infected with *Streptococcus pneumoniae, Hemophilus influenzae,* Chlamydia species, *Mycoplasma pneumoniae* or common viruses (Table 20-1).

Table 20-1   Causes of pneumonia

Cause	Normal Host	Abnormal Host
USUAL ORGANISM	Pneumococcus	Pneumococcus
	M. pneumoniae	Gram⁻ bacilli
	H. influenza	Anaerobic bacteria
	Viruses	*S. aureus*
	Chalamydia pneumonia, strain TWAR	*Moraxella catarrhalis*
UNUSUAL ORGANISM	Legionella	Enterococcus
	Mycobacterium	Group B streptococcus
	Group A streptococcus	Aspergillus
	Meningococcus	Nocardia
	B. anthracis	*P. carinii*
		Cytomegalovirus
		Mycobacteria

(Modified from Bradsher, RW: Overwhelming pneumonia. *Med Clin North Am* 67:1233, 1983)

Pneumococcal pneumonia. Most bacterial pneumonia in normal hosts is caused by *Streptococcus pneumoniae. S. pneumoniae,* also called pneumococcus, is an aerobic Gram-positive organism that tends to group in pairs. *S. pneumoniae* is the most frequent bacterial pneumonia requiring hospital admission. It also is the most common cause of pneumonia in the elderly and in patients with chronic diseases (discussed subsequently).

Pneumococcal pneumonia usually occurs during the winter months. Its onset is typically sudden and marked by shaking chills, high fever, pleuritic chest pain, dyspnea, tachypnea, a cough with **mucopurulent** or blood-streaked ("rusty") sputum. Respirations may be accompanied by grunting and nasal flaring. On physical exam, chest excursions may be decreased on the involved side, breath sounds are diminished, fine inspiratory crackles (rales) are heard, and a pleural friction rub may be present. Signs of consolidation, if they occur, appear later. These classical signs and symptoms may be suppressed in the young, elderly, or debilitated.

In many cases, the sputum Gram stain will reveal Gram-positive organisms which later culture out as pneumococci. Due to reports of relatively resistant strains of pneumococci, cultured organisms should be tested for penicillin susceptibility. Negative cultures do not rule out pneumococcal infection.

Typically, the patient's white blood count is elevated (**leukocytosis**). Blood cultures may be positive for pneumococci in 20% to 30% of patients. In the elderly, **bacteremia** is associated with increased mortality. Blood gases usually reveal a moderate to severe hypoxemia on room air, with accompanying hyperventilation. The pH may be higher than normal due to the hypocapnia.

The chest radiograph may be unremarkable, except for a vague haziness in the involved part of the lung. Consolidation, if it develops, may be well defined either in a lobar or patchy distribution (see accompanying box). Shadows in the costophrenic angles may appear in 10% to 20% of the patients, indicating pleural effusion (see later section).

Treatment of pneumococcal pneumonia involves antibiotic therapy, usually with penicillin G or erythromycin (Table 20-2). In addition, bed rest, pain medicine, adequate hydration, oxygen therapy, and pulmonary physical therapy, are prescribed. Compli-

Radiographic features of pneumonias

PATTERN	DESCRIPTION
Alveolar or acinar	Fluffy shadows that result from fluid accumulation in the distal airspaces of the lung; usually range from 0.5 to 1.0 cm in diameter and commonly are coalescent
Interstitial or reticular	Shadows that are a lacy network of linear markings that may reflect increased inflammatory material within the space surrounding the airspaces and/or vascular structures, but most commonly represent chronic changes such as fibrosis; linear changes may be the only abnormality or they may coexist with nodular shadows
Bronchopneumonia	Scattered fluffy shadows that tend to be patchy and follow the distribution of the central conducting airways; these may become confluent but rarely produce the "air-bronchogram" effect
Lobar pneumonia	Confluent shadows that usually terminate at pleural surfaces and usually but not always involve entire lobes or segments; a feature of lobar pneumonia is that the densities often surround the conducting airways to form a highly visible contrasting interface, the so-called "air bronchogram"
Necrotizing pneumonia	Pneumonia in which cavities are seen, that is, lung abscess; these lucencies may be apparent at the onset or may evolve as the inflammatory process advances; it is important not to confuse pneumonia in a patient with emphysema with necrotizing pneumonia

From Mitchell RS: Synopsis of clinical pulmonary disease, ed 4, St Louis, 1988, Mosby.

Table 20-2   Antibiotics used against organisms causing pulmonary infections

Infectious Agent	Primary Drugs	Secondary Drugs	Infectious Agent	Primary Drugs	Secondary Drugs
BACTERIA:			Bacteroides	penicillin	clindamycin metronidizole
Gram-Positive Bacteria:					
S. pneumoniae	penicillin	erythromycin vancomycin cephalosporin	Legionella pneumophila	erythromycin	rifampin ciprofloxacin
			N. meningitides (Meningococcal pneumonia)	penicillin	ciftriaxone
Group A beta-hemolytic streptococcus (S. pyogenes)	penicillin	vancomycin cephalosporin	Acid-Fast Bacteria:		
			M. tuberculosis	isoniazid rifampin pyrazinamide	ethambutol streptomycin
Group B streptococcus (S. agalactiae)	penicillin	vancomycin cephalosporin			
			M. avium intracellulare	isoniazid rifampin ethionamide clotazamine ciprofloxacin amikacin	clofazimine ansamycin
S. aureus					
penicillin sensitive	penicillin	cephalosporin vancomycin clindamycin			
penicillinase-producing	oxacillin nafcillin	cephalosporin vancomycin clindamycin	**OTHER:**		
			Mycoplama pneumoniae	erythromycin	tetracycline
methicillin-resistant	vancomycin	ciprofloxacin	Chlamydia pneumoniae	tctracycline	erythromycin
H. influenzae	ampicillin	amoxocillin-clavulanic acid cephalosporin	**FUNGI**		
			H. capsulatum	amphotericin B	ketoconazole
			C. immitis		fluconazole
Bacillus anthracis	penicillin	tetracycline erythromycin	B. dermatitidis		itraconazole
			P. carinii	TMP-SMX corticosteroids	pentamidine
Nocardia asteroides	sulfonamide	ampicillin+ erythromycin			
Gram-Negative Bacteria:			**VIRUSES**		
K. pneumoniae	gentamicin+ cephalosporin	tobramycin amikacin piperacillin ciprofloxacin	Influenza	amatidine	
E. coli			RSV	ribavirin	
S. marcensens			HIV	zidovudine (AZT)	dideoxycytidine (DDC) dideoxinocine (DDI)
P. vulgaris					
P. aeruginosa	tobramycin+ ticarcillin, piperacillin, azlocillin, or mezlocillin	ceftazidime+ amikacin ciprofloxacin	CMV	ganciclovir	foscarnet*
			Herpes simplex	acyclovar	foscarnet*
			Varicella zoster	acyclovar	
M. catarrhalis	amoxocillin-clavulanic acid	erythromycin tetracycline			

*Investigational

cations such as empyema, pleural effusion, and respiratory failure are treated as they arise.

The overall mortality rate for pneumococcal pneumonia is 4% for patients younger than 40 and 24% for those older than 40. Patients over 60 have death rates as high as 43%. Mortality also is increased in patients with multilobar involvement, and those in whom antibiotic therapy is delayed. Prevention of pneumococcal pneumonia by vaccination remains a highly desirable goal.

Hemophilus influenzae pneumonia. *Hemophilus influenzae* pneumonia is usually seen in children. Recently, *H. influenzae* has been recognized as an important cause of pneumonia in adults. Although infection is more common in abnormal hosts, the organism may be recovered from the oropharynx of healthy adults.

Physical findings associated with *H. influenzae* in adults are nondistinctive, resembling those seen with pneumococcal pneumonia. Due to its appearance (small, pleomorphic, coccobacillary), histologic evaluation is useful in identifying the presence of *H. influenzae.*

Mortality ranges from 10% to 20%, being highest when bacteremia is present. Bacteremia is most likely with the capsulated type B organism, which tends to strike debilitated patients. Nontypable *H. influenzae* is an important cause of morbidity and mortality in the elderly.

Most *H. influenzae* infections are responsive to ampicillin. Tetracycline, trimethoprim-sulfamethoxazole, amoxocillin-clavulanic acid, and first or second generation cephalosporins are alternative antibiotics (see Table 20-2).

Chlamydial and mycoplasmal pneumonias. Chlamydia species and *Mycoplasma pneumoniae* are among the most common agents causing community-acquired pneumonias. Both are considered "exotic" bacteria. Chlamydiae can only replicate within host cells, while *M pneumoniae* has no protective cell wall. These unusual features complicate identification and diagnosis.

Chlamydial pneumonia, caused by *Chlamydia pneumoniae,* is most common among otherwise healthy older children and young adults. The most common signs and symptoms are fever, nonproductive cough, and headache. Sinusitis, **pharyngitis,** and bronchitis may also occur. The full spectrum of clinical manifestations is now being defined.

Currently, definitive diagnosis is based on serologic tests, available mainly in research centers. Luckily, the organism is susceptible to common antibiotics, including tetracycline and erythromycin (see Table 20-2). Recovery is usually uneventful, although serious complications have been reported.

Pulmonary disease caused by *M. pneumoniae* ranges from mild bronchitis to full-blown adult respiratory distress syndrome. Since it is transmitted mainly by droplet nuclei, *M. pneumoniae* tends to spread quickly among people in close contact. Epidemics in military barracks, colleges, and schools are common.

Patients with mycoplasmal pneumonia complain of fever, **myalgia,** headache, minimally productive cough, and nonpleuritic chest pain. Pneumonia due to *M. pneumoniae* is often associated with massive pleural effusions, and acute interstitial lung disease. Serious nonpulmonary complications include pericarditis, pancreatitis, hemolytic anemia, and meningitis. Treatment consists of oral erythromycin or tetracycline for 2 to 3 weeks (see Table 20-2).

Viral pneumonias. Over 200 different viruses can cause respiratory tract infections. Viral pneumonias are much more common in infants and young children than in adults. Respiratory syncytial virus (RSV) and parainfluenza viruses are the main culprits in normal infants and children. Influenza is the most common viral pneumonia in adults.

RSV and parainfluenza viruses are paramyxoviruses. Other common paramyxoviruses cause the measles and mumps. Paramyxoviruses viruses are transmitted by direct person-to-person contact or via spread of droplet nuclei through the air.

There are three known serotypes of parainfluenza viruses, designated as types 1, 2, and 3. The most common specific illness caused by the parainfluenza viruses is childhood croup. Details on the clinical features and treatment of croup are provide in Chapter 35.

Because the population is usually exposed to the parainfluenza viruses during childhood, most adults have developed antibodies to them. Nonetheless, these viruses occasionally cause adult respiratory infections, especially viral laryngitis and pharyngitis.

Little is known about the development of parainfluenza infections. Vaccine development against parainfluenza viruses has been complicated by the possibility that antibody production might make the natural infection worse. Indeed, the severe disease caused by these viruses in newborn infants may be due to an immune response triggered by maternal antibody.

RSV also infects mainly infants and children. The most common disorder caused by RSV is bronchiolitis. Details on bronchiolitis also are provided in Chapter 35. In adults, RSV can cause colds and, less frequently, bronchopneumonia or bronchitis.

Another group of viruses, called the adenoviruses, can cause a variety of pulmonary-related infections. Most adenoviruses occur in children, causing about five percent of all lower respiratory tract illnesses in these patients. Childhood adenovirus infections have their highest incidence in the preschool years, and decline in frequency after age nine. Adenoviruses also are an important cause of respiratory disease in closely-quartered populations, such as on college campuses and the military quarters.

There are three primary types of adenoviruses respiratory infections: an acute, febrile, but generally self-limiting condition similar to influenza, a pertussis-like syndrome similar to that caused by *H. Influenza,* and pharyngoconjunctival fever. Overwhelming fatal pneumonias have been reported in both children and adults infected with some strains of the adenovirus. Respiratory infections caused by adenovirus are transmitted primarily by the fecal-oral route.

Influenza is an acute viral disease that produces fever, myalgia, headache, and malaise. The incidence of influenza varies widely, from sporadic occurrences during an interepidemic year to widespread **pandemic** outbreaks affecting millions.

Influenza is usually self-limiting, lasting a week or less. Among those with compromised immune systems, influenza can cause a progressive and sometimes fatal pneumonia. More often, however, influenza is complicated by bacterial superinfections, especially in elderly patients or those with underlying disease. These secondary bacterial infections usually involve *S. pneumoniae, H. influenzae* or *S. aureus.*

There are three **serotypes** of the influenza virus, designated as A, B, and C. The A virus is associated with pandemic influenza, whereas the B type tend to cause more localized epidemics. Influenza C infection in humans is sporadic and mild, being manifested only as pharyngitis and common colds.

Years ago, the diagnosis of viral pneumonia was based solely on clinical features (see accompanying box). Identification of the offending agent via viral cultures was available, but not practical.

Today, the diagnosis of viral pneumonia is based on both clinical and laboratory data. **Monoclonal antibodies** methods, immunofluorescence, and **ELISA** techniques have improved the sensitivity, specificity, and speed with which viral pneumonias can be diagnosed. Further advances are expected in the future as nucleic acid hybridization techniques are used to assess viral cultures and clinical specimens.

Treatment of most viral pneumonias includes bed rest, fluids to maintain adequate hydration, and pain medicine.

The same advances being made in diagnostic procedures are leading to an increasing number of anti-viral drugs. For RSV the agent is ribavirin, for influenza it is amantadine, and for herpes it is acyclovir (see Table 20-2). For example, early use of amantadine in influenza A can decrease the duration of fever and other systemic symptoms.

Patients who develop significant bacterial superinfections due to viral pneumonias should be hospitalized and started on a penicillinase-resistant penicillin. Thereafter, the offending bacterial agent is identified using one of the diagnostic methods previously described. Once the specific bacterial agent is uncovered, more specific antibiotic therapy is begun.

Of course, the best treatment for viral pneumonias is prevention. Prevention of viral pneumonias depends upon improved viral immunization practices. These are discussed in more detail under abnormal host pneumonias.

Unusual organisms

Less common causes of respiratory infections in normal hosts include *Legionella pneumophila, Mycobacterium tuberculosis, Bacillus anthracis,* group A beta-hemolytic streptococcus, the meningococcal bacteria, and the endemic fungi (see Table 20-1).

Legionnaires' disease. Legionnaires' disease is caused by *Legionella pneumophila,* a potentially life-threatening pneumonia. *L. pneumophila* is a Gram-negative organism that does not biochemically resemble any other known pathogen. Since its discovery in 1976, *L. pneumophila* has come to be recognized as a common cause of pneumonia. Between 3% and 15% of community-acquired pneumonias are Legionnaires' disease. *L. pneumophila* also accounts for as many as 13% of hospital-acquired pneumonias.

Among normal hosts, the organism is probably acquired by inhalation of contaminated aerosols produced by environmental reservoirs. These reservoirs include cooling systems, potable or domestic water systems, respiratory therapy devices, industrial coolants, and whirlpool spas. Hot water temperature (up to 50°C), stagnant water, sediment, and the presence of other microorganisms seem to enhance growth. In hospitalized patients, aspiration may be the key route of entry.

Legionnaires' disease is not very communicable—only 2% to 7% of exposed individuals develop infection. The incubation period is two to ten days. Three times as many males as females are affected with Legionnaires' disease, and age, cigarette smoking, and chronic medical disease (particularly **immunosuppression**) appear to be separate risk factors. Patients older than 55 and those with underlying diseases have a case fatality rate of 30%; however, even normally healthy persons have an alarming 5% mortality. Death is attributed to respiratory failure or shock.

The initial symptoms of Legionnaires' disease are comparable to influenza, that is general malaise, diffuse myalgia, and headache. Typically, these symptoms are followed within one to two days by a high fever and chills. Nausea, vomiting, and diarrhea may also occur early in the disease. Within 72 hours, a dry cough begins that is nonproductive or produces scanty mucoid sputum, which is sometimes blood-streaked. Dyspnea and hypoxia become marked as signs of consolidation develop. Pleuritic chest pain occurs in about every 1 out of 3 patients. Severe confusion or delirium may occur.

Laboratory tests may reveal leukocytosis, hyponatremia, and abnormal liver function. The chest X-ray usually shows patchy, often multilobar pulmonary consolidation, and, occasionally, small pleural effu-

---

Traditional clinical features used to diagnose common viral pneumonias

- Patient's age
- Patient's immune status
- Onset, severity and duration of symptoms
- Time of year
- Illness in other family members
- Community outbreaks

sions. The illness usually worsens for 4 to 7 days before improvement begins in those who recover.

Treatment involves IV erythromycin for 10 to 14 days, followed by oral therapy for an additional week (see Table 20-2). Rifampin may be added for serious cases. Supportive therapy includes the maintenance of a patent airway, the provision of adequate oxygenation, and the correction of fluid and electrolyte imbalances. Assisted ventilation and management of shock may be necessary for patients who develop cardiopulmonary failure.

Efforts to remove the offending organism from the environment include hyperchlorination, and superheating hot water systems (50° to 60°C). Ozone and UV light may also be effective. Additionally, cooling towers and evaporative condensers are being decontaminated and maintained with selected bacteriocidal agents.

Pulmonary tuberculosis. Pulmonary tuberculosis (TB) is an infection caused by the acid-fast bacillus *Mycobacterium tuberculosis*. Nearly eliminated in the US in the early 1980s, the number of TB cases increased by nearly 16% between 1985 and 1991. The greatest increase in TB is occurring among HIV-infected individuals. In addition, TB is on the rise in crowded urban populations, among the homeless, prison populations, migrant farm workers, and certain minorities and immigrants.

Infection normally occurs by inhaling organisms carried on droplet nuclei produced in the cough of an infected person. Inhalation is followed by replication of the organisms, local spreading through the lymph system, and further blood-borne dissemination throughout the body over 2 to 3 weeks. This first, or primary, infection is self-limiting, and normally escapes detection. Without detection or treatment, the organism remains in the body, in most cases contained by various host defense mechanisms for their lifetimes.

About 5% to 10% of infected individuals go on to develop the postprimary or chronic infection. This postprimary infection involves progressive pulmonary inflammation, turbercle formation and tissue **necrosis.** Malnutrition, diabetes, viral infections (including AIDS), end-stage kidney disease, chronic corticosteroid or immunosuppressive therapy, silicosis, and general debility all predispose development of the chronic infection.

The most frequent symptoms associated with chronic TB are cough, malaise, weight loss, and a low-grade fever. Night sweats, pleuritic pain, and a productive cough may or may not be present. In the presence of these symptoms, the appearance of blood in the sputum strongly suggests TB.

On physical examination, fine persistent crackles (rales) may be heard over the upper lobes. These are best heard during inspiration after a slight cough. Advanced disease may lead to retraction of the chest wall, deviation of the trachea, wheezes, and signs of pulmonary consolidation.

A chest X-ray helps disclose TB in many cases. Hilar lymph node enlargement associated with a small parenchymal lesion that heals with calcification is the usual picture of primary infection (Figure 20-1).

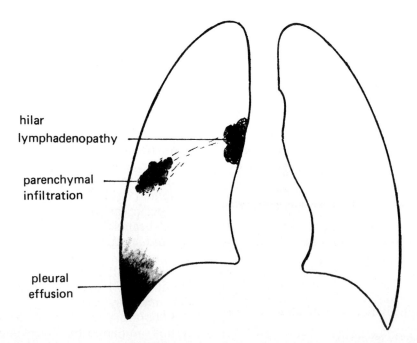

Fig. 20-1 Primary intrathoracic tuberculosis. (From Farzan, S: A concise handbook of respiratory diseases, ed. 2, East Norwalk, Conn, 1985, Appleton & Lange.)

However, many primary infections do not show X-ray abnormalities. The postprimary or chronic progressive form of TB typically reveals upper lobe infiltrations, with evidence of cavity formation (Figure 20-2). However, this tendency for upper lobe involvement is not always the case. When TB occurs secondary to an immune disorder, such as AIDS, the organisms may invade both the middle and lower lobes.

Skin testing can reveal a past or present infection. The tuberculin skin test is based on a delayed hypersensitivity (Type IV) reaction to a specific bacterial protein antigen. The Mantoux test is the most reliable, involving intracutaneous injection of purified protein derivative (PPD). A positive reaction is evident with **induration** of 10 mm or more in diameter. Unfortunately, the usefulness of the Mantoux test is limited by a high rate of false-negative reactions, especially among individuals infected with HIV. For this reason, persons with symptoms of TB should receive a chest X-ray, regardless of skin test results. If abnormalities are noted on X-ray, additional diagnostic testing should be performed.

To confirm the diagnosis of pulmonary TB, the bacillus must be recovered from the sputum, or gastric or tracheal washings. If there is no spontaneous sputum production, sputum induction using a heated saline aerosol or transtracheal aspiration may be needed. Cultures of pleural effusions or tissue biopsies may also confirm pulmonary TB.

Once the diagnosis is confirmed, antibiotic therapy is begun. Currently, this therapy consists of a 2 month induction phase of isoniazid (INH), rifampin (RIF), and pyrazinamide (PZA), followed by a 4 month continuation phase of INH and RIF (see Table 20-2). If drug-resistance is suspected, ethambutol (EMB)

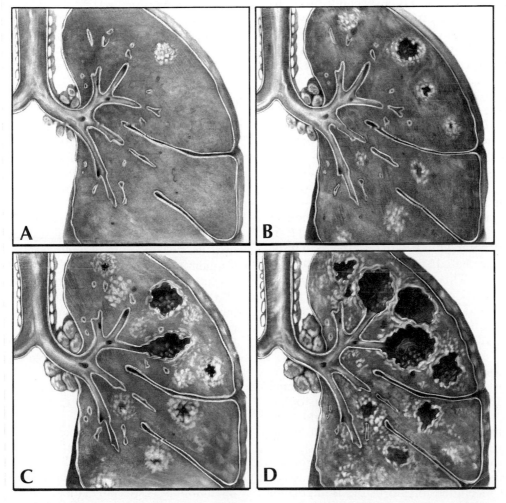

Fig. 20-2 Four stages of tuberculosis. **A,** Early primary infection. **B,** Cavity formed from a caseous tubercle and spread of primary lesions. **C,** Increased cavitation. **D,** Severe end-stage lung destruction. (From Des Jardins T: Clinical manifestations of respiratory disease, ed 2, St Louis, 1990, Mosby.)

and streptomycin (SM) may be included in the initial regimen, with the duration of therapy increased to as long as 12 months. When patients with infectious TB are hospitalized, they should initially be placed in AFB isolation (see Chapter 4) to protect employees and other patients. When patients are judged noninfectious, they may be moved to a private room or discharged. Three consecutive negative sputum smears on separate days or a negative culture virtually assures noninfectiousness.

The key factor determining the outcome of TB treatment is patient compliance with the drug regimen. In promoting and monitoring compliance, the physician, nurse, and respiratory care practitioner all play a major role. Noncompliance can not only lead to treatment failure (with increased disability and death), but also to continuing transmission and organism drug resistance. Multi-drug-resistant tuberculosis (MDR TB) is becoming an increasing problem, especially among hospitalized patients with the acquired immunodeficiency syndrome.

Contact with actively diseased patients is the greatest source of new cases of TB. Especially prone to developing TB in these situations are very young children and adolescent members of the patient's family. For this reason, household members and individuals having close contact with such patients should be skin tested. All contacts exhibiting a 5 mm or greater induration on skin test who have no history of reaction in the past should be considered infected with *M. tuberculosis* and immediately started on a preventive regimen, usually consisting of six months of isoniazid therapy.

There is a vaccine for TB, called Bacillus Calmette-Guerin (BCG). Unfortunately, immunity provided by BCG vaccine is highly variable, ranging from 0% to 76%. Several other factors also limit the usefulness of BCG vaccine. First, the risk of developing TB is already very low among those with negative skin tests. Second, once vaccinated, individuals will exhibit a positive skin test. This makes it difficult for the physician to discover early infections that can occur in these immunized individuals. For these reasons, BCG vaccination is recommended only where exposure to TB is great and the usual control measures are not possible.

Pulmonary mycoses. Fungal infections are called mycoses. The most common mycoses affecting normal people in the US are coccidioidomycosis, histoplasmosis, and blastomycosis (Figure 20-3). Several common features shared by these mycoses are identified in the accompanying box.

All three of these mycoses pose a common problem in the differential diagnosis of atypical pneumonia. For this reason, an epidemiologic history is important in patients with advanced pulmonary infections. Careful exposure and travel history frequently provide strong clues to aid diagnosis.

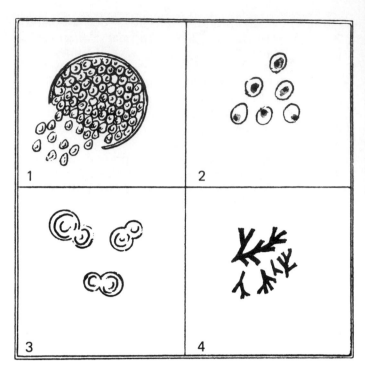

Fig. 20-3 Fungi commonly causing respiratory tract infection. **1,** *Coccidioides immitis;* **2,** *Histoplasma capsulatum;* **3,** *Blastomyces dermatitidis;* **4,** *Aspergillus fumigatus.* (From Farzan, S: A concise handbook of respiratory diseases, ed 2, East Norwalk, Conn, 1985, Appleton & Lange.)

Other diagnostic tests include sputum examination, culture, **serodiagnosis,** and tissue biopsy. *B. dermatitidis* and *C. immitis* may be seen in KOH-digested sputum, but microscopic identification of *H. capsulatum* is seldom possible. Culture of *H. capsulatum* and *B. dermatitidis* usually takes several weeks, and should not be attempted with *C. immitis.* Serodiagnosis also takes several weeks and is usually not helpful in directing therapy. In critically ill patients, invasive diagnostic tests, including tissue biopsy, are frequently needed to confirm the diagnosis.

Amphotericin B has been the primary therapy for all three mycoses (see Table 20-2). The recent availability of ketoconazole has changed the approach to treatment of some forms of fungal disease. However, ketoconazole has many adverse effects. Newer antifungal agents, such as fluconazole and itraconazole, hold promise for the future.

Abnormal hosts

An abnormal host has impaired host defenses. The box on page 460 lists examples of common clinical conditions in which host defenses are impaired.

Impaired host defenses predispose development of pneumonias, especially those of bacterial origin. Knowledge of which specific defense mechanism is impaired can give clues as to the organisms most likely to cause infection. For example, when the

Features shared by common mycoses

- Infections are endemic (occurring in circumscribed geographic areas); infecting agents are found in the soil and can be aerosolized;
- The fungal agent in each case exists in nature as a **mycelium** (mold) bearing infectious spores; these spores enter the host and then evolve to a yeast-like phase; the yeast-like phase is the tissue pathogen;
- Although local skin or mucous membrane inoculation is possible, the usual route of entry is the respiratory tract;
- Clinical manifestations and pathologic events are similar to TB; minimally symptomatic primary

infection is common, and chronic pulmonary or disseminated systemic infection is rare in normal hosts;
- The pathologic responses to these organisms are similar and consist of variable amounts of suppuration and granuloma formation; nodular densities are characteristic on X-ray (Figure 20-4);
- An intact cell-mediated immune response is needed to fight the infection; without it, the disease tends to spread systemically; immunosuppressive therapy and infection with HIV increase the risk of developing severe, progressive disease.

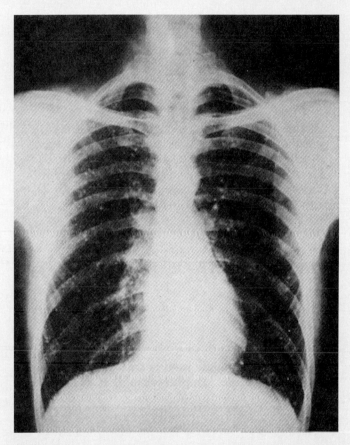

Fig. 20-4 Chest X-ray of a patient with histoplasmosis; granuloma are seen as small, round nodules throughout the lung fields. (From Des Jardins T: Clinical manifestations of respiratory disease, ed 2, St Louis, 1990, Mosby.)

problem is impaired humoral immunity (as with hypogammaglobinemia), usual organisms, such as *S. pneumoniae, H. influenzae,* or *P. aeruginosa* are the most likely pathogens. On the other hand, depressed cell-mediated immunity (as in AIDS) is more likely to result in unusual infections with atypical viruses, fungi, mycobacteria or *P. carinii.*

Usual Organisms

Common organisms causing pulmonary infections in abnormal hosts include *Staphylococcus aureus, S. pneumoniae,* Gram-negative bacilli, anaerobic bacteria, and influenza and respiratory syncytial viruses (see Table 20-1).

Staphylococcal pneumonia. Staphylococcal pneu-

Examples of conditions in which host defenses are impaired
AIDS
Alcoholism
Altered mental status
Antacid therapy
Antibiotic therapy
ARDS
COPD
Cytotoxic chemotherapy
Diabetes
Histamine blocker therapy
Immunosuppressive therapy
Increasing age
Leukemia
Other malignancy
Malnutrition
Prolonged mechanical ventilation
Renal failure/azotemia
Thoracoabdominal surgery
Tracheal intubation
Viral infections, especially HIV

monia is caused by *Staphylococcus aureus,* an aerobic Gram-positive cocci. *S. aureus* is an uncommon cause of community-acquired pneumonia, except during influenza epidemics, when its incidence rises to about 20%. It is most common in older debilitated patients and infants, especially after the administration of certain antibiotics. *S. aureus* also is a common cause of nosocomial pneumonia among postsurgical patients.

Staphylococcal pneumonia often begins with a mild cough, headache and generalized malaise. Depending on the host's resistance, it can abruptly change to a severe illness with high fever, chills, and a heavy cough productive of purulent or blood-streaked sputum. On physical examination, there may be signs of consolidation, pleural effusion, empyema, or even pneumothorax. The typical chest X-ray shows multilobar infiltrates, and may reveal areas of consolidation, **pneumatoceles,** abscesses, empyema, and pneumothorax (Figure 20-5).

Diagnosis of staphylococcal pneumonia normally is confirmed by culture of sputum or tracheal secretions. Cultures of the pleural fluid and blood may also be positive and leukocytosis is common. Blood gases usually reveal a severe hypoxemia on room air, which may manifest itself as a central cyanosis. The hypoxemia may cause hyperventilation and respiratory alkalosis.

Initial therapy consists of full systemic doses of a penicillinase-resistant antibiotic, such as oxacillin or nafcillin (see Table 20-2). Methicillin-resistant *S. aureus* should be treated with vancomycin. Supportive therapy includes treatment of hypoxemia with oxygen, maintenance of adequate hydration and electrolyte balance, and pulmonary physical therapy. Despite these measures, complications are common, and the mortality rate associated with staphylococcal pneumonia is as high as 32%.

Gram-negative bacillary (GNB) pneumonias. Gram-negative bacillary (GNB) pneumonias are a major cause of sickness and death both in the hospital and community. Mortality averages 50%, but can be as

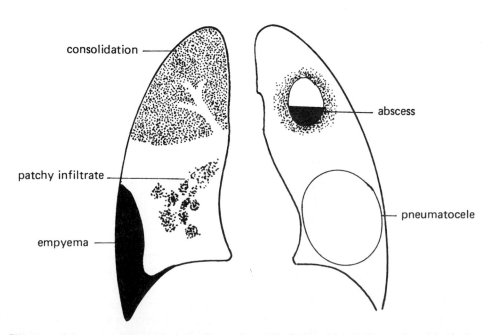

Fig. 20-5 Schematic representation of various radiographic findings in staphylococcal pneumonia. (From Farzan, S: *A concise handbook of respiratory diseases,* ed 2, East Norwalk, CN, 1985, Appleton & Lange.)

high as 70% to 80% with *Pseudomonas aeruginosa.* Healthy people occasionally may develop a GNB pneumonia, but most of these infections occur in compromised hosts. Pneumonia developing in patients who have been hospitalized longer than 3 to 4 days is more likely to involve hospital-acquired gram-negative bacteria.

The first step is colonization of the upper respiratory tract. Colonization is associated with severe illnesses, such as coma, **azotemia,** acidosis, and leukopenia. Once colonization occurs, impaired clearance mechanisms allow aspiration into the lungs. Once in the lungs, the organisms overwhelm compromised immune responses and cause actual infection (Figure 20-6).

The most common organisms causing GNB pneumonias are listed in the accompanying box. Identifying which specific organism is responsible for the infection is often difficult. Positive blood and pleural fluid cultures are valuable. The best information comes from semiquantitative cultures obtained by fiberoptic bronchoscopy, using either the protected brush technique or broncho-alveolar lavage (BAL).

Klebsiella pneumoniae is a gram-negative encapsulated bacillus. It is a common cause of pneumonia in elderly patients, especially those with pre-existing disease, such as COPD, diabetes, or alcoholism.

The onset of Klebsiella pneumonia is usually sudden. Patients typically have blood-tinged sputum and are tachypneic, cyanotic, and **jaundiced.** Laboratory findings include leukocytosis, with positive blood cultures occurring in about 25% of the cases. Examination of the sputum may or may not reveal encapsulated gram-negative rods. The chest X-ray typically shows lobar consolidation, with or without abscesses. Necrosis of lung tissue is common and occurs quickly.

Common causes of gram-negative bacillary pneumonias
Klebsiella pneumoniae
Moraxella catarrhalis
Escherichia coli
Pseudomonas aeruginosa
Serratia marcensens
Proteus vulgaris
Acinetobacter

Treatment is usually with cefotaxime and amikacin. Despite antibiotic therapy, mortality is high, ranging from 20% to 50%.

Moraxella catarrhalis is an aerobic Gram-negative diplococcus that is part of the normal flora upper airway. In patients with COPD, alcoholism, and other immunocompromising disorders, *M. catarrhalis* can cause bronchitis and pneumonia.

Patients with *M. catarrhalis* pneumonia have fever, cough, purulent sputum, and patchy lower lobe infiltrates on x-ray. The patient's history, combined with a positive sputum Gram stain and culture can aid diagnosis. Because most strains of *M. catarrhalis* are beta-lactamase-producing organisms, erythromycin, tetracycline, amoxicillin-clavulanic acid, or ciprofloxacin are recommended.

Pneumonias caused by *P. aeruginosa, E. coli, Serratia, Proteus,* and *Acinetobacter* occur mainly among hospitalized patients. The clinical features of these infections are similar; leukocytosis, hyperpyrexia, purulent sputum, and the appearance of bilateral

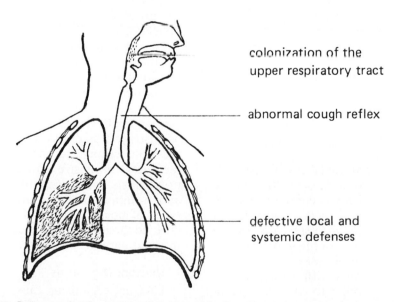

colonization of the upper respiratory tract

abnormal cough reflex

defective local and systemic defenses

Fig. 20-6 Pathogenesis of gram-negative pneumonia. (From Farzan, S: A concise handbook of respiratory diseases, ed 2, East Norwalk, CN, 1985, Appleton & Lange.)

pulmonary infiltrates and cavity formation on chest X-rays. However, since most of these patients are acutely ill to begin with, the onset of GNB pneumonia may be hard to distinguish from a general worsening of their underlying disease process.

Other findings are variable, but most similar to Staphylococcal pneumonia. Often associated with contaminated respiratory equipment, Pseudomonas can cause severe pneumonia, especially in immunosuppressed hosts. Pseudomonas also has a tendency to infect highly susceptible tissues, such as burn wounds or lung parenchyma affected by cystic fibrosis. Cyanosis, morning temperature spikes, and empyema are also common with Pseudomonas. Pseudomonas pneumonia commonly causes bilateral cavitation on X-ray.

E. coli pneumonia tends to infect mainly the lower lobes, due to spreads from the urinary or gastrointestinal tract. Proteus pneumonia commonly causes severe pleuritic chest pain. Serratia pneumonia is almost always associated with sepsis and empyema. Acinetobacter tends to cause a diffuse lower lobe bronchopneumonia, without consolidation or effusion. Acinetobacter infections are often traced to respiratory therapy equipment.

Initial antibiotic treatment of community-acquired GNB pneumonias involves a third-generation cephalosporin plus an aminoglycoside (gentamicin, tobramycin, amikacin). Because GNB pathogens causing nosocomial infections are frequently resistant to cephalosporins, an extended-spectrum penicillin (ticarcillin, piperacillin, azlocillin, or mezlocillin) should be combined with the aminoglycoside (see Table 20-2). Supportive therapy includes the maintenance of a patent airway, the provision of adequate oxygenation, and the correction of fluid and electrolyte imbalances. Despite aggressive intervention, the prognosis for patients with Gram-negative nosocomial pneumonias is generally poor.

Anaerobic bacteria. Anaerobic bacteria, especially *Bacteroides* and the fusospirochetes, cause severe pulmonary infections in abnormal hosts. Lung abscess, empyema, and necrotizing pneumonia are the three major pulmonary disorders caused by anaerobic bacteria. Risk factors include impaired consciousness, alcoholism, seizure disorders, periodontal disease, and cerebrovascular accidents.

Lung abscess is most commonly associated with aspiration of anaerobic bacteria. Colonization of the oral cavity with these organisms is common in alcoholic patients with severe tooth decay and infected gums. These so-called putrid abscesses are usually located in the posterior segments of the upper lobes or superior segments of the lower lobes.

Early in the process, patients with a lung abscess have signs and symptoms similar to any acute pneumonia: fever, chills, pleuritic chest pain, cough, and leukocytosis. The cough is often non-productive at onset. Consolidation due to pneumonitis surrounding the abscess is the most frequent finding.

In terms of laboratory findings, simple sputum cultures are usually not diagnostic, requiring alternative methods for collecting a specimen. On the X-ray, an early abscess may look the same as any localized pneumonitis. Later, a dense shadow may appear. Finally, after the abscess communicates with a bronchus and starts to drain, a central radiolucency appears, often with a visible air-fluid level (Figure 20-7).

If the abscess ruptures into a bronchus, the patient may suddenly cough up large amounts of sputum. Hemoptysis may also occur at this time. Fetid brown or gray sputum indicates a putrid infection caused by a mix of organisms, including anaerobes. Green or yellow musty sputum without an offensive odor indicates a nonputrid infection with a single pyogenic organism.

In the past, lung abscesses were treated by surgical drainage or resection. Today, this approach is a last resort, with antibiotic therapy the treatment of choice. Clindamycin, metronidizole and penicillin can be used (see Table 20-2). Although many of the newer cephalosporins possess anaerobic activity, none is better than penicillin.

In addition to antibiotic therapy, both postural drainage and therapeutic bronchoscopy can aid removal of abscess secretions. However, in order to avoid spreading the infection to healthy lung lobes or segments, postural drainage must be performed with extreme caution. In some patients, an artificial airway may be needed to aid clearance of secretions.

The prognosis for acute lung abscesses that are treated early is very good. Chronic lung abscess with severe associated disease has a mortality rate as high as 15% to 20%. Patients with a chronic lung abscess complicated by severe hemoptysis generally have a poor prognosis.

Nosocomial viral infections. Hospital-acquired viral infections are a growing problem. Influenza, RSV, parainfluenza viruses, and adenoviruses have all been implicated in nosocomial pneumonia outbreaks. The chronically ill, immunocompromised, elderly, and very young hosts are at highest risk. Hospital personnel also are at high risk for acquiring and transmitting these infections. In the case of influenza, control measures emphasize immunization and amantadine prophylaxis for susceptible patients and personnel, and isolation of those already infected. For other types of nosocomial viral infections, careful adherence to hand-washing procedures and isolation of infected patients are warranted.

Unusual Organisms

Unusual organisms causing pulmonary infections in abnormal hosts include Group B streptococcal pneumonia, *Hemophilus influenzae, Aspergillus fumi-*

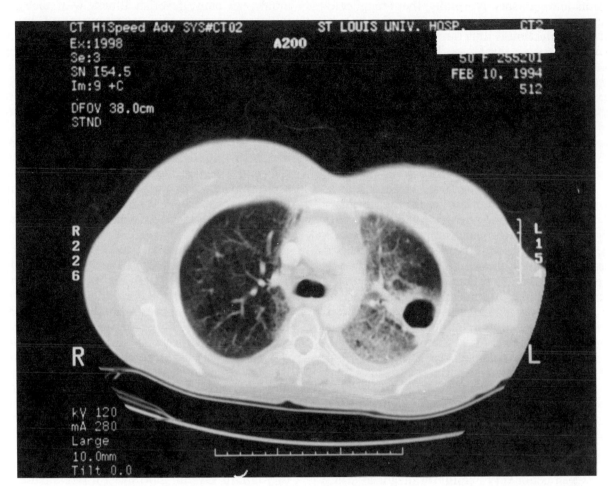

Fig. 20-7 Computer-assisted tomographic (CAT) scan of a cavity caused by an abscess. Pictured is a cross-section at the level of the carina, with the patient supine. The large cavity in the left lung resulted from an infection surrounding a cancerous tumor. The tumor necrosed leaving an abscess behind. A small amount of fluid is visible in the dependent portion of the cavity. The left lung shows tissue inflammation resulting from radiation therapy. (Courtesy Dept. of Radiology, St Louis University Health Sciences Center, St Louis)

gatus, Candida albicans, Nocardia asteroides, Pneumocystis carinii, cytomegalovirus (CMV), Varicella zoster and herpes simplex, *M. tuberculosis,* and *Mycobacterium avium intracellulare* (MAI) (see Table 20-1).

Group B streptococcal pneumonia. Group B streptococcal pneumonia is becoming more common. Most of these pneumonias are acquired in the hospital by elderly patients, with diabetes considered an important predisposing factor. The clinical picture consists of fever, leukocytosis, and X-ray evidence of diffuse infiltration. Pleural effusion and empyema are common. Treatment is with either penicillin or vancomycin (see Table 20-2). Mortality is high, with most patients dying of infection superimposed on underlying diseases.

***Hemophilus influenzae* pneumonia.** *Hemophilus influenzae* pneumonia was previously described as a source of infection in normal children and adults. In recent years, this organism has also become associated with pneumonia in compromised hosts, particularly those with chronic conditions such as alcoholism, chronic obstructive pulmonary disease, lung cancer, and ischemic vascular disease. Mortality is high, especially when the pulmonary infection is complicated with bacteremia. Most *H. influenzae* infections respond to ampicillin. Tetracycline, trimethoprim-sulfamethoxazole, amoxocillin-clavulanic acid, and first or second generation cephalosporins are alternative antibiotics (see Table 20-2).

Opportunistic fungal infections. Any of the mycoses that were previously described as infecting normal hosts can cause infection in compromised hosts. However, it is more common for compromised hosts to develop fungal infection with what are called the opportunistic organisms. Normally, these fungi colonize the skin and mucous surfaces of the normal human host. Infection is thus rare unless host defense mechanisms become impaired. The two most common causes of opportunistic fungal infections are *Aspergillus fumigatus* and *Candida albicans.*

Once established, *A. fumigatus* infection may manifest itself in one of three forms: invasive aspergillosis, allergic aspergillosis, or aspergilloma. Invasive aspergillosis is the opportunistic infection, found most often in immunocompromised hosts with chronic **granulocytopenia** (as in leukemia). Most of these patients have previously received high-dose steroids or broad-spectrum antibiotics for their primary illness.

Fungal mycelia first invade the pulmonary parenchyma, followed by blood-borne spread to other organs, especially the kidneys. Patients develop fever, and a pleural friction rub. On a chest X-ray, either a rounded pneumonia or multiple nodular densities appear. Cavitation may be seen on sequential films. Positive nasal cultures may be helpful in diagnosis, although biopsy is usually necessary. Progressive systemic invasion of the organism results in death if not treated quickly. Antibiotic treatment is usually with amphotericin B (see Table 20-2).

C. albicans pneumonia is an especially formidable problem in immunosuppressed patients. The infection often coexists with other pathogens, and pneumonia typically occurs late in the course of a critical illness. For this reason, the chest X-ray shows a mixed picture, which is not very helpful for diagnosis. Since it is part of the normal flora, isolation of *Candida* in the sputum is of little diagnostic value. Likewise, serologic testing and antigen assays are not very helpful. Reliable diagnosis requires tissue biopsy. As with invasive aspergillosis, amphotericin B is the primary therapy.

Nocardia asteroides. *Nocardia asteroides* is an aerobic Gram-positive species of actinomycetes. *N. asteroides* infections are rare except in organ transplant patients and those with hematologic malignancies. Culture of the sputum or pulmonary secretions obtained by bronchoscopy may help make the diagnosis. The typical X-ray shows cavitary lesions, nodules, and alveolar or interstitial infiltrates. Systemic spread via the blood is common, especially to the CNS. Antibiotic therapy with sulfonamide is the primary treatment (see Table 20-2). Due to the high rate of relapse, the antibiotic treatment may have to be prolonged. Even with early diagnosis and treatment, mortality is high.

***Pneumocystis carinii* pneumonia (PCP).** *Pneumocystis carinii* is an atypical fungi with both extra and intracellular life-stages. *P. carinii* causes severe pneu-

monia in immunosuppressed patients, almost exclusively those with AIDS. Symptoms of PCP may be insidious, with only exertional dyspnea. More commonly, an acute feverish illness with tachypnea is followed by the rapid development of interstitial infiltrates. There may also be chest pain, a variable amount of sputum production and lymphadenopathy. The chest X-ray typically shows a relatively symmetric, homogenous perihilar pneumonia that progresses to diffuse consolidation. Arterial blood gas analysis will usually show a large $P(A-a)O_2$, indicating the presence of physiologic shunting.

Fiberoptic bronchoscopy helps diagnose PCP in patients with AIDS. Sputum induction is a less invasive and effective alternative. Percutaneous needle aspiration may also provide diagnostic information. Once a specimen is obtained, the cysts typical of *P. carinii* can be seen in smears stained with methenamine-silver.

Current drug treatment of PCP consists of either trimethoprim sulfamethoxazole (TMP-SMX) or pentamidine isethionate, both by IV (see Table 20-2). Prior enthusiasm for pentamidine administration via the aerosol route (approved by the FDA in 1989) has recently waned. This is because clinical trials are confirming the superiority of TMP-SMX for preventing recurrent PCP infection. And when pentamidine is used, reduced dose IV therapy is proving better than the aerosol route for mild to moderate PCP. Interestingly, early adjunct use of corticosteroids has proved beneficial in decreasing mortality in patients with AIDS and severe PCP.

Even with the most aggressive treatment, many patients with PCP go on to develop full-blown respiratory failure. Overall mortality for AIDS patients with PCP is about 50%. If the patient has one or more complicating illnesses, such as Kaposi's sarcoma, PCP mortality increases to 70%.

Unusual viral infections. Immunocompromised hosts are susceptible to several viral pneumonias. These include infections caused by cytomegalovirus (CMV), as well as Varicella zoster and herpes simplex.

By early adulthood almost all individuals have been infected by CMV. The initial infection is usually asymptomatic. Thereafter, however, the virus remains dormant in the host. Reactivation tends to occur when the immune system falters.

In contrast to the normal host, symptomatic CMV infections are common in certain immunocompromised patients, particularly organ transplant recipients and patients AIDS. In transplant patients, an interstitial pneumonitis tends to occur in the second or third month after surgery. Patients exhibit severe hypoxemia and bilateral, symmetric interstitial infiltrates on chest X-ray. In AIDS patients, CMV infection tends to spread early and frequently coexists with other infections, particularly *P. carinii*. As with transplant recipients, the X-ray usually reveals bilateral interstitial infiltration, although nodular lesions have been described.

CMV pneumonia can be identified by culturing the virus from lung tissue specimens obtained by BAL, percutaneous needle aspiration, or open lung biopsy. However, the culture method is a lengthy and complex process, and not available in all settings. This method will probably be replaced by monoclonal antibody testing or DNA probes. Both techniques can provide rapid identification of CMV in tissue biopsy, cytologic specimens, or tissue culture.

Primary CMV infection can be prevented by screening of blood and organ donors. Immunoglobulin prophylaxis may help reduce the severity of infection. Reactivation of the virus can be delayed or stopped by IV acyclovir (see Table 20-2). Newer drugs with stronger anti-CMV activity, such as ganciclovir and foscarnet, may also prove useful. Future approaches will probably include recombinant or subunit vaccines or adoptive immunotherapy.

Normally, Varicella zoster and Herpes simplex viruses cause minor infection of the skin or mucous membranes. However, certain patient groups are at increased risk for spread of these viruses to the lungs or other organs. High risk groups include newborn babies, cancer patients, organ and bone marrow transplant recipients, and those deficiencies of cell mediated immunity.

Both viruses cause a patchy nodular pneumonia with scattered necrotic and hemorrhagic foci. Physical examination is often misleading and rapid progression of pneumonia can occur within hours. If given early in the course of a Varicella or Herpes infection, IV acyclovir can reduce both morbidity and mortality (see Table 20-2).

Mycobacterial pneumonias. Due to abnormalities of host defenses, persons with AIDS and other immunodeficiencies are especially vulnerable to mycobacterial pneumonias. Classical *M. tuberculosis* pneumonia is relatively common in patients with AIDS and in other compromised hosts, as are multiple-drug-resistant forms of this infection. A peculiar form of mycobacterial infection caused by *Mycobacterium avium intracellulare* (MAI) is also seen in AIDS patients.

TB is often the first infectious disease to appear in AIDS. In these patients, the clinical features of TB vary according to the stage of the HIV infection. Tuberculin skin tests commonly are negative. Early on, the clinical findings may be similar to those in HIV-negative persons. Late in the process, tuberculosis usually has atypical features. Chest X-rays may show infiltrates throughout the lung fields and cavities may not be present. Unlike TB in normal hosts, extrapulmonary and disseminated disease is common. Extrapulmonic disease occurs in the bone marrow, liver, lymph nodes, and spleen.

Like *M. tuberculosis,* MAI tends to spread systemically in AIDS patients. In contrast to TB, however, AIDS-related MAI disease tends to occur late rather than early, is **noncommunicable** and is not effectively treated with current drug treatments.

To help identify and prevent mycobacterial pneumonias in high risk groups, all patients who are HIV-positive or who are at risk for HIV infection should undergo Mantoux skin and anergy testing according to CDC protocol. Anergy testing should be accomplished at the time of PPD testing. Persons HIV-positive with a 5 mm or greater induration on skin testing but without active tuberculosis should be placed on 1 year of isoniazid prophylaxis.

In AIDS patients with *M. tuberculosis* pneumonia, the response to treatment is generally good. However, the standard length of therapy should be at least 9 months, using INH and rifampin usually supplemented by pyrazinamide in the first 2 months. Unfortunately, patients with MAI pneumonia do not respond as well to antibiotic therapy. Although a number of drugs, such as ansamycin and clofazimine, have been used to treat MAI infection (see Table 20-2), no regimen is uniformly successful and prognosis remains poor. The management of multiple-drug-resistant TB (MDR TB) emphasizes public health measures to ensure early diagnosis and ongoing compliance with the antibiotic regimen.

Those implementing infection-control measures for HIV-infected patients who have pulmonary findings should take tuberculosis into account until the disease is excluded. Medical personnel providing care for patients with tuberculosis should use universal blood and body substance precautions because of the possibility of undetected HIV infection in patients with tuberculosis. Health-care workers should be particularly alert to the need for preventing TB transmission in settings where cough-inducing procedures (such as sputum induction and aerosolized pentamidine treatments) are being performed. Other actions designed to reduce the risk of nosocomial TB transmission are listed in the accompanying box.

Procedures to prevent transmission of TB in the health-care setting

- Screening patients for TB
- Providing rapid diagnostic services
- Prescribing suitable antibiotics (including prophylaxis)
- Using physical measures to reduce air contamination
- Placing persons with active or suspected TB in isolation
- Screening health-care-facility personnel for TB
- Promptly investigating and controlling outbreaks

AIRWAY OBSTRUCTION

Airway obstruction may occur in the upper or lower airways. Acute upper airway obstruction is usually due to foreign bodies or trauma. A more common and chronic type of upper airway obstruction is obstructive sleep apnea.

Lower airway obstruction is a common pathophysiologic finding in asthma, chronic bronchitis, bronchiectasis, emphysema, and cystic fibrosis. Although each of these has distinct causes, significant overlap exists. Asthma, chronic bronchitis, and emphysema are often found in the same patient. The term COPD (chronic obstructive pulmonary disease) is often used to describe the finding of one or more of these diseases in a subject. The term reversible airway obstruction is used to describe the asthmatic component of airway obstruction.

Obstructive sleep apnea

Sleep apnea is cessation of breathing for 10 seconds or longer. It is diagnosed as 30 or more episodes of apnea per six hour intervals. Sleep apnea may be classified as obstructive, central, or mixed apnea. Obstructive sleep apnea is the type encountered most often in clinical practice.

Definition and pathophysiology

Obstructive sleep apnea (OSA) is defined as cessation of air movement for 10 seconds in spite of continued respiratory efforts (Figure 20-8). Obstructive apneic events are related to anatomic obstruction of the upper airway (see accompanying box). Muscular control of the upper airway is diminished. This allows the tongue or other oropharyngeal structures to obstruct the airway. The patient is initially quiet. Increasing respiratory efforts ensue, until the patient either resumes breathing or awakens. The stimuli to resume breathing appear to be hypoxemia or hypercapnia.

OSA is about eight times more common in males than in females, particularly in middle age. In men aged 40 to 65 years, the prevalence of OSA may be greater than 8%. The syndrome is often present in obese individuals. The short, thick neck may cause

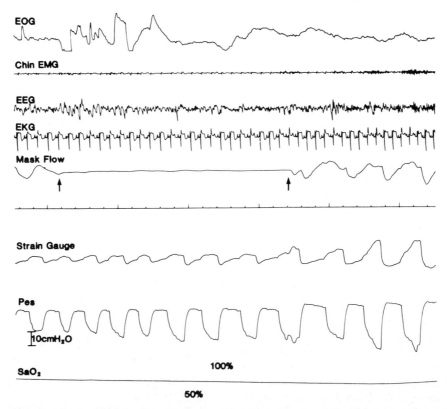

Fig. 20-8 Polysomnographic tracing of upper airway obstruction as seen in obstructive sleep apnea. Cessation of airflow (arrows) occurs despite continued respiratory efforts (strain gauge and esophageal pressure Pes). EOG = electro-oculogram, EEG = electroencephalogram, EMG = electromyogram, EKG = electrocardiogram, SaO$_2$ =pulse oximeter oxygen saturation. (From Mitchell RS, Petty TL, Schwartz MI: Synopsis of clinical pulmonary disease, ed 4, St Louis, 1988, Mosby.)

```
┌─────────────────────────────────────────┐
│        Factors related to upper airway   │
│        obstruction during sleep          │
│                                          │
│  ■ Obesity                               │
│  ■ Excessive pharyngeal tissue           │
│  ■ Enlarged tonsils or adenoids          │
│  ■ Goiter                                │
│  ■ Micrognathia                          │
│  ■ Myotonic dystrophy                    │
│  ■ Shy-Drager syndrome                   │
│  ■ Hypothyroidism (males)                │
│  ■ Acromegaly                            │
└─────────────────────────────────────────┘
```

pharyngeal narrowing that predisposes to obstruction. Some patients with OSA show evidence of upper airway abnormalities on pulmonary function studies. Patients with OSA often have histories of loud snoring and daytime sleepiness (hypersomnolence). Obstructive sleep apnea may also occur in subjects who are not obese but have related disorders that affect pharyngeal structures (see accompanying box). Approximately 20% of OSA patients also suffer from COPD. The underlying hypoxemia that accompanies COPD may influence the development of right heart failure in OSA.

Clinical features

The clinical features of sleep apnea include serious cardiac arrhythmias, systemic hypertension, pulmonary hypertension, cor pulmonale, and personality disorders. The diagnosis of obstructive sleep apnea includes a detailed history and physical examination, and pulmonary function studies to determine the presence of upper airway obstruction. Categorization of the type of sleep apnea (i.e., obstructive, central, or mixed) is made by polysomnographic sleep studies. The sleep study usually includes: (1) an EEG, (2) **electrooculogram** (EOG) to stage sleep, (3) airflow monitoring, (4) ECG to detect arrhythmias, (5) impedance **pneumography** or EMG to detect respiratory efforts, and (6) oximetry to detect desaturation. CT scanning of the upper airway may also help to identify the site of airway narrowing.

Management

Management of obstructive sleep apnea is multifaceted. Weight reduction provides some relief in the severity of the apnea, but may fail if weight loss is not maintained. Alteration of sleep posture also reduces the incidence of apnea in some subjects. Supplemental O_2 may be indicated to correct hypoxemia-induced arrhythmias and pulmonary hypertension. Protriptyline is a tricyclic antidepressant that markedly reduces REM sleep. Decreasing the amount of REM sleep often limits the number of apneic episodes. Central nervous system stimulants, such as methylphenidate, reduce daytime somnolence in subjects with either central or obstructive sleep apnea.

Surgical interventions for OSA include tracheostomy, palatopharyngoplasty, and mandibular advancement. Tracheostomy is used for emergency management of severe obstructive apnea. In palatopharyngoplasty, the posterior section of the palate and the uvula are **resected.** This shortens the soft palate. Tissues such as the tonsils and lateral posterior wall of the pharynx are removed to enlarge the airway. A small percentage of patients have mandibular malformations that result in OSA. Mandibular advancement can correct these abnormalities.

Mechanical support of ventilation, and of the airway in particular is commonly used to manage sleep apnea. Continuous positive airway pressure (CPAP) used at night prevents collapse of the airway when muscle tone is reduced. CPAP is effective only in OSA, not central apnea. Continuous mechanical ventilation is used for short term management when respiratory failure results from OSA or central apnea. If the problem is central in origin, negative pressure ventilation (using a chest cuirass or similar device) allows ventilation to be maintained without an artificial airway.

Asthma

Definition and pathophysiology

Asthma is a lung disease characterized by airway obstruction, inflammation, and hyperresponsiveness. Airway obstruction is caused by bronchospasm, mucosal edema, and excessive secretion of viscid mucus and is usually reversible (Figure 20-9 on page 468). In chronic asthma, bronchial smooth muscle hypertrophy may also be present.

Airway obstruction in asthma is triggered by inflammation. Inflammation causes release of chemical mediators such as histamine, slow-reacting substance of anaphylaxis (SRS-A), and eosinophil chemotactic factor (ECF-A) from airway cells (Figure 20-10 on page 468). These mediators cause infiltration of eosinophils and **neutrophils** and produce epithelial injury, smooth muscle hyperresponsiveness, and airflow obstruction. Over time, the inflammatory process may cause chronic airway irritation and increased sensitivity to inhaled allergens, environmental irritants, or infectious agents.

Airway hyperresponsiveness is the third key characteristic of asthma. The degree of airway hyperresponsiveness is a good indicator of the severity of asthma. Hyperresponsiveness is due mainly to inflammation, but may also be caused by imbalances in autonomic neural control or changes in smooth muscle function. Hyperresponsive airways exhibit an exaggerated bronchoconstrictor response to certain physical, chemical, and drug stimuli. Airway hyperresponsiveness may be genetically inherited at birth or

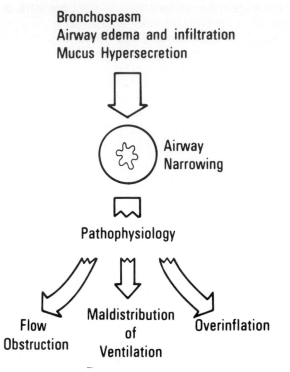

Bronchospasm
Airway edema and infiltration
Mucus Hypersecretion

Airway
Narrowing

Pathophysiology

Flow
Obstruction

Maldistribution
of
Ventilation

Overinflation

Fig. 20-9 Pathophysiology of asthma. (From Tisi GM: Pulmonary physiology in clinical medicine, ed 2, Baltimore, 1984, Williams & Wilkins.)

acquired later in life. Occupational asthma (due to on-the-job exposure to inhaled irritants) is a good example of the acquired variety. Occupational asthma may be the predominant occupational lung disease in the coming decade. Over 200 causative substances have been identified.

Asthma may also be categorized according to the causative agent involved. The term *extrinsic* or *atopic* asthma has been used to describe airway changes induced by an identified allergic response. *Intrinsic* or non-allergic asthma describes a similar response that is not triggered by a specific allergic or environmental agent.

Allergic asthma is associated with exposure to antigenic agents such as pollen or house dust. Individuals who are atopic display a positive response to skin allergy testing. Allergic asthma is common in children and adults under age 30.

Many other triggers which cannot be classified as allergic can cause an asthmatic response (Table 20-3). However, the pattern of inflammation and airway obstruction is nearly identical to that seen in allergic asthma. The mechanisms of cold air inhalation and exercise are probably related. In both, heat and water loss from the upper airway precipitates the asthmatic response.

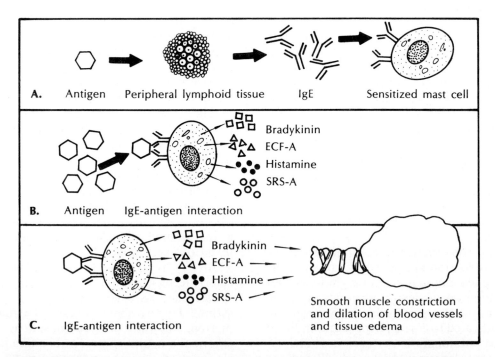

A. Antigen Peripheral lymphoid tissue IgE Sensitized mast cell

Bradykinin
ECF-A
Histamine
SRS-A

B. Antigen IgE-antigen interaction

Bradykinin
ECF-A
Histamine
SRS-A

Smooth muscle constriction and dilation of blood vessels and tissue edema

C. IgE-antigen interaction

Fig. 20-10 Immunologic mechanisms involved in asthma. **A,** Exposure to antigen sensitizes mast cells. **B,** Re-exposure to antigens cause mast cell to degranulate releasing mediators. **C,** Mediators produce inflammatory response characteristic of asthma. (From Des Jardins T: Clinical manifestations of respiratory disease, ed 2, St Louis, 1990, Mosby.)

Table 20-3 Asthma triggers

Allergic	Non-Allergic	Occupational
pollen	infections (viral)	tolune 2,4 diisocyanate
house dust mites	cold air	cotton dust
feathers	exercise	grain, flour
animal proteins	air pollution	wood dust
	tobacco smoke	insecticides
	drugs (aspirin)	animal, bird serum
	emotions, stress	

Diagnosis

To diagnose asthma, the physician must establish a history of reversible, episodic airway obstruction. This is done by careful attention to the results of the medical history, physical examination, and pulmonary function testing. Figure 20-11 on page 470 provides a general algorithm for differential diagnosis of asthma.

The box on page 471 outlines medical history topics that can help diagnose asthma. Elements of the physical examination useful in identifying chronic asthma include recurrent rhinitis, sinusitis or nasal polyps, evidence of pulmonary hyperinflation, wheezing, reduced breath sounds, or prolonged expiration, and eczema.

Simple pulmonary function studies, including the forced vital capacity, FEF_{25-75}, FEV_1 and FEV_1/FVC, follow the history and physical examination. These objective tests are essential in diagnosing asthma and assessing its severity. A normal VC with either a decreased FEV_1 or FEF_{25-75} indicates pure obstruction. When the FEV_1 is severely reduced with clear evidence of obstruction ($FEV_1/FVC < 75\%$), the vital capacity can also be reduced. When the FEF_{25-75} is the only abnormal finding, mild airflow obstruction is present, suggesting small airway disease.

Additional studies may also be useful in confirming a diagnosis of asthma. However, not all tests are appropriate for all patients. The accompanying box describes the common additional studies used in the differential diagnosis of asthma.

Management

As a chronic disorder, asthma should be managed rather than simply treated. The goals of asthma management are to: (1) maintain normal or near normal pulmonary function; (2) maintain normal activity levels; (3) prevent troublesome symptoms such as coughing or dyspnea; (4) prevent recurrent exacerbations, and (5) avoid the adverse effects of drug treatment.

To achieve these goals, a comprehensive management approach is required. Comprehensive asthma management includes ongoing assessment and monitoring of lung function, drug therapy, environmental

---

Additional studies used in differential diagnosis of asthma

- Complete blood count (CBC)
- Chest X-ray (useful in ruling out other causes of airway obstruction; a recent film is especially important for children)
- Sputum examination and stain for eosinophilia (sputum eosinophilia are highly characteristic of asthma; neutrophils predominate in bronchitic sputum)
- Nasal secretion and stain for eosinophils (neutrophilic nasal discharge is characteristic of sinusitis)
- Complete pulmonary function studies, including inspiratory and expiratory flow volume curve (these may reveal upper airway problems that simulate asthma)
- Determination of specific IgE antibodies to common inhalant allergens with skin (in vivo) or in vitro tests
- Rhinoscopy
- Sinus X-rays
- Bronchoprovocation with methacholine, histamine, or exercise challenge
- Provocative challenge with occupational allergens (chemicals)
- Evaluation of pH for gastroesophageal reflux

From: National Institutes of Health, National Asthma Education Program: Guidelines for the diagnosis and management of asthma, Bethesda Md, 1991, US Department of Health and Human Services [Publication No. 91-3042A].

---

control of allergens and irritants, and patient education.

Ongoing assessment and monitoring of lung function is usually provided by measurement of peak expiratory flow rate (PEFR). The PEFR is a simple, objective measure of airway obstruction that correlates well with the FEV_1 and can be easily performed by the patient. Daily self-monitoring of PEFR can: (1) help assess circadian (day-night) variations in lung function; (2) provide objective criteria for beginning, modifying or ending treatment; and (3) aid in identifying specific allergens that can worsen symptoms.

Interpretation of the PEFR is based on comparison to each patient's personal best or baseline value. This baseline value is usually the highest PEFR achieved after a period of maximum therapy. When the PEFR value is above 80% of the baseline, and no asthma symptoms are present, routine treatment continues. A PEFR between 50% to 80% of the norm indicates an acute worsening that may require a temporary increase in medication. A drop in PEFR below 50% of the baseline indicates an acute and severe attack that should be treated immediately with bronchodilator therapy.

Maintenance drug therapy for asthma includes beta-adrenergic bronchodilators, methylxanthines, corticosteroids, and mast cell inhibitors (refer to

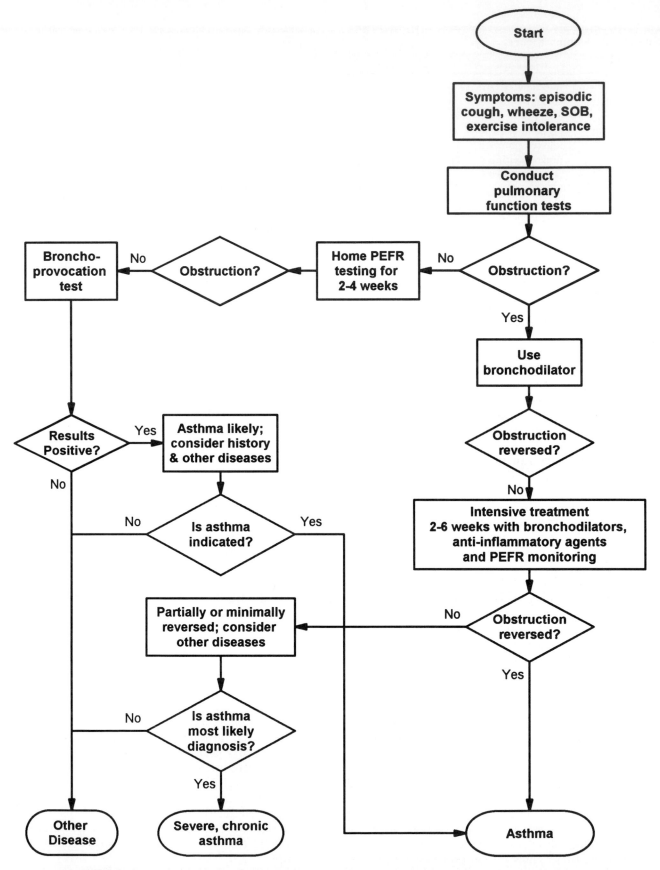

Fig. 20–11 Algorithm for the differential diagnosis of asthma. (Adapted from National Institutes of Health, National Asthma Education Program: Guidelines for the diagnosis and management of asthma, Bethesda Md, 1991, US Department of Health and Human Services.)

Topics in medical history helpful in diagnosing asthma

Topics to include in the history are:

I. Symptoms
  A. Cough, wheezing, shortness of breath, chest tightness, and sputum production (generally of modest degree)
  B. Conditions know to be associated with asthma, such as rhinitis, sinusitis, nasal **polyposis,** or atopic dermatitis

II. Pattern of symptoms
  A. Perennial, seasonal, or perennial with seasonal exacerbations
  B. Continuous, episodic, or continuous with acute exacerbations
  C. Onset, duration, and frequency of symptoms (days per week or month)
  D. Diurnal variations with special reference to nocturnal symptoms

III. Precipitating and/or aggravating factors
  A. Viral respiratory infections
  B. Exposure to environmental allergens (pollen, mold, house-dust mite, cockroach, animal dander, or secretory product, e.g., saliva or urine)
  C. Exposure to occupational chemicals or allergens
  D. Environmental change (e.g., moving to a new home, going on a vacation, and/or alterations in workplace, work processes, or materials used)
  E. Exposure to irritants, especially tobacco smoke and strong odors, air pollutants, occupational chemicals, vapors, gases, and aerosols
  F. Emotional expressions: fear, anger, frustration. crying, hard laughing
  G. Drugs (aspirin, beta blockers, nonsteroidal antiinflammatory drugs, others)
  H. Food additives (sulfites) and preservatives
  I. Changes in weather, exposure to cold air
  J. Exercise
  K. Endocrine factors (e.g., menses, pregnancy, thyroid diseases)

IV. Development of disease
  A. Age of onset, age at diagnosis
  B. Progress of disease (better or worse)
  C. Previous evaluation. treatment, and response
  D. Present management and response, including plans for managing acute episodes

V. Profile of typical exacerbation
  A. Prodromal signs and symptoms (e.g., itching of skin of the anterior neck, nasal allergy symptoms)
  B. Temporal progression
  C. Usual management
  D. Usual outcome

VI. Living situation
  A. Home age, location, cooling and heating (central with oil, electric, gas, or kerosene space heating), wood-burning fireplace
  B. Carpeting over a concrete slab
  C. Humidifier
  D. Description of patient's room with special attention to pillows, bed, floor covering, and dust collectors
  E. Animals in home
  F. Exposure to cigarette smoke, direct or sidestream, in home

VII. Impact of disease
  A. Impact on patient
    1. Number of emergency department or urgent care visits and hospitalizations
    2. History of life-threatening acute exacerbation, intubation, or oral steroid therapy
    3. Number of school or work days missed
    4. Limitation of activity, especially sports
    5. History of nocturnal awakening
    6. Effect on growth, development, behavior, school or work achievement, and lifestyle
  B. Impact on family
    1. Disruption of family dynamics, routines, or restriction of activities
    2. Effect on siblings and spouse
    3. Economic impact

VIII. Assessment of family's and patient's perception of illness
  A. Patient, parental, and spousal knowledge of asthma and belief in the chronicity of asthma and in the efficacy of treatment
  B. Ability of patient and parents or spouse to cope with disease
  C. Level of family support and patient and parents' or spouse's capacity to recognize severity of exacerbation
  D. Economic resources

IX. Family history
  A. IgE-mediated allergy in close relatives
  B. Asthma in close relatives

X. Medical history
  A. General medical history and history of other allergic disorders (e.g., chronic rhinitis, atopic dermatitis, sinusitis, nasal polyps, gastrointestinal disturbances, adverse reactions to foods, drugs); in children, history of early life injury to the airways (e.g., bronchopulmonary dysplasia, history of pulmonary infiltrates, documented pneumonia, viral bronchiolitis, recurrent croup, symptoms of gastroesophageal reflux, passive exposure to cigarette smoke); in adults, cigarette smoking history
  B. Detailed review of symptoms

From: National Institutes of Health, National Asthma Education Program: Guidelines for the diagnosis and management of asthma, Bethesda Md, 1991, US Department of Health and Human Services [Publication No. 91-3042A].

Chapter 21). Effective suppression of airway inflammation may reduce the need for bronchodilators. Management of the inflammatory response may also reduce morbidity and mortality associated with asthma. Desensitization to specific antigens may be useful in some forms of atopic asthma.

Patient and family education is an important adjunct in asthma management. Avoidance of environmental triggers requires understanding of the disease process by the patient. Individualized diagnosis and training in prevention of acute exacerbations are very beneficial.

Treatment during an acute attack

Most RCPs see asthmatic patients during an acute exacerbation of their condition. An acute asthma attack is characterized by chest tightness, severe dyspnea and audible expiratory wheezing. Cough may or may not be present. Sputum tends to be thick and mucoid, containing "plugs" and "spirals." On microscopic examination of the sputum, eosinophils are numerous. The differential blood count may also show eosinophilia.

Arterial blood gas results vary according to the stage of the attack (Table 20-4). Early on, hyperventilation caused by anxiety may cause respiratory alkalosis with a slight hyperoxemia. As the attack continues, respiratory alkalosis persists, but the V/Q imbalance worsens and the PaO_2 falls. If airway obstruction worsens, work of breathing increases. The $PaCO_2$ then rises, resulting in respiratory acidosis. This last stage of respiratory acidosis is a bad sign, indicating progression to status asthmaticus, and the potential need for intubation and artificial ventilation. Metabolic acidosis may also occur in conjunction with severe airflow obstruction. The metabolic component may be due to lactic acidosis and tissue hypoxia.

During the acute phase, the chest X-ray may show no abnormalities. In a severe episode, reversible hyperinflation may occur. Severe attacks may also be complicated by pneumothorax.

The principal goals in treating a patient suffering an acute exacerbation of asthma are to rapidly reverse airflow obstruction and correct hypoxemia. Figure 20-12 outlines a general treatment algorithm for the emergency management of acute asthma.

Acute airflow obstruction is treated mainly via liberal use of beta$_2$-agonists, as guided by serial PEFR measurements. Early use of systemic steroids may help those patients who fail to fully respond to adrenergic agents. Hypoxemia is treated with supplemental oxygen. Arterial blood gases should be monitored as needed.

Chronic bronchitis

Definition and pathophysiology

Chronic bronchitis is defined by its symptoms: a history of a productive cough for at least three months a year for two consecutive years. Pathologically, there is hypertrophy of the bronchial glands and an increase in the number of the goblet cells lining the respiratory tract mucosa, which typically is chronically inflamed.

Chronic bronchitics have severe V/Q imbalances. The result is usually a widened A-a gradient while breathing room air. Hypoxemia worsens with the extent of bronchial obstruction. Chronic hypoxemia may lead to secondary polycythemia. The combination of elevated Hb concentration and hypoxemia may result in cyanosis. Advanced chronic bronchitis is often accompanied by hypercapnia. The elevated $PaCO_2$ is compensated by renal retention and production of bicarbonate.

Chronic hypoxemia also favors development of cor pulmonale. V/Q mismatching causes vasoconstriction of pulmonary arterioles in hypoxic lung units. This increased pressure raises afterload on the right ventricle (RV), causing it to become enlarged. Radiographic evidence of an enlarged RV and pulmonary arteries is consistent with chronic bronchitis. Compromise of the RV is accompanied by distension of neck veins, an enlarged liver, and peripheral edema.

Management

Management of chronic bronchitis begins with removal of the predominant irritants. For many patients this irritant is cigarette smoke. Smoking cessation is imperative to halt the progression of the disease. Bronchitics who stop smoking often notice a transient increase in sputum production, followed by a gradual lessening. In some instances the pattern of chronic bronchitis "reverses" with an overall decrease in the volume of mucus produced each day. Avoidance of pulmonary infections is also essential. Annual immunization against viral influenza is recommended. Vaccination against bacterial pneumonias may be warranted. Early intervention with antibiotics is necessary if mucus production increases noticeably, or sputum color changes dramatically.

Adequate hydration promotes clearing of secretions. Mucolytic agents and expectorants may be indicated in some individuals, but their effectiveness has not been proven definitively. Bronchodilators may aid in mobilization of secretions in some patients.

Table 20-4 Arterial blood gases in asthma*

	Stages			
	1	2	3	4
PaO$_2$	↑	N	↓	↓
PaCO$_2$	↓	↓	↓	↑
pH	↑	↑	↑	↓

* ↑, increase; ↓, decreases; N, normal
From Tisi GM: Pulmonary physiology in clinical medicine, ed 2, Baltimore, 1984, Williams & Wilkins.

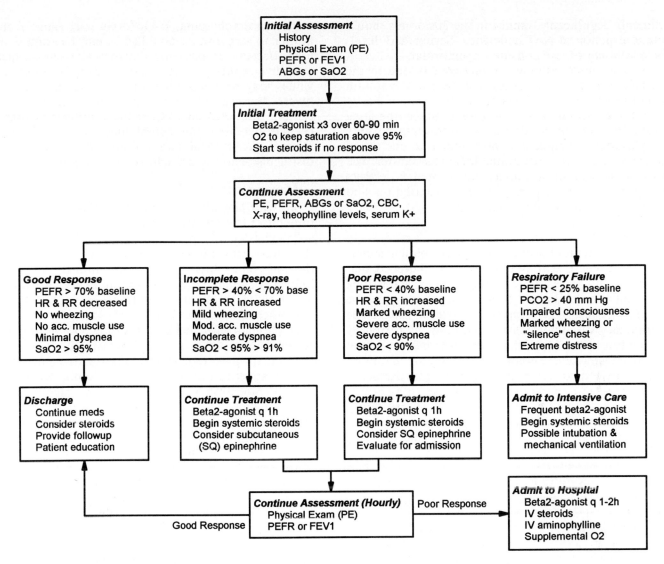

Fig. 20-12 General treatment algorithm for the emergency management of acute asthma in adults. (Adapted from National Institutes of Health, National Asthma Education Program: Guidelines for the diagnosis and management of asthma, Bethesda MD, 1991, US Department of Health and Human Services)

Oxygen therapy is indicated in patients whose PaO_2 is less than 55 torr at rest or during exercise. Oxygen is similarly indicated for individuals who have evidence of cor pulmonale. For chronic hypoxemia, oxygen supplementation should be continuous. Hypercapnic subjects who have completely compensated respiratory acidosis may ventilate only in response to hypoxemia. Oxygen therapy in these individuals must be titrated to provide an SaO_2 of 90%, without suppressing ventilation.

Emphysema

Definition and pathophysiology

Emphysema is defined anatomically as a destructive process of the lung parenchyma leading to permanent enlargement of the distal airspaces. Emphysema can be classified as either centrilobular (CLE), which mainly involves the respiratory bronchioles, or panlobular (PLE) which can involve the entire terminal respiratory unit. CLE is predominantly a disease of bronchitic patients who smoke cigarettes. PLE can occur in nonsmokers. As CLE progresses, it becomes increasingly difficult to distinguish it from PLE, at which point it may be labeled mixed or end-stage emphysema. In either case, bullae, or airspaces greater than 1 cm in size, may develop.

Emphysema may be due to an hereditary deficiency of the enzyme inhibitor called alpha-1 antitrypsin (AAT). AAT deficiency is an **autosomal recessive** disorder. Emphysematous changes are most severe in the homozygous state. In smokers who have the severest form of genetic deficiency (PiZ phenotype), dyspnea develops between ages 30 and 40. Death from emphysema is likely by age 50. The prognosis in nonsmokers is only slightly better. Adults who display clinically significant dyspnea in the 30s or 40s should raise suspicion of AAT deficiency. Serum AAT levels below 80 mg/dL are considered abnormal.

Airway obstruction in emphysema is due to the destruction of elastic tissues that normally maintain small airway patency. This results in a loss of elastic recoil (i.e., compliance increases). Since the lung tissue becomes more distensible, total lung capacity also increases. Diffusion is also impaired, due to the decrease in surface area available for gas transfer. The loss of alveolar surface area tends to match destruction of the capillary bed, so that ventilation and perfusion mismatching is minimal.

Diagnosis

Upon radiographic examination, the patient suffering from severe emphysema exhibits flattened diaphragms and increased **retrosternal** airspace (i.e. lung hyperinflation). Bullae, or large air sacs, may be visible on chest X-rays, especially near the apices. The pulmonary vasculature is attenuated at the periphery of the lung. These radiologic patterns may be useful for diagnosing severe emphysema. They are of limited sensitivity for detecting mild or moderate disease.

Patients with emphysema, like those with chronic bronchitis, tend to exhibit a decrease in expiratory flows. There is usually little or no response to bronchodilator therapy. Blood gas measurements can vary widely in emphysema. PaO_2 levels may range from normal to very low. Arterial $PaCO_2$ may be normal, or high. Because emphysema destroys alveolar surface area and capillary beds together, arterial blood gas values may be relatively normal in the presence of severe dyspnea. The emphysematous patient often exhibits an increased TLC, reduced diffusing capacity, and increased lung compliance. Table 20-5 summarizes the clinical and physiologic features that distinguish chronic bronchitis from emphysema.

Management

As with chronic bronchitis, smoking cessation is imperative to slow progression of the disease. Avoidance of other air pollutants is equally important. Respiratory infections can be extremely dangerous to the lung compromised patient. Immunization against influenza should be performed annually. Adequate nutrition is extremely important in patients with emphysema.

In patients with an FEV_1 less than 35% of predicted, mortality increases with decreasing body weight. Extreme dyspnea, particularly after eating can cause loss of appetite and weight loss. Malnourished patients demonstrate energy requirements significantly above predicted needs, especially during activity. The respiratory musculature may be affected by inadequate nutrition, as will skeletal muscle. Many emphy-

Table 20-5 Features that distinguish bronchial and emphysematous types of chronic obstructive lung disease

	Bronchial type B	Emphysematous type A
CLINICAL FEATURES		
History	Often recurrent chest infections	Often only insidiuos dyspnea
Chest exam	Noisy chest, slight overdistention	Quiet chest, marked overdistention
Sputum	Frequently copious and purulent	Usually scanty and mucoid
Weight loss	Absent or slight	Often marked
Chronic cor pulmonale	Common	Infrequent
Roentgenogram	Often evidence of old inflammatory disease	Often attenuated vessels and radiolucency
General appearance	"Blue bloater"	"Pink puffer"
PHYSIOLOGIC TESTS		
Lung volumes:		
TLC	Normal or slightly decreased	Increased
RV	Moderately increased	Markedly increased
RV/TLC	High	High
Lung compliance:		
Static	Normal or low	High
Dynamic	Very low	Normal or low
Airway resistance:		
Expiratory	Very high	High
Inspiratory	High	Normal
Diffusing capacity	Variable	Low
Chronic hypoxemia	Often severe	Usually mild
Chronic hypercapnia	Common	Unusual
Pulmonary hypertension	Often severe	Usually mild
Cardia output	Normal	Often low

From Burrows B, Knudson RJ, and Kettrl LJ: Respiratory insufficiency, St Louis, 1975, Mosby.

sema patients benefit from a high protein diet taken in small increments.

Bronchodilators, expectorants, antibiotics, and **inotropic** agents may be used to manage various aspects of dyspnea (see Chapter 21). Supplemental oxygen is indicated if the PaO_2 is less than 55 torr at rest or during exercise, or if evidence of cor pulmonale is present.

Chronic obstructive pulmonary disease (COPD)

Definition and pathophysiology

COPD is a widely used term to describe airway obstruction in patients who have emphysema, chronic bronchitis, asthma, or a combination of these (Figure 20-13). Bronchiectasis and bronchiolitis are also sometimes included as a components of COPD. Patients with COPD are characterized by dyspnea on exertion, with reduction of airflow on pulmonary function. Chronic bronchitis and emphysema, as described previously, are the most common components. Cigarette smoking is the most important common risk factor in the development of both emphysema and chronic bronchitis.

Airway reactivity (i.e. asthma) has been identified as a significant contributor to the pattern of obstruction in COPD. Increased airway reactivity is present in 15% to 70% of patients with chronic airflow obstruction. Both male and female smokers appear to have an increased incidence of hyperractive airways. This airway reactivity may be identified more readily by inhalation challenge testing than by simple response to bronchodilators.

Management

Treatment for the individual patient with COPD is based on the symptoms and their severity. First and foremost, patients must be encouraged to stop smoking. They should be taught to avoid other respiratory

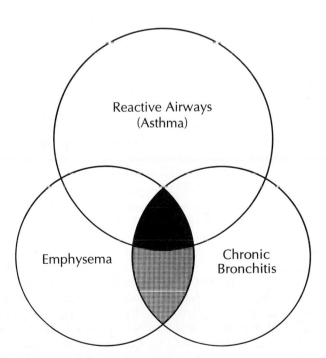

Fig. 20-13 Relationship of asthma, chronic bronchitis, and emphysema as components of chronic obstructive pulmonary disease (COPD). The exact proportions of overlap between these components is unclear; the diagram is not proportional. Many patients have features of emphysema and chronic bronchitis as a result of cigarette smoking (lightly shaded area). Hyperreactive airways may be common feature in many subjects who develop chronic bronchitis or emphysema. Some patients may display symptoms of all three disorders. (dark shaded area). (Redrawn from Burrows B, Knudson RJ, and Kettrl LG: Respiratory insufficiency, St Louis, 1975, Mosby.)

irritants. The use of mucolytics and expectorants is common, even though their effectiveness has yet to be proved. Bronchodilator therapy, either orally or by aerosol, is indicated when an asthmatic component exists. Failure of a single trial of bronchodilators should not preclude further trials. Many COPD patients demonstrate decreased symptoms (i.e. shortness of breath) in spite of minimal change in flow rates. Corticosteroids should be considered when there is evidence of airway reactivity. As with other chronic disorders, COPD patients tend to misuse medications. This includes overutilization during periods of respiratory distress. Many patients have difficulty using metered dose inhalers (MDI) correctly.

Patients with COPD may be treated with antibiotics empirically at the earliest sign of chest infection. Patients should be taught to look for signs of increased sputum production, increased cough, or fever. Bacterial infection often follows viral infection in patients with COPD. This is especially common in exacerbations of chronic bronchitis.

Breathing exercises (to increase efficiency of breathing) and bronchial hygiene (such as postural drainage) are frequently employed in severe cases of COPD (see Chapter 28). Due to the chronic nature of the component diseases, the best approach is a comprehensive pulmonary rehabilitation program. Pulmonary rehabilitation for COPD includes breathing retraining and physical reconditioning, along with education in self-care. More detail on pulmonary rehabilitation is provided in Chapter 37.

Bronchiectasis

Definition and pathophysiology

Bronchiectasis simply means dilation of the bronchi. It also implies the destruction of bronchial walls. There are three anatomic varieties of bronchiectasis. Saccular (cystic) bronchiectasis is the classic advanced form, characterized by irregular dilatations and narrowings. The term fusiform is used when the dilatations are especially large. Cylindrical, or tubular bronchiectasis is simply the absence of normal bronchial tapering. Cylindrical bronchiectasis is a manifestation of severe chronic obstructive lung disease rather than of true bronchial wall destruction.

Bronchiectasis is usually caused by repeated or prolonged episodes of pneumonitis, especially those complicating pertusis or influenza during childhood. Bronchiectasis may also be associated with bronchial obstruction caused by neoplasms, or the aspiration of a foreign body.

Bronchiectasis that involves most or all of the bronchial tree is usually genetic or developmental in origin. Cystic fibrosis, Kartagener's syndrome (bronchiectasis with dextrocardia and paranasal sinusitis), and agammaglobulinemia are all examples of inherited or developmental diseases associated with bronchiectasis (Figure 20-14).

Most cases of bronchiectasis are accompanied by severe chronic bronchitis. More advanced cases of bronchiectasis are often associated with anastomoses between the bronchial and pulmonary vessels. These anastomoses cause substantial right-to-left shunting, resulting in hypoxemia, pulmonary hypertension, and cor pulmonale.

Bronchiectasis is characterized by a chronic, loose cough, usually productive of large amounts of mucopurulent, often foul-smelling sputum. In advanced cases the sputum settles out into three distinctive layers: cloudy mucus on top, clear saliva in the middle, and purulent solid material on the bottom. Hemoptysis occurs in approximately 50% of all cases. Advanced untreated bronchiectasis is accompanied by frequent bronchopulmonary infections, chronic malnutrition, sinusitis, **clubbing,** cor pulmonale, and right heart failure. Physical signs are variable and not always helpful in diagnosis. Likewise, simple chest radiographs generally are insufficient to establish the diagnosis.

Bronchoscopy often reveals a deep velvety red mucosa, with pus in the areas of involvement. Cultures of sputum often show a variety of organisms, including common mouth flora, fusospirochetes, and anaerobic streptococci. Microscopic examination of the sputum may reveal necrotic elastic tissue, muscle fibers and epithelial debris.

Diagnosis

The diagnosis of bronchiectasis is confirmed by either CT scan or bronchography. Bronchography involves radiographic exposure of the lung after instillation of a contrast material, either iodized oil, iodine in water, or, more recently, powdered tantalum. Bronchography should only be performed after vigorous bronchial hygiene, postural drainage, and a course of antimicrobial therapy for at least a week. Bronchography should include every lung segment, but both lungs should not be studied at one time in patients with significantly impaired pulmonary function.

Management

The most important feature of the treatment of bronchiectasis is regular and vigorous bronchial hygiene, with postural drainage, generally continued for the rest of the patient's life. Antimicrobial therapy may be helpful in the management of acute exacerbations of bronchiectasis. However, prolonged antimicrobial therapy tends to allow drug-resistant organisms to multiply in the irreversibly ulcerated bronchi, and thus should be avoided.

Surgical resection of affected segments or lobes should be considered only when irreversible involvement of localized areas is clearly demonstrated. Re-

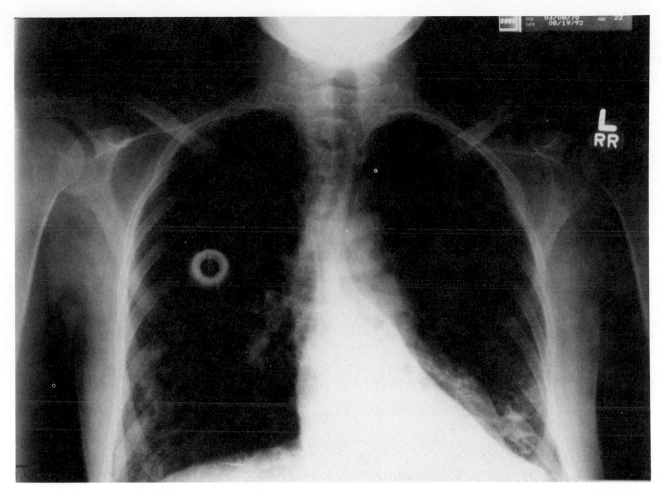

Fig. 20-14 Bronchiectasis. A slightly overexposed chest X-ray from a patient with cystic fibrosis. Near the left heart border is an almost completely consolidated portion of the left lower lobe. The dark patches are "air bronchograms"; bronchiectatic airways surrounded by consolidation and fluid. (Courtesy Dept. of Radiology, St Louis University Health Sciences Center, St Louis, MO)

section should be postponed until all efforts at medical management have failed.

Cystic fibrosis

Definition and pathophysiology

Cystic fibrosis (CF) is a genetically transmitted disorder that produces a suppurative pulmonary disease and pancreatic insufficiency. CF occurs once in approximately 2500 live births in Caucasians. About 5% of the Caucasian population carries the autosomal recessive trait that causes CF. The gene that produces CF has been identified. The gene makes a defective protein that affects transport of sodium and chloride within cells. As a result, mucus glands produce thick mucus. Mucus obstruction occurs in the airways, and in the pancreatic and biliary ducts.

CF was once considered only a pediatric disease. Advances in detecting and treating CF have increased the life expectancy to an estimated 40 years. Many CF patients, particularly those with a mild disease, now survive well into adulthood.

In infancy and early childhood, pancreatic insufficiency and related gastrointestinal disorders predominate. Abdominal cramping and bloating along with malabsorption is present in 85% of children with CF. Intestinal obstruction is a frequent complication. In later childhood and adolescence, respiratory symptoms and complications tend to increase in severity. Chronic bacterial bronchitis, especially *Staphylococcus aureus* infection, is common. In older children *Pseudomonas aeruginosa* becomes the major cause. CF patients also suffer from sinusitis. Pneumothorax is quite common in the presence of severe pulmonary impairment. Hemoptysis occurs in a small number of patients during acute exacerbations. Cor pulmonale frequently results from severe pulmonary involvement.

Diagnosis

Diagnosis of CF is based on elevated sweat chloride concentration in the presence of clinical signs and symptoms. Most (98%) individuals with CF have sweat chloride concentrations greater than 60 mEq/L. The rest have values between 50 and 60 mEq/L. A normal sweat chloride does not exclude the diagnosis of CF. Some patients may have a normal sweat chloride, but have clinical symptoms of the disease. In some instances the patient may be told that they do not have CF, because of the normal sweat chloride levels. Some patients with elevated sweat chlorides may have minimal respiratory or gastrointestinal symptoms. CF may not be diagnosed in these individuals, unless a sibling is also being evaluated.

Most CF patients are diagnosed in infancy or childhood, but as many as 20% are not recognized until after age 15. Late diagnosis is often due to the lack of significant pulmonary complications. Asthma and CF share several symptoms: chronic cough, bronchospasm, and sinusitis. Features that may help to delineate CF are chronic infection, clubbing of the fingers, hemoptysis, and an abnormal chest X-ray that does not improve. Adult CF patients are sometimes misdiagnosed with COPD, eosinophilic granuloma or sarcoidosis. Some adult cystics are diagnosed from non-respiratory findings such as intestinal obstruction or obstructive **azoospermia**.

Chest X-ray examination shows bronchiectatic changes and honeycombing in the majority of patients (Figure 20-15). In mild cases, hyperinflation and increased pulmonary vasculature are the only abnormalities. The upper lobes are often **hyperlucent.** In advanced CF the diaphragm becomes increasingly flattened as air trapping occurs. The heart silhouette is enlarged (cor pulmonale).

Management

Treatment of CF centers on management of the thick, tenacious mucus present in the lungs, and prevention of blockage in the pancreas and gastrointestinal tract. Mucolytics and expectorants are used together with bronchial hygiene, breathing exercises, and exercise therapy. Bronchodilators may be useful in relieving bronchospasm and improving the effectiveness of coughing. Corticosteroids can help relieve bronchospasm due to inflammation, both chronically and acutely. Antibiotics are commonly used on a continuous basis for many CF patients. Single drugs or a rotating regimen may be used to diminish exacerbations and reduce hospitalizations. IV antibiotics are indicated for severe deterioration. IV antibiotics may be given at home as effectively as in the hospital.

An enzyme preparation (rhDNase), administered by an aerosol route, has recently been approved for use in CF. This enzyme is genetically engineered to reduce mucus viscosity by digesting the extracellular DNA present in the secretions of CF patients. This

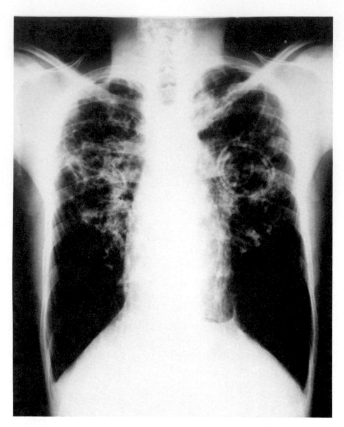

Fig. 20-15 Chest x-ray of a young adult cystic fibrosis patient. Bronchiectasis and "honey-combing" are evident throughout the lung fields. An indwelling catheter is superimposed over the left lung. (Courtesy Dept. of Radiology, St Louis University Health Sciences Center, St Louis, MO)

DNA comes from the nuclei of degenerating polymorphonuclear neutrophils. The secretions in CF patients are chronically infected, and attract neutrophils. By reducing the viscosity of the mucus, significant improvements in pulmonary function can be achieved. Use of Dnase (Pulmonzyme) results in an increase in FEV_1. Improvement in flows is also accompanied by reduced need for antibiotic therapy.

Now that the actual gene responsible for CF has been identified, more specialized forms of treatment are being developed. In addition, heart-lung and lung transplantation have evolved as an effective forms of treatment in CF patients who have severely compromised pulmonary function.

CF patients often suffer from malnutrition due to malabsorption. Infections and increased work of breathing can dramatically alter the individual's nutritional requirements. Proper diet and supplementation of vitamin A, D, E, and K are very important in maintaining body stores. Pancreatic enzymes may be administered to compensate for pancreatic insufficiency.

Oxygen therapy is indicated for either exercise-induced or resting hypoxemia. Supplemental O_2 reduces the tendency to develop cor pulmonale. It also alleviates dyspnea associated with exercise and may improve appetite and activity level.

SKELETAL, THORACIC AND PLEURAL DISORDERS

The most common conditions affecting the thorax are kyphoscoliosis, ankylosing spondylitis, and severe obesity. Pleural disorders include pleurisy, pleural effusion, empyema, pneumothorax, and hemothorax.

Kyphoscoliosis

Kyphosis is a condition in which the normal posterior curve of the spine is exaggerated. Scoliosis represents abnormal lateral curvature of the spine. Patients with kyphoscoliosis can develop pulmonary problems because of lung compression inside a distorted rib cage (Figure 20-16). Chronic pulmonary compression can lead to recurrent bronchial infections, and in some cases to respiratory failure.

Depending on the severity of the condition, patients may have normal lung function or show varying degrees of pulmonary restriction. In spite of thoracic deformities, patients with kyphoscoliosis often maintain near-normal ventilation through increased central drive and other compensatory mechanisms. Their specific airway conductance (sGaw) may be increased because of greater lung elastic recoil.

Blood gas measurements are variable. PaO_2 values may be reduced due to lung compression and low V/Q ratios. $PaCO_2$ levels are usually within normal limits. In severe cases there may be hypercapnia and respiratory failure.

Treatment is directed at preventing or minimizing recurrent infections and relieving any clinical significant hypoxemia. Periodic hyperinflation using intermittent positive pressure breathing (IPPB) has proved successful in increasing lung compliance. Surgical correction is necessary in many cases to reverse the abnormal spine curvature.

Ankylosing spondylitis

Ankylosing spondylitis is a condition in which the vertebral bodies and the costovertebral joints become fused. This causes a dramatic decrease in thoracic wall compliance. Because uniform diaphragmatic movement is retained, total lung capacity (TLC) and vital capacity (VC) are only slightly reduced. Harmful effects on ventilation are minor. Fibrous-cystic changes in the upper portions of the lung are apparent in some patients with ankylosing spondylitis.

Obesity

Severe obesity mechanically restricts ventilation, due to the increased mass of the thorax and abdomen. Obesity is also a component of a more general syndrome, consisting of chronic hypercapnia and hypox-

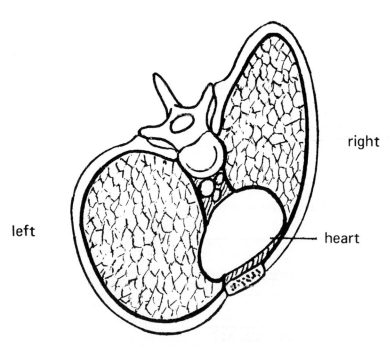

Fig. 20-16 Changes in the thorax resulting from scoliosis. Scoliosis causes rotation of the spine along its longitudinal axis, which in turn causes marked deformity of the rib cage. (From Farzan S: A concise handbook of respiratory diseases, ed 2, East Norwalk, CN, 1985, Appleton & Lange.)

emia, sleep apnea, and decreased respiratory center responsiveness to CO_2 (Figure 20-17). Complications, due primarily to chronic hypoxemia, include polycythemia, pulmonary hypertension, and cor pulmonale. Due to similarity with Charles Dickens' description of the fat boy in the Pickwick Papers, this condition is often referred to as the "Pickwickian Syndrome".

Weight reduction appears to relieve most of the symptoms. Weight loss either through diet or gastric surgery improves arterial oxygenation and reduces CO_2 retention. It is accompanied by increased lung volumes, lessening of polycythemia and reduction of apnea frequency. Oral progesterone therapy has been reported to stimulate ventilation in some patients. If weight reduction cannot be accomplished and sleep apnea is severe, tracheostomy may be necessary. More recently, continuous positive airway pressure (CPAP) by nose has been used to alleviate nocturnal airway obstruction (see Obstructive Sleep Apnea, this chapter, page 466).

Pleural disorders

Pleural disorders can cause pulmonary restriction through direct involvement of the pleural membranes, or as a result of space-occupying lesions. Pleurisy is an example of the former; pleural effusion, empyema, pneumothorax, and hemothorax are examples of the latter.

Pleurisy

Pleurisy is characterized by deposition of a fibrinous exudate on the pleural surface. Pleurisy is usually a complication of other disorders, such as pneumonia, pulmonary infarction, and pulmonary neoplasms. Pleurisy may also precede the development of some pleural effusions. Pleuritic chest pain, or pain that intensifies during inspiration, is the primary symptom. Referred pain may also occur. A pleural friction rub, with its characteristic grating sound, is usually heard on auscultation. Splinting of the involved side of the chest, with shallow respirations, is also common. Treatment is aimed at resolving the underlying disease process.

Pleural effusion

A pleural effusion is an abnormal collection of fluid in the pleural space. The balance of oncotic and hydrostatic forces in the pleural space favors the continuous movement of fluid from parietal to visceral pleural capillaries (Figure 20-18). Fluid may accumulate in the pleural space when either hydrostatic pressures increase or oncotic pressures decrease. The fluid originating in this manner is called a *transudate.*

Inflammatory processes, infiltrative diseases, or tumors may cause fluid accumulation in the pleural space without upsetting the balance of oncotic and hydrostatic forces. The rate of formation must over-

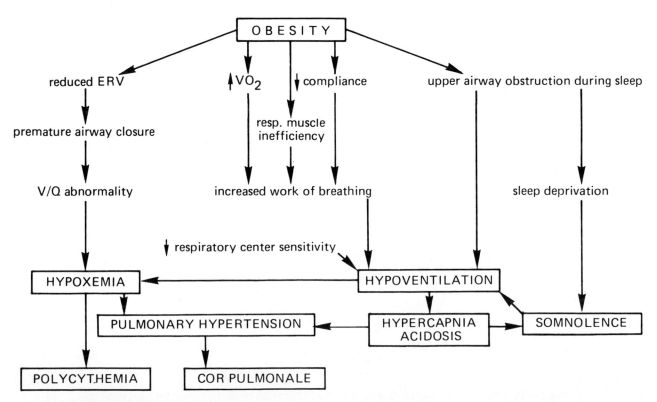

Fig. 20-17 Pathogenesis and pathophysiology of obesity-hypoventilation syndrome. (From Farzan S: A concise handbook of respiratory diseases, ed 2, East Norwalk, CN, 1985, Appleton & Lange.)

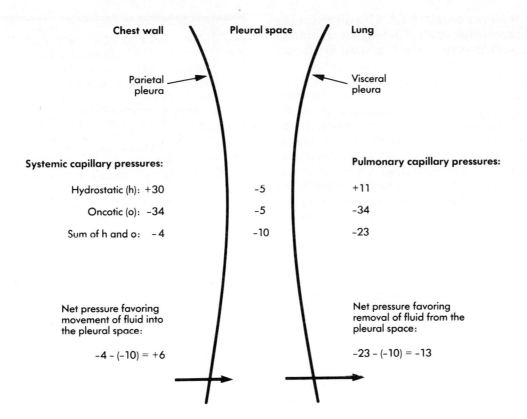

Chest wall   **Pleural space**   **Lung**

Parietal → pleura   Visceral ← pleura

Systemic capillary pressures:

Hydrostatic (h): +30   -5

Oncotic (o): -34   -5

Sum of h and o: - 4   -10

Pulmonary capillary pressures:

+11

-34

-23

Net pressure favoring movement of fluid into the pleural space:

-4 - (-10) = +6

Net pressure favoring removal of fluid from the pleural space:

-23 - (-10) = -13

Fig. 20-18 Normal pleural fluid movement. A physiologic balance between the systemic and pulmonary capillaries provides for continuous movement of fluid from parietal pleura capillaries into the pleural space and then into visceral pleura capillaries. All pressures are in cm H_2O. Pressure that tend to force fluid out of the capillaries are shown by a plus sign (+); pressure that act to hold fluid in the capillary or pleural space are assigned a minus sign (−). There is a net +6 cm H_2O pressure favoring fluid movement into the pleural space. In this diagram the surfaces are shown apart, but in healthy subjects they touch, separated only by a thin (and radiologically invisible) film of pleural fluid. (From Martin L: Pulmonary physiology in clinical practice: the essentials for patient care and evaluation, St. Louis, 1987, Mosby.)

whelm lymphatic clearance, which may be decreased by hydrostatic forces, or blocked by malignant infiltration. Pleural fluid originating in this manner is called an *exudate*. Exudates may be distinguished from transudates by their higher protein content. The accompanying box lists the various processes causing the two primary types of pleural effusions.

Patients with pleural effusions may be without symptoms. Chest or referred shoulder pain may be present. Depending on the severity of the effusion, dyspnea may range from mild to severe. With large effusions, pulmonary symptoms result from atelectasis due to compression and space-occupying effects of the fluid. Fever, sweats, cough, and expectoration may also be present. On physical examination there is decreased motion of the chest. Breath sounds are decreased or absent, as is vocal fremitus. Percussion of the chest wall is flat, and egophony may be noted on the affected side. If the effusion is large, the mediasti-

Diseases associated with exudative and transudative pleural effusions

EXUDATES	TRANSUDATES
Malignancy	Congestive heart failure
Carcinoma	Hypoproteinemic states,
Mesothelioma	including
Lymphoma	Nephrotic syndrome
Infection	Liver cirrhosis
Parapneumonic	Pneumothorax
Tuberculosis	Atelectasis
Fungal	Pulmonary embolism
Viral	(some cases)
Collagen-vascular	Peritoneal dialysis
Systemic lupus	Meigs' syndrome (benign
Rheumatoid arthritis	ovarian tumor)
Pulmonary embolism	
(some cases)	
Pancreatitis	
Subphrenic abscess	
Uremia	
Asbestosis	
Chylothorax	
Traumatic hemothorax	
Esophageal rupture	
Drug-induced effusion	
Postradiation therapy	
Sarcoidosis	
Idiopathic (undiagnosed)	

From Martin L; Pulmonary physiology in clinical practice: the essentials for patient care and evaluation, St Louis, 1987, Mosby.

num may shift away from the fluid. This displaces the trachea and the cardiac apex. Underlying atelectasis may cause a shift toward, instead of away from, the effusion.

There must be a fluid volume of at least 300 mL before a pleural effusion becomes evident on chest X-ray. Obliteration of the costophrenic angle is the earliest sign of pleural effusion. Movement of the fluid shadow, which pours into dependent areas of pleural space when the patient is placed on the involved side, may be helpful in demonstrating small effusions. Definitive diagnostic of pleural effusion is made by thoracentesis. Thoracentesis also provides specimens which are useful in identifying the underlying cause.

Treatment of pleural effusion is directed at resolution of the primary disease process. Small amounts of fluid can be removed by therapeutic thoracentesis. When the fluid volume is large, or continues to accumulate despite treatment, chest tube drainage may be necessary.

Pleural empyema

When pleural fluid is purulent or contains pyogenic organisms, it is called pleural *empyema*. Pleural empyema may result from the: (1) direct spread of a bacterial pneumonia, (2) rupture of a lung abscess into the pleural space, (3) invasion from a subdiaphragmatic infection, or (4) traumatic penetration. The most common infectious agents are anaerobic bacteria, *Staphylococcus, Streptococcus,* and certain gram-negative bacteria. Pleural pain and fever, in conjunction with the physical and X-ray signs of pleural effusion, are characteristic. Thoracentesis reveals a purulent exudate from which the causative organism may be cultured. As with lung abscess, empyema may become chronic.

Pneumothorax

Pneumothorax is a condition in which air enters the pleural space. This air leak may originate either from inside the lungs (through the airways), or through the chest wall. The accompanying box summarizes the major causes of the disorder.

Small pneumothoraces may go unnoticed. Pain may be experienced when the pneumothorax occurs, especially if parietal pleural irritation accompanies the air leak. With a large pneumothorax, the patient appears acutely dyspneic. On physical examination, chest expansion is reduced, and the percussion note is increased in resonance. Breath sounds and tactile fremitus are absent over the pneumothorax. The diagnosis can be confirmed by chest radiograph.

Gas pressure in a pneumothorax is slightly higher than in the pleural venous system. As a result, reabsorption of air from the pleural space usually occurs spontaneously. Small pneumothoraces resolve without treatment. Large pneumothoraces are usually treated by chest tube drainage.

Potential causes of pneumothorax

1. Air in the pleural space from the airways
   a. Idiopathic—occurs spontaneously without apparent reason: presumably caused by rupture of clinically inapparent bleb, cyst, or bulla
   b. Rupture or tear of esophagus or other mediastinal structure into the pleural space.
   c. Chronic lung disease (most commonly from severe emphysema, asthma, or interstitial fibrosis)
   d. Positive pressure ventilation, particularly with use of positive end-expiratory pressure (see Chapter 30)
   e. Infection, tumor, or foreign body causing a bronchopleural connection
2. Air in the pleural space from outside the chest wall
   a. Trauma
   b. During thoracentesis or pleural biopsy
   c. During insertion of central venous catheter

From Martin L; Pulmonary physiology in clinical practice: the essentials for patient care and evaluation, St Louis, 1987, Mosby.

In tension pneumothorax, air enters the pleural space on inspiration but cannot escape during expiration. This causes compression of the affected lung. (Figure 20-19). Tension pneumothoraces frequently occur when the air leak is from the airway through the visceral pleura. Continued breathing pushes air into

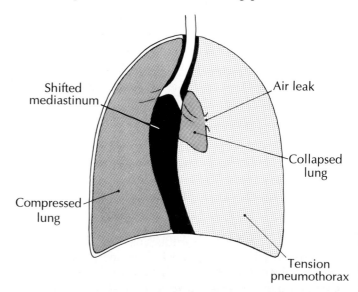

Fig. 20–19 Diagrammatic representation of a tension pneumothorax. An air leak, usually through a bronchus or ruptured alveolus, allows air to enter the pleural space. If air continues to leak in, as with a check valve type of lesion, gas in the pleural space becomes pressurized above atmospheric pressure. This positive pressure compresses the large vessels and the heart in the mediastinum. In addition the opposite lung is compressed. If the compression is untreated venous return to the heart may be compromised, leading to shock and even death.

the pleural space. This can occur easily in patients who are being ventilated with positive pressure. The trachea and mediastinal contents shift away from the affected side. Compression of the mediastinum can disrupt cardiac filling, resulting in a rapid fall in blood pressure and shock. A tension pneumothorax must be relieved immediately. Puncture of the chest wall with a large bore needle at the second anterior intercoastal space can relieve the pressure, converting the tension pneumothorax to a simple pneumothorax. Once the patient is stabilized, a chest tube can be inserted to control the pneumothorax.

Hemothorax

Hemothorax is characterized by pooling of blood in the pleural space. Hemothorax occurs commonly with chest trauma. It may also occur with tumors, tuberculosis, and pulmonary infarction. Physical findings in hemothorax are the same as those described for pleural effusion. Early removal of all blood from the pleural space is desirable. Although this may be accomplished by thoracentesis, chest tube drainage is usually necessary.

NEUROMUSCULAR CONDITIONS

Processes that interfere with the transmission of neural output to the respiratory muscles can result in restrictive impairments. Included in this category are disorders of the spinal cord, peripheral nerves, neuromuscular junctions, and respiratory muscles themselves. Some diseases, such as poliomyelitis, involve both the central control mechanism and peripheral neuromuscular apparatus.

Characteristic of these disorders is the inability to generate normal respiratory pressures. Although the FRC is maintained near normal levels, inspiratory muscle weakness causes a decrease in both the inspiratory reserve volume (IRV) and total lung capacity (TLC). Both the vital capacity (VC) and the maximum inspiratory pressure (PImax) are diminished. Expiratory muscle weakness may result in an increased residual volume (RV). Disorders affecting expiratory muscle may also reduce the maximum expiratory pressure (PEmax).

Muscle strength and VC can diminish substantially before producing respiratory failure. Severe hypoxemia and hypercapnia in these conditions indicates either progression of the primary process, or complications such as atelectasis. If respiratory pressures (i.e., PEmax and PImax) are preserved, hypoxemia and/or hypercapnia suggests a complication rather than progression of the primary process. In acute neuromuscular disorders, monitoring of maximum respiratory pressures may be superior to serial VC measurements, since VC may be reduced in either case.

Chronic neuromuscular disorders are associated with decreases in the compliance of both the lung and thorax. Decreased lung compliance may be due to microatelectasis, altered surfactant activity, or fibrotic changes resulting from recurrent infections. These secondary disorders cause a V/Q mismatching. Hypoxemia is greater than expected due to hypoventilation alone. Decreased chest wall compliance is probably due to gradual stiffening of the costochondral and costovertebral joints. Fibrotic changes or spasticity of the respiratory muscles may also decrease thoracic compliance. In chronic disease, measurement of VC may be a better indicator of function than is maximum respiratory pressure.

In mechanical disorders of the thorax an effective cough is usually well preserved. Expiratory muscle weakness in neuromuscular disorders interferes with a forceful cough. In cervical spinal cord injuries, paralysis of abdominal and intercostal muscles prevent spontaneous coughing altogether. Because such patients are unable to cough effectively, even minor increases in secretions can cause respiratory complications. Pneumonia is a common problem in patients suffering from neuromuscular disorders. Respiratory failure resulting from pneumonia is a frequent cause of death in this group.

Patients with neuromuscular disorders often breath rapidly, out of proportion to their decreased tidal volume. An increased minute ventilation ($\dot{V}E$) may result. $PaCO_2$ levels may be lower than normal (i.e., respiratory alkalosis or hyperventilation). The basis for the tachypnea is probably microatelectasis, which also accounts for the mild arterial hypoxemia commonly observed in these patients. Microatelectasis may be the result of the patient's inability to sigh. Failure to take periodic deep breaths may change alveolar surface forces and increase the tendency for alveolar collapse.

In progressive muscle weakness, tidal breathing decreases and dead space increases. Alveolar hypoventilation and worsening hypoxemia result. Artificial ventilatory support may be required to maintain the patient until the underlying cause can be treated.

Diaphragmatic paralysis

Neuromuscular disorders rarely progress to respiratory failure unless diaphragmatic weakness or paralysis is present. Diaphragmatic **paresis** or paralysis represents the end result of various neuromuscular disorders. Certain forms of diaphragmatic paralysis have unique clinical features.

Bilateral diaphragmatic paralysis

Bilateral phrenic nerve interruption can result in complete diaphragmatic paralysis. The most prominent clinical symptom of complete diaphragmatic paralysis is orthopnea. In the supine posture, the abdominal contents push the diaphragm up into the thorax. Negative pressure generated by the intercostal muscles pulls the diaphragm further into the thorax during inspiration. This produces paradoxic inward motion of the upper abdomen with thoracic expansion. The paradoxic motion impairs the normal distribution of ventilation to the lung bases, resulting in gas exchange abnormalities, atelectasis and hypoxemia.

In the upright position, patients often experience a dramatic increase in vital capacity, improvement in gas exchange, and alleviation of most symptoms. In this position, the weight of the abdominal contents offsets the negative intrapleural pressures, and the diaphragm no longer rises with inspiration.

Unilateral diaphragmatic paralysis

Most cases of unilateral diaphragmatic paralysis result from tumors invading one of the phrenic nerves. Compression or destruction of the phrenic nerve by surgery, trauma, or thoracic aneurysms may also cause unilateral paralysis. Isolated phrenic neuropathy or acute infectious neuritis also causes diaphragmatic paralysis, which is usually permanent. There is no effective treatment for permanent unilateral diaphragmatic paralysis. Reversible unilateral diaphragmatic paralysis is a rare complication of acute pneumonias, but may commonly occur following cardiac surgery.

Patients with unilateral diaphragmatic paralysis may exhibit a 15% to 20% reduction in both VC and TLC in the upright posture. There is greater impairment in the supine position.

In the absence of other diseases, most patients with unilateral diaphragmatic paralysis remain asymptomatic. This condition is most often diagnosed by chest X-rays. The paralyzed side maintains its normal contour but is displaced upward. On fluoroscopy, the paralyzed hemidiaphragm may descend somewhat on inspiration, mimicking normal contraction. However, with a sudden forceful inspiration (the sniff test) the paralyzed side rises further into the thorax, opposite to the direction of the normal side. This paradoxical motion is due to the sudden increase in intra-abdominal pressure and the sudden decrease of intrapleural pressure that occurs during the sniff.

Spinal cord disorders

The two most common restrictive conditions involving the spinal column are quadriplegia and disorders of the anterior horn cells.

Quadriplegia

Quadriplegia can result from acute cervical spinal cord trauma, spinal artery infarction, or compression (by tumor, hemorrhage, etc.). Such injuries usually cause profound respiratory compromise. Transection at or above the cord segments C3 to C5 results in complete cessation of all respiratory muscle activity. Injuries other than transection result in partial hemi-diaphragmatic paralysis. Transection below this level allows for use of only the diaphragm.

High cervical quadriplegics are unable to generate an adequate VC due to reduced inspiratory and expiratory muscle function. The expulsive phase of the cough cannot be generated. Since the stabilizing influence of the contracting intercostal muscles is lacking, the upper rib cage of the patient breathing solely with the diaphragm moves inward during inspiration, instead of expanding outward. The result is a diminished tidal volume. If portions of the lower cervical segments remain intact, there will be some accessory muscles activity, and less paradoxic motion. Paradoxic motion also diminishes as the condition becomes chronic, due to stiffening of the thorax.

When the quadriplegic patient is upright, the weight of the abdominal contents pulls downward on the diaphragm. Abdominal muscles, having lost their tone, cannot oppose this action, and the diaphragm shortens. The effectiveness of the quadriplegic's diaphragm is markedly diminished in the upright position. Abdominal binders can be used to offset lost abdominal muscle tone. This should be considered if the patient's VT falls when moved to the upright position.

A large percentage of patients with acute spinal cord injuries will require ventilatory support. The vital capacity in patients who have cervical spinal injuries is often 1.2 to 1.5 liters. PImax is also usually reduced. The requirement for ventilatory support is often temporary. After the initial phase of shock to the spinal cord passes, the chest wall becomes stiff, as described previously. The vital capacity may increase by a liter or more. Eighty percent of patients with injuries at or below the C4 level can eventually be weaned.

Anterior horn cell disorders

Poliomyelitis used to be the most common cause of impaired anterior horn cell function. Paralysis affects the lower extremities and trunk. Respiratory motor nuclei can be directly involved resulting in diaphragmatic or other respiratory muscle dysfunction. A syndrome of recurrent muscle weakness occurring 20 to 40 years after the initial bout of polio has been reported. This post-polio weakness syndrome progresses slowly, but may lead to progressive respiratory failure.

Amyotrophic lateral sclerosis (ALS) is now the most common cause of anterior horn cell dysfunction and its resultant respiratory muscle weakness. The disease most frequently presents as progressive muscle weakness in the distal extremities, especially in older adults. When the bulbar muscles are involved, the gag reflex may be impaired and aspiration can occur.

Respiratory symptoms generally do not occur until late in the course of ALS. Serial pulmonary function studies show a progressive loss of VC and TLC. The RV increases as respiratory muscle functions are lost. Respiratory failure may occur when an episode of bronchitis or aspiration pneumonia produces an acute complication. Supportive measures during the acute incident often return the patient to a stable condition. More than 50% of patients die of complications such as aspiration or pneumonia within 3 years of diagnosis.

Diseases affecting the peripheral motor nerves

The peripheral nerves may be affected by toxic agents, inflammatory processes, vascular disorders, malignancies, and metabolic or nutritional imbalances.

Polyneuritis

Polyneuritis describes widespread sensory and motor disturbances of peripheral nerves. It is most common in young or middle-aged men. Polyneuritis is characterized by the slow development of pain, tenderness, paresthesia, weakness, fatigability, and sensory impairment over a period of weeks. Muscular weakness is greatest in the distal extremities. Tendon reflexes are usually depressed or absent. Flaccid weakness and muscular atrophy may occur.

Guillain–Barré syndrome

In Guillain-Barré syndrome, patients often develop polyneuritis 1 to 2 weeks after a mild upper respiratory infection or episode of gastroenteritis. Less frequently, Guillain-Barré syndrome may occur in patients recently immunized against viral infections. The cause of this disorder is unknown. Either a hypersensitivity or autoimmune response of the nerves may be responsible. Guillain-Barré seems to be associated with carcinomas, herpes zoster infections, mononucleosis, and HIV seroconversion. This response is believed to lead to **demyelination** of the nerves and a mononuclear inflammatory reaction.

Early lower extremity weakness progresses within a few days to the upper extremities and face (hence the term *ascending paralysis*). Facial diplegia, **dysphagia,** or **dysarthria** may occur. Sensory changes are not usually present, but muscle tenderness and nerve sensitivity to pressure may occur. Weakness of trunk and extremity muscles may be severe, including flaccid paraplegia and marked respiratory muscle weakness. Daily bedside evaluation of VC and respiratory muscle strength (PEmax, PImax) is essential. At the height of the disorder, the cerebrospinal fluid usually shows a very high protein content with few or no white cells, an anomaly called *albuminocytologic dissociation.*

Treatment of patients with Guillain-Barré syndrome is usually symptomatic. Respiratory insufficiency requiring ventilatory support develops in about 25% of patients with Guillain-Barré syndrome. Patients should be intubated when they lose their ability to protect their airway. This may occur before frank respiratory failure. Early intubation, when the VC is 20 to 25 mL/kg, may reduce the risk of aspiration pneumonitis. Duration of ventilatory support averages 6 to 8 weeks, but periods of up to 30 months have been reported. Approximately 30% of patients requiring ventilatory support can be extubated within two weeks. The mortality for the Guillain-Barré syndrome is less than 5%. The majority of survivors recover completely. A small minority have persistent weakness and continue to be susceptible to recurrent respiratory failure due to respiratory infections.

Abnormalities of neuromuscular transmission

Abnormalities of neuromuscular transmission affect ventilation by disrupting the synapse between the motor end-plate and skeletal muscle cells. Myasthenia gravis is the classic example of this type of abnormality in neuromuscular transmission. Botulism and tetanus also affect the chemical activity occurring between the motor end-plate and skeletal muscle.

Myasthenia gravis

Myasthenia gravis is the most common disorder impairing neuromuscular transmission. It primarily affects young women and older men. The disease has a special affinity for muscles innervated by the bulbar nuclei. This includes muscles of the face, lips, eyes, tongue, throat, and neck. The cause of myasthenia gravis is unknown. Current evidence suggests that the primary mechanism is an autoimmune process causing rapid inactivation of acetylcholine at the myoneural junction.

The patient with myasthenia gravis exhibits pronounced fatigability of muscles, with consequent weakness and paralysis. Weakness of the extraocular muscles is apparent as diplopia and Strabismus. Speech and swallowing difficulties can occur after prolonged exercise of these functions. In patients with long-standing myasthenia, **myopathy** with severe diaphragmatic paresis may develop and lead to chronic respiratory failure.

Diagnosis of myasthenia gravis is made primarily from the history and physical findings. The diagnosis is confirmed using the Tensilon (edrophonium) test.

Tensilon exerts a direct stimulant effect on the neuro-muscular junction. Intravenous injection of 10 mg of Tensilon relieves weakness caused by myasthenia gravis within 20 to 30 seconds.

In most patients, initial treatment consists of anticholinesterase drug therapy with neostigmine methylsulfate. Subcutaneous or IM injection of neostigmine results in relief of symptoms within 10 to 15 minutes, lasting up to 4 hours. Encouraging short-term results have also been reported with the use of large amounts of adrenocorticotropic hormone (ACTH). Long-term ACTH injections and long-term oral prednisone have also been used with some success in chronic myasthenia. Beneficial effects in some patients have been reported upon surgical removal of the thymus gland.

Sudden onset of respiratory failure may occur as a result of an acute episode of the basic disease process (myasthenic crisis), or the excessive use of anticholinesterase drugs (cholinergic crisis). Respiratory failure may also follow initiation of ACTH or corticosteroid therapy. In the cholinergic crisis, mortality may be reduced by withdrawing anticholinesterase medications for about 72 hours after onset of respiratory difficulty. Positive pressure ventilatory support through an artificial airway is required.

Disorders of the muscles

The two most common muscular disorders causing pulmonary problems are muscular dystrophy and polymyositis.

Muscular dystrophy

Muscular dystrophies represent a group of hereditary disorders characterized by progressive degeneration of the skeletal muscles. The result is severe muscle weakness. The most common form is Duchenne's muscular dystrophy. Because Duchenne's muscular dystrophy occurs primarily as a result of an X-linked recessive trait, the disorder predominantly affects males. Other forms are autosomal and thus seen in both sexes.

Patients with muscular dystrophy are predisposed to pulmonary complications, and respiratory failure is a frequent cause of death. Children who have Duchenne's muscular dystrophy often develop significant kyphoscoliosis that combines with muscle weakness to cause severe respiratory failure. Inspiratory muscle weakness develops late in the progression of the disease and results in chronic alveolar hypoventilation. Chronic hypoventilation may also appear in patients with adequate muscle strength, suggesting a defect in the central respiratory control mechanism. Expiratory muscle weakness may impair cough in some patients. The weakness of the muscles of swallowing can lead to aspiration and recurrent pneumonias. Respiratory muscle weakness can be detected as marked decreases in both PEmax and PImax. Rapid, shallow tidal breathing is also characteristic.

Polymyositis

Polymyositis is a chronic inflammatory disease that affects the striated muscles. If associated with involvement of the skin, the disorder is known as dermatomyositis. In addition to the striated muscles and skin, other organs may be affected, including the lung and heart. A Type IV (delayed type or cell-mediated) hypersensitivity reaction may be responsible for this disorder.

Patients with polymyositis exhibit progressive weakness of the skeletal muscles of the extremities, as well as the cervical, pharyngeal, and trunk muscles. Direct involvement of the lungs in the disease process may result in inflammation and fibrosis. The primary respiratory complications are due to respiratory muscle weakness and difficulties in swallowing. For this reason, pneumonia is the most common cause of death in these patients. Corticosteroids and immunosuppressive drugs appear to slow progression of the disease, but increase the incidence of pulmonary infections by opportunistic organisms.

IMMUNOLOGIC DISORDERS

The immune system

The immune system has two interrelated components: cell-mediated immunity and humoral immunity. Key elements of the system include T lymphocytes, B lymphocytes, and circulating macrophages (Figure 20-20). T lymphocytes have receptors for both antigen-antibody complexes and complement. B lymphocytes have these receptors plus surface immunoglobins. The basic body immune response involves interaction between these lymphocytes and the macrophages.

Macrophages binds antigen to their cell membrane receptors, and engulf and lyse this foreign material. As they process foreign material, macrophages also secrete a variety of biochemical mediators.

This processing of antigen transforms the T lymphocytes into sensitized T cells. When re-exposed to antigen, sensitized T cells release cytotoxins and lymphokines. Cytotoxins help protect against intracellular pathogens, such as viruses and *Pneumocystis carinii*. The cytotoxic effect also functions in allographic tissue rejection and tumor resistance. Lymphokines activate additional macrophages and enhance their ability to kill microorganisms. The sensitization and subsequent action of the T cells is the primary mechanism in cell-mediated immunity.

Sensitization of T cell also produces T helper cells. T helper cells play a key role in humoral immunity. Humoral immunity involves interaction among anti-

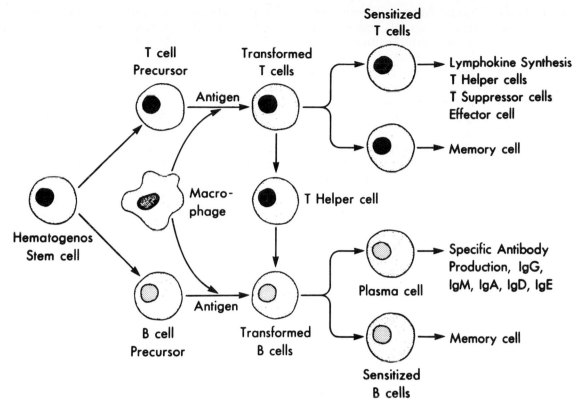

Fig. 20-20 Development of the humoral and cellular immune systems. Macrophage processing of antigen occurs prior to presentation to B lymphocytes and T lymphocytes, with T helper lymphocyte facilitation of immunologic production. (From Kryger MH, editor: Pathophysiology of respiration, New York, 1981, John Wiley & Sons.)

gen, T helper cells, macrophages, and B lymphocytes. This process transforms and sensitizes B cells. Once sensitized to a specific antigen, transformed B cells secrete immunoglobins. Only one kind of immunoglobin is produced by each lymphocyte, and each immunoglobin is specific to the original sensitizing antigen.

Immunoglobins play several key roles in host defense. Some immunoglobins serve as **opsonins,** stimulating phagocytic cells to engulf antigenic material. Others can fix complement, thereby initiating a complex series of enzymatic reactions that result in recruiting more phagocytes and lymphocytes to the affected area. Still others simply inhibit bacterial multiplication.

Excessive immune response (allergic reactions)

Allergic reactions represent an excessive response of the immune system to environmental antigens. Although such reactions may involve any organ system in the body, we will focus solely on allergic responses of the respiratory system.

Categories of allergic reactions

Allergic or *hypersensitivity* reactions may be classified into one of the four major types (Table 20-6, page 488). Of course, some hypersensitivity states may involve more than one category.

Type I (immediate-type hypersensitivity). Type I, or immediate-type hypersensitivity is produced when IgE antibodies fixed to mast cells react with antigens such as pollens, molds, or animal danders. Re-exposure to the allergen causes the release of histamine and other mediators of inflammation. This response is characteristic of extrinsic asthma, hay fever, anaphylaxis, and contact dermatitis.

Type II (cytotoxic hypersensitivity). Type II, or cytotoxic hypersensitivity is mediated by IgG or IgM antibodies. These antibodies react with antigen on target cells and activate complement, causing cellular lysis. Cytotoxic hypersensitivity occurs in Goodpasture's syndrome, poststreptococcal glomerulonephritis, and certain drug reactions.

Goodpasture's Syndrome consists of chronic, relapsing pulmonary hemosiderosis, often combined with fatal **glomerulonephritis.** In hemosiderosis, hemoglobin breaks down into hemosiderin, which deposits in the lungs. Clinical features of this syndrome include cough with recurrent hemoptysis, dyspnea, pulmonary infiltration, and anemia. Transbronchial biopsy via a flexible fiberoptic bronchoscope is a valuable diagnostic procedure. Identification of IgG deposits on the alveolar-capillary membrane by immunofluorescence is distinctive. Patients with Goodpasture's Syndrome have a poor prognosis. Immunosuppressive treatment with steroids and cyclophosphamide has been effective in some patients. There are several recent reports of patients with progressive respiratory and renal failure who improved after multiple plasma exchanges, a procedure called **plasmapheresis.** When the principal feature of the disease is renal failure, hemodialysis may be indicated.

Type III (immune complex hypersensitivity). Type III, or immune complex hypersensitivity may also be mediated by IgG or IgM antibodies. These antibodies form complexes with antigen and complement and cause the release of mediators that cause local tissue inflammation. Hypersensitivity pneumonitis (extrinsic allergic alveolitis), rheumatoid arthritis, and certain collagen vascular disorders, such as systemic lupus erythematosus, are examples of this process. In Type III allergic responses, prolonged exposure to antigen may result in a chronic inflammatory process and subsequent organ fibrosis.

As delineated in Table 20-6, hypersensitivity pneumonia is caused by exposure to a variety of organic dusts. Exposure in sensitized individuals causes both an interstitial and alveolar inflammatory process. IgG antibodies are usually present. Clinically, patients with hypersensitivity pneumonitis develop an acute fever, dry cough, dyspnea, and malaise within 5-6 hours after exposure to the offending antigen. Radiographic examination of the chest typically reveals a diffuse fine granular infiltration. Unlike Type I reactions, eosinophilia usually does not occur. A history of exposure is important in making the diagnosis. Treatment involves avoidance of exposure and, if symptoms are severe, corticosteroids. Repeated exposure may result in severe pulmonary fibrosis.

Type IV (delayed type or cell-mediated hypersensitivity). Type IV hypersensitivity is mediated by sensitized T lymphocytes. These T-cells react directly with antigen, producing inflammation through the action of lymphokines. The delayed type or cell-mediated hypersensitivity reaction is thought to contribute to acute and chronic transplantation reactions, tuberculosis, sarcoidosis, and other granulomatous diseases.

Sarcoidosis is a systemic inflammatory disease of unknown cause that primarily affects the lungs. In the lungs, a cell-mediated immune reaction causes inflammation and granuloma formation. Sarcoid granulomas look like those seen in tuberculosis, but do not show the central necrosis so common in mycobacterial disease. Both lymphocytes (T Helper cells) and macrophages are involved in the inflammatory process. Chronic inflammation leads to fibrosis and a restrictive pulmonary pattern, including decreased diffusing capacity.

Sarcoidosis tends to strike women more than men and blacks more than whites. Patients are often asymptomatic, although some exhibit coughing, wheezing, and dyspnea on exertion. Preliminary diagnosis generally occurs via the chest X-ray, which typically show bilateral hilar lymphadenopathy, with or without pulmonary infiltrates. Late in the disease process, the X-ray may show evidence of fibrosis and honeycombing. Lab tests are not helpful in establishing a diagnosis.

Sarcoidosis is usually self-limiting, but some patients progressively worsen over time. Treatment is with corticosteroids, both system and via the aerosol route.

Impaired immune response (immunodeficiency)

Deficiencies in the body's immune response, either humoral or cell-mediated, can compromise its ability to resist infection. Clinical conditions associated with a decreased immune response include alcohol intoxication, diabetes, uremia, hypogammaglobinemia, and **leukocytopenia.** Many therapeutic interventions, such as radiation therapy and the use of immunosuppressive drugs, also decrease patients' immune responses. More recently, the acquired immunodeficiency syn-

Table 20-6 Immunologic respiratory diseases

	Mechanism	Examples
Type I	IgE on cell reacts with allergen-releasing mediator	Asthma, hay fever
Type II	IgG or IgM directed against basement membrane; complement activated	Goodpasture's syndrome
Type III	Circulating antigen-antibody complexes deposited in lung; complement activated: inflammatory reaction	Hypersensitivity pneumonitis, collagen vascular diseases
Type IV	Cell-mediated (T lymphocyte) immunity: lymphokines: inflammatory reaction	Tuberculosis, granulomatous diseases

From Kryger MH, editor: Pathophysiology of respiration, New York, 1981, John Wiley & Sons.

Table 20-7   Hypersensitivity pneumonitis

Disease	Source of antigen	Precipitins
Air-conditioner and humidifier lung	Fungi in air conditioners and humidifiers	Thermophilic actinomycetes
Aspergillosis	Ubiquitous	*A fumagatis, A flavus, A niger, A nidulans*
Bagassosis (sugarcane workers)	Moldy bagasse	*Thermoactinomyces vulgaris*
Bird fancier's lung	Pigeon, parrot, hen droppings	Serum protein and droppings
Byssinosis	Cotton, flax, hemp workers	Unknown
Farmer's lung	Moldy hay	*Micropolyspora faeni, T vulgaris*
Malt worker's lung	Moldy barley, malt dusk	*A clavatus, A fumigatus*
Maple-bark pneumonitis	Moldy maple bark	*Cryptostroma corticale*
Mushroom worker's lung	Mushroom compost	*M faeni, T vlugaris*
Sequoiosis	Moldy redwood sawdust	*Graphium aurea basidium pullalans*
Wheat weevil disease	Infested wheat flour	*Sitophilus granarius*

From Mitchell RS: Synopsis of clinical pulmonary disease, ed 4, St Louis, 1988, Mosby.

drome, or AIDS, has come to our attention as an immune disorder of significant concern and growing magnitude.

Acquired immunodeficiency syndrome (AIDS)

First recognized in 1981, AIDS is caused by infection with the human immunodeficiency virus (HIV). HIV directly attacks the T-lymphocytes (including the T-Helper cells) of the immune system. Thus HIV primarily compromises the cell-mediated component of the immune system. However, because it also affects the T-Helper cells, HIV also compromises the humoral (antibody) component of host defense.

As of 1994, more than 360,000 cases of AIDS have been diagnosed in the United States. It is estimated that another 1-2 million persons in the US are infected with the HIV virus. Transmission occurs via mingling of blood or body fluids, as during unprotected anal or vaginal intercourse or by contaminated needles. Two population groups thus account for the vast majority of AIDS cases: homosexual or bisexual men, and heterosexual men or women who are intravenous drug abusers. AIDS has also been well documented among prisoners, central African immigrants, heterosexual partners of HIV-infected individuals, and children of HIV-infected mothers. Concern over the link between AIDS and blood transfusions has decreased since mandatory testing of whole blood and blood products for the HIV virus began in the mid-1980s.

Patients with suspected AIDS are seropositive for HIV, as determined by ELISA, Western blot testing, or (more recently) HIV antigen testing. Patients typically have chronic fever, severe fatigue, extensive weight loss, and lymphadenopathy. Lab data indicates a low T-Helper cell count, leukothrombocytopenia, and elevated serum globulins.

The clinical management of AIDS combines three approaches: preventive, therapeutic, and supportive. Because no current cure exists, and mortality exceeds 70 percent within two years of diagnosis, the main emphasis is still on prevention.

One major preventive effort has been to develop an HIV vaccine. However, many formidable barriers must be overcome before a safe and effective vaccine becomes widely available. The second element of prevention involves more traditional public health interventions. These methods include testing to protect blood and organ recipients, and education programs about the dangers of IV drug abuse and unprotected sex. Recommendations for preventing the spread of HIV within the hospital are discussed in Chapter 4.

Therapy for AIDS patients is divided into two categories: treatment aimed at the HIV infection itself and treatment aimed at the secondary infections and malignant disorders. The first drug that directly treats HIV infection, AZT (azidothymidine, or zidovudine), is approved by the FDA for treating symptomatic AIDS patients and those with helper T cell counts between 200 and 500/mm^3.

AZT is virostatic, not curative. Moreover, the drug can be quite toxic. As many as one-third of all AIDS patients exhibit significant side effects to AZT, with anemia and granulocytopenia being most common. These side effects often require a reduction in drug dosage or additional treatment with erythropoietin. Alternative FDA approved anti-HIV agents include dideoxycytidine (DDC) and dideoxinocine (DDI). Both appear to be less toxic than AZT. DDI can, however, cause severe diarrhea, pancreatitis and peripheral neuropathy. Monoclonal antibodies directed against the virus also are being studied, as are cloned cytokines.

The other therapeutic consideration in AIDS is treatment of the secondary infections and malignant diseases, which account for most of the morbidity and mortality. This aspect of AIDS was discussed in detail in the prior section on pneumonia in the compromised host.

The final aspect of AIDS management is social and supportive. Besides the economic cost, the personal and social costs of AIDS are immense. How and how well we address these economic, moral, and social issues may well shape the future direction of our health care delivery system.

INHALATIONAL LUNG DISEASES

Inhalational lung diseases are caused by organic or inorganic dusts, noxious fumes, or chemicals entering the respiratory tract. Exposure to organic dusts cause hypersensitivity pneumonitis (Table 20-7 page 489). Inorganic dusts, noxious fumes, and chemicals also cause serious respiratory problems.

Inhalation of inorganic dusts (pneumonconioses)

Pneumoconioses represent changes in the lung caused by the inhalation of an inorganic dust. A variety of inorganic materials may be inhaled into the lungs (see accompanying box). Iron and tin cause little or no tissue reaction and are categorized as *inert* pneumoconioses. Silica and others provoke a tissue reaction and are classified as *active* pneumoconioses.

Silicosis

Inhalation of silicon dioxide is responsible for silicosis. Silica-containing compounds, such as bauxite or silicates, may also cause the disease. Depending on intensity of exposure, silicosis may develop in as little as 18 months, or may take as long as 30 years to appear.

Common pneumoconioses

Inert pneumoconioses
  Iron: siderosis
  Tin: stannosis
  Barium: baritosis
  Cement
  Fiberglass
  Talc
Active pneumoconioses caused by silica or silica content (ie, fibrosis and other pathology producing)
  Silica
  Silicates, including kaolin
  Diatomaceous earth
  Asbestos
  Bauxite
Active pneumoconioses without silica
  Aluminum and aluminum oxide
  Coal
  Graphite
  Nickel carbonyl
  Tungsten carbide
  Beryllium
  Cadmium
  Cerium

From Mitchell RS: Synopsis of clinical pulmonary disease, ed 4, St Louis, 1988, Mosby.

Symptoms may be minimal. The patient usually exhibits a history of susceptibility to upper respiratory tract infections, bronchitis, and pneumonia. The most common complaint is dyspnea on exertion. Cough may be dry, but later becomes productive, frequently with blood-streaked sputum. Severe, occasionally fatal, hemoptysis may occur. Physical findings may be absent in patients with advanced silicosis. Lung biopsy is occasionally indicated to establish the diagnosis for purposes of insurance compensation.

Although not completely diagnostic, the chest X-ray may strongly suggest the diagnosis. Abnormalities are usually bilateral, symmetric, and predominantly in the hilar region. Small nodules tend to be of uniform density and size. Enlargement of hilar lymph nodes occurs early in the progression of the disease. Interstitial fibrosis is manifested by fine linear markings and reticulation.

There is no definitive treatment available for silicosis (or for any of the pneumoconioses). Prevention, by careful regulation of the workplace environment, is the only way to reduce the incidence of these disorders. Symptomatic or supportive treatment is indicated for chronic cough and wheezing.

Other pneumoconioses

Asbestosis and coal-workers' pneumoconiosis (CWP) are among the most common pneumoconioses other than silicosis. Asbestosis is caused by the inhalation of asbestos fibers. These fibers are hydrous silicates of magnesium, sodium, and iron. Asbestosis leads to fibrosis of lung tissue and often involves the visceral pleura. Asbestosis causes a restrictive ventilatory impairment, with dyspnea on exertion. Pleural plaques and pleural thickening are commonly identified on chest X-rays. Risk of lung carcinoma is increased in patients who smoke and have a history of asbestos exposure. Pleural mesothelioma is a very rare cancer found almost uniquely in individuals with a history of asbestos exposure.

Coal workers' pneumoconiosis (CWP) is due to exposure to coal dust, consisting mainly of carbon. Patients with CWP exhibit symptoms similar to silicosis. Many also have findings similar to COPD. As with silicosis, both conditions can lead to a progressive massive fibrosis (PMF).

Inhalation of noxious fumes and chemicals

There are hundreds of noxious fumes or chemicals capable of producing a pathologic response in the lung. Of these, carbon monoxide (CO), nitrogen dioxide (NO_2), and sulfur dioxide (SO_2) are the most common. Accidental exposure to high concentrations of these gases can cause acute injury to the lung.

Silo-filler's disease is caused by inhalation of NO_2 and SO_2 fumes emanating from agricultural silos that have been freshly filled. These fumes cause increased capillary permeability, resulting in a form of pulmonary edema. Immediately after exposure, the patient exhibits cough, dyspnea, and weakness. This may progress or be followed by a decrease in symptoms, which then reappear and become progressively worse. Diffuse crackles (rales) and rhonchi are heard, and the chest radiograph shows bilateral fluffy infiltrates that may coalesce into dense areas of pulmonary edema. Supplementary oxygen and ventilatory support may be necessary to correct the resulting hypoxemia. The morality rate can be as high as 30%.

PULMONARY NEOPLASMS

Pulmonary neoplasms may be either benign or malignant. Benign tumors are usually not life-threatening, unless they impinge upon a vital organ. They are not metastatic. Malignant tumors grow rapidly in a poorly organized fashion. They invade surrounding tissue and are metastatic. Malignant tumors most often arise in the bronchial mucosa and are referred to as bronchogenic carcinomas.

Bronchogenic tumors are divided into four major categories: (1) squamous cell carcinoma, (2) small-cell carcinoma (also called oat-cell carcinoma), (3) adenocarcinoma, and (4) large-cell carcinoma. Squamous cell carcinoma is the most common form, accounting for 30% to 50% of diagnosed cases. Small cell carcinoma is found in approximately 25% of cases. Adenocarcinoma and large cell carcinoma are each responsible for 15% to 35% of bronchogenic tumors.

Bronchogenic carcinoma is the most common intrathoracic malignancy. It occurs predominantly in men, but the incidence in women has increased markedly. Most cases occur in the cancer age group (40 to 70 years of age). The importance of hereditary and environmental factors in the cause of bronchogenic carcinoma is not known. Smoking accounts for 85% of lung cancers in men and 75% in women. The risk of lung cancer correlates directly with the number of cigarettes consumed per day. Other occupational hazards, such as asbestos exposure, have been linked to development of lung cancer.

Bronchogenic carcinoma is characterized by a persistent nonproductive cough, hemoptysis, and localized persistent wheeze. These clinical findings are associated with the bronchial irritation, erosion, and partial obstruction caused by the developing tumor. Pleural effusions may occur if the tumor invades the parietal pleura or mediastinum. The tumor itself, along with effusions, compress the surrounding lung tissue. Atelectasis is common.

Pulmonary infections occurring distal to the bronchial obstruction, such as pneumonia or lung abscess, frequently dominate the clinical picture and can mask the underlying neoplasm. If the lesion is large enough, there may be physical and radiographic signs of partial or complete bronchial obstruction with associated atelectasis and infection.

Diagnostic methods for bronchogenic carcinoma include X-rays, sputum analysis, and biopsy via bronchosope. A positive diagnosis of bronchogenic carcinoma can be made in 40% to 60% of cases on the basis of sputum cytology. Ideally, several fresh specimens should be studied. Forceps or brush biopsy obtained through the flexible fiberoptic bronchoscope (FFB) provides the diagnosis in 75% to 80% of bronchial tumor cases. The American Cancer Society does not recommend routine chest X-rays as the basis for detection of early lung cancers.

Early detection and surgical removal before metastasis occurs offer the best hope of cure. Small tumors can be resected. Larger tumors often require removal of a lobe (i.e., lobectomy) or of an entire lung (i.e., pneumonectomy). Preoperative pulmonary function testing (see Chapter 18) is used to identify surgical candidates who may be at risk of complications. Surgical resection may be impossible if the tumor involves other major thoracic structures. Endobronchial laser resection can be used for carcinomas that obstruct the major airways (see Chapter 22).

Radiation therapy is used in many cases, often in conjunction with surgical resection or chemotherapy. The ability to target specific areas for radiation allows tumors that cannot be surgically removed to be treated. Irradiation typically results in loss of pulmonary function. Chemotherapy for non-small cell carcinomas is palliative with poor response. Chemotherapy for small cell lung cancer is more effective.

CARDIOPULMONARY VASCULAR DISORDERS

The physiologic interrelationship among the heart, vasculature, and lungs necessitates an integrated approach to disorders characterizing these organ systems. Cardiac failure and pulmonary disorders associated with the cardiovascular system are frequently encountered in the critical care setting. Management of shock and various embolic disorders is often determined by understanding their pathophysiologies.

Cardiac failure

Cardiac failure may involve failure of either the left or right ventricles. Combined failure of both ventricles may occur, especially right heart failure following left-sided decompensation.

There are two categories of disorders associated with ventricular failure: (1) myocardial weakness or inflammation, and (2) excessive ventricular workload. The box on page 492 outlines these various disorders.

Etiology of ventricular failure

Myocardial weakness or inflammation
 Coronary artery disease
 Myocarditis
 Congestive cardiomyopathies
 Drugs
Excessive work load
 Increased resistance to ejection (afterload)
 Hypertension
 Stenosis of aortic or pulmonary valves
 Hypertrophic cardiomyopathy
Increased stroke volume
 Aortic insufficiency
 Mitral insufficiency
 Tricuspid insufficiency
 Congenital left-to-right shunts
Increased body demands
 Hypoxemia
 Anemia
 Thyrotoxicosis
 Pregnancy
 Arteriovenous fistula

Left ventricular failure

Left ventricular failure is commonly caused by systemic hypertension, coronary arterial disease, or aortic insufficiency. Less common is left ventricular failure caused by mitral valve insufficiency, hypertrophic cardiomyopathy, congestive cardiomyopathy, left-to-right shunts, congenital heart defects, and certain drugs. Infectious endocarditis may directly cause left ventricular failure, as well as aggravate other valve diseases. The term congestive heart failure (CHF) is often used synonymously with left ventricular failure.

Left ventricular failure is characterized by its symptoms: exertional dyspnea, cough, fatigue, and **nocturia.** In coronary arterial disease, angina pectoris is the predominant symptom. Exertional dyspnea is caused by pulmonary venous congestion, and the resultant decrease in lung compliance. Dyspnea also worsens when the patient assumes a recumbent position, due to increased pulmonary vascular engorgement. Paroxysmal nocturnal dyspnea (PND), often with a dry cough, may appear at any time. PND is associated with left ventricular failure due to severe hypertension, aortic stenosis or insufficiency, or myocardial infarction. Dyspnea due to left ventricular failure must be differentiated from other conditions causing shortness of breath. These include chronic pulmonary disease, obesity, severe anemia, **ascites,** and abdominal distention.

Nocturia is attributed to the excretion of edema fluid that occurs as kidney perfusion increases in the recumbent position. Nocturia may also reflect the decreased work of the heart at rest, or delayed effects of diuretics given during the day.

Physical examination of the patient with left ventricular failure usually discloses signs of left ventricular hypertrophy. The apical impulse is increased in strength with a leftward, downward displacement. A gallop rhythm, pulsus alternans, and an accentuated pulmonary component of the second sound (P2) may or may not be present. Physical signs of pleural effusion, though common, may not always be present.

The chest X-ray often reveals pulmonary venous congestion. This appears as increased blood flow to the upper lobes and Kerley B lines. Left ventricular enlargement is usually apparent on an X-ray. This may not be true if left ventricular failure is due to acute myocardial infarction or a cardiac arrhythmia. Left atrial enlargement is apparent in the case of mitral stenosis.

Right ventricular failure

The most common causes of right ventricular failure are mitral stenosis, pulmonary vascular hypertension, stenosis of the pulmonary valve, and right ventricular myocardial infarction associated with inferior myocardial infarction. Less common causes of right ventricular failure are tricuspid valve disease, infectious endocarditis involving the right side of the heart, and pulmonary hypertension in the adult respiratory distress syndrome (ARDS).

Right ventricular failure is characterized by anorexia, bloating, and right upper abdominal pain. These signs reflect hepatic and visceral congestion secondary to elevated venous pressure. Elevated jugular venous pressure, accompanied by abnormal systolic pulsation, is sometimes observed. Jugular venous pressure can be estimated by noting jugular filling during expiration above the clavicles with the patient sitting up at a 30° angle.

The liver is enlarged (i.e., hepatomegaly) and may be tender. Dependent edema usually subsides overnight in the early stages of this disorder, but eventually persists and worsens in severity. Pleural effusion, if it occurs, is more common on the right side. Coolness of the extremities and peripheral cyanosis of the nail beds, due to reduce peripheral blood flow, may be noted. Sinus tachycardia is usually present, and a right ventricular S3 sound may be heard.

In pure right-sided failure, the ECG indicates right ventricular hypertrophy. On radiographic examination of the chest, both right atrial and right ventricular enlargement may be seen. Specific chamber enlargement on X-ray is difficult to define when the right heart failure is secondary to left heart failure.

Treatment of ventricular failure

Treatment of heart failure is directed at the underlying cause. Supportive therapy includes decreasing myocardial workload, increasing the force and efficiency of myocardial contraction, and reducing the fluid retention.

Decreasing myocardial workload. Rest (either in bed or sitting in a chair) decreases the work of the heart and promotes diuresis. Oxygen therapy can also reduce myocardial workload, especially when hypoxemia is present. Left ventricular failure may be due to both a high filling pressure (more than 20 mm Hg) and low cardiac output. If so, vasodilator therapy can improve myocardial performance by reducing the impedance to left ventricular output, or afterload.

Increasing myocardial contractility. In patients with atrial fibrillation and a rapid ventricular rate, digitalis or one of its derivatives may be used to slow AV conduction. This prolongs diastolic filling time and increases cardiac output. Digitalis is less effective in hypertrophic states such as cardiomyopathy. In acute myocardial infarction, more potent inotropic agents, such as dobutamine are indicated (refer to Chapter 23).

Reducing fluid retention. Dietary restriction of sodium may be useful, but depends upon the severity of the failure. Diuresis is most easily accomplished with diuretics. Furosemide (Lasix), and ethacrynic acid, potent diuretics with a short duration of action, may be needed in acute conditions. Unfortunately, these agents, especially the thiazide diuretics, can cause significant potassium loss. For this reason, aldosterone antagonists such as spironolactone, which causes sodium diuresis without potassium loss are useful. Spironolactone can be combined with thiazides to neutralize their potassium–wasting effect.

Cardiopulmonary and pulmonary vascular disorders

In distinction to cardiac failure, several disorders involve the lung, heart, and pulmonary vasculature together. These include cor pulmonale, pulmonary edema, and pulmonary vascular hypertension.

Cor pulmonale

Cor pulmonale is right ventricular failure due to pulmonary parenchymal or vascular disease. The patient usually has chronic bronchitis or emphysema, with their characteristic signs and symptoms. Less common causes include pneumoconiosis, pulmonary fibrosis, kyphoscoliosis, and the obesity–hypoventilation syndrome. Obliteration of pulmonary capillaries, interstitial or alveolar fibrosis, and chronic hypoxemia combine to increase pulmonary artery pressure. This leads to right ventricular hypertrophy and eventual right heart failure (Figure 20-21).

Cor pulmonale may be acute, subacute, or, most commonly, chronic. Clinical features of cor pulmonale depend on the primary disease and its effects on the heart. The dominant symptoms of chronic cor pulmonale are respiratory. They include chronic productive cough, exertional dyspnea, wheezing, and fatigability. As with non-pulmonary right ventricular failure, dependent edema and right upper quadrant pain may appear. Chronic cor pulmonale may cause secondary polycythemia and cyanosis is a common finding. Other signs of chronic right heart failure include clubbing of fingers, distended neck veins, right ventricular heave or gallop, prominent lower sternal or epigastric pulsations, and hepatomegaly. Unless the patient is in shock, pulses are full and the extremities warm.

The ECG in cor pulmonale typically shows right ventricular dyspnea, with tall, peaked P waves, right axis deviation, and deep S waves in lead V6. Left axis deviation and low voltage may be noted in patients with pulmonary emphysema. Arrhythmias are frequent and nonspecific.

The chest X-ray will show an enlarged right ventricle, often accompanied by an engorged pulmonary artery circulation. Depending on the cause, interstitial or alveolar disease may also be apparent on the

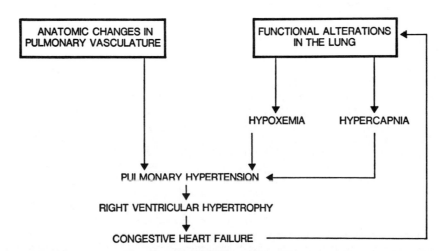

Fig. 20–21 Mechanisms of pulmonary hypertension and cor pulmonale. (Redrawn from Burrows B, Knudson RJ, Kettrl LJ: Respiratory insufficiency, St Louis, 1975, Mosby.)

chest film. In terms of laboratory findings, polycythemia is common. Typically, arterial blood gas analysis reveals an arterial oxygen saturation below 85%, with an elevated $PaCO_2$ values (i.e., greater than 45 torr).

Right ventricular failure may be differentiated from left ventricular failure by a history of respiratory disease, absence of orthopnea, and greater severity of cyanosis. The presence of bounding pulses and observation of warm extremities in the presence of edema also point to right-sided failure.

Pulmonary edema

Pulmonary edema is a condition in which excessive fluid volumes enter the pulmonary interstitium and alveoli. Acute pulmonary edema is normally accompanied by severe respiratory distress, tachypnea, and hypoxemia. It is considered a medical emergency. Appropriate treatment of pulmonary edema depends on identification of the cause.

A balance of oncotic and hydrostatic forces exists at the alveolar-capillary region. This equilibrium prevents fluid accumulation in the interstitial area (Figure 20-22). Pulmonary edema occurs when this balance is upset. The imbalance may be due to increased hydrostatic pressure, decreased oncotic pressure, or increased permeability of the capillary endothelial membrane (Table 20-8). Pulmonary edema due to increased hydrostatic pressures is classified as cardiogenic pulmonary edema. Pulmonary edema due to decreased oncotic pressure or increased capillary permeability is categorized as noncardiogenic pulmonary edema.

Cardiogenic pulmonary edema. Cardiogenic pulmonary edema may be caused by any disorder that elevates pulmonary capillary hydrostatic pressure high enough to cause fluid to leak into the alveolar interstitium or alveoli. Left ventricular failure is the most common cause of cardiogenic pulmonary edema. The causes and clinical manifestations of cardiogenic pulmonary edema are similar to those for left ventricular failure. The respiratory signs and symptoms in acute cardiogenic pulmonary edema are much more severe. The patient is extremely dyspneic and tachypneic. Hypoxemia may be evident as central cyanosis. Diffuse crackles and wheezes may be so prominent as to make cardiac auscultation difficult.

Treatment of cardiogenic pulmonary edema aims at decreasing left heart and pulmonary vascular pres-

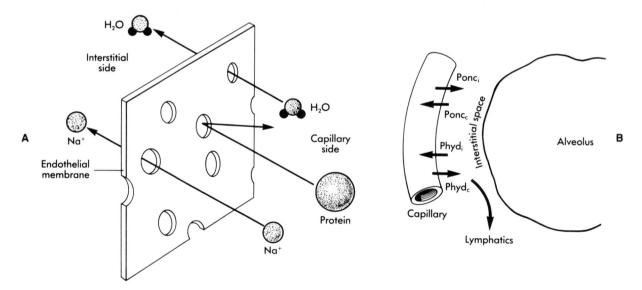

Fig. 20-22 A, Fluid transport from capillary to interstitial space. Intact endothelial membranes are permeable to water and small solutes (eg Na^+) but are impermeable to protein. In noncardiogenic edema, proteins leak through the damaged membranes, flooding the interstitium and alveolar spaces. **B,** Balance of colloid and hydrostatic forces in pulmonary capillaries. Colloid osmotic pressure is normally closely balanced against capillary hydrostatic pressure. Capillary hydrostatic pressure favors movement of fluid out of the capillary and is opposed by the hydrostatic pressure in the interstitial fluid. Colloid osmotic pressure of the plasma proteins tends to keep fluid in the capillary and is opposed by the osmotic pressure of proteins in the interstitial fluid. The exact pressures (oncotic and hydrostatic) within the pulmonary capillary are not known precisely, but the net result is a slight and continuous leak of fluid out of the capillaries and into the pulmonary interstitium, where it is picked up by interstitial lymphatics. Lymph flow from the lungs is approximately 10 to 20 mL/min. When this balance of forces is upset so that fluid movement overwhelms lymphatic drainage, pulmonary edema results. $Phyd_c$ = hydrostatic pressure in pulmonary capillary; $Phyd_i$ = hydrostatic pressure in pulmonary interstitium; $Ponc_c$ = oncotic pressure in pulmonary capillary; $Ponc_i$ = oncotic pressure in pulmonary interstitium. (From Martin L: Pulmonary physiology in clinical practice: the essentials for patient care and evaluation, St Louis, 1987, Mosby.)

Table 20-8 Mechanisms in the pulmonary capillary that influence movement of fluid into the pulmonary interstitium

Mechanism	Normal	Factor favoring excess fluid movement	Common clinical cause	Type of pulmonary edema
Hydrostatic pressure	6 to 12 mm Hg*	Increased value	Left ventricular failure	Cardiac
Oncotic pressure	20 to 25 mm Hg†	Decreased value	Liver cirrhosis	Noncardiac
Membrane permeability	—	Increased permeability	ARDS	Noncardiac

*Measured as pulmonary artery wedge pressure.
†Oncotic pressure can be qualitatively assessed by measurement of serum total protein or albumin, each of which correlates with the measured oncotic pressure. A low oncotic pressure is rarely, if ever, a sole cause of pulmonary edema; however, it is definitely a contributor factor in presence of another mechanism.
From Martin L: Pulmonary physiology in clinical practice: the essentials for patient care and evaluation, St Louis, 1987, Mosby.

sures. Elevating patients to the semi-Fowler's or sitting position decreases venous return to the heart. Morphine sulfate, given either intravenously or intramuscularly, relieves anxiety, increases venous compliance and decreases left ventricular preload. Oxygen should be administered in as high a concentration as possible. Oxygen relieves dyspnea, and lowers pulmonary vascular resistance by alleviating hypoxemia. Continuous positive airway pressure (CPAP) by mask may also improve oxygenation and help decrease venous return. Tourniquets, applied with sufficient pressure to obstruct venous but not arterial flow, and rotated every 15 minutes, also decrease venous return.

Diuresis using furosemide (Lasix) or thiazides is useful because of the potent and prompt diuretic action of these drugs. If abnormally high left ventricular afterload is a contributing factor, vasodilator therapy should be employed, using agents such as hydralazine (Apresoline) or prazosin (Minipress). Rapid digitalization is also of value in most patients.

Noncardiogenic pulmonary edema. Pulmonary edema in the absence of cardiac disease in previously healthy individuals can be caused by: (1) drugs such as nitrofurantoin or heroin, (2) the inhalation of smoke and other toxic substances, and (3) rapid ascent to high altitude. Pulmonary edema may also occur in some patients after severe central nervous system trauma. This so-called *neurogenic pulmonary edema* may be due to reflex stimulation of the adrenergic portion of the autonomic nervous system, causing a rapid shift of blood from the systemic to the pulmonary circulation.

The most common cause of acute noncardiogenic pulmonary edema is damage to the alveolar-capillary membrane. Extended inflammatory processes in the lung microvasculature and alveolar compartments is characteristic. Alterations in the alveolar surfactant may contribute to the increased capillary permeability. Damage to the alveolar-capillary membrane can be caused by many factors. All of these cause a severe disturbance in oxygen transfer from the alveoli into the pulmonary capillaries. These conditions, characterized by massive pulmonary capillary leakage with normal hydrostatic pressure, are grouped together under the name adult respiratory distress syndrome, or ARDS. Details on the causes, clinical manifestations and treatment of ARDS are provided in Chapter 29.

Pulmonary hypertension

Pulmonary hypertension is characterized by abnormally high pulmonary artery pressures. Pulmonary hypertension exists when the mean pulmonary artery pressure exceeds 22 mm Hg.

Table 20-9 summarizes the major causes of pulmonary hypertension and their underlying mechanisms. Lung and heart disease, in conjunction with hypoxemia, are the primary causes. Treatment of pulmonary hypertension is directed at the underlying cause; for

Table 20-9 Causes of pulmonary hypertension

Disease or condition	Underlying mechanism(s)
Lung diseases, including all forms of restrictive and obstructive lung conditions	Hypoxemia: loss of pulmonary blood vessels; acidosis
Heart disease, including left ventricular heart failure, mitral valve disease, congenital heart desease	Increased pulmonary capillary hydrostatic pressure
Pulmonary thromboembolic disease	Pulmonary artery narrowing; loss of pulmonary blood vessels
Pulmonary arteritis	Pulmonary artery narrowing; loss of pulmonary blood vessels
High altitude	Hypoxemia
Hypoventilation	Hypoxemia; acidosis
Chest wall deformity	Hypoxemia, acidosis: pulmonary artery narrowing
Idiopathic	Loss of pulmonary blood vessels: pulmonary artery narrowing

From Martin L: Pulmonary physiology in clinical practice: the essentials for patient care and evaluation, St Louis, 1987, Mosby.

example, reversal of left ventricular failure, or relief of hypoxemia.

One form of this disorder, called idiopathic or primary pulmonary hypertension occurs in the absence of other heart or lung diseases. Primary pulmonary hypertension is characterized by diffuse narrowing of the pulmonary arterioles without obvious reason. The clinical picture is similar to that of pulmonary hypertension from any other cause. Patients exhibit evidence of progressive right heart failure and low cardiac output, with weakness and fatigue. Edema and **ascites** become evident as the disorder progresses. Peripheral cyanosis is present, and syncope may occur with exertion. Late in the course of the disease, thrombi may develop as a result of the chronic low output failure. This predisposes the patient to pulmonary embolism.

There has been little effective treatment for primary pulmonary hypertension. Studies using a variety of oral vasodilators have shown promising results. These agents include phentolamine, nitrates, hydralazine, and selected calcium channel blockers. Of these agents, hydralazine and the calcium channel blocker niphedipine (Procardia) are probably the most effective. Lung transplantation may be a viable alternative in severe primary pulmonary hypertension that responds poorly to conventional therapies.

Shock

Shock is a condition in which perfusion to vital organs is inadequate to meet their metabolic needs. There are five general types of shock: hypovolemic, cardiogenic, septic (both hyperdynamic and hypodynamic), anaphylactic, and neurogenic. Table 20-10 differentiates among these categories according to their typical cardiopulmonary manifestations.

Common features of shock

Common to most forms of shock are certain endocrine and organ system responses. These are protective responses designed to assure continued perfusion to the vital organs.

Endocrine responses. Catecholamines, both epinephrine and norepinephrine, are elevated during shock. Elevation of catecholamine levels is a protective response that assures perfusion to vital organs. In hemorrhagic shock, increased catecholamines also promote hemostasis by facilitating blood coagulation. Although catecholamines dominate other hormones released during shock, their effects may be overcome by other factors. All forms of shock stimulate release of ACTH from the pituitary gland, increasing plasma levels of the glucocorticoids. Glucocorticoids have a mild inotropic effect on the heart, and may stabilize cell membranes to decrease movement of fluid from the intravascular space into the interstitium.

Organ system responses to shock. In response to shock, the kidneys conserve sodium and water. This occurs through the hormonal mechanisms described, and by the regulatory properties of the tubules themselves. The brain responds to shock with release of ACTH, ADH, and endorphins. The heart exhibits a decrease in myocardial contractility, due to decreased concentrations of calcium and increased levels of endorphins. Cardiac function during shock may be further compromised by: (1) decreased venous return, (2) increased afterload, and (3) decreased coronary blood flow.

The lungs respond to shock by increasing extravasation of protein and water into the interstitium, which may cause pulmonary edema. As previously discussed, increased extravasation of fluids in cardiogenic shock is due to increased pulmonary hydrostatic pressures. Increased extravasation of protein and water in septic and neurogenic shock, however, is due to increased capillary permeability.

Pulmonary edema due to cardiogenic or hypovolemic shock is easily managed, once the underlying problem is resolved. Pulmonary edema arising from septic or neurogenic shock is less readily cleared. In these cases, lung compliance decreases. Since perfusion of flooded alveoli continues, ventilation and perfusion becomes mismatched. The result is decreased arterial PO_2, increased shunting, and a widened A-a gradient.

Other responses. Shock can lead to disseminated intravascular coagulation, or DIC. This condition is characterized by platelet aggregation and fibrin deposition, with formation of thrombi throughout the microvasculature. These thrombi further complicate the patient's microcirculatory status, and may decrease the supply of oxygen and other nutrients to the tissues.

Hypovolemic shock

Hypovolemic shock is due to a decrease in intravascular fluid volume, resulting in decreased cardiac output and tissue perfusion. Decreased intravascular

Table 20-10 Cardiopulmonary response in shock

Type of shock	Pulmonary artery pressure	Systemic vascular resistance	Cardiac output
Hypovolemic	Decreased	Increased	Decreased
Septic (hyperdynamic)	Increased or decreased	Decreased	Increased
Septic (hypodynamic)	Decreased	Increased	Decreased
Cardiogenic	Increased	Increased	Decreased
Neurogenic	Decreased	Decreased	Increased or decreased
Anaphylactic	Decreased	Decreased	Increased or decreased

fluid volume may be due to hemorrhage, vomiting, diarrhea, or fluid loss in the bowel, peritoneal cavity, or interstitium.

In the early stages of hypovolemic shock, blood is diverted from organs that withstand ischemia well, such as the skin and skeletal muscle, to organs that withstand ischemia poorly, such as the kidneys, brain, and heart. Early in hypovolemic shock, the patient's mental status, pulse, blood pressure, and respiratory rate may all be normal. Careful examination often reveals postural changes in blood pressure, cool and clammy skin, flat neck veins, and concentrated urine.

If hypovolemia worsens, blood flow to the brain and heart eventually becomes insufficient to meet their metabolic needs. The patient may be anxious, agitated, confused, combative, or obtunded. Even in the supine position, the blood pressure is below normal. The pulse is rapid, weak and irregular, and the breathing pattern is deep and rapid.

Cardiogenic shock

Cardiogenic shock may be caused by myocardial disease, valvular disease, increased afterload, mechanical obstruction to venous return, or arrhythmias. Clinical signs and symptoms are those of severe acute left ventricular failure. The patient may be anxious, agitated, confused, combative, or obtunded. The patient usually has a rapid pulse, low blood pressure, and is tachypneic. Pulsus paradoxus may be present if the cause of the problem is pericardial tamponade. Unlike all other forms of shock, the neck veins are distended. Urine output is characteristically low.

Septic shock

Septic shock is due to the presence of bacteria in the blood stream (i.e., bacteremia). Common pathogens include gram-negative organisms associated with nosocomial infections. Among the most frequent causes of septic shock are urinary tract infections, artificial airways, IV related thrombophlebitis or contamination, postoperative infections, infected burns, and severe neutropenia, as may occur with cancer. The mortality rate for gram-negative sepsis is often over 50%. Sepsis may result in one of two forms of shock: hyperdynamic or hypodynamic (Table 20-10). Often hyperdynamic shock occurs first, followed by the more severe state of hypodynamic septic shock.

Anaphylactic shock

An anaphylactic reaction is an immediate and frequently fatal shock-like response. Anaphylaxis usually occurs within minutes after administration of foreign sera or drugs, especially penicillin and aspirin. Other drugs that can induce anaphylaxis are antisera such as tetanus antitoxin, protein-based drugs such as chymotrypsin or streptomycin, water-soluble iodine radiographic contrast media, and certain vaccines.

Symptoms of anaphylactic shock include apprehension, paresthesias, generalized urticaria or edema, choking, cyanosis, wheezing, cough, incontinence, low blood pressure, fever, dilation of pupils, loss of consciousness, and convulsions. Death may occur within 5 to 10 minutes.

Neurogenic shock

Neurogenic shock is due to generalized loss of vasomotor tone. Neurogenic shock may occur in spinal cord trauma, severe gastric dilatation, sudden pain, or the administration of a high spinal anesthetic. It leads to inadequate cardiac output and poor tissue perfusion. Patients suffering from neurogenic shock have rapid pulses and low blood pressures. The respiratory rate may be normal, as may the patient's mental status. The skin is usually warm and dry, and the neck veins are flat.

Treatment of shock

Management of shock involves fluid resuscitation, ventilatory and cardiac support, and drug therapy. Specific measures aim at correction of the underlying problem causing the inadequate perfusion. Special considerations are warranted in septic and anaphylactic shock.

Fluid resuscitation. The goal of fluid resuscitation in shock is to restore perfusion pressure to the vital organs. Fluid resuscitation is accomplished by IV administration of blood plasma, dextran, or isotonic electrolyte solutions in sufficient quantity to restore blood pressure, peripheral perfusion, and urine output. Central venous pressure (CVP) or pulmonary artery wedge pressure should be monitored to prevent fluid overload. Whole blood may be necessary in hypovolemic shock due to hemorrhaging.

Ventilatory and cardiac support. The first step is to establish an artificial airway and provide appropriate ventilatory support. Oxygen should be administered in as high a concentration as possible. In cases involving cardiac arrest, basic and advance cardiac life support measures are implemented (see Chapter 23). Support for a failing ventricle in cardiogenic shock may be provided by intra-aortic balloon counterpulsation.

Drug therapy. Hypovolemic shock and septic shock do not usually require drug therapy. Inotropic agents may be used to increase cardiac output in some patients. In cardiogenic or neurogenic shock, drug therapy is usually necessary. In cardiogenic shock, agents that reduce afterload on the left ventricle and increase its contractility are beneficial. In neurogenic shock, vasopressor agents may be of value. Diuretics reduce circulating fluid volume and decrease ventricular afterload. These are useful mainly in cardiogenic shock.

High dose corticosteroids have been used in septic shock, but their effectiveness remains uncertain. The best treatment for septic shock is early and aggressive intervention with appropriate antimicrobial drugs. Blood cultures should be taken whenever sepsis is suspected. Potential sources of infection, such as Foley catheters or IV infusions, should be identified. Quick elimination of these sources of bacteremia is often the most important step in management of septic shock.

In anaphylactic shock, epinephrine is administered immediately, usually followed by aminophylline. Hydrocortisone may also be useful in anaphylactic shock. Treatment is otherwise similar to that for neurogenic shock.

Embolic disorders

OEmbolic disorders, occur when a portion of the vasculature becomes blocked by abnormal material in the circulation. These disorders are a frequent cause of respiratory problems because the pulmonary circulation functions as a filter for the vascular system. Two types of embolism are common in management of patients receiving respiratory care: pulmonary thromboembolism and fat embolism.

Pulmonary thromboembolism

Seventy-five percent of pulmonary thromboemboli arise from clots occurring in the deep veins of the lower extremities. This event is common in older, bed-ridden patients and those having undergone extensive abdominal or pelvic surgery. Any sudden occurrence of pulmonary or cardiac distress in such patients should immediately suggest this diagnosis.

The clinical and laboratory features of pulmonary thromboembolism often depend on the size of the embolus. If obstruction occurs in a small terminal artery, clinical findings may be minimal or absent. Embolization of a medium-sized artery results in predominantly pulmonary symptoms and signs. Obstruction of a large artery is manifested predominantly by cardiac signs of acute right heart failure, with neck vein distention and liver engorgement. Massive embolism often progresses to shock, syncope, and sudden death.

Sudden onset of dyspnea is the most frequent symptom of pulmonary thromboembolism. Sudden dyspnea in any high-risk patient strongly suggests embolization of the pulmonary circulation. The patient with pulmonary thromboembolism often exhibits crackles (rales) and wheezing on auscultation. Signs of consolidation or pleural effusion may be present. Signs of consolidation are due to congestive atelectasis and infarction, which only occurs in about 10% of the cases. Pleuritic pain occurs mainly in those with severe embolization. Approximately one-third of these patients exhibit hemoptysis. Many of these respiratory signs and symptoms resemble those occurring in pneumonia. Table 20-11 lists key differences in the clinical presentation of these two disorders.

Cardiovascular signs may include tachycardia, accentuation of the second pulmonary sound, splitting of the second sounds of the aortic and pulmonary

Table 20-11 Pulmonary thromboembolism contrasted with bacterial pneumonia

	Thromboembolism	Pneumonia
SYMPTOMS		
Pain: Onset	Usually sudden	Sudden or gradual
Character	Often pleuritic	Usually pleuritic
Location	Usually lateralized	Usually lateralized
Severity	Variable	Variable
Cough	Uncommon until infarction	Usually present
Dyspnea	Mild to severe	Mild to severe
Sputum	More bloody	More purulent or rusty
Fever	None to moderate	Usually high
Chills	Rare	Common
Collateral history	Immobilization; previous phlebitis; postoperative, especially leg, hip, and pelvis; birth control medication; malignancy: CHF; prior PTE	Chronic alcoholism, COPD, bronchiectasis, diabetes, immunodeficient states
SIGNS		
Respiratory rate*	Rapid	Rapid
Pulse*	Rapid	Rapid
Chest examination	Often normal, especially early	Usually consolidated
Heart examination	Normal to frank failure	Usually normal
Extremities	Calf tenderness	Normal

From Mitchell RS: Synopsis of clinical pulmonary disease, ed 4, St Louis, 1988, Mosby.

valves, diastolic gallop, cyanosis, and elevated central venous pressure. Pulmonary signs, which may be transient, include tachycardia. Arterial blood gas analysis usually reveals hypoxemia with respiratory alkalosis. A normal PaO_2 generally excludes massive embolism.

The chest radiograph is usually negative. Areas of decreased pulmonary vascularity may be observed in massive embolism. Enlargement of a main pulmonary artery, elevation of a hemidiaphragm, and pleural effusion may be noted. Pulmonary densities due to congestive alelectasis or infarction may appear, but usually not until several days after the initial event.

Lung scans may be helpful in establishing the diagnosis. A normal perfusion scan generally rules out pulmonary embolism. Demonstration of normal ventilation of an area of lung that is not perfused strongly suggests pulmonary embolism. When either a major embolism is suggested or scanning is not definitive, pulmonary angiography can confirm the diagnosis.

Treatment of pulmonary thromboembolism depends upon its severity. Hypoxemia should be treated with oxygen, ideally 100%. Shock, if present, is managed with vasopressors. Intravenous heparin may be helpful in preventing further clotting. **Thrombolysis,** using urokinase or streptokinase, may help dissolve massive emboli of recent origin. Pulmonary embolectomy may be the only lifesaving measure for massive embolization. Pulmonary embolectomy requires cardiac bypass surgery. Pulmonary embolectomy may also be indicated if pulmonary hypertension results from chronic embolization.

Fat embolism

Fat embolism was originally thought to result from bone marrow embolization following long bone fracture. Bone fractures are just one of many potential types of trauma that can cause this disorder. Fat embolism syndrome manifests itself in neurologic dysfunction, respiratory insufficiency, and **petechiae** of the axilla, chest, and arms.

Following trauma, the blood concentration of fat macroglobules increases and peaks at about 12 hours. Blood levels return to normal within a few days. Increased concentration of fat macroglobules is greatest after fracture of the femur shaft. An increase also occurs after other types of fractures, and even has been observed after **laparotomy.** Other potential sources of fat macroglobules are: (1) coalescence of chylomicrons in response to stress or prolonged hypotension and (2) mobilization of subcutaneous fat. The fat globules are approximately 20 μm in diameter and are filtered by the lung. If present in large enough amounts, these globules block the pulmonary circulation and lead to right ventricular failure. Fat embolization may also occur in the brain, skin, and kidney. Brain embolization results in confusion, **nuchal** rigidity, and occasionally deep coma. Microembolization

of the capillaries in the skin produces the characteristic petechiae.

In the lung, breakdown of the trapped fat globules releases free fatty acids. These free fatty acids cause an increase in the level of kinins, which provoke local inflammatory reactions. Fatty acids may also cause **vasculitis,** and destroy pulmonary surfactant. The end result is pulmonary edema, decreased alveolar-capillary oxygen transfer, and severe hypoxemia. Free fatty acids may also cause thrombocytopenia and inhibit fibrinolysis, resulting in DIC.

Diagnosis of the fat embolism syndrome may be difficult. Fat globules in sputum and urine, along with elevated serum lipase values, are common after many forms of trauma. Patients with fat embolism syndrome exhibit a decreased hematocrit and platelet count, and may show changes in coagulation tests. Biopsy of the skin petechiae usually shows fat globules in the capillaries.

Once symptoms of the fat embolism syndrome develop, treatment is limited to supportive measures. Respiratory failure is managed as in the treatment of noncardiogenic pulmonary edema. Steroids in high doses may be beneficial.

RESPIRATORY COMPLICATION OF SURGERY

Respiratory complications are the primary cause of morbidity after major surgical procedures, and the second most important cause of postoperative death in elderly patients. Patients undergoing chest and upper abdominal operations are particularly prone to develop pulmonary complications. Surgery and anesthesia represent special hazards to those with a pre-existing chronic lung disease. The three most common respiratory complications associated with surgery are: atelectasis, pulmonary aspiration, and postoperative pneumonia.

Atelectasis

Atelectasis, is the most common postoperative pulmonary complication. It affects approximately 25% of patients recovering from abdominal surgery. Patients who have a reduced vital capacity as a result of either obstructive or restrictive lung disease are at particular risk. Abdominal or thoracic surgery almost always results in a further decrease in lung volumes. Atelectasis usually develops during the first or second postoperative day. It accounts for over 90% of the febrile episodes during this time period. The course of postoperative atelectasis is self-limiting in most patients, and recovery is uneventful.

Development of atelectasis involves obstruction of airways and other factors. Obstruction may result from an increase in the amount or tenacity of secretions caused by COPD, intubation, or anesthetic agents. Other factors that contribute to atelectasis include shallow breathing, splinting due to pain, and a transient decrease in surfactant production. Shallow breathing results in a progressive decrease in FRC. This pattern leads to alveolar collapse, particularly in the dependent portions of the lung. Since perfusion remains unchanged, a ventilation-perfusion mismatch causes arterial hypoxemia. Regions of atelectasis are especially prone to infection. If an area of the lung remains atelectatic for over 72 hours, pneumonia is almost certain.

Patients who develop atelectasis usually exhibit a fever of unknown origin and tachypnea. Physical examination may demonstrate elevation of the diaphragm on the affected side, scattered crackles (rales), and decreased breath sounds. These physical signs are not always present.

The best treatment for postoperative atelectasis is prevention. The likelihood of postoperative atelectasis can be minimized by early mobilization of the patient, frequent positional changes, and a vigorous regimen of deep breathing and coughing.

If atelectasis develops, treatment consists of airway clearance by chest percussion, coughing, and, if necessary, nasotracheal suction. Lung expansion therapy, including incentive spirometry and intermittent positive pressure breathing (IPPB) may be useful in facilitating deep breathing and re-expansion of atelectatic areas (see Chapter 27). Atelectasis due to obstruction of a large airway may require therapeutic bronchoscopy, a procedure that can usually be performed at the bedside with moderate sedation.

Pulmonary aspiration

Two thirds of all aspiration events follow thoracic or abdominal surgery. Of these, approximately 50% result in pneumonia. Nearly one third of patients with gross aspiration progressing to pneumonia die as a result of this condition.

In conscious, alert patients, protective mechanisms in the esophagus and pharynx normally prevent aspiration of oropharyngeal or gastric contents. Depression of the central nervous system by drug agents interferes with these defense mechanisms and increases the likelihood of aspiration. Other factors increasing the chances of aspiration are gastroesophageal reflux, food in the stomach, and supine or head down positioning. Some 80% of all patients with tracheostomies show evidence of one or more incidents of aspiration. This fact helps account for the high incidence of pulmonary infections among these patients.

The patient who suffers an aspiration episode typically exhibits tachypnea, crackles (rales), and signs of hypoxemia soon after the incident. Because the patients are often supine, the superior segments of the lower lobe are involved most often. Massive aspiration may progress quickly to cardiopulmonary arrest.

The extent of pulmonary injury caused by aspirated gastric contents is determined by the volume aspirated, the pH of the aspirate, and the frequency of the event. Aspirates with pH values of 2.50 or less cause immediate chemical pneumonitis. This chemical pneumonitis results in local edema and inflammation, and increases the likelihood of a secondary infection.

As with atelectasis, the best treatment for aspiration is prevention. The most important measures in the prevention of aspiration are to: (1) avoid general anesthesia in patients who have recently eaten, (2) properly position the patient before, during and after surgery, and (3) maintain a cuffed endotracheal tube in place until pharyngeal reflexes have completely returned.

If aspiration occurs, treatment involves reestablishing patency of the airway by vigorous suctioning. Bronchoscopy may be necessary. Corticosteroids may inhibit the inflammatory response of the lung parenchyma following massive aspiration of stomach contents.

Postoperative pneumonia

Some three fourths of hospital-acquired pneumonias occur in postoperative patients. In such patients, impairment of normal swallowing and respiratory clearance mechanisms allow bacteria to enter the lower respiratory tract. Atelectasis, aspiration, and copious secretions are important predisposing factors. Instrumentation of the respiratory tract, anesthesia, surgical pain, and use of narcotic-analgesics and sedatives all increase susceptibility of the host.

Risk of pneumonia is not the same for all surgical patients. Patients at greatest risk include the elderly, the severely obese, those with COPD or a history of smoking, and those with an artificial airway in place for prolonged periods of time. High risk patients can be identified by history and physical examination combined with spirometry.

It is not unusual for infecting bacteria to contaminate respiratory therapy equipment, such as ventilator circuits or nebulizers. *P aeruginosa* and *K pneumoniae* can thrive in the moist reservoirs of these devices, and have been the source of epidemic infections in critical care units.

Clinical manifestations of postoperative pneumonia are essentially those associated with the infecting organism. Fever, tachypnea, increased secretions, and physical changes characteristic of pulmonary consolidation are common findings. The chest X-ray often shows localized parenchymal consolidation.

Treatment of postoperative pneumonia consists of measures to aid the clearing of secretions, and the administration of antibiotics specific to the infecting organism.

Efforts to prevent postoperative pneumonia should start in the preoperative period. Such efforts should include evaluation of the patient's disease and risk factors. Concerted efforts should be made before elective surgery to have the patient stop smoking, improve nutrition, and correct gross obesity. In order to reduce exposure to antibiotic-resistant microorganisms, the preoperative hospital stay should be as short as possible. Training in deep breathing and effective coughing should be included as part of the preoperative regimen.

After surgery, early mobilization, vigorous respiratory care, and careful fluid and electrolyte balance are critical. If there is evidence of infection, bronchial hygiene measures and the administration of antibiotics specific to the offending organism should be instituted immediately.

BIBLIOGRAPHY

Aitken ML, Burke W, McDonald G, Shak S, Montgomery AB, Smith A: Recombinant human DNase inhalation in normal subjects and patients with cystic fibrosis, *JAMA* 267:1947, 1992.

Alberts WM, Brooks SM: Advances in occupational asthma, *Clin Chest Med* 13:281, 1992.

American Thoracic Society: Treatment of tuberculosis and tuberculosis infection in adults and children, *Am Rev Resp Dis* 134:355, 1986.

American Thoracic Society: Standards for the diagnosis and care of patients with chronic obstructive pulmonary disease (COPD) and asthma, *Am Rev Resp Dis* 136:225, 1987

American Thoracic Society: Indications and standards for cardiopulmonary sleep studies, *Am Rev Resp Dis* 139:559, 1989.

American Thoracic Society: Diagnostic standards and classification of tuberculosis, *Am Rev Respir Dis* 142:725-735, 1990.

American Thoracic Society: Control of tuberculosis in the United States, *Am Rev Respir Dis* 146:1623-1633, 1992.

Ampel NM, Wieden MA, Galgiani JN: Coccidioidomycosis: clinical update, *Rev Infect Dis* 11(6):897-911, 1989.

Atmar RL, Greenberg SB: Pneumonia caused by Mycoplasma pneumoniae and the TWAR agent, *Semin Respir Infect* 4:19, 1989,

Balmes JR: Surveillance for occupational asthma, *Occupat Med* 6:101, 1991.

Barnes DM: Strategies for an AIDS vaccine, *Science* 233:1149, 1986.

Barnes PF, Bloch AB, Davidson PT, Snider DE Jr: Tuberculosis in patients with human immunodeficiency virus infection, *N Engl J Med* 324:1644-1650, 1991.

Barnes PJ: A new approach to the treatment of asthma, *N Engl J Med* 321:1517, 1989.

Bartlett JG, et al: Bacteriology and treatment of primary lung abcess, *Am Rev Resp Dis* 109:510, 1974.

Baselski V: Microbiologic diagnosis of ventilator-associated pneumonia, *Infect Dis Clin N Amer* 7:331, 1993.

Baum GL, Wolinsky E: *Textbook of pulmonary diseases,* ed 4, Boston: 1989, Little, Brown.

Baydur A, Mili-Emile J: Respiratory mechanics in kyphoscoliosis, *Monaldi Arch Chest Dis* 48:69, 1993.

Bennett JV, Brachman PS (editors): *Hospital infections,* ed 3, Boston: 1986, Little, Brown.

Bernstein DI: Occupational asthma, *Med Clin North Am* 76:917, 1992.

Bjornson HS: Diagnosis and treatment of bacterial pneumonia in the intensive care unit: an overview, *Respir Care* 32(9):773-780, 1987.

Bloch AB, Rieder HL, Kelly GD: The epidemiology of tuberculosis in the United States, *Semin Respir Infect* 4(3):157-70, 1989.

Bodey GP, et al: Infections caused by *Pseudomonas aeruginosa, Rev Infect Dis* 5:279, 1983.

Boyars MC, Zwischenberger JF, Cox CS: Clinical manifestations of pulmonary fungal infections, *J Thor Imaging* 7:12, 1992.

Bradsher RW: Overwhelming pneumonia, *Med Clin North Am* 67(6):1233-50, 1983.

Bradsher RW: Blastomycosis, *Clin Infect Dis* 14(Suppl1):S82-90, 1992.

Buist AS: Asthma mortality: what have we learned? *J Allery Clin Immunol* 84:275, 1989.

Buist AS: Alpha 1-antitrypsin deficiency - diagnosis, treatment, and control: identification of patients, *Lung* 168(Suppl):543.

Burrows B, Knudson RJ, Kettrl LJ: *Respiratory insufficiency,* St Louis: 1975, Mosby.

Burrows B: Airways obstructive diseases: pathogenetic mechanisms and natural histories of the disorders, *Med Clin N Amer* 74:547, 1990.

Centers for Disease Control: Guidelines for preventing the transmission of tuberculosis in health care settings with special focus on HIV-related issues, *MMWR* 39:1, 1990.

Centers for Disease Control: National action plan to combat multidrug-resistant tuberculosis, *MMWR* 41(RR-11):5-48, 1992.

Clausen JL: The diagnosis of emphysema, chronic bronchitis, and asthma, *Clin Chest Med* 11:405, 1990.

Collins FS: Cystic fibrosis: molecular biology and therapeutic implications, *Science* 256:774, 1992.

Coolfont report: a PHS plan for prevention and control of AIDS and the AIDS virus, *Public Health Rep* 101:341, 1986.

Coombs RRA, Gell PGH, Lachmann PJ editors: *Clinical aspects of immunology,* ed 3, Oxford: England: 1975, Blackwell Scientific.

Coonrod JD: Pneumococcal pneumonia, *Semin Respir Infect* 4(1):4-11, 1989.

Cystic Fibrosis Foundation: Rationale for the use of human deoxyribonuclease I (rhDNase - Pulmozyme) in patients with cystic fibrosis, Cystic Fibrosis Foundation Volume IV, Section I, 1993.

Davies SF: Histoplasmosis: update 1989, *Semin Respir Infect* 5(2):93-104, 1990.

DeLorenzo LJ, Huang CT, Maguire GP, Stone DJ: Roentgenographic patterns of Pneumocystis carinii pneumonia in 104 patients with AIDS, *Chest* 91:323, 1987.

Des Jardins T: *Clinical manifestations of respiratory disease,* ed 2, St Louis: 1990, Mosby

Dhainaut JF, Brunet F: Right ventricular performance in adult respiratory distress syndrome, *Europ Resp Journal* 11(Suppl):490S, 1990.

Dierkesmann R: Indication and results of endobronchial laser therapy, *Lung* 168(Suppl):1095, 1990.

Dilworth JP, White RJ: Postoperative chest infection after upper abdominal surgery: an important problem for smokers, *Respir Med* 86:205, 1992.

Doebbeling BN, Wenzel RP: The epidemiology of *Legionella pneumophila* infections, *Semin Respir Infect* 2(4):206-221, 1987.

Donahoe M, Rogers RM: Nutritional assessment and support in chronic obstructive pulmonary disease, *Clin Chest Med* 11:487, 1990.

Dooley SW Jr, Castro KG, Hutton MD, et al: Guidelines for preventing the transmission of tuberculosis in health-care settings, with special focus on HIV-related issues, *MMWR* 39(RR17):1-29, 1990.

Dunn WF, Scanlon PD: Preoperative pulmonary function testing for patients with lung cancer, *Mayo Clin Proc* 68:371, 1993.

Elborn JS, Shale DJ, Britton JR: Cystic fibrosis: current survival and population estimates to the year 2000, *Thorax* 46:881, 1991.

Elliot CG: Pulmonary physiology during embolism, *Chest* 101(Suppl):163S, 1992.

Falk JL, O'Brien JF, Kerr R: Fluid resuscitation in traumatic hemorrhagic shock, *Crit Care Clin* 8:323, 1992.

Farzan S: *A concise handbook of respiratory diseases,* ed 2, East Norwalk, Conn: 1985 Appleton & Lange.

Feldman S, Stokes DC: Varicella zoster and herpes simplex virus pneumonias, *Semin Respir Infect* 2(2):84-94, 1987.

Fink JN: Hypersensitivity pneumonitis, *Clin Chest Med* 13(2):303-309, 1992.

Fink JN, deShazo R: Immunologic aspects of granulomatous and interstitial lung diseases, *JAMA* 258(20):2938-2944, 1987.

Fletcher EC: Chronic lung disease in the sleep apnea syndrome, *Lung* 168(Suppl):751, 1990.

Forshag MS, Cooper AD: Postoperative care of the thoracotomy patient, *Clin Chest Med* 13:33, 1992.

George RB, Owens MW: Bronchial asthma, *Dis Mon* 37:137, 1991.

Goble M: Drug-resistant tuberculosis, *Sem Respir Infect* 1:220-229, 1986.

Goedert JJ: Testing for human immunodeficiency virus, *Ann Intern Med* 105:609, 1986.

Gold JW. Overview of infection with the human immunodeficiency virus: infectious complications, *Clin Chest Med* 9:377-386, 1988.

Graman PS, Hall CB: Nosocomial viral respiratory infections, *Semin Respir Infect* 4(4):253-260, 1989.

Greenberg SB: Viral pneumonia, *Infect Dis Clin North Am* 5(3):603-621, 1991.

Gross NJ: Chronic obstructive pulmonary disease; current concepts and therapeutic approaches, *Chest* 97(Suppl):19S, 1990.

Haque AK: Pathology of common pulmonary fungal infections, *J Thor Imaging* 7:1, 1992.

Health and Public Policy Committee, American College of Physicians, and the Infectious Disease Society of America: Acquired immunodeficiency syndrome (position paper), *Ann Intern Med* 104:575, 1986.

Henderson FW: Pulmonary infections with respiratory syncytial virus and the parainfluenza viruses, *Semin Respir Infect* 2(2):112-121, 1987.

Horowitz ML, Schiff M, Samuels J, Russo R, Schnader J: Pneumocystis carinii pleural effusion. Pathogenesis and pleural fluid analysis, *Am Rev Resp Dis* 148:232, 1993.

Hudgel DW: Mechanisms of obstructive sleep apnea, *Chest* 101:541, 1992.

Hudgel DW: The role of upper airway anatomy and physiology in obstructive sleep apnea, *Clin Chest Med* 13:383, 1992.

Ingram RH, Fanta CH: *Neuromuscular processes.* In Scientific American Medicine, New York: 1988, Scientific American.

Kaliner MA: How the current understanding of the pathophysiology of asthma influences our approach to therapy, *J Allerg Clin Immunol* 92(Part 2):144, 1993.

Kaplan J, Staats BA: Obstructive sleep apnea syndrome, *Mayo Clin Proc* 65:1087, 1990.

Kaye MG, Fox MJ, Bartlett JG, et al.: The clinical spectrum of Staphylococcus aureus pulmonary infection, *Chest* 97(4):788-792, 1990.

Kearon C, Viviani GB, Kirkley A, Killian KJ: Factors determining pulmonary function in adolescent idiopathic thoracic scoliosis, *Am Rev Resp Dis* 148:288, 1993.

Kelly BJ, Luce JM: The diagnosis and management of neuromuscular diseases causing respiratory failure, *Chest* 99:1485, 1991.

Kimoff RJ, Cosio MG, McGregor M: Clinical features and treatment of obstructive sleep apnea, *Can Med Assoc J* 144:689, 1991.

Klotman ME, Hamilton JD: Cytomegalovirus pneumonia, *Semin Respir Infect* (2):95-103, 1987.

Lapp NL, Parker JE: Coal workers' pneumoconiosis, *Clin Chest Med* 13:243, 1992.

Larsen GL: Hypersensitivity lung disease, *Annu Rev Immunol* 3:59-85, 1985.

Leigh MW, Clyde WA Jr: Chlamydial and mycoplasmal pneumonias, *Semin Respir Infect* 2(3):152-158, 1987.

Levine SJ, White DA: *Pneumocystis carinii, Clin Chest Med* 9(3):395-423, 1988.

Levison ME, Kaye D: Pneumonia caused by gram-negative bacilli: an overview, *Rev Infect Dis* 7(Suppl)4:S656-65, 1985.

Levitz SM. Aspergillosis, *Infect Dis Clin North Am* 3(1): 1-18, 1989.

Martin L: *Pulmonary physiology in clinical practice:* the essentials for patient care and evaluation, St Louis: Mosby, 1987.

Mathewson HS. Treatment of pulmonary mycobacterial infections, *Respir Care* 35(5):427-429, 1990.

Matthay RA, Niederman MS, Weidemann HP: Cardiovascular-pulmonary interaction in chronic obstructive pulmonary disease with special reference to the pathogenesis and management of cor pulmonale, *Med Clin N Amer* 74:571, 1990.

Merigan TC: *Respiratory viral infections.* In Scientific American Medicine, New York: 1988 Scientific American.

Mitchell RS, Petty TL, Schwartz MI: *Synopsis of clinical pulmonary disease,* ed 4, St Louis: 1988, Mosby.

Moser KM, Auger Wr, Fedullo PF, Jamieson SW: Chronicthromboembolic pulmonary hypertension: clinical picture and surgical treatment, *Europ Resp Journal* 5:334, 1992.

Mountain RD, Heffner JE, Brackett NC, Sahn SA: Acid-base disturbances in acute asthma, *Chest* 98:651, 1990.

Muder RR, Yu VL, Fang GD: Community-acquired Legionnaires' disease, *Semin Respir Infect* 4(1):32-39, 1989.

Murphy TF, Sethi S: Bacterial infection in chronic obstructive pulmonary disease, *Am Rev Resp Dis* 146:1067, 1992.

National Institutes of Health, National Asthma Education Program: Guidelines for the diagnosis and management of asthma, Bethesda Md, 1991, US Department of Health and Human Services [Publication No. 91-3042A].

Nicotra MB, Rivera M: Chronic bronchitis: when and how to treat, *Semin Respir Infect* 3:61, 1988.

Partinen M, Telakivi T: Epidemiology of obstructive sleep apnea syndrome, *Sleep* 15(Suppl):S1, 1992.

Peterman TA, Curran JW: Sexual transmission of human immunodeficiency virus, *JAMA* 256:2222, 1986.

Quinones CA, Memon MA, Sarosi GA: Bacteremic *Hemophilus influenzae* pneumonia in the adult, *Semin Respir Infect* 4(1):12-8, 1989.

Ramsey BW, Farrell PM, Pencharz P: Nutritional assessment and management in cystic fibrosis: a consensus report, *Am J Clin Nutr* 55:108, 1992.

Remetz MS, Clemen MW, Cabin HS: Pulmonary and pleural complications of cardiac disease, *Clin Chest Med* 10:545, 1989.

Reynolds HY: Immunologic lung diseases (part 1), *Chest* 81(5):626-631, 1982.

Reynolds HY: Immunologic lung disease (part 2), *Chest* 81(6):745-751, 1982.

Robin ED, Cross CE, Zelis R: Pulmonary edema, *N Engl J Med* 288:239, 292, 1973.

Rose RM, Pinkston P, O'Donnell C, Jensen WA: Viral infection of the lower respiratory tract, *Clin Chest Med* 8(3):405-418, 1987.

Ruben FL, Cate TR: Influenza pneumonia, *Semin Respir Infect* 2(2):122-129, 1987.

Ruben FL, Nguyen ML: Viral pneumonitis, *Clin Chest Med* 12(2):223-35, 1991.

Sabanathan S, Eng J, Mearns AJ: Alterations in respiratory mechanics following thoracotomy, *J R Coll Surg Edinb* 35:144, 1990.

Sahn SA: The pathophysiology of pleural effusions, *Annu Rev Med* 41:7, 1990.

Sarosi GA: Community-acquired fungal diseases, *Clin Chest Med* 12(2):337-347, 1991.

Seale DD, Beaver BM: Pathophysiology of lung cancer, *Nurs Clin North Am* 27:603, 1992.

Seeger W, Gunther A, Walmrath HD, Grimminger F, Lasch HG: Alveolar surfactant and adult respiratory distress syndrome:

pathogenetic role and therapeutic prospects, *Clin Investigator* 71:177, 1993.

Shanley JD, Jordan MC: Viral pneumonia in the immuno-compromised patient, *Semin Respir Infect* 1(3):193-201, 1986.

Shepard JW, Olsen KD: Uvulopalatophyaryngoplasty for treatment of obstructive sleep apnea, *Mayo Clin Proc* 65:1260, 1990.

Snider GL: Emphysema: the first two centuries-and beyond, *Am Rev Resp Dis* 146:1615, 1992.

Spence TH: Pneumonia, in Civetta JM, Taylor RW, Kirby RR (editors): *Critical care,* ed 2, Philadelphia, 1992, JB Lippincott.

Spinelli A, Marconi G, Gorini M, Pizzi A, Scano G: Control of breathing in patients with myasthenia gravis, *Am Rev Resp Dis* 145:1359, 1992.

Sugerman HJ: Pulmonary function in morbid obesity, *Gastroenterol Clin Noth Am* 16:225, 1987.

Swartz MN: Clinical aspects of legionnaires' disease, *Ann Intern Med* 90:492, 1979.

Thomas PD, Hunninghake GW: Current concepts of the pathogenesis of sarcoidosis, *Am Rev Respir Dis* 135(3):747-760, 1987.

Thurlbeck WM: Pathophysiology of chronic obstructive pulmonary disease, *Clin Chest Med* 11:389, 1990.

Tisi GM: *Pulmonary physiology in clinical medicine,* ed 2, Baltimore: 1984, Williams & Wilkins.

US Department of Health and Human Services, Public Health Service: Prevention and control of influenza: Recommendations of the immunization practices advisory committee, *MMWR* 41(RR-9):1-17, 1992.

Volosky RL, Rubin FL: The re-emergence of tuberculosis: a previously forgotten disease becomes a problem for caregivers [editorial], *Respir Care* 38:880-883, 1993.

Wait MA, Estreta A: Changing clinical spectrum of spontaneous pneumothorax, *Am J Surg* 164:528, 1992.

Wentzel RP (editor): *Prevention and control of nosocomial infections,* Baltimore: 1987 Williams & Wilkins.

Wilson DO, Rogers RM, Wright EC, Anthonisen NR: Body weight in chronic obstructive pulmonary disease, *Am Rev Resp Dis* 139:1435, 1989.

Wright JL, Cagle P, Chrug A, Colby TV, Myers J: Diseases of the small airways, *Am Rev Resp Dis* 146:240, 1992.

5

Basic

Therapeutics

Pharmacology for Respiratory Care

■

James A. Peters

Barbara A. Peters

Respiratory pharmacology involves the use of chemical agents or drugs that affect the lungs. Generally, drugs are useful to the extent that they can maintain, enhance, or alter bodily function when a patient cannot cope with a particular disease. Determining when drugs are necessary is the responsibility of the physician. Administering and monitoring the effect of selected pulmonary drugs is the responsibility of the respiratory care practitioner (RCP).

Although competent RCPs should have general knowledge of most common drugs used in the care of their patients, they must have in-depth understanding of airway pharmacology. These drugs include bronchodilators, mucolytics, expectorants, steroids, and selected antimicrobial agents. Additionally, local anesthetics, such as xylocaine, are often used during arterial puncture and may also be nebulized before bronchoscopy.[1] Only by the intelligent and careful application of these potent chemicals can the desired therapeutic objectives be achieved without undo risk.

PRINCIPLES OF PHARMACOLOGY

A drug is a chemical substance that exerts a biologic effect.[2] Medically, a drug can be defined as a substance that is used for the treatment, diagnosis, or prevention of disease.[3] Pharmacology is the study of how drugs affect the body and how the body acts upon drugs. Specifically, pharmacology concerns six basic areas: (1) the chemical and physical properties of drugs, (2) the physiologic effects and site of action of drugs, (3) how drugs exert their effects or the "mechanism of action," (4) what the body does with drugs, i.e., the **absorption,** distribution, metabolism, and excretion of drugs, (5) dosages and routes of administration of drugs, and (6) side effects and toxicity. Understanding these six basic areas for each of the respiratory drugs one administers to patients is required for proper patient care.

Drug nomenclature

Practitioners will encounter many different drug names. Medications can be described by their chemical name, generic name, or their brand name. Table 21-1 lists the system of nomenclature of pharmacologic agents. In this text the generic name will be used, and if the brand name is mentioned it will appear in parentheses following the generic name.

Routes of administration

In order for a drug to exert a therapeutic effect, it must become available for absorption. Availability of a drug to the body depends on both its form (solid, liquid, or gas), and its route of administration.

There are three major routes available for the administration of therapeutic drug agents: (1) gastrointestinal (oral, nasogastric tube or rectal), (2) **parenteral** (injection, IV), and (3) topical. Topical includes not only medications directly applied to the skin but also applied directly to the lungs by inhalation. Selec-

Table 21-1 Naming of drugs

Name	Explanation	Example
Chemical name	Name based on chemical structure	1-(3,5-dihydroxyphenyl)-2-isopropylaminoethanol
Generic name	Common name; may reflect chemical name	Metaproterenol, orciprenaline
Brand name	The name that is used by the manufacturer	Alupent, Metaprel

Modified from Ziment I: Respiratory pharmacology and therapeutics, Philadelphia, 1978, WB Saunders.

tion of the "best" route for the administration of a drug depends on:
1. The available form(s) of the drug;
2. The desired rate of onset and duration of action of the drug;
3. The safety of the available route(s);
4. Whether a local or **systemic** (body-wide) effect is desired;
5. Whether or not the patient can swallow and retain an oral preparation;
6. The stability of the agent in gastrointestinal fluids;
7. The relative amount of the drug needed;
8. The convenience of the available route(s) administration

In general, the gastrointestinal route, specifically oral administration, is a safe, convenient, and economical way to administer most drugs. However, the majority of medications used in respiratory care are administered by inhalation and these have many of the same advantages of orally administered medications. Drug forms available for oral administration include pills, capsules, water solutions, alcohol elixirs, and emulsions. Rectal administration methods include suppositories and liquid solutions.

Parenteral routes are those involving drug administration by injection. This includes **subcutaneous, intramuscular,** and **intravenous** routes.

Topical routes include those methods whereby a drug agent is applied directly to the skin or mucous membranes. Lotions and ointments applied to the skin usually have only a local effect; whereas, skin patch **(transdermal)** medications like nicotine or estrogen use the skin circulation to deliver the drug to the rest of the body. The application of a drug agent to the mouth or nose can result in rapid absorption and subsequent local systemic effects.

Inhalation represents a special case of topical drug administration. In order to administer a drug agent by inhalation, it must first be either vaporized or placed in an aerosol suspension. Generally, this approach requires special equipment, such as aerosol generators or vaporizers (refer to Chapter 25). Metered-dose inhalers (MDI) are most commonly used to administer bronchodilators and at times a compressor pump is used to power a nebulizer of medication solution.

The immediate site of action by inhaled medica-

tions is in the airways. The secondary effects are systemic after absorption across the alveolar-capillary membrane. The dose received by inhalation depends on the depth of inhalation, how long the breath is held before exhalation, the concentration of the medication, and the number of breaths taken or duration of the treatment. The exact dose received is not certain since up to 80% of inhaled medicine is exhaled before deposition in the lungs. Some of the medication is swallowed and the remainder is retained in the lungs (10% to 20%). The use of devices (spacers) which attach to the mouthpiece of an MDI and add several inches of deadspace, can enhance the deposition of respirable sized particles. Some new breath actuated MDI devices have been introduced which should improve overall delivery of inhaled medication. Inhalation delivery of bronchodilator medications remains the most effective treatment for respiratory patients.

Drug administration

The safe use of drugs requires awareness of many different factors:
1. Mode of action
2. Side effects
3. Toxicity
4. Range of common dosages
5. Rate and route of excretion
6. Individual differences in response
7. Interaction with other drugs or food
8. Contraindications

Like any medication, respiratory drugs can cause undesirable effects. There is a small risk of bacteria or other contaminants riding the aerosolized particles into the lungs. This is more likely with improperly cleaned nebulizers. When medications are prepared for nebulization, the practitioner must observe proper handling and cleaning of the aerosolizing equipment. Disposable MDI's are less likely to carry this risk. Additionally, inhaled medications can leave an unpleasant taste in the mouth and in the case of inhaled steroids, can impair immunity.

To minimize problems associated with the delivery or use of medications one should follow recommended guidelines. The first concern is to make sure that the medication order is clear, understandable, and makes sense. The following box identifies the minimum requirements for a proper prescription for respiratory care related drugs. The practitioner should seek clarification from the physician if the order does not specify the necessary information.

Confirming drug prescription and administration information

1. Prescriptions should include:
   a. Patient's name
   b. Drug name
   c. Dose
   d. Frequency it is to be given
   e. Duration of administration (for some aerosol treatments)
   f. Route of administration
   g. Signature of physician
2. Before administering the prescribed drug the practitioner should double check:
   a. Patient's chart for order
   b. Patient's name band
   c. Check for medication allergies
   d. Medication labels
   e. Dates on medication
   f. Dosage
   g. Charted response to previous drug administration

When administering a medication, nothing should be taken for granted. The practitioner should always double check all information. If an error is suspected or a question arises, the practitioner should not proceed until satisfied that all is in proper order.

Although there are standard dosages routinely pre-scribed for patients, drug administration should always be individualized according to patients' needs. Individualized drug treatment is particularly important for the very young and very old. This is because adverse effects are more common in those patient populations.

BASIC PHARMACOKINETICS

It is well recognized that some drugs work better than others. The *efficacy* of a drug represents its peak or maximum biological effect. This is the most important feature of a medication since it determines whether or not a drug will have the effect one desires. On the other hand, the *potency* of a drug is its biological activity per unit weight, or the amount of drug required to produce a given effect.

Potency and Efficacy

Figure 21-1 illustrates the concepts of drug potency (the strength) and efficacy (the effectiveness) for two different drugs, labeled X and Y. Relative dosage is plotted on a horizontal logarithmic axis, with effect (measured as percent response) plotted on the vertical axis. Both drugs exhibit the typical "S" shaped dose-response curve, and both exert a comparable maximum effect (R_{max}). However, drug X achieves this maximum effect at a dosage some ten times lower than that required by drug Y. Thus drug X is said to be more *potent* than drug Y. Nonetheless, both drugs are capable of producing the same maximum effect and, therefore, have the same *efficacy*.

Figure 21-2 illustrates differences in efficacy between two drugs, labeled C and D. Clearly, drug C is

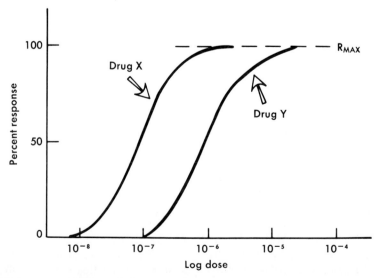

Fig. 21–1 Comparison of potency of two drug agents. (From Lehnert BE, Schachter EN: The pharmacology of respiratory care, St Louis, 1980, Mosby.)

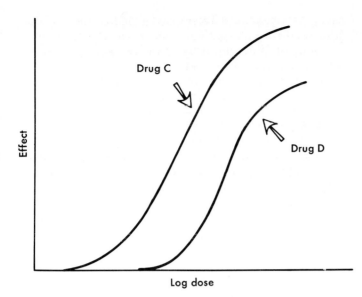

Fig. 21-2 Comparison of efficacy of two drug agents. (From Lehnert BE and Schachter EN: The Pharmacology of respiratory care, St Louis, 1980, Mosby.)

more potent than drug D, producing its effect at a substantially lower dose. In addition, the maximum effect of drug C (indicated by the highest portion of the dose-response curve) is greater than that of drug D. This indicates that drug C also has a greater efficacy than drug D. Although potency is important in determining the dosage of a particular agent, our primary goal is to use a drug that produces the desired effect with minimal side effects.

A *side effect* represents any effect produced by a drug other than its desired effect. Every drug has side effects. Some side effects can be significant health threats while others may be of no apparent concern. A "drug of choice" is a drug that best achieves the desired response with the fewest side effects. An example of a side effect is a respiratory drug that increases heart rate. This is an undesired response since a drug that was given for pulmonary purposes is producing a cardiovascular effect. Typically, the dose that can be given a patient is limited by the side effects it produces. Some people may have an increased *sensitivity* to a particular medicine and when given a normal dose show a marked reaction, but when given a small dose may respond quite favorably.

An increased sensitivity to a medication should not be confused with an allergic reaction to a medication. An allergic reaction is the most feared side effect from a medication since it can be life threatening. Allergies result when the immune system has been sensitized against a particular drug by a previous exposure. When the body is presented with the drug again the immune system responds causing the release of various biochemical agents. The severest form of allergy results in a *anaphylatic* reaction which can produce

marked respiratory distress and shock which without treatment can be fatal.

Because side effects can interfere and complicate the management of a patient's condition, careful monitoring of the patient is essential—especially after a drug is given for the first few times.

Also related to the body's response to chemical agents is the concept of *half-life* ($T_{1/2}$). Half-life is a measure of how rapidly a drug is inactivated or excreted from the body. Specifically, half-life refers to how much time it takes the body to decrease a given concentration of a drug to half its initial level. For example, if the $T_{1/2}$ of a drug is 2 hours, and its initial concentration after a given dose is 10 ng/mL of blood, then two hours later the concentration will drop to 5 ng/mL and 4 hours later it will be 2.5 ng/mL and so on. Half-life varies according to the chemical makeup of the pharmacologic agent, and determines how often a drug needs to be given to maintain a therapeutic level.

Half-life also varies according to the patient's condition. For example, the half-life of a drug administered to a geriatric patient may be prolonged because of compromised liver function. Likewise, a drug given to a premature infant may stay in the body longer because necessary enzyme systems are not yet fully developed. In these patients a smaller dose must be used or the drug must be given less frequently.

The liver is responsible for the metabolism and inactivation of most drugs. The kidneys, via the urine, is the major route for drugs, or their metabolites, to be eliminated from the body. Typically, enzymatic processes in the liver convert a drug to a less active form or help to make it more water soluble so it can be eliminated by the kidneys more readily. Enzymes capable of inactivating drugs are also found in other organ systems. For example, the stomach contains an enzyme capable of inactivating the bronchodilator isoproterenol, while an enzyme in the blood plasma can break down and inactivate the neuromuscular blocking agent succinylcholine.

The absorption, activity, and excretion of drugs are affected by both the chemical nature of the drug itself and the characteristics of the body fluids in which they exist. For example, drugs that are lipid soluble can readily diffuse across cell membranes. Those chemical agents that ionize (separate into positive and negative molecules or ions) are not lipid soluble and will not cross cell membranes. The degree of ionization of a drug will affect its cellular absorption and activity. *Un*ionized drugs cross membranes readily whereas ionized drugs do not.

For agents that form ions in solution, the degree of ionization is determined by both the surrounding pH (acidity or alkalinity) and the dissociation constant of the drug, or its pKa. The pKa of a drug is the pH at which it is 50% ionized. Drugs that are weak acids, such as salicylic acid (aspirin), have low dissociation constants (the pKa for salicylic acid is 3.5). On the other hand, drugs that are weak bases, such as quinine have high dissociation constants (the pKa for quinine is 8.2).

In general, when the pH of body fluids equals the pKa of the drug, we can expect 50% ionization. With weak acids, less ionization (and therefore greater absorption across cell membranes) will occur when the pH is lower (more acidic) than the pKa. The greater the acidity in the tissue, the more the free hydrogen ion (H^+) of a weak acid will be "pushed" back onto the drug thereby resulting in less ionization. In contrast, drugs that are weak bases tend to dissociate *less* when the environment is more alkaline (higher pH) than their pKa values. For example, in the stomach (with a strong acid, HCl, pH of about 1.0), salicylic acid (weak acid) remains mostly unionized and is therefore readily absorbed through the gastric mucosa. However, at this pH, quinine is almost completely ionized and poorly absorbed in the stomach. For these reasons, the acid-base status effects the uptake, distribution, bioavailability, and excretion of drugs.

Since the kidneys are the major route of excretion for most drugs, the plasma and urine pH, by their affect on drug ionization and lipid solubility, are important determinants of drug clearance from the body. In contrast to cellular absorption, urinary excretion is enhanced when a drug or drug metabolite is in ionized form (more water soluble) in the urine filtrate. Ionization of the agent minimizes its reabsorption back through the renal tubular cells, thereby facilitating its clearance in the urine. Of course, any compromise in kidney function can impair drug excretion and thereby lead to toxic drug levels. Patients with renal failure must have careful selection of medications so as to minimize toxic accumulation.

Weight, and more specifically, the percent body fat, as well as the size of a person, represents another influence on response to a given dose of a drug. A person with more body fat has greater storage sites for fat-soluble drugs. The larger a person, the greater the body water content and the more dilution will occur for a given dose of medication. This may result in drug concentration levels that may be less than effective. However, the size and amount of fat are less of a concern with drugs that are topically applied, such as those administered directly to the lungs by inhalation of aerosol.

Repeated use of a specific drug may result in a decreased response to the same dose. This phenomenon, known as *tolerance,* can be seen in asthmatic patients who have become "trigger happy" with their aerosol cartridge inhalers and dose themselves too frequently. They then find the medicine less effective than it otherwise would be for a given dose. For some drugs, tolerance can develop very rapidly, in minutes or hours. This rapid development of tolerance is called *tachyphylaxis.* Tolerance to medications is best addressed through patient education. Often, a combination of different drugs can be employed, thus minimizing the likelihood of tolerance to a specific drug. Drugs which work on the adrenergic system can be used in combination with those having anti-cholinergic action. These will be discussed in following sections.

Another factor that can alter the expected response to a given drug is *interaction* with other drugs. Since the average hospitalized patient receives about 10 different medications, the potential for undesired interactions resulting in adverse effects are very real.[4] It is difficult to predict what effect various drugs will have when combined together, hence the goal is to use as few drugs as is necessary as we monitor the patient for unwanted effects.

Drug interactions can result in *additive* effects, whereby the action of two drugs together equals the sum of their individual effects. Alternatively, administration of two or more drugs together can result in *potentiation,* whereby each increases the effect of the other, often in a greater than additive effect.[5] This is also referred to as *synergism* or the *multiplicative* effect. On the other hand, one drug may be able to block or *antagonize* the action of another agent, thereby lessening the effects or even rendering the first drug totally ineffective.

Additional factors that affect the response a patient has may be the time of administration, the pathologic state of the patient, genetic factors, and psychological factors.[6] For example, *when* a drug is given may influence the drug effect, since many body processes vary in a cyclic manner throughout the day (due to the body's diurnal or circadian rhythm). There may be some times during the day when a drug has greater effect than at other times. The pathologic condition of the patient is also important. Pathology of body systems such as the liver or kidneys may not allow inactivation or excretion of the drugs as expected, thus possibly leading to adverse side effects. Genetically, a person may lack certain enzymes that a particular drug requires to exert its effect. Last, the psychological state of the patient can play an important part in the effectiveness of the drug. Belief that a drug will work typically results in a better therapeutic outcome. In fact, some people can show improvement from taking an inert substance simply by believing that it will be beneficial for him. This *placebo effect* is real. Even the practitioner's attitude and confidence can have an impact on the outcome results, possibly making the difference between a good versus a marginal response to a given drug regimen.

Receptor theory of drug action

Drugs are thought to produce their effects either by acting directly at some specific receptor site, or by acting diffusely at many tissues. Those acting diffusely are termed *saturation-dependent* or nonreceptor drugs and include alcohol, hypnotics, anesthetics, and mucus–diluting agents such as water and saline. However, the majority of drugs act at receptor sites.

A *receptor* is a specific protein-related molecule embedded within and protruding out of cell membranes where reversible bonds can be formed with specific drugs. When a drug binds to the receptor, a molecular change occurs which is transmitted to the inside of the cell. This changes the biochemistry within the cell. Receptor-drug interaction has been likened to the action between a lock and a key. Receptors (the lock) are very specific as to what drugs (keys) will bond there. The shape, the size, and the **polarity** (electric charge) of the drug molecule has to be within the range of the receptor's specifications or no drug effect will occur. *Affinity* is the tendency a drug has to combine with a receptor.[5] If a drug has affinity and produces an effect, it is termed an *agonist.* A *partial agonist* is a drug that has affinity but cannot produce the full effect (results in only a *partial* effect).

In contrast, an *antagonist* is a drug that has affinity but produces no effect. An antagonist is capable of blocking any effect that an agonist would produce if the antagonist gets to the receptor first. This would be like putting a toothpick in a lock, thus not allowing the key to work. The toothpick fits inside the lock but is not able to open it. An antagonist can be *competitive* (forms reversible bond with receptor) or *noncompetitive* (forms irreversible bond), depending on the type of chemical bonds formed between the receptor and the drug.

The specificity of a drug is extremely important. Receptors will not respond to just any chemical that comes along. Only specific chemicals will have an effect on the receptor. This allows one to target a specific organ or a specific response by the body while at the same time limiting unwanted effects. The challenge of pharmacologists is to create medications which have only the effects one desires. Many of the most common bronchodilators have been derived from epinephrine which not only relaxes airway smooth muscles but has multiple effects all over the body. Pharmacologists have modified epinephrine and come up with drugs that work well on the airway cell receptors but have little affinity for cell receptors elsewhere in the body, such as the heart. The understanding of receptor-drug interactions has made this possible.

Pharmacodynamics of the nervous system

The nervous system and the endocrine system are the body's internal communication network. The nervous system is capable of rapid response and specific control, while the endocrine system is slower in its response and typically less precise in its effects. Both systems help regulate the body internally; this process of regulation is referred to as **homeostasis.** Both systems are similar in that pharmacologic agents can interact with them at receptor sites and thereby modify functions at selected tissue locations.

Looking closer at the nervous system we can classify it into several major divisions, as follows:

A. Central nervous system
B. Peripheral nervous system
  1. Somatic nervous system
  2. Autonomic nervous system
    (a) Sympathetic nervous system
    (b) Parasympathetic nervous system

The *central nervous system* (CNS) consists of the brain and spinal cord, and the *peripheral nervous system* consists of those nerve pathways that are outside of the CNS. These pathways can be functionally divided into the *afferent* pathways—those that conduct information to CNS—and the *efferent* pathways—those that conduct information away from the CNS.

The *somatic nervous system,* which is under conscious control, conducts impulses from the CNS to the skeletal muscles. The *autonomic nervous system,* in contrast, functions without conscious control, although **biofeedback** techniques can affect some of its functions. The autonomic system gets its name from the fact that it performs its many duties, minute by minute, whether we are awake or asleep, automatically. Among other things, the autonomic nerves govern the activities of the cardiac muscle, the smooth or involuntary muscles of all body systems (such as the **genitourinary,** pulmonary and cardiovascular systems), the sweat glands, and certain endocrine glands. Functioning of the autonomic nerve system is vital for maintaining homeostasis.

The autonomic division is itself divided into two competitive subdivisions, *sympathetic* and *parasympathetic* (Figure 21-3 on page 512). Most of the organ systems are innervated by both divisions. Balance between these two opposing divisions provides precise control of organ function. Generally, the effects of each subdivision of the autonomic nervous system on a given receptor organ are antagonistic to the other; inactivity of one allows the action of the other to dominate the organ response. Each thus exerts a constant action against the other, like two forces maintaining a steady pull on each end of a rope. This action is called *tone,* and it establishes a balance of influence on receptor function, providing fine control and rapid response.

The sympathetic division is designed mainly to maintain the safety of the entire organism, which expends energy. The parasympathetic division, on the other hand, is less dynamic in its response and is more concerned with preserving and restorating function. Table 21-2 on page 512 summarizes the major differ-

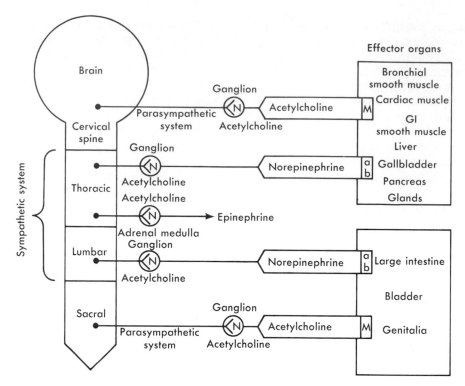

Fig. 21-3 Sympathetic and parasympathetic nervous system innervation. Note that there is dual innervation to effector organs. Acetylcholine is the transmitter at all ganglia and at parasympathetic sites. Their receptors are labeled N for nicotinic and M for musarinic. The transmitters for the sympathetic system at the effector organs are labeled a and b for alpha and beta respectively (see text).

ences between the sympathetic and parasympathetic components of the autonomic system.

Anatomy

Sympathetic fibers arise in the thoracic and lumbar spinal cord segments, traveling uninterrupted until they reach a *ganglion*. A ganglion is simply a relay point where many interconnections (synapses) are possible. The *preganglionic* sympathetic fibers are short and terminate at the ganglia, whereas *postganglionic*

fibers are long and terminate at various effector organs. The ratio of preganglionic to postganglionic fibers varies between 1:11 and 1:17. Thus a single preganglionic impulse can result in many outgoing impulses from a ganglion. This phenomenon tends to produce multiple effects at many different pathetic stimulation results in endocrine action via release of epinephrine from the adrenal gland into the blood. Thus, stimulation of the sympathetic system results in a diffuse response throughout the body.

Table 21-2   Differentiation between sympathetic and parasympathetic systems

	Sympathetic nervous system	Parasympathetic nervous system
Origin	Thoracolumbar	Craniosacral
Preganglionic fibers	Short	Long
Postganglionic fibers	Long, with many branches	Short, with few branches
Transmitter at ganglia	Acetylcholine	Acetylcholine
Receptor at ganglia	Nicotinic	Nicotinic
Transmitter at effector organ	Norepinephrine (acetylcholine at sweat glands, blood vessels of skeletal muscles)	Acetylcholine
Receptor at effector organ	Alpha, beta	Muscarinic
Major effect	Fight or flight	Feed or breed

The parasympathetic fibers originate from the brain and the sacral spinal cord segments and travel without synapsing until they reach the ganglia, which are located near the effector organs. The preganglionic fibers are long, and the postganglionic fibers are short (just the opposite of the sympathetic system). Their ratio is about 1:2, resulting in a more specific and localized response.

Chemical transmitters

The location where nerve fibers synapse, such as at the ganglia or at the effector organ, is called the *neuroeffector junction*. At these special sites, nerve impulses are passed along by a *chemical transmitter* or *mediator* (Figure 21-4). The chemical transmitter is released when a nerve impulse arrives and depolarizes the membrane that contains the transmitter. The transmitter then combines with the receptors of the ganglionic fibers or those of the effector organ. When the receptors are activated by the right chemical transmitter, the membrane depolarizes, producing a new impulse or resulting in a response at the **effector** organ. It is at these synaptic locations that autonomic-active drugs exert their effects.

The chemical transmitter at the ganglia of both the sympathetic and parasympathetic systems is *acetylcholine*. At effector organs, the sympathetic fibers release *norepinephrine*, whereas the parasympathetic fibers release acetylcholine. As long as the chemical transmitter is present it will exert its effect. For a drug to have the desired effect it must be similar to the chemical transmitter that normally exists at the ganglia or effector organ we want to influence. The chemical transmitter and its receptor identifies the type of nerve and its response.

Since nerve stimulation must be temporary, something must happen to the transmitter very soon after it is released or its action would continue. There are specific enzymes that destroy the transmitters as soon as they have exerted their effect. Norepinephrine (as well as epinephrine) is either: (1) reabsorbed back into the axon terminal that secreted it, (2) deactivated by catechol-o-methyl transferase (*COMT*) enzyme, or (3) deactivated by monoamine oxidase (*MAO*) enzyme. The parasympathetic transmitter, acetylcholine, is deactivated by *acetylcholinesterase*. The removal or deactivation of the transmitter makes it possible for the receptor sites to be stimulated again and again.

Sympathetic nerves that act through the release of norepinephrine (or epinephrine) are called *adrenergic*. Their name comes from the fact that the medulla of the adrenal gland releases adrenaline or epinephrine. Drugs that act like adrenaline are known as adrenergic agents. Since these drugs mediate the effects of the sympathetic nervous system, they are also frequently called *sympathomimetic* drugs, because they mimic the sympathetic system. Adrenergic drugs are also referred to as *catecholamines*. This name is derived from the plant *Mimosa catechu*, which has a chemical with a ring structure that is called a catechol. Drugs that resemble the chemical structure from this catechu plant and have an amino group attached are called catecholamines.[7] Epinephrine and norepinephrine have this same basic structure and therefore are catecholamines.

Cholinergic nerves produce and release their effects via acetylcholine. Drugs that have acetylcholine–like effects are called *cholinergic* agents. Since acetylcholine is the mediator in the parasympathetic nervous system at both the ganglia and the effector organ sites,

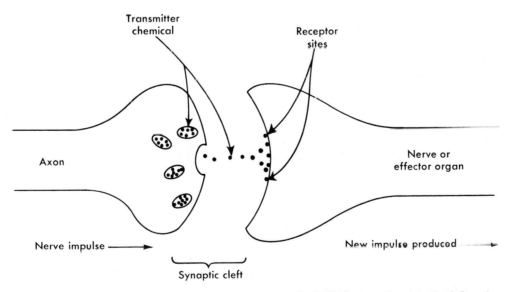

Fig. 21-4 The nerve impulse releases a chemical transmitter that flows across the **synaptic cleft** at the ganglion and effector organ. The chemical transmitter attaches to a receptor and initiates a new electrical impulse. Drugs can attach to the receptor sites, producing a response that is similar to the natural chemical transmitter released from the axon terminal.

drugs which have effects in these locations are called *parasympathomimetic* drugs.

Drugs that block the above effects can be referred to as *adrenergic blockers* or *cholinergic blockers* (or anticholinergics). Alternatively, the terms *sympatholytic* or *parasympatholytic* may be used to refer to drugs having antagonist effects on these two components. (*Lysis* or *lytic* refers to breaking something down, in the above case breaking down the sympathetic or parasympathetic effects).

Receptors

The receptors for these chemical transmitters are very specific. The receptors at the ganglia are called *nicotinic* receptors, named after the drug nicotine, which was found to exert a stimulating effect here. Nicotinic receptors are also found at skeletal muscles in the somatic nervous system. Acetylcholine is the transmitter chemical at the ganglia in both the sympathetic and parasympathetic systems. The receptors at the parasympathetic effector sites are called *muscarinic* receptors, named after a mushroom poison (muscarine) which was found to exert its stimulating effects here.

It is interesting to note that acetylcholine is the transmitter at both of these locations, but the receptors are slightly different. This can be understood with the lock and key explanation. In this case, the lock (receptors) are slightly different, but the key (acetylcholine) is a master key that can "unlock" both the nicotinic and muscarinic sites. However, drugs are designed to work selectively only at one site or the other, thus allowing us to achieve a more specific effect. Table 21-3 summarizes the effects seen when nicotinic and muscarinic receptors are stimulated.

The sympathetic nervous system receptors at the effector sites are of two basic types, *alpha* and *beta*. The characteristic effects of stimulating these two receptor sites are shown in Table 21-4. Beta receptors can be further differentiated into two sub-groups according to their abilities to hydrolyze fatty acids,

Table 21-3 Effects of nicotinic and muscarinic stimulation on various organ systems

Organ system	Nicotine effects	Muscarinic effects
Autonomic ganglia	Stimulated	—
Airways in lung	*	Constriction
Heart rate	*	Decreased
Blood pressure	*	Decreased
Blood vessels	*	Dilation
Gastrointestinal		
Tone	Increased	Increased
Motility	Increased	Increased
Sphincters	—	Relaxed
Salivary gland secretions	First increase,	Increase
Sweat glands	then decrease	Increase
Bronchial gland secretions		Increase
Eye	—	Pupil constriction; decreased accommodation
Skeletal muscle	Stimulated	—

Modified from Bergersen BS: Pharmacology in nursing, ed 14, St Louis, 1979, Mosby.
*Stimulation of nicotinic receptors at ganglia produces both sympathetic and parasympathetic effects. If muscarinic effects are blocked with atropine, then nicotinic stimulation results in sympathetic-like results.

stimulate the heart, dilate bronchi, and relax arterioles. Some beta stimulators primarily produce hydrolysis of fatty acids and cardiac stimulation, while others produce bronchodilation and arteriole relaxation. Receptors that affect primarily the heart are called *beta*$_1$ receptors, and those that primarily dilate bronchi are called *beta*$_2$ receptors. Drugs that primarily stimulate beta$_2$ receptors are the desired drugs to use for bronchodilation since fewer cardiac side effects accompany their use. One will often hear these medications referred to as *beta-adrenergic bronchodilators*.

Alpha–receptor stimulation in the cardiopulmo-

Table 21-4 Alpha and beta receptor effects in the cardiopulmonary system and elsewhere

	Alpha	Beta$_1$	Beta$_2$
Cardiopulmonary	Vasoconstriction	—	Vasodilation
	Slight bronchoconstriction	—	Bronchodilation
	Decrease in heart rate (reflex)	Increase in heart rate	—
	—	Increase in heart contraction	
Other effects	Enhancement of histamine release		Inhibition of histamine release
	Constriction of GI sphincters	Lypolysis	Skeletal muscle tremor
	Contraction of ureters	Relaxation of GI system	
	Dilation of pupils	Relaxation of uterus	
	Contraction of pilomotor muscles		
	Hepatic glycogenolysis		
	Contraction of uterus		

nary system results in vasoconstriction, slight bronchoconstriction and a reflex decrease in heart rate (refer to Chapter 10). As with beta receptors, alpha receptors can be further categorized according to their specific actions. *Alpha₁* receptor stimulation results in contraction of innervated smooth muscle such as in arterioles. *Alpha₂* stimulation inhibits the release of norepinephrine from the pre-synaptic area of nerves and also inhibits central (CNS) sympathetic outflow. Drugs can be chosen that will stimulate either or both of these alpha receptors. Generally, the predominant alpha effect is that associated with alpha₁ stimulation. Alpha₁ stimulating drugs have been used in respiratory care for decreasing mucosal congestion of the airways and nasal passages. The decongestant properties arise from the constriction of the blood vessels resulting in less fluid moving into a given area.

Cellular action

At the level of the smooth muscle cells, specific biochemical reactions occur in response to the release of chemical transmitters or pharmacologic agents (Figure 21-5). Beta₂ adrenergic drugs bind to the cell membrane receptor, *adenylate cyclase*. This enzyme, adenylate cyclase, catalyzes the conversion of

adenosine triphosphate (ATP) to cyclic adenosine monophosphate (cAMP) within the cell. The level or concentration of cAMP is important in mediating the effect of the drug that is bound to the receptor. cAMP exerts its effects through various enzyme systems (kinases), which result in the primary effect, relaxing the bronchial smooth muscle. Any drug that promotes an increase in cAMP levels will cause smooth muscle relaxation; any drug that decreases cAMP levels will cause smooth muscle constriction.

The level of cAMP is increased via activating the cellular adenylate cyclase receptor mechanism. Beta₂-adrenergic drugs increase cAMP by stimulating its production. However, cAMP levels can also be increased or maintained by simply blocking its inactivation. Normally, the enzyme *phosphodiesterase* hydrolyzes cAMP into an inactive form (5'AMP), thereby decreasing its concentration. Therefore, any drug that interferes with the action of phosphodiesterase will also increase cAMP levels. Drugs such as theophylline or caffeine inhibit *phosphodiesterase*. Stimulation of alpha receptors also decreases cAMP levels.

The action at the cholinergic receptors of smooth muscle is very similar, only the nucleotides are dif-

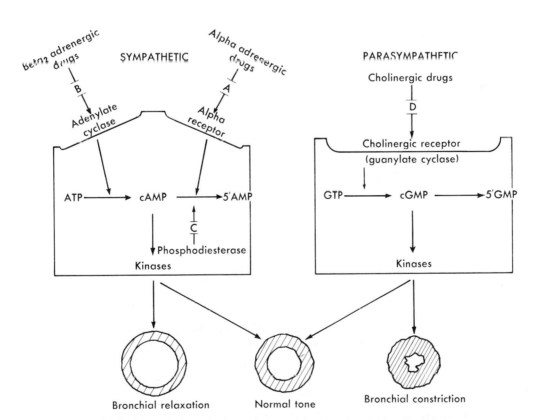

Fig. 21-5 Model of drug mechanism of action for adrenergic and cholinergic drugs. Note that drugs act at specific receptor sites, which then influences cAMP or cGMP levels. The amount of cAMP to cGMP determines the outcome on the bronchial smooth muscle. At *A,B,C,* and *D,* blocking agents can inhibit the function of the specific enzyme system.

ferent. In this case, guanosine triphosphate (GTP) is converted to cyclic guanosine monophosphate (cGMP). An increase in cGMP causes bronchoconstriction. Conversely, decreased production of cGMP results in bronchodilation. This could be accomplished using an anticholinergic drug (cholinergic blocker). As depicted in Figure 21-5, the bronchial smooth muscle tone is a function of the amount of cAMP and cGMP present at any given time. The level of cAMP and cGMP is a result of the sympathetic and parasympathetic nervous system activities, as well as the action of any drugs that may be present.

Obviously, antagonists can block these reactions at several key points. At point *A,* alpha effects can be blocked by drugs like phentolamine. Beta blockers like propranolol act at point *B,* whereas xanthines, such as theophylline, block phosphodiesterase at point *C.* Anticholinergic drugs, like atropine or ipratropium bromide, block cholinergic stimulation at point *D.*

GOALS OF RESPIRATORY PHARMACOLOGY

The primary purpose of respiratory pharmacology is to relieve or prevent the pathologic triad—bronchospasm, mucosal edema, and retained secretions. The agents used to relieve these symptoms can be called the treatment triad. These consist of bronchodilators, decongestants, and mucokinetic agents. The pathologic triad and treatment are outlined below:

Pathologic condition	Treatment
1. Bronchoconstriction	Bronchodilator (e.g., albuterol, ipratropium bromide)
2. Airway edema	Decongestant (e.g., racemic epinephrine)
3. Retained secretions	Hydration (e.g., water); mucolytics (e.g., acetylcysteine)

Figure 21-6 depicts the specific sites of action of the

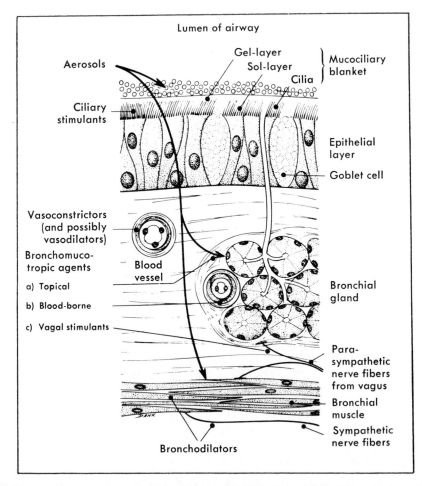

Fig. 21-6 Schema of anatomy showing important components of mucokinetic system. (From Ziment L: Secretions of the respiratory tract: physiology and pharmacology, New York, 1976, Projects in Health, Inc.)

various categories of pharmacologic agents used to relieve the pathologic triad. Bronchodilators increase airway patency by relaxing the spasm of the bronchial muscle, which is triggered by disease or irritation. Most decongestants (agents that relieve congestion) act by contracting the muscle fibers of the arterioles and small arteries, thereby reducing blood flow to the affected area and lowering the hydrostatic pressure that permits fluid to move into the tissues. Mucokinetic agents are used to loosen and mobilize secretions. Mucokinetic action may involve simple dilution of the mucus by direct application of liquid agents, stimulation of serous secretion within the airways (thereby decreasing thick mucus), or actual chemical breakdown of secretions. Bronchodilators and mucokinetic agents are discussed in detail in this chapter. Applicable decongestants are discussed.

Prevention of the pathologic triad is certainly the goal. It is always more of a challenge to treat the problem and make progress after a flare up of symptoms than to prevent or promote normal lung function. Pharmacologic prevention of the pathologic triad is directed at minimizing or blocking the underlying causes of airway bronchospasm and congestion. Immune reactions causing inflammation or infection are the primary factors in the development of the pathologic triad. Preventative treatment includes selected anti-inflammatory or antimicrobials agents. For the treatment of asthma the emphasis now is on treating the underlying inflammatory condition. Controlling the inflammation results in fewer exacerbations of bronchospasm.[8-11]

BRONCHODILATORS

Bronchodilation is most commonly achieved with adrenergic agents. Supplimenting this approval are selected anticholinergic drugs and the xanthines. Prostaglandins also are being studied for this purpose.

Adrenergic bronchodilators

Adrenergic bronchodilators are the most widely used of all drugs in respiratory care. Although our major focus will be on their effectiveness in relieving bronchial smooth muscle contraction, adrenergic bronchodilators are potent drugs with potential for multiple side effects. For this reason, the clinician must have full knowledge of the range of action of these agents and be able to recognize and respond to any untoward effects associated with their administration.

Some preparations of these drugs are administered orally, others by inhalation, some by injection, and some are effectively given by either route. Summarized in Table 21-4 are the general effects that adrenergic agents exhibit on the body as a whole. Table 21-5 on page 518, summarizes the common adrenergic agents in current use, providing information on their commercial preparations, dosages and quantitative estimation of their effects. This table can be referred to as each agent is discussed.

In addition to their effects on the bronchial smooth muscle and blood vessels, some adrenergic bronchodilators aid mucous transport. Studies following the parenteral use of the beta stimulant terbutaline, showed up to 110% of average tracheal mucous velocity in patients with chronic obstructive airway disease.[12] Mucociliary clearance was found to increase up to a maximum of 66% after using a terbutaline MDI.[13] There was no apparent increase in mucus flow in normal subjects. It is therefore possible that the effectiveness of catecholamines in the treatment of obstructive disease is enhanced by the dual action of bronchodilation and increased mucociliary clearance. Although the mechanism for the latter is not apparent, it may account for reports of increased mucus removal even though tests of airway patency show no improvement.

It also has been observed that some $beta_2$-adrenergic compounds, specifically fenoterol, can decrease lung recoil pressure.[14] In principle, this effect could result in less work of breathing for some patients. The decrease in lung recoil pressure appears related to the systemic action of the drug on the lung tissue, after absorption into the circulation. However, this action is of short duration (30 minutes or less).

It is well recognized that many of the effects of bronchodilators—especially side effects—occur as a result of the aerosolized drug being absorbed into the circulation. Studies indicate that only about 10% of the aerosolized drug actually deposits in the lung. The remainder is either exhaled or deposited in the mouth or oropharynx and swallowed.[15,16] Thus, plasma levels of the drug may be responsible for some of the drug action by way of absorption in the gastrointestinal tract, or by way of bronchial absorption.[17,18]

Studies have shown that when a spacer attached to a metered dose inhaler, there is less medication deposited in the oropharynx and more in the lungs. In fact, with a slow deep breath up to 16% of the drug deposited in the lungs; but with faster breaths only 13% of the medicine was retained in the lungs. Without the spacer, there was only 11% drug deposition.[19] Also, that nebulized solutions deposit more medicine in the lungs than do powdered forms.[20] With proper patient education and medication delivery equipment, side effects can be minimized and benefits increased.

Table 21-5 Adrenergic bronchodilators

Generic name	Brand name(s)	Available preparations	Single dose		Action			Duration (hours)
			Inhalation	Oral	alpha	beta₁	beta₂	
Epinephrine	Adrenalin Asthmanephrin	1:100 (1%) 10 mg/mL	0.25–0.5 mL	NA	+3	+4	+3	0.5 to 2 (Short)
Racemic epinephrine	Vaponefrin Micronephrin	1:44 (2.25%) 22 mg/mL	0.25–0.5 mL	NA	+2	+3	+2	0.5 to 2 (Short)
Ephedrine	Tedral Bronkotabs	15, 25, 50 mg tabs	NA	15–50 mg	+2	+3	+3	3 to 4 (Medium)
Isoproterenol	Isuprel	1:200 (0.5%) 5 mg/mL	0.25–0.5 mL	NA	—	+4	+4	0.5 to 2 (Short)
Metaproterenol	Alupent Metaprel	1:20 (5%) 50 mg/mL MDI (0.65 mg) 20 mg tabs	0.2–0.3 mL 2–3 puffs	20 mg	—	+2	+2	3 to 4 (Medium)
Isoetharine	Bronkosol Dilabron	1:100 (1%) 10 mg/mL	0.25–0.5 mL	NA	—	+1	+3	3 to 4 (Medium)
Albuterol	Ventolin Proventil Salbuterol	1:200 (0.5%) MDI (90 µg) 2, 4 mg tabs	0.5 mL 1–2 puffs	2 or 4 mg	—	+1	+4	4 to 6 (Long)
Terbutaline sulfate	Bricanyl Brethine Brethaire	2.5, 5 mg tabs 1:1000 IV/SC MDI (0.2 mg)	0.5 mL* 2 puffs	2.5 or 5 mg	—	+1	+4	3 to 7 (Long)
Bitolterol mesylate	Tornalate	MDI (0.37 mg)	2 puffs	NA	—	+3	+4	5 to 8 (Long)
Fenoterol	Berotec (Europe)	5, 10 mg tabs	NA	5 or 10 mg	—	+1	+4	8 to 10 (Long)
Pirbuterol	Maxair	MDI (0.2 mg)	2 puffs	—	—	+1	+4	4–6 (Long)

*Use of the parenteral form of terbutaline for inhalation under FDA investigation.

The commonly experienced side effects of adrenergic bronchodilators are summarized below:

Side effect	Cause
Increased heart rate	beta₁ stimulation
Arrhythmias, **palpitation**	beta₁ stimulation
Skeletal muscle tremor	beta₂ stimulation
Anxiety, nervousness, insomnia, nausea	beta₂ CNS stimulation
Decreased PaO₂ (occasional)	beta₂ vasodilation producing altered V̇/Q̇

All patients will experience one or more of these side effects while using adrenergic bronchodilators. Some patients will be more sensitive to adverse effects than others. The dose that is necessary to achieve adequate bronchodilation may result in excessive side effects. Thus termination of treatment might occur before therapeutic effects are achieved. Careful monitoring of respiratory patients is always essential, especially for those patients who are receiving heart medication or using other adrenergic drugs.

For hospitalized or home-care patients, monitoring by a respiratory care practitioner should occur when any *new* respiratory drugs are introduced into the patient's treatment program. Proper monitoring includes the following: assessment of pulse and respiratory rate before, during, and after the treatment; auscultation of the lungs before and after treatment; and observation for systemic symptoms of unwanted side effects, such as tremor, sweating, or fatigue.[21] A treatment should be terminated if pulse rate becomes excessive (increases more than 20/min) or should not even be started if a patient is experiencing a tachycardia. When a small-volume nebulizer is used to deliver the drug, the patient should be encouraged to breathe in a slow, relaxed manner with a moderate increase in tidal volume (refer to Chapter 25). All of the above monitored parameters should be charted, as well as any other patient response to the treatment. There are many individual variations that may modify these general recommendations, and specific problems or questions should be discussed with the patient's physician. It is understood that the safety profile of bronchodilators has been good. Over the last 10 years there has been less monitoring of patients using these drugs. The above recommendations are considered ideal and may not be necessary in all patients. Special care should be taken when starting a patient on a new drug, or when providing therapy to patients receiving other drugs, or those with other illnesses, or the elderly. In an out-patient setting it would be best to monitor the first use of a bronchodilator and use the opportunity to educate the patient in the proper use of the equipment.

Epinephrine

Epinephrine is the standard against which most sympathomimetics are judged. Epinephrine is a potent drug, and since it stimulates all types of adrenergic receptors, its use carries with it the risk of unwanted side effects. It performs important functions in regulating the body's metabolism and maintaining a state of alertness to cope with the environment. The health care practitioner sees this drug used frequently in the hospital for its effect on the circulation, during cardiopulmonary resuscitation (CPR), and to combat allergic reactions, for which it is administered by injection under the skin, into muscle, into veins, or even instilled directly into an endotracheal tube. It is almost completely inactivated in the stomach; thus oral use is not feasible. However, it has been used parenterally for many years for the relief of acute bronchial asthma.

Epinephrine is one of the most powerful bronchodilators and decongestants, whether given by injection or by aerosol. Indeed, its action by aerosol is both topical and systemic. Inhalation generally affords quicker response than does subcutaneous or intramuscular injection, although not exceeding the intravenous route. In studies comparing nebulized albuterol to subcutaneous epinephrine, there is no difference in effectiveness.[22,23] The aerosol route is certainly simpler and to be preferred over injection. In one study it was found that other beta-adrenergic bronchodilators resulted in a greater increase in FEV_1 than did the use of epinephrine.[24]

There are two major hazards to aerosolized epinephrine. First, the unwanted side effects may be a danger as well as a nuisance, and the effect on the cardiovascular system may outweigh its benefits. This is especially true in elderly patients or in those with known heart or vascular disease. Second, repeated use of epinephrine often leads to quicker development of tolerance—necessitating dangerously larger doses to achieve the desired therapeutic effect. A patient exhibiting this phenomenon is considered to be *epinephrine-fast*. Less commonly seen is a paradoxical response in which the symptoms of acute airway obstruction actually are made worse by these aerosols. It is believed that this adverse effect might be a result of the development of an allergy to some of the metabolic end-products of the drugs.[25]

If epinephrine is to be used as a bronchodilator-decongestant aerosol, nothing stronger than a 1% aqueous solution (1:100) should be considered safe. Two deep inhalations from 30 to 60 seconds apart are sufficient, and treatments should be spaced at least 4 hours apart. Because of the development of safer

preparations, some of which are described later in this chapter, the use of epinephrine aerosol is not very common.

Norepinephrine; levarterenol

This major sympathetic mediator, when administered therapeutically, is very limited in its action and, although not a bronchodilator, is included here for completeness. Levarterenol is exclusively an alpha-receptor stimulant (alpha agonist), with its primary effects being on the cardiovascular system. Given intravenously, its only clinical use is the support of blood pressure in certain types of severe shock.

Racemic epinephrine (Micronephrin, Vaponefrin)

This drug is a mixture of two **isomers** of epinephrine. It is less potent in its effects than epinephrine and therefore exerts fewer side effects, yet can achieve reasonable bronchodilation. It serves the purpose of relaxing bronchial smooth muscle and at the same time it decreases mucosal congestion by way of its alpha action. It has been recommended for laryngotracheobronchitis and croup,[26-29] and appears to be of value in recently extubated patients because of its decongestant action.

Ephedrine

The action of ephedrine is similar to the action of epinephrine, but it is not used with any regularity for bronchodilation. Although it is primarily used in an oral form, it has recently been reported to be effective when delivered by aerosol to a patient who had upper airway edema.[30]

Ephedrine is an **alkaloid** derived from the plant *Ephedra vulgaris,* an herb used by the Chinese for over 5,000 years. Ephedrine has a less intense but a longer lasting bronchodilating effect than epinephrine. Its longer duration of action is attributable to the fact that it is not inactivated by COMT or MAO. Also unlike epinephrine, it is a strong cerebral stimulant. A major advantage of ephedrine is its oral effectiveness, and it is used commonly in over–the–counter preparations with other bronchodilators, expectorants, or sedatives. Excessive use, as by patient self-administration, can cause marked mental excitation and elevation of blood pressure.

Isoproterenol (Isuprel)

A powerful beta stimulator (beta$_1$ and beta$_2$) with negligible alpha effects, isoproterenol has enjoyed wide use as an aerosol bronchodilator. Although much more selective in its effects than are epinephrine and ephedrine, its role as a bronchodilator is somewhat limited because of its stimulation of beta$_1$ receptors. The strong beta$_1$ effects of isoproterenol increase pulmonary blood flow proportionately more than ventilation, especially in poorly ventilated areas. This reduces the V/Q ratio in these areas and can cause or worsen hypoxemia. Further, strong beta$_1$ stimulation can increase the risk of cardiac arrhythmias, especially in the presence of hypoxemia.[31]

However, clinical experience with isoproterenol is extensive enough that it can still be used effectively as an inhalant, with reasonable safety. A major advantage of this aerosol is its somewhat better bronchodilating effect than that of epinephrine, with nearly complete absence of **vasopressor** action. In contrast to epinephrine, isoproterenol produces **vasodilation** and thus has negligible decongestant value. This effect tends to lower diastolic blood pressure, thereby encouraging an increase in heart rate. Other side effects are infrequent and mild. These include nausea, excitement, and tremors.[32]

It should be emphasized that adverse effects, or at least failure to achieve or sustain benefit, are commonly seen with most of the adrenergics now in use. Although unsatisfactory results may represent side effects, local airway irritation or the actual blockade of beta receptors by accumulated adrenergic metabolites may also be involved.[33] Isoproterenol is especially susceptible to the latter reaction, particularly if used too frequently or over too long a period of time. Metabolic by-products of isoproterenol can accumulate faster than enzymatic degradation can destroy them. Some of the metabolites block the beta receptor from bronchodilator action, and further administration of isoproterenol actually can increase bronchospasm.

Isoproterenol is available in aqueous concentrations of 1:100 and 1:200. For routine aerosol use the 1:200 strength is recommended. For intermittent short-term therapy, as in self-administration, two to four well-spaced inhalations at 4-hour intervals is a conservative program, although the general safety of the drug allows for considerable flexibility according to clinical need. For prolonged bronchodilation, especially as administered with mechanical ventilators, isoproterenol should be further diluted to concentrations of 1:400 or 1:600. With the availability of newer effective beta$_2$ bronchodilators, the use of isoproterenol is not very frequent.

Metaproterenol (Alupent, Metaprel)

A derivative of isoproterenol, metaproterenol has many of the same effects.[34,35] It can be taken orally or inhaled as an aerosolized powder from a pressurized cartridge, or a liquid form can be nebulized. It has beta$_1$ side effects when given by inhalation and comparable beta$_2$ effects when compared with isoproterenol, but with significantly increased duration of action. This medication is still commonly used and is shown to be effective and safe for most people.[36,37]

Isoetharine (Bronkosol, Bronkometer)

Isoetharine was one of the most commonly used bronchodilators but it has largely been replaced by other agents which are more selective and a little more effective. Although the profile of some newer bronchodilators appear to be more desirable, one clinical trial did not show any significant difference on effectiveness or hospital admission rates for asthmatics using isoetharine.[38] Isoetharine's bronchodilating effect is somewhat less than that of isoproterenol, but its cardiovascular side effects are also less intense.[39] It is mostly a beta$_2$ stimulator, with clinically insignificant beta$_1$ activity. In one test of cardiovascular response to a high dosage of IV isoetharine, patients exhibited decreases in systolic and diastolic blood pressure (beta$_2$ effect) and increase in heart rate (beta$_1$ effect), but no arrhythmias.[40] Isoetharine can be administered orally as well as by aerosol, and is reportedly more effective in conditions characterized by diffuse bronchospasm, as in bronchial asthma, than in those with obstructing secretions, as in chronic bronchitis.[41]

Albuterol (Proventil, Ventolin)

Albuterol (sometimes called salbutamol) is a selective beta$_2$ stimulant that has fewer side effects than isoproterenol but is as effective.[42-44] Presently, albuterol is the most commonly used beta$_2$ adrenergic bronchodilator. Nebulized albuterol appears to take longer to achieve bronchodilation but has a longer lasting effect because it is not metabolized by COMT.[45] A major asset is its effectiveness, whether given by mouth, intravenously, or in aerosol form. However, for many conditions the administration of the aerosolized drug appears to offer fewer side effects, and there are some indications that better results are achieved by this route in acute asthma.[46] The use of albuterol in infants with respiratory distress syndrome resulted in decreased airway resistance and improved lung compliance.[47]

The typical MDI dose is 90 μg per puff with two to three puffs recommended every four to six hours. When delivered via small volume nebulizer, the standard dosage is 2.5 mg QID. The solutions come in 0.083% (0.83 mg/mL), 0.5% (5 mg/mL) and 0.6% (6 mg/mL) concentrations.

Pirbuterol (Maxair)

This is a selective beta$_2$ adrenergic bronchodilator which is similar to albuterol. It has been found to have an effective onset of action by 15 minutes after inhalation and peak effectiveness realized by 60 minutes. This occurs without any notable side effects, even if administered at three times the recommended dose.[48] Other studies have shown it to be as safe or safer than metaproterenol.[49] Inhalation dose for adults and children over 12 years is 0.4 mg (two to three inhalations) which can be repeated every four to six hours.

Terbutaline sulfate (Bricanyl, Brethine, Brethaire)

Terbutaline is available in oral, parenteral and MDI preparations. Terbutaline is a specific beta$_2$ adrenergic with minimal beta$_1$ effects. It is twice as potent as metaproterenol and has a longer duration of action.[50] However, albuterol appears to have more potency and better blocking effect on bronchial hyper-responsiveness than terbutaline.[51] Compared with albuterol, terbutaline has been reported to be therapeutically equivalent but with slightly slower onset of action.[52,53] Bronchodilation with terbutaline appears to increase as the dose increases, but there is always greater potential for side effects when used at higher doses.[54] At or slightly above its recommended dosages terbutaline has proved safe.[55] Studies have shown that mucociliary clearance can increase by 50% with the use of inhaled terbutaline, which enhances its therapeutic effect.[13]

Bitolterol mesylate (Tornalate)

Bitolterol mesylate is a *pro-drug,* that is a chemical compound that is metabolized to an active form after deposition in the lung. Bitolterol is hydrolyzed in the lung tissue by esterases into the beta-adrenergic bronchodilator *colterol,* the active form. It exhibits preferential beta$_2$ effects. As a pro-drug, bitolterol has both a rapid onset of action and a comparatively longer duration of action (up to eight hours in some patients) than other comparable agents.[56] It is comparable to albuterol in many respects, but the increased duration of bronchodilation can provide a therapeutic advantage. Its airway hyper–responsive protective effects is similar to albuterol.[57] It is currently available only in an MDI preparation. The popularity of this medication will probably increase.

Fenoterol

Fenoterol is one of the newer beta adrenergic bronchodilators which has a dose response effect on bronchodilation and a fairly long duration of action.[58] Its long duration of action (about 8 hours) is accompanied by minimal beta$_1$ effects. However, a recent study using aerosolized fenoterol versus terbutaline reported a better overall clinical effect for terbutaline.[59] Studies find that fenoterol is effective at dilating both central and peripheral airways.[60,61] This is in contrast to studies showing that most beta adrenergic bronchodilators act mainly on the peripheral airways, while anticholinergics appear to exert their effects mainly on the central airways. This would give fenoterol an advantage in certain types of bronchoconstriction.

Salmeterol

This is another beta$_2$ adrenergic bronchodilator which is not yet available for general clinical use in the United States. It has bronchodilation capabilities similar to albuterol but with a duration of action of 12 hours or longer.[62-64] At 24 hours there is still some increased bronchodilation effects apparent.[65] The protective effects against exercise induced asthma (EIA) is equivalent to albuterol except the duration of protection is many hours longer.[66] It might also have some mild antiinflammatory effects. In clinical trials, salmeterol twice a day produced better control of asthma symptoms (as measured by change in FEV$_1$ and peak expiratory flow rates) than albuterol dosed four times a day and as needed.[67] The side effects and safety profile are similar to other bronchodilators. Regular use over a period of time may reduce salmeterol's protective effects against bronchoconstricting stimuli; however, the bronchodilating properties continue to be good.[68] If current testing continues to go well, salmeterol will become an important first line treatment in the management of asthma.

Anticholinergic (parasympatholytic) bronchodilators

Anticholinergic or parasympatholytic bronchodilators act at the muscarinic receptors of the parasympathetic nervous system. Normally, acetylcholine acts as the chemical transmitter at these postganglionic sites and result in smooth muscle contraction. In the lungs, this leads to bronchoconstriction. Agents which competitively block the action of acetylcholine will decrease intracellular levels of cGMP, thereby favoring smooth muscle relaxation. Thus bronchodilation from anticholinergic blockers is through a different pathway in the autonomic nervous system. For this reason, anticholinergics can be used either alone or in combination with beta adrenergics. When used together, they exert complimentary effects.

Atropine sulfate

Atropine is the model anticholinergic bronchodilator agent. Atropine is an alkaloid found in the plants Atropa belladonna and Datura stramonium. It has been used for many years in the treatment of airway disease. Inhalation of the smoke of stramonium leaves was an old favorite remedy for asthma prior to the modern pharmacologic era. The development and increased use of adrenergic drugs has gradually displaced atropine as a bronchodilator. Yet, anticholinergic agents have a useful role in the **pharmacopoeia** of respiratory care, especially in the treatment of reflex bronchoconstriction due to increased vagal tone.[69,70]

Related to other drugs such as scopolamine and hyoscyamine, atropine blocks the effect of parasympathetic stimuli by increasing the threshold of response of effector cells to acetylcholine. In principle, such action will elicit a response resembling stimulation of adrenergic receptors, since these are freed of competing and counteracting cholinergic stimulus. Although other parasympathetic nerves are affected, atropine inhibits vagal stimulation of the heart and respiratory tract, thereby elevating blood pressure and cardiac rate and dilating bronchi. In addition, atropine may act on the central nervous system, stimulating the respiratory centers to generate rapid, deep breathing.[70] Relative to the patient with airway obstruction, the two most important actions of atropine can be summarized as follows:

1. Reduction of secretions. Atropine inhibits secretions of nose, mouth, pharynx, and bronchi and, by reducing their fluid volumes, increases their viscosity. This property made atropine and related derivatives popular in compounds prescribed to relieve symptoms of the common cold and in preoperative medication to reduce the mucus-producing stimulus of anesthetics and airway instrumentation. However, this effect of atropine poses a potential threat to patients already handicapped by thick bronchial secretions, subjecting them to the risk of serious aggravation of their obstruction. This hazard has probably been the major impediment to the continued use of atropine in respiratory problems.

2. Bronchodilation. By blocking cholinergic influences on bronchial muscle, atropine potentiates beta-adrenergic dilation and widens the airways. Because there is no evidence that acetylcholine plays an active role in generating bronchospasm, atropine is a less effective dilator than either epinephrine, isoproterenol, or albuterol. Yet the beneficial effect of atropine on bronchoconstriction has been well demonstrated in airways that were subjected to dust inhalation and protected by the drug given parenterally.[71] Aerosol studies have employed 1% and 0.2% concentrations of atropine in equal parts of propylene glycol and water.[72]

With the proper administration of atropine aerosol, airway resistance can be significantly reduced in normal subjects as well as in obstructed patients. Bronchi are also protected against the induced bronchospasm of inhaled irritants such as carbachol and aluminum dust. Results are equally satisfactory with either the 0.2% or 2% solution. At times, atropine has been added in small amounts to sympathomimetic mixtures. One study has shown that an aerosol of isoproterenol and atropine methonitrate gives better bronchodilation than either one alone, combining the rapid onset and short duration of isoproterenol with the slower but more prolonged effect of atropine.[73]

Presently, atropine is combined with an adrenergic bronchodilator primarily when there is a need to reduce copious bronchial secretions.

Ipratropium bromide (Atrovent)

Ipratropium bromide (chemically N-isopropylnortropine) is an atropine-like agent originally developed in the 1960s. Like atropine, ipratropium bromide probably acts by antagonizing the action of acetylcholine and thereby inhibiting increases in intracellular cGMP.[74,75]

Ipratropium bromide is available currently only in MDI form, with a usual dose of approximately 36 μg (two inhalations) four times per day. At these dose levels, it produces bronchodilation about as effectively as does isoproterenol. Onset of its action is three to six times as long as that of isoproterenol, but its duration is four times greater.

In contrast to atropine, ipratropium bromide does not elicit any subjective drying of oral or **ocular** secretions. One study has suggested that atropine-like products acted predominantly on receptors in the larger airways, whereas beta$_2$-adrenergics favored the smaller (peripheral) airways.[76] Other investigators have found no difference in the pattern of response between ipratropium bromide and beta$_2$-adrenergics.[77,78] Ipratropium bromide is thus a useful adjunct to beta adrenergic therapy.[79]

Besides its centrally mediated anticholinergic effects,[80] ipratropium bromide also appears to lessen the effects of cell mediators that initiate bronchospasm (serotonin, histamine, PGF2 alpha and bradykinin), and even strengthens the smooth muscle relaxation effects of adrenergics.[81,82] Studies have shown that if ipratropium bromide is followed by metaproterenol in allergic asthmatics, there is significantly greater airway improvement over either agent used alone.[83] Ipratropium bromide may also useful in patients for whom adrenergic bronchodilators are contraindicated.[84] Moreover, the response to this bronchodilator is even greater in those asthmatics with a major psychogenic component to their asthma.[85] Ipratropium has also been shown to protect against histamine-induced bronchospasm.[86] Some clinicians have observed that ipratropium has been more effective in those with emphysema and chronic bronchitis.[87-89] For ventilator patients with acute exacerbations of COPD, bronchodilation with ipratropium is just as effective as albuterol and better than IV aminophylline, when given in-line with an MDI.[90] The bronchodilating effects of ipratropium are better than theophylline.[91] However, ipratropium does not promote mucociliary clearance as do beta adrenergic agents; in fact, one study has shown a mild decrease in mucus clearance.[92]

Xanthines

Xanthines are a group of organic vegetable compounds related to a naturally occurring precursor of uric acid. The three most important xanthines are caffeine, theophylline, and theobromine. We are all familiar with caffeine as the important ingredient of coffee, tea, cola drinks, and cocoa, but the xanthine group as a whole has some specific physiologic actions that make them valuable as pharmacologics. Although the relative effects of these three agents vary, all produce the following responses:

1. CNS stimulation
2. Bronchodilation
3. Pulmonary vasodilation
4. Smooth muscle relaxation
5. **Diuresis**
6. Coronary artery dilation
7. Cardiac stimulation
8. Skeletal muscle stimulation

Although caffeine and theobromine were used in the past for cardiac stimulation and diuresis, they have been replaced by more effective agents. However, the use of caffeine does result in some minor bronchodilation and protective effects against bronchospasm challenges.[93] Theophylline, on the other hand, still plays an important role in clinical therapeutics, although its use is frequently being relegated to a secondary or tertiary role. In addition to its use for bronchodilation, theophylline is employed in certain types and stages of congestive heart failure and is especially valuable in correcting **Cheyne-Stokes' breathing.** It has also received attention for its ability to decrease apneic episodes in premature infants.[94-96] There are various forms of theophylline such as aminophylline and oxtriphylline. The most common variant encountered is aminophylline, which is about 20% less potent than theophylline.

The value of theophylline can be appreciated from reviewing Figure 20-5. Unlike the adrenergics, which increase cAMP by stimulating its production, theophylline is thought to maintain cAMP levels by inhibiting phosphodiesterase, thereby decreasing its destruction. However, the actual mechanism of action is being re-evaluated since there is evidence now that inhibition of phosphodiesterase activity plays only a minor part in theophylline's smooth muscle relaxation. A suggested mechanism of action is by antagonism of adenosine at the receptor site.[97,98] It appears that bronchospasm can occur from adenosine's action at its receptor site, resulting in leukotriene and histamine release.[99] Theophylline may also competitively antagonize the prostaglandin PGF_2, a potent bronchoconstricting agent, and appears to have an effect on calcium movement across the cellular membranes of smooth muscle.

The bronchodilating action of theophylline provides a third and different mechanism for bronchospasm treatment—adding to what beta$_2$ adrenergics and anti-cholinergics can offer. For this reason, the practitioner will see theophylline or its various derivatives used in patients with diffuse bronchospasm, especially when the patient is refractory to some first-line drugs.

Acute bronchospasm has been commonly treated with intravenous administration of theophylline derivatives. Clinical findings in the last few years however, have shown no additional benefit to the use of theophylline if intravenous steroids and an inhaled beta adrenergic bronchodilator have been used.[100] Theophylline is actually being used less frequently for severe, acute bronchospasm without harm to patients.[101-103] There is indication that theophylline use in an acute situation will have more therapeutic effect if the patient has not been using it previously.[104] Intramuscular and rectal routes are sometimes used, but these are less effective. For overall treatment of patients prone to bronchospasm, oral theophylline or its derivatives have frequently been a part of the drug regimen (and still are) along with inhaled bronchodilators. Recent research suggests a mild interaction of theophylline and the lymphocytes (CD4, CD8) whereby it weakens the immune system's slow (late asthmatic response) response to bronchospasm.[105]

When theophylline is used, the goal is to maintain therapeutic plasma levels from 5 to 20 μg/mL. However, the therapeutic dose is very close to the toxic dose, and adverse effects are more likely. Thus it is common to give the least dose that appears to be effective—usually 5 to 15 μg/mL is sufficient to do the job. For this reason, prescribing physicians must periodically monitor serum theophylline levels on their patients in order to properly adjust the dosage and to minimize side effects.[106] The most common side effects, occurring at plasma levels of 20 to 30 μg/mL, are **anorexia,** nausea, and vomiting. Cardiovascular effects such as tachycardia, palpitations, and arrhythmias may be seen at plasma levels in excess of 30 μg/mL. CNS effects of nervousness, **insomnia,** and shakiness may be seen at or above therapeutic levels, with seizures possible when plasma levels reach 40 to 50 μg/mL. Because of the above mentioned side effects, patients with underlying heart disease, seizure disorders, or gastrointestinal problems are not the best candidates for use of this medication. Patients who develop theophylline toxicity often require hospitalization to assure proper management of their condition.

Variables that affect the half-life of the drug and therefore alter the dose or frequency of administration of theophylline are listed in Table 21-6 on page 524. Patients who smoke cigarettes have a shorter

Table 21-6 Variables affecting half-life of theophylline

SITUATIONS REQUIRING INCREASED DOSAGE	INCREASE*
1. Cigarette smoking	25–75%
2. Exposure to smog or hydrocarbons	10–25%
3. High caffeine intake	10–20%
4. Barbiturate or phenytoin use	10–15%
5. High-protein diet	10–15%
6. Suboptimal blood levels	—
7. Patients known to have high tolerance to theophylline	—
8. Children 2 months to 16 years	—
SITUATIONS REQUIRING DECREASED DOSAGE	**DECREASE***
1. Hepatic congestion or insufficiency	20–50%
2. Marked obesity	20–50%
3. Overt heart failure	20–30%
4. Marked hypoxemia	10–25%
5. Febrile illness	10–20%
6. Antibiotic use of erythromycin, troleandomycin, lincomycin, or clindamycin	10–20%
7. Cimetidine use	10–20%
8. Patients exhibiting toxic symptoms	—

*Approximate guidelines for dosage adjustments. Serum levels provide more accurate guidance. (Modified from information supplied by Irwin Ziment, MD. Used by permission.)

half-life of theophylline and therefore are required to take the medicine more often.[107] For those who discontinue smoking, the theophylline levels need to be monitored and the theophylline dosage readjusted to avoid toxicity. It has also been reported that certain upper respiratory tract viral infections can increase the half-life of theophylline.[108]

As an aerosol, aminophylline has been tried but is irritating to the pharynx, and can cause substantial wheezing and coughing. Moreover, most evidence indicates that aminophylline by aerosol has a minimal impact on forced expiratory flow rates in patients with acute obstructive disorders.[109,110]

Other bronchodilating agents

Eicosanoids

Eicosanoids (eicosa = twenty from Greek) are a family of compounds derived from the naturally occurring 20-carbon unsaturated fatty acid, arachidonic acid, produced in most every tissue of the body. The parent compounds of arachidonic acid are the essential fatty acids, linoleic and linolenic acid—both 18 carbon fatty acids, which are obtained from food. Arachidonic acid is the precursor for a number of biologically active compounds. The major categories of compounds presently recognized are prostaglandins, leukotrienes, thromboxanes, and lipoxins. These substances act like hormones at the local tissue level and typically have very short half-lives.

Thromboxanes are produced by platelets and promote vasoconstriction and platelet aggregation, and might also contribute to bronchospasm.[111] Lipoxins are more newly discovered and less understood but appear to influence the small vessels of the circulatory system and inhibit cytotoxic effects of natural killer cells. The interested student is referred to standard physiology texts for further discussion on these compounds.

Leukotrienes are important mediators of inflammatory responses in the body. Amino acid containing leukotrienes, LTC4, LTD4, and LTE4, are potent bronchoconstrictors and are activated by IgE allergic reactions. These leukotrienes are responsible for the slow-reacting substance of anaphylaxis.[112] They also are active players in asthma, adult respiratory distress syndrome, and some other diseases.[8,113-115] Research is developing leukotriene antagonists which may provide important bronchodilating medication in the future.[116-118] A current research agent is MK-571, which is an LTD4 receptor antagonist having a marked bronchodilator effect.[119]

Prostaglandins are important active substances which have a variety of physiological effects throughout the body. The first prostaglandins discovered were thought to have come from the prostate gland, hence the name. It is now known that prostaglandins are synthesized in all tissues, but the name persists. Of the many known prostaglandins, three are of substantial interest in respiratory pharmacology: PGE_1, PGE_2, and PGF_{2a}. Prostaglandin E_1 and E_2 cause relaxation of bronchial smooth muscle; prostaglandin F_{2a} causes contraction of bronchial smooth muscle.

Unlike the adrenergic or anticholinergic drugs previously discussed, prostaglandins do not act through autonomic control or mediator release. Instead, they appear to act directly on smooth muscle. PGE_1 and PGE_2 increase cellular adenyl cyclase and therefore cAMP, but by way of a pathway that cannot be blocked by sympathetic antagonists. Alteration of calcium influx into the cell also appears to be involved.[120] Prostaglandin F_{2a} is thought to act by way of direct stimulation of cGMP production.

Prostaglandins are produced *in vivo* during anaphylactic reactions and with pulmonary edema and embolism. Their synthesis is also increased by hypoxia, hypocapnia, and mechanical stimulation of the lung. This latter effect may help explain the hypotension sometimes associated with positive pressure ventilation.[121]

In general, aerosolized PGE_2 and PGE_1 have been shown to decrease airway resistance in asthmatic patients to a greater degree than isoproterenol, and PGE_2 has an additive effective to beta-adrenergic stimulation. Approaching the problems from a different direction, bronchodilation can also be achieved experimentally by the action of a substance known as polyphloretin phosphate, which inhibits the constrictor effect of PGF_{2a}. Continued research on the actions of the prostaglandins will no doubt help us better understand the mechanisms causing bronchospasm. This will help pharmacologists develop more effective treatments for airway obstruction.

MUCOKINETIC DRUGS

The mucociliary system represents the primary clearance and defense mechanism of the airway conducting zone of the lung (refer to Chapter 9). *Mucokinetics* is concerned with the movement of mucus in the respiratory tract, and the overall effectiveness of the mucociliary system.

The effectiveness with which the mucociliary system fulfills its important role in clearance and lung defense depends upon complex interactions between the mucus "blanket" and the cilia. The blanket consists of a high viscosity **mucopolysaccharide** gel layer that "floats" on top of a lower viscosity serous layer. Interestingly, although consisting mainly of water, the gel component of the mucus is relatively impervious to water (which is its primary constituent). This suggests that the gel layer serves not only to make surface transport easier, but also to prevent dehydration.[122]

In health, the composition of the mucus blanket represents a delicate balance between the secretions produced by the goblet cells and bronchial glands. The goblet cells are primarily responsible for production of the **mucopolysaccharide** gel layer, whereas the bronchial glands probably produce most of the watery secretions. Goblet cells are under local control, increasing their production mainly in response to irritant factors such as noxious gases or infectious agents. Although the bronchial glands can respond locally, they are primarily under central control, being stimulated to increase production mainly by vagal (parasympathetic) nerve stimulation.

The bronchial glands therefore can be affected by drugs that act either locally or systemically. The bronchial glands can be stimulated directly by topical cholinergic drugs, or systemically by agents that evoke a vagal response. Because cholinergic drugs (such as pilocarpine) have strong poisonous side effects, their use as mucokinetic agents is limited. On the other hand, oral expectorants like glyceryl guaiacolate or the iodides are commonly used as systemic agents evoking a vagal response by irritating the lining of the stomach.

Ciliary activity also is affected by chemical and physical agents, being increased by adrenergic drugs, and the methylxanthines.[13] On the other hand, ciliary activity is reduced by dehydration, cigarette smoke, ozone, alcohol, and anticholinergics such as atropine. Ipratropium bromide either does not effect or only mildly compromises clearance.[92,123]

Normal mucokinesis, then, depends on the proper composition of the gel and serous layers as well as optimum functioning of the cilia. Impairment of either of these systems can impair both pulmonary clearance and defense, increasing the likelihood of obstruction or infection. Mucokinetic therapy aims to maintain or improve functioning of the mucociliary mechanism, thereby promoting effective clearance of respiratory tract secretions and minimizing the possibility of infection. Aerosolized agents used to facilitate mucokinesis fall into four major categories: (1) diluting or hydrating agents, (2) wetting agents, (3) mucolytics, and (4) proteolytics.

Diluting or hydrating agents

Water

Of all the agents used to modify the character of respiratory tract secretions, none is more important, than water. Although water can be aerosolized or vaporized, *there is no substitute for adequate systemic hydration.* Generous consumption of water is necessary for optimum functioning of the respiratory system as well as the body in general. Water is one of the few agents that has no side effects unless taken in extremely large quantities. Only in small infants, patients with congestive heart failure, or excessive fluid retention is water restriction considered. Water is the first and most important agent to be considered when patients have difficulty mobilizing bronchial secretions. The aerosolization and vaporization of water is discussed in Chapter 25.

Saline

Saline (NaCl) is one of the most commonly used aerosols—either alone or with bronchodilators. Normal saline can be nebulized for diluting the mucus and enhancing clearance, or it can be instilled directly into the airway to aid suctioning.

Normal saline (0.9% NaCl) is considered a bland aerosol since its **osmolarity** approximates that of body fluids. However, as aerosolized normal saline particles enter the respiratory tract, the water in the droplets evaporates, resulting in a hypertonic solution (greater than 0.9%). Due to this increased tonicity, a normal saline aerosol can provoke bronchospasm in certain patients, particularly those with reactive airways. For these patients, the use of a supplementary bronchodilator may be necessary.

Half-normal saline (0.45% NaCl) is also used for mucosal hydration. Clinicians that prefer half-normal saline argue that evaporation of water from droplets of this hypotonic solution during its passage into the respiratory tract ultimately results in a solute concentration like that of normal saline. For this reason, half-normal saline is also often preferred with ultrasonic nebulization, since these small particles can face significant evaporation (refer to Chapter 25).

Hypertonic saline (1% to 15% NaCl) is the agent of choice for sputum induction. Its increased osmolarity is thought to result in increased movement of fluid into the mucosal blanket *(bronchorrhea)*. Moreover, its irritant properties promote coughing, which helps move the secretions. Since absorption of saline from the lungs into the circulation does occur, frequent use of the hypertonic saline in sodium-restricted patients is contraindicated.

Propylene glycol

Propylene glycol is both a solvent and hygroscopic agent. As a solvent for bronchodilators it helps stabilize aerosol droplets and can act as a mild preservative, inhibiting bacterial growth. In concentrations less than 5% it has a demulcent (soothing) effect on the respiratory mucosa. In concentrations of greater than 5% it is used to induce sputum. Its hydrating action is probably associated with its **hygroscopic** activity, i.e., by attracting water it dilutes the mucus. It should be noted that since it inhibits the growth of fungi and mycobacteria, it should not be used for sputum induction when the goal is to culture these organisms. In low concentrations, aerosolized propylene glycol appears to be safe.

Oral expectorants

Oral expectorants are included in our discussion of diluting agents because they promote dilution of mucus indirectly. Examples of oral mucokinetic agents are potassium iodide, commonly referred to as

SSKI (saturated solution of potassium iodide), guaifenesin (glyceryl guaiacolate), currently the most frequently used expectorant, and more common home remedies such as spices. These agents work by irritating the lining of the stomach, thereby stimulating the afferent fibers of the vagus nerve. Impulses sent to the CNS cause a vagal efferent response, stimulating bronchial glands to secrete more serous fluid. In concept, this action dilutes respiratory tract secretions, particularly the watery portion of the mucus blanket. This vagal activity occurs with apparently little or no bronchial constriction. Use of oral iodinated glycerol for management of mucous clearance has been shown to be well tolerated in COPD patients and helps improve respiratory symptoms.[124,125]

Wetting agents

Wetting agents are chemical substances designed to lower the surface tension of respiratory tract fluids. Some agents represent true detergents, interacting with the mucous to produce **emulsification** of the hydrophobic bonds between water and the mucopolysaccharide molecules. In concept, these agents should disperse the mucous into smaller particles, thereby improving water penetration and facilitating transport and removal. Other chemicals, such as ethyl alcohol, act by destabilizing the alveolar plasma exudates in acute pulmonary edema. Whereas the action of ethyl alcohol is generally well documented in the literature, the *in–vivo* effects of detergents are less well substantiated. For the sake of completeness, however, we discuss both categories of wetting agents.

Detergents

Presently, no detergent solutions designed for aerosol administration to the respiratory tract are currently on the market. In the past, aerosolized detergents like Alevaire and Tergemist were used clinically. These agents were late removed from the market due to unproven efficacy.

Ethyl alcohol

Whereas the detergent agents were developed to act directly on the mucus of the respiratory tract, ethyl alcohol is applied to destabilize the alveolar plasma exudates that can occur in cardiogenic pulmonary edema.

Cardiogenic pulmonary edema can be characterized by the accumulation of a thin watery exudate in the alveoli and bronchioles. The commonly observed "frothing" of this oozing is attributable, in part, to its surfactant content. The sufactant **lowers** the surface tension of the exudate. This results in the formation of stable bubbles which can obstruct ventilation. Contrary to popular opinion, ethyl alcohol does not lower the surface tension of this froth—this would only increase its stability. Instead, it probably changes the properties of the lecithin component of the surfactant, raising surface tension, and thereby destabilizing the froth.[126] Normally, 5 to 15 mL of 30 to 50% ethyl alcohol is vaporized, usually by positive pressure (to impede venous return and lower pulmonary vascular pressures). A minor and temporary side effect is irritation of the airway mucosa.

Mucolytics

N-acetylcysteine (Mucomyst)

In the search for agents effective in disrupting the mucoproteins responsible for the high viscosity of sputum in certain respiratory diseases, the action of the naturally occurring amino acid, L-cysteine, was studied. Although it was found to be an excellent mucolytic, it had substantial irritating properties. These were minimized by modifying the acid into an acetyl form, as it is now employed. It also has the advantage of being an antioxidant and has been shown to prevent the adverse effects that ozone has on mucociliary clearance.[123]

The chemical reaction between acetylcysteine and bronchial mucus has been extensively studied.[127] Acetylcysteine chemically replaces the disulfide bonds of mucoproteins with weaker sulfhydryl bonds. This actions disrupts the molecular structure, and lowers the viscosity of the mucus. This medicine is only indicated if purulent secretions are present.

Mucolysis is as effective with a 10% as with a 20% concentration. Whereas the stronger preparation can induce bronchospasm in some patients, the lesser strength is a negligible hazard.[128] Other studies have found both 10% and 20% to be harmless, neither producing significant bronchospasm.[129] One can now obtain commercial preparations of acetylcysteine premixed with selected beta-adrenergic bronchodilators. This combination can help minimize the bronchospasm that may occur in susceptible patients.

The possibility of damage to alveolar surfactant has been of concern with the inhalation of microaerosols of any kind, and especially ones with enzymatic action. Examination of both human and animal lung tissue after use of 10% acetylcysteine aerosol showed no change in surface activity.[130] Serious complications are rare. A burning sensation in the upper passages is occasionally reported, and nausea may be experienced. Some patients complain of the rotten-egg odor, but most adjust to it and appear to tolerate its use.

In general, the clinical response to this aerosol for the removal of mucoid secretions has been favorable. Indications for acetylcysteine covers a wide range, from the cystic fibrosis of childhood (in which it has scored considerable success), through the suppurative lung diseases, to the chronic bronchitis-emphysema of late adulthood.[131,132] Nevertheless, a small minority have felt that acetylcysteine, though effective *in vitro,* has not shown any benefit in patients and is of no clinical value.[133]

A practical point to note is the chemical reactivity between acetylcysteine and certain component parts of nebulization equipment, especially iron, copper, and rubber. Parts coming in contact with the amino acid (liquid or aerosol) should be made of glass, plastic, aluminum, chromed metal, silver, or stainless steel.

There is no critical dosage schedule for administering acetylcysteine aerosol; it is used according to individual needs. However, when using the premixed acetylcysteine and a bronchodilator, one must limit the frequency of administration with respect to the bronchodilator. It can be administered by hand nebulizer, compressor, or aerosol mask and in positive–pressure breathing devices, but the drug itself should not be put in a heated nebulizer. In addition to the aerosol route, acetylcysteine is often effectively used by direct instillation, especially to facilitate suctioning through tracheostomy or endotracheal tubes.

Sodium bicarbonate

Large mucoid molecular chains tend to break as the pH of their environment rises, and local bronchial alkalinity can reach a pH of 8.3 without untoward irritation or damage.[134] With the availability of more potent mucolytics such as acetylcysteine sodium bicarbonate aerosol is seldom used. For some patients, benefits can occasionally be seen with an aerosolized 2% sodium bicarbonate. For home use, a teaspoonful of the soda in a cup of sterile water makes a readily available solution.

Proteolytics

As the name indicates, members of this group *lyse* the protein material found in purulent sputum. High levels of protein, especially DNA, make the sputum viscous and difficult to expectorate. Early versions of these agents, including trypsin and bovine pancreatic dornase (Donavac) were geneally ineffective and are no longer marketed.

Recently, recombinant human deoxyribonuclease (rhDNase) has been cloned *in vitro* and successfully used with cyctic fibrosis (CF) patients. rhDNase greatly reduce the viscosity of purulent CF sputum, quickly transforming it from a viscous gel to a flowing liquid. This results in both objective improvements in lung function and less dyspnea. Aerosol inhalation of rhDNase is well tolerated by most patients, with no serious adverse reactions.

Surfactants

Surfactant deficiency is a common cause of respiratory distress in preterm infants. Over the last decade, the administration of artificial surfactant preparations has proved beneficial to these patients.[135] Aerosolized surfactant has not proved as therapeutic as direct instillation via endotracheal tube. But aerosolized delivery is being studied and may be a workable option in the future.[136] Instillation of surfactant is usually tolerated well but can be accompanied by bradycardia and oxygen desaturation, so careful monitoring is required.[135]

ADRENOCORTICOSTEROIDS

Adrenocorticosteroids have assumed a position of great importance in clinical therapeutics. Steroids can be life saving for patients experiencing an acute exacerbation of asthma, and are now recommended for regular use in asthmatics. Unfortunately, these powerful agents can cause many unwanted side effects. For these reasons, the RCP must have a good understanding of steroid use.

For the sake of convenience, we use the commonly employed expression "steroid," with the understanding that we mean adrenocorticosteroid. Like many familiar terms, it is not really correct, for steroids comprise a large group of organic compounds, many of which have physiologic properties unrelated to respiratory concerns. The steroids that concern us are potent hormones secreted by the cortex (outer layer) of the adrenal glands, as opposed to the sympathomimetic products of the adrenal medulla, already described. There are some five general groups of complex organic compounds produced in the adrenal cortex, of which the only group of importance to our present needs are the glucocorticoids. The name of this group derives from its involvement in carbohydrate metabolism, and its two most clinically useful members are cortisol and cortisone. Many commercial preparations and modifications of these two are available, with variable potencies and supposed specific responses.

Actions

The adrenal steroids exert a tremendous influence on body physiology, touching all organ systems. They have been referred to as "stress hormones" because they are secreted in greater amounts when the body is under stress, and severe trauma or prolonged critical illness may cause a depletion of their supply. In a complex way the steroids give support to the body to aid it through a crisis, and if they are acutely depleted or if their production is interrupted by abrupt destruction of the adrenals, the body functions deteriorate rapidly. On the other hand, a slow, chronic increase of cortical function does not produce a catastrophic picture but rather a multiplicity of signs and symptoms described as Cushing's syndrome.

A patient beginning to show evidence of excessive steroid action is often referred to as "Cushinoid." Some of the more common and important effects of hyperadrenalism are described below to illustrate the wide range of steroid action.[137-139]

Formation of glucose from body protein

When excessive, the formation of glucose from body protein can raise the blood sugar level high enough to produce "steroid diabetes" or to activate a latent, subclinical true diabetes. There can be associated protein loss with muscle wasting and weakness.

Depletion of bone calcium

Through a process of resorption, calcium is lost from bone. Structural thinning is such that fractures are frequent. This state of the bone is called *osteoporosis*.

Increase in fat production

Excessive amounts of fat are produced and are characteristically deposited in the subcutaneous tissues of the head and trunk. This results in a rounding of the facial contour, referred to as *moon face,* and an accumulation of fat at the base of the neck and upper back, called *buffalo hump.* These are two of the most prominent visible signs of a Cushinoid state.

Impaired immunologic response

Steroids inactivate circulating antibodies and thus can protect the body against the harmful effects of severe allergies. By the same token, however, this function lowers the body's resistance to infection, a point of significance especially with the prolonged use of steroids.

Reduction of inflammatory response

Steroids decrease the local vascular congestion and cellular infiltration that is the natural response to injury or infection. In addition, the deposition of fibrous tissue as part of the reparative process is inhibited. Of use in controlling the adverse effects of inflammation, this function also facilitates the spread of infection, since it interferes the usual process of localization. This is a serious threat to patients with infectious disorders.

Elevation of blood pressure

Steroids, through the mediation of certain electrolytes and other hormones, elevate the blood pressure. Of therapeutic significance, when the cardiovascular system no longer responds to sympathomimetics, as in certain states of shock, steroids often can help vasoconstrictors regain their pressor effects on the arterioles.

To complete the review of steroid action, mention should be made of the pituitary gland. The adrenal cortex is directly controlled by the anterior division of the pituitary gland, through a pituitary hormone called adrenocorticotropic hormone. The name itself describes a substance that stimulates *(-tropic)* the adrenal cortex and, not surprisingly, is almost always referred to as "ACTH." Administration of ACTH can be expected to elicit the same response as cortisol and cortisone, by stimulating the adrenal production of these substances. This presupposes that the adrenal cortex is in a functioning state, able to respond. Because the adrenals are likely to decrease their activity when steroids are given therapeutically, there is risk of adrenal atrophy with prolonged loss of function. Under such circumstances, ACTH may be given for periods of time to stimulate the adrenals to function and to prevent their atropy.

Use in respiratory care

In the treatment of respiratory diseases steroids are administered by inhalation, most commonly; orally for more significant exacerbations of bronchospasm; and by IV for serious bronchospasm. Steroids are used for their potent anti-inflammatory and anti-fibrogenic effects already mentioned, as well as for their ability to inhibit production and release of histamine (histamine produces bronchospasm) and to make beta$_2$ receptors more responsive to beta$_2$- adrenergics.[140,141] Thus, steroids not only help decrease the frequency of acute bronchospasm but also increase the effectiveness of adrenergic bronchodilators, especially in conditions where some tolerance has developed to them.[142] Aerosoloized steroids stimulate production of an intracellular protein, lipocortin, which inhibits synthesis of prostaglandins and leukotrienes.[143] The net result is to decrease inflammation and bronchospasm.[144]

Since it is now realized that the primary underlying pathology in asthma is airway inflammation, proper treatment requires targeting this inflammatory process.[9,145] Use of bronchodilators alone can remedy the bronchospasm, but if the inflammatory process is continuing, the patient's condition could be getting worse without it being apparent to the patient or doctor. Due to suppression of symptoms, less than sufficient therapy is employed until a severe exacerbation develops. This may be one of the reasons for the increased asthma mortality. Another proposed explanation for beta$_2$ adrenergic problems relates to an observed effect of high doses of adrenergic bronchodilator on increasing *cyclic adenosine monophosphate responsive element binding* protein (CREB). This CREB protein binds to the steroid receptor on the cell and diminishes the steroid anti-inflammatory effects.[146]

Aerosolized steroids, otherwise, can effectively treat underlying airway inflammation. The late phase response of allergic induced bronchospasm (due to SRS-A) can be mitigated or prevented by early use of inhaled steroids.[147] For significant bronchospasm, short courses (one to three weeks) of tapering oral steroids (prednisone) can provide dramatic improvement in the control of respiratory symptoms. Steroids do not replace bronchodilators, but should be used in addition to them.

Steroids are of particular value in the treatment of persons with asthma and with resistant allergies of the respiratory tract. The practitioner will witness dramatic responses to steroid therapy, but because of the wide spread action of the drug, various undesired effects can frequently accompany its use. Unlike other respiratory agents, which typically exert their side effects during or soon after the treatment, steroid side effects develop slowly (days to months) and without major symptoms. High doses of parenteral or enteral steroids may cause a psychological sense of well-being or anxiety.[148]

One possible side effect is a fungal infection, *candidiasis,* of the oropharynx or larynx, which can occur with the aerosol administration of steroids. Using the proper dosage can greatly minimize this complication. Having patients rinse their mouth out after treatments is also helpful in preventing this problem. Fortunately, for some of the more recently introduced steroids, candidiasis may be the only real side effect, since systemic absorption from the lung is minimal.

A summary of the steroids in current use in respiratory care is provided in Table 21-7. The following discussion highlights the major agents in this category.

Dexamethasone sodium phosphate (Decadron)

Dexamethasone is available in MDI preparations and can be used alone or mixed with a bronchodilator. The consensus is that this steroid is therapeutically active and effective throughout the entire respiratory tract from the nose to the bronchioles in the treatment of nasal allergies, allergic asthma, and some chronic obstructive states.[149,150] However, dexamethasone has definite systemic effects, readily detected by special urinary excretion tests. The systemic side effects have

Table 21-7 Commonly used steroids

Drug	Dose	Route
Beclomethasone (Vanceril, Beclovent)	2 inhalations tid/qid (42 µg/puff)	Aerosol
Flunisolide (AeroBid)	2 inhalations bid (250 µg/puff)	Aerosol
Triamcinolone acetonide (Azmacort)	2 inhalations tid (100 µg/puff)	Aerosol
	4–48 mg/day	Oral
Prednisone (Deltasone, Meticorten, Orasone)	5–60 mg/day	Oral
Dexamethasone (Dalalone, Decadron, Decaject, Hexadrol)	0.75–9 mg/day	Oral
	3 puffs tid/qid (84 µg/puff)	Aerosol
Methylprednisone Solu-Medrol	4–48 mg/day	Oral
	10–40 mg (initially)	IV
	40–120 mg (initially)	IM

limited the use of aerosolized dexamethasone in the lungs in favor of some newer products mentioned below.

Beclomethasone dipropionate (Vanceril, Beclovent)

After several years of use in Europe, the inhalant steroid beclomethasone became available in the United States in 1976. This drug was a significant step forward in the treatment of patients with bronchospasm. It is indicated in patients over six years of age with intrinsic, extrinsic, or mixed asthma who need chronic steroid therapy. Overall, beclomethasone appears to be an effective aerosolized steroid with minimal adverse effects that is of great therapeutic value to many patients.

Studies show that asthmatic symptoms decrease in about 80% of the cases concurrent with an improvement in pulmonary function. This occurs without the systemic side effects of oral steroids,[151-153] although Candidiasis may occur in a few. Most patients who have been dependent on oral steroids can switch to beclomethasone aerosol and maintain control of their asthmatic symptoms.[154,155] However, during acute exacerbations, oral steroids may be needed in previously steroid-dependent patients,[156] as well as in patients with pulmonary infiltration with eosinophilia.[157] Beclomethasone also has been reported to minimize the symptoms of perennial **rhinitis** that develop in people susceptible to various antigens such as pollen.[158-160]

Triamcinolone acetonide (Azmacort)

The steroid triamcinolone is a poorly soluble compound with good local and negligible systemic effects, which can be aerosolized for respiratory tract action. It is packaged as a suspension for intramuscular, intraarticular, or **intrabursal** injection, and in an MDI preparation. Studies show that in inhalations doses of about 100 μg each, four times per day, this agent allows most steroid-dependent asthmatics to stop oral steroids.[161,162] The majority of patients who are dependent on oral steroids can achieve a therapeutic effect with minimal side effects by using aerosolized triamcinolone.[163,164]

Flunisolide (AeroBid)

Flunisolide is another steroid packaged in the MDI form. It is well tolerated and effective in the treatment of steroid-dependent asthma.[165] This form of steroid is a bit more potent than the others so its recommended dosage is less: for adults and children, two inhalations (250 μg each) twice a day, for a total daily dosage of 1 mg.[166]

No matter which steroid is aerosolized, the actual dose administered is a matter of professional judgment and is the responsibility of the attending physi-

cian. In clinical practice, doubling or tripling the usual recommended dose during acute exacerbations may prevent the need for an oral "burst" of steroids and thereby stabilize the patient's condition before more aggressive measures are needed.[167] By and large, since steroid aerosols are usually packaged in metered dose inhalers (MDIs) for home use, the physician gives directions for use directly to the patient. However, should the practitioner be assigned to oversee the patient's treatment program, he or she should make certain that the physician gives specific orders. Whereas this should be the practice for any treatment, there are many instances in which established routines can be used, allowing the practitioner some flexibility to adjust techniques to individual needs. The great potency of the steroids and the possibility of adverse reactions demands that patients be properly instructed in their use. The many variables that influence the efficiency of aerosol treatment, such as function of the nebulizer, depth of ventilation, and ventilatory rate, make it impossible to precisely predict the systemic absorption of the drug. For this reason, astute clinical observation—in conjunction with more objective indicators such as pulmonary function tests—should be used to monitor and adjust the therapeutic dose schedule. Details on the proper use of metered dose inhalers are provided in Chapter 25.

Cromolyn sodium

Cromolyn sodium has proven effective for many years as an agent that helps prevent bronchospasm. It is an integral part of the treatment program for many asthmatics, but is not considered useful in acute, asthmatic attacks. It has been especially beneficial to many people in preventing exercise induced asthma (EIA).[168-171] Cromolyn may prevent EIA by minimizing airway cooling that occurs during rapid breathing, such as with exercise. This might be mediated by action on the bronchial vasculature.[172]

Cromolyn sodium acts by blocking the release of mediators such as histamine and leukotrienes C_4, D_4, E_4, which can cause bronchospasm (leukotrienes are the active agents in what was formerly called the slow-reacting substance of anaphylaxis, SRS-A, see discussion above).[173] These mediators are normally stored in special white blood cells called *mast cells*. When specific **antibody** receptors on the cells come in contact with specific antigens (pollen, dust, etc.) stored mediators are released (Figure 21-7).

For most of us this response merely attracts more white blood cells, dilates the local blood vessels, and results in more secretions at the site of irritation—all to help protect the body against the invasion of the foreign antigen. But people who are hypersensitive

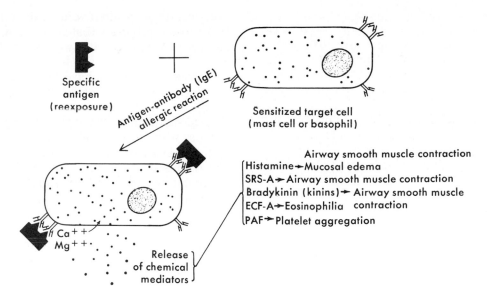

Fig. 21-7 Release of mediators from sensitized target cell in type I, IgE-mediated, immunologic reaction. (From Lehnert BE and Schachter EN: The pharmacology of respiratory care, St Louis, 1980, Mosby.)

(allergic) have exaggerated responses to these antigens. The result is excessive bronchospasm and secretions, with a marked increase in airway resistance.

As explained previously, steroids can decrease the allergic immune response and help prevent this reaction from occurring, but they also inhibit a multitude of other reactions in the prostaglandin and leukotriene pathways. Cromolyn sodium, on the other hand, primarily inhibits the mast cell response and does so with minimal side effects. However, it does not appear to work on everyone. It is effective in treating IgE-mediated reactions by stabilizing the mast cell membrane, but it is only effective if given *before* exposure to an offending antigen.[174] Cromolyn has been found to decrease symptoms in adults with chronic asthma, although these results vary.[175]

It must be emphasized that cromolyn sodium is only of value in preventing or moderating asthmatic attacks and is not effective once bronchospasm begins. However, one study stands alone in demonstrating some bronchodilatory effect of cromolyn in asthmatic patients.[176] More studies will undoubtedly further explore this new finding.

The regular use of cromolyn sodium inhalations during remission of symptoms can reduce the frequency and severity of attacks and lessen the amount of steriods previously needed to control symptoms.[177-179] Studies are now showing cromolyn sodium to be as effective as theophylline in the prophylactic treatment of asthmatics, when used on a regular basis. Cromolyn sodium has the added advantage of decreasing bronchial hyper-reactivity, thereby decreasing the frequency of asthmatic exacerbations.[180-182] Cromolyn sodium has also demonstrated clinical effectiveness in the reversal of histologic changes that occur with perennial rhinitis.[183-185]

For the prevention of bronchospasm, cromolyn sodium (Intal) is packaged as a 1% dry powder aerosol (administered by a SpinHaler rotary dispersion device) or in a 1% solution form for nebulization. A liquid nasal spray has been marketed for this purpose (Nasalcrom). Also available is a 4% solution (Opticrom) for allergic conjunctivitis. Currently under investigation, is the oral use of cromolyn sodium to help prevent severe food allergies.[186,187]

Nedocromil (Tilade)

Nedocromil is a newly introduced agent which is a pyranoquinoline dicarboxylic acid derivative with anti-inflammatory actions similar to cromolyn. Nedocromil appears to act primarily by stabilizing the mast cells.[174] Studies have shown it to be essentially as effective as cromolyn in prevention of bronchospasm.[188-190] It is also equally effective as cromolyn in the treatment of seasonal allergic rhinitis.[191] Nedocromil appears to inhibit release of substances (tachykinins) which can trigger bronchospasm.[192] It is recommended that it be taken on a regular basis, four inhalations per day (total dose 14 mg/day), in addition to bronchodilator therapy. The main side effect reported is an unpleasant taste in the mouth for some users.

Methotrexate

Methotrexate is an immunosuppressive drug which has been used in some cancers treatments. It is an oral medication used on occasion for those with chronic asthma.[11] It has been helpful in some, allowing one to decrease or discontinue the use of oral steroids.[193] Its main indication for trial use is for patients who are oral steroid dependent and cannot be tapered below a given amount without a bronchospasm flare-up.[194-196] Not all studies have found methotrexate to be beneficial.[197]

ANTIBIOTICS

Since the advent of the inhalation route for drug administration, interest has continued in using this approach to treat respiratory tract infections. This is especially true for those infections resistant to conventional therapy, such as lung abscess, necrotizing pnuemonias, and bronchiectasis.

In the mid-1940s sulfonamides were aerosolized, but the advent of penicillin and subsequent antibiotics stimulated extensive use of aerosols and the accumulation of a significant background of experience.[198-203] The rationale for aerosol therapy was based on the speculation that even with adequate blood levels of systemically administered antibiotics, the diffusion of the drug from blood into infected tissue for its direct antibacterial action was blocked by tissue reaction to the infection. It was believed that the presence of thick bronchial and alveolar exudates composed a formidable diffusion barrier, especially in localized lesions. Also, it was thought that interstitial edema and fibrosis of the diseased area were additional factors in preventing therapeutic antibiotic tissue levels. These observations were borne out by the frequent observation of active microbial growth in sputum while intensive systemic therapy was being administered.

Presently, the use of aerosolized antibiotics are uncommon, but on occasion one may see them used. Some of the underlying considerations in the use of aerosolized antibiotics follow. The ideal antibiotic for aerosol use has effective topical action and is poorly absorbed. Further, it is necessary that the infection being treated is accessible from the respiratory tract surface. From a practical point of view it can be generalized that aerosolized antibiotics play their greatest role in the treatment of stubborn gram-negative respiratory tract infections, where the nature of the infection and the frequently accompanying airway obstruction require long–term therapy. Large does of effective antibiotics can be used, self–administered at home if desired, with minimal hazard of untoward reactions. In the interest of economy, antibiotics should be aerosolized during inhalation only, using a small volume nebulizer. Table 21-8 lists those antibiotics that have been found suitable for aerosolization, with suggested doses for their use.[204]

Encouraging results have followed the use of aerosolized antibiotics in cystic fibrosis patients. Those using aerosolized gentamicin over a two year period showed significantly less lung deterioration compared to those who received only saline.[205] Another study of cystic fibrosis patients used an aerosol dose of carbenicillin and gentamicin. After a four month daily treatment period, there was significant improvement of pulmonary function values, and a dramatic drop in required hospitalizations.[206] These studies indicate that aerosol antibiotics appear to be an effective supplement to oral or IV antibiotic therapy in carefully selected patient categories.

However, the aerosol application of antibiotics is not a substitute for the systemic route. Although some patients respond dramatically, others show little or no benefit from this approach.[207,208] In view of the modifying factors listed previously and with variability of bacterial susceptibility encountered in systemic therapy, this is not surprising. However, the effectiveness of aerosolized antibiotics can be significantly increased by using a technique that deserves special mention.[209] The same exudates and secretions that impair drug diffusion from blood to tissue are able to interfere with the action of aerosolized particles, and they are probably responsible for many instances of therapeutic failure. The prior or concomitant use of bronchodilators will aid penetration of antibiotic particles but will not bring them into bacterial contact in the presence of thick secretions. Often, extensive therapy with heated water aerosol and chest physical therapy are essential to clear the airways for penetration and deposition of antibiotic aerosols.

Table 21-8 Antibiotics for aerosol use

Antibiotic	Aerosol dose
Carbenicillin	1–3 g
Neomycin*	50–400 mg
Bacitracin*	5000–200,000 units
Streptomycin	750–1000 mg
Chloramphenicol	200–400 mg
Kanamycin*	100–400 mg
Colymycin-M	25–150 mg
Polymyxin*	10–50 mg
Gentamicin*	40–120 mg
Amphotericin*	5–20 mg
Mycostatin*	100,000–400,000 units

From Miller WF: Fundamental principles of aerosol therapy, *Respir Care* 17:295, 1972.
*Poor or nonabsorbed in aerosol state.

In summary, aerosolized antibiotics are not intended to supplant the systemic route; rather they should be considered as a supplement in treating resistant, localized infections of the lung in selected patients. The use of antibiotics by inhalation is not frequently indicated; however, RCPs may occasionally be called on to administer these drugs by aerosol. When used in conjunction with techniques designed to enhance pulmonary clearance, aerosolized antibiotic agents may help reduce the amount of secretions and inhibit further bacterial growth. However, we must remember that the risk of distant spread of infection to other parts of the body can best be controlled by systemic administration of antibiotics.

ANTIVIRAL AGENTS

Antibiotics are not effective against viral illness. Recently, agents that are effective against some viruses, particularly those responsible for small airway infections (bronchiolitis) in children, have been studied.

A significant threat to a pediatric patient is infection with the respiratory syncytial virus (RSV). Studies with a synthetic nucleoside agent, ribavirin (Virazole), are demonstrating its effectiveness in the treatment of RSV infection, as well as in influenza A and B.[210-217] It has also been shown to be effective in adult patients, although RSV is not a common adult pathogen.[218]

Ribavirin appears to be the first broad spectrum antiviral agent showing antiviral properties against both DNA and RNA viruses, the two major groups of viruses. Studies of ribavirin's effectiveness against other viral infections such as viral hepatitis, Lassa fever, genital herpes, and herpes zoster, have demonstrated promising, but inconclusive results. Further studies are needed to justify ribavirin therapy for these indications.[219]

For the treatment of pediatric patients with respiratory syncytial virus, Ribavirin is supplied as a powder for reconstitution with sterile water. Administration is with a specialized microaerosol generator called the Small Particle Aerosol Generator-2 (SPAG-2), commercially available from the drug manufacturer (see Chapter 25). Treatment is carried out via an oxyhood, face mask, or mist tent for 12–18 hours per day over a period of at least three days. Using the recommended dosage and diluent in the aerosol generator, the average aerosol concentration of the drug is about 190 μg per liter of carrier gas. Adverse effects are relatively minor, and include rash and conjunctivitis.

Due to precipitation of the drug in the ventilator circuitry, attempts to apply the aerosol to children undergoing mechanical ventilation has posed serious problems, including jamming of the expiratory valve mechanisms. Recently, several clinicians have reported success in ribavirin administration during mechanical ventilation with special circuitry designed for this purpose.[220-221,215]

Precautions for health care workers must be taken so as to minimize exposure to exhaled ribavirin particles.[222,223] Special aerosol traps for collecting exhaled particles or adequately ventilated treatment rooms help decrease respiratory exposure to this medicine for those treating the patient.[224]

Despite some of these problems, ribavirin clearly is indicated for the treatment of specific viral infections of the lung in children, and may lead to more widespread use of similar agents in other viral disorders.

OTHER ANTIMICROBIALS

Among the opportunistic infections common in immunosuppressed patients, *Pneumocystis carinii* pneumonia (PCP) is a difficult to treat infection associated with a high mortality rate. Pneumocystis is a fungal-like organism which attaches to alveolar epithelial cells and involves the interstitial areas of the lungs. For the body to defend itself it requires proper function of macrophages and cytokines in order to prevent symptomatic infection. Hidden infection is common in man, but life threatening symptoms can occur in those whose immune systems are suppressed by steroids, cytotoxic drugs, radiotherapy, leukemia, severe malnutrition, or HIV. Treated conventionally, patients with PCP exhibit mortality rates between 30 to 50%.

The incidence of PCP infection has dramatically increased as the prevalence of HIV has increased and is one of the most common presenting infections of the Acquired Immune Deficiency Syndrome (AIDS).[225] In fact, patients with PCP for whom no other cause of immunodeficiency can be identified can be assumed to be an AIDS case.

The first agent proven to be of value in treating PCP infection was *pentamidine isethionate* (Pentam 300). Pentamidine isethionate is an aromatic diamidine compound that has been used extensively in the tropics for treatment of Trypanosoma and Leishmania infections. In the management of PCP infections in immunosuppressed children and adults, pentamidine can reduce mortality rates to about 3% in infants and 25% or less in children and adults.[225] Pentamidine probably interferes with the synthesis of DNA and RNA, but its actual mode of action is not fully understood.

Traditionally, pentamidine is administered via the intramuscular or intravenous route for 14 to 21 days. Approximately 50% of patients started on pentamidine require changing to another agent because of adverse effects. These adverse effects include altered glucose levels, anemia, neutropenia, azotemia, hypotension, and hyponatremia.[226] Due, in part, to these potent side effects, recent research has focused on the clinical effectiveness of aerosolized pentamidine (Nebupent).[227,228] After aerosol administration, the drug is almost exclusively recovered from the lung, with little extrapulmonary distribution. Moreover, aerosol administration delivers significantly higher concentrations of pentamidine to the air spaces than does intravenous delivery. This is especially so in patients with diffuse alveolar infiltrates and appears to be an effective adjunct to treatment that is better tolerated in many patients.[229-231] Typically, one of three dosing schedules are used: 30 mg or 150 mg every two weeks or 300 mg every four weeks for preventive treatment. On the highest dosage schedule, recurrence of PCP infection can be reduced by70%. Other dosing schedules have also shown to be effective.[232]

Adverse effects of aerosolized pentamidine include bronchospasm, which can be triggered in up to 26% of treated patients.[233] However, bronchoconstriction can be controlled with bronchodilator.[234] Other side effects include cough, fatigue, metallic taste, dyspnea, and some nausea at times. Aerosolized administration does appear safer than the parenteral route. It should be noted that proper aerosol techniques should be observed since health care workers in proximity to aerosol treatment can sustain low dose levels of pentamidine which can persist for weeks.[235]

Although pentamidine has emerged as a mainstay of therapy in the management of PCP in AIDS patients, trimethoprim-sulfamethoxazole, an orally dosed medicine which has been used for other infections for years, is also effective. In fact, trimethoprim-sulfamethoxazole is now considered the drug of choice for initial treatment since in low doses it offers better protection from disease than aerosolized pentamidine.[236] Because of the significance of PCP in immunosuppressed patients, continued research into these medications is vital.

NEW AND FUTURE THERAPEUTICS

Cystic fibrosis treatment now include efforts to correct a biochemical defect present in the lung. The gene which codes for normal chloride transport, but is defective in cystic fibrosis, appears to be correctable if replaced with a normal gene. It appears that this can be achieved using a virus which has been "inoculated" with a normal gene. The "therapeutic" virus is then delivered to the patient's lungs where it infects the cells with its genes, thereby providing the lung cells with the corrected gene. Further research and testing hopefully will result in a better treatment for cystic fibrosis patients.

CHAPTER SUMMARY

The primary purpose of respiratory pharmacology is to relieve or prevent the pathologic triad of bronchospasm, mucosal edema, and retained secretions. Bronchoconstriction and mucosal edema are treated by autonomic-active bronchodilating agents and are often accompanied by medications that prevent or lessen the inflammatory response due to allergic immunologic responses such as steroids and cromolyn sodium. Still in the experimental stage, prostaglandins may be of potential use in the relief of bronchospasm.

The clearance of retained secretions is approached using hydrating and wetting agents primarily. An occasional patient may benefit from a mucolytic. Associated with poor clearance of secretions and altered defense mechanisms, resistant infections of the lung may be treated with aerosolized antibiotic, antiviral, or other antimicrobial agents, as a supplement to the systemic route.

Effective use of these various drugs demands that the respiratory care practitioner have a sound background in the general principles of pharmacology, and in-depth knowledge of the mechanism of action, appropriate use, hazards, and side effects of all specific agents commonly applied in clinical practice. With an increasing emphasis on the self-administration of aerosolized drugs, RCPs must also develop the skills necessary to ensure patient compliance and understanding of proper usage and dose schedules.

REFERENCES

1. Hodgkin, J, Johnson, L, Lopez, B: An improved method for aerosolizing anesthetic for flexible bronchoscopy, *Resp Care* 21:134 137, 1976.
2. Goodman, LS, Gilman, A: *The pharmacological basis of therapeutics,* ed 6, New York, 1980, MacMillan.
3. Meyers, FH, Jawetz, E, Goldfien, A: *Review of Medical pharmacology,* ed 5, Los Altos, 1976, Lange Medical.
4. Issellbacher, KJ: *Harrison's principles of internal medicine,* ed 9, 1980, New York: McGraw Hill.
5. Goth, A: *Medical pharmacology: principles and concepts,* ed 11, St Louis, 1984, Mosby.
6. Bergersen, BS: *Pharmacology in nursing,* ed 14, St Louis, 1979, Mosby.
7. Harper, HA: Rodwell, VW, Mayes, PA: *Review of physiological chemistry,* Los Altos, 1977, Lange Medical.
8. Barnes, PJ: New aspects of asthma, *J Intern Med* 231(5):453, 1992.
9. Busse, W: Asthma in the 1990s. A new approach to therapy, *Postgrad Med* 92(6):177, 1992.
10. Canny, GJ, Levison, H: Childhood asthma: a rational approach to treatment [see comments], *Ann Allergy* 64(5):406, 1990.
11. Pueringer, RJ, Hunninghake, GW: Inflammation and airway reactivity in asthma, *Am J Med* 92(6A):32, 1992.
12. Santa Cruz, R, et al: Tracheal mucus velocity in normal man and patients with obstructive lung disease: effects of terbutaline, *Am Rev Respir Dis* 109:458, 1974.
13. Mortensen, J, Groth, S, Lange, P, Hermansen, F: Effect of terbutaline on mucociliary clearance in asthmatic and healthy subjects after inhalation from a pressurised inhaler and a dry powder inhaler, *Thorax* 46(11):817, 1991.
14. DeTroyer, A, Yernault, JC, Rodenstein, D: Influence of beta-2 agonist aerosols on pressure-volume characteristics of the lungs, *Am Rev Respir Dis* 118:987, 1978.

15. Ziment, I: Why are they saying bad things about IPPB? *Respir. Care.* 18:677, 1973.
16. Whelen, AM, Hahn, NW: Optimizing drug delivery from metered-dose inhalers, *Dicp* 25(6):638, 1991.
17. Davies, DS: Lung metabolism, Junod, AE, DeHaller, R, editors, New York, 1975, Academic Press.
18. Blackwell, EW et at: Metabolism of isoprenaline after aerosol and direct intrabronchial administration in man and dog, *Br J Pharmacol* 50:587, 1974.
19. Newman, SP, Clark, AR, Talaee, N, Clarke, SW: Pressurised aerosol deposition in the human lung with and without an "open" spacer device, *Thorax* 44(9):706, 1989.
20. Zainudin, BM, Biddiscombe, M, Tolfree, SE, Short, M, Spiro, SG: Comparison of bronchodilator responses and deposition patterns of salbutamol inhaled from a pressurised metered dose inhaler, as a dry powder, and as a nebulised solution, *Thorax* 45(6):469, 1990.
21. Smoker, JM, Tangen, MI, Ferree, SM, Hess, D, Rexrode, WO: A protocol to assess and administer aerosol bronchodilator therapy, *Respir Care* 31:780, 1987.
22. Kornberg, AE, Zuckerman, S, Welliver, JR, Mezzadri, F, Aquino, N: Effect of injected long-acting epinephrine in addition to aerosolized albuterol in the treatment of acute asthma in children, *Pediatr Emerg Care* 7(1):1, 1991.
23. Yamamoto, LG, Wiebe, RA, Anaya, C: Pulse oximetry and peak flow as indicators of wheezing severity in children and improvement following bronchodilator treatments, *Am J Emerg Med* 10(6):519, 1992.
24. Burgess, CD, Windom, HH, Pearce, N: Lack of evidence for beta-2 receptor selectivity: a study of metaproterenol, fenoterol, isoproterenol, and epinephrine in patients with asthma, *Am Rev Respir Dis* 143(2):444, 1991.
25. Keighley, JF: Iatrogenic asthma associated with adrenergic aerosols, *Ann Internm, Med* 65:985, 1966.
26. Singer, OP, Wilson, WJ: Laryngotracheobronchitis: 2 years' experience with racemic epinephrine, *Can Med Assoc J* 115:132, 1976.
27. Skolnik, NS: Treatment of croup. A critical review [see comments], *Am J Dis Child* 143(9):1045, 1989.
28. Kelley, PB, Simon, JE: Racemic epinephrine use in croup and disposition, *Am J Emerg Med* 10(3):181, 1992.
29. Wesley, CR, Cotton, E.K., Brooks, J.G: Nebulized racemic epinephrine by IPPB for the treatment of croup: a double-blind study, *Am J Dis Child* 132(5):484, 1978.
30. Gaffney, RJ, Harrison, M, Blayney, AW: Nebulized racemic ephedrine in the treatment of acute exacerbations of laryngeal relapsing polychondritis, *J Laryngol Otol* 106(1):63, 1992.
31. Editorial. Sympathomimetic bronchodilators (editorial), *Lancet* 1:535, 1971.
32. Sollman, R: *A manual of pharmacology,* Philadelphia, 1957 WB Saunders.
33. Eisenstadt, WS, Nichols, SS: Adverse effects of adrenergic aerosols in bronchial asthma, *Ann Allergy* 27:283, 1969.
34. McEvoy, JDS, Vall-spinosa, A, Paterson, JW: Assessment of orciprenaline and isoproterenol infusions in asthmatic patients, *Am Rev Respir Dis* 108:490, 1973.
35. Sobol, BJ: The rapidity of Alupent and isoproterenol, *Ann Allergy* 32:137, 1974.
36. Nussbaum, E, Eyzaguirre, M, Galant, SP: Dose-response relationship of inhaled metaproterenol sulfate in preschool children with mild asthma, *Pediatrics* 85(6):1072, 1990.
37. Nelson, MS, Hofstadter, A, Parker, J, Hargis, C: Frequency of inhaled metaproterenol in the treatment of acute asthma exacerbation, *Ann Emerg Med* 19(1):21, 1990.
38. Emerman, CL, Cydulka, RK, Effron, D, Lukens, TW, Gershman, H, Boehm, SP: A randomized, controlled comparison of isoetharine and albuterol in the treatment of acute asthma, *Ann Emerg Med* 20(10):1090, 1991.
39. Lands, AM et al: The pharmacologic actions of the bronchodilator drug isoetharine, *J Am Pharm Assoc* 47:744, 1958.
40. Shulman, M et al: Cardiovascular effects of isoetharine administered to surgical patients during cyclopropane anesthesia, *Br J Anaesth* 42:439, 1970.
41. El-Shaboury, AH: Controlled study of a new inhalant in asthma and bronchitis, *Br Med J* 5416:1037, 1964.
42. Kelman, GR et al: Cardiovascular effects of solbutamol, *Nature* 221:1251, 1969.
43. Owen, JA: A bronchodilator well-known in European, *Hosp Formulary* Aug:386, 1975.
44. Casaburi, R, Adame, D, Hong, CK: Comparison of albuterol to isoproterenol as a bronchodilator for use in pulmonary function testing, *Chest* 100(6):1597, 1991.
45. Snider, GL, Laguanda, R: Albuterol and isoproterenol aerosols. A controlled study of duration of effect in asthmatic patients, *JAMA* 221:682, 1972.
46. Bloomfield, P et al: Comparison of solbutamol given intravenously and by intermittent positive-pressure breathing in life-threatening asthma, *Br Med J* 6167(1):848, 1979.
47. Denjean, A, Guimaraes, H, Migdal, M, Miramand, JL, Dehan, M, Gaultier, C: Dose-related bronchodilator response to aerosolized salbutamol (albuterol) in ventilator-dependent premature infants, *J Pediatr* 120(6):974, 1992.
48. Tinkelman, DG, Lutz, C: Effect of increasing dosage of an inhaled beta-2 specific agonist on pulmonary function, tremor, and cardiovascular indices [published erratum appears in Ann Allergy, May 68(5):390, 1992]. *Ann Allergy* 68(1):23, 1992.
49. Tinkelman, DG, Brandon, ML, Grieco, M et al: Comparison of safety and efficacy of inhaled pirbuterol with metaproterenol, *Ann Allergy* 64(2 Pt 2):202, 1990.
50. Brogden, RN, Speight, TM, G.S., A: Terbutaline: a preliminary report of its pharmacological properties and therapeutic efficacy in asthma, *Drugs* 6:324, 1973.
51. Malo, JL, Ghezzo, H, Trudeau, C, Cartier, A, Morris, J: Duration of action of inhaled terbutaline at two different doses and of albuterol in protecting against bronchoconstriction induced by hyperventilation of dry cold air in asthmatic subjects, *Am Rev Respir Dis* 140(3):817, 1989.
52. Munzenberger, PJ, Papaioanou, HA, Massoud, N: A clinical comparison of terbutaline with albuterol administered by metered-dose inhaler, *Ann Allergy* 62(2):107, 1989.
53. Vilsvik, J, Schaanning, J, Stahl, E, Holthe, S: Comparison between Bricanyl Turbuhaler and Ventolin metered dose inhaler in the treatment of exercise-induced asthma in adults, *Ann Allergy* 67(3):315, 1991.
54. Mestitz, H, Copland, JM, McDonald, CF: Comparison of outpatient nebulized vs metered dose inhaler terbutaline in chronic airflow obstruction [see comments], *Chest* 96(6):1237, 1989.
55. Kelly, HW, McWilliams, BC, Katz, R, Murphy, S: Safety of frequent high dose nebulized terbutaline in children with acute severe asthma, *Ann Allergy* 64(2 Pt 2):229, 1990.
56. Pinnas, JL et al: Multicenter study of bitolterol and isoproterenol nebulizer solutions in nonsteroid using patients, *J Allergy Clin Immunol* 79:768, 1987.
57. Harris, JB, Ahrens, RC, Milavetz, G, Annis, L, Ries, R, Hendricker, C: Comparison of the intensity and duration of effects of inhaled bitolterol and albuterol on airway caliber and airway responsiveness to histamine, *J Allergy Clin Immunol* 85(6):1043, 1990.
58. Magnussen, H, Rabe, KF: The protective effect of low-dose inhaled fenoterol against methacholine and exercise-induced bronchoconstriction in asthma: a dose-response study [see comments], *J Allergy Clin Immunol* 90(5):846, 1992.
59. Trembath, PN et al: Comparison of four weeks' treatment with fenoterol and terbutaline aerosols in adult asthmatics, A double blind crossover study. *J Allergy Clin Immunol* 63(6):345, 1979.
60. Yanai, M, Ohrui, T, Sekizawa, K, Shimizu, Y, Sasaki, H, Takishima, T: Effective site of bronchodilation by antiasthma drugs in subjects with asthma, *J Allergy Clin Immunol* 87(6):1080, 1991.
61. Ohrui, T, Yanai, M, Sekizawa, K, Morikawa, M, Sasaki, H,

Takishima, T: Effective site of bronchodilation by beta- ad-renergic and anticholinergic agents in patients with chronic obstructive pulmonary disease: direct measurement of intrabronchial pressure with a new catheter, *Am Rev Respir Dis* 146(1):88, 1992.

62. Taylor, IK, O'Shaughnessy, KM, Choudry, NB, Adachi, M, Palmer, JB, Fuller, RW: A comparative study in atopic subjects with asthma of the effects of salmeterol and salbutamol on allergen-induced bronchoconstriction, increase in airway reactivity, and increase in urinary leukotriene E4 excretion, *J Allergy Clin Immunol* 89(2):575, 1992.

63. Simons, FE, Soni, NR, Watson, WT, Becker, AB: Bronchodilator and bronchoprotective effects of salmeterol in young patients with asthma [see comments], *J Allergy Clin Immunol* 90(5):840, 1992.

64. Derom, EY, Pauwels, RA, Van der Straeten, ME: The effect of inhaled salmeterol on methacholine responsiveness in subjects with asthma up to 12 hours, *J Allergy Clin Immunol* 89(4):811, 1992.

65. Verberne, AA, Hop, WC, Bos, AB, Kerrebijn, KF: Effect of a single dose of inhaled salmeterol on baseline airway caliber and methacholine-induced airway obstruction in asthmatic children, *J Allergy Clin Immunol* 91(1 Pt 1):127, 1993.

66. Anderson, SD, Rodwell, LT, Du Toit, J, Young, IH: Duration of protection by inhaled salmeterol in exercise-induced asthma, *Chest* 100(5):1254, 1991.

67. Pearlman, DS, Chervinsky, P, La Force, C et al: A comparison of salmeterol with albuterol in the treatment of mild-to-moderate asthma, *N Engl J Med* 327(20):1420, 1992.

68. Cheung, D, Timmers, MC, Zwinderman, AH, Bel, EH, Dijkman, JH, Sterk, PJ: Long-term effects of a long-acting beta 2-adrenoceptor agonist, salmeterol, on airway hyperresponsiveness in patients with mild asthma, *N Engl J Med* 327(17):1198, 1992.

69. Siminsson, BG, Jonson, B, Strom, B: Bronchodilatory and circulatory effects of inhaling increasing doses of an anticholinergic drug, ipratropium bromide (SCH 1000), *Scand J Respir Dis* 56:138, 1975.

70. Davison, FR: Handbook of materia medica, toxicology, and pharmacology, St Louis, 1949, Mosby.

71. Nadel, JA, Widdecombe, JG: Mechanism of bronchoconstriction with dust inhalation, *Clin Res* 10:91, 1962.

72. Dautreband, L et al: Effects of atropine microaerosols on airway resistance in man, *Arch Int Pharmacodyn* 139:198, 1962.

73. Chamberlain, DA et al: Atropine methonitrate and isoprenaline in bronchial asthma, *Lancet* 2:1019, 1962.

74. Storms, WW et al: Aerosol Sch 1000, *Am Rev Respir Dis* 111:419, 1962.

75. Gross, NJ: Sch 1000: a new anticholinergic bronchodilator, *Am Rev Respir Dis* 112:823, 1975.

76. Ingram, RH, McFadden, ER, Jr: Localization and mechanisms of airway responses, *N Eng J Med* 297(11):596, 1977.

77. Pare, PD, Lawson, LM, Brooks, LA: Patterns of response to inhaled bronchodilators in asthmatics, *Am Rev Respir Dis* 127(6):680, 1983.

78. Villate-Navarro, J et al: Comparative effects of turbutaline sulfate and ipratropium bromide on the respiratory system, *Med Clin (Barc)* 74(7):275, 1980.

79. Garmon, RG, Zemenick, RB: Acute severe asthma: part 2. Current therapy, *J Am Osteopath Assoc* 92(3):343, 1992.

80. Scano, G, Stendardi, L, Sergysels, R: Lung mechanics after aerosol and intravenous SCH 1000 in normal humans, *Int J Clin Pharmacol Ther Toxicol* 20(10):454, 1982.

81. Kitamura, S, Ishihara, Y, Sugiyama, Y et al: Effect of ipratropium bromide on the action of broncho-active agents, *Arzneimittelforsch* 32(2):128, 1982.

82. Nadel, JA: Parasympathetic regulation of lungs and airways: Chairman's summary, *Postgrad Med J* 51(Suppl 7):86, 1975.

83. Bruderman, I, Cohen-Aronovski, R, Smorzik, J: A comparative study of various combinations of ipratopium bromide and metaproterenol in allergic asthmatic patients, *Chest* 83(2):208, 1983.

84. Yeung, R, Nolan, GM, Levison, H: Comparison of the effects on inhaled SCH 1000 and fenoterol on exercise-induced bronchospasm in children, *Pediatrics* 66(1):109, 1980.

85. Rebuck, AS, Marcus, HI: SCH 1000 in psychogenic asthma. *Scand J Respir Dis* 103((suppl)):186, 1979.

86. Ihre, E, Larsson, K: Airways responses to ipratropium bromide do not vary with time in asthmatic subjects. Studies of interindividual and intraindividual variation of bronchodilatation and protection against histamine-induced bronchoconstriction, *Chest* 97(1):46, 1990.

87. Gross, NJ: Chronic obstructive pulmonary disease. Current concepts and therapeutic approaches. *Chest* 97(2 Suppl):19, 1990.

88. Braun, SR, McKenzie, WN, Copeland, C, Knight, L, Ellersieck, M: A comparison of the effect of ipratropium and albuterol in the treatment of chronic obstructive airway disease [published erratum appears in *Arch Intern Med* Jun, 150(6):1242], 1990. *Arch Intern Med* 149(3):544, 1989.

89. Simon, PM, Statz, EM: Drug treatment of COPD. Controversies about agents and how to deliver them, *Postgrad Med* 91(4):473, 1992.

90. Fernandez, A, Lazaro, A, Garcia, A, Aragon, C, Cerda, E: Bronchodilators in patients with chronic obstructive pulmonary disease on mechanical ventilation. Utilization of metered-dose inhalers, *Am Rev Respir Dis* 141(1):164, 1990.

91. Bleecker, ER, Britt, EJ: Acute bronchodilating effects of ipratropium bromide and theophylline in chronic obstructive pulmonary disease, *Am J Med* 91(4A):24, 1991.

92. Bennett, WD, Chapman, WF, Mascarella, JM: The acute effect of ipratropium bromide bronchodilator therapy on cough clearance in COPD, *Chest* 103(2):488, 1993.

93. Caffeine consumption decreases the response to bronchoprovocation challenge with dry gas hyperventilation. *Chest* 99(6):1374, 1991.

94. Gerhardt, T, McCarthy, J, Bancalari, E: Aminophylline therapy for idiopathic apnea in premature infants: effects on lung function, *Pediatrics* 62(5):801, 1978.

95. Brazier, JL, Renaud, H, Ribon, B, Salle, BL: Plasma xanthine levels in low birthweight infants treated or not treated with theophylline, *Arch Dis Child* 54(3):194, 1979.

96. Aranda, JV, Turmen, T: Methylxanthines in apnea of prematurity, *Clin Perinatol* 6(1):87, 1979.

97. Caffeine and theophylline as adenosine receptor antagonists in humans, *J Pharmacol Exp Ther* 258(2):588, 1991.

98. Chou, T: Wake up and smell the coffee. Caffeine, coffee, and the medical consequences, *West J Med* 157(5):544, 1992.

99. Bjorck, T, Gustafsson, LE, Dahlen, SE: Isolated bronchi from asthmatics are hyperresponsive to adenosine, which apparently acts indirectly by liberation of leukotrienes and histamine, *Am Rev Respir Dis* 145(5):1087, 1992.

100. Di Giulio, GA, Kercsmar, CM, Krug, SE, Alpert, SE, Marx, CM: Hospital treatment of asthma: lack of benefit from theophylline given in addition to nebulized albuterol and intravenously administered corticosteroid [see comments], *J Pediatr* 122(3):464, 1993.

101. Lam, A, Newhouse, MT: Management of asthma and chronic airflow limitation. Are methylxanthines obsolete? [see comments], *Chest* 98(1):44, 1990.

102. Johnston, ID: Theophylline in the management of airflow obstruction. 2. Difficult drugs to use, few clinical indications, *Bmj* 300(6729):929, 1990.

103. Spector, SL: Asthma and chronic obstructive lung disease: a pharmacologic approach, *Dis Mon* 37(1):1, 1991.

104. Janson, C, Boman, G, Boe, J: Which patients benefit from adding theophylline to beta 2-agonist treatment in severe acute asthma? *Ann Allergy* 69(2):107, 1992.

105. Ward, AJ, McKenniff, M, Evans, JM, Page, CP, Costello, JF: Theophylline—an immunomodulatory role in asthma? *Am Rev Respir Dis* 147(3):518, 1993.

106. Iwainsky, H, Sehrt, I: Theophylline therapy foundations and possibilities, *Z Erkr Atmungsorgane* 152(1):21, 1979.

107. Powell, JR et al: The influence of cigarette smoking and sex on theophylline disposition, *Am Re Respir Dis* 116:17, 1977.

108. Chang, KC, Bell, TD, Laver, BA, Chai, H: Altered theophylline pharmacokinetics during acute respiratory viral illness, *Lancet* 1(8074):1132, 1978.

109. Segal, MS: Aminophylline: A clinical overview, *Adv Asthma Allergy* 2:17, 1975.

110. Stewart, BN, Block, AJ: A trial of aerosolized theophylline in relieving bronchospasm, *Chest* 69:718, 1976.

111. Bureau, MF, De Clerck, F, Lefort, J, Arreto, CD, Vargaftig, BB: Thromboxane A2 accounts for bronchoconstriction but not for platelet sequestration and microvascular albumin exchanges induced by fMLP in the guinea pig lung, *J Pharmacol Exp Ther* 260(2):832, 1992.

112. Stechschulte, DJ: Leukotrienes in Asthma and Allergic Rhinitis, *New Eng J of Med* 323(25):1769, 1990.

113. Bernard, GR, Korley, V, Chee, P, Swindell, B, Ford-Hutchinson, AW, Tagari, P: Persistent generation of peptido leukotrienes in patients with the adult respiratory distress syndrome, *Am Rev Respir Dis* 144(2):263, 1991.

114. Drazen, JM, O'Brien, J, Sparrow, D et al: Recovery of leukotriene E4 from the urine of patients with airway obstruction, *Am Rev Respir Dis* 146(1):104, 1992.

115. Labat, C, Ortiz, JL, Norel, X et al: A second cysteinyl leukotriene receptor in human lung, *J Pharmacol Exp Ther* 263(2):800, 1992.

116. Cloud, ML, Enas, GC, Kemp, J et al: A specific LTD4/LTE4-receptor antagonist improves pulmonary function in patients with mild, chronic asthma, *Am Rev Respir Dis* 140(5):1336, 1989.

117. Robuschi, M, Riva, E, Fuccella, LM et al: Prevention of exercise-induced bronchoconstriction by a new leukotriene antagonist (SK&F 104353). A double-blind study versus disodium cromoglycate and placebo, *Am Rev Respir Dis* 145(6):1285, 1992.

118. Hui, KP, Barnes, NC: Lung function improvement in asthma with a cysteinyl-leukotriene receptor antagonist [see comments], *Lancet* 337(8749):1062, 1991.

119. Gaddy, JN, Margolskee, DJ, Bush, RK, Williams, VC, Busse, WW: Bronchodilation with a potent and selective leukotriene D4 (LTD4) receptor antagonist (MK-571) in patients with asthma, *Am Rev Respir Dis* 146(2):358, 1992.

120. Harvath, L, Robbins, JD, Russell, AA, Seamon, KB: cAMP and human neutrophil chemotaxis. Elevation of cAMP differentially affects chemotactic responsiveness, *J Immunol* 146(1):224, 1991.

121. Rau, JL: *Respiratory therapy pharmacology*, ed 2, St Louis, 1984, Mosby.

122. Dulfano, JJ, Adler, KB, Wooten, O: Physical properties of sputum: IV. Effects of 100 per cent humidity and water mist, *Am Rev Respir Dis* 107:130, 1973.

123. Allegra, L, Moavero, NE, Rampoldi, C: Ozone-induced impairment of mucociliary transport and its prevention with N-acetylcysteine, *Am J Med* 91(3C):67, 1991.

124. Petty, TL: The National Mucolytic Study. Results of a randomized, double-blind, placebo-controlled study of iodinated glycerol in chronic obstructive bronchitis [see comments], *Chest* 97(1):75, 1990.

125. Petty, TL: Chronic obstructive pulmonary disease—can we do better? *Chest* 97(2 Suppl):2, 1990.

126. Helmholz, FH: *Personal communication.*

127. Sheffner, AL: The mucolytic activity, mechanisms of action, and metabolism of acetylcysteine, *Pharmacotherapy* 1:47, 1964.

128. Hirsch, SR, Kory, RC: An evaluation of the effect of nebulized N-acetylcysteine on sputum consistency, *J Allerg* 39:265, 1967.

129. Moser, KM, Rhodes, PG: Acute effects of aerosolized acetylcysteine upon spirometric measurements in subjects with and without obstructive pulmonary disease, *Dis Chest* 49:370, 1966.

130. Thomas, PA, Treasure, RI: Effect of N-acetyl-L-cysteine on pulmonary surface activity, *Am Rev Respir Dis* 94:175, 1966.

131. Webb, WR: New mucolytic agents for sputum liquefaction, *Postgrad Med* 36:449, 1964.

132. Mucolytic agents: *Br Med J* 2:603, 1966.

133. Anderson, G: A clinical trial of muscolytic agent: acetylcysteine in chronic bronchitis, *Br J Dis Chest* 60:101, 1966.

134. Tainter, ML: Alevaire as a mucolytic agent, *N Engl J Med* 253:764, 1955.

135. Jobe, A: Pulmonary Surfactant Therapy, *NEJM* 328(12):861, 1993.

136. Aerosolized surfactant treatment of preterm lambs, *J Appl Physiol* 70(2):869, 1991.

137. Forsham, PH: The adrenal gland, *Clin Symp* 15:3, 1963.

138. Kleiner, IS, Orten, JM: Biochemistry, ed 7 1966, St Louis: Mosby.

139. Williams, RH: Textbook of endrocrinology, Philadelphia, 1962.

140. Aviado, DM, Carrillo, LR: Antiasthmatic addition and corticosteroids, *J Clin Pharmacol* 10:3, 1970.

141. Ellul-Micallef, R, Fenech, FF: Effect of intravenous prednisolone in asthmatics and diminished adrenergic responsiveness, *Lancet* 2:1269, 1975.

142. Mathewson, HS: Risks and benefits of aerosolized steroids, *Respir Care* 28:325, 1983.

143. Bone, R: Bronchial Asthma: Diagnostic and Treatment Issues, *Hospital Practice* Sept. 30:45, 1993.

144. Djukanovic, R, Wilson, JW, Britten, KM et al: Effect of an inhaled corticosteroid on airway inflammation and symptoms in asthma, *Am Rev Respir Dis* 145(3):669, 1992.

145. Barnes, PJ: A new approach to the treatment of asthma [see comments], *N Engl J Med* 321(22):1517, 1989.

146. Cotton, P: Asthma Consensus Is Unconvincing to Many, *JAMA* 270(3):297, 1993.

147. Fabbri, LM, Maestrelli, P, Saetta, M, Mapp, CE: Airway inflammation during late asthmatic reactions induced by toluene diisocyanate, *Am Rev Respir Dis* 143(3 Pt 2):S37, 1991.

148. Bender, BG, Lerner, JA, Poland, JE: Association between corticosteroids and psychologic change in hospitalized asthmatic children, *Ann Allergy* 66(5):414, 1991.

149. Norman, PS et al: Adrenal function during the use of dexameth-asone aerosols in the treatment of ragweed hay fever, *J Allerg* 40:57, 1967.

150. Fisch, BR, Grater, WC: Dexamethasone aerosol in respiratory tract disease, *J New Drugs* 2:298, 1962.

151. Clark, TJ: Corticosteroid treatment of asthma, *Schweiz Med Wochenschr* 110(6):215, 1980.

152. Chambers, WB, Malfitan, VA: Beclomethasone dipropionate aerosol in the treatment of asthma in steroid-independent children, *J Int Med Res* 7(5):415, 1979.

153. Datau, G, Rochiccioli, P: Cortiocotropic testing during long-term beclomethasone dipropionate treatment in asthmatic children, *Poumon Coeur* 34(4):247, 1978.

154. Richards, W et al: Steroid-dependent asthma treated with inhaled beclomethasone dipropionate in children, *Ann Allergy* 41(5):247, 1978.

155. Kass, I, Vijayachandra Nair, S, Patil, KD: Beclomethasone dipropionate aerosol in the treatment of steroid-dependent asthmatic patients. An assessment of 18 months of therapy, *Chest* 71(6):703, 1977.

156. Lee-Hong, E, Collins-Williams, C: The long-term use of beclomethasone dipropionate for the control of severe asthma in children, *Ann Allergy* 38(4):242, 1977.

157. Hudgel, DW, Spector, SL: Pulmonary infiltration with eosinophila. Recurrence in an asthmatic patient treated with becolmethasone dipropionate, *Chest* 72(3):359, 1977.

158. Neuman, I, Toshner, D: Beclomethasone dipropionate in pediatric perennial extrinsic rhinitis, *Ann Allergy* 409(5):346, 1978.

159. Brown, R, Ingram, RH, Mcfadden, RR: Effects of prosta-

glandin F2as on lung mechanics in nonasthmatic and asthmatic subjects, *J Appl Physiol* 44:150, 1978.

160. Girard, JP, Cuevas, M, Heimlich, EM: A placebo controlled double-blind trial of beclomethasone dipropionate in the treatment of allergic rhinitis, *Allergol Immunopathol* 6(2):109, 1978.

161. Bernstein, IL, Chervinsky, P, Falliers, CJ: Efficacy and safety of triamcinolone acetonide aerosol in chronic asthma. Results of a multicenter short-term controlled and long-term open study, *Chest* 81:20, 1982.

162. Grieco, MH, Dwek, T, Larsen, K, Rammohan, G: Clinical effects of aerosol triamcinolone acetonide acetonide in bronchial asthma, *Arch Intern Med* 138:1337, 1978.

163. Golub, JR: Long-term triamcinolone acetonide aerosol treatment in adult patients with chronic bronchial asthma, *Ann Allergy* 44(3):131, 1980.

164. Chervinsky, P, Petraco, AJ: Incidence or oral candidiasis during therapy with triamcinolone acetonide aerosol, *Ann Allergy* 43(2):80, 1974.

165. Slavin, RG, Izu, AE, Bernstein, IL et al: Multicenter study flunisolide aerosol in adult patients with steroid-dependent asthma, *J Allergy Clin Immunol* 66(5):379, 1980.

166. Corticosteroid aerosols for asthma. The Medical Letter 27:5, 1985.

167. Li, JT, Reed, CE: Proper use of aerosol corticosteroids to control asthma, *Mayo Clin Proc* 64(2):205, 1989.

168. Poppius, H, Muittari, A, Kreus, KE et al: Exercise asthma and disodium cromoglycate, *Br Med J* 4:337, 1970.

169. Chan-Yeung, M: The effect of SCH 1000 and disodium cromoglycate on exercise-induced asthma, *Chest* 71:320, 1977.

170. Briner, W, Jr., Bruno, PJ: Case report: 30-yr-old female with exercise induced anaphylaxis *Med Sci Sports Exerc* 23(9):991, 1991.

171. Obata, T, Matsuda, S, Akasawa, A, Iikura, Y: Preventive effect and duration of action of disodium cromoglycate and procaterol on exercise-induced asthma in asthmatic children, *Ann Allergy* 70(2):123, 1993.

172. Pichurko, BM, McFadden, ERJ, Bowman, HF, Solway, J, Burns, S, Dowling, N: Influence of cromolyn sodium on airway temperature in normal subjects, *Am Rev Resp Dis* 130(6):1002, 1984.

173. Woenne, R, Kattan, M, Levison, H: Sodium cromogylcate-induced changes in the dose-response curve of inhaled methacholine and histamine in asthmatic children, *Am Rev Respir Dis* 119(6):927, 1979.

174. King, HC: Mast cell stabilizers. Otolaryngol Head Neck Surg, 107(6 Pt 2):841, 1992.

175. Petty, TL, Rollins, DR, Christopher, K, Good, JT, Oakley, R: Cromolyn sodium is effective in adult chronic asthmatics, *Am Rev Respir Dis* 139(3):694, 1989.

176. Weiner, P, Greif, J, Fireman, E, Kivity, S, Topilsky, M: Bronchodilating effect of cromolyn sodium in asthmatic patients at rest and following exercise, *Ann Allergy* 53(2):186, 1984.

177. Mathison, DA et al: Cromolyn treatment of asthma, *JAMA* 216:1454, 1971.

178. Smith, JM: Prolonged use of disodium cromoglycate in children and young persons-ten years experience, *Schweiz Med Wochenschr* 110(6):183, 1980.

179. Turner-Warnick, M: Clinical practice with regard to management of the adult asthmatic with cromoglycate, *Schweiz Med Wochenschr* 110(6):183, 1980.

180. Furuwaka, CT, Shapiro, GG, Bierman, CW, Kraemer, MJ, Ward, DJ, Pierson, WE: A double-blind study comparing the effectiveness of cromolyn sodium and sustained-release theophylline in childhood asthma, *Pediatrics* 74(4):453, 1984.

181. Bernstein, IL: Cromolyn Sodium, *Chest* 87(1-Supp 1):68, 1985.

182. Selcow, JE, Mendelson, LM, Rosen, JP: Clinical benefits of cromolyn sodium aerosol (MDI) in the treatment of asthma in children, *Ann Allergy* 62(3):195, 1989.

183. Caballero, LM, Carbonell, AC, Climent P'erez, JL: Clinical and histological study to assess changes in the nasal mucosa in patients with chronic perennial rhinitis comparing sodium cromoglycate and placebo, *J Respir Dis* 59(3):160, 1978.

184. Goodman, ML, Irwin, JW: Disodium cromoglycate in anaphylaxis and pollinosis, *Ann Allergy* 40(3):177, 1978.

185. Frostad, AB: The treatment of seasonal allergic rhinitis with a 2% aqueous solution of sodium cromoglycate delivered by a metered dose nasal spray, *Clin Allergy* 7(4):347, 1977.

186. Jones, EAJ: Oral cromolyn sodium in milk induced anaphylaxis, *Ann Allergy* 54(3):199, 1985.

187. Stefanini, GF, Prati, E, Albini, MC et al: Oral disodium cromoglycate treatment on irritable bowel syndrome: an open study on 101 subjects with diarrheic type [see comments], *Am J Gastroenterol* 87(1):55, 1992.

188. Morton, AR, Ogle, SL, Fitch, KD: Effects of nedocromil sodium, cromolyn sodium, and a placebo in exercise-induced asthma, *Ann Allergy* 68(2):143, 1992.

189. Rebuck, AS, Kesten, S, Boulet, LP et al: A 3-month evaluation of the efficacy of nedocromil sodium in asthma: a randomized, double-blind, placebo-controlled trial of nedocromil sodium conducted by a Canadian multicenter study group, *J Allergy Clin Immunol* 85(3):612, 1990.

190. Greif, J, Fink, G, Smorzik, Y, Topilsky, M, Bruderman, I, Spitzer, SA: Nedocromil sodium and placebo in the treatment of bronchial asthma. A multicenter, double-blind, parallel-group comparison, *Chest* 96(3):583, 1989.

191. Schuller, DE, Selcow, JE, Joos, TH et al: A multicenter trial of nedocromil sodium, 1% nasal solution, compared with cromolyn sodium and placebo in ragweed seasonal allergic rhinitis, *J Allergy Clin Immunol* 86(4 Pt 1):554, 1990.

192. Verleden, GM, Belvisi, MG, Stretton, CD, Barnes, PJ: Nedocromil sodium modulates nonadrenergic, noncholinergic bronchoconstrictor nerves in guinea pig airways in vitro, *Am Rev Respir Dis* 143(1):114, 1991.

193. Dyer, PD, Vaughan, TR, Weber, RW: Methotrexate in the treatment of steroid-dependent asthma, *J Allergy Clin Immunol* 88(2):208, 1991.

194. Stempel, DA, Lammert, J, Mullarkey, MF: Use of methotrexate in the treatment of steroid-dependent adolescent asthmatics, *Ann Allergy* 67(3):346, 1991.

195. Guss, S, Portnoy, J: Methotrexate treatment of severe asthma in children, *Pediatrics* 89(4 Pt 1):635, 1992.

196. Mullarkey, MF, Lammert, JK, Blumenstein, BA: Long-term methotrexate treatment in corticosteroid-dependent asthma, *Ann Intern Med* 112(8):577, 1990.

197. Erzurum, SC, Leff, JA, Cochran, JE et al: Lack of benefit of methotrexate in severe, steroid-dependent asthma. A double-blind, placebo-controlled study [see comments], *Ann Intern Med* 114(5):353, 1991.

198. Olsen, A: Streptomycin aerosol in the treatment of chronic bronchiectasis: Preliminary report, *Proc Staff Meet Mayo Clin* 21:53, 1946.

199. Garthwaite, B, Barach, AL: Penicillin aerosol therapy in bronchiectasis, lung abscess, and chronic bronchitis, *Am J Med* 3:261, 1947.

200. Eastlake, C, Jr: Aerosol therapy in sinusitis, bronchiectasis, and lung abscess, *Bull NY Acad Med* 26:423, 1950.

201. Christie, HE et al: Aerosol therapy for lung abscess, *Can Med Assoc J* 62:478, 1950.

202. Melica, A et al: Oxytetracycline inhalation in the treatment of acute and chronic bronchial infection, *G Clin Med* 47:416, 1962.

203. Naumov, GP: Pathologic changes in upper respiratory passages and lungs following use of antibiotic electroaerosols, *Fed Proc* 25:654, 1966.

204. Stout, SA, Derendorf, H: Local treatment of respiratory infections with antibiotics, *Drug Intell Clin Pharm* 21:322, 1987.

205. Kun, P, Landau, LI, Phelan, PD: Nebulized gentamicin in children and adolescents with cystic fibrosis, *Aust Paediatr J* 20(1):43, 1984.

206. Battistini, A, Grzincich, GL, Grandi, F, Ferrara, D, Carchesio, L, Pistocchi, S: Aerosol administration inantibiotic therapy of cystic fibrosis, *Pediatr Med Chir* 5(4):161, 1983.
207. Pines, A et al: Gentamicin and colistin in chronic **purulent** bronchial infections, *Br Med J* 2:543, 1967.
208. Bilodeau, M et al: Studies of absorption of kanamycin by aerosol, *Ann NY Acad Sci* 132:870, 1966.
209. Spier, R et al: Aerosolized pancreatic dornase and antibiotics in pulmonary infection, *JAMA* 178:878, 1961.
210. Hall, CB, Walsh, EE, Hruska, JF, Betts, RF, Hall, WJ: Ribavirin treatment of experimental respiratory syncytial viral infection, *JAMA* 249:2666, 1983.
211. Knight, V, Bloom, K, Wilson, SZ et al: Ribavirin small-particle aerosol treatment of influenza, *Lancet* 2:945, 1981.
212. Knight, V: Aerosol treatment of influenza, *Cardiovasc Res Center Bull* 19:118, 1981.
213. McClung, HW, Knight, V, Gilbert, BE, Wilson, SZ, Quarles, JM, Divine, GW: Ribavirin aerosol treatment of influenza B virus infection, *JAMA* 249:2671, 1983.
214. Rimar, JM: Ribavirin for treatment of RSV infection, *MCN* 11:413, 1986.
215. Englund, JA, Piedra, PA, Jefferson, LS, Wilson, SZ, Taber, LH, Gilbert, BE: High-dose, short-duration ribavirin aerosol therapy in children with suspected respiratory syncytial virus infection, *J Pediatr* 117(2 Pt 1):313, 1990.
216. What is the clinical role of aerosolized ribavirin? Dicp 24(7–8):735, 1990.
217. Aerosol and intraperitoneal administration of ribavirin and ribavirin triacetate: pharmacokinetics and protection of mice against intracerebral infection with influenza A/WSN virus, *Antimicrob Agents Chemother* 35(7):1448, 1991.
218. Aylward, RB, Burdge, DR: Ribavirin therapy of adult respiratory syncytial virus pneumonitis, *Arch Intern Med* 151(11):2303, 1991.
219. Eggleston, M: Clinical review of ribavirin, *Infect Cont* 8:215, 1987.
220. Tiffin, NH, Warren, JB, Lee, RJ: Administration of ribavirin to a mechanically ventilated infant, *RRT* 23(1):10, 1987.
221. Demers, RR, Parker, J, Frankel, LR, Smith, DW: Administration of ribavirin to neonatal and pediatric patients during mechanical ventilation, *Respir Care* 31:1188, 1986.
222. Kacmarek, RM: Care-giver protection from exposure to aerosolized pharmacologic agents. Is it necessary? *Chest* 100(4):1104, 1991.
223. Harrison, R: Reproductive risk assessment with occupational exposure to ribavirin aerosol, *Pediatr Infect Dis J* 9(9 Suppl):S102, 1990.
224. Bradley, JS, Connor, JD, Compogiannis, LS, Eiger, LL: Exposure of health care workers to ribavirin during therapy for respiratory syncytial virus infections, *Antimicrob Agents Chemother* 34(4):668, 1990.
225. Salamone, FR, Cunha, BA: Update on pentamidine for the treatment of Pneumocystis carinii pneumonia, *Clin Pharm* 7:501, 1988.
226. Wharton JM, Coleman DL, Wofsy CB, et al: Trimethoprim sulfamethoxazole or pentamidine for Pneumocystis carinii pneumonia in the acquired immunodeficiency syndrome, *Ann Intern Med* 105:37, 1986.
227. Haverkos, HW: Assessment of therapy for pneumocystis carinii pneumonia, *Am J Med* 76:501, 1984.
228. Corkery, KJ, Luce, JM, Montgomery, AB: Aerosolized pentamidine for treatment and prophylaxis of Pneumocystis carinii pneumonia: An update, *Respir Care* 33:676, 1988.
229. Montgomery, AB, Debs, RJ, Luce, JM: Selective delivery of pentamidine to the lung by aerosol, *Am Rev Respir Dis* 137:477, 1988.
230. Sarti, GM: Aerosolized pentamidine in HIV. Promising new treatment for Pneumocystis carinii pneumonia, *Postgrad Med* 86(2):54, 1989.
231. Montgomery, AB, Debs, RJ, Luce, JM, Corkery, KJ, Turner, J, Hopewell, PC: Aerosolized pentamidine as second line therapy in patients with AIDS and Pneumocystis carinii pneumonia, *Chest* 95(4):747, 1989.
232. Murphy, RL, Lavelle, JP, Allan, JD: Aerosol pentamidine prophylaxis following Pneumocystis carinii pneumonia in AIDS patients: results of a blinded dose-comparison study using an ultrasonic nebulizer [see comments], *Am J Med* 90(4):418, 1991.
233. Katzman, M, Meade, W, Iglar, K, Rachlis, A, Berger, P, Chan, CK: High incidence of bronchospasm with regular administration of aerosolized pentamidine, *Chest* 101(1):79, 1992.
234. Quieffin, J, Hunter, J, Schechter, MT et al: Aerosol pentamidine-induced bronchoconstriction. Predictive factors and preventive therapy, *Chest* 100(3):624, 1991.
235. O'Riordan, TG, Smaldone, GC: Exposure of health care workers to aerosolized pentamidine, *Chest* 101(6):1494, 1992.
236. Carr, A, Tindall, B, Penny, R, Cooper, DA: Trimethoprim-sulphamethoxazole appears more effective than aerosolized pentamidine as secondary prophylaxis against Pneumocystis carinii pneumonia in patients with AIDS [see comments], *AIDS* 6(2):165, 1992.

Airway Care

Kim Simmons

CHAPTER LEARNING OBJECTIVES

1. Describe the hazards and complications and outline the procedure used in nasotracheal suctioning;
2. Compare and contrast rigid and flexible fiberoptic bronchoscopy, as used for both therapeutic and diagnostic purposes;
3. Differentiate among the four primary indications for insertion of an artificial airway;
4. Differentiate among the advantages, disadvantages, and methods of establishing tracheal airways via the oral, nasal, and tracheotomy route;
5. Describe the role and responsibilities of the respiratory care practitioner in the maintenance of artificial tracheal airways, including procedures for airway clearance and cuff care;
6. Identify the appropriate course of action in common artificial airway emergencies, to include tube obstruction, cuff leaks, and accidental extubation;
7. Differentiate between the methods and procedures used to extubate patients with oro- or nasotracheal tubes, versus those employed to remove a tracheostomy tube.

Respiratory care practitioners (RCPs) spend a great deal of time working with patients who have diseased lungs and impaired gas exchange. Adequate gas exchange is not possible if a patent airway is not provided, even with normal lungs. The importance of an adequate airway is demonstrated in the sequencing of CPR procedures, when the airway is given first priority (see Chapter 23). Airway care procedures are the responsibility of RCPs in many areas of the hospital setting. These areas include the general medical and surgical floors, in the critical care areas, as well as in the emergency room.

There are two broad areas of airway care in which RCPs must develop skills. First, the RCP must be proficient in airway clearance techniques, including those methods designed to ensure the patency of the patient's airway, natural or artificial. Second, the RCP must be able to insert and maintain artificial airways designed to support patients whose own natural airways are inadequate. This chapter will explore each of these areas.

AIRWAY CLEARANCE TECHNIQUES

Airway obstruction occurs secondary to retained secretions, foreign objects (such as tumors and aspirated food), and structural changes such as edema or traumatic injuries. Mechanical aspiration, or suctioning, allows the practitioner to remove retained secretions, blood or other semi-liquid fluids from the large airways.[2] This is accomplished by applying negative pressure to the airway through a catheter. Removal of foreign objects and suctioning below the carina are often done by bronchoscopy, which is performed by a physician. This technique often requires the assist-

ance of RCPs. Management of the structural changes and injuries will be discussed later in the section on artificial airways.

Airway aspiration (suctioning)

Retention of secretions increases airway resistance and the work of breathing, and may result in hypoxemia, hypercapnia, atelectasis, and infection. As described in Chapter 9, normal secretions are handled by the mucociliary escalator mechanism and swallowing. Difficulty in clearing secretions may be due to their thickness or amount, or to the patient's inability to generate an effective cough.

Indications

Retention of clearing secretions is the primary indication for suctioning. The most common clinical sign indicating retained secretions is abnormal breath sounds, especially course rhonchi occurring in the hilar region. If these sounds do not clear after coughing, the patient is having difficulty clearing secretions.

Disease processes which may require suctioning due to excess secretions include infectious disorders, COPD, and cystic fibrosis. Conditions which impair the cough mechanism, such as CNS depression or neuromuscular disease, can also cause retention of secretions and require suctioning.

Complications

There are several significant complications associated with suctioning. These complications are listed in the accompanying box and discussed in detail below.

Hypoxemia is a common complication of suctioning.[2,107,136] This is due to the fact that both air and secretions are removed during suctioning. In fact, greater decreases in oxygenation have been reported after suctioning than after an equal period of apnea.[14] Moreover, hypoxemia can lead to other complications, such as cardiac arrest and hypertension.[107]

To prevent hypoxemia, patients should always be preoxygenated prior to suctioning with 100% O_2. Where indicated, hyperinflated with a manual resuscitator should accompany preoxygenation.[2,20,107] Of course, one must use caution in preoxygenating patients with chronic hypercapnia, as this technique could decrease their stimulus to breath. Limiting the amount of time suction is applied also helps minimize hypoxemia.

Cardiac arrhythmias occur mainly as a result of hypoxemia.[2,107] Mechanical stimulation of the airway, particularly the area around the larynx, will also cause arrhythmias.[107] If the patient is connected to a cardiac monitor, the RCP should check it often for gross arrhythmias. Vagal stimulation, as the catheter enters the larynx or impacts the carina, can cause bradycardia or asystole. Tachycardia may result from patient agitation and hypoxemia. If any major change is seen in the heart rate or rhythm, the RCP should immediately stop suctioning and administer oxygen to the patient, providing manual ventilation as needed.

Hypotension during suctioning may be due to cardiac arrhythmias or severe coughing episodes that decrease venous return.[2,107] As with arrhythmias, if the patient becomes hypotensive, the procedure must be stopped and oxygenation and ventilation restored. Hypertension may be caused by hypoxemia or increased sympathetic tone due to stress, anxiety, pain, or changes in hemodynamics secondary to manual hyperventilation.[120,121]

Atelectasis is due to removal of too much air from the lungs.[2,107] This complication can be avoided by: limiting the amount of negative pressure used, keeping the duration of suctioning as short as possible, and providing hyperinflation before and after the procedure.

Using too large a suction catheter may also cause atelectasis. As long as the catheter is smaller than the airway, some of the air that is drawn into the catheter will come from the upper airway. On the other hand, if the catheter completely obstructs the airway, then suction will be applied to only the airway below the catheter. To avoid this complication, the external diameter of the catheter should never exceed one-half internal diameter of the airway.[128]

Airway trauma can occur as the tube is passed through the upper airway and the trachea.[2] The severity of trauma ranges from simple mucosal hemorrhage and nasal bleeding to laceration of nasal turbinates and pharyngeal perforation. This trauma occurs when a rigid catheter impacts on the walls of the airway. To avoid this complication, one should never use excessive force when advancing the catheter. Lubrication of the catheter will also ease its passage.

Mucosal trauma also occurs when the catheter adheres to the wall of the airway during suctioning.[107] As the catheter is withdrawn, mucosa is literally torn away from the underlying support structures. To avoid this problem, one should limit the amount of negative pressure used. In general, suction pressure should be set as low as possible, yet high enough to effectively clear secretions. For adults, this generally means using no more than -100 to -120 mmHg. For children, one should limit suction pressure to -80 to -100 mmHg. With infants, -60 to -80 mmHg is the limit.[11] In addition to limiting the suction pressure, one may use one of the many catheters designed to minimize mucosal trauma (Figure 22-1).

Contamination of the lungs with bacteria is another complication of suctioning. Contamination occurs when the catheter is passed through the upper airway.[2] Transient **bacteremia** has been reported with nasotracheal suctioning secondary to mucosal damage.[75] Immunosuppressed patients are likely to develop more serious complications. Sterile technique and gentle insertion help minimize this complication.

Increased intracranial pressure (ICP) have been

Complications of suctioning[1,2]

- Hypoxia/hypoxemia
- Cardiac arrhythmias
- Hypotension/hypertension
- Atelectasis
- Mucosal trauma
- Pulmonary hemorrhage/bleeding
- Infection (patient and/or caregiver)
- Elevated intracranial pressure
- Bronchoconstriction/bronchospasm
- Cardiac arrest
- Respiratory arrest

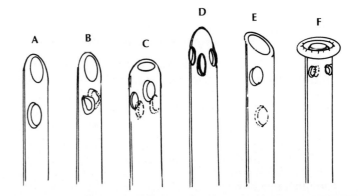

Fig. 22-1 Suction catheter tips used to minimize mucosal trauma.

reported during suctioning. An increase in ICP during suctioning is usually due to arterial hypertension or coughing.[2,15,106] These changes are only transient, with values normally returning to baseline within one minute. However, in patients who already have an elevated ICP, these changes could be significant. In these patients, aerosolized lidocaine given 15 minutes prior to suctioning may help reduce the rise in ICP.[15]

The presence of the catheter in the lower airway may stimulate normal protective mechanisms, resulting in coughing, laryngospasm, or bronchospasm.[2] The bronchospastic response may be particularly strong in patients with hyperactive airway disease. These patients should be assessed for the development of wheezes associated with suctioning.

Pushing the catheter into the oropharynx esophagus may illicit gaging and regurgitation.[2] The RCP should always be ready to reposition the patient and to suction the oropharynx if regurgitation occurs. Additionally, the practitioner should know the time at which the patient last ate or received a feeding. Nasogastric feedings may need to be stopped prior to suctioning to minimize the risk of regurgitation. This should be coordinated with nursing personnel.

Contraindications[2]

The most common contraindications against nasotracheal suctioning are listed in the accompanying box.[1,2] Epiglottitis and or croup are absolute contraindication for nasotracheal suctioning. Irritation caused by the catheter only worsens these upper airway disorders. Relative contraindications include situations in which catheter passage is difficult, such as occluded nasal passages or facial injuries. If a patient is already bleeding through the nose, or has a coagulopathy or bleeding disorder, suctioning may be delayed or performed with caution and extra lubrication. History of an irritable airway or laryngospasm is also considered a relative contraindication. Last, the presence of an upper respiratory tract infections may increase the chance of spreading pathogens further into the lungs, and is also a relative contraindication.

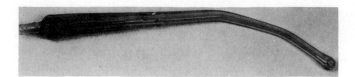

Fig. 22-2 Yankauer-type tonsil suction.

Procedure

Access to the trachea for suctioning can be gained through the nose, mouth, or an artificial airway. Nasotracheal suctioning will be discussed at this time.[2,107] Tracheal suctioning through the mouth should be avoided, as this causes gagging. Oropharyngeal secretions can be removed using a rigid tonsillar, or Yankauer suction tip (Figure 22-2). Suctioning through an artificial airway will be discussed in the section on airway maintenance.

Step 1: Assess the need for suctioning.[2] A patient should never be 'routinely' suctioned. The decision to suction a patient should be based on current physical findings, including coarse rhonchi, tactile fremitus, and an ineffective cough.

Step 2: Assemble and check the equipment.[2] Most suction catheter packages include the catheter, gloves, and a cup for rinsing the catheter. Additional equipment needed is listed in the accompanying box. If universal precautions are indicated, goggles, masks, and gowns may also be required. After connecting the catheter to the suction source, the practitioner should check the level of suction pressure. If no vacuum is generated at the thumbport, the practitioner should check for leaks in the tubing, at the collection container, or the regulator. In addition, if the collecting bottle is full, the float-valve will close and prevent vacuum transmission.

Step 3: Preoxygenate the patient.[9,107] For patients who can take a deep breath on their own, the RCP should initially apply the oxygen therapy device and instruct them to breathe slowly and deeply for about 30 seconds. For patients who cannot take a deep breath on their own, a manual resuscitator connected to an oxygen source should be used. Caution should

---

Contraindications for nasotracheal suctioning[1,2]

- Occluded nasal passages
- Nasal bleeding
- Epiglottitis or croup (absolute)
- Acute head, facial, or neck injury
- Coagulopathy or bleeding disorder
- Laryngospasm
- Irritable airway
- Upper respiratory tract infection

Equipment needed for nasotracheal suctioning

- Sterile suction catheter with thumb port
- Sterile glove(s)
- Goggles, mask, and gown (universal precautions)
- Sterile basin
- Sterile water or saline
- Sterile water soluble lubricating jelly
- Adjustable suction source
- Oxygen delivery system (mask and manual resuscitator)

be taken with chronically hypercapnic patients breathing on a hypoxic drive.

Step 4: Insert the catheter.[107] After the catheter has been lubricated, it should be inserted gently through the nostril, directing it toward the septum and the floor of the nasal cavity, without applying negative pressure. If any resistance is meet in the nose, gently twisting of the catheter should help. If resistance still occurs, the catheter should be withdrawn and inserted through the other nostril.

As the catheter moves into the lower pharynx, the patient should assume a "sniffing" position, by flexing the neck extending the atlanto-occipital joint (Figure 22-3). This position helps align the opening of the larynx with the lower pharynx, making catheter passage through the larynx more likely. Forward displacement of the tongue, which pulls the epiglottis upward and forward, may also aid catheter passage into the trachea (refer to Figure 26-3). The practitioner should continue to advance the catheter until the patient coughs, or a resistance is felt much lower in the airway.

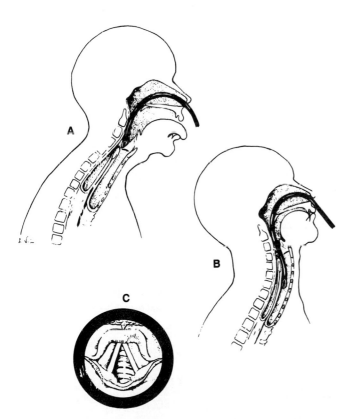

Fig. 22-3 Technique of nasotracheal suctioning. **A,** Optimal position of head in order to direct catheter tip anteriorly into the trachea. The neck is flexed and the head is extended. The tongue is protruded (and held there by a gauze 4 × 4). **B,** After the catheter has been advanced into the trachea, the tongue is released and the patient's head may be more comfortably positioned. **C,** View of the vocal cords from above. The cords are most widely separated during inspiration. (From Sanderson RG: The cardiac patient: a comprehensive approach, Philadelphia, 1972, WB Saunders.)

Step 5: Apply suction.[107] When the patient coughs, the RCP should apply suction, while withdrawing the catheter using a rotating motion. If an obstruction is felt, the RCP should pull the catheter back a few centimeters before applying suction. This maneuver will minimize mucosal damage. Since oxygenation has been shown to decrease after 5 seconds of suctioning, total suction time should not exceed 10 to 15 seconds.[2,107] If any cardiac disturbances result, the RCP should remove the suction catheter immediately and oxygenate the patient.

Step 6: Re-oxygenate and hyperinflate the patient.[2] The RCP should apply the oxygen device and proceed as in step 3. Patients unable to voluntarily take a deep breath must be hyperinflated and re-oxygenated with a manual resuscitator.

Step 7: Assess the patient. The patient should be assessed for any signs of hypoxemia including cyanosis, tachypnea, and tachycardia. If available, pulse oximetry and the ECG should be monitored. The presence of blood in the catheter or patient's nostrils should also be noted. Signs of increased intracranial pressure (ICP), such as complaints of headache, dizziness, or a change in level of consciousness should be observed. When available, ICP should also be monitored. However, this capacity is usually found only in critical care areas. Assuming no serious complications occur, the procedure should be repeated from step 3 to 7 until the patient's breath sounds have cleared or improved.

Since suctioning can cause serious complications, it should not be repeated unless it's effectiveness can be documented.[2] Effectiveness of the procedure can be evaluated by stimulation of a cough, removal of secretions, decreased work of breathing, and improved breath sounds. The stimulation of a cough, although not a goal of suctioning, does suggest the successful placement of the catheter.

Bronchoscopy

Bronchoscopy is the general term used to describe the insertion of a visualization instrument (**endoscope**) into the bronchi. Bronchoscopy is conducted for both therapeutic and diagnostic purposes. A detailed list of the diagnostic and therapeutic capabilities of bronchoscopy appears in the box on page 545.

There are two types of bronchoscopes in current use: rigid tube and flexible. Although RCPs most often assist in flexible fiberoptic bronchoscopy, an understanding of both types of devices is clinically useful.

Rigid tube bronchoscopy

The rigid bronchoscope is an open metal tube with a distal light source and a port for attaching oxygen or ventilating equipment (Figure 22-4, page 544).[90] The rigid bronchoscope is used most often by **otorhinolaryngologists** or thoracic surgeons. The tube is passed

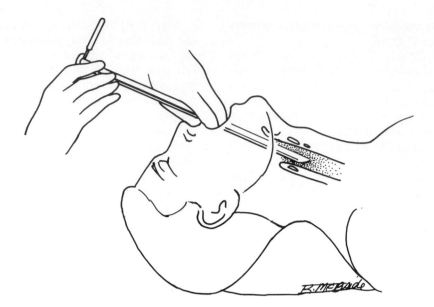

Fig. 22-4 Rigid tube bronchoscope.

through the mouth, down into the trachea and as far as the bronchi. A telescoping tube with mirrors is used to advance to and view segmental bronchi. Suctioning is via a metal tube passed through the bronchoscope. The large internal diameter of this suction tube allows for aspiration of thick **inspissated** secretions and large mucous plugs. A grasping forceps passed through the device allows removal of foreign bodies and biopsies of airway tumors.

Rigid bronchoscopy has several disadvantages. First, it is very uncomfortable for conscious patients. Moreover, it usually requires the assistance of an anesthesiologist and the use of an operating room.[33] Last, and most important, rigid bronchoscopy cannot access the smaller airways.

Flexible fiberoptic bronchoscopy (FFB)

In contrast, the flexible fiberoptic bronchoscope, or FFB, has gained popularity over the years due to both its versatility and ability to access very small airways.[63]

The typical FFB has a light transmission channel, a visualizing channel, and a multipurpose open channel (Figure 22-5). The open channel may be used for aspiration, tissue sampling, or oxygen administration. This type of bronchoscope is most often used by the **pulmonologist,** often with the assistance of a RCP.[27,129] The RCP prepares the patient by explaining the procedure, and administering an aerosolized local anesthetic to the patient's upper airway (in order to minimize gagging). The physician then inserts the

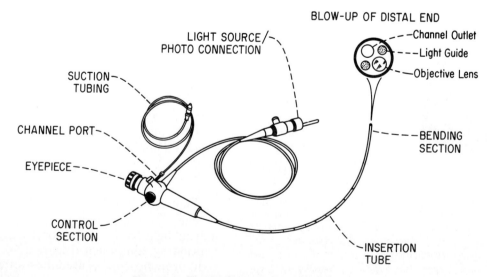

Fig. 22-5 Flexible fiberoptic bronchoscope.

Bronchoscopy: indications and therapeutic applications[61]

Diagnostic uses

Inspection of the lower airways

Mass, infiltrate, or other radiographic abnormality
Hemoptysis
Unexplained cough
Recurrent pneumonia or atelectasis
Localized wheezing
Symptoms or laboratory findings suggesting upper airway obstruction
Paralysis of recurrent laryngeal or phrenic nerve
Staging of known lung cancer
Positive sputum cytology without radiologic abnormality
Suspected tracheobronchial injury
Suspected bronchopleural fistula following lung surgery
Follow-up examination after therapeutic procedures (see below)

Bronchography (injection of contrast dye through broncho-scope to visualize airways radiographically)

Suspected bronchiectasis
Assessment of anatomy following surgery, laser treatment of obstructing tumor, or other procedure.

Acquisition of specimens for staining, culture, and/or patho-logic examination

Bronchoalveolar lavage (e.g., diagnosis of *P. carinii* pneumonia; assessment of interstitial lung disease)
Bronchial washings (e.g., sputum-negative suspected tuberculosis)
Protected catheter specimen brush (e.g., pneumonia undiagnosed by other methods)
Forceps biopsy or brushing of airway lesions or bronchial wall under direct vision
Transbronchial biopsy or brushing of distal airways and/or lung parenchyma under fluoroscopic guidance
Transbronchial needle aspiration or biopsy (e.g., to sample adjacent lymph nodes for metastasis)

Therapeutic uses

Facilitation of endotracheal intubation (passage of endotracheal tube over bronchoscope passed through vocal cords)
Removal of airway secretions (e.g., acute lobar atelectasis refractory to chest physiotherapy)
Removal of aspirated foreign bodies or other loose material from proximal bronchial tree.
Therapeutic bronchial or whole-lung lavage (e.g., in pulmonary alveolar proteinosis)
Palliative therapy of malignant tumors causing tracheal or bronchial obstruction
Brachytherapy (direct application of radiation therapy)
Laser phototherapy (vaporization of tumor tissue)
Fulguration using heater probes or bipolar electrodes

---

bronchoscope orally or nasally, using the head control to direct the tip to the location desired.

Therapeutic indications. As indicated in the accompanying box, there are five primary therapeutic indications for fiberoptic bronchoscopy. The role of the bronchoscope as an aid to endotracheal intubation will be discussed later. Removal of secretions to treat atelectasis is possible. However, the bronchoscope's open channel is quite small, and may become plugged if secretions are very thick. Wetting agents such as saline or mucolytics like acetylcysteine or sodium bicarbonate may be used to decrease the viscosity of the secretions.

Removal of foreign objects from the airway can be done using a variety of tools.[42,71] Forceps are used to remove small solid objects.[72] Large objects and organic material such as food can be retrieved with a basket.[81] This bronchoscope accessory has been used to remove objects as large as tweezers (9 cm) from mainstem bronchi.

Palliative bronchoscopic procedures for **nonresectable** lung cancer include both laser therapy and brachytherapy. Bronchoscopic laser therapy is indicated when endobronchial tumors obstruct the large airways. After the tumor is visualized, the laser energy is directed through a fiberoptic cable and fed into the bronchoscope. The laser can be set on low power to cause thermal necrosis and coagulation, or high power for vaporization.

Brachytherapy is the local application of ionizing radiation to treat tumors.[4] In this procedure, the bronchoscope is used to guide a catheter to the site of the tumor. The catheter is then left in place and attached to a source of **iridium**[192]. Brachytherapy can be combined with laser therapy. In this approach, the bronchoscope is passed to the area of the tumor. If the tumor is totally occludes the bronchus, the laser may be used to partially open the airway before insertion of the endobronchial catheter. If the airway is partially closed or the tumor is extrabronchial, the endobronchial catheter is put into position.

Complications. The complications of bronchoscopy are similar to those for suctioning (Table 22-1, page 546). However, the greater patient discomfort, longer duration, and the extent of airway penetration make this a more hazardous and complex procedure.

Hypoxemia is most severe in patients with underlying lung disease. To minimize this problem, all patients should receive oxygen before and during the procedure. When the nasal route is used to insert the bronchoscope, oxygen can be administered by a nasal catheter (in the opposite nares) or by a mask adapted to allow passage of the scope.

Hemodynamic changes (heart rate, blood pressure, and cardiac output) vary and may be related to differences in techniques or medications.

Bronchospasm also has been reported, and is most severe in asthmatic patients.[37,99] Premedication with

Table 22-1 Complications of fiberoptic bronchoscopy

Complication	Incidence (%)
Pneumonia	0.6
Pneumothorax	0.4
Airway obstruction	0.4
Respiratory arrest	0.2
Death	0.1
Vasovagal reaction	2.4
Fever	1.2
Cardiac dysrhythmia	0.9
Bleeding	0.7
Nausea and vomiting	0.2
ECG abnormality	0.2
Psychotic reaction	0.1
Aphonia	0.1

albuterol and ipratropium bromide may help relieve this problem, as will the use of sedatives or narcotic-analgesics which do *not* release histamine. Demerol and fentanyl are better for the asthmatic patient.

Procedure. [63,102] Key points to consider in planning and conducting bronchoscopy include premedication, equipment preparation, airway preparation, and monitoring. Also, to reduce the risk of aspiration due to gagging and loss of airway reflexes, the patient should refrain from food or drink for at least 8 hours prior to the start of the procedure. In addition, if the IV route is not already available, vascular access should be obtained prior to the start of the procedure.

Premedication. As previously mentioned, bronchoscopy is a very uncomfortable procedure. To decrease anxiety, the patient should be premedicated one to two hours in advance. The patient should be

Bronchoscopy equipment

For operator and assistant

Masks
Gloves
Gowns

For airway management

Endotracheal tubes
Bronchoscope adapter for endotracheal tube
Yankauer-type suction catheters
Suction pump
Suction tubing
Bite block
Adhesive tape
Water-soluble lubricant

Syringes, needles, and solutions

10- and 20-mL syringes, Luer-Lok
10- and 20-mL syringes, non-Luer-Lok
Needles, sharp tip
Needles, blunt-tip
Saline
Nonbacteriostatic saline

For obtaining specimens

Bronchoscope accessories
Specimen cups
Sputum traps

For handling specimens

Microscope slides
Viral and anaerobic transport media
Carbowax
Formalin

Miscellaneous items

Bronchoscope light source
Denture cups

Miscellaneous items continued

Emesis basins
Sunglasses, radio
Medicine cups
Cotton 4×4s and 2×2s

For patient support and monitoring

Pulse oximeter
Oxygen cannulae
ECG leads
Cardiac monitor

For anesthesia and sedation

Jackson forceps
Cotton balls
Heparin locks or caps
Intravenous catheters or "butterflies"
Alcohol wipes
Bandaids
Sterile swabs
Atomizer and accessories

Medications

Epinephrine 1:1000
Heparin lock flush solution
Sedatives (e.g., meperidine [Demerol], codeine, morphine, diazepam [Valium], midazolam [Versed])
Topical anesthetics (e.g., lidocaine [1, 2, & 4%], cocaine [4 or 10%], Cetacaine [solution of benzocaine and tetracaine], lidocaine jelly)

Paperwork

Consent forms
Specimen labels
Laboratory specimen forms
Radiology requisitions
Bronchoscopy charge slips
Physician's order forms

Reproduced with permission from Johnson NT, Pierson DJ: Pulmonary diagnostic procedures. In Pierson DJ, Kacmarek RM, editors: *Foundations of Respiratory Care*, New York, Churchill-Livingston, 1992. a"Crash" cart should be available in addition to listed items.

calm but alert enough to follow commands, such as taking a deep breath. Tranquilizers, such as the benzodiazepines (Valium, Versed) are frequently used for this purpose.

Another goal of premedication is to dry the patient's airway. This promotes anesthetic deposition, aids visibility, and can reduce procedure time. Atropine, given 1 to 2 hours prior to the procedure, is used to achieve this. Atropine may also help decrease vagal responses (such as bradycardia and hypotension) that can occur during bronchoscopy.

Narcotic-analgesics such as morphine or fentanyl may also be given.[63,102] In addition to reducing pain, these agents also help diminish laryngeal reflexes. However, narcotics should be withheld until those procedures requiring patient cooperation are completed. Of course, caution must be taken to avoid respiratory depression. Should it occur, naloxone (Narcan) must be available.

Additional narcotics and sedatives may be needed for patient comfort, and should be available. The need for antiarrhythmics, resuscitative drugs, narcotic antagonists, and IV fluids is harder to predict. Therefore, advance preparation will result in a more efficient and rapid response.

Equipment preparation. The RCP is often responsible for preparing equipment. The accompanying box provides a list of needed equipment. Special procedure rooms are often used for bronchoscopy and usually have most of the ancillary equipment already in place. All equipment must be thoroughly checked for function, tight connections, and integrity. This is especially true for small parts and connectors. Reports of aspirated pieces of equipment can be found in the literature.[66,104]

Airway preparation. The goals of airway preparation are to prevent bleeding; decrease cough and gagging, and decrease pain. Topical vasoconstrictors such as phenylephrine and cocaine are frequently used to prevent bleeding. Cocaine has the added advantage of increased sedation. Soaked cotton pledgets are introduced into the nostrils and advanced into the nasopharynx.

Airway anesthesia is achieved by topical anesthetics or nerve block.[41,47,60,69,84,101,126] Topical anesthetics are more common. The particular anesthetic and route of administration varies depending on experience and locale. Lidocaine, viscous lidocaine, lignocaine, and cocaine are often used. ELMA cream and lignocaine gel have been reported for use in the nasopharynx. However, they make affect visibility through the bronchoscope.

Lidocaine is commonly given by an atomizer to the nose, mouthwash to the oropharynx, and by nebulizer and bronchoscope (instillation) to the lower airways. Cocaine has also been given by intratracheal injection through the cricoid membrane and through the bronchoscope.[47] If lidocaine is nebulized, it is usually the RCP who performs this function. The use of nebulized lidocaine prior to bronchoscopy may limit the need for lidocaine instillations in the lower airways, and can make the procedure more pleasant for both patient and physician.[41,60,69]

Superior laryngeal nerve block will provide anesthesia in the upper larynx, but it does not affect the vocal cords. Transtracheal block through the cricoid membrane will anesthetize both the vocal cords and the trachea.[126]

Monitoring.[63] The RCP has an active role in monitoring the patient and should communicate any changes to the physician. Oxygenation should be monitored continuously via pulse oximeter. If desaturation occurs, the FiO_2 should be increased by an oxygen therapy device. Alternatively, the procedure can be temporarily halted, and oxygen can be given through the scope's open channel. The latter technique has the advantage of defogging the scope and diffusing any secretions. Suctioning for brief periods will help reduce the incidence or severity of hypoxemia.

Respiratory rate and depth should also be observed. Decreases in rate or depth may indicate oversedation. Continuous ECG and periodic blood pressure monitoring should also be routine. Arrhythmias and changes in blood pressure that occur are usually due to hypoxemia, vagal stimulation, pain, or anxiety. Prompt recognition of a problem and appropriate response will aid recovery.

Assisting with the procedure.[63] The physician inserts the bronchoscope into the airway and guides it by directing the tip by the thumb lever. While monitoring the patient, the RCP also may assist the physician by supplying syringes filled with anesthetic, vasoconstrictor, or mucolytic agents. Forceps or brushes are often inserted into the bronchoscope by the RCP. The physician then guides these devices to the desired area. In addition, sputum or tissue samples obtained by the physician may be collected by the RCP and prepared for laboratory analysis. Once the goals of the procedure have been achieved the bronchoscope is removed, the patient's recovery period begins.

Recovery. Hypoxemia that occurs during the procedure may persist after completion. Oxygen therapy should be maintained for up to 4 hours.[102] Adequate oxygenation via pulse oximetry should be confirmed before therapy is discontinued.

The risk of aspiration persists as long as the airway is anesthetized. Therefore, patients should remain in a sitting position and refrain from eating or drinking until sensation returns.[102]

Patients should also be assessed for the development of stridor or wheezes. The physician should be notified and appropriate aerosol therapy with racemic epinephrine or bronchodilators should be instituted.

In order to check for common complications (such

as pulmonary infiltrates or pneumothorax), some physicians order a chest X-ray after bronchoscopy.[85] Since abnormal findings are uncommon (about 8% with infiltrate and less than 1% with pneumothorax), the routine use of a follow-up X-ray is probably unwarranted.

Efficacy. In spite of the complexity of the procedure and the associated hazards, FFB is effective in most situations. The removal of aspirated foreign objects restores normal work of breathing and ventilation/perfusion ratios. Reversal of lobar collapse has been demonstrated with bronchoscopy, although not consistently.[8,33,64,95] Selective intrabronchial air insufflation may increase the success.[51,131] Reported improvement in patients' chest X-rays, PaO_2/FIO_2 and $P(A-a)O_2$ support the effectiveness of FFB as a treatment for lobar collapse.

Asthmatic patients may benefit from FFB if they are stable but refractory to current therapy.[73] Relief of dyspnea and improved cough have been reported when mucus plugs are removed. Symptomatic improvement correlated with improved pulmonary function (FEV_1 and FVC).

FFB with laser therapy or brachytherapy has improved the status of patients with cancer.[4,19,36,86,109] Clinical reports indicate decreases in work of breathing, dyspnea, and orthopnea due to widening of the airway lumen. At times, tumors that were previously classified as inoperable are made operable or require less extensive surgery. This technique has also been reported as "curative" when tumors are benign.[36]

Diagnostic use. The fiberoptic bronchoscopy is one of the most definitive tools for diagnosing lung cancer (see box on page 545). Moreover, as compared to transthoracic biopsy, FFB carries a much lower risk of pneumothorax. **Biopsy** of tumors in the airway parenchyma can often be obtained using a brush or forceps inserted through the bronchoscope. Bronchoalveolar lavage (BAL) also can be used to check for cancerous cells, infectious diseases, and parenchymal disorders. Diagnosis of airway changes such as granulomas, stenosis, fistulas, or tears can also be done with fiberoptic bronchoscopy.

INDICATIONS FOR ARTIFICIAL AIRWAYS

There are a variety of situations in which a patient's own airway is not adequate, and an artificial airway is required. The four basic indications for placement of an artificial airway are:[40,100,107,116]
1. To relieve airway obstruction;
2. To facilitate removal of secretions;
3. To protect the lower airways from aspiration;
4. To facilitate application of positive pressure ventilation.

Relieving airway obstruction

Airway obstruction can occur at any point in the airway, but is usually classified as either upper or lower in origin.[107] Upper airway obstruction occurs above the glottis, and includes the area of the nasopharynx, oropharynx, and larynx. Lower airway obstruction occurs below the vocal cords, and includes the area of the trachea, mainstem bronchi and the conducting airways.

Airway obstruction may also be classified by degree as either partial or complete. Partial airway obstruction varies in severity. A slight impairment may cause a mild increase in the work of breathing. More severe partial obstruction is associated with stridor and marked respiratory difficulty. Complete airway obstruction results in no air flow. However, exaggerated respiratory efforts, including retractions and the use of accessory muscles, may occur.

The causes of airway obstruction includes crushing injuries (secondary to trauma, edema, tumors), and anatomic or physiologic changes in muscle tone or tissue support. Decreased muscle tone in the upper airway results in collapse, whereas increased muscle tone in the larynx may lead to closure.

Artificial airways can bypass an obstructed airway and provide a clear passage for airflow. Such airways can bypass obstructions occurring in the upper airway, larynx and **extrathoracic** trachea. Normally, airway obstructions below the trachea must be dealt with by other means.

Although used to relieve acute airway obstruction, all artificial airways increase airway resistance.[13,50,100,108] The smaller the diameter of the airway, the longer the tube, and the greater the degree of curvature, the greater will be the resistance. Of course, the greater the resistance, the greater the resulting work of breathing.

Figure 22-6 clearly shows these relationships for four different sized endotracheal tubes, as compared to normal ("0 Tube"). As the graph shows, the work of breathing through a given sized tube (measured in joules/min) increases exponentially with increasing minute volume. Moreover, smaller tubes cause a dramatic increase in work, especially at higher minute volumes. Clearly, artificial airways impose additional work on the respiratory muscles, especially in patients with high ventilatory demands. This additional workload must be taken into account whenever an artificial airway is considered.

Secretion removal

As described in Chapter 9, normal airway secretions humidify inspired air and help clear small inhaled particles from the respiratory tract. If these secretions cannot be cleared, airway obstruction may result.

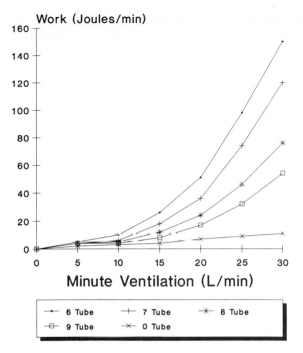

Fig. 22-6 Relationship between work of breathing, artificial airway size, and minute ventilation demonstrated in healthy volunteers. (Redrawn from Respiratory Care 33(2), 1988).

Airway obstruction increases the work of breathing and causes hypoxemia and hypercapnia. Moreover, stagnant secretions present an ideal medium for bacterial growth, which may cause infection. Artificial airways aid secretion removal mainly by providing more direct access to the airway.

Protecting the airway

Four reflexes help prevent aspiration of foreign material into the lower airway. These are the pharyngeal, laryngeal, tracheal and carinal reflexes.[107] The pharyngeal reflex produces a gag and swallowing response. The laryngeal response to stimulation is glottic closure. Stimulation of tracheal and carinal reflexes causes coughing.

Innervation for all these reflexes arises from the cranial nerves. The pharyngeal reflex is the only reflex innervated by two nerves: the glossopharyngeal (IXth cranial) and the vagus (Xth cranial). The remaining three reflexes are innervated by the vagus nerve.

Patients with CNS depression have varying degrees of decreased reflex response to stimulation. The loss of reflexes generally proceeds from the pharynx to the trachea, receding in the reverse order. For example, during induction of anesthesia, the first response to disappear is the gag reflex, with the last being the cough (carinal) reflex. This same sequence of reflexes can be used to evaluate the level of coma. As an example, the patient with only a carinal cough reflex is more obtunded than one who still exhibits a pharyngeal gag.

Some of the artificial airways that are placed into the trachea have a small cuff (a balloon-like structure) at their distal end. When inflated with air, this cuff seals the space between the sides of the tube and the walls of the trachea. This seal helps prevent liquid or particulate matter from the pharynx or larynx from getting into the lower trachea and lungs. The use of tracheal tube cuffs will be discussed in detail later in this chapter.

■ MINI CLINI ■

22-1

Artificial Airways and Work of Breathing

Problem: A mechanically ventilated patient with an artificial airway (endotracheal tube) in place has improved, and the attending physician wishes to wean the patient from mechanical ventilatory support. When this patient is removed from the ventilator and placed on a T-tube and allowed to spontaneously breathe through the endotracheal tube, he develops respiratory distress after 30 minutes, and must be returned to the ventilator. This failure to sustain spontaneous ventilation occurs despite conventional lung function tests and arterial blood gases which predict successful weaning from mechanical ventilatory support. Later

that day the patient extubates himself, and although health care personnel fear he will develop respiratory distress and require re-intubation, the patient does fine and has no further problems breathing spontaneously. What may explain this situation?

Discussion: Artificial airways always increase airways resistance and the work of breathing compared to the normal, non-intubated state. Especially in patients who have weak, easily fatigued respiratory muscles, the presence of an artificial airway may impose enough added work of breathing that the patient has difficulty maintaining spontaneous ventilation. Generally, when standard weaning criteria are met, the artificial airway should be removed as soon as possible after discontinuing mechanical ventilatory support; a major source of airway resistance is thus removed.

Positive pressure ventilation

Positive pressure ventilation is only feasible if a seal is maintained between the patient's airway and the ventilator. For short-term intermittent positive pressure breathing (IPPB) therapy, a temporary seal can usually be maintained by a cooperative patient using a mouthpiece and noseclips. Obviously, this arrangement is not practical for long-term mechanical ventilation, which may last for hours, days, or months. For this purpose, the usual approach is to place a cuffed artificial airway into the trachea.* Once in place, the tube cuff is inflated to provide a seal.

SELECTING AND ESTABLISHING AN ARTIFICIAL AIRWAY

In general, artificial airways are inserted either into the pharynx or into the trachea.

Pharyngeal airways

Pharyngeal airways prevent airway obstruction by keeping the tongue pulled forward and away from the posterior pharynx. This type of obstruction is common in the unconscious patient, due to a loss of muscle tone. By providing a clear passage into the lower pharynx, these airways also can aid suctioning. Since pharyngeal airways are used mainly in emergency life support, further details on both their use and that of other emergency airway equipment are provided in the next chapter.

Tracheal airways

Tracheal airways extend beyond the pharynx, into the trachea. There are two basic types of artificial airways which can be inserted into the trachea: endotracheal tubes and tracheostomy tubes. Endotracheal tubes are inserted either through the mouth or nose (oro- or nasotracheal), through the larynx and into the trachea. Tracheostomy tubes are inserted through a surgically created opening directly into the trachea. A summary of the advantages and disadvantages of each of these three approaches appears in Table 22-2.

Endotracheal (ET) tubes are semi-rigid tubes, most often made from polyvinyl chloride or related plastic polymers.[25,83] Figure 22-7, page 552, portrays a typical ET tube and its key components. The proximal end of the tube (1) is attached to a standard adapter with a 15 mm external diameter. The curved body of the tube (2) usually has length marking, indicating the distance (in cm) from the beveled tube tip (3). Other markings

may include the designation "I.T." and Z-79. I.T. is an abbreviation for implantation tested, meaning the tube material has been shown nontoxic to living tissue. Z-79 means the tube meets the design standards of the Z-79 Committee of the American National Standards Institute, or ANSI.

In addition to the beveled opening at the tip, there should be an additional side port or "Murphy eye" (3A) which ensures gas flow if the main port should become obstructed. The angle of the bevel (4) minimizes mucosal trauma during insertion. The tube cuff (5) is permanently bonded to the tube body. Inflation of the cuff seals off the lower airway, either for protection or to provide positive pressure ventilation. A small filling tube (6) leads from the cuff to a pilot balloon (7), used to monitor cuff status and pressure once the tube is in place. Finally, a spring loaded valve (8) with a standard connector for a syringe allows inflation and deflation of the cuff. Not shown, but included with most modern ET tubes, is a radiopaque indicator that is imbedded in the distal end of the tube body. This indicator allows for easy identification of tube position on X-ray.

As with ET tubes, tracheostomy tubes are generally made from plastic polymers, although some are still made from silver. Figure 22-8 on page 552, portrays a typical plastic tracheostomy tube and its key components.[83] The outer cannula (1) forms the primary structural unit of the tube, to which is attached the cuff (2) and a flange (3). The flange prevents tube slippage into the trachea, and provides the means to secure the tube to the neck. A removable inner cannula (4) with standard 15 mm adapter (5) is normally kept in place within the outer cannula, but can be removed for routine cleaning, or if it becomes obstructed. In order to prevent accidental removal, the inner cannula can be locked in place at the proximal end of the outer cannula (6). As with the ET tube, an inflation tube (7) leads from the cuff to a pilot balloon (9) and spring loaded valve (8). The tube is stabilized at the stoma site by cotton tape (10), which attaches to the flange, and is tied around the neck. An obturator with a rounded tip (11) is used for tube insertion. Prior to insertion, the obturator is placed within the outer cannula, with its tip extending just beyond the far end of the tube. This minimizes mucosal trauma during insertion, particularly the "snowplowing" effect that a rough tube edge can exert on the tracheal wall. Last, as with ET tubes, a radiopaque indicator (12) in the distal end of the tube helps confirms tube position on X-ray.

Oral ET tubes

The accompanying box lists the major advantages and disadvantages of oral intubation. The orotracheal or oral ET tube is the emergency airway of choice.[43,107,118] This is because oral intubation is the quickest and easiest means of establishing a tracheal

---

*Noninvasive approaches to positive pressure mechanical ventilation have recently been developed. These approaches generally use form-fitting nasal masks, and have been used for periods of several days to weeks. See Chapter 38 for details.

Table 22-2   Advantages and Disadvantages of Tracheal Airway Routes

	Advantages	Disadvantages

Oral intubation	Tube insertion is faster, easier, less traumatic, and more comfortable
	Larger tube is tolerated
	  Easier suctioning
	  Probable less airflow resistance
	  Probable decreased work of breathing
	  Easier passage of fiberoptic bronchoscope
	Reduced risk of the tube kinking
	Avoidance of nasal and paranasal complications, including epistaxis and sinusitis
		Aesthetically displeasing, especially long term
		Greater risk of self-extubation or inadvertent extubation
		Greater risk of mainstem bronchus intubation
		Risk of tube occlusion by biting or trismus
		Risk of injury to lips, teeth, tongue, palate, and oral soft tissues
		May require additional use of oral airway
		Great risk of retching, vomiting, and aspiration

Nasal intubation	Less retching and gagging
	Greater comfort in long-term use
	Less salivation
	Improved ability to swallow oral secretions
	Improved communication
	Improved mouth care and oral hygiene
	Avoidance of occlusion of orotracheal tube by biting, trismus
	Easier nursing care
	Avoidance of oral complications of oral intubation
	Less posterior laryngeal ulceration
	Better tube anchoring; less chance of inadvertent extubation
	Reduced risk of mainstem bronchus intubation
	Some patients can swallow liquids, providing a means of nutritional support
	Blind nasal intubation does not require muscle relaxants or sedatives
	May avert "crash" oral intubation
		Pain and discomfort, especially with inadequate preparation
		Nasal and paranasal complications, including epistaxis, sinusitis, and otitis
		More difficult to perform
		Spontaneous breathing is required for blind nasal intubation
		Smaller tuber is necessary
		  Greater suctioning difficulty
		  Probable increased airflow resistance
		  Probable increased work of breathing
		  Difficulty passing fiberoptic bronchoscope
		Small risk of transient bacteremia

Tracheotomy	Avoidance of laryngeal and upper airway complications of translaryngeal intubation Greater comfort Facilitation of feeding, mouth care, suctioning, and speech Psychologic benefit (improved motivation) Easier passage of fiberoptic bronchoscope Easier reinsertion Aesthetically less objectionable Facilitation of weaning from ventilator Elimination of risk of mainstem bronchus intubation Probable reduced work of breathing Better anchoring (reduced risk of decannulation) Improved ability to place a curved-tipped suction catheter in the left mainstem bronchus Improved mobility (transfer out of ICU to ward or extended-care facility)	Greater expense (additional charges of $2000–$3000) Requirement for use of operating room in most cases Need for general anesthesia in most cases Permanent scar More severe complications, including tracheal stenosis Greater mortality rate Delayed decannulation Increased frequency of aspiration Greater bacterial colonization rate Persistent open stoma after decannulation, reducing cough efficiency

*Reproduced with permission from Stauffer JL, Silvestri RC: Complications of endotracheal intubation, tracheostomy, and artificial airways, *Respir Care* 27(4): 417-434, 1982.

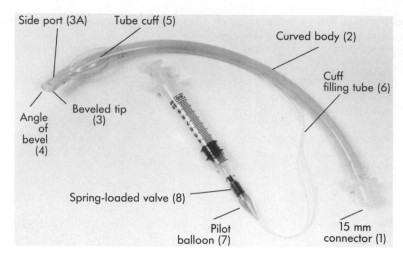

Fig. 22-7 Typical endotracheal tube.

airway. In addition, oral ET tubes offer less airway resistance than nasal tubes. This is due to their larger inner diameter, shorter length and decreased curvature.

In spite of these advantages, oral ET tubes have several drawbacks, especially when used for long periods. Patient discomfort and gagging are common in conscious patients. For this reason, oral ET tubes are used mainly for short-term airway management of unconscious patients, such as during general anesthesia. Accidental extubation, or removal, of an oral ET tube is also a common problem. Most commonly, extubation occur when an unrestrained patient pulls the tube out. Extubation may also occur when the tape used to secure the tube loosens. Dislocation of the tube, up or down in the trachea, may be related to the loosening of the tape, or motion of the patient's head and neck.

Provision of oral hygiene is particularly difficult with oral ET tubes, as is oral provision of liquids. Damage to the lips, teeth, gums, and pharynx may occur either during the intubation procedure itself or over time due to irritation and pressure necrosis.

Oral intubation procedure. The procedure of placing an oral ET tube is called orotracheal intubation. This skill can be safely performed by any appropriately trained physician, RCP, nurse, or paramedic.[65,127] Familiarity with upper airway anatomy and proper

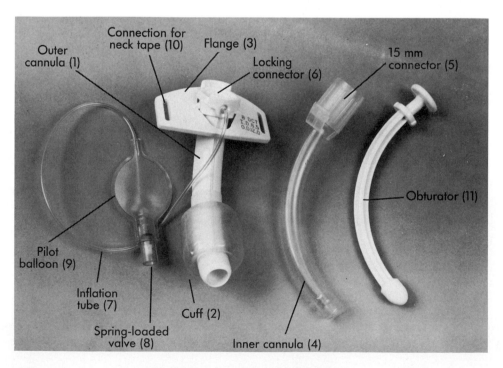

Fig. 22-8 Parts of a tracheostomy tube.

selection of equipment are essential parts of this training. A description of the basic steps in orotracheal intubation is discussed below.[40,107,141] Proficiency in this technique can only be developed with extensive training. Typically, this training involves manikin practice and application on anesthetized patients under the guidance of an anesthesiologist, or other appropriately skilled individual.

Step 1: Assemble and check equipment. The accompanying box lists the equipment necessary for intubation. The laryngoscope blade should be attached to the handle and the light source checked for secure attachment and brightness.[62] If the light does not function, first check to see that the bulb is tight. If the scope still does not light, check the batteries or replace the bulb.

Suction equipment should be assembled and suction pressure checked prior to intubation, since vomitus or secretions may obscure the pharynx or glottis. See the prior section on suctioning for guidance on troubleshooting this equipment.

The RCP should select an appropriate size tube, but have available at least one size larger and one size smaller. Table 22-3 provides guidelines for the selection of orotracheal tubes according to patient age, and includes recommended maximum suction catheter sizes to be used with each tube. Note that ET tube sizes are normally expressed in metric units, corresponding to the internal diameter of the tube. The French scale, still common with suction catheters, is based on the external diameter of tubes and catheters. To convert French to metric units, simply divide the French size by 3.14. For example, a 12 French suction catheter has an external diameter of about 4 mm.

Table 22-3   Pediatric to adult endotracheal tube sizes

Age	Tube Size (mm)	Suction Catheter
Premature	2.5	5 French
Newborn	3.0	6
6 months	3.5	6
18 months	4.0	8
3 years	4.5	8
5 years	5.0	10
6 years	5.5	10
8 years	6.0	10
12 years	6.5	12
16 yrs/small adult female	7.0	14
Adult females (average)	8.0	14
Adult males	9.0	14

After selecting the correct size tube, the RCP should inflate the cuff and check it for leaks. This can be done with either a pressure manometer, or by submerging the inflated cuff in a cup of sterile water. A leak exits if either pressure can't be held or bubbles escape under water. Of course, you must be sure to deflate the cuff prior to insertion. To ease insertion, the outer surface of the tube should be lubricated with a water soluble gel. Last, some clinicians insert a **stylet** into the tube to add rigidity and maintain shape during insertion. The tip of the stylet must never extend beyond the ET tube tip.

Step 2: Position the patient. The mouth, pharynx, and larynx must be aligned in order to visualize the glottis and insert the tube. This alignment is accomplished by combining moderate cervical flexion with extension of the atlanto-occipital joint. To achieve this position, one or more towels are placed under the patient's head, the neck is flexed, and then the head is tilted backward with the hand (Figure 22-9, page 554).

Step 3: Preoxygenate the patient. A patient in need of intubation is often apneic or in respiratory distress. Adequate ventilation and oxygenation by bag and mask should be provided prior to intubation. 100% oxygen provides the patient with a reserve during the intubation procedure. No longer than 30 seconds should be devoted to any intubation attempt. If intubation fails, the patient should immediately be ventilated and oxygenated for 3 to 5 minutes before a repeat attempt.

Step 4: Insert the laryngoscope. The RCP uses the left hand to hold the laryngoscope, with the right hand used to open the mouth (Figure 22-10, page 554). The laryngoscope is then inserted into the right side of the mouth, and moved toward the center, displacing the tongue to the left. The tip of the blade is then advanced along the curve of the tongue until the epiglottis is visualized.

Step 5: Visualize the glottis. The arytenoid cartilage and epiglottis should come into view as the blade

Equipment necessary for endotracheal intubation

- Oxygen flowmeter and tubing
- Suction apparatus
  Flexible suction catheters
  Yankauer (tonsillar) tip
- Manual resuscitation bag and mask
- Oropharyngeal airway(s)
- Laryngoscope (2) with assorted blades
- Endotracheal tubes (3 sizes)
- Tongue depressor
- Stylet
- Stethoscope
- Tape
- Syringe
- Lubricating jelly
- Magill forceps
- Local anesthetic (spray)
- Towels (for positioning)
- CDC barrier precautions (gloves, gowns, masks, eyewear)

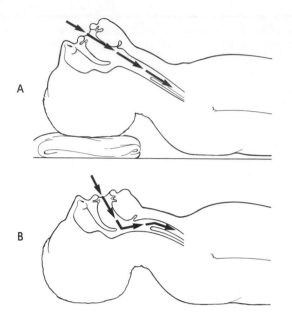

Fig. 22-9 A, Correct preintubation head position. **B,** Incorrect preintubation head position.

reaches the base of the tongue (Figure 22-11). If these structures are not visible, it is likely that the blade has been advanced too far and may be in the esophagus. If this is the case, the practitioner should maintain upward force on the laryngoscope, slowly withdrawing it until the larynx comes into view.

Step 6: Displace the epiglottis. The technique used to move the epiglottis depends on the type of blade used (Figure 22-12). The curved or MacIntosh blade lifts the epiglottis indirectly as the tip of the blade is advanced into the vallecula and the laryngoscope is lifted up and forward (Figure 22-12, *A*). The straight or Miller blade lifts the epiglottis directly as the tip of the blade is advanced beyond it and the laryngoscope is lifted up and forward (Figure 22-12, *B*).

In lifting the tip of the blade, the RCP should avoid levering the laryngoscope against the teeth, as this can damage the teeth and gums. The practitioner can avoid this problem by keeping the wrist fixed and moving the handle of the laryngoscope in the direction it is pointing when the epiglottis is visualized.

Step 7: Insert the tube. Once the glottis is visualized and the epiglottis moved, the tube is inserted from the right side of the mouth and advanced without obscuring the glottic opening (Figure 22-13, page 556). The tip of the tube should be seen passing between the cords and then advanced until the cuff has passed the cords by 2 to 3 centimeters.[40]

Once the tube is in place, the RCP stabilizes the tube with the right hand, using the left hand to remove the laryngoscope and the stylet. The RCP should then inflate the cuff to seal the airway and immediately provide ventilation and oxygenation.

Step 8: Confirm tube placement.[70,116] The first step used to assess proper placement is auscultation. The practitioner should listen for equal and bilateral breath sounds as the patient is being bagged. Air movement or gurgling sounds over the epigastrium indicate possible esophageal intubation. In addition, the RCP should observe the chest wall for adequate and equal chest expansion. These movements, combined with auscultation, are often reinforcing. For example, decreased breath sounds on the left and

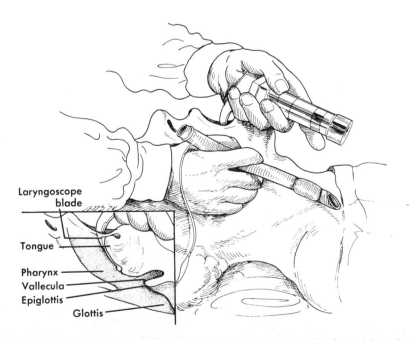

Laryngoscope blade
Tongue
Pharynx
Vallecula
Epiglottis
Glottis

Fig. 22-10 To achieve orotracheal intubation, rescuer, with laryngoscope in left hand, introduces blade into right side of mouth, displacing tongue to the left. (From Ellis PD, Billings DM: Cardiopulmonary resuscitation: procedures for basic and advanced life support, St Louis, 1980, Mosby.)

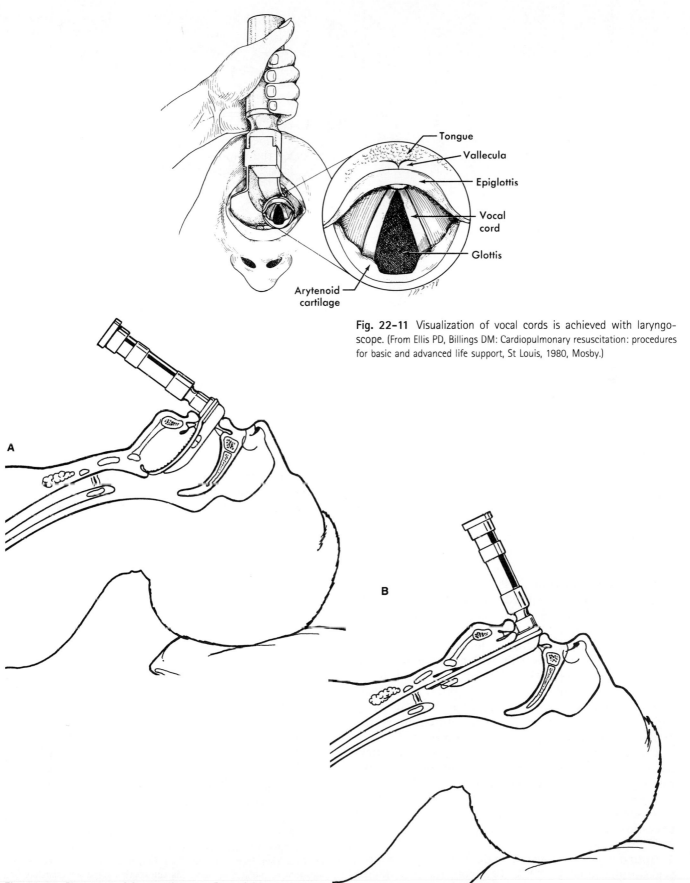

Tongue
Vallecula
Epiglottis
Vocal cord
Glottis
Arytenoid cartilage

Fig. 22-11 Visualization of vocal cords is achieved with laryngoscope. (From Ellis PD, Billings DM: Cardiopulmonary resuscitation: procedures for basic and advanced life support, St Louis, 1980, Mosby.)

A

B

Fig. 22-12 Placement of **A,** curved, versus **B,** straight, laryngoscope blade.

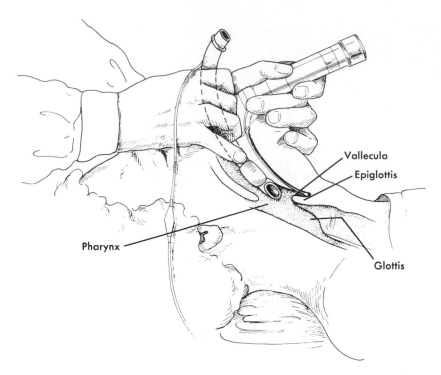

Fig. 22-13 Insertion of endotracheal tube. (From Ellis PD, Billings DM: Cardiopulmonary resuscitation: procedures for basic and advanced life support, St Louis, 1985, Mosby.)

decreased chest wall movement on the same side would indicate intubation of the right mainstem bronchus. Right mainstem intubation can be corrected by slowly withdrawing the tube, while listening for the return of right-side breath sounds.

Capnometry, or exhaled CO_2 analysis, can also help determine proper tube placement. Most bedside capnometry is provided by an infrared gas analyzer (see Chapter 17). Since inspired air contains about only about 0.04% CO_2, and end-tidal gas about 6% CO_2, proper placement of an ET tube in the respiratory tract will cause carbon dioxide levels to abruptly rise during end expiration. This will be evident on the capnogram (Figure 22-14). On the other hand, if the tube is in the esophagus, the "end-expired" CO_2 levels will remain near zero. The major problem in using capnometry to confirm tracheal intubation is the expense and availability of the equipment.

Colorimetric CO_2 analysis is an inexpensive alternative to infrared capnometry. Functioning much like pH paper, a colorimetric system has an indicator that changes color when exposed to different CO_2 levels. A disposable colorimetric system designed exclusively to confirm tube placement during intubation is shown in Figure 22-15.

Both devices are effective in detecting most esophageal intubations.[5,30,80,94,96,97] The colorimetric device has the advantage of portability and single patient usage. However, its use in cardiac arrest victims needs careful attention as color changes may be slight. The lower exhaled CO_2 levels during CPR may be due to low pulmonary blood flow. Generally, the end-tidal CO_2 increases with the return of spontaneous circulation.[80,133] Unfortunately, end tidal CO_2 analysis is not a reliable indicator of mainstem bronchial intubation.

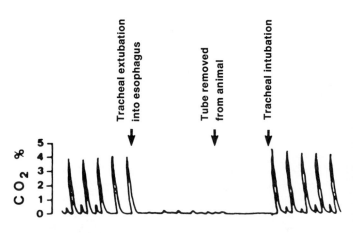

Fig. 22-14 Capnogram tracing showing changes in expired %CO_2 with proper and improper placement of endotracheal tube in test animals. (From Murray IP, Modell JH: Early detection of endotracheal tube accidents by monitoring carbon dioxide concentrations in respiratory gas, *Anesthesiology* 59:344-346, 1983).

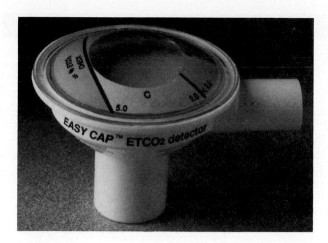

Fig. 22-15 A disposable colorimetric CO_2 detector for confirming tracheal intubation. (Courtesy of Nellcor, Hayward CA).

biting down on the tube (Figure 22-17, page 558). After the tube is stabilized, a chest X-ray should be taken to confirm its position.

Complications of oral intubation include damage to the teeth and gums, and laceration of the lips, tongue, pharynx, larynx, and esophagus.[69,82] The most serious complications are acute hypoxemia, hypercapnia, bradycardia and cardiac arrest.[40,67,118,137] Proper technique, adequate prior ventilation and oxygenation of the patient, and adherence to strict intubation time limits will help minimize these hazards. In addition, sedation and anesthesia (similar to that used with bronchoscopy) can reduce complications and facilitate intubation in the semi-comatose or combative patient.[9,40,43,116] Paralysis is not needed if the patient can be adequately sedated.[43] A variety of alternative techniques are available to help with difficult intubations.[40,74] However, a discussion of these techniques is beyond the scope of this chapter.

Nasal ET tubes

Nasal ET, or nasotracheal tubes are more difficult to insert than orotracheal tubes. Nonetheless, nasotracheal insertion is the route of choice in many clinical situations. Situations in which nasotracheal intubation is the preferred route include patients with cervical spine or **maxillofacial** injuries who are in need of a short-term artificial airways.

Once in place, nasotracheal tubes offer several distinct advantages over the oral route. Since the tape used to hold the tube is placed mainly on the nose and upper cheeks, tube stability is enhanced and oral hygiene is facilitated. Also, nasotracheal tubes are better tolerated by both conscious and semi-conscious patients. Due to smaller tubes, better tube stability

Proper tube placement in the trachea can be confirmed without a chest X-ray using a fiberoptic laryngoscope. After assuring patient reoxygenation, the RCP inserts a fiberoptic laryngoscope directly into the ET tube (Figure 22-16). Visualization of the carina distal to the tip of the ET tube assures proper placement in the trachea. More precise placement is possible by moving the laryngoscope from the tube tip to the carina, while measuring this distance.

Step 9: Stabilize the tube. The RCP should not secure the tube until placement is confirmed by auscultation. After confirming placement and while holding it in position, the RCP secures the tube to the skin above the lip and on the cheeks using tape. Normally, a bit block, oropharyngeal airway, or similar device will be needed to prevent the patient from

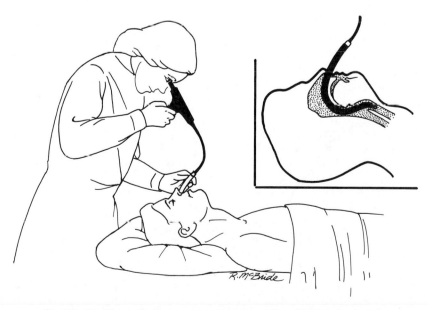

Fig. 22-16 Fiberoptic laryngoscopy used to confirm ET tube placement.

Capnometry and Endotracheal Tube Placement

Problem: At a Code Blue in the emergency room a patient is intubated by a respiratory care practitioner. A capnometer is attached to the endotracheal ET tube to confirm placement in the trachea. The end-expired CO_2 is 0% as the patient is ventilated with a manual resuscitator. At this time, no one is performing cardiac compressions. Should the therapist conclude that the ET tube is not in the trachea?

Discussion: Not necessarily. If the patient is in cardiac arrest, no blood is perfusing the alveoli, and therefore, no CO_2 is entering alveoli. The result is an end-tidal CO_2 of 0%. Once cardiac compressions begin (and they should begin immediately in confirmed cardiac arrest!) and if compressions are effective, one should see an increase in end-tidal CO_2 as blood begins to perfuse the alveoli, and CO_2 diffuses out of the blood.

Of course, there are other simple ways to confirm ET tube placement in the trachea, e.g. bilateral breath sounds upon auscultation, and chest excursions. A rise in end-tidal CO_2 however, is a sure indication that the ET tube is in the lungs, since the only source of CO_2 is the alveolus.

and less pressure on the glottis, nasotracheal intubation may also be associated with fewer complications than oral intubation.[117]

However, there are several disadvantages to the nasal route for intubation. Since passage through the node requires a smaller and longer tube, airway resistance will be higher.[50] Since regular switching between nares is not practical, necrosis of the nasal septum and external meatus may occur. In addition, the tube may block drainage from either the sinuses or eustachian tubes. This can cause sinusitis or **otitis media,** which—in some critically ill patients—has lead to sepsis.[56] Nosebleed is not usually a problem until extubation. Oral feedings are still very difficult, but patients can sip water in small quantities.

Nasal intubation procedure. Nasotracheal intubation is performed either blindly or by direct visualization.[40] The direct visualization approach requires either a standard or fiberoptic laryngoscope. For the blind technique to work, the patient must be breath-

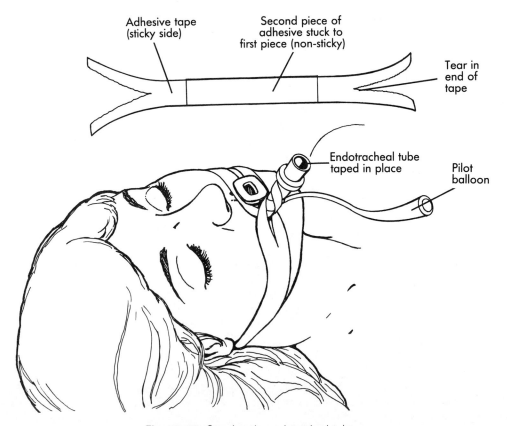

Fig. 22-17 Securing the endotracheal tube.

ing spontaneously. Equipment assembly, patient positioning and preoxygenation are essentially the same as with oral intubation. Sprays of 0.25% racemic epinephrine and 2% lidocaine may also be needed to provide local anesthesia and vasoconstriction of the nasal passage.

Direct visualization. The equipment needed for nasal intubation by direct visualization is the same as for oral intubation, with the addition of Magill forceps. The tube should be lubricated to aid passage. Insertion, with the bevel directed toward the septum, proceeds inferiorly and posteriorly. When the tip of the tube is in the oropharynx, the RCP should open the mouth, insert the laryngoscope, and visualize the glottis. With the right hand, the RCP uses the Magill forceps to grasp the tube just above the cuff and direct it between the cords (Figure 22-18). Flexion of the neck will help advance the tube past the cords. The average depth of tube insertion from the external naris is 25 cm for adult males and 23 cm for females.[40] Confirmation of position and stabilization follow, as with the oral route.

Alternatively, either a fiberoptic bronchoscope or laryngoscope to guide tube passage.[141] With the bronchoscopic method, the distal end of the scope is passed through the ET tube and directed into the trachea. Once placement is assured, the RCP slides the ET tube down over the scope into proper position. The procedure is similar with a fiberoptic laryngoscope. However, since directional control of the scope is limited, positioning of the head and neck are used to help guide the tube.

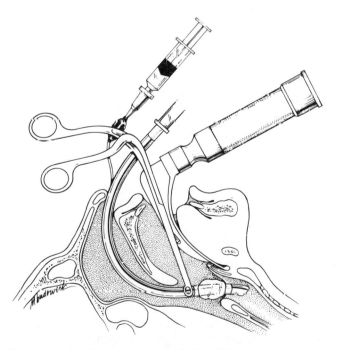

Fig. 22–18 Nasal intubation using the Magill forceps. (From Finucane BT, Santora AH: Principles of airway management, Philadelphia, 1988, FA Davis.)

Blind Passage. During blind nasal intubation, the patient should be either in the supine or sitting position.[141] As with direct visualization, the tube is inserted through the nose. As the tube approaches the larynx, the RCP listens through the tube for air movement. The breath sounds become louder and more tubular when the tube passes through the larynx. Successful passage of the tube through the larynx usually is indicated by a harsh cough, followed by vocal silence. If the sounds disappear, the tube is moving toward the esophagus. Failure to advance the tube through the larynx can be corrected by tube, head, and neck manipulations. Confirmation of tube placement and stabilization should follow.

A flexible light wand may be used to aid blind nasotracheal intubation.[141] The light wand is a battery powered stylet with a bulb at its distal tip. The wand is passed through the mouth into laryngopharynx. Once passed beyond the glottis, the wand light is visible through the neck. If it is midline, placement in the trachea is confirmed. An ET tube is then passed over the light wand into proper position.

Complications associated with nasotracheal intubation include damage to the nasal septum resulting in bleeding, or trauma to the nasopharynx, oropharynx or larynx. Hypoxemia, hypercapnia, bradycardia and cardiac arrest also can occur, but are generally less likely than with the oral route. That fewer serious problems are reported for nasal intubation does not necessarily mean that this approach is safer. It may simply mean that patients who undergo nasal intubation are more stable than those requiring the oral route.

Tracheostomy tubes

Because it enters the trachea directly, a tracheostomy tube is the most efficient artificial airway. A 'trach' tube is also the device of choice for overcoming upper airway obstruction or trauma. As compared to oral or nasal tracheal tubes, tracheostomy tubes offer the advantages of lower airway resistance, less movement of the tube within the trachea, greater patient comfort, and the ability to provide oral feedings. Moreover, since a tracheostomy tube is shorter than either an oral or nasal tube, deeper and more efficient suctioning is possible.

Nonetheless, tracheostomy tubes have several disadvantages. First, insertion requires a surgical procedure (tracheotomy). The surgical and anesthesia risks of tracheotomy are greater than endotracheal intubation, with a reported mortality rate up to 5%. Complications occurring during or immediately after tracheotomy tend to be more serious than those seen with intubation. Of course, neither the incidence nor potential seriousness of complications should deter tracheotomy when it is needed.

Indications. The primary indication for trache-

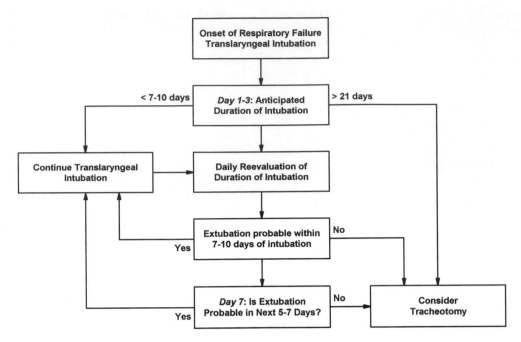

Fig. 22-19 An approach to timing tracheotomy in patients intubated and mechanically ventilated for respiratory failure. (From Heffner JE: Timing of tracheotomy in ventilator-dependent patients, *Clin Chest Med* 12(3):611-625, 1991.)

otomy is the prolonged need for an artificial airway. Depending on the literature source, "prolonged" is defined anywhere between 10 days to 3 weeks.[10,51,68,77,100,116]

The key clinical question is exactly how long an ET tube can remain in place before laryngeal damage occurs. If this period were known for sure, we could easily avoid problems by switching from ET to trach tube at the appropriate time. Unfortunately, there are no firm timelines. Some investigators report a strong correlation between the length of intubation and the occurrence of complications.[117,140] But other studies find no significant relationship.[38,68,135]

As with most other interventions, the decision as to when to switch from ET to trach tube should be individualized.[57,77,100] Pertinent factors that should be considered in making this decision are summarized in the accompanying box. Figure 22-19 provides a decision-making algorithm useful in timing tracheotomy in critically ill patients.

Of course, not all patients are switched from ET tubes to trachs. Tracheostomy is occasionally the airway of first choice. Examples include repeated unsuccessful intubations, obstruction above the cricoid, laryngectomy, and neuromuscular disease.

Complications. One of the most common complications occurring during tracheotomy is hemorrhage.[87,117] The area is extremely vascular with the jugular veins, carotid arteries and thyroid isthmus near the trachea. Air leaks including pneumothorax, **pneumodiastinum,** and subcutaneous emphysema

---

Factors to consider in switching from ET tube to tracheostomy

1. The projected time the patient will need an artificial airway
2. The patient's tolerance of the endotracheal tube
3. The patient's overall condition (including nutritional, cardiovascular, and infection status)
4. The patient's ability to tolerate a surgical procedure
5. The relative risks of continued endotracheal intubation versus tracheostomy

---

may occur.[87,117,139] Alternatively, high negative intrathoracic pressure secondary to an occluded airway may pull air into these potential spaces. Incorrect placement of the tube in the space between the skin and the trachea will also cause air leaks.

Tracheoesophageal fistula and vocal cord paralysis secondary to recurrent laryngeal nerve injury have also been reported as complications of tracheotomy.[87] Both of these problems can be minimized by careful technique and ensuring midline entry into the trachea.

There are also reports of cardiopulmonary arrest during tracheotomy. This serious complication may be due to a strong vagal reflex during airway manipulation, development of a tension pneumothorax, or failure to rapidly secure the airway.[87]

After the procedure, hemorrhage, wound infection, and acute tube occlusion secondary to blood, secretions or tissue can occur. Should the tube become dislodged within the first few days after surgery, it may be very difficult to replace. This is because a new stoma tends to easily close.[31,87] To avoid this problem, traction sutures should be placed during the initial procedure. Should extubation occur, these sutures can then be used help pull the stoma open and toward the skin. If attempts to reinsert the tube fail, the patient should be intubated immediately with an oral or nasal ET tube.

Although a trach tube bypasses the larynx, patients still can exhibit diminished glottic closure and dysphasia. These problems can increase the likelihood of aspiration. Trach patients may need intravenous feeding until normal swallowing reflexes return.

Late (weeks or months) complications of tracheostomy include tracheal stenosis, tracheoesophageal fistula, tracheoinnominate artery fistula, and airway bacterial colonization.[77,143] Some of these problems are common to ET tubes, and will be discussed later in this chapter.

Tracheotomy procedure. Tracheotomy should be performed by a skilled surgeon as an elective procedure when the patient's airway is already stabilized. Mortality and morbidity are lower with elective tracheotomy than when this procedure is performed on an emergency basis. The RCP may be asked to assist in tracheotomy, especially if performed at the bedside. For this reason we will briefly describe the procedure.[77,139]

A local anesthesia is used and the patient mildly sedated, conditions permitting. If an ET tube is in place, it should not be removed until just prior to the insertion of the trach tube. This ensures a patent airway and provides additional stability to the trachea during the procedure. Tracheostomy with **electrocautery** should be considered in patients with a bleeding disorder.[132]

The incision is made either horizontally or vertically in the neck over the second or third tracheal ring. The vertical incision requires opening of fewer tissue planes, and affords easier insertion and removal of the airway. The vertical incision also allows for more tube movement with swallowing. A horizontal incision produces less disfigurement, but may cause improper angulation of the tube within the trachea.

Once the skin and subcutaneous tissue have been incised, the platysma muscles are divided and the thyroid gland is located. The thyroid isthmus, which overlies the second and third tracheal rings, must be divided and ligated. Careful surgical technique is required as the thyroid is a highly vascular structure. Entrance into the trachea is made through either a horizontal incision between rings, or a vertical one through the second and third rings (Figure 22-20). As little cartilage as possible should be removed, in order to promote better closure after extubation.

Once the stoma is created and the tracheostomy tube is selected and prepared for insertion, the ET tube may be removed. The lumen of the trachea can be evaluated to ensure that the trach tube is the correct size. In general, the tube size is correct if it occupies between two-thirds to three-quarters of the internal tracheal diameter. Table 22-4, page 562, lists

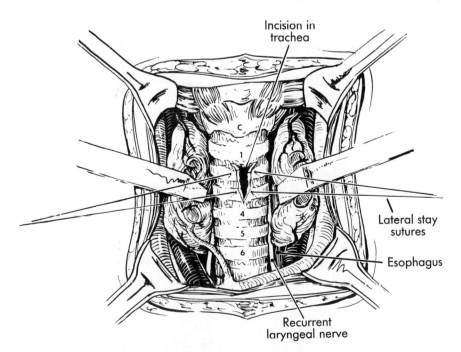

Fig. 22-20 Tracheal incision. (From Crews ER, Lapuerta L: A manual of respiratory failure, Springfield, IL, 1972, Charles C Thomas, Publisher.)

Table 22-4 Approximate tracheostomy tube sizes

Jackson size	Internal diameter	External diameter	French size
00	2.5	4.5	13
0	3.0	5.0	15
1	3.5	5.5	16.5
2	4.0	6.0	18
3	4.5–5.0	7	21
4	5.5	8	24
5	6.0–6.5	9	27
6	7.0	10	30
7	7.5–8.0	11	33
8	8.5	12	36
9	9.0–11.0	13	39
10	10.0	14	42
11	10.4–11.0	15	45
12	11.5	16	48

the various trach tube sizes, using Jackson, internal diameter, external diameter, and French scales. Table 22-5 provides guidelines for selecting a tracheostomy tube according to a patient's age, using the Jackson size for reference. Within an age category, the exact size tube chosen depends on the patient's height and weight.

Insertion of the tube, inflation of the cuff and securing of the tube follow. Tracheostomy tube ties should be secure enough to prevent movement of the tube but allow for one finger width of play to decrease skin necrosis.[31] Wound edges should not be excessively tight as this will promote accumulation of subcutaneous or mediastinal air.[77]

AIRWAY TRAUMA ASSOCIATED WITH TRACHEAL TUBES

Artificial airways do not exactly conform to patients' anatomy. The result is pressure on soft tissues, which can result in ischemia and ulceration.[12,82] In addition, artificial airways tend to shift position as the patient's head and neck move or as the tube is manipulated.[12] This can result in friction-like injuries. Occasional reaction to the materials composing the tube may also cause problems.

Depending on the type of tube, damage to the patient's airway can occur anywhere from the nose

Table 22-5 Pediatric to adult tracheostomy tube sizes

Age	Jackson reference
Premature	000–00
Birth to 6-mo	0
6–18 mo	1
18 mo to 4–5 yr	1–2
4–5 yr to 10 yr	2–3
10 to 14 yr	3–5
14 yr to adult	5–9+

down into the lower trachea. Nasal and oral damage were discussed previously. In this section, we will review laryngeal and tracheal trauma associated with tracheal tubes. Figure 22-21 shows the common injuries associated with both ET and tracheostomy tubes.

The four most common sites of injury caused by ET tubes are: (1) the posteromedial portion of the vocal cords, (2) the posteromedial portion of the arytenoid cartilages, (3) the posterolateral aspect of the cricoid cartilages, and (4) the trachea, from rings three through seven.[10] Occasionally the anterior tracheal wall also may be affected. Since tracheostomy tubes do not pass through the larynx, injury due to these airways is limited to tracheal sites.

The severity of damage may range from swelling, edema, and minor bleeding to permanent anatomical airway changes.[10,68,118,122,138,140] The reported incidence of these complications may vary due to the method of evaluation and the time elapsed before followup. For example, slight changes in the mucosa may not result in symptoms, but can be detected by bronchoscopy. Thus, the reported incidence of these problems would be higher when assessed by bronchoscopy. In contrast, some forms of airway damage may take weeks, months, or years to develop. If patient followup is done before damage becomes evident, the reported incidence will be lower.

Because injury often cannot be assessed while an artificial airway is in place, the patient's airway should always be evaluated carefully after extubation. Techniques commonly used to diagnose airway damage include physical examination, simple neck radio-

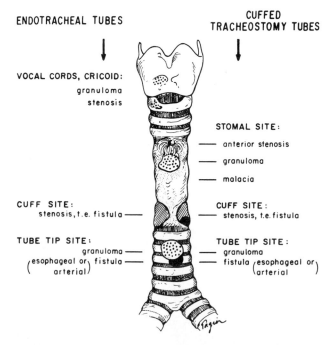

Fig. 22-21 Tracheal injuries produced by cuffed endotracheal and tracheostomy tubes. (From Grillo HC: Surgery of the trachea, *Curr Probl Surg*, July 1970.)

graphy, air **tomography,** fluoroscopy, laryngoscopy, bronchoscopy, and pulmonary function studies.[122,138]

Laryngeal lesions

The most common laryngeal injuries associated with ET intubation are glottic edema, vocal cord inflammation, laryngeal and vocal cord ulcerations, and vocal cord polyps and granulomas. Less common and more serious are vocal cord paralysis, laryngeal web, and laryngeal stenosis.

Glottic edema and vocal cord inflammation are transient changes that occur secondary to pressure from the ET tube, or trauma during intubation.[82,117] The reported incidence of these problems varies from 20% to 30%.

The primary concern with glottic edema and vocal cord inflammation is not while the patient is intubated, but after extubation. Since swelling can worsen over 24 hours after extubation, patients should be evaluated periodically for the delayed development of glottic edema.

The most common symptoms of glottic edema and vocal cord inflammation are hoarseness and stridor. Hoarseness occurs in nearly three-quarters of all extubated patients. Generally, hoarseness is benign and usually resolves over a few hours to days.

Stridor is a high-pitched noise heard during inspiration. Because it is associated with increased airway resistance and work of breathing, stridor is a more serious symptom than hoarseness. In adults, the presence of stridor indicates that the diameter of the anatomic airway is 5 mm or less.

Stridor is often treated with racemic epinephrine (2.25% Vaponephrine) via aerosol.[82,116] The goal of the treatment is to reduce glottic or airway edema by mucosal vasoconstriction. A steroid may also be added to the aerosol to further reduce inflammation.

In order to reduce laryngeal edema in patients who have had prolonged intubation, or those who have failed prior extubation due to glottic edema, IV steroids may be given 24 hours prior to extubation.[82] If stridor continues and is unresponsive to treatment, structural changes that narrow the airway should be suspected.

Laryngeal and vocal cord ulcerations have been reported in 20% to 50% of extubated patients.[118] These changes have been reported after as little as seven hours of intubation, and are generally acute in nature. The primary symptom is hoarseness, which usually resolves spontaneously. No therapy is indicated.

Vocal cord polyps and granulomas may occur as the tissues heals after ulceration.[68,118] Polyps and granulomas may take weeks or months to form. Some authors report these changes as uncommon, while others report incidence rates as high as 42%. Early symptoms include difficulty in swallowing, hoarseness, and stri-

dor. Case reports indicate that these symptoms tend to resolve spontaneously in most patients. Long-term complications include dry cough, difficulty in raising sputum, orthopnea, and lower respiratory tract infections. If symptoms are severe, the polyps or granulomas may need to be removed surgically.

Vocal cord paralysis due to the either tube pressure on the cords or the recurrent laryngeal nerve has been reported.[122] Incidence varies from about 3% to 5% of previously intubated patients. The primary symptom is a stridor that does not resolve with racemic epinephrine treatments. However, obstructive symptoms may resolve within 24 hours, and full movement of the cords can return over several days. If the obstructive symptoms do not resolve, tracheotomy may be indicated. For some patients, unilateral vocal cord paralysis increases the chance of aspiration.[82]

A laryngeal web is the result of necrotic tissue forming fibrin and incorporating cellular debris.[107,118] This "membrane" may occupy varying amounts of the glottic lumen. A laryngeal web may take days or months to form. Symptoms include stridor or abrupt total airway obstruction. If the web is pliable, treatment consists of aspirating the web with a suction catheter. Otherwise, laser laryngoscopy may be indicated.

Laryngeal stenosis has been reported due to intubation or tracheotomy when performed too close to the first tracheal ring.[82] The normal tissue of the larynx is replaced by scar tissue, which causes stricture and decreased mobility. The symptoms of laryngeal stenosis are similar to those for vocal cord paralysis, namely, stridor and hoarseness. Since laryngeal stenosis does not resolve spontaneously, surgical correction is usually necessary. Occasionally, a permanent tracheostomy may be required.

Tracheal lesions

Whereas laryngeal lesions occur only with oral or nasal ET tracheal tubes, tracheal lesions may occur after use of any tracheal airway. The most common tracheal lesions caused by artificial airways are tracheal granulomas, tracheomalacia, and tracheal stenosis.[82,118] Less common, but more serious complications are tracheoesophageal and tracheoinnominate fistulas.

Tracheal granulomas usually form in the trachea near the tracheal tube tip. They are probably related to tube movement.[10] Another site of granuloma development is the tracheal stoma itself. This may be due to a foreign body reaction.[68,122] Case reports indicate a 30% acute incidence of tracheal granulomas, with 10% of the patients going on to demonstrate chronic changes associated with tracheal stenosis.

Tracheomalacia and tracheal stenosis occur either separately or together. Tracheomalacia is the softening of the cartilaginous rings, which causes collapse of the trachea during inspiration. Processes similar to those causing mucosal ulceration may lead to **debridement** of the epithelium, and exposure and necrosis of the tracheal rings.[10] The extent of tracheomalacia depends on the degree of damage to the cartilage.

Tracheal stenosis is a narrowing of the lumen of the trachea, which can occur as the tracheal rings start to heal. Fibrous scarring causes the airway to narrow. In patients with ET tubes, this type of damage most often occurs where the tracheal wall was in contact with the inflated cuff. However, tracheal stenosis has been reported to affect segments of the trachea larger than those normally in contact with the tube cuff. This type of tracheal stenosis is circumferential and may be submucosal or transmural.

In patients with tracheostomy tubes, stenosis may occur either at the cuff site or at the tip of the tube. Stenosis at the stoma site is more common. Typically, stenosis at the stoma occurs when the sides of the incision pull together during healing. Usually the posterior wall of the trachea is unaffected.[10,117,122,143] Stenosis at the stoma site may be caused by too large a stoma, infection of the stoma, movement of the tube, or frequent tube changes.[143]

Signs of possible tracheal damage prior to extubation include difficulty in sealing the trachea with the cuff, and evidence of tracheal dilation on chest X-ray.[82,89] Post-extubation signs and symptoms depend on the severity of the damage. These signs and symptoms may develop acutely within minutes, but more commonly become evident over a 2 to 3 month period.[68,138] Difficulty with expectoration may be seen in mild cases. Dyspnea at rest indicates more severe damage than dyspnea on exertion. Stridor will occur if the tracheal lumen is less than 5 mm in diameter.[138] Occasionally, patients are diagnosed and treated for asthma without improvement in symptoms.[122] Tomography, fluoroscopy and pulmonary function studies, especially flow volume loops, maybe helpful in quantifying the severity of the damage. Flow-volume loops are also helpful in distinguishing between tracheomalacia and tracheal stenosis.[122,138,143] Tracheomalacia will appear as a variable obstruction with different inspiratory and expiratory patterns. Tracheal stenosis will appear as a fixed obstructive pattern, with flattening of both the inspiratory and expiratory limbs of the flow-volume loop (Figure 22-22).

Treatment depends on the severity, especially the length and circumference of the damage.[82,122] If the patient has been treated for asthma using steroids, they should be discontinued as soon as possible, since they may promote infection and delay healing. Laser therapy may be useful if the lesion is small. Resection and end-to-end anastomosis may be indicated when the damage involves less than three tracheal rings. More involved damage may require staged repair.

A tracheoesophageal or T-E fistula is a direct communication between the trachea and esophagus. Tracheoesophageal fistula may occur in infants as a congenital defect. As a complication of artificial airways, tracheoesophageal fistula has an incidence of between 1% to 5%, and has been reported with both tracheostomy and ET tubes. If it occurs soon after tracheotomy, incorrect surgical technique may be the cause. Later development is related to sepsis, malnutrition, tracheal erosion from the cuff and the tube,

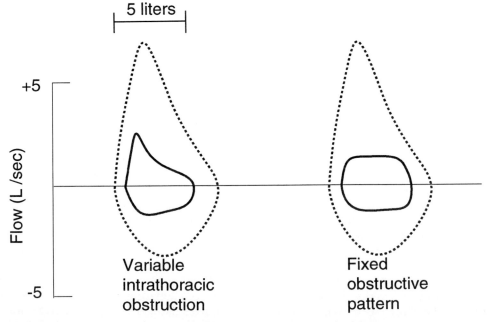

Fig. 22-22 Variable intrathoracic (left) versus fixed obstructive pattern (right) flow-volume loops. Dotted lines are normals for comparison. Tracheomalacia is typically seen as a variable obstruction, while tracheal stenosis most often presents with a fixed pattern.

and esophageal erosion from nasogastric tubes.[16,82,142] Diagnosis can be made by a history of recurrent aspiration and abdominal distention as air is forced into the esophagus during positive pressure ventilation. Direct examination of the trachea and esophagus by bronchoscopy and endoscopy will confirm the diagnosis. Treatment involves the closure of the defect in the trachealis muscle and the wall of the esophagus.

A tracheoinnominate fistula is a direct connection between the trachea and the innominate artery. Tracheoinnominate fistula is a rare complication, but is the most common cause of delayed hemorrhage after tracheotomy.[77] This potentially life-threatening complication occurs if the tracheal tube is placed too low, thereby rubbing against and eroding the innominate artery. Diagnosis may be made by pulsation of the tracheostomy tube prior to the onset of hemorrhage. Once hemorrhage begins, hyperinflation of the cuff may slow the bleeding, but the patient must be taken to surgery.[143] Even with proper corrective action, only 25% of patients who develop this serious complication survive.

Prevention

As we have seen, damage to the larynx and the trachea ranges from acute inflammation to chronic structural changes such as stenosis. Not all patients develop long term complications, and the reasons for these differences are not fully understood. The amount of time before intubation causes damage also varies greatly from patient to patient. Nonetheless, there are several actions and precautions that we know can minimize the development of trauma due to tracheal airways.

Many studies suggest that tube movement is a primary cause of injury.[11,18,116] Several methods can be used to limit tube movement. Sedation to keep patients comfortable may prevent them from trying to extubate themselves. Nasotracheal tubes are easier to stabilize and may move less than orotracheal tubes. Patients with tracheostomy tubes should have respiratory therapy equipment attached through the use of swivel adapters so the tubing may move without moving the airway.[77,122] If the tracheostomy patient requires oxygen therapy, tracheostomy collars are preferred to T-tubes or Briggs adapters.[31]

Once in place, ET and tracheostomy tubes should not be changed unless necessary. Selection of the correct size airway is also important.[10] It has been suggested that an ET tube one size smaller than can be fit through the opening of the glottis should be used. The patient should be discouraged from unnecessary coughing or efforts to talk, which will prevent the cords from closing around the tube.[18] Pressure necrosis from the cuff on ET or tracheostomy tubes may be reduced by limiting cuff pressures to that needed to minimize aspiration or provide ventilation.[10,122,138] If the airway has been placed to provide access for suctioning or to bypass an obstruction, it may not be necessary to inflate the cuff at all.

Infected secretions have been implicated in the development of **tracheitis** and mucosal destruction, and infection of the tracheotomy stoma has been linked to tracheal stenosis.[68,138] Therefore, sterile techniques should be used when working with these tubes. Good tracheostomy care, including aseptic cleaning of the stoma with hydrogen peroxide, should be carried out routinely. Soiled tracheostomy dressings should also be changed as needed.

It should be realized that the most serious complications of tracheal airways occur in less than 10% of the patients requiring intubation. This relatively small risk should never deter action when a tracheal airway is needed. However, once the airway is established, only sound techniques of airway management and maintenance can minimize the possibility of serious complications.

AIRWAY MAINTENANCE

Once a tracheal airway is in place, the RCP must attend to several aspects of airway maintenance. Among the critical responsibilities in this area are: (1) securing the tube and maintaining its proper placement, (2) providing for patient communication, (3) assuring adequate humidification, (4) minimizing the possibility of infection, (5) facilitating clearance of secretions, (6) providing appropriate cuff care, and (7) troubleshooting airway-related problems. Although each of these topics will be discussed in a separate section, it is important to realize that certain aspects of airway maintenance are interrelated. For example, not checking to see if the patient needs to be suctioned could result in an obstructed tube, which may, in turn, require troubleshooting.

Securing the airway and confirming placement

ET tubes, nasal or oral, are often secured with tape. The tape is secured to one side of the face, then wound around the tube and airway once or twice before securing the end to the skin again (refer to Figure 22-17). Silk tape is adequate if the period of intubation is short, such as during surgery. However, this type of tape is easily loosened by oral secretions which may result in movement of the tube. Cloth tape seems to be better for longer use, and may adhere to the skin better after application of **tincture of benzoin**. Some practitioners recommend applying benzoin to the tube itself so the tape will be more securely attached to the tube. Disadvantages of taping tubes in place include allergic reactions to the tape and damage to the skin when removing soiled or loose tape.

Alternatively, some manufactures have developed tube holder systems which use straps and plastic adapters to stabilize the tube.[125] Case reports demonstrate that the incidence of skin damage, tube movement, and self extubations with these stabilizing devices are less than with traditional taping methods. However, of and by themselves, these devices cannot prevent airway trauma.

Tracheostomy tubes may be held in place through the use of cloth ties that are threaded through the flanges of the tube. Two separate pieces may be used and tied together on the side of the patient's neck. Another method uses one long piece of cloth tie that goes through one flange and around the patient's neck, and threading through the other flange before being tied. An alternative to cloth ties is a strip of foam rubber with Velcro attachments that are threaded through the flanges. This system is easier to change and does not cause skin necrosis as often as cloth ties. Whichever material is used, the ties should be loose enough to fit one finger's width between the ties and the patient's neck. This will also help minimize skin damage.

Proper placement of ET and tracheostomy tubes may be assessed on chest X-ray. The tip of the tube should be 3 to 7 cm above the carina or between T2 and T4.[18,45,82,116] This position will minimize the chance of the tube moving down into the mainstem bronchi or up into the larynx. There are two important points to remember when assessing tube position on X-ray. First, on an AP film, the esophagus is behind the trachea. Therefore, esophageal intubation may be missed. If a tube is suspected of being located in the esophagus, a lateral film will help. Second, the position of an ET tube will change with head and neck position (Figure 22-23).[26] Flexion of the neck moves the tube toward the carina, and extension will pull the tube toward the larynx. Therefore, when reviewing a film for tube placement, the practitioner should check the position of the head and neck. If the tube is malpositioned, the RCP should remove the old tape and reposition the tube, using the cm markings as a guide. This often requires two people to prevent extubation.

As an alternative to using chest films to confirm tube placement, a practitioner trained in fiberoptic laryngoscopy or bronchoscopy may confirm the position of the tube visually.[91] Using this method, the fiberoptic scope is inserted into the tube, and the carina directly visualized. By moving the scope from the tube tip to the carina, and measuring the distance of laryngoscope displacement, the exact distance of insertion can be determined.

Providing for patient communication

One of the most frustrating aspects of providing care to a patient with a tracheal tube is their impaired ability to talk. Phonation requires moving vocal cords and airflow between them. ET tubes prevent vocal cord movement and do not allow for exhaled air to pass between the cords. Standard tracheostomy tubes allow for vocal cord movement but no airflow.

The experienced practitioner may use lip reading, but this technique is very difficult in patients with orotracheal tubes, due to the tape around the mouth that is used to secure the tube. As an alternative, the alert patient may write their messages on paper or some other writing surface. This sounds simple, but may be made difficult by restricted hand movement due to restraints and arterial or IV line placement in the hand or forearm. Moreover, it is often difficult for critically ill patients to hold up their heads to see a writing pad. A better solution is a letter, phrase, or

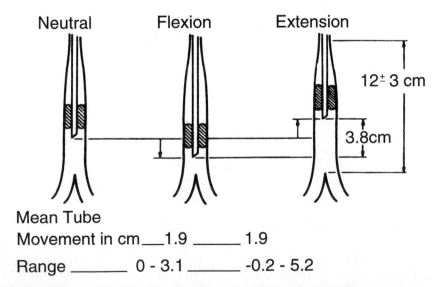

Fig. 22-23 Effect of neck flexion and extension on endotracheal tube position. (From Conrardy PA, et al: Alterations of endotracheal tube position: flexion and extension of the neck, *Crit Care Med* 4:8-12, 1976).

picture board.[6] These communication adjuncts allow patients to communicate by simple pointing. The use of large but simple drawings are particularly important for patients who cannot clearly see print.

In conscious patients for whom long-term tracheostomy is indicated, consideration should be given to a "talking" tracheostomy tube (Figure 22-24).[34,44] These specialized airways provide a separate inlet for compressed gas, which escapes above the tube, thereby allowing phonation. There are some problems associated with these tubes. The continuous gas flow through a new tracheostomy may promote the development of air leaks. High flow rates may irritate the glottis secondary to drying. Secretions may occlude the speaking gas outlets. While not life-threatening, it can be frustrating for the patient and practitioner.

For spontaneously breathing patients with intact upper airway reflexes, a one-valve attached to the tracheostomy tube allows for inspiration through the tracheostomy tube and exhalation through the larynx. Speech is coordinated with exhalation through the larynx.

Assuring adequate humidification

Although tracheal tubes provide an airway to conduct gas to and from the lungs, they do not function as well as our natural airways. Specifically, artificial tracheal airways bypass the normal humidification, filtration, and heating functions of the upper airway. It has been shown that decreased humidity in the inspired air will cause secretions to thicken.[110] Cool air may also decrease ciliary function. Singly or in combination, these conditions may impair the mucociliary escalator and result in retention of secretions. If a patient is intubated to help clear secretions, failure to provide adequate humidification will compound the problem. Tenacious secretions may plug tracheal tube and render it useless. In fact, a plugged tracheal tube constitutes an emergency situation, the management of which will be discussed later in this chapter.

In order to prevent these problems, the inspired air should be provided to the airway as near to body temperature and humidity (BTPS) as possible. Devices capable of providing saturated gas at or near body temperature include heated humidifiers and heated jet type nebulizers.[24,34,116] These devices should provide saturated gas to the airway at a temperature between 32°C and 36°C. This may require a higher temperature at the humidification device, since heat loss will occur as gas moves toward the patient (refer to Chapter 25). The selection of humidification device should be based on patient needs and assessment the airway, to include the volume and thickness of secre-

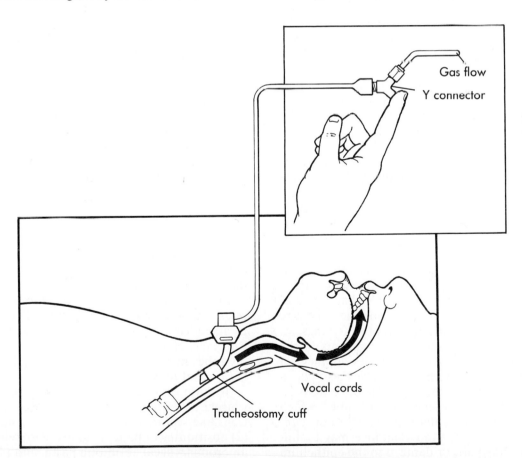

Fig. 22-24 "Talking" tracheostomy tube.

tions, and the history of mucus plugging or tube occlusions.

Minimizing nosocomial infections

Patients with tracheal airways are very susceptible to bacterial colonization of the lower respiratory tract. Colonization refers to the presence of bacteria without a physiologic or immunologic response. The presence of bacteria does not always equate with infection.

Typically, when infection occurs, there will be changes in the patient's sputum (color, consistency, or amount), breath sounds (wheezes, crackles or rhonchi) or chest X-ray (infiltrates or atelectasis).[76] Additional changes associated with bacterial infection include fever, increased heart rate, and leukocytosis. The reported incidence of nosocomial pneumonia in patients having artificial airways with or without mechanical ventilation range from 12% to 40%.

Tracheal tubes increase the possibility of pulmonary infection by several routes.[29,76,110] Bacteria can easily enter into the lower airway around the tube or through its lumen. Endotracheal intubation introduces organisms into the lower airway as the tube passes through the mouth or nose. Pathogenic bacteria may be found in the mouth, especially if the patient is receiving antibiotics which have eliminated the normal flora. Since the glottis is propped open by the ET tube and the cuff may not completely seal the airway, aspiration of the pharyngeal contents around the tube may occur in up to 70% of intubated patients. Last, anything that passes through the tube, such as suction catheters, saline, or aerosolized medications, may carry bacteria into the lower airway.

Bacteria may be found adhering to the inner walls of the tubes within a substance called gylcocalyx. This material, composed of polysaccharides and the bacteria which produce it, forms a film on the surface of artificial devices such as tracheal airways. This material seems to protect the bacteria from antibiotics and phagocytosis by macrophages. Common respiratory pathogens such as *Pseudomonas aeruginosa, Staphylococcus aureus, Staphylococcus epidermis,* and Acinteobacter are excellent producers of gylcocalyx.[76,114] Although the presence of gylcocalyx has been demonstrated, its role in the development of pneumonia is still not well understood. It is possible that pieces of this film may be broken off as suction catheters are passed through the tube and down into the lungs.

The introduction of pathogenic organisms in the lower airway is only one factor in the development of pulmonary infection. Retained secretions also play a major role. Impaired mucociliary clearance may occur secondary to the presence of the tube[76] which blocks the mucociliary escalator proximal to the cuff. Also responsible for impaired clearance may be improperly humidified air, or damage to the epithelium from improper suctioning technique. Mucosal damage results in a surface that bacteria may attach to thereby, decreasing its clearance.[29]

Impaired clearance may also be due to the patient's inability to cough effectively. There are two major factors that impair coughing in intubated patients. First pain, sedation, muscle fatigue, or impaired neuromuscular reflexes may compromise thoracic compression, thereby lowering the velocity of the expired air. Inability to close the glottis has a similar effect. In spite of these factors, many patients with ET tubes are able to generate an effective "huff." Patients with tracheostomy tubes seem better able to perform this maneuver, possibly because the airway is shorter.

The presence of a nasogastric (NG) tube and the use of antacids is also associated with the development of nosocomial infection.[76] The NG tube increases the likelihood of gastric reflux, impairs swallowing and can serve as a conduit for bacteria to move into the oropharynx. The use of antacids may raise the pH of the GI tract and permit the overgrowth of normal flora. These two factors can increase oropharyngeal colonization with abnormal flora.

Another factor which may further contaminate the upper airway is improper handling of oropharyngeal (Yankauer) suction devices. Often found lying in the patient's bed, these devices are used without sterile technique. Once the oropharynx becomes contaminated, any secretions which are aspirated around the tracheal tube further increase the likelihood of pulmonary infection.

Bacteria that do gain access to the lower airways are normally handled by the body's immune system, including antibodies, alveolar macrophages and **polymorphonuclear cells.**[53] However, the patient's own defense mechanism may not be adequate due to chronic illness, malnutrition, or immunosuppression.

In order to minimize the development of contamination and/or pneumonia, RCPs should try to prevent introducing organisms into the airway. This is done by: (1) adhering to sterile technique during suctioning, (2) ensuring that only aseptically clean or sterile respiratory equipment is used for each patient, and (3) consistently washing hands between patient contacts (refer to Chapter 4).[76]

In addition, efforts should be made to prevent retention of secretions. Suctioning, chest physiotherapy and adequate humidification are useful to this end. Routinely changing the inner cannula on tracheostomy tubes may also help minimize bacterial contamination and infection.

Techniques to decrease the consequences of pharyngeal aspiration include: (1) use of ulcer medications like sucralfate that maintain normal gastric pH, (2) positioning of patients to decrease reflux, (3) using an oropharyngeal antibiotic paste, and (4) suctioning above the tracheal tube cuff.[29,76,79,105]

Facilitating clearance of secretions

The primary means to aid secretion clearance in patients with tracheal airways is tracheobronchial aspiration, or tracheal suctioning.[1] The indication, hazards, and equipment needed for suctioning through tracheal tubes is basically the same as that for nasotracheal suctioning. Indications for suctioning which are more specific to patients with artificial airways and/or mechanical ventilation are listed in the accompanying box.[1]

Procedure

Alterations in the procedure for tracheobronchial aspiration are as follows:[1]

Step 1: Assess the patient. If breath sounds are clear, one pass of the suction catheter should be done periodically to ensure the tip of the tube does not become plugged. Very thick secretions may not move with airflow and thus may not create any adventitious sounds. However, routine suctioning is not recommended.

Step 2: Assemble the equipment. The equipment for tracheal aspiration is the same as for nasotracheal suctioning, with the addition of sterile saline for

instillation. In concept, instillation of small volumes of saline directly into the airway may help promote a cough, thin secretions and aid in their removal. However, there are conflicting reports in the literature regarding the efficacy of this method.[3,48] A new catheter design allows for continuous irrigation with suctioning. One study has suggested increased removal with the design.[61] If the secretions are very tenacious, instillation of acetylcysteine or sodium bicarbonate (2%) tends to be more effective than normal saline. This may require a physician's order. Last, careful attention should be given to the size of the suction catheter. The outer diameter of the catheter should not exceed one-half of the internal diameter of the tracheal tube.

Step 3: Preoxygenate and hyperinflate the patient. Hyperinflation can easily be accomplished via a manual resuscitator. If the patient is on a ventilator, increasing ventilator volume, increasing ventilator sigh rate, or activating the manual sigh button will provide hyperinflation.[1] However, stacking of breaths or insufficient expiratory time should be avoided. Patients with COPD may need to be hyperinflated without increasing the FIO_2. Other patients should receive 100% oxygen for at least 30 seconds. This may be accomplished by manual resuscitator or ventilator. If using a ventilator to provide 100% oxygen, it is important to allow adequate "washout-time". This will ensure the delivery of 100% oxygen prior to the disconnection of the patient.[17]

Step 4: Insert the catheter. Insert the catheter carefully. When an obstruction is felt or a strong cough elicited, the RCP should withdraw the catheter and apply suction.

Step 5: Apply suction. Use the same technique previously described for nasotracheal suction.

Step 6: Re-oxygenate and hyperinflate. The increased FIO_2 should be maintained for at least 1 minute.[1]

Step 7: Assess the patient. Assess the effectiveness of the procedure and the occurrence of any untoward effects. The box, page 570 outlines the key variables to monitor prior to, during, and after suctioning.[1] Take any corrective steps necessary. Repeat Steps 3 through 7 as needed until improvement is seen or any severe reactions occur.

Tracheal suctioning is judged effective if breath sounds improve, work of breathing decreases, or oxygen saturation or blood gases improve. In addition, if the patient is on a volume-cycled ventilator, both the peak inspiratory pressure and measured airway resistance should decrease. Patients receiving pressure-controlled ventilation should show an increase in tidal volume.[1]

Given their already unstable condition, patients receiving ventilatory support are especially prone to develop hypoxemia during suctioning.[1,107] Much research has been done to find better methods to

---

Indications for tracheal suctioning[1]

1. The need to remove retained pulmonary secretions as evidenced by one of the following:
   Coarse breath sounds by auscultation or 'noisy' breathing
   Increased peak inspiratory pressures during volume-controlled mechanical ventilation or decreased tidal volume during pressure-controlled ventilation.
   Patient's inability to generate an effective spontaneous cough.
   Visible secretions in the airway
   Changes in monitored flow and pressure graphics
   Suspected aspiration of gastric or upper airway secretions
   Clinically apparent increased work of breathing
   Deterioration of arterial blood gas values
   Radiologic changes consistent with retention of pulmonary secretions
2. The need to obtain a sputum specimen to rule out or identify pneumonia or other pulmonary infection or for sputum cytology
3. The need to maintain the patency and integrity of the artificial airway
4. The need to stimulate a patient cough in patients unable to cough effectively secondary to changes in mental status or the influence of medication
5. Presence of pulmonary atelectasis or consolidation, presumed to be associated with secretion retention

> ### Parameters to monitor prior to, during, and after tracheal suctioning:[1]
>
> 1. Breath sounds
> 2. Oxygen saturation
>   Skin color
>   Pulse oximeter, if available
> 3. Respiratory rate and pattern
> 4. Hemodynamic parameters
>   Pulse rate
>   Blood pressure, if indicated and available
>   EKG, if indicated and available
> 5. Sputum characteristics
>   Color
>   Volume
>   Consistency
>   Odor
> 6. Cough effort
> 7. Intracranial pressure, if indicated and available
> 8. Ventilator parameters
>   Peak inspiratory pressure and plateau pressure
>   Tidal volume
>   Pressure, flow, and volume graphics, if available
> FIO_2
> 9. Arterial blood gases, if indicated and available

from the circuit.[1] Some studies have suggested that the use of these catheters can decrease the severity of hypoxemia during suctioning.[22,34,92] This may occur secondary to maintenance of PEEP levels and rapid restoration of gas flow. However, even when these closed system catheters are used, the FIO_2 should be increased prior to suctioning.

In terms of infection control, clinical studies indicate that as long as the suction system is changed every 24 to 48 hours and flushed appropriately, bacterial colonization and infection are unlikely.[92] In addition, since the system is closed, contaminated droplet nuclei are not disseminated when the patient huffs or coughs.[23,35] The extra weight the in-line catheter adds to the circuit may need extra support to lessen tension on the tracheal tube.[88] Another concern of practitioners is the catheter "feels" different and may not remove secretions as efficiently. This has yet to be studied.

Another factor to be considered is the influence of in-line catheters on ventilator function.[28,54] The presence of the catheter in the airway increases resistance and may cause the pressure limit to be reached. The resultant decrease in tidal volume may lead to hypoxemia. Therefore, the pressure limit may need to be

prevent this complication. Although the current literature is controversial, there are a few consistent guidelines.

First, hyperoxygenation prior to suctioning will minimize the drop in PaO_2 in most patients. Hyperoxygenation combined with hyperventilation provides even more protection.[20,46] However, hyperventilation may agitate some patients.[78] Hyperoxygenation and hyperventilation have been reported to be more effective when done through the ventilator, as opposed to a manual resuscitator.[21,119] This appears especially true for patients on high levels of support, such as positive end-expiratory pressure (PEEP). Moreover, manual resuscitators cannot always provide 100% oxygen or deliver a consistent tidal volume, and maintaining sterile technique and PEEP levels is difficult with some of these devices.[21]

Insertion of the catheter through an adapter that does not require ventilator disconnection may also be helpful in preventing hypoxemia. This technique is recommended for patients receiving high levels of support, especially PEEP levels greater than 10 cm H_2O.

Two alternative suction catheter design may also be considered to minimize hypoxemia: (1) the closed system multi-use catheter, and (2) the double lumen catheter.

As pictured in Figure 22-25, the closed system multi-use suction catheter is incorporated directly into the ventilator circuit. Once in place, suctioning can be performed without disconnecting the patient

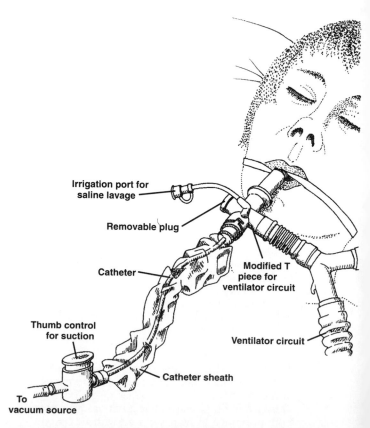

Fig. 22-25 A closed system multi-use suction catheter. (From Sills JR: Respiratory Care certification guide, St Louis, Mosby, 1991.)

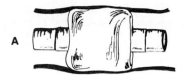
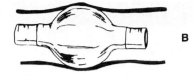

Fig. 22-26 Diagram comparing shapes of high residual volume, low-pressure cuff, **A,** and low residual volume, high-pressure cuff, **B.** (From McPherson SP: Respiratory therapy equipment, ed 4, St Louis, 1989, Mosby.)

increased. In the assist/control mode, the reduced airway pressure which occurs during the application of suction pressure, may result in auto cycling and inadequate I/E ratio.

The second catheter design is a double lumen device that can provide both suction pressure and oxygen delivery.[34,113,124] When the valve on this catheter is closed, suction pressure is delivered to the airway; when the valve is opened, oxygen is delivered. Again the reduction in PaO_2 and SaO_2 is usually attenuated. Factors that affect the efficient use of this device are the ratio of suction catheter to tracheal tube size, oxygen insufflation flow rate, and the circumference of the tracheal tube to vent excess insufflation flow.[128]

Providing cuff care

Tracheal tube cuffs are used to seal the airway for mechanical ventilation or to prevent or minimize aspiration. As previously mentioned, tracheal stenosis and tracheomalacia are associated with cuff use. The pathogenesis of these problems is related to the amount of cuff pressure transmitted to the tracheal wall. If cuff pressure exceeds the mucosal perfusion pressure, ischemia, ulceration, necrosis and exposure of the cartilage may result.

The importance of cuff pressure

How much pressure is transmitted from the cuff to the tracheal wall depends on the diameter, thickness, and compliance of the cuff. Inflated cuffs were the major cause of airway damage in the 1960's when small volume, high pressure cuffs were common. Since the 1970's, high residual volume, low pressure cuffs have become the norm (Figure 22-26). The full inflated diameter of these cuffs is greater than the diameter of the trachea. This means that the cuff does not have to be fully inflated to seal the airway, and less internal cuff pressure is needed. Thus, when properly used, these cuff should transmit less pressure to the tracheal wall than their small volume, high pressure counterparts. Although the use of high residual volume, low pressure cuffs has lessened the incidence of tracheal damage, this type of injury has not been eliminated.

Measuring cuff pressure

One of the most important aspects of airway care is the measurement of cuff pressure. The perfusion pressure of the tracheal mucosa ranges from 30 mm Hg at the arterial side, to 18 mm Hg at the venous side. Maximum recommended levels of cuff pressures thus range from 20 to 25 mm Hg.[82,107]

Cuff pressure can be measured with a three-way stopcock, syringe and pressure manometer (Figure 22-27). With the stopcock opened to the syringe, manometer and cuff, air is added or removed while the RCP observes the pressure changes on the manometer. It is important to realize most manometers are calibrated in cm H_2O, and not mm Hg. Thus the "acceptable range" of 20 to 25 mm Hg equates to between 24 cm to 30 cm H_2O.

The cuff does not have to be inflated to these levels if the trachea can be sealed with less pressure. Overinflation of a high volume, low pressure cuff is equivalent to using a high pressure cuff.[82,122] This problem is common if the tube chosen is too small for that patient's trachea. Another cause for high cuff pressures is high airway pressures generated by mechanical ventilation.[49] Distention of the lumen of the tube occurs when pressure is the highest and will push on the trachea. Over time, this may cause tracheal dilation.

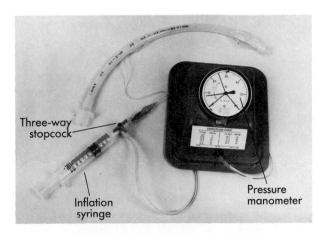

Fig. 22-27 Measuring cuff pressure by way of in-line pressure monitor.

■ MINI **C** LINI ■

22-3

Measuring Cuff Pressure

Problem: A three-way stopcock, syringe and pressure manometer (see Fig. 26-28) are used to measure the cuff pressure of a patient's endotracheal tube. You connect the stopcock to the cuff pilot tube, the syringe and the pressure manometer, and rotate the stopcock valve such that there is communication between the cuff and the pressure manometer. In this position, the stopcock is closed to the syringe. You now observe the pressure registered by the manometer and record it as the endotracheal tube's cuff pressure; however, you are told by an observing respiratory care practitioner that the pressure you have recorded is not the pressure that actually existed in the cuff. Is your colleague correct?

Discussion: Your colleague is correct. When you opened the stopcock to allow cuff pressure to communicate with the manometer, some of the gas in the cuff left the cuff to fill the connecting tubing; this lowered the pressure in the cuff. To accurately assess the pressure that first existed in the cuff, you would need to perform the following procedures: (1) Position the stopcock so that it is closed to the pilot tube; then connect it to the pilot tube. (2) Attach the syringe (all air expelled) and manometer to the stopcock and position the stopcock to allow communication between the cuff and syringe. (3) Aspirate all cuff gas and record the volume (**do this only after suctioning secretions from above the cuff**). (4) Re-inject the gas into the cuff. (5) Close the stopcock to the syringe and allow manometer and cuff to communicate. (6) Close the stopcock to the manometer and aspirate the gas from the cuff again; this volume will be less than that in Step 3 because some cuff gas in now in the manometer connecting tubing. (7) Note the difference in gas volume between Step 3 and 6; this is the volume of cuff gas now occupying the connecting tube. (8) Re-inject the volume into the cuff, close the stopcock to the syringe, remove the syringe and withdraw the plunger until a volume equal to the difference noted in Step 7 is obtained. (9) Inject this additional volume into the cuff-manometer system and note the pressure; the pressure registered is the actual pressure that originally existed in the cuff.

If you are only interested in obtaining a cuff pressure that allows a minimal leak, you can simply position the stopcock so that all 3 channels communicate, and then add or withdraw air with the syringe until a minimal leak is obtained. At this point, the manometer pressure can be recorded as actual cuff pressure because all pressures are at equilibrium.

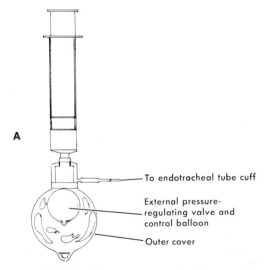

A

— To endotracheal tube cuff

— External pressure-regulating valve and control balloon

— Outer cover

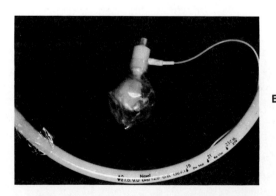

B

Fig. 22-28 A, Lanz external pressure-regulating valve and control balloon regulate cuff pressure. **B,** Endotracheal tube with pressure-regulating valve. (From McPherson SP: Respiratory therapy equipment, ed 4, St Louis, 1980, Mosby.)

Cuff Inflation

Two alternative inflation techniques are used: (1) the minimal occluding volume (MOV), and (2) the minimal leak technique (MLT). Periodic deflation of the cuff for 5 to 10 minutes every hour has also been suggested, although the adequacy of this method is questionable.

Minimal occluding volume (MOV) technique.[107,116] In the MOV technique, the RCP slowly inflates the cuff until the air flow heard escaping around the cuff during a positive pressure breath ceases. Because the airways expand during the application of positive pressure, pressure on the trachea during inspiration is less than during expiration. The amount of ischemia that may result using the MOV technique depends on both the cuff pressure used and the rate of the positive pressure breaths.

Minimal leak technique (MLT).[10,116] The MLT method is similar to the MOV method, in that air is slowly injected into the cuff until the leak stops. However, once a seal is obtained, the RCP removes a small amount of air, allowing a slight leak at peak inflation pressure. Because this leak occurs during the positive pressure breath, pharyngeal secretions tend to be blown up at peak inflation, minimizing the likelihood of aspiration.

Some authors suggest that pressure monitoring is not needed if the MLT approach is used.[93] However, a minimal leak may be obtained at cuff pressures of 25 mm Hg in some patients. This is common at high ventilator pressures or if the tube is too small for the patient's airway. For this reason, cuff pressure measurements should still be conducted, regardless of the inflation method used.[117]

Alternative cuff designs

Several different types of cuffs have been designed to minimize mucosal trauma.[83,107] The Lanz tube incorporates an external pressure regulating valve and control reservoir designed to limit the cuff pressure to between 16 and 18 mm Hg (Figure 22-28). The Kamen-Wilkinson foam cuff is another alternative which is designed to seal the trachea with atmospheric pressure in the cuff. Prior to insertion, the foam cuff must be deflated. Once in position, the pilot tube is opened to the atmosphere, and the foam allowed to expand against the tracheal wall. Expansion of the cuff stops when the tracheal wall is encountered.

Minimizing the likelihood of aspiration

When judging the adequacy of a tracheal seal, the RCP must also take into account the potential for aspiration. The use of minimal leak technique and high volume cuffs does not absolutely prevent aspiration.[130] Also, aspiration is reported to be more common in spontaneously breathing patients than in those receiving positive pressure ventilation. This may be due to the movement of pharyngeal secretion around the cuff during the negative pressure phase of a spontaneous inspiration. Aspiration has also been reported to be more common with tracheostomy tubes than with ET tubes.

The **methylene blue** test can help determine whether or not this "leakage" type of aspiration is occurring.[39,130] Methylene blue may be added to the patient's feedings or swallowed by the patient in a small amount of water. Once the dye is introduced, the patient's trachea is suctioned through the artificial airway. If blue-tinged secretions are obtained when performing suctioning, aspiration is occurring.

If aspiration is confirmed, efforts must be made to minimize it. Oropharyngeal suctioning (above the tube cuff) should be performed as needed. In order to decrease the possibility of aspiration with feedings, the head of the bed should be elevated (where possible). Also, the feeding tube can be inserted into the **duodenum,** with its position confirmed by X-ray. The use of slightly higher cuff pressure during and after feeding may also minimize aspiration.

There are reports in the literature that suggest aspiration around a cuff will occur even with all precautions taken. There are also reports of feeding tubes being advanced past inflated cuffs into the trachea.[52,88,115]

Troubleshooting airway emergencies

The areas discussed so far are routine aspects of airway care. Three emergency situations that may occur include tube obstruction, cuff leaks, and accidental extubation. Clinical signs frequently encountered under these circumstances include various degrees of respiratory distress, changes in breath sounds, and air movement through the mouth.

Decreased breath sounds are a common finding in airway emergencies. The RCP must try to identify specific indicators for each of these problems, such as the inability to pass a suction catheter (obstruction), the ability to fully pass a catheter (extubation), or air flow around the tube (leaky cuff). Replacement airways should be kept at the bedside, as well as a manual resuscitator, mask, and gauze pads (for tracheotomized patients).

Tube obstruction

Obstruction of the tube is one of the most common causes of airway emergencies. Tube obstruction can be caused by: (1) kinking of or biting on the tube, (2) herniation of the cuff over the tube tip, (3) jamming of the tube orifice against the tracheal wall, and (4) mucus plugging (Figure 22-29, page 574).

Depending on whether the tube obstruction is partial or complete, different clinical signs will be present.[82] With partial airway obstruction in the spontaneously breathing patient, there will be decreased breath sounds and decreased air flow through the tube. If the patient is receiving positive pressure ventilation via a volume-cycled ventilator, peak inspiratory pressures will rise, often causing the pressure limit alarm to sound. With complete tube obstruction, the patient will exhibit severe distress, no breath sounds will be heard, and there will be no gas flow through the tube.

If the tube is kinked or jammed against the tracheal wall, the obstruction often can be relieved by moving the patient's head and neck.[82,107] If this does not relieve the obstruction, a herniated cuff may be blocking the airway, and the RCP should deflate the tube cuff. If these steps fail to overcome the obstruction, the practitioner should try to pass a suction catheter through the tube.[43] How far one can insert the catheter helps determine the site of obstruction. If a catheter is inserted near to or just past the end of the tube and does not cause coughing, a herniated cuff or mucus plug is the likely problem. In the case of mucus plugging, the RCP should attempt to aspirate the plug before considering more drastic action.

In situations involving tracheostomy tubes with an inner cannula, the RCP should remove the inner cannula and check to see if the plug is lodged in the tube. If it is, the patient can be ventilated through the outer cannula with a bag and mask, or the inner cannula can be replaced with a backup one.

If the obstruction cannot be cleared using the above techniques, the airway must be removed and replaced. In patients having undergone recent tracheotomy (four or five days), the stoma may not be well established, and may close when the tube is removed. Ideally, suture ties left in place by the surgeon can be used to pull open the stoma.

Once an obstructed airway has been removed, first priority must be given to restoring adequate ventilation and oxygenation. For patients with a tracheotomy stoma this may require sealing the wound with a gauze pad, like that used to temporarily close chest wounds in the field. Only after adequate ventilation and oxygenation are assured should airway reinsertion be undertaken.

Cuff leaks

A leak in the cuff, pilot tube, or one-way valve is a problem mostly for patients receiving mechanical ventilation. This will cause a system leak, with a resultant loss of delivered volume and a decrease in peak inspiratory pressure.

A small cuff leak can be detected by noting decreasing cuff pressures over time. A large leak, such as occurs with a blown cuff, has a more rapid onset. Breath sounds will be decreased, but the spontaneously breathing patient will have air movement through the tube. With positive pressure breaths air flow can often be felt at the mouth. Under such circumstances, the practitioner should try to re-inflate the cuff, while checking the pilot tube and valve for leaks.[112]

Similar findings can occur when an ET tube is positioned too high in the trachea, either near the glottic opening or in the esophagus.[82,103] Before presuming a cuff leak, the RCP should attempt to advance the tube slightly and reassess the leak and equality of breath sounds in both lung fields.

Leaks at the valve or in the pilot tube can be bypassed using a needle and stopcock placed in the pilot tube distal to the leak. This will allow the cuff to be reinflated and avoid emergency reintubation. A blown cuff requires extubation and reintubation.

Accidental extubation

Partial displacement of an airway out of the trachea can be detected by noting decreased breath sounds, decreased air flow through the tube, and the ability to pass a catheter to its full length without meeting an obstruction or eliciting a cough. With positive pres-

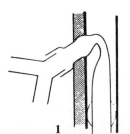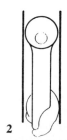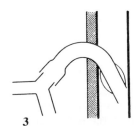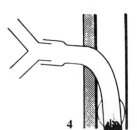

Fig. 22-29 Causes of tube obstruction. See text for details. (From Sykes MK, McNichol MW, Campbell EJM: Respiratory failure, Philadelphia, 1969, FA Davis.)

sure ventilation, air flow through the mouth or into the stomach may be heard and peak inspiratory pressures may be lowered. The RCP should completely remove the tube and provide ventilatory support as needed until the patient can be reintubated.

EXTUBATION

For most patients, endotracheal intubation is a temporary measure which will eventually be followed by extubation. Patients who are not candidates for extubation are those with permanent tracheostomies and those requiring permanent ventilatory support.

Indications

Extubation is indicated when the need for an artificial airway no longer exists. Specifically, if inserted to overcome an airway obstruction, the airway should be removed when the obstruction has been cleared. Alternatively, if inserted to aid secretion clearance, the airway should be removed when the patient can handle his or her own secretions. In terms of protecting the lower airway, if the patient is conscious and the pharyngeal reflex has returned to normal, an artificial airway is no longer indicated. Last, if the airway was inserted to provide positive pressure ventilation, it should be removed when the patient no longer needs ventilatory support.

Procedure

Since the RCP play a key role in extubation, and because the techniques differ somewhat, we will review the procedures for removing oro- or naso- tracheal and tracheostomy tubes separately.

Oro- or nasotracheal tubes

The following procedure is recommended for oro- or nasotracheal extubation:[82,107]

Step 1: Assemble equipment needed for the procedure, including suctioning apparatus, suction kits, oxygen and aerosol therapy equipment, manual resuscitator and mask, aerosol nebulizer with racemic epinephrine and normal saline (if ordered), and an intubation tray.

Step 2: Suction the ET tube and through the pharynx to above the cuff. This will help avoid aspiration of secretions after the cuff is deflated. The RCP should dispose of this kit and prepare another for use, or prepare a rigid tonsillar (Yankauer) suction tip. Patients will often cough after the tube is pulled and may need help with clearance.

Step 3: Oxygenate the patient well after suctioning. Extubation is a stressful procedure that can cause hypoxemia.

Step 4: Deflate the cuff. Remove all the air possible. Some practitioners then cut the valve off the pilot tube

to ensure that any remaining air is easily displaced during removal.

Step 5: Remove the tube. There are two techniques that are used to remove the tube. In the first method, the RCP gives a large breath with the manual resuscitator, and removes the tube at peak inspiration (when the cords are maximally abducted).[116] In the second method, the practitioner has the patient cough, pulling the tube during the expulsive expiratory phase. This also results in maximal abduction of the cords.

Step 6: Apply appropriate oxygen and humidity therapy, if ordered. Patients who have been receiving mechanical ventilation may still require some oxygen therapy, usually at a higher FiO_2. Other patients may require some oxygen, since this is a stressful procedure. If humidity therapy is indicated, most clinicians suggest a cool mist after extubation. A heated mist may only increase the swelling that normally occurs after extubation, thereby worsening airway obstruction.

Step 7: Assess the patient. The RCP should check for good air movement by auscultation. Stridor or decreased air movement after extubation indicate upper airway problems. The patient's respiratory rate, heart rate, color, and blood pressure should be assessed. The RCP should also be on the lookout for nose bleeding following nasotracheal extubation. The patient should be encouraged to cough, with assistance as needed.

Step 8: Reassess the patient often. Laryngeal edema may worsen with time and stridor may develop. Racemic epinephrine should be kept available. Arterial blood should be sampled and analyzed as needed.

The major complication associated with extubation is laryngospasm. Post-extubation laryngospasm is usually a transient event, lasting a matter of seconds. Should this occur, oxygenation may be maintained with a high FiO_2, and the application of positive pressure. If laryngospasm persists, a neuromuscular blocking agent may have to be given, which will necessitate manual ventilation or reintubation.

Another complication common after extubation is glottic edema. When stridor is heard immediately after extubation, the RCP should be wary of further problems, as the swelling can dramatically worsen. If stridor is present, a racemic epinephrine treatment may be given to lessen the swelling. In children, post-extubation edema is often subglottic, and may require reinsertion of the airway.

Since the vocal cords have had limited function during the intubation period, they may not fully close as needed once the airway has been removed. To avoid aspiration, oral feedings, except sips of cool water or ice chips, should be withheld for 24 hours post-intubation.[82]

Tracheostomy decannulation

There are several approaches to removing tracheostomy tubes.[44] Since patients with trachs often have problems with aspiration or secretions, a weaning process is used rather than abrupt removal of the tube. Weaning is done using either fenestrated tubes, progressively smaller tubes, or tracheostomy buttons.

Prior to extubation, a comprehensive patient assessment is required. The patient should have sufficient muscle strength to generate an effective cough. Ideally, there should be no active pulmonary infection and the volume and thickness should be acceptable. Patency of the upper airway should be assessed via bronchoscopy. Since deadspace will be increased when the tube is removed, adequate nutrition and muscle strength must be present.[44] After removal of the tube, the stoma will close on its own in a matter of days. The particular decannulation technique used will depend on the patient's needs and the experience and preferences of the attending physician.

Fenestrated tracheotomy tubes. A fenestrated tracheotomy tube is a double cannulated tube that has an opening in the posterior wall of the outer cannula above the cuff (Figure 22-30). Removal of the inner cannula opens the fenestration. Plugging of the proximal opening of the tube's outer cannula, accompanied by deflation of the cuff, allows for assessment of upper airway function. Removal of the plug allows access for suctioning. If the need for mechanical ventilation occurs, the inner cannula can be reinserted.

One problem associated with this type of tracheostomy tube is malposition of the fenestration, such as between the skin and the stoma, or against the posteri-or wall of the larynx.[111] Customizing the fenestration can help avoid this problem.[59,123] Proper fenestration placement is shown in Figure 22-31. Proper placement can be confirmed using fiberoptic bronchoscopy.

Case reports have demonstrated granular tissue formation in some patient using a fenestrated trach tube. This tends to occur on the anterior tracheal wall, above the tube fenestration. This granular tissue may occlude the fenestration, cause bleeding (especially with tube changes), or result in airway obstruction upon decannulation. Given the location of this granular tissue, these problems may be due to poor positioning of the fenestration within the airway.

Progressively smaller tubes. A second airway weaning technique is to use smaller and smaller tracheostomy tubes. As with fenestrated tubes, this approach maintains the airway, but allows for increasing use of the upper airway. This technique is also indicated in patients whose airway is too small for the fenestrated tubes that are currently available. The use of progressively smaller tubes may also allow for better healing of the stoma.

The problem with these techniques is the continued presence of a tube within the lumen of the airway.[7,44] The presence of the tube (cuffed or uncuffed) increases airway resistance. In patients with pre-existing obstructive disorders, this added airway resistance may be too much to bear, resulting in failed extubation. These tubes can also impair coughing by preventing full compression.

Tracheal buttons. The tracheal button also may be used to maintain a tracheal stoma.[44,134] Unlike the fenestrated tube, the tracheal button fits from the skin

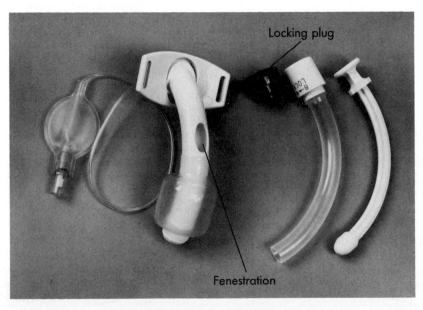

Fig. 22-30 Fenestrated tracheostomy tube.

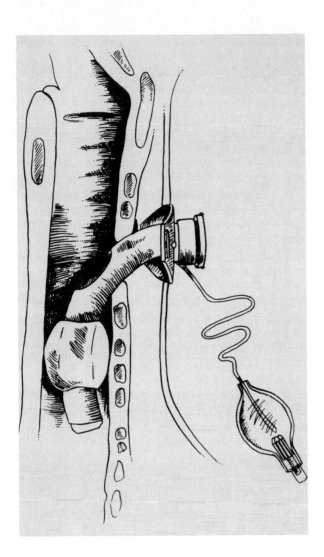

to just inside the anterior wall of the trachea (Figure 22-32). Therefore, the problem of added resistance is avoided. Since the tracheal button has no cuff, its use is limited to relieving airway obstructing and aiding the removal of secretions. Adapaters can be used that allow suctioning through the button. An optional one-way valve on the external end of the button allows for inspiration with less deadspace, and expiration with speech.

After tracheostomy decannulation, the patient should be assessed for vocal cord responses.[44] The problems seen with the cords may be related to laryngeal injury during intubation. Alternatively, decreased vocal cord responsiveness may occur secondary to the loss of laryngeal stimulation when the upper airway was bypassed. Vocal cord abnormalities can result in either aspiration or acute airway obstruction. A replacement trach tube and suctioning equipment should be available. If no complications develop, the stoma will close spontaneously over a few days. Surgery may be needed if there is any infection.

Fig. 22-31 Proper positioning of a fenestrated tracheostomy tube. (From Snyder GM: Individualized placement of tracheostomy tube fenestration and in situ examination with the fiberoptic laryngoscope, *Respir Care* 28(10): 1297, 1983.)

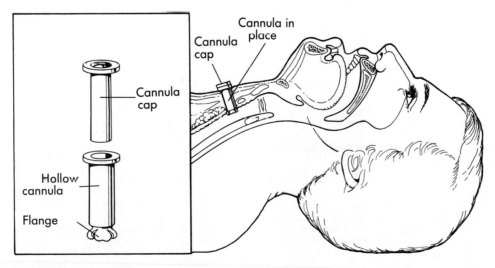

Fig. 22-32 Tracheostomy button.

CHAPTER SUMMARY

Maintaining patients' airways is one of the most important functions of the RCP. Airway clearance, including suctioning and assisting with bronchoscopy, is the most common responsibility of respiratory care personnel. Proficiency in airway clearance methods requires knowledge of both the indications and complications associated with these procedures.

The ability to recognize the need for an airway, to select the most appropriate device, and to insert or assist in its insertion are of equal importance. Maintenance of inserted artificial airways is also a major responsibility of RCPs. In this role, the practitioner must ensure that the patients' needs are addressed on an individual basis, and that any immediate or long-term risks to the patient are minimized.

Last, RCPs assume an important role in deciding when and how best to remove an artificial airway. It is toward this goal, of restoration of normal airway function, that the practitioner must always strive.

REFERENCES

1. AARC clinical practice guideline: Endotracheal suctioning of mechanically ventilated adults and children with artificial airway, *Respir Care* 38(5): 500-504, 1993.
2. AARC clinical practice guidelines: Nasotracheal suctioning, *Respir Care* 37(8): 898-901 1992.
3. Ackerman MH: The use of bolus normal saline instillations in artificial airways; Is it useful or necessary? *Heart Lung* 14(5): 505-506, 1985.
4. Allen MD, et al: Combined laser therapy and endobrochonial radiotherapy for unresectable lung carcinoma with bronchial obstruction, *Am J Surg* 150(1): 71-77, 1985.
5. Anton WR, et al: A disposable end-tidal CO_2 detector to verify endotracheal intubation, *Ann Emerg Med* 20(3): 271-5, 1991.
6. Appel-Hardin SJ: Communicating with intubated patients, *Crit Care Nurse* 4(6): 26-27, 1984.
7. Beard B, Monaco FJ: Tracheostomy discontinuation Impact of tube selection on resistance during tube occlusion, *Respir Care* 38(3): 267-270, 1993.
8. Bellomo R, Tai E, Parkin G: Fibreoptic bronchoscopy in the critically ill A prospective of its diagnostic and therapeutic value, *Anaesth Intensive Care* 20(4): 464-469, 1992.
9. Benumof JL: Management of the difficult adult airway. With special emphasis on awake tracheal intubation, *Anesthesiology* 75(6): 1087-1110, 1991.
10. Berlaud JF: Prolonged endotracheal intubation vs tracheostomy, *Crit Care Med* 14(8): 742-745, 1986.
11. Birdstal C: What suction pressures should I use? *Am J Nurs* 866, 1985.
12. Bishop MJ: Mechanisms of laryngotracheal injury following prolonged tracheal intubation, *Chest* 96(1): 185-186, 1989.
13. Bolder PM, et al: The extra work of breathing through adult endotracheal tubes, *Anesth Analg* 65(8): 853-9, 1986.
14. Boutros AR: Arterial blood oxygenation during and after endotracheal suctioning in the apneic patient, *Anesthesiology* 32(2): 114-118, 1970.
15. Brown B, Peeples D: The effects of hyperinflation and lidocaine intracranial pressure response to endotracheal suctioning, *Heart Lung* 21(3): 286, 1992.
16. Bugge-Asperheim B, Birkeland S, Storen G: Tracheo-oesophageal fistula caused by cuffed tracheal tubes, *Scand J Thor Cardiovasc Surg* 15: 315-319, 1981.
17. Campbell RS, Branson RD: How ventilators provide tempo-rary O_2 enrichment: What happens when you press the 100% suction button, *Respir Care* 37(8): 933-937, 1992.
18. Carroll PF: Artificial airways equals real risks, *Nursing* 16(8): 56-59, 1986.
19. Cavalrere S, Foccoli P, Farina PL: Nd YAG laser bronchoscopy. A five year experience with 1, 396 applications in 1,000 patients, *Chest* 94(1): 15-21, 1988.
20. Chulay M: Arterial blood gas changes with a hyperinflation and hyperoxygenation suctioning intervention in critically ill patients, *Heart Lung* 17(6): 654-61, 1988.
21. Chulay M, Graeber GM: Efficacy of a hyperinflation and hyperoxygenation suctioning intervention, *Heart Lung* 17(1): 15-22, 1988.
22. Clark AP, et al: Effects of endotracheal suctioning on mixed venous oxygen saturation and heart rate in critically ill adults, *Heart Lung* 19(5): 552-557, 1990.
23. Cobley M. Atkins M, Jones PL: Environmental contamination during tracheal suction. A comparison of disposable conventional catheters with a multiple-use closed system device, *Anesthesia* 46(1): 957-961, 1991.
24. Cohen IL, et al: Endotracheal tube occlusion associated with the use of heat and moisture exchanges in the intensive care unit, *Crit Care Med* 16(3): 277-9, 1988.
25. Colice GL: Technical standards for tracheal tubes, *Clin Chest Med* 12(3): 433-448, Sept 1991.
26. Conrardy PA, et al: Alteration of endotracheal tube position flexion and extension of the neck, *Crit Care Med* 4(2): 8-12, 1976.
27. Coppolo DP, et al: A role for the respiratory therapist in flexible fiberoptic bronchoscopy, *Respir Care* 30(5): 323-327, 1985.
28. Craig KC, Benson MS, Pierson DJ: Prevention of arterial oxygen desaturation during closed-airway endotracheal suction effect of ventilator mode, *Respir Care* 29(10): 1013-1018, 1984.
29. Craven DE, Steiger KA: Nosocomial pneumonia in the intubated patient. New concepts on pathogenesis and prevention, *Infect Dis Clin North Am* 3(4): 843-66, 1989.
30. Day SL, Wooton L, MacIntrye N: Rapid analysis of exhaled CO_2 to assess endotracheal tube placement, *Respir Care* 37(10): 1161-1165, 1992.
31. Darvich-Kodjouri C: Care of the patient with a new tracheostomy, *Am Rev Respir Care* 10(6): 42-48, 1987.
32. Dellinger RP: Fiberoptic bronchoscopy in adult airway management, *Crit Care Med* 18(8): 882-7, 1990.
33. Dellinger RP, Bandi V: Fiberoptic bronchoscopy in the intensive care unit, *Crit Care Clinic* 8(4): 755-72, 1992.
34. Demers B: The impact of technology on the risks associated with endotracheal suctioning and airway management. The changes a decade has wrought, *Respir Care* 34(5): 339-341, 1989.
35. Deppe SA, et al: Incidence of colonization, nosocomial pneumonia, and mortality in critically ill patients using a trach care closed-suction system vs an open-suction system prospective, randomized study, *Crit Care Med* 18(12): 1389-1393, 1990.
36. Dierkesman R: Indication and results of endobronchial laser therapy, *Lung* 168 Suppl 1095-1102, 1990.
37. Djukanovic R, et al: The safety aspects of fiberoptic bronchoscopy, bronchoalveolar lavage, and endobronchial biopsy in asthma, *Am Rev Respir Dis* 143(4pt 1): 772-7, 1991.
38. El-Naggar M, et al: Factors influencing choice between tracheostomy and prolonged translaryngeal intubation in acute respiratory failure a prospective study, *Anesth Analg* 55:195-201, 1976.
39. Elpern EH, Jacobs ER, Bone RC: Incidence of aspiration in tracheally intubated adults, *Heart Lung* 16(5): 527-531, 1987.
40. Finucane BT, Santora AH: *Principles of airway management,* FA Davis, Philadelphia 1988
41. Foster WM, Hurewitz AN: Aerosolized lidocaine reduces dose of topical anesthetic for bronchoscopy, *An Rev Respir Dis* 164(2): 520-2, 1992.

42. Fulginiti J, et al: Retrieval of an aspirated bullet fragment by flexible bronchoscopy in a mechanically ventilated patient, *Chest* 103(2):626–627, 1993.

43. Gallagher TJ: Endotracheal intubation, *Crit Care Clin* 8(4): 665–676, 1992.

44. Godwin JE and Heffner JE: Special critical care considerations in tracheostomy management, *Clin Chest Med* 12(3): 573–583, 1991.

45. Goodman LR, et al: Radiographic evaluation of endotracheal tube position, *Am J Roetgenol* 127(3): 433–434, 1976.

46. Goodnough SK: The effects of oxygen and hyperinflation on arterial oxygen tension after endotracheal suctioning, *Heart Lung* 14(1): 11–17, 1985.

47. Graham DR, et al: Comparison of three different methods used to achieve local anesthesia for fiberoptic bronchoscopy, *Chest* 102(3): 704–7, 1992.

48. Gray JE, MacIntyre NR, Kronenberger WG: The effects of bolus normal-saline instillation in conjunction with endotracheal suctioning, *Respir Care* 35(8): 785–790, 1990.

49. Guyton D, Banner MJ, Kirby RR: High-volume, low pressure cuffs. Are they always low pressure? *Chest* 100(4): 1076–1081, 1991.

50. Habib MP: Physiologic implications of artificial airways, *Chest* 96(1): 180–184, 1989.

51. Haenel JB, et al: Efficacy of selective intrabronchial air insufflation in acute lobar atelectasis, *Am J Surg* 164(5): 501–5, 1992.

52. Hand RW, et al: Inadvertent transbronchial insertion of narrow bone feeding tubes in the pleural space, *JAMA* 251(18): 2396–2397, 1984.

53. Harada RN, Repine JE: Pulmonary host defense mechanism, *Chest* 87(2): 247–252, 1985.

54. Harshbarger SA, Hoffman LA, Trillo TG, Pensky MR: Effects of a closed tracheal suction system on ventilatory and cardiovascular parameters, *Am J Crit Care* 1(3): 57–61, 1992.

55. Hart TP, Manhutte CK: Evaluation of a closed-system directional tip suction catheter, *Respir Care* 37(11): 1260–5, 1992.

56. Heffner JE: Airway management in the critically ill patient, *Crit Care Clin* 6(3): 533–550, 1990.

57. Heffner JE: Timing of tracheotomy in ventilator-dependent patients, *Clin in Chest Med* 12(3): 611–625, 1991.

58. Heffner JE, Miller S, Sahn SA: Tracheostomy in the intensive care unit: part 2: Complications, *Chest* 90(3): 430–436, 1986.

59. Herranz MF: Individualized fenestration of tracheostomy tubes, *Respir Care* 29(12): 1246, 1984.

60. Issac PA, et al: A jet nebulizer for delivery of topical anesthesia to the respiratory tract. A comparison with cricothyroid puncture and direct spraying for fiberoptic bronchoscopy, *Anaesthesia* 45(1): 46–8, 1990.

61. Isea JO, et al: Controlled trial of a continuous irrigation suction catheter vs conventional intermittent suction catheter in clearing bronchial secretion from ventilated patients, *Chest* 103(4): 1227–1230, 1993.

62. Johnson JD, Love JD: Lights out; a preventable complication of endotracheal intubation, *Chest* 87(5): 701–702, 1985.

63. Johnson NT, Pierson DJ: Pulmonary diagnostic procedures, in, *Foundations of respiratory care,* DJ Pierson and Kacmarek RM editors, Churchill-Livingstone New York 1992.

64. Jolliet P, Chevrolet JC: Bronchoscopy in the intensive care unit, *Intensive Care Med* 18(3): 160–9, 1992.

65. Kacmarek RM: The role of the respiratory therapist in emergency care, *Respir Care* 37(6): 523–32, 1992.

66. Kamholz SL, Rothman NI, Underwood PS: Fiberbronchoscopic retrieval of iatrogenically introduced endobronchial foreign body, *Crit Care Med* 7(8): 346–348, 1979.

67. Kaplan JD, Schuster DP: Physiologic consequences of tracheal intubation, *Clinics Chest Med* 12(3): 425–432, 1991.

68. Kastamos N, et al: Laryngotracheal injury due to endotracheal intubation incidence, evolution, and predisposing factors. A prospective long-term study, *Crit Care Med* 11(5): 362–367, 1983.

69. Keane D, McNicholas WT: Comparison of nebulized and sprayed topical anaesthesia for fibreoptic bronchoscopy, *Eur Respir J* 5(9): 1123–5, 1992.

70. Kovac AL: Upper airway trauma and obstruction. A review of causes, evaluation and management, *Respir Care* 38(4): 351–361, 1993.

71. Kurtz CP, Sakurai H, Yoo OH: Successful retrieval of fractured tracheostomy cannula by flexible fiberoptic bronchoscopy, *Mt Sinai J Med* 57(6): 371–3, 1990.

72. Lan RS, et al: Use of fiberoptic bronchoscopy to retrieve bronchial foreign bodies in adults, *Am Rev Respir Dis* 140(6): 1734–7, 1989.

73. Lang DM, et al: Safety and possible efficacy of fiberoptic bronchoscopy with lavage in the management of refractory asthma with mucous impaction, *Ann Allergy* 67(3): 324–30, 1991.

74. Lechman MJ, Donahoo JS, Macvaugh H: Endotracheal intubation using percutaneous retrograde guidewire insertion followed by antegrade fiberoptic bronchoscopy, *Crit Care Med* 14(6): 589–590, 1986.

75. Lefrock JL, et al: Transient bacteremia associated with nasotracheal suctioning, *JAMA* 236(14): 1610–1612, 1976.

76. Levine SA, Neederman MS: The impact of tracheal intubation on host defenses and risks for nosocomial pneumonia, *Clin Chest Med* 12(3): 523–543, 1991.

77. Lewis RJ: Tracheostomies: indications, timing, and complication, *Clin Chest Med* 13(1): 137–149, 1992.

78. Lookinland S, Appel PL: Hemodynamic and oxygen transport changes following endotracheal suctioning in trauma patients, *Nurs Res* 40(3): 133–139, 1991.

79. Mahul P, et al: Prevention of nosocomial pneumonia in intubated patients respective role of mechanical subglottic secretion drainage and stress ulcer prophylaxis, *Intensive Care Med* 18(1): 20–5, 1992.

80. Matthews PJ, Matthews LM, Mitchell RR: Airway monitoring and ventilation what the future holds, *Nursing* 22(2): 48–51, 92.

81. McCullough P: Wire basket removal of a large endobronchial foreign body, *Chest* 87(2): 270–271, 1985.

82. Mcculloch TM, Bishop MJ: Complications of translaryngeal intubation, *Clin Chest Med* 12(3): 507–521, 1991.

83. McPhearson SP, Spearman CB: *Respiratory therapy equipment,* ed 4, Mosby, St. Louis 1990.

84. Middleton RM, Shah A, Kirkpatrick MB: Topical nasal anesthesia for flexible bronchoscopy. A comparison of methods in normal subjects and in patients undergoing transnasal bronchoscopy, *Chest* 99(5): 1093–6, 1991.

85. Milam MG, Evins AE, Sahn SA: Immediate chest roentgenography following fiberoptic bronchoscopy, *Chest* 96(3): 477–479, 1989.

86. Mohsenefor Z, Jasper AC, Koerner SK: Physiologic assessment of lung function in patients undergoing laser photoresection of tracheobronchial tumors, *Chest* 93(1): 65–69, 1988.

87. Myers EN, Carrau RL: Early complicators of tracheostomy incidence and management, *Clin Chest Med* 12(3): 589–595, 1991.

88. Nakao MA, Killan D, Wilson R: Pneumothorax secondary to inadvertent placement of a nasoenteric tube past a cuffed endotracheal tube, *Crit Care Med* 11(3): 210–211, 1983.

89. Neff TA, Clifford D: A new monitoring toll-the ratio of the tracheostomy tube cuff diameter to the tracheal air column (C/T ratio), *Respir Care* 28(10): 1287–1290, 1983.

90. Netter FH: The Ciba collection of medical illustrations, vol 7 Respiratory system, *CIBA,* Summit New Jersey 1979

91. Nielsen, LH, et al: Fiberoptic bronchoscopic evaluation of tracheal tube position, *Eur J Anaesthesiol* 8(4): 277–9, 1991.

92. Noll ML, Hix CD, Scott G: Closed tracheal suction systems effectiveness and nursing implications, *AACN Clin Iss Crit Care Nurs* 1(2): 318–326, 1990.

93. Off D, et al: Efficacy of the minimal leak technique of cuff inflation in maintaining proper intracuff pressures for patients with cuffed artificial airways, *Respir Care* 28(9):1115–1120, 1983.

94. O'Flaherty D, Adams AP: The end-tidal carbon dioxide detector. Assessment of a new method to distinguish oesophageal from tracheal intubation, *Anaesthesia* 45(8): 653–5, 1990.

95. Olopade Co, Prakash UB: Bronchoscopy in the critical-care unit, *Mayo Clin Proc* 64(10): 1255–63, 1989.

96. Orrato JP, et al: Multicenter study of a portable hand-size, colorimetric end-tidal carbon dioxide detection device, *Ann Emerg Med* 21(5): 518–523, 1992.

97. Owen RL, Cheney FW: Use of an apnea monitor to verify endotracheal intubation, *Respir Care* 30(1): 974–976, 1985.

98. Panacek EA, et al: Selective left endobronchial suctioning in the intubated patient, *Chest* 95(4): 885–7, 1989.

99. Peacock AJ, Benson-Mitchell R, Godfrey R: Affects of fibreoptic bronchoscopy on pulmonary function, *Thorax* 45(1): 38–41, 1990.

100. Plummer AL, Gracey DR: Consensus conference on artificial airways in patients receiving mechanical ventilation, *Chest* 96(1): 178–180, 1989.

101. Randell T, et al: Topical anaesthesia of the nasal mucosa for fibreoptic airway endoscopy, *Br J Anaesth* 68(2): 164–167, 1992.

102. Reed AP: Preparation of the patient for awake flexible fiberoptic bronchoscopy, *Chest* 101(1): 244–253, 1992.

103. Richard RR, McCall J, Burford JG: Air movement around an endotracheal tube cuff, *Respir Care* 28(8): 1039–1040, 1983.

104. Roach JM, Ripple G, Dillard TA: Inadvertent loss of bronchoscopy instruments in the tracheobronchial tree, *Chest* 101(2): 568–569, 1992.

105. Rodriguez-Roldan JM, et al: Prevention of nosocomial lung infection in ventilated patients use of an antimicrobial pharyngeal non- absorbable paste, *Crit Care Med* 18(11): 1239–1242, 1990.

106. Rudy EB, et al: The relationship between endotracheal suctioning and changes in intra-cranial pressure: A review of the literature, *Heart Lung* 15(5): 488–494, 1986.

107. Shapiro B, et al: *Clinical applications of respiratory care,* ed 4 Mosby, St. Louis, 1991.

108. Shapiro M: Work of breathing through different sized endotracheal tubes, *Crit Care Med* 14(12): 1028–1031, 1986.

109. Shea JM, et al: Survival of patients undergoing Nd YAG laser therapy compared with Nd YAG laser therapy and brachytherapy for malignant airway disease, *Chest* 103(4): 1028–1031, 1993.

110. Shehleton ME, Nield M: Ineffective airway clearance related to artificial airways, *Nurs Clin North Am* 22(1): 167–178, 1987.

111. Siddharth P, Mazzarella L: Granuloma associated with fenestrated tracheostomy tubes, *Am J Surgery* 150 279–280, 1985.

112. Sills J: An emergency cuff inflation technique, *Respir Care* 31(3): 199–201, 1986.

113. Smith RM, Benson MS and Schoene RB: Efficacy of oxygen insufflation in preventing arterial oxygen desaturation during endotracheal suctioning of mechanically ventilated patient, *Respir Care* 32(10): 865–869, 1987.

114. Sottile FD, et al: Nosocomial pulmonary infection possible etiologic significance of bacterial adhesion to endotracheal tubes, *Crit Care Med* 14(4): 265–270, 1986.

115. Stark P: Inadvertent nasogastric tube insertion into the tracheo-bronchial tree, *Radiology* 142(1): 239–240, 1982.

116. Stauffer JL: Medical management of the airway, *Clin Chest Med* vol 12(3): 449–482, 1991.

117. Stauffer JL, Olson DE, Petty TL: Complications and consequences of endotracheal intubation and tracheotomy. A prospective study of 150 critically ill adults, *Am J Med* 701(1): 65–76, 1981.

118. Stauffer JL, Silvestri RC: Complications of endotracheal intubation, tracheostomy, and artificial airways, *Respir Care* 27(4): 417–434, 1982.

119. Stone KS: Ventilator versus manual resuscitation bag as the method for delivery hyperoxygenation before endotracheal suctioning, *AACN Clin Iss Crit Care Nurs* 1(2): 289–299, 1990.

120. Stone KS, Bell SD, Preusser BA: The effect of repeated endotracheal suctioning on arterial blood pressure, *Appl Nurs Res* 4(4): 152–158, 1991.

121. Stone KS, Preusser BA, Groch KF, Karl JI, Gonyon DS: The effect of lung hyperinflation and endotracheal suctioning on cardiopulmonary hemodynamics, *Nurs Res* 40(2): 76–80, 1991.

122. Streitz JM, Shaphay SM: Airway injury after tracheostomy and endotracheal intubation, *Surg Clin North Am* 71(6): 1211–1230, 1991.

123. Synder GM: Individualized placement of tracheostomy tube fenestration and in-situ examinations with the fiberoptic laryngoscope, *Respir Care* 28(10): 1294–1298, 1983.

124. Taft AA, Meshoe SC, Denisan FA, Lain DC, Chaudhay BA: A comparison of two methods of preoxygenation during endotracheal suctioning, *Respir Care* 36(11): 1195–1201, 1991.

125. Tasota FJ, et al: Evaluation of two methods used to stabilize oral endotracheal tubes, *Heart Lung* 16(2): 140–146, 1987.

126. Teale C, et al: Local anaesthesia for fibreoptic bronchoscopy comparison between intratracheal cocaine and lidnocaine, *Respir Med* 84(5): 407–408, 1990.

127. Thalman JJ, Rinaldo-Gallo S, MacIntyre, NR: Analysis of an endotracheal intubation service provided by respiratory care practitioners, *Respir Care* 38(5): 469–473, 1993.

128. Tiffin NH, Keim MR, Trewen TC: The effects of variations in flow through an insufflating catheter and endotracheal tube and suction catheter size on test lung pressures, *Respir Care* 35(9): 889–897, 90.

129. Treanor S, Benitez WD, Raffin TA: Respiratory therapists as fiberoptic bronchoscopy assistants, *Respir Care* 30(5): 321–322, 1985.

130. Treloar DM, Stechmiller J: Pulmonary aspiration in tube-fed patients with artificial airways, *Heart Lung* 13(6): 667–671, 1984.

131. Tsao TC, et al: Treatment for collapsed lung in critically ill patients. Selective intrabronchial air insufflation using the fiberoptic bronchoscope, *Chest* 97(2): 435–438, 1990.

132. Turnbull AD, Carlon G: Airway management in the thrombocytopenic cancer patient with acute respiratory failure, *Crit Care Med* 7(2): 76–77, 1979.

133. Varon AJ, Morrina J, Civetta JM: Clinical utility of colometric end-tidal CO_2 detector in cardiopulmonary resuscitation and emergency intubation, *J Clin Monit* 7(4): 289–293, 1991.

134. Venus B: Five year experience with Kistner tracheostomy tube, *Crit Care Med* 8(2): 106–110, 1980.

135. Via-Reque E, Rottenborg C: Prolonged oro-or nasotracheal intubation, *Crit Care Med* 9(9): 637–639, 1981.

136. Walsh JM, Vandewarf C, Hoschert D, Fahey PJ: Unsuspected hemodynamic alterations during endotracheal suctioning, *Chest* 95(1): 162–165, 1989.

137. Watson CB: Tracheal intubation in the emergency setting, *Respir Ther* 16(4): 20–2, 24–5, 50, 1986.

138. Weber AL, Grillo HC: Tracheal stenosis an analysis of 151 cases, *Radiol Clin North Am* 16(2): 291–308, 1978.

139. Wenig BL, Applebaun EL: Indications for and techniques of tracheostomy, *Clin Chest Med* vol 12(3): 545–553, 1991.

140. Whited RE: A prospective study of laryngotracheal sequelae in long-term intubation, *Laryngoscope* 94(3): 317–377, 1984.

141. Wilson, Roger S: Upper airway problems, *Respir Care* 37(6): 533–550, 1992.

142. Wissing DR, Romero MR, Payne K: An unusual complication of prolonged intubation, *Respir Care* 32(5): 359–360, 1987.

143. Wood DE, Mathesen DJ: Late complications of tracheostomy, *Clin Chest Med* 12(3): 597–609, 1991.

Emergency Life Support

■

Craig L. Scanlan

William Goerlich

CHAPTER LEARNING OBJECTIVES

1. Identify the major categories of sudden death, including specific causes of respiratory and cardiac arrest;
2. Differentiate between the goals, methods, procedures and personnel resources of basic and advanced cardiac life support;
3. Describe the procedures used to determine unresponsiveness, breathlessness, and pulselessness in a victim suspected to have suffered respiratory and/or cardiac arrest;
4. Outline the basic life support procedures used to restore the airway and provide ventilatory and circulatory support to adults, children, and infants;
5. Describe the procedures used to evaluate the effectiveness of basic life support measures;
6. Distinguish between the single and double rescuer protocols used in basic life support;
7. Identify, apply and troubleshoot the key adjunct equipment used in advanced cardiac life support to maintain and restore ventilation and oxygenation;
8. Differentiate among the common cardiac arrhythmias and their clinical significance;
9. Describe the appropriate use of drug and electrical therapies in advanced cardiac life support;
10. Identify the role of the respiratory care practitioner in postresuscitative patient care;
11. Describe the common complications, hazards, and pitfalls associated with basic and advanced cardiac life support equipment and procedures.

Emergency life support involves a variety of methods and procedures designed to deal with sudden, life-threatening events caused by cardiac or respiratory failure. Respiratory care practitioners (RCPs) play a vital role in emergency life support.[1] In the hospital setting, RCPs normally serve as key members of the resuscitation team. In addition to managing the airway, practitioners often participate in circulatory support, drug and electrical therapy, and postresuscitative care.

In the community, RCPs frequently serve as certified cardiopulmonary resuscitation instructors, extending their knowledge to lay personnel through organizations such as the American Heart Association or Red Cross.

Both roles require mastery of an extensive knowledge base and the development of an array of sometimes difficult manual skills. Although no substitute for supervised practice under simulated conditions, this chapter provides the foundation knowledge needed to apply both basic and advanced life support techniques in a variety of settings, and with various patient groups. The practitioner is encouraged to obtain further competencies by completion of formal courses in cardiopulmonary resuscitation (CPR), Advanced Cardiac Life Support, Pediatric Advanced Life Support, and Neonatal Resuscitation.

CAUSES AND PREVENTION OF SUDDEN DEATH

Sudden death is a common event both inside and outside the hospital. Among adults, coronary heart disease is the primary cause of sudden death, accounting for some 500,000 fatalities annually.[2]

Accidents are the leading cause of sudden death among persons aged 1 to 37 in the United States and the 4th leading cause of death overall.[3] Trauma due to motor vehicle accidents, drowning, electrocution, burns, suffocation, and drug intoxication are the major factors involved in accidental death among adults.[4]

Among children, accidents are the leading cause of sudden death, causing about 44% of the fatalities in the 1 to 14 year old age group.[5] A particularly serious cause of sudden death in children is obstruction of the airway by foreign bodies.[6,7] Foreign body obstruction accounts for over 3,000 deaths annually, most of which occur in children under 5 years of age.[3]

Among newborn infants, nearly 6% require special

life support in the delivery room. This figure rises to over 80% for infants with birth weights less than 1500 grams.[4]

Although not all these deaths are preventable, early use of life support methods can reduce this alarming toll of sudden death. Provision of CPR by bystanders can at least double the survival rate of victims of cardiac or respiratory arrest.[8] Moreover, early intervention can decrease the subsequent likelihood of neurologic impairment by as much as 10 fold.[8] Comprehensive implementation of emergency life support on a community-wide basis throughout the nation could save between 100,000 and 200,000 lives per year.[4,9-11]

Emergency life support involves a variety of methods and procedures designed to deal with sudden, life-threatening events caused by cardiac or respiratory failure.[10-14] Emergency life support traditionally consists of two related phases: *Basic Life Support* or BLS, and *Advanced Cardiac Life Support or ACLS.*[4]

Basic life support aims either to: (1) prevent cardiac or respiratory arrest through prompt identification and intervention, or (2) support failed circulation and respiration via cardiopulmonary resuscitation (CPR).[4] Basic life support should be started by any person present at the time the incident occurs. Trained individuals should begin CPR as soon as possible and the local emergency medical system must be activated immediately.[4]

Advanced cardiac *life support* includes the essential elements of BLS, but provides additional measures not used by lay personnel. These measures include supporting oxygenation and ventilation with adjunct equipment, starting an **IV** route, administering drugs, monitoring cardiac function, controlling arrhythmias and providing postresuscitative care.[4] While BLS can be initiated and conducted by lay personnel, ACLS requires physician supervision, either in person or by way of telecommunication.

DETERMINING THE NEED FOR EMERGENCY LIFE SUPPORT

The primary indications for emergency life support are respiratory and cardiac arrest. The most common causes of respiratory arrest are drug overdose, drowning, suffocation, stroke, electrocution, smoke inhalation, acute airway obstruction by a foreign body, and airway obstruction due to unconsciousness or coma (refer to accompanying box on causes of respiratory failure).[4]

Like respiratory arrest, cardiac arrest has many potential causes. The most frequent causes of cardiac arrest are electrical disturbances or arrhythmias associated with myocardial ischemia or acute myocardial infarction.

If respiratory arrest occurs first, the heart will

normally continue to beat for a few minutes. Such patients frequently have a pulse. However, without ventilation, body stores of oxygen are rapidly used up. The resulting tissue hypoxia quickly impairs both cardiac and neural function. However, rapid recognition and treatment of respiratory arrest can prevent a secondary cardiac arrest and decrease the likelihood of permanent brain damage.

If, on the other hand, the primary event is cardiac arrest, no oxygen is circulated and tissue hypoxia occurs almost immediately. A secondary respiratory arrest quickly follows as the brainstem is deprived of its oxygen supply.

When ventilation and circulation both cease, a condition of *clinical death* exists.[12] With early treatment, clinical death is reversible. However, should tissue hypoxia be prolonged, irreversible cell damage occurs, resulting in *biological death.*

Exactly how much time can elapse before clinical death becomes biological death is unknown. Generally, biological death occurs four to six minutes after ventilation and circulation cease. However, many factors may extend this time period, including hypothermia and certain drugs. In fact, some organs can sustain periods of anoxia of 15 minutes or more. The primary exception is the brain. Although other organs may be successfully resuscitated after prolonged periods of anoxia, brain death may occur much more rapidly, resulting in irreversible loss of cerebral function.

Thus, the goal of emergency life support is to reverse clinical death by restoring ventilation and circulation before brain death can occur. Emergency life support should be initiated whenever the signs of clinical death are recognized and continue until the patient is declared dead by a physician. Since firm evidence regarding brain death is seldom available during resuscitation, the decision to stop emergency life support is as much a moral and ethical judgement as a clinical one.

BASIC LIFE SUPPORT

Basic life support aims to restore ventilation and circulation to victims of airway obstruction, and respiratory and cardiac arrest, all without using equipment.[4,15,16] These skills can be used by a single practitioner to restore ventilation and circulation until the victim is revived or until ACLS equipment and personnel are available.

In sequence, the steps in BLS are: (1) initial assessment to determine unresponsiveness, (2) activation of the emergency medical system, (3) airway restoration, (4) ventilation, and (5) restoration of circulation. The last three steps are the traditional 'ABCs' of resuscitation: (A)irway, (B)reathing, and (C)irculation.

Each of the ABCs start with an assessment phase.[4] The first phase determines unresponsiveness, the second determines breathlessness, and the third pulse-lessness.

Determining unresponsiveness

Basic life support begins when an otherwise conscious victim is found in an unresponsive or collapsed state. Since many hospitalized patients exhibit decreased levels of consciousness, practitioners can avoid needless intervention by being fully aware of their patient's mental status (see Chapter 16).

When coming upon a collapsed victim outside the hospital setting who appears unconscious, you should first look for any obvious head or neck injuries. If such injuries are apparent, great care should be taken in subsequent manipulation of the neck and in any effort to move the individual.[4,14]

Whatever the location, you quickly assess the individual's level of consciousness by tapping or gently shaking the shoulder and shouting "Are you OK?." If this fails to stir the victim, the practitioner should call for help and activate the emergency medical system.[4]

Getting help and activating the emergency medical system

Once you confirm that the victim is unresponsive, you must immediately call for help and activate the emergency medical system. Outside the hospital, this may mean having someone call 911 or the local EMS service. Within the hospital, specific protocols exist for 'calling a code.' All RCPs must be familiar with their institution's protocols for handling these emergency situations.

Restoring the airway

After calling for help and activating the emergency medical system, you must try to securing an open airway. First, you should quickly inspect the victim to see if there is any neck or facial trauma. If spinal cord trauma is suspected, you must carefully position the neck in a neutral in-line position and modify procedures requiring hyperextension.[4] Also, when victims are found lying on their side or stomach, you will have to move them to a supine position before beginning airway procedures. To do so, use the 'log-roll' technique (rolling the patient as a unit so that the head, shoulders and body move simultaneously without twisting, Figure 23-1).[4] Last, you should try to ensure that the victim is positioned on a hard flat surface.

The most common cause of airway obstruction is loss of muscle tone, which causes the tongue to fall back into the pharynx, thereby blocking air flow.[4,17-19] Movement of the lower jaw and extension of the neck pulls the tongue from the posterior pharyngeal wall and opens the airway. One of two procedures is used. The head-tilt/chin-lift method is the primary procedure recommended for the lay public when spinal

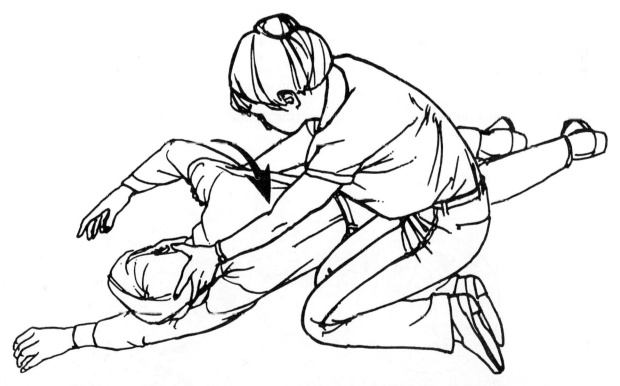

Fig. 23-1 Log-roll technique to move prone-lying victim to supine position needed for basic life support.
(From: Guidelines for cardiopulmonary resuscitation and emergency cardiac care, *JAMA* 268: 2171-2302, 1992.)

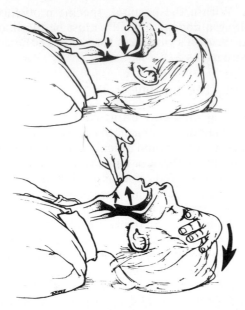

Fig. 23-2 Opening the airway. *Top:* Airway obstruction produced by tongue and epiglottis. *Bottom:* Relief by head tilt-chin lift. (From American Heart Association: Standards for cardiopulmonary resuscitation and emergency cardiac care, *JAMA* (suppl) 255:2843-2989, 1986. Copyright 1986, American Medical Association.)

trauma is not suspected.[4,20] A second method is the jaw thrust, used mainly by trained clinicians.[20,21] One of these maneuvers will usually open the airway.

Head-tilt/chin-lift

For most situations, the head-tilt/chin-lift is the easiest and most effective procedure to open the airway. This method allows dentures to remain in place, thereby making mouth-to-mouth ventilation easier.[20] The head-tilt/chin-lift technique is also the least fatiguing method to maintain an open airway. The procedure is as follows (Figure 23-2):

1. Position the victim on his back.
2. Place one hand on the victim's forehead and apply a firm pressure with the palm to tilt the head backward. Place the fingers of the other hand under the bony part of the patient's lower jaw near the chin and brings the mandible forward. Be sure to avoid pressure on the soft tissues of the chin since this might obstruct the airway.

Jaw thrust maneuver

The jaw thrust is also called the mandible thrust or triple airway maneuver. The jaw thrust is effective, but is more fatiguing and technically more difficult than the head tilt/chin lift method.[21]

The jaw thrust should be used when spinal cord trauma is suspected. When using the jaw thrust, you can support the neck and keep the airway open with minimal movement, thus preventing further spinal cord damage.[4] However, the position required for the jaw thrust makes single rescuer mouth-to-mouth ventilation and external cardiac compression difficult. Thus, the jaw thrust is used only when two or more trained rescuers are present. The procedure is as follows (Figure 23-3):

1. Place the victim on his or her back as previously described, and kneel at the victim's head.
2. Place the finger tips behind the angles of the lower jaw in front of the earlobes and displace the mandible forward and upward while at the same time tilting the head backward without extending the neck. Be careful not to compress the area below the angle of the mandible, as this is where the carotid is located. Carotid pressure may cause bradycardia.

One of these airway procedures may be the only life-saving measure required. Once the airway is cleared and opened, you should immediately assess the victim's ventilation.

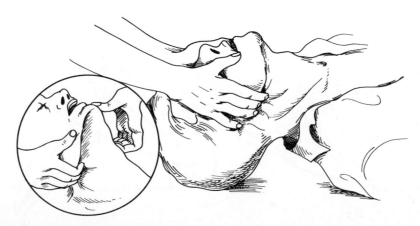

Fig. 23-3 Jaw-thrust maneuver. (From Ellis PD, Billings DM: Cardiopulmonary resuscitation: procedures for basic and advanced life support, St Louis, 1980, Mosby.)

Restoring ventilation

Determining breathlessness

Before you attempt to provide artificial ventilation, you should assess for the presence of breathing. To determine breathlessness, place your ear over the victim's airway while simultaneously observing for spontaneous chest movement (Figure 23-4). Breathlessness exists if you see no chest movement and hear or feel no breath sounds.[4,16] This should take no longer than 3 to 5 seconds.

Providing artificial ventilation

During respiratory arrest, you must provide oxygen within 4 to 6 minutes, or biological death will follow. You can restore the oxygen supply by exhaling into the victim's mouth, nose, or tracheal stoma. These procedures can be used for any victim, with appropriate modification for the patient's size, age, and respiratory rate.

Mouth-to-mouth ventilation. You can restore oxygenation through mouth-to-mouth ventilation by inflating the victim's lungs with exhaled air. To do so, you double your tidal volume by taking deep breaths and exhale directly into the victim's mouth. Exhaled air provides about 18% oxygen and 2% carbon dioxide, sufficient to achieve an arterial oxygen tension (PaO_2) of between 50 to 60 torr.[16]

You confirm adequate ventilation by noting a rise and fall of the chest wall and by hearing and feeling air escape during passive exhalation. A tidal volume of between 800 and 1200 mL is required for most adults. Children require proportionally smaller volumes. In these victims, a volume sufficient to cause a rise and fall of the chest wall should be used.

You should initially give two slow deep breaths, 1.5 to 2 seconds each. You must avoid excessive volumes or too fast an inspiratory rate, since this can push air into the stomach and cause gastric distention. An amount sufficient to cause a rise and fall of the chest should be used to gauge the volume needed in both children and adults.

The procedure for adults is as follows (Figure 23-5):
1. Place the victim on his or her back on a hard flat surface. Use the log roll technique.
2. Kneel at the patient's side and open and clear the airway as previously described. Pinch the victim's nose with the thumb and index finger close to the nares to prevent air escape during ventilation.
3. Take a deep breath and, while making a seal over the victim's mouth, exhales slowly but forcibly for 1 to 1.5 seconds for each breath.[22] A good seal over the patients mouth is essential. If you cannot get a good seal using this method, you should attempt mouth-to-nose ventilation.
4. Remove your mouth and allow the victim to exhale passively. Provide a second breath after this deflation pause.[22]
5. After successfully delivering two slow breaths, you should immediately assess the circulatory status.

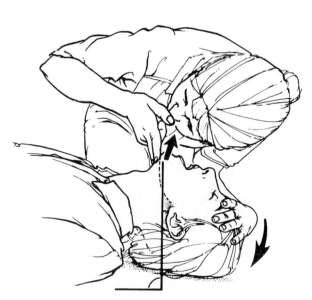

Fig. 23-4 Determining breathlessness. (From American Heart Association: Standards for cardiopulmonary resuscitation and emergency cardiac care, *JAMA* (suppl) 255:2843-2989, 1986. Copyright 1986, American Medical Association.)

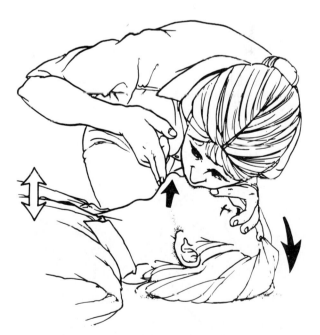

Fig. 23-5 Adult mouth-to-mouth ventilation. (From American Heart Association: Standards for cardiopulmonary resuscitation and emergency cardiac care, *JAMA* (suppl) 255:2843-2989, 1986. Copyright 1986, American Medical Association.)

6. Should your initial attempt to ventilate fail, reposition the victim's head and repeat the effort.[4,16] If a second attempt at ventilation fails, proceed with methods described later under foreign body airway obstruction.

7. Assuming your mouth-to-mouth ventilation is successful and the patient remains apneic, continue the effort at a rate of one breath every 5 seconds to maintain the minimum adult rate of 12/min.[4,16]

Although airway maneuvers for children and infants are similar for those in adults, there are several key differences. Anatomic differences in the infant's airway make it especially susceptible to occlusion by the tongue.[23-27] You should thus only slightly extend the infant's head or tilt it back gently into a neutral position when using the head-tilt-chin lift maneuver. You must also avoid closing the mouth or pushing on the soft tissues under the chin, since these can cause obstruction of the airway.

The procedure for children and infants is as follows (Figures 23-6 and 23-7):

1. If the patient is an infant (under age 1) create an air tight seal by placing your mouth over the infant's nose and mouth (Figure 23-6).[23-27]

2. Ventilate a child between 1 and 8 years old using the same technique as with adults (Figure 23-7).[27-30]

3. Provide an initial slow breath (1 to 1.5 seconds per breath) sufficient to cause a rise in the chest.

In infants, small puffs of air from the cheeks are usually sufficient to achieve this end.[23-27]

4. Remove your mouth and allow the victim to exhale passively. Provide a second breath after this deflation pause.

5. After successfully delivering two slow breaths, you should immediately assess the circulatory status.

6. Should you initial attempt to ventilate fail, reposition the victim's head and repeat the effort. You may need to move a child's head through a wide range of positions to secure an open airway. Remember that hyperextension of a child's neck can actually cause obstruction and should be avoided. If a second attempt at ventilation fails, proceed with methods described later under foreign body airway obstruction.

7. Assuming your mouth-to-mouth ventilation is successful and the patient remains apneic, continue to provide one breath every 3 seconds (20/min).[4,16,24,30]

Mouth-to-nose ventilation. There are situations in which mouth-to-mouth ventilation cannot be performed. These include **trismus** (involuntary contraction of the jaw muscles), and traumatic jaw or mouth injury. There are also times when it is difficult to maintain a tight seal with the lips using the mouth-to-mouth method. In these situations, you should use mouth-to-nose ventilation. The procedure is as follows (Figure 23-8):[17,31]

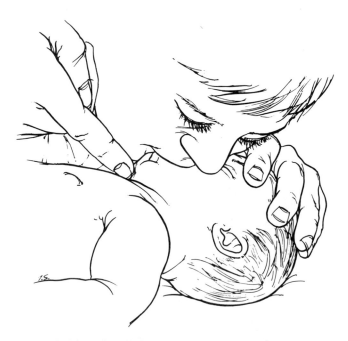

Fig. 23-6 Mouth-to-mouth and nose seal for infants. (From American Heart Association: Standards for cardiopulmonary resuscitation and emergency cardiac care, *JAMA* (suppl) 255:2843-2989, 1986. Copyright 1986, American Medical Association.)

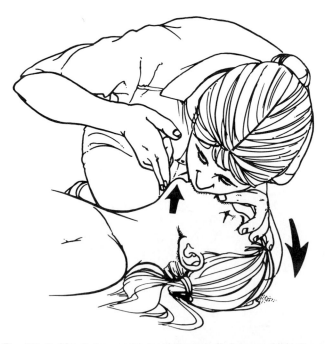

Fig. 23-7 Mouth-to-mouth ventilation applied to a child. (From American Heart Association: Standards for cardiopulmonary resuscitation and emergency cardiac care, *JAMA* (suppl) 255:2843-2989, 1986. Copyright 1986, American Medical Association.)

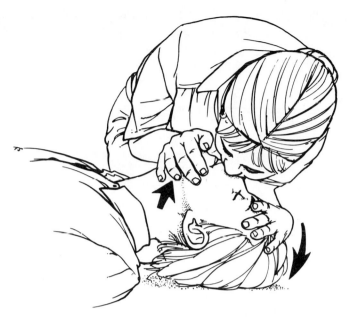

Fig. 23-8 Mouth-to-nose ventilation. (From American Heart Association: Standards for cardiopulmonary resuscitation and emergency cardiac care, *JAMA* (suppl) 255:2843-2989, 1986. Copyright 1986, American Medical Association.)

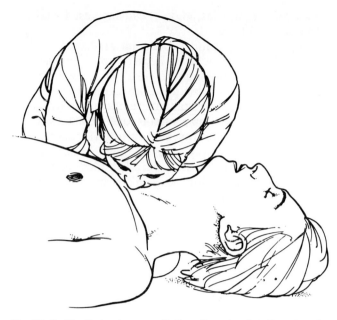

Fig. 23-9 Mouth-to-stoma ventilation. (From American Heart Association: Standards for cardiopulmonary resuscitation and emergency cardiac care, *JAMA* (suppl) 255:2843-2989, 1986. Copyright 1986, American Medical Association.)

1. Place the victim on his or her back.
2. Use the head-tilt/chin-lift maneuver to establish the airway, being sure to completely close the mouth.
3. Inhale deeply and exhale into the patient's nose. You may need to apply greater force than with mouth-to-mouth ventilation because the nasal passageways are smaller.
4. Remove your mouth from the nose to allow the patient to exhale passively. If the patient does not exhale through the nose (due to nasopharyngeal obstruction from the soft palate), open the victim's mouth or separate the lips to facilitate exhalation.
5. After successfully delivering two slow breaths, you should immediately assess the circulatory status.
6. If the victim remains apneic, maintain ventilation at the rate appropriate for his or her age.

Mouth-to-stoma ventilation. You can ventilate patients with tracheostomies or laryngectomies directly through the stoma or tube.[4,16] These patients can be identified by an obvious stoma or a **tracheostomy** or **laryngectomy** tube in place. Some patients wear a Medic Alert tag or bracelet that tells you a stoma is present. If no chest expansion occurs during mouth-to-mouth ventilation, you should look for the presence of a stoma.

The procedure for mouth-to-stoma ventilation is as follows (Figure 23-9):
1. Place the victim on his or her back with the neck in vertical alignment. You usually do not need to

extend the neck or seal the nose or mouth, since oropharyngeal structures are bypassed by the stoma.
2. Ensure that the stoma is clear of any obstructing matter and breathe directly into the stoma (or tube). If the victim has a cuffed tracheostomy tube in place, you should inflate the cuff, to prevent air escape around the tube. If the tube is uncuffed, you may need to seal off the mouth and nose with the hand or, if available, a tight fitting face mask.
3. After delivering two slow breaths, you should immediately assess the victim's circulatory status.
4. If the victim remains apneic, maintain ventilation at the rate appropriate for his or her age.

Evaluating the effectiveness of ventilation

Without accessory equipment, you can confirm adequate ventilation by observing the rise and fall of the victim's chest. You should also feel resistance as the victim's lungs expand, and hear and feel air escaping during exhalation. You should also note the victim's skin color; a return of normal color, particularly in the nailbeds and mucous membranes, indicates effective oxygenation. Also, you should carefully observe the victim every minute or so to see if spontaneous breathing returns.

Hazards and complications

The most common complications that occur with emergency ventilation are: (1) worsening existing neck or spine injuries, and (2) causing gastric distention and vomiting.

Worsening neck and spine injuries. As previously described, you can worsen neck or spine injuries by inappropriately moving the head or extending the neck. You can avoid this pitfall by carefully assessing the victim for head, neck, or spine injuries. If this type of injury is apparent, you should carefully support the head and avoid side-to-side motion. Moreover, you should open the airway using the jaw thrust maneuver, rather than the head-tilt/chin-lift. If the jaw thrust is unsuccessful in establishing an airway, a *slight* head tilt should be tried.[4]

Gastric distention and vomiting. During prolonged mouth-to-mouth ventilation, air enters the esophagus and stomach.[32] Thus some gastric distention is usual, particularly in children. Severe gastric distention puts pressure on the diaphragm, thus restricting lung expansion during inspiration. Gastric distention can also increase vagal tone and cause reflex bradycardia and hypotension.[14]

Most important, however, is the fact that severe gastric distention promotes **regurgitation.** Since the unconscious patient lacks normal upper airway reflexes, regurgitated stomach contents can easily be aspirated into the lungs. Massive aspiration of stomach contents into the lungs is nearly always a fatal event.

You can minimize gastric distention by breathing smoothly and avoiding rapid bursts of air during ventilation.[22,32-34] Using the least amount volume needed to produce lung expansion, as evaluated by the rise and fall of the chest, helps prevent excess air from entering the stomach. Mouth-to-nose ventilation also appears to decrease the likelihood of gastric distention. This is probably because the high resistance passages of the nose allow less of the inflation pressure to reach the hypopharynx.[17] Last, downward pressure applied to the cricoid cartilage may effectively compress the esophagus between the larynx and vertebral column, thereby preventing regurgitation.[33,34] Of course, this last technique should only be performed by trained health professionals, and is limited to situations involving two or more rescuers.[4]

If gastric distention is impairing ventilation, efforts should be made to manually expel the accumulated air.[4] To perform this procedure, all rescue efforts (including external cardiac compression) should be temporarily halted. The victim should be turned to his or her side, facing away from the practitioner. You can then apply gentle pressure with the flat of the hand between the umbilicus and lower rib cage to expel air and gastric contents (Figure 23-10).

Suction equipment should be available while attempting this procedure. If advanced life-support equipment and personnel are available, stomach contents may also be removed using a nasogastric tube.

Occasionally the victim may vomit during rescue

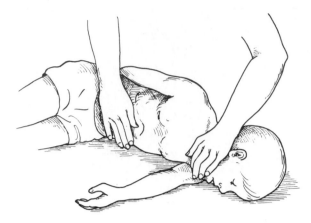

Fig. 23-10 Relieving gastric distention with gentle pressure on abdomen. (From Ellis PD, Billings DM: Cardiopulmonary resuscitation procedures for basic and advanced life support, St Louis, 1980, Mosby.)

attempts. If vomiting occurs, the practitioner should immediately turn the victim onto his side, wipe out the mouth, and resume the resuscitation effort.[4]

Restoring circulation

Determining pulselessness

After you give two slow breaths, you should immediately determine whether or not a pulse is present. Do not attempt to restore circulation until after you confirm pulselessness.

You determine pulselessness by palpating a major artery. In adults and children over one year old, the carotid artery in the neck should be palpated. To locate the carotid artery, maintain the head tilt with one hand while sliding the fingers of your other hand into the groove created by the trachea and the large neck muscles (Figure 23-11). The carotid artery area must be palpated gently to avoid compression of the artery or pushing on the carotid sinus. Because the pulse may be slow, weak, or irregular, you should allow about 8 to 10 seconds to confirm the presence or absence of a pulse.[4]

In infants, the brachial artery is preferred for assessing pulselessness. To palpate the brachial artery, grasp the infant's arm with your thumb outward, slide your fingers down toward the anticubital fossa and press gently to feel for a pulse. Alternatively, you can palate the femoral artery of the adult, child, or infant.

In hospital critical care settings, bedside monitoring equipment may provide supporting or confirming information regarding the respiratory or circulatory status of a patient. However, information obtained from these devices should never substitute for careful manual assessment of the patient.

If the patient has a pulse but is not breathing, you should begin ventilation immediately, using the appropriate rate. If no pulse is palpable, then external

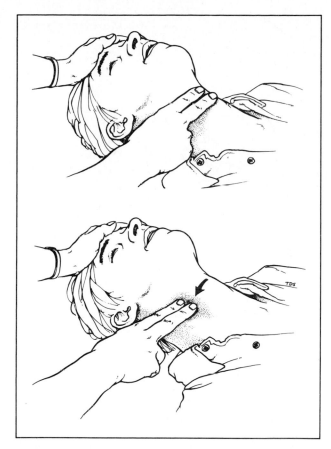

Fig. 23-11 Determining pulselessness. (From American Heart Association: Standards for cardiopulmonary resuscitation and emergency cardiac care, *JAMA* (suppl) 255:2843-2989, 1986. Copyright 1986, American Medical Association.)

chest compressions must be interposed with ventilatory support.

Providing chest compressions

Even without equipment, you can restore circulation using external chest compressions. In this procedure you manually compress the lower half of the sternum (for the adult patient) in a serial fashion. Cardiac output produced by external chest compressions is about one–fourth normal,[35] with arterial systolic pressures between 60 to 80 mm Hg.[4] Blood flow during chest compression is probably due to both the pump action of the heart and changes in the intrathoracic pressure.[35,36]

Chest compressions must be delivered to all pulseless patients. You modify the position, rescue technique, and compression rate according to the age and size of the victim.[37] You judge the need to modify the technique by the size of the victim and the effectiveness of the compression, as determined by palpating the pulse during compressions.

Adults. The procedure for adults is as follows (Figures 23-12 and 23-13, page 590):

1. Place the victim supine on a firm surface. Chest compressions are more effective when the victim is on a firm surface. You should thus place the victim on the ground or floor. When victims are in bed or on a litter, place a board or tray under them. A cardiac arrest board is ideal, but you may have to use a removable bed piece or food tray.
2. Expose the patient's chest to identify landmarks for correct hand position. If the victim is fully

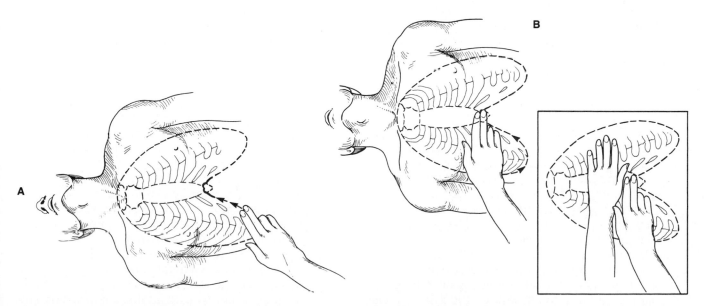

Fig. 23-12 Xiphisternal junction. **A,** Locating junction. **B,** hand position. (From Ellis PD, Billings DM: Cardiopulmonary resuscitation: procedures for basic and advanced life support, St Louis, 1980, Mosby.)

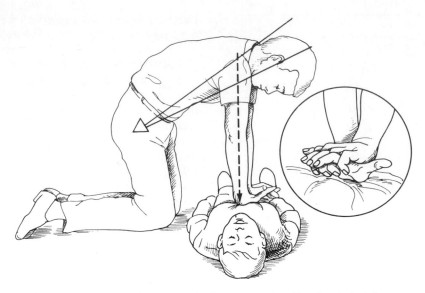

Fig. 23-13 Practitioner's position for external cardiac compression. Note interlocked fingers to prevent pressure on rib cage. (From Ellis PD, Billings DM: Cardiopulmonary resuscitation: procedures for basic and advanced life support, St Louis, 1980, Mosby.)

clothed, you should quickly remove or cut off any clothing or underwear.

3. Choose a position close to the patient's upper chest so that the weight of the body can be used for compression. If the patient is on a bed or litter, stand next to the bed or litter with the patient close to that side of the bed. If the bed is high or you are short, you may need to lower the bed, stand on a stool or chair, or kneel on the bed next to the victim. If the patient is on the ground, kneel at his or her side.

4. Identify the lower half of the sternum. Locate the lower margin of the patient's rib cage that is closest to you. Palpate upward along the ribs to the midline, locating the notch where the ribs meet the sternum in the center of the lowest part of the chest (See Figure 23-12). Place two fingers on the junction, and the heel of the other hand next to the two fingers. Then place the other hand on top of the hand on the sternum, and lock your elbows.

5. Perform compression with the weight of the body exerting force on the outstretched arms, elbows held straight. Your shoulders should be positioned *above* the patient so that the thrust of each compression is straight down onto the sternum, using your upper body weight and the hip joints as a fulcrum (Figure 23-13). Do not let the hands leave the chest.

6. Compress the sternum 1-1/2 to 2 inches (3.8 cm to 5.0 cm). Apply compressions regularly, rhythmically, and without bouncing or rolling the patient at a rate of 80 to 100/min.[37,38] The compression phase of the cycle should be equal in duration to the upstroke phase.[39]

7. If CPR must be interrupted for transportation or advance life-support measures, chest compression should resume as quickly as possible. Compressions should not cease for more than 5 seconds (30 seconds if intubating the victim).[37] This is particularly important if drugs are being administered.

Children. Children older than 8 years of age, especially if large, should receive chest compressions as outlined for adults. The procedure for younger children (1 to 8 years old) is as follows (Figure 23-14):[4,40,41]

1. Place the victim in the supine position on a firm surface. Small children may require additional support under the upper body. This is particularly true when chest compressions are given with mouth-to-mouth ventilation, since extension of the neck raises the shoulders. The head should be no higher than the body.

2. Identify the lower third of the sternum. Because the liver and spleen of younger children lie higher in the abdominal cavity special care must be taken to ensure proper positioning. Palpate upward along the rib cage toward the midline until you reach the notch where the sternum and ribs meet. Place the heel of the hand you will use for compression two fingerbreadths above this point. Use the other hand to maintain head position and maintain an airway.

3. Compress the chest about 1 to 1-1/2 inches at a rate of 100/min. Generally, the heel of one hand is sufficient to achieve compression in these small children. As with adults, compression and relaxation times should be equal in length and delivered smoothly.

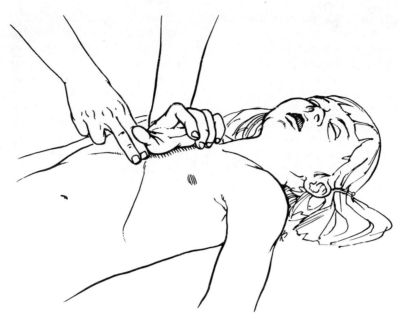

Fig. 23-14 Locating hand position for chest compressions in child. (From American Heart Association: Standards for cardiopulmonary resuscitation and emergency cardiac care, *JAMA* (suppl) 255:2843-2989, 1986. Copyright 1986, American Medical Association.)

Infants. The procedure for infants (up to 1 year old) is as follows (Figure 23-15):[4,40,41]

1. Use the lower third of the sternum for compression in the infant. Proper placement is determined by imagining a line across the chest connecting the nipples. Place your index finger along this line on the sternum. Then place your middle and ring fingers next to the index finger. Raise your index finger and perform compressions with the middle and ring fingers. Use the other hand to maintain the infant's head position and airway.

2. Compress the sternum is between 1/3 to 1/2 the total depth of the chest (about 1/2 to 1 inch) at a rate of 100/min. Compression and upstroke phases should be equal in length and delivered smoothly. Your fingers should remain on the chest at all times.

Neonates. In neonates, life-threatening emergencies are frequently due to hypoxia and hypothermia. Rapid correction of these problems may forestall the need for CPR. However, chest compressions are indicated if the neonate's heart rate falls below 60/min or remains between 60 to 80/min for

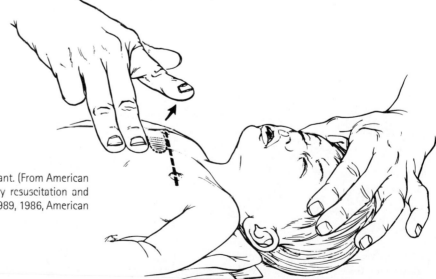

Fig. 23-15 Position for chest compression in infant. (From American Heart Association: Standards for cardiopulmonary resuscitation and emergency cardiac care, *JAMA* (suppl) 255:2843-2989, 1986, American Medical Association.)

more than 30 seconds despite adequate ventilation with 100% oxygen.

You may perform neonatal chest compression using a 'wrap-around' technique (Figure 23-16). With this method, you encircle the neonate's chest with both hands and position your thumbs on the sternum. The other fingers of both hands support the neonate's back. You position your thumbs just below the **intermammary** line, making sure not to compress the xiphoid or lower portion of the sternum. You compress the sternum 1/2 to 3/4 inch at a rate of 120/min. Compression should be performed smoothly, with downstroke and upstroke times about equal. After every third compression, the neonate should receive a breath of 100% oxygen.

Judging the effectiveness of chest compressions

The single best indicator of the effectiveness of chest compressions is the presence of a pulse during compression. The pulse should be palpable with each compression.

Hazards and complications

External cardiac compression is not without hazards, and you must make every attempt to minimize these by using correct technique. Complications associated chest compression include gastric perforation, laceration of the liver, contusion of the lung, fractured ribs, sternum, or spine, **pneumothorax, hemothorax,** fat emboli, **cardiac tamponade,** and ruptured heart.[43-48]

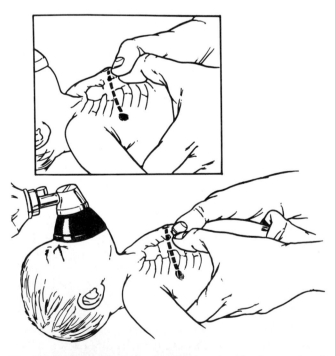

Fig. 23-16 Neonatal chest compression using the 'wrap-around' technique. (From Guidelines for cardiopulmonary resuscitation and emergency cardiac care, *JAMA* 268: 2171-2302, 1992.)

These complications are most often linked to improper hand position. Placement of the hands too far to either the left or right can cause fractured ribs or laceration of the lung; incorrect placement on the left can also injure the heart itself. If you place the hands too high on the sternum, you can fracture the sternum; too low a placement can cause a fractured xiphoid or lacerations of the liver. Correct identification of landmarks and proper hand placement will minimize the likelihood of these complications.

Chest compressions in special circumstances

Several unique circumstances exist which require modification of the normal procedures for applying cardiac compressions. These situations include near drownings, electrical shock, and patients with pacemakers or prosthetic heart valves.

Drowning. When cardiac arrest occurs following as a result of drowning, the victim must be moved as quickly as possible to a firm surface. Cardiac compressions cannot be given while a victim is in the water.

Electrical shock. Electrical shock can cause either cardiac or respiratory arrest. Cardiac arrest is due to ventricular fibrillation. Respiratory arrest occurs secondary to paralysis of the ventilatory muscles. Initially, the victim must be removed from contact with the source of electricity and assessed. The rescuer must pay special attention to dangers that can harm him/her. Do not touch a victim who is still connected to an electric source. Turn the power off. If cardiac arrest has occurred, the practitioner should administer CPR immediately.

Pacemakers. Individuals with pacemakers may suffer cardiac arrest due to battery failure or other mechanical difficulties. CPR for these victims is similar to the procedure previously described.

Artificial heart valves. Chest compressions can damage the heart of a patient who has recently undergone surgery to implant an artificial valve (especially mitral or tricuspid valves). However, the patient will die if nothing is done. For this reason, external cardiac compressions should be done until a qualified surgeon can perform emergency **thoracotomy** and internal cardiac compression.

Cardiopulmonary resuscitation

Although respiratory and cardiac arrest may occur separately, most often they happen together. For this reason, you will usually combine artificial ventilation with cardiac compressions. The two combined together are aptly called cardiopulmonary resuscitation, or CPR. CPR can be administered by one person alone, or by a team of two or more individuals.

Single-practitioner CPR

If you are the only person present, you will initially have to assess the situation, determine unresponsiveness, and call for help by yourself. You then initiate the ABCs, as previously described. You open and clear the airway, assess breathing, and give two slow breaths if the victim is apneic. If you cannot ventilate the victim, you should repeat the process once again. If your second attempt to ventilate fails, you should assume that the airway is obstructed and proceed as outlined later in this chapter.[4,16]

Assuming the initial attempt to ventilate is successful, you go on to check the pulse. If a pulse is present, but there is no spontaneous breathing, you should continue to ventilate the patient using the methods previously described. If there is no pulse, you initially should deliver 15 chest compressions, at the rate of 80 to 100/min (adults). Compressions should follow the timing of "one and two and three and four" until the 15 compressions are administered. At this point, you should position yourself at the victim's head, open the airway, and administer two slow deep breath as was done before. You then return to the chest and administer another cycle of 15 compressions followed by 2 more breaths (15:2 ratio).[4,16]

After 4 cycles of compressions and ventilations, you reassess the patient. To do so, palpate the carotid pulse for 3 to 5 seconds and observe for spontaneous breathing. If there is no pulse or breathing, you continue CPR, stopping only to reassess the victim every few minutes. If the pulse returns, the patient's ventilatory status is assessed and supported as needed.

With infants and children, the cycle consists of 5 compressions to every one breath and is timed by counting "one and two and three and four and five" (a rate of 80 to 100/min), followed by one breath. The infant and child's pulse and ventilatory efforts should be assessed after 20 cycles (about 1 minute) and every few minutes thereafter.

Two-practitioner CPR

When two persons are available, assessment, rescue, and evaluation can be shared. One practitioner ventilates and evaluates the effectiveness of CPR. The other administers cardiac compressions. To facilitate movement, each practitioner should assume the appropriate rescue position on opposite sides of the victim. In the adult patient, the compression to ventilatory ratio is 5:1 and the timing for compressions are set at "one and two and three and four and five" (a rate of 80 to 100 times per minute).[4,16]

When two people provide support, the individual providing compressions briefly pauses (1.5 to 2 seconds) after the fifth compression so that the second practitioner can administer the ventilation. The cycle is then repeated. After the first minute, the pulse is reassessed. If there is no pulse, CPR is continued.

Reassessment should then be performed every few minutes thereafter. If a pulse returns, the airway must be maintained and ventilations supported as needed.

To provide rest for the individual delivering cardiac compressions, the practitioners may change positions. The individual doing cardiac compressions calls for the change, saying in sequence with compression, "We/will/change/next/time," or words to this effect. The individual providing ventilation gives a breath at the end of the next compression cycle and moves quickly into position for cardiac compression. The individual previously responsible for compressions moves to the head, and checks for a pulse. If no pulse is found, he or she should give one breath. The cycle then continues with the two practitioners in their new positions.[4,16]

Rescue attempts should continue until either: (1) advanced life support is available, (2) the practitioner(s) note spontaneous pulse and breathing, or (3) a physician pronounces the victim dead. A cardiopulmonary emergency presents a crisis for the victim and his family, and appropriate support and intervention should be provided for both. Victims who survive CPR should be transported quickly to tertiary care facilities, ideally only after advanced life support is instituted.

Evaluating the effectiveness of CPR

It is important that you continue to judge both the effectiveness of CPR and the victim's response. Because successful CPR depends on adequate circulation, it is imperative that you develop an effective technique for compression depth, rhythm, and rate. With ineffective compressions, blood flow is minimal and biological death ensues. If the compression cycle does not allow for an adequate relaxation phase, venous return and stroke volume may be decreased, creating a situation similar to cardiac tamponade. Compression rates should be appropriate for the victim's age. If possible, you should quickly assess the effectiveness of the compressions every minute, with a more comprehensive assessment conducted every 4 to 5 minutes.

The presence of a pulse is the most reliable indicator of effective cardiac compressions. In adults and children, you can use the carotid or femoral pulse. In infants and neonates, the brachial pulse is easier to palpate.[4] The pulse should be palpable with each compression. If one practitioner is present, he or she can palpate the pulse every minute. If two or more practitioners are available, they can monitor the pulse continuously.

Skin color is a parameter that is readily observed but imprecise in judging the effectiveness of CPR. However, if normal color returns, you can assume that oxygenation has improved.

You can estimate the effectiveness of cerebral oxygenation by observing pupil responses to light. However, pupil responses may be altered by drugs or diseases, making this sign somewhat unreliable. To check pupillary responses, open the eyelids and observe the pupils for size and their response to light. Pupils that are constricted and respond to light indicate adequate cerebral oxygenation. Pupils that are dilated but react to light indicate poor oxygenation. Dilated and nonreactive pupils are a bad sign. The likelihood of irreversible brain death is high if pupils have been dilated and fixed for 15 to 30 minutes or longer.

The return of consciousness and the presence of tears are a good sign, indicating restoration of cerebral blood flow and oxygenation. The lacrimal glands are supplied by the internal carotid artery and, if blood supply is adequate, tears will be present. Additionally, reflexes such as swallowing or vomiting may return as the victim regains neurologic function.

Contraindications to CPR

There are few contraindications against CPR, since the pulseless apneic patient will die within 4 to 6 minutes without intervention. Fear of further harm should never influence the decision to begin CPR. CPR is contraindicated only when the patient is obviously dead (as noted by such findings as **rigor mortis**). In the hospital, CPR is contraindicated when a valid 'Do Not Resuscitate' (DNR) order is in effect,[49] or if a properly executed living will (advanced directive) specifically requests that CPR not be initiated. (See Chapter 5.)

Health concerns and CPR

Recent concerns have arisen among both the lay public and health professionals regarding possible transmission of infectious diseases—especially AIDS—during CPR.[50-51] In one survey, 45% of the physicians and 80% of the nurses indicated that they would refuse to provide mouth-to-mouth ventilation for a stranger.[52] In general, these concerns are unwarranted.[53] Moreover, the reluctance of lay personnel and health professionals to initiate CPR poses a clear danger to the effectiveness of early intervention in life-threatening emergencies for the public as a whole.

Personnel with a duty to provide CPR should follow the guidelines established by the Center for Disease Control (CDC) and the Occupational Safety and Health Administration (OSHA). These recommendations include the use of latex gloves, masks and goggles.[54-55] Mechanical 'barrier' aids to ventilation (masks, filters, valves) have also been suggested, as much to allay fear as to protect the rescuer.[56] However, these devices require training to use properly, are not universally available, and are not as effective as mouth-to-mouth ventilation.

Although blood or body fluids technically can be exchanged via mouth-to-mouth ventilation, CDC surveillance reports on job-related AIDS have never reported such an incident.[57] Other infectious diseases such as herpes simplex and tuberculosis may present a higher risk, but few cases have been reported. While the degree of risk is believed to be low, health care providers who perform mouth to mouth ventilation on a person suspected of having tuberculosis should receive follow up evaluation using standard approaches. Moreover, any practitioner who might hesitate to provide mouth-to-mouth ventilation to a victim in need should always carry (and know how to use) an appropriate barrier device for this purpose.

Last, equipment contaminated with blood or other body fluids during a resuscitation effort should always be discarded in appropriate receptacles or thoroughly cleaned and disinfected following hospital protocols.

Dealing with an obstructed airway

Early recognition of foreign body airway obstruction is critical. Foreign bodies may cause either partial or complete obstruction. Partial obstruction may allow nearly adequate air exchange, in which case the patient remains conscious and coughing. As long as air exchange is present, the patient should be reassured and allowed to clear their own airway by coughing.

If partial obstruction continues or air exchange worsens, the EMS system should be activated. Poor air exchange exists when the patient has a weak or ineffective cough, increased inspiratory difficulty, or becomes cyanotic.

With a completely obstructed airway, the patient frequently clutches at his or her throat. This is known as the universal distress signal for foreign body obstruction. The person with a complete obstruction cannot talk, cough or breath, and is in dire need of emergency intervention.

If your attempts to open a victim's airway are unsuccessful, or if you observe a foreign body in the mouth or pharynx, you can use several procedures to obtain a clear passageway.

For adults and children, the procedure of choice for clearing a foreign body is the abdominal thrust or Heimlich maneuver.[58-63] For infants with an obstructed airway, back blows are attempted first and, if unsuccessful, are followed by chest thrusts.[4,23,62,63] Backblows are not used in the adult choking victim. Chest thrusts however, may be used with female victims in the advanced stages of pregnancy and in markedly obese individuals in place of abdominal thrusts.[4] Both procedures normally are followed by a manual check and removal of any obstructing foreign material.

Abdominal thrusts (Heimlich Maneuver)

Forceful thrusts applied to the epigastrium can dislodge an obstruction caused by a food bolus, vomitus, or other foreign body. Quick thrusts to the abdomen rapidly displace the diaphragm upward, thus increasing intrathoracic pressure and creating expulsive expiratory airflow. Like a normal cough, this expulsive airflow may be sufficient to expel the foreign body from the airway. The procedure for performing abdominal thrusts in adults and children is as follows (Figure 23-17):

1. If the victim is sitting or standing, stand behind him or her and wraps your arms around the victim's waist. Make a fist with one hand and place the thumb side midline on the abdomen slightly above the navel and well below the tip of the xiphoid process (Figure 23-17, *A*). Grasp the fist with the other hand and delivers a quick upward and inward thrust. Each thrust should be a separate and distinct movement. The process is repeated and continued until the obstruction is removed or the patient loses consciousness.

2. When the victim has collapsed or is unconscious, the abdominal thrust can be delivered with the victim in the lying position (Figure 23-17, *B*). Place the victim in the supine position, face upward, so that the foreign body can be easily expelled. If the victim vomits, quickly turn the victim's head to the side and wipe out the mouth. Kneel astride the victim's hips and place the heel of one hand on the abdomen between the umbilicus and xiphoid, and the other hand on top. Then rock forward to give a quick upward thrust, repeating it 5 times, or as needed.

3. An alternative approach is to kneel near the victim's hips with the shoulders over the victim and, using the same hand position, press on the epigastrium. This position is preferred if you also must perform mouth-to-mouth ventilation or external cardiac compression, since you can easily change position. If two practitioners are available, one can give the abdominal thrusts while the other manages the airway and retrieves the foreign body.

4. A conscious victim who is alone can attempt to dislodge the foreign body with self-administered abdominal thrusts. He may be able to press a fist into the abdomen or push the abdomen against a firm surface such as a counter top, sink, chair back, railing, or tabletop.

After each cycle of abdominal thrusts, you should check the oral cavity by 'sweeping' it with two or three fingers. After removal of any foreign material, you should again attempt to ventilate the patient. If ventilation can be provided, breathing and circulation are assessed, and appropriate intervention taken. If you cannot ventilate the patient, then you should institute another cycle of thrusts, followed by an airway check and an attempt to ventilate. This procedure is repeated until the airway is open and the patient can be ventilated.

Back blows and chest thrusts

Because the Heimlich maneuver can easily cause abdominal injury when applied to infants, a combination of back blows with chest thrusts is used to clear

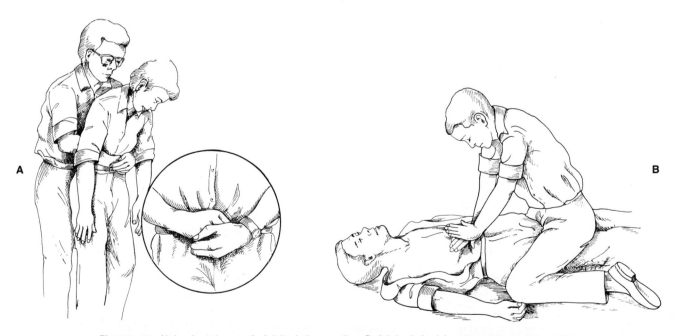

Fig. 23-17 Abdominal thrusts. **A,** Adult victim standing. **B,** Adult victim lying. (From Ellis PD, Billings DM: Cardiopulmonary resuscitation: procedures for basic and advanced life support, St Louis, 1980, Mosby.)

foreign bodies from the upper airway of these victims.[4] Back blows alone may create sufficient force to dislodge trapped objects.[62,63] If back blows are ineffective, chest thrusts are administered. Back blows, followed by 5 chest thrusts and inspection of the airway is continued until the airway is restored.[4] The procedure is as follows (Figure 23-18):

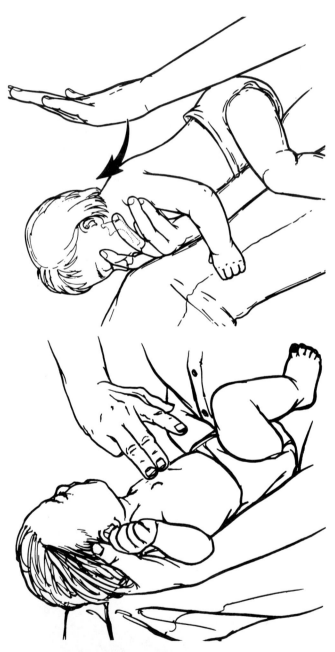

Fig. 23-18 Use of back blows and chest thrusts to clear foreign bodies from infant airways. (From: Guidelines for cardiopulmonary resuscitation and emergency cardiac care, *JAMA* 268: 2171-2302, 1992.)

1. You can administer back blows to infants more efficiently if you hold the child straddled over one arm with the head lower than the body.
2. Use the flat portion of the hand to gently but quickly deliver five back blows between the shoulder blades.
3. If the back blows do not clear the infant's airway, you should turn the infant over and institute a series of five chest thrusts. Like the abdominal thrust, the chest thrust creates a rapid rise in intrathoracic pressure, thereby aiding expulsion of the foreign body. Chest thrusts for infants are performed in the same manner and at the same location as that used for cardiac compressions, but at a slower rate.
4. As with adults, you should try to clear the airway between attempts to expell the foreign body. To do so, first visually inspect the oral cavity, and remove any foreign matter you can see. Deep blind finger sweeps of an infant or child's mouth is not recommended.

Evaluating the effectiveness of foreign body removal

After each airway restoration maneuver, you must determine whether the foreign body has been expelled and the obstructed airway cleared. If the foreign body is not dislodged, you should repeat the appropriate sequence (abdominal thrusts for adults and children; back blows and chest thrusts for infants) until successful.[4,16]

Successful removal of an obstructing body is indicated by: (1) confirmed expulsion of the foreign body, (2) clear breathing and the ability to speak, (3) a return of consciousness, and (4) a return of normal color.

If successive attempts to clear the airway by these means fail, more aggressive techniques are indicated, if available. These include: (1) direct laryngoscopy and foreign body removal with Magill forceps, (2) transtracheal catheterization, (3) cricothyrotomy, and (4) tracheotomy. Obviously, these methods require specially trained personnel and equipment, and are aptly categorized as advanced life support techniques. Transtracheal catheterization and cricothyrotomy are discussed later in this chapter. Laryngoscopy, bronchoscopy, and tracheotomy were described in Chapter 22.

Hazards and complications

The major hazard associated with abdominal thrusts is possible damage to internal organs, such as laceration or rupture of abdominal or thoracic viscera.[64,65] This complication can be avoided by properly placing the arms and fist below the xiphoid and lower margin of the ribs.[4]

Vomiting is another complication associated with abdominal thrusts, and one that is impossible to avoid. Vomiting itself is a minor problem. It is the aspiration of vomitus into the lung that represents the hazard. Aspiration can only be prevented using the accessory airway equipment and procedures discussed later under advanced life support.

Manual removal of foreign material from the upper airway also can be hazardous. The problem here is the possibility of forcing the object deeper into the airway.[4] This hazard can be minimized by attempting to remove only those objects actually within reach.

ADVANCED CARDIAC LIFE SUPPORT

Advanced cardiac life support extends BLS capabilities by providing additional measures beyond immediate ventilatory and circulatory assistance. These measures include using accessory equipment to support ventilation and oxygenation, monitoring the ECG, establishing an IV route for drug administration, and applying selected drug agents and electrical therapies. If advanced life support is successful, an individualized regimen of postresuscitative care usually follows.[4]

The initiation of basic life support should never be delayed while awaiting advanced capabilities. Quick intervention is the primary factor determining success in any resuscitation effort. Moreover, the use of advanced cardiac life support measures should never interfere with or delay continuity in the provision of BLS. Last, any accessory equipment employed in a resuscitation effort must be in good working order. Assurance of proper equipment functions requires periodic performance testing according to prescribed standards and regulations.[4]

During advanced cardiac life support in the hospital, the RCP assumes primary responsibility for supporting oxygenation, establishing and maintaining the airway, and providing ventilation. Practitioners must thus demonstrate high levels of proficiency in these advanced life support skills.

Support for oxygenation

Although expired air ventilation provides an acceptable level of oxygenation, low cardiac output, pulmonary shunting and V/Q abnormalities during CPR lead to hypoxia. Hypoxia, in turn, results in anaerobic metabolism and metabolic acidosis. Metabolic acidosis impedes the action of certain drugs and can diminish the effectiveness of electrical therapies. For these reason, the highest possible concentration of oxygen should be applied as soon as possible.[4]

During advanced cardiac life support, supplemental oxygen is normally given through accessory devices designed to support ventilation. Thus, the ability of these devices to provide high FIO_2s is a key factor in judging their performance. The performance of these devices will be discussed in a subsequent section.

Airway control

Accessory equipment designed to provide airway control during advanced cardiac life support includes a variety of masks and artificial airways. When the airway cannot be secured by any of these means, it may be necessary to surgically establish a **percutaneous** route.

Masks

A well-fitting mask used with expired-air oxygen can maintain adequate ventilation during CPR.[66-68] Mask-to-mouth ventilation generally is easier to perform and provides higher tidal volumes than via a bag-valve-mask, but less than mouth-to-mouth ventilation.[68]

Used for this purpose, an ideal mask should be made of transparent material, be capable of tightly sealing against the face, provide an inlet for supplemental oxygen, and employ a standard 15/22 mm connection.[4] Moreover, it should be available in various sizes to accommodate adults, children and infants. One-way valves, if provided, should be simple, dependable, and jam-free.

The use of masks to support ventilation presumes that the airway can be maintained by conventional basic life support techniques. Application of the mask-to-mouth technique is best done with the practitioner positioned at the head of the victim, using the jaw-thrust maneuver to maintain the airway (Figure 23-19). Obviously, this approach is only possible when a second person is available to provide chest compressions.

Mask-to-mouth ventilation with supplemental oxygen represents a viable alternative to bag-valve-mask methods of airway maintenance and ventilation. Moreover, since masks can serve as barrier devices, fear of disease transmission can be minimized and rapid response ensured. Thus, in the absence of highly trained personnel, mask-to-mouth ventilation should

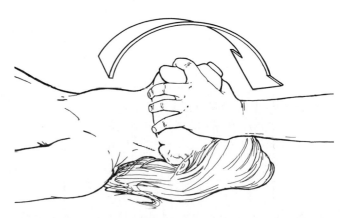

Fig. 23-19 Proper placement of hands to hold resuscitator mask to patient's face and perform head-tilt maneuver.

be considered the procedure of choice until an artificial airway can be properly placed.[4]

Artificial airways

After appropriate use of basic life support methods to secure the airway, the practitioner may use an artificial airway to achieve one or more of the following goals: (1) to restore airway patency, (2) to maintain adequate ventilation, (3) to isolate and protect the airway from aspiration, (4) to provide access for clearance of secretions, and (5) to provide an alternate route for administration of selected drugs.[4,69]

Which airway should be used in a given situation depends on careful assessment of the status of the victim, together with an in-depth knowledge of the capabilities and limitations of the equipment at hand.[70]

Pharyngeal airways. Pharyngeal airways can help restore airway patency and maintain adequate ventilation, particularly when using a bag-valve-mask device. A properly placed pharyngeal airway also may help provide access for suctioning. Pharyngeal airways should only be used after BLS methods have successfully opened and cleared the airway.

Pharyngeal airways restore airway patency by separating the tongue from the posterior pharyngeal wall. Two types of pharyngeal airways are used in clinical practice: the oropharyngeal airway and the nasopharyngeal airway.

Oropharyngeal airways come in many different sizes to fit adults, children, and infants. Figure 23-20 shows the two most common oropharyngeal airway designs: the Guedel airway (Figure 23-20, *A*) and the Berman airway (Figure 23-20, *B*). Both types

have an external flange: (1), a curved body, (2) that conforms to the shape of the oral cavity, and (3) one or more channels. The Guedel airway has a single center channel, while the Berman type uses two parallel side channels.

In order to choose the correct size airway, the practitioner places the devices on the side of the patient's face with the flange even with the patient's mouth. The correct size airway measures from the corner of the patient's mouth to the angle of the jaw following the natural curve of the airway.

Because inserting an oropharyngeal airway can provoke a gag reflex, vomiting, or laryngeal spasm, these devices generally are contraindicated in conscious or semi-conscious patients.[4] They are also contraindicated when there is trauma to the oral cavity, mandibular, or maxillary areas of the skull. Moreover, these airways should never be placed when either a space-occupying lesion or foreign body already obstructs the oral cavity or pharynx.

Two techniques may be used to inserted an oropharyngeal airway.[14] In the first method, you displace the tongue away from the roof of the mouth with a tongue depressor. You then slip the curved portion of the airway over the tongue, following the curve of the oral cavity.

In the second approach, you apply the jaw-lift technique to help displace the tongue. Your rotate the oropharyngeal airway 180° before insertion. In this manner the airway itself helps separate the jaws and further displace the tongue. As the tip of the airway reaches the hard palate, you rotate it by 180°, aligning it as before in the pharynx.

In either approach, incorrect placement can dis-

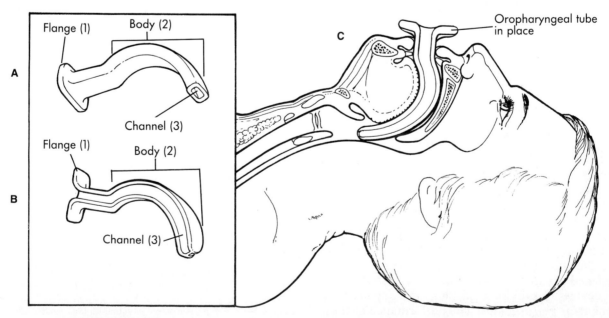

Fig. 23-20 Oropharyngeal airways. **A,** Guedel airway. **B,** Berman airway. **C,** Airway in place.

place the tongue further back into the pharynx and worsen the obstruction. For this reason, oropharyngeal airways must be inserted carefully, and only by trained personnel.

As shown in Figure 23-20, *C*, when properly inserted, the tip of an oropharyngeal airway lies at the base of the tongue above the epiglottis, with its flange portion extending *outside* the teeth. Only in this position can this device properly maintain airway patency.

Nasopharyngeal airway airways are inserted through the nose instead of the mouth. As shown in Figure 23-21, a properly inserted nasopharyngeal airway provides a passageway from the external nares to the base of the tongue, at a point just behind the epiglottis. Like the oropharyngeal type, the nasopharyngeal airway helps restore airway patency by separating the tongue from the posterior pharyngeal wall.

Generally, the nasopharyngeal airway is indicated when placement of an oropharyngeal airway is not possible. The nasopharyngeal airway is also used when you cannot separate the jaws of a victim, as may occur with seizures.

A nasopharyngeal airway should *not* be used when there is trauma to the nasal region, or the nasal passages are blocked by space-occupying lesions or foreign objects. Moreover, due to the very small size of the nasal passageway in children and infants, the use of nasal airways is generally limited to adults.[4]

Most nasal airways are made from either rubber or plastic polymers, and sized by external diameter in French units, with 26 to 32 French being the common size range for adults. Anatomically, the length of the airway is more critical than its diameter. You can estimate the needed length by measuring the distance from the patient's earlobe to the tip of their nose.

To insert a nasopharyngeal airway, you should tilt the head slightly backward. You should lubricate the airway with a water-soluble agent to ease insertion. Once lubricated, you position the airway perpendicular to the frontal plane of the face, and slowly advance it through the inferior meatus of either the right or left nasal cavity, making sure that the bevel edge faces the septum. If you feel an obstruction during insertion, gentle twisting may facilitate placement. If you meet continued resistance, the most likely cause is a deviated nasal septum. In this case, you should simply attempt passage through the other naris or try a smaller diameter tube.[14]

Once the airway is inserted, you should try to quickly visualize and confirm its correct position, using a tongue depressor if necessary. Breath sounds must be present. A properly positioned nasopharyngeal airway is usually stabilized by its own flange.

Esophageal obturator airway (EOA). As shown in Figure 23-22, page 600, the esophageal obturator airway, or EOA, consists of a cuffed hollow tube tipped with a soft plastic obturator at its distal end. The tube, which passes through a mask, has several holes in its upper portion. Some EOAs are modified to include a gastric tube which can be extended beyond the distal tip into the stomach. This modified version is called the esophageal gastric tube airway, or EGTA.[4]

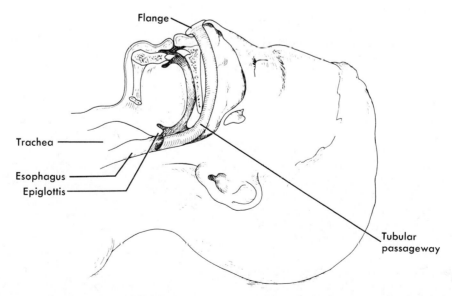

Fig. 23-21 Nasopharyngeal airway provides long passageway extending from external naris to base of tongue just above epiglottis. (From Ellis PD, Billings DM: Cardiopulmonary resuscitation: procedures for basic and advanced life support, St Louis, 1980, Mosby.)

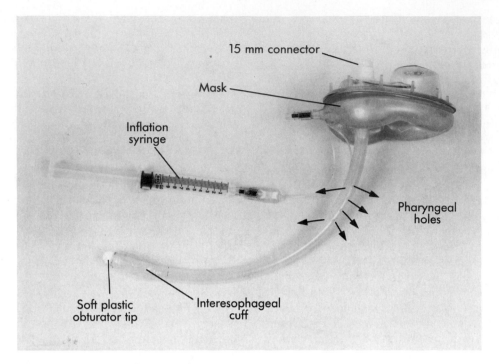

Fig. 23-22 Parts of esophageal obturator airway.

In concept, the EOA is inserted blindly into the esophagus, thereby blocking it off. With the esophageal cuff inflated and the mask tightly sealed to the victim's face, air under pressure is diverted out the pharyngeal holes in the tube and into the trachea and lungs (Figure 23-23).[71-74]

In practice, the EOA's effectiveness depends on the adequacy of the seal obtained with its face mask. Even among highly trained personnel an adequate seal is difficult to obtain. Thus the level of ventilation provided by the EOA is generally less than that realized with endotracheal intubation.[73]

Moreover, the use of the EOA has been associated with several potentially life-threatening complications. The most common complication of EOA use is inadvertent insertion into the trachea.[73] Obviously, if not immediately recognized, this complication will quickly result in asphyxia. Additional reported complications of EOA use are aspiration, esophageal laceration, and rupture.[75-77]

Additional field studies have shown that the intubation success rate with the EOA is only about 80%, and that patients with this airway in place are consistently underventilated.[78] Based on the numerous reports of problems and complications, the Committee on Trauma of the American College of Surgeons has recommended against use of the EOA/EGTA.[79]

Nonetheless, the EOA is still being used in some prehospital settings. Thus the RCP may still encounter this type of airway adjunct already placed in patients being admitted to the emergency room. For this reason, emphasis here is on proper removal of the device, rather than its insertion.

Removal of the EOA is frequently followed by immediate regurgitation of stomach contents.[4] Use of the EGTA decreases the likelihood of regurgitation, but does not eliminate it.

In unconscious or semiconscious patients, the EOA should not be removed until a cuffed endotracheal tube is in place.[79] In this manner, the lower airway can be protected from the possible aspiration of stomach contents that can occur with regurgitation.

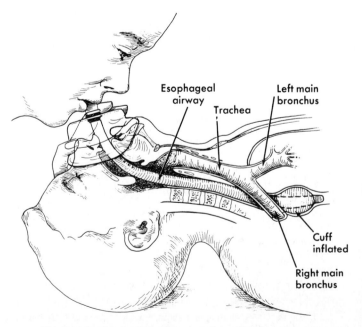

Fig. 23-23 Esophageal obturator airway (EOA) in place.

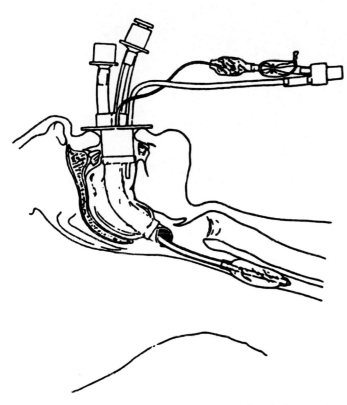

Fig. 23-24 Pharyngeal-tracheal lumen airway (PTLA). See text for description (From Reines HD: Airway management options, *Respir Care* 37(7): 695-705, 1992.)

Pharyngeal-tracheal lumen airway and esophageal tracheal combitube. Two other airway devices similar in concept to the EOA/EGTA are the pharyngeal-tracheal lumen airway (PTLA) and esophageal tracheal combitube (ETC).

The PTLA attempts to minimize accidental tracheal intubation and occlusion that may occur with the EOA/EGTA, while also providing for better ventilation (since a mask is not needed).[77] The PTLA is a 'tube-within-a-tube' that is inserted blindly into the oropharynx (Figure 23-24). If the longer tube enters the trachea, a balloon is inflated and the patient ventilated as if an endotracheal tube were in place. If the longer end enters the esophagus, then a balloon is inflated to occlude the esophagus. In this latter case, the patient is ventilated via the pharynx through the shorter outer tube. An additional large balloon at the proximal of the PTLA occludes the pharynx, making a mask unnecessary. Of course, the potential for aspiration after removal of the PLTA is the same as with the EOA/EGTA.[77] However, initial studies indicate a higher intubation success rate and better ventilation with the PTLA than with the EOA.[80]

Like the PTLA, the ETC is also a double lumen tube. However, the two ETC tubes run parallel to each other, rather than one inside the other. The ETC is advanced blindly beyond the pharynx into either the esophagus or trachea.[81] Regardless of placement, infla-

tion of a pharyngeal balloon seals off this passageway, thus avoiding the need for a mask. A distal balloon seals off the other passage (either esophagus or trachea). If the tube is in the esophagus, ventilation is provided through a lumen with pharyngeal holes (like the EOA). If the tube ends up in the tracheal, the other lumen is used, as with an endotracheal tube. Preliminary studies on the ETC indicate adequate function during cardiopulmonary resuscitation, surgery, and intensive care.[81-82]

Endotracheal intubation. Endotracheal intubation is the preferred method for securing the airway during CPR. Once positioned properly, an endotracheal tube can maintain a patent airway, prevent aspiration of stomach contents, permit suctioning of the trachea and mainstem bronchi, facilitate ventilation and oxygenation, and provide a route for drug administration.[4,69]

However, attempts to intubate the trachea must never interfere with providing adequate ventilation and oxygenation by other means. Thus endotracheal intubation should be performed only by highly trained personnel. Moreover, intubation attempts during resuscitation should never last more than 30 seconds. Adequate ventilation and oxygenation must be provided between attempts.[4]

Figure 23-25, page 602, show a cuffed orotracheal tube properly positioned in the trachea, being used with a manual bag-valve device to provide ventilation and oxygenation. With this arrangement, ventilation no longer need be synchronized with chest compressions. Instead, adequate ventilation and oxygenation can be provided with 12 to 15 asynchronous breaths per minute.[83]

RCPs can and should be trained in endotracheal intubation techniques, as applied in both emergency life support and prolonged mechanical ventilation situations. Details on the necessary equipment, procedure, and short and long-term complications of endotracheal intubation are provided in Chapter 22.

Percutaneous routes

Situations sometimes arise in which the airway cannot be secured by endotracheal intubation. These include upper airway or laryngeal trauma, foreign body obstruction, and laryngospasm. In such cases, restoration of ventilation and oxygenation may depend on establishing an alternative airway route, one below the site of obstruction. Typically, these methods surgically establish direct access to the trachea via a percutaneous route, through the skin of the anterior neck.

The two most common methods of percutaneous airway access are transtracheal catheterization and cricothyrotomy. Obviously, because such methods carry significant risks, they should be performed only by skilled personnel and then only after all other methods have failed.

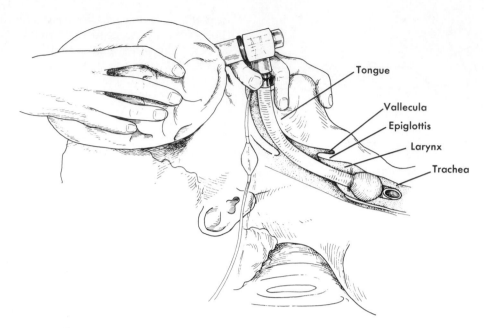

Fig. 23-25 Orotracheal tube in place being used with bag-valve resuscitator.

Transtracheal catheterization. As shown in Figure 23-26, *A*, transtracheal catheterization involves puncture of the cricothyroid membrane with a 12 to 16 gauge needle surrounded by a plastic catheter. Alternatively, the membrane immediately below the first tracheal ring may be used as the point of entry. In either case, the needle is guided at a 45° angle caudally into the trachea. Aspiration of air into the attached syringe confirms proper placement.

Once positioned in the trachea, the catheter is advanced over the needle until the hub reaches the puncture site where it is stabilized. Ventilation is provided by connecting the catheter to either a 50 psi oxygen source with a valve mechanism[84] or a jet ventilator designed for this purpose. When "on," oxygen flows into the trachea under positive pressure, causing lung inflation. When "off," flow ceases and the patient exhales normally through the nose and mouth (Figure 23-26, *B*).

Transtracheal catheterization is an extremely delicate procedure. Misplacement of the catheter into the esophagus can cause inadequate ventilation, gastric

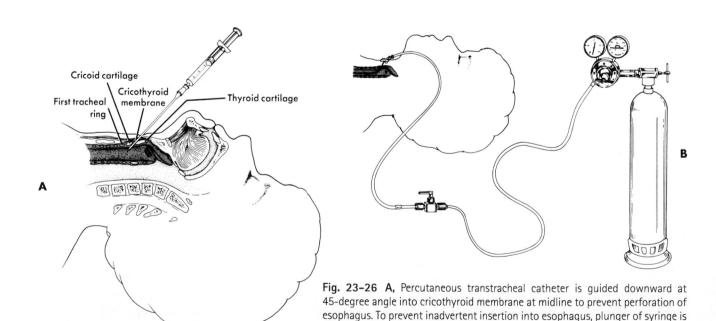

Fig. 23-26 A, Percutaneous transtracheal catheter is guided downward at 45-degree angle into cricothyroid membrane at midline to prevent perforation of esophagus. To prevent inadvertent insertion into esophagus, plunger of syringe is aspirated continually. **B,** Ventilation via high-pressure oxygen.

insufflation, and regurgitation. Puncture of one of the many arteries in the region can cause hemorrhage. Subcutaneous and mediastinal emphysema are also possible with incorrect placement. Nonetheless, when performed by trained personnel, transtracheal catheterization is a quick means of providing oxygenation and ventilation when other methods fail.

Cricothyrotomy. A cricothyrotomy is a surgical procedure that opens a passageway through the cricothyroid membrane (refer to Figure 23-27). Once the opening is established, an endotracheal tube can be inserted directly into the trachea. As with transtracheal catheterization and insufflation, cricothyrotomy represents a procedure of last resort when trying to secure an obstructed airway.

Since cricothyrotomy establishes a larger opening than that possible with transtracheal catheterization, suctioning of the lower airway is possible with this method. On the other hand, cricothyrotomy can be more time-consuming than transtracheal catheterization. Moreover, incorrectly performed cricothyrotomy can cause permanent damage to the vocal cords or thyroid gland. For these reasons, cricothyrotomy should only be attempted by specially trained and experienced medical professionals.

Ventilation

Accessory equipment used to support ventilation in advanced life support includes manual and oxygen-powered resuscitators.[85] Manual resuscitators, also called bag-valve devices or bag-valve-masks (BVMs), are available for adults, children and infants. Oxygen-powered resuscitators, on the other hand, are strictly limited to adult application.[4]

Bag-valve-mask units (BVMs)

BVMs are devices that combine a self-inflating bag with a nonrebreathing valve mechanism.[85,86] These devices may be used in conjunction with a face mask, endotracheal tube, or esophageal obturator airway. All are capable of providing ventilation with air. When supplied with a supplementary oxygen source, BVMs can provide up to 100% oxygen. Although initially designed as adjuncts for emergency life support, BVMs are used extensively in other respiratory care settings, particularly in the areas of airway management and continuous mechanical ventilation.

Design. Design, performance and testing standards for BVMs have been established by various organizations, including the American Heart Association, American Society for Testing and Materials, and the

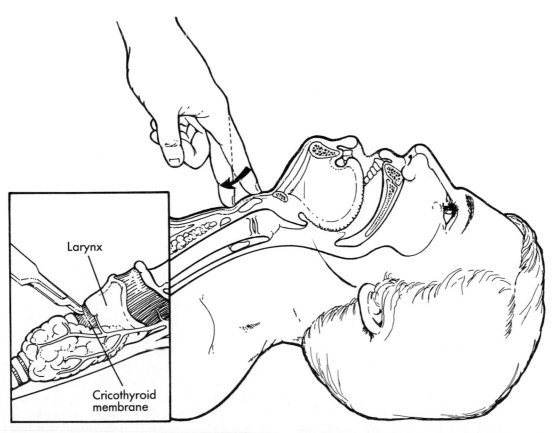

Larynx

Cricothyroid membrane

Fig. 23-27 Cricothyroidotomy.

International Standards Organization.[4,87,88] The 'ideal' adult BVM should be self filling, have standard connectors (15/22 mm) and be easy to clean and sterilize (or disposable). It should have a true nonrebreathing, low resistance, non-jamming valve system that can accept at least 15 L/min oxygen input. At oxygen input flows of 15 L/min, rates of 12/min and tidal volumes between 600 and 800 mL, it should provide an FIO_2 in excess of 0.85.

The ideal BVM should also perform satisfactorily under all common environmental conditions (including temperature extremes) and be available in adult and pediatric sizes. Generally, adult and pediatric BVMs should *not* have any pressure relief valve. Neonatal resuscitators should be equipped with a 40 cm H_2O 'pop-off.' This pop-off should provide an audible signal (to alert the user that gas is being vented), an override mechanism, and a visual indicator of on/off status.

Figure 23-28 provides a schematic of a typical manual resuscitator, showing gas movement and valve action during both the inhalation/compression and exhalation/relaxation phases. Key components shown in this schematic are the nonrebreathing valve

(on the left), the bag itself (heavy black lines in the center), the oxygen inlet and bag inlet valve (to the right of the bag), and the oxygen reservoir tube (far right).

During exhalation (Figure 23-28, *A*), gas flows out from the patient's lungs through the nonrebreathing valve and out to the atmosphere. At the same time (as the bag expands), the intake valve opens and 100% oxygen flows into the bag from both the reservoir and oxygen inlet.

During the inhalation phase (Figure 23-28, *B*), the bag is manually compressed, causing bag pressure to rise. This increase in bag pressure simultaneously closes the inlet valve and opens the nonrebreathing valve, forcing gas into the patient. While the bag inlet valve is closed, oxygen coming in through the oxygen inlet goes into the reservoir tube, where it is stored for the next breath.

Of course this schematic shows only one of many possible designs used by BVM manufacturers. Different BVMs employ different designs and have different capabilities. Several bench studies conducted with these devices show a rather wide range of capability, with some BVMs not meeting accepted standards.[89-95] For this reason, great care must be taken in selecting a BVM for hospital-wide use.

Use. The individual responsible for ventilating a patient with a BVM should position themselves at the top of the victim's head. Ideally, an oral airway should be inserted and the head-tilt used to keep the airway open (assuming no neck injuries). While using one hand to keep the head extended and mask tightly sealed to the patient's face, the RCP uses the other hand to compress the bag (Figure 23-29). For adults, bag compression should deliver a volume of 10 to 15 mL/kg at a moderate flow (lasting about 2 seconds).

Unfortunately, single-rescuer BVM ventilation is consistently less effective than mouth-to-mouth or mouth-to-mask technique ventilation.[96-100] Extensive training is required to effectively apply this method, and some individuals with small hands simply cannot achieve good ventilation using a face mask. Effective ventilation is more likely when two practitioners are available, one to hold the mask and one to squeeze the bag.[4,101] When a partner is not available and you cannot adequately ventilate a patient with a BVM, you should immediately switch to the mouth-to-mouth technique.

In addition to providing adequate ventilation, BVMs should provide a high FIO_2. Although all BVM units on the market theoretically can deliver 100% oxygen, the actual FIO_2 provided at the bedside depends on several factors. These factors include oxygen input flow, reservoir volume, delivered stroke volume and rate, and bag refill time.[91-93] As a general guideline, to achieve the highest possible FIO_2 with a bag-valve-mask unit, you should always: (1) use an oxygen reservoir, (2) provide the highest acceptable

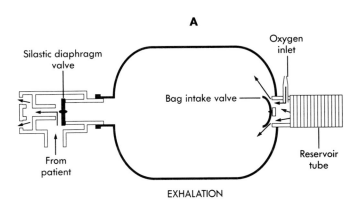

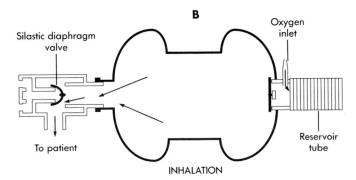

Fig. 23-28 Schematic of a typical BVM relaxation device showing **A**, exhalation/relaxation phase, and **B**, inhalation/compression phase. (From McPherson, SP: Respiratory Therapy equipment, ed 4, St Louis, 1990, Mosby.)

■ MINI **C** LINI ■

23-1

Ventilation During CPR

Problem: You are observing a "Code Blue" in progress in the intensive care unit. The patient is pulseless and cardiac compressions are being administered. You notice that the respiratory care practitioner is ventilating the patient via an endotracheal tube at a considerably higher minute ventilation than one would normally establish on a mechanical ventilator for a patient of this size. Is the increased minute ventilation needed?

Discussion: In cardiopulmonary arrest, the absence of blood flow and oxygenation leads to severe tissue hypoxia, anaerobic metabolism, and lactic acid formation. Both bicarbonate and non-bicarbonate blood buffers work to buffer the lactic acid, and in the case of bicarbonate buffer, carbon dioxide is produced as a by-product:

$$H^+ + HCO_3 \rightarrow H_2CO_3 \rightarrow H_2O + CO_2.$$

Thus, in cardiopulmonary arrest, carbon dioxide is produced not only by tissue metabolism but also by lactic acid buffering. Therefore, artificial ventilation administered during a "Code Blue" should produce larger than "normal" minute ventilation to accommodate the additional carbon dioxide production and to compensate for metabolic lactic acidosis. If sodium bicarbonate is given intravenously, more carbon dioxide would be produced as lactic acid is buffered. This situation would also call for greater alveolar ventilation.

---

oxygen input flow, (3) deliver an appropriate tidal volume over a 2 second period (when using a mask), and (4) assure the longest possible bag refill time.[4,86,101]

Hazards and troubleshooting. BVMs are relatively simple and safe advanced life support devices. However, three major hazards associated with their use bear emphasis. The first and most common problem is unrecognized equipment failure. The second major hazard (occurring only with mask ventilation) is gastric distention. The last major hazard is pulmonary **barotrauma.**

Regarding unrecognized equipment failure, your knowledge of how BVMs operate should help you understand the operational testing and troubleshooting of these devices. First, since these devices provide essential life-support capability, they should never be placed at the bedside or applied to a patient without first confirming their proper operation.

To quickly confirm that a BVM is in proper working order, conduct a simple pressure test. Occlude the patient side of the nonrebreathing valve outlet and vigorously try to compress the bag. If the inlet and outlet valves are in place and properly working, you will encounter a strong resistance to compression and no gas will leak out of the bag. If you can easily compress the bag or gas quickly leaks out, the device is not working properly, and should immediately be replaced.

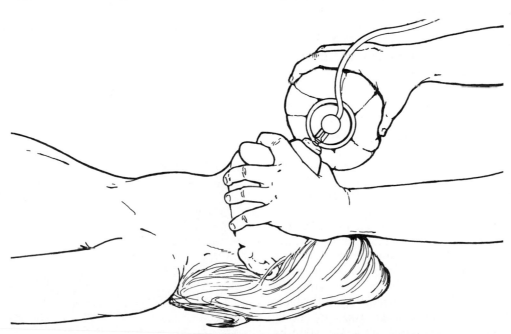

Fig. 23-29 Ventilation using a bag-valve mask and head-tilt/chin-lift method.

Even properly working bags can fail while in use on a patient. Most often, this is due to valve failure or obstruction with foreign material. The telltale signs of BVM failure are a either: (1) a rapid and dramatic *decrease* in the pressure required to compress the bag (usually signalling oxygen inlet valve failure), or (2) an inability of the patient to fully exhale (indicating a jammed or malfunctioning nonrebreathing valve). Whatever the cause of failure, you should never waste time to repair the device. Either replace it immediately or switch to an alternative method of ventilation until a working BVM is available.

Gastric distention is another common hazard encountered when using a bag-valve device with a face mask. As previously discussed under mouth-to-mouth ventilation, gastric distention can be minimized by providing low to moderate inspiratory flows. With a BVM applied to an adult, this means using a full 2 seconds to deliver the tidal volume.[100] Additionally, downward pressure on the cricoid cartilage may reduce gastric insufflation, but should only be used on unconscious victims.[103,104] Pressure is applied using the thumb and forefinger to both sides of the cartilage, just lateral to the midline. Too much cricoid pressure can worsen the situation by causing tracheal compression and obstruction.

Even when these measures are used, some gastric distention is likely. Only by isolating the lower airway with a cuffed endotracheal tube can the problems associated with gastric distention be avoided.

Barotrauma has long been recognized as a potential hazard when using BVMs.[105] However, with the full bag volume of adult BVMs generally no more than 2000 mL, the potential for barotrauma when applied to adults is small. Obviously, using adult BVM on a small child or infant is contraindicated. Moreover, some 'pediatric' BVMs have bag volumes over 500 mL, clearly enough to cause barotrauma if applied to small children or infants. This is why current standards for neonatal BVMs include a required pressure pop-off.[87,88]

However, BVM pressure relief pop-off valves are not without problems. Despite manufacturer's specifications, pressures as high as 106 cm H_2O have been reported with some pediatric pop-off valves.[106,107] In addition, when gas does vent through the BVM pressure relief, both tidal volume and FIO_2 are significantly lower.[85,106] Based on these problems, the best equipment for a trained practitioner to use when ventilating a small child or infant probably is a BVM with an in-line pressure manometer instead of a pressure pop-off.[85] When properly used, this setup generally assures safe and consistent pressure delivery. Alternatively, adjustable volume-controlled manual resuscitators are being developed for use with neonates, and may soon be available.[108]

Oxygen-powered resuscitators

Oxygen-powered resuscitators are manually triggered valves that are powered by compressed oxygen (Figure 23-30). These devices can be used with a mask, an endotracheal tube, an esophageal airway, or a tracheostomy tube. The practitioner provides ventilation by pressing the actuator button or trigger while gauging its adequacy by observing chest movement.

Although simple in concept, oxygen-powered resuscitators present many problems. First, most of these devices deliver high initial flows. High flows increase the likelihood of gastric distention when used with a mask.[109-112] Even in intubated patient, high flow can lead to maldistribution of ventilation and intrapulmonary shunting.

In addition, the flow delivered by these devices varies inversely with airway pressure. Some oxygen-powered resuscitators will stop delivering gas at high airway pressures.[4] This is most likely when the victim has high airway resistance or low compliance, or is receiving in chest compressions.

In addition, oxygen-powered resuscitators seem very prone to malfunction and failure.[85] Failure rates as high as 25% have been reported in the field, with the most common defects being: (1) inadequate inflation pressures, (2) excessive inflation pressures, (3) failure to allow exhalation, and (4) insufficient flow (demand mode).[111] Regarding excessive inflation pressures, there are reports of valve failure and delivery of up to 3,500 cm H_2O pressure to the airway![111,113-115]

Obviously, preventive maintenance can help overcome these problems. In addition, the RCP should quickly check the function of an oxygen-powered resuscitator before applying it to a patient. This can be done simply by inflating a test lung or plastic bag with the device, while observing for proper inflation and deflation. Even with these precautions, the RCP

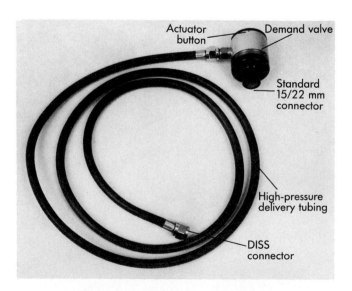

Fig. 23-30 Gas-powered resuscitator.

may still encounter failure of one of these devices at the bedside. Quick recognition of the problems is essential. You can detect inadequate or excessive inflation pressures, or failure to allow exhalation by carefully observing chest movement and auscultating the lungs. You can recognize insufficient flow (demand mode) by observing abnormal patient efforts during spontaneous breathing attempts. If any of these problems are identified, the practitioner should discontinue use of the oxygen-powered resuscitator and provide alternative ventilation and oxygenation.

Based on both clinical demands and past reports of problems, performance and safety standards for oxygen-powered resuscitators have been strengthened.[4,87,88] Ideal characteristics for these devices are provided in the accompanying box.

Unfortunately, few of the oxygen-powered resuscitators in current use meet these criteria. In addition, due to the high trigger pressures and low flows occurring with these devices when operating in the demand mode, they should not be used on spontaneously breathing patients.[4] Last, oxygen-powered resuscitators should never be used to replace the oxygen reservoirs on bag-valve-mask devices.[116]

In summary, oxygen-powered resuscitators are useful but potentially hazardous devices. When considering their use as adjunct equipment in ACLS, the following guidelines apply: (1) they should not be used on pediatric patients, (2) they should be used only on intubated adult patients (due to problems with gastric inflation), (3) personnel using these devices should be trained to recognize malfunctions and institute BVM ventilation should malfunction occur, and (4) units should be inspected and tested before and after each use and regularly maintained.[4,85,117,118]

Ideal characteristics of an oxygen-powered resuscitator[4,87,88]

- Provides a constant flow of 100% oxygen at less than 40 L/min
- Limits inspiratory pressure to 60 cm H_2O via a relief valve
- Allows inspiratory pressure limit up to 80 cm H_2O (under medical direction)
- Sounds an audible alarm whenever the relief valve is activated
- Operates under common environmental conditions and temperature extremes
- Provides demand flow without increasing the work of breathing
- Has a standard 15-mm/22-mm coupling for airways and attachments
- Is rugged, break-resistant, compact and easy to hold
- Has a trigger positioned so that both hands of the rescuer can remain on the mask to hold it in position

---

Transport ventilators

Automatic transport ventilators, or ATVs, have been used both in and outside the hospital setting for nearly 20 years.[119,120] In the US, their acceptance as adjunct equipment for advanced life support has been slow, due mainly to concerns over synchronizing ventilation with chest compressions. According to the American Heart Association, these concerns are unfounded.[4] In patients who are not intubated, one can easily interpose compressions between ATV breaths. And in intubated patients, one does not have to synchronize ventilation with compressions.

Several different models of ATVs are available.[121-125]

When compared with bag-valve ventilation during transport within the hospital, ATVs can better maintain a constant minute ventilation and adequate arterial blood gases.[126,127] Comparable results with bag-valve devices occur only when tidal and minute volumes are constantly monitored.[128]

Outside the hospital, ATVs are at least as good as other devices in providing ventilation and oxygenation to intubated patients.[121,129,130] In addition, both bench studies and animal research suggests that ATVs are better than other methods for ventilating unintubated patients in respiratory arrest.[100] Specifically, when compared to mouth-to-mask, bag-valve-mask, and manually triggered devices, ATVs tends to provide better lung inflation with less gastric insufflation. This is due to the lower inspiratory flow rates and longer inspiratory times provided by ATVs.[4]

ATVs have many advantages over other methods of providing ventilation and oxygenation during emergency life support. These include: (1) freeing the practitioner for other tasks when the patient is intubated, (2) allowing the practitioner to use both hands to maintain the mask position and airway in unintubated patients, and (3) providing a constant tidal volume, rate, and minute ventilation.

Disadvantages of ATVs are few. Most ATVs are pneumatically powered and thus require a high pressure oxygen source to work. Regardless of power source, the practitioner using an ATV must assure that a bag-valve-mask device is always available as a backup in case of power failure. In addition, several ATVs cannot be used on children less than 5 years old.

Perfusion support

Advanced life support techniques designed to enhance perfusion include both alternative compression techniques and adjunct equipment and procedures.

Alternative compression techniques

Recently, several manual techniques that aim to improve perfusion during CPR have been introduced. These include intermittent abdominal compression

---

Ideal characteristics of an automatic transport ventilator[4]

- Functions as constant inspiratory flow generator
- Has a lightweight standard 15 mm/22 mm connector
- Has a breathing circuit with a low compression factor
- Has a pressure manometer to monitor airway pressure
- Is lightweight (2 to 5 kg), compact, and rugged
- Works under all common environmental conditions and temperature extremes
- Normally limits inspiratory pressure to 60 cm H_2O
- Allows inspiratory pressure limit up to 80 cm H_2O (under medical direction)
- Sounds an audible alarm when inspiratory pressure limit reached
- Consumes a minimal amount of gas (at a minute volume of 10 L/min, the device should run for at least 45 minutes on an E cylinder)
- Delivers 100% oxygen ($FIO_2 = 1.0$)
- Provides inspiratory times of 2 seconds (adults) and 1 second (children)
- Provides inspiratory flows of about 30 L/min (adults) and 15 L/min (children)
- Provides at least two rates, 10/min (adults); 20/min (children)
- Has an alarm to indicate loss of source gas
- Has an alarm to indicate patient disconnection
- If a demand flow valve is incorporated, it should deliver a peak inspiratory flow rate on demand of at least 100 L/min at −2 cm triggering pressure to minimize the work of breathing.

CPR (IAC-CPR),[131-136] simultaneous ventilation and compression (with or without abdominal binding),[137-142] active chest compression-decompression,[143] and high-frequency chest compression.[144-146]

During intermittent abdominal compression CPR (IAC-CPR), the patient's abdomen is compressed during the relaxation phase of chest compression. Survival rates among patients resuscitated with IAC-CPR tend to be higher than with standard CPR in the hospital setting. However, IAC-CPR performed outside the hospital has not shown major advantages.[131,132]

Additional new approaches take advantage of the entire thorax as a pump during CPR. These methods include simultaneous ventilation and abdominal binding with chest compression.[137-142] Although research has shown that these methods can improve hemodynamics over standard CPR,[137,138] improvement in actual resuscitation outcomes has not been demonstrated.[139] For this reason, the American Heart Association does not currently recommended simultaneous ventilation and compression CPR for treatment of patients in cardiac arrest.[4]

Active compression-decompression CPR is performed with a hand-held suction device applied to the mid-sternum.[143] The device is used to compress the sternum in the usual way (100 compressions/min, with a compression depth of 1.5 to 2 inches and a 50% duty cycle). During the relaxation phase, however, the chest is actively decompressed by pulling upward on the suction device. Animal research indicates that active compression-decompression CPR provides higher coronary and systemic arterial pressures than standard CPR.[143] Further research is needed before this technique becomes adopted for use on humans.

High-frequency CPR is the last of the new alternative CPR techniques proposed to improve perfusion during cardiac arrest. In animal studies, increasing the compression rate to 120/min appears to improve both perfusion pressures and resuscitation outcomes.[144-146] Human trials are needed to determine how well this method works for cardiac arrest victims.[4]

In summary, there are several new approaches being proposed to improve perfusion during cardiac arrest. Of these, intermittent abdominal compression CPR (IAC-CPR) appears to be best researched among human subjects and thus is closest to acceptance as an adjunct technique in advanced cardiac life support.

Adjunct equipment and procedures

The primary noninvasive equipment used to support perfusion during cardiac arrest is the mechanical chest compressor. Additional noninvasive approaches include the CPR vest and the pneumatic antishock garment. Invasive methods include internal cardiac compression, cardiopulmonary bypass, and intra-aortic balloon counterpulsation.

Mechanical compressors. Several types of mechanical compressors are available to provide chest compressions. Properly applied, these devices can provide an optimum pattern of chest compression and eliminate the rapid fatigue that occurs with manual techniques.[147] Although models for children and infants have been marketed, the American Heart Association currently recommends that manual compressors be used only with adults.[4] The hazards of mechanical compressors are essentially the same as those common to manual chest compression, including the potential for separation of the ribs at the costochondral junction, sternal fractures, and organ lacerations. The major drawback in their use is the potential for delay or interruption in the application of manual chest compression while setting up or adjusting the apparatus.

The manually operated chest compressor consists of a simple, reliable, and low-cost lever device that easy to set up and use (Figure 23-31). Ideally, the user should be able to adjust the movement of the plunger head from 1.5 to 2.0 inches.[4]

The pneumatic mechanical chest compressor is

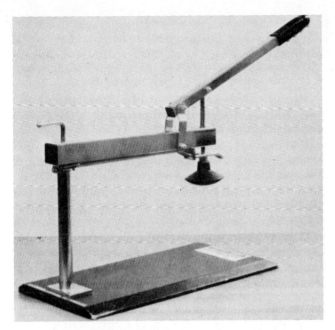

Fig. 23-31 Portable hand pump for external cardiac massage designed by Dr. James J. Lally. The plunger can be adjusted according to the individual's size. (From Stephenson HE Jr: Cardiac arrest and resuscitation, ed 4, St Louis, 1974, Mosby.)

powered by compressed gas and provides user-adjustable rates, plunger displacements, and compression-to-relaxation ratios (Figure 23-32). Most pneumatic mechanical chest compressors are also capable of providing ventilation via an automatically-cycled, pressure limited valve similar in design to the oxygen powered resuscitators previously described. These compressor-ventilators are most effective when used in conjunction with a cuffed endotracheal tube.

Both these devices produce hemodynamic results

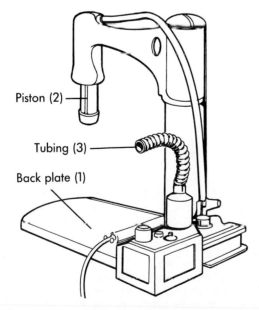

Piston (2)

Tubing (3)

Back plate (1)

Fig. 23-32 Pneumatically powered chest compressor.

comparable to manual chest compression[145,147,148] However, mechanical compressors can limit mobility when the victim must be transported, and constant monitoring by trained personnel is essential in maintaining the correct position of the plunger.

CPR vest. Looking much like a large blood pressure cuff, the CPR vest is a pneumatically-powered gas bladder that encircles the patient's thorax. Intermittent positive pressure applied to the vest increases intrathoracic pressure, thus taking advantage of the thoracic-pump mechanism for enhancing blood flow. Although research has shown that the CPR vest can improve patient hemodynamics during cardiac arrest, actual patient outcome data is limited.[139-141] For this reason, the American Heart Association does not yet recommend routine use of the CPR vest for cardiac arrest victims.[4]

Pneumatic antishock garment (MAST). The pneumatic antishock garment (also called Military Anti-Shock Trousers, or MAST) was developed for field treatment of hypovolemic shock due to massive blood loss. When inflated, this device applies continuous pressure to the lower extremities and abdomen, thereby compressing the large veins, increasing peripheral resistance, and raising the mean arterial blood pressure. Despite its usefulness in treating hypovolemic shock, no evidence exists to support its application in cardiac arrest.[4,149]

Internal (open-chest) cardiac massage. Open-chest cardiac massage involves surgical exposure of the pericardium by thoracotomy and direct manual compression of the heart by a surgeon's hand (Figure 23-33, on page 610). This technique can provide near-normal perfusion to the brain and heart.[150-155] Moreover, if applied within the first 25 minutes of cardiac arrest, direct cardiac massage can improve survival.[153,154] However, due to its many complications, the routine use of this method is not justified.[4]

Open-chest cardiac massage is indicated in patients with penetrating chest trauma who develop cardiac arrest. Other indications include: (1) cardiac arrest caused by hypothermia, pulmonary embolism, pericardial tamponade, or abdominal hemorrhage, (2) chest deformity where closed-chest CPR is ineffective, (3) penetrating abdominal trauma with deterioration and cardiac arrest, and (4) blunt trauma with cardiac arrest.[156,157]

Extracorporeal circulation. Emergency treatment of patients in cardiac arrest has been provided by portable heart-lung machines or pump-oxygenators. The bypass pump is connected via the femoral artery and vein, making a thoracotomy unnecessary. Oxygenation is provided by a membrane element, as with standard ECMO. Although feasible in selected patients,[158-161] this approach is confined to centers where it is available. In addition, the time required to institute cardiopulmonary bypass limits its use as an emergency support measure.

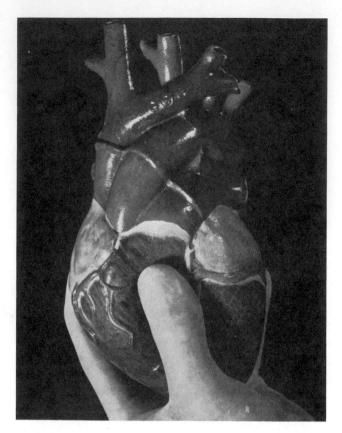

Fig. 23-33 With apex of heart cupped in practitioner's palm, fingers are extended toward base of heart posteriorly and thumb is extended toward base of heart anteriorly for internal cardiac compression. (From Stephenson HE Jr: Cardiac arrest and resuscitation, ed 4, St Louis, 1974, Mosby.)

Intra-aortic balloon counterpulsation. Intra-aortic balloon counterpulsation is a mechanical procedure that increases mean aortic pressures and coronary blood flow to the myocardium during diastole. This is done by placing a gas-actuated balloon in the descending aorta. Synchronous inflation of the balloon after left ventricular contraction provides a forceful counterpulsation. This counterpulsation boosts back flow into the aortic arch and coronary arteries (Figure 23-34). Since this counterpulsation only augments existing left ventricular function, the intra-aortic balloon cannot, by itself, provide adequate perfusion in the event of true cardiac arrest.

Currently, this device is used mainly to provide interim support for: (1) patients with mechanical failure of the left ventricle that is surgically correctable, or (2) patients exhibiting poor ventricular function after coronary bypass surgery.

Restoration of cardiac function

Perfusion support techniques can only restore circulation temporarily. Advanced cardiac life support must go beyond simple perfusion support and try to identify, remove, or relieve the underlying cause of cardiac failure. This is done by combining electrocardiographic (ECG) monitoring with drug and electrical therapies.

Electrocardiographic (ECG) monitoring

Because most cases of cardiac arrest are due to arrhythmias, ECG monitoring should be started as soon as the needed equipment and personnel arrive.[4] This may be done with either standard ECG equipment or the quick-look paddles now available on most defibrillators.

Given their important role in ACLS, RCPs must be skilled in arrhythmia recognition. Although the experienced RCP may be able to quickly interpret gross arrhythmias appearing on ECG monitors at the bed-

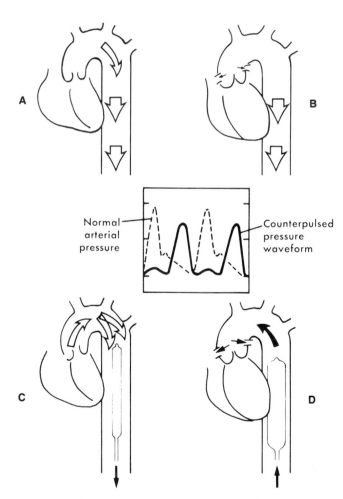

Fig. 23-34 Physiology of counterpulsation. Diagram of normal cardiac cycle pressure flow sequence compared with counterpulsed pressure flow sequence. **A,** Normal systole, characterized by antegrade volume flow and peak intra-aortic pressures. **B,** Normal diastole, showing continued antegrade volume flow and adequate intra-aortic pressure for coronary perfusion. **C,** Balloon deflation before systole, allowing antegrade volume flow from the aortic arch (systolic unloading). **D,** Counterpulsed diastole, mechanically boosting volume flow retrograde to the aortic arch, heightening diastolic pressure and coronary perfusion. (From Shroeder JS, Daily EK: Techniques in bedside hemodynamic monitoring, St Louis, 1976, Mosby.)

II

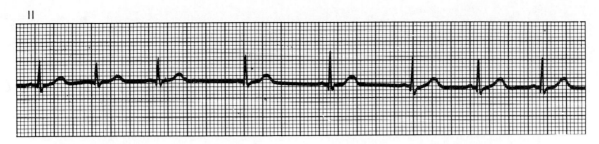

Fig. 23-35 Sinus arrhythmia. (From Conover MH: Cardiac arrhythmias: exercises in pattern interpretation, ed 2, St Louis, 1978, Mosby.)

side, these skills only develop after much practice with actual rhythm strips.

Comprehensive examination of ECG rhythm strips proceeds through four systematic steps. First, one calculates the heart rate, using the number of R-R intervals in a 6 second time period and then multiplying by 10. Then, again using the R-R interval, one determines the regularity of the rhythm. Next, one determines the presence or absence of P waves, their shape, and the duration of the P-R interval. Last, one inspects the QRS complex and measures its duration.[162-165]

When monitoring a patient's ECG, the clinician must always be aware of the old adage "treat the patient, not the monitor." Judgments about the patient's clinical condition should always direct the course of any therapy. As such, the RCP must always be aware of the patient's clinical condition. Moreover, the RCP should always be on guard for factors predisposing patients to develop cardiac arrhythmias, such as acidosis and hypokalemia.

Without attempting an exhaustive analysis, we will review the most common arrhythmias, with an emphasis on those that are life-threatening. Table 23-1, page 612 summarizes these arrhythmias and their key features, categorized by the site at which they originate.[162-165]

Sinus arrhythmia (Figure 23-35). Sinus arrhythmia is the most frequent and least harmful of all arrhythmias. It tends to occur most frequently in the young, but can be found at almost any age. Its key feature is an irregular but rhythmic change in cardiac rate usually synchronous with the respiratory cycle.[162-165] Typically, the heart rate increases during inspiration and decreases during expiration. Otherwise the overall rate, P waves, P-R interval, and QRS complex are normal. Presumably, sinus arrhythmia is caused by alterations in the strength of vagal (parasympathetic) tone on the sinus node. This condition has no pathologic implications, and no treatment is indicated.

Sinus tachycardia (Figure 23-36). In sinus tachycardia, the sinus node discharges at rates between 100 to 160 per minute. Typically, the rhythm is regular, and the P waves, P-R interval, and QRS complex are normal.[162-165]

Sinus tachycardia is caused by many factors. Sympathetic stimulation (fear, anxiety, pain, adrenal release of epinephrine, adrenergic drugs) is the most common cause. Parasympathetic inhibition, like that caused by atropine and its derivatives, has a similar effect. Increased metabolic demand, such as may occur with fever, trauma, or **hyperthyroidism,** can also increase the rate of sinus node discharge. Sinus tachycardia can also be caused by hypoxemia, hypercapnia and hypotension. In fact, any condition causing decreased blood pressure can result in tachycardia. This is why this arrhythmia is commonly seen in conditions such as shock, congestive heart failure, acute myocardial infarction, and pulmonary embolism.

V₁

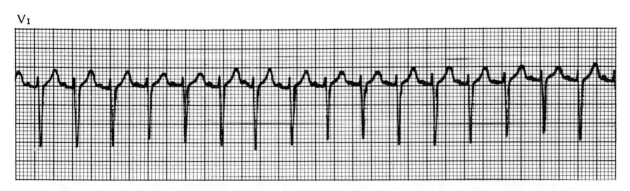

Fig. 23-36 Sinus tachycardia. (From Conover MH: Cardiac arrhythmias: exercises in pattern interpretation, ed 2, St Louis, 1978, Mosby.)

Table 23–1   Summary of common cardiac arrhythmias

Arrhythmia	Category	Rate	Rhythm	P waves	PR interval	QRS complex	Treatment	Comments
Sinus arrhythmia	Benign	60–100/min	Irregular	Normal	Normal	Normal	None	Heart rate periodically increases and decreases
Sinus tachycardia	Minor	100–160/min	Regular	Normal	Normal	Normal	Remove underlying cause	May result from sympathetic stimulation or para-sympathetic inhibition; also increased metabolic rates, hypoxemia
Sinus bradycardia	Minor	40–60/min	Regular	Normal	Normal	Normal	Remove underlying cause; atropine	May result from excessive parasympathetic stimulation
Sinoatrial arrest	Minor	60–100/min; lower with missed beats	Regular except missed beat	Normal	Normal	Normal	None unless frequent; treat underlying cause, pacer may be needed	May result from excessive parasympathetic stimulation
Premature atrial contractions	< 6 min/minor > 6/min major	60–100/min	Regular except PAC	PAC p-wave abnormal	PAC PR may be < 0.12	Normal	< 6/min none; > 6/min antiarrhythmics such as quinidine or procainamide	Caused by atrial irritability; no compensatory pause (compare with PVCs)
Paroxysmal supraventricular tachycardia	Major	160–250/min	Regular	May be hidden or abnormal	Difficult to assess	Normal; some may be widened	Cartoid artery massage; adenosine, verapamil, adrenergic antagonists, digitalis, procainamide; synchronous cardioversion	Caused by atrial irritability; may compromise ventricular filling
Atrial flutter	Major	atrial: 200–400/min ventricular; 60–150/min	Depends on conduction (regular or irregular)	"F" waves saw-tooth pattern	Difficult to assess	Normal	Adrenergic antagonists, Beta blockers, digitalis, quinidine, procainamide; synchronous cardioversion	Ratio of blocked to trans-mitted impulses may be constant at 2:1, 3:1, or 4:1
Atrial fibrillation	Major	atrial: > 350/min ventricular: variable	Markedly irregular	Indistinguish-able; uneven baseline	Indistinguish-able	Normal	Synchronous cardioversion, procainamide; digitalis, propranolol	May compromise ventricular filling, resulting in pulse deficit

	Severity	Rate	Rhythm	P wave	PR	QRS	Treatment	Comments
First degree atrioventricular block	Major	60–100/min	Regular	Normal	PR > 0.20	Normal	None	Delayed AV nodal conduction; may be caused by ischemia or digitalis
Second degree atrioventricular block (Mobitz type 2)	Major	60–100/min	Regular	Normal; some not conducted	Normal or prolonged; fixed PR	Normal; some dropped at regular ratio (3:2, 4:3, etc)	Electrical pacemaker	Most often caused by ischemia; may progress to 3rd degree
Second degree atrioventricular block (Wenckebach type)	Major	60–100/min	Irregular	Normal; some not conducted	Progressive increase in PR time	Normal; some dropped at regular ratio (3:2, 4:3, etc)	Pacer, atropine, isoproterenol, epinephrine	Most often caused by ischemia; may progress to 3rd degree
Third degree atrioventricular block	Major; can be lethal	atrial may be normal ventricular: < 40/min	Regular but AV separate	Normal	Cannot be determined	Usually normal; may be widened	Electrical pacemaker, atropine, dopamine, epinephrine	May result in episodes of cerebral ischemia
Premature ventricular contractions	< 6/min major > 6/min major	60–100/min	Regular except PVC	Normal; none with PVC	Normal; none with PVC	>0.12 sec; distorted	Antiarrhythmics such as lidocaine	indicates ventricular irritability; compensatory pause is normal RT wave leads to ventricular tachycardia
Ventricular tachycardia	Major; can be lethal	140–200/min	Usually regular	Absent or hidden	Absent or hidden	Continuous PVCs; same amplitude	Lidocaine countershock	May compromise ventricular filling & cause shock; can resolve itself
Torsade de pointes	Major; can be lethal	140–200/min	Usually regular	Absent or hidden	Absent or hidden	Continuous PVCs; changing axis and amplitude	Magnesium; procainamide, countershock	A more serious form of ventricular tachycardia
Ventricular fibrillation	Lethal	Cannot be determined	Cannot be determined	Absent	Absent	Chaotic; no defined pattern	Defibrillation	No cardiac output

II

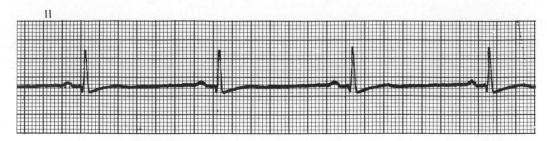

Fig. 23-37 Sinus bradycardia. (From Conover MH: Cardiac arrhythmias: exercises in pattern interpretation, ed 2, St Louis, 1978, Mosby.)

Sinus tachycardia is the body's response to some underlying condition. As such, sinus tachycardia should be viewed more as a symptom than a pathology. Thus treatment should be directed at the underlying cause.

Sinus bradycardia (Figure 23-37). In sinus bradycardia, the sinus node discharges at rates less than 60/min. Typically, the rhythm is regular, and the P waves, P-R interval, and QRS complex are normal.[162-165]

As with sinus tachycardia, various factors can contribute to a decreased rate of sinus node discharge, not all of which are abnormal. For example, heart rates less than 60/min are not uncommon in highly conditioned athletes.

In the clinical setting, however, sinus bradycardia is most often caused by an increased level of parasympathetic tone. The most common factors increasing parasympathetic tone are vagal stimulation and administration of adrenergic blocking agents. Hypothermia and increased intracranial pressure may also slow the sinus node.

Decisions to treat sinus bradycardia revolve around two key questions: (1) are there serious signs and symptoms? (2) are the signs and symptoms related to the slow heart rate? Serious signs and symptoms include ischemic chest pain, shortness of breath or CHF, decreased consciousness, hypotension, or PVCs in the setting of acute myocardial infarction. If a decision to treat sinus bradycardia is made, atropine, a parasympatholytic, is the drug of choice.[166] In addition to atropine, transcutaneous pacing may be required. Should atropine and pacing fail, the use of

sympathetic agents such as dopamine or epinephrine may be considered.[4]

Sinus arrest (Figure 23-38). As the name implies, sinus arrest causes cardiac standstill. Although sinus arrest can be prolonged, it usually shows up on the ECG as an intermittent dropped beat.[162-165] Thus the underlying rate is normal, the rhythm is regular (except for the missed beats), and P waves, P-R intervals and QRS complexes are all normal.

The basic defect in sinoatrial arrest is failure of the sinus node to initiate an impulse. Most often, this is due to strong vagal impulses. Although this is usually a temporary problem, prolonged or recurrent failure of the SA node to discharge can lead to severe bradycardia or cardiac arrest. Sinus arrest may accompany the early stages of anesthesia or certain bodily manipulations that elicit a strong vagal reflex. Strong vagal reflexes are common during endoscopic procedures (including bronchoscopy, laryngoscopy, and endotracheal intubation), and whenever thoracic organs are manipulated during surgery. Prolonged or recurrent sinus arrest that adversely effects cardiac output is normally treated with electrical therapy (see following section). Alternatively, drugs such as atropine[167] or epinephrine may also be used.

Premature atrial contractions (Figure 23-39). As described in Chapter 10, any area of the heart can initiate an action potential. Localized areas of the atria, A-V junction, and ventricles are the most common sites for such independent excitation. Because they occur away from the normal focus of stimulation, these independent discharges are referred to as *ectopic foci.*

II

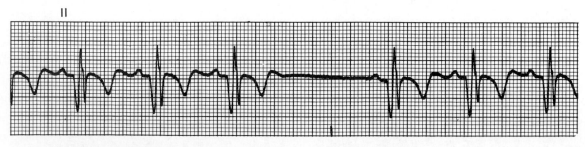

Fig. 23-38 Sinus arrest. (From Conover MH: Cardiac arrhythmias: exercises in pattern interpretation, ed 2, St Louis, 1978, Mosby.)

II

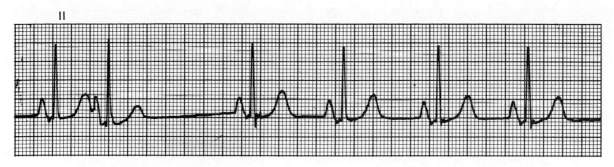

Fig. 23–39 Premature atrial contraction. (From Conover MH: Cardiac arrhythmias: exercises in pattern interpretation, ed 2, St Louis, 1978, Mosby.)

The underlying cause of any premature contraction is increased myocardium excitability.[162-165] Although strong sympathetic stimulation is the most common cause, increased myocardium excitability is also associated with hypoxemia, hypercapnia, and acidosis.

A premature atrial contraction (PAC) typically occurs at normal cardiac rates. Because the action potential arises from other than the sinus node, the P wave is often abnormal in shape. Although a normal QRS follows the abnormal P wave, (the P-R interval can vary) there usually is a slight delay before the next normal sinus discharge. However, this delay is normally shorter than the compensatory pause seen with premature ventricular contractions.[61] Thus, except for the PAC itself, the rhythm is regular.

Although PACs usually do not cause serious signs or symptoms, they do indicate the presence of an irritable focus which can interfere with normal cardiac function. Thus treatment is directed at the underlying cause. For example, if hypoxemia is suspected as a contributing factor, then supplemental oxygen would be indicated. Antiarrhythmic drugs are indicated only when PACs are multifocal in origin or occur at a rate of more than 6/min.

Supraventricular tachycardia (SVT) (Figure 23-40). The term supraventricular tachycardia is commonly used to describe any tachycardia *not* of ventricular origin. This grouping can include sinus tachycardia,

atrial tachycardia, junctional tachycardia, atrial flutter, and atrial fibrillation (with rates above 100). These individual supraventricular arrhythmias should be identified by ECG and treated accordingly.

A more specific form of SVT involves rapid impulse formation due to a re-entry mechanism that develops in the atria and/or AV junction. Normally, a single impulse from the SA node transverses the atria and continues down into the ventricles, causing depolarization and contraction. In re-entry, an ectopic focus disrupts this normal conduction. The impulse not only moves down to the ventricles, but also returns back to the atria. This pattern repeats itself over and over in a self-perpetuating or circular manner.

Typically, this form of SVT results in heart rates between 160 and 220/min. The rhythm is regular, which distinguishes it from rapid atrial fibrillation. However, due to its rapid rate, P waves may not be seen. If identifiable, the P waves look abnormal. In addition to the rate and regular rhythm, SVT is characterized by a normal QRS complex. At very high SVT rates, the ventricles may not have enough time to completely fill. Incomplete ventricular filling can result in decreased cardiac output and congestive failure.

The treatment of SVT varies according to the clinical situation. If the patient with SVT is ill or

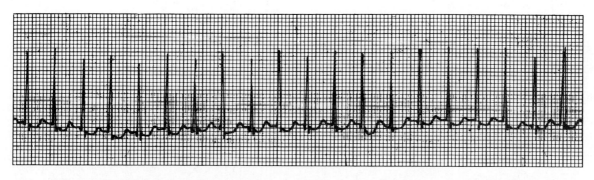

Fig. 23–40 Paroxysmal supraventricular tachycardia. (From Conover MH: Cardiac arrhythmias: exercises in pattern interpretation, ed 2, St Louis, 1978, Mosby.)

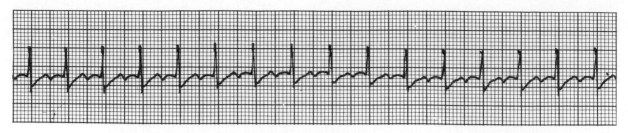

Fig. 23-41 Atrial flutter with 2:1 atrioventricular conductions. (From Conover MH: Cardiac arrhythmias: exercises in pattern interpretation, ed 2, St Louis, 1978, Mosby.)

unstable, the treatment of choice is immediate synchronized electrical cardioversion (described subsequently). If the patient is stable, other interventions are tried before considering cardioversion. The most common nonelectrical treatment for SVT is vagal stimulation via carotid artery massage or the **Valsalva maneuver.** If these attempts are ineffective and the patient remains stable, drugs such as adenosine or verapamil may halt SVT.[168] Other second line drugs include digoxin and beta blockers.

Atrial flutter (Figure 23-41). Atrial flutter is named for the flutter-like or sawtooth pattern seen on the ECG. Atrial flutter is caused by either a rapid circular movement of a stimulus or a repetitive single ectopic focus exciting the atria. These impulses occur with a clock-like regularity at rates between 250 to 300/min. True P waves are absent, being replaced by the characteristic "F" or flutter waves.

Because the AV node usually does not transmit more than 180 impulses per minute, many of the atrial impulses are blocked. The ratio of blocked to transmitted impulses often occurs at a constant ratio, such as 2:1, 3:1, or 4:1.[162-165] Actual ventricular rates vary with the degree of block, normally ranging between 60 to 150/min. Depending on conduction, the ventricular rate may be either regular or irregular. In rare cases, the AV node will transmit all or most of the atrial impulses, resulting in ventricular rates as high as 300/min. Ventricular rates this high always result in acute cardiac failure.

Flutter is usually caused by disease, and, even with

a partial block, the ventricular rate may be high enough to compromise cardiac filling and emptying. In the stable patient, supplemental oxygen and close observation may be the best immediate approach. In the patient with symptoms, efforts are made to control the ventricular rate and restore a normal sinus rhythm. Drug agents, including beta blockers and calcium channel blockers (such as verapamil), can help achieve these goals. However, when atrial flutter causes hemodynamic instability, synchronized electrical cardioversion is indicated.

Atrial fibrillation (Figure 23-42). Atrial fibrillation is among the most common major arrhythmias. In atrial fibrillation the atria are subject to a completely uncontrolled, irregular barrage of impulses at rates above 350/min. The AV node transmits as many of these impulses as it can, resulting in a chaotic and irregular ventricular response. P waves and P-R intervals are present, being replaced by irregular undulations of the isoelectric baseline.

During atrial fibrillation, some ventricular contractions are too weak to be palpated at peripheral locations. This causes a difference between the cardiac rate determined by auscultation over the precordium, and that palpated at a peripheral artery. This phenomenon is called a *pulse deficit,* and is a cardinal clinical sign of atrial fibrillation.[162-165]

Fairly normal activity is not incompatible with atrial fibrillation, as long as the ventricular rate is controlled. However, atrial fibrillation can impair ventricular filling. In fact, without the ventricular

V₁

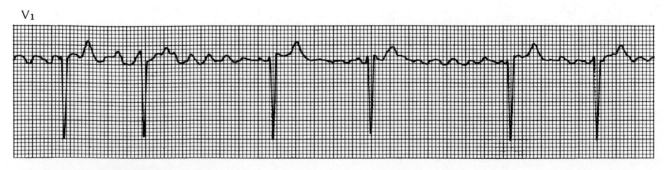

Fig. 23-42 Atrial fibrillation. (From Conover MH: Cardiac arrhythmias: exercises in pattern interpretation, ed 2, St Louis, 1978, Mosby.)

priming that normal atrial contractions provide, atrial fibrillation can decrease cardiac output by as much as 25%. In addition, retention of blood in the atria raises the risk of blood clotting and thrombus formation, with subsequent embolization.

Generally, treatment for atrial fibrillation is indicated when the patient has either a high ventricular rate or clinical signs of decreased cardiac output. As with atrial flutter, treatment options include selected drugs (beta blockers, calcium channel blockers) and electrical cardioversion.

Atrioventricular block (Figure 23-43, 23-44, 23-45). Myocardium disorders caused by inflammation, infarction or ischemia can impair or block sinus impulse conduction through the A-V node or the bundle

of His.[162-165] A similar effect is caused by the toxic reaction of the myocardium to digitalis or its derivatives. Arrhythmias caused by impaired or blocked sinus impulse conduction through the A-V node or the bundle of His are collectively called atrioventricular (A-V) block.

Depending upon the severity of the conduction disturbance, three levels of A-V block are recognized. In order of their relative severity, these are termed first degree, second degree, and third degree heart block.

If the only abnormality is a prolonged P-R interval (greater than .20 seconds), the block is considered as first degree and is caused by a consistent delay in conduction across the AV node (Figure 23-44). If

V₁

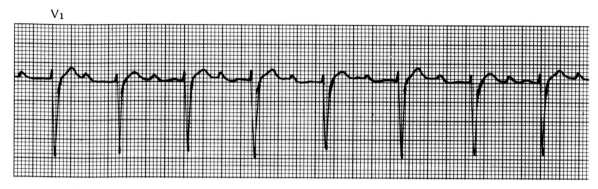

Fig. 23-43 First-degree heart block. (From Conover MH: Cardiac arrhythmias: exercises in pattern interpretation, ed 2, St Louis, 1978, Mosby.)

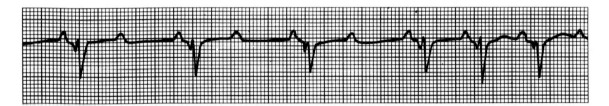

Fig. 23-44 Second-degree heart block (Mobitz type II). (From Conover MH: Cardiac arrhythmias: exercises in pattern interpretation, ed 2, St Louis, 1978, Mosby.)

V₁

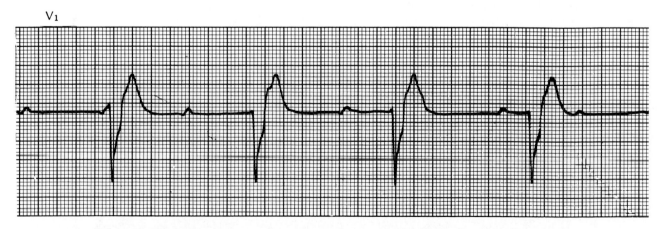

Fig. 23-45 Third-degree heart block. (From Conover MH: Cardiac arrhythmias: exercises in pattern interpretation, ed 2, St Louis, 1978, Mosby.)

some atrial impulses are conducted but others are dropped—resulting in two or three times as many P waves as QRS complexes—the block is termed second degree (See Figure 23-45). If no atrial impulses are conducted to the ventricles, the block is considered third degree, or "complete" (Figure 23-46).[162-165]

Were it not for the ability of myocardial tissue below the AV node to develop its own impulses, third degree heart block always would be lethal. Fortunately, all myocardial tissue has the ability to generate action potentials, and thus serve as the heart's pacemaker. However, ventricular pacemaker tissue tends to discharge at much slower rates than the sinus node, typically 20 to 40/min. This rate may not always be sufficient to provide adequate blood flow. In addition, third degree AV block tends to be unstable and can deteriorate into ventricular standstill. Acute unconsciousness may occur without warning, resulting in Stokes-Adams syncope (fainting). Convulsions and death may accompany such episodes.

First degree A-V block generally causes no symptoms and is not treated. External pacing is the treatment of choice for the symptomatic patient with second and third degree AV block. Pharmacologic intervention may be indicated until a pacemaker is available. Appropriate drug agents include atropine (in certain cases), dopamine, and epinephrine.[4]

Premature ventricular contractions (Figure 23-46). A premature ventricular contraction, or PVC, occurs when an ectopic focus in the ventricles spontaneously depolarizes. Since a PVC starts at the opposite end of the conduction chain, its path through the ventricles is grossly abnormal. The result is a widened and distorted QRS complex, and often an irregular T wave. Rates are generally normal, and the rhythm is regular, with the exception of the premature beat. P waves and P-R intervals are normal in sinus beats, but missing during the premature depolarization.

The distinguishing feature of premature ventricular contractions is the longer than normal refractory period they impart to myocardial fibers.[162-165] Because the extra ectopic stimulus occurs out of phase, it interferes with the usual sequence of excitability and refractoriness and causes a lag before the next contraction. This is called a *compensatory pause*. A full compensatory pause exists when the interval between the premature beat and the next normal one is twice as long as the interval between two normal beats.

PVCs indicate increased irritability of the ventricles. This may be due to either an increase in sympathetic stimulation or local factors. Among the most common local factors increasing ventricular irritability are hypoxia and electrolyte disturbances.

Symptoms may be absent, or the patient may complain of palpitations or a thumping in the chest. The patient may actually be aware of the absence of heart action during the compensatory pause, as well as the difference in contractile force between normal and some abnormal beats.

The clinical significance of PVCs generally depends on their frequency and the presence or absence of underlying disease. Infrequently occurring unifocal PVCs are commonly observed in clinical practice, and may not require treatment. In patients with myocardial ischemia or infarction, aggressive treatment is indicated if the PVCs: (1) are frequent (greater than six per minute), (2) originate from multiple foci, (3) occur close to the T wave, or (4) occur in pairs.[162-165]

Treatment of PVCs includes correction of any underlying electrolyte imbalances (most notably hypokalemia and hypomagnesemia), and the use of selected antiarrhythmic agents, especially lidocaine (discussed subsequently).[168]

Ventricular tachycardia (Figure 23-47). Ventricular tachycardia ('V-Tach') occurs when one or more irritable foci within the ventricle discharge at rapid rates, creating the appearance of a prolonged chain of PVCs. Rates typically range from 140 to 220/min, and are usually regular. Due to the dissociation of atrial and ventricular conduction, P waves may be buried in the QRS complex and therefore not easily seen.[162-165] A variant of ventricular tachycardia, called torsade de pointes, is characterized by gradual alteration in the

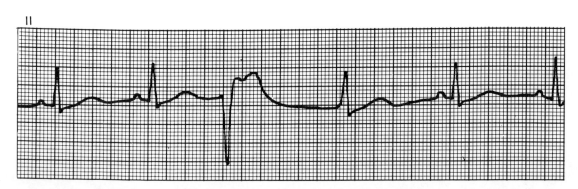

Fig. 23-46 Premature ventricular contraction. (From Conover MH: Cardiac arrhythmias: exercises in pattern interpretation, ed 2, St Louis, 1978, Mosby.)

V₁

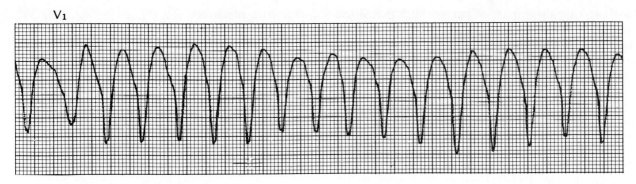

Fig. 23-47 Ventricular tachycardia. (From Conover MH: Cardiac arrhythmias: exercises in pattern interpretation, ed 2, St Louis, 1978, Mosby.)

amplitude and direction of the electrical activity of the ventricles.[169]

Although it may come and go in brief episodes or paroxysms, ventricular tachycardia is always a sign of serious underlying pathology, and should be treated immediately. Short, self-limiting runs of V-Tach are generally managed with lidocaine. If lidocaine does not work, first procainamide and then bretylium may be used.[168]

In patients with sustained V-Tach who exhibit hypotension, ischemic chest pain, shortness of breath, decreased consciousness, or signs of pulmonary edema, immediate synchronized cardioversion is indicated. Patients with sustained V-Tach in full cardiac arrest are treated similarly to patients with ventricular fibrillation (described below). Torsade de pointes is best treated by electrical pacing.[4] However, magnesium sulfate may be used to treat this form of ventricular tachycardia.

Ventricular fibrillation (Figure 23-48). Ventricular fibrillation ('V-Fib') represents a rapid, sustained, and uncontrolled depolarization of the ventricles. During V-Fib, the ECG is characterized by irregular, widened, and poorly defined QRS complexes. Rather than exhibiting coordinated contractions, the ventricles quiver in a totally disorganized manner. Thus, cardiac output during ventricular fibrillation is essentially zero. The rapid fall in cardiac output produces an acute cerebral hypoxia, often manifested by convulsions. For this reason, V-Fib is uniformly fatal if not corrected immediately.

Many conditions can cause ventricular fibrillation. The most common causes include electric shock, anesthesia, mechanical irritation of the heart, severe hypoxia, myocardial infarction, and large doses of digitalis or epinephrine.

Regardless of cause, ventricular fibrillation constitutes a true emergency situation. Patient survival depends on immediate provision of advanced cardiac life support, especially electrical defibrillation. Early defibrillation is the major determinate of survival in cardiac arrest due to V-Fib.[4]

Drug intervention

Although the full scope of drug use in ACLS is beyond the scope of this chapter, RCPs must have general knowledge of both the various drug categories and specific agents used in emergency situations.[168]

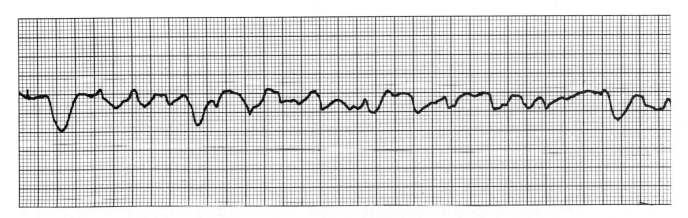

Fig. 23-48 Ventricular fibrillation. (From Conover MH: Cardiac arrhythmias: exercises in pattern interpretation, ed 2, St Louis, 1978, Mosby.)

We will provide a summary of current pharmacologic management of emergency cardiovascular problems.

Routes of administration. Unless a central vein is already cannulated, the ideal route for drug administration in emergency situations is a peripheral intravenous (IV) line.[4] IV drugs should be given by rapid bolus injection, followed by a 20-mL bolus of IV fluid and elevation of the extremity.[170]

Selected drugs (epinephrine, lidocaine, and atropine) may also be given via an endotracheal tube.[171,172] Higher doses in larger volumes are necessary if this route is used. For intratracheal installation, 2 to 2.5 times the usual IV dose should be given, diluted in 10 mL of normal saline or distilled water.[173]

The intraosseous route is also an option, especially in small children or infants. Direct intracardiac injection is indicated only for epinephrine, and then only if no other route is available.[4]

Major drug categories and agents. Table 23-2, on pages 622-623, summarizes the major drug categories and primary agents currently used in advanced cardiac life support. These include oxygen, IV fluids, analgesics, drugs that control heart rate and rhythm, drugs that improve cardiac output and blood pressure, sodium bicarbonate, diuretics, and thrombolytic agents.

Oxygen. Control of hypoxemia is a high priority during advanced cardiac life support. The highest possible oxygen concentration, preferably 100%, should be given as soon as possible in all resuscitation attempts.[4] Of course, control of hypoxemia can also help prevent cardiac arrest.

IV fluids. Volume expansion is critical in patients with hypovolemia. Intravenous fluids are also used to provide a route for drug administration. Normal saline (0.9%) is the fluid of choice for IV therapy in cardiac arrest.

Analgesics. Morphine sulfate is the primary analgesic agent used in ACLS. Besides being effective against the pain and anxiety common with myocardial infarction, morphine increases venous capacitance, decreases venous return, and causes a mild dilation of the arterial vasculature.[174] These secondary actions of morphine are particularly useful in the treatment of acute pulmonary edema and pulmonary vascular congestion.[4] Occasionally, other analgesics, such as meperidine, are used. This is especially true in the setting of right ventricular infarct where a sudden reduction in venous return (which can result from morphine) could adversely effect cardiac output.

Drugs that control heart rate and rhythm (antidysrhythmics). There are four major classes of antidysrhythmic drugs, plus a miscellaneous category.[175]

Class I antidysrhythmics lower the resting membrane potential (thus decreasing irritability), slow the rate of depolarization, and prolong the refractory period of myocardial tissue. The most common agents in this class are lidocaine and procainamide HCl. Based on its proven safety and efficacy, lidocaine is the drug of choice for PVCs, V-Tach and V-Fib.[168] Procainamide HCl is recommended when lidocaine is contraindicated or is ineffective in controlling ventricular ectopic beats.[4]

Class II drugs block beta-adrenergic receptors, thereby decreasing the SA node discharge rate, slowing conduction through the AV node, and decreasing heart rate. Propranolol, acebutolol and esmolol are good examples of Class II agents.

Class III drugs prolong the duration of the action potential without changing the resting membrane potential. Bretylium tosylate and amiodarone HCl are the most commonly used drugs in this class. Bretylium is used to treat V-Fib if lidocaine and procainamide HCl prove ineffective.[176]

Class IV agents inhibits calcium ion influx across the cell membrane during depolarization. This decreases SA node discharge rate and conduction velocity through the AV node. The calcium-channel blockers verapamil and diltiazem are the model drugs in this category. Verapamil is used to treat SVTs that don't respond to adenosine (see below).[168] Verapamil and diltiazem have generally replaced digoxin in the treatment of supraventricular arrhythmias.[177]

Miscellaneous antidysrhythmics include adenosine, which slows AV node conduction, and digoxin, which decreases conduction velocity and prolongs the AV node's effective refractory period. Adenosine is a relatively new drug that depresses AV node conduction, making it effective in terminating some forms of SVT.[178-180]

Drugs that improve cardiac output and blood pressure. Drugs in this category affect either the rate and strength of cardiac contractions or the tone of the peripheral vasculature. They include epinephrine, norepinephrine, dopamine, dobutamine, isoproterenol, atropine, calcium, nitroglycerine, and sodium nitroprusside.

Drugs that affect heart rate are called *chronotropic agents.* Those that alter the strength of cardiac contractions are referred to as *inotropic drugs.* Positive "trops" tend to increase heart rate or contractility. This effect may occur indirectly via parasympathetic blockade, or directly through beta-adrenergic stimulation.[181] Negative trops decrease heart rate or contractility by blocking beta adrenergic stimulation (refer to Chapter 21).

This same mechanism is responsible for many vasoactive drugs, which effect the smooth muscle via alpha or beta-adrenergic stimulation or blockade. Alternatively, some vasoactive agents exert their effect directly on smooth muscle.

Due to its strong alpha-adrenergic effects, epinephrine HCl is one of the most important drugs used in ACLS.[182] Because early administration of epinephrine can increase cardiac output, it is the first drug given during cardiac arrest. The initial IV dose is a 1 mg bolus. If the initial dose of epinephrine is ineffective, higher doses (5 mg or 0.1 mg/kg) may be considered.[183-184] In addition, time between epinephrine doses can now be as little as 3 minutes. Epinephrine can be given effectively by endotracheal tube in doses 2 to 2.5 times the IV dose. With both positive inotropic and chronotropic effects, epinephrine is also used to treat hypotension associated with certain bradycardias.

Norepinephrine is a naturally occurring agent related to epinephrine. Primarily an alpha-adrenergic agent, norepinephrine causes intense vasoconstriction, thus making it useful in treating hypotension due to vasodilation (not hypovolemia). Unfortunately, norepinephrine also causes marked renal and **mesenteric** vasoconstriction, with possible ischemia.[168]

Dopamine is a naturally occurring chemical that is the precursor of norepinephrine.[4] Its effects are dose-dependent. At low doses, dopamine increases both renal and mesenteric blood flow. In moderate doses, dopamine has beta-adrenergic effects, increasing both the heart's rate and contractility, thereby increasing systolic pressure. At high doses, dopamine has alpha effects similar to epinephrine, but is less effective at improving hemodynamics during cardiac arrest.[185] Dopamine may be used to treat hypotension caused by bradycardias either during or after resuscitation.[168]

Dobutamine is a synthetic beta-adrenergic catecholamine with potent positive inotropic effects. Although dobutamine is useful in treating heart failure, its is not generally used during resuscitation.

Isoproterenol is a pure beta-adrenergic agent with potent positive inotropic and chronotropic effects. Because it also causes peripheral vasodilation, the increase in blood pressure seen with isoproterenol occurs at the expense of the heart, which must beat faster and harder to keep pressures up. In addition, isoproterenol increases myocardial workload and oxygen consumption. Last, isoproterenol can exacerbate ischemia and cause arrhythmias in patients with heart disease. For these reasons, isoproterenol has limited uses in advanced cardiac life support, being used mainly to treat torsade de pointes when it does not respond to magnesium.

Atropine is a parasympatholytic drug used to treat sinus bradycardia, sinus arrest, certain AV nodal blocks, and asystole. Atropine's positive chronotropic properties are the result of cholinergic (parasympathetic) blockade.[166-167]

In addition to their antidysrhythmic properties, Class II agents like propranolol can reduce heart rate and contractility. These beta-adrenergic blocker are thus useful in reducing cardiac workload after an acute myocardial infarction, and may help decrease the incidence of ventricular fibrillation and infarct size in these patients. While beta blockers are sometimes used to treat SVTs, they are clearly third line drugs. Beta blockers are contraindicated in patients with bradycardias, hypotension, and congestive heart failure. Also, beta blockers should be withheld from patients with hyperreactive airways predisposing to bronchospasm.[168]

Calcium (chloride or gluconate) exerts a positive inotropic effect on isolated myocardial tissue, but its ability to enhance the heart's contractility during arrest has not been shown. Currently, high levels of calcium are considered detrimental.[4] Calcium may be helpful in the presence of confirmed **hyperkalemia, hypocalcemia** or calcium channel blocker overdose.[187] Otherwise calcium should not be used.[4]

Nitroglycerin and sodium nitroprusside cause vasodilation by relaxing vascular smooth muscle. Both agents can reduce cardiac workload by decreasing the peripheral arterial pressure (afterload) and reducing the volume of blood returning to the heart (preload). Taken **sublingual**, nitroglycerin is highly effective in the treatment of painful coronary artery spasms (angina). Nitroglycerin may also be given by IV in emergency situations to treat congestive heart failure. Nitroglycerin is preferred over sodium nitroprusside in patients with coronary artery disease, because nitroprusside can worsen ischemia.[186]

Sodium bicarbonate. Buffer agents such as sodium bicarbonate ($NaHCO_3$) have limited use in resuscitation. Adequate alveolar ventilation and rapid restoration of blood flow are the mainstay in controlling acid-base disturbances during cardiac arrest.[188] In most cases, the harmful effects of $NaHCO_3$ administration during CPR outweigh any potential benefits.[4]

Harmful effects of $NaHCO_3$ administration during CPR include: (1) impaired oxygen unloading (due to a left shift of the oxyhemoglobin curve), (2) **hyperosmolarity,** (3) hypernatremia, (4) depression of myocardial and cerebral function, (5) inactivation of simultaneously given catecholamines, and (6) a paradoxical intracellular acidosis.[189] For these reasons, the routine use of $NaHCO_3$ early in resuscitation is not recommended. After extended periods of cardiac arrest, $NaHCO_3$ may be helpful. Bicarbonate is also indicated for arrest patients who have *pre-existing* metabolic acidosis (not hypoxic lactic acidosis), hyperkalemia, or an overdose with acidic drugs.[4]

Diuretics. One of the most commonly used diuretics is furosemide (Lasix). Furosemide causes diuresis by inhibiting sodium reabsorption in the kidneys (predominately in the loop of Henle). Furosemide also has a venodilating effect, which reduces venous return to the heart (preload) thereby decreasing cardiac work. Furosemide is used to treat patients with acute pulmonary edema, and may be useful in the management of cerebral edema after cardiac arrest.[4]

Thrombolytic agents. Thrombolytic agents such as streptokinase, urokinase and t-PA (tissue plasminogen activator) breakdown blood clots. This action is useful in treating patients with acute myocardial infarction when the coronary artery blockage is caused or worsened by a clot. When promptly admin-

Table 23-2 Drug agents used in advanced life support

Drug	Indications	Contraindications	Preparation	Route	Dosage	Pharmacologic effects
Lidocaine HCl	Ventricular tachycardia, hyperexcitable myocardium, multifocal PVCs, ventricular fibrillation	Heart block, asystole, PEA	Variable	IV bolus IV drip Intracardiac Endotracheal	1–1.5 mg/kg bolus every 5 to 10 minutes up to 3 mg/kg	Raises electrical stimulation threshold Depresses ventricular electrical activity
Procainamide HCl	Ventricular tachycardia, hyperexcitable myocardium, multifocal PVCs, ventricular fibrillation	Heart block, asystole, PEA	100 mg/mL (10 mL unit)	IV bolus IV drip	20 mg/minute to maximum of 17 mg/kg 1–4 mg/min drip	Raises electrical stimulation threshold Depresses ventricular electrical activity May cause hypotension
Bretylium tosylate	Ventricular tachycardia, hyperexcitable myocardium, multifocal PVCs, ventricular fibrillation	Heart block, asystole, PEA	50 mg/mL (10 mL unit)	IV bolus	5 mg/kg IV bolus In VF repeat 10 mg/kg after 5–10 minutes In UT 5–10 mg/kg diluted in 50 mL over 8–10 minutes	Raises electrical stimulation threshold Depresses ventricular electrical activity May cause hypotension
Atropine sulfate	Idioventricular rhythms, nodal bradycardia, pulseless electrical activity (PEA), escape rhythms, sinus arrest, asystole	Sinus, atrial, and ventricular tachycardia	0.1 mg/mL (10 mL unit)	IV bolus Endotracheal	0.5–1 mg IV repeated every 3–5 minutes to a maximum of 3 mg	Increased heart rate Increased force of contractions (mainly affects atrial activity)
Dobutamine HCl	Depressed myocardial contractility	Hypertension, PVCs, atrial fibrillation, hypertrophic aortic stenosis	250 mg powder (reconstitute)	IV drip	2.0–20 µg/kg/min	Increased force of contractions Increased heart rate Enhanced atrioventricular conduction
Calcium salts (gluconate, chloride)	Hypocalcemia hyperkalemia	Concurrent digitalis use (relative)	100 mg/mL (10% solution)	IV (not to be mixed with other drugs)	chloride: 2–4 mg/kg gluconate: 5-8 mL(10%)	Increased force of contractions Increased ventricular excitability May suppress sinus node
Dopamine HCl	Hypotension	Ventricular tachycardia, frequent PVCs	40 mg/mL (5 mL unit)	IV drip	5.0–20 mg/kg/min	Increased renal, splanic flow at low doses (4 to 6 µg/kg/min) beta-adrenergic effects at moderate doses (60 to 10 µg/kg/min) alpha-adrenergic effects at high doses (above 10 µg/kg/min)
Sodium nitroprusside	Hypertension	Hypotension CHF	50 mg powder (reconstitute)	IV drip only	0.1–10 µg/kg/min	Direct peripheral vasodilation

Drug	Indications	Contraindications/Cautions	Concentration	Route	Dose	Action
Epinephrine HCl	Cardiac standstill, ventricular fibrillation, asystole, EMD, sinus arrest, idioventricular rhythm	Ventricular tachycardia, frequent PVCs	0.1 mg/mL (1:10,000)	IV bolus Intracardiac Endotracheal	1 mg every 3–5 minutes in cardiac arrest	Increased heart rate; Increased force of contractions; Vasoconstriction; Increased coronary perf pressures; Increased myocardial irritability; Increased myocardial O_2 consumption
Propranolol HCl	Angina pectoris, myocardial infarction (MI), supraventricular arrhythmias, ventricular tachycardia	Hypotension, CHF, reactive airway disease	1 mg/mL	IV bolus	0.1 mg/kg (not to exceed 1 mg/min)	Decreased heart rate; Decreased stroke volume; Decreased myocardial O_2 consumption; Increased LVEDP
Verapamil HCl	Angina pectoris, MI, supraventricular arrhythmias, mild hypertension	Hypotension, CHF, 2nd- or 3rd-degree heart block, Atrial fibrillation with Wolf-Parkinson-White syndrome	2.5 mg/mL (5 mL unit)	IV bolus	2.5–5 mg IV over 2 minutes	Decreased heart rate; Prolonged atrioventricular conduction; Decreased myocardial contractility; Coronary artery vasodilation; Peripheral vasodilation
Isoproterenol HCl	Idioventricular rhythms, bradycardia, heart block	Ventricular tachycardia frequent PVCs	0.2 mg/mL (1:5000)	IV drip with dextrose	2–10 ug/min	Increased heart rate; Increased force of contractions; Vasodilation; Possible decrease coronary perfusion
Adenosine	SVT	Use with caution if patient has asthma	3 mg/mL	Rapid IV over 1–2 seconds followed by 20 mL saline flush	6 mg	Conductor decrease AV node
Tissue plasminogen activator (t – PA)	Acute coronary occlusion	Active internal history of CVA/trauma	20 mg powder (reconstitute)	IV	100 mg over 3 hours	Lysis of thrombi clot in coronary artery
Streptokinase	Acute coronary occlusion	Active internal history of CVA/trauma	1.5 million IV powder (reconstitute)	IV	1.5 million IV over 1 hour	Lysis of thrombi clot in coronary artery
Norepinephrine	Cardiogenic or vasogenic shock	hypovolemia	4 mg/4 mL	IV drip	.5–1.0 micrograms per minute titrated to effect	Alpha adrenergic stimulation
Diuretics Lasix (furosemide)	CHF pulmonary edema	hypovolemia	100 mg/10 mL	IV	20–100 mg IV	Diuresis/venodilation

■ MINI CLINI ■

23-2

Problem: You are taking care of a mechanically ventilated, post myocardial infarction patient in the coronary intensive care unit. You have noticed the occurrence of 15 to 20 bizarre ventricular complexes on the ECG during the last minute as shown in the figure below.

Classify the abnormal complex and indicate the proper drug therapy.

Discussion: The ECG below reveals a premature ventricular contraction

Treating Cardiac Arrhythmias

(PVC). This means that an irritable focus in the ventricle has fired prematurely, i.e. this focus reached its membrane threshold potential earlier than the cells in the SA node, and thus initiated ventricular depolarization. (This irritability could be due to local myocardial hypoxia or electrolyte imbalances.) Because the PVC's are occurring at a rate greater than six per minute, aggressive treatment is indicated. Underlying electrolyte imbalances must be corrected, adequate oxygenation must be maintained, and antiarrhythmic drugs should be infused. Lidocaine is the drug of choice for PVC's.

II

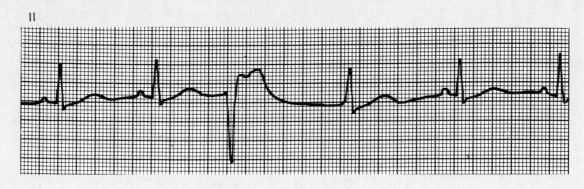

istered, these agents can help restore circulation through blocked coronary arteries, thus limiting myocardial death. Administration must be within 6 hours of chest pain.[4]

Electrical therapy

There are three general types of electrical therapy used in emergency cardiac care: (1) unsynchronized countershock, or defibrillation, (2) synchronized countershock, or cardioversion, and (3) electrical pacing.

Countershock (defibrillation and cardioversion). When an electrical shock of appropriate strength is applied to the myocardium, all myocardial fibers simultaneously depolarize. In concept, once all cells depolarized, those that spontaneously fire at the fastest rate should be able to regain control and pace the heart. Normally, it is the sinus node that spontaneously depolarizes most quickly. After electric shock, the sinus node should discharge first, and thus capture all parts of the myocardium as the depolarization wave travels through the still silent heart.

Defibrillation is an unsynchronized shock used to simultaneously depolarize the myocardial fibers. It is the definitive treatment for both ventricular fibrillation and pulseless ventricular tachycardia. If one of these arrhythmias is present and the proper equip-

ment and trained personnel are available, the patient should be defibrillated immediately.

Currently, the American Heart Association recommends an initial energy level of 200 joules for defibrillation of adult victims, with 2 joules per kilogram for children and infants.[4] If this level does not restore orderly ventricular depolarization, the second shock should be 200 to 300 joules.[190] Third and subsequent shocks should at 360 joules for adults, or about 4 joules per kilogram for children and infants.[190,191]

Electrode paddle size and placement are important in assuring that the full energy of the countershock is applied. For adults, paddles should be 10 cm in diameter, with 8 cm being adequate for older children. Electrode paddles for infants should be 4.5 cm in size.

Normally, one paddle is placed below the clavicle and just to the right of the upper portion of the sternum, with the other positioned on the midaxillary line to the left of the left nipple. Alternatively, one paddle may be placed on the left precordium, with the other positioned posteriorly under the patient, behind the heart. Paddles should be prepared with conducting gel and applied with firm pressure (about 25 lbs).

Cardioversion is similar to defibrillation, with two major exceptions. First, the countershock is synchronized with the heart's electrical activity (the R wave).

Synchronization is necessary because electrical stimulation during the refractory phase (part of the T wave) can cause ventricular fibrillation or ventricular tachycardia. Second, the energy used during cardioversion is usually less than that applied during defibrillation.

Cardioversion is considered when a patient with an organized arrhythmia producing a high ventricular rate exhibits signs or symptoms of cardiac decompensation. These so-called 'tachyarrhythmias' include SVT, atrial flutter, atrial fibrillation, and V-Tach.

If the arrhythmia is not causing serious signs or symptoms, drug therapy is used first. On the other hand, if the patient shows hypotension, exhibits signs of decreased consciousness or pulmonary congestion, or complains of chest pain, cardioversion is indicated.

Electrical pacing. Another application of electrical therapy uses intermittently-timed, low energy discharges to replace or supplement the heart's natural pacemaker. There are two primary types of electrical pacing. First, the electrical discharge can be delivered from an external power pack through wires inserted into the patient's chest wall (transcutaneous or transthoracic pacing). Alternatively, wire electrodes may be floated through the large veins and implanted directly inside the heart (transvenous pacing). Because it can be started quickly, transcutaneous pacing is the method used most often in emergency cardiac care.

Pacemaker therapy is used to treat sinus bradycardias that produce serious signs and symptoms and do not respond to atropine. Electrical pacing is also used to manage second (type II) and third degree heart block. Electrical pacing can also be used to treat some tachyarrhythmias. In these cases, the pacemaker is set to discharge faster than the underlying rate. After a few seconds, the pacemaker is stopped to allow the heart's intrinsic rate to return. This is called over-drive pacing. Although over-drive pacing has shown promise in treating certain SVTs and V-Tach, pharmacologic intervention (when the patient is stable) and cardioversion (when the patient is unstable) remain the treatments of choice.

Since defibrillation can cause damage to permanent pacemakers, care should be taken not to place the electrode paddles near these devices. After a patient with a permanent pacemaker undergoes either cardioversion or defibrillation, the device should be checked for proper function.[4]

Monitoring during advanced cardiac life support

Although extensive monitoring is used in most critical care settings, monitoring during emergency life support is usually limited to ECG, pulse, blood pressure, and intermittent arterial blood gas samples.[192] Recently, several approaches designed to enhance knowledge of patient status during CPR have been developed or proposed. These include methods to better monitor ventilation, oxygenation, and airway status. Table 23-3 summarizes the utility, feasibility, and long-term costs of these approaches to emergency monitoring.[192]

Electrocardiography (ECG) is the most common and among the most useful monitors during advanced cardiac life support. The ECG provides the basis for selecting various drug and electrical therapies during CPR, and helps indicate patient response to these interventions. However, the RCP must remember that an acceptable ECG rhythm does not necessarily mean that cardiac output is adequate.[192] Other indices of perfusion, such as pulse, blood pressure and capnography, are needed to confirm adequate cardiac output.[193]

Given the importance of monitoring tidal volume and respiratory rate in critically ill patients receiving ventilatory support, it is surprising to note that these parameters are not commonly assessed during CPR. With numerous studies indicating large variations in tidal volume delivery during bag-valve-mask and bag-mask ventilation,[96-99,101,126,127] monitoring of this simple ventilatory parameter during CPR would seem essential. Most current bag-valve-mask devices can be easily connected to a portable spirometer, making the procedure relatively simple.[194] In fact, all than may be needed is a simple indicator to tell the practitioner whether the tidal volume is too large or too small (above or below 800 mL for adults).[192]

Given the tendency of rescuers to apply too high a rate, monitoring the frequency breathing is probably just as important.[192] High rates can promote gastric

Table 23-3 Comparison of factors for consideration when using monitors during resuscitation[192]

Monitor	Useful	Feasible	Initial Cost	Long-Term Cost
ECG	Yes	Yes	High	Low
Tidal volume	Yes (adults)	?	High	Low
Airway pressure	Yes (neonates)	Yes	Low	Low
Transcutaneous PO$_2$	Yes	No	High	Moderate
Conjunctival PO$_2$	Yes	No	High	Moderate
Pulse oximetry	No	?	High	Moderate
Art blood gases	?	Yes	High	Moderate
Ven blood gases	Yes	No	High	Moderate
Capnography	Yes	No	High	Moderate
Colorimetric CO$_2$ Indicator	?	Yes	Low	Moderate
Lighted stylet	?	?	Moderate	Moderate
Esophageal detector device	?	Yes	Low	Low
Magnetic tube marker	?	?	Moderate	Moderate

■ MINI CLINI ■

23-3

Route of Drug Administration

You are working in a small rural hospital and are called to the emergency room where a victim is in cardiac arrest. You are able to intubate the patient and ventilate with a manual bag-valve-mask (BVM) unit at 100% inspired oxygen concentration. Nurses are performing cardiac compressions and attempting unsuccessfully to start a peripheral IV line. The ECG monitor reveals a fine ventricular fibrillation pattern. Electrical defibrillation is unsuccessful on the first two attempts. Immediate administration of epinephrine is indicated, but attempts to secure an IV route continue to be unsuccessful. What action is appropriate at this time?

Discussion: Because of its strong inotropic and alpha-adrenergic effects, epinephrine should be the first drug given in cardiac arrest, and should be administered as soon as possible. Epinephrine can convert fine fibrillation to coarse, vigorous fibrillation and improve the chances for successful electrical defibrillation. In the above case, because an intravenous route is not available, epinephrine should be directly instilled into the endotracheal tube at 2 to 2.5 times the IV dose diluted in 10 ml of normal saline or distilled water. This is an effective route of administration. In addition, lidocaine can be administered via the endotracheal tube.

---

insufflation in nonintubated patients.[22] In addition, high rates can lower delivered oxygen concentrations, due to decreased bag refill time.[102] Last, fast rates may not increase the victim's alveolar ventilation, especially when physiologic deadspace is high.[192]

It is not currently practical to monitor the tidal volume delivered to infants during CPR.[192] For this reason, and due to the unreliability of the pressure pop-offs or relief valves on most infant resuscitators,[106] airway pressure should be monitored during infant CPR.[87,195] When airway pressure is not monitored, peak inflation pressures tend to be higher than when a manometer is placed in line.[196] Unfortunately, some aneroid manometers tend to underestimate actual airway pressures at the high rates common during infant CPR.[197]

Tissue oxygenation, and thus the adequacy of perfusion, can be monitored by any one of several methods. Noninvasive methods include the transcutaneous PO_2 ($P_{TC}O_2$), conjunctival PO_2, and pulse oximetry. Invasive methods include arterial and mixed venous blood gases.

The transcutaneous PO_2 ($P_{TC}O_2$) is a relatively sensitive indicator of perfusion during cardiac arrest.[198] When perfusion decreases, the $P_{TC}O_2$ falls; when blood flow is restored, the $P_{TC}O_2$ rises.[192] However, $P_{TC}O_2$ is technically difficult to apply during CPR. In addition, electrodes used during transcutaneous PO_2 monitoring require an equilibration period of 10 to 15 minutes before accurate data can be obtained. For these reasons, transcutaneous PO_2 monitoring has limited applicability during emergency life support.

Like the $P_{TC}O_2$, the conjunctival PO_2 can indicate the adequacy of perfusion, especially cerebral blood flow.[199] With the onset of cardiac arrest, conjunctival PO_2 normally drops to zero. When a functional cardiac rhythm returns, the conjunctival PO_2 rises.[192] Unfortunately, the conjunctival PO_2 monitor has the same technical limitations as the transcutaneous PO_2 system. In addition, conjunctival PO_2 is not an accurate indicator of cerebral oxygenation when epinephrine is administered.[192]

Pulse oximetry has been recommended as a tool for monitoring oxygenation and perfusion during CPR.[200] Because the pulse oximeter uses pulsatile flow as the basis for its measurements, it would seem ideally suited for this task. Unfortunately, noise and limb motion during CPR often result in false oximeter readings.[192,201] Thus the pulse oximeter has limited utility as a monitoring tool during CPR.

Arterial blood gases are one of the more common invasive measures made during CPR. Unfortunately, animal studies show that arterial blood gas and pH measures do not accurately reflect tissue acid-base status during CPR.[202] While the arterial blood may show respiratory alkalosis, mixed venous blood is typically high in CO_2 with a low pH.[192] In fact, arterial blood tends to indicate the effectiveness of ventilation, while the mixed venous blood reflects cardiac output during CPR. Thus, although arterial blood gases can help predict outcomes (respiratory alkalosis is a bad sign), their overall role as a monitoring tool during CPR is limited.[203] Mixed-venous blood gases, on the other hand, provide both **prognostic** and therapeutic data. Unfortunately, mixed-venous blood gases can only be obtained during CPR in patients who already have a pulmonary artery catheter in place.

Capnography is typically used during CPR to help confirm endotracheal tube placement (see Chapter 22). However, end-tidal CO_2 levels ($P_{ET}CO_2$) can be a sensitive indicator of pulmonary blood flow and cardiac output, especially if ventilation is held constant.[192] Specifically, a fall in cardiac output causes a fall in $P_{ET}CO_2$. Conversely, if whole body perfusion rises, the $P_{ET}CO_2$ tends to climb.[204] $P_{ET}CO_2$ also correlates well with coronary perfusion pressure, a critical parameter during CPR.[192] Thus, despite its relative expense, capnography appears to be a promising tool for assessing both airway placement and perfusion status during emergency life support. However, more research is needed before this approach is recommended for widespread adoption.[192]

Other monitoring tools used during CPR include several airway devices designed to aid in or confirm endotracheal intubation (see Table 23-3). The uses of these adjuncts is described in Chapter 22.

In summary, there are a number of both invasive and noninvasive approaches to monitoring during CPR. Although many of these tools provide useful data, their impact on patient survival has yet to be fully evaluated.

Postresuscitative patient care

The post-cardiac arrest patient may exhibit an optimal response, in which case he or she will regain consciousness, be responsive and breathe spontaneously. More often, however, the patient will require support of one or more organ systems.

If the patient is conscious and breathing spontaneously following resuscitation, supplemental oxygen, maintenance of an IV infusion, and continuous cardiac and hemodynamic monitoring may be all that is necessary. A 12-lead ECG, a chest X-ray, arterial blood gases, and a clinical chemistry profile should be obtained as soon as possible.[4] Ideally, the patient should be placed under close supervision and observation, preferably in an intensive care or coronary care unit.

On the other hand, patients who remain unconscious, are apneic, or are hemodynamically unstable must be placed in a special care unit. Only in this setting can underlying organ system insufficiency or failure be properly identified and managed. Organs most likely to exhibit failure after resuscitation are the lung, heart and vasculature, and kidneys. CNS failure is an ominous sign, and generally indicates a failed resuscitation attempt.

Respiratory management

If the patient remains apneic or exhibits irregular breathing after resuscitation, mechanical ventilation should be instituted via a properly positioned endotracheal tube, with an initial oxygen concentration of 100%. Arterial blood gases, preferably obtained through an arterial line, should be analyzed as needed until the oxygenation and acid-base status of the patient stabilizes. Arterial blood gas analysis will also help differentiate between pulmonary and non-pulmonary (or cardiac) causes of hypoxemia and tissue hypoxia, if present.[4] Details on the selection and use

of mechanical ventilators, and appropriate patient monitoring procedures are provided in Section VII of this text.

Cardiovascular management

A 12-lead ECG, chest X-ray, clinical chemistry profile, and cardiac enzyme results should be reviewed, along with current and past drug histories. Where feasible, a flow-directed, balloon-tipped pulmonary artery catheter should be inserted and connected to a thermal dilution cardiac output computer.[4] This will provide needed data on the adequacy of vascular volumes, left ventricular performance, and overall tissue perfusion. On this basis, sound judgments can be made regarding the need for fluid therapy, and the selection and use of appropriate drugs.

Renal management

Ideally, the bladder should be catheterized, and fluid input and output carefully monitored. Renal function tests, including urine sediment, electrolytes, blood urea nitrogen (**BUN**), and creatinine should be monitored. If these data suggests renal failure, **nephrotoxic** drugs or agents excreted through the kidneys should be given with care. If renal failure is confirmed, **hemodialysis** may be indicated.[4]

CNS management

Significant advances are being made in limiting CNS damage associated with poor cerebral perfusion and oxygenation.[203-207]

However, current non-experimental approaches to CNS 'resuscitation' are limited to maintaining arterial blood pressure, while simultaneously lowering intracranial pressures and preventing seizures.[4] Elevation of the head aids cerebral vascular drainage, while drug agents such as phenobarbital can decrease seizures. Since tracheobronchial suction and mechanical ventilation can both elevate intracranial pressures, RCPs responsible for these procedures must exercise due care in their use.[4] Special techniques may be needed to minimize both the cardiovascular and cerebrovascular consequences of mechanical ventilation.

CHAPTER SUMMARY

The prompt action of a respiratory care practitioner can restore ventilation and circulation to victims of respiratory arrest and cardiac arrest. All RCPs should be skilled in the basic methods of airway maintenance, foreign body removal, artificial ventilation, and external chest compression. The practitioner must be able to modify and evaluate the effectiveness of these procedures, taking into account both the age of the victim and the clinical circumstances.

In addition to providing basic life support, RCPs are key members of the in-hospital advanced cardiac life support team. In this role, the practitioner assumes a vital role in managing the airway and providing effective oxygenation and ventilation. Practitioners may also participate in providing circulatory support, drug and electrical therapy, and postresuscitative care. By applying this expertise in an appropriate, proficient, and systematic manner —and sharing it through the education of lay personnel—RCPs can help reduce the alarming toll of sudden death currently affecting our population.

REFERENCES

1. Kacmarek RM: The role of the respiratory therapist in emergency care, *Respir Care* 37(6):523–530, 1992.
2. Morbidity and Mortality Chartbook on Cardiovascular, Lung, and Blood Diseases 1990. Bethesda, Md: National Heart, Lung and Blood Institute; 1990.
3. National Safety Council: *Accident facts,* Chicago, 1992, National Safety Council.
4. American Heart Association: Guidelines for cardiopulmonary resuscitation and emergency cardiac care: Recommendations of the 1992 National Conference, *JAMA* (Suppl.), 268:16, 2135–2302, 1992.
5. Division of Injury Control, Center for Environmental Health and Injury Control, Centers for Disease Control. Childhood Injuries in the United States, *AJDC* 144:627–646, 1990.
6. Singer J: Cardiac arrest in children, *J. Am. Coll. Emerg. Phys.* 6:198–205, 1977.
7. Eisenberg M, Bergner L, Hallstrom A: Epidemiology of cardiac arrest and resuscitation in children, *Ann. Emerg. Med.,* 12:672–674, 1983.
8. Guerci AD, Weisfeldt ML. Mechanical-ventilatory cardiac support, *Crit Care Clin,* 2(2):209–220, 1986.
9. Committee on Trauma, American College of Surgeons: *Early care of the injured patient,* ed 4, Philadelphia, 1990.
10. Goldberger E: *Treatment of Cardiac Emergencies,* ed 5, St Louis, 1990, Mosby.
11. Grant H, Murray R, Bergeron D: *Emergency Care,* ed 5, Bowie, MD, 1990, Robert J. Brady Co.
12. Huszar R: *Emergency cardiac care,* Bowie, M, 1974, Robert J. Brady Co.
13. Schwartz GR, Cayten GC, et al: *Principals and Practices of Emergency Medicine* ed 3, 1992, Philadelphia, Lea and Fibiger.
14. Ellis PD, Billings DM: *Cardiopulmonary resuscitation: procedures for basic and advanced life support,* St. Louis, 1980, Mosby.
15. Shapter R (editor): Cardiopulmonary resuscitation: basic life support, *Clinical Symposia* 26:7, 1974.
16. *Instructors Manual for Basic Life Support,* Dallas, 1987, American Heart Association.
17. Ruben H, Elam JO, Ruben AM, et al: Investigation of upper airway problems in resuscitation, *Anesthesiology* 22:271–279, 1961.
18. Boidin MP: Airway patency in the unconscious patient, *Br. J. Anaesth.* 57:306–310, 1985.
19. Morikawa S, Safar P, Decarlo J: Influence of head position upon airway patency, *Anesthesiology* 22:265, 1961.
20. Guildner C: Resuscitation: opening the airway, a comparative study of techniques for opening an airway obstructed by the tongue, *J. Am. Coll. Emerg. Phys.* 5:558–590, 1976.
21. Safar P, Lind B: Triple airway maneuver, artificial ventilation and oxygen inhalation by mouth-to-mask and bag-valve-mask techniques, in Proceedings of the 1973 National Conference on CPR, Dallas, American Heart Association, 1975.
22. Melker R: Recommendations for ventilation during cardiopulmonary resuscitation. Time for change?, *Crit Care Med* 13:882–883, 1985.
23. Zideman D: ABCs of resuscitation. Resuscitation of infants and children, *Br Med J* (Clin Res Ed) 292(6535):1584–1588, 1986.
24. Milner AD: Resuscitation of the newborn, *Arch Dis Child* 66(1 Spec No):66–69, 1991.
25. Lamb FS, Rosner MS: Neonatal resuscitation, *Emerg Med Clin North Am* 5(3):541–557, 1987.
26. Sinkin RA, Davis JM: Cardiopulmonary resuscitation of the newborn, *Pediatr Rev* 12(5):136–141, 1990.
27. Zaritsky A: Cardiopulmonary resuscitation in children, *Clin Chest Med* 8(4):561–571, 1987.
28. Rockney RM, Alario AJ, Lewander WJ: Pediatric advanced life support: Part I. Airway, circulation and intravascular access, *Am Fam Physician* 43(4):1223–1230, 1991.
29. Fredrickson JM: Overview of advanced life support for pediatric patients, *J Emerg Nurs* 16(1):17–24, 1990.
30. Outwater KM, Ludwig S, Peterson MB: Pediatric resuscitation, *J Emerg Nurs* 15(6):466–74, 1989.
31. Safar P, Redding J: 'Tight jaw' in resuscitation, *Anesthesiology,* 20:701–702, 1959.
32. Ruben H, Knudsen EJ, Carugati G: Gastric inflation in relation to airway pressure, *Acta. Anaesth. Scand.,* 5:107–114, 1961.
33. Sellick BA: Cricoid pressure to control regurgitation of stomach contents during induction of anesthesia, *Lancet,* 2:404–406, 1961.
34. Melker RJ: Alternative methods of ventilation during respiratory and cardiac arrest, *Circulation,* 74(6 Pt 2):IV63–65, 1986.
35. Jackson RE, Freeman SB: Hemodynamics of cardiac massage, *Emerg Med Clin North Am* 1(3):501–513, 1983.
36. Babbs CF: New versus old theories of blood flow during CPR, *Crit Care Med* 8:191–195, 1980.
37. Vaagenes P, et al: On the technique of external cardiac compression, *Crit Care Med* 6:176–180, 1978.
38. Rudikoff M, et al: Importance of compression rate during external cardiac massage in man, *Circulation* Suppl. 54:II-225, 1976.
39. Taylor G, et al: Importance of prolonged compression during cardiopulmonary resuscitation in man, *N Engl J Med* 296:1515–1517, 1977.
40. Orlowski JP: Optimum position for external cardiac massage in infants and children, *Crit Care Med* 12:224, 1984.
41. Ludwig S, Kettrick RG, Parker M: Pediatric cardiopulmonary resuscitation, *Clin Pediatr* 23:71, 1984.
43. Krischer JP, Fine EG, Nagel, EL, et al: Complications of Cardiac Resuscitation, *Chest* 92:287–291, 1987.
44. Bjork RJ, Snyder BD, Campion, DC, et al: Medical complications of cardiopulmonary arrest, *Arch Intern Med* 142:500–503, 1982.
45. Atcheson SG, Fred HL: Complications of cardiac resuscitation, *Am Heart J* 89:263–264, 1975.
46. Enarson D, et al: Flail chest as a complication of cardiopulmonary resuscitation, *Heart & Lung* 6:1020–1022, 1977.
47. Custer JR, Polley TZ Jr, Moler F: Gastric perforation following cardiopulmonary resuscitation in a child: report of a case and review of the literature, *Pediatr Emerg Care* 3(1):24–27, 1987.
48. Hargarten KM, Aprahamian C, Mateer J: Pneumoperitoneum as a complication of cardiopulmonary resuscitation, *Am J Emerg Med* 6(4):358–61, 1988.
49. Council on Ethical and Judicial Affairs, American Medical Association: Guidelines for the appropriate use of do-not-resuscitate orders, *JAMA* 265:1868–1871, 1991.
50. Cardiopulmonary resuscitation, AIDS, and public panic [editorial], *Lancet* 340(8817):456–457, 1992.
51. Michael AD, Forrester JS: Mouth-to-mouth ventilation: the dying art, *Am J Emerg Med* 10(2):156–161, 1992.
52. Brenner BE, Kauffman J: Reluctance of internists and medical nurses to perform mouth-to-mouth resuscitation, *Arch Intern Med* 153(15):1763–1769, 1993.
53. Stirba C: Cardiopulmonary resuscitation in patients with acquired immunodeficiency syndrome, *Arch Intern Med* 49(10):2380, 1989.

54. Centers for Disease Control: Update: universal precautions for prevention of transmission of human immunodeficiency virus, hepatitis B virus, and other bloodborne pathogens in health-care settings, *Morb Mortal Wkly Rep* 37(24):377–82, 387–8, 1988.

55. Goldsmith MF: OSHA bloodborne pathogens standard aims to limit occupational transmission, *JAMA* 267(21):2853–2854, 1992.

56. Madama VC: Safe mouth-to-mouth resuscitation requires adjunct equipment, caution, *Occup Health Saf* 60(1):56, 58, 64, 1991.

57. From the Centers for Disease Control and Prevention. Surveillance for occupationally acquired HIV infection—United States, 1981–1992, *JAMA* 268(23):3294, 1992.

58. Heimlich HJ, et al: Food choking and drowning deaths prevented by external subdiaphragmatic compression, *Ann Thorac Surg* 20:188, 1975.

59. Heimlich HJ: A life saving maneuver to prevent food choking, *JAMA* 234:398, 1975.

60. Heimlich HJ: Death from food-choking prevented by a new life-saving maneuver, *Heart & Lung* 5:755–758, 1976.

61. Heimlich HJ: The Heimlich maneuver: where it stands today, *Emerg Med* 10(7):89–93, 1978.

62. Day RL, Crelin ES, DuBois AB: Choking: the Heimlich abdominal thrust vs back blows: An approach to measurement of inertial and aerodynamic forces, *Pediatrics* 70:113–119, 1982.

63. Day RL, DuBois AB: Treatment of choking, *Pediatrics,* 71:300, 1983.

64. van der Ham AC, Lange JF: Traumatic rupture of the stomach after Heimlich maneuver, *J Emerg Med* 8(6):713–715, 1990.

65. Palmer E: The Heimlich maneuver misused, *Curr Prescribing* 5:45–49, 1979.

66. Safar P: Pocket mask for emergency artificial ventilation and oxygen inhalation, *Crit Care Med* 2:273–276, 1974.

67. Harrison RR, Maull KI, Keenan, RL, et al: Mouth-to-mask ventilation: A superior method of rescue breathing, *Ann Emerg Med* 12;765–768, 1982.

68. Hess D, Ness C, Oppel A, Rhoads K: Evaluation of mouth-to-mask ventilation devices, *Respir Care* 34(3):191–195, 1989.

69. Reines, HD: Airway management options, *Resp Care* 37(7):695–705, 1992.

70. Stauffer JL: Medical management of the airway, *Clin Chest Med* 12(3):449–482, 1991.

71. Don Michel TA, Gordon, AS: Esophageal obturator airway: a new adjunct for artificial respiration. In Proceedings of the national conference on standards for CPR and ECC. Washington, DC, 1973, American Heart Association.

72. Schofferman J, O'Neil P, Lewis AJ: The esophageal obturator airway: a clinical evaluation, *Chest* 69:67–71, 1976.

73. Bryson T, Benumof JI, Ward CF: The esophageal obturator airway: a clinical comparison to ventilation with a mask and oropharyngeal airway, *Chest* 74:537–539, 1978.

74. Don Michel TA, Gordon, AS: The esophageal obturator airway: a new device in emergency cardiopulmonary resuscitation, *Br Med J* 281:1531–1534, 1980.

75. Donen N, Tweed WA, Dashfsky S, et al: The esophageal obturator airway: An appraisal, *Can Anaesth Soc J* 30:194–200, 1983.

76. Pilcher DB, DeMeules JE: Esophageal perforation following use of esophageal airway, *Chest* 69:377–380, 1976.

77. McCabe CJ, Brown BJ: Esophageal obturator airway, ET tube, and pharyngeal-tracheal lumen airway, *Am J Emerg Med* 4(1):464–471, 1986.

78. Bass RR, Allison EJ, Hunt RC: The esophageal obturator airway: a reassessment of its use by paramedics, *Ann Emerg Med* 11:358–360, 1982.

79. Committee on Trauma: *Advanced Trauma Life Support,* Chicago, 1989, American College of Surgeons.

80. Bartlett RL, Martin SD, McMahan JM, et al: A comparison of the pharyngeotracheal lumen airway and the endotracheal tube, *J Trauma* 32(3):280–284, 1992.

81. Frass M, Frenzer R, Zdrahal F, et al: The esophageal tracheal combitube: preliminary results with a new airway for cardiopulmonary resuscitation, *Ann Emerg Med* 16:768–772, 1987.

82. Frass M, Frenzer R, Meyer G, et al: Mechanical ventilation with the esophageal tracheal combitube (ETC) in the intensive care unit, *Arch Emerg Med* 4:219–225, 1987.

83. Melker R, Cavallaro D: Synchronous and asynchronous ventilation during cardiopulmonary resuscitation, *Ann Emerg Med* 12:142, 1983.

84. Attia RR, Battit GE, Murphy JD: Transtracheal ventilation, *JAMA* 234:1152–1153, 1975.

85. Barnes TA: Emergency ventilation techniques and related equipment, *Respir Care* (7):673–90, 1992.

86. McPherson SP: *Respiratory therapy equipment,* ed 4, St. Louis, 1990, Mosby.

87. American Society for Testing and Materials: Standard specifications for performance and safety requirements for resuscitators intended for use with humans (F-920–85), Philadelphia, 1985, American Society for Testing and Materials.

88. International Standards Organization: Internation standard ISO 8382:1988 (E)—Resuscitators intended for use with humans, New York, 1988, American National Standards Institute.

89. White RD, Gilles BP, Polk BV: Oxygen delivery by hand-operated emergency ventilation devices, *J Am Coll Emerg Phys* 2:105–108, 1973.

90. Emergency Care Research Institute: Evaluation: manually operated infant resuscitators, *Health Devices* 3:164, 1974.

91. Steinbach RB, Carden E: Assessment of eight adult resuscitator bags, *Respir Care* 20:69, 1975.

92. Emergency Care Research Institute: Evaluation: manual resuscitators, *Health Devices* 8:133, 1979.

93. Barnes TA, Watson ME: Oxygen delivery performance of four adult resuscitation bags, *Respir Care* 27:139–146, 1982.

94. Barnes TA, Potash R: Evaluation of five disposable operator-powered adult resuscitators, *Respir Care* 34:254–261, 1989.

95. Barnes TA, McGarry W: Evaluation of ten disposable manual resuscitators, *Respir Care* 35:960–968, 1990.

96. Elling R, Politis J: An evaluation of emergency medical technicians' ability to use manual ventilation devices, *Ann Emerg Med* 12:765–768, 1983.

97. Hess D, Baran C: Ventilatory volumes using mouth-to-mouth, mouth-to-mask, and bag-valve-mask techniques, *Am J Emerg Med* 3:292–296, 1985.

98. Cummins RO, Austin D, Graves JR, Litwin PE, Pierce J: Ventilation skills of emergency medical technicians: a teaching challenge for emergency medicine, *Ann Emerg Med* 15:1187–1192, 1986.

99. Johannigman JA, Branson RD, Davis K Jr, Hurst JM: Techniques of emergency ventilation: a model to evaluate tidal volume, airway pressure, and gastric insufflation, *J Trauma* 31:93–98, 1991.

100. Fuerst RS, Banner MJ, Melker RJ: Inspiratory time influences the distribution of ventilation to the lungs and stomach: implications for cardiopulmonary resuscitation, *Ann Emerg Med* In press.

101. Jesudian MC, Harrison RR, Keenan RL, Maull KI: Bag-valve-mask ventilation: two rescuers are better than one: preliminary report, *Crit Care Med* 13:122–123, 1985.

102. Priano LL, Ham J: A simple method to increase F_IO_2 of resuscitator bags, *Crit Care Med* 6:48, 1978.

103. Sellick BA: Cricoid pressure to control regurgitation of stomach contents during induction of anaesthesia, *Lancet* 2:404–406, 1961.

104. Wraight WJ, Chamney AR, Howells TH: The determination of an effective cricoid pressure, *Anaesthesia* 38:461–466, 1983.

105. Klick JM, Bushnell LS, Bancroft, ML: Barotrauma as a potential hazard of manual resuscitators, *Anesthesiology* 49:363, 1978.

106. Finer NN, Barrington KJ, Al-Fadley F, Peters KL: Limitations of self-inflating resuscitators, *Pediatrics* 77:417–420, 1986.
107. Kissoon N, Connors R, Tiffin N, Frewen TC: An evaluation of the physical and functional characteristics of resuscitators for use in pediatrics, *Crit Care Med* 1992; 20(2):292–6.
108. Pasquet EA, Frewen TC, Kissoon N, Gallant J, Tiffin N: Prototype volume-controlled neonatal/infant resuscitator, *Crit Care Med* 16:55–57, 1988.
109. Emergency Care Research Institute: Evaluation: gas-powered resuscitators, *Health Devices* 8:24, 1978.
110. Pearson SW, Redding JS: Evaluation of the Elder demand valve resuscitator for use by first-aid personnel, *Anesthesiology* 28:623–624, 1967.
111. Osborn HH, Kayen D, Home H, Bray W: Excess ventilation with oxygen-powered resuscitators, *Am J Emerg Med.* 1984;2:408–413.
112. Melker RJ, Banner MJ: Positive pressure and spontaneous ventilation characteristics of demand-flow valves: implications for resuscitation, *Ann Emerg Med.* In press.
113. Emergency Care Research Institute: Hazard: demand valve resuscitators, *Health Devices* 5:145–146, 1976.
114. Pradis IL, Caldwell EJ: Traumatic pneumocephalus: a hazard of resuscitators, *J Trauma* 19:61–63, 1979.
115. Fasi TH, Lucas, BG: An evaluation of some mechanical resuscitators for use in the ambulance service, *Ann R Coll Surg Engl* 62:291–293, 1980.
116. Campbell TP, et al: oxygen enrichment of bag-valve-mask units during positive pressure ventilation: a comparison of methods, *Ann Emerg Med* 17:232–235, 1988.
117. Phillips GD, Showronski GA: Manual resuscitators and portable ventilators, *Anaesth Intensive Care* 14:306–313, 1986.
118. Emergency Care Research Institute: Inspection and preventive maintenance procedure: pulmonary resuscitators (gas powered). *Health Devices* 17(11):348–54, 1988.
119. Downs JB, Marston AW: A new transport ventilator: an evaluation, *Crit Care Med* 5(2):112–114, 1977.
120. Harber T, Lucas BG: An evaluation of some mechanical resuscitators for use in the ambulance service, *Ann R Coll Surg Engl* 62:291–293, 1980.
121. Branson RD, McGough EK: Transport ventilators, *Probl Crit Care* 4:254–274, 1990.
122. Nolan JP, Baskett PJF: Gas-powered and portable ventilators: an evaluation of six models, *Prehosp Disaster Med* 7:25–34, 1992.
123. Johannigman JA, Branson RD, Campbell R, Hurst JM: Laboratory and clinical evaluation of the MAX transport ventilator, *Respir Care* 35(10):952–959, 1990.
124. McGough EK, Banner MJ, Melker RJ: Variations in tidal volume with portable transport ventilators, *Resp Care* 37:233–239, 1992.
125. Branson RD: Intrahospital transport of critically ill, mechanical ventilated patients, *Respir Care* 37(7):775–803, 1992.
126. Braman SS, Dunn SM, Amico CA, Millman RP: Complications of intrahospital transport in critically ill patients, *Ann Intern Med* 107:469–473, 1987.
127. Gervais HW, Eberle B, Konietzke D, Hennes HJ, Dick W: Comparison of blood gases of ventilated patients during transport, *Crit Care Med* 15:761–763, 1987.
128. Weg JG, Hans CF: Safe intrahospital transport of critically ill ventilator-dependent patients, *Chest* 96:631–635, 1989.
129. Melker RJ: A clinical evaluation of the pneuPAC ventilator. Presented at the Fourth World Congress on Intensive and Critical Care Medicine; July 1985; Jerusalem, Israel.
130. Hurst JM, Davis K Jr, Branson RD, Johannigman JA: Comparison of blood gases during transport using two methods of ventilatory support, *J Trauma* 29:1637–1640, 1989.
131. Mateer JR, Stueven HA, Thompson BM, Aprahamian C, Darin JC: Prehospital IAC-CPR versus standard CPR: paramedic resuscitation of cardiac arrests, *Am J Emerg Med* 3:143–146, 1985.
132. Sack JB, Kesselbrenner MB, Bregman D: Survival from in-hospital cardiac arrest with interposed abdominal counterpulsation during cardiopulmonary resuscitation, *JAMA* 267:379–385, 1992.
133. Barranco F, Lesmes A, Irles JA, et al: Cardiopulmonary resuscitation with simultaneous chest and abdominal compression: comparative study in humans, *Resuscitation* 20:67–77, 1990.
134. Berryman CR, Phillips GM: Interposed abdominal compression-CPR in human subjects, *Ann Emerg Med* 13:226–229, 1984.
135. Babbs CF, Blevins WE: Abdominal binding and counterpulsation in cardiopulmonary resuscitation, *Crit Care Clin* 2(2):319–32, 1986.
136. Ward KR, Sullivan R J, Zelenak RR, Summer WR: A comparison of interposed abdominal compression CPR and standard CPR by monitoring endtidal PCO2, *Ann Emerg Med* 18:831–837, 1989.
137. Rudikoff MT, Maughan WL, Eftton M, Freund P, Weisfeldt ML: Mechanisms of blood flow during cardiopulmonary resuscitation, *Circulation* 61:345–352, 1980.
138. Niemann JT, Rosborough JP, Niskanen RA, Alferuess C, Criley JM: Mechanical 'cough' cardiopulmonary resuscitation during cardiac arrest in dogs, *Am J Cardiol* 55:199–204, 1985.
139. Krischer JP, Fine EG, Weisfeldt ML, Guerci AD, Nagel E, Chandra N: Comparison of prehospital conventional and simultaneous compression-ventilation cardiopulmonary resuscitation, *Crit Care Med* 17:1263-1269, 1989.
140. Swenson RD, Weaver WD, Niskanen RA, Martin J, Dahlberg S: Hemodynamics in humans during conventional and experimental methods of cardiopulmonary resuscitation, *Circulation* 78:630–639, 1988.
141. Kern KB, Carter AB, Showen RL, et al: Comparison of mechanical techniques of cardiopulmonary resuscitation: survival and neurologic outcome in dogs, *Am J Emerg Med* 5:190–195, 1987.
142. Martin GB, Carden DL, Nowak RM, Lewinter JR, Johnston W, Tomlanovich MC: Aortic and fight atrial pressures during standard and simultaneous compression and ventilation CPR in human beings, *Ann Emerg Med* 15:125–130, 1986.
143. Cohen TJ, Tucker KJ, Redberg RF, et al: Active compression-decompression resuscitation: a novel method of cardiopulmonary resuscitation, *Am Heart J* 124(5):1145–50, 1992.
144. Feneley MP, Maler GW, Kern KB, et al: Influence of compression rate on initial success of resuscitation and 24 hour survival after prolonged manual cardiopulmonary resuscitation in dogs, *Circulation* 77:240–250, 1988.
145. Kern KB, Sanders AB, Raife J, Milander MM, Otto CW, Ewy GA: A study of chest compression rates during cardiopulmonary resuscitation in humans: the importance of rate-directed chest compressions, *Arch Intern Med* 152:145–149, 1992.
146. Wolfe JA, Maier GW, Newton JR Jr, et al: Physiologic determinants of coronary blood flow during external cardiac massage, *J Thorac Cardiovasc Surg* 95(3):523–32, 1988.
147. Taylor GJ, Rubin R, Tucker M, et al: External cardiac compression: A randomized comparison of mechanical and manual techniques, *JAMA* 240:644–646, 1978.
148. McDonald JL: Systolic and mean arterial pressures during manual and mechanical CPR in humans, *Ann Emerg Med* 11:292–295 1982.
149. Mahoney BD, Mirick MJ: Efficacy of pneumatic trousers in refractory prehospital cardiopulmonary arrest, *Ann Emerg Med* 12:8–12, 1983.
150. Del Guercio LRM, Feins NR, Cohn JD, et al: Comparison of blood flow during external and internal cardiac massage in man, *Circulation* 31(suppl I):I171–I180, 1965.

151. Sanders AB, Keru KB, Ewy GA, Atlas M, Bailey L: Improved resuscitation from cardiac arrest with open-chest massage, *Ann Emerg Med* 13:672–675, 1934.

152. Sanders AB, Kern KB, Atlas M, Bragg S, Ewy GA: Importance of the duration of inadequate coronary perfusion pressure on resuscitation from cardiac arrest, *J Am Coll Cardiol* 6:113–118, 1985.

153. Kern KB, Sanders AB, Badylak SF, et al: Long-term survival with openchest cardiac massage after ineffective closed-chest compression in a canine model, *Circulation* 75:498–503, 1987.

154. Geehr EC, Lewis FR, Auerbach PS: Failure of open-heart massage to improve survival after prehospital nontraumatic cardiac arrest [letter], *N Engl J Med* 314:1189–1190, 1986.

155. Kern KB, Sanders AB, Janas W, et al: Limitations of open-chest cardiac massage after prolonged, untreated cardiac arrest in dogs, *Ann Emerg Med* 20:761–767, 1991.

156. Rosenthal RE, Turbiak TW: Open-chest cardiopulmonary resuscitation, *Am J Emerg Med* 4(3):248–258, 1986.

157. Eldor J, Frankel DZ, Davidson JT: Open chest cardiac massage: a review, *Resuscitation* 16(3):155–162, 1988.

158. Hartz R, LoCicero J III, Sanders JH Jr, et al: Clinical experience with portable cardiopulmonary bypass in cardiac arrest patients, *Ann Thorac Surg* 1990;50:437–441.

159. Angelos MG, Gaddis M, Gaddis G, Leasure JE: Cardiopulmonary bypass in a model of acute myocardial infarction and cardiac arrest, *Ann Emerg Med* 1990;19:874–880.

160. Tisherman SA, Safar P, Abramson NS, et al: Feasibility of emergency cardiopulmonary bypass for resuscitation from CPR-resistant cardiac arrest: a preliminary report, *Ann Emerg Med* 1991;20:491. Abstract.

161. Reedy JE, Swartz MT, Raithel SC, Szukalski EA, Pennington DG: Mechanical cardiopulmonary support for refractory cardiogenic shock, *Heart Lung* 19(5 Pt 1):514–23, 1990.

162. Goldberger E: *Essentials of Clinical Electrocardiography,* Philadelphia, 1990, JB Lippincott.

163. Fassler M, Steuble B: *Electrocardiogram Interpretation and Emergency Intervention,* Springhouse, 1991, Springhouse Corp.

164. Marriott HJL: *Practical Electrocardiography,* ed 8, Baltimore, 1988, Williams and Wilkins.

165. Catalano J: *Guide to ECG Analysis,* Philadelphia, 1993, JB Lippincott.

166. Scheinman MM, Thorburn D, Abbott JA: Use of atropine in patients with acute myocardial infarction and sinus bradycardia, *Circulation* 52:627–633, 1975.

167. Stueven HA, Tonsfeldt DJ, Thompson BM, Whircomb J, Kastenson E, Aprahamian C: Atropine in asystole: human studies, *Ann Emerg Med* 13(9, Part 2):815–817, 1984.

168. Mathewson HS, Conyers, D: Advanced cardiac life support update: Uses of drugs, *Respir Care* 38(9):1020–1023, 1993.

169. Fontaine G, Frank R, Grosgogeat Y: Torsades de pointes: definition and management, *Mod Concepts Cardiovasc Dis* 51:103–108, 1982.

170. Emerman CL, Pinchak AC, Hancock D, Hagen JF: The effect of bolus injection on circulation times during cardiac arrest, *Am J Emerg Med* 8:190–193, 1990.

171. Hahnel J, Lindner KH, Ahnefeld FW: Endobronchial administration of emergency drugs, *Resuscitation* 17(3):261–72, 1989.

172. Raehl CL: Endotracheal drug therapy in cardiopulmonary resuscitation, *Clin Pharm* 5(7):572–9, 1986.

173. Aitkenhead AR: Drug administration during CPR: what route? *Resuscitation* 22:191–195, 1991.

174. Zelis R, Mansour EJ, Capone RJ, Mason DT, Kleckner R: The cardiovascular effects of morphine: the peripheral capacitance and resistance vessels in human subjects, *J Clin Invest* 54:1247–1258, 1974.

175. Jost P: The role of antidysrhythmics in cardiac arrest, *Crit Care Nurs Q* 10(4):63–67, 1988.

176. Olson DW, Thompson BM, Darin JC, Milbrath MH: A randomized comparison study of bretylium tosylate and lidocaine in resuscitation of patients from out-of-hospital ventricular fibrillation in a paramedic system, *Ann Emerg Med* 13(9, Part 2):807–810, 1984.

177. Ellenbogen KA: Role of calcium antagonists for heart rate control in atrial fibrillation, *Am J Cardiol* 69:36B–40B, 1992.

178. DiMarco JP, Sellers TD, Berne RM, West GA, Belardinelli L: Adenosine: electrophysiologic effects and therapeutic use for terminating paroxysmal supraventricular tachycardia, *Circulation* 68:1254–1263, 1983.

179. McCabe JL, Adhar GC, Menegazzi JJ, Paris PM: Intravenous adenosine in the prehospital treatment of paroxysmal supraventricular tachycardia, *Ann Emerg Med* 21:358–361, 1992.

180. Parker RB, McCollam PL: Adenosine in the episodic treatment of paroxysmal supraventricular tachycardia, *Clin Pharm* 9:261–271, 1990.

181. Brown CG, Werman HA: Adrenergic agonists during cardiopulmonary resuscitation, *Resuscitation* 19(1):1–16, 1990.

182. Hebert P, Weitzman BN, Stiell IG, Stark RM: Epinephrine in cardiopulmonary resuscitation, *J Emerg Med* 9(6):487–495, 1991.

183. Callaham ML: High-dose epinephrine therapy and other advances in treating cardiac arrest [clinical conference], *West J Med* 152(6):697–703, 1990.

184. Gonzalez ER, Ornato JP: The dose of epinephrine during cardiopulmonary resuscitation in humans: what should it be? *DICP* 25(7–8):773–777, 1991.

185. Lindner KH, Ahnefeld FW, Bowdler IM: Comparison of ephinephrine and dopamine during cardiopulmonary resuscitation, *Intensive Care Med* 15:432–438, 1989.

186. Jaffe AS, Roberts R: The use of intravenous nitroglycerin in cardiovascular disease, *Pharmacotherapy* 2:273–280, 1982.

187. Dembo DH: Calcium in advanced life support, *Crit Care Med* 9:358, 1981.

188. Bishop RL, Weisfeldt ML: Sodium bicarbonate administration during cardiac arrest, *JAMA,* 235:255–260, 1976.

189. Federiuk CS, Sanders AB, Kern KB, et al: The effect of bicarbonate on resuscitation from cardiac arrest, *Ann Emerg Med* 20:1173–1177, 1991.

190. Adgey AA: Electrical energy requirements for ventricular defibrillation, *Br Heart J* 40:1197–1199, 1978.

191. Chameides L, Brown GE, Raye JR, et al: Guidelines for defibrillation in infants and children, *Circulation* 56(suppl): 502A–503A, 1977.

192. Hess D, Eitel D: Monitoring during resuscitation, *Respir Care* 37(7):739–765, 1992.

193. Waxman K: Noninvasive monitoring in emergency resuscitation, *Ann Emerg Med* 15:1434–1436.

194. Ornato JP, Bryson BL, Donovan PJ, et al: Measurement of ventilation during cardiopulmonary resuscitation, *Crit Care Med* 11:79–82, 1983.

195. Kauffman GW, Hess DR: Modification of the infant Laerdal resuscitation bag to monitor airway pressure, *Crit Care Med* 10:112–113, 1982.

196. Goldstein B, Catlin EA, Vetere JM, Arguin LJ: The role of in-line manometers in minimizing peak and mean airway pressure during hand-regulated ventilation of newborn infants, *Respir Care* 34:23–27, 1989.

197. Bizzle TL, Kotas RV: Positive pressure hand ventilation: potential errors in estimating inflation pressures, *Pediatrics* 72:122–125, 1983.

198. Tremper KK, Waxman K, Bowman R, Shoemaker WC: Continuous trancutaneous oxygen monitoring during respiratory failure, cardiac decompensation, cardiac arrest and CPR: trancutaneous oxygen monitoring during arrest and CPR, *Crit Care Med* 8:377–381, 1980.

199. Rutherford WF, Panacek EA, Griffith JK, et al: Prediction of changing cerebral blood flow by the use of the conjunctival/arterial oxygen tension index, *Crit Care Med* 17:1328–1332, 1989.

200. Narang VPS: Utility of the pulse oximeter during cardiopulmonary resuscitation, *Anesthesiology* 65:239–240, 1986.
201. Moorthy SS, Dierdorf SF, Schmidt SI: Erroneous pulse oximetry data during CPR, *Anesth Analg* 70:334–341, 1990.
202. Sanders AB, Otto CW, Kern KB, et al: Acid-base balance in a cannine model of cardiac arrest, *Ann Emerg Med* 17:667–671, 1988.
203. Weil MH, Rackow EC, Trevino R, et al: Difference in acid-base stae between venous and arterial blood during cardiopulmonary resuscitation, *N Engl J Med* 315:153–156, 1986.
204. Weil MH, Bisera J, Trevino RP, Rackow EC: Cardiac output and end-tidal carbon dioxide, *Crit Care Med* 13:907–909, 1985.
205. Bircher NG: Brain resuscitation, *Resuscitation* 18(Suppl): S1–11, 1989.
206. Bircher NG: Neurologic management following cardiac arrest, *Crit Care Clin* 5(4):773–84, 1989.
207. Henneman EA: Brain resuscitation, *Heart Lung* 15(1):3–11, 1986.

24

Production, Storage, and Delivery of Medical Gases

■

Robert Thalken

It is from the humble beginning of the hospital "oxygen service" that the present skilled technology of respiratory care evolved. Although respiratory care practitioners have assumed many more challenging duties, assuring the safe and uninterrupted supply of medical gases is still a key responsibility.

In this chapter, we will consider the production and storage of medical gases, and the devices used to control their delivery in the clinical setting. We will call upon some previously discussed principles as we describe both the gaseous and liquid forms of medical gases. Much of the information in this chapter is drawn from two primary sources, with which all RCPs should be familiar. These sources are the codes of the National Fire Protection Association and the publications of the Compressed Gas Association. In addition, the reader can find useful information in the many brochures and publications available from gas and equipment manufacturers.

AGENCIES

Many agencies are involved in the control of manufacturing and safe use of medical gases and devices employed in respiratory care. Because more detailed information is available from other sources, we provide only a general description of these various agencies.

The agencies discussed in this chapter can be divided into two general groups: those that *recommend* standards and procedures, and those that actually *regulate* by statutory authority. The key recommending and regulating agencies associated with respiratory care are described in the box on page 634.

Recommending agencies

Recommending agencies are usually made up of individuals or formal organizations involved in some aspect of technology. Through consensus of their members, they establish and encourage *voluntary* compliance with pertinent standards. A good example of a recommending agency is the Compressed Gas Association (CGA). The CGA consists of equipment manufacturers and distributors, as well as others involved in the production of compressed and liquefied gases.[1]

Practitioners involved in respiratory care can and should provide input to recommending bodies. The most direct method for input is through the American Association for Respiratory Care (AARC). The AARC maintains active communication with key national standards agencies affecting respiratory care practice via liaison personnel or actual committee representation.

Regulating agencies

Regulating agencies are federal, state, and local bodies that have the *statutory authority* to enforce laws controlling the manufacture and safe use of gases, drugs, and devices. A good example of a regulatory agency is the Food and Drug Administration (FDA). Among its many responsibilities, the FDA sets purity standards for medical gases and oversees requirements for medical devices.[2-4]

Regulating and recommending agencies involved with medical gases

Recommending agencies
Compressed Gas Associations (CGA)

The CGA is made up of companies involved in the compressed gas industry. It has created standards and safety systems for compressed gas systems.

National Fire Protection Association (NFPA)

The NFPA is an agency involved in improved methods of fire protection and prevention, including creating standards for the storage of flammable and oxidizing gases.

International Standards Organization (ISO)

The ISO is the international agency for standardization covering most areas of technology.

American National Standard Institute (ANSI)

ANSI is a private nonprofit organization that coordinates the voluntary developments of national standards in the United States and represents U.S. interests in the area of international standardization.

Z-79 Committee

Z-79 is the American National Standards Committee on standards for anesthesia and ventilatory devices. These devices include anesthesia machines, reservoir bags, tracheal tubes, humidifiers, nebulizers, and other oxygen related equipment.

Regulating agencies
Department of Transportation (DOT)

The department of the federal government given the responsibility in 1970 for compressed gas cylinders, which were previously regulated by the Interstate Commerce Commission (ICC).

Dept of Health and Human Services (HHS)

This department of the federal government was formerly called the Department of Health, Education and Welfare (HEW). HHS has created many agencies that are involved in health delivery. As an example, the Food and Drug Administration (FDA) is an agency that requires a certain level of purity for medical gases.

Food and Drug Administration (FDA)

The FDA is an agency of HHS and requires a certain level of purity for medical gases.

Bureau of Medical Devices (BMD)

The BMD is an agency of FDA and was formed in 1976 to classify, provide standards for, and regulate medical devices.

Occupational Safety and Health Agency (OSHA)

OSHA is an agency of the federal Department of Labor and is responsible for occupational safety.

Table 24-1 Medical gases

Laboratory gases	Therapy gases	Anesthetics
Carbon dioxide	Air	Nitrous oxide
Helium	Helium/oxygen	
Nitrogen	Oxygen	
	Oxygen/carbon dioxide	
	Oxygen/nitrogen	
	Oxygen/nitric oxide*	

*Investigational (research) use only.

Regulatory agencies often adopt the voluntary standards developed by recommending agencies as their legal requirements. As an example, a local county government might adopt the NFPA standards for the storage of bulk oxygen. Under such circumstances, the voluntary standards of a recommending agency become the statutory requirements of a governmental regulating body.

Because both voluntary standards and legal requirements are under constant review and revision, no text can possibly assure complete and up-to-date coverage. Health care institutions and their professional staff share responsibility to maintain current knowledge in these areas, and, where applicable, to assure ongoing compliance.

CHARACTERISTICS OF MEDICAL GASES

Of all the many gases that are produced and used commercially, we are interested in the few that are called medical gases (Table 24-1). Of these, we will focus on the therapeutic gases, generally excluding laboratory and anesthetic gases. From a safety point of view, however, RCPs should be familiar with all gases used in the clinical setting, especially those posing a fire risk.

In regard to fire risk, medical compressed gases are classified as either nonflammable (will not burn), nonflammable but will support **combustion,** or flammable (will burn readily).[1] According to this classification, the common medical gases are grouped as follows:

Nonflammable: nitrogen, carbon dioxide, helium
Support combustion: oxygen, nitrous oxide, air, oxygen-nitrogen, oxygen-carbon dioxide, helium-oxygen, nitric oxide
Flammable: cyclopropane, ethylene*

The rest of this section provides details on the characteristics and production of the gases and gas mixtures commonly used in respiratory care.

---

*Cyclopropane and ethylene were once common anesthetic agents, but are no longer in use. They are included here only for completeness.

Oxygen (O₂)

Characteristics

Oxygen is a colorless, odorless, transparent, and tasteless gas.[1] It exists naturally as free molecular oxygen and as a component of a host of chemical compounds. Oxygen comprises almost 50% by weight of the earth's crust and occurs in all living matter in combination with hydrogen as water. At STPD, oxygen has a density of 1.429 g/L, being slightly heavier than air (1.29 g/L). Oxygen is not very soluble in water. At room temperature and one atmosphere pressure, only 3.3 mL of oxygen can dissolve in 100 mL of water. Nonetheless, this small amount is sufficient for all aquatic life.

As indicated previously, *oxygen is nonflammable* but it greatly accelerates combustion. A match would be consumed in an instant if lit in an oxygen rich environment. Burning speed increases with either: (1) an increase in the oxygen percent at a fixed total pressure, or (2) with an increase in total pressure of a constant gas concentration. Thus both oxygen concentration and partial pressure influence the rate of burning.[5]

Production

Oxygen is produced by one of several methods. Chemical methods for producing small quantities of oxygen include electrolysis of water and the decomposition of sodium chlorate ($NaClO_3$). Most medical grade oxygen is mass-produced by fractional distillation of atmospheric air.[1] Low-flow oxygen for home use is produced by physical separation from air.

Fractional distillation. Fractional distillation is the most common and least expensive method for producing oxygen. The process involves several related steps. First, atmospheric air is filtered to remove pollutants, water and carbon dioxide. The purified air is then converted to a liquid by compressing it to high pressure, and then cooling the mixture by rapid expansion (the Joule-Thompson effect).

The resulting mixture of liquid oxygen and nitrogen is heated slowly in a distillation tower. Nitrogen, with its boiling point of −195.8° C (−320.5° F), escapes first, followed by the trace gases of argon, krypton, and xenon. The remaining liquid oxygen is then transferred to specially insulated cryogenic (low temperature) storage cylinders. Alternatively, the oxygen is converted directly to gas for storage under high pressure in metal cylinders.

This method produces oxygen which is about 99.5% pure. The remaining 0.5% is mostly nitrogen and trace argon. FDA standards require an oxygen purity of at least 99.0%.[6]

Physical separation. Two methods are used to separate oxygen from air.[7] The first method uses molecular "sieves" composed of inorganic sodium aluminum silicate pellets. These pellets absorb nitrogen and water vapor from the air, thus providing a concentrated mixture of over 90% oxygen for patient use. The second method uses a semipermeable plastic membrane to filter nitrogen (but not water vapor) from **ambient** air. This system can produce an oxygen mixture of about 40%. These devices, called oxygen concentrators, are used primarily for oxygen supply in the home care setting. For this reason, details on their principles of operation and appropriate use will be covered in Chapter 38.

Air

Atmospheric air is a colorless, orderless naturally occurring gas mixture consisting of 20.095% oxygen, 78.084% nitrogen and about 1% 'trace' gases, mainly argon. At STPD, the density of air is 1.29 g/L, which is used as the standard for measuring specific gravity of other gases. Oxygen and nitrogen can be mixed to produce a gas with an oxygen concentration equivalent to air (19.5% to 23.5%).[7] However, air for medical use is usually produced by filtering and compressing atmospheric air.[1,8]

Figure 24-1 depicts a typical large medical air compressor system. These systems use an electrical motor to power a piston in a compression cylinder. On its downstroke, the piston draws air in through a filter system via an inlet valve. On its upstroke, the piston compresses the air in the cylinder (closing the inlet valve), and delivers it via an outlet valve to a reservoir tank. Air from the reservoir tank is then reduced to the desired working pressure by a pressure reducing valve before being delivered to the piping system.

For medical gas use, air must be dry and free of oil or particulate contamination.[9] Drying is achieved by

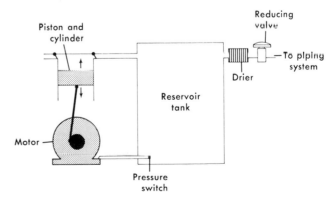

Fig. 24-1 Large air-compressor system for piping system. Compressor sends gas to reservoir at higher than line pressure. When preset pressure level is reached, pressure switch shuts compressor off. Gas leaves reservoir and passes through dryer to remove moisture, and reducing valve reduces gas to desired line pressure. When reservoir pressure has dropped to near line pressure, pressure switch turns compressor back on. (From McPherson SP, Spearman CB: Respiratory therapy equipment, ed 3, St Louis, 1985, Mosby.)

several methods, the most common of which is refrigeration (to produce condensation). To avoid oil or particulate contamination, most medical air compressors use Teflon piston rings, as opposed to the carbon rings or oil lubrication used in nonmedical air compressors. Large medical air compressors must be capable of maintaining high flows (at least 100 L/min) at the standard working pressure of 50 psig for all equipment in use.

Smaller compressors are available for bedside or home use. These compressors use a diaphragm or turbine to compress the air, and generally do not have a reservoir. This design limits both the pressure and flow capabilities of these devices. For this reason, small compressors must never be used to power equipment that needs unrestricted flow at 50 psig, such as pneumatically-powered ventilators (see Chapter 31). However, small diaphragm or turbine compressors are ideal for powering devices such as small volume medication nebulizers (Chapter 25).

Carbon dioxide (CO_2)

At normal atmospheric temperatures and pressure, CO_2 is a colorless and odorless gas with a specific gravity of 1.53 (about 1.5 times heavier than air). Carbon dioxide does not support combustion or maintain animal life. For medical use, carbon dioxide usually is produced by heating limestone in contact with water. The gas is recovered from this process, and liquefied by compression and cooling.[1] The FDA purity standard for carbon dioxide is 99.0%.[6]

Mixtures of oxygen and 5% to 10% carbon dioxide were once used for various therapeutic purposes, including treatment of singultus (hiccups) and atelectasis. Today, the therapeutic use of carbon dioxide mixtures is limited. CO_2 mixtures are still used in membrane oxygenators (heart-lung machines) and to calibrate blood gas analyzers. However, most medical carbon dioxide is used for diagnostic purposes in the clinical laboratory.

Helium (He)

Helium is second only to hydrogen as the lightest of all gases, with a density at STPD of 0.1785 g/L. Helium is odorless and tasteless and inert (thus nonflammable). It is a good conductor of heat, sound and electricity, but is poorly soluble in water. Although present in small quantities in the atmosphere, helium is commercially produced from natural gas by liquefication to purity standards of at least 95%.[6] Free helium can also be liberated from uranium ore by heating.

Being both chemically and physiologically inert, helium cannot support life. Thus breathing 100% helium can cause severe hypoxemia and death. When mixed with oxygen, however, helium can be used therapeutically. Some clinical centers use 'heliox' to treat severe cases of large airway obstruction, such as life-threatening asthma. In these cases, helium's low density decreases the effort required to breathe.

Nitrous oxide (N_2O)

Nitrous oxide is a colorless gas with a slightly sweet odor and taste that is used clinically as an anesthetic agent. Like oxygen, nitrous oxide can support combustion. However, nitrous oxide cannot support life and will cause death if inhaled in pure form. For this reason, inhaled nitrous oxide must always be mixed with at least 20% oxygen. Nitrous oxide is produced by thermal decomposition of ammonium nitrate.

Nitrous oxide's use as an anesthetic agent is based on its CNS depressant effect. However, only dangerously high level of N_2O provide true anesthesia. This is why nitrous oxide/oxygen mixtures are almost always used in combination with other anesthetic agents.

Long-term human exposure to nitrous oxide has been associated with a form of neuropathy. In addition, epidemiologic studies have linked chronic nitrous oxide exposure with an increased risk of fetal disorders and spontaneous abortions. Based on this knowledge, the National Institute for Occupational Safety and Health (a division of OSHA) has set an upper exposure limit for hospital operating rooms of 25 **ppm** nitrous oxide.[1]

Nitric oxide (NO)

Nitric oxide is a colorless, nonflammable and toxic gas which supports combustion. Nitric oxide is produced by oxidation of ammonia at high temperatures in the presence of a catalyst. In combination with air, nitric oxide forms brown fumes of nitrogen dioxide (NO_2). Together, these two gases are strong respiratory irritants which can cause chemical pneumonitis and a fatal form of pulmonary edema.[1] Exposure to high concentrations of nitric oxide alone can cause methemoglobinemia (see Chapter 12).

While not yet FDA approved, nitric oxide is being used experimentally to treat certain forms of pulmonary hypertension. In very low concentrations (80 to 100 ppm) mixed with oxygen, nitric oxide dilates the pulmonary blood vessels. This effect has proved beneficial in treating persistent pulmonary hypertension of the newborn (PPHN)[10] and the Adult Respiratory Distress Syndrome (ARDS).[11] However, more research is needed before this potentially hazardous gas becomes accepted for its therapeutic value.

STORAGE OF MEDICAL GASES

Gas cylinders

The containers used to store and ship compressed or liquid medical gases are high pressure cylinders. The design, manufacture, transport, and use of these cylinders are carefully controlled by both industrial standards and federal regulations. Gas cylinders are made of seamless steel and are classified by the DOT according to their fabrication method. DOT type '3A' cylinders are made from carbon steel, while DOT type '3AA' containers are manufactured using a steel alloy that is **tempered** to produce higher strength.[1]

Markings and identification

Medical gas cylinders are marked by metal stampings on their shoulders that supply specific information (Figure 24-2).[12,13] Although the exact location and order of these markings may vary, the practitioner should be able to identify several key items of information.

The letters ICC (Interstate Commerce Commission) or DOT are followed by the cylinder classification (3A or 3AA) and the normal filling pressure in pounds per square inch. Below this one normally finds the letter size of the cylinder (E, G, etc.), followed by its serial number. A third line provides a mark of ownership, often followed by the manufacturers' stamp or a mark identifying the inspecting authority.

On the opposite surface of the cylinder one normally finds an abbreviation indicating the method of cylinder manufacture. Also in this vicinity are series of symbols that include data on the cylinder's original safety test, and dates of all subsequent tests.

These safety tests occur every 5 or 10 years, as specified in DOT regulations.[12,14] During these tests, cylinders are pressurized to five-thirds of their service pressures. While under pressure, cylinder leakage, expansion, and wall stress are determined. The notation "E.E.," followed by a number indicates the cylinder's elastic expansion in cubic centimeters under these test conditions.

Subsequent to hydrostatic pressure testing, cylinders are inspected internally and cleaned. A plus (+) sign appearing immediately after the test date means that the cylinder is approved for filling to 10% above its service pressure. For example, an approved cylinder with a service pressure of 2015 psi can be filled to about 2200 psi.

In addition to these permanent marks, all cylinders are color coded and labeled to identify their contents.[15,16] Table 24-2, page 638 lists the color codes for medical gases as adopted by the Bureau of Standards of the US Department of Commerce.[17] For comparison, the color codes adopted by the Canadian Standards Association also are included. As can be seen, color codes are not internationally standardized. For this reason, the color of a cylinder must be used only as a guide. As with any drug agent, you must always positively identify the cylinder contents by carefully reading its label. Moreover, based on reports of improperly mixed therapeutic gases,[18] the specified oxygen percentage in a gas mixture should be verified by analysis prior to administration.

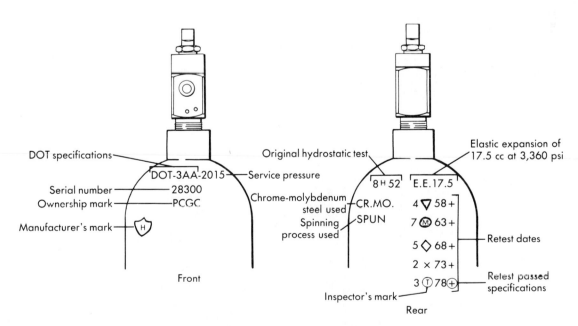

Fig. 24-2 Typical markings for cylinders containing medical gases. Front and back views are for illustration purposes only; exact location and order of markings are variable.

Table 24-2   Color codes medical gas cylinders

Gas	USA	Canada
Oxygen	Green	White*
Carbon dioxide	Gray	Gray
Nitrous oxide	Blue	Blue
Cyclopropane	Orange	Orange
Helium	Brown	Brown
Ethylene	Red	Red
Carbon dioxide/oxygen	Gray/green	Gray/white
Helium/oxygen	Brown/green	Brown/white
Nitrogen	Black	Black
Air	Yellow*	Black/white
Nitrogen/oxygen (other than air)	Black/Green	Pink

*Historically, vacuum systems are identified as white in the USA and yellow in Canada. For this reason, the CGA recommends that white not be used for any cylinders in the US or yellow in Canada.

Cylinders sizes and contents

Letter designations are used for different size cylinders (Figure 24-3). Table 24-3 provides a listing of the most common cylinder sizes and contents for the gases which RCPs use most often.

Sizes AA through E are referred to as "small cylinders" and are used most often for anesthetic gases and portable oxygen supply. You can easily identify these small cylinders by their unique connecting mechanism. Small cylinders use a connector called a *yoke,* while large cylinders (F to H & K) have a threaded outlet from their valves. More detail on

these different connectors is provided later in this chapter.

Filling (charging) cylinders

How a cylinder is filled depends on whether the contents are kept in the gaseous or liquid state. Among gases that can be stored as liquids, some can be kept in liquid form at room temperature, while others must be maintained in a cryogenic (low temperature) state. Cryogenic storage of gases as liquids will be discussed in a following section.

Compressed gases. A gas cylinder normally is filled to its service pressure (the pressure stamped on its shoulder) at 70°F. However, as previously described, approved cylinders can be filled to 10% in excess of the service pressure.

Liquefied gases. Gases with critical temperatures above room temperature can be stored as liquids at room temperature (see Chapter 7). These gases includes carbon dioxide and nitrous oxide. Rather than using a filling pressure, cylinders of these gases are filled according to a specified *filling density.* The filling density is the ratio between the weight of liquid gas put into the cylinder and the weight of water the cylinder could contain if full. For example, the filling density for carbon dioxide is 68%. This allows the manufacturer to fill a cylinder with liquid CO_2 up to 68% of the weight of water that a full cylinder could hold. The filling density for nitrous oxide is 55%.

Cylinder pressures for these liquid gases are much

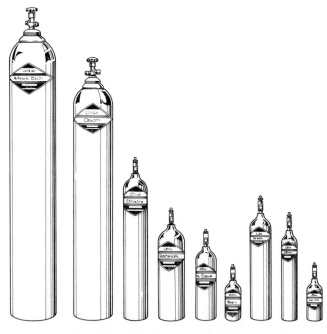

Fig. 24-3   Cylinder sizes by letter code.

Table 24-3 Common Cylinder Sizes and Gases Used in Respiratory Therapy

Cylinder sizes	Gas (cylinder pressure at 21.11°C [70°F] [psig*])					
	Carbon dioxide (840)	Helium (1650 to 2000)	Nitrous oxide (745)	Oxygen (1800 to 2400)	Helium-oxygen mixtures (1650 to 2000)	Carbon dioxide mixtures (1500 to 2200)
D:						
Contents weight (lb)	4.0	0.1	4.0	1.0	—	—
Gas volume at 21.11°C (70°F) and 14.7 psia†						
Cubic feet	33.0	10.6	34.5	12.6	11.0	12.6
Liters	934.0	300.0	975.0	356.0	310.0	356.0
E:						
Contents weight (lb)	6.6	0.2	6.6	2.0	—	—
Gas volume at 21.11°C (70°F) and 14.7 psia						
Cubic feet	56.0	17.0	57.0	22.0	18.0	22.0
Liters	1,585.0	480.0	1,610.0	622.0	510.0	622.0
G:						
Contents weight (lb)	50.0	1.5	56.0	16.0	—	—
Gas volume at 21.11°C (70°F) and 14.7 psia						
Cubic feet	425.0	146.0	485.0	186.0	150.0	186.0
Liters	12,000.0	4,130.0	13,750.0	5,260.0	4,250.0	5,260.0
H-K:						
Contents weight (lb)	—	—	64.0	20.0	—	—
Gas volume at 21.11°C (70°F) and 14.7 psia						
Cubic feet	—	—	557.0	244.0	—	—
Liters	—	—	15,800.0	6,900.0	—	—

From the Standard for Nonflammable Medical Gas Systems (NFPA 56 F), 1973, copyright National Fire Protection Association, Boston, Mass.
* Pounds per square inch gauge.
† Pounds per square inch absolute.

lower than for those stored as in the gas phase. Because the liquid does not fill the entire volume of a cylinder, the space above the liquid surface contains gas in equilibrium with the liquid. *The pressure in a liquid filled cylinder thus equals the pressure of the vapor at any given temperature.*

The pressure in a cylinder thus depends on the state of its contents. In a gas-filled cylinder, the pressure represents the force required to compress the gas into its smaller volume. In contrast, the pressure in a liquid-filled cylinder is the vapor pressure needed to keep the gas liquefied at that temperature.

Measuring cylinder contents

Due to these differences in the physical state of matter, different methods are needed to measure the contents of compressed and liquid gas cylinders.

Compressed gas cylinders. For gas-filled cylinders, the volume of gas in the cylinder is directly propor-

tional to its pressure at a constant temperature. If a cylinder is full at 2200 psig, it will be half full when the pressure drops to 1100 psig. Thus, in order to know how much gas is contained in a compressed gas cylinder, you need only measure its pressure.

Liquid gas cylinders. In a liquid gas cylinder, the measured pressure is the vapor pressure above the liquid. *This pressure bears no relationship to the amount of liquid remaining in the cylinder.* As long as some liquid remains (and the temperature remains constant), the vapor pressure—and thus the gauge pressure—stays constant.

Only when all the liquid is gone and the cylinder contains just gas will the pressure fall in proportion to a reduction in volume. Thus monitoring the gauge pressure of liquid gas cylinders is only useful after all the liquid vaporizes. The only accurate method to determine the contents of a liquid-filled cylinder is to weigh it.

Figure 24-4 compares the behavior of compressed

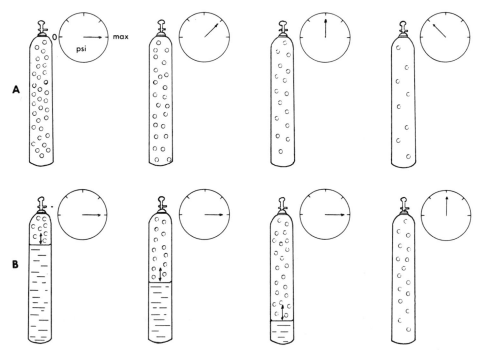

Fig. 24-4 The content of a gas-filled cylinder, **A,** is directly proportional to the gas pressure. As gas is withdrawn, for example, a pressure drop of 50% indicates a loss of 50% of the contained gas. In a liquid-gas cylinder, **B,** gauge pressure measures only the vapor pressure of gas in equilibrium with the liquid phase, and this remains constant at a given temperature as long as liquid is present. Only when all the liquid phase has vaporized, as the cylinder nears depletion, does the gauge pressure drop proportionately to the terminal volume of remaining gas.

Table 24-4 Gas volume conversion factors

Liters	Cubic feet	Gallons
28.316	1	7.481
1	0.03531	0.2642
3.785	0.1337	1

gas and liquid gas cylinders during use. Of course, the vapor pressure of liquid gas cylinders varies with the temperature of their contents. For example, the pressure in a nitrous oxide cylinder at 70°F is 745 psig; at 60°F, the pressure drops to 660 psi. As the temperature rises toward the critical point, more liquid vaporizes and the cylinder pressure rises. Should a cylinder of nitrous oxide warm to 97.5°F (its critical temperature) the entire contents will convert to gas. Only at this temperature and above will the cylinder gauge pressure accurately reflect cylinder contents.

Estimating the duration of compressed gas cylinder flow

When using a cylinder of therapeutic gas, you must be able to predict how long its contents will last at a given flow. You can estimate a cylinder's duration of flow if you know the following facts: (1) the gas flow, (2) the cylinder size, and (3) the cylinder pressure at the start of therapy.

For a given flow, the more gas a cylinder holds, the longer it will 'last.' Conversely, for a given contents, the higher the flow, the shorter time until emptying. Thus, a cylinder's duration of flow is directly proportional to its contents and inversely proportional to its flow. Mathematically, these relationships can be expressed in a simple formula:

$$\text{Duration of Flow} = \frac{\text{Contents}}{\text{Flow}}$$

Unfortunately, the units commonly used in the US to measure these quantities are not the same. Cylinder contents are generally specified in cubic feet or gallons, while gas flow normally is measured in liters. Table 24-4 provides the factors needed to convert among these units.

Rather than memorizing various size cylinder contents and constantly converting between metric and English units, you can quickly calculate duration of flow using cylinder factors. Cylinder factors are derived for each common gas and cylinder size using the following formula:

$$\text{Cylinder Factor (L/psig)} = \frac{\text{Cubic feet in full cylinder} \times 28.3}{\text{Pressure of full cylinder in psig}}$$

The numerator of the equation uses the English-metric conversion constant (28.3) to convert cubic feet to liters. Dividing the resulting volume by the pressure in a full cylinder yields the cylinder factor. As you can see, the cylinder factor represents the liters of gas that leave a given cylinder for every 1 psig drop in gauge pressure. Table 24-5 provides cylinder factors for the therapeutic medical gases and common cylinders sizes. The factors for O_2, O_2/N_2, and air will be used in the vast majority of situations.

Once the factor for a given gas and cylinder are known, calculating the duration of flow is a simple matter of applying the following equation:

$$\text{Duration of Flow (min)} = \frac{\text{Pressure (psig)} \times \text{Factor}}{\text{Flow (L/min)}}$$

As an example, let's estimate the duration of a G cylinder of oxygen with a gauge pressure of 800 psi providing a flow of 8 L/min. Referring to Table 24-5, you find the oxygen G cylinder factor of 2.41. Applying the prior equation:

$$\text{Duration of Flow (min)} = \frac{800 \times 2.41}{8}$$
$$= 241 \text{ minutes (about 4 hours)}$$

Of course, you should always give yourself a wide margin of safety when estimating cylinder duration of flow. This is especially important if you cannot be present during use and must schedule yourself to return with a fresh cylinder. For example, some clinicians always return 30 to 40 minutes before the appointed time; others compute duration of flow to 300 to 500 psig instead of 0 psig (empty). Assuming one's calculations are correct and there is no change in flow, both these method assure an uninterrupted supply.

Bulk oxygen

Because of the huge volumes of oxygen used in the average size hospital, we need to look briefly at large bulk storage systems. Bulk oxygen storage consists of any system capable of holding more than 13,000 cubic feet of gas ready for use.[1] These systems usually are

Table 24-5 Factors to calculate cylinder duration of flow (min)

Gas	D	E	G	H&K
$O_2,O_2/N_2$,air	0.16	0.28	2.14	3.14
O_2/CO_2	0.20	0.35	2.94	3.84
He/O_2	0.14	0.23	1.93	2.50

located outside, but may be placed in a special building designed for this purpose. Safety standards for bulk oxygen systems are published by the NFPA and are subject to further control by local community fire and building codes.[9]

Not all respiratory care departments oversee their hospital's bulk oxygen system. Nonetheless, RCPs are responsible for assuring an uninterrupted supply of oxygen to their patients. Given the numerous reports of bulk supply system failures,[19-21] RCPs must be familiar with bulk units in general, and, more specifically, the system used in their institution.

Bulk oxygen systems store either gaseous or cryogenic liquid oxygen at a central source. Gaseous oxygen then flows from the central source to the hospital floors via a piping system, with outlets conveniently located by each patient's bed.

The advantages of a centrally located bulk oxygen supply over portable cylinders are many. First, despite the large initial investment in equipment, the long-term cost of bulk oxygen is far cheaper. Second, a bulk oxygen system is less prone to interruption. Third, the inconvenience and hazard of moving and storing multiple cylinders is eliminated. Fourth, pressure regulation is achieved in one step at the central station, with the gas piped to the bedside already reduced to the standard pressure of 50 psig. This eliminates the need for separate pressure-reducing valves at each outlets. Last, because it is a low pressure system, a bulk oxygen supply is much safer to use than high-pressure cylinders.

Gaseous bulk oxygen

There are three general systems that provide large central supplies of gaseous oxygen. These include: (1) standard cylinder manifolds, (2) fixed cylinders, and (3) trailer units.

Standard cylinder manifolds. The cylinder manifold is the most common gaseous bulk oxygen system. Cylinder manifolds are also used to supply bulk nitrous oxide to most operating rooms.

A manifold system consists of a series of large compressed oxygen cylinders (normally H or K size) banked together in series (Figure 24-5).[1] Manifolds usually have sides: a "primary bank" and a "reserve bank." When the primary system falls to a set pressure, a control valve automatically switches over to the reserve bank. At this time, the cylinders in the depleted primary bank should be taken 'off-line' and replace by fresh ones. These fresh cylinders now become the reserve bank.

Normally, a manifold system also contains pressure reducing valves and an alarm. The alarm should sound when reserve switch-over occurs, and also should warn of impending depletion or malfunction.

Fixed cylinders. Fixed cylinders consist of large banks of up to 75 cylinders permanently fixed at a stationary site. When empty, they are refilled on site by a truck carrying liquid oxygen. Before being pumped into the cylinders, the liquid oxygen is converted to gas by warming. Fixed cylinders may serve as a reserve supply for a fixed station liquid bulk system.

Trailer units. Very large cylinders mounted on trailers can be towed to a facility and connected to the piping system. For heavy oxygen usage, trailers with up to 30 large cylinders are available. Replacement is a simple matter of switching trailers. Like other compressed systems, trailer gas is at 2200 psig pressure. Trailer units are useful as a replacement supply in the event of primary system failure or when maintenance is needed.

Liquid bulk oxygen

Due to their economy, safety and convenience, liquid oxygen is the bulk delivery system of choice for most hospitals. Moreover, a liquid oxygen delivery system minimizes storage space requirements. At its boiling point of $-297.3°F$ ($-183°C$), one cubic foot of liquid O_2 equals 860.6 cubic feet of gaseous oxygen at ATPD. This allows a small volume of liquid to provide a very large amount of oxygen in gaseous form.

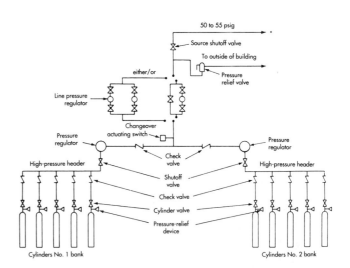

Fig. 24-5 Alternating supply system is composed of primary and secondary supplies, which alternate to charge piping system. (From McPherson SP, Spearman CB: Respiratory therapy equipment, ed 3, St Louis, 1985, Mosby. Reproduced by permission from Standard for nonflammable medical gas systems [NFPA no. 56F], Copyright 1973, National Fire Protection Association, Boston, Mass.)

The major physical difference between oxygen and those gases previously described is that its critical temperature of $-181.1°F$ ($-118.8°C$) is well below room temperature. For this reason the methods used to produce and store liquid oxygen are much more complex than those used for other liquid medical gases.

The method for producing liquid oxygen (compression, cooling and fractional distillation of air) was described previously. One produced, the liquid oxygen must be kept well below its critical temperature, or it will revert back to its gaseous form. To keep oxygen in liquid form, it is stored in special containers under relatively low pressure (less than 250 psig).[1]

All liquid oxygen containers are constructed on the principle of a large thermos bottle. They consist of inner and outer steel shells, separated by a vacuum. The vacuum effectively prevents conduction of heat to the liquid, maintaining it below its critical temperature without refrigeration. To convert the liquid to gas, these systems all include a vaporizer. A liquid oxygen vaporizer usually consists of coiled uninsulated metal tubing that exposes the liquid to ambient temperatures. This passive warming is sufficient to vaporize the liquid oxygen into its gaseous form. Containers also have a safety vent that allows vaporized liquid oxygen to escape if warming causes cylinder pressures to rise.

There are two types of liquid oxygen containers: the liquid oxygen cylinder and the permanent station or stand tank.

Liquid oxygen cylinders. Liquid oxygen cylinders are used as a primary supply when gas usage is too large for a gaseous manifold system but too small to require a permanently installed stand tank. Smaller cylinders of this type are also used for oxygen supply in private homes.[11]

Large liquid oxygen cylinders hold the equivalent of 3000 cubic feet of gas, about equal to 12 standard size H/K cylinders.[1] Two or more liquid cylinders can be banked together like compressed gas cylinders. Large liquid cylinder manifolds are common in small hospitals or larger nursing homes.

Small liquid oxygen cylinders are designed primarily for home use. These cylinders come in several different sizes. Depending on their size, they may hold between 2/3 to 1-1/2 cubic feet of liquid oxygen (equivalent to about 500 to 1200 cubic feet of gaseous oxygen). Small liquid oxygen cylinders are refilled on site by transferring liquid oxygen from a large cylinder.[22] Chapter 38 details the use of these small liquid oxygen cylinders in the home setting.

Fixed stations (stand tanks). Fixed stations are large cylindrical or spherical containers with capacities up to the gaseous equivalent of 130,000 cubic feet (Figure 24-6). As with small cryogenic cylinders, the liquid oxygen is converted to gas by vaporizers. These systems are designed to ensure an uninterrupted gas supply and are refilled from service tank trucks according to schedules designed for each hospital. All medical liquid bulk systems incorporate pressure reducing valves to lower pressure to 50 psig.

Bulk oxygen safety precautions

Detailed standards for design, construction, placement and use of bulk oxygen systems are published by the NFPA[9] and summarized in other sources.[7] Among the key provisions in these standards is the requirement for a reserve or backup gas supply. The NFPA standard requires that the reserve supply be equal to the average daily gas usage of the hospital. To meet this requirement, most larger institutions have a second smaller liquid stand tank. Smaller institutions use a bank of fixed compressed gas cylinders.

Total failure of hospitals' bulk oxygen supply systems have been reported, with major problems occurring in as many as one third of all hospitals.[19-21] Such situations presents immediate danger to any patient receiving oxygen or gas-powered ventilatory support. For this reason, the respiratory care department must be prepared. Established protocols should provide a quick means to identify affected patients, secure equipment, and respond according to a predetermined priority scheme. Practitioners should be familiar with this departmental protocol and their role in addressing such an emergency.

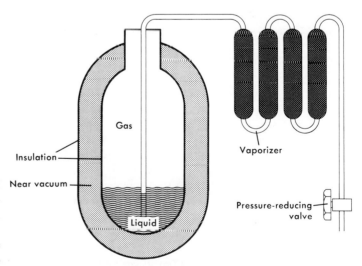

Fig. 24-6 A liquid-oxygen stand tank (fixed station). (From McPherson SP, Spearman CB: Respiratory therapy equipment, ed 3, St Louis, 1985, Mosby.)

DISTRIBUTION AND REGULATION OF MEDICAL GASES

Before medical gases can be administered to a patient, they must be delivered to the bedside and reduced to a workable pressure. This is the primary function of gas distribution and regulation systems.

Modern hospital gas distribution systems deliver bulk oxygen and compressed air to patient rooms and special care areas via an elaborate piping network. Included in this network may be a vacuum source and—for surgical areas—nitrous oxide. However, whenever patients are transported or other gases are required, cylinders must still be used as the gas source.

Gas pressures are regulated either within the piping network or directly at the cylinder source. In either case, various safety systems are used to minimize the likelihood of administering the wrong gas to a patient.

Whether by central supply or cylinder, patient safety is always the primary aim in delivering medical gases. For this reason, RPCs must be proficient in the use of both type of systems.

Central piping systems

Structural standards for piping systems are established by the NFPA and are described in more detail elsewhere.[9] Figure 24-7 show a simple central piped gas system. Normally, the gas pressure in a central piping system is reduced to the standard working pressure at the bulk source or storage location. A main alarm warns of pressure drops or interruptions in flow from the source. Zone valves throughout the system can be closed for system maintenance or in case of fire. Wall outlets at the delivery sites provide connections to the system for various equipment. Normally, oxygen and air are provided to the delivery outlets at 50 psig with unrestricted flow. Since delivery outlets may include not only oxygen, but also air, vacuum, and possibly nitrous oxide, special safety connectors are used to prevent misconnections.

Safety indexed connector systems

With the large number of compressed gases in current use, one of the greatest risks in medical gas therapy is giving the wrong gas to a patient. Certainly, care on the part of the practitioner in reading labels and other identifiers is one important deterrent to such an accident. However, human error is always a potential risk. For this reason, the industry has developed special connectors, called *indexed safety systems,* for gas delivery and regulation equipment.

The purpose of a safety system is to make certain connections between cylinders and delivery systems impossible. For example, when properly used, such a system should prevent you from connecting a cylinder of nitrous oxide to a system for giving oxygen. We will describe only the key elements of the indexed safety systems in common use; you are encouraged to become familiar with their details as provided in the applicable CGA publications.[23-25]

There are three basic indexed safety systems in-

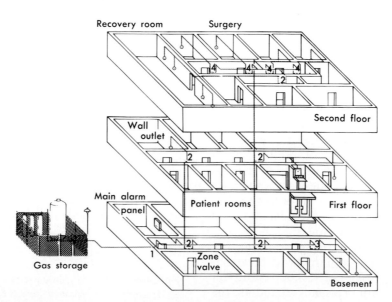

Fig. 24-7 A hospital piping system. Numbers indicate zone valves. (From McPherson SP, Spearman CB: *Respiratory therapy equipment,* ed 3, St Louis, 1985, Mosby. Courtesy Puritan-Bennett Corp, Los Angeles, Calif.)

volved in the delivery and regulation of medical gases: (1) the American Standard Compressed Gas Cylinder Outlet and Inlet Connections, or American Standard Safety System (ASSS) for short, (2) the Diameter-Index Safety System (DISS), and (3) the Pin-Index Safety System (PISS).

American standard safety system (ASSS)

Adopted in the US and Canada, the American Standard Safety System provides standards for threaded *high pressure* connections between compressed gas cylinders and their attachments. Specifications for 62 listed gases are explained in detail in the applicable CGA publication.[23]

The ASSS standards apply only to large cylinders with threaded valve outlets (sizes F through H/K). They provide specifications for the mating nipples and hexagonal nuts by which pressure regulators are attached to the valve. Figure 24-8 illustrates a cutaway of a joined threaded outlet and nipple. The gas channel through the nipple of the regulator is aligned with the channel through the threaded outlet. The two parts are secured by a hexagonal nut that is attached to the nipple by a shoulder and flange mechanism.

By varying the size (or "bore") of the cylinder outlet and nipple for each gas, the ASSS standards should make misconnections impossible. For example, it should not be possible to connect CO_2 cylinders to an oxygen bank.

There are two fundamental divisions of the ASSS: thread position and thread direction. Thread position may be internal or external. Thread direction may be right-handed or left-handed. Each division is further segmented by varying the number, pitch, and diameter (bore) of the threads. In general, left-handed threads are used for fuel gases, and right-handed threads are used for nonfuel (including medical) gas-

es. Most of the valve outlets have external threads, and their corresponding nipples have internal threads.

Because the are only 26 different connections for the 62 listed gases and mixtures, each gas may *not* have its own unique connection. This means that some gases share identical connections.

In catalogs of cylinder equipment, the practitioner will see the connection specifications listed for each type of cylinder and gas. A typical description for a large cylinder of oxygen is as follows:

CGA-540 × 0.903-14NGO-RH-Ext

This tells us that the connection for the threaded outlet of this cylinder is listed by the CGA as connection No. 540, that the outlet has a thread diameter (bore) of 0.903 inch, that there are 14 threads per inch, and that the threads are right handed (RH) and external (Ext).

Generally, you will use but one or two outlet connections, since most of the small number of different gases you employ are grouped within a few connector sizes. However, practitioners should be familiar with the classification scheme in general, since expanding instrumentation and scope of services in the future may bring them into contact with other gases and gas systems.

Pin-indexed safety system (PISS)

Pin-indexing is part of the American Standard listing just described, but applies only to the valve outlets of small cylinders, up to and including size E.[23] These cylinders use a *yoke* type connection.

Figure 24-9, page 646 illustrates the general structure of cylinder valves and the yoke used with small cylinders. Figure 24-9, *A* is a cross-section of a small cylinder valve, similar in principle to cylinder valves in general. The valve stem (*1*) connects to a threaded valve plunger (*2*). The cylinder outlet (*3*) is separated from the gas channel (*7*) by the valve seat (*4*). Turning of the stem via a handgrip (*not shown*) opens and closes the valve seat, permitting or restricting gas outflow.

An emergency pressure release (*5*) allows gas to escape should pressures within the cylinder rise to dangerous levels. A pair of borings in the valve body of small cylinders (*6*) represent part of the Pin-Index Safety System. Finally, the valve is attached to the body of the cylinder by a threaded connection (*8*).

Figure 24-9, *B* shows a yoke connector for the A through E size cylinders. The hand screw is used to hold the yoke firmly onto the valve. The small receiving nipple (*background*) fits into the gas outlet (*3*) and is normally sealed with a single nylon washer or bushing. The two pins (*foreground*) are positioned to mate with the borings in the valve stem (*6*) of the Pin-Indexed Safety System. Failure to properly tighten the hand screw or use a nylon bushing will cause a

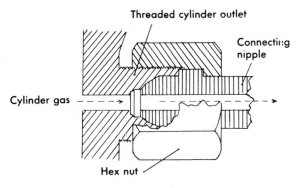

Fig. 24-8 This sketch illustrates the structure of a typical American Standard connection, such as might be used to attach a reducing valve to a large high-pressure cylinder. The hexagonal nut is held onto the nipple of the reducing valve by a circular collar, seen as a cross-sectional projection on the nipple. As a hex nut is tightened on the threaded cylinder outlet, the end of the nipple is snugly seated into the conical outlet. (Modified from CGA Phamphet V-1, connection no. 540, Compressed Gas Association, Inc. New York.)

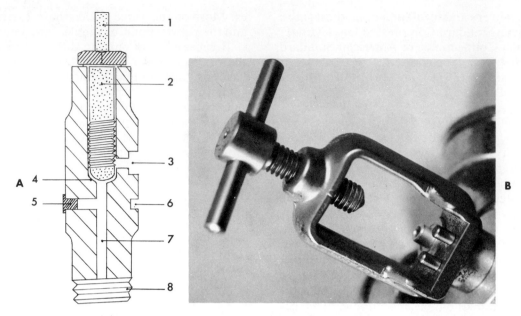

Fig. 24-9 A, Diagrammatic sectional sketch of a small cylinder valve. **B,** Photograph of the yoke connector used with small cylinders. (See text for description.)

leak when the cylinder valve stem is opened. There is also a report of an oxygen regulator fire caused when two yoke bushings (instead of one) were used to seal the connection.[26]

Like the ASSS, the PISS is designed to prevent the wrong cylinder from being attached to a given appliance. The exact position of the two holes drilled in the face of the valve and the two pins on the yoke vary for each gas. Unless the pins and holes align perfectly, the yoke nipple will not seat in the recess of the valve. Six hole/pin positions comprise the total system and because of overlapping, adjacent holes cannot be used **inadvertently.** There are therefore ten possible combinations, of which nine are used.

Figure 24-10 is a composite drawing of the location of all six possible holes and the numbers by which they are indexed. Table 24-6 lists the gases included in the PISS system, including their index positions.

Diameter-Indexed safety system (DISS)

Whereas the ASSS and PISS deal with high pressure connections between cylinders and equipment, the DISS was established to prevent accidental interchange of *low pressure* (less than 200 psig) medical gas connectors.[24] Specifically, the DISS is used in respiratory care to connect equipment to a low pressure gas source. Typically, DISS connection are found in one of three places: (1) at the outlet of pressure reducing valves attached to cylinders, (2) at the wall outlets of

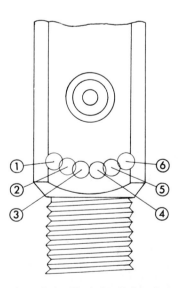

Fig. 24-10 Location of the Pin-Index Safety System holes in the cylinder valve face, varies pairs of which constitute indices for different gases. (See text for the complete pairings.) (Modified from CGA Pamphlet V-1, Pin-Index Safety System, Compressed Gas Association, Inc, New York.)

Table 24-6   Pin-Indexed Gases

Gas	Index hole position
O_2	2-5
O_2/CO_2 (CO_2 not over 7%)	2-6
He/O_2 (He not over 80%)	2-4
C_2H_4	1-3
N_2O	3-5
$(CH_2)_3$	3-6
He/O_2 (He over 80%)	4-6
O_2/CO_2 (CO_2 over 7%)	1-6
Air	1-5

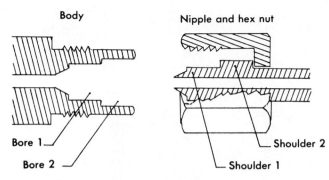

Fig. 24-11 Schematic illustration of components of a representative DISS connection. The two shoulders of the nipple allow the nipple to unite only with a body that has corresponding borings. If the match is incorrect, the hex nut will not engage the body threads. (Modified from CGA Pamphlet V-5, DISS connection no. 1100, Compressed Gas Association, Inc, New York.)

Table 24-7   DISS Connection Numbers and Assigned Gases

Connection number	Gas	Connection number	Gas
1020	Unassigned	1120	Unassigned
1040	N_2O	1140	C_2H_4
1060	He	1160	Air
	He/O_2 (O_2 20%)	1180	He/O_2 (He 80% or less)
1080	CO_2	1200	O_2/CO_2 (CO$_2$ 7% or less
	O_2/CO_2 (CO$_2$ 7%)	1220	Suction
1100	$(CH_2)_3$	1240	O_2 (standard)

central piping systems, and (3) at the inlet of flowmeters, nebulizers, ventilators and other pneumatic equipment.

As shown in Figure 24-11, the DISS connection consists of an externally threaded body and a mated nipple with hex nut. As the two parts are joined, the shoulders of the nipple and bores of the body mate, with the union held together by a hand-tightened hex nut. Indexing is achieved by varying the dimensions of the borings and shoulders.

There are 11 indexed DISS connections plus one for oxygen, for a total of 12 (Table 24-7).[24] It should be noted that the standard threaded oxygen connector (0.5625 inch in diameter and 18 threads per inch), became commonplace *before* the DISS was adopted. Although technically not part of the system, oxygen has been given a DISS number of 1240.

Although you will generally use oxygen or air from a central outlet, you may need to administer mixtures of helium and oxygen or carbon dioxide and oxygen, which have DISS connections. To avoid stocking a large variety of pressure regulators and connectors for special gas use, you can use adapters to convert among various DISS connections. Of course, using adapters to bypass a safety system carries with it the increased risk of misconnection. For this reason, practitioners should exercise extreme caution when adapting equipment connections. Misconnections can and still do occur, with unfortunate patient consequences.[27]

Quick-connect systems

Quick-connect systems are a variation of the standard DISS connections, designed specifically to provide easy attachment of equipment to wall station outlets of piping systems.[5] Various manufacturers have designed specially shaped connectors for each gas (Figure 24-12). Because the connector for each gas has a distinct shape, it will not fit an outlet for another gas. Unlike the DISS system, however, each manufacturer has independently developed its own system. For this reason, connectors from different manufacturers cannot be used with each other. As long as a single quick-connect system is used throughout a hospital, this incompatibility is seldom a problem.

In summary, various safety systems help prevent inadvertent misconnections between medical delivery systems and equipment. Figure 24-13, page 648 summarizes the use of and relationships among the ASSS, PISS, and DISS systems as applied to cylinder gases. Proficiency in the proper use of these systems is a basic skill of RCPs.

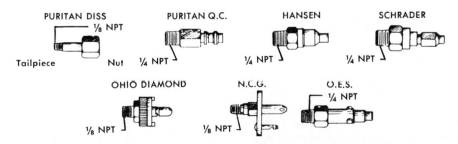

Fig. 24-12 Common brands of quick connects. (From McPherson SP, Spearman CG: Respiratory therapy equipment, ed 3, St Louis, 1985, Mosby. Courtesy Putitan-Bennett Corp, Los Angeles, Calif.)

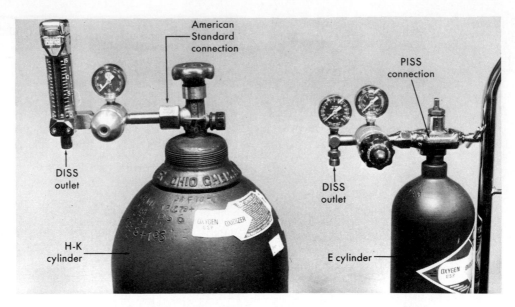

Fig. 24-13 Comparison of safety systems used for compressed gases. Note that the DISS connections are for outlets that have reduced pressures (less than 200 psig), while the American Standard connection is shown for a large cylinder and the PISS connection is shown for a small cylinder.

Regulating gas pressure and flow

Whatever the source of medical gas, to administer it to a patient, you must be able to regulate its pressure and flow. When the goal is simply to reduce gas pressure, a *reducing valve* is employed. A *flowmeter* is a device that controls the flow of a gas. A device that controls both pressure and flow is called a *regulator*.

For cylinder gases such as oxygen or compressed air, the high pressure leaving the cylinder must first be reduced to a lower "working" pressure. In the US, this working pressure is standardized at 50 psig. For bulk delivery systems with individual station outlets, built-in reducing valves drop the pressure to 50 psig. This standard pressure may then be applied directly to power devices such as ventilators (refer to Chapter 31). However, when the goal is to control the delivery of medical gas to a patient (as described in Chapter 26), a device to meter flow must also be used.

High-pressure reducing valves

There are three types of high pressure reducing valves: the preset reducing valve, the adjustable reducing valve, and the multiple-stage reducing valve.[7] Although these valves all function on the same principle, their design features and use are different enough to deserve individual description.

Preset reducing valve. Figure 24-14 portrays the basic design features of a high-pressure preset reduc-

ing valve. High-pressure gas (2200 psig for oxygen) enters the valve through (*A*), with the inlet pressure displayed on the pressure gauge (*B*). The body of the

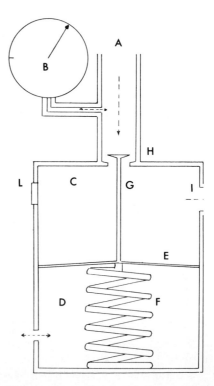

Fig. 24-14 Diagram of preset, high-pressure—reducing valve. (See text for details.)

valve is divided into a high pressure chamber (*C*) and an ambient pressure chamber (*D*) by a flexible diaphragm (*E*). Attached to the diaphragm in the ambient pressure chamber is a spring (*F*) which is fixed to the other side of the chamber. Also attached to the diaphragm, but in the high pressure chamber, is a valve stem (*G*) that seats on the high pressure inlet (*H*). Gas flows through the valve inlet (*H*) into the high pressure chamber, and on to the gas outlet (*I*). The pressure chamber is supplied with a safety vent (*L*) preset to 200 psig to release pressure in the event of malfunction.

The spring tension is calibrated to "give" when the pressure on the diaphragm exceeds 50 psig. When this happens, the valve stem is pushed forward and closes the high pressure inlet, thus preventing further entry of gas into the reducing valve. However, as long as gas is allowed to escape from the pressure chamber through the outlet (*I*), the inlet valve will remain open and permit gas flow. Thus, the regulator maintains a balance between outlet flow and inlet pressure. Automatic adjustment of the diaphragm-spring combination keeps the pressure in the high pressure chamber at a near constant 50 psig, thus the name "preset." Preset reducing valves are normally used in conjunction with high pressure gas cylinders to lower the pressure to the standard 50 psig used with most respiratory care equipment.

Adjustable reducing valve. Although most respiratory care equipment is designed to function at the standard 50 psig, some devices need variable pressures. In order to provide variable outlet pressures from a high pressure gas source, you need an *adjustable* reducing valve. Figure 24-15 shows the basic design features of a high-pressure adjustable reducing valve. As with the preset design, the inlet valve (*H*) remains open until the gas pressure exceeds the spring tension, thus displacing the diaphragm and blocking further gas entry. However, while the preset reducing valve provides a fixed pressure, the adjustable reducing valve allows you to change outlet pressures. You can change outlet pressures using a threaded hand control (*K*) attached to the end of the diaphragm spring. By changing the tension on the valve spring, you can vary pressures over a wide range, usually between 0 to 100 psig.

The most common application of the adjustable reducing valve is in combination with a Bourdon type flow gauge, to be described later. When we combine a flow meter with a reducing valve, we call the device a regulator.

Multiple-stage reducing valve. As the name suggests, the multiple-stage reducing valve reduces pressure in two or more steps. Multiple-stage reducing valves can be either preset or adjustable, and can be combined with a flow metering device as a true regulator. You may have occasion to use two-stage reducing valves, but rarely three-stage units.

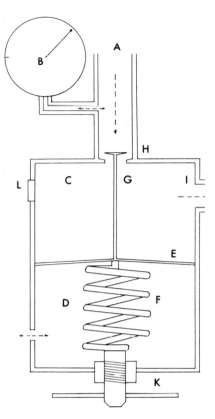

Fig. 24-15 Diagram of an adjustable, high-pressure reducing valve. (See text for details.)

Figure 24-16, page 650, shows the internal workings of a two-stage pressure reducing valve. Gas from a cylinder inlet initially enters a first stage pressure reduction chamber. Usually, the diaphragm spring tension of the first stage is factory preset to an intermediate pressure between 200 to 700 psig. Then the second stage lowers this pressure to the working level (in three-stage units, the second stage lowers the pressure to about half of the first). Since each pressure chamber will have one safety relief vent, you can usually determine the number of stages in a reducing valve by noting the number of relief vents present.

Because pressure is reduced in multiple steps, these reducing valves are able to provide more precise and smooth flow control. However, multiple-stage reducing valves regulators are larger and more costly than single stage reducing valves. For this reason, they are indicated only when minimal fluctuations in pressure and flow are critical factors, as in research activities. For routine hospital work, the simpler single-stage reducing valves are quite satisfactory.

Proper use of high-pressure reducing valves. When you open a cylinder that is attached to a high-pressure reducing valve, gas is rapidly decompressed then recompressed. Since the recompression phase is adiabatic, high temperatures are generated. These rapid pressure and temperature changes are potentially

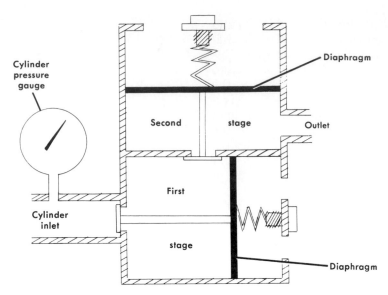

Fig. 24-16 Multistage reducing valve. Double-stage reducing valve is functionally two single-stage reducing valves working in tandem. Gas enters first stage (first reducing valve), and its pressure is lowered. Gas then enters second stage (second reducing valve), and pressure is lowered to desired working pressure (usually 50 psig). A three-stage reducing valve would have one more reducing valve in series. (From McPherson SP, Spearman CB: Respiratory therapy equipment, ed 3, St Louis, 1985, Mosby.)

hazardous. Rapid pressure swings can cause failure of reducing valve components.[28] Failed components can become high velocity projectiles, endangering practitioner and patient alike. Rapid temperature changes can ignite combustible materials.[29] Ignition of combustible materials in the presence of 100% oxygen can cause an explosion. The accompanying box provides guidelines to minimize the risk associated with setting up oxygen cylinders with a high-pressure reducing valves or regulator.[7]

Low-pressure gas flowmeters

It is not enough that you simply reduce the pressure of gases used in the clinical setting. As with drugs, administration of medical gases to patients requires some knowledge of the "dosage" being delivered. This is accomplished, in part, by metering the rate of gas flow to the patient through a device called a *flowmeter.*[7]

When a high pressure gas cylinder is used to provide medical gas for patient use, *both* a reducing valve and a flowmeter are combined into a regulator. However, when gas is provided through a central supply system, the pressure has already been reduced to 50 psig by the time it reaches the outlet stations. This eliminates the need for pressure reducing devices at the bedside and requires only a device to regulate flow.

■ MINI **C**LINI ■

24-1

Leaky Connections

Problem: Following standard procedure, you attach a pressure-reducing valve to an oxygen cylinder. Upon opening the cylinder valve, you hear gas leaking at or near the connection.

Solution: A leak usually indicates that the connection between the pressure-reducing valve and cylinder outlet is not tight. If the cylinder outlet is a standard ASSS threaded connector, either the connection is cross-threaded or not properly seated and tightened. To fix this problem, close the cylinder valve, and remove and reattach the pressure-reducing valve, being careful to properly thread the connection and tighten with a wrench. If the cylinder outlet is a pin-indexed connector, close the cylinder valve, and remove the pressure-reducing valve. Check to make sure that the nylon washer is present, in good condition and properly fitted. Then reattach the pressure-reducing valve, being careful to properly seat connection and hand tighten. If the leak continues after these corrective actions, chances are that the pressure-reducing valve is malfunctioning and should be replaced.

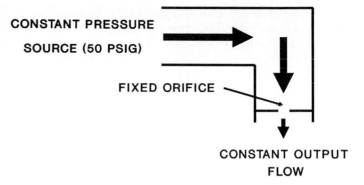

Fig. 24-17 Flow restrictor.

Procedure for set-up of an oxygen cylinder and regulator

The following steps are recommended for proper connection of a cylinder before use:

1. Secure the cylinder according to the CGA guidelines. Verify the contents from the label that also matches the color code and valve indexing.
2. Remove the protective cap or wrap and inspect the cylinder valve to be certain that it is free of dirt, debris, and oil.
3. Warn those present that you are about to "crack" the cylinder valve and that it will make some noise. Then turn the cylinder valve away from any people present, stand to the side, and quickly open and close the valve. This maneuver will remove any dust or small debris from the cylinder valve outlet.
4. Inspect the inlet of the device to be attached for debris, dirt, or oil. Check the label of the device to be certain it is specified for high-pressure service and that it is intended for use with the gas to be administered. Oxygen-reducing valves and regulators should also have a label stating: OXYGEN—USE NO OIL.
5. Once the inlet of the reducing valve or regulator has been found free of contaminants, securely tighten (but DO NOT force) the device onto the cylinder outlet. When making connections, use appropriate wrenches that are oil and grease free. Never use pipe wrenches. Use only cylinder valve connections that conform to American Standard and Pin Index Safety System (ANSI) B57.1. Low-pressure threaded connections must comply with the DISS or they must be noninterchangeable low-pressure quick connects. Never connect fixed or adjustable orifices or metering devices directly to a cylinder without a pressure-reducing valve.
6. Be certain that the regulator or reducing valve is in the off or closed position, and then slowly open the cylinder valve to pressurize the reducing valve or regulator that is attached. Once the pressurization has occurred, open the cylinder valve completely and then turn it back one-fourth to one-half turn to prevent a condition known as "valve freeze," where the valve cannot be turned.

There are three primary types of flowmeters used in respiratory care: the flow restrictor, the Bourdon gauge, and the Thorpe tube. The Thorpe tube itself has two different designs: pressure compensated or not pressure compensated (uncompensated). Although uncompensated Thorpe tubes are rarely used, you probably will apply all of these flow metering devices at one time or another. For this reason, we will compare and contrast the principles underlying each of the four.

Flow restrictors. The flow restrictor is the simplest and least expensive type of flow metering device. As shown in Figure 24-17, a flow restrictor consists solely of a fixed orifice, calibrated to delivery a specific flow at a constant pressure (50 psig).

The operation of the flow restrictor is based on the principle flow resistance, as described in Chapter 7. Specifically, we may quantify the flow of gas through a tube using the following equation:

$$R = \frac{P_1 - P_2}{\dot{V}}$$

rearranging the equation to solve for flow ($\dot{V}$) yields the following:

$$\dot{V} = \frac{P_1 - P_2}{R}$$

where $\dot{V}$ is the volumetric flow per unit time, P_1 is the pressure at the *upstream* point (point 1), P_2 is the pressure at the *downstream* point (point 2), and R is the total resistance to gas flow.

By design, a flow restrictor must always be used with a source of constant pressure (usually 50 psig). As long as the source pressure remains fixed, $P_1 - P_2$ should also stay constant. With a fixed size orifice, the resistance to gas flow (R) also remains constant. With both the numerator and denominator of the above equation fixed, the resulting flow will also be a constant value for any given orifice size.

With a constant driving pressure and constant gas density, the actual flow through an orifice is proportional to the square of its internal diameter:[30]

$$\dot{V} \approx diameter^2$$

Thus, as long as the downstream pressure (P_2) remains negligible, a given sized orifice attached to a 50 psig gas source will always produce a constant flow of known value. A flow restrictor is thus classified as a fixed orifice, constant pressure flow metering device.[31]

Commercially produced flow restrictors designed for clinical use are calibrated at 50 psig. A selection of models is available, each providing a specific preset flow. Typically, these devices are used to provide calibrated *low flows* of oxygen, in the range of 1/2 to 3 L/min.

In addition to low cost and simplicity, flow restrictors provide added safety, especially in patients requiring precise low flows of oxygen (refer to Chapter 26). Since the flow through the device is fixed, neither the patient or practitioner can inadvertently alter the prescribed liter flow. Moreover, the accuracy of flow restrictors is gravity-independent, meaning that they can be used in any position. As we shall see, this is an important advantage when using oxygen in transport situations.

However, flow restrictors have many disadvantages. With flow fixed, a new restrictor is needed whenever the flow must be changed. To overcome this problem, some manufacturers make restrictors with a selection of orifice sizes, which you can set using a rotary dial. However, these devices can cost as much as other flowmeters that can provide a continuous range of flow.

Last, the accuracy of a flow restrictor depends on a constant and specific pressure difference across the orifice. For example, should the source pressure drop below 50 psig, or should the downstream pressure rise, the flow through a restrictor will be less than that designated. Although large drops in upstream (source) pressure are rare, rises in downstream pressure (distal to the restrictor) are more common. Downstream pressure rises whenever you connect a device with high flow resistance to the restrictor. This includes jet nebulizers and some types of humidification equipment (described in Chapter 25). With such equipment, the oxygen flow will be less than the set value. For this reason, flow restrictors must never be used with any equipment that creates high flow resistance.

Bourdon gauge. A Bourdon gauge is a low pressure flow metering device *always* used with an adjustable high pressure reducing valve. Like the flow restrictor, the Bourdon gauge uses a fixed orifice. Unlike the flow restrictor, however, the Bourdon gauge operates under variable pressures, as adjusted via the pressure reducing valve. The Bourdon gauge is thus classified as a fixed orifice, variable pressure flow metering device.[31]

As depicted in Figure 24-18, outflow resistance in a Bourdon gauge is created by a calibrated orifice of fixed size (*A*). The gauge itself is located proximal to the calibrated orifice by a connector (*B*). Inside the gauge is a curved, hollow, closed tube (*C*) that responds to pressure changes by changing shape. The force of gas pressure tends to straighten the tube, causing its distal end to move. This motion is transmitted to a gear assembly and indicator needle (*D*). A numbered scale is calibrated to read the needle movement in units of flow (L/min).

As with the flow restrictor, the Bourdon gauge's fixed orifice assures that the output flow is proportional to the driving pressure. However, the Bourdon gauge provides a continuous range of flows, which you adjust by altering the pressure on the attached reduc-

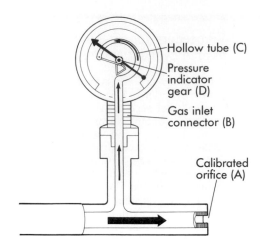

Fig. 24-18 Components of a Bourdon pressure gauge.

ing valve. Thus, *although the gauge actually senses pressure, it is calibrated to display flow.*

Also like the flow restrictor, a Bourdon gauge's accuracy is not affected by gravity. Thus, this device is ideal when you cannot keep the flowmeter in an upright position. This situation is common when you transport patients with a portable oxygen source. In these cases, keeping the oxygen supply (usually E cylinders) upright is seldom convenient, and movement of both the oxygen supply and patient is common. Combined with its continuous range of flows, this makes the Bourdon gauge the metering device of choice for patient transport.

The main disadvantage of the Bourdon gauge is its variable accuracy against downstream pressure changes. Since the Bourdon gauge really indicates pressure, any major increase in pressure distal to the orifice will alter its reading. Specifically, if resistance distal to the orifice increases, the pressure difference across it will decrease. This will cause a lower output flow. But since the flow reading is based on pressure proximal to the orifice (which stays constant), the gauge will show a flow *higher* than that actually delivered.[7] Indeed, because the gauge records valve chamber pressure, it will register flow even when the outlet is completely blocked (Figure 24-19)! Thus, if you need accurate flows when using a device that creates high resistance, the Bourdon gauge should not be selected. Instead, you should use a compensated Thorpe tube.

Thorpe tube flowmeter. The Thorpe tube flowmeter is always attached to a 50 psig source, either a preset pressure reducing valve or a bedside station outlet. As compared to the flow restrictor and Bourdon gauge, the Thorpe tube is classified as a variable orifice, constant pressure flow metering device.[31]

Figure 24-20 shows how the Thorpe tube flowmeter works. The key component in this meter is a tapered transparent tube with a float. The diameter of the tube increases from bottom to top (exaggerated here for

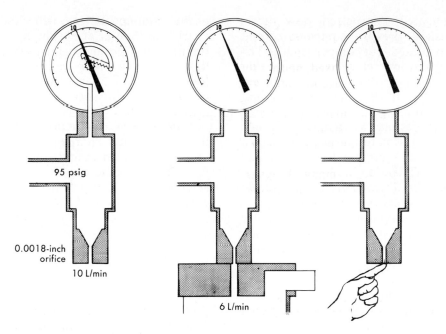

Fig. 24-19 Bourdon regulator with resistance downstream. If resistance is placed on Bourdon regulator, postrestriction pressure is no longer constant, as it will be somewhat higher than atmospheric pressure. Pressure greadient is then decreased; because only prerestriction pressure and not actual pressure gradient is monitored, the reading will be erroneously high. (From McPherson SP, Spearman CB: Respiratory therapy equipment, ed 3, St Louis, 1985, Mosby. Courtesy Puritan-Bennett Corp. Los Angeles, Calif.)

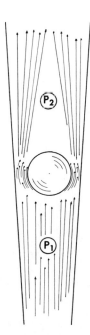

Fig. 24-20 The position of the float in the Thorpe tube-type flowmeter is based on a balance between the force of gravity and the pressure difference (P1 − P2) across it, as determined by the variable-sized orifice created between the float and the tube wall.

clarity). While in use, the float is suspended against the force of gravity by the flow of gas. Its position is noted against an adjacent scale, which is normally calibrated in liters per minute.

While the Bourdon gauge actually measures pressure, the Thorpe tube truly measures flow. The Thorpe tube's ability to measure flow is based on the complex interaction of the forces of fluid dynamics and gravity.[30] When gas begins to flow through the tube, a pressure difference ($P_2 - P_1$) is created across the float. As the float rises in the widening tube, the space available for flow around it increases (equivalent to increasing the orifice). With an increase in the orifice size, *resistance to flow decreases.* This decreased resistance allows higher flow for a given pressure difference. Ultimately, the float stabilizes when the pressure difference across the float (an upward force) equals the opposing downward force of gravity.

Any increase in input flow initially disrupts this balance, creating an increase in the pressure difference across the float. With the upward pressure difference greater than the downward force of gravity, the float rises. However, as the float rises, the available "orifice" increases in diameter. Flow resistance around the float drops, and the pressure difference once again equilibrates with gravity. The float position thus stabilizes at a higher level, proportionate to the greater flow around it.

As previously indicated, Thorpe tube flow meters are of two basic designs: pressure compensated and not pressure compensated (uncompensated). The term pressure compensation refers to a design that prevents a change in downstream resistance (often called "back pressure") from affecting its flow calibration. For medical gas administration, all manufacturers now supply only pressure compensated Thorpe tubes. However, some gas metering devices used in ventilators and anesthesia equipment are still of the uncompensated design. Therefore it is important that you understand the effect of pressure compensation on the accuracy of these devices.

As we have seen, increased downstream resistance is common when a flowmeter is connected to certain types of equipment. Practically all therapy gas equipment creates some flow restriction. Devices such as jet nebulizers produce very high downstream resistance. Depending on their design, Thorpe tube flowmeters respond to resistance in one of two different ways.

Uncompensated Thorpe tube. The uncompensated Thorpe tube flowmeter is calibrated in L/min, but at *atmospheric pressure* (without restriction).[7] Gas from a 50 psig source flows into the meter at a rate controlled by a needle valve located *before* the flow tube (Figure 24-21, *A*). When you attach flow restricting equipment to the meter, downstream resistance increases, raising pressure in the flow tube. As long as this pressure does not exceed 50 psig, gas will continue to flow through the tube. However, the added downstream resistance increases the pressure in the flow tube above atmospheric. At higher pressures, a

greater amount of gas will flow through a given restriction than at atmospheric pressure. Thus, with the float at a given height, *more* gas will be flowing through the tube than indicated on the scale. Therefore, *with a restriction to outlet flow, an uncompensated Thorpe tube displays less gas flow than the patient actually receives.*[7]

Compensated Thorpe tube. In contrast, the scale of the compensated Thorpe tube flowmeter is calibrated at 50 psig instead of atmospheric pressure.[7] Also, its flow control needle valve is placed *after* the flow tube (Figure 24-21, *B*). Thus, the entire meter operates at a constant pressure of 50 psig. Knowing that the compensated Thorpe tube operates at 50 psig helps identify it. When a compensated Thorpe tube is connected to a 50 psig gas source with the flow valve closed, the float will 'jump,' then return to zero as the meter is pressurized.

Because the entire meter operates at a constant pressure, an increase in downstream resistance causes pressure to rise only in that portion of the circuit distal to the needle valve. As long as the downstream pressure does not exceed 50 psig (in which case flow will cease), the float's position will accurately reflect actual outlet flow. For this reason, the pressure compensated Thorpe tube is the preferred instrument in most clinical situations.

The only factor limiting the use of the pressure compensated Thorpe tube is gravity. Since its accuracy depends on being kept in an upright position, it is not the ideal choice for patient transport. In these cases, the gravity-independent Bourdon gauge is a satisfactory alternative.

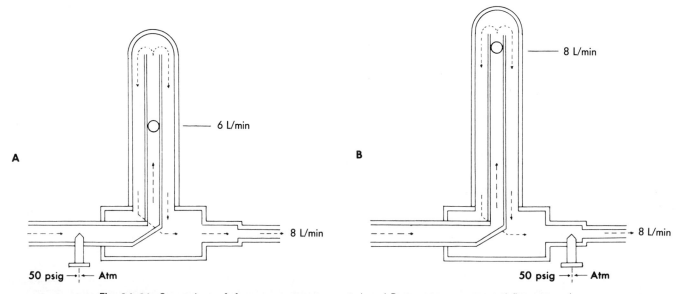

Fig. 24-21 Comparison of, **A**, pressure-uncompensated, and **B**, pressure-compensated flowmeters. In the former, the flow-control valve is proximal to the meter, and the gauge records less than the actual output. In the later, location of the valve distal to the meter correlates the gauge reading with the output. (See text for detailed explanation.)

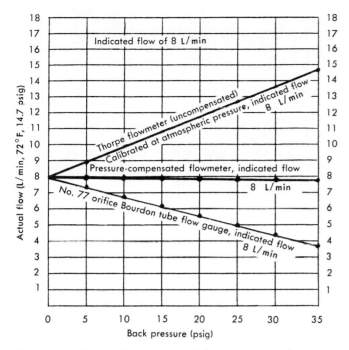

Fig. 24-22 Comparative accuracy of flow-metering devices. (From McPherson SP, Spearman CB: Respiratory therapy equipment, ed 3, St Louis, 1985, Mosby. Modified from Puritan-Bennett Corp, Los Angeles, Calif.)

Figure 24-22 summarizes the effects of downstream resistance or "back pressure" on the Bourdon gauge, pressure compensated, and uncompensated Thorpe tube type flow metering devices.

CHAPTER SUMMARY

Although RCPs have assumed many more challenging duties, assuring the safe and uninterrupted supply of medical gases is still a key responsibility. Thus your ability to provide quality respiratory care depends, in part, on your knowledge of medical gases storage and distribution.

Beyond ensuring compliance with various regulatory standards, the RCP selects and applies appropriate devices to regulate gas pressure and control gas flow. Although safety systems exist to minimize errors in medical gas delivery, they are no substitute for the careful application of clinical knowledge. Only in this manner can safety and quality be assured.

REFERENCES

1. Compressed Gas Association: *Handbook of compressed gas,* ed 3, New York, 1990, Van Nostrand Reinhold.
2. Bancroft ML, Steen JA: Health device legislation: an overview of the law and its impact on respiratory care, *Resp Care* 23:1179, 1978.
3. Code of Federal Regulations, Title 21 CFR Parts 200–299 (Food and Drugs), United States Government Printing Office, Washington, DC 20402.
4. Safe Medical Devices Act of 1990, Public Law 101–629.
5. National Fire Protection Association: Fire hazards in oxygen-enriched atmospheres (NFPA 53M). Quincy, MA, 1990, National Fire Protection Association.
6. The United States Pharmacopeia/National Formulary, United States Pharmacopeial Convention, Inc., 12601 Twinbrook Parkway, Rockville, MD 20852.
7. McPherson SP: *Respiratory therapy equipment,* ed 4, St. Louis, 1990, Mosby.
8. Compressed Gas Association: Compressed Air for Human Respiration (CGA G-7)/ANSI Z86.1), Arlington, VA, Compressed Gas Association.
9. National Fire Protection Association: Health care facilities (NFPA/ANSI 99). Quincy, MA, 1990, National Fire Protection Association.
10. Bone RC: A new therapy for the adult respiratory distress syndrome, *N Engl J Med* 328(6):431–2, 1993.
11. Roberts JD, Polaner DM, Lang P, Zapol WM: Inhaled nitric oxide in persistent pulmonary hypertension of the newborn, *Lancet* 340(8823): 818–9, 1992.
12. Department of Transportation, *Code of Federal Regulations,* Title 49 CFR, Parts 100–199. Washington, DC, US Government Printing Office.
13. Compressed Gas Association: Method of marking portable compressed gas containers to identify the material contained (CGA C-4). Arlington, VA, Compressed Gas Association.
14. Compressed Gas Association: Methods for hydrostatic testing of compressed gas containers (CGA C-1). Arlington, VA, Compressed Gas Association.
15. Compressed Gas Association: Standard color marking of compressed gas containers for medical use (CGA C-9). Arlington, VA, Compressed Gas Association.
16. Compressed Gas Association: Guide to the preparation of precautionary labeling and marking of compressed gas containers (CGA C-7). Arlington, VA, Compressed Gas Association.
17. Compressed Gas Association: Characteristics and safe handling of medical gases (P-2). Arlington, VA, 1989, Compressed Gas Association.
18. Cylinders with unmixed helium/oxygen, *Health Devices* 19(4):146, 1990.
19. Anderson WR: Oxygen pipeline supply failure: a coping strategy, *J Clin Monit* 7(1):39–41, 1991.
20. Feeley TW, Hedley-Whyte J: Bulk oxygen and nitrous oxide delivery systems: design and dangers, *Anesthesiology* 44(4):301–305, 1976.
21. Bancroft ML, duMoulin GG, Headley-Whyte J: Hazards of bulk oxygen systems, *Anesthesiology* 52:504, 1980.
22. Compressed Gas Association: Transfilling of liquid oxygen to be used for respiration (CGA P-2.6), Arlington, VA, Compressed Gas Association.
23. Compressed Gas Association: Compressed gas cylinder valve outlet and inlet connections (ANSI/CGA V-1), Arlington, VA, Compressed Gas Association.
24. Compressed Gas Association: Diameter index safety systems (CGA V-5), Arlington, VA, Compressed Gas Association.
25. Compressed Gas Association: Standard for flowmeters, pressure reducing regulators, regulator/flowmeter and regulator/flowgauge combinations for the administration of medical gases (ANSI/CGA E-7), Arlington, VA, Compressed Gas Association.
26. Oxygen regulator fire caused by use of two yoke washers, *Health Devices* 19(11 Spec No):426–427, 1990.
27. Mismating of precision brand medical gas fittings, *Health Devices* 19(9):333–334, 1990.
28. Allberry RA: Minireg failure [letter], *Anaesth Intensive Care,* 17(2):234–235, 1989.
29. West GA, Primeau P: Nonmedical hazards of long-term oxygen therapy, *Respir Care* 28(7):906–12, 1983.
30. Grant WJ: *Medical gases: their properties and uses,* Chicago, 1978, Year Book Medical Publishers.
31. Ward, JJ: Equipment for mixed gas an oxygen therapy, in Barnes TA, editor: *Respiratory care practice,* Chicago, 1988, Year Book Medical Publishers.

Humidity and Aerosol Therapy

■

Jim Fink

CHAPTER LEARNING OBJECTIVES

1. Identify the primary indications for humidity and aerosol therapy;
2. Differentiate among the various types of humidification devices, and the key factors affecting their performance;
3. Relate the physical properties of aerosols to their penetration and deposition in the human lung;
4. Compare and contrast the major categories of aerosol delivery devices according to their principles of operation and appropriate clinical use;
5. Given appropriate clinical and patient data, select the most appropriate aerosol delivery system to achieve the intended objectives;
6. Identify the major hazards associated with humidity and aerosol therapy.

The respiratory system is responsible for a number of functions in addition to gas exchange. One function of the upper airway is to ensure that inspired gases are warmed and adequately humidified. When the upper airway is bypassed, e.g., after placement of an endotracheal tube, inspired gases must be artificially humidified. Another function of the upper airway is to protect the lungs by filtering inspired gas, an aspect that we must understand if we are to effectively target medications to the airway and lungs. In order to appropriately deliver humidified gases and aerosols, the respiratory care practitioner (RCP) must understand basic concepts of humidification and aerosol systems and be knowledgeable in selection of appropriate equipment and development of therapeutic strategies. This chapter will review how inspired gases are normally humidified, describe currently available techniques for providing humidification to patients whose normal airway mechanisms are compromised, and describe techniques for delivering aerosol therapy.

CLINICAL INDICATIONS FOR HUMIDITY AND AEROSOL THERAPIES

Humidity and aerosol therapy are provided both to ensure maintenance of normal physiologic conditions and as therapy for pathologic conditions. In this chapter we shall view aerosol therapy as both a mode of humidification and as a mechanism for delivery of medications to the lung.

Maintaining normal physiologic conditions

The primary goal for humidity therapy is to provide adequate humidification and heat the inspired gas to approximate normal inspiratory conditions at the point of entry into the airway. Heat and humidity assure normal operation of the mucociliary transport system. The circumstances under which the gas is administered to a patient should be humidified and warmed are numerous (see accompanying box).

Inspired gases should be humidified to assure normal physiologic conditions, as well as to treat abnormalities of the respiratory tract. The most common situation in which gases are humidified is during administration of medical gases. Administration of dry gases at flows exceeding 4 L/min to the airways is known to pose a hazard, accounting for heat and water loss and, if prolonged, causing structural damage. As the airway is exposed to relatively cold dry air, ciliary motility is reduced, airways become more irritable, mucus production increases, and pulmonary secretions become thick and encrusted in the airways. The hazard is particularly great when the normal humidifying capability of the upper airways is lost, as

---

Indications for delivery of humidified gases and aerosols

Primary indications for humidifying inspired gas

1. Administration of medical gases
2. Delivery of gas to the bypassed upper airway
3. Thick secretions in nonintubated patients

Additional indications for warming inspired gases

1. Hypothermia
2. Reactive airway response to cold inspired gas

Primary indications for aerosol administration

1. Delivery of medication to the airway
2. Sputum inductions

occurs with endotracheal intubation[1]. Cytologic studies demonstrate damage to tracheal epithelium within two hours of administration of dry gases via endotracheal tube, while gases at 60% relative humidity produced no damage.[2] Even when room air is being breathed through an artificial airway, external humidification of the inspired gas should be assured. The loss of the humidifying capabilities of the upper airway causes the *Isothermal Saturation Boundary (ISB)* to shift toward the lower airways. This approaches critical importance when differences between ambient and tracheal temperatures exceed 10° C and the burden of regulating heat and water falls upon the more distal airways, less accustomed to humidifying inspired gases.

The appropriate level of humidification and temperature to achieve when administering medical gases varies according to the method of delivery. Gas delivered to the nose or mouth should be heated and humidified to 22° C at 50% relative humidity (RH) with an absolute humidity (AH) of 10 mg/L. Gas delivered to the hypopharynx, such as when administered by nasal catheter, should range from 29 to 32° C at 95% RH (AH 28 to 34 mg/L)[3]. When gas is delivered directly into the trachea through an endotracheal tube or tracheotomy tube, it should be warmed to 32 to 35° C at 100% RH (AH 36 to 40 mg/L).

The delivery of warmed, humidified inspired gases can also be used to prevent and treat a variety of pathologic conditions. Heated, humidified inspired gas is advocated for the treatment of upper airway inflammation, hypothermia, airway hyperactivity associated with breathing cold, dry gases, and prevention and treatment of thick, tenacious pulmonary secretions.[4]

Upper airway inflammation

The use of cool humidified gases, often with bland aerosols, are advocated in the treatment of upper airway inflammation due to croup, epiglottitis, and post extubation swelling, etc.[5] The cool mist is thought to promote localized vasoconstriction, reduce swelling, and relieve the discomfort associated with upper airway inflammation.

Hypothermia

Delivery of warm, humidified gases can also be used to treat hypothermia. For the hypothermic patient, rewarming and reduction of further heat loss can be aided by heating the inspired gases.[6]

Airway hyperreactivity to cold inspired gas

Patients may react with severe bronchospasm to breathing cold inspired gas. For example, there is evidence that some asthmatics have increased airway resistance when breathing cold air.[7] The cause of the bronchospasm is most likely due to a shift of the ISB to more distal airways with associated stimulation of mast cells in that area. This response can be reduced by warming the inspired gases or providing gas humidified with > 20 mg/L H_2O at 23° C.[8]

Treatment of thick secretions

Humidification of inspired gas has been advocated in patients with thick, tenacious secretions, whether they have intact upper airways or not. Currently no studies support the role of external humidifiers in improving the character and mobilization of thick secretions. The most effective method for improving the character of pulmonary secretions is systemic hydration. Nonetheless, humidification has been advocated for the patient with tenacious secretions that are difficult to clear.[9,10] Heating the humidifier may also help improve the character and expectoration of the secretions.

In addition to humidification, aerosol therapy with bland solutions such as distilled water and hypertonic saline are used to stimulate cough, as well as secretion production. Such therapy has been used for diagnostic sputum induction.

Delivery of medication to the airway

Aerosol therapy is also used to deliver drugs to the airway. The indication for aerosol drug delivery is largely based on the indications for the drug and the targeted site of delivery. Table 25-1, page 658, lists the wide variety of drugs and current clinical indications for aerosol drug delivery.[11]

DEFINITIONS

Humidity

Humidity is molecular water in air. The actual content or amount of water in a given volume of air is termed *absolute humidity* (AH) and is typically expressed in mg/L.

Relative humidity (RH) is the content of water vapor expressed as a percentage of the maximum capacity of vapor that can be held at the same temperature. Relative humidity is calculated by dividing the amount of water in the air (content) by the capacity (amount of water vapor that a gas can hold at any given temperature) of the air to hold water when totally saturated at a given temperature.

$$\text{Relative humidity (RH)} = \frac{\text{Content}}{\text{Capacity}}$$

At normal atmospheric pressure a gas cannot be more than 100% saturated. The greater the tempera-

Table 25-1   Clinical indications for various drugs delivered by aerosol to the airway

Nasal delivery		Lung delivery	
Clinical indication	Drug	Clinical indication	Drug
Allergies	Steroids	Asthma	Steroids
			Cromolyn Sodium
			Atropine
			Bronchodilators
Osteoporosis	Calcium	Influenza, RSV	Ribavirin
Diabetes	Insulin		Insulin
		Pneumocystis	Pentamidine
Bone disease	Calcitonin	Fungal infection	Amphotericin
Hormone deficiency	Growth hormone	Cystic fibrosis	Antibiotics, Dynase
HIV related neuropathy	Peptide T		
Migraine	Ergotamine	Immunization	Vaccines
Post-operative pain	Butorphanol	Sarcoidosis	Steroid

Adapted from Dolovich M. Physical principles underlying aerosol therapy. Journal of Aerosol Medicine 1989:2(2);171–186.

ture of a gas, the greater its ability to hold water vapor. Table 25-2 shows the capacity of air to hold water at 100% saturation across a range of temperatures. As temperature decreases and capacity falls to equal content, water condenses or "rains out" of the gas, forming dew. This is called the *dew point,* and indicates the point at which gas is 100% saturated. For example, on a hot summer day in Florida the temperature is 34° C with 80% relative humidity which means the water content, or AH, is 30 mg/L. This is the capacity of gas at 30° C. As the sun goes down and the air cools below 30° C, dew forms. The lower the temperature, the more water condenses from the air. As the temperature rises, the same *absolute* humidity results in a decreasing *relative* humidity. The temperature-humidity curve becomes steeper above 20° C, allowing relatively large volumes of water to be exchanged with relatively small changes in temperature.

Two heat exchange mechanisms are important in conditioning inspired air, heat transfer by evaporation and by convection. The heat loss by evaporation from the respiratory system is defined as the latent heat of vaporization of water. Energy is required for the water to change from a liquid to a vapor state. The specific heat of air is 1008 J/kg. The specific heat of water is 4200 J/kg, more than four times greater than air. Latent heat of vaporization (and latent heat of condensation) of water is 2450 J/kg. Water is able to act as a heat reservoir in the respiratory tract because of these differences in energy requirement between heat of evaporation and heat of convection. Convection is the heat transfer from the mucosa to the inspired air. While both evaporation and convection cool the mucosa, heat loss due to evaporation of water is a bigger factor than the heat loss due to convection.

Under normal conditions about 250 ml water and 1470 J of heat are lost from the lung each day. Approximately 495 ml of water and 28,468 J of heat are required to change room air from its usual temperature of about 24° C and RH 50% to alveolar conditions. In order to accomplish this, 245 ml of water and 27,000 J of heat must be reclaimed and returned to the upper respiratory tract every day.[12]

Aerosol

An aerosol is a suspension of solid or liquid particles in gas. Aerosols exist all around us as pollen, spore, dust, smoke, smog, fogs, mists, and viruses (Figure 25-1).[13] We can also create aerosols for therapeutic uses by physically shattering or shearing matter or liquid into small particles and dispersing it into a suspension. This can be accomplished using gas jets, spinning disks, ultra high frequency sound, or discharge of small quantities of freon.

The particle size of an aerosol depends on the device used to generate it and the substance being aerosolized. The equipment used to produce aerosols and nebulizers, generally produce aerosols consisting

Table 25-2   Saturated water vapor content at various temperatures

Temperature		Content
°C	°F	mg/L
0	32	4.9
10	50	9.4
15	59	12.8
20	68	17.3
25	77	23.0
30	86	30.4
35	95	39.6
37	98.6	43.9
40	104	51.1
45	113	65.6
50	122	83.2

of particles of varying diameters and shapes, referred to as *heterodisperse*. An aerosol in which particles are of uniform size (GSD ≤ 1.2μm) are called *monodisperse*. *Monodisperse* aerosols are rarely used in respiratory care.

Aerosols can be described in terms of the characteristics of the particles they contain. Frequency distribution curves of particle diameter, particle count, and particle mass are used to determine the mean and standard deviation of aerosol characteristics. The aerodynamic diameter of particles takes into account variability in particle shapes and density, determined by an aerosol's sedimentation velocity in air compared to the diameter of a unit density sphere. The *mean mass aerodynamic diameter* (MMAD) defines the distribution of particle diameter around which the mass of particles is equally distributed with 50% of particles heavier and 50% lighter. The geometric standard deviation (GSD) is a measure of the variability of the particle diameters within the aerosol (set at one standard deviation on the curve at 15.87% and 84.13% of the mean); the higher the GSD, the more larger and smaller particles are present. As the GSD increases the MMAD increases because larger particles carry more mass.[11]

Optimal delivery of aerosol to the lung depends on the size of the particles, inhalation technique, and pulmonary function of the patient. Even under the best of circumstances, <20% of an aerosol actually deposits in the lungs. Aerosol droplets with a MMAD ≤ 5 μm tend to deposit in the lung. Most particles > 5 μm impact on the upper airway. The depth of penetration into the bronchial tree is inversely proportional to particle size down to a size of less than 1 μm (Table 25-3, page 660). Particles less than 1 μm are so light and stable that many do not deposit in the lungs. Even

when they do settle in the lung these particles carry very small quantities of medication.

Size	Relative Volume
1 μm	1
2 μm	8
3 μm	27
4 μm	64
5 μm	125
10 μm	1000

Aerosols with a MMAD of 0.8 to 2.0 μm are targeted to the lung parenchyma. Particles less than 0.8 μm are often exhaled, and of such small volume that they often contribute little to therapeutic effect.

Aerosol particles often change size due to evaporation or hygroscopic properties. Since these changes occur as a factor of time, the process is referred to as particle *aging*. The rate of particle growth is inversely proportional to the size of a particle. Small particles grow faster than larger particles. The rate of aging depends on the initial size of the particle, the time in suspension, and external conditions to which the particle is subjected.

Small particles get even smaller when inhaled with ambient gas at room temperature. As the inspired air is heated enroute to the lungs, the capacity of the gas to hold water increases and *evaporation* of water in the particle reduces its size. Aerosols of water soluble materials when introduced into a heated and humidified ventilator circuit may grow due to **hygroscopic** properties. In short, most particles will age, due to changes in temperature and humidity encountered enroute to the lungs. There is a natural tendency to assess a nebulizer's generation of aerosol by visually observing the mist produced. The unaided human eye cannot identify particles less than 1,000 μm in diameter (equivalent to a median sized grain of sand). What

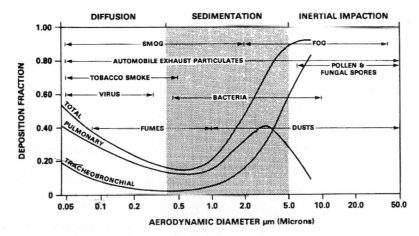

Fig. 25-1 Chart demonstrating the range of particle diameters over which diffusion, sedimentation and inertial impaction occur as well as the range of particle diameters of some commonly encountered aerosols. (Adapted from Newhouse MT, Dolovich M Aerosol therapy in children. In Basic mechanisms of pediatric respiratory disease: cellular and integrative. Toronto BC Decker, 1991. Used by permission.)

Table 25-3 Effect of particle size on deposition of aerosol to the airway

Particle size (μm)	Percent Deposition in			% Total deposition	% Cleared (exhaled)
	Upper airway (oropharynx)	Conducting zone	Alveolar region		
1	0	0	16	16	84
2	0	2	40	42	58
3	5	7	50	62	38
4	20	12	42	74	26
5	37	16	30	83	17
6	52	21	17	90	10
7	56	25	11	92	8
8	60	28	5	93	7

we see when observing the output of a nebulizer is the defraction of light as it passes through the particles, rather than the particles themselves. Consequently, the manufacturer who brings us a nebulizer with an optimal particle size, may get a less than enthusiastic reception from clinicians "looking" for an effective mist production. The best way to determine the output of a nebulizer is by measuring it directly. Two major methods of doing this are use of a laser counter, and a staged cascade impactor.

PHYSIOLOGIC CONTROL OF HEAT AND MOISTURE EXCHANGE

A primary function of the upper respiratory tract is to assure heat exchange and humidification. A variety of mechanisms exist to accomplish these goals. The normal airway conditions gas during both inspiration and exhalation. During inspiration the airway heats and humidifies gas. By the time inspired gas reaches the lung parenchyma it is fully saturated to 100% relative humidity (RH) at body temperature. The point at which this occurs is called the isothermic saturation boundary (ISB).[14] Above the ISB, temperature and humidity decrease during inspiration and increase during exhalation. Below the ISB, there are no fluctuations in temperature or relative humidity. The point of ISB is normally approximately 5 cm below the carina at the level of the third generation airways. A number of factors can cause the ISB to shift further down the airways. The ISB shifts distally with decreased environmental temperature and humidity, mouth breathing, and increased tidal volume, as a result of endotracheal intubation which bypasses the upper airway completely. The ISB will, however, never fall to the level of the respiratory bronchioles or alveoli.

Normal heat and moisture exchange within the airways is a complex mechanism.[2] During normal inspiration, turbulent flow of inspired gases ensures adequate contact of air with the mucosa. As inspired gas warms, water vapor is transferred to it by evaporation of fluid from the mucosal lining. Warming and humidification continue until the inspired gas is fully saturated at body temperature. The latent heat of vaporization remains as water vapor and does not contribute to warming of gases. Loss of latent heat of vaporization does cause the mucosa to cool. At the end of inspiration, the temperature of the nasal mucosa is 31° C because of loss of heat by turbulent convection and loss of latent heat of vaporization.[15]

During normal exhalation, heat is transferred to the cooler tracheal and nasal mucosa by convection. As gases cool, they hold less water vapor; condensation occurs, causing water to accumulate on the tracheal surfaces, where it is reabsorbed by the mucus. Heat is transferred back to the mucosa, resulting in warming and rehydration. Latent heat and water are held until the next inspiration.

The extent of heat exchange and humidification of inspired gases is influenced by the efficiency of the nose and mouth. During normal breathing, air flow in the nose is turbulent, heat is transferred by turbulent convection over the turbinates and conchae and direct contact of air with the respiratory mucosa. When breathing through the mouth, air flow is more laminar, requiring heat transfer by radiation. Because air is a poor conductor of heat, the mouth is less efficient than the nose in heating inspired air.

The nose is also an active humidifier, while the mouth is not. The respiratory mucus layer in the nose is kept moist by secretions from mucus glands, goblet cells, and transudation of fluid through cell walls. The nasal mucosa has the greatest concentration of mucus glands and is quite vascular, providing an excellent source of heat and water, capable of supplying nearly 1 liter of fluid to inspired air each day. Heat is transferred from the rich capillary beds close to the mucosal surface. Because the nasal mucosa is cooled during inspiration, it is also able to reclaim significant quantities of heat and water on exhalation. The mucosa lining the sinuses, trachea, and bronchi also aid in heating and humidifying inspired gases.

The structure of the nose appears to be engineered with extraordinary heat and humidity maintaining abilities and also functions as an organ of thermoregulation. Under conditions where the environmental temperature is greater than body temperature, the blood flow to the turbinates increases and heat is lost through the nose.

The benefits of nose-breathing on heat and humidity over mouth breathing are probably overstated. Sara and Currie[16] evaluated the temperature and humidity of inspired gas in normal patients and those who had undergone tracheotomy. In the upper trachea, gas inspired through the nose had a temperature of 34° C with an absolute humidity (AH) of 34 mg/L, compared with gas inspired through a tracheotomy which had a temperature of 31° C with AH of 26 mg/L. Primiano, et al[17] measured temperature and water vapor continuously at the oropharynx during oral and nasal breathing of room air at 22° C with relative humidity (RH) 15% to 39%. At the pharynx the temperature difference between inspired and expired gas was 4° C during nose and 7° C during mouth-breathing. Inspired gas increased 5° C during mouth-breathing and 9° C during nose-breathing. Expired gas temperature from the nose was 1° to 2° C less than body temperature, while that obtained during mouth-breathing was 2° to 3° C less. During both mouth and nose-breathing the difference between inspired and expired temperature was 10° to 11° C. During inspiration with nose-breathing RH was ≈95% at the oropharynx, while during mouth-breathing RH was ≈75%. On exhalation the RH values were similar between the 2 groups, ≈95% RH at the pharynx and ≈90% RH at the airway opening. These data suggest that the normal airway is capable of conditioning inspired gas to meet the needs of the lung no matter how it is delivered to the small airways. Medical gases delivered to the upper airway, therefore do not require humidification beyond standard ambient conditions, although some authors have recommended otherwise.

The upper airway and lungs also serve the function of protecting the airway by filtering particulates from inhaled gas as it travels to the lung parenchyma. The upper airway effectively filters out most particles > 10μm. The nose offers more efficient filtering than does the mouth. Further filtration occurs at more distal levels within the tracheobronchial tree.

As with any mechanical system, the upper airway has limitations. It functions most efficiently under normal physiologic conditions. When presented with dry, cold inspired gases, as is the case when administering medical gases which contain no water vapor, the ISB is shifted further down the respiratory tract and ciliary function and mucus production are compromised. The lower gas temperature further down in the airways reduces ciliary activity within as few as 10 minutes. Once compromised, ciliary function can take several weeks to recover. Respiratory secretions become thicker, contributing to mucus plugging and inability to maintain normal bronchopulmonary hygiene.

GENERAL PRINCIPLES OF EQUIPMENT OPERATION

An understanding of the methods used to humidify inspired gases is essential to the RCP. The first concept that must be understood is the difference between a humidifier and a nebulizer. A *humidifier* is a device that adds molecular water to gas. In contrast, a *nebulizer* is a device that produces an aerosol or suspension of particles in gas. While the theoretical difference between humidifiers and nebulizers is clear-cut, the clinical selection of one type of device versus another has significant overlap and is not based on definitive scientific data. Some humidifiers create aerosols, while some nebulizers add humidity to gas. Nebulizers have been employed to humidify gas, and, in the case of anesthesia devices, humidifiers or vaporizers have been used to administer anesthetic agents.

Humidifiers

General principles

Three variables affect the ability of a device to humidify gas: temperature, surface area, and time of contact. These factors are applied to various degrees in the design of virtually every commercially available humidification device.

Temperature. The greater the temperature, the more water vapor gas will hold. Failure to add heat to a humidifier significantly reduces its efficiency and output. Unheated humidifiers become less efficient as evaporation occurs within the humidifier and the water in the reservoir cools. Cooling occurs because: (1) compressed gas cools as it expands (as it is delivered through the humidifier), and (2) water evaporation also results in cooling. Consequently, unheated humidifiers may operate at temperatures more than 10° C below ambient temperature. As gas leaves a 10° C humidifier at 100% RH (absolute humidity 9.4 mg/L) it is only 43% RH at a room temperature of 24° C, and 21% RH at body temperature. Heated humidifiers actively replace heat lost from vaporization and compensate for cooling from gas expansion as shown in Figure 25-2, page 662.

Temperature is such a critical factor that if enough heat can be added to the humidifying system, the effects of small surface area or short contact time can usually be overcome.

Surface area. The greater the ratio of surface contact area to gas volume, the more efficient the humidifier. As the surface area available for direct contact between water and gas increases, there is more opportunity for evaporation to occur. The simplest use of surface area is to pass gas over a body of water, but this often results in a relatively low ratio. Several ways to optimize the surface area ratio in humidifiers include bubble diffusion, aerosol generation of water droplets, and integration of passover with wick technologies.

The bubble diffusion technique breaks up a stream of gas into bubbles that then rise through a column of water, causing diffusion of water into the gas. The smaller the gas bubble, the greater the ratio of surface area to relative gas volume, bringing more gas into contact with water. Although a large bubble has a greater surface area than a small bubble, a smaller relative volume of the gas in the bubble comes in contact with the water.

A corollary of this technique is to create an aerosol of water droplets in the gas stream. The smaller the particles and the greater the mist density (number of particles per volume of gas), the more surface area that is available for contact and subsequent evaporation.

Finally, passing gas over the surface of water will increase the humidity in the gas (Figure 25-3). The device used can be as simple as blowing the gas over a pan of water, or as elaborate as those with vanes or wicks to optimize the surface interface. The larger the

gas volume above the surface of the water and the smaller the surface area of the reservoir, the less efficient the humidifier, due to the low ratio of surface area to volume. The wick-type humidifier is a variant of the passover humidifier that uses a porous absorbent paper (wick) extending above the surface of the water reservoir. Gas comes in contact with the water-saturated wick as well as the surface of the water.

Hygroscopic condenser humidifiers, also known as heat and moisture exchangers (HME) incorporate a large network or surface of hygroscopic paper, or filter material. By bringing the stream of gas into contact with water-laden surfaces of the filter material, a very high surface-to-volume ratio is created.

Contact time. The longer the gas is in contact with water, the greater the opportunity for evaporation. For the bubble diffusion humidifier, the deeper the water above the gas outlet, the greater the time of contact as the bubbles rise to the surface. As soon as the gas escapes from the water reservoir and ends contact with the fluid surface, humidification ceases. Low gas flows through the humidifier tend to provide greater contact time than high flows. Aerosols suspended in the gas stream have extended contact (and opportunity for evaporation) as the gas travels to the patient and enters the lungs.

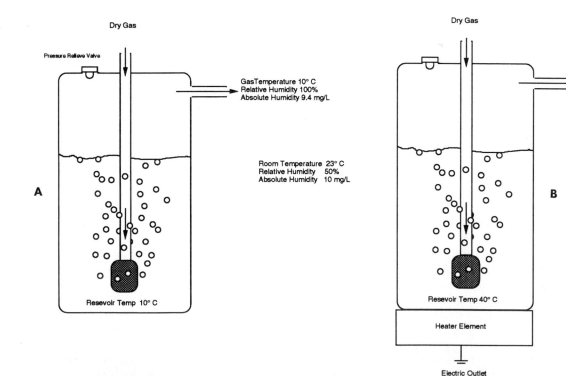

Fig. 25-2 The effects of reservoir temperature on humidity output with (**A**) unheated and (**B**) heated bubble type humidifiers. (From Fink J, Cohen N: Humidity and aerosols. In Eubank D, Bone R: Principles and applications of cardiorespiratory care equipment, St Louis, 1994, Mosby.)

Temperature 20°C. AH 17.3 mg/L

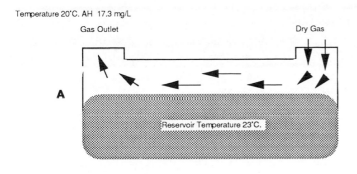

Temperature 35°C. AH 40 mg/L

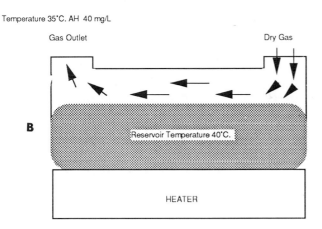

Fig. 25-3 Effect of temperature on humidity output with a simple passover humidifier when unheated (**A**) and heated (**B**). (From Fink J, Cohen N: Humidity and aerosols. In Eubank D, Bone R: Principles and applications of cardiorespiratory care equipment, St Louis, 1994, Mosby.)

Types of humidifiers

Humidifiers can be classified into 3 general types, defined primarily by the method of contact between the water and gas. Humidifier types include bubble-type humidifiers, passover humidifiers, and jet nebulizer-humidifiers. Heat and moisture exchangers (HME) are also classified as humidifiers.

Bubble-type humidifier. As previously described, in the bubble humidifier gas is directed under the surface of water and diffused to form bubbles (Figure 25-2). The larger the bubble the greater the surface contact for the individual bubble, but the lower volume of gas actually in contact with the water. The deeper the water the longer the contact. Bubble humidifiers are commonly used with simple oxygen administration devices (i.e., cannulas, catheters, simple masks, reservoir rebreathers, and high concentration Venturi masks) and without heaters to bring gas to ambient levels of humidity. The dry medical gas is directed into a water-filled reservoir where the stream of gas is broken up (diffused) into bubbles which gain humidity as they rise through the water. While some designs use series of small holes in a tube running beneath the surface of the water, others incorporate some form of

diffuser. The diffusers can be made of plastic foam, sintered metal, or mesh.

Bubble humidifiers are most efficient when used with gas flows of 5 L/min or less. They produce a water vapor content ranging from 10 mg/L to 20 mg/L.[18] The higher the flow, the lower the vapor content (due to the cooling of the reservoir). While heating the reservoir might improve efficiency of these units, the devices generally are connected to small-bore tubing that are obstructed by condensate as the humidified gas cools enroute to the patient. The condensate in the tubing counteracts any efficiencies gained by heating with this configuration.

To protect against obstructed or kinked tubing, bubble humidifiers should incorporate a pressure relief valve that provides an audible and visible alarm when high pressures develop in the humidifier. The alarm serves the dual purpose of indicating that the flow of gas from the device has been interrupted and protecting the humidifier from being damaged by the excessive pressure. The pop-off device is often a gravity or spring-loaded valve that releases pressures above 2 psi. The popoff valve should automatically resume normal position when pressures return to normal.[19]

At high flows bubble humidifiers produce particulates that can transmit or carry bacteria such as *Pseudomonas aeruginosa* from the reservoir of the humidifier to the patient.[22-29] The aerosol droplets carry the bacteria[30]; molecules of water cannot carry bacteria. Any device that produces aerosols, therefore, must be changed or cleaned regularly during routine use and consistently between patients to assure that pathogens in the reservoir do not contaminate the patient.[31]

The majority of patients who receive supplemental oxygen therapy should have the inspired gases humidified. Some of the key factors associated with different types of humidification devices are itemized in Table 25-4, page 664. Some practitioners have not used humidifiers for patients requiring supplemental oxygen at low flow rates or for short periods of time. Recently, the American College of Chest Physicians (ACCP) have suggested that simple bubble humidifiers are not necessary when delivering fresh gas flows of 4 L/min or less.[32] Their recommendation is based on the absence of data demonstrating the clinical value of added humidification when low flows of gas are administered. Based on their recommendations, humidifiers are often not added to low flow oxygen delivery systems in such settings as recovery rooms, where the oxygen administration time is usually short. Eliminating the use of humidifiers for low flow oxygen reduces costs for routine administration. The cost savings, however, are not so great that supplemental humidification should be withhheld from patients who experience nasal dryness or irritation associated with unhumidified inspired gases. Howev-

Table 25-4 Comparison of humidification an aerosol delivery systems

Factor	Unheated humidifier	Heated humidifier	Heated wick	Gas driven nebulizer	Mechanical nebulizer	HME
Output (mg/L)	15–20	35–50	35–50	20–40	40–1000	20–35
Temperature (° C)	15–20	34–40	30–40	15–20	15–25	22–28
Maintain body temp	–	+++	+++	––	–––	+
Electric hazard	no	yes	yes	no	yes	no
Infection	+	+	+	–––	–––	+
Over heating	++	––	–	+	+	+
Hypothermia	–	++	++	–	–	–
Overhydrate	+	–	–	–	–––	+
Underhydrate	––	+	+	+	++	––
Inc. inspir resistance	+	+	++	–	––	–––

+ = positive attribute
– = negative attribute

er, all patients receiving low flow gas should be monitored for complaints for dryness or irritation. When either exists, a humidifier should be added to the inspired delivery system.[33]

Humidifiers are added to the oxygen delivery system for most nonintubated and all intubated patients. Commercially available humidifiers are either unheated or add heat to increase the humidity output. The unheated bubble type humidifiers are capable of humidifying dry medical gas to an absolute humidity between 10 mg and 13 mg/L when used at flows between 2 and 10 L/min.[34] Unheated bubble humidifiers are less efficient at flows above 5 L/min and are of limited effectiveness at flows above 10 L/min. When flows greater than 10 L/min are required, another type of humidifying device should be selected. Table 25-5 describes the absolute humidity achieved when oxygen is bubbled through 4 commercially available disposable bubble type humidifiers. Note that the absolute humidity increases as the flow rate is reduced.

Unheated humidifiers should meet the recommendations contained in the American National Standards Institute (ANSI) Z-79.9, section 3.1.1.1.[19] The recommendation is that a fluid output of 10 mg/L should be provided by the humidifier. The minimum level of 10 mg/L is felt to be the lowest acceptable humidity level needed to minimize mucosal damage to the upper airway under a variety of use environments. In addition, 10 mg/L of water will provide approximately 50% relative humidity at 72°F ambient conditions, enhancing the dissipation of static electricity in order to prevent fires.

Passover-type humidifier. The passover-type humidifier directs gas over the surface of a body of water. The passover wick-type humidifier incorporates a wick of absorbent paper or cloth that draws water from the reservoir, saturating the fabric or paper which then contacts the gas stream. The pass-

over/barrier humidifier utilizes a hydrophobic barrier which allows water molecules to cross from the water reservoir into the gas stream.

Jet nebulizer. Jet nebulizers use a jet of compressed gas that passes through a restricted orifice. This creates a low pressure area at the orifice which draws fluid up from a reservoir. The fluid is then sheared or shattered into droplets by the airstream. Some devices, as shown in Figure 25-4, direct the mist into mechanical **baffles,** reducing the size of the particles that leave the nebulizer.

When used for humidification, jet nebulizers can deliver between 26 mg and 35 mg H_2O/L when unheated. Heating these nebulizers can deliver 33 mg to 55 mg H_2O/L.[35-38] While jet humidifiers can increase water content, they pose an increased risk of infection from bacteria that might colonize the reservoir. Consequently, these devices should always be filled with sterile fluids or medications changed daily.[31] Recommendations for adding fluids to the reservoir include discarding residual fluids from the reservoir prior to filling.

One commercially available jet nebulizer, the Puritan Bubble/Jet® humidifier is designed to function as either a bubble humidifier or a jet humidifier. The dry source gas is directed either through the connecting tubing to the diffuser at the bottom of the reservoir, or

Table 25-5 Absolute humidity provided by 4 commercially available bubble type humidifiers

L/min	Aerwey	Aquapak	McGaw	Travenol
2	17.2	17.6	20.4	20.4
4	16	17.7	18.4	19.5
6	15.6	16.9	16.9	16.2
8	14.6	14.9	14.9	15.7

Absolute humidity in mg/L for four unheated bubble humidifier at increasing liter flowrates. (Data from Darin et al: *Respir Care* 27:41, 1981)

through a jet that draws fluid from the reservoir, creating a mist. As a bubble humidifier, an adapter is used to connect to small bore oxygen tubing. The large bore outlet without the adapter fits the larger bore aerosol tubing, which is used to avoid obstruction from aerosol rain-out.

Jet nebulizers, when used as humidifiers, are identical to the large volume nebulizers described below. No data support the use of a jet nebulizer as opposed to any other type of heated humidifier.

Heated humidifiers. A variety of devices are commercially available to provide heated humidity. Selection of a heated humidifier should be based on many key factors. The following criteria are based on ANSI standards,[19] AARC Clinical Practice Guidelines[38] and reports from the ECRI.[39,40] Key features include the following:

- *Over temperature protection.* Gas temperature delivered to the patient should not be settable to above 40° C. When temperatures $\geq$ 40° C are reached audible and visual alarms should indicate an over temperature condition and interrupt power to the heater.
- *Audible and visual alarms* should indicate when remote temperature sensors are disconnected, absent, or defective and power to the heater should be interrupted to protect from overheating.
- *Temperature overshoot should be minimized.* Overshoot can occur with any humidifier, producing gas hotter than 40° C with short term overshoot common. Servo controlled units can overshoot when the unit is allowed to warm-up without flow through the circuit, the patient airway temperature probe is not inserted in the circuit (or becomes dislodged during operation), or when flow is increased, decreased, or interrupted during normal operation. Non servo-controlled units can overheat gas when temperature controls are set too high or gas flow is abruptly reduced.

- *Indicators for delivered gas temperature should be accurate* to within 3° C of the indicated value.
- *Humidifier temperature output should not vary more than 2° C* from the set value (at the patient).
- *Warm-up time should not take more than 10 to 15 minutes.*
- *Water level should be readily visible* in either the humidifier or remote reservoir.
- *Humidifiers should be able to withstand ventilation pressures of $\geq$ 100 cmH₂O.*
- *Internal compliance should be relatively stable* so that changes in water level do not make significant changes in the delivered tidal volume. ECRI[39] recommends that the compliance be less than that of the intended patient (< 1 mL/cm H₂O for neonates) and vary less than 0.3 mL/cm H₂O from high to low water level.
- *The humidifier should not be too hot to touch during operation.* Readily accessible surfaces should not be hotter than 37.5° C. A warning label should warn of any metal surface that can reach 50° C and is accessible when changing the humidification chamber or during disassembly.
- *Operator or feed system must not be able to overfill humidifier* to the point that water can block gas flow through the humidifier or ventilator circuit. Humidifiers should not be damaged by spilled fluids.
- *Electromagnetic Interference (EMI) from other devices should not affect humidifier performance.* The unit should not be damaged between 95 and 135 V rms.
- *Fuses or circuit breaker should be clearly labeled and easy to reset or replace.* The unit should have adequate overcurrent protection to prevent ventilator shutdown, or loss of power to other equipment on the same branch circuit due to internal equipment failures.
- *Misassembling the unit in a way that would be hazardous to the patient should be impossible.* Direction of gas flow should be indicated on interchangeable components for which proper direction is essential.
- *The humidifier should be assembled and filled in a manner that minimizes the introduction of infectious materials or foreign objects.*
- *Service and operation manuals should be provided with the humidifier and should cover all aspects of use and service.*

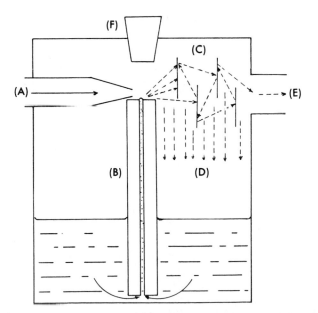

Fig. 25-4 Jet nebulization occurs when gas flow (*A*) passes through restricted orifice over capillary tube (*B*) creating a negative pressure which draws fluid up where it is sheared off and directed into baffles (*C*) where large particles rain out and return to the reservoir (*D*) and small particles proceed out toward the patient (*E*). A variable air entrainment port (*F*) is used to blend in room air and increase total flow to the patient.

Table 25-6 provides a brief summary of a few critical factors in commercial heated humidifiers such as reservoir size and the ability to maintain a fixed volume when used with neonates.

Reservoir and feed systems

As the inspired gases are humidified, water must be added to the humidifier. The system used to replace the water in the humidifier should be designed for ease of operation, to assure continuity of therapy, and to minimize disruption of ventilatory support for patients requiring mechanical ventilation. Continuous feed systems provide consistent water replacement and allow replenishment without operator intervention. These systems often rely on gravity, usually with a pole-mounted reservoir external to the humidifier mechanism.

A number of methods are available for regulating continuous feed systems. They include flotation controls, level-compensated reservoirs, and optical sensors. For the flotation-type systems, as water level raises, a float is lifted to occlude the flow of water. ALP, 3M/Bird, Anamed, and Fisher Paykel manufacture flotation-type feed systems.

In level-compensated systems (manufactured by Hudson/RCI and Marquest) an external reservoir is aligned horizontally with the humidifier, maintaining relatively consistent water levels across the external reservoir to the humidifier chamber (See Figure 25-5).

Optical sensors have also been used to control the water level of continuous-feed systems. Travenol mar-keted a humidifier with a feed system with an optical sensor which triggered a solenoid tube clamp from the water reservoir to the heated chamber. The optical sensor monitored the water level in the fluid chamber. As the water level falls, the system electronically opens a solenoid tube clamp, allowing water to flow into the chamber. As the water level rises to the predetermined level, the sensor closes the clamp and flow ceases.

Another system (Inspiron) incorporates a hydrophobic barrier, a membrane that allows water vapor, but not water to pass through it (Figure 25-6). With the barrier in place, the chamber cannot overfill from the gravity feed water source unless the barrier is disrupted or broken.

A number of intermittent feed systems are also available. The least sophisticated intermittent system utilizes a bottle of water which is poured into the humidifier. This type of system, as manufactured by Puritan Bennett and Fisher Paykel, requires interruption of humidifier operation (and mechanical ventilation, if used) to open the humidifier and pour water into the reservoir. These systems may use a bag with line feed that must be manually switched to fill the humidifier.

The Marquest chamber pour-type system does not require disruption of ventilation allowing filling without interruption through use of an internal level reservoir (Figure 25-7, page 668). The gravity water-feed system does require manual filling but uses a valve that is closed prior to opening and filling the

Table 25-6 Summary of heated humidifiers

Brand	Method/ heater type	Chamber volume	Auto feed?	Servo controlled?
Emerson	Passover Plate	2000 mL large Variable	No	No
Cascade II	BTH Immersion	900 mL-large Variable	No	Yes
Bird	Wick/passover Wrap around	20 mL-small Fixed	Yes	No
Fisher Paykel	Wick/passover Plate	230–280 mL Variable	Limited	Yes
RCI Concha	Wick Wrap around	182–72 mL Fixed (peds)	Yes	Yes
Inspiron	Passover/filter Plate	10 mL small Fixed	Yes	No
Marquest	Passover Plate	370 mL Fixed	Yes	Yes
Bournes	BTH/passover Plate	Medium Variable	No	No
Mona Loa	Passover/wick Immersion	20 mL Fixed	Yes	Yes
HPD Medical	Wick/passover Plate	230–350 mL Variable	Limited	Yes
Anamed Heated Wick	Heated wick Heated wire	No chamber Fixed	No	Yes

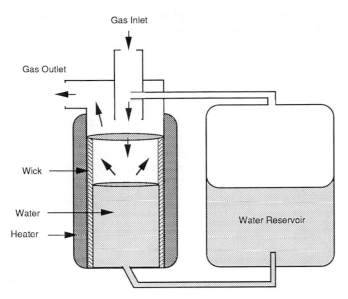

Gas Inlet

Gas Outlet

Wick

Water

Heater

Water Reservoir

Fig. 25-5 Schematic of the Hudson RCI Concha Column wick type humidifier with level reservoir feed system. (From Fink J, Cohen N: Humidity and Aerosols. In Eubank D, Bone R: Principles and Applications of Cardio respiratory Care Equipment, St Louis, 1994, Mosby.)

humidifier without disconnecting or interrupting humidifier operation.

Intermittent feed systems have several disadvantages. As the water level in manual feed systems falls, ventilator circuit compliance changes. Since gas is less compressible than water, changing water volume in a fixed volume container alters the compressible volume in both the humidifier and ventilator circuit. As a result, when water level changes during use, so too does the delivered volume. This problem is of greatest concern with mechanically ventilated newborns and pediatric patients. Those systems that are open are considered to be more susceptible to contamination of the reservoir. Finally, the humidifier chamber can become empty, if not checked regularly. For humidifiers which do not have alarms for low water levels, the humidity and temperature of gas delivered to the patient will be adversely affected.

Heating systems

To improve the water output of the humidifiers, the water in the humidifier should be heated. Heated water humidifiers are particularly useful for patients with bypassed upper airways and/or those receiving mechanical ventilatory support. Active humidifiers use electricity to heat water and/or gas. There are three methods of heating the water. The heating element may be located in: (1) the base of the humidifier, usually as a heating plate located under the reservoir or "wrapped around" all or part of the humidifier chamber; (2) a yolk or collar heater that sits between the water reservoir and active heating chamber, and (3) immersion heaters, with the heating element actually immersed into the water reservoir. Some systems incorporate a combination of one or more heating technique.

All heaters have controllers that regulate electric power to the heater element. Heated humidifiers are defined as either servo-controlled or non servo-controlled. Servo-controlled units monitor the temperature of gas delivered to the patient, adjusting the power to the heater based on the difference between the temperature setting and the temperature monitored by a thermistor probe placed downstream from the humidifier, at or near the patient airway connection. When the set temperature of the heater is greater than the distal temperature, the controller applies more power to the heater. As the distal temperature nears or exceeds the set temperature, power is reduced.

Thermistor probes at the airway are best placed in the inspiratory limb of the ventilator circuit far enough from the patient "wye" to reduce the influence of exhaled gas temperature which may be higher than that delivered by the humidifier. These probes should not be placed inside heated environments such as isolettes, where the surrounding air temperature fools the heater into thinking it can reduce or stop adding heat to the humidifier.

Non servo-controlled units monitor the temperature of the heater, providing power to the heater element based on the setting of the temperature control knob. The patient's airway temperature does not influence the temperature of the heater. Both types of units have alarms and alarm-activated heater shutdown. Each individual heater has distinct advantages and disadvantages regarding performance, cost,

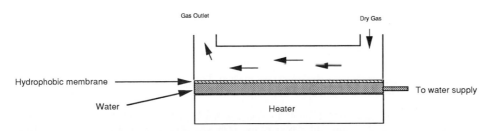

Gas Outlet   Dry Gas

Hydrophobic membrane

Water

Heater

To water supply

Fig. 25-6 Schematic of the Vapophase humidifier showing how the hydrophobic membrane separates water from the gas flow. (From Fink J, Cohen N: Humidity and aerosols. In Eubank D, Bone R: Principles and applications of cardiorespiratory care equipment, St Louis, 1994, Mosby.)

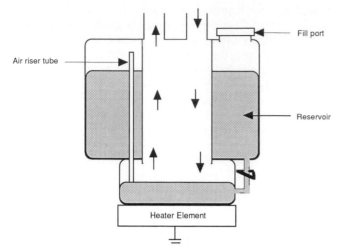

Fig. 25-7 The Marquest SCT 2000 humidifier has a passover humidifier that incorporates a reservoir that surrounds the humidifier chamber. The reservoir can be filled without interrupting ventilation. (From Fink J, Cohen N: Humidity and aerosols. In Eubank D, Bone R: Principles and applications of cardiorespiratory care equipment, St Louis, 1994, Mosby.)

safety, and ease of use which should be taken into account when selecting a system to purchase.

The American National Standards Institute (ANSI) Z-79.9 recommends that heated humidifiers have a water output level of at least 30 mg/L (100% RH at 30° C).[19] This is considered to be the minimum level of humidity required to avoid mucosal damage and drying of secretions for those patients whose upper airway has been bypassed by an endotracheal or tracheotomy tube. ECRI recommends that humidifiers have an output of 37 mg H₂O/L for inspired gas (85% RH at body temperature or 100% RH at 34° C).[39]

One problem with heated humidifier systems is that once heated, the gas cools as it passes through tubing enroute to the patient. With standard circuit tubing, the ambient environment conducts heat away from the tubing and gas, reducing the temperature of the gas. As the gas cools, its ability to hold water vapor is reduced and condensation "rain out" occurs. The amount of condensate is proportional to the temperature differential, and is affected by the ambient temperature, the gas flow, the selected patient airway temperature, and the length, diameter, and thermal mass of the breathing circuit.

One solution to the temperature drop and condensate in the tubing is to heat the inspired gas as shown in Figure 25-8. Gas can be heated to as much as 50° C as it leaves the humidifier, providing 83 mg/L of water. If the gas temperature falls to 37° C at the patient connection, 44 mg/L water will be delivered. The remaining 40 mg/L of water (more than half of the total water coming out of the humidifier) will condense in the inspiratory limb of the circuit. This large amount of essentially "wasted" water carried in the humidified gas is costly, making the delivery system very inefficient. In addition to the direct cost of the lost water, the tubing must be frequently drained to avoid the condensate in the circuit occluding the flow of gas through the circuit, or inadvertently "drowning" the patient. This condensate often becomes contaminated with bacteria from the patient's sputum.[41] When draining the tubing, it should be positioned so that the drainage is *away* from the patient's airway to avoid accidental lavage.

Condensate also poses a risk to the staff, because when the circuit is disconnected, the RCP can be sprayed with contaminated fluid in the eyes or other mucus membranes. When heated humidifier systems are used, universal infection control practices must be observed, using gloves and goggles as splash guard to minimize risk of exposure to contaminated secre-

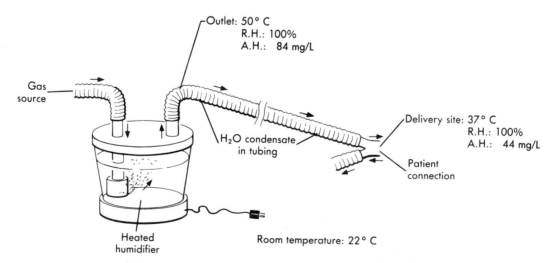

Fig. 25-8 Gases leaving the humidifier at 50° C cool as much 8° C within one foot of standard aerosol tubing, and condensation forms. The gas remains 100% saturated, but the cooling gas has reduced capacity to hold water and condensation form. Note that almost half of the original water is "lost" to condensate in this example.

tions. In addition, condensate should always be treated and disposed of as contaminated waste.[42,44]

Water traps may be placed in both the inspiratory and expiratory limbs to aid drainage of condensate from the ventilator circuit, reducing the obstruction to gas flow in the circuit. Water traps should be located a dependent points in the circuit, to allow drainage by gravity. The water traps selected should minimize changes in circuit compliance and allow emptying without disrupting ventilation.

The best way to reduce condensation is to keep it from forming. This is done by maintaining the gas at a constant temperature within the circuit itself. Several mechanisms can be used to accomplish this, including increasing the thermal mass of the circuit itself, utilizing a coaxial circuit with the inspiratory limb surrounded by the expiratory limb, or adding heated wires to the circuit. Increasing the passive thermal mass of the circuit serves to insulate the gas inside the tubing from the cool ambient air outside. This is done by using thicker walled tubing, or wrapping the tubing with insulating material. These systems tend to reduce temperature drop in the inspiratory limb, but fail to eliminate significant condensate formation.

An alternative is to surround the inspiratory limb of the circuit with the expiratory limb. This technique uses the patient's warm exhaled gas as a heated air bath surrounding the inspiratory limb. This principle is the basis of the Baines-type anesthesia circuit. These "coaxial" circuits have never gained favor for use in long-term support because of concerns about potential increases in imposed airway resistance and work of breathing.

The most practical method to prevent condensation has been to install heated wires into the inspiratory limb of the circuit. This has become the most common approach to reduce condensation with standard heated water humidifiers. Reusable or disposable heated-wire loops are inserted into the tubing to heat the gas and reduce the temperature differential between humidifier and patient. Most heated wire circuits utilize dual servo-controls with two temperature probes, one monitoring the temperature of gas leaving the humidifier and the other placed at or near the patient airway (Figure 25-9). The controller regulates the differential between humidifier output and patient airway. When heated wire circuits are used, the humidifier operates at a lower temperature (32° C to 36° C) than with conventional circuits (45° C to 50° C). The reduction in condensate in the tubing results in less sterile water use, reduced need for drainage, and less infection risk for both patient and workers.

Many humidifiers with heated wire capability include a "relative humidity" control that regulates the temperature differential between humidifier and circuit temperature. It is important to realize that with these systems, the temperatures do not reliably reflect absolute or relative humidity, but only the tempera-

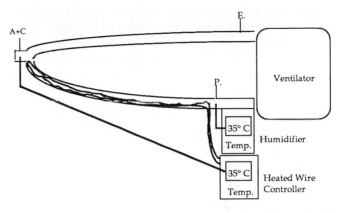

Fig. 25-9 Heated wire in inspiratory limb of ventilator circuit maintains temperature and 40 mg/L absolute humidity from humidifier (*P*) to patient (*A*). Ambient cooling of exhaled gas to 28° C enroute to exhalation valve (*E*) resulting in > 10 mg/L raining out in tubing. (From Fink J, Cohen N: Humidity and aerosols. In Eubank D, Bone R: Principles and applications of cardiorespiratory care equipment, St Louis, 1994, Mosby.)

ture differential between the 2 sites. If the humidifier is cooler than the gas in the inspiratory limb, the absolute humidity remains the same, while relative humidity decreases. Under these circumstances, the circuit will have no condensate, so the RCP cannot be certain that the gas is being humidified at all. Similarly, when the humidifier is minimally hotter than the gas in the circuit, RH increases or stays the same, with minimal reduction in absolute humidity; little or no condensate forms in the circuit. To assure that the inspired gas is being humidified, the temperature differential should be adjusted to the point that a few drops of condensation form near the patient's airway connector. This minimal condensate is the most reliable indicator that gas is fully saturated. If no condensate is visible, the RH could be anywhere between 99% and 0%, and clinicians would have no way of knowing the exact value without a hygrometer.

Few RCPs would be comfortable setting up or monitoring a ventilator without periodically analyzing oxygen or monitoring volumes, but few clinicians measure relative humidity in their critical care practice. A battery operated digital hygrometer/thermometer can be purchased for less than $300, and can prove valuable in assuring proper humidification of delivered medical gas.

An unusual variant of the heated wire circuit is one that has no humidifier reservoir (Figure 25-10, page 670). The Adult Respiratory Wick Humidification System (Anamed) humidifies the gas while enroute within the inspiratory limb of the ventilator circuit. This is accomplished with a cloth wick and wire heating element which run parallel in the inspiratory limb of the disposable ventilator circuit, ending with a disposable internal thermistor probe placed just before the patient wye. A water pump is used to prime the circuit by pressurizing a soaker hose within the wick. A wick well positioned at the lowest point of the circuit collects excess water and acts as a reservoir to keep the wick wet. The manufacturer claims that the wick needs to be primed only once every two to four hours. The heated wire controller has a single connection, and the use of the internal probe reduces the potential for leaks secondary to loose or disconnected probes. To reduce work of breathing for patient inspiratory efforts, the inspiratory limb has a 2 mm greater internal diameter than standard adult circuits, Figure 25-10.

Heat and moisture exchanger

The heat and moisture exchanger (HME) is also classified as a humidifier. It is often referred to as an "artificial nose." Like the nose, the HME captures exhaled heat and moisture, and uses it to heat and humidify the next inspiration. Unlike the nose, it is a passive humidifier that does not add heat or water to the system. The role of the HME is to conserve heat and moisture from expired gas and to return them to the patient during the next inspiration. The ideal HME should have a low compliance, add little dead space to a ventilator circuit, add minimal weight, incorporate standard connections, add minimal resistance to flow, and operate at 70% efficiency. Efficiency is defined as the ratio of the absolute humidity of exhaled gas to the humidity returned to the patient by the HME.[20,36]

Heated and moisture exchangers have been in clinical use since the 1950's. They work in one of three ways. *Condenser* humidifiers allow expired water vapor to condense onto the relatively cool surface of the condenser. The condenser element is usually constructed of metallic gauze, corrugated metal, or parallel metal tubes to provide high thermal conductivity. On inspiration, air cools the condenser to room temperature. On exhalation, the fully saturated gas cools as it enters the condenser and water rains out. The air then has 100% RH at considerably lower temperature; the temperature of the condenser itself is increased. On the next inspiration, cool dry air is warmed by the condenser by evaporation of water from the surface. Condenser humidifiers are usually only about 50% efficient under ideal conditions.

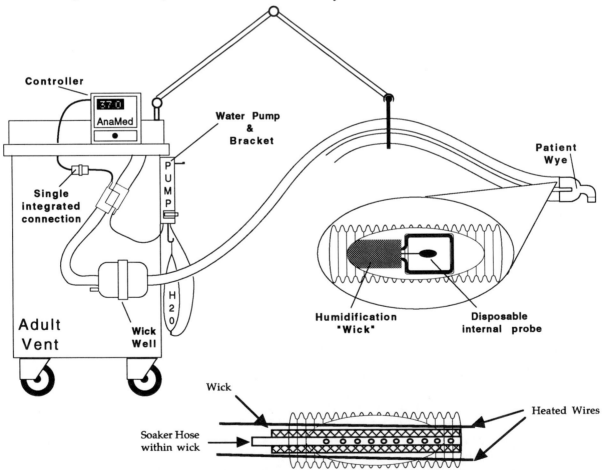

Fig. 25-10 The heated wick humidification system from Anamed heats a cotton wick in the inspiratory limb of the ventilator circuit. A pump pushes water through a "soaker hose" within the wick. A well is placed at the low point of the circuit allowing any condensate or overfill to be reabsorbed by the wick during operation.

Hygroscopic condenser humidifiers (Figure 25-11) contain materials such as paper, wool, or foam which are of low thermal conductivity. The material is then impregnated with a hygroscopic chemical such as calcium chloride or lithium chloride. The chemicals help to capture the exhaled water on expiration, reducing the relative humidity of the exhaled gas to less than 100%; more water is available to humidify the next inspiration. During exhalation, warm saturated gas precipitates water on the cool condenser element, while water molecules bind to the salt without transition from vapor to liquid state, and thus without generation of latent heat. During inspiration, the lower water vapor pressure in the inspired gas liberates water molecules from the hygroscopic compound, without cooling due to vaporization. The efficiency of these devices can be as high as 70%.

Hydrophobic condenser humidifiers (Figure 25-12) use a water repellent element with a large surface area and low thermal conductivity. Low thermal conductivity means that heat from conduction and latent heat of condensation is not dissipated. During exhalation, the condenser temperature rises to about 25° C, due to conduction and latent heat of condensation. On inspiration, cool gas and evaporation cools the condenser down to 10° C. This large temperature change results in more water being conserved to be used in humidifying the next breath. These devices are about 70% efficient. Hydrophobic humidifiers can also act as efficient microbiologic filters.

A number of characteristics of heat and moisture exchangers must be taken into account when selecting the device for humidification. The efficiency of heat and moisture exchangers falls as tidal volume, inspiratory flow, or FIO_2 increase.[46] Resistance through the HME is also important. When the HME is dry, resistance across the device is minimal. After several

hours of use, however, resistance increases. Ploysongsang, et al, demonstrated that extended use of the HME in a lung model resulted in increased resistance, due to water absorption.[47,48] For some patients, the increased work of breathing imposed by the HME may not be well-tolerated, particularly if the underlying lung disease causes increased work of breathing.

Heat and moisture exchangers are also considered bacteriostatic. HMEs eliminate condensation from the ventilator circuit and *may* reduce the circuit as a potential source of infection. Several authors have shown that the Siemens hydrophobic condenser humidifier prevents contamination of ventilator circuits and does not produce aerosols that could carry bacteria.[49] Other researchers evaluating a number of HMEs were not able to confirm their safety with respect to nosocomial infection risk, demonstrating that many of the devices produced or passed aerosols that carry bacteria. Of the Siemens, Engstrom, Pall, and Portex

Hydrophobic Condenser

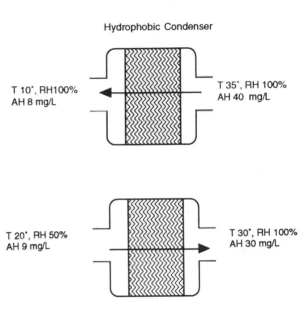

Hydrophobic Membrane Filter

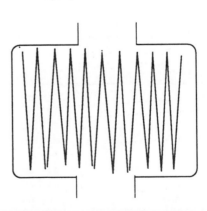

Fig. 25-12 Hydrophobic humidifier

Hygroscopic Condenser

Expiration

T 22°, RH100%
AH 22 mg/L

T 35%, RH 100%
AH 40 mg/L

Inspiration

T 20°, RH50%
AH 9 mg/L

T 28°, RH 100%
AH 27 mg/L

Fig. 25-11 Hygroscopic humidifier

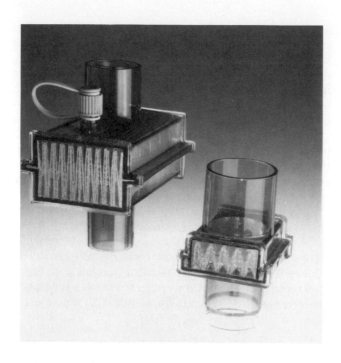

Fig. 25-13 Pall HMEs

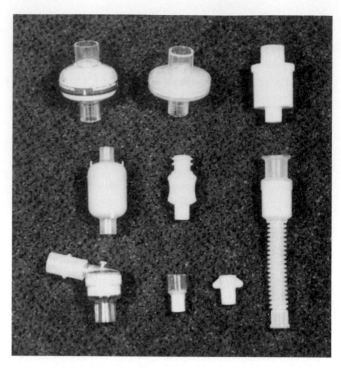

Fig. 25-14 Examples of heat and moisture exchanges (HMEs). (From Fink J, Cohen N: Humidity and aerosols. In Eubank D, Bone R: Principles and applications of cardiorespiratory care equipment, St Louis, 1994, Mosby.)

hydrophobic condenser humidifiers only the Pall humidifier (Figure 25-13) satisfactorily removed spores from the gas stream. Hedley, et al concluded that the pleated membrane filter provides a wider margin of safety than either hygroscopic or composite devices.[50]

Heat and moisture exchangers provide an inexpensive alternative to humidifiers when used for short-term ventilation of adult patients who do not have complex humidification needs, such as might be required for a brief period of time in a recovery room, emergency department, during transport, or to complete a radiologic procedure. The HME does not provide sufficient heat or humidification for long term management. When a HME is to be used, a device appropriate for the individual patient, based on size

and tidal volume should be selected. Table 25-7 itemizes dead space, measured output, and materials used in several available HMEs. HMEs come in a wide variety of shapes and sizes as demonstrated in Figure 25-14. Pall has recently introduced an HME for side-stream capnography. Several HME devices have been designed for application of low flow oxygen to the patient with bypassed upper airway.

Heat and moisture exchangers are contraindicated for a variety of clinical situations.[38] They should not be used as part of the ventilator circuit for patients with thick, copious, or bloody secretions, patients

Table 25-7 Commercially available heat and moisture exchangers

Brand	Dead space	(Output (mg/L)	Material
Pall Conserve	98 mL	23	Hydrophobic ceramic fiber
Siemens Servo 150	92 mL	25	Cellulose sponge and felt
Intertech	75 mL	26	Hydrophobic filter media
Engstrom Edith	89 mL	26	Hygroscopic polypropylene
Mallinckrodt Nose	61 mL	21	Hygroscopic plastic foam
Airlife HumidAir	41 mL	24	Hygroscopic synthetic felt
Terumo Breathaid	11.5 mL	14	Altern. aluminum/cellulose fiber
Portex Humid Vent-1	10 mL	23	Hygroscopic paper roll

(From Fink J, Cohen N: Humidity and aerosols. In Eubank D, Bone R: Principles and applications of cardiorespiratory care equipment, St Louis, 1994, Mosby.)

with a large leak around an endotracheal tube, such as might occur with a large bronchopleurocutaneous fistula, or leaking endotracheal tube cuff. In this situation, if the exhaled tidal volume is less than 70% of the delivered tidal volume, incomplete rebreathing will impair HME humidification. The HME is also contraindicated for patients with body temperatures less than 32° C, and patients with minute ventilations greater than 10 L/min.

Hazards associated with use of the HME include hypothermia, under hydration and impaction of pulmonary secretions, potential increase in resistive work of breathing through the HME or as a result of mucus plugging of the airways, hypoventilation due to increased added dead space, and inaccurate low-pressure alarm with ventilator disconnection due to the high resistance when ventilating through the HME. In addition, the heat and moisture exchangers must be removed from the patient circuit during aerosol administration, unless the MDI or SVN is placed between the HME and the patient.

Infection control implications of equipment selection

Aerosol and condensate from ventilator circuits are known sources of patient contamination. Advances in circuit and humidifier technology have reduced the risk of contamination and nosocomial infection. Use of the wick or passover humidifier minimizes aerosolization of water from the heated reservoir. Heated wire circuits reduce production and pooling of condensate within the circuit. Rhames, et al demonstrated that bubble type humidifiers such as the Puritan Bennett Cascade® humidifier produce aerosols that can carry bacteria.[30] Wick humidifiers do not. In addition, Gilmour, et al demonstrated that temperatures at which wick humidifiers operate can kill bacteria within the chamber.[52] In a study evaluating contamination of ventilator circuits which incorporate wick humidifiers with heated wire circuits, Fink, et al demonstrated that the contamination of ventilator circuits occurs from the patient to the circuit, rather than vice versa.[53] In no case did they find the reservoir infected with any organism that was not previously identified in patient sputum. The probable explanation for these findings is that since no aerosols are generated, there is no apparent route of transmission for bacteria from the humidifier to the patient.

In 1979 the Center for Disease Control (CDC) recommended that ventilator circuits and nebulizers be changed every 24 hours to reduce risk of nosocomial infection in critically ill patients. The frequent changes recommended by the CDC were based in large part on data using non heated circuits and heated bubble type humidifiers or large reservoir nebulizers. In 1994, draft guidelines from the CDC states that insufficient data exists to support a recommendation limiting the time that a ventilator circuit should be used. The change in CDC recommendations was largely based on the following information.

Dreyfus and coworkers compared 48 hour ventilator circuit changes with no circuit changes in patients who required over 96 hours of ventilation. They used wick and cascade humidifiers and nonheated wire circuits. They found no difference in incidence of pneumonia or duration of ventilatory support between the two groups. They concluded that the frequency of ventilator circuit change had no effect on the rate of nosocomial pneumonia.[54]

Boher, et al. evaluated the impact of seven day ventilator circuit changes on the incidence of nosocomial lower respiratory tract infection rates. They compared the incidence of infection with 7 day circuit changes to historical controls whose circuits were changed every 48 hours. The study used wick type humidifiers without heated wire circuits. They noted that infection rates decreased from 18 per 1000 ventilator days with 48 hour circuit changes to 13 per 1000 ventilator days with 7 day changes.[55] Krauss, et al had similar findings with nonheated wire circuits (from 16/1000 to 11/1000). Using heated wire circuits in adults, pediatrics, and neonates Alfredson, et al, documented a decrease in infection rates from 11.9 (with 2 to 3 day circuit changes) to 4.8/1000 ventilator days) (7 day changes) in a population of neonates, pediatrics, and adults.[56] These results suggest that extended use of ventilator circuits have not only been no worse than more frequent changes, but actually reduced infection rates. It remains unclear why these dramatic reductions in rates have occurred.

Frequent ventilator circuit changes have themselves been identified as a risk factor for nosocomial pneumonia and death. Craven, et al found that patients who had the circuit changed every 24 hours were at greater risk than those whose circuit was changed every 48 hours. They speculated that the increased manipulation of the airway or tubing may have resulted in flushing contaminated condensate into the airway or increased leakage of bacteria around the endotracheal tube into the trachea.[57]

As a result of these studies, many institutions are now decreasing the frequency of ventilator circuit changes. Since 1990, the policy at the University of California, San Francisco has been to change ventilator circuits weekly or when the circuit becomes grossly contaminated with secretions or blood. This change has resulted in significant savings in equipment and personnel time. In 1993, the cost of changing the ventilator circuit every 7 days averaged $1,350/ventilator/year compared with $9,500/vent/year with the circuit changed daily.

PHYSICS OF AEROSOL DELIVERY

Mechanisms of deposition

Deposition of inhaled particles in the lung is caused by a combination of mechanisms. These include impaction due to inertia, sedimentation due to gravity, and diffusion due to Brownian motion. The relative importance of each factor depends on the size, shape, location, and motion of the particle (Figure 25-15).

Inertial impaction is the deposition of particles by collision with a surface. This is the primary mechanism for deposition of particles over 5μm in diameter. The larger the particle size, the greater the inertia (Figure 25-16). Turbulent flow, complex convoluted passageways, bifurcation of the airways, and inspiratory flows greater than 30 L/min increase the impaction of particles in the larger airways. Most particles over 10 μm in diameter deposit in the nose or mouth. Particles between 5 to 10 μm in diameter tend to deposit in proximal airways before reaching bronchioles ≤ 2 mm in diameter. High inspiratory flows (greater than 30 L/min cause greater deposition in the upper airway.

Gravitational sedimentation occurs when particles slow and settle out of suspension. Gravitational sedimentation is a time-dependent mechanism affecting particles down to 1 μm in diameter.

Sedimentation is the primary mechanism for deposition of particles 1 to 5μm in diameter in the central airways. Breath-holding, by increasing residence time in the lung, affects deposition through gravitation sedimentation, especially in the last 6 generations of the airway. A 10 second breath-hold has been reported to provide optimal particle deposition.[58-59]

Diffusion and *Brownian movement* are primary

mechanisms for deposition of particles less than 3μm in diameter into the lung parenchyma. Particle deposition in this size range is reported to be divided between central and peripheral airways.[60] Optimal deposition of particles smaller than 3μm in diameter occurs when inspiratory flow is less than 60 L/min and tidal volume is less than 1 liter. The overall significance of tidal volume to aerosol deposition and clinical response to medication has not been well-established. Bigger breaths theoretically capture more aerosol, but this relationship has not been conclusively demonstrated.

Effects of nebulizer design

Design characteristics of nebulizers affect the size and density of particles generated. Aerosol particle size can be reduced by incorporating baffles (surfaces that remove aerosol particles from suspension due to inertial impaction) into the design of the nebulizer. Baffles are used to produce optimal size particles by allowing large particles to impact on the baffle surface, while leaving smaller particles in suspension. The internal walls of the nebulizer, an object placed in line with the jet gas flow, the surface of a one-way valve, or the internal walls of a spacer or drying chamber can all serve as baffles. Well-designed baffle systems add to the efficiency of jet and mechanical nebulizers by removing large particles from suspension.

Baffling can also occur unintentionally, affecting the aerosol output and deposition. Unintentional baffles can be created by the angles within the aerosol tubing, interfaces with other devices outside of the aerosol generator, and from the surfaces of the upper airway itself. Tubing, spacers, settling chambers, holding chambers, and one-way valves placed between the nebulizer and the patient also allow sedimentation of

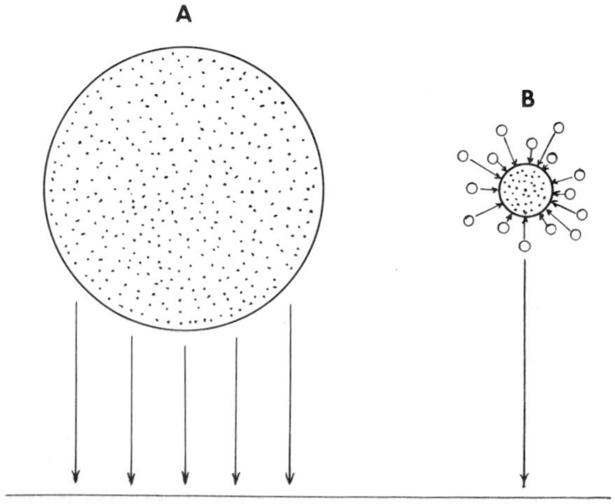

Fig. 25-15 Effect of mass on particle size. Large particles **(A)** are more susceptible to force of gravity than smaller particles **(B)** which are more affected by the bombardment of molecules, depositing by diffusion.

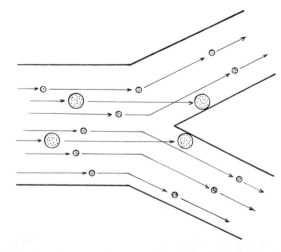

Fig. 25-16 Inertial impaction of large particles whose masses tend to maintain their motion in straight lines. As airway direction changes, the particles deposit on nearby walls. Smaller particles are carried around corners by the airstream and fall out less readily.

larger particles, reducing MMAD and output of the aerosol. The drying chamber used in the ICN Pharmaceutical Small Particle Aerosol Generator (SPAG) produces a consistent small MMAD with very low GSD. Large particles that are not baffled by the nebulizer, or connecting tubing, will be deposited in the nose or upper airway.

Factors affecting drug distribution

The goal of aerosol drug delivery is to apply the physical properties of gas to deliver a known concentration of drug to the lung. Dosing of aerosolized medication to the lung remains an imprecise science. *In vitro* and *in vivo* models have been established to define deposition of particles of various size within the lung. These models establish the relationship between particle size and aerosol deposition under optimal circumstances. It is less clear how much, if any, drug is delivered to the targeted areas of the lung in disease states and during acute exacerbations of underlying lung dysfunction.

The factors which affect delivery of drug to the lung by aerosol generators include inspiratory flow rate, respiratory rate, caliber of intrinsic airways, nose versus mouth-breathing, mask versus mouthpiece delivery, type and ease of use of the nebulizer, drug formulation, humidity, and patient characteristics including age, ability to coordinate inspiratory effort, and comprehension.

Inspiratory flows

High inspiratory flows are associated with greater deposition of drug within the upper airways due to impaction. Recent data suggests that high flows result in improved drug distribution. This is certainly the case with dry powder inhalers in which decreased inspiratory flows effect the actuation of dry powdered inhalers and results in reduced drug available for inhalation. In addition, high flows result in preferential distribution of gas to the larger airways and non gravity dependent areas of the lung.

Respiratory rate

Tachypnea can reduce residence time of drug within the lung, allowing less opportunity for deposition. This becomes of greater significance in patients with reduced FRC and ERV.

Inspiratory pattern

Large tidal volumes may cause greater drug deposition. However this relationship has yet to be confirmed in clinical trials.

Airway caliber

Decreased size of the airways, as occurs in patients with severe bronchospasm, restricts flow of aerosol to targeted distal airways. Under this circumstance, the aerosol is deposited into the larger, more proximal airways. In these clinical situations, administration of larger drug doses may be required.

Inhalation by mouth versus nose

The nose is a much more effective filter than the mouth. As a result, nasal inhalation filters most particles greater than 10 μm. Mouth-breathing provides less effective filtration, allowing greater deposition of aerosol within the lung.

Mask vs mouthpiece delivery

Inhalation through the mouth provides more respirable particles to the lung than inhalation through the nose. The desire to provide optimal drug delivery, however, should be tempered by the importance of patient comfort. The choice of mask or mouthpiece should consider patient comfort, rather than aerosol deposition alone. This is especially true when the patient is primarily mouth-breathing, as is often the case with asthmatics during moderate to severe bronchospasm. It appears to be a normal mechanism, during states of increased work of breathing, for patients to bypass the nose, thereby reducing 50% of the anatomically imposed work of breathing through the upper airway. In such cases, the patient will breathe primarily through their mouth until such time as the airway resistance is reduced, along with the need for a bronchodilator.

Nebulizer type

Continuous nebulization, producing aerosol continuously throughout the patient's respiratory cycle, is not very efficient in delivering medication to the patient. This is because aerosol that is produced between inspirations is largely lost to the atmosphere. Demand nebulizers, which actuate in coordination with inspiration, are more efficient in delivering medication. However, these devices increase nebulization time as much as four-fold for the same volume of medication.

The ease or difficulty of use of the aerosol delivery system effects the speed and reliability of self-administration. Systems with multidose convenience appear to be the easiest for patients to use.

Drug formulation

The drug formulation can influence drug delivery. Almost any solution can be nebulized, but the physical characteristics of the solution can affect particle size and nebulizer output. Formulations of dry powders are limited to only a few preparations. Metered dose inhalers have a greater variety of available formulations, but incorporating new drugs into metered dose inhalers is a lengthy process; therefore the drugs are not always available in the most desirable or therapeutically optimal form.

Humidity

Humidity affects both wet and dry aerosols. Droplets of solutions can either evaporate or grow depending on the water content and temperature of the gas around them. Powder will clump or aggregate in high humidity, thereby reducing delivered doses.

Patient characteristics

Small infants breath mainly via the nose, have tiny airways, small inspired volumes, high respiratory rates, and are unable to cooperate to achieve ideal drug delivery. Older children are also often unable or unwilling to cooperate. Elderly patients may not be able to physically manipulate devices or to understand or cooperate with techniques to optimize aerosol delivery.

Actuation of the aerosol device during inspiration is mandatory with some nebulizers, particularly metered dose inhalers. Poor patient coordination will drastically reduce the delivered dose.

The patient's ability to understand the therapy and its goals significantly affects the therapeutic efficacy of any treatment. Patients need not only to understand the basic administration technique, but also must be able to keep track of dosing requirements and recognize undesirable side effects and techniques utilized to reduce them.

AEROSOL GENERATORS

General principles

Aerosol generators are commonly used by RCPs to deliver medications to the airway and lungs, and to humidify inspired gas. A variety of methods are used to generate aerosols for therapeutic uses. The most common methods include jet nebulizers, meter dose inhalers (MDI), dry powder inhalers (DPI), and ultrasonic nebulizers. Spinning disk nebulizers are rarely used in clinical respiratory care, being more frequently used as room humidifiers.

Aerosol drug therapy

Aerosols are frequently used to provide delivery of medications to the lung. The airways of the respiratory tract provide an ideal route for drug administration. In many cases aerosols are superior in terms of efficacy and safety to the same systemically administered drugs used to treat pulmonary disorders.[61] Aerosols deliver a high drug concentration to the airway directly, while providing very low systemic doses and minimizing systemic side effects. As a result, aerosol drug delivery has a high therapeutic index. Drugs can be delivered by aerosol using small volume nebulizers, large volume nebulizers, or metered dose inhalers. Ribavirin has been delivered by a specially manufactured device. The small-particle aerosol generator (SPAG) has been used to administer ribavirin.

Types of aerosol generators

Jet nebulizer

Jet nebulizers utilize the Bernoulli principle; a high pressure gas is driven through a restricted orifice (jet) positioned to intersect the top of a tube whose base is immersed in solution (Figure 25-17). The resulting effect produces an area of low pressure which draws the solution up a capillary tube into the jet stream, which shatters the fluid into droplets. If properly designed, the stream of gas directs the droplets to impact against a baffle, the internal walls of the nebulizer, and/or the surface of the solution. Impaction removes the large particles from suspension and allows them to return to the reservoir, while smaller particles remain suspended in the gas and exit from the nebulizer. Droplet size and nebulization time are inversely proportional to gas flow through the jet. The higher the flow rate to the nebulizer, the smaller the particle size generated and the greater the time needed to nebulize the solution.

Small volume nebulizer

Small volume nebulizers (SVNs) are frequently used to deliver medication, particularly bronchodilators. A variety of different SVNs are available. Each has specific characteristics, particularly with respect to output which results in differences in delivery of drug to the lung (Table 25-8, page 678). Despite these differences, no studies have been done to date which demonstrate significant differences in clinical response based on SVN design. Similarly, no studies have reported that the clinical response differs depending on the flows provided during the treatment.[62-63] The lack of difference may be real or may represent how studies of nebulizer efficiency are performed. Each of the studies used high doses of drugs. The large doses may mask any inefficiencies of the nebulizers themselves. One study did demonstrate that the dose delivered to stable asthmatics did make a difference.[64]

Device selection may be of greater importance for administration of drugs other than bronchodilators, particularly to ensure efficient delivery of expensive drugs. Such substances include anti-viral agents, alpha$_1$-antitrypsin, artificial surfactants and pentamidine. Nebulizers with a MMAD less than $2\mu m$ should be used for targeting delivery to the lung parenchyma. SVNs such as the Respirgard II® utilize one way valves as auxiliary baffles to create desired particle size. Other specialty nebulizers such as the Vortran HEART and ICN SPAG-2 are described later in the chapter. The accompanying box itemizes factors that effect the efficacy of SVNs.

The amount of drug nebulized by a SVN increases as diluent is increased. Typical SVNs will deliver more drug as an aerosol when the volume in the nebulizer is 4 ml as opposed to 2 ml with a constant nebulizer flow of 6 to 8L/min. Particle size decreases as flowrate

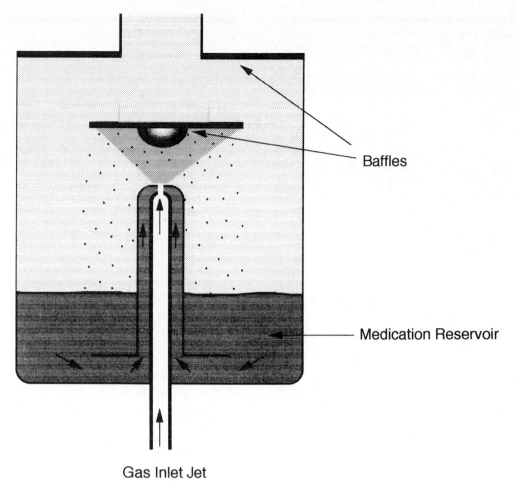

Baffles

Medication Reservoir

Gas Inlet Jet

Fig. 25-17 Components of a jet nebulizer. (From Fink J, Cohen N: Humidity and aerosols. In Eubank D, Bone R: Principles and applications of cardiorespiratory care equipment, St Louis, 1994, Mosby.)

increases. This has not been shown to correlate with differences in clinical responses at varying diluent volumes and flowrates.[65] Another characteristic of SVNs which is important to consider is the dead space volume. Dead space volume is the residual volume of medication that remains in the nebulizer after the nebulizer runs dry. It varies from 0.5 mL to 1.0 mL. The greater the dead space volume, the more drug is wasted and the less efficient is the delivery system.

Many of the commercially available SVNs function only when kept in an upright position. Others are designed to operate in a variety of positions. This can be accomplished by directing a jet across the opening of multiple capillary tubes extending from a variety of points across the medication chamber. With this design, at least one capillary tube will be submerged in the medication no matter what the position of the nebulizer. The jet draws medication from the reservoir and directs the spray into an opposing baffle.

Humidity and temperature affects the performance of SVNs. They each affect particle size and the concentration of drug remaining in the nebulizer.

Evaporation of water and adiabatic expansion of gas can reduce the temperature of the aerosol to as much as 5° C below ambient temperature. As gas warms to room temperature, the particle size will be reduced. The aerosol particles entrained into a warm, fully saturated gas stream, such as a ventilator circuit, may increase in size.

SVNs will deliver the medication effectively only when used properly. Because the nose is such an efficient filter of particles over 5μm, clinicians have long recommended that aerosol be inhaled through the mouth. Nose-breathing filters out large particles and deposits more medication in the upper airway. Despite these theoretical differences, there appears to be no difference in clinical response between treatments given by mouthpiece or by mask when the patient is mouth-breathing. The selection of delivery method, (mask or mouthpiece) should be made based on patient preference and comfort.

The ventilatory pattern does influence deposition of aerosols into the lower respiratory tract from small volume nebulizers; in most situations, however, normal tidal breathing is encouraged during a treatment.

Table 25-8 Differences in particle size and output between various SVN and other nebulizer types

	MMAD	GSD
JET NEBULIZERS		
Respirgard II	0.93	±1.8
Centimist	1.1	±2.2
Aerotech II	2.0	±2.5
Fan JET	4.3	±2.5
Vortran HEART	3.5–2.2	±1.8–2.1
MedicAid Sidestreatm	2.75–3.0	
6 L/min	6.0	
12 L/min	3.7	
ULTRASONIC NEBULIZERS		
FISO Neb	5.0	±2.0
Green Machine	>12.0	
Portasonic	1.6	±2.2
Pulmosonic	4.2	±2.3
DeVilbiss 900	2.8	±2.1

	MMAD	Output
MDI	2.4	
Rotahaler (DPI)	2.6	
Jet Nebulizer	2–5.0	0.25–0.4 mL/min
Baffled Jet Nebulizer	0.25–4.0	0.1–1.0 mL/min
Ultrasonic Nebulizer	1.6–12	6 mL/min
Hydrosphere	1.2–4.0	7 mL/min

(Adapted from Fallot, *Respir Care* 1991;36(9):1011. With permission.)

Factors affecting SVN performance

Nebulizer design

Brand
Lot
Tolerances in manufacturing between:
   Lots
   Individual units
Baffles
   Internal
   One way valves
   Angles enroute to patient
Residual volume
Position dependency
Reservoirs or extension
Trigger ports
Use of vents

Gas source—wall, cylinder. compressor

Pressure
Gas density
Flow rate through nebulizer
Humidity
Temperature

Characteristics of drug nebulized

Viscosity
Surface tension
Homogeneity
Volume fill

Slow inspiratory flows seem to be the most valuable maneuver to improve deposition. Deep breathing and breath-holding during nebulizer therapy do not appear to augment the deposition of drug compared with tidal breathing alone.[66]

Continuous nebulization during the entire respiratory cycle results in considerable waste of drug. In between inspirations, the drug is lost to the environment. With a normal inspiratory:expiratory (I:E) ratio of 1:3, only 25% of the nebulized drug delivered to the face will get into the airway.

Techniques to minimize drug loss have been utilized. Intermittent nebulization, using a patient-controlled finger port to direct gas to the nebulizer only during inspiration, provides greater opportunity to deposit more drug in the lung. It does, however, increase the duration of treatment by as much as three to five times and requires considerably more patient hand breath coordination than continuous nebulization. Drug delivery can be significantly enhanced by the use of a valved storage chamber (such as the Mizer), which holds aerosol that is generated during exhalation. The simple addition of a 50 mL tube as an expiratory reservoir to a nebulizer also improves drug delivery with a small volume nebulizer.

With the large number of SVNs available on the market, it is clear that not all nebulizers are created equal. In fact, not all SVNs work at all.[67] Care should

be taken to evaluate the SVN you use the same way you would comparatively evaluate ventilator performance.

SVN with during mechanical ventilation. Aerosol administered by SVN to intubated and ventilated patients tends to deposit in the tubing of the ventilator circuit; less medication is delivered to the patient. Deposition in the lung of ventilated patients has been measured in a range of 1.5% to 3.0%.[67-68] McIntyre estimated the deposition by this route to be only about 3% of the delivered dose[68], while Fuller et al found that deposition of drug by small volume nebulizer is 1.5%.[70]

When delivering medications by SVN to intubated, mechanically ventilated patients, the clinician must identify the most appropriate location for the nebulizer. Hughes and Saez[71] found that the optimal placement of the nebulizer is in the inspiratory limb at the manifold of the ventilator circuit, about 18 inches from the patient wye. They demonstrated that the worst position for the nebulizer was between the patient and the wye connector of the circuit, particularly when using continuously nebulized medication, when the drug that is nebulized after inspiration is complete is driven down the expiratory limb of the ventilator circuit and lost to the patient. The box on page 679 outlines the optimum techniques to use.

Optimal technique for use of SVN with mechanical ventilation

1. Assess patient for need
2. Establish dose to compensate for decreased delivery
2. Place drug in neb to fill vol ≥ 4 ml.
3. Place SVN in inspiratory line ≥ 18 inches from the patient wye.
4. Gas flow to nebulizer at 6 to 8 L/min
   a. Use ventilator if it meets flow needs and cycles on inspiration only; otherwise
   b. Use continuous flow from external source adjust volume or pressure limit to compensate for flow
5. Turn off flowby or continuous flow while nebulizing
6. Tap neb periodically until all medication is nebulized
7. Remove neb from circuit, rinse with sterile water and run dry
8. Return ventilator to previous settings
9. Monitor patient for adverse response
10. Assess outcome

Large volume nebulizer

Large volume nebulizers can also be used to administer bronchodilators and active medications to the lung. The large volume nebulizer is particularly useful when traditional dosing strategies are ineffective in treating severe bronchospasm. In the treatment of acute exacerbations of asthma with bronchodilators, a variety of methods are used to optimize treatment. When the patient does not respond to standard dosage, the frequency of administration is often increased, up to every 15 minutes. An alternative method of therapy to frequent SVN treatments is to provide continuous nebulization, providing a nebulizer with adequate solution to operate continuously and deliver a controlled rate of medication. The large volume nebulizer can be used to provide continuous therapy. The continuous therapy not only assures that the drug is delivered frequently enough to optimize bronchodilation, but can also be delivered without patient interruption. The bronchodilator can be delivered while the patient sleeps.

Vortran's High Output Extended Aerosol Respiratory Therapy (HEART®) nebulizer has been used for providing continuous aerosol therapy with bronchodilators and other medications. This nebulizer has a 240 ml reservoir and produces particles between 3.5 and 2.2 μm MMAD. The actual output and particle size vary based on the pressure at which the nebulizer operates and the flow rate.[72] The one problem with using a large volume nebulizer for continuous treatment is that the concentration of drug increases over time as evaporation occurs. The patient receiving continuous bronchodilator therapy must be closely monitored for signs of drug toxicity.

The HEART® nebulizer can also be used with the Vortran signal actuated nebulizer (VISAN®) for mechanically ventilated patients, providing a high output of respirable particles on demand. The VISAN® provides synchronous operation with aerosol produced at high flows during inspiration, actuated by an electronic signal from the ventilator, so that timing is synchronized with inspiration. The device has a temperature bath to provide thermal control and a built-in air-controlled magnetic stirrer under the nebulizer reservoir to provide for uniform nebulization of suspension, colloids, and liposomes over extended periods.[72]

Another method for continuous delivery of bronchodilator by large volume nebulizer is to use an IV infusion pump to drip premixed bronchodilator solution into a standard SVN. The cost and availability of infusion pumps make this an expensive device, but appears to be capable of providing a dose each hour that is equivalent to treatments every 15 minutes by a small volume nebulizer using standard dosing.[73-81]

Small-particle aerosol generator

The small-particle aerosol generator (SPAG®), is a jet-type aerosol generator manufactured by ICN Pharmaceuticals specifically for administration of ribavirin (Virazole®). Ribavirin is an antiviral that has been recommended for treatment of high risk infants and children with respiratory syncytial virus (RSV) infections.[82] The effectiveness of this drug has been questionable. Few studies have demonstrated that ribavirin is useful therapy,[83] although recent data suggest that it is useful for ventilated infants with RSV.[84-85] The SPAG® (Figure 25-18, page 680) was specifically designed to facilitate administration of ribavirin. The device is unique in clinical respiratory care practice in that it incorporates a drying chamber with its own flow control to produce a stable aerosol. The SPAG reduces medical gas source from the normal line pressure 50 psig to as low as 26 psig; it has a variable regulator, which is adjustable by the clinician. The regulator is connected to two flow meters controlling flow to the nebulizer and drying chamber respectively. The nebulizer is located within the reservoir jar containing the medication, directing the aerosol output directly into the wall of the reservoir. As the aerosol leaves the medication reservoir/nebulizer and enters the long cylindrical drying chamber, a flow of dry gas is added to the aerosol. The dry gas serves to reduce particle size through evaporation and to transport the particles to the patient. Nebulizer flow should be maintained at about 7 lpm with total flow from both flowmeters not less than 15 lpm. The drying chamber helps to make the output almost monodisperse with aerosol particles mostly between 1.2 to 1.4 μm. The SPAG II® nebulizer tends to operate consistently even with back pressure and may be used with masks, hoods, tents or ventilator circuits.

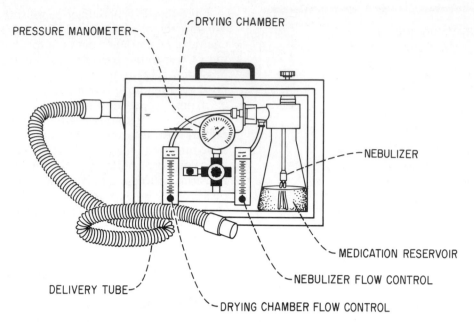

PRESSURE MANOMETER

DRYING CHAMBER

NEBULIZER

MEDICATION RESERVOIR

NEBULIZER FLOW CONTROL

DELIVERY TUBE

DRYING CHAMBER FLOW CONTROL

Fig. 25-18 Small particle aerosol generator

Concerns of exposure of this drug to care providers has resulted in measures to contain and scavenge aerosols escaping from the direct vicinity of the patient.[86-92]

SPAG in ventilated patients. Ribavirin has been used most successfully to treat patients who require intubation and mechanical ventilatory support.[93] Unfortunately, the manufacturer of the drug suggests that it not be given through a ventilator circuit, because of concern about drug accumulation and occlusion of the circuit. Demers, et al described a system for use with ventilator circuits that utilizes filters on the expiratory limb of the circuit and incorporates a water seal pop-off and one way valve between the SPAG and humidifier outlet.[94] Kacmarek and Kratohvil[95] describe a system which incorporates a one way valve connecting the SPAG to the inspiratory limb of the circuit of a Sechrist ventilator. The connection is made distal to the humidifier to prevent back flow of the aerosol during positive pressure breaths. They also reduce the inspiratory flow by 7.5 L/min. A Pall filter was placed in the expiratory limb proximal to the exhalation valve. When using either of these techniques to deliver ribavirin to mechanically ventilated patients, care should be taken to ensure that there is no leak around the cuff of the endotracheal tube. Gas leaking around the cuff will contaminate the environment during positive pressure breaths.

Nasal spray pump

The spray pump is the most common device used for nasal aerosol administration sympathomimetic, anitmuscarinic, antiallergic, and anti-inflammatory drugs. The spray pump generates lower internal pressures than SVN, producing larger particles which are better targeted for nasal deposition. Deposition with the nasal spray pump is mostly in the anterior nose, with clearance to the nasopharynx. 100 μL puffs appear to deposit more medication than 50 μL puffs, and deposition occurs to a greater surface area with a 35 degree spray angle than with 60 degrees.

The spray pump with available aqueous based formulations is rapidly replacing the CFC based MDIs used for nasal administration which are scheduled to be banned by 1996.

Metered dose inhaler

Metered dose inhalers (MDI) are freon-powered nebulizers which provide multidose convenience through use of a metering device (Figure 25-19). They are pressurized canisters containing a drug in the form of a micronized powder, suspended with a mixture of two or more chlorofluorocarbon (CFC) propellants (freons) along with a dispersal agent. MDIs are the most widely used form of aerosol device for administration of bronchodilators, anticholinergics, and steroids; more formulations of these drugs are now available for use by MDI than for use with other types of other nebulizers.

A variety of dispersal agents are used to improve drug delivery by keeping the drug in suspension. The most common dispersal agent is surfactant. The surfactants, commonly soya lecithin, sorbitan trioleate, and oleic acid help to both keep the drug suspended in the freon and lubricate the valve mechanism. The dispersal agents are usually present in amounts at least equal to or greater than the quantity of drug to be administered. The high concentration of the dispersal

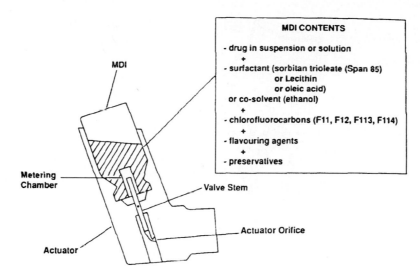

Fig. 25-19 Metered dose inhaler (MDI) with ingredients. (From Newhouse MT, Dolovich M: Aerosol therapy in Children. In *Basic mechanisms of pediatric respiratory disease: cellular and integrations,* 1991, Toronto, BC Decker.)

agent has clinical significance. Some patients develop severe cough or wheezing caused by the propellant or surfactant, so care must be exercised when initiating therapy by MDI.[97]

The majority of the spray from most MDIs, up to 60% to 80% by weight, consists of the chlorofluorocarbon with only 1% active drug. The large quantity of CFCs is also of clinical importance. Adverse reactions to CFCs have been reported when administered in much larger doses than encountered with even aggressive therapy. Anecdotal reports of adverse response to freon has been reported in adults and children.[97-99]

The output volume of MDIs varies from 30 to 100 μL, which contains 50 μg to 5 mg of drug, depending on the drug administered.[100-101] Most MDIs use a 50 μL metering chamber to control drug delivery. Increasing the volume of the chamber does not improve drug delivery. More of the additional drug is lost at the actuator mouthpiece due to the lower rate of evaporation of the greater amount of propellant released and is therefore not available to the patient.[102]

Aerosol production from an MDI takes approximately 20 m/sec. Aerosolization of the liquid released from the metered dose canister begins as the propellants vaporize or "flash" and continues as the propellant evaporates. The velocity of the liquid spray leaving the MDI is about 15 m/sec. The speed falls to less than half the maximum velocity within 0.1 sec as a cloud develops and moves away from the actuator orifice.[103] The particles produced from the "flashing" of propellants are initially 35 μm and rapidly decrease in size due to evaporation as the particle moves away from the nozzle.[104]

The particle size influences the delivery of drug by MDI. Due to the velocity of the jet, approximately 80% of the dose impacts and deposits in the oropharynx, especially when the canister is fired from inside the mouth.[102,105] Manufacturers of MDIs can adjust the particle size delivered by the device to influence drug targeting and subsequent absorption.

The particle size and spray pattern produced by MDIs are determined by a variety of factors. A primary determinant is the vapor pressure of the canister. For most metered dose inhalers, propellant vapor pressure varies from about 300 to 500 kPa at 20° C, creating a heterodisperse aerosol with MMADs of 3 to 6 μm and a GSD of 2 μm.[11] The higher the vapor pressure, the smaller the particle size.

The major determinant of the vapor pressure is the composition of the chlorofluorocarbons. The rate of evaporation of the CFC determines the coarseness of the spray. The slower the rate of evaporation, the coarser the spray. Finer sprays can be produced by using greater quantities of CFC 12 or more volatile compounds. Raising the temperature of the canister also increases the pressure and reduces the particle size.

Other variables which can be adjusted to change the particle size include the size of the valve stem and actuator orifice (Figure 25-20, page 682), the drug concentration, and addition of cosolvents. The smaller the valve stem size and the actuator orifice size, the finer the spray. Higher drug concentrations produce coarser aerosols. Ethanol has also been used as a cosolvent for drug delivery.[11] Its use results in a coarser spray, which may facilitate delivery of some drugs. The chlorofluorocarbons evaporate more slow-

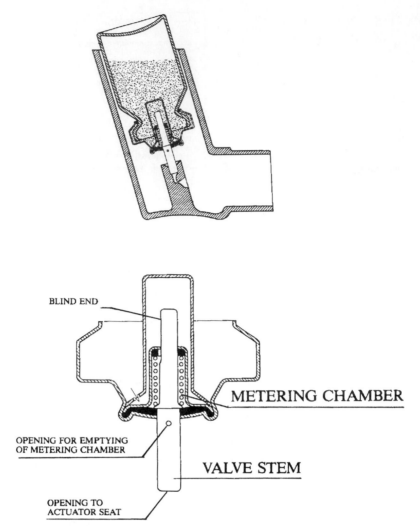

Fig. 25-20 MDI Valve (From Fink J, Cohen N: Humidity and aerosols. In Eubank D, Bone R: Principles and applications of cardiorespiratory care equipment, St Louis, 1994, Mosby.)

ly in the presence of alcohol. The alcohol concentration must be taken into account when selecting a metered dose inhaler for drug delivery. Concentrations of alcohol can be over 35% in some products. The alcohol can be a respiratory irritant for some patients.

Effect of ban on CFCs in MDIs. In 1974 it was determined that CFCs in the stratosphere were being converted by ultra violet radiation into chlorine, a potent green house gas that was destroying the ozone layer. In 1984 pictures of the hole in the ozone layer over Antarctica resulted in an international treaty to ban the importation and production of CFCs worldwide by 1996. The CFCs in MDIs only represented 0.5% of total CFC use at that time. Hydrofluorocarbons (HFC) do not contain chlorine, have higher vapor pressure, and lower solubility than CFCs. As suitable replacements for CFCs were identified, pharmaceutical companies began a minimum 8 year cycle of testing and meeting FDA criteria to prove compa-

rable efficacy of the new MDI. Of the 25 million COPD patients in America, most rely on MDI for one or more medications. As it was determined that SVN was more expensive, less portable, and required more time to administer than MDI, and DPI was too flow dependent for small children and during severe exacerbations, the international committee has extended the time limit for eliminating CFC based MDI for administration targeted to the lung.

Delivery characteristics. The MMAD of most MDIs is between 3 and 6 μm[106] with a deposition in the lung of about 10%.[107-108] As much as 80% of the dose is deposited in the mouth and may be a factor in systemic absorption as opposed to direct aerosol delivery to the lung since the MDI delivers a significant amount of drug to the mucous membranes of the mouth and stomach. Unfortunately, the actual amount of drug delivered to an individual patient is unpredictable because of significant interpatient variability.[105]

A number of studies have documented the clinical efficacy of metered dose inhalers.[109-112] MDIs have been demonstrated to be at least as effective as other nebulizers used for drug delivery. As a result, MDIs are often the preferred method for delivering bronchodilators to spontaneously breathing as well as intubated, ventilated patients.[113-114]

The MDI has become a common method by which to deliver drugs to the lung. The device is now available to administer all commonly used bronchodilators and steroids. The successful administration of medications by MDI is very technique dependent. The patient must coordinate actuation of the MDI with early inspiration. The usual recommended method of delivery is to have the patient slowly exhale to residual volume prior to inspiration and to close the lips tightly around the MDI actuator. Actuate the MDI immediately after beginning a slow inspiratory flow (<0.75 L/sec) ending with a breath hold of 10 seconds. This is reported to optimize lung deposition.[115-118]

Dolovich and others have shown increased deposition in the lung when the MDI is placed 4 cm from an open mouth position.[108] This technique improves lung deposition, while decreasing oral deposition. The lung volume at which the aerosol is inhaled, beginning at residual volume, functional residual capacity, or 80% of total lung capacity apparently does not significantly affect the amount of aerosol deposited in the lung or the clinical response to the bronchodilator.[119] It is possible that for patients with unstable airways, exhaling down to residual volume could result in closure of airways with reduction of distribution of the next inhaled breath of aerosol to the lung. If true, the preferred technique might be for normal exhalation to functional residual capacity before inspiration and actuation of the MDI. The accompanying box outlines the optimal technique as described above.

Oral deposition of drug delivered by MDI, as with SVN, can account for as much as 80% of the dose. The medication may be swallowed or absorbed by the mucous membranes, producing greater systemic side effects. The worst reported side effect of oral deposition with MDI is increased oral thrush or opportunistic yeast infections associated with use of inhaled steroids. Rinsing the mouth post steroid administration is recommended to reduce effects of oral deposition. Unfortunately, deposition preferentially occurs at the point of greatest turbulence which is the larynx, which can not be effectively reached by gargling.

Improper MDI inhalation technique has been reported to range from 24% to 67% of previously instructed patients. This seems to correlate with findings that fewer than 65% of physicians and nurses involved in outpatient instruction of patients with MDI performed properly at least four of seven steps of administration.[120] Proper patient instruction is essential and rather time consuming, requiring 10 to 28 minutes for initial instruction. Repeated instruction improves performance, but must occur several times.[121-122] Even with the best instruction, some patients, especially infants, young children, and patients in acute distress may be unable to coordinate proper administration; under these circumstances, accessory devices such as holding chambers should be considered.

Vitalograph has developed the Aerosol Inhalation Monitor (AIM) (Figure 25-21) to help teach patients the closed-mouth MDI administration technique. Using placebo aerosols, AIM monitors and provides visual feed back on: coordinated inspiration with firing (depth charges are dropped and descend), appropriate inspiratory flow rates, duration of inspiration (depth charges blow up submarines), and breath holding (diver rises to the surface.) Proper sequence and timing results in a merry tune.

Optimal technique for use of MDI without accessory device

1. Warm MDI to hand or body temperature
2. Assemble apparatus (make sure there are no objects or coins in device that could be aspirated or obstruct out flow)
3. Shake canister vigorously and hold canister upright, placing actuator 4 cm (two fingers) a way from open mouth (aimed directly into mouth)
4. After a normal exhalation, begin to inspire slowly (0.5 L/min.), while actuating MDI. Continue inspiration to total lung capacity.
5. Hold breath for 10 seconds.
6. Wait 1 minute between actuations.

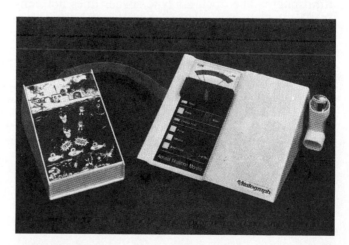

Fig. 25-21 AIM Vitalograph Aerosol Inhalation Monitor used to teach children and adults the closed-mouth technique of MDI administration. (From Fink J, Cohen N: Humidity and aerosols. In Eubank D, Bone R: Principles and applications of cardiorespiratory care equipment, St Louis, 1994, Mosby.)

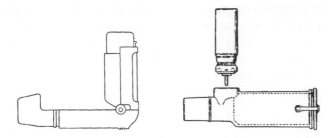

Fig. 25-22 Examples of MDI Spacers (From Fink J, Cohen N: Humidity and aerosols. In Eubank D, Bone R: Principles and applications of cardiorespiratory care equipment, St Louis, 1994, Mosby.)

Accessory devices with MDI. Accessory devices have been used in conjunction with the MDI to reduce oropharyngeal deposition and reduce or eliminate the need for hand-breath coordination. These devices have markedly improved the therapeutic efficacy of MDIs and broadened their usefulness in acute and critical care environments. Accessory devices have been the critical factor making MDI consistently equivalent to treatment with small volume nebulizers.

The accessories which appear to be most effective are spacers and holding chambers. The spacer, such as an open-end straight tube, baggy, PVC tube, Open Spacer Synchronizer® , or Optihaler® (Figure 25-22) provides space for the aerosolized medication or "plume" to expand and the chlorofluorocarbons to evaporate, allowing larger particles to impact on the walls of the device, reducing oropharyngeal deposition.[124] Spacer devices still require considerable coordination of actuation with breathing pattern. Exhalation immediately following actuation will clear the aerosol from the device, wasting the dose to the atmosphere. The open air type spacer does not contain the aerosol at all, depending entirely on coordinated patient technique for drug delivery.[125]

Holding chambers (Nebuhaler® , Aerochamber® , DHD Ace® shown in Figure 25-23) are similar to spacers in allowing the plume to develop and reducing oropharyngeal deposition. The key difference is the addition of a valve or enclosure, which permits the aerosol to be drawn from the chamber on inspiration, but prevents the remaining aerosol in the chamber from being cleared on exhalation. The use of the chamber allows patients with small tidal volumes to empty aerosol from the chamber with successive breaths. With the holding chamber in use, the patient can exhale into the mouthpiece or mask as the MDI is actuated, without blowing away any of the medication. The InspirEase™ is an exception; it does not have a one-way valve.

The DHD ACE® (Figure 25-23) uses a mouthpiece with a one-way valve and inspiratory orifice at one end and a flow indicator attached to the other end of the chamber, allowing the device to do double-duty as an accessory device for nonintubated and ventilated patients. While the chamber works well in ventilated patients, this configuration has not been studied and reported on in the literature.

The use of spacers and holding chambers has improved utilization of metered dose inhalers for delivery of bronchodilators. Larger doses of the medication are delivered to the lower respiratory tract, with a greatly improved therapeutic ratio. Spacers and holding chambers tend to reduce oral deposition, reduce bad taste of medication and reduce the "cold Freon" effect which causes many children to stop inhalation with MDI actuation. Both accessory devices provide comparable advantages for the patient that can coordinate MDI discharge with optimal breath control.[126] A holding chamber which incorporates an appropriately sized mask is available for use with

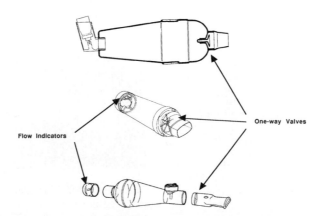

Flow Indicators

One-way Valves

Fig. 25-23 Examples of MDI holding chambers. (From Fink J, Cohen N: Humidity and aerosols. In Eubank D, Bone R: Principles and applications of cardiorespiratory care equipment, St Louis, 1994, Mosby.)

infants, children, and adults (Figure 25-24, *A*). These units allow effective administration to patients who are unable to use a mouthpiece device, due to size, age, coordination, or mentation (Figure 25-24, *B*).[126-134] The use of the MDI with the holding chamber may be as effective a method of delivering drugs as small volume nebulizers.[135-145] Additional comparative studies will be helpful to more clearly define the clinical situations where one technique may be superior to the other.

The accessory devices used with the metered dose inhalers do cause a reduction in MMAD of the original spray through evaporation and impaction of the larger particles on the wall or valves of the device.[146] The smaller particle size results in a 10- to 15-fold decrease in the dose of drug delivered to the pharynx.[108] The use of the holding chamber is particularly helpful when administering steroids, since the total dose required will be less and systemic side effects can be minimized.[147-148] Even with a holding chamber in use, however, respirable particles do settle out and deposit within the device. The accompanying box outlines the optimum technique for MDI use with a holding chamber.

In order to eliminate hand-breath coordination in MDI administration, the autohaler (3M) was developed to allow flow triggered actuation of an MDI in response to patient inspiratory effort (Figure 25-25,

Optimal technique for use of MDI with holding chamber

1. Assess need.
2. Warm MDI to hand or body temperature.
3. Assemble apparatus (make sure there are no objects or coins in device that could be aspirated or obstruct out flow).
4. Shake canister vigorously and hold canister upright.
5. Place holding chamber in mouth or place mask over nose and mouth encouraging patient to breath through mouth.
6. Breath normally and actuate at the beginning of inspiration (Note: Larger breaths with breath holding may be encouraged in patient who can cooperate, but this has not shown to increase clinical response to inhaled bronchodilators.)
7. Allow 30 to 60 seconds between actuations.
8. Monitor patient for adverse response.
9. Assess outcome.

page 686). A MDI canister is spring loaded in preparation for firing by cocking a lever at the top of the unit. When the patient takes a breath in, a vane is moved when generated flow is between 30 to 60 L/min, the canister is pressed down into the actuator, and the MDI is fired. While this device addresses hand breath

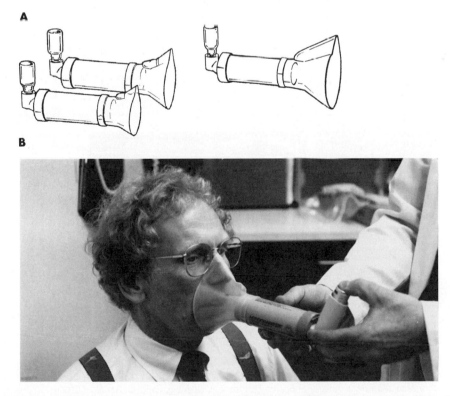

Fig. 25-24 Different size masks used with MDI and holding chamber (**A**). Adult patient receiving medication via holding chamber with mask (**B**). (From Fink J, Cohen N: Humidity and aerosols. In Eubank D, Bone R: Principles and applications of cardiorespiratory care equipment, St Louis, 1994, Mosby.)

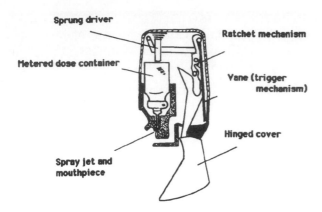

Fig. 25-25 Diagram of the original autohaler from Riker/3M that has been available for several years in Europe.

coordination with bronchodilator administration, it has yet to be seen whether such devices may require use of a spacer/holding chamber to reduce pharyngeal deposition. Because the autohaler, as marketed in the United States, can only be breath actuated, it would seem that a patient during acute exacerbation may not be able to generate sufficient flows to fire the MDI. The ability to manually fire the MDI, independent of patient ability to generate specific flow rates, would allow broader application for those patients with periodic life threatening increase in airway obstruction.

MDI administration to intubated patients. Spacers are also used to optimize drug delivery by metered dose inhalers to intubated, mechanically ventilated patients. Three basic styles of adapter are available (Figure 25-26), including elbow, inline, and chamber devices.

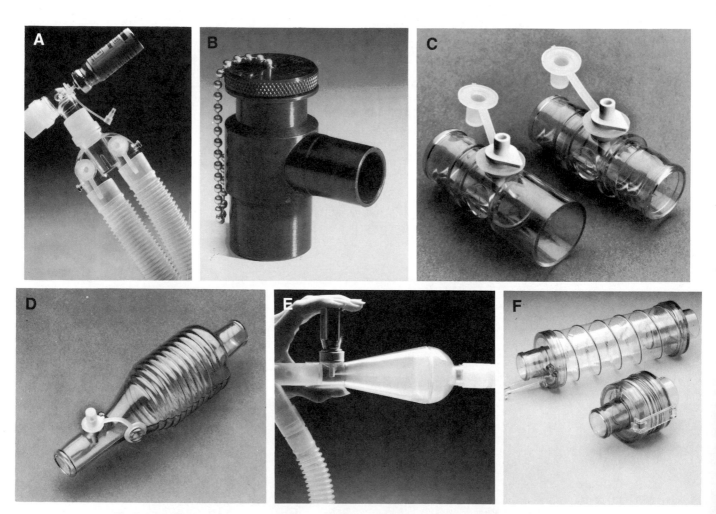

Fig. 25-26 Metered dose inhaler adaptors. **A,** Metered dose inhaler elbow. (Courtesy of IPI, Chicago, IL.) **B,** Bronchodilator-Tee. (Courtesy of Boehringer Laboratories, Norristown, Pa.) **C,** Metered dose inhaler inspiratory limb adaptor. (Courtesy of Baxter-Pharmaseal, Valencia, Calif.) **D,** Aerosol suspension chamber. (Courtesy of Baxter-Pharmaseal.) **E,** Aerosol Cloud Enhancer. (Courtesy of DHD, Diemolding Healthcare Division, Canastota, N.Y.) **F,** Aerovent. (Courtesy of Monaghan, Plattsburgh, N.Y.) (From Opt Holt T: Aerosol generators and humidifiers. In Core textbook of respiratory care practice, ed 2, St Louis, 1994, Mosby.)

The elbow style device allows the MDI to be actuated directly into the airway, either endotracheal or tracheotomy tube. The actuation is directed into a very constricted space; the majority of the chlorofluorocarbons and medication impact onto the walls of the artificial airway prior to evaporation and "aerosolization" of the medication. The result is a small percentage of respirable particles delivered beyond the tip of the airway into the lung.[149]

Inline devices allow the MDI to be actuated in line with the inspiratory limb of the ventilator circuit tubing. While the tubing is generally wider than the internal diameter of an endotracheal tube, it is still narrower than the space required for plume development, and there is still a large percentage of medication trapped in the tubing; the delivered dose of respirable particles is low.

Chamber style devices are designed to allow an aerosol "plume" to develop. Within this cloud the chlorofluorocarbons evaporate before the bulk of the medication contacts the surface of the chamber or ventilator tubing. The use of the chamber device may result in less impaction of the medication on the walls of circuit tubing or airway compared with the other devices used with ventilated patients.

One question which frequently arises when using drugs delivered by MDI to ventilated patients is the dose of drug required. Many studies have suggested that the dose of drug delivered per puff from the MDI is less when administered to the ventilated patient compared with the dose delivered to the nonintubated, spontaneously breathing patient. Bishop, et al used a bench model and determined that application of drug by metered dose inhaler to an endotracheal tube using the Monaghan AeroVent® chamber, Instrumentation Industries RTC-22® spacer, or the Intermedical Intec 172275® spacer resulted in less drug being delivered compared to the drug delivered to a "normal airway." They estimated that if deposition of drug delivered by MDI to the normal airway is 10%, then these adapters might be expected to deposit only

1% using the Intec® chamber, 3% with the RTC-22® chamber, and 6% with the AeroVent® chamber of dose in the lung.[150]

Using a similar bench model, Ebert, et al confirmed that chamber style MDI devices produced greater volume of respirable particles than the in-line or elbow style devices (Figure 25-27).[151] Fuller, et al, using the AeroVent® chamber to deliver medication by metered dose inhaler to intubated, ventilated patients demonstrated a 5.5% deposition of drug delivered by MDI compared to 1.5% deposition when delivered by a small volume nebulizer.[70]

It may be reasonable to assume that all intubated or ventilated patients receive a significantly smaller percentage of medication in the lung than the nonintubated patient, and that to deliver comparable amounts of medication to the lung, larger doses (up to ten fold) may be required. A number of studies have demonstrated that the dose required is larger to achieve the same therapeutic endpoint for medications delivered by MDI to intubated versus nonintubated patients. Since the specific dose required is unpredictable, our practice is to titrate the dosage of bronchodilator delivered to ventilated patients using an MDI, usually with albuterol and to incorporate a AeroVent® adapter. Individual puffs are given at 15 to 30 second intervals, up to 20 puffs. The patient's response is monitored to determine clinical response and onset of side effects. If the patient demonstrates no side effects, but continued clinical signs of increased airway resistance, repeated doses are administered by the protocol until the desired clinical response is achieved or toxicity develops. Utilizing a similar technique, only 60% of adult patients demonstrated any significant response to the bronchodilator when given up to 40 puffs. The patients had an optimal clinical response at approximately 24 puffs as shown in Figure 25-26. Adverse reactions (tachycardia or PVCs) occurred in only 4 of 120 patients; all were minor and required no treatment. This evaluation suggests that more medication is required for

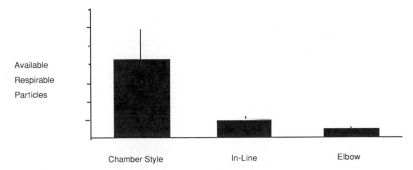

Fig. 25-27 Comparison of available respirable particles delivered to an intubated bench model using chamber, in-line and elbow style adapters. (Adapted from Ebert J, Adams AB, Green-Eide B: An evaluation of MDI spacers and adapters: their effect on respirable volume of medication, *Respir Care* 37: 962-968, 1992.)

clinical improvement for ventilated patients, but that the higher doses were tolerated with minimal adverse reaction.[152]

Dhand, et al demonstrated measurable responses in sedated patients with 10 puffs of albuterol (using a chamber style adapter),[153] while Manthous reported no measurable response with up to 100 puffs (using an elbow style adapter).[154]

Effective delivery of aerosol with MDI in the ventilator circuit can vary from 2% to 40% in in vitro models.[155] Fink, et al demonstrated a variety of factors including mode of ventilation, spontaneous volumes, flow patterns, and humidity. Using an *in vitro* model, spontaneous volumes of 500 mL resulted in greater deposition than an 800 mL control mode breath in a humidified circuit. Figure 25-28 shows the effect of humidity and modes of ventilation on aerosol delivered from an MDI with chamber style adapter to the lower respiratory tract of a spontaneously breathing lung model. These factors are considered in recommended techniques for MDI administration during mechanical ventilation, itemized in the accompanying box.

Dry powder inhaler

The dry powder inhaler (DPI) is another form of metered dose inhaler. Inhalation of drug in a crystalline or powder form has become increasingly popular because this delivery system is relatively inexpensive, does not depend on the use of chlorofluorocarbons and does not require the hand-breath coordination required of metered dose inhalers. Aerosols of dry powder are created by drawing air though an aliquot of the powder. High inspiratory flows required for optimal performance result in pharyngeal impaction of drugs in a manner similar to metered dose inhalers. The clinical efficacy of drugs delivered by DPI appears to be similar to the results with metered dose inhalers, particularly when the MDI is used without an accessory chamber.[156]

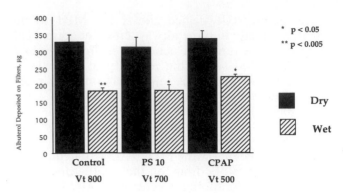

Fig. 25-28 Comparison of deposition of 12 puffs (1080 μg) of albuterol during three modes of ventilation with dry and wet ventilator circuits in a bench model.

A variety of factors influence drug delivery by DPI. DPIs are breath-actuated. Relatively high inspiratory flows are required to release the powder as respirable particles.[157-158] The required high inspiratory flows make the dry powder inhalers small children or any patients who are so compromised that they cannot achieve flow rates of 0.5 to 1 liter per second or greater. DPIs are usually restricted to use for prophylactic and maintenance therapy. They are not acceptable for use during an acute bronchospastic episode and are generally not recommended for infants or children less than 6 years of age.[159] For maintenance therapy, however, a DPI is preferred by many patients, both adult and older children.[156]

Although hand-breath coordination is not as important an issue with DPI versus MDI, coordination in the use of the device can influence drug delivery. Exhalation into the device can result in loss of drug delivered to the lung. Some devices also require assembly, which can be cumbersome or difficult for some patients.

High humidity can also affect drug availability from DPI.[156] The hygroscopic powder will clump if exposed to a relative humidity >50%, creating larger particles which are not as effectively inhaled. Drugs delivered by DPI are carried in lactose or glucose. The drug particle size is from 1 to 2 μm, while the carrier has a particle size of approximately 20 to 25 μm. Most of the carrier impacts in the oropharynx, where it can cause irritation. DPI may not reliably be used for patients with artificial airways, either endotracheal or tracheotomy tubes.

Several DPIs use individual doses administered as gelatin capsules that are punctured prior to inhalation (Spinhaler®, Rotohaler®, Figure 25-29) or from individual blister packets of drug (diskhaler). The Turbo-haler® is a multidose preloaded powder system with 200 doses of drug, terbutaline sulfate or budesonide. The accompanying box outlines the optimum technique for use of a DPI.

Technique for administration of MDI in ventilator circuit

1. Assess need for bronchodilator
2. Establish ventilator dose of ≥ 8 puffs
3. Shake MDI and warm to hand temperature
4. Place MDI in adapter in ventilator circuit
5. Actuate: chamber style adapter—fire at end expiration immediately before inspiration. other adapters—actuate at beginning of inspiration
6. Wait ≥ 15 second between actuations
7. If patient can take a spontaneous breath ≥ 500 mL, coordinate actuation with beginning of deep spontaneous breath and encourage breath hold of 4 to 10 seconds.
8. Monitor for adverse response
9. Assess outcome

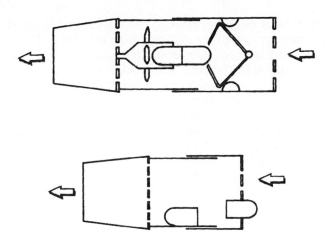

Fig. 25-29 Diagram of Spinhaler® and Rotohaler® administration devices for single dose dry powder inhaler.

Ultrasonic nebulizer

An ultrasonic nebulizer (USN) uses a piezo-electric crystal vibrated at a high-frequency (greater than 1 MHz) to create an aerosol. The crystal transducer, composed of substances, such as quartz-barium titanate, converts electricity into sound. The beam of sound is focused in the liquid above the transducer, creating waves in the liquid immediately above the transducer. If the frequency is high enough, and the amplitude of the signal strong enough, the oscillation waves crest, disrupting the surface of the liquid, creating a "geyser" of droplets.

Large volume USNs usually have the transducer built into an apparatus that includes multiple electronic components as shown in Figure 25-30. The devices use relatively inexpensive medication cups for individual patient use, eliminating the need to steri-

lize the entire apparatus between patients. They use water as a couplant between the transducer and the medication being nebulized. The medication cup, with a flexible diaphragm on the bottom, is seated into a couplant chamber filled with enough water to allow a firm water seal between transducer and cup. This water conducts the sound energy to the diaphragm or cup bottom, which in turn vibrates the medication to produce an aerosol. The water used as couplant must be changed regularly and the unit cleaned to minimize contamination from direct physical contact with the nebulizer and medication cups between treatments.

USNs tend to have higher output rate (0.5 to 7.0 mL/min) and higher mist density than conventional jet nebulizers. The particle or droplet size (MMAD) delivered by an ultrasonic nebulizer is related to the frequency at which the crystals vibrate. The frequency is usually specific to the device selected and is rarely adjustable by the user. The particle size is inversely proportional to frequency. For example the DeVilbiss Portasonic® operates at a frequency of 2.25 MHz and

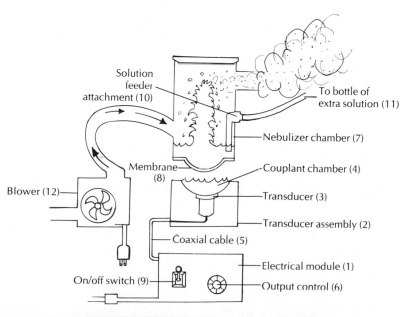

Fig. 25-30 Components of an ultrasonic nebulizer.

produces a MMAD of 2.5 μm while the DeVilbiss Pulmosonic® operates at 1.25 MHz and produces a much less respirable particle range of 4 to 6 μm MMAD. The amplitude of the signal affects the output from the nebulizer. The greater the amplitude, the greater the output from the nebulizer, up to the limit of the device design. Increases beyond that specific upper limit will not improve the device output.

Particle size and aerosol density are also affected by the source and flow of gas that conducts the aerosols from the nebulizer to the patient. If the nebulizer is producing a steady output of particles, the greater the flow of gas through the chamber, the more dilute the same number of particles will be in the larger volume of gas. The faster the flow of gas, the greater chance that large particles are driven out of the nebulizer before they can coalesce with other particles and settle out. Low flows are associated with smaller particles and higher density of mist. High flow rates yield larger particles and less density. Unlike jet nebulizers, the temperature of the solution placed in the ultrasonic nebulizer increases during use. As the temperature increases, the drug concentration will also rise, increasing the likelihood of undesired side effects.

The larger commercial units utilize low flow blowers which can deliver either air or other compressed gases via a flowmeter. A blender can be added to the delivery system to more precisely control the delivered gas concentration. Aerosol tubing, mask, or mouth piece can be used to administered the ultrasonically-nebulized solution.

Smaller USNs have been designed primarily for individual use. They do not use water-filled couplants. Medication is placed directly into the manifold in direct contact with the transducer. The transducers are connected by cable or connector to a power source, often battery-powered to increase portability. The small nebulizers, which incorporate the transducer manifold at the patient airway, rely upon the patient's inspiratory flow rate to evacuate the aerosol from nebulizer to the lung.

A variety of USNs are available. The particle size and output from the nebulizers varies considerably from one device to another. Some are capable of producing particle sizes up to 12 μm.

The primary use for the USN is to induce sputum for diagnostic purposes. Small volume ultrasonic nebulizers have also been promoted for bronchodilator therapy in nursing homes or other extended care facilities as an alternative to pneumatically driven small volume nebulizers. The small volume USN may offer some advantage since most have less dead space than small volume nebulizers, reducing the need for a large quantity of diluent to assure delivery of drugs. The contained portable power source adds a great deal of convenience in mobility. Both theoretical

advantages of the ultrasonic devices are outweighed by the high cost of the device, which may be up to ten times the cost of a pneumatic nebulizer and one hundred times the cost of a treatment administered by metered dose inhaler or dry powder inhaler.

USNs have also been used to administer undiluted bronchodilators to patients with severe bronchospasm.[160] Since the nebulizers have minimal dead space, the treatment time is shortened. Use of undiluted bronchodilator is not new and is typically included in manufacturers product dosing information found in the Physician's Desk Reference. Because the USN manifold is prohibitively expensive, however, some RCPs have suggested a technique with the use of a one way valve between the medication chamber and mouthpiece so that multiple patients can be treated consecutively without concern about infection. It is yet to be confirmed that a simple one-way valve manifold is adequate protection against contamination of the medication chamber; in addition, contact with infectious secretions on the outside of the nebulizer manifold could result in transmission of pathogens from one patient to another.

USNs have also found a place as room humidifiers, often used as an alternative to steam vaporizers and centrifugal nebulizers in the home setting. When used for this purpose, it is important to remember that any ultrasonic nebulizer with an open water reservoir can become contaminated and transmit airborne pathogens. Care should be taken to assure that these units are cleaned on a regular basis and that water is discarded from the reservoir periodically between cleanings. The recommended cleaning cycle is about once every 6 days.[161]

As suggested, the primary limitation to the use of USNs is the cost of the devices. The cost varies from $150 to over $1,000. The cost of the ultrasonic nebulizers is considerably greater than the cost of acquisition and operation of other available nebulizers.

The use of USNs is associated with a number of potential complications. They include over hydration, bronchospasm, infection, and disruption of the drug structure when used to administer medications.[162-163]

Over hydration can occur due to the large fluid output from the nebulizers and their potential to deliver small particles to the lung parenchyma directly. Over hydration is of greatest risk after prolonged treatment of newborns, small children, and other patients with fluid and electrolyte imbalances. In addition to over hydration of the patient, pulmonary secretions can also swell after treatment with an ultrasonic nebulizer.

Bronchospasm can also occur after treatment with an ultrasonic nebulizer. The delivery of cold, high density aerosols have been associated with increased airway resistance and irritability in a number of patients. In addition, sterile water administered through the ultrasonic nebulizer is known to be more irritating than normal saline.[164]

Medications administered by USN can become more concentrated during the treatment. This occurs because the solvent evaporates at a rate faster than the drug. Ultrasonic nebulizers have also been known to disrupt the structure of medications. Those nebulizers with an acoustic output of greater than 50 watts/cm^2 cause changes in the structure of aerosolized medications. If the power output of the nebulizer is 50 watts/cm^2 or less and the aerosol output is less than 2 ml/minute, the nebulizers are reported to be safe when used to deliver medications.[163]

Device selection for aerosol drug administration

The MDI with holding chambers is the most convenient, versatile and cost-effective way to deliver aerosol and should be the first choice for delivery when the required drug formulation is available. The DPI is a viable alternative with the subset of medications available in those patients that can generate the required flows. As the need to deliver multiple doses makes administration more time consuming, the SVN or continuous nebulizer becomes a viable alternative. Table 25-9 presents a comparison of devices used to deliver bronchodilators to the lungs.

Selection of the appropriate aerosol delivery devices depends largely on the drug to be delivered, the volume of output required, and the intended site of action. Particles $\leq$ 1.8 μm are targeted to the lung parenchyma, and devices such as the SPAG or a well baffled SVN may be the nebulizer of choice. Bland aerosol may best be targeted with MMAD $\geq$ 5 μm to the upper airway, 1 to 5 μm for sputum inductions, and 2 to 10 μm for heated bland aerosol for treating bypassed upper airway.

Bland aerosol therapy

Aerosol therapy is used to provide humidification, to obtain samples of pulmonary secretions for diagnosis, and to provide pharmocologic therapy, including bronchodilators, steroids, and antibiotics directly to the airways. Aerosol therapy with bland solutions such as saline is used for therapeutic and diagnostic purposes. Large volume, ultrasonic nebulizers, Babbington nebulizers, and mist tents are commonly used for these purposes.

Large volume nebulizers

Large volume pneumatic nebulizers, with reservoir volumes greater than 100 mL, are commonly used to aerosolize solutions such as saline for prolonged periods of time. These devices have also been used to provide continuous administration of active medications, such as bronchodilators.

Large volume nebulizers with bland solutions are

Table 25-9 Comparison of characteristics of types of nebulizers for administration of medications to the lung

	MDI holding chamber	SVN	DPI	USN	MDI Alone
Flow independent	+++	+++	-	+++	-
Volume independent	+++	+++	--	+++	-
Coordination independent	+++	+++	+	++	-
Low oral deposition	+++	-	-	-	-
Ease of use	+++	+++	+++	++	++
Portable	+++	+	+++	+	+++
Quick to administer	+++	+	+++	+	+++
Low cost	++	-	++	---	+++
Low infection risk	+++	---	+++	---	+++
Effective with:					
Severe asthma	+++	+++	+	+	+
Small children	+++	+++	-	++	-
Ventilators	+++	++	--	-	-
Unusual meds	--	+++	--	+	--

+ = Positive characteristic
− = Negative characteristic

primarily indicated to provide humidification of medical gases for patients with bypassed upper airways, as treatment of upper airway inflammation using cold mist for local vasoconstriction, and to induce sputum production most often for diagnostic purposes.

Although bland aerosol therapy using large volume nebulizers has been advocated as a method to hydrate the dehydrated patient, little data document the benefit of this method of fluid delivery. Most often parenteral fluid administration by the oral or intravenous route is superior and is associated with less risk, particularly for infection, and has a lower cost. For delivery of humidified inspired gases, large volume nebulizers offer little advantage over alternative methods.

Most large volume nebulizers operate utilizing the 50 psig gas source regulated by a flowmeter. The total gas flow delivered through large volume nebulizers is dependent upon the design of the delivery system. Venturi entrainment is utilized with most of these units to provide the desired FiO$_2$ using oxygen as a gas source and air entrainment. Oxygen flow through the flowmeter is generally limited to between 10 to 15 L/min. Total flow is dependent on the flow rate of driving gas and the selected FiO$_2$ (the aperture size through which air is entrained). Any back pressure in this Venturi system (e.g., mask CPAP) will reduce total flow and, hence, increase the FiO$_2$.

In general, large volume pneumatic nebulizers are high flow devices, intended to provide enough flow to meet and exceed patient inspiratory flow rates. The high flows are generated because of the entrainment of room air superimposed on the high flow from the wall oxygen source. Table 25-10 shows the total gas flow developed at various FIO_2s at oxygen flows of 10 and 15 L/min with no back pressure. When the patient's inspiratory flow becomes exceedingly high, however, as can occur with a severe infiltrative pneumonia, the nebulizer may not be able to provide sufficient flow to guarantee a desired inspired oxygen concentration. For example, if a patient has an inspiratory flow rate of 50 L/min and the patient requires an FIO_2 of .60, the nebulizer will not provide sufficient flow to the patient. The maximum flow that will be provided is 20 to 30 L/min. If the patient is not to entrain more room air from around a mask, additional flow would have to be provided by adding additional nebulizers. As the required FIO_2 increases, the flow provided from each nebulizer falls due to less air entrainment. In order to assure the desired FIO_2, the number of nebulizers which must be added becomes unwieldy. In these clinical situations, high flow nebulizers, such as the Misty Ox Gas Injector Nebulizer®, or a heated humidifier with a blender should be used.

Although there are a variety of large volume nebulizer designs, they all provide similar humidification.[34,35] When large volume nebulizers are used to provide drug solutions, such as bronchodilators, the concentration of the drug will increase with continued delivery due to the preferential evaporation of diluent.

One problem with the large volume nebulizer when used for continuous therapy is the noise generated by the high flows. The American Academy of Pediatrics recommends that sound levels remain below 58 dB to avoid hearing loss for patients in incubators and hoods. This level is exceeded by a number of nebulizers on the market. Environmental sound pollution is also an issue in nursing units with a large volume of patients in close proximity, such as post-anesthesia recovery units.

Another potential concern with the use of large volume nebulizers is the potential for over-hydration when they are used for prolonged periods of time. This is particularly problematic when these devices are used for infants and small children. When large volume nebulizers are used in these clinical situations, the patients must be closely monitored for clinical signs of fluid overload. Large volume nebulizers can precipitate airway irritability and increase airway resistance, particularly if the nebulizers deliver cold aerosols.

Disposable large volume nebulizers are manufactured by a number of companies; each offers slight modifications as to reservoir size, air entrainment options, and heater design and availability. The relative humidity provided at body temperature ranges from 58% to 74% for disposable units when cold and 75% to 96% when heated.

These devices utilize either immersion, bottom plate, wrap around, or yolk collar heaters (Figure 25-31); they rarely have sophisticated servo-control systems to monitor and control the temperature of the aerosol delivered to the patient. Most systems do not shut down with low water levels and can overheat when empty. Disposable large volume nebulizer heaters can malfunction; for example, they can operate cold without warning the practitioner when the heating element malfunctions or heat to the point of inflicting thermal injury, again without alarming.

Examples of disposable large volume nebulizers are discussed in the following paragraphs.

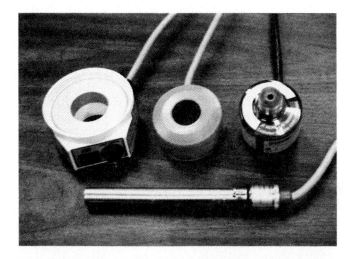

Fig. 25-31 Types of heaters used with nebulizers and humidification systems. The TheraMist Heater (Pegasus) *(left)* sits at the base of the humidification chamber above the water bottle. The Travenol 2M8021 Nebulizer heater *(center)* fits around a metal collar on the neck of the nebulizer. The AquaTherm (Hudson/RCI) *(right)* heats water en route to the nebulizer. The Puritan Immersion Heater *(bottom)* extends directly into the reservoir. (From Fink J, Cohen N: Humidity and aerosols. In Eubank D, Bone R: Principles and applications of cardiorespiratory care equipment, St Louis, 1994, Mosby.)

Table 25-10	Total gas flow developed by large volume air-entertainment nebulizers		
FIO_2	AIR/OXYGEN	Total flow @ 10 L/min	15 L/min
0.24	25.0/1	260	390
0.30	8.0/1	90	135
0.35	4.6/1	46	69
0.40	3.2/1	32	48
0.60	1.0/1	20	30
0.70	0.6/1	16	24
0.80	0.34/1	13.4	20
0.9	0.14/1	11	16
1.0	0/1	10	15

$$\text{Liters of Air/L of Oxygen} = \frac{1.0 - FIO_2}{FIO_2 - 0.21}$$

RCI Aquapak nebulizer®. RCI Aquapak® nebulizer uses a heater positioned between the reservoir and the nebulizer. Water is heated as it passes through the heater. This type of heater is thought to be self-sterilizing, creating enough heat to kill pathogens, or at least not contributing to the pathogen load of the patient. The sterility of this device, however, is not well-documented. It is unclear whether sterility can be guaranteed in situations where the heater is used with high flows that might overwhelm the heater's capabilities.

Professional medical products Prefil® nebulizer. This servo-controlled heater (Figure 25-32) uses a continuous temperature feedback to control an automatic safety shut-off to safeguard against the possibility of tracheal burns. LED display of delivered aerosol temperature is used with Prefil® large volume disposable nebulizer.

Mistyox HIgh FiO₂ high flow nebulizer®. The Mistyox® nebulizer uses a turboheater™, which sits with a detachable, easy to clean chamber, between the reservoir bottle and the nebulizer manifold. Gas leaves the nebulizer and is routed into the heater chamber where it contacts the heater plate, and exits to the patient. This unit can produce up to 60 L/min total flow at FiO₂, utilizing high flow flowmeters.

Inspiron®. The Inspiron® nebulizer utilizes an immersion heater which enters through the top of the nebulizer and directly contacts the solution in the reservoir.

Baxter/Travenol®. The Baxter/Travenol® nebulizer incorporates a collar heater that rests around the

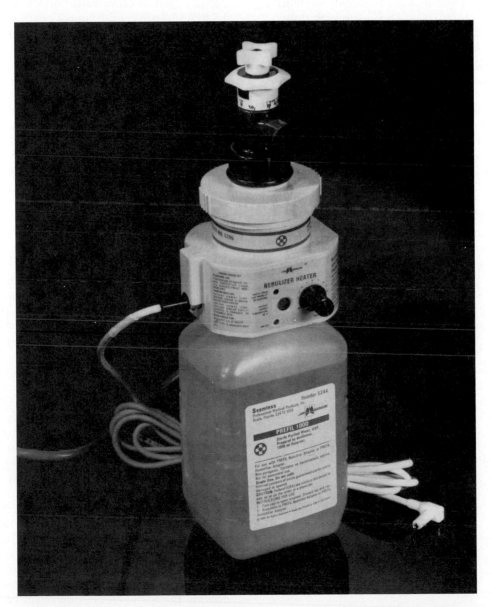

Fig. 25-32 Seamless (Dart) allows adjustment and servo-control of temperature.

metal neck of the nebulizer body, between the manifold and the reservoir. There is no contact between heater and aerosol.

Misty Ox Gas Injector Nebulizer®. The Misty Ox Gas Injector Nebulizer® (GIN) is a high flow nebulizer that does not depend upon entrainment ports to increase total flow or mix oxygen. To develop high flows, the GIN uses two flowmeters, one source of gas operates the nebulizer, while generating near "flush" flows of 40 L/min, while a secondary gas source feeds into the side of the manifold with similar flow rates. This device can develop total flows over 80 L/minute with stable oxygen concentrations. The GIN can also be used with CPAP circuits because the back-pressure imposed by the circuit will not effect the delivered oxygen concentration. This device uses the Turbo-heater™ system. Limitations of the device include the requirement for two gas flow sources and the relatively high sound levels generated with the high flows.

ALP High Efficiency Nebulizer system. The ALP High Efficiency Nebulizer has a unique design using a lightweight probe heater element which extends from the electronic heat controller at the wall plug, reducing weight and bulk at the nebulizer. The probe element inserts into a sleeve at the nebulizer. Water is drawn from the reservoir, around the outside of the heater sleeve and onto the jet interface, making no direct contact with the heater. Large particles that coalesce in the nebulizer can drain back into the reservoir.

Babbington nebulizer

The Babbington nebulizer (Figure 25-33) employs a high-pressure gas source directed into a glass sphere

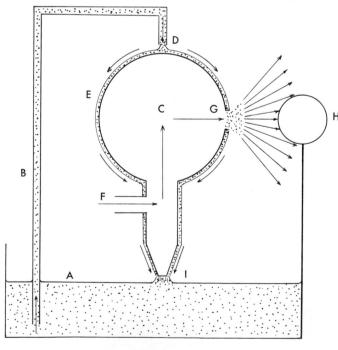

Fig. 25-33 Babbington nebulizer.

with a slit from which the gas exits. The outside of the sphere is continuously bathed with a thin layer of liquid. As the gas leaves the sphere it ruptures the film of water, sending particles toward an impactor baffle. A small stream of gas is directed up a siphon tube, acting to pump solution from the reservoir to a holding chamber from which liquid drips onto the sphere. Three models have been produced in the United States, Solosphere®, Hydrosphere® and Maxicool®. They are no longer commercially available.

Solosphere®, as its name implies, has a single sphere and can be used with a heater base. The Hydrosphere® and Maxicool® both have two spheres and produce considerably higher output. They have been commonly used for tent applications. All have air entrainment capabilities, high density output and an MMAD ≈ 4 μm. The Solosphere provides a high density mist of consistent particle size. It can deliver 15 to 63 L/min by face mask or tracheotomy collar. It can be used as an alternative to standard pneumatic large volume nebulizers.

The Hydrosphere provides 15 to 135 L/min flows, compared to the Maxicool which can generate flows of from 30 to 257 L/min when the source gas is provided at 50 psig. These units are most commonly used with closed or open-top mist tents, where their high flow output flushes heat and carbon dioxide from the enclosed environment. They typically run cool enough so that they do not need ice or refrigeration for tent applications.

Mist tent

Mist tents have been used for the last 40 years for a variety of applications. They have been commonly used for the treatment of croup and have adopted the label "croup" tent. The cool aerosol is purported to promote peripheral vasoconstriction of the airway, reducing airway resistance.

Two potential areas of concern when using a mist tent include increasing CO_2 concentrations within the tent and the tendency of the tents to retain heat from the body, raising the temperature within the tent. The CO_2 within the tent can be minimized by assuring adequate fresh gas flow to the tent. The temperature problem is handled differently by each manufacturer. Most systems provide some mechanism to reduce the temperature in the tent to below room temperature. Some, like the Maxicool®, utilizes high fresh gas flows to cool the tent. Others, like the jet type nebulizers used in some tents have lower flows and must incorporate a cooling device. Air-Shields Croupette® uses ice to cool the aerosol delivered to the patient. The Ohmeda Ohio Pediatric Aerosol Tent uses a large reservoir jet nebulizer with a "damper" to effect circulation to the tent, while a refrigeration unit communicates directly with the inside of the tent, cooling the air. The cooling effect of the unit causes considerable rainout, which is drained to a collection bottle outside of the tent. The Mistogen CAM-2® Tent uses a Freon refrigeration device to cool water which circulates through a cooling panel. The Mistogen CAM-3® utilizes the Peltier-effect based thermoelectric system, in which electric current passes through a semiconductor augmenting heat absorption and release. As warm air is taken from the tent, heat is transferred and released in the room while cool air is returned to the tent.

HAZARDS OF AEROSOL THERAPY

While aerosol therapy can be a clinically valuable tool when properly applied, certain hazards and considerations are associated with its use. *Foremost among these potential hazards is the risk of infection.* Other potential risks include the pulmonary and systemic effects of the "bland" solutions aerosolized, reactivity of the airway to particulate aerosols, medication side effects (including the potential for drug reconcentration), and the omnipresent problem of electrical shock (previously discussed).

Infection

Whereas the *potential* for humidification devices to spread bacteria has been demonstrated, aerosol generators have long been known to be a primary source for nosocomial infections.[27-30] The organisms most commonly associated with contamination of aerosol generators are gram negative bacilli, particularly *Pseudomonas aeruginosa.* More recently, disturbing case reports of nosocomial infection by Legionella pneumophila (the cause of the highly virulent Legionnaires' Disease) have been disseminated.[166]

That aerosol generators spread bacteria via the airborne route has been clearly demonstrated. In a recent study using canine models with *Pseudomonas aeruginosa* pneumonia, dogs were divided into three groups: a control group, a group supported by mechanical ventilation with heated humidification, and a group breathing a continuous heated aerosol. Careful air sampling revealed that the control animals did not spread the organism at all. Animals supported by mechanical ventilation exhaled contaminated aerosols, but organisms could not be recovered at distances greater than 2 feet from the source. On the other hand, contaminated aerosols were recovered *at distances as great as 15 feet* from the animals breathing the heated aerosol.[17]

Various procedures have been recommended for reducing contamination and infection for respiratory care equipment. Recent guidelines promulgated by the Center for Disease Control recommend that humidification and nebulization reservoir systems should: (1) start sterile, and (2) be changed or replaced with disinfected or sterile water (*not* tap or simple distilled water) every 24 hours. More detail on procedures for infection control are provided in Chapter 4.

Pulmonary and systemic effects

Given the rapid absorption of fluid that can occur through the lung, even "bland" acrosols present potential risks. Excess water can cause overhydration, and excess normal saline has the potential to cause fluid and electrolyte imbalances and hypernatremia.[168] Research on animal models has shown that inhalation of water aerosols for as little as 72 hours results in focal tissue abscesses, localized inflammation, weight gain, increased respiratory rates, and decreased serum osmolarity. Aerosolized normal saline (0.9%) administered over the same period resulted in atelectasis and pulmonary edema.[169] Although not directly generalizable to humans, such findings minimally suggest that *indiscriminate use of continuous aerosol therapy should be avoided.* Beyond this, it is clear that careful preassessment of the need and potential risks of continuous aerosol therapy should be conducted prior to its implementation, especially among those at potential risk from these pulmonary and systemic effects. Patients presumably at risk include all infants, those with preexisting fluid and electrolyte imbalances, those with high potential for fluid and electrolyte imbalances, and any patient with diagnosed atelectasis or pulmonary edema.

A related problem is the patient who exhibits difficulty in evacuating mobilized secretions. Care should always be taken to ensure that patients are capable of clearing secretions once they are mobilized by aerosol therapy. Proper coughing techniques, controlled deep breathing, and postural drainage and percussion should accompany aerosol therapy to promote secretion evacuation from the bronchial tree (refer to Chapter 28). For those patients unable to clear secretions adequately, mechanical tracheobronchial aspiration or fiberoptic bronchoscopy may be indicated.

Airway reactivity

It has been shown that high density bland aerosols produced by ultrasonic nebulization and less dense aerosol of water can cause reactive bronchospasm and increase airway resistance, especially in patients with preexisting respiratory disease.[64] Administration of bronchodilators before high density mist therapy and avoidance of use of water can help prevent this problem. Apparently heated jet aerosols do not produce the same increase in airway resistance. Cool mists can also increase airway reactivity.

It is well known that common mucolytics such as acetylcysteine can produce significant bronchospasms in sensitive persons. Therefore, it is generally recommended that a bronchodilator drug also be used to prevent or minimize this occurrence.[170]

Based on this knowledge, the potential for inducing bronchospasm should always be considered a possibility when giving high density bland aerosols or nebulized drug agents to which the airway may be sensitive. Monitoring patients for reactive bronchospasm should include peak flow measurements before and after therapy auscultation for adventitious breath sounds, observation of the patient's breathing pattern and overall appearance; and most essentially, communicating with the patient during therapy.

Drug reconcentration

During the baffling and recycling of solutions undergoing nebulization, as droplets are continuously returned to the fluid reservoir, the potential exists for the solute concentration of the solution to increase. Under such conditions, the patient is subjected to increasingly higher concentrations of the agent during the course of therapy, thereby posing a risk of drug toxicity. It was at first believed that this phenomenon occurred only in jet nebulizers, but an excellent study has demonstrated that drug reconcentration can occur in both jet and ultrasonic nebulizers.[171]

One of the drugs used was the mucolytic acetylcysteine. When subjected to 30 minutes of ultrasonic nebulization using ambient air as the carrier gas, acetylcysteine concentrations rose from 20.5% to 40.1%. When control of temperature and humidity ensured full water vapor saturation of the carrier gas, reconcentration did not occur. Table 25-11 vividly illustrates these differences. The conclusion drawn was that under conditions of low humidity in the carrier gas, evaporation of solvent (water) occurs at a faster rate than the heavier drug solute, thereby progressively raising the concentration of the residual solution.

Obviously, this problem is only of potential significance when medications are being nebulized over

periods in excess of 10 to 15 minutes, and then only if the total dosage available for nebulization exceeds that prescribed. Although these conditions seldom pertain to current practices, practitioners should still be wary of the possibility for and consequences of drug reconcentration.

METHODS TO CONTROL ENVIRONMENTAL CONTAMINATION

A variety of techniques are available to protect the environment, staff, and other patients from contamination during respiratory therapy procedures. Nebulized medication that escapes into the atmosphere from the nebulizer or is exhaled by the patient becomes a form of second hand exposure to health care providers and others in the vicinity of the treatment.

Much recent attention has been raised regarding risk to health care workers by exposure to some of the aerosolized medications, particularly ribavirin and pentamidine. Concerns have also been expressed about potential teratogenicity of these agents. The risk imposed by continuous exposure to aerosolized antibiotics, steroids, and bronchodilators has also been raised, although no studies have demonstrated any significant risk. Although the risk has not been demonstrated, practitioners should be careful when administering any aerosolized agents.

The greatest risks for health care workers at the present time is associated with the administration of ribavirin and pentamidine and from respiratory-transmitted diseases, particularly tuberculosis. Conjunctivitis, headaches, bronchospasm, shortness of breath, and rashes have been reported in health care workers administering ribavirin and pentamidine.[91] When treating patients with ribavirin or pentamidine, the treatment should be provided in a private room or booth, tent, or specially designed station to minimize environmental contamination. If the treatment is provided in a private room, the room should have negative pressure ventilation with adequate air exchanges (at least 6 per hour) to clear the room of residual aerosols before the next treatment, or a tent, to minimize environmental exposure. HEPA filters should be used to filter room or tent exhaust or the aerosol should be scavenged to the outside.

Chambers and booths

Booths or stalls should be used for sputum inductions and aerosolized medication in any area in which multiple patients are treated. They should be designed to provide adequate air flow to draw aerosol and droplet nuclei from the patient to an appropriate filtration system, or exhaust directly to the outside. Booths and stalls should be adequately cleaned between patients.

A variety of booths and specially designed stations

Table 25-11 Drug reconcentration during ultrasonic nebulization

Aerosolization time (minutes)	Percent acetylcysteine	
	Ambient air	Humidified air
0	20.5	20.5
5	21.7	20.4
10	23.0	20.2
15	26.4	20.1
20	29.0	20.2
25	32.8	20.6
30	40.1	20.5

(Modified from Glick RV: Drug reconcentration in aerosol generators. *Initial Ther* 15:179, 1970.)

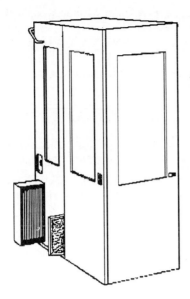

Fig. 25-34 Emerson treatment booth provides containment of aerosol during therapy.

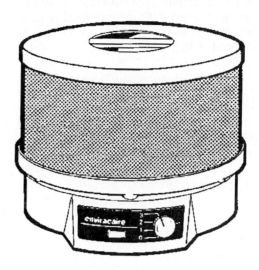

Fig. 25-35 Enviracare room HEPA filter provides local exhaust ventilation.

are now available for delivery of pentamidine or ribavirin.

The Emerson containment booth (Figure 25-34) is a good example of a system that completely isolates the patient during aerosol administration drawing all gas through a prefilter and HEPA filter.

In areas where proper air exchanges do not exist, devices such as the Enviracare (Figure 25-35) have been used to provide local exhaust ventilation through a HEPA filter medium. Little data exists supporting efficacy of these devices, although they are recently enjoying some popularity in home use.

The AeroStar Aerosol Protection Cart (Respiratory Safety Systems, San Diego, CA) is one such portable patient isolation station for administration of hazardous aerosolized medication (Figure 25-36). It has been used frequently during sputum induction and for pentamidine treatment. The patient compartment is collapsible with swing out counter, and three polycarbonate walls. Captured aerosols are removed by a HEPA filter. A prefilter is used to retain larger dust particles and prevent early loading of the more expensive HEPA filter. A Minihelic pressure gauge is used to monitor HEPA filter performance.

Filters and nebulizers used in treatments with pentamidine and ribavirin should be treated as hazardous wastes and disposed of accordingly. Goggles, gloves, and gowns should be used to serve as splatter shields and to reduce exposure to medication residues and body substances. The staff should be screened for adverse effects of exposure to the aerosol medication. The risks and safety procedures should be reviewed regularly.

In addition to the risks associated with aerosol medication administration, risk of tuberculosis transmission has become of great concern recently due to

an increase in case numbers and development of multidrug resistant strains of the organism.[173-174] Tuberculosis is transmitted in the form of droplet nuclei 0.3 to 0.6 μm that carry the TB bacilli. Consequently protection from aerosols that can transmit TB requires the same protection that should be exercised to reduce exposure to other aerosols in the 1 to 10 μm range. Known or suspected TB patients should be

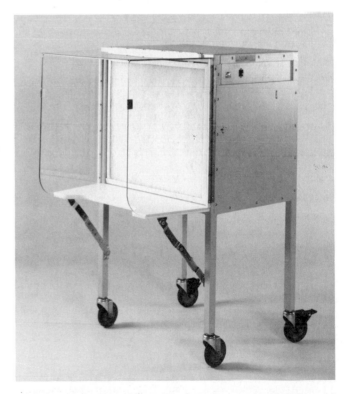

Fig. 25-36 BioSafety Systems AeroStar draws gas from patient and through a HEPA filter.

placed in private rooms with negative pressure ventilation which exhausts to the outside. If environmental isolation is not possible or the health care worker must enter the patient room, personal protective equipment should be used.

Personal protective equipment

Personal protective equipment is recommended when caring for any patient with a disease which can be spread by respiration. The greatest risk is for communication of tuberculosis or chicken pox. While environmental controls should be instituted when caring for these patients, universal precautions and respiratory isolation techniques should also be implemented.

A variety of masks and respirators have been recommended for use when caring for a patient with tuberculosis or other respiratory-transmitted diseases. Traditional surgical masks, particulate respirators, disposable and reusable HEPA filters, and powered air purifying respirators (PAPR) have all been utilized. Unfortunately no data are available to determine the most effective and clinically most useful device to protect the health care worker or others.

REFERENCES:

1. Ingelstedt S: Studies on the conditioning of air in the respiratory tract, *Acta Otolaryngol Suppl* 131:1, 1956
2. Chalon J, Loew DAY, Malbranche J: Effects of dry air and subsequent humidification on tracheobronchial ciliated epithelium, *Anesthesiology* 37:338–34, 1972.
3. Chatburn, RL, Primiano FP: A Rational Basis for Humidity Therapy, *Resp Care* 32(4):249–3, 1987.
4. Ward JJ, Helmholtz HF: Applied Humidity and Aerosol Therapy. In Burton GG, Hodgkin JE, Ward JJ: *Respiratory Care: a guide to clinical practice,* ed 3, Lippincott, Philadelphia, 1991.
5. Scanlan C: Humidity and Aerosol Therapy. In Scanlan CL, Spearman CB, Sheldon RL, editors: *Egan's Fundamentals of Respiratory Care,* ed 5, St Louis, 1990, Mosby.
6. Anderson S, Herbring BG, Widman B: Accidental profound hypothermia, *Br J Anaesth* 42:653, 1970.
7. Wells RE, Walker JEC, Hickler RB: Effects of cold air on respiratory airflow resistance in patients with respiratory-tract disease, *N Eng J Med* 263:268, 1960.
8. Walker JEC, Wells RE Jr, Merrill EW: Heat and water exchange in the respiratory tract, *Am J Med* 30:259–267, 1961.
9. Shapiro BA, Kacmarek RM, Cane RD, et al: *Clinical Application of Respiratory Care,* ed 4, St Louis, 1991, Mosby.
10. Kacmarek RM: Humidity and Aerosol Therapy. In Pierson DJ, Kacmarek RM *Foundations of Respiratory Care,* editors: New York, 1992, Churchill Livingston. 793–824.
11. Dolovich M: Physical principles underlying aerosol therapy, *Journal of Aerosol Medicine* 1989:2(2);171–186.
12. Kapadia FN, Shelley MP: Normal Mechanisms of Humidification. Recent Advances in Humidification: *Problems in Respiratory Care.* 1991:4(4):395–402.
13. Newhouse MT, Dolovich M: *Aerosol therapy in children. basic mechanisms of pediatric respiratory disease: Cellular and Integrative,* 1991, B.C. Decker.
14. Shelley MP, Lloyd GM, Park GR: A review of the mechanisms and the methods of humidification of inspired gas, *Intensive Care Medicine* 14: 1–9, 1988.
15. McFadden ER Jr, Pichurke BB, Bowman HF, et al: Thermal mapping of the airways in humans, *J Appl Physiol* 2:564–570, 1985.
16. Sara C, Currie T: Humidification by nebulization, *Med J Aust* 1:174–179, 1965.
17. Primiano FP Jr, Montague FW Jr, Saidel GM: Measurement system for water vapor and temperature dynamics, *J Appl Physiol* 56:1679–1685, 1984.
18. Gray HSJ. Humidifiers. In Shelly MP, Branson RD; MacIntyre NR: *Problems in Respiratory Care:* recent advances in humidification, 4(4):423–34, 1991.
19. American National Standards Institute. American national standards for Nebulizer and Humidifiers, *ANSI Z* 79.9–1979, 1979.
20. Seigel D, Romo B: Extended use of prefilled humidifier reservoirs and the likelihood of contamination, *Respir Care* 35:806–810, 1990.
21. Reinarz JA, Pierce AK, Mays BB, Sandford JP: The potential role of inhalation therapy equipment in nosocomial pulmonary infection, *J Clin Invest* 44:831–9, 1965.
22. Hoffman MA, Finberg L: Pseudomonas infections in infants associated with a high-humidity environment, *J Pediatr* 46:626–30, 1955.
23. Macpherson CR: Oxygen therapy—an unsuspected source of hospital infections? *JAMA* 167:1083–6, 1958.
24. Sever JL: Possible role of humidifying equipment in spread of infections from the newborn nursery, *Pediatrics* 24:50–3, 1959.
25. Schulze T, Edmondson EB, Pierce AK, Sanford JP: Studies of a new humidifying device as a potential source of bacterial aerosols, *Am Rev Respir Dis* 96:517–519, 1965.
26. Phillips I: Pseudomonas aeruginosa respiratory tract infections in patients receiving mechanical ventilation, *J Hyg* (Camb). 65:229–35, 1967.
27. Pierce AK, Edmondson EB, McGee G, Ketcherside J, Loudon RG, Sanford JP: An analysis of factors predisposing to gram-negative bacillary necrotizing pneumonia, *Am Rev Respir Dis* 94:309–315, 1966.
28. Pierce AK, Sanford JP, Thomas, GD, Leonard JS: Long-term evaluation of inhalation therapy equipment and the occurrence of necrotizing pneumonia, *N Engl J Med* 282:10;528–531, 1970.
29. Pierce AK, Sanford JP: Bacterial contamination of aerosols, *Arch Intern Med* 131:156–159, 1973.
30. Rhame FS, Streifel A, McComb C, Boyle M: Bubbling humidifiers produce microaerosols which can carry bacteria, *Infection Control* 7:403–406, 1986.
31. Guideline for the prevention of nosocomial pneumonia and guideline ranking scheme. Guidelines for prevention and control of nosocomial infections. Centers for Disease Control, Atlanta. 1982.
32. American College of Chest Physicians—NHLBI: National Conference on oxygen therapy, *Respir Care* 29:922, 1984.
33. Darin J: The need for rational criteria for the use of unheated bubble humidifiers, (editorial) *Respir Care* 27(8):945–947, 1982.
34. Darin J, Broadwell J, MacDonnell R: An evaluation of water-vapor output from four brands of unheated prefilled humidifiers, *Respir Care* 27:41, 1981.
35. Mercer TT, Goddard RF, Flores RL: Output characteristics of several commercial nebulizers, *Ann Allergy* 23:314–326, 1965.
36. Klein EF, Shah DA, Shah NJ, Modell JH, Desautels D: Performance characteristics of conventional prototype humidifiers and nebulizers, *Chest* 64:690–696, 1973.
37. Hill TV, Sorbello JG: Humidity outputs of large-reservoir nebulizers, *Respir Care* 32:225–260, 1987.
38. AARC Clinical Practice Guidelines: Humidification during mechanical ventilation, *Respir Care* 37(8):887–890, 1992.
39. ECRI: Heated Humidifiers, *Health Devices* 16 (7):223–250, 1987.
40. ECRI: Single Product review: Marquest SCT 2000 Heated Humidifier, *Health Devices* 20 (1):23–27, 1991.
41. Craven DE, Goularte TA, Make BJ: Contaminated condensate in mechanical ventilator circuits. A risk factor for nosocomial pneumonia, *Am Rev Resp Dis* 129:625–628, 1984.

42. Craven DE, Goularte TA, Make BJ: Contaminated condensate in mechanical ventilator circuits. A risk factor for nosocomial pneumonia, *Am Rev Resp Dis* 129:625–628, 1984.

43. Centers for Disease Control. UPdate: Universal precautions for prevention of transmission of human immunodeficiency virus, Hepatitus B virus, and other blood borne pathogens in health care settings, *MMWR* 37:377–388, 1988.

44. Boyce JM, White RL, Spruill EY, Wall M: Cost-effective application of the Centers for Disease Control guidelines for prevention of nosocomial pneumonia, *Am J Infect Control* 13:228–232, 1985.

45. Branson RD, Hurst JM: Laboratory evaluation of moisture output of seven airway heat and moisture exchangers, *Resp Care* 32:741–747, 1987.

46. Shelly MP: Inspired Gas Conditioning, *Resp Care* 37(9): 1070–1080, 1992.

47. Ploysongsang Y, Branson D, Rashkin MC, Hurst JM: Effect of flowrate and duration of use on the pressure drop across six artificial noses, *Respir Care* 343:902–907, 1989.

48. Nishimura M, Nishijima MK, Okada T, Taenaka N, Yoshiya I: Comparison of flow-resistive work load due to humidifying devices, *Chest* 97:600–604, 1990.

49. Cadwallader HL, Bradley CR, Ayliffe GAJ: Bacterial contamination and frequency of changing ventilator circuitry, *J Hosp Infection* 15:65–72, 1990.

50. Hedley RM, Allt-Graham J: A comparison of the filtration properties of heat and moisture exchangers, *Anaesthesia* (England) 47(5):414–420, 1992.

51. AARC Clinical Practice Guidelines: Humidification during mechanical ventilation, *Respir Care* 37(8):887–890, 1992.

52. Gilmour IJ, Boyle MJ, Streifel A: Humidifiers kill bacteria, *Anesthesiology* 75:A498, 1991.

53. Fink J, Mahlmeister M, York M, Cohen NH: Patterns of contamination of ventilator circuits: Implications for frequency of circuit changes in critically ill patients. In press.

54. Dreyfuss D, Djedaini K, Weber P, Brun P, Lanore J, Rahmani J, Boussougant Y, Coste F: Prospective study of nosocomial pneumonia and of patient and circuit colonization during mechanical ventilation with circuit changes every 48 hours versus no change, *Am Rev Resp Dis* 143:738–743, 1991.

55. Boher M, Lohse S, Glasby C, Friel M, Quan S, Mandel R: Impact of 7-day circuit changes on nosocomial lower respiratory tract infections, *Am J Inf Control* 20:103, 1991.

56. Alfredson T, Earl A, Larson R, Cronin J, Hauptman D, Fahey PJ: Effect of extending ventilator circuit changes from 2–3 to every 7 days. In Press.

57. Craven DE, Kunches LM, Kilinsky V, Lichtenberg DA, Make BJ, McCabe WR: Risk factors for pneumonia and fatality in patients receiving continuous mechanical ventilation, *Am Review of Respir Dis* 133:792–796, 1986.

58. Heyder J, Gebbart J, Rudolf G, Stahlhofen W: Physical factors determining particle deposition in the human respiratory tract, *J Aerosol Sci* 11:505–515, 1980.

59. Newman SP, Bateman JRM, Pavia D, Clarke SW: The importance of breath-holding following the inhalation of pressurized aerosol bronchodilators. In Baran D, editor: *Recent advances in aerosol therapy: first Belgian symposium on aerosols in medicine.* Brussels 1979.

60. Yu CP, Nicolaides P, Soong TT: Effect of random airway sizes on aerosol deposition, *Am Ind Hyg Assoc J* 40:999–1005, 1979.

61. Svedmyr N: Clinical advantages of the aerosol route of drug administration, *Respir Care* 36(9):922–930, 1991.

62. Hadfield JW, Windebank WJ, Bateman JRM: Is driving gas flow clinically important for nebulizer therapy? *Br J Dis* 80:550–54, 1986.

63. Douglas JG, Leslie MJ, Crompton GK, Grant IWB: A comparative study of two doses of salbutomol nebulized at 4 and 8 L/min in patients with chronic asthma, *Br J Dis* 80:55–58, 1986.

64. Johnson MA, Newman SP, Bloom R, Talaee N, Clarke SW: Delivery of albuterol and ipratropium bronide from two neb

65. Hess D, Horney D, Snyder T: Medication-delivery performance of eight small-volume, hand-held nebulizers: Effects of diluent volume, gas flowrate and nebulizer model, *Respir Care* 34:717–723, 1989.

66. Zainuddin BM, Tolfree SEJ, Short M, Spiro SG: Influence of breathing pattern on lung deposition and bronchodilator response to nebulized salbutamol inpatients with stable asthma, *Thorax* 43:987–991, 1988.

67. Alvine GF, Rodgers P, Fitzsimmons KM, Ahrens RC: Disposable jet nebulizers: How reliable are they? *Chest* 101:316–319, 1992.

68. Dahlback M, Wollmer P, Drefeldt B, Johnson B: Controlled aerosol delivery during mechanical ventilation, *J Aerosol Med* 4:339–347, 1989.

69. MaIntyre NR, Silver RM, Miller CW, Schuler F, Coleman RE: Aerosol delivery in intubated, mechanically ventilated patients, *Crit Care Med* 13:81–84, 1985.

70. Fuller HD, Dolovich MB, Posmituck G, Pack WW, Newhouse MT: Pressurized aerosol versus jet aerosol delivery to mechanically ventilated patients: comparison of dose to the lungs, *Am Rev Respir Dis* 141:440–444, 1990.

71. Hughes JM, Saez J: Effects of nebulizer mode and position in a mechanical ventilator circuit on dose efficiency, *Respir Care* 32:111–1135, 1987.

72. Raabe OG, Lee, JIC, Wong GA: A signal actuated nebulizer for use with breathing machines, *J Aerosol Med* 2(2):201–210, 1989.

73. Colacone A, Wolkove N, Stern E, Afilalo M, Rosenthal TM, Kreisman H: Continuous nebulization of albuterol (salbutamol) in acute asthma, *Chest* 97:693–697, 1990.

74. Moler FW, Hurwitz ME, Custer JR: Improvement in clinical asthma score and $PaCO_2$ in children with severe asthma treated with continuously nebulized terbutaline, *J Allergy Clin Immunol* 81:1101–09, 1988.

75. Portnoy J, Aggarwal J: Continuous terbutaline nebulization for the treatment of severe exacerbations of asthma in children, *Ann Allergy* 60:368–71, 1988.

76. Robertson C, Smith F, Beck R, Levison H: Response to frequent low doses of nebulized salbutamol in acute asthma, *J Pediatr* 106:672–74, 1985.

77. Schuh S et al: High- versus low dose, frequently administered nebulized albuterol in children with severe acute asthma, *Pediatrics* 83:513–18, 1989.

78. Rebuck AS, Chapman KR, Abboud R, Pare PD, Kreisman H, Wolkove N, et al: Nebulized anticholinergic and sympathomimetic treatment of asthma and chronic obstructive airway in the disease in the emergency room, *Am J Med* 82:59–64, 1987.

79. Ba M, Thivierge RL, Lapierre JG, Gaudreault P, Spier S, Lammare A: Effects of continuous inhalation of salbutamol in acute asthma (abstract), *Am Rev Respir Dis* 135:A–326, 1987.

80. Amado M, Portnoy J, King K: Comparison of bolus and continuously nebulized terbutaline for treatment of severe exacerbations of asthma (abstract), *Ann Allergy Clin Immunol* 81:318, 1988.

81. Amado M, Portnoy J: A comparison of low and high doses of continuously nebulized terbutaline for treatment of severe exacerbations of asthma (abstract), *Ann Allergy* 60:165, 1988.

82. Committee on Infectious Diseases, American Academy of Pediatrics: Ribavirin therapy of respiratory syncytial virus, *Pediatrics* 475–478, 1987.

83. Kacmarek RM: Ribavirin and pentamidine aerosols: caregiver beware! (editorial), *Respir Care* 35:1034–6, 1990.

84. Herbert MF, Gugliemo, BJ: What is the clinical role of aerosolized ribavirin? *DICP* 24:735–8, 1990.

85. Smith DW, Frankel LR, Mathers LH, Tang ATS, Ariagno RL, Prober CG: A controlled trial of aerosolized ribavirin in infants receiving mechanical ventilation for severe respiratory syncytial virus infections, *N Eng J Med* 325:24–29, 1991.

86. Harrison R: Assessing exposures of health care personnel to aerosols of ribavirin—California, *MMWR* 37:560–568, 1988.

87. Harrison R: Reproductive risk assessment with occupational exposure to ribavirin aerosol, *Pediatric Infect Dis J* 9(suppl):S102–5, 1990.

88. Arnold SD, Buchan RM: Exposure to ribavirin aerosol, *Appl Occup Environ Hyg* 6:271–279, 1991.

89. Rodriguez WJ, Bui RH, Connor JD, Kim HW, Brandt CA, Parrott RH, et al: Environmental exposure of primary care personnel to ribavirin aerosol when supervising treatment of infants with respiratory syncytial virus infections, *Antimicrob Agents Chemother* 31:1143–1146, 1987.

90. Diamond SA, Dupuis LL: Contact lens damage due to ribavirin exposure (letter), *DICP* 23:428–9, 1989.

91. Waskin H: Toxicology of antimicrobial aerosols: a review of aerosolized ribavirin and pentamidine, *Respir Care* 36(9):1026–36, 1991.

92. Massachusetts Department of Labor and Industries, Division of Occupational Hygiene: *Ribavirin alert* DOH #1558, 1989.

93. Adderley RJ: Safety of ribavirin with mechanical ventilation, *Pediatr Infect Dis J* 9 (Suppl):S112–4, 1990.

94. Demers RR, Parker J, Frankel LR, Smith DW: Administration of ribavirin to neonatal and pediatric patients during mechanical ventilation, *Respir Care* 31:1188, 1986.

95. Charney W, Corkery KJ, Kraemer R: Engineering administration controls to contain the delivery of aerosolized ribavirin: results of simulation and application to one patient, *Respir Care* 35:1042–8, 1990.

96. Kacmarek RM, Kratohvil J: Evaluation of a double-enclosure double-vacuum unit scavenging system for ribavirin administration, *Respir Care* 37:37–45, 1992.

97. Des Jardins, T: Freon-propelled bronchodilator use as a potential hazard to asthmatic patients, *Respir Care* 21 (1)50 –57, 1980.

98. Breeden CC, Safirstein BH: Albuterol and spacer-induced atrial fibrillation, *Chest* 98:762–3, 1990.

99. Silverglade A: Cardiac toxicity of aerosol propellants. *JAMA* 222(7);827–8, 1972.

100. Moren F: Aerosol dosage forms and formulations. In Moren F, Newhouse MT, Dolovich MB, editors: *Aerosols in medicine: principles, diagnosis and therapy.* Amsterdam: Elsevier. 1985.

101. Hallworth GW: The formulation and evaluation of pressurized metered dose inhalers. In Ganderton D, Jones T, editors: *Drug delivery to the respiratory tract.* Chichester, England: Ellis Horwood. 1987.

102. Newhouse MT, Dolovich M: Aerosol Therapy in Children. Basic Mechanisms of Pediatric Respiratory disease: Cellular and Integrative, 1991, BC Decker.

103. Dhand R, Malik SK, Balakrishan M, Verma SK: High speed photographic analysis of aerosols produced by metered dose inhalers, *J Pharm Pharmacol* 40:429–430, 1988.

104. Wiener MV: How to formulate aerosols to obtain the desired spray pattern, *Soc Cos Chem* 9:289–297, 1958.

105. Newman SP: Aerosol generators and delivery systems, *Respir Care* 36:939–951, 1991.

106. Kim CS, Trujillo D, Sackner MA: Size aspects of metered-dose inhaler aerosols, *Am Rev Respir Dis* 132:137–142, 1985.

107. Newman SP, Pvia D, Moren F, Sheahan NF, Clarke SW: Deposition of pressurized aerosols in the human respiratory tract, *Thorax* 36:52–55, 1981.

108. Dolovich M, Ruffin RE, Roberts R, Newhouse MT: Optimal delivery aerosols from metered dose inhalers, *Chest* 80 (supp):911–15, 1981.

109. Jenkins SC, Heaton RW, Fulton TJ, Moxham J: Comparison of domicilliary nebulized salbutomol and salbutomol from a metered-dose inhaler in stable chronic airflow limitation, *Chest* 91:804–7, 1987.

110. Cissik JH, Bode FR, Smith JA: Double-blind crossover study of five bronchodilator medications and two delivery methods in stable asthma. Is there a best combination for use in the pulmonary laboratory? *Chest* 90 (4):489–493, 1990.

111. Shim CS, Williams MH Jr: Effect of bronchodilator administered by canister versus jet nebulizer, *J. Allergy Clin Immunol* 73:387–90, 1984.

112. Mestitz H, Coplan J, McDonald C: Comparison of outpatient nebulized vs metered dose inhaler terbutaline in chronic airflow obstruction, *Chest* 96:1237–1240, 1989.

113. AARC Clinical Practice Guidelines: Selection of aerosol delivery device, *Respir Care* 37(8):891–7, 1992.

114. Faculty and Working Group: American Association for Respiratory Care. Aerosol Consensus Conference Statement— 1991, *Respir Care* 36:916–921, 1991.

115. Newman SP, Pavia D, Clarke SW: Simple instructions for using pressurized aerosol bronchodilators, *J Royal Soc Med* 73:776–779, 1980.

116. Riley DJ, Liu RT, Edelman NH: Enhanced responsed to aerosolized bronchodilator therapy in asthma using respiratory maneuvers, *Chest* 76:501–507, 1979.

117. Grainger JR: Correct use of aerosol inhalers, *Can Med Assoc J* 116:584–585, 1977.

118. Woolf CR: Correct use of pressurized aerosol inhalers, *Can Med Assoc J* 121:710–711, 1979.

119. Riley DJ, Weitz BW, Edelman NH: The responses of asthmatic subjects to isoproterenol inhaled at differing lung volumes, *Am Rev Respir Dis* 114:509–515, 1976.

120. Guidry GG, Brown WD, Stogner SW, George RB: Incorrect use of metered dose inhalers by medical personnel, *Chest* 1010(1):31–3, 1992.

121. Crompton GK: Problems patients have using pressurized aerosol inhalers, *Europ J Respir Dis (Suppl)* 119:101–4, 1982.

122. De Blaquiere P, Christensen DB, Carter WB, Martin TR: Use and misuse of metered-dose inhalers by patients with chronic lung disease: a controlled randomized trial of two instruction methods, *Am Rev Respir Dis* 140:910–916, 1989.

123. Allen SC, Prior A: What determines whether an elderly patient can use a metered dose inhaler correctly? *Br J Dis Chest* 80:45–9, 1986.

124. Kim CS, Eldridge MA, Sackner MA: Oropharyngeal deposition and delivery aspects of metered-dose inhaler aerosols, *Am Rev Respir Dis* 135:157–164, 1987.

125. Tschopp JM, Robinson S, Caloz JM, Frey JG: Bronchodilating efficacy of an open-spacer device compared to three other spacers, *Respir Care* 37:61–64, 1992.

126. Lee N, Rachelefsky G, Kobayashi RH, et al: Efficacy and safety of albuterol administered by power driven nebulizer (PDN) versus metered dose inhaler (MDI) with Aerochamber and mask in infants and young children with acute asthma, *American Academy of Pediatrics Abstract* Nov 1990.

127. Kraemer R, Frey U, Sommer CW, Russi E: Short-term effect of albuterol, delivered via a new auxiliary device, in wheezy infants, *Am Rev Respir Dis* 144:347–351, 1991.

128. Hodges IGC, Milner AD, Stokes GM: Assessment of a new device for delivering aerosol drugs to asthmatic children, *Arch Dis Child* 56:787–9, 1981.

129. Lee H, Evans HE: Evaluation of inhalation aids of metered dose inhalers in asthmatic children, *Chest* 91:366–369, 1987.

130. Gurwitz G, Levison H, Mindorf C, Reilly P, Worsley G: Assessment of a new device (Aeroschamber) for use with aerosol drugs in asthmatic children, *Ann of Allergy* 50: 166–170, 1983.

131. Barbera JM, Sly RM, Eby DM, Middleton HB: Responses to a bronchodilator aerosol delivered by Aerochamber to young children, *Ann of Allergy* 52:224, 1984.

132. Katz R, Rachelefsky G, Rohr A, Wo J, Gracey V, et al: Use of tube spacer, Aerochamber (A) to improve the efficacy of a metered dose inhaler (MDI) in asthmatic children, *J Allergy Clin Immunol* 77:185, 1986.

133. Konig P, Gayer D, Kantak A, Kreutz C et al: A trial of metaproterenol by metered-dose inhaler and two spacers in preschool asthmatics, *Pediatr Pulmonol* 5:247–51, 1988.

134. Conner WT, Dolovich MB, Frame RA, Newhouse MT: Reliable salbutamol administration in 6- to 36-month old children by means of a metered dose inhaler and aerochamber with mask, *Pediatr Pulmonol* 6:263–267, 1989.

135. Madsden EB, Bundgaard A, Hidinger KG: Cumulative dose-response study comparing terbutaline pressurized aerosol administered via a pear shaped spacer and terbutaline in a nebulized solution, *Euro J Clin Pharm* 23:27–30, 1982.

136. Morgan MDL, Sing BV, Frame MH, Williams SJ: Terbutaline aerosol given through pear spacer in acute severe asthma, *Br Med J* 285:849–850, 1983.

137. Berenberg MJ, Baigelman W, Cupples LA, Pearce L: Comparison of metered-dose inhaler attached to an Aerochamber with an updraft nebulizer, *J of Asthma* 22(2):87–92, 1985.

138. Newhouse MT, Dolovich MB: Control of asthma by aerosols, *N Eng J Med* 315:870–874, 1986.

139. Newman SP, Woodman G, Clarke SE, Sackner MA: Effect of inspirease on the deposition of metered-dose aerosols in the human respiratory tract, *Chest* 89(4):551556, 1986.

140. Newhouse MT, Dolovich MB: Aerosol therapy: Nebulizer vs metered dose inhaler, *Chest* 91:799–800, 1987.

141. Mestitz, H, Copland JM, McDonald CF: Comparison of outpatient nebulized vs metered dose inhaler terbutaline in chronic airflow obstruction, *Chest* 96(6):1237–40, 1989.

142. Berry RB, Shinto RA, Wong FH, Despars JA, Light RW: Nebulizer vs spacer for bronchodilator delivery in patient hospitalized for acute exacerbations of COPD, *Chest* 96:(6)1241–1246, 1989.

143. Hodder RV: Metered dose inhaler with spacer is superior to wet nebulization for emergency room treatment of acute severe asthma, *Chest* 94 (Suppl):52S, 1988.

144. Gervais A, Begin P: Bronchodilatation with a metered-dose inhaler plus an extension, using tidal breathing vs jet nebulization, *Chest* 92(5): 822–4, 1987.

145. Summer W, et al: Aerosol bronchodilator delivery methods relative impact on pulmonary function and cost of respiratory care, *Arch Int Med* 149:618–622, 1989.

146. Dolovich M, Chambers C, Mazza M, Newhouse MT: Relative efficient of four metered dose inhaler (MDI) holding chambers (HC) compared to albuterol MDI. Presented at American Lung Association American Thoracic Society 1992 International Conference at the Symposium on Aerosol delivery systems.

147. Salzman GA, Pyszczynski DR: Oropharyngeal candidiasis in patients treated with beclomethasone dipropionate delivered by metered-dose inhaler alone and with Aerochamber, *J. Allergy Clin Immunol* 81:424–8, 1988.

148. Toogood JH, Baskerville J, Jennings B, Lefcoe NM, Johansson SA: Use of spacer to facilitate inhaled corticosteroid treatment of asthma, *Am Rev Respir Dis* 129:723–9, 1984.

149. Crogan SJ, Bishop MJ: Delivery efficiency of metered dose aerosols given via endotracheal tube, *Anesthesiology* 70:1008–1010, 1989.

150. Bishop MJ, Larson RP, Buschman DL: Metered dose inhaler aerosol characteristics are affected by the endotracheal tube actuator/adapter used, *Anesthesiology* 1263–1265, 1990.

151. Ebert J, Adams AB, Green-Eide B: An evaluation of MDI spacers and adapters: Their effect on the respirable volume of medication, *Respir Care* 37:862–868, 1992.

152. Fink JB, Cohen N, Covington J, Mahlmeister M: Titration for optimal dose response to bronchodilators using MDI and spacer in 120 ventilated adults (abstract), *Respir Care.*

153. Dhand, R, Jubran A, Tobin MJ: Response to bronchodilator administration by metered dose inhaler in mechanically ventilated patients with COPD (abstract), *Am Rev Respir Dis* 145:A895, 1993.

154. Manthous CA, Hall JB, Schmidt GA, Wood LDH: Metered-dose inhaler versus nebulized albuterol in mechanically ventilated patient, *Am Rev Respir Dis* 148:1567–70, 1993.

155. Fink J, Dhand R, Jenne J, Tobin M: Effect of Humidity and simulated patient effort and aerosol deposition during mechanical ventilation: a laboratory bench study. In press.

156. Pederson S: How to use a rotohaler, *Arch Dis Child* 61:11–14, 1986.

157. Pederson S, Hansen OR, Fuglsang G: Influence of inspiratory flowrate upon the effect of a Turbuhaler, *Arch Dis Child* 65:308–310, 1990.

158. Engel T, Heinig JH, Madsen F, Nikander K: Peak inspiratory flowrate and inspiratory vital capacity of patients with asthma measured with and without a new dry powder inhaler device (Turbuhaler), *Eur Respir J* 3:1037–1041, 1990.

159. Hansen OR, Pederson S: Optimal inhalation technique with terbutaline Turbuhaler, *Eur Respir J* 2:637–639, 1990.

160. Ballard RD, Bogin RM, Pak J: Assessment of bronchodilator response to a B-adrenergic delivered from an ultrasonic nebulizer, *Chest* 100:410–415, 1991.

161. Chatburn RL, Lough MD, Klinger JD: An in-hospital evaluation of the sonic mist ultrasonic room humidifier, *Respir Care* 29:893–899, 1984.

162. Doershuk CF, Mathews LW, Gillespie CT, Lough MD, Spector S: Evaluation of jet type and ultrasonic nebulizers in mist tent therapy for cystic fibrosis, *Pediatrics* 41:723–732, 1968.

163. Boucher RGM and Kreuter J: Fundamentals of the ultrasonic atomization of medicated solutions, *Ann Allergy* 26:59, 1968.

164. Lewis RA, Ellis CJ, Fleming JS, Balachandran W: Ultrasonic and jet nebulizers: differences in the physical properties and fractional deposition on the airway responses to nebulized water and saline aerosols (abstract), *Thorax* 39:712, 1984.

165. Fallat RJ, Kandal K: Aerosol exhaust: escape of aerosolized medication into the patient and caregiver's environment, *Respir Care* 36(9):1008–16, 1991.

166. Kaan, JA, Simoons-Smit, AM, and McLaren, DM: Another source of aerosol causing nosocomial Legionnaires' disease, *J. Infect* 11:145–148, 1985.

167. Christopher, KL, Saravolatz, LD, Bush, TL, and Conway, WA: The potential role of respiratory therapy equipment in cross infection. A case study using a canine model for pneumonia, *Am Rev Respir Dis* 128:271–275, 1983.

168. Lyons, HA: Use of therapeutic aerosols, *Am J Cardiol* 12:462, 1969.

169. Stehlin, CS, and Schare, BL: Systemic and pulmonary changes in rabbits exposed to long-term nebulization of various therapeutic agent, *Heart Lung* 9:311–315, 1980.

170. Ziment, I: *Respiratory pharmacology and therapeutics,* Philadelphia, 1978, Saunders.

171. Glick, RV: Drug reconcentration in aerosol generators, *Inhal Ther* 15:179, 1970.

172. Reykus JF: There's more to respirators than meets the eye. *Occupational Health and Safety* Oct: 50–58, 1989.

173. ECRI: Tuberculosis, Part II: Respirators and Recommendations, *Technology for Respiratory Therapy* 13(1):1–4, 1992.

174. Dooley SW, Castro KG, Hutton MD, Mullan RJ, Polder JA, Snider DE, Jr: Guidelines for preventing the transmission of tuberculosis in health-care setting, with special focus on HIV-related issues, *MMWR* 1190;39 (no. RR-17).

26

Medical Gas Therapy

■

Craig L. Scanlan

Robert Thalken

Gas therapy is the most common mode of respiratory therapy in both the acute and long-term care settings. Indeed, the origins of respiratory care as a specialized field parallel the introduction of O_2 therapy as a legitimate treatment modality.

Since that time, major changes have occurred in both our understanding of the physiological effects of the various medical gases, and in the technology employed to deliver them. Of particular importance is the growing acceptance of the premise that medical gases must be treated the same as any drug. "Dosages" must be chosen, responses monitored, and changes made according to predetermined goals.

In this context, the respiratory care practitioner (RCP) must possess more than just technical knowledge of equipment. In consultation with the physician, the skilled clinician should be able to determine the desired goals of gas therapy, select the proper mode of administration, monitor the patient's response to the prescribed regimen, and recommend changes in the approach taken according to individual patient needs.

OXYGEN THERAPY

Oxygen is the most widely used—and abused—medical gas. Although less common today than in the past, abuse of oxygen is based mainly on a lack of clarity regarding its capabilities and hazards. Recent efforts to better define the proper use of O_2 therapy include the National Heart, Lung and Blood Institute National Conference on Oxygen Therapy,[1] and the American Association for Respiratory Care's clinical practice guidelines on O_2 therapy in the acute care hospital[2] and in the home and or extended care facility.[3]

As the primary member of the health care team responsible for its use, the RCP must be well versed in both the goals and objectives of O_2 therapy, and its hazards and limitations.

Goals of oxygen therapy

The overall goal of O_2 therapy is to maintain adequate tissue oxygenation while minimizing cardiopulmonary work. Specific clinical objectives for oxygen therapy include the following:
1. To correct documented arterial hypoxemia or suspected tissue hypoxia;
2. To decrease the symptoms associated with chronic hypoxemia;
3. To prevent or minimize the increased cardiopulmonary work load associated with compensatory responses to hypoxemia.

Correcting hypoxemia

In adults, children and infants older than 28 days, documented hypoxemia exists when the arterial PO_2 is less than 60 torr and/or the arterial saturation of hemoglobin with oxygen (SaO_2) is less than 90%.[1,2] In neonates (infants 28 days old or younger), hypoxemia exists when the PaO_2 is less than 50 torr, the SaO_2 is less than 88% or the capillary oxygen tension (PcO_2) is less than 40 torr.[4] Whenever hypoxemia is documented, O_2 therapy is indicated.

In addition, there are certain situations in which O_2 therapy may be indicated without firm evidence of hypoxemia. These include conditions in which tissue hypoxia is suspected. Examples include severe dyspnea, carbon monoxide poisoning, cyanide poisoning or shock.[1,5,6] Oxygen also may be given without laboratory documentation to patients suffering from conditions where hypoxemia is common. Hypoxemia is common in conditions such as severe trauma,[7] acute myocardial infarction[8] and post-anesthesia recovery.[9]

Regardless of specific cause, only hypoxemia caused by hypoventilation, diffusion defects, or moderate V/Q imbalances can be corrected with simple O_2 therapy (see Chapter 15). Hypoxemia due to physiologic shunting does not respond well to simple oxygen therapy. In these situations, special modes of airway pressure therapy, such as PEEP or CPAP, are indicated (refer to Section 7).

Decreasing the symptoms of hypoxemia

In addition to actually relieving hypoxemia, O_2 therapy can help relieve the hypoxemic symptoms common to patients with certain lung disorders. Specifically, patients with **COPD** and some forms of interstitial lung disease tend to report less dyspnea when breathing supplemental oxygen than when breathing air.[10] In addition, O_2 therapy may improve mental function among patients suffering from chronic hypoxemia.[11]

Minimizing cardiopulmonary workload

The cardiopulmonary system compensates for hypoxemia by increasing ventilation and cardiac output. In cases of acute hypoxemia, supplemental oxygen can decrease demands on both the heart and lungs. For example, hypoxemic patients breathing air can only achieve acceptable arterial oxygenation by increasing their ventilation. Increased ventilatory demand increases the work of breathing. In these cases, supplemental oxygen can reduce both the high ventilatory demand and work of breathing.

Likewise, patients with arterial hypoxemia can maintain acceptable oxygen delivery to the tissues only by increasing their cardiac output. If O_2 therapy can increase arterial oxygen content, the heart will not have to pump as much blood per minute to meet tissue demands. This reduced workload is particularly important when the heart is already stressed by disease, as in myocardial infarction, or as a result of increased metabolism, as in severe trauma or infection.

Hypoxemia also causes pulmonary vasoconstriction and pulmonary hypertension. Pulmonary vasoconstriction and hypertension increase workload on the right heart. In patients with chronic hypoxemia, this increased workload can lead to right ventricular failure (cor pulmonale). Oxygen therapy can reverse the pulmonary vasoconstriction and hypertension, thus decreasing right ventricular workload.[12,13]

Guiding principles of oxygen therapy

Like any drug, oxygen has both good and bad biologic effects.[14] As such, we should always give the minimum dose needed to obtain the desired result, and no more. In terms of dosage and depending on equipment, oxygen usually is ordered either in liters per minute or as a concentration. When a concentration is pre-

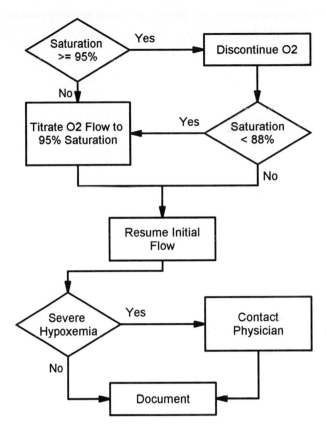

Fig. 26-1 Protocol for assessing oxygen therapy using pulse oximetry. (From Smoker JM, Hess DR, et al: A protocol to assess oxygen therapy, *Respir Care* 31(1):35–39, 1986.)

scribed, it may be either a percent, such as 24%, or a fractional concentration (FiO_2), such as 0.24.

Once the desired result is achieved, we maintain the dosage and continue to monitor the patient's response. Changes in the patient's response require adjustment in dosage. As soon as the patient can maintain adequate arterial oxygenation without supplemental O_2, therapy should be discontinued. Using this dose-response approach, we provide the *least* amount of oxygen needed to overcome hypoxemia, thus minimizing its harmful effects.

A simple protocol which applies these concepts to guide O_2 therapy decision-making appears in Figure 26-1.[15] As indicated, this protocol is based on ongoing assessment of the patient's hemoglobin saturation, as measured by pulse oximetry (**SpO_2**).

The criterion used to rule out hypoxemia (and thus discontinue therapy) is an SpO_2 of 95% or higher.* If the patient's SpO_2 falls below 88%, the oxygen flow or

---

*When using pulse oximetry to monitor a patient's response to O_2 therapy, it is wise to use an SaO_2 of 95% (instead of 90%) as the criterion measure for discontinuing oxygen therapy. This higher standard is needed to account for the relative imprecision of pulse oximetry measures (± 4%) and the tendency of these devices to read higher than actual saturations with dark-skinned individuals. For more details see Chapter 17.

Basic monitoring of oxygen therapy[2]

- Clinical assessment including but not limited to cardiac, pulmonary, and neurologic status
- Assessment of physiologic parameters (PaO_2 or saturation) in conjunction with the initiation of therapy; or
  Within 12 hours of initiation with $FIO_2 < 0.40$
  Within 8 hours, with $FIO_2 \geq 0.40$ (including postop)
  Within 72 hours in acute myocardial infarction
  Within 2 hours for any patient diagnosed as COPD
  Within 1 hour for the neonate

FIO_2 is **titrated** until the SpO_2 equals or exceeds 95%. Should it be impossible to maintain an adequate SpO_2 (88% or higher) with simple O_2 therapy, the patient's physician should be contacted and informed of the severity of the hypoxemia. In either case, the RCP documents the therapy, including the patient's response and any changes made.

As is evident, ongoing assessment is the key to rational O_2 therapy. Depending on the objectives and clinical situation, this assessment may range in complexity from simple observation to complex and costly monitoring techniques.[16] However, all patients receiving oxygen should undergo an initial bedside assessment. Ideally, this assessment should include evaluation of their cardiac, pulmonary, and neurologic status before and after beginning treatment. Thereafter, either arterial PaO_2 or SpO_2 should be measured Within an appropriate time interval (see preceding box).

Harmful effects of oxygen

Oxygen is essential for human life. However, too much oxygen can be harmful.[17,18] The accompany box lists the major harmful effects of excessive oxygen in humans.

Harmful effects of excessive oxygen in humans

- Oxygen toxicity[19-25]
- Oxygen-induced hypoventilation[26-31]
- **Retinopathy** of prematurity (retrolental fibroplasia)[32-39]
- Absorption atelectasis[40-43]
- Depression of ciliary and/or leukocyte function[44,45]
- Altered surfactant production/activity[46-48]

Oxygen toxicity

The classic description of pulmonary O_2 toxicity was written by Lorrain Smith in 1897. He accurately described the typical congestion, inflammation, and edema that we now know follows long-term exposure to high PO_2s.

Despite this understanding, O_2 toxicity in humans remains an incompletely defined phenomenon.[25] This is mainly because patients who require high FIO_2s are acutely ill and often require other treatments, such as positive pressure ventilation. Since positive pressure ventilation itself can cause lung damage, the separate effect of high FIO_2s is difficult to determine. Nonetheless, both animal research and clinical experience demand that we treat O_2 as a hazardous drug, especially when given in high concentrations over long time periods.

Oxygen toxicity is a syndrome that primarily involves the lungs and CNS. Oxygen's harmful effects are determined mainly by two factors: (1) the PO_2, and (2) the exposure time (Figure 26-2). The higher the PO_2 and the longer the exposure, the greater the likelihood of damage to the lungs or CNS.

As indicated in Figure 26-2, CNS effects (including tremors, twitching, and convulsions) tend to occur only when breathing oxygen at pressures greater than one atmosphere (hyperbaric pressures). On the other hand, pulmonary effects can and do occur at PO_2 levels commonly used in clinical practice. For this reason, we will emphasize the pulmonary effects of high PO_2s.

The physiologic responses of normal humans to breathing 100% O_2 at sea level is summarized in Table 26-1.[49] Early on, subjects complain of substernal chest pain and tightness. Mild inflammation of the tracheobronchial tree also occurs, but pulmonary function tests are normal during the first 12 hours. Between 12 and 24 hours, the vital capacity tends to decrease. This is followed by a decrease in lung compliance and exercise PO_2, with a widening $P(A-a)O_2$. Finally, between 30 and 72 hours, the diffusing capacity of the lung ($DLCO$) begins to fall.[50,51]

These changes occur much faster under hyperbaric conditions.[20,21] Subjects exposed to only 12 hours of 100% O_2 at two atmospheres pressure complain of cough, substernal chest tightness and burning, and dyspnea. Accompanying these clinical symptoms are a decrease in vital capacity, residual volume, and lung compliance.[19]

Clinical picture. The clinical picture of patients exposed to high PO_2s for prolonged periods is like that seen in diffuse bronchopneumonia.[52] Patchy **infiltrates** are observed on chest X-rays, usually most prominent in the lower lung fields. On autopsy, the alveolar region is edematous and filled with an **exudate** of large cells.

As with pneumonia, the alveolar exudate and consolidation occurring with O_2 toxicity create areas with

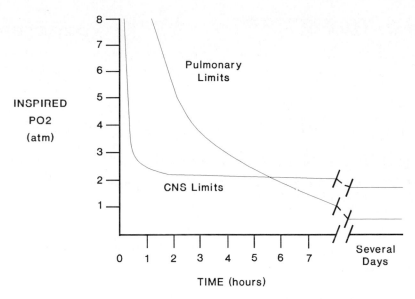

Fig. 26-2 Relationship between PO_2 and exposure time responsible for oxygen toxicity. (From Lambertsen CJ: In DiPalma JR, editor: Drill's pharmacology in medicine, New York, 1971, McGraw-Hill. Used by permission of McGraw-Hill.)

Table 26-1 Physiologic responses to exposure to 100% inspired oxygen

Exposure Time (Hours)	Physiologic Response
0–12	Normal pulmonary function
	Tracheobronchitis
	Substernal chest pain
12–24	Decreasing vital capacity
24–30	Decreasing lung compliance
	Increasing $P(A-a)O_2$
	Decreasing exercise PO_2
30–72	Decreasing diffusing capacity

Adapted from Jenkinson SG: Oxygen toxicity in acute respiratory failure, *Respir Care* 28:614–617, 1983.

low V/Q ratios and physiological shunting. Thus begins a vicious cycle, whereby attempts to relieve the hypoxemia by raising the FiO_2 only worsens the toxic effects (Figure 26-3).[53] However, if the patient can be kept alive while the FiO_2 is lowered, the pulmonary lesion will sometimes resolve.

Pathological changes in the alveolar region. The first observable effect of exposure to high PO_2s on the lung is damage to the capillary **endothelium**. This is followed by interstitial edema, which thickens the alveolar-capillary membrane. Early on, Type I alveolar cells are destroyed, while Type II cells actually increase in number.[18,25] Destruction of basement membranes and an exudative phase follows. Capillary beds swell and, in some cases, are destroyed.[19,25] In the end stages, hyaline membranes form in the alveolar region, followed by the development of pulmonary fibrosis and hypertension.[19,25]

Biochemical basis. Oxygen's toxic effect on the lung is probably due to overproduction of oxygen free radicals. Oxygen free radicals are normal by-products of cellular metabolism. The most important oxygen free radicals are the superoxide anion, the hydroxyl free radical, and the oxygen singlet (Figure 26-4, page 706).[54] These highly reactive species can produce oxidation reactions that inhibit **enzyme** functions or actually injure or kill cells. Normally, however, these radicals are detoxified by one of several enzymatic pathways or antioxidant reactions (Figure 26-4). Enzymes that detoxify oxygen free radicals include superoxide dismutase, glutathione peroxidase, and cata-

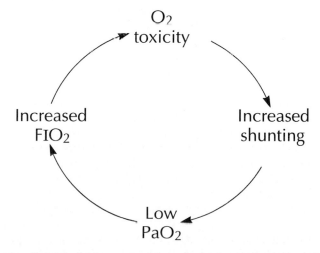

Fig. 26-3 The vicious cycle that can occur in treating hypoxemia with high FiO_2s. High FiO_2s can be toxic to the lung parenchyma and cause further physiologic shunting. Increased shunting worsens the hypoxemia, necessitating higher FiO_2s. (Adapted from Flenley DC: Long-term oxygen therapy—state of the art, *Respir Care* 28:876-884, 1983.)

OXYGEN RADICALS · ENZYME DEFENSES

$$O_2 \xrightarrow{e^-} O_2^{-\cdot}$$ (Superoxide anion) · Superoxide Dismutase

$$O_2 \xrightarrow{e^-} O_2^{-\cdot} \xrightarrow{e^- + 2H^+} H_2O_2$$ (Hydrogen peroxide) · Glutathione Peroxidase

$$O_2^{-\cdot} + O_2^{-\cdot} + H_2 \rightarrow O_2 + H_2O_2$$ (Hydrogen peroxide) · Catalase

$$O_2^{-\cdot} + H_2O_2 \xrightarrow{Fe} O_2 + 2\cdot OH$$ (Hydroxyl radical)

Fig. 26-4 Oxygen radicals that are produced during a hyperoxic exposure and the enzymatic defenses that act to eliminate the radicals. (Adapted from Jenkinson SG: Oxygen toxicity in acute respiratory failure, *Respir Care* 28:614-617, 1983.)

lase. Other nonspecific cellular antioxidants that defend against oxygen free radicals are vitamin E, vitamin C, and beta-carotene.[54] Normal antioxidant defenses are adequate to protect human cells when breathing air, but apparently are overwhelmed during exposure to high PO_2s.[49]

In concept, lung exposure to high PO_2s increases free radical production. As the normal detoxification systems are overwhelmed, cell damage occurs, followed by infiltration of neutrophils and macrophages. These scavenger cells then release inflammatory mediators that worsen the initial injury.[25]

High PO_2s also cause release of additional free radicals from neutrophils and platelets. These secondary sources of free radicals may produce the capillary endothelial damage previously described.[49]

Defense and tolerance. Various animal studies have identified factors that alter the lung's tolerance to high PO_2s. For example, superoxide dismutase levels increase with inhalation of moderate FIO_2s. If later the same lung is re-exposed to a high PO_2, the harmful effect is less than there would have been without the initial exposure. This phenomenon is known as *tolerance.*

The accompanying box summarizes the other major factors affecting the development of pulmonary O_2 toxicity in animal models.[25] Exactly how these factors alter the process is not fully known. However, changes in cellular immune responses and free radical production and detoxification are implicated. Unfortunately, use of this knowledge to help forestall or prevent O_2 toxicity in humans has not yet proven successful.[25]

How much oxygen is safe? Exactly what levels of oxygen are safe is still the subject of heated debate. Most studies indicate that FIO_2s up to 0.50 can be breathed for extended periods without major lung damage.[19,42] Contrary to these observations is research showing protein leakage into the alveoli after exposure to FIO_2s between 0.30 and 0.50 for only two days.[56] In addition, there are autopsy reports on patients who received long-term low-flow home O_2 therapy showing evidence of O_2 toxicity.[57] In contrast, early US astronauts were exposed to the 100% O_2 at

---

Factors altering development of oxygen toxicity[25]

Hastened onset or increased severity-
- Increased age
- Steroid administration
- Catecholamines (e.g., epinephrine)
- Protein malnutrition
- Vitamin C, E or A deficiency
- Trace metal deficiency (selenium, copper)
- Elevated serum iron
- Bleomycin or adriamycin (chemotherapy)
- Paraquat herbicide exposure
- Hyperthermia

Delayed onset or decreased severity-
- Moderate oxygen administration
- Adrenalectomy
- Endotoxin exposure
- Prior lung damage
- Antioxidants (e.g., vitamin E)
- Glutathione
- Hypothermia
- Immaturity

1/3 atmosphere for extended periods without any harmful effects. In combination, these reports suggests that a safe upper limit for PIO_2 is around 250 to 280 torr (33% to 37% O_2 at sea level).

Rather than applying strict cut-offs, one can weigh both FIO_2 and exposure time in assessing the risks of high PO_2s. Using this approach, exposure to 100% O_2 for more than 24 hours should be avoided if at all possible. High FIO_2s are acceptable, however, if the concentration can be lowered to 70% within 2 days and 50% or less in 5 days.[58] Obviously, the goal should always be to use the lowest possible FIO_2 compatible with adequate tissue oxygenation.

Regardless of approach, supplemental O_2 must never be withheld from the severely hypoxic patient. Although the toxic effects of high FIO_2s can be serious, the alternative is certain death due to tissue hypoxia.

Oxygen–induced hypoventilation

The effect of supplemental O_2 on ventilation is well documented.[28] When a *normal* subject breathes 100% O_2, the peripheral chemoreceptors remain essentially inactive. However, because blood oxygen levels are high, there is less reduced hemoglobin available to carry carbon dioxide. This causes a slight rise in $PaCO_2$, which, in turn, stimulates the medullary respiratory center. Increased respiratory center output results in a 5% to 20% *increase* in minute ventilation.

In contrast, in COPD patients with chronic hypoxemia and hypercapnia, breathing moderate to high FIO_2s can *reduce* the minute ventilation by as much as 14% to 18%.[29-30] This reduction in ventilation is accompanied by a rise in $PaCO_2$, which can average as high as 23 torr.[30]

Mechanism. For years, a worsening of hypoventilation in COPD patients who breathe high FIO_2s was attributed to suppression of the hypoxic peripheral chemoreceptor reflex (Chapter 14). Specifically, since the central response to CO_2 in these patients is blunted, it was postulated that their primary stimulus to breathe was via oxygen lack, as sensed by the peripheral chemoreceptors. In theory, high blood O_2 levels suppress these peripheral chemoreceptors, thereby depressing ventilatory drive.[27,28]

Recent research tends to challenge these long-held assumptions. First, the response of COPD patients with chronic hypoxemia and hypercapnia to supplemental O_2 is extremely variable.[31] Second, the fall in minute ventilation that can occur when these patients breathe high FIO_2s is often followed by a slow increase in $\dot{V}E$ back to pretreatment levels.[30] Last, the rise in $PaCO_2$ that is observed in some patients is due mainly to impaired gas exchange, not depression of ventilation.[30,31] Apparently, O_2 administration in these patients further disrupts the V/Q balance, causing an increase in the VD/VT ratio and thus the $PaCO_2$.[31]

Avoidance. Regardless of mechanism then, hypoventilation is a potential hazard of O_2 therapy in patients with chronic lung disease. As with O_2 toxicity, however, this harmful effect should never stop us from giving oxygen to a patient in need. Preventing hypoxia should always be the first priority.

In order to prevent hypoxia but avoid hypoventilation in these patients, we should aim for an arterial PO_2 between 50 to 60 torr. Generally, this approach provides adequate oxygenation, while minimizing the likelihood of hypoventilation.[26-28,59-60]

PO_2s between 50 to 60 torr can be achieved safely in most patients with chronic hypercapnia using low FIO_2s. FIO_2s between 0.24 and 0.30 carry few risks, and can be delivered by several different methods. Continuous monitoring of oxygen saturation decreases this risk further. Although the $PaCO_2$ may rise slightly, it usually levels off after an hour or so. Should the $PaCO_2$ continue to rise and the pH fall below 7.25, the patient is probably developing hypercapnic respiratory failure unrelated to O_2 therapy. In these cases, ventilatory support may be required (see Chapter 29).

As important as the level of blood oxygenation is in these patients, the need for continuous therapy is even more critical. If O_2 therapy is stopped—even for short periods such as meals—the PaO_2 may fall rapidly below pretreatment levels, causing profound hypoxia.[27] For this reason, the RCP must assure that both the patient and all involved caregivers understand the importance of continuous therapy. Moreover, the equipment needed to assure continuous therapy always must be available.

Retinopathy of prematurity (ROP)

Retinopathy of prematurity (formerly called retrolental fibroplasia) is an abnormal **ocular** condition that occurs in some premature or low birth–weight infants who receive supplemental O_2. The disease was established as a specific entity in the early 1950's, when it was observed that some premature infants given oxygen developed eye damage that caused permanent blindness.[32]

Although excessive oxygen is not the only factor associated with ROP, it is the best documented.[33] Excessive blood oxygen levels produce retinal vasoconstriction, which leads to necrosis of the blood vessels. Thereafter, new vessels form and increase in number. Hemorrhage of these new vessels causes scarring behind the eye's retina. Scarring can lead to retinal detachment and blindness.[36,37]

Because premature infants often need supplemental oxygen, the risk of ROP poses a serious management problem. The American Academy of Pediatrics recommends keeping the arterial PaO_2 below 80 torr as the best way to minimize the risk of ROP.[2,61]

It should be noted that oxygen-induced eye damage may not be limited to newborn infants. Near total blindness was reported in a 32-year-old man following prolonged exposure to supplemental oxygen that produced PaO_2s between 250 and 300 torr.[62] The apparent cause of visual loss in this case was retinal arterial constriction.

Absorption atelectasis

FIO_2s above 0.50 are believed to present a significant risk of absorption atelectasis.[40-42] Normally, nitrogen is the primary gas in both the alveoli and blood. Breathing high levels of oxygen depletes both alveolar and blood nitrogen within several minutes. Removal of nitrogen from the blood greatly lowers the total pressure of gases in the venous system. This creates a large pressure gradient for diffusion of gases between the venous blood and any body cavity with a total gas pressure at or near atmospheric.

In the lung, the large pressure gradient between the pulmonary capillary blood and alveoli when breathing high FIO_2s is of no major consequence unless the respiratory zone becomes obstructed. If this occurs, a large oxygen diffusion gradient is established (Figure 26-5, *A*). With no source for repletion, oxygen rapidly diffuses into the blood. *Should oxygen continue its outward movement,* the total pressure in the alveolus will keep falling until it collapses.[43]

Because collapsed alveoli are perfused but not ventilated, absorption atelectasis increases the physiologic shunt.[41] Moreover, because surface tension forces make it hard to reopen collapsed alveoli, special modes of ventilatory support, such as continuous positive airway pressure (CPAP), may be needed to restore the normal V/Q relationship in the affected areas (refer to Chapters 29 and 30).

The risk of absorption atelectasis is increased when patients breathe at low tidal volumes as a result of sedation, surgical pain or CNS dysfunction. In these cases, poorly ventilated alveoli may become unstable when they loose oxygen faster than it can be replaced.[43] This can result in a more gradual shrinking of the alveoli, and may lead to complete collapse, even when not breathing supplemental oxygen (Figure 26-5, *B*). In the alert patient this is not as great a risk, since the natural "sigh" mechanism periodically hyperinflates the lung.

Other harmful effects

Both animal and human experiments have shown that ciliary clearance rates in the tracheal are markedly slowed by exposure to 100% oxygen.[44,45] In addition, high PO_2s can interfere with the production of pulmonary surfactant.[46-48] The primary mechanism appears to be disruption or inactivation of the methyltransferase pathway for lecithin synthesis.

In addition to its association with ROP, excessive oxygen in infants can cause constriction of the cerebral vessels and ductus arteriosus. In infants, cerebral vasoconstriction can increase the likelihood of cerebral bleeding, while closure of the ductus (a normal event in healthy infants) can be a concern in infants with ductus-dependent heart lesions.[2] Last, supplemental O_2 can worsen the lung damage seen in patients suffering from paraquat poisoning[63] and those receiving chemotherapy with bleomycin.[64]

Oxygen delivery equipment

O_2 delivery systems have evolved over time according to both available technology and our changing knowledge of physiologic needs. Devices such as the nasal catheter have remained basically unchanged, while various cannulas, masks, and enclosures have been refined and developed to better meet specific clinical objectives.[65]

Today, the RCP can choose from a wide array of systems for administering oxygen and other therapeutic gases. Given the practitioner's role in the selection of these devices, it is essential that he or she know the capabilities and limitations of these systems, and be skilled in their application under a variety of clinical conditions.[66,67]

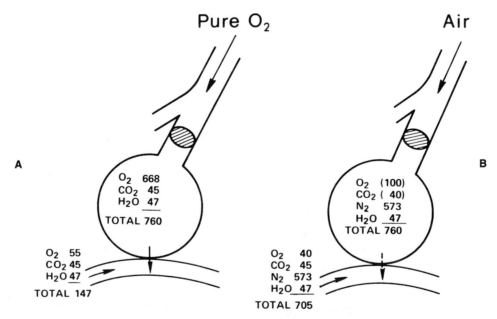

Fig. 26–5 Reasons for atelectasis of alveoli beyond blocked airways when oxygen is breathed, **A,** and when air is breathed, **B.** Note that in both cases, the sum of the gas partial pressures in the mixed venous blood is less than in the alveoli. In **B,** the PO_2 and PCO_2 are shown in parentheses because these values change with time. However, the total alveolar pressure remains within a few mm Hg of 760. (From West JB: Respiratory physiology: the essentials, ed 3, Baltimore, 1985, Williams & Wilkins.)

General performance characteristics

The ideal oxygen system should deliver *any* desired FIO_2 under all clinical conditions. In addition, it should be comfortable enough for patients to tolerate for prolonged periods. Generally, this ideal is achieved only with expensive and complex equipment, and sometimes requires an artificial airway. Although less than ideal, simpler and cheaper O_2 therapy systems are usually satisfactory under all but the most demanding situations.

In clinical practice, we judge oxygen systems according to both the FIO_2 they deliver and the stability of this FIO_2 under changing patient demands. Using these criteria, we can categorize O_2 therapy equipment into one of two major categories: variable-performance devices and fixed-performance devices (Table 26-2).[68]

A variable-performance device delivers oxygen at a flow that provides only a portion of the patient's inspired gas needs.[67-70] Because the device provides only part of the inspired gas, the delivered oxygen is diluted with room air. Thus, as the patient's ventilatory pattern changes, so too does the FIO_2. In fact, the FIO_2 delivered by a variable-performance device can vary widely from breath to breath and minute to minute. Because the flow delivered by variable-performance equipment is always less than that needed by the patient, these devices are also called *low-flow systems*.

A fixed-performance oxygen therapy device provides *all* the patient's inspired gas needs, thus assure a precise and stable FIO_2.[69,70] When the device is applied correctly, the patient's FIO_2 is constant, regardless of ventilatory pattern.[67]

We can fully meet patients' inspired gas needs by matching either their inspiratory flow or volume. As long as the flow coming from the device equals or exceeds the patient's flow, only the prescribed mixture will be breathed. Fixed-performance devices that provide a constant FIO_2 by meeting or exceeding the patient's flow are called *high flow systems*.

Instead of matching the patient's flow, we can provide a *volume* of oxygen (or oxygen mixture) equal to the patient's inspired volume. Typically, this requires a reservoir system that holds and gathers oxygen while the patient is exhaling. When the patient inhales, all the inspired gas comes from the reservoir. Assuming that the system is leak-free and prevents rebreathing, this approach will also assure a precise and stable FIO_2. Fixed-performance devices that provide a constant FIO_2 by meeting the patient's inspired volume needs are called *reservoir systems*.

Figure 26-6, page 710 demonstrates the key differences between these various oxygen delivery systems. As is evident, the patient's inspiratory flow exceeds that provided by the low-flow system *(A)*, resulting in dilution with room air. Moreover, the greater the patient's inspiratory flow, the more air is breathed, and the less the FIO_2. In contrast, the flow delivered via the fixed–performance high-flow system *(B)* always exceeds the patient's flow, resulting in a stable and precise FIO_2. The same result can be achieved with a reservoir system *(C)*. However, this requires that: (1) the reservoir volume always exceeds the patient's tidal volume, and (2) there are no air leaks in the system.

Based on their performance characteristics, we will describe the application of low-flow, reservoir and high–flow oxygen delivery systems. Due to their unique features, a fourth category of delivery systems called enclosures will be discussed separately.

Low-flow systems

Typical low-flow systems provide supplemental oxygen directly to the airway at flows of 15 L/min or less. Since a normal adult's inspiratory flow exceeds 15 L/min, the oxygen provided by a low flow device will be diluted with air. How much air dilution occurs depends on the difference between the O_2 flow and the patient's inspiratory flow. Thus any factor that changes the patient's inspiratory flow will alter the FIO_2.

The most common low-flow O_2 therapy device is the nasal cannula. A nasal catheter is also available but rarely used. Recently, low flow oxygen conserving devices have been developed to decrease oxygen waste during long-term therapy, especially in the home (refer to Chapter 38).

Nasal cannula. The nasal cannula (Figure 26-7, page 710) is a disposable plastic appliance consisting of two tips or prongs about 1 cm long connected to a

---

Table 26-2   Oxygen therapy systems

Category	Description	FIO$_2$	Examples
Variable-performance (Low-flow system)	Provides only a portion of inspired gas needs	Varies with patient min ventilation	Nasal cannula Nasal catheter Simple mask
Fixed-performance (High-flow systems)	Meets the patient's inspired *flow* needs	Constant	Air-entrainment mask (low FIO$_2$)
Fixed-performance (Reservior systems)	Meets the patient's inspired *volume* needs	Constant	Leak-free nonrebreathing mask

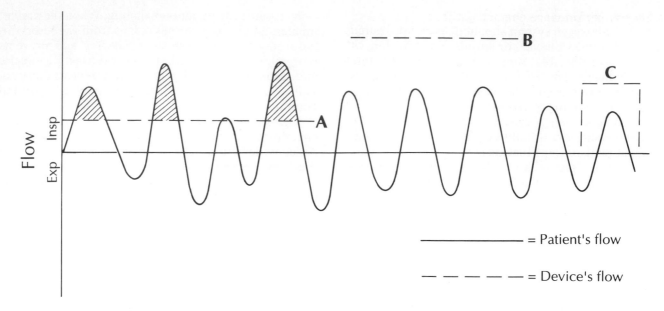

Flow

Insp

Exp

A

B

C

——————— = Patient's flow

— — — — — = Device's flow

Fig. 26-6 Differences between oxygen delivery systems. With the low-flow system, *A*, the patient's inspiratory flow often exceeds that delivered by the device, causing dilution with room air (shaded areas). The high-flow system, *B*, always exceeds the patient's flow, and thus provides a stable FiO$_2$. The same result can be achieved with the reservoir system, *C*, which stores a reserve volume (flow x time) that equals or exceeds the patient's tidal volume.

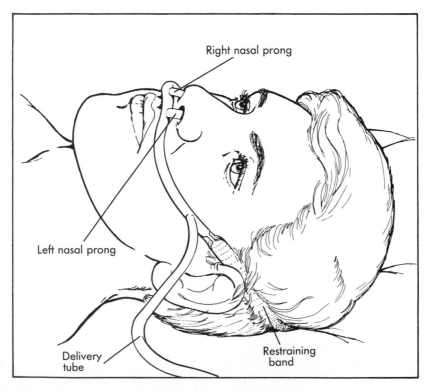

Right nasal prong

Left nasal prong

Delivery tube

Restraining band

Fig. 26-7 Nasal cannula.

small-bore oxygen supply tube. The prongs are insert-ed directly into the vestibule of the nose. The supply tubing is attached either directly to an oxygen flow-meter, or—if humidification is required—to a simple bubble humidifier (Chapter 25). In general, additional humidification is required only when the flow exceeds 4 L/min.[71-73]

The nasal cannula can be used on both adults and children. Special models have been developed for infants. Cannulas are easy to apply, lightweight, inex-pensive and disposable. In addition, cannulas are among the best tolerated of all O_2 therapy devices.

As variable-performance devices, however, cannu-las are limited to stable patients who are not acutely ill. Generally, the nasal cannula is not suitable for critically ill patients, especially those whose inspirato-ry flows vary widely.[67] In addition, cannulas tend to be very unstable and are easily dislodged from a restless patient. Also, flows above 6 to 8 L/min (even when humidified) can produce patient discomfort, includ-ing nasal dryness and bleeding.[67] Nasal conditions such as deviated septum, mucosal edema, excessive mucous drainage, and **polyps** may interfere with ade-quate oxygen delivery. Last, unintentional application of PEEP (positive end-expiratory pressure) has been reported with the use of a nasal cannula in infants.[74]

Nasal catheter. While cannula prongs only project into the nasal vestibule, a nasal catheter is inserted through the nasal passage until its tip rests in the oropharynx (Figure 26-8). Oxygen is delivered through several small holes at the catheter tip. Since the nose is being totally bypassed, it is generally a good idea to use a bubble humidifier with a nasal catheter.

Successful O_2 therapy by catheter requires proper insertion and maintenance. Before introduction, the RCP should lubricate the distal 1/3 to 1/2 of the catheter using small amounts of either a water-soluble or petroleum-based jelly. One should then initiate a low flow of oxygen through the catheter and connect-ing tubing. Then quickly test for system leakage by obstructing or 'pinching-off' the catheter. If no leaks are present, the bubble humidifier pressure relief should sound.

The RCP then gently advances the catheter along the floor of either nasal passage until it reaches the oropharynx. Position in the oropharynx should be confirmed visually using a tongue depressor and flash-light. Once the catheter tip is visualized below the uvula, it should be retracted upward until just out of sight, and then fastened to the bridge of the nose with adhesive tape. Incorrect catheter placement below the uvula can provoke gagging or swallowing of gas, which together can increase the possibility of **aspira-tion** of stomach contents.

If direct visualization is not possible, the RCP can use a "blind" procedure. Using this method, the depth of insertion is estimated by placing the catheter on the side of the patient's face and measuring the distance from tip of the nose to the ear lobe. The RCP then inserts the catheter through the nose into the orophar-ynx an equivalent distance.

Under no circumstances should a catheter be forced through the nose. If significant resistance is felt during insertion, one should simply use the opposite naris. The same disorders affecting the nasal cannula (previously described) may block catheter passage. Attempts to force it through will only damage the mucosa and may worsen these conditions. In fact, a case report has linked trauma due to a nasal catheter as a cause of **pneumocephalus**.[75]

The presence of a catheter also increases nasal secretions. In addition, dry or **inspissated** secretions can cause the catheter to stick to the nasal mucosa. To avoid these problems, catheters should be removed and fresh ones inserted in the opposite naris at least every 8 hours.

In general, whenever an oxygen catheter is ordered, a nasal cannula will suffice. Indeed, due to their complexity of use, patient discomfort and associated hazards, oxygen catheters have been largely replaced by cannulas. Most current usage is limited to special situation (like bronchoscopy) in which a cannula cannot be used. In addition, catheters are still com-monly used for long-term O_2 therapy in infants.

Performance characteristics. In terms of relative performance, most studies indicate that the nasal cannula and catheter provide similar levels of blood oxygenation.[76-79]

Even so, various bench and human studies have reported wide ranges of delivered oxygen from nasal devices.[79-81] Table 26-3, page 712, summarizes these findings, as compared to the 'theoretical' FIO_2 at various flows for a nasal cannula.[67] The theoretical FIO_2 is based on a formula that take into account the

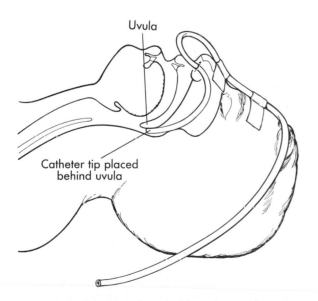

Uvula

Catheter tip placed behind uvula

Fig. 26-8 Placement of nasal catheter in nasopharynx.

Table 26-3   Oxygen concentrations delivered by the nasal cannula

Flow (L/min)	Theoretical FiO$_2$	Measured FiO$_2$		
		Gibson et al[79]	Shacter et al[80]	Ooi et al[81]
1	0.24	0.22	0.23	0.25–0.38
2	0.28	0.21–0.22	0.24	0.29–0.52
3	0.32	0.22–0.24	0.25	0.33–0.61
4	0.36	—	0.26	0.38–0.70
5	0.40	0.24–0.25	—	—
6	0.44	—	—	0.44–0.83
8	0.48	—	—	0.50–0.90
10	0.52	0.30–0.46	—	—
15	0.56	0.35–0.61	—	—

(From Branson RD: The nuts and bolts of increasing arterial oxygenation: devices and techniques, *Respir Care* 38: 672-686, 1993.)

O_2 flow and the patient's tidal volume, I:E ratio, rate of breathing, and anatomic reservoir.[68] This formula predicts an average 4% increase in inspired oxygen concentration for every liter of supplemental O_2 administered *at normal tidal volumes and rates.*

As Table 26-3 shows, the FiO$_2$s actually delivered by cannula are very different from those predicted. Moreover, even at a given flow, some studies reveal large variations in the delivered FiO$_2$. These differenc-es in FiO$_2$ at a constant flow are due to changes in the patient's rate or depth of breathing. This effect can be seen clearly in Figure 26-9.[80] For a given rate of breathing, increases in O_2 flow increase the FiO$_2$. However, an increase in rate of breathing decreases the FiO$_2$.

Of course, these observations prove that low-flow systems provide variable FiO$_2$s. The actual FiO$_2$ received depends mainly on the patient's inspiratory flow. Inspiratory flow, in turn depends on the tidal volume, rate (thus minute ventilation) and I:E ratio. High tidal volumes, fast rates, large minute ventilations or short inspiratory times (low I:E ratios) all cause greater air dilution, and thus a lower FiO$_2$ for a given O_2 input flow. Conversely, small tidal volumes, slow breathing rates, low minute ventilations or long inspiratory times (high I:E ratios) result in less air dilution, and thus a higher FiO$_2$. In addition, breathing with the mouth open may lower the FiO$_2$ delivered by nasal cannula.[82] Table 26-4 summarizes these relationships for low-flow oxygen delivery systems.

These relationships confirm that precise bedside measurement of the FiO$_2$ delivered by low-flow systems is not practical. Without knowing the patient's exact FiO$_2$, the RCP must rely on assessing the actual response to O_2 therapy. The RCP assesses the response to oxygen therapy by combining astute bedside obser-

■ MINI **C**LINI ■

26-1

FiO$_2$ Produced By a Nasal Cannula

Problem: A patient with COPD suffering an acute **exacerbation** is placed on a nasal cannula at 2 L/min oxygen. The patient has a respiratory rate = 20/min. You measure the tidal volume at 250 mL. and with a stopwatch, you measure inspiratory time at one second. You are told by a respiratory care practitioner colleague that at 2 L/min, the cannula cannot deliver FiO$_2$ greater than 28%. Is your colleague correct?

Discussion: Your patient is breathing at a rate of 20/min which allows 3 seconds per respiratory cycle. Your measurement reveals that inspiratory time is one second in length. During one second a tidal volume of 250 mL is inspired. Let us evaluate the oxygen composition of that 250 mL inspired volume: First, during one second, the cannula provides 33.3 mL of 100% O_2 (i.e. 2 L/min converts to 33.3 mL/sec: 2000 mL/60 sec = 33.3). We can assume this 33.3 mL of O_2 is part of the 250 mL inspired. Second, the tidal volume is generally exhaled before expiratory time ends,

which means an end expiratory pause occurs. Lets assume that the tidal volume was exhaled in the first 1.5 seconds, leaving 0.5 seconds of essentially no expired gas flow. This allows the nasal and oral pharynx to partially fill with oxygen during the last 0.5 seconds of expiratory time: 33.3 mL/sec × 0.5 sec. = 16.65 mL of 100% O_2. This 16.65 mL O_2 will become part of the 250 mL tidal volume inspired. Finally, the remainder of the tidal volume is entrained room air which contains 21% oxygen. The 250 mL tidal volume is the sum of its components as described above: 33.3 mL O_2 from the cannula, 16.65 mL O_2 from nasal/oral reservoir, and 200.05 mL entrained room air.

The inspired oxygen fraction would be computed thus:

nasal cannula output = 33.3 mL O_2
oxygen in nasal and
oral anatomic reservoir = 16.65 mL O_2
21% of the remaining
    200.05 mL = 42.0 mL O_2
Total oxygen volume = 91.95 mL O_2
Tidal volume = 250 mL
FiO$_2$ = 91.95/250 = 37%

Thus, even at 2 L/min, a cannula on a shallowly breathing patient will deliver surprisingly high FiO$_2$. If the intent is to deliver 25% to 28% O_2 to this patient, then the patient is receiving considerably more oxygen than expected. A fixed performance system (high flow system) is more appropriate in this patient. (**Note:** although one would rarely perform the above calculation in the clinical setting, the calculation illustrates the point that low inspired oxygen concentrations are not guaranteed by low-flow cannulas. This emphasizes the need to assess the **outcome** of O_2 therapy via blood gases.)

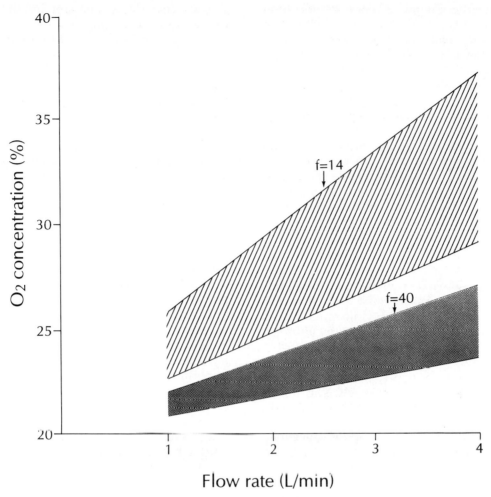

Fig. 26-9 The effect of input flow and rate of breathing on the oxygen concentration delivered by nasal cannula. Oxygen concentration is directly proportional to input flow but inversely related to rate of breathing. (From Schachter EN, Littner MR, Luddy P, Beck GJ: Monitoring of oxygen delivery systems in clinical practice, *Crit Care Med* 8(7): 405-409, 1980.)

Table 26-4 Factors affecting FIO_2 delivery by low-flow oxygen systems

Increases FiO₂	Decreases FiO₂
Higher O_2 input	Lower O_2 input
Mouth-closed breathing*	Mouth-open breathing*
Lower inspiratory flow	Higher inspiratory flow
Lower tidal volume	Higher tidal volume
Slow rate of breathing	Fast rate of breathing
Small minute ventilation	Large minute ventilation
Long inspiratory time	Short inspiratory time
High I:E ratio	Low I:E ratio

*cannula only

vation with laboratory testing. As specified in the previous section on Guiding Principles, appropriate lab tests include either arterial blood gases (for the PaO_2) or pulse oximetry (for the SpO_2).

Appropriate use. Because flows greater than 6 to 8 L/min are uncomfortable for most patients, nasal devices are not suitable when the desired FIO_2 exceeds 40% to 45%.[76] In addition, low-flow nasal devices should not be used on unstable patients with changing minute volumes.[67] If higher concentrations or stable FIO_2s are needed, either a reservoir or high-flow system should be used.

However, for patients with stable minute volumes who need only low to moderate FIO_2s, low-flow nasal devices are the ideal delivery system. In addition, low-flow nasal devices are the system of choice for many home care patients who require long-term O_2 therapy. In terms of specific device, the nasal cannula is always the first choice for the cooperative and alert patient.

Oxygen conserving devices. Oxygen conserving devices are special low-flow delivery systems modified to reduce the oxygen waste that occurs during patient exhalation.[83] Because they can lower the cost of O_2 delivery, conserving devices are used mainly in the home care setting. For this reason, oxygen conserving devices are covered in Chapter 38 (Respiratory Home Care).

Problem solving and troubleshooting. Common problems with low-flow oxygen delivery systems include inaccurate flows, system leaks and obstructions, device displacement, obstruction of a single naris, and skin irritation.

Inaccurate oxygen flows have been reported as a problem among both adults and infants. In infants with chronic respiratory failure, accurate delivery of low-flow oxygen is essential. An analysis of 27 low-flow meters used with such infants found that delivered flows differed significantly from set flows, particularly at the 250 mL/min (1/4 L/min) setting.[84] Among adults, an assessment of the accuracy of O_2 delivery systems in two medical units showed that only 90 of 206 patients (44%) were receiving oxygen as prescribed. This discrepancy was due to inaccurate flow metering, with errors ranging from 15% at 8 L/min to 40% at 1 and 2 L/min.[85]

Given the increasing trend to assess the *outcomes* of O_2 therapy via either blood gases or pulse oximetry, assuring the absolute accuracy of oxygen 'input' flows is not usually essential. Nonetheless, respiratory care services should regularly test new and existing O_2 delivery equipment for gross error. Testing should be done with either a calibrated laboratory flowmeter or using a water-sealed bell spirometer. Where accuracy is deemed most critical (as with infants receiving long-term low-flow therapy), a specific range of acceptable flow error should be set (e.g., $\pm$ 5%). Equipment not meeting this standard should either be taken out of service entirely or identified by label as not for use under the specified conditions.

System leaks and obstructions can also lead to inaccurate flows, even when metering devices are working properly. Leaks occur most often at connection points in the system, particularly when a humidifier is used. Common leak sites include connections between the flowmeter and humidifier, the humidifier top and jar, and the humidifier outlet and tubing connection.

If a humidifier is in use, the RCP can check for leaks by crimping the delivery tubing while gas is flowing through the system. If the system is leak-free, gas pressure will rise quickly and cause the humidifier relief valve to sound. If a large leak is present, pressure will not rise and the relief valve will not sound. Once a leak is confirmed, the RCP should check and tighten all connections.

The effect of an outflow obstruction is basically the same as crimping the delivery tubing; pressure will rise and the humidifier relief valve will sound. In fact, the most common cause of outflow obstructions in O_2 systems is crimped or twisted delivery tubing. This common problem occurs when the patient rolls over in bed or moves to a new position. The solution is simple: reposition the patient and the delivery tubing to prevent obstruction.

When using flows below 2 L/min (without a humidifier), leaks and obstructions are more difficult to confirm. In these cases, the RCP can at least verify that flow is being delivered by immersing the cannula prongs into water and observing bubbling. More quantitative assessment would require a calibrated laboratory test system.

Although nasal devices are among the most comfortable and convenient O_2 delivery systems, there are also among the most prone to displacement. Obviously, should a nasal cannula be displaced entirely off the face, the patient will receive no supplemental oxygen at all. However, even minor displacement, such as one prong shifting out of the nose, can have major consequences. For example, a mean fall in PaO_2 of 22 torr has been observed in healthy volunteers when switched from breathing with two prongs to a single prong.[86] In sick patients with marginal oxygenation, this large a drop in PaO_2 could result in severe hypoxia.

For these reasons, whenever setting up oxygen on a new patient, the RCP should always explain the importance of keeping the device in proper position. For agitated patients who cannot understand or follow instructions, hand restraints may be needed to assure continuous therapy. In addition, clinical experience suggests that the 'over-the-ear' type cannulas tend to be more stable than those with a simple head strap. Last, whenever at the bedside, the RCP should always check patients for proper positioning of their O_2 appliance.

As described in Chapter 9, conditions causing obstruction of one nasal passage are quite common. In these cases, patients receiving O_2 therapy with a two-prong nasal cannula will receive only 1/2 the prescribed flow. The result will be much like that previously described for normal individuals breathing through a single prong.

Depending on the FIO_2 desired, there are several solutions to this problem. Obviously, masks provide O_2 both nasally and orally, and would be appropriate for short duration therapy. As discussed subsequently, specific masks can be selected to deliver a range of FIO_2s. On the other hand, if a low FIO_2 is desired and patient long-term comfort is a consideration, a single prong cannula can be used.[87]

Although modern nasal cannulas are made from non-reactive plastics, constant traction and movement of these devices can result in skin irritation. Moreover, some sensitive patients can exhibit allergic reactions to these materials.[88] If left untreated, such irritation can result in necrosis and permanent tissue damage. To avoid these problems, the RCP should make sure that the device is tight enough to avoid displacement, but not so tight as to cause skin irritation. Should any swelling, **erythema** or bleeding be observed above the lips, on the cheeks, or about the ears, the RCP should immediately contact the patient's nurse and assist in planning a treatment regimen to prevent further injury. For the RCP, this may mean recommending an alternate delivery device, or using small cotton pads to minimize pressure on sensitive points.

Reservoir systems

As compared to low-flow systems, reservoir devices usually provide a higher FIO_2 for a given oxygen input. In principle, this is achieved by extending the patient's anatomic reservoir. When the patient's inspiratory flow exceeds the oxygen flow into the device, the reservoir volume is tapped.

The most common reservoir systems are face masks. Face mask performance varies according to three key factors: (1) the O_2 input flow, (2) the reservoir volume, and (3) the amount of air leakage. Variations in these factors determine whether a given mask operates as a fixed or variable performance device. A mask can guarantee a fixed oxygen concentration of gas only if: (1) the reservoir volume is large enough to meet all inspired volume needs, and (2) no air enters the system during inspiration. If these conditions are not met, the mask will deliver a variable FIO_2.

Although the RCP will find minor variations between brands of masks used in their work settings, these devices share many common features. In general, oxygen mask are the device of choice when moderate to high FIO_2s are needed quickly and for a relatively short time. Thus masks are the first choice in emergency situations. Although most patients can tolerate an oxygen mask for several hours, prolonged therapy usually requires alternative approaches.

To achieve maximum performance, masks must be tightly sealed to the patient's face. Of course, this adds to the patient's discomfort. Another source of discomfort is the heat build-up that occurs within masks. Temperatures rise because the mask impedes the normal radiant heat loss from around the face and mouth. Last, an oxygen mask can be a hazard on a patient who is prone to vomit. Since a mask can block the flow of vomitus, aspiration back into the lung can occur. For this reason, masks must be used cautiously on unconscious patients.

There are three types of masks in common clinical use: the simple mask, the partial rebreathing mask, and the nonrebreathing mask.

Simple mask (Figure 26-10). The simple mask is a disposable plastic unit with neither valves nor a reservoir bag. Exhaled air is vented directly through holes in its body. If O_2 input is interrupted, air is drawn in through these holes and around the mask edge.

Simple masks are used at flows between 5 and 12 L/min. A minimal flow of 5 L/min is needed to ensure

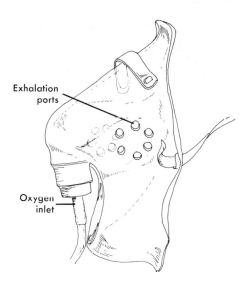

Fig. 26-10 Simple mask. Oxygen is delivered to cone-shaped face piece from which patient both inhales oxygen and draws in room air through exhalation ports. On exhalation, gas exits exhalation ports. (From McPherson SP: Respiratory therapy equipment, ed 3, St Louis, 1985, Mosby.)

that the mask volume is replenished with oxygen at the end of exhalation. At flows less than 5 L/min, the mask volume acts as deadspace and causes CO_2 rebreathing.[89,90]

Because its reservoir volume is small, and because air easily enters through the numerous holes during inspiration, a simple mask functions as a low–flow system. Thus the FIO_2 delivered by a simple mask depends on the O_2 input flow, the mask (reservoir) volume, air leakage, and the patient's breathing pattern.[91,92]

In terms of input flow, FIO_2s provided by simple masks range from 0.38 to 0.46 at 6 L/min[76] to 0.82 to 0.88 at 15 L/min.[79] Regarding breathing pattern and air leaks, FIO_2s ranging from 0.36 to 0.77 have been reported under varying conditions.[93-95] Table 26-5 summarizes the findings of a controlled laboratory study which assessed the impact of O_2 input flow, minute ventilation and leaks on the FIO_2 provided by a simple mask.[95] As expected, the lower the input flow, the higher the minute ventilation and the greater the air leakage, the lower the FIO_2.

Table 26-5 FIO_2 Delivered via simple face mask[67,91]

Flow (L/min)	Loose-fitting mask Minute ventilation (L)			Tight-fitting mask		
	5	12	20	5	12	20
			FIO_2			
2	0.36	0.31	0.28	0.47	0.31	0.27
4	0.46	0.37	0.33	0.60	0.41	0.33
6	0.47	0.40	0.35	0.72	0.50	0.40
8	0.46	0.42	0.38	0.77	0.59	0.46

Breathing frequency = 15 breaths/min

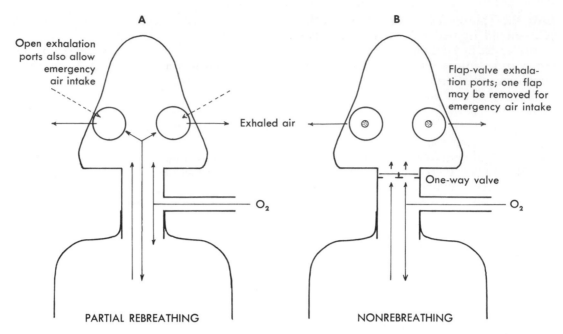

Fig. 26-11 Diagrammatic illustrations of the difference between, **A,** disposable partial rebreathing oxygen mask and, **B,** disposable nonrebreathing mask. In both, oxygen flows directly into the mask during inspiration and into the reservoir bag during exhalation. However, the early portion of exhaled air in **A** returns to the bag to be rebreathed with incoming oxygen in the next breath. Terminal air escapes through exhalation ports. In **B** all exhaled air is vented through a port in the mask, and a one-way valve between the bag and mask prevents rebreathing.

Based on these data, and considering its convenience and relative comfort, the simple mask is the device of choice whenever moderate FIO_2s (0.40-0.60) are needed for a short time. Applicable situations includes the immediate postoperative recovery state, and temporary therapy while awaiting definitive plans.

Partial rebreathing mask (Figure 26-11, *A*). The partial rebreathing mask provides added reservoir volume via a 1 liter bag. In concept, the partial rebreather conserves oxygen by having the patient rebreathe some exhaled air.

As shown in Figure 26-11, *A*, source oxygen flows into the neck of the mask, passing directly into the mask itself during inspiration. During exhalation, source oxygen enters the bag. When the patient exhales, about the first third of the exhaled air returns into the bag, where it mixes with source oxygen. Since this portion of exhaled represents the anatomic deadspace, it contains mostly oxygen and little CO_2. As the bag fills with both source oxygen and exhaled air, rising system pressure directs the remaining exhaled air (with its high CO_2 content) out the mask's exhalation ports. As long as the oxygen inflow prevents the bag from collapsing during inhalation (usually at least 6 L/min) reservoir contamination with CO_2 is negligible.[96]

At flows between 6 and 10 L/min, and when properly adjusted to minimize leaks, the partial rebreather provides FIO_2s between 0.35 to 0.60.[77]

Higher concentrations are probably provided at higher flows.[67] The fact that higher FIO_2s are uncommon with this system indicates significant air dilution. This dilution occurs mainly through the exhalation ports, which in most disposable devices consist of numerous holes in the mask body.* For this reason, the partial rebreather functions as a low-flow system, providing variable FIO_2s that are not much different from the simple mask.

Nonrebreathing mask (Figure 26-11, *B*). The unique feature of the nonrebreathing mask is its series of one-way valves. As in the partial rebreather, source oxygen flows either into the bag or mask during exhalation. In the nonrebreather, however, a one-way valve between the bag and mask prevents exhaled gas from returning into the bag. Instead, exhaled gas is diverted out to the atmosphere through one or more additional one-way exhalation valves in the mask body.

In concept, a leak-free nonrebreathing mask with competent valves and enough flow to prevent bag collapse during inspiration should deliver 100% source gas. Although this may have been true of the original nondisposable BLB design,[97] today's disposable versions do not match up to this ideal.[67] Indeed, laboratory studies with healthy volunteers indicate

---

*In some partial and nonrebreathing masks, the open ports in the mask body are a safety feature that allows air breathing if the oxygen source fails. For this reason, they should never be closed off or obstructed.

that a typical disposable nonrebreathing mask delivers FiO₂s between 0.57 to 0.70, with an average of only 0.63.[76]

Disposable nonrebreathers fail to provide high fixed FiO₂s because of large air leaks. Besides the typical loose fit, one of the two exhalation ports on most nonrebreathers is usually not covered with a one-way valve. As with the partial rebreather, this allows air breathing should source oxygen fail or the patient's needs suddenly exceed the available input flow. However, it also allows air dilution during periods of high inspiratory flow. *Common disposable nonrebreathing masks should therefore be considered variable performance systems.*

Despite these limitations, the nonrebreather is the system of choice for short-term administration of high concentrations of oxygen. It is also the best choice when the need arises to administer therapeutic gas mixtures, such as helium-oxygen (discussed subsequently).

Should FiO₂s above 0.70 be needed, the ideal solution would be one of the high-flow, fixed-performance devices discussed in the next section. If such a system is not readily available, some clinicians suggest combining a nasal cannula (set at 15 L/min or higher) with a disposable nonrebreathing mask. By literally 'flooding' the patient's airway with oxygen, this approach probably does provide a higher FiO₂ than that achieved with a nonrebreather alone.

High-flow systems

High-flow systems supply a given oxygen concentration at a flow that equals or exceeds the patient's inspiratory flow, thus ensuring a stable FiO₂. In order to meet variations in patients' inspiratory demands, a high-flow device should provide at least 60 L/min total flow;[92] under some conditions 100 L/min or more may be needed.

There are two major categories of high-flow devices: (1) air entrainment systems, and (2) blending systems. Air entrainment systems direct a high pressure oxygen source through a jet, entraining room air at fixed ratios. Blending systems take separate pressurized air and oxygen sources as input, then mix these gases either manually or via a precision valve. Regardless of approach, as long as the gas flow meets or exceeds the patient's peak inspiratory flow, both systems function as fixed performance devices, assuring a constant FiO₂.

Air entrainment and blending systems do differ in regard to the range of available FiO₂s. Because entrainment devices must dilute the source gas with air, they *always* provide less than 100% oxygen. The more air they entrain, the higher their total output flow and the lower the delivered FiO₂s. Since total output flow is inversely proportional to FiO₂, high flows are possible only when delivering low oxygen concentrations.

Thus air entrainment devices function as true high-flow systems only at low FiO₂s.

On the other hand, because blending systems mix high pressures air and oxygen, a full range of FiO₂s (0.21 to 1.0) is available at high flows. When used with an appropriate humidifier and airway appliance, a blending device thus approaches our earlier definition of an "ideal" gas delivery system.

As with any oxygen delivery device, choosing the appropriate high flow system requires matching of clinical objectives with patient needs and equipment performance.

Air entrainment systems. All air entrainment systems employ a restricted **orifice** or jet nozzle through which oxygen flows at high velocity. Lateral shear forces cause air entrainment through ports located near the jet site.[98] The amount of air entrained at these ports is directly proportional to the *velocity* of oxygen at the jet. The smaller the jet, the greater the velocity of oxygen, and the more air entrained.

Air entrainment systems are indicated when the objective is to provide a controlled low FiO₂, generally between 0.24 to 0.40. When set to deliver more than 35% to 40% oxygen, most air entrainment devices cannot provide sufficient flow to meet patients' inspiratory needs. Whenever the flow output from a device is less than the patient's inspiratory flow, air dilution occurs and system performance becomes variable. To appreciate these relationships, one must fully understand the basic principles of gas mixing and air entrainment.

Principles of air entrainment. The delivered oxygen concentration (**FDO₂**)* and total flow provided by an air entrainment device are a function of three key variables: (1) the oxygen input flow through the jet, (2) the device's air to oxygen ratio, and (3) the amount of flow resistance downstream from the mixing site.[98,99]

In terms of oxygen input, several studies have shown that the FDO₂ provided by most air entrainment devices remains within 1% to 2% of that specified, regardless of input flow.[99,100] Some exceptions do exist, and variations up to 6% have been measured under changing jet flow.[100] For these reasons, RCPs who give oxygen via air entrainment systems should be thoroughly familiar with the particular device they are using, including its specific performance capabilities.

The air-to-oxygen ratio of air entrainment devices is a constant value for each jet/port size used for a given FDO₂. Calculation of both the FDO₂, and the air-to-oxygen ratio needed to obtain a given FDO₂ is based on the a modification of the dilution equation for solutions, as discussed in Chapter 13.

---

*The distinction between delivered oxygen fraction (FDO₂) and actual inspired oxygen fraction (FiO₂) is important especially for air entrainment devices. Ideally, FiO₂ should equal FDO₂, *meaning that the device is supplying all the patient's oxygen needs. If the FiO₂ is less than the FDO₂, the patient is* drawing in additional room air.

In diluting any solution, the initial volume times the initial concentration equals the final volume times the final concentration. Mathematically:

$$V_1C_1 = V_2C_2$$

Given that a gas mixture is a solution, we can apply this equation to mixing oxygen with other gases. For example, if we dilute 2 liters of 100% oxygen with 2 liters of nitrogen (0% oxygen), use of the above equation would yield a final oxygen concentration of 50%:

$$V_1C_1 = V_2C_2$$
$$(2 \text{ liters}) \times 100\% = (4 \text{ liters}) \times C_2$$
$$C_2 = \frac{2 \text{ liters}}{4 \text{ liters}} \times 100\%$$
$$= 50\%$$

In clinical practice we more commonly combine *two* gases of different O_2 concentrations (air and oxygen) to derive a third mixture. Modification of the simple dilution equation to allow the mixing of two "solutions" to derive a third is as follows:

$$V_FC_F = V_1C_1 + V_2C_2$$

Here V_1 and V_2 are the volumes of the two gases being mixed, C_1 and C_2 the respective concentration of the applicable gas in these volumes (usually oxygen), and V_F and C_F the final volume and concentration of the resulting mixture. Depending on the values known, we can use various forms of this equation to compute: (1) the final concentration of a mixture of air and oxygen, (2) the air-to-oxygen ratio needed to obtain a given FIO_2, or (3) the amount of oxygen we need to add to a volume of air to obtain a given FIO_2.

A common clinical problem requires the RCP to determine what FIO_2 results from mixing a given volume of air and oxygen. For example, let us assume that you need to know the FIO_2 that would result from mixing 3 volumes of air ($FIO_2 = 0.21$) with one volume of oxygen ($FIO_2 = 1.0$).

First we rearrange the above equation to solve for the final concentration of oxygen (C_F):

$$C_F = \frac{V_1C_1 + V_2C_2}{V_F}$$

Then we substitute the values for V_1 and C_1 (the air) and V_2 and C_2 (the oxygen):

$$C_F = \frac{(3 \times 0.21) + (1 \times 1.0)}{4}$$
$$C_F = \frac{1.63}{4}$$
$$C_F = 0.41$$

Thus, when we mix 3 volumes of air with one volume of oxygen, we obtain a gas mixture with an FIO_2 of about 0.40.

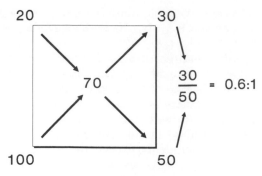

Fig. 26-12 "Magic box."

There are other clinical situations in which the RCP needs to compute the air-to-oxygen ratio needed to achieve a given FIO_2. To accomplish this task, a different arrangement of the general mixing equation is used:

$$\frac{V_1}{V_2} = \frac{(C_2 - C_F)}{(C_F - C_1)}$$

As applied to mixing air and oxygen, V_1 represents the volume of air (with an oxygen concentration of 21%) (C_1); V_2 represents the volume of pure oxygen ($C_2 = 100$); and C_F the oxygen percentage desired (O_2%). Therefore:

$$\frac{\text{Liters air}}{\text{Liters } O_2} = \frac{(100 - O_2\%)}{(O_2\% - 21)}$$

For example, suppose you need to produce an oxygen concentration of 70% by mixing air with pure oxygen. We would compute the air-to-oxygen ratio needed to achieve this concentration as follows:

$$\frac{\text{Liters air}}{\text{Liters } O_2} = \frac{(100 - O_2\%)}{(O_2\% - 21)}$$
$$\frac{\text{Liters air}}{\text{Liters } O_2} = \frac{(100 - 70)}{(70 - 21)}$$
$$= \frac{30}{49}$$
$$\approx \frac{0.6}{1.0}$$

Thus, to obtain a final mixture of 70% oxygen, you would mix about 0.6 liters of air with every 1.0 liter of oxygen.

In order to avoid these computations, many RCPs use a simple aid referred to as the "magic box" (Figure 26-12).[101] To use this aid, draw a box and places 20 at the top left* and 100 at the bottom left. Then place the desired oxygen percentage is in the middle of the box (in this case 70%). Next, subtract diagonally from lower left to upper right (disregard

---

*20 is used for ease of estimation; for accuracy in computing ratios needed for concentration of 30% or below, you must use 21.

the sign). Then subtract diagonally again from upper left to lower right (disregard the sign). The resulting numerator (30) is the value for air, with the denominator (50) being the value for oxygen.

By convention, air-to-oxygen ratios are always expressed with the denominator (liters of oxygen) set to 1. To reduce 30:50 to a ratio of X:1, simply divide the numerator (30) by the denominator (50). The resulting number (0.6) divided by 1 is the air-to-oxygen ratio:

$$\frac{30}{50} = \frac{0.6}{1.0}$$

Note that the ratio derived by the "magic box" is the same as that previously computed using the general mixing equation. Based on computations using the general mixing equation, Table 26-6 lists the approximate air-to-oxygen ratios for several common oxygen percentages.

Knowing the air-to-oxygen ratio for a given F_DO_2 allows the RCP to derive another essential parameter, the total output flow. In order to calculate total flow output of an air entrainment system, you must know both the oxygen input flow and the system's air-to-oxygen ratio.

Since total output flow is the sum of oxygen input and air entrained, your first step is to add the air-to-oxygen ratio 'parts.' For example, if the ratio is 1:3, there are $1 + 3 = 4$ total parts (1 liter air; 3 liters oxygen). Next, you simply multiply the sum of the ratio parts times the O_2 input flow in L/min. The result is the total output flow in L/min.

For example, let's compute the total output flow of an air entrainment device designed to deliver 28% and set up with an oxygen input of 6 L/min:

ratio at 28% = 10:1 (Table 26-6)

sum of air-to-oxygen ratio parts = 10 + 1 = 11

total output flow = sum of ratio parts × input flow

total output flow = 11 × 6 = 66 L/min

Thus a 28% air entrainment device set up with an oxygen input flow of 6 L/min has a total output flow of 66 L/min.

The other major factor determining the F_DO_2 provided by an air entrainment device is downstream flow resistance. In the presence of flow resistance distal to the jet, the volume of air entrained will always decrease. With less air being entrained, total flow output decreases and F_DO_2 rises.

Although the delivered oxygen concentration rises, the actual F_IO_2 received by the patient may *decrease,* especially on devices set to deliver 30% to 50% O_2.[99] This is due mainly to the decrease in total output flow. As the total output flow falls below that needed to meet the patient's inspiratory needs, room air must be inhaled. A similar event occurs if the air intake ports surrounding the jet become occluded. Under both

Table 26-6 Approximate air-to-oxygen ratios for oxygen concentrations in common use

% Oxygen	Approximate air-to-oxygen ratio*	Total ratio parts†
100	0:1	1
80	0.3:1	1.3
70	0.6:1	1.6
60	1:1	2
50	1.7:1	2.7
45	2:1	3
40	3:1	4
35	5:1	6
30	8:1	9
28	10:1	11
24	25:1	26

*Assuming 20.9% oxygen in air.
†Total flow of mixed air and oxygen can be calculated by multiplying the total ratio parts times the oxygen flow rate (L/min).

conditions, these high-flow systems begin to behave like low-flow devices.

The two most common systems in this category are the air entrainment mask (AEM) and the air entrainment nebulizer. In general, AEMs are indicated for alert patients with normal humidification mechanisms intact. Air entrainment nebulizers, on the other hand, are used to deliver O_2 when either the upper airway is bypassed or a humidity deficit is causing problems with airway clearance.

Air entrainment mask (AEM). The use of an oxygen mask to provide controlled F_IO_2s via air entrainment was first reported in 1941 by Barach and Eckman.[102,103] Barach's system provided relatively high F_IO_2s (above 40%) using adjustable air entrainment ports to control the amount of air mixed with oxygen. Some 20 years later, Campbell developed an entrainment mask that provided controlled low F_IO_2s, calling it a "Venti-mask."[104]

Principle. As the name "Venti-mask" suggests, the operating principle behind these devices has often been attributed to the Venturi principle. This is incorrect.[98,99] Rather than using an actual Venturi tube to entrain air, these devices employ a simple restricted orifice or jet through which oxygen flows at high velocities. Air is entrained by shear forces at the boundary of jet flow, not by low lateral pressures. The smaller the orifice, the greater the velocity of oxygen and the more air entrained. Figure 26-13, page 720, depicts a typical AEM, designed to deliver a range of low to moderate F_IO_2s (0.24-0.40). As can be seen, the mask consists of a jet orifice or nozzle, around which is an air entrainment port (upper drawing). The body of the mask has several large ports which allow escape of both excess flow from the device and exhaled gas from the patient. In this design, the F_IO_2 is regulated by selecting and changing the jet adapter. The smallest jet provides the highest oxygen velocity and thus the most air entrainment and the lowest F_IO_2 (0.24).

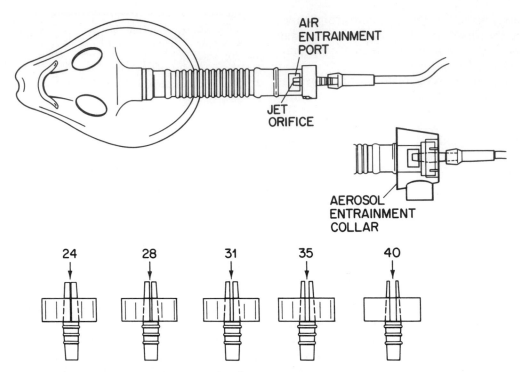

Fig. 26-13 Typical air entrainment mask (AEM). FiO$_2$ is regulated by changing jet adapter. Aerosol collar allows high humidity or aerosol entrainment from an air source. (From Kacmarek RM: In-hospital O$_2$ Therapy. In Kacmarek RM, Stoller J (editors): *Current Respiratory Care*, Toronto, 1988, BC Decker.)

Conversely, the largest jet provides the lowest oxygen velocity and thus the least air entrainment and the highest FiO$_2$ (0.40). Other AEM designs may vary both jet and entrainment port size to provide even a broader range of FiO$_2$s. Note also the aerosol entrainment collar that fits over the air entrainment ports (to be discussed subsequently).

In order to assure a controlled FiO$_2$ at flows high enough to prevent air dilution, an AEM's total output flow must exceed the patient's *peak* inspiratory flow.[99] During normal quiet breathing, peak inspiratory flows seldom exceed 30 L/min, but this can easily double or triple in acutely ill patients. As a general rule of thumb, a total output flow of at least 60 L/min should be established; higher flows may be needed for patients with high minute ventilations or breathing rates.

Accuracy. Studies assessing the accuracy of AEMs provide a mixed picture. Early laboratory studies found small but measurable difference between AEMs' set and delivered FdO$_2$s. These differences increased when using an aerosol entrainment collar (discussed subsequently).[105]

When comparing FdO$_2$ to actual patient FiO$_2$, however, larger differences have been reported, especially with devices set above 40%.[76] With AEMs set above 40%, the actual FiO$_2$ was always lower than the FdO$_2$. This was because the subjects' peak inspiratory flows exceeded the total output flow provided by the devices at these higher settings.

A subsequent laboratory study of the Hudson Multivent AEM concluded that FiO$_2$s were predictable only at the 24% setting using the recommended flows.[106] Predictable function at the 26% and 28% settings could be achieved, but only by increasing the oxygen input flow above the recommended setting. At settings above 30%, FiO$_2$s were unpredictable, regardless of oxygen input flow. For example, at the 0.50 setting, the device studied provided an FiO$_2$ of only 0.39.

A more recent laboratory study of the same device concluded that this AEM was not likely to deliver the set oxygen concentration, and that the FiO$_2$ provided was unpredictable.[107] In addition, it was reported that route of breathing (oral or nasal) had no effect on FiO$_2$, but mask position did. Specifically, rotation of the mask in the coronal plane produced large changes in FiO$_2$. With the mask parallel to the coronal plane of the model, the FiO$_2$ was about 10% less than set. When the mask was angled 10 degrees toward the face, the actual FiO$_2$ was about 20% less than set. Finally, when the mask was angled 10 degrees away from the face, the resulting FiO$_2$ was only about half the set value. These differences were attributed to localization of the oxygen stream in the center of the mask.[105]

Mask design, especially volume, also appears to effect performance. Most studies have reported that in order to function as true fixed-performance devices, AEMs should have large volumes (300 mL or more).[108,109] In addition, some researchers have criticized the 'aviation-style' masks typically used in the US, because gas is delivered to the side of the nose and mouth (the original Campbell design delivered gas directly to the nose and mouth). However, one contrary report concludes that AEM volume is important only when patient demand exceeded total flow.[110] Consistent with all prior studies, however, was the conclusion that AEM performance changes from fixed to variable whenever the patient's inspiratory flow exceeds the total gas flow delivered by the device.

Appropriate use. Air-entrainment masks can ensure stable FiO_2s to most patients who require less than 35% oxygen. Thus COPD patients who may hypoventilate when exposed to high FiO_2s are candidates for AEM usage. The AEM is also a good choice for patients with high or changing ventilatory demands who need a stable low FiO_2s.

AEMs are generally best used for short periods when precise control over FiO_2 is needed, such as during acute exacerbations of COPD. Due to their size, discomfort, and appearance, they are less well tolerated for long-term therapy than nasal cannulas. Moreover, unlike cannulas, these masks must be removed for eating and drinking. As previously discussed, even a short break in O_2 therapy can cause rapid drops in PaO_2. In order to ensure continuity of therapy when patients must remove their masks, the RCP should make available a cannula set at a flow which produces an equivalent FiO_2 or SpO_2.

Problem-solving and troubleshooting. The most common clinical problems with AEMs are: (1) providing sufficient total output flow to ensure a stable FdO_2, (2) providing FdO_2s different from the present levels, and (3) providing extra humidification.

Providing sufficient total output flow to ensure a stable FdO_2 is mainly of concern with AEMs set to deliver 30% or more oxygen. With these masks, the RCP can assure higher output flows by raising the oxygen input flow, even if this means exceeding the manufacturer's specifications. As a rule of thumb, you should try to assure a minimum total output flow of at least 60 L/min. For example, when setting-up a 35% AEM (mixing at a 5:1 ratio), you would set the oxygen input flow to at least 10 L/min.

If the need arises to provide an FdO_2 different from those available via an AEM, you can bleed additional oxygen into the entrainment port. By adding a secondary oxygen flow, any FdO_2 can be achieved. An equation to compute these various FdO_2s is provided in the literature.[111]

If high flows causes mucosal drying, the inspired gas mixture provided by an AEM can be humidified.[105,112] While a simple bubble humidifier can be used, very little increase in humidification occurs because of the relatively large amounts of air entrained.[67] A better solution is to add aerosol to the entrained air through the accessory aerosol collar

(see Figure 26-13). Obviously, to maintain the set FdO_2, this aerosol must be delivered by an air–powered nebulizer. As an added benefit, aerosol collars help prevent accidental blockage of the AEM's entrainment ports, such as may occur with bedsheets. However, with the addition of aerosol particles to room air, entrained volume falls and FdO_2 increases slightly.[67]

Air entrainment nebulizers. Pneumatically powered air entrainment nebulizers share most of the features of AEMs, but have added capabilities. Specifically, these devices provide additional humidification and heat control. Humidification is provided by using the oxygen jet not only to entrain air, but also to produce an aerosol. Temperature control is provided by either an immersion or 'hot-plate' heater. In combination, these added features allow delivery of particulate water (in excess of BTPS needs) to the airways (see Chapter 25).

Appropriate use. With their added humidification and heat control, air entrainment nebulizers have been the traditional device of choice for delivering O_2 to patients with artificial tracheal airways (see Chapter 22).[113] Typically, this is done using either a T-tube (Brigg's adapter) or tracheostomy mask. Alternatively, an oxygen mixture with aerosol can be delivered to patients with intact upper airways using either an aerosol mask or face tent (Figure 26-14).[114]

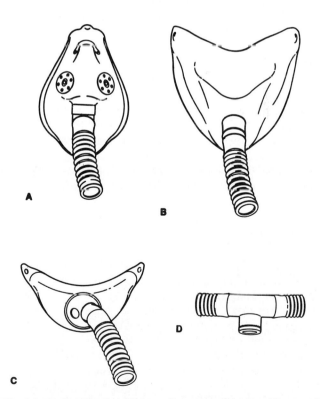

Fig. 26-14 Devices for delivery of oxygen mixtures with aerosol; aerosol maks; face tent; tracheostomy collar; T tube. (From Kacmarek RM: In-hospital O_2 Therapy. In Kacmarek RM, Stoller J (editors): *Current Respiratory Care,* Toronto, 1988, BC Decker.)

Performance. Whereas AEMs can vary both jet and entrainment port size to obtain a given F_DO_2, gas-powered nebulizers have a fixed orifice. Thus air to oxygen ratios can be altered only by varying air entrainment port size. Permanent nebulizers typically have fixed entrainment settings, such as 100, 70, and 40%. Disposables nebulizers usually have 6 to 8 settings that provide F_DO_2s between 0.28 to 1.0.[67]

As with AEMs, air entrainment nebulizers perform as fixed-performance devices only when their output flows meet or exceed the patient's inspiratory demands. Unlike AEMs, however, the RCP cannot easily increase nebulizer output flows by raising the oxygen input. With most nebulizers systems, the extremely small size of the jet (needed for aerosol production) limits the maximum oxygen input flow to between 12 and 15 L/min at 50 psig. Thus, for example, the total output flow of an air entrainment nebulizer set to deliver 40% O_2 will range between 48 and 60 L/min. Although this may be adequate for most patients, it is not sufficient for those with very high inspiratory flows or minute volumes.

In addition, the actual FIO_2 received by patients may be affected by the choice of airway appliance. For example, the FIO_2s delivered by face tent are consistently lower than the nebulizer F_DO_2s, especially at the 70% and 100% settings.[115] How much of these differences is due to changes in nebulizer output flow (as opposed to the appliance itself) is not known.

For these reasons, air entrainment nebulizers should be treated as fixed-performance devices only when they are set to deliver 40% oxygen or less. Even at the 40% setting, however some variance in F_DO_2 may occur.[76,77,79] Certainly, when a nebulizer is used to deliver 40% or more oxygen, the RCP should determine whether its flow is sufficient to meet patient needs.

There are two ways to assess the adequacy of flow provided by an air entrainment nebulizer. The first method is simple visual inspection. With this approach (generally used only with a T-tube), the RCP sets up the device to deliver the highest possible flow at the prescribed FIO_2. After connecting the system to the patient, the RCP then visually observes the mist output at the expiratory side of the T-tube. As long as one can still observe mist escaping *throughout* inspiration, flow is adequate to meet patient needs, and the delivered FIO_2 is assured.

The second way to assess the adequacy of nebulizer flow is to actually compare it with the patient's peak inspiratory flow. You can estimate a patient's peak inspiratory flow during tidal breathing using the following formula:[116]

$$\text{peak inspiratory flow} = \frac{\pi V_T}{2T_I}$$

where V_T is the average tidal volume, T_I is the inspiratory time, and π and 2 are constants. Alternatively, if minute ventilation is used instead of tidal volume, the following formula should be used:[116]

$$\text{peak inspiratory flow} = \frac{\pi \dot{V}_E(T_I+T_E)}{2T_I}$$

where $\dot{V}_E$ is the minute ventilation, T_I is the inspiratory time, T_E is the expiratory time, and π and 2 are constants.

Once the patient's peak inspiratory flow is known, the RCP then computes the device's total output flow, using the methods previously described for AEMs. As long as the nebulizer's total output flow exceeds the value computed for the patient, a stable FIO_2 is assured. On the other hand, if the patient's peak flow exceeds that provided by the nebulizer, the device will function as a low-flow system, with variable FIO_2.

The simplest approach to achieving high F_DO_2s when oxygen is being delivered to patients via T-tube

---

■ MINI C L I N I ■

26–2

Computing Minimum Flow Needs

Problem: A doctor orders 40% oxygen via air entrainment nebulizer to a patient with a tidal volume of 0.5 L and an inspiratory time of 1 sec. What is the minimum nebulizer input flow needed to assure the prescribed FIO_2?

Solution: First compute the patient's inspiratory flow:

$$\text{peak inspiratory flow} = \frac{\pi \times V_T}{2T_I}$$

$$\text{peak inspiratory flow} = \frac{3.14 \times 0.5}{2}$$

$$\text{peak inspiratory flow} = 0.79 \text{ L/sec} \times 60 = 47.10 \text{ L/min}$$

Thus, to assure the prescribed FIO_2, the air entrainment nebulizer must provide a total flow of at least 47.10 L/min to this patient. To compute the minimum nebulizer input flow need-ed, simply sum the air/oxygen ratio for 40% and divide the result into the total flow needs:

sum the air/oxygen ratio (3:1) for 40%

$$3 + 1 = 4$$

divide the result into the total flow needs:

$$\frac{47.10}{4} = 11.78 \approx 12 \text{ L/min}$$

Thus the minimum nebulizer input flow needed to assure the prescribed FIO_2 for this patient is 12 L/min.

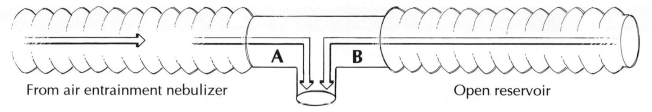

Fig. 26-15 The use of an open volume reservoir to enhance delivered oxygen concentrations with a T-tube. 50 to 150 mL of aerosol tubing are connected to the expiratory side of the T-tube. When the patient inhales, gas at the set FiO$_2$ is drawn first through the inspiratory side of the circuit *(A)*. If the patient's flow exceeds nebulizer flow, gas will then be drawn from the reservoir side *(B)*. Only after the reservoir volume is fully tapped will room air be entrained and the FiO$_2$ decreases.

is to add an open volume reservoir to the system. To add an open volume reservoir, you simply connect 50 to 150 mL of aerosol tubing to the *expiratory* side of the T-tube (Figure 26-15). During exhalation, both system flow and the patient's expired gases discharge out through this reservoir. During the following short pause between exhalation and inspiration, system flow fills this reservoir with source gas at the set FdO$_2$. When the patient then inhales, gas at the set FdO$_2$ is drawn initially from the system through the inspiratory side of the circuit. Should the patient's flow exceed nebulizer flow, however, gas will then be drawn from the reservoir. Only after the reservoir volume is fully tapped will room air be entrained and the FiO$_2$ lowered.

Given its simplicity, adding an open volume reservoir to the expiratory side of T-tubes has become standard procedure in most clinical settings. Unfortu-

nately, this approach can only be used with intubated patients. Even then, the small reservoir size limits its ability to assure stable FiO$_2$s (especially above 40%), and larger reservoirs can cause rebreathing.

One of four additional approaches can be used to achieve a high and stable FiO$_2$ for patients receiving O$_2$ therapy via air entrainment systems. The first is to combine an inspiratory volume reservoir (usually a compliant 3 to 5 liter anesthesia bag) with a one-way expiratory valve.[119] In this system, when patient flow exceeds nebulizer flow, a drop in system pressure closes the expiratory valve. With the expiratory valve closed, inhalation of room air is impossible. Instead, any additional gas must be drawn from the inspiratory reservoir, at the set FdO$_2$. Although such a system assures delivery of the set oxygen concentration, it can pose a significant hazard. Should source flow stop for any reason, the patient would not be able to draw

---

Problem-solving and troubleshooting. When used as oxygen delivery systems, air entrainment nebulizers present many clinical problems. The most common problems these devices pose to the RCP are: (1) inaccurate FdO$_2$s, (2) getting FdO$_2$s below 28%, and (3) maintaining FdO$_2$s at high flows.

In terms of accuracy, the FdO$_2$ delivered by most air entrainment nebulizers is usually higher than set. The reason for this difference is the added downstream resistance created by the delivery tubing.[113] In general, this effect is worst at high mixing ratios (low FdO$_2$s), or when the tubing becomes blocked with water. Even in the latter situation, however, tube blockage must exceed 70% before changes in FdO$_2$ occur.[117]

Assessing Patient Flow vs. Nebulizer

The worst case scenario occurs when the delivery tubing become completely obstructed with condensed water. With complete obstruction, resistance is so high that no air is entrained. In this case, the oxygen input simply escapes out the air entrainment port and is never delivered to the patient. To avoid these problems and assure as accurate a FdO$_2$ as possible, the RCP should always check the delivery tub-

ing of air entrainment nebulizers and keep it clear of condensate.

Even with no water in the nebulizer's tubing, flow resistance makes it hard to provide less than 28% oxygen with these systems. Should the prescribing physician require an FiO$_2$ below 0.28, you can use compressed air to drive the nebulizer and then bleed oxygen into the delivery tubing via a connector.[118] Using an oxygen analyzer, you then carefully adjust the O$_2$ input flow until the desired percent is achieved.

The last and most common problem RCPs encounter with air entrainment devices is how to maintain high FdO$_2$s for patients with high inspiratory flows. The common methods for achieving this goal are summarized in the box, page 724.

■ MINI CLINI ■

26-4

Air Entrainment Nebulizers: Total Flow Vs. Patient Demand

Problem: Your patient is breathing oxygen via an endotracheal tube T-adaptor attached to an air entrainment nebulizer set to deliver 40% O_2. The oxygen flowmeter powering the nebulizer is set at 12 L/min, which is the maximum flow the nebulizer can accommodate. You notice that the aerosol mist almost, but never quite disappears during inspiration. Arterial blood gases reveal an unacceptably low PaO_2 and the physician asks you to increase FIO_2 to 0.50. Because the air entrainment control can be set to deliver an FIO_2 of 0.50 you make this change. You "T" in an oxygen analyzer at the nebulizer outlet and measure 50% O_2. Is the patient receiving an $FIO_2 = 0.50$?

Discussion: Probably not. At 40%, the air: O_2 entrainment is 3 parts of air entrained for each liter of oxygen. With an oxygen flow of 12 L/min, 12×3, or 36 liters of air are entrained and added to the 12 liters of oxygen each minute for a total flow output of 48 L/min. Since the mist almost disappeared during each inspiration, we can assume that we were essentially matching the patient's inspiratory flow demand. When FIO_2 is switched to the 50% setting, the air: O_2 entrainment changes to 1.66 liters of air entrained by each liter of oxygen flow. At 12 L/min oxygen flow, 12×1.66, or 19.92 liters of air are entrained each minute and added to the 12 liters per minute of oxygen flowing through the nebulizer jet for a total flow output of 31.92 L/min. Obviously, this patient's inspiratory flow demands are no longer being met, and room air is being entrained through the open side of the endotracheal T-adaptor. The patient's FIO_2 must now be less than 50%. Blending systems capable of delivering high flows at any oxygen concentration would be the ideal systems for delivering FIO_2s greater than 50%.

room air directly into the system, and could suffocate. For this reason, oxygen delivery systems using this approach must be equipped with an emergency inlet valve that allows room air breathing in the event of source gas failure.

The second and most common approach to providing a high and stable FIO_2 is to connect two or more nebulizers together with a "Y" adaptor (Figure 26-16).[67,114,120] For example, while a single air entrainment nebulizer set at 60% (1:1 ratio) with a maximum input flow of 15 L/min has a total output flow of only 30 L/min, connecting two of these devices together doubles the total output flow to 60 L/min (the 'minimum' needed for a high flow device).

Unfortunately, recent research has challenged the conventional wisdom of this approach. Table 26-7 summarizes the results of a laboratory study that measured simulated FIO_2s at different breathing patterns while using an aerosol face mask with two jet nebulizers in tandem.[121] As can be seen, 60% oxygen was achieved only when tidal volumes were below 500 mL. 80% oxygen could not be provided at *any* combination of patient rate or tidal volume. Last, at the 100% setting, most 'patients' received less than 80% O_2, with some getting as little as 50%!

The third option for providing a high and stable FIO_2 via an air entrainment system is like that previously described for achieving a low FIO_2. In this case, however, you power the nebulizer with oxygen, not air. The nebulizer should be set to a *lower* FIO_2 than that prescribed (thus generating higher flows). You then bleed supplemental oxygen into the delivery tubing, which raises both the FIO_2 and total output flow. Last, using an O_2 analyzer, you carefully adjust the oxygen input flow until the desired FIO_2 is achieved.[114]

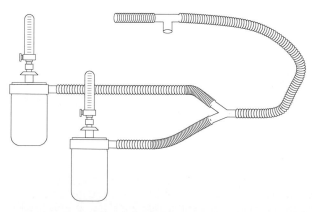

Fig. 26-16 Use of two nebulizers in parallel to provide high FIO_2 at high flow.

Methods to provide high FIO_2s to patients with high inspiratory flows (air entrainment systems)

- Add open reservoir to expiratory side of T-tube
- Provide inspiratory reservoir with one-way expiratory valve
- Connect two or more nebulizers together in parallel
- Set nebulizer to low FDO_2; bleed-in O_2; analyze/adjust
- Use specialized flow generator

The last means for delivering high FiO₂s at high flows with air entrainment are specialized systems like the Downs flow generator. These devices are essentially Pitot-tubes (see Chapter 8) with high input flow capabilities. This design provides higher FDO₂s at high flows, while minimizing the effect of downstream resistance on FDO₂. Two models are available. The fixed flow generator attaches directly to an oxygen flowmeter and provides an FDO₂ of 0.33. The adjustable flow generator attaches to a 50 psig oxygen source and provides FDO₂s between 0.33 and 1.0 with flows exceeding 100 L/min.[122]

Blending systems. Whereas air entrainment systems must dilute oxygen with air at atmospheric pressure, a blending device mixes high pressure (50-psig) oxygen and air to obtain a specific FDO₂. This allows precise control over both FDO₂ and total flow output. Moreover, most blending systems can provide flows well in excess of 60 L/min, thus qualifying them as true fixed-performance delivery devices. Blending is done either manually or via a proportioning valve.

Mixing gases manually. When gases are mixed manually, you set separate air and oxygen flowmeters to achieve a desired FDO₂ at the needed flow. To compute the needed oxygen flow, you apply the following equation (a modified form of the general mixing equation):[114,123]

$$O_2 \text{ flow} = \frac{\text{Total flow} \times (FDO_2 - 0.21)}{0.79}$$

For example, if you needed to provide a patient with 50% oxygen at a total flow of 60 L/min, you would compute the needed O₂ flows as:

$$O_2 \text{ flow} = \frac{\text{Total flow} \times (FDO_2 - 0.21)}{0.79}$$

$$O_2 \text{ flow} = \frac{60 \times (0.50 - 0.21)}{0.79}$$

$$O_2 \text{ flow} = \frac{60 \times 0.29}{0.79}$$

$$O_2 \text{ flow} = \frac{17.40}{0.79}$$

$$O_2 \text{ flow} = 22 \text{ L/min}$$

Once the oxygen flow is computed, you can easily determine the air flow:

$$\text{Air flow} = \text{Total flow} - \text{oxygen flow}$$
$$\text{Air flow} = 60 - 22$$
$$\text{Air flow} = 38 \text{ L/min}$$

Thus to provide a patient with 50% oxygen at a total flow of 60 L/min, you would blend 22 liters of oxygen with 38 liters of air.

Manual gas blending is used with gas injection nebulizers. Unlike those using air entrainment, gas injection nebulizers require pressurized air *and* oxygen as source gases, and two high flow (0 to 70 L/min)

Table 26-7 Simulated FIO₂ via face mask from two nebulizers in parallel[115]

VT (mL)	Breaths/minute			
	20	25	30	35
	Nebulizer setting (%) 60–80–100	Nebulizer setting (%) 60–80–100	Nebulizer setting (%) 60–80–100	Nebulizer setting (%) 60–80–100
	FIO₂ at Airway			
200	60–78–91	60–77–90	60–75–86	60–73–84
300	60–76–84	60–72–80	60–68–78	58–64–74
400	60–70–78	60–55–72	57–63–68	55–59–65
500	59–68–70	56–62–67	54–59–63	52–56–50
600	57–68–64	55–62–60	52–58–56	50–54–54
700	56–66–60	54–60–58	50–56–54	48–53–52
800	54–62–56	51–58–52	48–54–50	—

flowmeters. One gas powers the nebulizer jet, while the other is 'injected' at a specific flow to achieve a given FDO₂. FDO₂s in the 0.70 to 0.75 range at flows of 60 L/min or more are provided when O₂ powers the nebulizer at 40 L/min and air is injected. Conversely, FDO₂s between 0.65 and 0.70 are available at higher flows (90 to 100 L/min) when air powers the nebulizer and oxygen is injected.

Oxygen blenders. Instead of manually mixing air and O₂, a proportioning valve can be used. When combined with appropriate pressure reduction regulators and an alarm system, such a device is called an *oxygen blender.*

Figure 26-17 shows the major components found

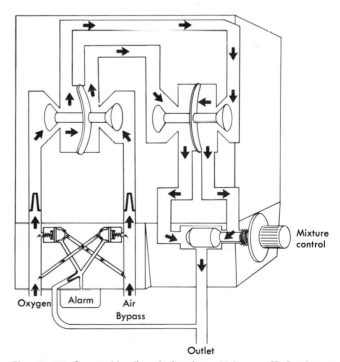

Fig. 26-17 Oxygen blending device. (From McPherson SP: Respiratory therapy equipment, ed 3, St Louis, 1985, Mosby.)

in a typical oxygen blender. Air and oxygen enter the blender and pass through two pressure regulating valves in series. These regulators exactly match the air and oxygen pressures. Gas then flows to a precision proportioning valve. Since the two gas pressures at this point are equal, varying the size of the air and oxygen inlets provides precise control over their relative concentrations. Last, an alarm system provides an audible warning when either source gas fails or drops below a specified level. Usually, this alarm system also provides a 'cross-over' or bypass feature whereby failure of one gas source causes the blender system to switch to the other. For example, should the air source fail when delivering 60% oxygen, the alarm will sound and the blender will switch over to deliver 100% oxygen.

Appropriate use. Most patients' oxygen needs can be met with simple modification to air entrainment nebulizer systems. However, when those devices cannot provide high enough FDO_2s at high flows, the RCP should consider a blending system.

Blending systems can be either open or closed. An open system is equivalent to a T-tube, but with higher FDO_2s at higher flows. In general, an open system should provide the specified FDO_2 at flows greater than 100 L/min.

Alternatively, the RCP can select a closed system (Figure 26-18).[121] In this system, the prescribed gas mixture is provided by either a set of air/oxygen high-flow flowmeters (manual mixing) or by a high-flow blender. The gas mixture is then warmed and humidified, ideally by a servo-controlled heated humidifier. Gas then flows through large-bore tubing into a inspiratory volume reservoir, which includes a fail-safe inlet valve. Last, gas is delivered to the patient via a close airway appliance, in this case a mask with one-way expiratory valves. Such a device is capable of assuring an FIO_2 of up to 1.0, even in patients with minute ventilations in excess of 30 L/min.[121]

Problem-solving and troubleshooting. Problems with high-flow blending systems include failure or inaccuracy of the mixing system, variable flow output, nonrebreathing valve malfunction, and inadequate humidification. Additional problems and hazards associated with the humidification devices used in these systems are covered in Chapter 25.

There are several reports of failure or inaccuracy of oxygen blenders.[124,125] Although it is impossible to prevent equipment failure, the RCP must always assure that several conditions are met before applying any life-supporting device to a patient.

First, you should always check to assure that the equipment has undergone proper testing and preventive maintenance, according to the manufacturer's specifications and hospital protocol. Second, when first setting up a device—and before applying it to the patient—you should perform whatever tests are needed to confirm its proper operation (see accompanying box). Last, you should check and confirm the FDO_2 by calibrated O_2 analyzer, at least once per shift.[2] As always, should the device not perform according to expectations, you should immediately replace it.

Another clinical problem the RCP can encounter with O_2 blenders is variation in output flow with changes in either source pressure or FDO_2.[126,127] Specifically, some blenders may provide inadequate flow output when source pressures fall below 50 psig, or when the FDO_2 is either very low or very high. Only knowledge of the specific device(s) in use and clinical testing of output flow under usage conditions can prevent problems in this area.

A problem seen only with *closed* high-flow blending systems is failure of the nonrebreathing valves. As with any spontaneous breathing system, failure of a nonrebreathing valve can have catastrophic results.[128,129] Without safety provisions, should an inspiratory valve jam shut, the patient can suffocate. Should an expiratory valve jam, inhalation can still occur, but exhalation will be blocked. This can lead to rebreathing or result in pulmonary **barotrauma.**

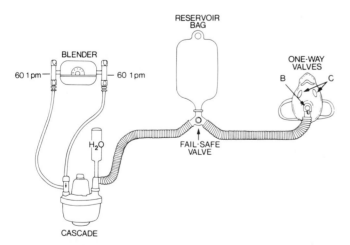

Fig. 26-18 High-flow nonrebreathing face mask with reservoir bag. Air and oxygen flowmeters each capable of 0-100 L/min flow. (From Foust GN, Potter WA, Wilons MD, et al: *Chest* 99:1346, 1991. Used by permission.)

Procedure for confirming operation of an oxygen blender

1. Confirm that inlet pressure of air and oxygen are within manufacturer's specifications;
2. Test low air and oxygen alarms by disconnecting each source; also confirm safety bypass or cross-over system;
3. Analyze oxygen concentration at 100%, 21% and specified FDO_2.

The same problems can occur when nonrebreathing valves are misassembled at the factory.[130] The only sure way to avoid these problems is to: (1) always inspect and test all breathing valves before application to a patient, and (2) always include fail-safe relief valves in the delivery system. A fail-safe inspiratory valve is mandatory. Fail-safe expiratory valves are optional.

The last major problem with blending systems is providing adequate humidification at high flows. If a jet nebulizer is used with an oxygen blender, flows are limited by both the restricted orifice and the need to set the device at the 100% source gas setting. Simple bubble humidifiers also can restrict flow, and tend to lose efficiency at higher flow rates.[114] Low resistance cascade or wick-type heated humidifiers can provide as much as 90% relative humidity at 37° C, with continuous flows in excess of 60 L/min.[131]

Enclosures

The concept of enclosing a patient in a controlled O_2 atmosphere is among the oldest approaches to oxygen therapy. Indeed, whole rooms were once used for this purpose.[65] With today's simpler airway devices, enclosures are generally used only with infants and children. The primary types of oxygen enclosures in current use with infants and children are tents, incubators and hoods.

Oxygen tents. Oxygen tents were once the most common method for O_2 therapy with both adults and children. Today, their use with adults is rare, but they are still used with children. In general, tents are air-conditioned or cooled by ice to provide a comfortable temperature within a plastic sheet canopy (Figure 26-19).

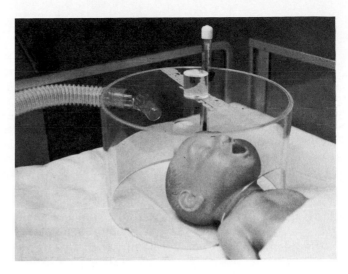

Fig. 26-20 Infant oxygen hood.

The major problem with these systems is that frequent opening and closing of the canopy causes wide swings in oxygen concentration. Moreover, constant leakage makes high FIO_2s impossible. For example, O_2 input flows of 12 to 15 L/min can only provide 40 to 50% oxygen in large tents. Comparable FIO_2s can be achieved in smaller pediatric or "croup" tents with flows between 8 and 10 L/min. Due to these limitations, tents are used primarily to provide pediatric aerosol therapy to children with croup or cystic fibrosis.

Hoods. An oxygen hood is the best method for providing controlled O_2 therapy to infants.[132] As depicted in Figure 26-20, an 'oxyhood' covers only the head, leaving the infant's body free for nursing care. Oxygen is delivered to the hood via either a heated air entrainment nebulizer or a blending system with a heated humidifier. A minimum flow of 7 L/min should be set in order to prevent accumulation of carbon dioxide.[133] Depending on the size of hood, flows of 10 to 15 L/min may be needed to maintain stable high oxygen concentrations. Higher flows are generally not needed and may produce harmful noise levels.[134]

With premature infants, it is especially important to assure that the gas mixture is properly warmed and humidified, and not directed toward the patient's face or head. Low temperatures or convection cooling created by high flows over the head causes heat loss and cold stress. In premature infants, cold stress can increase oxygen consumption and even cause apnea.[132]

For these reasons, the temperature of gases provided to an infant in an oxyhood should be precisely set to maintain a *neutral thermal environment* (NTE). The NTE temperature varies according to an infant's age and weight. For example, the NTE temperature

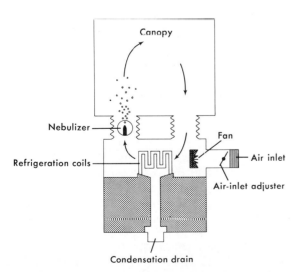

Fig. 26-19 Adult oxygen tent incorporating refrigeration coils for cooling. (From McPherson SP: Respiratory therapy equipment, ed 3, St Louis, 1985, Mosby.)

for newborns weighing under 1200 grams is 35° C. For older infants weighing 2500 grams or more, the NTE is lower, about 30° C.[135] More detail on the importance of temperature regulation in infants is provided in Chapter 35.

Incubators. Incubators are plexiglass enclosures that combine servo-controlled convection heating with supplemental O_2 (Figure 26-21). In older models, humidification was provided via a blow-over water reservoir located under the patient platform. However, due to the high infection risk associated with this design, these systems are no longer in common use. When supplemental humidity is needed, it is usually provided via an external heated humidifier or nebulizer.

Supplemental oxygen can be provided by directly connecting the incubator to a flowmeter with heated humidifier. In some units, a filtered air entrainment device limits the FDO_2 to about 0.40. However, leaks and frequent opening of the incubator dilute the oxygen levels well below 40%. On the other hand, blockage of the inlet filter can cause less air entrainment and a higher O_2 concentration.

Given the highly variable FDO_2s provided by these devices, the best way to control oxygen delivery to infants in an incubator is with an oxyhood. To do so, the oxyhood is placed over the infant's head, *inside* the incubator. When using this setup, the RCP must be sure to assess the FDO_2 and gas temperature within the oxyhood, not in the incubator. Ideally, incubator or oxyhood FDO_2 should be monitored continuously (see following section).[136]

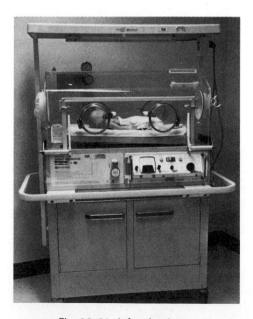

Fig. 26-21 Infant incubator.

Because hoods provide better FDO_2 control, and because servo-controlled radiant heating warmers are generally more convenient, plexiglass incubators are not as popular as they used to be. However, these devices are still the best choice for providing stable infants with a neutral thermal environment.

Problem-solving and troubleshooting. The most common problems with oxygen therapy enclosures are variations in FDO_2s, fire risk, temperature regulation, and infection control.

Variations in FDO_2s occur most often when an infant or child must be removed for a therapeutic or diagnostic procedure. To avoid this problem, the RCP must be prepared to provide an equivalent FDO_2 by alternative means. For example, if an infant must be removed from an 40% oxyhood for a neurologic exam, a simple neonatal size O_2 mask could be substituted.

Any enclosure with an oxygen-enriched atmosphere poses an increased risk of fire. For this reason, the RCP must ensure that all electrical appliances with the potential to spark—such as call bells and electric toys—are kept out of the enclosure.

Temperature regulation has always been a concern with these devices. In pediatric tents, cooling is needed to overcome the radiant heat build-up from the patient's body. Ideally, enclosure temperature should be in the 18 to 22° C range. If the temperature is too warm, the patient will be extremely uncomfortable. Too cool a temperature can cause excessive condensation and aerosol rain-out.

Unlike pediatric aerosol tents, incubators are warmed above room temperature. Modern systems control the temperature inside the incubator via a servo mechanism hooked to a **thermistor** probe placed on the infant's abdomen. Several recent reports of electrical malfunction of these systems are cause for concern.[137,138] Only careful ongoing confirmation of incubator temperature via a separate thermometer can avoid this problem.

Due to their size and complexity, oxygen therapy enclosures are among the most difficult systems to properly clean and disinfect. Tent canopies are always disposable, as are some oxyhoods. Incubators remain a problem source of nosocomial infections. Reusable tent parts, especially nebulizer components, should be cleaned and sterilized according to the methods described in Chapter 4. Nondisposable hoods and incubators should be carefully washed and wiped-down with a broad-spectrum surface disinfectant between patients.

A less common problem unique to infant oxyhoods has to do with proper head positioning. Specifically, flexion contractures of the neck have been reported in infants receiving oxyhood therapy.[139] Problem such as these can be easily prevented by careful positioning of the infant's head. Too much flexion (or extension) of the neck should be avoided.

Monitoring delivered oxygen concentrations

Rationale and approach

Traditionally, oxygen therapy monitoring has emphasized the delivered concentration, or FDO_2. This focus on 'input' is historically based. After all, it was not until the late 1960's that the clinical capability to easily measure arterial PO_2s even existed. Prior to then, monitoring was limited to observational assessment of the patient's response to a given FDO_2.

Today, focus has shifted to assessing the *outcomes* of oxygen therapy. Monitoring now emphasizes the physiologic results of oxygen therapy, such as the PaO_2 or arterial hemoglobin saturation.

There is no doubt that this change in emphasis has provided a more objective approach to oxygen therapy. One must never forget, however, that proper assessment of any outcome requires knowledge of the input. Specifically, to properly assess the effect of O_2 therapy on a patient, you must know how much of this drug you are giving. Only by comparing the input (FDO_2) to outcome (PaO_2 or SpO_2) can you determine how severe the problem is, and what the course of therapy should be. In addition to the obvious patient benefit, FDO_2 assessments provide essential data for quality assurance on equipment function.

For these reasons, RCPs must regularly analyze the FDO_2s provided by oxygen delivery systems. Depending on the objectives of the therapy and the patient's status, monitoring can be continuous or intermittent. At a minimum, all O_2 delivery systems should be checked at least once per day, and after any change in prescribed settings.[2] As indicated in the accompanying box, some systems require more frequent checks. For newborns, the standard practice appears to be continuous analysis of FDO_2, with a system check at least every 4 hours.

Oxygen analyzers

Delivered O_2 concentrations are measured by calibrated oxygen analyzers. There are three basic types of oxygen analyzers commonly used at the bedside: the physical analyzer, the electrical analyzer, and the electrochemical analyzer.[140,141] In order to effect use these devices, the RCP must understand how they work.

Physical analyzer. The physical analyzer takes advantage of oxygen's *paramagnetic* susceptibility. Because oxygen molecules are paramagnetic, they are attracted to the strongest portion of a magnetic field. Diamagnetic gases (such as nitrogen) are less affected by magnetic fields.

The physical analyzer consists of a small glass dumbbell that is filled with nitrogen and suspended on a quartz fiber in a magnetic field (Figure 26-22). When oxygen is not present, the force on the quartz fiber is exactly counterbalanced by the magnetic field. When O_2 molecules enter the system, this field is disrupted. This upsets the balance and rotates the glass dumbbell. A small mirror attached to the quartz fiber reflects a beam of light onto a translucent scale calibrated in both oxygen percent and PO_2 (torr).

A major advantage of this analyzer is its ability to detect and measure oxygen in any mixture of gases. Since the number of O_2 molecules in the measuring chamber is determined by the partial pressure, the physical analyzer actually measures the PO_2, and not the oxygen concentration. However, the indicator scale for this type analyzer is calibrated in *both* oxygen percent and PO_2 (Figure 26-23, page 730). For this reason, the percent concentration reading will only be accurate at sea level. When used at higher altitudes, the PO_2 reading is accurate, but the percent concentration will read low. Thus the physical analyzer scale must be recalibrated when used above sea level.

Also, since the instrument is calibrated to measure the PO_2 in the dry state, water vapor must be removed before analysis. This is done via a drying chamber

---

Monitoring delivered oxygen concentrations[2]
All oxygen delivery systems should be checked at least once per day. More frequent checks by calibrated analyzer are necessary in systems:
■ Prone to FDO_2 changes (eg, hoods, high-flow blending systems)
■ Applied to patients with artificial airways
■ Delivering a heated gas mixture
■ Applied to unstable patients are those with $FIO_2 \geq 0.50$

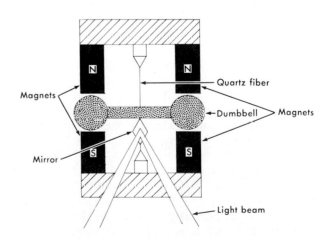

Fig. 26-22 Physical oxygen analyzer principle of operation. (From McPherson SP: Respiratory therapy equipment, ed 3, St Louis, 1985, Mosby.)

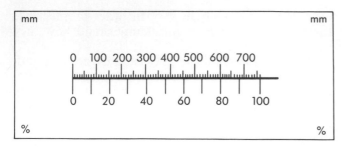

Fig. 26-23 Calibrated scale for physical analyzer showing oxygen percentage and mmHg.

filled with blue silica gel crystals that absorb water vapor. Also in the drying chamber is anhydrous cobalt chloride, which turns pink when saturated with water. The color change from blue to pink tells the user that the crystals in the drying chamber should be changed.

Because the physical analyzer generates no heat, it can be used with flammable gases. However, because gas flow through the chamber moves the dumbbell, this analyzer can only be used with static gas samples.[141]

Electric analyzer. The electric oxygen analyzer is based on the principle of *thermal conductivity.* All gases conduct heat, but to varying degrees. A gas's coefficient of thermal conductivity indicates how well it conducts heat (refer to Chapter 7). Because oxygen conducts heat better than nitrogen, changes in the proportions of these two gases alter the overall thermal conductivity of the mixture. The change in thermal conductivity of an O_2/N_2 mixture is directly proportional to the amount of oxygen present.

The electrical analyzer measures changes in thermal conductivity using a battery-powered Wheatstone bridge (Figure 26-24). One limb of the bridge is exposed to the test gas, with the other limb acting as a variable resistor (for calibration).

To calibrate the instrument before use, one draws air into the sample chamber, and then balances the bridge by adjusting a **rheostat** until the scale reads 21%. Introducing additional O_2 into the chamber draws more heat away from the sample wires, lowers their electrical resistance, and increases the current flow. This creates an "imbalance" in current across the two limbs of the bridge, which is measured by a **galvanometer.** Although actually measuring a difference in potential, the galvanometer reads the oxygen percent.

Since the comparison is based on the relative amounts of O_2 and N_2 in the mixture, the electrical analyzer measures the concentration of oxygen in nitrogen, not its partial pressure. For this reason, if you try to measure a mixture other than oxygen in nitrogen, you will get a false reading. The electrical analyzer can, however, be scaled to measure other gas mixtures. The helium analyzer used on many pulmo-

nary function devices is a good example of an electrical analyzer calibrated for other gas mixtures.

Because water vapor's thermal conductivity differs from both oxygen and nitrogen, electrical analyzers must be provided with a constant level of humidity. This is done by either drying the sample (like the physical analyzer), or saturating it with water vapor. Electrical analyzers that saturate the gas sample use hydrated silica gel crystals (pink) for this purpose.

A final consideration is the circuit resistance that electrical analyzers generate. This can produce enough heat to ignite flammable gases. For this reason, electrical analyzers should *never* be used to measure oxygen concentrations in a flammable gas mixture.

Electrochemical analyzers. Electrochemical analyzers are of two types: the polarographic (Clark) electrode, and the galvanic fuel cell. While physical and electrical analyzers provide only intermittent sampling capability, electrochemical analyzers allow continuous monitoring of oxygen concentrations.

Both the polarographic electrode and the galvanic fuel cell measure the partial pressure of oxygen. This is done via a reduction-oxidation (REDOX) reaction. The REDOX reaction occurs in an electrolyte gel across an **anode** and a **cathode,** separated from the air by a semipermeable membrane. Oxygen diffuses through the membrane at a rate proportional to its PO_2. It then migrates to the anode, where it is chemically reduced to hydroxyl ions. These hydroxyl ions then migrate to the cathode, where they oxidize a metal (usually lead or silver). The REDOX reaction thus results in current flow between the anode and cathode which is directly proportional to the PO_2. Current is measured on a galvanometer calibrated in percent oxygen.

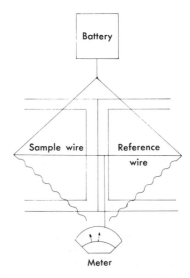

Fig. 26-24 Electrical oxygen analyzer. (From McPherson SP: Respiratory therapy equipment, ed 3, St Louis, 1985, Mosby.)

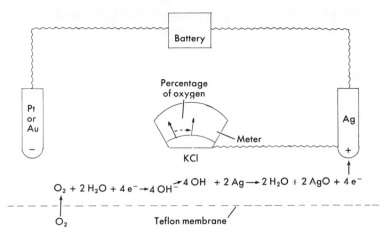

Fig. 26-25 Example of diagram for polarographic (Clark-type) electrode for gaseous oxygen measurement. (From McPherson SP: Respiratory therapy equipment, ed 3, St Louis, 1985, Mosby.)

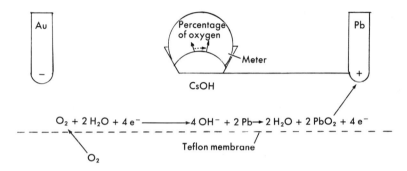

Fig. 26-26 Example of diagram for galvanic fuel cell for gaseous oxygen analysis. (From McPherson SP: Respiratory therapy equipment, ed 3, St Louis, 1985, Mosby.)

The polarographic analyzer electrode is basically the same as that in blood gas analyzers (see Chapter 17). The probe has a platinum or gold anode and a silver cathode (Figure 26-25). A small battery-generated current maintains electrode polarity and speeds the reaction, thus providing a relatively fast response time.

The galvanic fuel also employs a gold anode, but usually has a lead cathode. However, unlike the Clark electrode, current flow is sustained solely by the chemical reaction itself (Figure 26-26). Thus, unless accessories such as warning alarms are provided, the galvanic fuel cell needs no external electrical power. Unfortunately, this advantage carries a cost: galvanic fuel cells tend to have slower response times than Clark electrodes. Table 26-8 provides a summary of the principles and features of the oxygen analyzers used in respiratory care.

Table 26-8 Comparison of oxygen analyzers

	Physical (paramagnetic)	Electrical (thermal conduction)	Electrochemical (polarographic)	Electrochemical (galvanic cell)
Parameter measured	Partial pressure	Oxygen concentration	Partial pressure	Partial pressure
Accurate with other gases?	Yes	Oxygen and nitrogen only	Yes	Yes
Sampling technique	Intermittent/static sample	Intermittent/static sample	Continuous/dynamic	Continuous/dynamic
Use with flammable gases?	Yes	No	Yes	Yes
Oxygen consumption	No	No	Yes	Yes

Problem-solving and troubleshooting

Essentially all clinical oxygen analysis is now made with electrochemical devices. For accurate results, these devices must be properly calibrated. While variations in procedure exist among equipment, all electrochemical devices use a two-point calibration.

A typical two-point calibration involves exposing the sensor to two levels of oxygen. In the most common procedure, the RCP first exposes the electrode or fuel cell to air. If the reading on air is not 21%, the RCP adjusts the device's 'offset' control until it reads 21%. Then the RCP exposes the sensor to 100% oxygen. If the device reads 100% at this concentration, the analyzer is properly calibrated and can be used to assess F_DO_2. If the device does not read 100% at this concentration, a separate gain control on some systems may allow recalibration.

Failure to read (or calibrate to) 100% when exposed to 100% oxygen indicates analyzer malfunction. The most common causes of analyzer malfunction are: (1) low batteries, (2) sensor depletion, and (3) electronic failure.

Since a low battery condition is so common, the first step in troubleshooting these devices should be to replace the batteries. If the analyzer still does not calibrate with fresh batteries, the problem is probably a depleted sensor.

In terms of sensor depletion, spent fuel cells must be replaced. Clark electrodes, however, can be 'recharged,' usually by cleaning the anode and cathodes and replacing the electrolyte solution.

If the analyzer still fails to calibrate after battery and sensor replacement, the most likely problem is an internal failure of its electrical system. In this case, the RCP should make sure the device is taken out of service and sent for repair or replacement. Failure to recognize malfunction or take defective equipment out of service can have disastrous consequences.[142]

Inaccurate readings can also occur with electrochemical analyzers due to either condensed water vapor or pressure fluctuations. Galvanic cells are particularly sensitive to condensation. When used continuously, these systems should ideally be placed in the delivery circuit *proximal* to any heated humidifier or nebulizer.

Fuel cell and Clark electrode readings are also affected by **ambient** pressure changes. Under conditions of low pressure (high altitude), these devices read lower than the actual oxygen concentration. Conversely, higher pressures, as occur during positive pressure ventilation, cause these devices to read higher than the actual F_DO_2. Of course, these observations are consistent with the fact that both devices actually measure the PO_2, but use a percent concentration scale.

Selecting a delivery approach

With the wide variety of techniques available for giving oxygen, it is obvious that there is no one best method. Although the decision to give oxygen is a medical one, it is not always easy for the physician to know exactly which approach is the best for a given patient. For this reason, the RCP should be involved in the initial selection of an appropriate delivery system. Ideally, the RCP also should be responsible for ongoing oversight of the prescribed therapy. This responsibility should include making recommenda-

---

■ MINI C LINI ■

26-5

Effect of Water Vapor on a Polarographic Oxygen Analyzer

Problem: Assume that a polarographic oxygen analyzer is calibrated to read 100% when analyzing dry pure oxygen from a flowmeter attached to a 50 psi wall outlet. If this unit's sensor is then placed in a ventilator circuit where gas is 100% saturated with water vapor at 37°C, will the device still record 100% O_2?

Discussion: A polarographic analyzer is sensitive to the number of oxygen molecules that diffuse through its sensing membrane. The device thus measures PO_2, although it is calibrated to register in concentration (percentage) units. A dry gas sample of 100% O_2 would have a partial pressure of 760 torr at sea level. A polarographic analyzer calibrated to register 100% when analyzing this sample interprets a $PO_2 = 7.6$ torr as 1%

oxygen. If this analyzer is then used to analyze a sample of 100% oxygen at 37°C and 100% saturated with water vapor, it is actually exposed to a different PO_2. This saturated gas sample's PO_2 is 1.0 (760−47) = 713 torr. (The partial pressure of water vapor at 37°C, 100% relative humidity is 47 torr; because barometric pressure is 760 torr, PO_2 must be 713 torr). The analyzer still "sees" 7.6 torr PO_2 as 1% oxygen. Because actual PO_2 is 713 torr, the analyzer will register 713/760 or 93.8% oxygen. This discrepancy can be corrected by simply calibrating the analyzer on 100% saturated gas.

tions—based on sound patient assessment—changing or discontinuing the treatment regimen.

When selecting or recommending a change in oxygen delivery system, the RCP should always remember the 'three Ps': *Purpose*, *Patient*, and *Performance*. The goal is always to match the performance characteristics of the equipment to both the objectives of therapy (purpose) *and* the patient's special needs.

Purpose

The general purpose or objective for all O_2 therapy is to raise the FiO_2 sufficiently to correct arterial hypoxemia. Other objectives, including decreasing hypoxic symptoms and minimizing increased cardiopulmonary work, follow from this primary purpose.

Patient

Key patient considerations in selecting O_2 therapy equipment for use in the acute care setting are summarized in the accompanying box. Knowledge of these factors will help guide the RCP in selecting the appropriate equipment. For example, in a moderately hypoxemic adult patient with an endotracheal tube in place, our selection will generally be limited to either an air-entrainment nebulizer or O_2 blender/humidifier system connected to a T-tube (Brigg's adapter). On the other hand, an infant with moderate hypoxia and a normal airway usually will require an oxygen enclosure (hood or enclosed incubator).

Equipment performance

As previously described, oxygen systems vary according to both the actual FDO_2 and the stability of the FiO_2 under changing patient demands. As a general rule, the more critically ill the patient, the greater the need for stable, high FDO_2s. Conversely, less acutely ill individuals generally will require lower, less exact FDO_2s.

General goals and patient categories

Based on overall consideration of these 'three Ps,' general goals can be set for several major patient categories.

In emergency situations where tissue hypoxia is suspected, patients should be given as high an FiO_2 as possible, ideally 100%. This can be achieved via either a true high-flow or closed reservoir system. The goal is the highest possible blood oxygen content. Clinical examples include respiratory/cardiac arrest, severe trauma, shock, carbon monoxide poisoning and cyanide poisoning. Carbon monoxide and cyanide poisoning may require hyperbaric oxygen therapy (discussed subsequently).

In the critically ill adult patient with moderate to severe hypoxemia, either a reservoir or high-flow system capable of at least 60% oxygen should initially be chosen. Thereafter, changes in FDO_2 (and device) should be based on assessment of physiologic parameters, with the goal being a PaO_2 above 60 torr or a hemoglobin saturation above 90%.

Among more stable, but acutely ill adults suffering from mild to moderate hypoxemia, systems capable of low to moderate oxygen concentrations should be chosen. In these cases, stability of FiO_2 is not critical. Applicable devices include the nasal cannula at moderate flows or a simple mask. Common examples include patients in the immediate post-op phase or those recovering from acute myocardial infarction.

Adult patients with chronic lung disease and an accompanying acute-on-chronic hypoxemia present a special case. In this group, the goal is to ensure adequate arterial oxygenation without depressing ventilation. Adequate oxygenation for these patients generally means an SaO_2 in 85% to 90% range, with PaO_2s between 50 and 60 torr.[60,104,143,144] Normally this is achieved with either low-flow nasal oxygen or a low concentration (24% to 28%) AEM. The less stable the patient, the greater the need for the high-flow AEM.

Patients with COPD or diffuse interstitial lung disease who have hypoxic-related conditions that may improve with oxygen are candidates for long-term continuous low-flow O_2 therapy.[145-149] Examples of hypoxic-related conditions that may improve with oxygen therapy are listed in the accompanying box.

These patients typically receive oxygen therapy in the home setting. Here, considerations of patient comfort, cost, and convenience are paramount. For this reason, oxygen conserving devices, such as pulsed delivery systems and transtracheal catheters, are the

---

Key patient factors when selecting oxygen therapy equipment
■ Severity/cause of hypoxemia
■ Patient age group (infant, child, adult)
■ Degree of consciousness/alertness
■ Presence/absence of a tracheal airway
■ Stability of the minute ventilation

Hypoxic-related conditions that may improve with oxygen therapy
■ Pulmonary hypertension
■ Recurring congestive heart failure (CHF)
■ Chronic cor pulmonale
■ Erythrocytosis
■ Impaired cognitive processes
■ Nocturnal restlessness
■ Morning headache

first choice.[83] The need for continuous long-term O_2 therapy in general, and oxygen conserving devices in particular, are covered in Chapter 38 (Respiratory Home Care).

Last, children and infants requiring oxygen therapy deserve special consideration. This is due to both the unique hazards associated with oxygen delivery to these patients, and their poor tolerance for airway appliances. These considerations are detailed in Chapter 35.

HYPERBARIC OXYGEN THERAPY

Hyperbaric oxygen therapy (HBO) is the therapeutic use of oxygen at pressures greater than one atmosphere.[150] Pressures during HBO usually are expressed in multiples of atmospheric pressure absolute, or **ATA.** One ATA equals 760 torr or 101.32 kPa. Most HBO is conducted at pressures between 2 and 3 ATA.[151,152]

Physiologic effects

The known physiologic effects of HBO are summarized in the accompanying box.[150,153] These effects are due mainly to either high pressure or high oxygen tensions in body fluids and tissues (hyperoxia).

In conditions like air embolism and decompression sickness, high pressure exerts a physical effect on air or nitrogen bubbles trapped in the blood or tissues.[154] According to Boyle's Law, high pressure reduces the size of these bubbles and thus minimize their potential harm. With pressure crucial in these cases, HBO treatments may be conducted at pressures of 6 ATA or more.[151]

The second beneficial effect of HBO is hyperoxia. Breathing room air, only a small amount of oxygen dissolves in the plasma (about 0.3 mL/dL). At 3 ATA, plasma contains nearly 7 mL/dL dissolved oxygen, a level exceeding average resting tissue uptake.

O_2 supply to the tissues affects the immune system, wound healing, and vascular tone. A tissue PO_2 of at least 30 mm Hg is necessary for normal cellular function. Lower PO_2s are often seen in damaged and infected tissues. Increasing oxygen supply to the tissues can help restore both white blood cell function and antimicrobial activity.[155,156]

Hyperoxia also effects the cardiovascular system. HBO causes generalized vasoconstriction and a small drop in cardiac output. Although these changes may decrease blood flow to a region, this is more than offset by the increase in O_2 content. In conditions such as burns, cerebral edema, and crush injuries, vasoconstriction may be helpful, reducing edema and tissue swelling while maintaining tissue oxygenation.[157]

Last, hyperoxia helps form new capillary beds, a process called **neovascularization.** Although its exact mechanism is unknown, neovascularization is an

essential component of tissue repair, especially in radiation-induced injuries.[151]

Methods of administration

HBO is administered via either a multiplace or a monoplace chamber. A multiplace chamber is a large tank capable of holding up to a dozen or more people (Figure 26-27, *A*). Since patients are directly cared for by medical staff inside the tank, multiplace chambers have air-locks that allows entry and egress without altering the pressure. Normally, the multiplace chamber is filled with air. Only the patient breathes 100% oxygen (via mask or other device). Because multiplace chambers can achieve pressures of 6 ATA or more, they are ideal for decompression sickness and air embolism.[151]

The typical monoplace chamber consists of a transparent Plexiglas cylinder large enough only for a single patient (Figure 26-27, *B*). During therapy, the cylinder oxygen concentration is kept at 100%. Thus, the patient need not wear a mask. Due to the high O_2 concentration, most electronic equipment cannot be used in a monoplace chamber. In addition, many ventilators do not function properly under these conditions.[158,159] However, monitoring systems and ventilators can be specially adapted to allow treatment of the critically ill under hyperbaric pressures.[150]

Indications

HBO has long been accepted as the primary treatment for decompression sickness suffered by divers.[154] Other indications for HBO are listed in the accompanying box.[150,151,160] The two most common acute conditions that the RCP will see treated with HBO are air embolism and carbon monoxide poisoning.

Air embolism

Air embolism is a complication that can occur with certain cardiovascular procedures, lung biopsy, hemodialysis, and central line placement.[161-165] If air bubbles reach the cerebral or cardiac circulation, they can cause severe neurologic symptom or sudden death.

Physiologic effects of hyperbaric oxygen therapy[150,153]
Bubble reduction (Boyle's Law)
Hyperoxygenation of blood and tissue (Henry's Law)
Vasoconstriction
Enhanced host immune function
Neovascularization

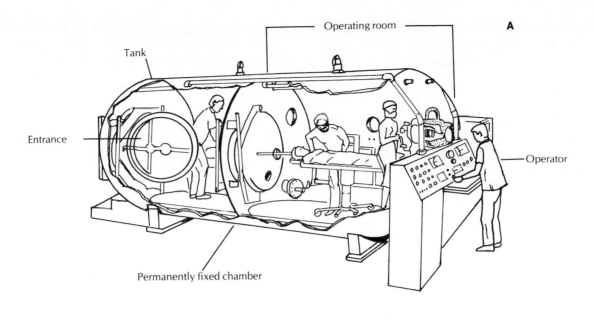

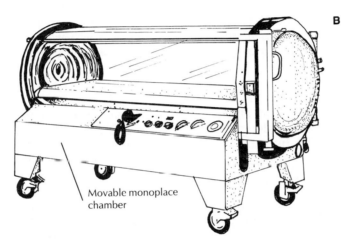

Fig. 26-27 A, Fixed hyperbaric chamber. **B,** Monoplace chamber.

Indications for hyperbaric oxygen therapy[150,151,160]

Acute conditions
  Decompression sickness
  Air or gas embolism
  Carbon monoxide and/or cyanide poisoning
  Acute traumatic ischemias (compartment
    syndrome; crush injury)
  Clostridial gangrene
  Necrotizing soft-tissue infection
  Ischemic skin grafts or flaps
  Exceptional blood loss

Chronic conditions
  Enhanced healing of problem wounds
  Refractory osteomyelitis
  Radiation necrosis

HBO decreases the air bubbles' volume and helps oxygenate local tissues. Typical treatment for air embolism involves immediate pressurization in air to 6 ATA for 15 to 30 minutes. This is followed by decompression to 2.8 ATA with prolonged oxygen treatment.[151]

Carbon monoxide poisoning

Carbon monoxide (CO) poisoning accounts for half of all poisonings deaths in the U.S. Patients suffering from carbon monoxide poisoning improve quickly when treated with HBO.[166-170] This is because HBO is the fastest way to remove carbon monoxide from the blood. If a patient breathes air, it takes over five hours to remove just half of the blood's carboxyhemoglobin. Breathing 100% oxygen reduces this 'half-life' to 80 minutes. The half-life of carboxyhemoglobin under HBO at 3 ATA is only 23 minutes.[171] The

---

**Criteria for HBO therapy for
acute carbon monoxide
poisoning[151]**

History of unconsciousness
Presence of neuropsychiatric abnormality
Presence of cardiac instability or cardiac ischemia
Carboxyhemoglobin level > 25% (lower levels in
children and pregnant women)

---

box above lists current criteria for selecting patients
with acute carbon monoxide poisoning for treatment
with HBO.[151]

Complications and hazards

The common complications of HBO are listed in the
box below.[151] These complications are due to either
high pressure or oxygen toxicity. The most frequent
problems involve barotrauma to closed body cavities,
such as the middle ear or sinuses.[172] Pneumothroax
and air embolism are also possible during HBO
treatment, but are rare in patients with normal
lungs.[173]

As previously discussed, oxygen at high pressures
can be **neurotoxic.** Early signs of impending CNS
toxicity include twitching, sweating, **pallor,** and restlessness. This is usually followed by seizures and
convulsions. However, CNS toxicity is rarely seen
with the pressures and treatment times commonly
used for clinical HBO therapy.[160]

In terms of pulmonary oxygen toxicity, HBO treatments do not normally exposes patients to high PO_2s
long enough to cause damage. However, HBO may
have an additive effect on critically ill patients who
receive high FIO_2s between HBO treatments.[151]

**Major complications of
hyperbaric therapy[151]**

Barotrauma

Ear or sinus trauma
Tympanic membrane rupture
Pneumothorax
Air embolism

Oxygen toxicity

Central nervous system toxic reaction
Pulmonary toxic reactions

Other

Fire
Sudden decompression
Reversible visual changes
Claustrophobia

Avoiding fires and sudden decompression are primary safety concerns. Only 100% cotton material
should be used to avoid static electrical discharge. No
alcohol or petroleum-based products should be used,
and the patient must not wear sprays, makeup, or
deodorant.

Problems-solving and troubleshooting

Although fire hazards restrict the use of certain electronic equipment, some monitors and ventilators
with solid-state circuitry can be used within the
chamber, allowing intensive care of critically ill patients.[150]

In regard to ventilator use, reductions in delivered
tidal volumes should be expected and corrected.[150] If
not accounted for, this problem can lead to respiratory hypercapnia and acidosis. Hypercapnia, in turn,
can worsen CNS toxicity, due to cerebral vasodilation.

Last, pressure and flow regulating equipment used
in a hyperbaric chamber must either be specifically
designed for operation at chamber pressures or appropriately modified for this use.

OTHER MEDICAL GAS THERAPIES

Although oxygen is the primary medical gas used by
the RCP, three other gas mixtures bear mention.
These include carbon dioxide (CO_2), helium (He), and
nitric oxide (NO). Carbon dioxide is included here for
historical completeness only, having been replaced by
other approaches. Helium therapy is undergoing renewed emphasis as an adjunct tool in certain forms of
airway obstruction. Last, nitric oxide, though still
under investigational use, show promise as a potent
pulmonary vasodilator.

Carbon dioxide therapy

Today, the therapeutic use of CO_2 is rare. CO_2 therapy
was once used to: (1) improve cerebral blood flow, (2)
stimulate deep breathing, and (3) treat refractory
singulation (hiccup, hiccough). These early uses for
CO_2 inhalation have been replaced by safer and more
effective modes of respiratory care.

Helium therapy

Helium's value as a therapeutic gas is based solely on
its low density. As detailed in Chapter 7, when flow is
turbulent, driving pressure is proportional to the
square of the flow time a constant related to gas
density. Since flow in the large airways is mainly
turbulent, use of a low density gas mixture in place of
air or O_2 will lower the driving pressure needed to
move gas in and out of this area. With less pressure
required to move gas through the large airways, the

patient's work of breathing will decrease. However, this effect is limited to large airway obstruction. Flow in the small airways is viscosity-dependent, not density-dependent.

Helium has been used as an adjunct tool in managing large airway obstruction for nearly 60 years.[174] Barach described the rationale for using helium in 1935 for decreasing the work of breathing,[175] and was still recommending its use for asthma in 1976.[176] Subsequently, helium-oxygen therapy has been shown effective in managing certain patients with COPD,[177] acute upper airway obstruction of various origin,[178-182] postextubation stridor in pediatric trauma patients,[183] and refractory viral croup.[184]

Guidelines for use

Because helium is inert and unable to support life, it must always be mixed with at least 20% oxygen. The most common combination is 80% helium and 20% oxygen. For practical purposes, this mixture is comparable to air, with helium used in place of nitrogen. However, while air has a density of 1.293 gm/L, the density of an 80% helium mixture is 0.429 gm/L. For a comparable flow through obstructed large airways, this low density mixture can dramatically lower the work of breathing.[174]

Although it is possible to mix helium and oxygen at the bedside, it is much safer and convenient to use commercially prepared cylinders of premixed gases. In addition to the 80/20 combination, a mixture of 70% He/30% O_2 is commonly available (density = 0.554 gm/L). This mixture provides additional oxygen which is helpful in treating the hypoxemia that can occur with large airway obstruction.

Due to helium's high diffusibility, mixtures of this gas generally should be given via either a closed system (such as a nonrebreathing mask) or a small-volume reservoir device, like a simple mask.[185] Due to leakage, low-flow nasal devices are ineffective for delivering helium mixtures. Large volume enclosures, such as hoods, are also unsatisfactory. This is because helium tends to concentrate at the top of these devices. Helium mixtures can also be given through cuffed tracheal airways via positive-pressure ventilators.[179]

When given by mask, the RCP should realize that a typical hospital oxygen flowmeter will not be accurate with a helium-oxygen mixture. Flowmeters calibrated for helium do exist, but they are not required. Instead, correction factors can be used. For example, the correction for an 80/20 helium-oxygen mixture is 1.8. This means that for every 10 L/min indicated flow, 10 × 1.8 or 18 L/min of the 80/20 mixture actually leave the flowmeter. Thus to deliver a specific flow from a 80/20 helium-oxygen source, the RCP would set the flowmeter to the desired flow *divided* by 1.8. Thus if a flow of 9 L/min of an 80/20 helium-oxygen mixture were needed, the RCP would set the flowmeter to 9/1.8 or 5 L/min. Factors for any other mixture can be

calculated if needed. The factor for a 70/30 helium-oxygen mixture is 1.6.

Problem-solving and troubleshooting

The low density of helium mixtures makes them poor vehicles for aerosol transport. High density bland water aerosols are difficult to delivered with helium mixtures, as are aerosolized drugs.

The low density of helium mixtures also make coughing less effective. An expulsive cough depends, in part, on the development of turbulent flow in the large airways. Since helium promotes laminar flow, clearance of secretions by coughing is impaired. Assuming the patient can develop an effective cough, this problem can be rectified by washing out the helium before coughing.

The most common side effect of helium is a benign one. When breathing helium mixtures, the spoken word is badly distorted at a pitch so high as to make it almost unintelligible. This is of importance only to the conscious, nonintubated patient, who should be warned of the effect and reassured that it will disappear immediately after stopping therapy.

A more serious problem are reports of hypoxemia associated with breathing helium mixtures.[186,187] Although these problems may have been caused by using too low an oxygen concentration (20%), there is another possibility. Specifically, some commercial cylinders of helium/oxygen have been found to contain these gases in an 'unmixed' or separated state.[188] The only way to avoid this potential hazard is to analyze the *oxygen* concentration coming from the cylinder before administering the gas mixture to a patient.

Nitric oxide therapy

While not yet FDA approved, nitric oxide is being used experimentally to treat certain forms of pulmonary hypertension. In very low concentrations (< 40 ppm) mixed with oxygen, nitric oxide selectively dilates the pulmonary blood vessels. This effect has proved beneficial in treating persistent pulmonary hypertension of the newborn (PPHN)[189] and the Adult Respiratory Distress Syndrome (ARDS).[190] However, more research is needed before this potentially hazardous gas becomes accepted for its therapeutic value.[191]

Even if approved for clinical use, nitric oxide will present several major technical issues.[191] First will be the problem of how to deliver nitric oxide/oxygen mixtures without producing other poisonous gases like nitrogen dioxide (NO_2). The second major problem will be how to accurately measure the concentration of NO and its by-products. RCPs will no doubt participate in overcoming these problems, and thus aid in the introduction of this promising new therapeutic gas.

CHAPTER SUMMARY

Medical gas therapy represents a major responsibility of the RCP. The safe and effective use of medical gases demands careful consideration of the patient's underlying disease process as the basis for determining an appropriate approach. Based on this foundation knowledge, the practitioner must be capable of matching a chosen modality to the patient's needs, and monitoring the patient's response according to the therapeutic goals chosen, with due consideration for potential hazards and contraindications.

REFERENCES

1. Fulmer JF, Snider GL: American College of Chest Physicians —National Heart, Lung and Blood Institute National Conference on Oxygen Therapy, *Chest* 86:224–247, 1984.
2. American Association for Respiratory Care: Clinical Practice Guideline—Oxygen Therapy in the Acute Care Hospital, *Respir Care*, 36(12):1410–1413, 1991.
3. American Association for Respiratory Care: Clinical Practice Guideline—Oxygen Therapy in the home or extended care facility, *Respir Care*, 37(8):918–922, 1991.
4. American Academy of Pediatrics, American College of Obstetricians and Gynecologists: *Guidelines for perinatal care*, ed 2, 1988.
5. Winter PM, Miller JN: Carbon monoxide poisoning, *JAMA* 1976;236:1502–1504.
6. Holland MA; Kozlowski LM: Clinical features and management of cyanide poisoning, *Clin Pharm* 5(9):737–41, 1986.
7. Snider GL, Rinaldo JE. Oxygen therapy in medical patients hospitalized outside of the intensive care unit, *Am Rev Respir Dis* 122(5, Part 2):29–36, 1980.
8. Maroko PR, Radvany P, Braunwell E, Hale SL: Reduction of infarct size by oxygen inhalation following acute coronary occlusion; *Circulation* 52:360–368, 1975.
9. Fairley HB: Oxygen therapy for surgical patients, *Am Rev Respir Dis* 122(5, Part 2):37–44, 1980.
10. Swinburn CR, Mould H, Stone TN, et al: Symptomatic benefit of supplemental oxygen in hypoxemic patients with chronic lung disease, *Am Rev Respir Dis* 143(5 Pt 1):913–915, 1991.
11. Block AJ: Neuropsychologic aspects of oxygen therapy, *Respir Care* 28(7):885–888, 1983.
12. Continuous or nocturnal oxygen therapy in hypoxemic chronic obstructive lung disease: a clinical trial. Nocturnal Oxygen Therapy Trial Group, *Ann Intern Med* 93(3):391–398, 1980.
13. MacNee W, Wathen CG, Flenley DC, Muir AD: The effects of controlled oxygen therapy on ventricular function in patients with stable and decompensated cor pulmonale, *Am Rev Respir Dis* 137(6):1289–1295, 1988.
14. Ryerson EG, Block AJ: Oxygen as a drug: clinical properties, benefits, modes, and hazards of administration, In Burton GG, Hodgkin JE, Ward JJ: Respiratory Care: *A Guide to Clinical Practice*, ed 3, Philadelphia, 1991, JB Lippincott.
15. Smoker JM, Hess DR, Frey-Zeiler VL, et al: A protocol to assess oxygen therapy, *Respir Care* 31(1):35–39, 1986.
16. Hess D: Techniques and devices for monitoring oxygenation, *Respir Care* 38(6):646–669, 1993.
17. Lodato RF: Oxygen toxicity, *Crit Care Clin* 6(3):749–765, 1990.
18. Fisher AB: Oxygen therapy: side effects and toxicity, *Am Rev Respir Dis* 122(5, Part 2):61–69, 1980.
19. Winter PM, Smith G: The toxicity of oxygen, *Anesthesiology* 37:210, 1972.
20. Pratt PC: Pathology of oxygen toxicity, *Am. Rev. Respir. Dis* 110(2):51, 1974.
21. Clark JM: The toxicity of oxygen, *Am. Rev. Resp. Dis.* 110(2):40, 1974.
22. Frank L, Massaro D: Oxygen toxicity, *Am J Med* 69:117–126, 1980.
23. Bryan CL, Jenkinson SG: Oxygen toxicity, *Clin Chest Med* 9(1):141–152, 1988.
24. Jackson RM: Molecular, pharmacologic, and clinical aspects of oxygen-induced lung injury, *Clin Chest Med* 11(1):73–86, 1990.
25. Durbin, GD, Wallace, KK: Oxygen toxicity in the critically ill patient, *Respiratory Care*, 38(7):739–750.
26. Mithoefer JC, Karetsky MS, Mead GD: Oxygen therapy in respiratory failure, *N Engl J Med* 277:947–949, 1967.
27. Cullen, JH, and Kaemmerlen, JT: Effect of oxygen administration at low rates of flow in hypercapnic patients, *Am Rev Respir Dis* 95:116, 1967.
28. Hodgkin, JE, editor: *Chronic obstructive pulmonary disease: current concepts in diagnosis and comprehensive care*, Park Ridge, IL, 1979, American College of Chest Physicians.
29. Aubier M, Murciano D, Fournier M, Milic-Emili J, Pariente R, Derenne JP: Central respiratory drive in acute respiratory failure of patients with chronic obstructive pulmonary disease, *Am Rev Respir Dis* 122(2):191–199, 1980.
30. Aubier M, Murciano D, Milic-Emili J, Touaty E, Daghfous J, Pariente R, Derenne JP: Effects of the administration of O_2 on ventilation and blood gases in patients with chronic obstructive pulmonary disease during acute respiratory failure, *Am Rev Respir Dis* 122(5):747–754, 1980.
31. Sassoon CS, Hassell KT, Mahutte CK: Hyperoxic-induced hypercapnia in stable chronic obstructive pulmonary disease, *Am Rev Respir Dis* 135(4):907–911, 1987.
32. Kensey V, Jacobus J, Hemphill, F: Retrolental fibroplasia and the use of oxygen, *AMA Arch Ophthalmol* 56:481, 1956.
33. Kinsey VE, Arnold HJ, Kalina RE, et al: PaO_2 levels and retrolental fibroplasia: a report of the cooperative study, *Pediatrics* 60(5):655–668, 1977.
34. Hildebrand WL, Hilliard J, Schreiner R, et al: Use and abuse of oxygen in the newborn, *Am Fam Physician* 18(3):125–132, 1978.
35. Yu VY, Hookham DM, Nave JR: Retrolental fibroplasia—controlled study of 4 years' experience in a neonatal intensive care unit, *Arch Dis Child* 57(4):247–252, 1982.
36. George DS, et al: The latest on retinopathy of prematurity, *MCN* 13:254–258, 1988.
37. Flynn JT: Retinopathy of prematurity, *Pediatr Clin North Am* 34(6):1487–1516, 1987.
38. Flynn JT, Bancalari E, Bachynski BN, et al: Retinopathy of prematurity. Diagnosis, severity, and natural history, *Ophthalmology* 94(6):620–629, 1987.
39. Garner A: The role of hyperoxia in the aetiology of retinopathy of prematurity. *Doc Ophthalmol* 74(3):187–193, 1990.
40. Douglas ME, Downs JB, Dannemiller FJ, et al: Changes in pulmonary venous admixture with varying inspired oxygen, *Anesth Analg* 55:688, 1976.
41. Shapiro BA, Cane RD, Harrison RA, Steiner MC: Changes in intrapulmonary shunting with administration of 100 percent oxygen, *Chest* 77(2):138–141, 1980.
42. Register SD, Downs JB, Stock MC: Is 50% oxygen harmful? *Crit Care Med* 15:598, 1987.
43. West JB: *Pulmonary pathophysiology—the essentials*, ed 4, Baltimore, 1992, Williams & Wilkins.
44. Laurenzi GA, et al: Adverse effect of oxygen on tracheal mucus flow, *N Engl J Med* 279–333, 1978.
45. Sackner MA, Landa J, Hirsch J, Zapata A: pulmonary effects of oxygen breathing: a 6-hour study in normal men, *Ann Intern Med* 82:40–43, 1975.
46. Gilder H, McSherry CK: Mechanisms of oxygen inhibition of pulmonary surfactant synthesis, *Surgery* 76(1):72–79, 1974.
47. King RJ, Coalson JJ, Seidenfeld JJ, et al: O_2- and pneumonia-induced lung injury. II. Properties of pulmonary surfactant, *J Appl Physiol* 67(1):357–365, 1989.
48. Holm BA, Notter RH, Siegle J, Matalon S: Pulmonary physiological and surfactant changes during injury and recovery from hyperoxia, *J Appl Physiol* 59(5):1402–1409, 1985.

49. Jenkinson SG: Oxygen toxicity in acute respiratory failure, *Respir Care* 28:614–617, 1983.
50. Welch BE, Morgan TE, Clammon HG: Time concentration effects in relation to oxygen toxicity in man, *Fed Proc* 22:1053, 1963.
51. Caldwell PRB, Lee WL, Schildnaut HS, et al: Changes in lung volumes, diffusing capacity and blood gases in men breathing oxygen, *J Appl Physiol* 21:1477, 1966.
52. Hyde RW, Rawson AJ: Unintentional iatrogenic oxygen pneumonitis—response to therapy, *Ann Int Med* 71:517, 1969.
53. Flenley DC: Long-term oxygen therapy—state of the art, *Respir Care* 28:876–884, 1983.
54. Fridovich L: The biology of oxygen radicals, *Science* 20:875–880, 1978.
56. Griffith DE, Holden WE, Morris JF, et al: Effects of common therapeutic concentrations of oxygen on lung clearance of ^{99m}Tc DTPA and bronchoalveolar lavage albumin concentrations, *AM Rev Respir Dis* 134:233–237, 1986.
57. Petty, TL, Stanford, RE, and Neff, TA: Continuous oxygen therapy in chronic airway obstruction: observations on possible oxygen toxicity and survival, *Ann Intern Med* 753–762, 1971.
58. Steinberg KP, Pierson DJ: Clinical approaches to the patient with acute oxygenation failure, in Pierson DJ and Kacmarek RM (eds): *Foundations of respiratory care,* 1992, New York, Churchill Livingstone.
59. Mithoefer JC: Indications for oxygen therapy in chronic obstructive pulmonary disease, *Am Rev Respir Dis* 110 (part 2):35, 1974.
60. Hutchinson DCS, et al: Controlled oxygen therapy in respiratory failure, *B Med J* 2:1157, 1964.
61. American Academy of Pediatrics, American College of Obstetricians and Gynecologists: *Guidelines for perinatal care,* ed 2, Evanston, IL, 1988.
62. Kobayashi, and Murakami: Blindness of an adult caused by oxygen, *JAMA* 219:741, 1972.
63. Fairshter RD, Rosen SM, Smith WR, et al: Paraquat poisoning: new aspects of therapy, *Q J Med* 45:551–565, 1976.
64. Ingrassia TS, Ryu JH, Trastek VF, Rosenow EC: Oxygen-exacerbated bleomycin pulmonary toxicity, *Mayo Clin Proc* 66:173–178, 1991.
65. Leigh, JM: The evolution of oxygen therapy apparatus, *Anaesthesia* 29:462, 1974.
66. Demers, RR: Oxygen delivery systems for use in acute respiratory failure, *Respir Care,* 28:553–560, 1983.
67. Branson RD: The nuts and bolts of increasing arterial oxygenation: devices and techniques, *Respir Care* 38(6):672–686, 1993.
68. Shapiro BA, Harrison RA, Trout, CA: *Clinical application of respiratory care,* ed 4, Chicago, 1991, Mosby.
69. Leigh JM: Variation in performance of oxygen therapy devices, *Anesthesia,* 25:100, 1970.
70. Leigh JM: Variation in performance of oxygen therapy devices, *Ann Royal Coll Surg* 52:234, 1973.
71. Estey W: Subjective effects of dry versus humidified low-flow oxygen, *Respir Care* 25:1143–1144, 1980.
72. Levine ER: Low-flow oxygen without humidity, *Respir Ther* 16(4):11, 50, 1986.
73. Campbell E, Baker D, Crites-Silver P: Subjective effects of oxygen for delivery by nasal cannula: a prospective study, *Chest* 86:241–247, 1988.
74. Locke RG, Wolfson MR, Shaffer TH, et al: Inadvertent administration of positive end-distending pressure during nasal cannula flow, *Pediatrics* 91(1):135–8, 1993.
75. Frenckner B, Ehren H, Palmer K, Noren G: Pneumocephalus caused by a nasopharyngeal oxygen catheter, *Crit Care Med* 18(11):1287–1288, 1990.
76. Redding JS, McAfee DD, Parham AM: Oxygen concentrations received from commonly used delivery systems, *South Med J* 71:169, 1978.
77. Kory RC, et al: Comparative evaluation of oxygen therapy techniques, *JAMA,* 179:767, 1962.
78. Poulton TJ, Comer PB, Gibson RL: Tracheal oxygen concentrations with nasal cannula during oral and nasal breathing, *Respir Care* 25:739, 1980.
79. Gibson RL, et al: Actual tracheal oxygen concentrations with commonly used oxygen equipment, *Anesthesiology,* 4:471, 1976.
80. Schachter EN, Littner MR, Luddy P, Beck GJ: Monitoring of oxygen delivery systems in clinical practice, *Crit Care Med* 8(7): 405–409, 1980.
81. Ooi R, Joshi P, Soni N: An evaluation of oxygen delivery using nasal prongs, *Anaesthesia* 47(7):591–593, 1992.
82. Dunlevy CL, Tyl SE: The effect of oral versus nasal breathing on oxygen concentrations received from nasal cannulas, *Respir Care* 37:357–360, 1992.
83. O'Donohue, W: Oxygen conserving devices, *Respir Care* 32: 37–42, 1987.
84. Williams GR, Masters IB, Harris MA: Errors in low flow oxygen delivery systems, *Aust Paediatr J,* 25(6):370–371, 1989.
85. Jeffrey AA, Ray S, Douglas NJ: Accuracy of inpatient oxygen administration, *Thorax* 44(12):1036–1037, 1989.
86. Hess D, D'Agostino D, Magrosky, S, et al: Effect of nasal cannula displacement on arterial oxygen tension, *Respir Care* 29(1):21–24, 1984.
87. Petty, TL, Nett, LM, Lakshminarayan, S: A single nasal prong for continuous oxygen therapy [letter], *Chest* 64:146–147, 1973.
88. Toome, BK: Allergic contact dermatitis to a nasal cannula [letter], *Arch Dermatol* 125(4):571, 1989.
89. Jensen AG, Johnson A, Sandstedt S: Rebreathing during oxygen treatment with face mask. The effect of oxygen flow rates on ventilation, *Acta Anaesthesiol Scand* 35(4):289–292, 1991.
90. Campkin NT, Ooi RG, Soni NC: The rebreathing characteristics of the Hudson oxygen mask, *Anaesthesia* 48(3):239–242, 1993.
91. Collis JM, Berthune DW: Oxygen by face mask and nasal catheter, *Lancet* 1:787, 1967.
92. Goldstein RS, Young J, Rebuck AS: Effect of breathing pattern on oxygen concentration received from standard face masks, *Lancet* 2(8309):1188–1190, 1982.
93. Bethune DW, Collis JM: The evaluation of oxygen masks. A mechanical method, *Anaesthesia* 22(1):43–54, 1967.
94. Bethune DW; Collis JM: An evaluation of oxygen therapy equipment. Experimental study of various devices on the human subject, *Thorax* 22(3):221–225, 1967.
95. Milross J, Young IH, Donnelly P: The oxygen delivery characteristics of the Hudson Oxy-one face mask, *Anaesth Intensive Care* 17(2):180–184, 1989.
96. Committee on Public Health: A report: effective administration of inhalation therapy with special reference to ambulatory and emergency oxygen treatment, *Bull NY Acad Med* 38:135, 1962.
97. Boothby WM, Lovelace WR, Vihlein A: The BLB oxygen inhalation apparatus: improvements in design and efficiency by studies on oxygen percentages in alveolar air, *Proc Mayo Clin* 15:194–206, 1940.
98. Scacci, R: Air entrainment masks: jet mixing is how they work: the Bernoulli and Venturi principles are how they don't, *Respir Care,* 24:928, 1979.
99. McPherson, SP: Oxygen percentage accuracy of air-entrainment masks, *Respir Care,* 19:658, 1974.
100. Friedman SA, et al: Effects of changing jet flows on oxygen concentrations in adjustable entrainment masks (abstract), *Respir Care,* 25:1266, 1980.
101. Riggs JH: *Respiratory facts,* Philadelphia, 1988, FA Davis.
102. Barach AL, Eckman M: A mask apparatus which provides high concentrations with accurate control of the percentage of oxygen in the inspired air and without the accumulation of carbon dioxide, *J Aviation Med* 12:39, 1941.
103. Barach AL, Eckman M: A physiologically controlled oxygen mask apparatus, *Anesthesiology* 2:421, 1941.
104. Campbell, EJM: A method of controlled oxygen administration which reduces the risk of carbon dioxide retention, *Lancet* 1:12, 1960.

105. Cohen JL, et al: Air-entrainment masks: A performance evaluation, *Respir Care* 22:277, 1977.

106. Woolner DF, Larkin J: An analysis of the performance of a variable venturi-type oxygen mask, *Anaesth Intensive Care* 8(1):44–51, 1980.

107. Hunter J, Olson LG: Performance of the Hudson Multi-Vent oxygen mask, *Med J Aust* 148(9):444–447, 1988.

108. Fracchia G, Torda TA: Performance of venturi oxygen delivery devices, *Anaesth Intensive Care* 8(4):426–430, 1980.

109. Cox D, Gillbe C: Fixed performance oxygen masks. Hypoxic hazard of low-capacity drugs, *Anaesthesia* 36(10):958–964, 1981.

110. Hill SL, Barnes PK, Hollway T, Tennant R: Fixed performance oxygen masks: an evaluation, *Br Med J* (Clin Res Ed) 288(6426):1261–1263, 1984.

111. Lyew MA, Holland AJ, Metcalf IR: Combined air and oxygen entrainment. Effect on the percentage output of fixed performance masks, *Anaesthesia* 45(9):732–735, 1990.

112. Spier WA, et al: Oxygen concentration delivered by venturi masks with in-line humidification, *JAMA* 216:879, 1971.

113. Farney RJ, et al: Oxygen therapy: appropriate use of nebulizers, *Am Rev Respir Dis* 115:567, 1977.

114. McPherson SP: *Respiratory therapy equipment,* ed 4, St Louis, 1990, Mosby.

115. Monast RL, Kaye W: Problems in delivering desired oxygen concentrations from jet nebulizers to patients via face tents, *Respir Care* 29(10):994–1000, 1984.

116. Bar ZG: Predictive equation for peak inspiratory flow, *Respir Care* 30(9):766–770, 1985.

117. Klein EF, Mon BK, and Mon MJ: Oxygen accuracy with venturi nebulizer systems (abstract), *Crit Care Med* 7:186, 1979.

118. Durham J, Miller WF: Controlled oxygen administration with adequate humidification, *Inhal Ther* 14:87, 1969.

119. Hartmann-Andersen F, Andersen PK, Olsen JE: Admixture of atmospheric air in the T-piece used as a weaning system, *Acta Anaesthesiol Scand* 25(1):63–6, 1981.

120. Kacmarek RM: Methods of oxygen delivery in the hospital, In Christopher, KL, editor: The current status of oxygen therapy, *Probl Respir Care* 3:563–574, 1990.

121. Foust GN, Potter WA, Wilons MD, Golden EB: Shortcomings of using two jet nebulizers in tandem with an aerosol face mask for optimal oxygen therapy, *Chest* 99:1346–1351, 1991.

122. Fried JL, Downs JB, Davis JEP, Heenan TJ: A new venturi device for administering continuous positive airway pressure (CPAP), *Respir Care* 26:133–136, 1981.

123. Atlas, G: Calculating F_DO_2 for mixtures of air and oxygen [letter], *Respir Care* 37(5):477–478, 1992.

124. Emergency Care Research Institute: Inaccurate O_2 concentrations from oxygen-air proportioners, *Health Devices* 18(10):366–367, 1989.

125. Karmann U, Roth F: Prevention of accidents associated with air-oxygen mixers, *Anaesthesia* 37(6):680–682, 1982.

126. Scott LR, et al: Performance characteristics of five models of air-oxygen blenders under various simulated clinical conditions, *Respir Care* 31(1):31–34, 1986.

127. Emergency Care Research Institute: Air proportioners, *Health Devices* 14:263–267, 1985.

128. Munford BJ, Wishaw KJ: Critical incidents with nonrebreathing valves, *Anaesth Intensive Care* 18(4):560–563, 1990.

129. Smith J, Conway B, Mackenzie CF, Matjasko J: Nonrebreathing valve competence, *Crit Care Med* 15(4):328–330, 1987.

130. Disposable T-tube oxygenators: do not use before inspecting or testing, *Health Devices* 21(3–4):137–138, 1992.

131. Poulton TJ, Downs JB: Humidification of rapidly flowing gas, *Crit Care Med* 9(1):59–63, 1981.

132. Klaus MH, Fanaroff AA, editors: *Care of the high risk neonate,* ed 3, Philadelphia, 1986, Saunders.

133. Gale R, Redner-Carmi R, Gale J: Accumulation of carbon dioxide in oxygen hoods, infant cots, and incubators, *Pediatrics* 60(4):453–456, 1977.

134. Dawes GW, Williams TJ: The oxygen hood as a noise factor in infant care, (abstract) *Respir Care,* 24:12, 1979.

135. Scopes J, and Ahmed I: Ranges of critical temperatures in sick and premature newborn babies, *Arch Dis Child* 41:417, 1966.

136. Hildebrand WL, Hilliard J, Schreiner R, et al: Use and abuse of oxygen in the newborn, *Am Fam Physician* 18(3):125–32. 1978.

137. Emergency Care Research Institute: Air-Shields Vickers C-86 infant incubators, *Health Devices* 17(10):314–315, 1988.

138. Nobel JJ: Infant incubators, *Pediatr Emerg Care* 7(6):365–366, 1991.

139. Oelberg DG, Adcock EW: Oxygen hoods: an unusual cause of neonatal flexion contractures, *Am J Dis Child* 137(2):182, 1983.

140. Wilson RS, and Taver MB: Oxygen analysis: advances in methodology, *Anesthesiology* 37:112, 1972.

141. Bageant RA: Oxygen analyzers, *Respir Care* 24:410, 1979.

142. Baker AJ, Hall R: Malfunction of Hudson electrochemical oxygen sensor [letter], *Anaesth Intensive Care* 17(4):516–518, 1989.

143. O'Donohue WJ, Baker JP: Controlled low-flow oxygen for respiratory failure, *Chest,* 63:818, 1973.

144. Bone RC, Pierce AK, Johnson RL: Controlled oxygen administration in acute respiratory failure in chronic obstructive pulmonary disease: A reappraisal, *Am J Med* 65:896, 1978.

145. Petty TL, et al: Outpatient oxygen therapy in chronic obstructive pulmonary disease a review of 13 years' experience and an evaluation of modes of therapy, *Arch Intern Med* 139:28, 1979.

146. Nocturnal Oxygen Therapy Trial Group: Continuous or nocturnal oxygen therapy in hypoxemic chronic obstructive lung disease, *Ann Intern Med* 93:391, 1980.

147. Anthonisen NR: Home oxygen therapy in chronic obstructive pulmonary disease, *Clin Chest Med* 7(4):673–678, 1986.

148. O'Donohue WJ: Home oxygen therapy. Why, when and how to write a proper prescription, *Postgrad Med* 87(2):59–61, 1990.

149. Tiep BL: Long-term home oxygen therapy, *Clin Chest Med* 11(3):505–521, 1990.

150. Weaver LK: Hyperbaric treatment of respiratory emergencies, *Respir Care* 37(7):720–734, 1992.

151. Grim PS, Gottlieb LJ, Boddie A, Batson E: Hyperbaric oxygen therapy, *JAMA* 263(16):2216–2220, 1990.

152. NHLBI workshop summary: Hyperbaric oxygenation therapy, *Am Rev Respir Dis* 144(6):1414–21, 1991.

153. Hyperbaric Oxygen Therapy: A Committee Report Bethesda, MD: Undersea and Hyperbaric Medical Society, 1986.

154. Francis TJ, Dutka AJ, Hallenbeck JM: Pathophysiology of decompression sickness. In: Bove AA, Davis JC, editors: *Diving Medicine* Philadelphia, Pa, 1990 Saunders.

155. Forman HJ, Thomas MI: Oxidant production and bactericidal activity of phagocytes, *Ann Rev Physiol* 48:669–680, 1986.

156. Knighton DR, Halliday B, Hunt TK: Oxygen as an antibiotic: the effect of inspired oxygen on infection, *Arch Surg* 119:199–204, 1984.

157. Nylander G, Lewis D, Nordstrom H, Larsson J: Reduction of postischemic edema with hyperbaric oxygen, *Plast Reconstr Surg* 76:596–601, 1985.

158. Blanch PB, Desautels DA, Gallagher TJ: Deviations in function of mechanical ventilators during hyperbaric compression, *Respir Care* 36(8):803–814, 1991.

159. Youn BA, Houseknecht R, DeAntonio A: Review of positive-end expiratory pressure and its application in the hyperbaric environment, *J Hyperbaric Med* 6(2):87, 1991.

160. Davis JC, Dunn JM, Heimbach RD: Hyperbaric medicine: patient selection, treatment procedures, and side effects. In Davis JC, Hunt TK, eds: *Problem Wounds: The Role of Oxygen.* New York, Elsevier Science Publishing, 1988.

161. Thomatis L, Nemiroff M, Riahi M, et al: Massive arterial air embolism due to rupture of pulsatile assist device: successful treatment in the hyperbaric chamber, *Ann Thorac Surg* 32:604–608, 1981.
162. Peirce EC II: Specific therapy for arterial air embolism, *Ann Thorac Surg* 29:300–303, 1980.
163. Cianci P, Posin JP, Shimshak RR, Singzon J: Air embolism complicating percutaneous thin needle biopsy of lung, *Chest* 92:749–750, 1987.
164. Baskin FE, Wozniak RL: Hyperbaric oxygenation in the treatment of hemodialysis associated air embolism, *N Engl J Med* 293:184–185, 1975.
165. Murphy BP, Hartford FJ, Cramer FS: Cerebral air embolism resulting from invasive medical procedures: treatment with hyperbaric oxygen, *Ann Surg* 201:242–245, 1985.
166. Myers RAM, Snyder SK, Linberg S, Cowley RA: Value of hyperbaric oxygen in suspected carbon monoxide poisoning, *JAMA* 246:2478–2480, 1981.
167. Norkool DM, Kirkpatrick JN: Treatment of acute carbon monoxide poisoning with hyperbaric oxygen: a review of 115 cases, *Ann Emerg Med* 14:1168–1171, 1985.
168. Goldbaum LR, Ramirez RG, Absalom KB: What is the mechanism of carbon monoxide toxicity? *Aviat Space Environ Med* 46:1289–1291, 1975.
169. Jackson DL, Menges H: Accidental carbon monoxide poisoning, *JAMA* 243:772–774, 1980.
170. Kindwall EP: Carbon monoxide poisoning treated with hyperbaric oxygen, *Respir Ther* 5:29–33, 1975.
171. Peterson JE, Stewart RD: Absorption and elimination of carbon monoxide by inactive young men, *Arch Environ Health* 21:165–175, 1970.
172. Bassett BE, Bennett PB: Introduction to the physical and physiological bases of hyperbaric therapy. In Davis JC, Hunt TK, editors, *Hyperbaric Oxygen Therapy*. Bethesda, MD: Undersea and Hyperbaric Medical Society, 1977.
173. Bond GF: Arterial gas embolism. In Davis JC, Hunt, TK, eds. *Hyperbaric Oxygen Therapy*. Bethesda, Md: Undersea and Hyperbaric Medical Society, 1977.
174. Egan DF: Therapeutic uses of helium, *Conn Med* 31:355, 1967.
175. Barach, AL: The use of helium in the treatment of asthma and obstructive lesions of the larynx and trachea, *Ann Intern Med* 9:739, 1935.
176. Weiss EG, Segal MS, editors: *Bronchial asthma: Mechanisms and therapeutics*, Boston, Little, Brown & Co, 1976.
177. Ishikawa, Segal, MS: Re-appraisal of helium-oxygen therapy on patients with chronic lung disease, *Ann Allergy* 31:536, 1973.
178. Lu TS, et al: Helium-oxygen in the treatment of upper airway obstruction, *Anesthesiology* 45:678, 1976.
179. Motley HL: Helium-oxygen therapy, *Respir Care* 18:668, 1973.
180. Boorstein JM, Boorstein SM, Humphries GN, Johnston CC: Using helium-oxygen mixtures in the emergency management of acute upper airway obstruction, *Ann Emerg Med* 18(6):688–690, 1989.
181. Skrinskas GJ, Hyland RH, Hutcheon MA: Using helium-oxygen mixtures in the management of acute upper airway obstruction, *Can Med Assoc J* 128(5):555–558, 1983.
182. Curtis JL, Mahlmeister M, Fink JB, et al: Helium-oxygen gas therapy. Use and availability for the emergency treatment of inoperable airway obstruction, *Chest* 90(3):455–457, 1986.
183. Kemper KJ, Ritz RH, Benson MS, Bishop MS: Helium-oxygen mixture in the treatment of postextubation stridor in pediatric trauma patients, *Crit Care Med* 19(3):356–359, 1991.
184. Nelson DS, McClellan L: Helium-oxygen mixtures as adjunctive support for refractory viral croup, *Ohio State Med J* 78(10):729–730, 1982.
185. Stillwell PC, Quick JD, Munro PR, Mallory GB: Effectiveness of open-circuit and oxyhood delivery of helium-oxygen, *Chest* 95(6):1222–1224, 1989.
186. Ravenel SD: Hypoxemia following inhalation of helium-oxygen [letter], *J Pediatr* 109(2):392–393, 1986.
187. Bull WW, Koren G, England S, et al: Hypoxia associated with helium-oxygen therapy in neonates, *J Pediatr* 106(3):474–476, 1985.
188. Emergency Care Research Institute: Cylinders with unmixed helium/oxygen, *Health Devices* 19(4):146, 1990.
189. Roberts JD, Polaner DM, Lang P, Zapol WM: Inhaled nitric oxide in persistent pulmonary hypertension of the newborn, *Lancet* 340(8823):818–9, 1992.
190. Bone RC: A new therapy for the adult respiratory distress syndrome, *N Engl J Med* 328(6):431–2, 1993.
191. Miller CC, Miller JW: Pulmonary vascular smooth muscle regulation: the role of inhaled nitric oxide gas, *Respir Care* 37(10):1175–1185.

27

Lung Expansion Therapy

∎

Craig L. Scanlan
Alan Realey
Linda Earl

Lung expansion therapy include a variety of respiratory care modalities designed to increase lung volume. Historically, intermittent positive pressure breathing, or IPPB, was used extensively for this purpose. More recently, incentive spirometry, continuous positive airway pressure (CPAP) and positive expiratory pressure (PEP) have been introduced as alternative lung expansion methods.

Ongoing research on these methods continues to demonstrate mixed results. Clearly, some patients benefit, while others don't. Current evidence suggests that benefits should be expected only when patients are carefully selected and the approach chosen is administered and closely monitored by a skilled clinician.

In this context, the respiratory care practitioner (RCP) plays a vital role. In consultation with the prescribing physician, the RCP should assist in identifying those patients most likely to benefit from lung expansion therapy, recommend and initiate the appropriate therapeutic approach, monitor the patient's response, and alter the treatment regimen according to individual need.

PHYSIOLOGY AND CLINICAL APPLICATION

Physiology

All modes of lung expansion therapy increase lung volume by increasing the transpulmonary pressure gradient.[1,2] As detailed in Chapter 11, the transpulmonary pressure gradient (P_L) represents the difference between the alveolar pressure (Palv) and the pleural pressure (Ppl):

$$P_L = Palv - Ppl$$

With all else constant, the greater the transpulmonary pressure gradient, the more the alveoli expand.

As depicted in Figure 27-1, the transpulmonary pressure gradient can be increased by either: (1) decreasing the surrounding pleural pressure (Figure 27-1, *A*), or (2) increasing the alveolar pressure (Figure 27-1, *B*). A spontaneous deep inspiration increases the transpulmonary pressure gradient by decreasing the pleural pressure. On the other hand, positive pressure increases the transpulmonary pressure gradient by raising the pressure inside the alveoli.

All lung expansion therapies use one of these two approaches. Incentive spirometry (IS) enhances lung expansion via a spontaneous and sustained *decrease* in pleural pressure. Positive airway pressure techniques use the opposite approach. They *increase* alveolar pressure. Positive pressure lung expansion therapies may apply pressure during inspiration only (IPPB), during expiration only (PEP and EPAP), or during both inspiration and expiration (CPAP).

Although all these approaches are used in lung expansion therapy, it should be clear that those methods which decrease pleural pressure are more normal than those that raise alveolar pressure. As discussed in Chapter 10, negative pleural pressures aids venous return to the right heart. On the other hand, positive pressure impedes venous return, and can actually decrease cardiac output. Moreover, positive pressure can compress the lung's vascular beds and increase pulmonary vascular resistance. Other physiologic effects of positive pressure, especially those associated with long-term ventilatory support, are discussed in Chapter 30.

Clinical application

The primary use of lung expansion therapies is to prevent or treat atelectasis. Atelectasis can occur in any patient who cannot take deep breaths. Patients

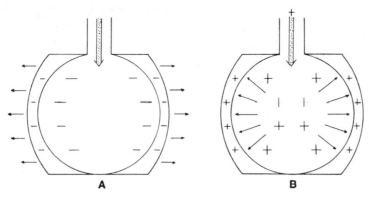

Fig. 27-1 Transpulmonary pressure gradients with spontaneous inspiration (**A**) and positive pressure inspiration (**B**).

who have difficulty taking deep breaths without assistance include those with neuromuscular disorders, those who are heavily sedated, and patients who have undergone upper abdominal or thoracic surgery.

Postoperative patients are at highest risk for atelectasis.[3] As many as 70% of patients who have undergone upper abdominal surgery exhibit clinical signs of postoperative atelectasis.[4,5] Factors contributing to postop atelectasis include shallow breathing, a failure to take deep breaths, and a transient decrease in surfactant production. In combination, these factors cause a progressive decrease in functional residual capacity (Figure 27-2). The decrease in FRC leads to alveolar collapse, most often in the basal or dependent portions of the lung.[6] Since perfusion remains unchanged, a V/Q mismatch results, causing arterial hypoxemia (Figure 27-2). Pain further restricts ventilation.[7] Compounding the effects of the pain itself is the tendency of postop patients to voluntarily contract or "splint" muscles in the incisional area. Splinting further decreases tidal volumes and hinders deep breathing. The result is a decrease in ventilatory reserve, as measured by the vital capacity (Figure 27-2).

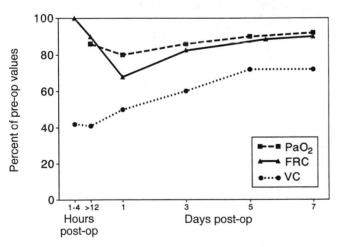

Fig. 27-2 Changes in oxygenation, FRC and vital capacity after upper abdominal surgery. (From Craig DB: Postoperative recovery of pulmonary function, *Anesth Analg* 60:46–52, 1981.)

Most postoperative patient also have problems coughing effectively. An ineffective cough impairs normal clearance mechanisms and increases the likelihood of infection. Some forms of lung expansion therapy may also help improve clearance of secretions.

Patients with neuromuscular disorders which restrict use of the diaphragm also may benefit from lung expansion therapies. Loss of the normal sigh mechanism in these patients often results in a progressive loss of lung volume, a decrease in pulmonary compliance, a drop in ventilation-perfusion (V/Q) ratios, and arterial hypoxemia.

INCENTIVE SPIROMETRY

Incentive spirometry (IS) has been the mainstay of lung expansion therapy for well over a decade. Incentive spirometry is designed to mimic natural sighing by encouraging patients to take slow, deep breaths.[8-10] Incentive spirometry is performed using devices which provide visual cues to the patients that the desired flow or volume has been achieved.[9,11-13]

The desired volume and number of repetitions to be performed is initially set by the RCP or other qualified caregiver. The inspired volume goal is set on the basis of predicted values, or observation of initial performance.

Physiologic basis

The basic maneuver of IS is a sustained, maximal inspiration (SMI). An SMI is a slow, deep inhalation from the FRC up to (ideally) the total lung capacity, followed by a 5 to 10 second breath hold. An SMI is thus functionally equivalent to performing an inspiratory capacity maneuver, followed by a breath hold.

Figure 27-3, page 744, compares the alveolar and pleural pressure changes occuring during a normal spontaneous breath and a sustained maximal inspiration during incentive spirometry.

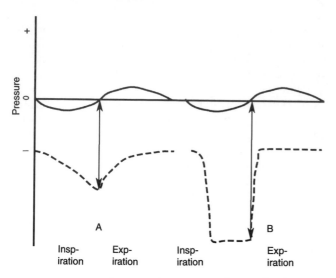

Fig. 27-3 Alveolar (solid lines) and pleural (dotted lines) pressure changes during (A) spontaneous breathing and (B) sustained maximum inspiration (IS). Note the difference in transpulmonary pressure gradients (arrowed lines).

During the inspiratory phase of spontaneous breathing, the drop in pleural pressure caused by expansion of the thorax is transmitted to the alveoli. With alveolar pressure now negative, a pressure gradient is created between the airway opening and the alveoli. This transrespiratory pressure gradient (Prs) causes gas to flow from the airway into the alveoli.

Alveolar expansion during spontaneous inspiration (equivalent to the change in volume) is proportional to the difference between the alveolar and pleural pressures at end inspiration:

$$\text{Alveolar expansion} \approx \text{Palv} - \text{Ppl (end inspiration)}$$

The difference between the alveolar and pleural pressures at end inspiration is called the transpulmonary pressure gradient (PL). Thus:

$$\text{Alveolar expansion} \approx \text{PL (end inspiration)}$$

It is useful to think of the alveolar expansion occurring during spontaneous inspiration as based on an "outside-in" model of pressure changes. Pressure drops *outside* the lung (pleural space) are transmitted *in* to the alveoli.

During spontaneous expiration, as the lungs and chest wall recoil, pleural pressure become less negative, and alveolar pressure rise above atmospheric. This reverses the transrespiratory pressure gradient. With alveolar pressure now greater than pressure at the airway opening, gas flows out from the alveoli to the atmosphere.

As can be seen in Figure 27-3, *B*, a sustained maximal inspiration causes the pleural pressure to drop well below normal. This increases the transpulmonary pressure gradient, which is sustained for a few seconds with a breath hold. By increasing the trans-

pulmonary pressure gradient and further expanding the alveoli, atelectasis can often be successfully treated or prevented.[14,15]

Indications

Indications for incentive spirometry are listed in the box above.[16]

The primary indication for IS is to treat existing atelectasis.[17] IS may also be used as a preventive measure when conditions exist that make the development of atelectasis likely.[9] Clinical conditions predisposing to atelectasis include upper abdominal and thoracic surgery, and any major surgery on COPD patients that requires general anesthesia.[5,13-15,18,19] Last, patients with neuromuscular disorders which restrict use of the diaphragm may benefit from IS.[20]

Contraindications

Incentive spirometry is a simple and relatively safe modality. For this reason, contraindications are few (see box below).

Of course, because it requires patient participation, IS cannot be performed on unconscious patients or those otherwise unable to cooperate.[17] In addition, if a patient is unwilling or unable to follow directions (as with very small children), IS should not be attempted. Last, IS is only effective in patients who can generate a

---

Indications for incentive spirometry[16]

- Presence of pulmonary atelectasis
- Presence of conditions predisposing to atelectasis:
  - Upper abdominal surgery
  - Thoracic surgery
  - Surgery in patients with COPD
- Presence of a restrictive lung defect associated with quadraplegia and/or dysfunctional diaphragm

---

Clinical situations contraindicating incentive spirometry[16]

- Unconscious patients or those unable to cooperate
- Patients who cannot properly use IS device after instruction
- Patient unable to generate adequate inspiration, eg:

  VC < 10 mL/kg or
  IC < 1/3 predicted normal

minimally adequate inspiration.[16] If this is not possible, IS is deferred and other more suitable treatment options must be considered, such as IPPB.

Hazards and complications

Given its normal physiologic basis, incentive spirometry presents few major hazards and complications. Those that can occur are listed in the box below.[16]

Acute respiratory alkalosis occurs when the patient performs IS too rapidly. Dizziness is the most frequently reported untoward effect. This problem is easily corrected with repeat instruction and close follow-up.

Cardiovascular side effects do not normally occur as the maneuver mimics physiologic breathing and no positive airway pressure is employed. One exception to this generalization occurs when maximal inspiration is maintained against a closed glottis, and the abdominal muscles are contracted. This **Valsalva-like maneuver** increases pleural pressures and can cause a vagal response that decreases the cardiac rate. Proper patient instruction can correct or prevent this problem.

Discomfort secondary to pain is usually the result of inadequate pain control. This problem can be rectified by assuring appropriate analgesia. In addition, pain medication should be coordinated with IS activity.

Pulmonary barotrauma occurs when the elastic limits of lung tissue are exceeded. Typically, this occur when a high transpulmonary pressure gradients causes gross overdistension (too high a volume at too high a pressure). Although IS does increase the transpulmonary pressure gradient, the volume and pressure changes that occur are generally not enough to cause gross overdistension in otherwise healthy lungs. The exception is lung tissue that is already overdistended, as in emphysema. In these patients, pulmonary barotrauma is a real possibility that the RCP must always be on guard against.

Hypoxemia is never caused by incentive spirometry *per se*. Hypoxemia only occurs when O_2 therapy via mask is interrupted to perform IS. If hypoxemia

is likely, the O_2 mask should be changed to a nasal cannula at the proper flow for the duration of the IS treatment. Likewise, IS alone rarely causes bronchospasm, but may exacerbate a pre-existing condition.

Fatigue due to repetitive IS maneuvers is possible, especially in patients with pre-existing respiratory muscle weakness. Fatigue may also be due to the high work of breathing imposed on the patient by some IS devices.[21] Signs of fatigue in spontaneously breathing patients include tachypnea and paradoxical abdominal-chest movement. Fatigue may also be recognized by a progressive drop in IS volumes during a therapy session. Should fatigue occur, the RCP should adjust the treatment accordingly.

Equipment

Part of incentive spirometry's appeal is the relative simplicity and low cost of the equipment. Although recent advances in technology have made available some very sophisticated approaches, there is no evidence that these devices produce any better outcomes than their lower cost, disposable counterparts.

Indeed, no one has ever shown that equipment of any sort is needed to achieve the goals of IS. Traditional prescriptions for the patient to "deep breath and cough," if aggressively followed, may well be as effective as the use of a given IS device with cooperative patients.[9,10,11,17]

However, the use of IS equipment as a substitute for this traditional regimen has a sound practical basis. First, IS equipment helps in setting and monitoring progress toward measurable goals, thereby providing some degree of patient motivation (the "incentive" of incentive spirometry). Second, once a patient is properly instructed in the method, the treatment regimen can be conducted without direct supervision, thus making this approach more cost-effective than the one-on-one intervention otherwise required.

IS devices can generally be categorized as volume or flow-oriented. Volume-oriented devices actually measure and visually indicate the volume achieved during the SMI. Flow-oriented devices, on the other hand, measure and visually indicate inspiratory flow. This flow is equated with volume by assessing the duration of inspiration or time (flow $\times$ time = volume).

Volume-oriented devices

A typical volume-oriented disposable IS device is shown in Figure 27-4, page 746. This device is a true volume displacement incentive spirometer. A corrugated large-bore breathing hose and mouthpiece connect the patient to a flexible plastic bellows. During inspiration, as the patient draws air through the

---

Hazards and complications of incentive spirometry[16]
■ Hyperventilation and respiratory alkalosis
■ Discomfort secondary to inadequate pain control
■ Pulmonary barotrauma
■ Hypoxemia (with interruption of therapy)
■ Exacerbation of bronchospasm
■ Fatigue

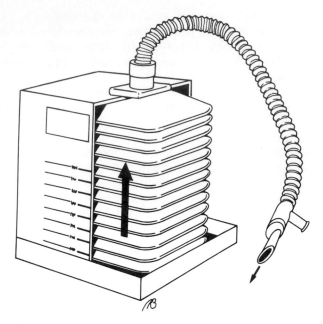

Fig. 27-4 Volume incentive breathing exerciser. (From Euganks DH, Bone RC: *Comprehensive Respiratory Care, a Learning System,* ed 2, St. Louis, 1990. Mosby. Used by permission.)

breathing hose, the bellows rises. An indicator on the device enclosure indicates the volumetric displacement. Once it reaches its maximum displacement for a given breath, the patient is told to hold the bellows in place for 5 to 10 seconds (the end-inspiratory hold). After completion of the maneuver, the patient removes the mouthpiece, allowing gravity to return the bellows to its initial starting position.

Flow-oriented devices

Whereas volume-oriented IS devices actually measure volume, flow-oriented devices provide only an indirect indicator of the patient's inspired volume. Typically, this is achieved with calibrated flow indicators which function on the same principle as a Thorpe-tube flowmeter.

Figure 27-5 shows an example of a flow-oriented IS device. Ping-pong like balls: (1) are enclosed in three connected plastic flow tubes, (2) as the patient inhales through the mouthpiece, (3) a pressure drop and (4) causes the ball in the first tube to rise to a level equivalent to the flow around it. Each tube is calibrated such that full displacement of its ball equals a specific flow, as indicated on the wall of the tube (600, 900, and 1200 cc/sec in the device pictured in Figure 27-4). As flow exceeds the maximum for the first tube, the ball in the second tube rises, followed by that in the third tube. To maintain an end-inspiratory hold with this type of device, the patient is instructed to keep the indicator balls elevated to full displacement for as long as possible.

Inspired volume is estimated as the product of inspired flow times time:

$$V \text{ (liters)} = \frac{\dot{V} \text{ (cc/sec)} \times time \text{ (sec)}}{1000}$$

For example, if a patient were to maintain displacement of the balls in the first and second chamber of this device for 3 seconds, the estimated inspired volume would be calculated as:

$$V \text{ (liters)} = \frac{[900 \text{ cc/sec} \times 3 \text{ sec}]}{1000}$$
$$V \text{ (liters)} = 2.7 \text{ liters}$$

Obviously, given the relative lack of precision of such devices and the errors inherent in the bedside measurement of these short time intervals, volume measurements derived from flow-oriented incentive spirometers should be treated only as rough estimates of actual inspired volume. To overcome this problem, many manufacturers now provide hybrid IS devices that are flow-oriented, but include a relatively accurate volume accumulator.

There is no conclusive evidence to support the use of one type or brand of IS device over others.[22] For this reason, the decision as to which equipment is best currently must be based on empirical assessment of patient acceptance, ease of use, and cost.

Administering incentive spirometry

As with IPPB, the successful application of IS involves three phases: planning, implementation, and followup. Since many of the components of this process are similar to those previously described, we only will highlight the key points and differences in approach.

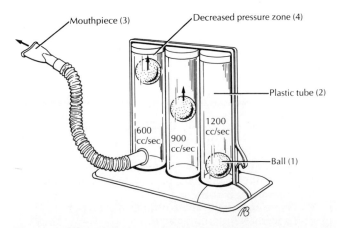

Fig. 27-5 Flo-oriented incentive spirometer. (From Eubanks DH, Bone RC: *Comprehensive respiratory care,* St Louis, 1985, Mosby.)

Clinical situations indicating a need for incentive spirometry

- Surgical procedure involving upper abdomen or thorax
- Conditions predisposing to development of atelectasis including immobility, poor pain control, and abdominal binders
- Presence of neuromuscular disease involving respiratory muscles

---

Preliminary planning

During preliminary planning, the need for IS should be determined, and desired therapeutic outcomes should be set. In terms of need, the box above lists the clinical situations indicating a need for incentive spirometry.[16]

Once the need is established, planning for IS should focus on selecting explicit therapeutic outcomes. The box below lists potential outcomes that can be considered for patient receiving incentive spirometry.[16]

Obviously, the outcomes applicable to a given patient depend on the diagnostic information that supports the need for IS. In this regard, the baseline patient assessment is critical. Ideally, patients scheduled for upper abdominal or thoracic surgery should been screened prior to undergoing this procedure. Assessment conducted at this point will help identify patients at high risk for postoperative complications and allow determination of their baseline lung volumes and capacities. Moreover, this approach provides an opportunity to orient high risk patients to the procedure *before* undergoing surgery, thereby increasing the likelihood of success when incentive spirometry is provided after surgery.

Potential outcomes of incentive spirometry

Absence of or improvement in signs of atelectasis:

Decreased respiratory rate
Remission of fever
Normal pulse rate
Resolution of abnormal breath sounds
Normal chest X-ray
Improved PaO_2 and decreased $P(A-a)O_2$
Increased VC and peak expiratory flows
Restoration of pre-op FRC or VC

Improved inspiratory muscle performance:

Attainment of preoperative flow and volume levels
Increased forced vital capacity (FVC)

Implementation

Successful incentive spirometry requires effective patient teaching. In instructing a patient to use an incentive spirometer, the RCP should set an initial goal that is attainable, but requires some moderate effort. Setting too low an initial goal results in little incentive and an ineffective maneuver, at least initially. The patient should be instructed to inspire slowly and deeply in order to maximize the distribution of ventilation.

A common problem in initial instruction is that the patient may tend to inspire very rapidly, using the accessory muscles of ventilation to aid the work of the diaphragm. Correct technique will emphasize diaphragmatic breathing at a slow to moderately inspiratory flows. Demonstration is probably the most effective way to ensure patient understanding and cooperation. By using oneself as an example, both the operation of the device and the proper breathing technique can be easily explained, and much trial and error avoided.

Upon maximal inspiration, the patient should be instructed to sustain the breath for 5 to 10 seconds. Many patients have difficulty with this aspect of the maneuver. Adding a one-way valve (which prevents exhalation) to the IS device can increased both inspired volume and breath-hold time, even in uncoached patients.[23] However, the safety of this modification has not been assessed.

A normal exhalation should follow the breath-hold, and the patient should be given the opportunity to rest as long as needed prior to the next SMI maneuver. Some patients in the early postoperative stage may need to rest for as much as 30 seconds to a minute between maneuvers. This rest period helps avoid a common tendency among some patients to repeat the maneuver at rapid rates, thereby causing respiratory alkalosis. The goal is not rapid, partial lung inflation but intermittent, maximal inspiration.

The exact number of sustained maximal inspirations needed to reverse or prevent atelectasis is not known, and surely varies according to the patient's clinical status. However, because normal individuals average about 6 sighs per hour, an IS regimen should probably aim to ensure a minimum of 5 to 10 SMI maneuvers each hour.[16,24]

Followup

As always, assessing the patient's performance is vital to ensuring goals achievement. To do so, the RCP should make return visits to monitor treatment sessions until correct technique and appropriate effort are achieved. Suggested monitoring activities for IS are outlined in the box on page 748.[16]

Once the patient has demonstrated mastery of technique, IS may be performed with minimal supervision.[12,17,25] Even when self-administered, records of progress, as related to the patient's clinical status,

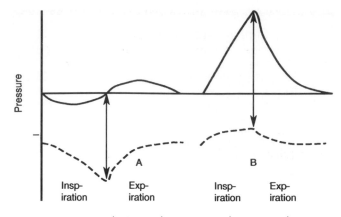

Fig. 27-6 Alveolar (solid lines) and pleural (dotted lines) pressure changes during (A) spontaneous breathing and (B) IPPB. Note the difference in transpulmonary pressure gradients (arrowed lines).

must be maintained throughout the course of treatment. The result of this assessment can guide the physician and RCP in revising the respiratory care plan or terminating treatment once its goals are achieved.

INTERMITTENT POSITIVE PRESSURE BREATHING (IPPB)

Intermittent Positive Pressure Breathing, or IPPB, was introduced as a clinical modality by Motley in 1947.[26] Since that time, IPPB has had a volatile history. During its early years, IPPB enjoyed widespread use and acclamation. Physicians and RCPs alike used IPPB for a broad range of clinical conditions. Although clinical evidence supporting it use was lacking, IPPB became the predominant mode of respiratory care by 1970.

Subsequently, IPPB can under attack as both an unvalidated and overused treatment modality.[27-30] In 1980, the Respiratory Care Committee of the American Thoracic Society (ATS) prepared guidelines for the use of IPPB, supporting its rational application in certain clearly defined clinical situations.[31] Later that decade, the American Association for Respiratory Care (AARC) disseminated a statement asserting the effectiveness of IPPB in several, very specific clinical situations.[32] Most recently, the AARC has established a clinical practice guideline for IPPB therapy.[33]

Clearly, IPPB should neither be totally condemned nor universally applied. Like so many other respiratory care modalities, the effectiveness of IPPB requires that: (1) patients be carefully chosen, (2) the indications for therapy be specifically defined, (3) the goals of therapy be clearly understood, and (4) the treatment be properly administered by a trained RCP.

Definition and physiologic principle

IPPB refers to the application of inspiratory positive pressure to a spontaneously breathing patient as an intermittent or short-term therapeutic modality.[33] On an intermittent basis, IPPB "treatments" usually last 15 to 20 minutes, and may be given several times each day.[31,34] Short-term use is for purposes of assisting ventilation, and may be provided over a period of several hours, such as overnight. This chapter will emphasize the intermittent use of IPPB as a treatment modality. Chapter 38 provides details on the short-term use of intermittent positive pressure breathing for ventilatory assistance in the home.

Figure 27-6 compares the alveolar and pleural pressure changes occuring during a normal spontaneous breath and IPPB. As can be seen in Figure 27-6, *B* IPPB reverses the normal spontaneous pressure gradients. Instead of negative alveolar pressure causing gas flow into the lungs, positive pressure at the airway opening creates the needed gradient. As with spontaneous breathing, gas flows from the airway into the lungs. However, alveolar pressures *rise* during the inspiratory phase of IPPB.

This rise in alveolar pressure increases P_L and expands the alveoli. Because alveolar pressure is greater than pleural pressure during IPPB, positive pressure is transmitted from the alveoli to the pleural space, causing pleural pressure to rise somewhat during inspiration. Depending on the mechanical properties of the lung, pleural pressure may actually exceed atmospheric pressure during a portion of inspiration.

As compared to spontaneous breathing and incentive spirometry, alveolar expansion occurring during IPPB is based on "inside-out" pressure changes. Pressure increases *in* the lung are transmitted *out* to the surrounding pleural space and thoracic structures.

As with spontaneous breathing, the recoil force of the lung and chest wall, stored as potential energy during the positive pressure breath, causes a passive exhalation. As gas flows from the alveoli out to the airway opening, alveolar pressure drops to atmospheric level, while pleural pressure is restored to its normal subatmospheric range (Figure 27-6, *B*).

Indications for IPPB

In the past, IPPB therapy was administered for a host of reasons, some well founded and others without any sound clinical or physiologic basis. Today, this cavalier approach is no longer acceptable. As previously stated, the use of IPPB must be supported by **corroborating** patient data that clearly indicates a potential benefit. Substantiated indications for IPPB are listed in the box above.[33,35]

Improving lung expansion

In regard to improving lung expansion, there are two major patient groups for which IPPB can be helpful. First, IPPB may be useful for patients with clinically diagnosed atelectasis not responsive to other therapies, such as incentive spirometry and chest physiotherapy.[3,17] This includes patients with atelectasis who cannot cooperate with other therapies.[33]

In concept, a correctly administered IPPB treatment should provide these patients with augmented tidal volumes, achieved with minimal effort. In fact, an aggressive respiratory therapy regimen which includes IPPB has been shown to be as effective as therapeutic bronchoscopy in treating patients with lobar atelectasis.[11] The optimal breathing pattern to reinflate collapsed lung units with IPPB consists of slow, deep breaths that are sustained or held at end-inspiration. This type of inspiratory maneuver increases the distribution of inspired gas to areas of the lung with low compliance, specifically, the atelectatic areas.

Although the application of IPPB to treat atelectasis is well substantiated, its use prophylactically to prevent the occurrence of this postoperative complication is not well supported.[35,36]

Providing short-term ventilatory support

There are two general situations in which IPPB can be used to provide short-term ventilatory support. The first is acute hypercapnic respiratory failure. The second is for patients with chronic disorders that cause muscle weakness.

IPPB is an alternative to tracheal intubation and continuous mechanical ventilation for some patients with acute hypercapnic respiratory failure.[32,37-39] Patients most likely to benefit from this approach are those with pre-existing COPD whose condition acutely worsens.

The augmented tidal volumes provided by IPPB can increase minute ventilation, thereby lowering the arterial PCO_2 and reversing respiratory acidosis. IPPB with supplemental O_2 can also improve arterial oxygenation. In addition, bronchodilators may be given at appropriate intervals to decrease airway resistance. In combination with aggressive bronchial hygiene measures, increased tidal volumes and bronchodilation may contribute to improved clearance of pulmonary secretions.[39]

In this manner, the patient suffering from an acute exacerbation of COPD can be stabilized sufficiently to treat the underlying problem without committing to long-term ventilatory support. Stabilization of such patients may require continuous treatment for several hours or more. However, given the poor outcomes and high cost of long-term ventilatory support in these patients, early and aggressive intervention with IPPB during an acute exacerbation of chronic lung disease represents a sound clinical decision.

Short-term noninvasive intermittent positive pressure ventilation (NIPPV) is also of use in selected chronic disorders that cause muscle weakness.[40-45] For example, night-time NIPPV in these patients rests their respiratory muscles, allowing greater daytime strength and endurance.[46,47]

Aiding delivery of aerosolized drugs

Using IPPB to help deliver aerosolized drugs is still somewhat controversial.[48-50] Currently, the AARC recommends a careful, closely supervised trial of IPPB for this purpose *only* when other treatment modalities, such as MDI or nebulizer, have failed.[33] Applicable patient groups include those with severe bronchospasm, as in acute asthma, status asthmaticus, and exacerbated COPD, and those whose conditions impair the deep breathing needed to assure adequate aerosol deposition.[33]

In these patients, IPPB may help maintain a breathing pattern more conducive to aerosol drug deposition.[39] However, just as with MDIs and SVNs, the dose of any aerosolized drug delivered via IPPB circuit is unpredictable. Indeed, incorrectly applied IPPB may be a less effective vehicle for aerosolized administration of drugs than other simpler methods, even in patients not able to maintain an optimal breathing pattern.[48,51] For this reason, the decision to use IPPB as an alternative method for giving aerosolized drugs should be based on clear evidence that the patient is unable to properly use a SVN or MDI.

Contraindications for IPPB

There are several clinical situations in which IPPB should not be used (see accompanying box).[33] With the exception of untreated tension pneumothorax, most of these contraindications are relative. As with all procedures, a sound knowledge of the patient's

---

Clinical situations contraindicating IPPB therapy[33]

- Tension pneumothorax
- Intracranial pressure (ICP) > 15 mm Hg
- Hemodynamic instability
- Active hemoptysis
- Tracheoesophageal fistula
- Recent esophageal surgery
- Active untreated tuberculosis
- Radiographic evidence of bleb
- Recent facial, oral, or skull surgery
- Singulation (hiccups)
- Air swallowing
- Nausea

---

condition—tempered with common sense—should guide the RCP in the decision-making process. Thus, a patient with any of the listed conditions should be carefully evaluated before a decision is made to begin IPPB therapy.[33]

Tension pneumothorax

Without a functioning chest tube, a tension pneumothorax is a life-threatening situation. Under such circumstances, IPPB can cause further compression of the heart and great vessels, resulting in complete cardiopulmonary collapse. Patients with less severe air leaks, such as subcutaneous emphysema, are prone to develop pneumothoraces and should be carefully evaluated for IPPB therapy.

Increased intracranial pressure

IPPB's effect on venous return is not limited to the thorax. Positive pressure in the thorax also can retard cerebral venous return. Because the brain is enclosed in a "fixed" container, impedance to the outflow of blood engorges the cerebral circulation, and can increase **intracranial** pressure (ICP). In instances where increased intracranial pressures are problematic, such as after **neurosurgery** or brain trauma, IPPB generally is contraindicated.

Hemodynamic instability

Patients who are hemodynamically unstable are poor candidates for IPPB. Marked hypotension and cardiovascular insufficiency are thus relative contraindications to IPPB. In these situations, it is essential that the RCP weigh the benefits of therapy against the potential hazards for each patient.

Active hemoptysis

Hemoptysis is usually a medical emergency in which there is no logical rationale for lung expansion therapy of any kind. If active bleeding is occurring from pulmonary tissue, positive pressure may only worsen the situation.

Tracheoesophageal (T-E) fistula and esophageal surgery

T-E fistula is a rare congenital condition normally corrected by surgery as soon as it is diagnosed. Moreover, most patients with a T-E fistula (neonates) are seldom, if ever, candidates for IPPB. However, if positive pressure were applied to the airway of these patients, gas could enter the esophagus, resulting in gastric insufflation. In reality, this problem is associated mainly with the long-term ventilatory support of infants awaiting surgical intervention, and normally is addressed by endotracheal intubation. In adults, recent esophageal surgery may also contraindicate IPPB.

Active tuberculosis

It has been suggested that IPPB may cause the spread of localized pulmonary infections such as TB. In addition, IPPB could rupture the cavities that are seen in the advances stages of untreated TB. Likewise, the fragility of emphysematous blebs (as identified by X-ray) may contraindicate IPPB.

In addition to these specific clinical situations, IPPB should never be used when a less complex or less expensive modality can be used as effectively.[33,39] Last, IPPB should never be administered when there is a lack of adequate, skilled supervision.[39] Many of the reported failures associated with IPPB are due to this problem. Successful IPPB depends upon careful planning, effective patient teaching, and skillful application under the watchful eye of a knowledgeable RCP. IPPB is strictly contraindicated when these most basic conditions cannot be met.

Hazards and complications of IPPB

As with any clinical intervention, certain hazards and complications are associated with IPPB. These potential problems should be addressed in the initial stages of planning for IPPB. In addition, hazards and complications must be considered throughout the course of therapy as part of the process of assessing the patient for unwanted side effects. The major hazards and complications of IPPB are listed in the box on page 751.[33,52] The following discussion highlights some of these key problems and the related responsibilities of the RCP.

Increased airway resistance

IPPB therapy is associated with increased airway resistance in some subjects, especially those patients with hyperreactive airways. In known asthmatics and others with increased potential for bronchospasm, a bronchodilator should always be given along with the IPPB treatment. Bland aerosols alone are not recommended as these may result in bronchospasm in some.

Pulmonary barotrauma

The high pressures and high volumes associated with some forms of IPPB therapy can cause lung tissue damage, referred to as *pulmonary barotrauma.* The likelihood of this problem is probably highest in patients with COPD, especially those with bullous emphysema. In these patients, air under pressure may cause pneumothorax, **pneumomediastinum, pneumopericardium** or **subcutaneous** emphysema. Again, careful preassessment and ongoing monitoring are vital in preventing barotrauma.

Nosocomial infection

It is well documented that respiratory care equipment can be a source of hospital-acquired infections. In the hospital, RCPs responsible for IPPB therapy should implement CDC universal precautions,[53] and, where appropriate, follow the guidelines for prevention of tuberculosis transmission.[54] More specific guidance regarding infection control with IPPB is provided in the discussion of the actual procedure.

Hypocapnia and respiratory alkalosis

There is often a tendency for patients to breathe more rapidly than desired during IPPB. Since tidal volumes are also being augmented, a large increase in minute ventilation can occur, causing respiratory alkalosis. In general, keeping the respiratory rate between 6 to 8/min helps avoid this problem. Nonetheless, it is vital that the RCP remain with the patient throughout the treatment and be on guard for the signs and symptoms hypocapnea. These signs and symptoms include dizziness and numbness or tingling of the extremities (parasthesia).

Hypoventilation, hyperoxia and respiratory acidosis

In some patients with chronic hypercapnia, abrupt lowering of the $PaCO_2$ during IPPB therapy may result in a period of post-treatment hypoventilation and respiratory acidosis. Likewise, hyperoxia may decrease ventilation in sensitive patients. In both cases, the rising CO_2 levels after therapy may worsen any pre-existing hypoxemia.

Worsened V/Q imbalance and hypoxemia

Hypoxemia can also occur during IPPB therapy when air is the source gas. This is probably due to the maldistribution of ventilation and perfusion caused by positive pressure ventilation.[55,56]

Impaired venous return

As previously discussed, positive intrathoracic pressure can impede venous return. Decreased venous return can cause a fall in cardiac output. Normal individuals compensate for this effect by increasing venomotor tone. However, if compensation is not possible, or if the patient is already hypotensive, IPPB can dramatically lower cardiac output. For this reason, RCPs administering IPPB should conduct a preliminary bedside assessment of the patient's cardiovascular status and monitor high risk patients throughout the treatment for the signs and symptom of compromised cardiovascular function.

Gastric distension

When positive pressure is applied to the pharynx, the esophagus can open and gas can pass directly into the stomach. The pressure at which this occurs is called the *esophageal opening pressure.* The esophageal opening pressure is somewhere between 20 to 25 cm H_2O. Pharyngeal pressures exceeding this range may cause gastric distension.

Gastric distension is uncommon in the alert and cooperative patient receiving IPPB therapy. It is the neurologically obtunded patient that is at highest risk. Moreover, the problem occurs most often during IPPB therapy given by mask.

Gastric distension by itself is a minor inconvenience. The real problem with excess air in the stomach is the potential for vomiting and aspiration. Proper instruction and supervision of cooperative patients, and the avoidance of pressures higher than needed to achieve the desired goal, should help prevent this hazard. For the obtunded patient receiving IPPB by mask a nasogastric tube must be in place.

Air trapping and auto-PEEP

In some patients, especially those with COPD, IPPB can cause or worsen air trapping. When due to mechanical ventilation, air trapping is often referred to as auto-PEEP or intrinsic PEEP (see Chapter 30). PEEP stands for positive end-expiratory pressure. Air trapping or auto-PEEP exists when the pressure remaining in the alveoli at end-expiration is greater than zero.

Air trapping causes overdistention of the lung tissue and can increase the incidence of pulmonary barotrauma. Because it increases pleural pressure, air trapping can also directly impair cardiovascular performance. In addition, air trapping can compress pulmonary blood vessels and increase pulmonary vascular resistance. Last, air trapping impairs inspiratory muscle action and increases the work of breathing.

Air trapping is most likely when insufficient time is provided for exhalation. Mechanically retarding exhalation—thereby lengthening the expiratory phase and preventing early small airway closure—may help, but is not always successful. Moreover, expiratory retard raises pleural pressures, increasing the possibility of detrimental cardiovascular effects and pulmonary barotrauma. The best way to avoid air trapping during IPPB is to allow sufficient time for exhalation. Generally, this can be achieved by using low rates (6 to 8/min) and long expiratory times (at least 4 to 5 seconds).

Psychological dependence

Some patients may come to rely on the psychological benefits of IPPB even in the absence of proven physiologic effect. Many patients who have been using IPPB for years clearly would receive the same benefits by means of simpler and less costly approaches. However, habit and psychological attachment preclude changing the treatment regimen without considerable resistance. Patience and understanding must be displayed in dealing with such patients.

IPPB equipment

The accompanying box lists the basic equipment needed to provide a short-term IPPB treatment.[33] The key piece of equipment is the IPPB device.

IPPB can be administered by any device that can provide intermittent positive pressure to the airway. This includes devices designed solely for IPPB, volume-, pressure-, or time-limited ventilators, or manual resuscitator (bag-valve-mask assemblies). In this section, we will focus on IPPB devices.

IPPB devices are mechanical ventilators and function according to the principles described in Chapter 31. However, machines designed solely for IPPB treatments generally are much simpler in design and function. In this section, we will discuss the general features of IPPB devices, and look at a few representative examples. More detailed descriptions of the design and function of the many IPPB devices in current use is available elsewhere.[57]

General features

IPPB devices are usually powered by either a 50 psig pressure source or an electrical compressor. All IPPB devices are patient-triggered. A patient-triggered device "turns on" or begins gas delivery by sensing and responding to the small effort (negative pressure) made by the patient at the beginning of inspiration. In this manner, the patient determines when inspiration under positive pressure begins. Typically, inspiration ends when a predetermined pressure is reached at the airway. IPPB devices that end inspiration according to a preset pressure are termed *pressure-cycled*.

All IPPB devices also incorporate either a true venturi or air entrainment jet to enhance flow. An IPPB breathing circuit generally includes a nebulizer (for aerosol administration), and an exhalation valve. The exhalation valve closes during machine inspiration, thereby forcing gas under pressure into the lungs. At the end of inspiration, the exhalation valve opens and allows expired gases to escape to the atmosphere.

Breathing valve

All patient-triggered IPPB devices have a breathing valve that responds directly to pressure differences generated during breathing. Typically, these valves not only initiate gas flow at the beginning of inhalation, but also terminate inhalation once the preset pressure is reached.

Although differing somewhat in design, these valves all function alike. As a patient begins inspiration, the valve senses the drop in pressure and opens to allow gas flow under pressure. As gas continues to flow during inspiration, pressure at the airway and in the system rises. This increase in pressure also is sensed by the valve, which closes when the pressure reaches a certain critical level, which is preset by the RCP.

The amount of negative pressure needed to open the breathing valve and begin inhalation is determined by the *sensitivity* of the device. Depending on the design, sensitivity may be fixed or adjustable. The pressure level required to close the valve, thereby initiating exhalation, is called the *cycling pressure*. The cycling pressure is always adjustable, typically up to 30 to 60 cm H_2O. Because ventilators are categorized mainly according to the mechanism ending inspiration (refer to Chapter 31), these devices are commonly referred to as *pressure-cycled ventilators*.

The two most common valve designs used in patient-triggered IPPB equipment are the sliding

---

Basic equipment needed for short-term IPPB therapy[33]

- IPPB device, ventilator or manual resuscitator
- IPPB breathing circuit and connecting tubing
- Nebulizer (SVN or MDI with accessory adapter)
- Mouthpiece, flange (lip seal), nose clips, mask, or ET tube adapter
- Tissues and emesis basin/container for expectorated sputum
- Gloves, goggles, gown, and mask as indicated
- Hand-held spirometer or other volume-measuring device
- Oral and/or endotracheal suction equipment

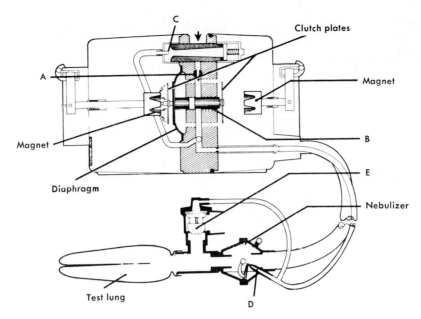

Fig. 27-7 Structure of Bird Mark 7. (Courtesy Bird Corp, Palm Springs, Calif. From McPherson SP: Respiratory therapy equipment, ed 3, St Louis, 1985, Mosby.)

alignment valve and the rotary alignment valve. Bird IPPB devices use the sliding valve, while Bennett equipment incorporates the rotary type. For purposes of comparison, we will provide a brief overview of the function of each.

Sliding alignment valve (Bird). A typical Bird ventilator (the Mark 7) is shown in Figure 27-7. 50 psig source gas flows into the top of the unit (downward arrow), immediately encountering a variable flow control valve (*A*). Distal to the flow control valve is the *sliding alignment valve* (*B*). As depicted in the figure, the valve is shifted to the left, such that its center passage is misaligned with the source gas stream, blocking further flow (the "off" position).

Connected to either end of the valve are metallic plates, each close to a permanent magnet. The distance between the magnets and the plates can be varied by threaded controls levers to either side of the device.

The left and right sides of the device are separated by a flexible diaphragm, which is attached to the alignment valve. Because the left side of the device is open to the atmosphere, it is called the *ambient chamber*. The right side, or *pressure chamber*, is continuous with the breathing circuit and patient airway (test lung in this example).

When the patient begins to inhale, negative pressure is transmitted through the breathing circuit back to the pressure chamber. This creates a pressure difference across the flexible diaphragm that tends to pull it—and the attached alignment valve—to the right. However, the attractive force between the left metallic plate and its magnet opposes movement of the diaphragm, in direct proportion to the distance between the two. If the negative pressure in the

pressure chamber is great enough to overcome this magnetic force, the diaphragm will move to the right, aligning the center passageway of the valve with the main stream of gas, and initiating the inspiratory cycle.

Exactly how much negative pressure must be generated by the patient to begin inspiration (the sensitivity of the device) is determined by the distance between the ambient chamber plate and magnet, as set by the RCP. The closer the plate and magnet, the greater the negative pressure—and patient effort—needed to move the diaphragm and open the valve.

Once the sliding alignment valve opens, source gas normally takes two routes. Some goes directly to a venturi jet (*C*), while the rest is diverted to the mainstream nebulizer jet (*D*) and exhalation valve chamber (*E*). Pressurization of the exhalation valve forces it closed, preventing gas from escaping during inspiration.

As pressure in the pressure chamber rises during inspiration, the flexible diaphragm tends to bow back toward the left. However, its movement is opposed by the attraction between the pressure chamber plate and magnet. Exactly how much positive pressure is needed to end inspiration (the cycling pressure) is determined by the distance between the pressure chamber plate and magnet. As with the sensitivity adjustment, this distance can be adjusted by the RCP. The closer the pressure chamber plate and magnet, the greater the positive pressure needed to move the diaphragm back to the left and close the alignment valve.

Once the alignment valve moves back to the left, source gas flow stops, and the exhalation valve (*E*) opens. This allows the patient to exhale passively, until the next inspiratory cycle begins.

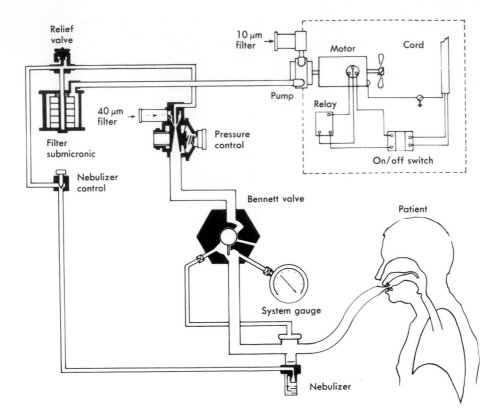

Fig. 27-8 Frunctional diagram of AP series ventilators. (Courtesy Puritan-Bennett Corp, Los Angeles. From McPherson SP: Respiratory therapy equipment, ed 3, St Louis, 1985, Mosby.)

This design gives the RCP precise control over sensitivity, flow, and end-inspiratory cycling pressure. Limited control over FIO_2 is provided by a valve which optionally diverts source gas away from the venturi (the "air-mix" control). If the device is powered by 100% oxygen, bypassing the venturi results in 100% oxygen delivery to the patient. However, bypassing the venturi greatly lowers the device's total flow output. Moreover, even when the venturi is used, FIO_2s are extremely variable and generally higher than one might assume.

High FIO_2s occur even on air-mix because: (1) oxygen accumulates in the ambient chamber at high pressures, and (2) nebulizer flow (a large component of the total flow) is 100% source gas. Adding an oxygen blender and reservoir system provides exact FIO_2 control, but this approach is expensive, complicated, and requires a source of compressed air.

Rotary alignment valve (Bennett). A typical Bennett IPPB device (the AP-5) is shown in Figure 27-8. Unlike the Bird Mark 7, the Bennett AP-5 has a self-contained power source, a small electrical compressor (boxed in dotted lines). Compressor output first passes through a submicronic filter, and then follows two pathways. Part of the compressor output goes to a nebulizer control valve, which allows adjustment of nebulizer flow. The rest of the gas flows to the diluter-regulator.

The diluter-regulator serves has two key components. Its built-in venturi entrains air, thereby enhancing the device's output flow. In addition to the venturi, a simple adjustable spring-loaded pressure reducing valve provides precise control over system pressures.

Gas at the set pressure (0 to 30 cm H_2O for the AP-5) then passes to the Bennett valve. The Bennett valve consists of a counterweighted hollow drum and attached vane that can rotates within a special housing (Figure 27-9). Inspiration is triggered when the patient creates a small pressure difference across the drum vane (about -0.5 cm H_2O). This small pressure difference rotates the drum. Drum rotation aligns two openings with the main stream of pressurized gas coming from the diluter-regulator. With the valve now open, gas is allowed to flow into the breathing circuit and on to the patient.

As the drum rotates open, pressurized gas flows to a balloon-like exhalation diaphragm in the breathing circuit. When inflated, this exhalation diaphragm occludes the breathing circuit's exhalation port, thereby preventing escape of gas.

As gas continues to flow through the system during inspiration, pressure distal to the valve increases. Because the proximal pressure is constant, the pressure difference across the valve decreases throughout inspiration. As this pressure gradient decreases, the opposing force of the drum's counterweight slowly rotates the valve back toward the closed position. As the valve slowly closes, system flow decreases throughout inspiration. When the pressures across the valve begin to equalize, flow decreases to a critical minimum value of about 1 to 3 L/min. At this point, the force of gravity on the counterweight overcomes the small difference in pressure across the valve. The valve closes and flow ceases.

When the Bennett valve closes, pressurized gas in the exhalation diaphragm is released. Deflation of the exhalation diaphragm opens the exhalation port, allowing expired gases to escape out to the atmosphere. This cycle is repeated when the patient again initiates an inspiratory effort.

Like the Bird IPPB device, the Bennett design allow the RCP control over the end-inspiratory cycling pressure. However, unlike the Bird IPPB devices, the Bennett design provides no direct way to control flow. More advanced models in the Bennett Series do offer a choice between 100% source gas and air dilution (allowing some variation in total output flow). In addition, the PR-2 line incorporates a simple flow control mechanism. Even so, the flow output of the Bennett type IPPB device is determined mainly by the initial pressure setting. The greater the preset system pressure, the greater the initial flow.

Due to the design of their valves, Bennett IPPB devices also differs from Bird systems in regard to sensitivity control. While Bird ventilators provide a wide range of sensitivity settings, the pressure needed to trigger a Bennett device is designed into the valve assembly. More advanced models in the Bennett series do allow some adjustment of sensitivity. In the clinical application of IPPB, however, this difference is of minor practical importance.

Like the Bird devices, modifications to this basic Bennett design provide for automatic (time) cycling to begin inspiration, thereby allowing their use in long-term ventilatory support. However, simple devices

---

Clinical situations indicating a need for IPPB[33]

- Clinical diagnosis of atelectasis
- Reduced lung volumes, eg:
    Vital capacity < 10–15 mL/kg
    Inspiratory capacity < 40% predicted
- Reduced expiratory flows (precluding effective cough), eg:
    FEV_1 < 65% predicted
    FVC < 70% predicted
- Neuromuscular disorders or **kyphoscoliosis** with associated decreases in lung volumes and capacities
- Fatigue or muscle weakness with impending respiratory failure
- Presence of acute severe bronchospasm or exacerbated COPD that fails to respond to other therapy

---

like the Bird and Bennett IPPB systems are generally not used for long-term ventilatory support.

Administering IPPB

Effective IPPB requires careful preliminary planning, individualized patient assessment and implementation, and thoughtful follow-up. In all three phases of the process, the RCP should work closely with the prescribing physician to determine patient need, select the appropriate therapeutic approach, and assess patient progress toward predefined clinical outcomes. Only by assuring that these elements are combined as part of the overall respiratory care plan can the RCP expect to achieve desired results.

Preliminary planning

During preliminary planning, the need for IPPB should be determined, and desired therapeutic outcomes should be set.

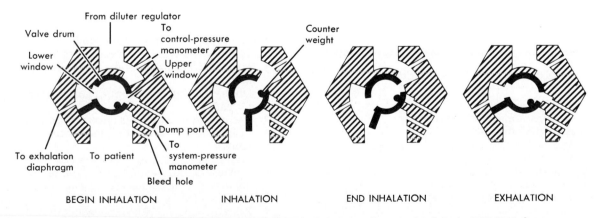

Fig. 27-9 Bennett valve. (From McPherson SP: Respiratory therapy equipment, ed 3, St Louis, 1985, Mosby.)

Determining need. A patient in need of IPPB must requires this therapy to meet one or more of the indications previously described. Common clinical situations consistent with these indications are described in the box on page 755.[33]

Setting goals or outcomes. Obviously, the outcomes chosen for a given patient should be based on diagnostic information that supports the need for IPPB therapy. In addition, therapeutic outcomes should be as explicit and measurable as possible. Outcomes must also be consistent with the therapeutic indications, previously described. Outcomes which are inconsistent with these indications are generally inappropriate. The box below lists potential accepted and desired outcomes of IPPB therapy.[33]

Obviously, not all these outcomes apply to every patient. As an example, for a patient exhibiting clinical signs and symptoms of postoperative atelectasis, we might set the following outcomes:

1. A spontaneous inspiratory capacity 70% of predicted
2. Improvement in the chest X-ray
3. Remission of ausculatory signs of atelectasis

Evaluating alternatives

A key component in early planning must be consideration of alternative therapies. Specifically, before staring IPPB, the RCP and prescribing physician must determine whether simpler and less costly methods might be as effective in achieving the desired outcomes.[39] If this is the case, further consideration of IPPB should be postponed until the patient's response to the simpler therapy is assessed.

Baseline assessment

Prior to beginning therapy, the RCP should conduct a baseline patient assessment. This information will help individualize the treatment and allows objective evaluation of the patient's subsequent response to therapy. Together with the patient's medical history, this baseline assessment also alerts the RCP to possible problems or hazards associated with administering IPPB to a specific patient.

The baseline assessment should include both a general evaluation of the patient's clinical status, and a specific assessment related to the chosen therapeutic goals. The general assessment, common to all patients for whom IPPB is ordered, should include: (1) measurement of vital signs, (2) observational assessment of the patient's appearance and sensorium, and (3) chest auscultation. The more focused assessment should be individualized according to the identified clinical goals.

Obviously, assessment for different therapeutic outcomes require different baseline information. In the situation just cited above, the RCP would obtain a baseline measure of the patient's inspiratory capacity at the bedside. For patients in impending respiratory failure receiving IPPB to forestall intubation and mechanical ventilatory support, arterial blood gas information would be a critical component of the assessment plan. On the other hand, if IPPB is selected to enhance delivery of a bronchodilator aerosol, bedside assessment of forced expiratory flows would be an integral part of the evaluation. Only in this manner can the therapy be individually tailored according to the patient's status and needs.

Implementation

Implementation of the IPPB involves infection control, equipment preparation, patient orientation, and careful adjustment of the treatment parameters according to the patient's response.

Infection control. Standard considerations to avoid transmission of infection between RCP and patient during IPPB therapy are outlined in the accompanying box.

Equipment preparation. Although all IPPB equipment should undergo a regular schedule of preventive maintenance and calibration, it is the RCP's responsibility to ensure that all components are in proper working order prior to any patient use. Most respiratory care departments have standard protocols for this purpose.

Potential outcomes of IPPB therapy

- Improved inspiratory or vital capacity
- Increased FEV_1 or peak flow
- Enhanced cough and secretion clearance
- Improved chest X-ray
- Improved breath sounds
- Normalized arterial blood gases+
- Favorable patient subjective response

+For treating respiratory failure only.

Infection control precautions for IPPB therapy:[33]

- Use proper handwashing technique
- Follow CDC universal precautions
- Follow CDC guidelines for preventing spread of TB
- Observe all infection control guidelines posted for patient
- Use only sterile diluents and medications
- Eisinfect all reusable equipment between patients
- Change nebulizers or high-level disinfect at conclusion of dose administration, or every 24 hours with continuous use, or more often when visibly soiled
- Rinse nebulizers with sterile water only

Because pressure-cycled IPPB devices will not end inspiration if leaks in the system occur, it is iportant to check the patency of the patient's breathing circuit prior to each use. This can be done by aseptically occluding the patient connector and manually triggering a breath at a low flow setting. If the system pressure rises and the machine cycles off, the circuit is free of any major leak.

Patient orientation. Successful IPPB therapy depends mainly on the effectiveness of initial patient orientation. Before the first treatment, the RCP must carefully explain to the patient the purpose of the therapy. This explanation should be tailored to the patient's level of understanding, and address, at a minimum, the following points: (1) why the physician ordered the treatment, (2) what the treatment does, (3) how it will feel, and (4) what the expected results are. In order to confirm patient understanding, the attempt to answer all questions thoroughly.

The IPPB device must not be brought to the bedside until the RCP feels the patient adequately understands the procedure and the importance of cooperation. Once the RCP decides to bring the equipment to the bedside, a simple functional description may allay any fear or anxiety associated with the use of such an unfamiliar device.

A simulated demonstration of the procedure can be particularly useful in this regard. This can be done effectively with a test lung or, if deemed necessary, by self-application using a separate breathing circuit kept for this purpose. For some patients, an effective demonstration can make the difference between success and failure in implementing the treatment regimen.

Patient positioning. For best results, the patient should be positioned in as close to an upright posture as possible. Slouching should be discouraged because it will impair diaphragm movement and decrease inspired volumes. A very obese patient should ideally be positioned standing upright next to the bed, but this is often not practical.

Initial application. In order to eliminate airway leaks in the alert patient, an initial trial of noseclips may be needed until the technique is understood and the treatment can be performed without them. The mouthpiece must be inserted well past the lips and a tight seal must be encouraged to prevent gas leakage from the site. A flanged mouthpiece may be needed for some patients. The use of a mask is fraught with hazards and is suggested only for alert and cooperative patients otherwise unable to accomplish the treatment without leakage from the system.

The machine should be set so that a breath can be initiated with minimal patient effort. A sensitivity or trigger level of -1 to -2 cm H_2O is adequate for most patients. Initially, system pressure is set to between 10 to 15 cm H_2O. Resulting volumes should be measured and the pressure adjusted accordingly after the treat-

ment has begun. If the device has a flow control, the RCP should begin the treatment will a low to moderate flow, and adjust it according to the patient's breathing pattern. Generally, the goal will be to establish a breathing pattern consisting of 6 to 8 breaths/min, with an expiratory time of at least three to four times longer than inspiration of (I:E ratio of 1:3 to 1:4 or lower). Obviously, these setting may need to be adjusted according to individual needs and patient response. Moreover, careful monitoring of the breathing pattern—and coaching to maintain it—must be conducted throughout the treatment.

Adjusting parameters. Once the treatment begins and the patient's basic ventilatory pattern is established, setting should be individually adjusted and monitored according to the goals of the therapy. Examples of this individualized approach to IPPB administration include the different strategies characterizing the treatment of atelectasis, the management of respiratory failure, and the administration of aerosolized drugs.

Treating atelectasis. When used to treat atelectasis, IPPB therapy should be volume oriented. In these situations, arbitrary pressure settings are not acceptable and tidal volumes must be monitored. A tidal volume goal must be set for each individual patient and the therapy delivered on the basis of these goals.

There are various ways of determining these volume goals. Most clinical centers strive to achieve an IPPB tidal volume of 10 to 15 mL/kg of body weight, or at least 30% of the patient's predicted inspiratory capacity. If the initial volume fall short of this goal and the patient can tolerate it, the pressure is gradually raised until the goal is achieved. Pressures as high as 30 to 35 cm H_2O may be needed to achieve this end.[58]

To achieve the largest inspiratory volumes during IPPB, the RCP should encourage the patient to breathe actively during the positive pressure breath.[58] However, no definitive studies exist that demonstrate the need to have the patient actively participate in inspiration. Regardless of approach, IPPB is only useful in the treatment of atelectasis if the volumes delivered exceed those volumes achieved by the patient's spontaneous efforts.[59,60-62]

Treating respiratory failure. When IPPB is used as a preliminary measure to treat hypercapneic respiratory failure, the goal is to stabilize or prevent further decline in lung function. Assessment of this outcome is based on astute observation, bedside measurement of lung mechanics, and serial analysis of ABGs. Absolute volume adjustments in these situations are less important than ensuring that: (1) alveolar ventilation is sufficient to meet metabolic needs, (2) adequate oxygenation is maintained, and (3) sufficient mechanical reserves exit to avert long-term mechanical ventilation. Treatment should thus focus on achieving a breathing pattern that minimizes the work of breathing, and maintaining acceptable PO_2, PCO_2 and pH levels.

Delivering aerosolized drugs. The first choice for aerosol drug administration to spontaneously breathing adults is an MDI.[63-65] A small volume jet nebulizer (SVN) can be equally effective, and may be required with some patients. Only when these first-line strategies fail should IPPB be considered for this purpose.[33]

Standard drug dosages for delivery via IPPB are the same as for SVNs, but may be as much as 10 times higher than the MDI dose.[66,67] This is due to the small percentage of the aerosol output that actually deposits in the airway with IPPB.[48,68] In any case, the standard drug dosage is only a starting point. For maximum benefit, dosages should be individually titrated according to the patient's clinical response.[66-67]

When using IPPB to deliver aerosolized drugs, the device should be set to deliver a slow, deep breath. In addition, the RCP should encourage the patient to sustain a breath hold at end-inspiration, ideally for five or more seconds. Of course, the limits of comfort and tolerance for the individual patient must not be exceeded.

As previously discussed, when the objective of aerosol drug administration is bronchodilation, the RCP must assess the effect of the treatment on relevant pulmonary function measures. In this case, forced expiratory flows should be measured and documented again *after* therapy. How long one must wait after therapy before making these measurements depends on the pharmacodynamics of the specific drug;

in general, 5 to 10 minutes after conclusion of the IPPB session is sufficient.

Discontinuation and followup

Depending on the goals of therapy and the condition of the patient, IPPB treatments typically last from 15 to 20 minutes. Followup activities include post-treatment assessment of the patient, record-keeping, and equipment maintenance.

Post-treatment assessment. At the end of a treatment session, the RCP should repeat the initial patient assessment. As with the baseline assessment, this followup evaluation has two components. The general followup evaluation of the patient's clinical status should focus on determining any pertinent changes in vital signs, sensorium, and breath sounds, with emphasis on identifying possible untoward effects. The more specific followup assessment provides information relevant to evaluating progress toward achieving the chosen goals of therapy.

Treatment frequency should be determined by assessing patient response to therapy. For acute care patients, orders should be re-evaluated based on patient response to therapy at least every 72 hours or with any change of patient status.[33]

Record-keeping. A succinct but complete account of the treatment session, including the results of pre- and post-assessment, must be entered in the patient's medical record according to the approved institutional protocol. Any untoward patient responses must also immediately be reported to responsible personnel, to include at least the prescribing physician and attending nurse.

> ## Monitoring IPPB therapy[33+]
>
> **Machine performance:**
>
> Sensitivity
> Peak pressure
> Flow setting
> FIO_2
> Inspiratory time
> Expiratory time
> I:E ratio
>
> **Patient response**
>
> Breathing rate and expired volume
> Peak flow or $FEV_1/FVC\%$
> Pulse rate and rhythm (from EKG if available)
> Sputum—quantity, color, consistency and odor
> Mental function
> Skin color
> Breath sounds
> Blood pressure
> SpO_2 (if hypoxemia is suspected)
> ICP (in patients for whom ICP is important)
> Chest X-ray
> Subjective response to therapy

+Above items should be chosen as appropriate for the specific patient.

Monitoring and troubleshooting

As indicated in the accompanying box, monitoring of IPPB therapy involves both machine performance and patient response.[33] Information derived from monitoring helps the RCP make adjustments to therapy and can aid in the identification of common problems.

Machine performance. In terms of machine performance, large negative pressure swings early in inspiration indicate an incorrect sensitivity or trigger setting. In this case, the RCP should increase the sensitivity or alter the trigger level until only -1 to -2 cm H_2O are needed to trigger the device into inspiration.

Should system pressure drop *after* inspiration begins, or fail to rise until the very end of the machine breath, the problem is too low a flow. In this situation, the RCP should increase the flow (as tolerated) until system pressure rises quickly and holds near the preset value.

The opposite situation can also occur. Too high a flow will cause the device to cycle off prematurely. A lower flow setting will usually resolve this common problem. Alternatively, an IPPB device may cycle off prematurely when air flow is obstructed. Kinked tubing, an occluded mouthpiece or active resistance to inhalation by the patient are the most common causes of this problem. Checking the circuit and properly instructing the patient are the best ways to prevent or correct these problems.

Leaks pose a different problem. In the presence of leaks, a pressure-cycled IPPB device will not reach its preset cycling pressure, and will thus not cycle off. This problem is evident when inspiration continues well beyond the expected time.

To troubleshoot leaks, the RCP should differentiate between the machine and patient interface. Machine leaks most commonly occur at connection points, such as the nebulizer or exhalation valve. In addition, a torn or improperly seated exhalation valve diaphragm will cause a large system leak. Leaks at the patient interface usually occur at the mouth (loose seal around mouthpiece) or through the nose. If the problem is mouth leaks, additional instruction may help. If not, a flanged mouthpiece may be needed. Leaks through the nose are easily corrected with noseclips.

Patient response. In monitoring the patient's response, the RCP must take into account the intended purpose of the therapy and the patient's clinical conditions. These factors will dictate exactly what must be monitored for a given patient. Should *any* significant problem arise indicating an adverse response, we recommend that RCPs always follow the "triple-S" rule: stop, stay, stabilize. **Stop** the treatment (it may be causing the adverse response); **stay** with the patient (call for help if needed); don't leave until the patient's condition is **stabilized.**

POSITIVE AIRWAY PRESSURE THERAPY

Like IPPB, positive airway pressure adjuncts use positive pressure to increase the transpulmonary pressure gradient and enhance lung expansion. Unlike IPPB, positive airway pressure therapy require no complex machinery. Indeed, some methods do not even need a source of pressurized gas.

Definitions and physiologic principle

There are three current approaches to positive airway pressure therapy: positive expiratory pressure (PEP), expiratory positive airway pressure (EPAP), and continuous positive airway pressure (CPAP).[69] As discussed here, all approaches are intermittently applied as treatment modalities. Continuous use of CPAP is discussed in Chapter 30.

During PEP therapy, the patient exhales against a fixed-orifice flow resistor. With a flow resistor, expiratory pressures depend on the patient's expiratory

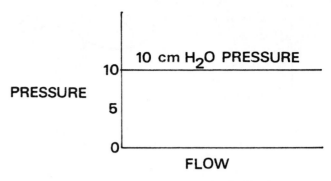

Fig. 27-10 Characteristics of a true threshold resistor.

flow. The higher the expiratory flow through a given-sized orifice, the greater the expiratory pressure. Patients are taught to actively but not forcefully exhale through the flow resistor to maintain a pressure between 10 to 20 cm H_2O.[70-74] PEP does not require a source of pressurized gas.[69] Like pursed-lip breathing, PEP increases pressure within the airways. This back pressure helps keep the airways open throughout exhalation. By preventing airway collapse during expiration, PEP helps move secretions into the larger airways, and may contribute to resolving atelectasis.

EPAP therapy is similar to PEP therapy, except a threshold resistor replaces the flow resistor. The pressure generated by a threshold resistor is independent of flow (Figure 27-10). The threshold resistor can be set to provide specific expiratory pressures independent of flow, usually between 10 to 20 cm H_2O.[75-77] Because the mechanical properties of threshold resistors differ from flow resistors, the physiologic effects of EPAP are not the same as PEP.[78] As with PEP therapy, EPAP does not require a source of pressurized gas.[69]

Figure 27-11 compares the alveolar and pleural

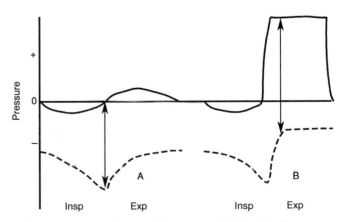

Fig. 27-11 Alveolar (solid lines) and pleural (dotted lines) pressures during **(A)** spontaneous breathing and **(B)** EPAP. Note difference in transpulmonary pressure gradients (arrows).

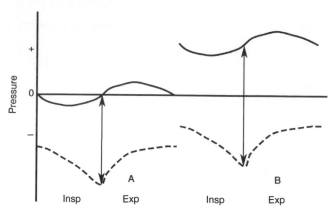

Fig. 27-12 Alveolar (solid lines) and pleural (dotted lines) pressures during **(A)** spontaneous breathing and **(B)** CPAP. Note difference in transpulmonary pressures (arrows).

pressure changes occurring during a normal spontaneous breath (Figure 27-11, *A*) and EPAP (Figure 27-12, *B*). As can be seen in Figure 27-11, *B*, the inspiratory phase of EPAP is similar to spontaneous breathing. As expiration begins, however, airway and alveolar pressures quickly rise to the preset EPAP level. This increases the transpulmonary pressure gradient during exhalation, which prevents airway closure and elevates the FRC.

While PEP and EPAP create *expiratory* positive pressure only, CPAP maintains a positive airway pressure throughout both inspiration and expiration.[79-89] Figure 27-12 compares the alveolar and pleural pressure changes occurring during a normal spontaneous breath (Figure 27-12, *A*) and CPAP (Figure 27-12, *B*). As can be seen, CPAP elevates and maintains high alveolar and airway pressures *throughout* the full breathing cycle. This increases transpulmonary pressure gradient throughout both inspiration and expiration.

Typically, the patient on CPAP breathes through a pressurized circuit against a threshold resistor, with pressures maintained between 5 to 20 cm H_2O.[69] To maintain system pressure throughout the breathing cycle, CPAP requires a source of pressurized gas.

Exactly how CPAP helps resolve atelectasis is unknown. However, the following factors probably contribute to its beneficial effects: (1) the recruitment of collapsed alveoli via an increase in FRC, (2) a decreased work of breathing due to increased compliance or abolition of auto-PEEP, (3) an improved distribution of ventilation through collateral channels (e.g., pores of Kohn), and (4) an increase in the efficiency of secretion removal.[62,80,90]

Indications

Positive airway pressure adjuncts are used mainly for two purposes: to mobilize secretions and treat atelec-

tasis. PEP therapy was originally developed as an aid to mobilize secretions, but has been applied to treat atelectasis. EPAP and CPAP are primarily used to treat atelectasis.

Specific indications for positive airway pressure therapies are listed in the accompanying box.[69] We will limit discussion to the use of positive airway pressure therapies for reducing air trapping and preventing or reversing atelectasis. The use of these modalities to help mobilize retained secretions is discussed in Chapter 28.

In terms of reducing air trapping in obstructive lung diseases, PEP therapy has been shown to improve the distribution of ventilation, increase the FRC and opens up lung regions that are otherwise closed off in cystic fibrosis.[71] In asthma and COPD, CPAP reduces the load on the inspiratory muscles, improves their efficiency, and decreasing the energy cost of breathing.[91-93]

In regard to postoperative complications, both PEP and CPAP have been shown to increase the FRC, lower the $P(A-a)O_2$, and decrease the incidence of atelectasis in patients having undergone major surgery.[81,94,95]

Even though evidence exists to support the use of CPAP therapy in the treatment of postoperative atelectasis, the duration of beneficial effects appears limited. Indeed, the corresponding increase in FRC may be lost within 10 minutes after the end of the treatment.[81,86,87] For this reason, it has been suggested that CPAP should be used on a continuous, not intermittent basis.[84]

CPAP by mask has also been used to treat cardiogenic pulmonary edema.[96] In such patients, CPAP reduces venous return and cardiac filling pressures, and improves compliance and decreases the work of breathing.

Contraindications

No absolute contraindications to the use of intermittent PEP, EPAP, or CPAP therapy have been reported in the literature. Nonetheless, there are several factors that the RCP should evaluate before a decision is made to initiate positive airway pressure therapy (see box on page 761).[69,74,88]

Indications for positive airway pressure therapy[69]

- To reduce air trapping in asthma and COPD
- To prevent or reverse atelectasis
- To aid in mobilization of retained secretions
- To optimize bronchodilator delivery

Hazards and complications

Most hazards and complications associated with positive airway pressure therapy are caused by either the increased pressure or the apparatus itself (see accompanying box). The increased work of breathing caused by the apparatus can lead to hypoventilation and hypercapnia.[88] In addition, since none of these modalities augment spontaneous ventilation, patients with an accompanying ventilatory insufficiency may hypoventilate during application. Although barotrauma is a potential of any positive airway pressure therapy, no documented cases have been reported. This is probably due to the population of patients using such therapy, and the techniques employed.[74]

Equipment

Equipment needed for PEP therapy includes a form-fitting face mask, a one way T-valve assembly, a pressure manometer, and an adjustable flow resistor (Figure 27-13).[74] A mouthpiece can be used instead of a mask for some patients. For patients requiring aerosolized bronchodilator therapy, a SVN can be added to the system.[99]

There are two approaches to EPAP therapy. The simplest approach is to use the same equipment as used for PEP therapy, but replace the flow resistor with a threshold resistor. This type of EPAP system requires no pressurized source gas.

Alternatively, a pressurized gas source can be used

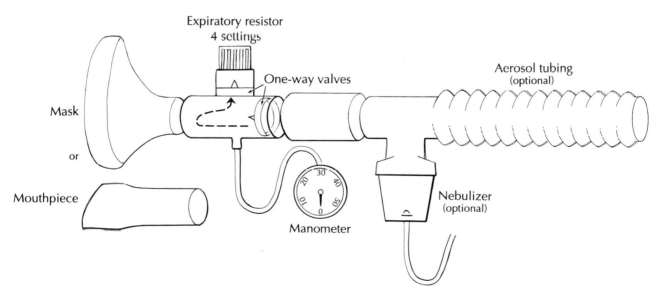

Fig. 27-13 Equipment needed for positive expiratory pressure (PEP) therapy. (Redrawn from Malmeister MJ, Fink JB, Hoffman GL: Positive expiratory pressure mask therapy: theoretical and practical considerations and a review of the literature, *Respir Care* 36:1218-1229, 1991.)

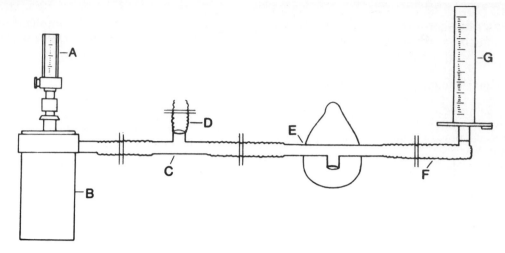

Fig. 27-14 Continuous-flow EPAP system. See text for description. (From Branson Rd, Hurst JM, Dellayen CB: Mask CPAP: state of the art, *Respir Care* 30:846-857, 1985.)

to provide EPAP (Figure 27-14). Pressurized gas from a flowmeter (*A*) flows continuously into a large volume aerosol generator (*B*), into the inspiratory limb of a breathing circuit. Attached to a T-piece in the inspiratory limb of the circuit (*C*) is an aerosol reservoir (*D*), open to the atmosphere. This reservoir provides extra volume if the patient's inspiratory flow exceeds that of the system. The patient breaths in and out through a mask attached to a T-piece (*E*). On the inspiratory side of the T-piece is a one-way inspiratory valve (not shown). This valve allows the patient to draw gas from the inspiratory limb, but prevent exhalation back into that side of the circuit. The expiratory limb of the circuit (*F*) is connected to a threshold resistor, in this case a water column (*G*).

With gas flowing continuously through the circuit, the pressure in the EPAP system is proportional to the height of the water column. EPAP pressure can be varied by adding or removing water from this column. Other types of threshold resistors that can be used for either EPAP or CPAP are listed in the box below.

Threshold resistors for EPAP/CPAP
■ Underwater columns
■ Spring-loaded diaphragms or disks
■ Gravity-weighted balls
■ Balloon valves with preset pressure
■ Reverse venturi systems
■ Electromechanical valves

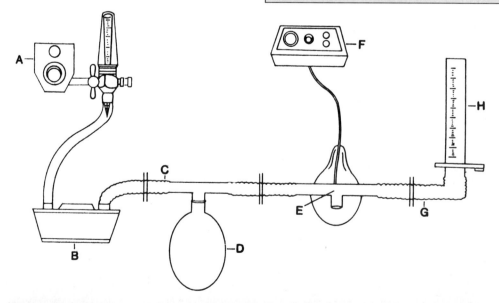

Fig. 27-15 Continuous-flow CPAP circuit. See text for description. (From Branson RD, Hurst JM, Dellayen CB: Mask CPAP; state of the art, *Respir Care* 30:846-857, 1985.)

Equipment used to deliver CPAP varies substantially in design and complexity.[88,100] For purposes of illustration, the key elements of a simple continuous flow CPAP circuit is shown in Figure 27-15. A breathing gas mixture from an oxygen blender (*A*) flows continuously through a humidifier (*B*) into the inspiratory limb of a breathing circuit (*C*). A reservoir bag (*D*) provides reserve volume if the patient's inspiratory flow exceeds that of the system. The patient breaths in and out through a simple valveless T-piece connector (*E*). A pressure alarm system with manometer (*F*) monitors the CPAP pressure at the patient's airway. The alarm system can warn of either low (usually due to a disconnection) or high system pressure. The expiratory limb of the circuit (*G*) is connected to a threshold resistor, in this case a water column (*H*).

As can be seen, the CPAP circuit is essentially the same as the EPAP circuit, with the exception of the closed reservoir and monitoring system. Because it is a closed system, the CPAP circuit should also have an emergency inlet valve (not shown). This emergency inlet valve ensures that atmospheric air is available to the patient should the primary gas source fail.

Administering positive airway pressure therapy

As with all respiratory care, effective positive airway pressure therapy requires careful planning, individualized patient assessment and implementation, and thoughtful follow-up.

Planning

During planning, the need for positive airway pressure therapy should be determined, and desired therapeutic outcomes should be set. The box below lists the common clinical findings indicating a need for positive airway pressure therapy intended to treat atelectasis.[69]

Outcome measures indicating successful application of these modalities for treating atelectasis are basically the opposite of these findings. Specifically,

an improvement in breath sounds, an improvement in vital signs, resolution of abnormal X-ray findings, and the restoration of normal oxygenation would all indicate that the therapy had achieved its goal.[69]

Procedures

For PEP therapy, the patient should be seated comfortably with elbows resisting on a flat surface. The mask is placed snugly over the nose and mouth. Using diaphragmatic breathing, the patient inhales a volume 2 to 3 times larger than the normal tidal volume. The patient then slowly (not forcefully) exhales to the FRC through the flow resistor, keeping the positive expiratory pressure between 10 and 20 cm H_2O. This procedure is repeated for 10 to 20 breaths, at which time the mask is removed and the patient performs 2 to 3 "huff" coughs.[74]

This sequence is repeated 4 to 6 times for each PEP therapy session (10 to 20 minutes). Common strategies for PEP vary from twice to four times daily, with frequency determined by assessment of patient response to therapy.[69] During acute exacerbations, therapy should be performed at increasing intervals rather than extending the length of the therapy sessions.

Whether used on an intermittent or continuous basis, CPAP is a complex and potentially hazardous approach to patient management. As with all therapies, the appropriate CPAP level for a given patient must be determined on an individual basis.[80] Initial application and monitoring require a broader range of knowledge and skill than that required for simpler modes of lung expansion therapy. For this reason, detailed discussion on administering CPAP and managing patients receiving this form of therapy is covered in Chapters 29 to 34.

Monitoring and troubleshooting

As with other lung expansion therapies, monitoring of positive airway pressure involves both the equipment performance and patient response (see box on page 765).[33]

CPAP poses a real danger of hypoventilation. Experience with long-term CPAP clearly demonstrates that patients must be able to maintain adequate excretion of carbon dioxide on their own if the therapy is to be successful.

For these reasons, patients receiving CPAP must be closely and continuously monitored for untoward effects. In addition, it is vital that the CPAP device be equipped with means to monitor the pressure delivered to the airways, and alarms to indicate the loss of pressure due to system disconnect or mechanical failure. These are essential components of any CPAP device.

The most common problem with positive airway pressure therapies is system leaks. When using a mask, a tight seal must maintained in order to keep pressure levels above atmospheric. Any significant

---

Clinical findings indicating a need for positive airway pressure therapy to treat atelectasis[69]

- Change in breath sounds consistent with atelectasis
- Change in vital signs—increase in breathing rate, tachycardia, fever
- Abnormal chest X-ray indicating with atelectasis, mucus plugging, or infiltrates
- Deterioration in arterial oxygenation or SpO_2

leaks in the system will result in the loss of positive airway pressure. Because a tight seal requires a tight fitting mask, pain and irritation may occur in some patients, especially if the therapy is prolonged.

The development of the new nasal CPAP units has addressed some of the comfort issues as well as correction of leakage associated with CPAP, however its use intermittently for this purpose has not been well documented.

More serious a problem with CPAP is the possibility of gastric insufflation and aspiration of stomach contents. As with IPPB by mask, this potential hazard can be eliminated by use of a nasogastric tube.

In CPAP system, the RCP must also ensure that the flow is adequate to meet the patient's needs. Generally, the flow is initially set to 2 to 3 times the patient's minute ventilation. Thereafter, flow adjustments are made by carefully observing the airway pressure. Flow is adequate when the system pressure drops no more than 1 to 2 cm H_2O during inspiration.[88]

SELECTING AN APPROACH

The best approach for achieving a given clinical goal is always the safest, simplest and most effective method for a given patient. Selecting an approach for lung

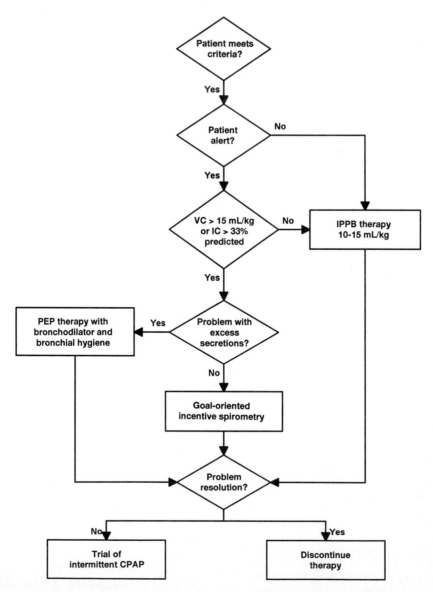

Fig. 27–16 Example protocol for selecting an approach for lung expansion therapy (see text for details.)

<table>
<tr><td>

Monitoring positive airway pressure therapy[69+]

Equipment performance:

Inspiratory pressure (CPAP only)
Expiratory pressure
Source gas flow setting (CPAP only)
FiO_2 (CPAP only)
Nebulizer (if used)

Patient response

Breathing rate and pattern
Minute volume (CPAP only)
Peak flow or $FEV_1/FVC\%$
Pulse rate and rhythm (from EKG if available)
Sputum—quantity, color, consistency and odor
Mental function
Skin color
Breath sounds
Blood pressure
SpO_2 (if hypoxemia is suspected)
Blood gas analysis (if indicated)
ICP (in patients for whom ICP is important)
Chest X-ray
Subjective response to therapy

</td></tr>
</table>

+Above items should be chosen as appropriate for the specific patient.

expansion therapy thus requires in-depth knowledge of both the methods available and the specific condition and needs of the patient being considered for therapy.

Figure 27-16 presents a sample protocol for selecting an approach to lung expansion therapy. As indicated in the algorithm, the patient must first meet the criteria for therapy by having one or more of the indications previously specified. For patients meeting the inclusion criteria, the RCP first determines the degree of alertness. Since an obtunded patient cannot be expected to cooperate with IS or PEP/EPAP therapy, IPPB at 10 to 15 mL/kg is initiated with appropriate monitoring.

If, on the other hand, the patient is alert, a bedside assessment is conducted. This assessment should include measurement of either the inspiratory or vital capacity, and evaluation of the volume and consistency of the patient's secretions.

For the patient having no difficult with secretions, if the VC exceeds 15 mL/kg of lean body weight, or the IC is greater than 33% of predicted, incentive spirometry is given. If either the VC or IC is less than these threshold levels, IPPB is initiated, with the pressure gradually manipulated from the initial setting to deliver the at least 15 mL/kg.

If excessive sputum production is a compounding factor, a trial of PEP therapy is substituted for IS. Based on patient response, bronchodilator therapy and bronchial hygiene measures may be added to this regimen.

If monitoring fails to show improvement and atelectasis persists, a trial of CPAP should be considered. Because the evidence on the effectiveness of CPAP is still contradictory,[87,101] its current use should be limited to treating atelectasis after alternative approaches have been tried without success.

CHAPTER SUMMARY

Lung expansion therapy includes a variety of modalities designed to increase lung volume. When applied to achieve rationally selected goals among carefully chosen patients, lung expansion therapy is an important component of comprehensive respiratory care.

In the past, IPPB was applied to patients without much attention to careful planning, implementation or followup. Later, this modality was nearly abandoned, with little consideration for the possible benefits of its use with carefully chosen patients. Over time, other approaches to lung expansion therapy have developed, including incentive spirometry, intermittent CPAP, and PEP therapy. With these developments has come a more scientific approach to their use. Continuing investigation into the safety and efficacy of these modalities is providing the basis for rational delivery of lung expansion therapy.

As our understanding of these approaches grows, it is apparent that positive outcomes can be achieved only with careful planning, implementation and followup. In this context, the RCP will continue to play a primary role.

REFERENCES

1. Ingram RH: Mechanical aids to lung expansion, *Am Rev Resp Dis* 122:23–25, 1980.
2. Martin RJ, Roger RM, Grant BA: The physiologic basis for the use of mechanical aids to lung expansion, *Am Rev Respir Dis* 122:105–107, 1980.
3. Marini JJ: Postoperative atelectasis: pathophysiology, clinical importance, and principles of management, *Respir Care* 29(5):516–528, 1984.
4. Hughes RL: Improving postoperative tidal volumes, *Respir Care* 26(10):985–986, 1981.
5. Indihar RJ, Forsberg DP, Adams AB: A prospective comparison of three procedures used in attempts to prevent postoperative pulmonary complications, *Respir Care* 27(5):564–568, 1982.
6. Meyers JR, Lembeck L, et al: Changes in functional residual capacity of the lung after operation, *Arch Surg* 110(5):576–583, 1975.
7. Sabanathan S, Eng J, Mearns AJ: Alterations in respiratory mechanics following thoracotomy, *J R Coll Surg Edinb* 35(3):144–150, 1990.
8. Bartlett RH, Krop P, et al: Physiology of yawning and its application to postoperative care, *Surg Forum* 21:223–224, 1970.
9. Craven JL, Evans GA, et al: The evaluation of incentive spirometry in the management of postoperative pulmonary complications, *Br J Surg* 61:793–797, 1974.
10. Petz TJ: Physiologic effects of IPPB, blow bottles and incentive spirometry, *Curr Rev Respir Ther* 1:107–111, 1979.
11. Darin J: Effectiveness of hyperinflation therapies for the prevention and treatment of postoperative atelectasis, *Curr Rev Respir Ther* 12:91–95, 1984.

12. Scuderi J, Olsen GN: Respiratory therapy in the management of postoperative complications, *Respir Care* 34:281–291, 1989.

13. Dohi S, Gold MI: Comparison of two methods of postoperative respiratory care, *Chest* 73:592–595, 1978.

14. Iverson LIG, Ecker RR, et al: A comparative study of IPPB, the incentive spirometer, and blow bottles: the prevention of atelectasis following cardiac surgery, *Ann Thorac Surg* 35:197–200, 1978.

15. Celli BR, Rodriguez KS, Snider GL: A controlled trial of intermittent positive pressure breathing, incentive spirometry, and deep breathing exercises in preventing pulmonary complication after abdominal surgery, *Am Rev Respir Dis* 130:12–15, 1984.

16. American Association for Respiratory Care: Clinical practice guideline: incentive spirometry, *Respir Care* 36(12):1402–1405, 1991.

17. Bartlett RH: Respiratory therapy to prevent pulmonary complications of surgery, *Respir Care* 29(6):667–679, 1984.

18. Jung R, Wright J, et al: Comparison of three methods of respiratory care following upper abdominal surgery, *Chest* 78:31–35, 1980.

19. Stock MC, Downs JB, et al: Prevention of postoperative pulmonary complications with CPAP, incentive spirometry, and conservative therapy, *Chest* 87:151–157, 1985.

20. Walker J, Cooney M, Norton S: Improved pulmonary function in chronic quadriplegics after pulmonary therapy and arm ergometry, *Paraplegia* 27:278–283, 1989.

21. Mang H, Obermayer A: Imposed work of breathing during sustained maximal inspiration: comparison of six incentive spirometers, *Respir Care* 34:1122–1128, 1989.

22. Lederer DH, Vandewater JM, Indech RB: Which breathing device should the preoperative patient use? *Chest* 77:610–613, 1980.

23. Baker WL, Lamb VJ, Marini JJ: Breath-stacking increases the depth and duration of chest expansion by incentive spirometry, *Am Rev Respir Dis* 141(2):343–346, 1990.

24. McConnell EA: Teaching your patient to use an incentive spirometer, *Nursing* 23(2):18, 1993.

25. Rau JL, Thomas L, Haynes RL: The effect of method of administering incentive spirometry on postoperative pulmonary complications in coronary artery bypass patients, *Respir Care* 33(9):771–778, 1988.

26. Motley HL, Werko L, et al: Observations on the clinical use of intermittent positive pressure, *J Aviat Med* 18:417–435, 1947.

27. Pierce AK, Saltzman HA: Conference on the scientific basis for respiratory therapy, *Am Rev Resp Dis* 110(2):1, 1974.

28. Pierce AK: Scientific basis of in-hospital respiratory therapy, *Am Rev Respir Dis* 122(2):1, 1980.

29. O'Donohue, WJ: IPPB past and present, *Respir Care* 27(5):588–589, 1982.

30. Demers RR: IPPB treatments: indications and alternatives, *Respir Care,* 23(8):758–759, 1978.

31. The Respiratory Care Committee of The American Thoracic Society: Guidelines for the use of intermittent positive pressure breathing, *Respir Care* 25(3):365–370, 1980.

32. American Association For Respiratory Care: The pros and cons of IPPB: AARC provides an assessment on its effectiveness, *AARC Times* 10(10):48–50, 1986.

33. American Association for Respiratory Care: Clinical practice guideline. Intermittent positive pressure breathing, *Respir Care* 38(11):1189–1195, 1993.

34. Kittredge P: What is not an IPPB treatment? *Respir Care* 23(3):262–263, 1978.

35. Handelsman H: Intermittent positive pressure breathing (IPPB) therapy. *Health Technol Assess Rep* (1):1–9, 1991.

36. Pontoppidan H: Mechanical aids to lung expansion in nonintubated surgical patients, *Am Rev Respir Dis* 122(2):109, 1980.

37. Brochard L, Isabey D, et al: Reversal of acute exacerbations of chronic obstructive lung disease by inspiratory assistance with a face mask, *N Engl J Med* 323(22):1523–1530, 1990.

38. Elliott MW, Steven MH, et al: Non-invasive mechanical ventilation for acute respiratory failure, *BMJ* 300(6721):358–360, 1990.

39. Ziment I: Intermittent positive pressure breathing, in Burton, GG, Hodgkin JE, editors: *Respiratory care: A guide to clinical practice,* ed 2, Philadelphia, 1984, JB Lippincott.

40. Ellis ER, Grunstein RR, et al: Noninvasive ventilatory support during sleep improves respiratory failure in kyphoscoliosis, *Chest* 94(4):811–815, 1988.

41. Rodenstein DO, Stanescu DC, et al: Adaptation to intermittent positive pressure ventilation applied through the nose during day and night, *Eur Respir J* 2(5):473–478, 1989.

42. Bach JR, Alba AS: Management of chronic alveolar hypoventilation by nasal ventilation, *Chest* 97(1):52–57, 1990.

43. Heckmatt JZ, Loh L, Dubowitz V: Night-time nasal ventilation in neuromuscular disease, *Lancet* 335(8689):579–582, 1990.

44. Branthwaite MA: Assisted ventilation 6. Non-invasive and domiciliary ventilation: positive pressure techniques, *Thorax* 46(3):208–212, 1991.

45. Piper AJ, Parker S, et al: Nocturnal nasal IPPV stabilizes patients with cystic fibrosis and hypercapnic respiratory failure, *Chest* 102(3):846–50, 1992.

46. De Troyer A, Deisser P: The effects of intermittent positive pressure breathing on patients with respiratory muscle weakness. *Am Rev Respir Dis* 124(2):132–137, 1981.

47. Goldstein RS, De Rosie JA, et al: Influence of noninvasive positive pressure ventilation on inspiratory muscles. *Chest* 99(2):408–415, 1991.

48. Dolovich MB, Killian D, et al: Pulmonary aerosol deposition in chronic bronchitis: intermittent positive pressure breathing versus quiet breathing, *Am Rev Respir Dis* 115(3):397–402, 1977.

49. Intermittent positive pressure breathing therapy of chronic obstructive pulmonary disease. A clinical trial. *Ann Intern Med* 99(5):612–20, 1983.

50. Gonzalez ER, Burke TG: Review of the status of intermittent positive pressure breathing therapy, *Drug Intell Clin Pharm* 18(12):974–976, 1984.

51. Kacmerek RM, Hess D: The interface between patient and aerosol generator, *Respir Care* 36:952–976, 1991.

52. Shapiro BA, Peterson J, Carne RD: Complications of mechanical aids to intermittent lung inflation, *Respir Care* 27(4):467–470, 1982.

53. Centers for Disease Control: Update: Universal Precautions for prevention of transmission of human immunodeficiency virus, hepatitis B virus, and other blood-borne pathogens in health-care settings, *MMWR* 37:377–388, 1988.

54. Centers for Disease Control: Guidelines for preventing the transmission of tuberculosis in health-care settings, with special focus on HIV-related issues, *MMWR* 37(RR-17), 1–29, 1990.

55. Bynum LJ, Wilson JE, Pierce AK: Comparison of spontaneous and positive-pressure breathing in supine normal subjects, *J Appl Physiol* 41(3):341–347, 1976.

56. Chevrolet JC, Martin JG, et al: Topographical ventilation and perfusion distribution during IPPB in the lateral posture, *Am Rev Respir Dis* 118(5):847–854, 1978.

57. McPherson SP: *Respiratory therapy equipment,* ed 4, St Louis, 1990, Mosby.

58. Welsh MZ, Shapiro BJ, et al: Methods of intermittent positive pressure breathing, *Chest* 78:463–467, 1980.

59. Morrison J: A proposal for the more rational use of IPPB, *Respir Care* 24:318–322, 1976.

60. O'Donohue WJ: Maximum volume IPPB for the management of pulmonary atelectasis, *Chest* 76:683–687, 1979.

61. Powers WE, Morrison J: Evaluation of inspired volumes in postoperative patients receiving volume-oriented IPPB, *Respir Care* 23:39–41, 1978.

62. O'Donohue WJ: Measures for lung expansion in postoperative patients, *Respir Care* 26:987–989, 1981.

63. American Association for Respiratory Care: Clinical practice

guideline. Selection of aerosol delivery device, *Respir Care* 37(8):891–897, 1992.

64. Pedersen JZ, Bundgaard A: Comparative efficacy of different methods of nebulising terbutaline. *Eur J Clin Pharmacol* 25:739–742, 1983.
65. Weber RW, Petty WE, Nelson HS: Aerosolized terbutaline in asthmatics: comparison of dosage strength, schedule, and method of administration, *J Allergy Clin Immunol* 63:116–121, 1979.
66. Tashkin DP: Dosing strategies for bronchodilator aerosol delivery, *Respir Care* 36(9):977–988, 1991.
67. Nelson HS, Spector SL, et al: The bronchodilator response to inhalation of increasing doses of aerosolized albuterol, *J Allergy Clin Immunol* 72:371–375, 1983.
68. Newman SP: Aerosol deposition considerations in inhalation therapy, *Chest* 88(2, Suppl):152S–160S, 1985.
69. American Association for Respiratory Care: Clinical practice guideline: Use of positive airway pressure adjuncts to bronchial hygiene therapy, *Respir Care* 38(5):516–521, 1993.
70. Tomescn P, Stovring S: Positive expiratory pressure (PEP) as lung physiotherapy in cystic fibrosis: a pilot study, *Eur J Respir Dis* 65:419–422, 1984.
71. Groth S, Staranger G, et al: Positive expiratory pressure (PEP-mask) physiotherapy improves ventilation and reduces volume of trapped gas in cystic fibrosis, *Bull Eur Physiopathol Respir* 21:339–343, 1985.
72. Oberwaldner B, Evans JC, Zach MS: Forced expirations against a variable resistance: a new chest physiotherapy method in cystic fibrosis, *Pediatr Pulmonol* 2(6):358–367, 1986.
73. Steen HJ, Redmond AO, et al: Evaluation of the PEP mask in cystic fibrosis, *Acta Paediatr Scand* 80(1):51–56, 1991.
74. Malmeister MJ, Fink JB, Hoffman GL: Positive expiratory pressure mask therapy: theoretical and practical considerations and a review of the literature, *Respir Care* 36:1218–1229, 1991.
75. Katz JA: PEEP and CPAP in perioperative respiratory care, *Respir Care* 29(6):614–629, 1984.
76. Schlobohm RM, Falltrick RT, et al: Lung volumes, mechanics, and oxygenation during spontaneous positive-pressure ventilation: the advantage of CPAP over EPAP, *Anesthesiology* 55:416–422, 1981.
77. Douglas ME, Downs JB: Cardiopulmonary effects of PEEP and CPAP, *Anesth Analg* (Cleve) 57:346–350, 1978.
78. Lieberman JA, Tarnow J, Cohen NH: Comparison of a fixed-orifice and threshold-resistor for the delivery of positive expiratory pressure to nonintubated patients (abstract), *Chest* 102(Suppl):97S, 1992.
79. Garrard CS, Shah M: The effects of expiratory positive airway pressure on function residual capacity in normal subjects, *Crit Care Med* 6:320–322, 1978.
80. Andersen JB, Olesen KP, et al: Periodic continuous positive airway pressure, CPAP, by mask in the treatment of atelectasis: a sequential analysis, *Eur J Respir Dis* 61:20–25, 1980.
81. Paul WL, Downs JB: Postoperative atelectasis: intermittent positive pressure breathing, incentive spirometry, and face-mask positive end-expiratory pressure, *Arch Surg* 116:861–863, 1981.
82. Carlsson C, Sonden B, Thylen U: Can postoperative continuous positive airway pressure (CPAP) prevent pulmonary

complications after abdominal surgery? *Intensive Care Med* 7:225–229, 1981.
83. Covelli HD, Weled BJ, Beekman JF: Efficacy of continuous positive airway pressure administered by face mask, *Chest* 81(2):147–150, 1982.
84. Williamson DC, Modell JH: Intermittent continuous positive airway pressure by mask, *Arch Surgery* 117:170–972, 1982.
85. Stock MC, Downs JB: Administration of continuous positive airway pressure by mask, *Acute Care* 10:184–188, 1983.
86. Stock MC, Downs JB, Corkran ML: Pulmonary function before and after prolonged continuous positive airway pressure by mask, *Crit Care Med* 12:973–974, 1984.
87. Stock MC, Downs JB, Cooper RB, et al: Comparison of continuous positive airway pressure, incentive spirometry, and conservative therapy after cardiac operations, *Crit Care Med* 12:969–972, 1984.
88. Branson RD, Hurst JM, Dellayen CB: Mask CPAP: state of the art, *Respir Care* 30:846–857, 1985.
89. Lindner KH, Lotz P, Ahnefeld FW: Continuous positive airway pressure effect on functional residual capacity, vital capacity and its subdivisions, *Chest* 92(1):66–70, 1987.
90. Andersen JB, Qvist J, Kann T: Recruiting collapsed lung through collateral channels with positive end expiratory pressure, *Respir Dis* 260–266, 1979.
91. Martin JG, Shore S, Engel LA: Effect of continuous positive airway pressure on respiratory mechanics and pattern of breathing in induced asthma, *Am Rev Respir Dis* 126:812–817, 1982.
92. Mansel JK, Stogner SW, Norman JR: Face-mask CPAP and sodium bicarbonate infusion in acute, severe asthma and metabolic acidosis, *Chest* 96:943–944, 1989.
93. Petrol BJ, Calderini E, Gottfried SB: Effect of CPAP on respiratory effort and dyspnea during exercise in severe COPD, *J Appl Physiol* 69(1):179–188, 1990.
94. Campbell T, Ferguson N, McKinlay RGC: The use of a simple self-administered method of positive expiratory pressure (PEP) in chest physiotherapy after abdominal surgery, *Physiotherapy* 72:498–500, 1986.
95. Rickstcn SE, Bengtsson A, et al: Effects of periodic positive airway pressure by mask on postoperative pulmonary function, *Chest* 89:774–781, 1986.
96. Perel A, Williamson DC, Modell JH: Effectiveness of CPAP by mask for pulmonary edema associated with hypercarbia, *Intensive Care Med* 9(1):17–19, 1983.
97. Strumpf DA, Harrop P, et al: Massive epistaxis from nasal CPAP therapy, *Chest* 95(5):1141, 1989.
98. Viale JP, Annat G, et al: Additional inspiratory work in intubated patients breathing with continuous positive airway pressure systems, *Anesthesiology* 63(5):536–539, 1985.
99. Anderson JB, Klausen NO: A new mode of nebulized bronchodilator in severe bronchospasm, *Eur J Respir Dis* 63(Suppl):97–100, 1982.
100. Freid JL, Downs JB, et al: A new venturi device for administering continuous positive airway pressure (CPAP), *Resp Care* 26:133–136, 1981.
101. Carlson C, Sondem B, Tyhler V: Can post-operative continuous positive airway pressure prevent pulmonary complications after abdominal surgery? *Inten Care Med* 7:225–229, 1981.

Chest Physical Therapy

■

Craig L. Scanlan

Chest physical therapy (CPT) represents a collection of diverse techniques designed to help clear airway secretion, improve the distribution of ventilation, and enhance the efficiency and conditioning of the respiratory muscles.[1,2] These methods include positioning techniques, chest percussion and vibration, directed coughing, and various breathing and conditioning exercises.[3,4]

As with many of respiratory care methods, various CPT procedures were often introduced without scientific assessment for one purpose, then applied to treat other sometimes dissimilar conditions in the hope that they would help.[5] This approach resulted in the widespread and indiscriminate application of CPT to patients with many different cardiopulmonary disorders. For example, in the late 1970s, over 55% of the patients admitted to a single critical care recovery unit received some form of this therapy.[6] With the decrease in popularity of other respiratory care methods (such as IPPB) during the early 1980s, CPT use continued to grow at a rapid pace.[7]

Seldom during this period was the efficacy of chest physical therapy questioned. It was not until recently that CPT methods have been studied scientifically.[8] Results of these studies indicate that selected methods of CPT are effective with certain patients under specific clinical conditions. This scientific approach has recently been reiterated by the American Association for Respiratory Care (AARC) in the development of Clinical Practice Guidelines for several CPT methods.[9,10,11]

Thus, chest physical therapy can be a valuable component of comprehensive respiratory care, but only if used when indicated. Successful outcomes require careful patient evaluation and selection, a clear definition of therapeutic goals, rigorous application of the appropriate methods, and ongoing assessment and followup.[9,10,11]

GOALS OF CHEST PHYSICAL THERAPY

The five primary goals of chest physical therapy are summarized in the accompanying box.[1-3]

Preventing the accumulation of secretions is a prophylactic goal, most often applied to high risk surgical

---

Goals of chest physical therapy

■ To prevent the accumulation of secretions
■ To improve the mobilization of secretions
■ To promote more efficient breathing patterns
■ To improve the distribution of ventilation
■ To improve cardiopulmonary exercise tolerance

---

patients or those with neurologic conditions which can impair respiratory tract clearance. *Improving the mobilization of secretions* applies mainly to patients with pre-existing disorders that cause an abnormal increase in the volume or viscosity of secretions, such as cystic fibrosis. The *promotion of more efficient breathing patterns* is an appropriate goal when structural or functional abnormalities impair efficient use of the respiratory muscles. *Improving the distribution of ventilation* is a legitimate goal of CPT when ventilation-perfusion abnormalities impair pulmonary gas exchange. Last, *improving cardiopulmonary exercise tolerance* represents a long-term goal associated with comprehensive patient rehabilitation programs, as discussed in depth in Chapter 37.

The importance of identifying a specific goal or goals for a given patient cannot be overemphasized. Without a clear goal in mind, it is difficult to justify the use of CPT. Moreover, only by identifying the goals of therapy can one select the best mode of CPT, and assess its effects. To set rational goals, one must understand the clinical indications for CPT.

INDICATIONS FOR CHEST PHYSICAL THERAPY

Recent reviews on the effectiveness of CPT in groups of patients with similar conditions have refined our understanding of the indications for this mode therapy.[8,12] In general, these conditions may be grouped into those representing *acute* clinical disorders, and those of a more *chronic* nature.[8,13] A separate category, the *preventive* use of CPT, also warrants examination.[1,3] Current well substantiated indications for CPT are summarized in Table 28-1.

Chest physical therapy for acute conditions

Among the acute conditions for which scientific evidence currently supports the application of chest physical therapy are: (1) acutely ill patients with copious secretions,[14] (2) patients in acute respiratory failure with clinical signs of retained secretions (audible abnormal breath sounds, deteriorating ABGs, chest radiographic changes),[15] (3) patients with acute lobar atelectasis,[16-18] and patients with V/Q abnormalities due to lung infiltrates or consolidation.[19-21]

Acute conditions for which research has shown that chest physical therapy is *not* beneficial include: (1) acute exacerbations of COPD,[22-24] (2) pneumonia without clinically significant sputum production,[25-27] and (3) uncomplicated asthma.[4,5,8,28]

Chest physical therapy for chronic conditions

There are two broad categories of chronic conditions for which scientific evidence currently supports selected CPT techniques. These include: (1) conditions causing chronic production of large volumes of sputum, and (2) COPD accompanied by inefficient breathing patterns and/or decreased exercise tolerance.

Chronic production of large volumes of sputum

Chest physical therapy has been shown effective in aiding secretion clearance and improving pulmonary function in chronic conditions associated with copious sputum production. These conditions include

Table 28-1 Indications for chest physical therapy

Category	Indications
Acute conditions	Copious secretions
	Acute respiratory failure with retained secretions
	Acute lobar atelectasis
	V/Q abnormalities caused by unilateral lung disease
Chronic conditions	Copious secretions
	COPD with inefficient breathing patterns or decreased exercise tolerance
Preventative use	Postoperative respiratory complications
	Neuromuscular disorders?
	Exacerbations of COPD?

? indicates unproven benefit.

cystic fibrosis,[29-32,33] bronchiectasis,[34,35] and certain patients with chronic bronchitis.[36-38] In general, sputum production must exceed 25 to 30 mL per day for CPT to significantly improve secretion removal.[39]

Chronic obstructive pulmonary disease

The theoretical objectives for chest physical therapy in these patients is to reduce dyspnea and respiratory disability while improving exercise tolerance and the activities of daily living.[40]

In order to acquire a new, more efficient breathing pattern, simple physical conditioning methods (such as walking, climbing stairs, etc.) are combined with breathing retraining and ventilatory muscle exercise, using a variety of manual or mechanical techniques.[40-42] With a few exceptions, most studies indicate that these methods have an immediate objective benefit on blood gases and alveolar ventilation, due to a reduced respiratory rate and increased tidal volume.[40] Maximum exercise capacity, maximum work

---

■ M I N I **C** L I N I ■

28-1

Goals of Chest Physical Therapy

Problem: A physician orders chest physical therapy as a treatment for all patients with chronic bronchitis who are hospitalized because it provides a needed form of "pulmonary hygiene" which will be helpful in facilitating airway secretion clearance. Why is this rationale not always appropriate?

Discussion: The utilization of chest physical therapy (CPT) requires that there be a specific goal or goals which the clinician hopes to achieve. Using a general term such as "pulmonary hygiene" for a hospitalized patient with chronic bronchitis neither provides the RCP a clear clinical indication for the therapy nor a means for evaluating the effectiveness of the therapy. In order to determine what the goals of therapy should be, the physician and clinician providing the therapy should understand what the indications for CPT are. Only then would there be a method for determining the best course of action in facilitating airway secretion clearance.

rate, and respiratory muscle endurance may also be improved over the short-term.[43]

However, long-term results are contradictory and more difficult to interpret.[40,44] While some studies have noted both clinical and functional improvements with fewer relapses and hospital admissions, others studies have not been able to show any patient benefit. Unfortunately, such long-term studies often lack control groups, or suffer from imprecise definition of the clinical state being managed. Clearly, more research is needed before the appropriate indications for CPT in long-term rehabilitation are clearly delineated.[40,44]

Preventive use of chest physical therapy

Chest physical therapy has been suggested as a preventive or prophylactic mode of respiratory care in a variety of patient disorders.[1,3] These include patients at high risk for developing postoperative respiratory complications, patients with neurological disorders that compromise respiratory tract clearance, and patients with chronic lung disease likely to develop acute exacerbations of their disorder. Current evidence presents a mixed picture regarding the benefits of prophylactic CPT.

Preventing postoperative respiratory complications

The three most common respiratory complications associated with surgery are atelectasis, pulmonary aspiration, and postoperative pneumonia.[45] Among those at highest risk for developing these complications are patients with chronic obstructive pulmonary disease.[46] Chest physical therapy, *when used in combination with other respiratory care modalities designed to promote lung expansion,* has been shown effective in decreasing the incidence of postoperative respiratory complications in these and other selected high risk patients.[47-49] CPT immediately after surgery also lowers the risk of postoperative pulmonary complications in the elderly, with a regimen of *preoperative* therapy further decreasing the incidence of postoperative atelectasis in these patients.[50] However, the benefits of CPT alone in reducing complications in other surgical patients are questionable.[51] In general, For this reason, the routine use of CPT after surgery is not supported.[12]

Preventing respiratory problems in neuromuscular dysfunction

Patients with neuromuscular dysfunction are at increased risk for secretion retention.[52] Typically, the underlying disease process impairs coughing. Although lung function may remain normal, neuromuscular disease also predisposes to breathing at low lung volumes, a pattern which increases the likelihood of alveolar collapse. As ventilatory reserve decreases, the risk of progressive atelectasis and secretion retention is increased. In concept, prompt recognition and treatment of abnormal respiratory function in neuromuscular disorders should help prevent problems related to ineffective airway clearance. Although this is a logical assumption supported by numerous case reports, there currently are no comparative studies that demonstrate the benefits of prophylactic CPT in these patients.

Preventing exacerbations of chronic lung disease

Although CPT is still used extensively to prevent acute exacerbations of chronic lung disease, firm evidence to support this application in scanty. Only in the long-term management of cystic fibrosis have comparative studies shown the potential effect of CPT in preventing acute deterioration in patient status. Specifically, when CPT is administered to patients with cystic fibrosis on a regular basis, little or no functional improvement is realized. However, periods *without* CPT tend to result in a progressive worsening of the patient's functional status, which can be reversed with renewal of regular CPT.[53]

PATIENT ASSESSMENT

Effective chest physical therapy requires proper initial and ongoing patient assessment. Obviously, all the key elements involved in determining the need for respiratory care apply, as detailed in Section IV of the text. Formulation of the respiratory care plan thus depends on the results of initial physical assessment, laboratory testing (including pulmonary function tests), and radiologic evaluation.

As an essential element of CPT, initial and follow-up assessment enables the RCP to:[3]

1. Understand the underlying medical or surgical condition as it relates to the patient's altered respiratory status;
2. Select and plan an appropriate treatment regimen;
3. Evaluate the effectiveness of the selected treatment regimen;
4. Recommend changes in the treatment regimen;
5. Identify the appropriate point to discontinue treatment;
6. Formulate a discharge and home care plan for those in need of continued care outside the institutional setting.

Factors to consider in the initial assessment of need for CPT are listed in the accompanying box. In regard to the bedside assessment, an ineffective cough, absent or increased sputum production, a labored breathing pattern, decreased breath sounds or crackles or rhonchi, tachypnea, tachycardia, or fever indicate a potential problem with retained secretions.

In combination, comprehensive review and evaluation of these various factors will determine the likelihood of successful outcomes. Such assessment, when incorporated into the respiratory care planning process, clearly distinguishes the "bang, breathe and cough" approach from an effective and individually tailored treatment plan.[3]

CHEST PHYSICAL THERAPY METHODS

There are five primary methods used in chest physical therapy. These methods include: therapeutic positioning, chest percussion and vibration, coughing and related expulsion techniques, breathing retraining, and conditioning exercises. Appropriate use of these techniques requires an understanding of their underlying principles, relative efficacy, and methods of application.

Therapeutic positioning

Therapeutic positioning involves using gravity to achieve specific clinical objectives. The three primary objectives of therapeutic positioning are to: (1) promote lung expansion and prevent retention of secretions (turning), (2) improve arterial oxygenation (dependent positioning), (3) help mobilize secretions (postural drainage), and (4) relieve dyspnea (relaxation positioning).

Turning

Turning is the rotation of the body around the longitudinal axis.[9] Turning is also referred to as kinetic therapy or continuous lateral rotational therapy.[54,55] Patients may turn themselves or be turned by a caregiver or using a special rotational bed.[9]

Indications. The primary purpose of turning is to promote lung expansion,[19-21,56-58] improve oxygenation,[57,59] and prevent retention of secretions.[55] Other benefits include a reduction in venostasis,[60,61] and prevention of skin ulcers.[62] Specific indications for turning patients with disorders affecting the respiratory system are listed in the accompanying box.[9,54]

Contraindications. There are only two absolute contraindications to turning: unstable spinal cord injuries and traction of arm abductors.[55,54,63] Relative contraindications include severe diarrhea, marked agitation, a rise in ICP, large drops in blood pressure (> 10%), worsening dyspnea, hypoxia, and cardiac arrhythmias.[55,54,63]

Efficacy. Turning can help reduce the incidence of major pulmonary complications (including atelectasis and pneumonia) among critically ill patients, especially those who are comatose or immobile.[64-66] Turning may also shorten ICU stays and result in fewer ventilator days among selected patients.[67] In general, the benefits of turning are probably greatest in patients with less severe illnesses.[67] This is because prevention of pulmonary complications has a greater impact on outcomes among these patients.[55]

Technique. Patients may turn themselves or be turned by a caregiver or using a special rotational bed.[9] Special rotational beds, such as the Roto-Rest Bed (Kinetic Concepts, Inc, San Antonio, TX) rotate continuously on their long axis through a 124° arc every 3 to 4 minutes (Figure 28-1, page 772).[54] **Trendelenburg** and reverse Trendelenburg positions can be used, and any position locked along the rotation arc.

Hazards and complications. Common hazards associated with turning include "plumbing" problems and adverse patient responses.

"Plumbing" problems include ventilator discon-

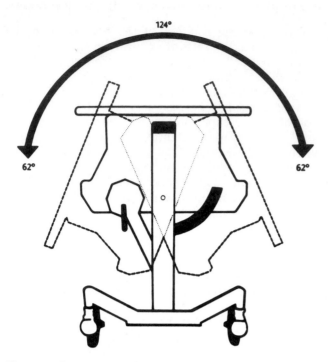

124°

62°   62°

Fig. 28-1 Rotation arc of Roto-Rest Bed. (Courtesy of Kinetic Concepts, Inc, San Antonio, Texas.)

nection, accidental extubation, accidental aspiration of ventilator circuit condensate, and disconnection of vascular lines or urinary catheters.[54] Adverse patient responses include patient intolerance, cardiac arrhythmias, increased ICP, or worsening dyspnea and hypoxemia.[54]

Dependent positioning

Using positioning solely to enhance the distribution of ventilation in patients with significant V/Q imbalances is now a widely accepted clinically maneuver.[7] Problems that can be treated with this simple approach include acute localized conditions, such as unilateral pneumonias, and conditions resulting in a more generalized decrease in lung volume, such as the adult respiratory distress syndrome (ARDS).

In concept, dependent positioning at first seems illogical. In normal subjects, both the side-lying (lateral decubitus) and head-down position result in a *decrease* in functional residual capacity, of about 18% and 27% respectively.[68] This is due to displacement of the dome of the dependent diaphragm further up into the thorax than in the sitting or standing position.

However, this diaphragmatic displacement and lower FRC places the dependent zones of the lung on a steeper portion of the pressure-volume curve, resulting in a greater change in volume for a given pressure change, and thus better ventilation.[69,70] Thus, as in the upright position, the "down" portion of the lung always receives the best ventilation and also the best blood flow.

Unilateral lung disease. The effects of side-lying positioning on V/Q ratios in patients with unilateral lung disease clearly support the application of dependent positioning to improve oxygenation in these patients. In patients with unilateral chest infiltrates, the PaO_2 tends to fall significantly when the "bad" lung is down.[71,72] This fall in PaO_2 is due to the increase in shunting that occurs as gravity increases perfusion through collapsed lung units. Because these units are collapsed, most of the ventilation would tend to go to the upper lung, further worsening the V/Q relationship.

Logically, the opposite of this effect, that is *placing the good lung in the dependent or down position,* may be used to enhance oxygenation in patients with unilateral lung disease.[20,21,73] Coincidently, placement of the good lung down is also the position of choice for most postural drainage.

However, in conditions such as lung contusions that cause internal pulmonary bleeding, the nonaffected lung may have to be placed in the up position. This will help prevent blood that has accumulated in the diseased lobes or segments from entering the good lung.[6] Placement of the diseased lung in a *down* position is also indicated in the presence of a completely or partially filled lung abscess, and with unilateral pulmonary interstitial emphysema (PIE).[73]

Generalized decreases in lung volume. The benefits of positioning in patients with a generalized decrease in lung volume associated with the adult respiratory distress syndrome (ARDS) also have been reported.[19] In this study, patients receiving mechanical ventilation were turned from the supine to the prone position. In addition, support was provided to the upper thorax and pelvis, thereby allowing the abdomen to protrude. Once placed in this position, patients exhibited a mean increase in arterial oxygen tension of 69 torr (range, 2 to 178 torr), without a change in tidal volume, inspired oxygen concentration, or level of positive end-expiratory pressure (PEEP). No significant change in mean arterial carbon dioxide tension, respiratory frequency, or effective compliance was observed after positioning.

This maneuver alone made it possible to reduce the FIO_2 in 4 of the 5 patients who required mechanical ventilation of the lungs, and to defer intubation in the one patient who was breathing spontaneously. Arterial PO_2 decreased in 12 of 14 instances after patients were turned from prone to supine.

The physiologic basis for this positioning effect is less clear than with unilateral lung disease. Improved arterial oxygenation due to a reduction in abdominal restriction to the movement of the diaphragm is unlikely, since no change in effective compliance of the lungs/thorax was observed. Clearly, the switch to the prone position somehow improves the V/Q relationship, but exactly how this occurs remains uncertain. Studies of prone positioning in infants suggest

---

Indications for postural drainage[9]

- Difficulty clearing secretions:
  sputum production greater than 25 to 30 mL/day (adult)
  retained secretions in patients with artificial airways
- Presence of atelectasis due to mucus plugging
- Diagnosis of diseases such as cystic fibrosis, bronchiectasis, or cavitating lung disease
- Presence of foreign body in airway

Contraindications to postural drainage

- Absolute contraindications:
  head and neck injury until stabilized
  active hemorrhage with hemodynamic instability
- Relative contraindications:
  intracranial pressure (ICP) > 20 mm Hg
  patients in whom increased ICP is to be avoided (eg, neurosurgery, aneurysms, eye surgery)
  recent spinal surgery or acute spinal injury
  empyema
  bronchopleural fistula
  cardiogenic pulmonary edema
  large pleural effusions
  pulmonary embolism
  aged, confused, or anxious patients who do not tolerate position changes
  rib fracture, with or without flail chest
  surgical wound or healing tissue
  uncontrolled hypertension
  distended abdomen
  esophageal surgery
  active hemoptysis
  uncontrolled airway at risk for aspiration

---

that a decrease in asynchronous chest wall movement may be responsible.[74] These findings cannot, however, be generalized to adults.

Postural drainage

Postural drainage involves the use of gravity to help move respiratory tract secretions from lung lobes or segments into the central airways.[3,9] This is done by simply placing the segmental bronchus to be drained in a vertical position relative to gravity.[75,76]

Efficacy. Assessing the efficacy of postural drainage alone is difficult because most studies combine this method with other modes of chest physical therapy.[77] Moreover, several different criteria have been used to judge its effectiveness. These include the volume and consistency of sputum produced, the clearance of radioactive albumin particles, and various measures of pulmonary function.

Despite these limitations, the current literature supports the following conclusions:

1. Postural drainage does *not* facilitate mucociliary clearance in normal subjects;[78]
2. Postural drainage does *not* improve pulmonary function in patients with stable chronic lung disease who produce scanty amounts of secretions;[79,80]
3. Postural drainage is most effective in conditions characterized by excessive sputum production (30 mL or more per day);[8,39,81]
4. To be effective, postural drainage probably requires head-down positions in excess of 25 degrees;[8,36,78]
5. Adequate systemic and airway hydration is a prerequisite for effective mucociliary clearance in general, and postural drainage in particular.[82]

Indications. Based on these conclusions, specific indications for postural drainage have been identified (see box above).[9]

Contraindications. Postural drainage is not risk free. Prior to initiating postural drainage, potential benefits must be weighed against potential risks. Contraindications to postural drainage are listed in the accompanying box.[9]

Technique. Based on a preliminary assessment of the patient, and a substantiation of the need, the RCP, in consultation with the ordering physician, identifies the appropriate lobe(s) and segments for drainage. Also based on the preliminary assessment, the RCP determines the potential need for modification of the position(s) chosen. Modification of head-down positions may be required in patients with unstable cardiovascular status, hypertension, cerebrovascular disorders, and orthopnea.[9,75]

Treatment times should be scheduled either before or at least 1-1/2 to 2 hours *after* meals or tube feedings.[3] If the patient assessment indicates that pain may hinder treatment implementation, consideration also should be given to coordinating the treatment regimen with prescribed pain medication.

Before positioning, the procedure (including adjunctive techniques) is explained to the patient. As necessary, clothing around the waist and neck should be loosened.[3] Also, any monitoring leads, IV tubing, and oxygen therapy equipment connected to the patient should be inspected and adjusted to ensure continued function during the procedure. Vital signs, including pulse, respirations, and blood pressure, should be taken before initiation of the procedure. Auscultation should also be conducted prior to initiating drainage. These simple assessments will serve as baseline measures for monitoring the patient's response during the procedure, and can assist in determining its effect after completion.[75]

Figures 28-2 through 28-10 depict the primary positions used to drain the various lung lobes and segments.[75] In head-down positions in general, the foot of the bed must be elevated above the head by at least 16 to 18 inches to achieve the desired 25 degrees angle. In the ambulatory care setting, a "tilt-table" may be used in lieu of a hospital bed. A tilt-table allows precise positioning at head-down angles up to 45 degrees. When angles this large are used, shoulder supports must be provided to prevent the patient from sliding off the table. Modifications of these positions for infants and children are discussed in Chapter 35.

Once the patient is positioned, the RCP should confirm his or her comfort and ensure proper support of all joints and boney areas with pillows or towels. Stippled areas in Figures 28-2 through 28-10 indicate the anatomic location for percussion and vibration, if ordered to accompany the procedure.

The indicated position should be maintained for a minimum of 3 to 15 minutes if tolerated, and longer if good sputum production results.[9] Between positions, pauses for relaxation and breathing control are useful and can help prevent hypoxemia.[83] During the procedure, the RCP should continually observe the patient for signs of ill effects. Other parameters that may need to be monitored during postural drainage are listed in the accompanying box.[9] Since postural drainage positioning predisposes patients to arterial desaturation, pulse oximetry should be considered a routine component of monitoring during postural drainage.[84]

The RCP should also ensure appropriate coughing technique, both during and after positioning. When using the head-down positions, strenuous coughing should be avoided, since this will markedly raise intracranial pressure. Rather, the patient should use the forced expiration technique (described later). In general, total treatment time should not exceed 30 to 40 minutes. Both the patient and the RCP should understand that postural drainage does not always result in the immediate production of secretions.

More often, secretions are simply mobilized toward the trachea for easier removal by coughing. If the procedure causes vigorous coughing, the patient should sit up until the cough subsides.

After the procedure, the RCP should restore the patient to the pretreatment position, and ensure his or her stability and comfort. Immediate post-treatment assessment should include repeat vital signs, chest auscultation, and patient questioning regarding his or her subjective response to the procedure.

Outcome assessment. Specific outcome criteria indicating a positive response to postural drainage are listed in the accompanying box.[9] In general, achievement of one or more of these outcomes indicates that the therapy is achieving its objectives and should be continued. Not all criteria are required to justify continuing postural drainage.[9]

Because secretion clearance is affected by patient hydration, one may need to wait for at least 24 hours after optimal systemic hydration has been achieved to see any evidence of increased sputum production.[9] In the interim, tracheobronchial clearance can be enhanced in some patients by applying particulate water to the airway with an unheated jet nebulizer.[85]

In assessing outcomes, the RCP also should be aware that breath sounds may actually seem to 'worsen' following therapy.[9] Typically, the RCP may initially note diminished breath sounds and crackles before therapy that change over to coarse rhonchi after treatment. This is due to the loosening of secretion and their movement into the larger airways, an intended purpose of the therapy. These coarse rhonchi should clear after coughing or suctioning.

In terms of the patient's subjective response to therapy, the patient should be encouraged to report on any pain, discomfort, shortness of breath, dizziness, or nausea during or after therapy.[9] Any of these adverse effects may be grounds for either modifying or stopping treatment. On the other hand, patient reports of easier clearance or increased volume of secretions after therapy support continuing therapy.[9]

Moderate changes in vital signs during treatment should be expected. Should the patient develop brady-

continue text from page 779

Parameters to monitor during postural drainage[9]

- Sputum production (quantity, color, consistency, odor)
- Cough effectiveness
- Pulse rate, dysrhythmia, and EKG if available
- Blood pressure
- Breathing pattern and rate
- Breath sounds
- Skin color
- Arterial saturation (SpO_2)
- Intracranial pressure (ICP) (if monitored)
- Mental function
- Subjective response, i.e., pain, discomfort, dyspnea

Outcome criteria indicating successful postural drainage[9]

- Increase in sputum production
- Improvement in breath sounds
- Restoration of normal vital signs
- Resolution of abnormal chest X-ray
- Normalization in ABG values or oxygen saturation
- Improved in ventilator variables (indicating decreased resistance or increased compliance)
- Patient's positive subjective response to therapy

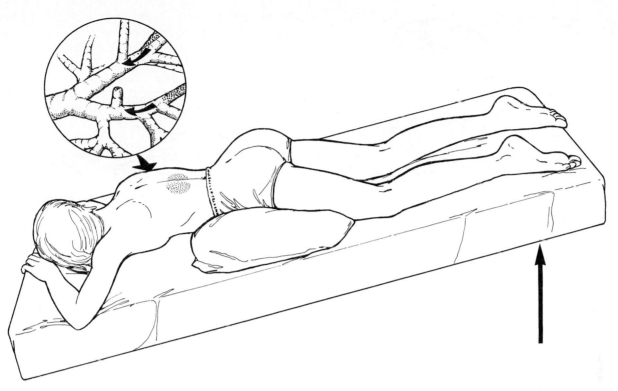

Fig. 28-2 Position for drainage of posterior basal segment of lower side.

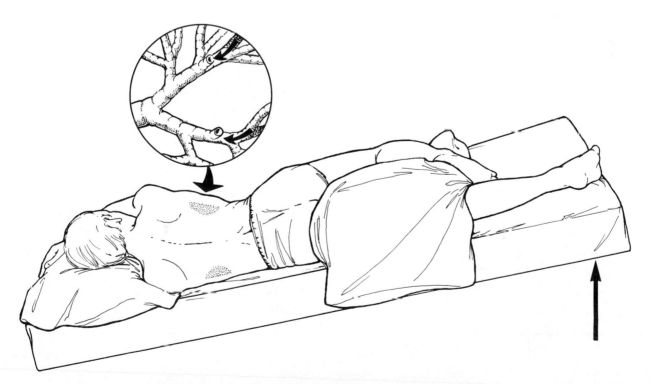

Fig. 28-3 Position for drainage of lateral basal segment of lower lobe.

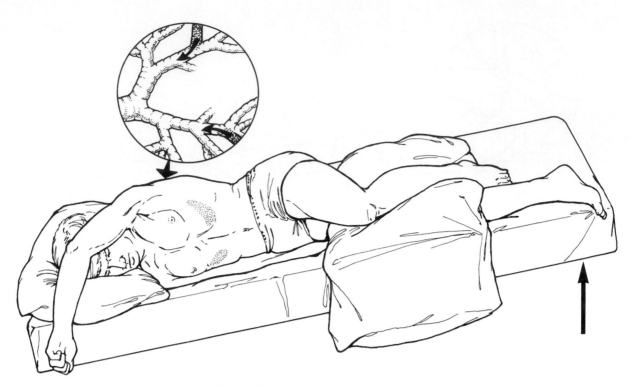

Fig. 28-4 Position for drainage of anterior basal segment of lower lobe.

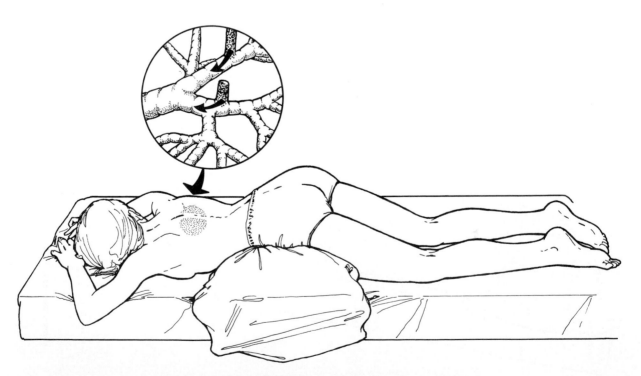

Fig. 28-5 Position for drainage of superior segment of lower lobe.

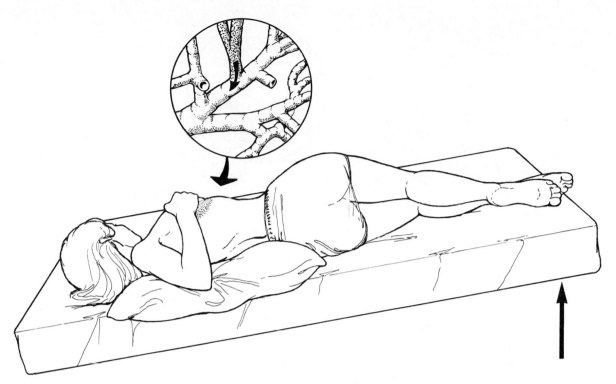

Fig. 28-6 Position for drainage of lateral and medial segments of middle lobe.

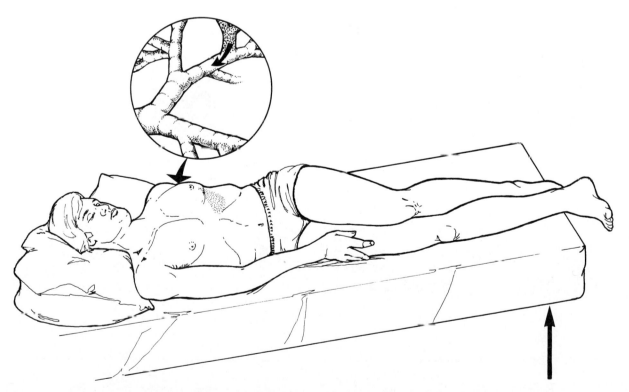

Fig. 28-7 Position for drainage of superior and inferior lingular segment.

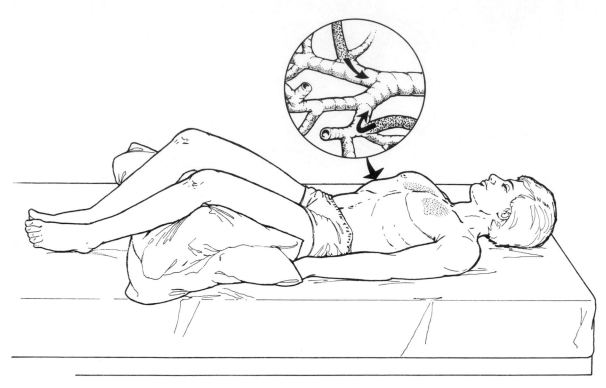

Fig. 28-8 Position for drainage of anterior segment of upper lobe.

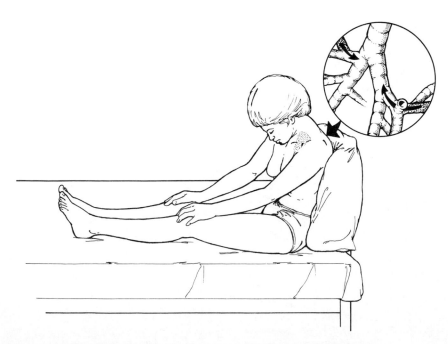

Fig. 28-9 Position for drainage of apical segment of upper lobe.

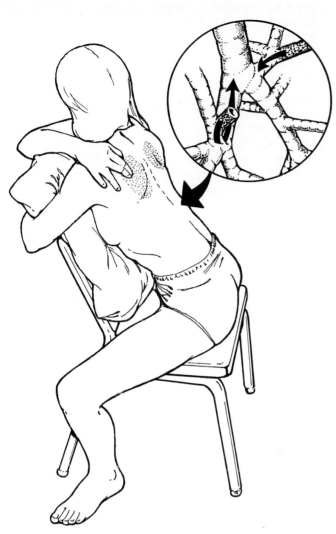

Fig. 28-10 Position for drainage of posterior segment of upper lobe.

cardia, tachycardia, or irregularities in pulse or blood pressure, postural drainage should be stopped.[9]

Documentation and follow-up. Charting should include specification of position(s) used, time in position, patient tolerance, subjective and objective indicators of treatment effectiveness (including the amount and consistency of sputum produced), and any untoward effects observed. Since the effects of the procedure may not be immediately evident, the RCP should make a return visit within 1 to 2 hours after treatment, or followup with the patient's nurse.

Relaxation positioning

Relaxation positioning is a simple technique designed to help relieve dyspnea in patients with COPD or those with acute shortness of breath due to an asthma. Figures 28-11 and 28-12 shows the relaxation positions useful in both the sitting and standing positions.

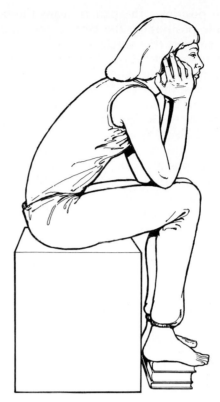

Fig. 28-11 Resting position, patient seated while leaning on hands.

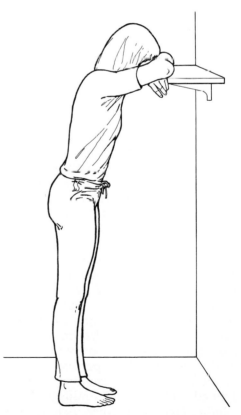

Fig. 28-12 Resting position, patient standing while leaning on elbows that have been placed on wall or chest-high object.

In both positions, the patient leans the body forward, while positioning the elbows and upper arms against a support (the thighs or wall). This position has two major effects. First, the forward flexion about the waist relaxes the abdominal muscles, thereby facilitating descent of the diaphragm. Second, fixing the upper arms allows the patient to make more efficient use of the accessory muscles of inspiration, especially the pectoralis groups (refer to Chapter 9). In combination with a purposefully slower breathing pattern, this posture can help reduce the work of breathing, increase tidal volumes, and decrease the subjective sensation of dyspnea.[86]

In reality, many patients with COPD have already learned to assume these relaxation positions when they experience dyspnea. When properly reinforced by the RCP and combined with other maneuvers designed to improve diaphragmatic activity and slow the breathing pattern, the full benefits of these positional techniques can be realized.

Percussion and vibration

Percussion and vibration both involve application of mechanical energy to the chest wall using the either the hands or various electrical or pneumatic devices. Both methods are designed to augment secretion clearance.[87] In theory, percussion should help jar retained secretions loose from the tracheobronchial tree, making them easier to remove by coughing or suctioning. Vibration, on the other hand, is designed to aid movement of secretions toward the central airways during exhalation.

Efficacy

As with postural drainage, assessing the efficacy of percussion and vibration is difficult, since most studies combine this method with others.[8] Moreover, the patients studied often have very different clinical problems. In addition, there is no consensus as to what is the "right" force or frequency for percussion and vibration.[3,51,88] Nonetheless, there are some potentially positive finding in the literature.

In a study of ten patients with a variety of disorders (including atelectasis, pleural effusion, and pneumonia) mechanical vibration, when combined with positional changes and suctioning, improved arterial oxygen saturation at 30 and 60 minutes after therapy.[89] Of course, whether the vibration alone caused these improvements could not be determined.

In a more specific study, patients with cystic fibrosis treated with mechanical percussion and postural drainage did produce significantly more sputum than those treated with postural drainage alone.[90] More recent studies confirm that percussion and vibration can increase the volume of sputum production in selected patients.[91-94] Used together with postural drainage, vibration also has proved useful as an adjunct to hyperinflation and suction in treating the early stages of acute lobar atelectasis.[95]

Indications

For these reasons, and in light of current knowledge, the widespread use of these methods cannot be justified.[8] However, since percussion and vibration methods may increase the volume of sputum production in some patients, their selective use may be appropriate. Specifically, percussion and vibration should be considered as an adjunct to postural drainage and coughing only when these methods alone fail to mobilize secretions.[9,94]

Contraindications. As with postural drainage, potential risks are associated with percussion and vibration. Relative contraindications to percussion and vibration are listed in the accompanying box.[9]

Percussion technique

Percussion, when indicated, is applied over the surface landmarks of the area being drained (Figures 28-2 to 28-10). Manual percussion is accomplished with the hands in a cupped position, with fingers and thumb closed. In this manner, a cushion of air is trapped between the hand and chest wall. The striking force may be against the bare skin, although a thin layer of cloth, such as a hospital gown or bedsheet, does not significantly impair transmission of the energy wave.

The RCP, holding his or her arm with the elbow partially flexed and wrist loose, rhythmically strikes the chest wall in a waving motion, using both hands alternately in sequence (Figure 28-13). Slower, more relaxing rates are better tolerated by patient and RCP alike.[1] It is not a difficult technique to master, but skill and experience are needed to determine the appropriate force and to maintain a rhythmic pattern.

Contraindications for percussion and vibration[9]

- Subcutaneous emphysema
- Recent epidural spinal infusion or spinal anesthesia
- Recent skin grafts, or flaps, on the thorax
- Burns, open wounds, and skin infections of the thorax
- Recently placed transvenous or subcutaneous pacemaker
- Suspected pulmonary tuberculosis
- Lung contusion
- Bronchospasm
- Osteomyelitis of the ribs
- Osteoporosis
- Coagulopathy
- Complaint of chest-wall pain

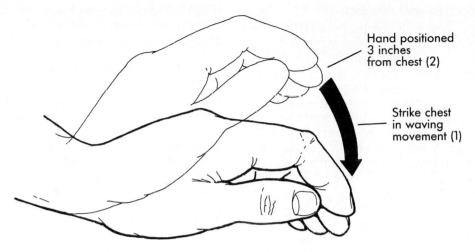

Hand positioned
3 inches
from chest (2)

Strike chest
in waving
movement (1)

Fig. 28-13 Movement of cupped hand at wrist to percuss chest.

Ideally, the percussion should proceed back and forth in a circular pattern over the localized area for a period of 3 to 5 minutes. Naturally, care must be exercised by the RCP to avoid tender areas or sites of trauma or surgery, and percussion must never be performed directly over boney prominences, such as the clavicles or vertebrae.

Vibration technique

When indicated, chest vibration is often used together with percussion, but limited to application during exhalation. Typically, the RCP lays one hand on the patient's chest over the involved area and places the other hand on top of the first (Figure 28-14). Alternatively, the hands may be placed on either side of the chest. After the patient take a deep breath, the RCP exerts slight to moderate pressure on the chest wall, and initiates a rapid vibratory motion of the hands throughout expiration.

Mechanical percussion and vibration

Various electrical and pneumatic devices have been developed to generate and apply the energy waves used during percussion and vibration. Although no substitute for a skilled RCP, these devices do not tire and can deliver consistent rates, rhythms, and impact forces.[96] However, there is currently no firm evidence to indicate that these devices are any more effective than manual techniques.[9]

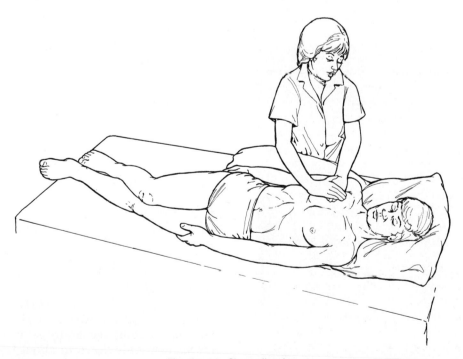

Fig. 28-14 Chest vibration.

High frequency chest wall compression

High frequency chest wall compression (HFCC) is a new mechanical technique for augmenting secretion clearance that is showing some promise.[97] The HFCC device (ThAIRapy System, American Biosystems) has two components: (1) a variable air-pulse generator, and (2) a non-stretch inflatable vest that covers the patient's entire torso (Figure 28-15). Small gas volumes are alternately injected into and withdrawn from the vest by the air-pulse generator at a fast rate, creating an oscillatory motion against the patient's thorax.

Patients perform 30 minute therapy sessions at oscillatory frequencies between 5 and 25 Hz. The ideal frequency for a given patient is that which produces the highest flows and the largest volumes per chest compression during tidal breathing. Depending on need and response, between 1 and 6 therapy sessions may occur per day.

Although it is to early to draw firm conclusions, preliminary studies indicate that HFCC has the potential to increase secretion clearance over traditional CPT methods, at least in cystic fibrosis patients.[97,98] HFCC also appears to be at least as good as CPT in promoting secretion clearance in mechanically ventilated patients.[99] Last, cystic fibrosis patients using HFCC have show long-term improvements in actual pulmonary function (FVC and FEV_1).[100]

Coughing and related procedures

Although generally taken for granted, the cough is one of our most important protective reflexes.[101] By rid-

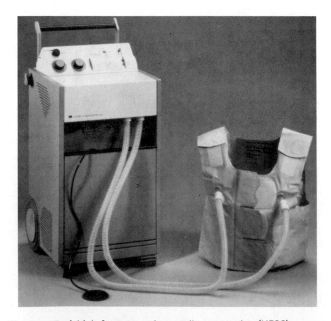

Fig. 28-15 A high frequency chest wall compression (HFCC) system. (Courtesy of American Biosystems.)

ding the larger airways of excessive mucus and foreign matter, the cough complements normal mucociliary clearance, and helps ensure airway patency.

Mechanism of normal cough

Normally, a cough begins when sensory endings of certain nerves become irritated. These nerves may include vagal fibers in the larynx, trachea or larger bronchi; or afferent fibers of the glossopharyngeal nerve in the pharynx. A cough can also be induced by stimulation of nerve endings in the mucous membranes of the esophagus, pleural surface, and auditory canal. Once generated, these impulses travel to the cough center in the medulla, which reflexly stimulates the muscles of the chest and larynx to initiate the cough sequence.[102,103]

Figure 28-16 depicts the sequence of events occurring during a normal cough. There are four distinct phases. In the initial *irritation* phase, an abnormal stimulus provokes sensory fibers to send afferent impulses to the cough center. This stimulus normally is either inflammatory, mechanical, chemical, or thermal. Infection is a good example of cough stimulation due to an inflammatory process. Foreign bodies can provoke a cough through mechanical stimulation. Chemical stimulation can occur when irritating gases are inhaled. Finally, cold air may cause thermal stimulation of sensory nerves and produce a cough.

Once these afferent impulses are received and processed, the cough center stimulates the respiratory muscles to initiate a deep *inspiration* (the second phase). In normal adults, this inspiration averages one to two liters.

During the third or *compression* phase, efferent nerve impulses cause glottic closure and a forceful contraction of the expiratory muscles. Lasting about 0.2 sec, this compression phase results in a rapid rise in pleural and alveolar pressures, often in excess of 100 mm Hg.

At this point the glottis opens, initiating the *expulsion* phase. With the glottis open, a large pressure gradient is established between the alveoli and airway opening. Together with the continued contraction of the expiratory muscles, this pressure gradient causes a violent, expulsive flow of air from the lungs, with velocities often as high as 500 miles per hour! Because the nasopharynx is closed off when the glottis opens, foreign material expelled from the respiratory tract enters the mouth, where it can be expectorated or swallowed.

In terms of clinical use, it is important to realize that a cough also may be initiated voluntarily, without the presence of irritating stimuli. This is in contrast to the sneeze, which generally cannot be induced without local irritation. Also critical to understand is the fact that a cough generally is an effective clearance mechanism only down to about the sixth or seventh branching of the tracheobronchial tree.[1] Thus, retain-

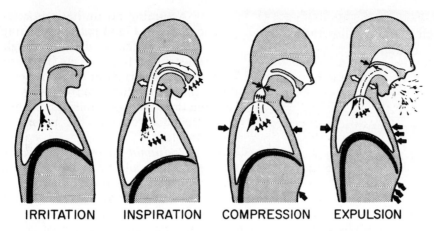

IRRITATION   INSPIRATION   COMPRESSION   EXPULSION

Fig. 28-16 The cough reflex. (From Cherniack RM and Cherniack L: Respiration in health and disease, ed 3, Philadelphia, 1983, WB Saunders.)

ed secretions beyond this level must first be mobilized into the larger airways by other methods if they are to be effectively cleared. Last, and of utmost concern in the clinical setting, is the fact that *interference with any one of its four phases can result in an ineffective cough,* thereby impairing the patient's ability to clear respiratory tract secretions. Table 28-2 provides examples of factors which can impair the normal cough reflex, according to the phase affected.

Directed cough

Directed cough is a deliberate maneuver that is taught, supervised, and monitored.[10] Directed cough aims to mimic the features of an effective spontaneous cough, to help to provide voluntary control over reflex, and to compensate for physical limitations that can impair this reflex.[10]

Efficacy. Cough has little direct effect on secretion clearance in individuals who cannot produce sputum.[104] Coughing may indirectly enhance mucus clearance in normal individuals by stimulating the mucoc-

iliary apparatus.[105] However, in patients with copious secretions, directed coughing is as least as good at clearance as more complicated methods.[8,36] Vigorous directed coughing alone has been shown to provide radioaerosol clearance as good as that resulting from a combination of postural drainage, percussion and vibration administered by a skilled therapist, although the more comprehensive treatments did produce a greater volume of sputum.[30]

However, current knowledge suggests that coughing and other modes of CPT may differ in regard to where they act. Directed coughing is most effective in clearing secretions from the central, but not peripheral airways.[37,106] This difference is consistent with our understanding of the physiology of the normal cough mechanism, as previously discussed.

Indications. Indications for directed cough are listed in the accompanying box.[10] As is evident, directed cough may be used alone or in combination with other bronchial hygiene therapies. In addition, directed cough may be used to help obtain sputum specimens for diagnostic analysis.

Table 28-2 Mechanisms impairing the cough reflex

Phase	Examples of impairments
Irritation	Anesthesia
	CNS depression
	Narcotics-analgesics
Inspiration	Pain
	Neuromuscular dysfunction
	Pulmonary restriction
	Abdominal restriction
Compression	Laryngeal nerve damage
	Artificial airway
	Abdominal muscle weakness
	Abdominal surgery
Expulsion	Airway compression
	Airway obstruction
	Abdominal muscle weakness

Indications for directed cough[10]

- The need clear retained secretions from the central airways
- The presence of atelectasis
- To help prevent postoperative pulmonary complications
- As a routine part of bronchial hygiene in patients with cystic fibrosis, bronchiectasis, chronic bronchitis, necrotizing pulmonary infection, or spinal cord injury
- As a component of other bronchial hygiene therapies
- To obtain sputum specimens for diagnostic analysis

Contraindications to directed cough[10]

- Inability to control infection spread by droplet nuclei (eg, *M. tuberculosis*)
- Presence of an elevated ICP or known intracranial aneurysm
- Presence of reduced coronary artery perfusion (eg, acute MI)
- Acute unstable head, neck, or spine injury

Contraindications. The few clinical situations in which directed cough is contraindicated are listed in the box above.[10] As always, these contraindications must be weighed against the potential benefits of directed cough for each patient.

Technique. The first step in applying directed cough is to establish a need. Clinical situations indicating a need for directed cough are listed in the box below.[10]

Once the clinical need is established, the RCP should then assess the patient to determine if any factors exist which could limit the success of directed cough. For example, an effective directed cough regimen is generally not possible with obtunded, paralyzed, or uncooperative patients.[10] In addition, some patients with advanced COPD or severe restrictive disorders (including neurologic, muscular, or skeletal abnormalities) may not be able to generate an effective spontaneous cough.[10] Likewise, pain or fear of pain caused by coughing may limit the success of directed cough. Last, systemic dehydration, thick, tenacious secretions, artificial airways, or the use of CNS depressants or antitussives can thwart efforts to implement an effective directed cough regimen.

Should one or more of these limitations exist, it is the responsibility of the RCP to recommend alternative means to help remove secretions. Alternative secretion clearance strategies are discussed subsequently.

Clinical situations indicating a need for directed cough[10]

- Spontaneous cough that fails to clear secretions from the airway
- Ineffective spontaneous cough as judged by:
  - clinical observation
  - evidence of atelectasis
  - results of pulmonary function testing
- Postoperative upper abdominal or thoracic surgery patient
- Long-term care patients who retain airway secretions
- Presence of artificial tracheal airway

Assuming no limitations exist, directed coughing can begin. Good patient teaching is critical in developing an effective directed cough regimen. The three most important aspects involved in patient teaching are: (1) instruction in proper positioning, (2) instruction in breathing control, and (3) exercises to strengthen the expiratory muscles.[101] These activities are modified according to the patient's underlying clinical problem.

Positioning. To generate an effective cough, the patient should be properly positioned. Patients must be taught to assume a position which aids exhalation and allows easy thoracic compression.[1,101] Due to abdominal muscle tension, it is difficult to generate an effective cough in the supine position.[101] Rather, the patient should be placed in a sitting position, with shoulder rotated inward, the head and spine slightly flexed, and the forearms relaxed or supported. In order to provide abdominal and thoracic support, the feet should be supported. If the patient is unable to sit up, the head of the bed can be raised, with the knees slightly flexed, and the feet braced on the mattress.

Breathing control. Breathing control measures help ensure that the inspiration, compression, and expulsion phases of the cough are maximally effective and coordinated. For effective inspiration, the patient should be taught to inspire slowly and deeply through the nose, using the diaphragmatic method (discussed subsequently). In patients with copious amounts of sputum, such breaths alone may stimulate coughing by loosening secretions in the larger airways.

After the patient is able to achieve a satisfactory deep inspiration, he or she is told to bear down against the glottis, in much the same manner as would occur during straining at stool. In patients with pain, or those subject to bronchiolar collapse, it is probably best that they be shown how to "stage" their expiratory effort into two or three short bursts. For these patients, this method is generally less fatiguing and more effective in producing sputum than a single violent expulsion.[1,101]

Effective breathing control is best taught via demonstration. Using demonstration, the RCP can go through the various phases of the cough sequence, emphasize the correct technique, and point out common errors, such as simple throat clearing.

Strengthening the expiratory muscles. At times, proper positioning and breathing control alone may not assure an effective cough. More often than not, this limitation is due to weak expiratory muscles. Expiratory muscle weakness is common in patients with COPD who suffer from a general lack of muscle conditioning, and patients having undergone long-term ventilatory support, during which muscles may atrophy from lack of use. In either case, an effective cough cannot be developed until these muscles are reconditioned. Details on expiratory muscle conditioning are provided later in this chapter.

Modifications in technique. As previously discussed, several factors can limit the success of directed cough. To overcome these limitations, the RCP needs to modify the normal directed cough routine, according to the needs of the individual patient. Good clinical examples of the need to modify directed cough are seen in the surgical patient, the patient with COPD, and the patient with a restrictive neuromuscular disorder.

Surgical patients. In patients undergoing surgery, *preoperative* training in breathing control can help prepare the patient for the postoperative regimen. This can minimize the anxiety over pain that commonly impairs an effective cough in these patients. In addition, the postoperative regimen can be enhanced by coordinating the coughing sessions with prescribed pain mediation, and assisting the patient in "splinting" the operative site. This may initially be accomplished by the RCP, using the hands to support the area of incision. Later, the patient can be taught to use a pillow to splint the site. The *forced expiration technique,* or FET (to be discussed subsequently) may also be of value in these patients.

COPD patients prone to bronchiolar collapse. In some patients with COPD, the high pleural pressures during a forced cough may compresses the smaller airways and limit the cough's effectiveness. In this case, the patients should be placed in the sitting relaxation positioned previously described.[101] The RCP then instructs the patient to slowly inhale through the nose while concurrently moving to a full upright position. The goal is a moderate, as opposed to full inspiration. This reduces the volume of air to be removed by the patient and results in less of a rise in pleural pressure.

To compensate for characteristic loss of expulsive force, the patient is told to exhale with moderate force through pursed lips, while bending forward.[101] This forward flexion of the thorax enhances expiratory flow by upward displacement of the abdominal contents. After 3 to 4 repetitions of this maneuver, the patient is encouraged to bend forward and initiate short staccato-like bursts of air. This technique relieves the weak patient of the strain of a prolonged hard cough, and the staccato rhythm at a relatively low velocity minimizes airway collapse. This technique has a modification called "huffing" whereby the patient is instructed to make the sound of "huff, huff, huff" rapidly with the mouth open, the sound audibly coming from the throat.[107,108]

Alternatively, either the forced expiration technique or autogenic drainage may be used in these patients. Both these clearance mechanisms are discussed subsequently.

Patients with neuromuscular conditions. Patients with neuromuscular conditions present the RCP with a special challenge in cough management. Depending on the nature of the neuromuscular disorder, the normal reflex reaction to irritation may be impaired or absent, deep inspiration may be impossible, glottic closure may be incomplete, or expiratory muscles may not be able to contract. In cases where one or more of these factors causes significant retention of secretions, an artificial airway normally is indicated (refer to Chapter 22). This allows direct access to the central airways for secretion removal via suctioning.

Whether an artificial airway is present or not, these patients typically are unable to generate the forceful expulsion needed to move secretions toward the trachea.[109,110] In these cases, manually assisted directed cough may be required.

Manually assisted cough is the external application of mechanical pressure to the **epigastric** region or thoracic cage, coordinated with forced exhalation.[10] In this technique, the patient takes as deep an inspiration as possible, assisted as needed by the application of positive pressure via self-inflating bag or IPPB device. At the end of the patient's inspiration, the RCP begins exerting pressure on the lateral costal margin or epigastrium, increasing the force of compression throughout expiration. This mimics the normal cough mechanism by generating an increase in the velocity of the expired air,[111] and may be helpful in moving secretions toward the trachea, where the can be removed by suctioning.

Manually assisted directed cough with pressure to the lateral costal margins is contraindicated in patients with osteoporosis or flail chest.[10] Manually assisted cough using epigastric pressure is contraindicated in unconscious patients with unprotected airways, in pregnant women, and in those with acute abdominal pathology, abdominal aortic aneurysm, or hiatal hernia.[10]

Forced expiration technique

The forced expiration technique (FET) is a modification of the normal directed cough. The FET consists of one or two forced expirations from mid-to-low lung volume *without closure of the glottis,* followed by a period of diaphragmatic breathing and relaxation.[112] The goal of the this method is to help clear secretions with less change in pleural pressure and less likelihood of bronchiolar collapse.[8]

To help keep their glottis open during an FET, patient should be taught to phonate or "huff" during expiration. The period of diaphragmatic breathing and relaxation following the forced expiration is essential in restoring lung volume and minimizing fatigue.

Comparative clinical studies on the effectiveness of this method have demonstrated favorable results. In general, when self-applied by patients with copious secretions, the FET results in better sputum production in less time than traditional therapist-supervised intervention.[31] Moreover the FET has been shown to provide better **radioaerosol** clearance than directed coughing, especially when combined with postural drainage.[35] This evidence suggests that the ideal chest physical therapy regimen in patients with copious secretions may well be postural drainage combined with the forced expiration technique.[113]

Autogenic Drainage

Autogenic drainage represents another modification of directed coughing, developed and popularized in European cystic fibrosis centers.[114,115] Autogenic drainage begins with low-lung-volume breathing, inspiratory breath holds, and controlled exhalation. Over the treatment session, patients progress to increase their inspired volumes and expiratory flows.[116] The principle is to balance expiratory force, intrabronchial pressure, and the stability of the bronchial walls to obtain maximal expiratory airflow without causing airway collapse.[12]

Studies of the effectiveness of autogenic drainage are limited. In CF patients, autogenic drainage has been shown to have produced significantly more sputum than coughing alone.[117] However, other CPT techniques were deemed more effective than autogenic drainage. In asthmatic patients, use of autogenic therapy over an 8-month period resulted in significant improvements in respiratory function (FEV_1), as compared to psychotherapy alone.[118]

Unfortunately, the technique is difficult to teach patients (especially children), and is probably of little value in the treatment of the critically ill.[119] A simplified approach has been developed to make the procedure easier to teach and learn,[120] but this modification has not undergone testing by clinical trials.

Mechanical exsufflation

Some 40 years ago, peak expiratory flows similar to those seen with a spontaneous cough were obtained with mechanical exsufflators.[121,122] These devices were used clinical to clear secretions from patients unable to cough, especially those with neuromuscular disorders like polio.[123] Their use continued up until the mid-1960s, when artificial tracheal airways and suctioning became the method of choice for secretion clearance in patients unable to cough.[55]

Recently, a mechanical insufflation-exsufflation device has been reintroduced and applied to ventilator-assisted patient with neuromuscular disorders.[124,125] In these patients, the device can generate peak expiratory flows in the normal range (mean of 7.5 L/s). This flow far exceeds that generated by manually assisted directed coughing. No significant complications have yet been reported with use of this device. However, clinical trail data is currently unavailable, and the utility of these devices has not yet been proved in critically ill patients.

Positive airway pressure adjuncts

Positive airway pressure adjuncts are used to mobilize secretions and treat atelectasis.[11] Positive airway pressure adjuncts include continuous positive airway pressure (CPAP), expiratory positive airway pressure (EPAP), and positive expiratory pressure (PEP). The use of these methods to treat atelectasis was reviewed in Chapter 27. Here we will focus on the use of these methods as adjuncts in secretion clearance, with an emphasis on PEP therapy.

As adjuncts for secretion clearance, positive airway pressure methods must never be used alone. Positive airway pressure methods are always combined with directed cough or other airway clearance techniques.[11]

Indications

The accompanying box lists the indications for positive airway pressure therapy. Refer to Chapter 27 for contraindications.

Assessment of need

Clinical situations indicating a need for positive airway pressure therapy in general and PEP therapy in particular are the same as those previously described for directed postural drainage and coughing. In general, PEP is most effective as an adjunct in secretion removal in disease states characterized by excessive sputum production (> 30 mL/day).[9,113]

PEP equipment

Equipment for PEP therapy includes a form-fitting face mask, a one way T-valve assembly, a pressure manometer, and an adjustable flow resistor (Figure 28-17).[126] A mouthpiece can be used instead of a mask for some patients. For patients requiring aerosolized bronchodilator therapy, a SVN can be added to the system.[127]

PEP technique

During PEP therapy, the patient exhales against a fixed-orifice flow resistor. With a flow resistor, expiratory pressures depend on the patient's expiratory flow. The higher the expiratory flow through a given-sized orifice, the greater the expiratory pressure. Patients are taught to actively but not forcefully exhale through the flow resistor to maintain a pressure between 10 to 20 cm H_2O.[127-131] This sequence is

---

Indications for positive airway pressure therapy[11]

- To reduce air trapping in asthma and COPD
- To prevent or reverse atelectasis
- To aid in mobilization of retained secretions
- To optimize bronchodilator delivery

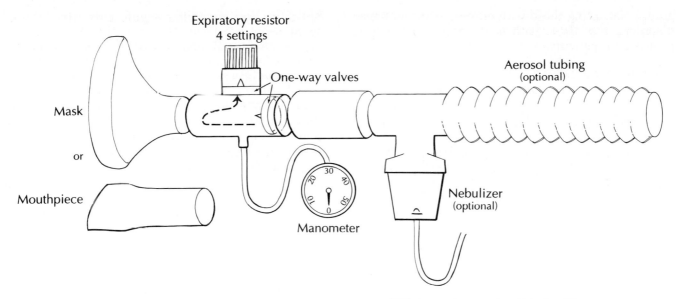

Fig. 28-17 Equipment needed for positive expiratory pressure (PEP) therapy. (Redrawn from Malmeister MJ, Fink JB, Hoffman GL: Positive expiratory pressure mask therapy: theoretical and practical considerations and a review of the literature, *Respir Care* 36:1218-1229, 1991.)

repeated 4 to 6 times for each PEP therapy session (10 to 20 minutes). Common strategies for PEP vary from twice to four times daily, with frequency determined by assessment of patient response to therapy.[11] During acute exacerbations, therapy should be performed at decreasing intervals rather than extending the length of the therapy sessions.

Like pursed-lip breathing, PEP increases pressure within the airways. This back pressure helps keep the airways open throughout exhalation. By preventing airway collapse during expiration, PEP helps move secretions into the larger airways for expectoration via coughing or swallowing.[132]

Efficacy

The efficacy of PEP therapy is best studied and documented in cystic fibrosis patients. In these patients, PEP therapy is as good or better in mobilizing secretions as postural drainage,[133] the forced expiratory technique (FET),[134] or autogenic drainage.[117] PEP therapy also can provide significant improvements in lung function over the course of in-patient treatment for CF.[129,135] However, when applied to patients with chronic bronchitis, PEP has no demonstrable effect on regional lung clearance.[136]

Breathing exercises

Breathing exercises represent a broad category of activities designed to achieve a variety of purposes, including the following:[137]

1. To promote greater use of the diaphragm and decreased use of the upper rib cage and other accessory muscles of inspiration;

2. To increase awareness of the muscles of respiration and to suppress the tendency for hurried and gasping respiration;
3. To provide patients with the tools necessary to better handle the distressful symptom of dyspnea;
4. To identify and provide a means by which inefficient and inappropriate muscle use can be diminished or eliminated;
5. To improve the efficiency of alveolar ventilation by increasing tidal volume, slowing the rate of breathing, prolonging the expiratory time and promoting better distribution of ventilation to perfusion;
6. To improve the strength and endurance of the respiratory muscles;
7. To improve the effectiveness of the cough;
8. To improve the delivery of therapeutic aerosols;
9. To teach patients to coordinate their breathing with body motions and the activities of daily living;
10. To relieve exertional dyspnea so that patients can improve their overall cardiopulmonary fitness and general exercise tolerance.

Our analysis will focus first on the application of specific inspiratory and expiratory breathing exercises, followed by a discussion of more general conditioning activities. Integration of these exercises and conditioning activities into a comprehensive rehabilitation program are discussed in Chapter 37. Although emphasis is placed on the application of these techniques to patients with chronic obstructive pulmonary disease, where appropriate, mention will be made of their potential use among other patient groups, including those with chronic neuromuscular disorders, and those with acute problems, such as postsurgical patients.

Inspiratory breathing exercises

There are three primary types of inspiratory breathing exercises: diaphragmatic (abdominal) breathing, lateral costal breathing, and inspiratory resistive breathing.

Diaphragmatic (abdominal) breathing exercises. As discussed in prior chapters, chronic obstructive pulmonary disease, especially those forms characterized by loss of elastic tissue, pulmonary distention, and air trapping, result in grossly inefficient use of the diaphragm and excessive dependence on the accessory muscle of inspiration.[138] The primary purpose of diaphragmatic or "abdominal" breathing exercises is to promote greater use of the diaphragm and decreased use of the accessory muscles of inspiration. Initially, this is accomplished by developing an increase awareness of diaphragmatic activity by the patient, followed by exercises designed to increase the strength of this primary muscle of inspiration. Long term benefits to the patient may include an increased efficiency of alveolar ventilation, achieved by virtue of an increased tidal volume, slower rate of breathing, and increased exercise tolerance.

Efficacy. Three questions are critical in addressing the effectiveness of diaphragmatic breathing exercises. First, we must ask whether it is possible to voluntarily alter one's breathing pattern from mainly accessory to mainly diaphragmatic breathing. Second, if it is possible to voluntarily change the nature of inspiratory muscle use, we must know whether or not this change affects the pattern of ventilation or its distribution. Lastly, we must know whether or not such exercises can improve overall muscle strength and endurance.

In regard to the ability of diaphragmatic breathing exercises to alter the pattern of breathing, the evidence is clear.[139] In patients with chronic obstructive pulmonary disease, diaphragmatic breathing exercises have been shown to increase the relative contribution of this muscle to ventilation from about 40% (during uncoached spontaneous breathing) to about 67%.[139]

The impact of diaphragmatic breathing exercises on the pattern of ventilation and its distribution is more controversial. There is general consensus that diaphragmatic breathing exercises can result in increased tidal volume, and slower rates of breathing.[137] However, studies of the effect of diaphragmatic breathing exercises on the distribution of ventilation provide mixed results. In normal subjects, breathing mainly with the intercostal and accessory muscles results in a greater distribution of the inspired air to the upper lung regions, as compared to either normal or diaphragmatic breathing. At low inspiratory flows, the distribution of ventilation with diaphragmatic breathing does not differ significantly from normal spontaneous breathing. However, at higher inspiratory flows, a normal breathing pattern causes a maldistribution of ventilation to the upper lung regions, not unlike that occurring during intercostal and accessory muscles use.[140] Unfortunately, similar studies in patients with chronic obstructive lung disease have shown no systematic difference in the overall distribution of ventilation between spontaneous and augmented diaphragmatic breathing.[139]

Research result also provide a mixed picture regarding the impact of diaphragmatic breathing exercises on muscle strength and endurance. In one study of patients with chronic obstructive bronchitis with moderate disability, three weeks of controlled diaphragmatic breathing produced no beneficial effects on exercise performance (walking) or the perceived strain of exercise, as compared to a placebo treatment.[141] However, several other studies have demonstrated positive results in the application of inspiratory breathing retraining, most often when included as a component of general conditioning exercise activity.[43,142-145] Although the outcome measures in these studies vary somewhat, the following general benefits of inspiratory muscle breathing retraining were realized: a decrease in respiratory rate and increase in tidal volume, PaO_2, and oxygen consumption during exercise: an increased maximum sustainable ventilatory capacity (**MSVC**): and an increased maximum 12 minute walking distance.

Technique. Changing the breathing pattern is a slow and difficult process, requiring the utmost patience on the part of the RCP. This is because it is often very difficult for a patient who has come to rely extensively on the thoracic accessory muscles to revert back to diaphragmatic breathing. Indeed, many patients may never be able to fully accomplish this changeover.

Before starting a breathing exercise, the RCP should ensure that the patient is relaxed both mentally and physically. Before teaching any new breathing exercise, the RCP also should demonstrate it on him or herself, explaining both the purpose of each maneuver, and how best the patient can accomplish it.

The best position for initiating diaphragmatic breathing exercises is similar to that used for cough training, that is a 45 degree sitting position, with shoulders rotated inward, the head and spine slightly flexed, the forearms relaxed or supported, and the knees bent. In order to minimize use of the upper thoracic respiratory muscles, a modification of the Jacobeson relaxation exercise may be employed.[1] In this technique, the patient is asked to shrug the shoulders, and holds them up for a short period. Alternatively, the RCP asks the patient to tighten the muscles of the arms and chest, then relax.

Once the patient is properly prepared, the RCP places a hand on the patient's upper abdomen, in the epigastric region below the xiphoid process (Figure 28-18). The patient is then encouraged to inhale slowly through the nose, taking air into the abdomen, with an effort forceful enough to lift the RCP's hand. As the patient initiates the effort, the RCP provides progressive resistance to the outward movement of the epigastric region, releasing the pressure at the end of inspiration.

The patient's awareness of the effort should be confirmed, and the exercise repeated (with rest as necessary) until satisfactory movement is achieved. Because of the physical work involved, the initial time tolerated by the patient may be short, but as performance improves, the exercise may be extended to 30 minutes three to four times daily. Ideally, the patient can be taught to perform the exercise on him or herself, using progressive epigastric pressure in the same manner as applied by the RCP.

During this early learning phase, the RCP must be on guard for common errors, including arching of the patient's back or simple protrusion of the abdomen.[137] Both these maneuvers mimic true diaphragmatic breathing, but are readily recognized. If a patient persists in these ineffective action despite appropriate instruction and feedback, the RCP should consider use of the lateral costal breathing exercises (discussed next) as an alternative.

In patients who can tolerate head-down positions, it may be possible to enhance this exercise using a Trendelenburg position in bed or on a tilt-table. In this variation, the patient is positioned in a 20° head-down tilt. As with the standard procedure, diaphragmatic action is taught and confirmed with progressive hand pressure. In subsequent treatment sessions, resistance to inspiration is provided by a weight placed over the epigastric region. Initially, this weight may be as little as 5 pounds, but with strengthening of the diaphragm, the load may be progressively increased in 5 pound increments up to 20 to 30 pounds, as tolerated.

Once the patient masters diaphragmatic breathing in the sitting position, the RCP should assist the ambulatory patient in applying this technique while standing, and, subsequently, as a component of the walking regimen.

Lateral costal breathing exercises. Lateral costal breathing exercises are intended to augment abdominal breathing. This modification of the diaphragmatic technique consists of expanding and contracting the costal margin, which increases mobility of the diaphragm and, in theory, increases ventilation to the lung bases. Lateral costal breathing exercises are a viable alternative to the diaphragmatic method, especially in patients having undergone abdominal surgery. As such, lateral costal breathing exercises have an effect comparable to the diaphragmatic technique on alveolar ventilation, muscle strength and endurance, and the patterns of breathing.

Technique. The RCP places his or her hands over the costal margins so that they almost cup the lower rib edges (Figure 28-19, page 790). At the end of exhalation, the RCP begins application of pressure. The patient is instructed to breathe around the waist and push the hands away, to direct attention to this area. As inhalation begins, the RCP gradually increases the manual pressure to the expanding ribs, while encouraging a slow, deep breath. Finally, the patient is taught to use his or her own hands to mobilize the lower ribs.

Inspiratory resistive breathing. Research conducted in the mid 1970s clearly demonstrated that both respiratory muscle strength and endurance of healthy subjects could be increased by a six week training program involving resistive breathing exercises.[146] Subsequently, this technique was introduced and successfully applied as a simple alternative to traditional breathing exercises in patients with pulmonary disease.[147-152]

In concept, inspiratory resistive breathing represents the simple imposition of an additional workload

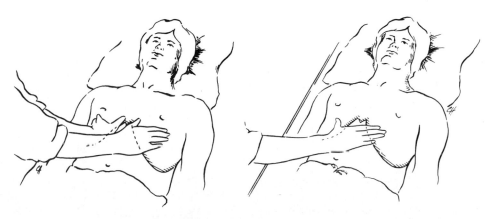

Fig. 28–18 Placement of therapist's hand for diaphragmatic breathing. (From Frownfelter D: Chest physical therapy and pulmonary rehabilitation: an interdisciplinary approach, ed 2, St Louis, 1987, Mosby.)

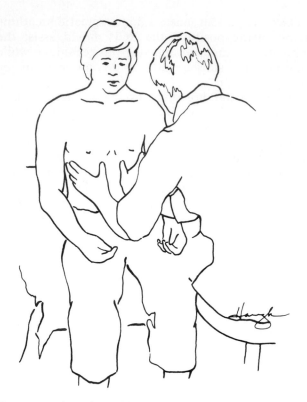

Fig. 28–19 Lateral costal breathing exercises. (From Frownfelter D: Chest physical therapy and pulmonary rehabilitation: an interdisciplinary approach, ed 2, St Louis, 1987, Mosby.)

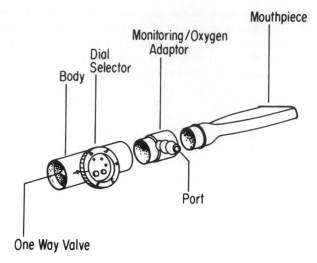

Fig. 28-20 Flow-resistive breathing device.

on the inspiratory muscles (mainly the diaphragm) during breathing. Over time, this increased workload should increase both the strength and endurance of these muscles. In turn, the increased strength and endurance of the inspiratory muscles should improve the patient's exercise tolerance.

The first device designed for this purpose was a simple adjustable flow resistor combined with a one-way valve (Figure 28-20). During inspiration, the patient breathes through a restricted orifice of variable size. Flow resistance across this orifice creates a pressure difference between the atmosphere and mouth, thereby increasing the load placed on the inspiratory muscles. During expiration, gas flows unimpeded out the exhalation valve. Because the pressure difference during inspiration varies directly with the rate of flow, the load placed on the inspiratory muscles with this type of device is greater when the patient breathes fast, and less when the patient breathes more slowly.

More recently, a threshold resistor has become commercially available for this purpose (Figure 28-21). Rather than using a restricted orifice to increase the pressure differential, the threshold resistive breathing device uses an adjustable spring-loaded valve. This assures a relatively constant load regardless of how fast or slowly the patient breathes.[153] With this device, it is possible to set a specific load in terms of the negative inspiratory pressure (cm H_2O) necessary to open the valve.

Efficacy. In clinical trials using comparison groups, various researchers have shown that an inspiratory resistive breathing exercise training program can result in significant patient benefits. Among the positive

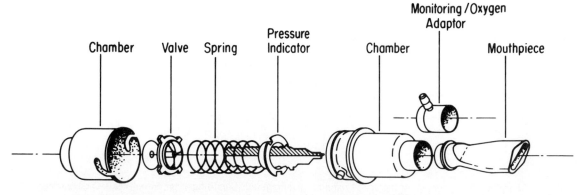

Fig. 28-21 Threshold (spring-loaded) resistive breathing device.

outcomes generally reported are: decreased dyspnea and respiratory frequency, increased inspiratory muscle strength, and increased respiratory muscle endurance.[146-152] However, these benefits tend to occur without a change in either resting pulmonary function or overall exercise performance, as assessed by cycle ergometer exercise, stair climbing, walking distance or treadmill walking.[154] Moreover, some studies have failed to show any significant benefit at all.[154,155]

Recently, it has been suggested that variations in the breathing strategy used during inspiratory resistive exercise may have a profound effect on its outcomes. Specifically, analysis of the breathing patterns used by patients has shown that a reduction in the peak mouth pressure, breathing frequency, and external resistive work, combined with a longer inspiratory time, is the most beneficial approach.[155]

Related to the general concern over variations in patient's breathing strategies has been a lack of validated clinical guidelines for prescribing inspiratory resistive exercises.[156] However, with the availability of the threshold resistive device, this situation is changing. A recent clinical study has shown that a resistive load of 30% of the maximum inspiratory pressure, or **PImax**, represents the minimum load necessary to effect an increase in inspiratory muscle strength and endurance.[157] Moreover, the use of this minimum load over a two month training program *did* result in an increase in general exercise tolerance, as measured by the maximum 12 minute walking distance.

Technique. Based on these findings, it is evident that the success of this method depends on proper patient evaluation, training and followup, as conducted by a knowledgeable RCP.

In terms of evaluation, in addition to the general assessment of the patient (previously described), the RCP initially should measure the patient's maximum inspiratory pressure, using a calibrated pressure manometer like that depicted in Figure 28-22. Once the PImax is obtained, the RCP can compare the patient's value to established norms, as delineated in Table 28-3.[158] This preliminary measure of inspiratory muscle strength thus helps in establishing initial loads and provides the basis for the subsequent monitoring of patient progress.

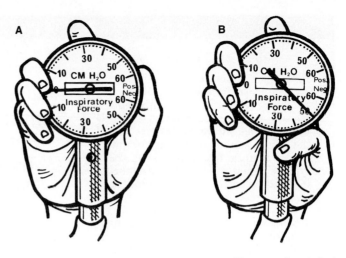

Fig. 28-22 An inspiratory force measurement. The gauge is attached to the patient's airway, **A,** The patient is instructed to take a deep breath while the clinician obstructs the airway by closing the open port on the gauge, **B,** The negative pressure detection, measured here as −50 cm of water, is the patient's maximum inspiratory force. (From Pilbeam SP: Mechanical ventilation: physiological and clinical applications, ed 1, St Louis, 1986, Multi-media Publishing.)

In preparation for exercise training, the patient should be instructed to assume a position which relaxes the abdominal muscles, such as that used for cough training. Instruction in diaphragmatic breathing should ideally *precede* the application of the inspiratory resistive exercises, thereby assuring appropriate emphasis on the use of this muscle of respiration.

If using a flow resistive device, the RCP initiates instruction at the maximum orifice setting, while measuring the inspiratory pressure generated through the monitoring/oxygen adapter (a second adapter may be necessary if the patient is receiving supplemental oxygen). The RCP encourages the patient to inhale and exhale slowly through the device, at a rate of no more than 12 to 15 per minute. If the generated inspiratory pressure is less than 30% of the measured PImax, the next smaller orifice is selected, with this procedure repeated until the 30% effort is consistently achieved.

Once the appropriate effort is achieved, the patient is instructed to begin exercise with the device in one or two regular daily sessions of 10 to 15 minutes duration. As the level of resistance becomes more tolerable over time, the patient progressively increases the *duration* of the sessions to 30 minutes. A self-maintained log of treatment times can help motivate the patient and assist the RCP in subsequent progress monitoring.

At this point, the patient should be re-evaluated by the RCP, to include measurement of the PImax. If the patient exhibits an increase in the PImax, the level of resistance should be increased (by decreasing the size

Table 28-3   Normal maximum inspiratory pressure (cm H$_2$O) by age and sex

Age group	Mean (± SD) PImax from residual volume	
	Male	Female
9-18	−96 ± 35	−90 ± 25
19-50	−127 ± 28	−91 ± 25
51-70	−112 ± 20	−77 ± 18
>70	−76 ± 27	−66 ± 18

From Rochester DF and Hyatt RE: Respiratory muscle failure, *Med Clin North Am* 67:573-579, 1983.

■ M I N I C L I N I ■

28–2

Failure of an Inspiratory Resistive Training Program

Problem: A patient is using an inspiratory muscle training device which incorporates a variable orifice flow resistor. After several months of routine training, the RCP observes that the device is not improving the patient's exercise tolerance. Could the type of inspiratory muscle trainer being used be partly responsible for the lack progress noted?

Discussion: The basic concept of inspiratory muscle training devices are that they impose a certain amount of inspiratory pressure at the mouth which must be overcome by respiratory muscles during breathing. This additional workload is thought to help improve both the strength and endurance of the muscles of inspiration. There are two types of inspiratory muscle trainers; a variable orifice flow resistor and the threshold resistor. The main limitation of the flow resistor device is that since the pressure generated at the mouth varies directly with the rate of flow during inspiration, changes in breathing pattern can effect the load placed on the inspiratory muscles. The threshold resistor on the other hand, uses a spring-loaded valve to maintain a relatively constant inspiratory muscle load regardless of inspiratory flow rate. In this clinical situation, the lack of patient progress noted by the RCP may be attributed to either the use of the flow resistor training device itself or failure of the training method to demonstrate clinical benefit.

of the orifice) to the new 30% level, with session time restored back to 10 to 15 minutes, and the exercise progression and followup repeated. If, on the other hand, the PImax is not increased, the RCP should attempt to determine the cause by questioning the patient and inspecting the log. In many cases, a failure to demonstrate an improvement in PImax can be attributed to simple noncompliance with the exercise regimen.

When using a threshold resistive device, the technique is essentially the same, except that loads can be set directly on the device. As with the flow resistive device, once the initial load is determined, the patient progressively increases the *duration* of the session. On re-evaluation by the physician or RCP, the load may be increased, with the patient then repeating the cycle of increasing session time.

Expiratory breathing exercises

There are two primary types of expiratory breathing exercises: pursed-lip breathing and forced exhalation abdominal breathing. The former technique is used exclusively in patients with chronic obstructive pulmonary disease who are prone to early airway collapse. The latter method has been used in these patients, but may also be useful as an adjunct to cough training in other groups with expiratory muscle dysfunction.

Pursed-lip breathing. Pursed-lip breathing is a simple maneuver that many patients with chronic pulmonary disease adopt without instruction. The espoused purpose of pursed-lip breathing is to prevent the air trapping caused by bronchiolar collapse, especially that associated with pulmonary emphysema.[159]

By increasing expiratory flow resistance, pursed-lip breathing has two primary effects. First, pursed-lip breathing increases upstream pressures in the tracheo-bronchial tree during exhalation.[160] This causes the equal pressure point (EPP) to move further up toward the larger airways, thereby decreasing the likelihood of bronchiolar collapse.[161] Second, pursed-lip breathing decreases expiratory flow rates. This decreases the frequency of breathing and prolongs the expiratory time.[159,162]

Efficacy. Patients with chronic obstructive pulmonary disease who breath through pursed lips tend to exhibit both an increase in alveolar ventilation and an improvement in the V/Q ratio as indicated by a decrease in the $P(A-a) O_2$.[163] Whether these beneficial effects are due mainly to the movement of the EPP or to the decrease in respiratory rates is not known for sure. The fact that simple deep breathing at slow rates alone may have similar effects in these patients suggests that it is the pattern of breathing that is of primary importance.[162] However, the changes in airway pressure generated during pursed-lip breathing may help diminish feelings of dyspnea by altering tension relationships of the respiratory muscles.[164]

Technique. In preparation for training in pursed-lip breathing, the patient should be placed in a comfortable position. The RCP instructs the patient to inhale slowly through the mouth. During exhalation, the patient is taught to purse the lips as if whistling, controlling the velocity of exhaled air to the slowest that is consistent with comfortable ventilation. Ideally, this should lower the rate of breathing and increase the expiratory time such that it is at least two to three times longer than inspiration. Efforts should be made to avoid strenuous expiratory efforts, as this may simply increase the tendency toward bronchiolar collapse. The technique should be reinforced as needed, and the patient encouraged to apply this method whenever dyspnea is sensed.

Forced exhalation abdominal breathing. Forced exhalation abdominal breathing exercises are designed to strengthen the contractile force of the abdominal wall muscles. This technique is useful in patients with poor muscle conditioning that limits exercise capacity, or those with an ineffective cough due to a specific weakness of the expiratory muscles.

Forced exhalation abdominal breathing exercises are best taught with the patient in the supine position, with a pillow under the patient's head and the knees drawn up comfortably to relax the anterior abdominal wall. The principles of technique are illustrated in Figure 28-23. The patient's hand is placed on the epigastrium, in order to focus attention to this area (*A*). Much of the success of therapy will depend on the degree to which the RCP can keep the patient's mind on this epigastric movement. Exercise is always started in the same manner, by exhaling from the resting level. At the same time the patient is instructed to pull in the upper abdomen gradually, with conscious force, prolonging exhalation as long as possible (*B*). At end-exhalation the patient is told to inhale easily through the nose, letting the upper abdomen balloon out (*C*), and the cycle is repeated. The patient is advised to think of all breathing as taking place in the abdomen rather than in the chest; therefore, as the patient inhales, the abdomen should swell, lifting up the hand, and as he or she exhales, the hand should fall with the receding abdomen.

During the maneuver, the RCP must keep reminding the patient to concentrate on all respiratory movement as taking place in the area in contact with the hand, and to disregard the chest completely. Many patients, trying hard to cooperate, will suddenly forget the sequence they were taught, contracting the epigastric wall during inhalation and attempting to relax it during exhalation.

The RCP encountering this problem will find two techniques useful in correcting the breathing pattern. The first is the steady repetition over several breathing cycles of "inhale, abdomen out, exhale, abdomen in" to help fix the rhythm in the patient's mind. The second is the placement of a hand over the patient's hand on the abdominal wall to exert gentle but firm pressure, depressing the epigastrium during the prolongation of exhalation. Much practice may be required for this seemingly simple procedure, but as proficiency is acquired, the patient is encouraged to make a positive effort to use the diaphragm and abdominals, rather than the upper thoracic accessory muscles.

To vary the forced exhalation exercise, the patient may be taught to do it in the seated position, employing the added techniques of forward bending as shown in Figure 28-24, page 794. The patient relaxes in straight-backed chair, sitting upright to commence the maneuver. With the arms hanging loosely by the side to promote relaxation of the thoracic skeletal muscles, he or she slowly exhales through pursed lips while slowly bending forward and retracting the upper abdomen (Figure 28-24, *A*). When properly timed, flexion of the trunk should be complete at the moment of end-expiration. The body is then raised while the patient inhales through the nose, letting the abdomen distend as the lungs fill. When inhalation is completed, the patient should be back in the upright position. To aid exhalation, the forward bending uses the flexion of the trunk to compress the abdomen and elevate the diaphragm. This exercise is especially helpful to the patient having difficulty clearing secretions, because it tends to stimulate their mobility and facilitate their removal by cough.

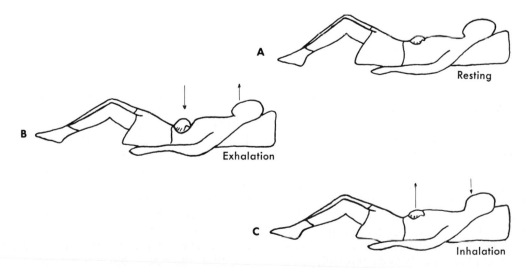

Fig. 28-23 Forced-exhalation abdominal breathing. (See text for description.)

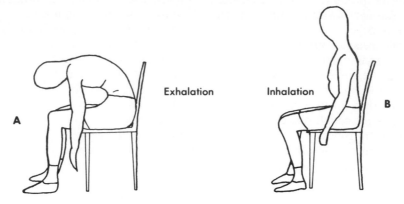

Fig. 28-24 Forced-exhalation abdominal breathing, seated. (See text for description.)

Coordinating breathing with walking

The ultimate objective of all breathing exercises is to increase the patient's tolerance for physical activity. Of all the major complaints expressed by patients with chronic obstructive pulmonary disease, none is more important than the inability to walk comfortably. This may manifest itself as difficulty in walking from room to room within the home, or a hesitancy to leave the home at all. In the hospital, the RCP will observe that many patients breathe with ease while resting in bed or chair, but revert to severe thoracic or paradoxical ventilation as soon as they start to walk. Improving walking tolerance generally does more to increase the patient's morale than any other therapeutic intervention.

The primary purpose of walking exercises is to help minimize dyspnea during exertion, thereby increasing the patient's tolerance for increased activity. Ideally, this is achieved by coordinating physical exertion with the rhythm of breathing, using the prolonged phase of exhalation as the period of maximum effort. This implies that the patient has mastered the act of diaphragmatic breathing and fully understands its purpose.

To prepare for walking exercise, the patient must first practice diaphragmatic breathing in the standing relaxation position, as previously described (Figure 28-12). The patient is then instructed to begin movement while breathing slowly, taking two steps during inhalation and three steps during exhalation. This rhythm helps the patient to maintain a ventilatory ratio in which exhalation time exceeds that devoted to inhalation. Moreover, it lets the patient perform the most exertion when it is easier, during the relatively passive expiratory phase. Because this exercise is developed so that it can be done smoothly, the patient will find that walking will consume much less energy than when his or her breathing was haphazard.

Patients who master this coordinated walking technique will find it applicable to many other activities. For example, it will greatly help the patient in climbing stairs, which ordinarily is one of the most difficult chores for those with severe chronic obstructive pulmonary disease. In this adaptation of the method, the patient learns to manage two or three steps during exhalation, while resting during inhalation.

Graded exercises

Somewhat as the culmination, or end objective, of the breathing exercises just described, a system of graded exercises is used to increase the patient's overall physical conditioning. Graded exercises are designed to gradually increase the patient's overall physical conditioning over an extended period of time. This progressive approach minimizes the likelihood of ill effects and allows careful progress monitoring by the RCP.

A patient is ready for this aspect of physical therapy only after any acute exacerbation of the disease process is under control and he or she has mastered the basic breath control techniques previously discussed.

Whereas techniques in performing progressive exercises may vary, the general principles are the same. Pulmonary and cardiac function, including blood gas analysis, are assessed before starting the program, and are repeated according to the needs of each treatment schedule. Whether a treadmill or an exercise bicycle is used is less important than the ability to vary patient workload in a quantitative fashion. We will limit our discussion here to the use of the treadmill.

The first exposure of the patient to exercise is tentative, to judge response and tolerance, and to teach the proper technique. Supplemental oxygen is normally given to the patient as needed, usually via a nasal cannula. Initially, the treadmill adjusted to 0% grade and a rate not to exceed 1 mph. The RCP must give encouragement to those patients who initially are apprehensive, and assure them that they can step off the moving surface at any time. During the first trial the RCP must see that the patient is using the diaphragm to breathe, since it is under such conditions of stress that he or she is likely to revert to thoracic or paradoxical breathing, and this cannot be permitted if the exercise regimen is to be successful.

Graded exercises are scheduled on a regular basis, usually daily, over a period of weeks to months. The pitch of the walking surface, its speed, and the duration of exercise are increased in increments tailored to each patient. These are good criteria for evaluating progress. For example, if a patient walks 10 minutes at 0% grade and 1 mph initially, and later walks 15 minutes at 2% grade and 1.5 mph, this represents significant improvement.

Even more important is the gradual reduction in the need for supplemental oxygen as the intensity of the exercise increases. It may seem paradoxical that increasing exercise of a patient with respiratory insufficiency should lower the oxygen requirement, but the physiologic reason for this is the foundation for this aspect of rehabilitation. We must remember that patients with chronic obstructive pulmonary disease often become sedentary, resulting in a progressive deterioration of the skeletal muscles. Since poorly conditioned skeletal muscle consumes more oxygen per minute for a given workload than does properly conditioned muscle, this progressive deterioration places disproportionately high energy demands on the patient—demands which can not always be met.

The clinical improvement from a graded exercise program is attributed to two factors.[165,166] First, although pulmonary function tests may show little functional change, exercise improves the patient's respiratory muscle strength and endurance, thereby increasing maximum ventilatory capacity. Second, physical conditioning will lower the maximum oxygen consumption for a given workload, thereby increasing the dyspnea threshold. Together, both factors greatly increase the patient's exercise tolerance.

Although the program just described would have to be conducted under the constant supervision of trained personnel in a rehabilitation facility, there may be instances in which such supervision is not practical or possible.[167,168] With proper selection, many patients can profit from a well planned program of graded exercise at home. One of the many valuable services of the RCP is the training and followup supervision of patients for such programs.

Graded exercises with oxygen also can be done at home, but should be attempted only if both the patient's attending physician and RCP consider the patient responsible and intelligent enough to follow directions accurately.[169] Home exercise can be provided by an exercise cycle, or by level walking, if space permits. Supportive oxygen, supplied in small liquid or compressed gas cylinders, can be carried by the walking patient with a shoulder sling. According to the patient's capabilities, an individualized schedule of graded walking can be developed. However, such a schedule must be reviewed frequently to assess re-

sults, and modified, as necessary. More details on the proper use and integration of graded exercise activity within an organized rehabilitation program is provided in Chapter 37.

COMPLICATIONS AND ADVERSE EFFECTS OF CHEST PHYSICAL THERAPY

When they occur, the complications and adverse effects of CPT can be significant and severe. However, either these problems are infrequent or are significantly under-reported.[7] Among the major complications of CPT, pulmonary hemorrhage, rib fractures, and cardiac arrhythmias are potentially the most severe. Lesser adverse effects include increased intracranial pressure, hypoxemia, decreased cardiac output, and increased airway resistance.

Hemorrhage

Massive pulmonary hemorrhage leading to death has been cited as a major complication of chest physical therapy.[7,170] In case reports of this fatal complication, the underlying cause was attributed to either a pulmonary abscess or bronchopleural fistula. Moreover, hemoptysis or bleeding of bright red blood was always observed prior to the incident. Based on these reports, one should logically avoid CPT when active hemoptysis is present.

Fractured ribs

Fractured ribs are often identified as a complication of CPT, most often attributed to percussion and vibration. However, only one report of this potential problem appears in the medical literature, and then only associated with the management of an infant with hyaline membrane disease, a condition in which rib fractures are common anyway.[7,171] For this reason, the likelihood of properly performed chest physical therapy causing rib fractures should be considered small, and the presence of rib fractures should not be considered an absolute contraindication to percussion and vibration. If, as the literature suggests, percussion and vibration should not be used extensively, the possibility of this complication is even more remote.

Cardiac arrhythmias

Among critically ill patients, about one in three develops a cardiac arrhythmia during conventional CPT, with 10% developing a serious rhythm disturbance.[172] Major arrhythmias during CPT cause a significantly drop in blood pressure and respiratory rate, with an increase in heart rate. Increased age and the presence of acute cardiac disorders are associated with increased risk of arrhythmias. For these reasons, when CPT is ordered for older patients and patients with acute cardiac disease, the ordering physician and RCP should carefully weigh the risk of arrhythmias against the benefits of treatment.[172]

Increased intracranial pressure

Obviously, both coughing and the use of any head-down position in CPT poses the risk of increased intracranial pressure (ICP). Increases in **ICP** averaging as high as 23 mm Hg have been reported in patients with head injuries when placed in a Trendelenburg position.[173] Although this effect is blunted by certain anesthetic agents and high oxygen concentrations, any form of CPT that could raise ICP must be applied with extreme caution to high-risk patients. In the absence of ICP monitoring, CPT should be attempted in these patients only when benefit clearly outweighs the risks.[7]

Hypoxemia

The fact that CPT can decrease PaO_2 was clearly demonstrated some 20 years ago.[174] Subsequent studies have shown that this fall in arterial oxygenation is most likely in patients with cardiovascular instability, or those with profuse bronchial secretions.[175,176]

As previously discussed, arterial hypoxemia also is worsened in patients with unilateral lung disease when they are positioned with the bad lung down.[20,21,71] Tyler has found PaO_2 differences as great as 100 torr between right and left side-lying positions in such patients, although the average drop was less than 17 torr.[177] The factor most associated with the effect of CPT on oxygenation appears to be the baseline PaO_2.[7] In general, *the higher the PaO_2 before chest physical therapy, the greater will be the drop in this measure during treatment.*

In patients with chronic obstructive pulmonary disease, measurements of arterial oxygen saturation (SaO_2) during CPT indicate only a small risk of hypoxemia in this group. In a series of patients being managed for *acute* exacerbations of COPD, none exhibited a significant change in arterial oxygen saturation during CPT.[178] In stable COPD patients being managed on an out-patient basis, only one of 15 exhibited a clinically significant fall in SaO_2 (from 94% to 67%).[179] Moreover, this decrease in saturation occurred only after bronchodilator administration, but not during CPT alone.

Thus, the potential risk of hypoxemia during CPT is real, but generally predictable and small. This risk can be minimized by provision of supplemental oxygen or an increase in the delivered FIO_2 during chest physical therapy.

Impaired cardiac output

Decreases in cardiac output of as much as 50% have been reported in some patients receiving a CPT regimen that included an artificial cough using positive pressure hyperinflation.[180] These changes occurred only in those who were unconscious or too ill to resist the treatment procedure. Impaired venous return due to increased intrathoracic pressure was the probable cause of this effect, along with failure of the normal cardiovascular compensatory mechanisms.[7]

In a group of patients recovering from mitral valve surgery, CPT (consisting of percussion, vibration, and costal breathing, followed by coughing) causes a mean drop in cardiac output of 14%, and an average decrease in mixed venous PO_2 of 9 torr (from 41 to 32 torr).[181] Although the fall in mixed venous PO_2 observed in this study suggests that tissue oxygenation can be compromised during CPT procedures, contrary results have been reported.[7]

As with arterial oxygenation, the likelihood of CPT adversely affecting cardiac output and oxygen delivery is probably related to the relative cardiovascular stability of the patient. The probability of an adverse cardiovascular effect is therefore greatest when CPT is applied to those with hypovolemia, those in shock due to any cause, or those who have lost the compensatory mechanisms normally responsible for regulating blood pressure and flow.

Impaired coronary and cerebral perfusion

Impaired cardiac and cerebral perfusion are rare adverse effects of CPT. Impaired perfusion is probably due to spikes in intrathoracic pressure during coughing paroxysms. Abrupt increases in intrathoracic pressure can reduce coronary blood flow velocity in some patient and thus compromise cardiac function.[182]

Reduced cerebral perfusion is also associated with coughing paroxysms.[183] The increase in intrathoracic pressure due to coughing causes thoracic venous congestion and increases cerebral venous pressures. The result can be reduce cerebral perfusion leading to light-headedness or confusion, or syncope.[183]

Increased airway resistance

It is logical to assume that CPT should *improve* airway caliber and lower airway resistance. Indeed, chest physical therapy applied to patients with either chronic bronchitis or cystic fibrosis has been shown to increase expiratory flowrates after therapy.[184,185] However, this improvement appears to be substantially less among those patients who exhibited signs of bronchospasm during therapy, such as wheezing.

That CPT may actually *increase airway resistance*

in some patients has also been demonstrated. In a study of patients with chronic bronchitis during an acute exacerbation of their illness, nearly half exhibited a fall in FEV_1 immediately following CPT, with restoration back to baseline values within 30 minutes after therapy.[23] Importantly, subjects exhibiting the greatest fall in FEV_1 tended to have the most reactive airways, as judged by their response to bronchodilators. Moreover, administration of a bronchodilator prior to CPT abolished this adverse response in all patients.

Likewise, although chest physical therapy has been shown to result in an overall improvement in the specific **airway conductance** (the inverse of airway resistance) among a *group* of patients, about one in five exhibited a fall in this measure of airway caliber.[186] Why airway resistance increased in these patients remains unclear, since neither a failure to clear sputum nor **hyperreactivity** of the airways was considered a contributing factor.

Apparently, CPT can cause an increase in airway resistance in some patients. The primary mechanism responsible for this adverse effect is probably reversible bronchospasm occurring in patients with hyperreactive airways. Ideally, these patients can be identified in advance by virtue of a positive response to bronchodilator agents. For these individuals, the administration of a bronchodilator before therapy may minimize or abolish this adverse response.

Neurologic symptoms

Headache, paresthesia, numbness, and visual disturbances (including retinal hemorrhage) have all been reported as adverse effects of chest physical therapy.[183] These effects are probably due to the reduced cerebral perfusion previously described and limited to situation in which the patient experiences sever paroxysms of coughing.

CHAPTER SUMMARY

Chest physical therapy represents a collection of physical techniques designed to facilitate clearance of airway secretion, improve the distribution of ventilation, and enhance the efficiency and conditioning of the muscle of respiration. It was not until recently that rigorous scientific methods have been applied to study the effectiveness of these methods in groups of patients with similar conditions. Results of these studies indicate that selected methods of CPT are effective with certain patients under specific clinical circumstances.

Among the conditions for which scientific evidence currently supports the application of chest physical therapy are: (1) acutely ill patients with copious secretions, (2) patients in acute respiratory failure with clinical signs of retained secretions, (3) patients with acute lobar atelectasis, (4) patients with V/Q abnormalities due to lung infiltrates or consolidation, (5) patients with chronic conditions characterized by production of large volumes of sputum, and (6) patients with chronic obstructive pulmonary disease who exhibit inefficient breathing patterns and/or decreased exercise tolerance.

There are five primary methods employed in chest physical therapy. Used alone or in combination, these methods include: therapeutic positioning, chest percussion and vibration, coughing and related expulsion techniques, breathing retraining, and conditioning exercises. Each method differs according to its underlying principle, relative efficacy, and method(s) of application. The appropriate selection and application of these techniques depends first and foremost on proper initial and ongoing assessment of the patient, including the results of initial physical assessment, laboratory testing (including pulmonary function tests), and radiologic evaluation.

The complications and adverse effects of CPT can be significant and severe. However, either these problems are infrequent or are significantly under-reported. Among the major complications of CPT, pulmonary hemorrhage, cardiac arrhythmias, and rib fractures are potentially the most severe. Lesser adverse effects include increased intracranial pressure, hypoxemia, decreased cardiac output, and increased airway resistance. Recognition of the potential for these problems, and careful preliminary respiratory care planning can minimize their likelihood and ensure the safe and effective provision of chest physical therapy.

REFERENCES

1. Frownfelter D: *Chest physical therapy and pulmonary rehabilitation: an interdisciplinary approach,* ed 2, St Louis, 1987, Mosby.
2. American Physical Therapy Association, Cardiopulmonary Section: Definition of chest physical therapy, American Physical Therapy Association, 1982.
3. Frownfelter D Barnes, TA: Chest physical therapy and airway care, In *Respiratory care practice,* St Louis, 1988, Mosby.
4. Rochester D, Goldberg S: Techniques of respiratory physical therapy, *Am Rev Respir Dis* 122(suppl): 133–146, 1980.
5. Murray J: The ketchup-bottle method, *N Eng J Med* 300:1155–1157, 1979.
6. MacKenzie CF, Ciesla N, et al: *Chest physiotherapy in the intensive care unit,* Baltimore, 1981, Williams and Wilkins.
7. Tyler ML: Complications of positioning and chest physiotherapy, *Respir Care* 27:458–466, 1982.
8. Kirilloff LH, Owens GR, et al: Does chest physical therapy work? *Chest* 88:436–444, 1985.
9. American Association for Respiratory Care: Clinical practice guideline: postural drainage therapy, *Respir Care* 36(12): 1418–1426, 1991.
10. American Association for Respiratory Care: Clinical practice guideline: directed cough, *Respir Care* 38(5): 495–499, 1993.
11. American Association for Respiratory Care: Clinical practice guideline: use of positive airway pressure adjuncts to bronchial hygiene therapy, *Respir Care* 38(5):516–521, 1993.
12. Eid N, Buchheit J, Neuling M, Phelps H: Chest physiotherapy in review, *Respir Care* 36(4):270–282, 1991.
13. Sutton P, Pavia D, et al: Chest physiotherapy: A review, *Eur J Respir Dis* 63:188–201, 1982.

14. Connors AF, Hammon WE, Martin RJ, et al: Chest physical therapy: the immediate effect on oxygenation in acutely ill patients, *Chest* 78:559–564, 1980.

15. MacKenzie CF, Shin B, and McAslan TC: Chest physiotherapy: The effect on arterial oxygenation, *Anesth Analg* 57:28–30, 1978.

16. Marini JJ, Pierson DJ, and Hudson LD: A prospective comparison of fiberoptic bronchoscopy and respiratory therapy, *Am Rev Respir Dis* 119:971–978,, 1979.

17. Marini JJ: Postoperative atelectasis: Pathophysiology, clinical importance, and principles of management, *Respir Care* 29:515–522, 1984.

18. Hammond WE, Martin FJ: Chest physical therapy for acute atelectasis, *Phys Ther* 61:217–220, 1981.

19. Douglas WW, Rehder K, Beynen FM, et al: Improved oxygenation in patients with acute respiratory failure: the prone position, *Am Rev Respir Dis* 115:559–566, 1977.

20. Dhainaut JF, Bons J, et al: Improved oxygenation in patients with extensive unilateral pneumonia using the lateral decubitus position, *Thorax* 35:792–793, 1980.

21. Syracuse DC, Hyman AI, King TC: Postural influences on arterial blood gases in patients with unilateral pulmonary consolidation, *Surg Forum* 30:173–174, 1979.

22. Anthonisen P, Riis P, Sogaard-Anderson T: The value of lung physiotherapy in the treatment of acute exacerbations in chronic bronchitis, *Acta Med Scand* 175:715–719, 1964.

23. Campbell AH, O'Connell JM, Wilson F: The effect of chest physiotherapy upon the FEV_1 in chronic bronchitis, *Med J Aust* 1:33–35, 1975.

24. Newton D, Stephenson A: Effects of physiotherapy on pulmonary function, *Lancet* 2:228–230, 1978.

25. Graham W, Bradley D: Efficacy of chest physiotherapy and intermittent positive pressure breathing in the resolution of pneumonia, *N Eng J Med* 299:624–627, 1978.

26. Britton S, Bejstedt M, Vedin L: Chest physiotherapy in primary pneumonia, *Br Med J* 290:1703–1704, 1985.

27. Stapleton T: Chest physiotherapy in primary pneumonia (letter), *Br Med J* 291:143, 1985.

28. Wissing DR, Boggs PB, George RB: Use of respiratory care procedures in the management of hospitalized asthmatics, *Ann Allergy* 61:407–419, 1988.

29. De Boeck C, Zinman R: Cough versus chest physiotherapy, *Am Rev Respir Dis* 129:182–184, 1984.

30. Rossman CM, et al: Effects of chest physiotherapy on the removal of mucous in patients with cystic fibrosis, *Am Rev Respir Dis* 126:131, 1982.

31. Pryor S, Webber B, et al: Evaluation of the forced expiration technique as an adjunct to postural drainage in treatment of cystic fibrosis, *Br Med J* 2:417–418, 1979.

32. Zach MS, Oberwaldner B: Chest physiotherapy—the mechanical approach to antiinfective therapy in cystic fibrosis, *Infection* 15:381–384, 1987.

33. Reisman J, Rivington-Law B, Corey M, et al: Role of conventional therapy in cystic fibrosis, *J Pediatr* 113:632–636, 1988.

34. Mazzocco MC, Owens GR, et al: Chest percussion and postural drainage in patients with bronchiectasis, *Chest* 88:360–363, 1985.

35. Sutton P, Parker R, Webber B, et al: Assessment of the forced expiration technique, postural drainage, and directed coughing in chest physiotherapy, *Eur J Respir Dis* 64:62–68, 1983.

36. Oldenburg FA, Dolovich MB, Montgomery JM, et al: Effects of postural drainage, exercise, and cough on mucous clearance in chronic bronchitis, *Am Rev Respir Dis* 120:739–745, 1979.

37. Bateman JR, Newman SP, et al: Is cough as effective as chest physical therapy in the removal of excessive bronchial secretions? *Thorax* 36:683–687, 1981.

38. Bateman JR, Newman SP, Daunt KM, et al: Regional lung clearance of excessive bronchial secretions during chest physiotherapy in patients with stable chronic airways obstruction, *Lancet* 1:294–279, 1979.

39. Sergysels R: Can respiratory kinesitherapy palliate the functional sequelae of chronic obstructive bronchopathies? *Rev Fr Mal Respir* 11:605–608, 1983.

40. Gimenez M: Technics and results in respiratory kinesitherapy of chronic obstructive bronchopneumopathies, *Rev Fr Mal Respir* 11:525–43, 1983.

41. Faling LJ: Pulmonary rehabilitation—physical modalities, *Clin Chest Med* 7:599–618, 1986.

42. Make, BJ: Pulmonary rehabilitation: myth or reality? *Clin Chest Med* 7:519–540, 1986.

43. Casciari RJ, Fairshter RD, et al: Effects of breathing retraining in patients with chronic obstructive pulmonary disease, *Chest* 79:393–398, 1981.

44. Housset B, Tetard C, Derenne JP: Respiratory physiotherapy and respiratory mechanics of chronic respiratory insufficiency, *Rev Fr Mal Respir* 11:915–921, 1983.

45. Bartlett RH, et al: Studies on the pathogenesis and prevention of postoperative pulmonary complications, *Surg Gynecol Obstet* 137:925, 1973.

46. Tarhan S, et al: Risk of anesthesia and surgery in patients with chronic bronchitis and chronic obstructive pulmonary disease, *Surgery* 74:720, 1973.

47. Bartlett RH: Respiratory therapy to prevent pulmonary complications of surgery, *Respir Care* 29:667–679, 1984.

48. Kigin CM: Chest physical therapy for the postoperative or traumatic injury patient, *Phys Ther* 61:1724, 1981.

49. Vraciu J, Vraciu R: Effectiveness of breathing exercises in preventing pulmonary complications following open heart surgery, *Phys Ther* 57:1367–1370, 1977.

50. Castillo R, Haas A: Chest physical therapy: comparative efficacy of preoperative and postoperative in the elderly, *Arch Phys Med Rehabil* 66:376–379, 1985.

51. Torrington KG, Sorenson DE, Sherwood LM: Postoperative chest percussion with postural drainage in obese patients following gastric stapling, *Chest* 86:891–895, 1984.

52. Hoffman LA: Ineffective airway clearance related to neuromuscular dysfunction, *Nurs Clin North Am* 22:151–166, 1987.

53. Desmond KJ, Schwenk WF, Thomas E, et al: Immediate and long-term effects of chest physiotherapy in patients with cystic fibrosis, *J Pediatr* 103:538–542, 1983.

54. Hess D, Agarwal NN, Myers CL: Positioning, lung function, and kinetic bed therapy, *Respir Care* 37(2): 181–197, 1992.

55. Judson MA, Sahn SA: Mobilization of secretions in ICU patients, *Respir Care* 39(3): 213–226, 1994.

56. Miller RD, Fowler WS, Helmholz F: Changes of relative volume and ventilation of the two lungs with change to the lateral decubitus position, *J Lab & Clin Med* 47(2):297–304, 1956.

57. Zack MB, Pontoppidan H, Kazemi H: The effect of lateral positions on gas exchange in pulmonary disease. A prospective evaluation, *Am Rev Respir Dis* 110:49–55, 1974.

58. Piehi MA, Brown RS: Use of extreme position changes in acute respiratory failure, *Crit Care Med* 4:13–14, 1976.

59. Chulay M, Brown J, Summer W: Effect of postoperative immobilization after coronary artery bypass surgery, *Crit Care Med* 10:176–179, 1982.

60. Green BA, Green KL, Klose KJ: Kinetic nursing for acute spinal cord injury patients, *Paraplegia* 18(3): 181–186, 1980.

61. Becker DM, Gonzalez M, et al: Prevention of deep venous thrombosis in patients with acute spinal cord injuries: use of rotating treatment tables, *Neurosurgery* 20(5):675–677, 1987.

62. Green BA, Green KL, Klose KJ: Kinetic therapy for spinal cord injury, *Spine* 8(7):722–728, 1983.

63. Sahn SA: Continuous lateral rotational therapy and nosocomial pneumonia, *Chest* 99(5):1263–1267, 1991.

64. Gentilello L, Thompson DA, et al: Effect of a rotating bed on the incidence of pulmonary complications in critically ill patients, *Crit Care Med* 16(8):783–786, 1988.

65. Fink MP, Helsmoortel CM, et al: The efficacy of an oscillating bed in the prevention of lower respiratory tract infection in critically ill victims of blunt trauma: a prospective study, *Chest* 97(1):132–137, 1990.

66. deBoisblanc BP, Castro M, et al: Effect of air-supported, continuous, postural oscillation on the risk of early ICU pneumonia in nontraumatic critical illness, *Chest* 103(5):1543–1547, 1993.

67. Summer WR, Curry P, Haponik EF, Nelson S, Elston R: Continuous mechanical turning of intensive care unit patients shortens length of stay in some diagnostic-related groups, *J Crit Care* 4:45–53, 1989.

68. Marini JJ, Tyler M, Hudson L, et al: Influence of head-dependent positions on lung volume and oxygen saturation in chronic airflow obstruction, *Am Rev Respir Dis* 129:101–105, 1984.

69. Clauss RH, Scalabrini BY, Ray JF, et al: Effects of changing body position upon improved ventilation-perfusion relationships, *Circulation* 37(suppl):214–217, 1968.

70. Kaneko K, Mille-Emili J, Dolowich MB: Regional distribution of ventilation and perfusion as a function of body position, *J Appl Physiol* 21:767–777, 1966.

71. Zack MB, Pontoppidan H, Kazemi H: The effect of lateral positions on gas exchange in pulmonary disease: A prospective evaluation, *Am Rev Respir Dis* 110:49–55, 1974.

72. Remolina C, et al: Positional hypoxemia in unilateral lung disease, *N Eng J Med* 304:523–525, 1981.

73. Demers RR: Down with the good lung—(usually) (editorial), *Respir Care* 32:849–850, 1987.

74. Martin RJ, Herrell N, Rubin D, Fanaroff: An Effect of supine and prone positions on arterial oxygen tension in the preterm infant, *Pediatrics* 63:528–531, 1979.

75. Harris JA, Jerry BA: Indications and procedures for segmental bronchial drainage, *Respir Care* 20:456, 1975.

76. Tecklin JS: Positioning, percussing, and vibrating patients for effective bronchial drainage, *Nursing* 79 9:64–71, 1979.

77. Zausmer E: Bronchial drainage: Evidence supporting the procedures, *Phys Ther* 48:586–591, 1968.

78. Wong JW, Keens TG, Wannamaker EM, et al: Effects of gravity on tracheal transport rates in normal subjects and in patients with cystic fibrosis, *Pediatrics* 60:146–152, 1977.

79. March H: Appraisal of postural drainage for chronic obstructive pulmonary disease, *Arch Phys Med Rehab* 52:528–530, 1971.

80. May D, Munt P: Physiologic effects of chest percussion and postural drainage in patients with stable chronic bronchitis, *Chest* 79:29–32, 1979.

81. Loring M, Denning C: Evaluation of postural drainage by measurement of sputum volume and consistency, *Am J Phys Med* 50:215–219, 1971.

82. Chopra SK, Taplin GV, Simmons DH, et al: Effects of hydration and physical therapy on tracheal transport velocity, *Am Rev Respir Dis* 115:1009–1014, 1974.

83. Pryor JA, Webber BA, Hodson ME: Effect of chest physiotherapy on oxygen saturation in patients with cystic fibrosis, *Thorax* 45(1):77, 1990.

84. Ross J, Dean E, Abboud RT: The effect of postural drainage positioning on ventilation homogeneity in healthy subjects, *Phys Ther* 72(11):794–799, 1992.

85. Conway JH, Fleming JS, et al: Humidification as an adjunct to chest physiotherapy in aiding tracheobronchial clearance in patients with bronchiectasis, *Respir Med* 86(2):109–14, 1992.

86. Barach AL: Chronic obstructive lung disease: postural relief of dyspnea, *Arch Phys Med Rehabil* 55:494, 1974.

87. Radford R, et al: A rational basis for percussion - augmented mucociliary clearance, *Respir Care* 27:556–563, 1982.

88. Sutton PP, Lopez-Vidriero MT, Pavia D, et al: Assessment of percussion, vibratory-shaking and breathing exercises in chest physiotherapy, *Eur J Respir Dis* 66:147–152, 1985.

89. Holody B, Goldberg H: The effect of mechanical vibration physiotherapy on arterial saturation in acutely ill patients with atelectasis or pneumonia, *Am Rev Resp Dis* 124:372–375, 1981.

90. Denton R: Bronchial secretions in cystic fibrosis: the effects of treatment with mechanical percussion vibration, *Am Rev Respir Dis* 86:41–46, 1962.

91. Pavia D, Thompson M, Phillipakos D: A preliminary study of the effects of a vibrating pad on bronchial clearance, *Am Rev Respir Dis* 113:92–96, 1976.

92. Wollmer P, Ursing K, et al: Inefficiency of chest percussion in the physical therapy of chronic bronchitis, *Eur J Respir Dis* 66:233–239, 1985.

93. Gallon A: Evaluation of chest percussion in the treatment of patients with copious sputum production, *Respir Med* 85(1):45–51, 1991.

94. van der Schans CP, Piers DA, Postma DS: Effect of manual percussion on tracheobronchial clearance in patients with chronic airflow obstruction and excessive tracheobronchial secretion, *Thorax* 41:448–452, 1986.

95. Stiller K, Geake T, et al: Acute lobar atelectasis. A comparison of two chest physiotherapy regimens, *Chest* 98(6):1336–1340, 1990.

96. Eubanks DH, Bone RC: Comprehensive respiratory care, St Louis, 1985, Mosby.

97. Hansen LG, Warwick WJ: High-frequency chest compression system to aid in clearance of mucus from the lung, *Biomed Instrum Technol* 24(4):289–294, 1990.

98. Kluft J, Fink R, et al: Comparison of bronchial drainage treatments by sputum quantity, *Pediatr Pulmonol* 8(suppl):S299, 1992.

99. Whitman J, Van Beusekom R, et al: Preliminary evaluation of high-frequency chest compression for secretion clearance in mechanically ventilated patients. *Respir Care* 38(10):1081–1087, 1993.

100. Warwick WJ, Hansen LG: The long-term effect of high-frequency chest compression therapy on pulmonary complications of cystic fibrosis, *Pediatr Pulmonol* 11(3):265–271, 1991.

101. Langerson J: The cough: Its effectiveness depends on you, *Respir Care* 24:142–149, 1979.

102. Leith DL: Cough, in Brain JD, Proctor DF, Reid LM: editors: *Respiratory defense mechanisms*, New York, 1977, Marcel Dekker.

103. Irwin RS, et al: Cough: A comprehensive review, *Arch Intern Med* 137:1189, 1977.

104. Camner P: Studies on the removal of inhaled particles from the lungs by voluntary coughing, *Chest* 80(6, Suppl):824–827, 1981.

105. Bennett WD, Foster WM, Chapman WF: Cough-enhanced mucus clearance in the normal lung, *J Appl Physiol* 69(5):1670–1675, 1990.

106. Hasani A, Pavia D, et al: The effect of unproductive coughing/FET on regional mucus movement in the human lungs, *Respir Med* 85 Suppl A:23–26, 1991.

107. Petty TL: Chronic obstructive pulmonary disease, New York, 1978, Marcel Dekker.

108. Hietpas BG, Roth RD, Jensen WM: Huff coughing and airway patency, *Respir Care* 24:710–713, 1979.

109. Black LF, Hyatt RE: Maximal static respiratory pressures in generalized neuromuscular disease, *Am Rev Respir Dis* 103(5):641–650, 1971.

110. Szeinberg A, Tabachnik E, et al: Cough capacity in patient with muscular dystrophy, *Chest* 94:1232–1235, 1988.

111. Braun SR, Giovannoni R, O'Connor M: Improving the cough in patients with spinal cord injury, *Am J Phys Med* 63(1):1–10, 1984.

112. Partridge C, Pryor J, Webber B: Characteristics of the forced expiratory technique, *Physiotherapy* 75(3):193–194, 1989.

113. Pavia D: The role of chest physiotherapy in mucus hypersecretion, *Lung* 168 Suppl:614–621, 1990.

114. Chevalier J: Autogenic drainage. In: Lawson D, Ed. *Cystic Fibrosis*: horizons, Chichester, 1984, John Wiley.

115. Schoni MH: Autogenic drainage: a modern approach to physiotherapy in cystic fibrosis, *J R Soc Med* 82 Suppl 16:32–37, 1989.

116. Dab I, Alexander F: The mechanism of autogenic drainage studied with flow volume curves, *Monogr Paediatr* 10:50–53, 1979.

117. Pfleger A, Theissl B, Oberwaldner B, Zach MS: Self-administered chest physiotherapy in cystic fibrosis: a comparative study of high-pressure PEP and autogenic drainage, *Lung* 170(6):323–330, 1992.

118. Henry M, de Rivera JL, et al: Improvement of respiratory function in chronic asthmatic patients with autogenic therapy, *J Psychosom Res* 37(3):265–270, 1993.

119. Anderson JB, Falk M: Chest physiotherapy in the pediatric age group, *Respir Care* 36(6):546–552, 1991.

120. Lindemann H, Boldt A, Kieselmann R: Autogenic drainage: efficacy of a simplified method, *Acta Univ Carol [Med] (Praha)* 36(1–4):210–212, 1990.

121. Barach AL, Beck GJ, Smith W: Mechanical production of expiratory flow rates surpassing the capacity of human coughing, *Am J Med Sci* 226:241–248, 1953.

122. Barach AL, Beck GJ: Exsufflation with negative pressure, *Arch Intern Med* 93:825–841, 1954.

123. Cherniack RM, Hildes JA, Alcock AJW: The clinical use of exsufflator attachment for tank respirators in poliomyelitis, *Ann Intern Med* 40:540–548, 1954.

124. Bach JR, Smith WH, et al: Airway secretion clearance by mechanical exsufflation for post-poliomyelitis ventilator-assisted individuals, *Arch Phys Med Rehabil* 74(2):170–177, 1993.

125. Bach JR: Mechanical insufflation-exsufflation, *Chest* 104:1553–1562, 1993.

126. Malmeister MJ, Fink JB, Hoffman GL: Positive expiratory pressure mask therapy: theoretical and practical considerations and a review of the literature, *Respir Care* 36:1218–1229, 1991.

127. Anderson JB, Klausen NO: A new mode of nebulized bronchodilator in severe bronchospasm, *Eur J Respir Dis* 63(Suppl):97–100, 1982.

128. Tomesen P, Stovring S: Positive expiratory pressure (PEP) as lung physiotherapy in cystic fibrosis: a pilot study, *Eur J Respir Dis* 65:419–422, 1984.

129. Groth S, Staranger G, et al: Positive expiratory pressure (PEP-mask) physiotherapy improves ventilation and reduces volume of trapped gas in cystic fibrosis, *Bull Eur Physiopathol Respir* 21:339–343, 1985.

130. Oberwaldner B, Evans JC, Zach MS: Forced expirations against a variable resistance: a new chest physiotherapy method in cystic fibrosis, *Pediatr Pulmonol* 2(6):358–367, 1986.

131. Steen HJ, Redmond AO, et al: Evaluation of the PEP mask in cystic fibrosis, *Acta Paediatr Scand* 80(1):51–56, 1991.

132. Falk M, Kelstrup M, et al: Improving the ketchup bottle method with positive expiratory pressure (PEP) in cystic fibrosis, *Eur J Respir Dis* 65:423–432, 1984.

133. Lannefors L, Wollmer P: Mucus clearance with three chest physiotherapy regimes in cystic fibrosis: a comparison between postural drainage, PEP and physical exercise. *Eur Respir J* 5(6):748–753, 1992.

134. Mortensen J, Falk M, et al: The effects of postural drainage and positive expiratory pressure physiotherapy on tracheobronchial clearance in cystic fibrosis, *Chest* 100(5):1350–1357, 1991.

135. Oberwaldner B, Theissl B, et al: Chest physiotherapy in hospitalized patients with cystic fibrosis: a study of lung function effects and sputum production, *Eur Respir J* 4(2):152–158, 1991.

136. van Hengstum M, Festen J, et al: Effect of positive expiratory pressure mask physiotherapy (PEP) versus forced expiration technique (FET/PD) on regional lung clearance in chronic bronchitis. *Eur Respir J* 4(6):651–654, 1991.

137. Barrascout AR: Chest physical therapy and related procedures, in Burton GG, Hodgkin JE (eds.): *Respiratory care: a guide to clinical practice,* ed 2, Philadelphia, 1984, JB Lippincott.

138. Grassino A, Bellemare F, LaPorta D: Diaphragm fatigue and the strategy of breathing in COPD, *Chest* 85(suppl 6):515–545, 1984.

139. Grimby G, Oxhoj H, Bake B: Effects of abdominal breathing on distribution of ventilation in obstructive lung disease, *Clin Sci Mol Med* 48:193–199, 1975.

140. Fixley MS, Roussos CS, Murphy B, et al: Flow dependence of gas distribution and the pattern of inspiratory muscle contraction, *J Appl Physiol* 45:733–741, 1978.

141. Williams IP, Smith CM, McGavin CR: Diaphragmatic breathing training and walking performance in chronic airways obstruction, *Br J Dis Chest* 76:164–166, 1982.

142. Levine S, Weiser P, Gillen J: Evaluation of a ventilatory muscle endurance training program in the rehabilitation of patients with chronic obstructive pulmonary disease, *Am Rev Respir Dis* 133:400–406, 1986.

143. Belman M, Mittman C: Ventilatory muscle training improves exercise capacity in chronic obstructive pulmonary disease patients, *Am Rev Respir Dis* 121:273–280, 1980.

144. Pardy RL, Rivington RN, et al: Inspiratory muscle training compared with physiotherapy in patients with chronic airflow limitation, *Am Rev Respir Dis* 123:421–425, 1981.

145. Weiner P, Azgad Y, Ganam R: Inspiratory muscle training combined with general exercise reconditioning in patients with COPD, *Chest* 102(5):1351–1356, 1992.

146. Leith DE, Bradley M: Ventilatory muscle strength and endurance training, *J Appl Physiol* 41:508–516, 1976.

147. Anderson JB, Dragsted L, Kann T, et al: Resistive breathing training in severe chronic obstructive lung disease: a pilot study, *Scand J Respir Dis* 60:151–156, 1979.

148. Sonne LJ, Davis JA: Increased exercise performances in patients with severe COPD following inspiratory resistive training, *Chest* 81:436–439, 1982.

149. Asher MI, Pardy RL, Coates AL, et al: The effects of inspiratory muscle training in patients with cystic fibrosis, *Am Rev Respir Dis* 126:855–859, 1982.

150. Keens TG, Krastins IRB, Wannamaker EM, et al: Ventilatory muscle endurance training in normal subjects and patients with cystic fibrosis, *Am Rev Respir Dis* 116: 853–860, 1977.

151. Falk P, Eriksen AM, et al: Relieving dyspnea with an inexpensive and simple method in patients with severe chronic airflow limitation, *Eur J Respir Dis* 66:181–186, 1985.

152. Chen H, Dukes R, Martin BJ: Inspiratory muscle training in patients with chronic obstructive pulmonary disease, *Am Rev Respir Dis* 131:251–255, 1985.

153. Clanton TL, Dixon G, et al: Inspiratory muscle conditioning using a threshold loading device, *Chest* 87:62–66, 1985.

154. McKeon JL, Turner J, Kelly C, et al: The effect of inspiratory resistive training on exercise capacity in optimally treated patients with severe chronic airflow limitation, *Aust NZ J Med* 16:648–62, 1986.

155. Belman MJ, Thomas SG, Lewis MI: Resistive breathing training in patients with chronic obstructive pulmonary disease, *Chest* 90:662–669, 1986.

156. Sobush DC, Dunning M: Providing resistive breathing exercise to the inspiratory muscles using the PFLEX device. Suggestion from the field, *Phys Ther* 66:542–544, 1986.

157. Larson JL, Kim MJ, Sharp JT: Inspiratory muscle training with a threshold resistive breathing device in patients with chronic obstructive pulmonary disease, *Am Rev Respir Dis* 133:A100, 1986.

158. Rochester DF, Hyatt RE: Respiratory muscle failure, *Med Clin N Am* 67:573–579, 1983.

159. Evans TW, Howard P: Whistle for your wind, *Br Med J* 289:449–450, 1984.

160. Ingram RH, Schilder DP: Effect of pursed lips expiration on the pulmonary pressure-flow relationship in obstructive lung disease, *Am Rev Respir Dis* 95:381–388, 1967.

161. Martin L: *Pulmonary physiology in clinical practice, the essentials for patient care and evaluation,* St Louis, 1987, Mosby.

162. Thoman RL, Stoker GL, Ross JC: The efficacy of pursed lips breathing in patients with chronic obstructive pulmonary disease, *Am Rev Respir Dis* 3:100–106, 1966.

163. Mueller RE, Petty TL, Filley GF: Ventilation and arterial blood gas changes induced by pursed-lip breathing, *J Appl Physiol* 28:784, 1970.
164. Howell JBL: Breathlessness in pulmonary disease. In Howell JBL, Campbell EJM editors: *Breathlessness,* Oxford, England, 1966, Blackwell Scientific.
165. Pierce AK, et al: Responses to exercise training in patients with emphysema, *Arch Intern Med* 113:28, 1964.
166. Barach AL, Petty TL: Is chronic obstructive lung disease improved by physical exercise? *JAMA* 234:854, 1975.
167. Haas A, et al: *Pulmonary therapy and rehabilitation: principles and practices,* Baltimore, 1979, Williams & Wilkins.
168. Lertzman MM, Cherniack RM: Rehabilitation of patients with chronic obstructive pulmonary disease, *Am Rev Respir Dis* 114:1145, 1976.
169. Pierce AK, Paez PN, Miller WF: Exercise therapy with the aid of a portable oxygen supply in patients with emphysema, *Am Rev Respir Dis* 91:653, 1965.
170. Hammon WE, Martin RJ: Fatal pulmonary hemorrhage associated with chest physical therapy, *Phys Ther* 59:1247–1248, 1979.
171. Puorhit DM, Caldwell C, Lerkoff AH: Multiple rib fractures due to physiotherapy in a neonate with hyaline membrane disease, *Am J Dis Child* 129:1103–1104, 1975.
172. Hammon WE, Connors AF Jr, McCaffree DR: Cardiac arrhythmias during postural drainage and chest percussion of critically ill patients, *Chest* 102(6):1836–1841, 1992.
173. Moss E, Gibson JS, Mcdowall GD: The effects of nitrous oxide, Althesin and thiopental on intracranial pressure during chest physiotherapy in patients with severe head injuries, in Shulman, K, Mararow, A, Miller, JD, et al: editors: *Intrcranial pressure IV,* New York, 1980, Springer-Verlag.
174. Halloway R, Adams EB, Desai SD, et al: Effect of chest physiotherapy on blood gases of neonates treated with intermittent positive pressure respiration, *Thorax* 24:421–426, 1969.
175. Gormenzano J, Branthwait MA: Effects of physiotherapy during intermittent positive pressure ventilation: Changes in arterial blood gas tensions, *Anaesthesia* 27:258–263, 1972.
176. Gormenzano J, Branthwaite MA: Pulmonary physiotherapy with associated ventilation: Arterial blood gas tension changes following pulmonary physiotherapy with IPPB, *Anaesthesia* 27:249–257, 1972.
177. Tyler ML, Hudson LD, Grose BL, et al: Prediction of oxygenation during chest physiotherapy in critically ill patients (abstract), *Am Rev Respir Dis* 121(part 2):218, 1980.
178. Buscaglia A, St. Marie M: Oxygen saturation during chest physiotherapy for acute exacerbation of severe chronic obstructive pulmonary disease, *Respir Care* 28:1009–1013, 1983.
179. Moody LE, Martindale CL: Effect of pulmonary hygiene measures on levels of arterial oxygen saturation in adults with chronic lung disease, *Heart & Lung* 7:315–319, 1978.
180. Laws AK, McIntyre RW: Chest physiotherapy: A physiologic assessment during intermittent positive pressure ventilation in respiratory failure, *Can Anaesth Soc J* 16:487–493, 1969.
181. Barrell SE, Abbas HM: Monitoring during physiotherapy after open heart surgery, *Physiotherapy* 64:272–273, 1978.
182. Kern MJ, Gudipati C, et al: Effect of abruptly increased intrathoracic pressure on coronary blood flow velocity in patients, *Am Heart J* 119:863–870, 1990.
183. Stern RC, Horwitz SJ, Doershuk CF: Neurologic symptoms during coughing paroxysms in cystic fibrosis, *J Pediatr* 112:909–912, 1988.
184. Feldman J, Traver GA, Taussig LM: Maximal expiratory flows after postural drainage, *Am Rev Respir Dis* 119:239–245, 1979.
185. Tecklin JS, Holsclaw DS: Evaluation of bronchial drainage in patients with cystic fibrosis, Phys Ther 1975; 55: 1081–1084.
186. Cochrane GM, Webber BA, Clarke SW: Effects of sputum on pulmonary function, *Br Med J* 2:1181–1183, 1977.

6

Acute and Critical Care

29

Respiratory Failure and the Need for Ventilatory Support*

■

Timothy B. Op't Holt
Craig L. Scanlan

CHAPTER LEARNING OBJECTIVES

1. Define respiratory failure and distinguish between its two primary types;
2. Compare and contrast the concepts of acute and chronic respiratory failure;
3. Identify the common causes of respiratory failure according to their effect on the respiratory apparatus;
4. Differentiate among the six primary pathophysiologic processes underlying respiratory failure, and the mode(s) of ventilatory support indicated in each;
5. Compare and contrast the justification for ventilatory support in selected special circumstances;
6. Recognize the limitations of quantitative approaches in assessing patients' needs for ventilatory support.

Prior to 1960, the term respiratory failure did not appear in the medical literature.[1] Since then, advances in life support and monitoring techniques have refined our ability to define and manage this now common clinical problem.

In simple terms, respiratory failure occurs when the lung can no longer fulfill its primary function of gas exchange. This means that the process of *external* respiration, or the exchange of O_2 and CO_2 between the alveoli and the capillaries is inadequate.[2] Despite this simple definition, abnormal gas exchange can occur in a wide range of clinical disorders. These condtions range from the simple, such as a drug overdose, to the complex, such as the Adult Respiratory Distress Syndrome.

Like failure of any other organ systems, respiratory failure is a life-threatening event that demands immediate treatment. Given the range of clinical disorders causing respiratory failure, it is not surprising that treatment strategies are also numerous. Depending on the underlying problem, treatment can range from simple oxygen therapy to full-blown ventilatory support.

Thus respiratory failure is really a complex clinical concept. Of course, effective management of respiratory failure requires an in-depth understanding of its causes and clinical manifestations. This chapter will focus on the etiology, pathophysiology and clinical features of respiratory failure, with special emphasis on identifying the need for ventilatory support.

*Portions adapted with permission from Pierson DJ: Indications for mechanical ventilation in acute respiratory failure, *Respir Care* 28:570–577, 1983.

BASIC CONCEPTS IN RESPIRATORY FAILURE

If respiratory failure is defined as inadequate gas exchange at the lung, then it should reveal itself as abnormal arterial blood gases. The first objective criteria for diagnosing respiratory failure were based on blood gases. In 1965, Campbell defined respiratory failure as a condition in which the patient's PaO_2 was below 60 torr *or* the $PaCO_2$ was above 50 torr while breathing air at sea level.[3]

This simple definition provided by Campbell is still used today. However, we now know that the absolute blood gas values signaling respiratory failure may be above or below these levels, depending on the clinical circumstances. For example, whether a PaO_2 of 60 torr indicates respiratory failure depends, in part, on the patient's age, the FIO_2, and the barometric pressure.[4] Likewise, an arterial PCO_2 above 50 torr may or may not signal respiratory failure.

For respiratory failure to exist, these abnormal blood gases must be due to a pulmonary or respiratory–related problem. For example, hypoxemia due to intracardiac shunting or hypercapnia due to metabolic alkalosis do not indicate respiratory failure.[5]

Problems of oxygenation versus problems of ventilation

Campbell's early definition of respiratory failure made it clear that oxygenation and ventilation are two separate processes. Thus, problems with oxygen exchange can occur separately from problems with ventilation.

Based on this knowledge, we can define two broad types of respiratory failure: (1) that associated with abnormal oxygenation, and (2) that due to inadequacies in ventilation.[1,6-9] Respiratory failure caused by abnormalities of oxygenation is called *hypoxemic respiratory failure*. Respiratory failure due to inadequate ventilation is called ventilatory or *hypercapnic respiratory failure*.[2] Table 29-1 on page 806 compares and contrasts these two major types of respiratory failure.

As shown in Table 29-1, the primary findings in hypoxemic respiratory failure are a lower PaO_2 and a high $P(A-a)O_2$. Moreover, the $PaCO_2$ in hypoxemic respiratory failure is either normal or low.

Mechanisms responsible for hypoxemic respiratory failure include all causes of arterial hypoxemia except hypoventilation and a low FIO_2 (see Chapter 15). Specifically, hypoxemic respiratory failure can be caused by a diffusion impairment, a low $\dot{V}/\dot{Q}$ ratio, or intrapulmonary shunting. Of these, only a low $\dot{V}/\dot{Q}$ ratio and shunting are common in clinical practice.

The hallmark of hypercapnic respiratory failure is a high $PaCO_2$. As with hypoxemic respiratory failure, the PaO_2 while breathing air is low. However, this low PaO_2 is *not* due to an oxygenation disturbance in the lung. The PaO_2 is low simply because the excess carbon dioxide displaces oxygen out of the alveoli (refer to Chapter 12). That oxygen exchange across the lung is normal in hypercapnic respiratory failure is confirmed by a normal $P(A-a)O_2$. Thus the underlying process leading to pure hypercapnic respiratory failure is alveolar hypoventilation.

Of course hypoxemic and hypercapnic respiratory failure can occur together. If this is the case, the PaO_2 would be low, and both the $PaCO_2$ and the $P(A-a)O_2$ would be increased (Table 29-1).[8] In this combined form of respiratory failure, hypoventilation co-exists with either a $\dot{V}/\dot{Q}$ inequality or shunt.[1]

■ MINI CLINI ■

29-1

Classification and Treatment of Respiratory Failure

Problem: Two patients present with the following arterial blood gases at sea level:

Patient A	Patient B
pH = 7.45	pH = 7.21
PCO_2 = 33 mmHg	PCO_2 = 72 mmHg
HCO_3 = 22 mEq/L	HCO_3 = 28 mEq/L
PO_2 = 40 mmHg	PO_2 = 53 mmHg
FIO_2 = .21	FIO_2 = .21

These blood gases are compatible with which types of respiratory failure? What is the $P(A-a)O_2$ for each patient? In which patient would administration of 100% oxygen yield important information that would affect therapy decisions?

Discussion: The $PaCO_2$ of 33 mmHg in patient A tells us that the hypoxemia cannot be due to hypoventilation (simple displacement of oxygen by carbon dioxide). Patient A is clearly not a case of hypercapnic respiratory failure. Patient B, on the other hand, has obvious hypercapnia ($PaCO_2$ = 72 mmHg) and hypoxemia. However, the hypoxemia of 53 mmHg is easily explained by the fact that patient B is hypoventilating; that is, the PaO_2 has fallen by essentially the same amount that the $PaCO_2$ has risen. Patient B

clearly has a ventilatory problem, and is an example of acute hypercapnic respiratory failure (acute, because of the low pH; no compensatory retention of bicarbonate is present). To clarify the oxygenation status of these patients, $P(A-a)O_2$ can be calculated as follows:

Patient A: PAO_2 = .21 (760−47) − 33/.8
= 108 mmHg
PaO_2 = 40
$P(A-a)O_2$ = 108−40 =
68 mmHg on room air
(normal $P(A-a)O_2$ = 5−10
mmHg on room air)

Patient B: PAO_2 = .21 (760−47) − 72/.8
= 60 mmHg
PaO_2 = 53 mmHg
$P(A-a)O_2$ = 60−53 =
7 mmHg on room air

The $P(A-a)O_2$ of 7 mmHg in patient

B indicates normal oxygen transfer across the lung. The $P(A-a)O_2$ of 68 mmHg in patient A indicates an obvious oxygenation defect; oxygen transfer across the lung is inefficient. Thus, patient A has pure hypoxemic respiratory failure, and patient B has pure hypercapnic respiratory failure.

Administering 100% O_2 would yield clinically important information only in patient A because we already know that oxygen transfer is normal in patient B. Giving patient A 100% oxygen would allow us to assess the response of PaO_2 to oxygen therapy, and thus the kind of oxygenation defect. If PaO_2 rises to near maximal values on 100% O_2 then V/Q mismatch is the cause of hypoxemia, and simple oxygen therapy is rational. If PaO_2 responds poorly, then shunt is the cause of hypoxemia. Some form of positive end expiratory pressure (PEEP or CPAP) may be effective in reexpanding airless alveoli. The rational therapy in the case of patient B is intubation and mechanical ventilation, unless some more conservative means of increasing ventilation is effective. Correcting patient B's ventilation will automatically restore PaO_2 to normal.

Table 29-1 Hypoxemic and hypercapnic respiratory failure

Type of respiratory failure	Blood gas changes		
	PaO₂*	PaCO₂	P(A-a)O₂
Hypoxemic	Low	Normal to low	High
Hypercapnic	Low	High	Normal
Combined	Low	High	High

*In each case, PaO_2 is lower than predicted for the FIO_2. When breathing high FIO_2, PaO_2 can be adequate, eg, 90 to 100 torr in the face of severe oxygenation failure.

From Martin L: Pulmonary physiology in clinical practice, St Louis, 1987, Mosby.

Acute versus chronic respiratory failure

Our concept of respiratory failure must also take into account the duration of the problem, and whether any compensatory response has occurred. The term acute respiratory failure indicates that the gas exchange abnormality developed too rapidly for compensation to occur. Thus acute respiratory failure is a life-threatening event which usually requires drastic intervention, including some form of ventilatory support.[1,9,10]

On the other hand, chronic respiratory failure develops over a period of weeks to months. This gives the body time to compensate for the problem.[1] Compensatory responses to chronic hypoxemia include various mechanisms to improve oxygen transport, as discussed in Chapter 15. The primary compensation for chronic hypercapnia is renal buffering of hydrogen ions, as described in Chapter 14.

■ MINI C LINI ■

29-2

Acute-On-Chronic Respiratory Failure

Problem: A 55-year-old patient presents to the emergency room in obvious respiratory distress, complaining of shortness of breath and increased sputum production over the last week. He is alert and oriented. The patient has a temperature of 100.5°F, is using accessory muscles to breathe, respiratory rate is 25/min, and heart rate is 120/min. The patient has a history of heavy cigarette smoking and was previously diagnosed as having chronic obstructive pulmonary disease (COPD). Current arterial blood gases on room air are:

pH = 7.33
PCO₂ = 70 mmHg
HCO₃⁻ = 36 MEq/L
PO₂ = 35 mmHg

What type of respiratory failure, if any, does this represent and what kind of therapy is indicated?

Discussion: The history and current blood gases imply that under normal stable conditions, this patient probably has chronic hypercapnic respiratory failure; that is, compensated respiratory acidosis. The HCO₃ of 36 mEq/L is the key to this interpretation; the kidneys require days to retain this much bicarbonate. This renal bicarbonate retention must have been a compensatory response to high PaCO₂. We can reasonably conclude that stable blood gases on room air would probably be similar to the following:

pH = 7.38
PCO₂ = 59 mmHg
HCO₃⁻ = 34 mEq/L
PO₂ = 55 mmHg

These blood gases are compatible with chronic hypercapnic respiratory failure; a compensated respiratory acidosis exists. The probable scenario is that this patient developed a pulmonary infection which exacerbated his compromised ability to ventilate and caused acute CO₂ retention. The emergency room blood gases are compatible with acute ventilatory (hypercapnic) failure superimposed on an underlying chronic (compensated) ventilatory failure. The low PaO₂ cannot be explained by hypoventilation alone; that is, simple displacement of oxygen by the high PaCO₂ does not account for a PaO₂ as low as 35 mmHg. There must be an additional factor which helps cause the low PaO₂, such as V/Q mismatch or intrapulmonary shunt. Therefore, this patient is suffering from a combined hypoxemic-hypercapnic respiratory failure, sometimes called "acute-on-chronic" respiratory failure. The P(A-a)O₂ is above normal, confirming an oxygenation defect.

$$PAO_2 = .21 (713) - 70/.8 = 62 \text{ mmHg}$$
$$P(A-a)O_2 = 62-35 = 27$$
mmHg gradient on room air

Appropriate therapy in this alert, oriented patient would be conservative but vigorous therapy aimed at improving ventilation. Oxygen therapy is reasonable because an oxygenation defect exists. Antibiotics are indicated to treat the infection causing the exacerbation. Increased airway secretions indicate the need for vigorous bronchopulmonary hygiene therapy (chest physical therapy, aerosol therapy, bronchodilator therapy, and naso tracheal suctioning). This should improve ventilation, reduce PaCO₂, and increase the pH. Oxygen therapy should be used to bring the PaO₂ to approximately 60 mmHg (or about 90% HbO₂ saturation). During oxygen therapy, the PaCO₂ and pH should be closely monitored to insure that O₂ therapy does not induce further hypoventilation and acidosis. In some cases, IPPB may be used to forestall the need for invasive and hazardous mechanical ventilation.

Of course, a patient with chronic respiratory failure may acutely worsen. This so-called *acute-on-chronic* form of respiratory failure generally involves patients with a preexisting chronic pulmonary disorder, such as COPD (MiniClini 29-2).[11] Typically, these patients have compensated for both the hypoxemia and hypercapnia caused by their disease. However, any acute exacerbation of the process can cause a rapid deterioration in respiratory status. This usually involves both a rise in the $PaCO_2$ and fall in PaO_2, signaling a combined form of respiratory failure. Therapy must be directed to treat the underlying cause of the acute failure and to return the patient's blood gas status to its previous compensated values.[12]

Respiratory failure versus respiratory insufficiency

Although the terms respiratory failure and respiratory insufficiency are interchanged, it is useful to draw a distinction between their meanings. While respiratory failure is always accompanied by abnormal arterial blood gases, respiratory insufficiency is not. Instead, respiratory insufficiency represents a condition in which breathing is accompanied by abnormal signs and symptoms, such as dyspnea or paradoxical breathing. Signs and symptoms like these usually signal an increased work of breathing. Thus, a patient with respiratory insufficiency may have normal or near normal blood gases, but at the expense of an increased work of breathing.[13]

Because respiratory insufficiency can lead to respiratory failure, RCPs must always take into account the full clinical picture of the patient, as opposed to just assessing lab data. Early recognition of respiratory insufficiency, before full-blown respiratory failure develops, may avert the need for ventilatory support. This is especially true in managing patients with acute-on-chronic respiratory failure.[11]

ETIOLOGY OF RESPIRATORY FAILURE

As previously discussed, a wide diversity of clinical disorders can disrupt gas exchange and cause respiratory failure.[1,5,8]

Major categories of respiratory failure

The causes of respiratory failure can be categorized by how they impair breathing or gas exchange. Figure 29-1 depicts the key functional divisions of the respiratory system. According to this scheme, an abnormality affecting any one of these areas can cause inadequate gas exchange and respiratory failure. The box on page 808 list some of the more common causes

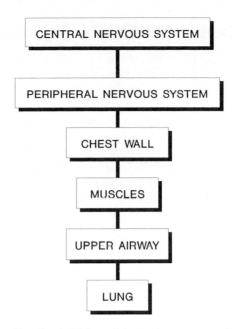

Fig. 29-1 Functional divisions of the respiratory system. Dysfunction in any one division can cause respiratory failure. (Redrawn from *Respir Care* 24:4, April 1979.)

of respiratory failure, categorized by the division of the respiratory system affected.

In general, most disorders of the nervous system or muscles cause a reduction in alveolar ventilation, and thus a primary hypercapnic respiratory failure. Disorders of the chest wall and pleura have variable effects on respiration. As restrictive disorders, these abnormalities reduce lung volumes, including tidal volume. However, if the patient can compensate for a reduced tidal volume with an increased rate, adequate alveolar ventilation can be maintained. Indeed, some patients with restrictive disorders tend to hyperventilate.

Nonetheless, reduced tidal volumes can cause progressive atelectasis (or lung collapse). Moreover, some chest wall or pleural disorders actually compress lung tissue (as in kyphoscoliosis) or worsen the distribution of ventilation (as in flail chest). These problems can also lead to atelectasis or areas of low $\dot{V}/\dot{Q}$. Thus restrictive disorders can also cause hypoxemic respiratory failure.

Upper airway disorders typically cause either partial or complete airway obstruction. Partial or complete airway obstruction results in both a hypoxemic and hypercapnic respiratory failure.

Last, severe intrinsic lung diseases can cause either a combined or purely hypoxemic respiratory failure. A good example of combined respiratory failure due to intrinsic lung disease is COPD. Adult respiratory distress syndrome is a good example of an intrinsic lung disorder causing a pure hypoxemic respiratory failure.

Differences in etiology according to age

The most common causes of respiratory failure vary according to age.[1] In newborn infants, the most common cause of respiratory failure is an intrinsic lung disorder called neonatal respiratory distress syndrome or hyaline membrane disease. Common causes of respiratory failure in infants 1 to 24 months old are immature immune defenses (causing infection) and small airway obstruction (resulting from infection). In older children, respiratory failure is most often caused by status asthmaticus, cystic fibrosis, or foreign body aspiration. More detail on the conditions causing respiratory failure in infants and children is provided in Chapter 35. The rest of this chapter will focus on respiratory failure in the adult.

Interrelationship among problems

Of course, two or more of these problems may coexist at the same time, or be complicated by related conditions. Motor vehicle trauma resulting in both brain injury and flail chest, or a heroin drug overdose that also results in pulmonary edema are good examples of situations in which two problems, both capable of leading to respiratory failure, coexist.

An excellent example of complications caused by related conditions is the interrelation between heart disease and respiratory failure. Respiratory failure may complicate an acute myocardial infarction directly, as with pulmonary edema, or indirectly, due to decreased cerebral perfusion. On the other hand, a myocardial infarction may complicate respiratory failure by decreasing oxygen transport to the tissues and increasing the metabolic demands on the heart.[14]

Last, critical illness in general increases the risk of respiratory failure. Critically ill patients are prone to develop complications such as nosocomial pneumonias, sepsis, embolization, electrolyte imbalances, and renal failure.[1] Such complications can themselves lead to respiratory failure.

The adult respiratory distress syndrome (ARDS)

Nowhere is the relationship among the various factors involved in respiratory failure more apparent than with the Adult respiratory distress syndrome (ARDS). As the term suggests, ARDS is not a disease, but rather a remarkably uniform pattern of features characterizing the lung's response to injury.[15] The accompanying box lists the broad range of disorders that can lead to ARDS.

Causes of respiratory failure

Central nervous system

Drug overdose (e.g., opiates, barbiturates, tranquilizers, alcohol)
Obesity-related hypoventilation (Pickwickian syndrome)
Primary alveolar hypoventilation syndrome **(Ondine's curse)**
Central sleep apnea syndrome
Stroke
Tumors
Brain, brainstem, or spinal cord trauma
Multiple sclerosis
Syringomyelia
Myxedema
Metabolic imbalances (hyperglycemia, hyponatremia, etc.)
Infections (meningitis, encephalitis, etc.)

Peripheral nervous system

Poliomyelitis (also acts centrally)
Amyotrophic lateral sclerosis
Guillain-Barre syndrome
Botulism poisoning
Tetanus
Drugs (curare, succinylcholine)

Chest wall (including pleura)

Kyphoscoliosis
Ankylosing spondylitis
Morbid obesity

Flail chest
Restrictive pleural diseases

Muscles

Muscular dystrophy
Polymyositis
Myasthenia gravis
Muscle fatigue or atrophy

Upper airway

Epiglottitis
Laryngotracheitis
Trauma
Tracheal stenosis
Internal or external (compressing) tumors
Foreign body
Micrognathia

Intrinsic lung diseases

COPD
Asthma
Cystic fibrosis
Pneumonia
Pulmonary emboli (thromboemboli, fat emboli, etc.)
Interstitial/parenchymal lung diseases (including fibrosis)
Oxygen toxicity
Pulmonary edema
ARDS

Conditions associated with ARDS

Pulmonary-related conditions

Infections (viral, bacterial, fungal)
Aspiration
    Gastric contents
    Near-drowning
    Hydrocarbon fluids
Inhaled Toxins
    Oxygen
    Smoke inhalation
    Chemicals (NO_2, Cl_2, NH_3, phosgene)
Trauma
    Lung contusion
    Chest trauma
Other
    Radiation pneumonitis
    Postperfusion (cardiopulmonary bypass)
    High altitude pulmonary edema

Nonpulmonary conditions

Shock of any cause
Drug overdose
Disseminated intravascular coagulation
Massive blood transfusion
Sepsis
Fat embolism
Hemorrhagic pancreatitis
Uremia
Anaphylaxis
Nonthoracic trauma
Neurogenic pulmonary edema
Eclampsia

Pathophysiology

Despite the wide range of problems associated with ARDS, the sequence of pathologic changes occurring in the lung is similar.[16] These changes occur in three phases: the acute or exudative phase (up to 6 days); the subacute or proliferative phase (4 to 10 days); and the chronic phase (8 days and on). Structural changes associated with chronic pulmonary hypertension may also develop in the chronic phase.

Figure 29-2 on page 810, depicts the events occurring during the acute phase of ARDS. As evident, the common denominator is alveolar-capillary membrane damage. Regardless of cause, such damage increases membrane permeability. This results in leakage of fluid and protein into the interstitial space and alveoli (Figure 29-3, page 810).[17-21] As this protein-rich edema fluid collects in the alveoli, hyaline membranes form (Figure 29-3), and surfactant activity becomes impaired.[22-25] Alveoli not filled with exudate become unstable and collapse. This results in progressive atelectasis, as evident in the characteristic chest X-ray over changes over time (Figure 29-4, page 811).

In combination, the noncardiac pulmonary edema, hyaline membrane formation and atelectasis severely impair gas exchange, especially oxygenation. Since the hypoxemia is due to severe physiologic shunting, it does not respond well to oxygen therapy. This so-called *refractory hypoxemia* is one of the primary clinical hallmarks of ARDS.

Pulmonary edema, atelectasis, and surfactant loss also reduce lung volumes and compliance. As shown in Figure 29-5, page 812, these changes increase the pressure differences needed to produce the same tidal volume. With a larger pressure difference needed to move a given volume of gas, the patient's work of breathing progressively increases. This increased work of breathing manifests itself at the bedside in dyspnea, tachypnea, and signs of respiratory muscle fatigue, such as paradoxical breathing.

Patients surviving the acute phase of ARDS go on to the proliferative phase. In this phase, metaplasia of the alveolar cells occurs, with early evidence of fibrosis.[16] Progression to the chronic phase is marked by more extensive fibrosis and pulmonary vascular changes.

Management

With the exception of treating infectious causes, the management of ARDS has been limited to supportive measures. Specifically, since this syndrome was first described in the late 1960's, mechanical ventilation with PEEP (positive end-expiratory pressure) has been the mainstay of treatment.

Limits of supportive management. Unfortunately, despite over 25 years experience in managing ARDS, the mortality rate still remains extremely high (60% to 80%). Over the last 10 years, various new modes of ventilatory support have been developed to help combat ARDS. These include inverse ratio ventilation, high frequency ventilation, alternating positive airway pressure, prone position ventilation, and differential lung ventilation.[26-30] Most of these modes have shown some good physiologic effects. However, none have proven effective in lowering mortality rate.

Treating the causes. Instead of trying to treat the pathophysiologic effects of ARDS, focus is now shifting to identifying and treating the biochemical causes. Recent research suggests that ARDS is the end result of an inflammatory process gone wild. The normal inflammatory process helps limit and repair injury. However, there are times when this normal process gets out of control and goes berserk.[31] Instead of limiting injury, this so-called rogue inflammation actually worsens it.

Figure 29-6, page 812 shows how rogue inflammation may cause lung injury. Although the exact biochemical triggers are not known, infection and trauma play key roles. Also, the exact the sequence of events, mediators involved, and their interactions may vary greatly among patients. Nonetheless, a general description of what is currently known about this process is useful.

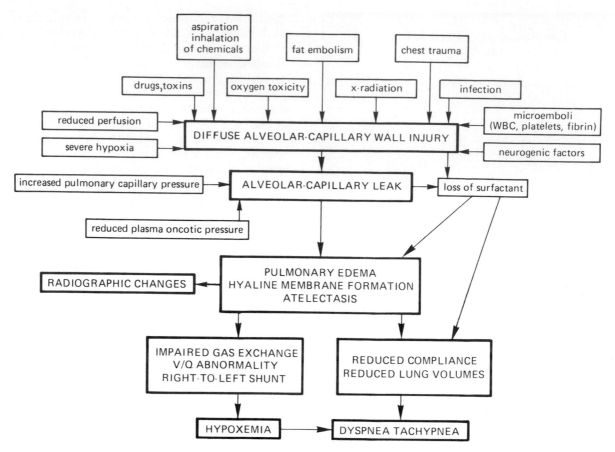

Fig. 29-2 Pathogenesis and pathophysiology of adult respiratory distress syndrome. (From Farzan S: A concise handbook of respiratory diseases, ed 2, East Norwalk, Conn, 1985, Appleton & Lange.)

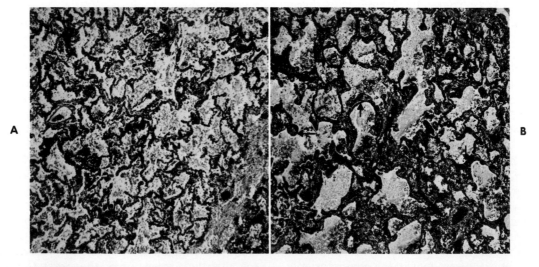

Fig. 29-3 Characteristic early light microscopic abnormalities in ARDS caused by viral pneumonia. **A,** Alveolar filling with proteinaceous and cellular debris. **B,** Abnormalities after 48 to 72 hours, showing hyaline membranes *(arrows)* in addition to alveolar filling. (From Moser KM and Spragg RG: Respiratory emergencies, ed 2, St Louis, 1982, Mosby.)

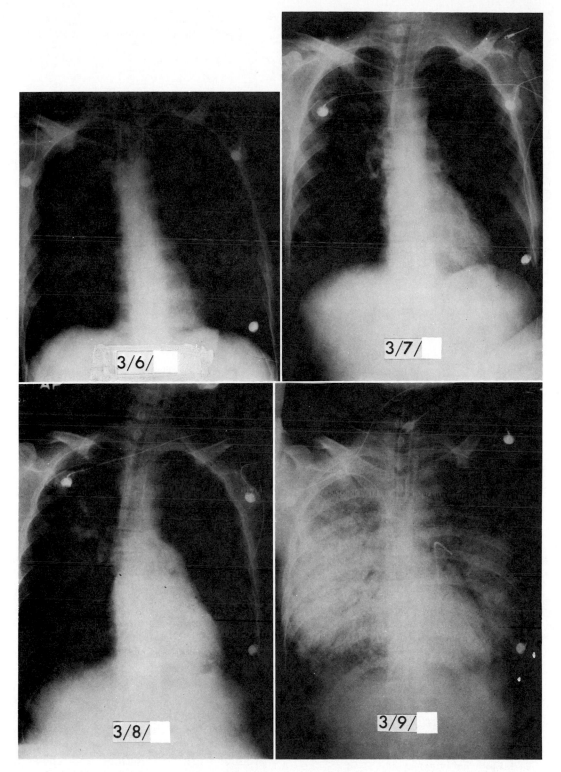

Fig. 29-4 Characteristic roentgenographic changes as ARDS develops. (From Moser KM and Spragg RG: Respiratory emergencies, ed 2, St Louis, 1982, Mosby.)

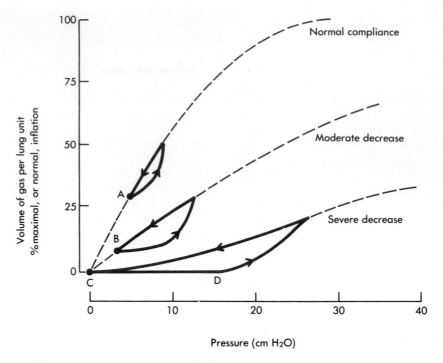

Fig. 29-5 Conceptualization, based on data from several sources, of the relationship of unit lung volume to transpulmonary pressure. *Solid lines* represent inflation and deflation curves during constant tidal volume; *dashed lines* represent deflation curves over full range of transpulmonary pressures. As ARDS increases in severity and compliance progressively decreases, functional residual capacity decreases from point *A* to *B* to *C*. At *C* the unit is collapsed. Before it can be reinflated, a critical opening pressure (*D*) must be exceeded. Thus, with ARDS of increasing severity, the pressure required to produce the same tidal volume progressively increases. (From Moser KM and Spragg RG: Respiratory emergencies, ed 2, St Louis, 1982, Mosby.)

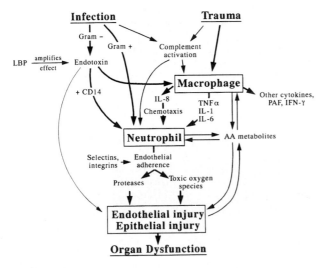

Fig. 29-6 Possible sequence of events producing lung inflammation and injury. LBP = lpoplysaccharide − binding protein; IL − 1= interleukin − 1; IL − 6 = interleukin − 6; IL − 8 = interleukin − 8; TNFa = tumor necrosis factor-alpha; PAF = platelet activating factor; AA = aachidonic acid; IFNg = interferon-gamma. (From Hudson LD: Pharmacologic approaches to respiratory failure, *Respir Care* 38:754-764, 1993.)

Infection or trauma activate complement, a normal blood component. Complement activation promotes adherence of neutrophils (**polymorphonuclear lymphocytes**) to the capillary endothelium. As these activated neutrophils gather and adhere to the capillary endothelium, damaging enzymes and oxygen radical are released. These factors injure both the capillary endothelium and alveolar epithelium (Type I cells). This allows protein-rich fluid to escape into the interstitium and alveoli, leading to the typical clinical picture of ARDS, previously described.

That patients with low neutrophil counts (**neutropenia**) can also develop ARDS suggests that this white blood cell is not the only culprit.[32] Macrophages may also play a key role in this process. Macrophages produce various **cytokines** and **chemotaxic** factors which attract neutrophils to the inflamed area. In addition, macrophage activity results in the production of arachidonic acid, which is also a source of injury.

ARDS is also associated with increased blood levels of certain hormones and other chemical mediators.[15,33] These substances include histamine, **bradykinin, serotonin,** and certain prostaglandins. These agents have potent vasoactive properties, including the ability to cause constriction of the pulmonary venous circulation, and the tendency to increase capillary endothelial permeability.

Pharmacologic approaches. Based on our better knowledge of the biochemistry of ARDS, numerous drug agents are being developed and tested. Most general anti-inflammatory drugs, such as corticosteroids and prostaglandin E_1, have shown little benefit. Other agents, including nitric oxide, surfactant, nonsteroidal anti-inflammatory drugs (NSAIDs), antiendotoxin antibodies, and anticytokines are undergoing clinical trials and may prove effective.[31,34] Of all these agents, RCPs will be most closely involved with nitric oxide and surfactant replacement. The potential use of nitric oxide, a potent pulmonary vasodilator, is discussed in Chapter 26. We will briefly discuss surfactant use in ARDS here.

Surfactant replacement. In ARDS, Type II cell damage occurs. This damage alters surfactant composition and synthesis. Altered surfactant function increases alveolar surface tension, and decreases pulmonary compliance. These changes result in localized alveolar collapse, decreased FRC, and increased physiologic shunting.

In concept, surfactant replacement should limit lung injury by two mechanisms. First, it should restore lung mechanics by replacing depleted endogenous surfactant. Second, surfactant administration may also help eliminate harmful free oxygen radicals.[35]

Recent research confirms some beneficial effects. In two different studies, ARDS patients treated with aerosolized surfactant showed improved compliance, had lower $P(A-a)O_2$s, FIO_2s, and shunting and exhibited lower mortality than those not receiving surfactant.[35,26] In another study, instillation of surfactant resulted in a transient increase in PaO_2 and improved gas exchange.[37]

Although the use of surfactant in ARDS appears promising, there remain may questions and unresolved problems. Key questions involve safety, efficacy, patient selection, and timing. Problems include method of administration, dose in relation to volume and concentration, and cost.[38]

INDICATIONS FOR VENTILATORY SUPPORT

Clearly, the causes of respiratory failure are extremely diverse, and often interrelated. Current management focuses on general supportive measures. Management options tend to emphasize common patterns of pathophysiology, as opposed to specific diseases.

By definition, acute respiratory failure is the primary indication for instituting ventilatory support. However, despite over three decades and millions of patient hours of experience, there is still no consensus on the best approach to ventilatory support.

Modes of ventilatory support

As defined in the accompanying box,[39,40] the primary modes of ventilatory support in current use are: (1) continuous mandatory ventilation (CMV), either in the control or assist/control mode, (2) intermittent mandatory ventilation (IMV), (3) pressure support ventilation (PSV),[41] and (4) continuous positive airway pressure (CPAP).

Variation in these four modes are based on how breath size is determined, and what occurs during expiration. The size of machine-provided breaths (CMV and SIMV only) can be regulated by controlling either the delivered volume or pressure. Thus, during volume-controlled SIMV, breaths of a given volume are periodically applied to the airway, with the patient breathing spontaneously between machine breaths. On the other hand, during pressure-controlled CMV, a set amount of pressure is applied to the airway during every inspiration.

Key modes of ventilatory support

Continuous mandatory ventilation (CMV): The application of positive pressure at the airway opening during *every* inspiration. Two major variations of CMV are based on whether the machine or patient initiates or triggers the breath:

Control mode CMV (machine-triggered): continuous mandatory ventilation in which the frequency of breathing is determined by the ventilator according to a preset cycling interval, *without* initiation by the patient.

Assist/control mode CMV (machine- or patient-triggered): continuous mandatory ventilation in which the *minimum* frequency of breathing is predetermined by the ventilator controls, but the patient can trigger breaths at a faster rate.

Intermittent mandatory ventilation (IMV): Periodic ventilation with positive pressure, with the patient breathing spontaneously between breaths. As with CMV, these breaths may be machine-triggered only (control mode IMV) or machine or patient-triggered (synchronous IMV, SIMV).

Pressure support ventilation (PSV): Patient-triggered, pressure-limited, flow-cycled ventilation designed to augment a spontaneously generated breath. The patient has primary control over the frequency of breathing, the inspiratory time, and the inspiratory flow.

Continuous positive airway pressure (CPAP): The maintenance of a pressure above atmospheric at the airway opening throughout a spontaneous breathing cycle.

Regarding what occurs during expiration, airway pressure may either be allowed to fall back to atmospheric (0 cm H_2O), or be kept elevated. During continuous positive airway pressure (CPAP), pressure remains elevated continuously. However, elevated or positive end-expiratory pressure (PEEP) may be combined with any of the other three modes. Thus, for example, during volume-controlled CMV with PEEP, a set volume is applied to the airway during every inspiration, with pressure maintained above atmospheric during expiration.

One additional variable to consider is the airway itself. Traditionally, positive pressure ventilation has always been provided through either endotracheal or tracheostomy tubes (see Chapter 22). Recently, oronasal or nasal masks have been successfully used as the route for positive pressure ventilatory support.[42-44] This approach is called *noninvasive intermittent positive pressure ventilation* (NIPPV). As the name suggests, NIPPV is not a separate mode of ventilatory support, but simply a different route applicable for any of the existing modes. More details on these various modes of ventilatory support is provided in Section VII.

Parameters indicating the need for ventilatory support

A common assumption in clinical practice is that patient management will become more effective once we know the right indicators or measures. Over the last three decades, many measures have been suggested as indicating the need for ventilatory support. Table 29-2 provides a summary of these indicators as synthesized from various sources.[5,45-51] These measures vary from simple bedside observations to complex determinations requiring research equipment. Moreover, many of the most common indicators are measured or are used differently by different clinicians.

Confounding the use of these measures is the fact that some patients with severe chronic disorders exhibit marked abnormal values on some indicators, yet are perfectly stable. In these cases, common sense tells us that ventilatory support is not needed. This illustrates the limitations of applying strict numerical criteria to determine when to initiate ventilatory support.

Table 29-2 Some measurements used in determining the need for ventilatory support*

Measurement	Values Normal	Values Ventilatory support indicated†
Tidal volume (V_T) (mL/kg)	5-8	<5
Vital capacity (VC) (mL/kg)	65-75	<10; <15
Forced expiratory volume in one second (FEV_1) (mL/kg)	50-60	<10
Functional residual capacity (FRC) (% of predicted value)	80-100	<50
Respiratory rate (f) (breaths/min)	12-20	>35
Maximum inspiratory pressure (MIP) (cm H_2O)	80-100	<20; <25; <30
Minute ventilation ($\dot{V}_E$) (L/min)	5-6	>10
Maximum voluntary ventilation (MVV) (L/min)	120-180	<20; <(2 × $\dot{V}_E$)
Dead space fraction (V_D/V_T) (%)	0.25-0.40	>0.60
$PaCO_2$ (torr)	35-45	>50; >55
PaO_2 (torr)	75-100 (breathing air)	<50 (air); < 70 (mask O_2)
Alveolar-to-arterial PO_2 gradient [$P(A-a)O_2$], breathing 100% O_2 (torr)	25-65	>350; >450
Arterial/alveolar PO_2 ratio (PaO_2/PAO_2)	0.75	<0.15
Arterial PO_2/inspired O_2 fraction ratio (PaO_2/FIO_2) (torr)	350-450	<200
Intrapulmonary right-to-left shunt fraction ($\dot{Q}s/\dot{Q}T$) (%)	≤5	>20; >25; >30

Adapted from Pierson DJ: Indications for mechanical ventilation in acute respiratory failure, *Respir Care* 28:5, 1983.
*Adapted in part from references 5, 23-29.
†Multiple cut-off values indicate different recommendations by different sources.

Nonetheless, an analysis of the physiologic bases underlying these numerous indicators is useful. Table 29-3 rearranges these measures according to the six main physiologic processes they assess. We will first review each of these major processes. We will then look at the application of ventilatory support in several special clinical situations, including its preventative or prophylactic use.

Inadequate alveolar ventilation

Arterial PCO_2 reflects alveolar ventilation. By definition, when the $PaCO_2$ is elevated, hypoventilation is present. When alveolar hypoventilation produces severe respiratory acidosis, acute hypercapnic respiratory failure is present.[52]

Importance of pH. On the other hand, hypoventilation that develops slow enough for renal compensation to occur poses no immediate threat of life. For example, two patients might have the following arterial blood values:

	Patient A	Patient B
$PaCO_2$	60	60
HCO_3	25	36
pH	7.25	7.38

Although both patients have the same level of hypercapnia, only one (Patient A) exhibits acute respiratory failure. Patient B, on the other hand, has a compensated respiratory acidosis, and thus is suffering from chronic hypercapnic respiratory failure. This distinction is of fundamental importance in respiratory care, and emphasizes the need to use both $PaCO_2$ and pH as indicators for ventilatory support.

From the foregoing it is clear that the $PaCO_2$ alone is not an adequate indicator for initiating ventilatory support. The threshold value shown in Table 29-2 are valid only when they represent a sudden change from a patient's usual state, something that can be detected only by examining the pH as well.

Table 29-3 Indications for ventilatory support, classified by physiologic mechanism

Mechanism	Best available indicators
Inadequate alveolar ventilation	$PaCO_2$ and pH
Inadequate lung expansion	V_T; VC; f
Inadequate respiratory muscle strength	MIP; MVV; VC
Excessive work of breathing	V_E required to keep PCO_2 normal; V_D/V_T, f
Unstable ventilatory drive	Breathing pattern, clinical setting
Severe hypoxemia	$P(A-a)O_2$; PaO_2/P_AO_2; PaO_2/FiO_2; $\dot{Q}s/\dot{Q}_T$

Adapted from Pierson DJ: Indications for mechanical ventilation in acute respiratory failure, *Respir Care* 28:5, 1983.

When CO_2 retention develops acutely, how far must the arterial pH fall before life is threatened? In one study of complications occurring during mechanical ventilation, mortality and morbidity rose in patients whose pH values fell below 7.30.[53] Thus most clinicians aim to keep the pH above 7.25 to 7.30.

Although pH is a better indicator of acute hypercapnic respiratory failure than is $PaCO_2$, trends in these values are more important still. Worsening respiratory acidosis over minutes or hours, particularly in the face of vigorous therapy, is an indication for ventilatory support, regardless of the specific pH value used as a threshold.

Significance of an elevated $PaCO_2$. Since an elevated $PaCO_2$ increases ventilatory drive in normal subjects, the very existence of hypoventilation suggests other problems with the respiratory apparatus. Specifically, the presence of acute respiratory acidosis indicates one of three major problems. Either: (1) the patient is not normally responding to the elevated $PaCO_2$, (2) the patient is responding normally, but the signal is not getting through to the respiratory muscles, or (3) despite normal neural response mechanisms, the lungs and chest bellows are simply incapable of providing adequate ventilation, due to parenchymal disease or muscular weakness.[54]

Modes of ventilatory support. In pure hypercapnic respiratory failure, the selection of ventilatory support mode depends, in part, on the cause of alveolar hypoventilation. When the problem is due to a decreased ventilatory drive, as in an uncomplicated drug overdose, simple CMV is usually sufficient. However, when the problem is due to a restrictive disorder of the lungs or chest bellows, and the patient is responding normally to the elevated $PaCO_2$, CMV may cause patient-machine asynchrony ("fighting" the ventilator)[55] and increase the work of breathing.[56,57]

Moreover, the high rate of spontaneous breathing seen in these patients may cause a rapid swing to respiratory alkalosis once they are placed in the assist/control mode of CMV. For this reason, some authorities suggest that IMV is the mode best able to normalize alveolar ventilation in these cases.[55]

Inadequate lung expansion

Even when alveolar ventilation is adequate, some patients may not be able to maintain normal lung expansion. Inadequate lung expansion may occur during general anesthesia, after upper abdominal surgery, following spinal cord injuries, and in acute restrictive lung disease, such as ARDS. The inability to maintain normal lung expansion may lead to atelectasis and pneumonia.

Bedside assessment. Measurements used to gauge the need for ventilatory support when the problem is inadequate lung expansion include tidal volume (V_T), vital capacity (VC), respiratory rate (f), and functional residual capacity (FRC). Although useful in research, bedside FRC measurement in critically ill patients is not yet practical.

Spontaneous VT is the most direct measure of end–expiratory lung expansion. A value of 5 mL/kg or less in an acutely ill patient may indicate the need for ventilatory assistance. Experimental support for this belief comes from studies of normal patients under general anesthesia. These patients developed progressive hypoxemia and loss of lung compliance.[58,59] Both problems were reversed by intermittent deep breaths. The same ill effects have been observed in patient receiving controlled ventilation with physiologically normal tidal volumes (5 to 7 mL/kg.)[60] These studies were largely responsible for the development of automatic sigh mechanisms now found on most mechanical ventilators.

High vs low tidal volumes. Subsequent studies showed that CMV with supernormal tidal volumes (10 to 15 mL/kg) without intermittent sighs effectively prevented both hypoxemia and loss of lung compliance.[61,62] These observations were the basis for routinely using supernormal tidal volumes in acutely ill patients with inadequate lung expansion.

Although some early laboratory studies tended to support this notion,[63,64] recent work suggests that supernormal tidal volumes (and the pressure needed to deliver them) may be harmful.[65] This has lead to the recommendation to use smaller tidal volumes (as low as 5 mL/kg) in order to keep the peak alveolar pressures below 35 cm H_2O.[66] Instead of supernormal tidal volumes, PEEP and/or CPAP are used to maintain the FRC.

Modes of ventilatory support. Thus, in patients with inadequate lung expansion, efforts should be made to maintain positive airway pressure throughout the ventilatory cycle. If alveolar ventilation is adequate, simple CPAP should suffice. On the other hand, if inadequate lung expansion coexists with inadequate alveolar ventilation, then CMV with PEEP or IMV with PEEP is indicated (MiniClini 29-3). In either case, alveolar pressures should be kept below 35 cm H_2O.

Inadequate respiratory muscle strength

For effective ventilation to occur, the respiratory muscles must be capable of bearing the load imposed on them (refer to Chapter 11). As shown in Figure 29-7, there exists a range of workloads within which the respiratory muscles function optimally.

Fatigue vs atrophy. Subnormal workloads lead to muscle atrophy, or an actual loss of muscle mass and contractile force. A good example of respiratory muscle *atrophy* occurs in patients with spinal cord trauma, such as quadriplegics. On the other hand, workloads in excess of a muscle's energy utilization capabilities can lead to *fatigue*. Fatigue represents a reversible decrease in the force developed by a muscle during sustained or repeated contractions.

Respiratory muscle fatigue may occur whenever the elastic or resistive workload is excessive, as in pulmonary fibrosis (excessive elastic work), or asthma (excessive resistive work).[67]

Whether by atrophy or fatigue, respiratory muscle strength may be inadequate to support normal levels of ventilation. Thus, respiratory muscle weakness can lead to inadequate lung expansion, loss of lung

---

■ MINI **C**LINI ■

29-3

Indications for CPAP Vs. CMV with PEEP

Problem: A patient in the ICU is severely tachypneic and hypoxemic. The respiratory rate is 30/min. On approximately 50% oxygen by mask at sea level, the patient's PaO_2 = 50 mmHg, $PaCO_2$ = 30 mmHg, pH = 7.51, HcO_3^- = 23 mEq/L. The patient is in distress but alert and able to cooperate and follow instructions.

What is this person's $P(A-a)O_2$?

What type of respiratory failure is this?

What is appropriate initial therapy?

Discussion: First, the patient does not have hypercapnic respiratory failure as is confirmed by the $PaCO_2$ of 30

mmHg. The patient does have a serious oxygenation defect, confirmed by the $P(A-a)O_2$.

PAO_2 = .50 (713) − 30/.8 = 318 mmHg
$P(A-a)O_2$ = 318 − 50 = 268 mmHg

The high $P(A-a)O_2$ indicates the presence of severe intrapulmonary shunt. Shunts this severe can only

occur when significant airway closure and atelectasis are present. The mode of therapy should be aimed at re-inflating collapsed alveoli and keeping them open throughout the breathing cycle. In this patient, alveolar ventilation is obviously not impaired ($PaCO_2$ = 30 mmHg). Therefore, continuous positive airway pressure (CPAP) alone may be effective in reducing shunt. (CPAP does not ventilate the patient; all breaths are patient-initiated and spontaneous.) CPAP may be applied non-invasively by mask, as would be indicated in this alert, cooperative patient. If hypercapnia and acidemia develop, then mechanical ventilation with PEEP would be indicated.

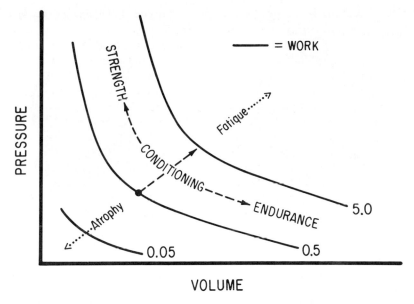

Fig. 29-7 In this representation of the relationships between the quantity and quality of workloads placed on ventilatory muscles, the isopleths represent three rates of work. A subnormal work rate (0.05 kg·m·mm^{-1}) can result in atrophy, whereas a supranormal work rate (5 kg·m·mm^{-1}) can condition or, if high enough, fatigure muscles. Note that the quality of a constant workload can be characterized by the relationship between the muscle pressure generation *(pressure)* and the muscle contraction distance *(volume change)*. A high-pressure low-volume change workload emphasizes isometric conditioning and improves strength; low-pressure high-volume change workload emphasizes isobaric conditioning and improves endurance. (Redrawn from Problems in pulmonary disease, Winter 1986.)

compliance, hypoventilation, atelectasis, and pneumonia.

Bedside assessment. As shown in Table 29-3, the most commonly measures of respiratory muscle strength are the maximum inspiratory pressure (MIP),[68] maximum voluntary ventilation (MVV), and VC.

Although the threshold value varies, the MIP is a readily available measurement that can be taken on any patient (Figure 29-8, page 818). Patients who can generate MIPs in excess of 30 cm H_2O probably have sufficient muscle strength for continued spontaneous ventilation. A value less negative than 30 cm H_2O is compatible with adequate lung inflation in some persons with chronic neuromuscular conditions. However, low MIP values in acutely ill patients implies little reserve and the threat of progressive ventilatory insufficiency.

The MVV maneuver can be performed at the bedside with a hand-held mechanical or electronic spirometer. The MVV is useful in assessing ventilatory reserve, but it requires cooperation and cannot be performed by most critically ill patients.

As with most of the parameters listed in the tables, these traditional measures have not been investigated prospectively as criteria for initiating ventilatory support. Data justifying their use come mainly from studies of ventilator weaning.[69,70]

Supplementing these methods of assessing the strength of the respiratory muscles are a variety of new quantitative research methods, some of which may soon be available at the bedside. These new methods are discussed Chapter 33.

Modes of ventilatory support. The best mode of ventilatory support for patients with inadequate respiratory muscle strength is a matter of considerable controversy. In general, if the cause of respiratory muscle weakness is fatigue, it seems logical to have a mechanical ventilator assume most of the work of breathing, as with occurs with CMV in the assist/control mode. How long this may be needed varies with the degree of fatigue. However, fatigued respiratory muscles typically take anywhere from 24 to 48 hours to fully recover. During this period, the ongoing need for ventilatory support should be carefully monitored. Since the respiratory muscles are resting during this time, care must be taken to avoid progression to a state of atrophy.

On the other hand, if the cause of weakness is atrophy, it seems reasonable to progressively load the respiratory muscles by allowing the patient to breathe spontaneously, as occurs during IMV.[55] The problem with this approach is the increased work of breathing imposed by artificial airways, ventilator circuits, and demand valve systems.

Pressure support ventilation (PSV) is an adjunct to

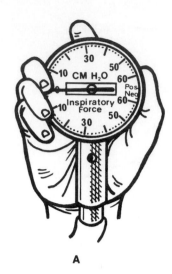
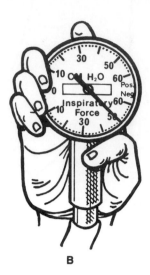

A   B

Fig. 29-8 An inspiratory pressure measurement. The gauge is attached to the patient's endotracheal tube, **A,** The patient is instructed to take in a deep breath while the clinician obstructs the airway by closing the open port on the gauge. **B,** The negative pressure deflection, measured here as − 50 cm H_2O, is the patient's inspiratory pressure. (From Pilbeam SP: Mechanical ventilation: physiological and clinical applications, St Louis, 1986, Mosby.)

ventilatory support or may be substituted for CMV or IMV in patients with respiratory muscle weakness.[41,71,72] Besides overcoming the imposed work of breathing, PSV may help recondition the respiratory muscles, thereby aiding weening from ventilatory support.[56,73-75]

Excessive work of breathing

Respiratory muscle weakness may be a primary cause of respiratory failure, as with atrophy. However, most respiratory muscle weakness is due to fatigue. Fatigue, in turn, is caused most often by an excessive work of breathing. Whether due to an increase in elastic or frictional load, patients with excessive work of breathing can develop both hypoventilation and $\dot{V}/\dot{Q}$ imbalances (due to inadequate lung expansion).

Bedside assessment. Clinically, a rapid rate of breathing is a cardinal sign of an high work of breathing. Sustained rates above 35 breaths/min in the adult usually indicate a need for ventilatory support. Other clinical signs of an increased work of breathing include tachycardia, a widened paradoxical pulse, diaphoresis (perspiration), a distressed facial expression, accessory muscle use, paradoxical rib cage/abdominal movements, and a positive Hoover's sign (inward motion of the lower rib cage during inspiration, suggesting hyperinflation).[76]

Overall workload is reflected in the minute volume ($\dot{V}E$), as compared to the $PaCO_2$ (see Table 29-3). In general, a $\dot{V}E$ of 10 L/min or less represents an acceptable ventilatory demand for most adult patients.

Minute volumes above 10 L/min are difficult for most adults to sustain, particularly if the process causing the acute episode continues for a period of days.

The $\dot{V}E$ needed to maintain **normocapnia** is determined by two factors: CO_2 production ($\dot{V}CO_2$), which reflects metabolic needs, and the dead space fraction (VD/VT), which indicates the efficiency of ventilation. An increase in either can produce excessive ventilatory demand for a given patient.

A VD/VT of 0.6 or greater is sometimes cited as an indication for ventilatory support. This criterion was first applied in patients with ARDS.[5] Of course, ARDS is characterized not only by increased VD/VT, but also by severe hypoxemia and poor lung expansion. It is thus uncertain whether the VD/VT ratio provides additional relevant information in these patients. Moreover, the fact that some stable COPD patients have VD/VT values greater than 0.6 support our emphasis on clinical judgment is deciding when to initiate ventilatory support.

Modes of ventilatory support. When increased work of breathing is due to poor lung expansion and decreased compliance, modes of ventilatory support which increase the FRC should be used. Generally, CMV with PEEP or IMV with PEEP are the strategies of choice. CPAP is contraindicated until the overall work of breathing can be decreased.

There is much less agreement on how to best ventilate patients in whom excessive work of breathing is due to increased resistance to air flow. When the problem is acute and patient-ventilator synchrony cannot be achieved (as in some cases of status asthmaticus), control mode CMV (with paralysis or sedation) may be needed.[66] Even when patient-ventilator synchrony is not a problem, many of these patients develop dynamic hyperinflation (auto-PEEP; intrinsic PEEP) and are at high risk for pulmonary barotrauma. Thus the issue of mode (usually CMV vs IMV) takes a back seat to the prevention of these potential complications. To decrease the likelihood of dynamic hyperinflation and barotrauma in these patients, the goal should be to provide the lowest minute volume that produces acceptable gas exchange and leads to the longest expiratory time.[66] In some cases, this may mean accepting an elevated $PaCO_2$, as long as the pH can be kept above 7.30.[77,78]

In either case, the RCP must remember that too narrow endotracheal tube can impose an additional burden on the ventilatory apparatus.[79] Especially when the $\dot{V}E$ is high, patients who can breathe comfortably through an 8 mm tube may be unable to do so through a 6 mm or 7 mm tube without ventilatory assistance. In this circumstance, PSV can help the patient overcome the added work associated with breathing through a small tube.

Unstable ventilatory drive

As shown in Table 29-3, there are no objective bedside indicators to confirm an unstable ventilatory drive. However, most patients at high risk can be identified in advance. These patients include those suffering from head injury, drug overdose, or cerebrovascular accident. In addition, patients whose neurological status is unstable or deteriorating, whose measured intracranial pressure (ICP) is increasing, or who have apneic episodes or irregular ventilatory patterns, fall into this category.

Modes of ventilatory support. At present, it is probably best to select a mode that provides full ventilatory support to these patients. Although this traditionally implies CMV, IMV with a base rate equal to that used with CMV is also satisfactory. For patients who stabilize after the first 24 hours and have no other reasons for mechanical ventilation, or in those with stable patterns of irregular breathing, such as Cheyne-Stokes respiration, mechanical ventilation is not indicated. Deliberate hyperventilation to diminish brain swelling is a separate indication that will be discussed later.

Severe hypoxemia

The sixth major physiologic problem for which ventilatory support may be needed is severe hypoxemia. As we have seen, hypoxemic respiratory failure is defined in terms of degree of hypoxemia.[8,9,80] Yet the relationship between ventilatory support and oxygenation is unclear in many patients.[52]

Bedside assessment. Table 29-2 lists four different measures of hypoxemia that have been used to assess the need for ventilatory support. Most of these relate degree of arterial hypoxemia against either the FIO_2 or PaO_2.

The most commonly used and accepted measure of the severity of hypoxemia is the alveolar–to–arterial oxygen tension gradient, or $P(A-a)O_2$. As described in Chapter 12, the alveolar PO_2 in the alveolar–to–arterial oxygen tension gradient is calculated using the alveolar air equation:

$$PAO_2 = FIO_2(PB - PH_2O) - \frac{PaCO_2}{R}$$

Unless the respiratory exchange ratio (R) is measured at the bedside with a metabolic cart, R is assumed to be 0.8. A $P(A-a)O_2$ of 350 torr or greater during breathing of 100% O_2 indicates severe hypoxemia. Patients with this high a $P(A-a)O_2$ usually (but not always) require some form of ventilatory support.

The degree of hypoxemia can also be judged using the arterial–to–alveolar PO_2 ratio (called the a/A ratio), or the PaO_2-to-FIO_2 (P/F) ratio. Using the latter, one finds that a patient with a PaO_2 of 80 torr breathing 40% O_2 would have a PaO_2/FIO_2 ratio of 200. This value is used by many as a threshold to indicate the need for ventilatory support with PEEP or CPAP.

The actual shunt fraction, or $\dot{Q}s/\dot{Q}T$, also is used to indicate the severity of hypoxemia in acute respiratory failure. Consensus as to what exact value (0.20, 0.25, or 0.30) should be used is undecided.

Modes of ventilatory support. Hypoxemia causing shunts as large as these can occur only in the presence of significant atelectasis. Thus the mode of ventilatory support chosen in these cases must be able to recruit, open and keep open collapsed alveoli.

CMV with PEEP or IMV with PEEP have been the mainstays of treatment used to correct this type of hypoxemia. More recently, several new and novel approaches to ventilatory support have been tried. These include high frequency ventilation, inverse ratio ventilation, and airway pressure release ventilation.[27,28,66] All aim to improve oxygenation while keeping mean airway pressures lower than with CMV.

Of course, the treatment of severe hypoxemia need not involve mechanical ventilation at all. Continuous positive airway pressure (CPAP) also can help lower shunting and improve oxygenation in selected patients.[55] Unfortunately, patients with severe hypoxemia often have other problems, such as alveolar hypoventilation, or respiratory muscle fatigue. In these situations, CPAP is contraindicated.

Prophylactic (preventive) ventilatory support

In addition to the six general indications listed in Table 29-3, some suggest that ventilatory support should be considered whenever one or more of these problems might develop. This approach is based on the premise that instituting ventilatory support prior to a problem's development can prevent its bad effects. Unfortunately, little substantiating information currently exists to justify prophylactic use of ventilatory support.

The most obvious potential use of prophylactic mechanical ventilation is in the immediate post-operative period. We know that immediately after some type of surgery (particularly upper abdominal procedures), vital capacity may fall to one third or less than normal. We also know that hypoxemia, atelectasis, and pneumonia are frequent complications in the postoperative period (see Chapter 20). Together, these factors suggest that mechanical ventilation could be used to maintain adequate alveolar expansion and thus prevent these problems from occurring.

Despite the logic of this approach, studies of prophylactic mechanical ventilation in the post-op setting have failed to show any significant benefit.[81] Given its many hazards and complications,[82-85] clinicians should be cautious in applying ventilatory support unless the need is well documented.

Special uses for ventilatory support

The literature contains many descriptions of various modes of ventilatory support in diverse clinical situations. Among those most often cited are closed head injuries, flail chest, obstructive lung disease, and sleep apnea.

Closed head injury

A separate indication for mechanical ventilation is to deliberately hyperventilate patients with closed head injuries. Only patients with elevated **ICPs** should be considered for this approach.[66] The goal is usually to lower the $PaCO_2$ to between 25 and 30 torr.[86,87] Because hypocapnia and alkalosis both help reduce cerebral blood flow, hyperventilation (using control mode CMV) can reduce brain swelling and intracranial pressure (ICP) in these patients.

Generally, the clinical benefits of hyperventilation diminish after a day or two. This is because the brain's acid-base balance gradually returns to normal, even in the presence of peripheral alkalosis. For this reason, patients' $PaCO_2$s should gradually be restored to normal over 24 to 48 hours.[66]

Flail chest

Traumatic flail chest is another specific condition that has been cited as an indication for mechanical ventilation.[88]

Flail chest traditionally has been defined as a condition in which three or more ribs are broken in two or more locations. The result is an unstable or flailing chest wall that often moves paradoxically with breathing efforts. Significant impairment of gas exchange can occur, particularly of oxygenation. In concept, mechanical ventilation can help stabilize the flail segment, thereby improving gas exchange and aiding healing of the bones.

Over the last 30 years, an increasing body of evidence suggests that most patients with flail chest do *not* require mechanical ventilation. Several studies have found that such patients can be managed in much the same way as trauma patients in general.[89-92] This is consistent with the notion that it is not the flail segment but the associated lung contusion, aspiration of gastric contents, and other injuries that determine the course of illness. In the absence of other indications, only rarely is the disruption of thoracic integrity itself severe enough to require ventilatory support.[93,94]

Obstructive lung disease

For acute **exacerbations** of asthma and COPD, most clinicians take a more conservative approach to mechanical ventilation. There are two main reasons for this. First, patients with severe obstructive diseases are especially prone to complications of mechanical ventilation, and to difficult weaning once the acute episode resolves. Second, and more important, is the fact that early, aggressive intervention with more conservative therapy can avoid the need for mechanical ventilation in many of these patients.

While mild to moderate acute respiratory alkalosis is the rule in acute asthma attacks, a $PaCO_2$ value rising to or above normal despite treatment is regarded as an ominous sign,[95] even if usual criteria for hypercapnic respiratory failure (e.g., $PCO_2 > 50$, pH < 7.30) have not yet been met. In the past, mechanical ventilation has often been initiated in such cases. This approach was based on the notion that progression to life-threatening respiratory acidosis was predictable once the $PaCO_2$ began to climb.

Clinical studies tend to refute this conventional wisdom. Hypercapnia does indicate the severity of an asthma attack. However, intubation and mechanical ventilation can be avoided in many patients, even when the $PaCO_2$ climbs to 60 torr or higher.[96]

The key is whether the patient remains alert and cooperative during therapy.[97-99] If the patient becomes lethargic or looses consciousness, or if severe dyspnea persists, the rate of breathing stays excessively high (> 40 breaths/min), or signs of fatigue become apparent (such as the use of accessory muscles), mechanical support may be warranted.[100]

Acute respiratory failure occurring during an exacerbation of COPD is usually reversible through aggressive application of the same modes of therapy used in long-term management.[52,101,102] A combination of judicious oxygen therapy, bronchodilator administration, corticosteroids, respiratory stimulants, appropriate antibiotics, and vigorous bronchial hygiene measures can enable the clinician to avoid mechanical ventilation in most instances.[102,103] As in status asthmaticus, the main indications for intubation are uncontrollable, progressive respiratory acidosis despite vigorous therapy, in combination with an altered mental status. The latter may consist either of stupor or of uncontrollable agitation that makes sedation mandatory and renders adequate nursing and respiratory therapy care impossible.

Recently, the use of NIPPV has been advocated to avoid having to intubate patients with acute-on-chronic respiratory failure. Since it is well known that once intubated and ventilated, these patients are difficult to wean from mechanical ventilation, this alternative has been well received.

In several studies, the majority of patients with ventilatory failure and/or severe hypoxemia have been successfully ventilated using either simple PSV or bi-level PSV (BiPAP®) by mask.[42-44,104] These studies indicate that in selected patients with obstructive lung disease, NIPPV can restore pH and $PaCO_2$ to acceptable levels without the need for intubation. Moreover, patient comfort is high and complications are low. NIPPV is also being used in obstructive and central sleep apneas (see below).

Sleep apnea

Sleep apnea is a general term pertaining to episodic cessation of breathing during sleep (see Chapter 20). Since brief periods of apnea are normal during sleep, the sleep apnea syndrome is strictly defined as the occurrence of five or more apneic periods per hour, each lasting at least 10 seconds. Moreover, these episodes must result in clinically perceptible signs or symptoms, such as polycythemia or day-time **hypersomnolence.**[8]

Currently, there are two recognized forms of the sleep apnea syndrome: central sleep apnea and obstructive sleep apnea. As the name implies, central sleep apnea is most likely due to a defect in the central nervous system's respiratory control mechanism. Typically, patients with central sleep apnea do not make efforts to breath during the apneic periods. Patients with the central sleep apnea syndrome may be of any age, weight or sex. Increasingly, NIPPV is being used to provide ventilatory support for patients with central sleep apnea.[105,106]

Obstructive sleep apnea, on the other hand, is characterized by occlusion of the oropharynx, accompanied by continuing efforts to breathe. Obstructive sleep apnea is associated with a number of well defined factors, with obesity in men being the most common finding (see the accompanying box).

Until recently, treatment for moderately severe sleep apnea syndrome was limited to weight reduction for obesity, the use of respiratory stimulants, or mechanical devices, such as tongue retainers. Sleep apnea not responsive to these methods was sometimes treated surgically with either tracheostomy or **uvulopalatopharyngoplasty,** a procedure involving shortening of the soft palate, and removal of the uvula and tonsils.

Factors that increase risk for obstructive sleep apnea
Obesity (particularly in men)
Alcohol (only in men and when consumed before bedtime)
Irregular work shift (eg, night shift)
COPD
Large tonsils
Craniofacial deformities (eg, acromegaly)
Enlarged tongue
Hypothyroidism
Chest wall deformities
Tranquilizers (particularly when added to any other risk factor)

From Martin L: Pulmonary physiology in clinical practice, St Louis, 1987, Mosby.

Over the last decade, continuous positive airway pressure (CPAP) has emerged as an alternative treatment for obstructive sleep apnea. As depicted in Figure 29-9, the continuous positive airway pressure, usually administered via a nasal device, distends the oropharynx, thereby preventing occlusion by the tongue and soft palate.[107]

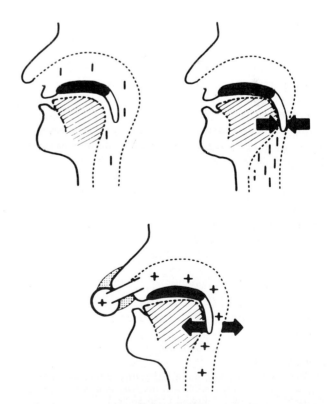

Fig. 29-9 Nasal constant positive airway pressure for obstructive sleep apnea. The positive airway pressure can prevent pharyngeal collapse *(arrows)*.

Comparative studies indicate that CPAP is the most successful, least hazardous, and best tolerated of all sleep apnea treatments.[108] BiPAP® is also effective in OSA in that it may allow for a decrease in the CPAP level if a high CPAP level is not tolerated.[109]

CPAP also has been used with success in central sleep apnea disorders.[110,111] Exactly why CPAP should be effective in this type of sleep apnea is not entirely clear. However, recent research suggests that upper airway collapse may also play a role in central sleep apnea. Specifically, central sleep apnea may be due, in part, to a reflex inhibition of respiration caused by activation of the supraglottic mucosal receptors during upper airway closure.[111]

CHAPTER SUMMARY

Although simple in concept, respiratory failure is a complex clinical phenomenon. The best way to comprehend respiratory failure is to understand the various patterns of underlying pathophysiology.

Numerous measures exist to help quantify the nature and severity of respiratory failure. However, these criteria cannot and should not substitute for sound bedside judgment.

Sound bedside judgment should be based on assessment of the patient's baseline status, the severity of pre-existent lung disease (or the presence of related chronic cardiovascular problems), and the nature of the acute episode itself.

Based on these considerations, one would probably try to avoid ventilatory support of a patient with an acute asthma attack who could be expected to improve within hours. However, in the face of severe chest trauma or progressive neuromuscular disease, the need to begin ventilatory support is more apparent. In any case, the hazards of mechanical ventilation must be weighed against the expected benefits for each person.

Were clinical judgment based solely on a list of numbers, every patient would be treated the same. To avoid this formula approach, most good clinicians shun strict numeric criteria. Instead, they emphasize the importance of serial observations and the patient's medical history in deciding whether to apply ventilatory support.[12] Nonetheless, objective measures can provide a physiological framework for the application of sound clinical judgment to this fundamental aspect of respiratory care.

REFERENCES

1. Bryan CL: Classification of respiratory failure. In Kirby RR, Smith RA, Desautels DD, editors: *Mechanical ventilation,* New York, 1985, Churchill Livingstone.
2. Shapiro BA, Harrison RA, Walton JR: *Clinical Application of Blood Gases,* ed 3, St Louis, 1982, Mosby.
3. Campbell EJM: Respiratory failure, *Br Med J* 1:1451, 1965.
4. Petty TL: Acute respiratory failure. In Petty TL editor: *Intensive and Rehabilitative Respiratory Care,* Philadelphia, 1982, Lea & Febiger.
5. Pontoppidan H, Geffin B, Lowenstein E: *Acute respiratory failure in the adult,* Boston, 1973, Little, Brown.
6. Martin L: Respiratory failure, *Med Clin North Am* 61:1369, 1977.
7. Balk R, Bone RC: Classification of acute respiratory failure, *Med Clin North Am* 67:551, 1983.
8. Martin L: *Pulmonary physiology in clinical practice, the essentials for patient care and evaluation,* St Louis, 1987, Mosby.
9. Bone RC: Acute respiratory failure: Classification, differential diagnosis, and introduction to management. In Burton GG, Hodgkin JE editors: *Respiratory Care: A Guide to Clinical Practice,* ed 2, Philadelphia, 1984, JB Lippincott.
10. Demling RH, Nerlich M: Acute respiratory failure, *Surg Clin North Am* 63:337, 1983.
11. Demers RR, Irwin RS: Management of hypercapnic respiratory failure: a systemic approach, *Respir Care* 24:328–335, 1979.
12. Schmidt GA, Hall JB: Acute on chronic respiratory failure, *JAMA* 261:3444–3453, 1989.
13. Shapiro BA, Harrison RA, Trout CA: *Clinical applications of respiratory care,* ed 3, St Louis, 1985, Mosby.
14. Suter PM: Cardiopulmonary interactions in acute respiratory failure, Update in intensive care and emergency medicine series, vol 2, New York, 1987, Springer-Verlag.
15. Lake KB: Adult respiratory distress syndrome (high permeability pulmonary edema). In Burton GG, Hodgkin JE editors: *Respiratory Care: a guide to clinical practice,* ed 2, Philadelphia, 1984, JB Lippincott.
16. Meyrick B: Pathology of the adult respiratory distress syndrome, *Crit Care Clin* 2(3):405–28, 1986.
17. Shale DJ: The adult respiratory distress syndrome—20 years on, *Thorax* 42:641–645, 1987.
18. Biondi JW, Hines RL, Barash PG, et al: The adult respiratory distress syndrome, *Yale J Biol Med* 59:575–597, 1986.
19. Brandstetter RD: The adult respiratory distress syndrome—1986, *Heart & Lung* 15:155–164, 1986.
20. Bernard GR, Brigham KL: The adult respiratory distress syndrome, *Annu Rev Med* 36:195–205, 1985.
21. Fein A, Wiener-Kronish JP, Niederman M, Matthay MA: Pathophysiology of the adult respiratory distress syndrome. What have we learned from human studies?, *Crit Care Clin* 2(3):429–453, 1986.
22. Mason RJ: Surfactant in adult respiratory distress syndrome, *Eur J Respir Dis* 153(suppl.):229–236, 1987.
23. Hallman M, Maasilta P, Sipila I, Tahvanainen J: Composition and function of pulmonary surfactant in adult respiratory distress syndrome, *Eur Respir J Suppl* 3:104s–108, 1989.
24. Holm BA, Matalon S: Role of pulmonary surfactant in the development and treatment of adult respiratory distress syndrome, *Anesth Analg* 69(6):805–18, 1989.
25. Seeger W, Pison U, Buchhorn R, et al: Surfactant abnormalities and adult respiratory failure, *Lung* 168(suppl.):891–902, 1990.
26. Marini JJ: Lung mechanics in the adult respiratory distress syndrome, Recent conceptual advances and implications for management, *Clin Chest Med* 11(4):673–90, 1990.
27. MacIntyre NR: New forms of mechanical ventilation in the adult, *Clin Chest Med* 9(1):47–54, 1988.
28. Stoller JK, Kacmarek RM: Ventilatory strategies in the management of the adult respiratory distress syndrome, *Clin Chest Med* 11(4):755–772, 1990.
29. Schuster DP: A physiologic approach to initiating, maintaining, and withdrawing mechanical ventilatory support during acute respiratory failure, *Am J Med* 88(3):268–78, 1990.
30. Hinson JR, Marini JJ: Principles of mechanical ventilator use in respiratory failure, *Annu Rev Med* 43:341–61, 1992.

31. Husdon LD: Pharmacologic approaches to respiratory failure, *Respir Care* 38(7):754–764, 1993.

32. DalNogare AR: Southwest Internal Medicine Conference: Adult respiratory Distress Syndrome, *Am J Med Sci* 298(6):413–430, 1989.

33. Hechtman HB, Valeri CR, Shepro D: Role of humoral mediators in adult respiratory distress syndrome, *Chest* 86:623–627, 1984.

34. Goldstein G, Luce JM: Pharmacologic treatment of the adult respiratory distress syndrome, *Clin Chest Med* 11(4):773–787, 1990.

35. Holm BA, Matalon S: Role of pulmonary surfactant in the development and treatment of adult respiratory distress syndrome, *Anesth Analg* 69:805–818, 1989.

35. Wiedemann H, Baughmann R, deBoisblanc B, et al: A multicenter trial in human sepsis induced ARDS of an aerosolized synthetic surfactant (Exosurf), *Am Rev Respir Dis* 145:184, 1992.

36. Weg J, Reines H, Balk R, et al: Safety and efficacy of an aerosolized surfactant (Exosurf), in human sepsis induced ARDS, *Chest* 100:137S, 1991.

37. Richman PS, Spragg RG, Merritt TA, et al: Administration of porcine-lung surfactant to humans with ARDS: Initial experience (abstract), *Am Rev Respir Dis* S135:A5, 1987.

38. Lewis JF, Jobe AH: Surfactant and the adult respiratory distress syndrome, *Am Rev Respir Dis* 147:218–233, 1993.

39. Pulmonary terms and symbols: A report of the ACCP-ATS Joint Committee on Pulmonary Nomenclature, *Chest* 67:583, 1975.

40. American Association for Respiratory Care: Consensus conference on the essentials of mechanical ventilators, *Respir Care* 37:999–1130, 1992.

41. Kacmarek RM: the role of pressure support ventilation in reducing the work of breathing, *Respir Care* 33:99–120, 1988.

42. Wysocki M, Tric L, Wolff M, et al: Noninvasive pressure support ventilation in patients with acute respiratory failure, *Chest* 103:907–913, 1993.

43. Pennock BE, Crawshaw L, Kaplan PD, et al: Additional experience with BiPAP/nasal mask in patients with acute respiratory failure, *Am Rev Respir Dis* 145:, 1992.

44. Meduri GU, Conoscenti CC, Menashe P, Nair S: Noninvasive face mask ventilation in patients with acute respiratory failure, *Chest* 95:865–870, 1989.

45. Pierce AK: Acute respiratory failure. In Guenter CA and Welch MH (editors): *Pulmonary medicine* Philadelphia, 1982, JB Lippincott.

46. Mclees BD: Critical care medicine, in Wyngaarden, Smith LH, Jr, editors: *Cecil's textbook of medicine,* ed 16, Philadelphia, 1982, WB Saunders.

47. Geer RT: Mechanical ventilation. In Fishman, AP, editor: *Pulmonary diseases and disorders,* New York, 1980, McGraw-Hill.

48. Jay SJ: Acute respiratory failure. In Stein JH, editor: *Internal medicine,* Boston, 1983, Little, Brown.

49. Caprio GS, Riley MA: The mechanically ventilated patient. In Morrison ML editor: *Respiratory intensive care nursing,* ed 2, Boston, 1979, Little, Brown.

50. Stauffer JL: Establishment and care of the airway. In Petty TL editor: *Intensive and rehabilitative respiratory care,* ed 2, Philadelphia, 1982, Lea & Febiger.

51. Peters RM: Work of breathing and abnormal mechanics, *Surg Clin N Am* 54:955–966, 1974.

52. Pierson DJ: Acute respiratory failure. In Sahn SA, editor: *Pulmonary emergencies,* New York, 1982, Churchill-Livingstone.

53. Zwillich CW, Pierson DJ, Creagh CE, et al: Complications of assisted ventilation, *Am J Med* 57:161–169, 1974.

54. West JB: Causes of carbon dioxide retention in lung disease, *N Engl J Med* 284:1232, 1971.

55. Downs JB: Ventilatory patterns and modes of ventilation in acute respiratory failure, *Respir Care* 28:586–591, 1983.

56. Marini JJ, Capps JS, Culver, BH: The inspiratory work of breathing during assisted mechanical ventilation, *Chest* 87:612–618, 1985.

57. Marini JJ, Rodgiguez, RM, Lamb V: The inspiratory workload of patient-initiated mechanical ventilation, *Am Rev Respir Dis* 134:902–909, 1986.

58. Bendixen HH, Bullwinkel B, Hedley-White J, Laver MB: Atelectasis and shunting during spontaneous ventilation in anesthetized patients, *Anesthesiology* 25:297–301, 1964.

59. Egbert LD, Laver MB, Bendixen HH: Intermittent deep breaths and compliance during anesthesia in man, *Anesthesiology* 24:57–60, 1963.

60. Bendixen HH, Hedley-White J, Laver MB: Impaired oxygenation in surgical patients during general anesthesia with controlled ventilation: a concept of atelectasis, *N Engl J Med* 269:991–996, 1963.

61. Sykes MK, Young WE, Robinson BE: Oxygenation during anesthesia with controlled ventilation, *Br J Anaesth* 37:314–325, 1965.

62. Visick WD, Fairley HB, Hickey RF: The effects of tidal volume and end-expiratory pressure on pulmonary gas exchange during anesthesia, *Anesthesiology* 39:285–290, 1973.

63. Ruiz BC, Calderwood HW, Modell JH, Brogdon JE: Effect of ventilatory patterns on arterial oxygenation after near-drowning with fresh water: a comparative study in dogs, *Anesth Analg* 52:570–576, 1973.

64. Modell JH, Calderwood HW, Ruiz BC, et al: Effects of ventilatory patterns on arterial oxygenation after near-drowning is sea water, *Anesthesiology* 40:376–384, 1974.

65. Parker JC, Hernandez LA, Peevy KJ: Mechanisms of ventilator-induced lung injury, *Crit Care Med* 21:131–143, 1993.

66. American College of Chest Physicians: ACCP consensus conference—mechanical ventilation, *Chest* 104:183–1859, 1993.

67. Macklem PT: Respiratory muscle dysfunction, *Hosp Pract* 21(3):83–90, 95–96, 1986.

68. Black LF, Hyatt RE: Maximal static respiratory pressures in generalized neuromuscular disease, *Am Rev Respir Dis* 103:641–647, 1971.

69. Sahn SA, Lakshminarayan S: Bedside criteria for discontinuation of mechanical ventilation, *Chest* 63:1002–1005, 1973.

70. Pierson DJ: Weaning from mechanical ventilation in acute respiratory failure: concepts, indications, and techniques, *Respir Care* 28:646–660, 1983.

71. Brochard L, Pluskwa F, Lemaire F: Improved efficacy of spontaneous breathing with inspiratory pressure support, *Am Rev Respir Dis* 136:411–415, 1987.

72. MacIntyre NR: Respiratory function during pressure support ventilation, *Chest* 89:677–683, 1986.

73. Fiastro JF, Quan BF, Habib MP: Pressure support compensation for inspiratory work due to endotracheal tubes and demand CPAP (abstract), *Chest* 89:441S, 1986.

74. MacIntyre NR: Weaning from mechanical ventilatory support: volume assisting intermittent breaths versus pressure assisting every breath, *Respir Care* 33:121–125, 1988.

75. Brochard L, Pluskwa F, Lemaire F: Pressure support (PS) of spontaneous breathing (SB) assists weaning from mechanical ventilation (abstract), *Am Rev Respir Dis* 134:A122, 1986.

76. Schuster DP: A physiologic approach to initiating, maintaining, and withdrawing mechanical ventilatory support during acute respiratory failure, *Am J Med* 88:268–278, 1990.

77. Darioli R, Perret C: Mechanical controlled hypoventilation in status asthmaticus, *Am Rev Respir Dis* 129:385–387, 2984.

78. Kacmarek RM, Hickling KG: Permissive hypercapnia, *Respir Care* 38:373–387, 1993.

79. Sahn SA, Lakshminarayan S, Petty TL: Weaning from mechanical ventilation, *JAMA* 235:2208–2212, 1976.

80. Murray JF: Pathophysiology of acute respiratory failure, *Respir Care* 28:531–540, 1983.

81. Shackford SR, Virgilio RW, Peters RM: Early extubation versus prophylactic ventilation in the high risk patient: a comparison of postoperative management in the prevention of respiratory complications, *Anesth Analg* 60:76–80, 1981.

82. Zwillich CW, Pierson DJ, Creagh CE, et al: Complications

of assisted ventilation: A prospective study of 354 consecutive episodes, *Am J Med* 57:161–169, 1974.

83. Stauffer JL, Olson DE, Petty TL: Complications and consequences of endotracheal intubation and tracheotomy, A prospective study of 150 critically ill adult patients, *Am J Med* 70:65–76, 1981.

84. Johanson W.G: Infectious complications of respiratory therapy, *Respir Care* 27:445, 1982.

85. Bone RC: Complications of mechanical ventilation and positive-end expiratory pressure, *Respir Care* 27:402–407, 1982.

86. Crockard HA, Coppel DL, Morrow WFK: Evaluation of hyperventilation in treatment of head injuries, *Br Med J* 4:634–640, 1973.

87. Becker DP, Miller JD, Ward JD, et al: The outcome from severe head injury with early diagnosis and intensive management, *J Neurosurg* 47:491–502, 1977.

88. Avery EE, Morch ET, Benson DW: Critically crushed chests: A new method of treatment with continuous mechanical hyperventilation to produce alkalotic apnea and internal pneumatic stabilization, *J Thorac Surg* 32:291–311, 1956.

89. Cullen P, Modell JH, Kirby RR, et al: Treatment of flail chest: use of intermittent mandatory pressure and positive end-expiratory pressure, *Arch Surg* 110:1099–1103, 1975.

90. Trinkle JK, Richardson JD, Franz JL, et al: Management of flail chest without mechanical ventilation, *Ann Thorac Surg* 19:355–363, 1975.

91. Shackford SR, Smith DE, Zarins CK, et al: The management of flail chest: a comparison of ventilatory and nonventilatory treatment, *Am J Surg* 132:759–762, 1976.

92. Shackford SR, Virgilio RW, Peters RM: Selective use of ventilator therapy in flail chest injury, *J Thorac Cardiovasc Surg* 81:194–201, 1981.

93. Parham AM, Yarbrough DR, Redding JS: Flail chest syndrome and pulmonary contusion, *Arch Surg* 113:900–903, 1978.

94. Management of the stove-in chest with paradoxical movement, *Br Med J* 2:1242, 1977.

95. Rebuck AS, Read J: Assessment and management of severe asthma, *Am J Med* 51:788–798, 1971.

96. Bondi E, Williams MH, Jr: Severe asthma: course and treatment in the hospital, *NY State J Med* 77:350–353, 1977.

97. Williams MH Jr.: Life-threatening asthma, *Arch Intern Med* 140:1604–1604, 1980.

98. Fish JE, Summer WR: Acute lower airway obstruction: asthma. In Moser KM, Spragg RG editors.: *Respiratory emergencies,* ed 2, St Louis, 1982, Mosby.

99. Scoggin CH: Acute asthma and status asthmaticus. In Sahn, SA editor: *Pulmonary emergencies,* New York, 1982, Churchill-Livingstone.

100. Hagedorn SD: Acute exacerbations of COPD, *Postgrad Med* 91:105–112, 1992.

101. Light, RW: Conservative treatment of hypercapnic acute respiratory failure, *Respir Care* 28:561–566, 1983.

102. Martin TR, Lewis SW, Albert, RK: The prognosis of patients with chronic obstructive pulmonary disease after hospitalization for acute respiratory failure, *Chest* 82:310–314, 1982.

103. Hudson LD, Pierson DJ: Comprehensive respiratory care for patients with chronic obstructive pulmonary disease, *Med Clin North Am* 65:629–645, 1981.

104. Brochard L, Isabey D, Piquet J, et al: Reversal of acute exacerbations of chronic obstructive lung disease by inspiratory assistance with a face mask, *N Engl J Med* 323:1523–1530, 1990.

105. Restrick LJ, Fox NC, Braid G, et al: Comparison of nasal pressure support ventilation with nasal intermittent positive pressure ventilation in patients with nocturnal hypoventilation, *Eur Respir J* 6(3):364–370, 1993.

106. Guilleminault C, Stoohs R, Schneider H, et al: Central alveolar hypoventilation and sleep. Treatment by intermittent positive pressure ventilation through nasal mask in an adult, *Chest* 96(5):1210–1212, 1989.

107. Sullivan CE, Berthon-Jones M, Issa FG, et al: Reversal of obstructive sleep apnea by continuous positive airway pressure applied through the nares, *Lancet* 1:862, 1981.

108. Katsantonis GP, Schweitzer PK, Branham GH, et al: Management of obstructive sleep apnea: comparison of various treatment modalities, *Laryngoscope* 98:304–309, 1988.

109. Sanders MH, Kern N: Obstructive sleep apnea treated by independently adjusted inspiratory and expiratory positive airway pressures via nasal mask. Physiologic and clinical implications, *Chest* 98(2):317–324, 1990.

110. Hoffstein V, Slutsky AS: Central sleep apnea reversed by continuous positive airway pressure, *Am Rev Respir Dis* 135:1210–1212, 1987.

111. Issa FG, Sullivan CE: Reversal of central sleep apnea using nasal CPAP, *Chest* 90:165–171, 1986.

Physics and Physiology of Ventilatory Support

■

Craig L. Scanlan

Christina Blazer

No aspect of respiratory care is as challenging, or as potentially rewarding, as the successful application of ventilatory support to patients in respiratory failure. As with all respiratory care interventions, the success of ventilatory support depends first and foremost on the respiratory care practitioner's (RCP) understanding of both its underlying principles and physiologic effects.

PHYSIOLOGIC BASIS OF VENTILATORY SUPPORT

All modes of ventilatory support inflate the lungs by increasing the transpulmonary pressure gradient (PL). As detailed in Chapter 11, PL is the difference between the alveolar pressure, Palv, and the pleural pressure, Ppl:

$$P_L = Palv - Ppl$$

With all else constant, alveolar inflation volume is directly proportional to PL.

As shown in Figure 30-1, page 826, PL can be increased by either decreasing pleural pressure (Figure 30-1, A), or increasing alveolar pressure (Figure 30-1, B). A spontaneous inspiration increases PL by decreasing pleural pressure. Negative pressure ventilation exerts a similar effect by decreasing the pressure around the chest wall during inspiration. On the other hand, positive pressure ventilation increases PL by raising the alveolar pressure during inspiration.[1]

A third type of ventilatory support, called continuous positive airway pressure, or CPAP, keeps alveolar pressures elevated *throughout* both inspiration and expiration. Since CPAP keeps airway pressure constant throughout breathing, gas flow in and out of the lung depends on *spontaneously* generated changes in pleural pressure, just like normal breathing.

Negative pressure ventilation (NPV)

In concept, negative pressure ventilation (NPV) is similar to spontaneous breathing. During spontaneous inspiration, muscle contraction expands the thorax, which, in turn, decreases pleural pressure. This drop in pressure is transmitted to the alveoli, creating a transrespiratory pressure gradient (Prs). Prs is the difference between the pressure at the airway opening (Pao) and the alveolar pressure (Palv):

$$Prs = Pao\ (0) - Palv\ (negative)$$

The change in alveolar volume during spontaneous inspiration is proportional to the size of the transpulmonary pressure gradient (PL):

$$Alveolar\ expansion \approx P_L\ (end\ inspiration)$$
$$\approx Palv - Ppl$$

During spontaneous ventilation, the inspiratory drop in pleural pressure is due to active muscle contraction. NPV decreases pleural pressure during inspiration by exposing the chest to subatmospheric pressure. This negative pressure at the body surface

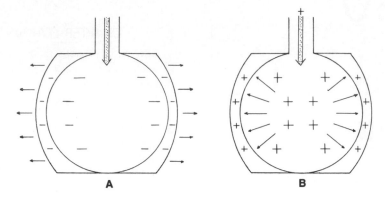

Fig. 30-1 Diagrammatic illustration of the difference between inspiratory forces of, **A,** negative pressure and, **B,** positive pressure ventilation.

(Pbs) is transmitted first to the pleural space and then to the alveoli:

$$\downarrow \text{Pbs} \rightarrow \downarrow \text{Ppl} \rightarrow \downarrow \text{Palv}$$

Since the airway remains exposed to atmospheric pressure during NPV (Pao = 0), a Prs like that generated during spontaneous inspiration is created. Thus, gas flows from the relatively high pressure at the airway opening (zero) to the relatively low pressure in the alveoli (negative). As with spontaneous breathing, alveolar expansion during NPV is determined by the size of the transpulmonary pressure gradient.

During expiration in *both* spontaneous breathing and NPV, the lungs and chest wall passively recoil back to their resting end-expiratory levels. As this occurs, pleural pressure becomes less negative, and alveolar pressure rises above atmospheric. This reverses the transrespiratory pressure gradient. As Palv becomes greater than Pao, gas flows from the alveoli out to the airway opening.

Positive pressure ventilation (PPV)

As depicted in Figure 30-2, *PPV reverses the pressure gradients seen during spontaneous breathing.* Gas flows into the lungs because pressure at the airway opening is positive, while alveolar pressure remains at zero:

$$\text{Prs} = \text{Pao (positive)} - \text{Palv (0)}$$

As during spontaneous breathing, gas flows from the airway opening into the alveoli. However, alveolar pressure *rises* during PPV. This rise in Palv expands the alveoli. As compared to spontaneous inspiration or NPV, however, the pressure gradient is reversed. Because Palv is greater than Ppl during PPV, positive pressure is transmitted from the alveoli to the pleural space, causing pleural pressure to rise during inspiration. Depending on the lung's mechanical properties, pleural pressure may actually exceed atmospheric pressure during a portion of inspiration.

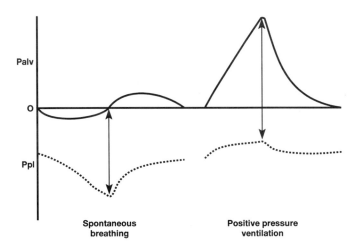

Fig. 30-2 Pressure gradients during spontaneous breathing (left) and positive pressure ventilation, or PPV (right). As during spontaneous breathing, gas flows from the airway opening into the alveoli. However, alveolar pressure rises during PPV. This rise in Palv expands the alveoli. As compared to spontaneous breathing, however, the pressure gradient is reversed. Because Palv is greater than Ppl during PPV, positive pressure is transmitted from the alveoli to the pleural space, causing pleural pressure to rise during inspiration.

As with spontaneous breathing, the recoil force of the lung and chest wall, stored as potential energy during the positive pressure breath, causes a passive exhalation. As gas flows from the alveoli out to the airway opening, alveolar pressure drops to atmospheric level, while pleural pressure is restored to its normal subatmospheric range.

Continuous positive airway pressure (CPAP)

Like NPV and PPV, CPAP increases PL and causes alveolar expansion. However, unlike both NPV and PPV, airway pressure with CPAP is basically constant throughout breathing (Figure 30-3). Since airway pressure does not change, CPAP does not provide ventilation. In order for gas to move into the lungs during CPAP, the patient must spontaneously create

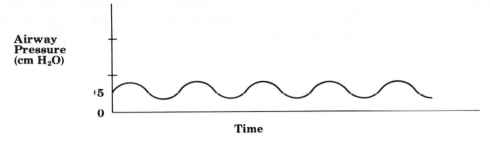

Fig. 30-3 CPAP. (From Pilbeam SP: Mechanical ventilation: physiological and clinical applications, St Louis, 1986, Mosby.)

a transrespiratory pressure gradient. Thus, while NPV and PPV create the pressure gradients needed for gas flow into the lungs, CPAP only maintains alveoli at greater inflation volumes.

As we shall see, CPAP can be combined with PPV. In this approach, airway pressure is kept positive throughout both inspiration and expiration, as with CPAP. However, during inspiration, additional positive pressure is applied to the airway, above the CPAP level (Figure 30-4).

During the expiratory phase, airway pressure is allowed to return to the CPAP level. Because positive airway pressure is maintained during expiration, this approach is commonly called CMV with positive end-expiratory pressure, or CMV with PEEP.

Because PPV is the most common ventilatory support strategy in current use, we will emphasize the physical principles and physiologic effects underlying this approach.

PHYSICAL PRINCIPLES OF POSITIVE PRESSURE VENTILATION

The physical principles underlying PPV are best understood using an orderly framework of analysis. Given the broad diversity of ventilatory support modes that have evolved over the last 20 years, developing such a system is no small task. Fortunately, Chatburn recently developed just such a framework.[2] His system is based on the systematic

description of breath types and control, phase, and conditional variables.

Breath types and support level

Most modern ventilators can provide two major types of breaths: spontaneous or mandatory. A *spontaneous breath* is initiated *and* ended by the patient. Any breath either initiated *or* terminated by the ventilator is called a *mandatory breath*. "Patient breath" is a common synonym for a spontaneous breath, while the term "machine breath" is equivalent to a mandatory breath.

When all breaths received by the patient are mandatory, we are providing *full* ventilatory support, or continuous mandatory ventilation (CMV). If only some breaths are mandatory, while the rest are spontaneous, the level of ventilatory support is considered *partial*. Partial ventilatory support is also called intermittent mandatory ventilation, or IMV.

Control variables

A control variable is a physical parameter that can be manipulated by a ventilator. As detailed in Chapter 31, a ventilator can have control over either pressure, volume, flow, or time. In general, only one of these variables can be controlled at any given instant.

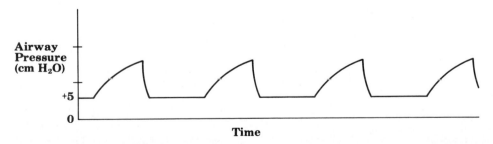

Fig. 30-4 CPAP combined with CMV (CMV with PEEP). (From Pilbeam SP: Mechanical ventilation: physiological and clinical applications, St Louis, 1986, Mosby.)

Phase variables

Any breath, whether spontaneous or mandatory, can be described in detail by answering four simple questions (see accompanying box).[3]

The variable causing a breath to begin is the *trigger variable*. To describe what happens during inspiration, we must know whether the breath is pressure or flow-generated, and what *limit variable* is in effect. The variable causing a breath to end is the *cycle variable*. To describe what happens during expiration, we must know what *baseline variable* is in effect.

Trigger variable

On most modern adult ventilators, either the machine or patient can initiate a breath. If the machine initiates the breath, the trigger variable is usually time. If the patient initiates the breath, pressure, flow, or volume may serve as the trigger variable.[4] Manual or operator-initiated triggering is also available on most ventilators.

Time triggering. When triggering by time, a ventilator initiates a breath according to a predetermined time interval, without regard to patient effort.[5,6] Time triggering is often called *controlled ventilation.*

Controlled ventilation places essentially all ventilatory parameters in the hands of the clinician. For this reason, controlled ventilation is the only strategy that can provide precise and consistently predictable physiologic results. However, controlled ventilation is poorly tolerated by most conscious patients, often requiring sedation or paralysis to be successful.

Specific systems for setting a controlled breathing rate vary from ventilator to ventilator.[5,7] The most common approach is via a rate control that divides each minute into equal time segments, allotting one time segment for each full breath. When a rate control is used, inspiratory and expiratory times will vary according to other control settings, such as flow and volume. An alternative approach is to provide separate timers for inspiration and expiration. Changing either or both of these timers will alter the breathing rate. Last, on some ventilators, the clinician sets an expiratory time only, with the inspiratory time and rate determined by other parameters, such as flow and volume.

Ventilatory support phase variables[3]

To describe a spontaneous or mandatory breath, one breaks the breath down into its four phases, and answers the following questions:
1. What causes the breath to begin?
2. What happens during inspiration?
3. What causes the breath to end?
4. What occurs during expiration?

Patient triggering. With patient triggering, the patient's inspiratory effort triggers the ventilator to begin inspiration. To do so, the ventilator must "sense" the patient's effort. This is done by measuring either pressure, flow or volume.

Currently, the most common patient trigger variable is pressure. With pressure being the trigger variable, a patient's inspiratory effort causes a drop in pressure within the ventilator circuit. When this pressure drop reaches the pressure sensing mechanism, the ventilator triggers on and begins gas delivery.

On most ventilators, the clinician can adjust the pressure drop needed to trigger a breath. This adjustable mechanism is called the *sensitivity* or *trigger-level* control.[7] How fast the ventilator mechanism responds to patient effort is called the *response time*. A ventilator's response time is measured as the msec between the onset of patient effort and the start of machine flow. Unlike sensitivity, response time is not normally adjustable. Figure 30-5 demonstrates the concepts of sensitivity and response time for a pressure-triggered system.

Ideally, both the pressure drop needed to trigger a ventilator and its response time should be as small as possible. Either a large pressure drop or a delay in flow delivery can increase a patient's work of breathing.[4]

Using flow as the trigger variable is a bit more complex. A ventilator that uses flow triggering typically provides a continuous low flow of gas through its circuit (Figure 30-6). The ventilator measures both input and output flow. Between breaths, input flow equals output flow. Should the patient begin to inhale, output flow momentarily drops below input flow, triggering the machine to provide a breath.

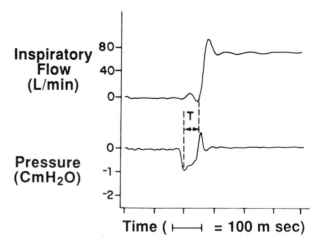

Fig. 30-5 Tracing of pressure and flow during initiation of a pressure-triggered mechanical breath. Sensitivity is measured as the pressure drop needed to initiate flow, in this case about 1 cm H_2O. Response time (T) is measured as the time interval between this 1 cm H_2O pressure drop and the actual start of flow, here about 70 msec. (From: Capps JS, Ritz R, Pierson DJ: An evaluation in four ventilators, of characteristics that affect work of breathing, *Respir Care* 32(11):1017-1024, 1987.)

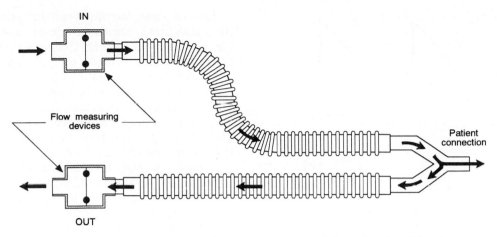

Fig. 30-6 Schematic representation showing essential features of flow triggering. Triggering occurs when the patient inspires from the circuit and increases the difference between input and output flow.

To adjust the sensitivity of a flow-triggered system, the RCP usually sets both a base continuous flow and a trigger flow level. Typically, the trigger flow level is set to 1 to 3 L/min (below baseline). For example, if you set the base continuous flow at 10 L/min and the trigger at 2 L/min, the ventilator will trigger when the output flow falls to 8 L/min or less.

When compared to pressure, using flow as the trigger variable decreases a patient's work of breathing.[8,9] However, ventilators that use a flow-triggering mechanism tend to be highly susceptible to circuit leaks or movement caused by turbulence or gas flow through condensed water. Either of these conditions can cause **spurious** breaths, which can disrupt patient-ventilatory synchrony and increase the work of breathing. Using volume as the trigger can help overcome this problem, but currently only the Drager Babylog uses true volume triggering.[2]

Pure patient triggering is often referred to as *assisted ventilation.* When in effect, the patient is solely responsible for triggering inspiration and determining the rate of breathing.[5,6] Of course, this approach is basically the opposite of controlled ventilation, with the patient having full control over breathing. Unfortunately, pure patient triggering provides no back-up mechanism to ventilate a patient who stops breathing. For this reason, time and patient triggering are often combined.

Patient or time triggering. The combination of time or patient triggering is often called *assist-control ventilation.* In this approach, a minimum trigger rate is set according to a predetermined time interval, for example 10 breaths/min. However, the patient can override this minimum by triggering breaths at a faster rate.[5,6]

Figure 30-7, page 830, diagrams typical pressure waveforms seen during time and pressure (patient) triggered CMV. Pressure is graphed on the vertical axis, with time being the horizontal axis. Note that during pressure triggering, each positive-pressure breath begins with a slight pressure drop, indicating patient effort sensed by the machine. Moreover, the time between pressure-triggered breaths is somewhat variable. When breaths are purely time-triggered, however, the time between breaths is constant. Patient inspiratory effort, even if it were to occur, would not influence the predetermined rate.

Nature of the inspiratory phase

During the inspiratory phase of ventilatory support, spontaneous or mandatory breaths are delivered to the patient, with resulting changes in pressure, volume, and flow. We will analyze: (1) how pressure is generated and applied during inspiration, and (2) how the imposition of limits affect the parameters of ventilation.

Generation and application of positive pressure. There are two major ways ventilators apply positive pressure to the airway: pressure generation and flow generation.[3,10-12]

Pressure generation. A pressure generator develops a pressure pattern which is not influenced by changes in lung or thorax mechanics. On the other hand, the flow delivered by a pressure generator can and does change with both patient effort and lung mechanics.

The most common application of pressure generation is the constant pressure generator. The theory underlying a constant pressure generator is shown in Figure 30-8, page 830. In Figure 30-8, *A* bellows, *B* is connected to a pair of elastic lungs, *L*. The bellows and lungs are separated by a closed valve, *V*. A weight, *W* on top of the bellows creates a constant force per unit area, or pressure.

Opening the valve creates a pressure gradient between the bellows and the lungs, and gas will flow from the area of higher pressure, the bellows, to the area of lower pressure, the lungs. As gas flows into the lungs, their pressure rises (Figure 30-8, *B*). However,

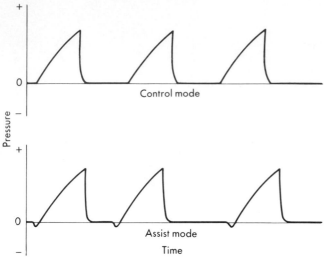

Fig. 30–7 Pressure waveforms for CMV during control mode (top) and assist mode (bottom). Note regular time intervals for control mode while time intervals for assist mode are more variable. Slight negative pressure "triggers" assist breaths.

the pressure in the bellows remains constant. Thus, as the pressure in the lungs rises, the pressure gradient between lungs and bellows falls. Because flow is proportional to the pressure gradient, it decreases as well.

In this case, airway pressure remains constant throughout the breath (a square wave), while flow tapers (Figure 30-9, *A*). Changes in compliance or resistance will not change the pressure waveform, but will alter flow. Decreased compliance causes more rapid filling of the alveoli, with a more rapid tapering of flow and thus a shortened inspiratory time (Figure 30-9, *B*). Increased resistance will slow flow into the lungs, slowing the taper of the flow wave and lengthening inspiration (Figure 30-9, *C*).

A useful analogy for the constant pressure generator is sipping soda pop through a straw. The pressure available to "push" the liquid into your mouth is constant (atmospheric pressure). However, changes in your sipping effort will alter the flow through the straw. The harder you sip, the greater the flow; the less effort you apply, the less liquid reaches your mouth. Likewise, when a ventilator breath is pressure generated, the patient can get more or less flow simply by increasing or decreasing his or her effort. The characteristics of a constant pressure generator are summarized in the box on page 832.

Although the constant pressure generator is the most common application of pressure generation, there are other possibilities. For example, rather than being constant throughout inspiration, pressure could

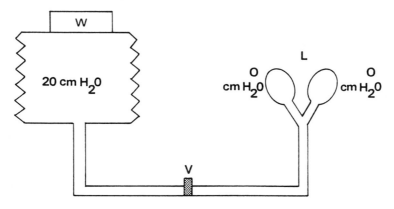

Fig. 29-7   Mechanical properties of constant pressure generator.

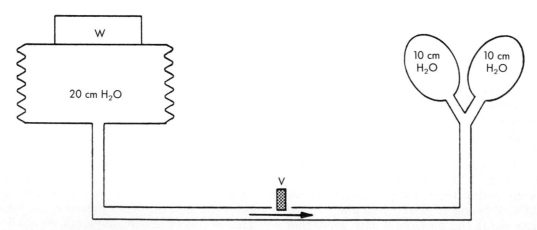

Fig. 30–8 Mechanical properties of a constant pressure generator. Top, constant pressure generator at mid-inspiration.

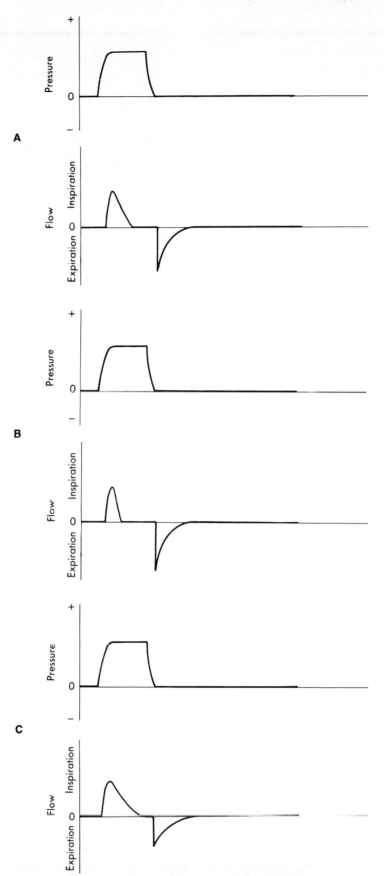

Fig. 30-9 Pressure and flow waveforms for a constant pressure generator. **A** represents "normal" conditions while **B** illustrates a decrease in CL and **C** shows an increase in Raw.

Characteristics of a constant pressure generator
1. The pressure pattern throughout inspiration is constant (a square wave);
2. The pressure pattern is not affected by the patient's lung mechanics;
3. The flow delivered varies with patient effort and lung mechanics;
4. Flow starts out high early in inspiration and progressively decreases throughout the breath.

Characteristics of a constant flow generator
1. The flow throughout inspiration is constant (a square wave);
2. The flow pattern is not affected by the patient's effort or lung mechanics;
3. The delivered pressure varies with patient effort and lung mechanics;
4. Pressure increases linearly throughout inspiration.

increase or decrease in a fixed or predictable way. Although still pressure generation, a device using this approach is referred to as a nonconstant pressure generator.

Flow generation. If flow is not affected by changes in lung or thorax mechanics, a ventilator is classified as a flow generator. In this case, the pressure pattern varies with changes in patient effort and lung mechanics.

The most common application of flow generation is the constant flow generator. The theory underlying a constant flow generator is shown in Figure 30-10. The large pressure difference between the bellows and lungs would create unacceptably high pressure and flows if a restricted orifice, *R*, did not limit flow and pressure changes.

Since the pressure gradient changes very little, flow remains constant throughout inspiration, creating a rectangular waveform (square wave). Pressure in-

creases progressively throughout inspiration (Figure 30-11, *A*). With decreased compliance (Figure 30-11, *B*), flow remains constant, while pressure rises to a higher level than normal (if volume remains constant.) The characteristics of a constant flow generator are summarized in the box above.

A good analogy for the constant flow generator would be taking a drink from your garden hose. In this case, the flow is dictated by the spigot setting. Because the water pressure at the source is so high, flow will remain constant at this setting, regardless of your efforts to draw in more or less water. If you are very thirsty and the spigot setting is too low, you will not get enough water. Conversely, if the spigot setting is too high, flow will exceed your ability to swallow. Likewise, when a ventilator breath is flow generated, the patient gets whatever flow the machine is set to deliver. Of course, this may be too much, too little, or just right; increasing or decreasing inspiratory effort

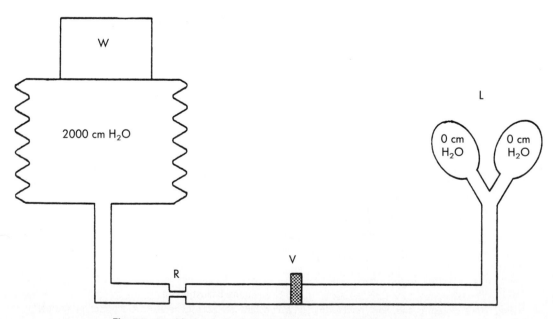

Fig. 30-10 Mechanical principles underlying constant flow generator.

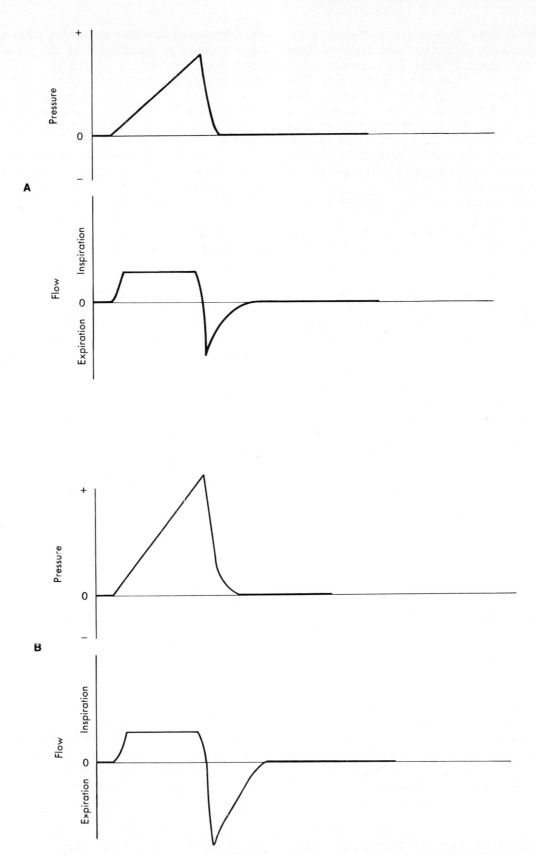

Fig. 30–11 Pressure and flow waveforms for a constant flow generator under different patient conditions. **A** shows typical wave forms for "normal" conditions. **B** illustrates a decrease in CL. Note that in **B** the inspiratory flow pattern remains unchanged while inspiratory pressure increases and expiratory flow increases.

will not alter the flow.

As with pressure generation, the constant flow generator is only one possibility. For example, rather than being constant throughout inspiration, flow could change in a predictable way. For example, flow could increase or decrease throughout inspiration, or rise then fall (like a sine wave). As long as the *pattern* of flow remains the same (uninfluenced by the patient), these variations are still considered flow generation.[3,12,13] For clarity, however, they are called *nonconstant flow generation.*

Limit variables. A limit variable is a parameter that can reach and maintain a preset level before inspiration ends, but does not terminate inspiration. Either pressure, flow, or volume can serve as a limit variable.[2]

Unfortunately, there is another, sometimes confusing use of the term "limit." Often, limit is incorrectly used to describe a ventilator's backup or safety mechanism to normal cycling. Typically, these mechanisms are output alarms which may also end inspiration. For example, all modern volume-cycled ventilators incorporate a pressure alarm mechanism. Normally, the pressure alarm is set to a level above that needed to deliver the present volume. Should the pressure required to deliver the volume rise to the preselected level, the ventilator automatically cycles to end inspiration. Some ventilators, such as the Bear 2, also can place an upper threshold on the inspiratory time or I:E ratio. This alarm mechanism serves to override volume cycling when the inspiratory time become dangerously long. In both examples, when the alarm threshold is reached, inspiration ends. Of course, this is different from a true limit variable, which does not terminate inspiration when reached. For clarification then, it is best to refer to these threshold alarms as backup cycling mechanisms rather than limits.

Pressure as a limit variable. There are two primary ways to have pressure serve as the limit variable. By definition, a ventilator that acts as a constant pressure generator during inspiration limits the applied pressure. The two most common applications of this approach are pressure support ventilation (PSV) and pressure control ventilation (PCV).

In each case, the ventilator acts as a constant pressure generator, limiting airway pressure to a value preset by the clinician. Once reached, this pressure limit is maintained throughout inspiration and never exceeded. Inspiration ends when another variable, such as time (PCV) or flow (PSV) reaches its cycle threshold.

We also can set pressure as a limit variable when using a flow generator. Typically, this type of pressure limiting requires a mechanical or electromechanical pressure relief valve (Figure 30-12). In such a system, inspiratory flow causes airway pressure to rise. If the pressure limit is reached before inspiration ends, then the remaining flow escapes out the relief valve, while the pressure is maintained at the preset limit. In this case, pressure is limited by the relief valve, but inspiration ends only when another variable, such as time, reaches its cycle threshold. This approach, called *time-cycled, pressure-limited ventilation,* is the most common type of ventilatory support for infants.

Flow as a limit variable. Flow serves as a limit variable whenever a ventilator acts as a flow generator. In this case, the clinician-set peak flow is the limit variable. Typically, this preset flow is reached and maintained until a cycle variable, such as volume or time, ends inspiration.

Volume as a limit variable. The most common application of volume as a limit variable is the volume or inflation-hold maneuver. The option to provide an inflation-hold is found on most ventilators used in critical care. During this maneuver, a preset volume is reached, but inspiration does not end until a preset time interval (the pause time) has elapsed. Thus the volume, having been reached and maintained or held, serves as a limit variable.

When an inflation-hold is activated, rather than allowing immediate exhalation, the ventilator exhalation valve remains closed for a predetermined time interval.[3] During this time interval, the inspired volume is held in the patient's lungs, with no gas flow allowed into or out of the system. With no gas flow, pressure in the ventilator and tubing system attempts to equilibrate with the alveolar pressure. This equilibration between the system and alveolar pressures manifests itself as a pressure drop at the airway, as recorded on the ventilator's pressure manometer. When pressure equilibration is complete, a pressure "plateau" can be observed (Figure 30-13).

The inflation-hold is used for both therapeutic and diagnostic purposes. Its role as a treatment modality remains controversial (see the next section). However, the use of an inflation-hold to monitor pulmonary mechanics is well established.[14,15] Specifically, by applying an inflation-hold, the clinician can measure both inspiratory airway resistance and total lung/thorax compliance. More detail on this monitoring technique is provided in Chapter 33.

Clinical importance of the inspiratory phase

Manipulation of inspiratory variables (trigger, control, limit) has two major physiologic impacts. First, by altering trigger, control, and limit variables, we can affect patient-ventilator interaction and the work of breathing. Second, alteration of these variables can affect the distribution of ventilation in the lung, and thus the efficiency of gas exchange.

Patient-ventilator interaction. As shown in Figure 30-14, various combinations of trigger, control, and limit variables modify patient-ventilator interaction. At one extreme is time-triggered, flow-limited ventila-

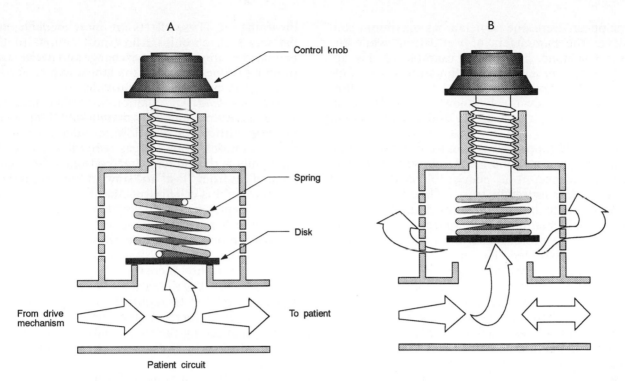

A   B

Control knob

Spring

Disk

From drive
mechanism

To patient

Patient circuit

Fig. 30-12 A, Pressure-limiting device consisting of spring-loaded valve. **B,** When pressure within patient circuit exceeds valve set by tension of spring, disk lifts and excess pressure is vented to atmosphere.

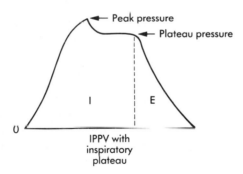

Peak pressure

Plateau pressure

I   E

0

IPPV with
inspiratory
plateau

Fig. 30-13 Pressure plateau seen when using an inflation-hold (volume-limited breath). (From Martin L: Pulmonary physiology in clinical practice, St Louis, 1987, Mosby.)

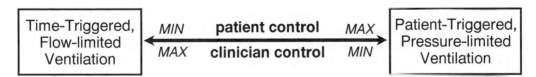

| Time-Triggered, Flow-limited Ventilation | MIN / MAX | **patient control** / **clinician control** | MAX / MIN | Patient-Triggered, Pressure-limited Ventilation |

Fig. 30-14 The range of patient and clinician control with various modes of ventilation. With time-triggered, flow-limited ventilation, the clinician has maximum control over the parameters of ventilation, while the patient has none. The classic example of this approach is volume cycled, flow-limited control mode CMV. At the other extreme is patient-triggered, pressure-limited ventilation. This approach gives the patient maximum control, which tends to enhance patient-ventilator synchrony.

tory support. Here, the clinician has maximum control over the parameters of ventilation, while the patient has none. The classic example of this approach is volume cycled, flow-limited control mode CMV. In this mode, when each breath occurs, how long it lasts, and how much (volume) it delivers are all predetermined by the clinician and outside patient control.

Although this approach assures a consistent minute volume and thus maximum control over $PaCO_2$ and acid-base balance, it is poorly tolerated by most patients. This is especially true if either the flow fails to match patient needs, or the inspiratory time exceeds patient demand. If the flow is too low, inspiratory time may be prolonged to the point that patient synchrony is disrupted. The result is "flow hunger," and an increased work of breathing. In these cases, sedation or paralysis may be required to minimize patient effort and normalize the work of breathing. Conversely, if flow is too high, peak pressures will increase, and poor gas distribution may result.

At the other extreme (see Figure 30-14) is patient-triggered, pressure-limited ventilatory support. This approach gives the patient significant control over both time and volume parameters, and results in a high degree of patient-ventilator synchrony.

Gas Exchange. Various inspiratory factors also affect pulmonary and exchange. The primary inspiratory factors affecting gas distribution and exchange are the flow pattern, flow rate, and presence or absence of an inflation-hold.

Flow pattern. Most modern positive pressure ventilators provide an assortment of inspiratory flow patterns. In mechanical and computer models, a decelerating flow pattern (as produced by a constant pressure generator) improves gas distribution to lung units with high time constants.[16-18] Similar findings in humans have been reported.[19] When compared to a constant flow pattern, the decelerating flow waveform has been shown to reduce peak pressure, inspiratory work, V_D/V_T ratio, and $P(A-a)O_2$, without affecting hemodynamic performance.[20] Moreover, in an animal model of acute lung injury, a decelerating flow waveform was shown to improve oxygenation better than a constant flow pattern.[21]

However, nitrogen washout analysis of lung models has failed to show significant differences in gas distribution among available flow patterns.[22] Similar analysis in humans has not confirmed the superiority of any one flow pattern in promoting efficient gas distribution.[23] Likewise, in an animal lung model with high airway resistance, no flow pattern was identified as having a unique advantage for gas exchange.[24]

Flow rate. In most spontaneously breathing subjects, low inspiratory flows improve gas distribution. During ventilatory support, the reverse is true. High ventilator flows not only improve gas exchange,[25] but also decrease air trapping,[26] and minimize the work of breathing.[27,28] These effects are most evident among patients with chronic airflow obstruction. In these patients, the improved gas exchange and decreased air trapping is due mainly to the longer expiratory time that high inspiratory flows provide.

Inflation-hold. An inflation-hold also affects gas exchange. By momentarily maintaining lung volume under conditions of zero flow, an inflation-hold provides additional time for gas redistribution between lung units with different time constants. This movement of gas from "fast" to "slow" filling spaces during inflation-hold is called **pendelluft.**[16,17]

In concept, pendelluft should improve gas distribution and oxygenation. As applied clinically, however, an inflation-hold has a greater impact on the efficiency of ventilation than on oxygenation.[29] In both animal and human studies, increasing the inflation-hold time decreases the V_D/V_T ratio, $PaCO_2$, and inert gas washout time.[23,29] In addition, adding an inflation-hold effectively increases the total inspiratory time, thereby shortening the time available for exhalation (see the following section on inspiratory-expiratory ratios).

Patient effect on inspiration phase. Just as alterations in the inspiratory phase can affect the patient, so too can the patient affect the inspiratory phase. As we have seen, flow patterns delivered by pressure generators can change with changes in the mechanical properties of the patient's lungs. The reverse is also true. Changes in lung mechanics can alter how some ventilators behave during inspiration.

The primary difference between a flow generator and a pressure generator is the available driving pressure. As long as the available driving pressure is at least three times greater than the airway pressure, a ventilator can function as a true flow controller. In clinical practice, only a few ventilators can generate the high pressures needed to perform as flow generator. Indeed, many ventilators categorized as flow generators develop only moderate driving pressures. Although these devices can maintain constant flows against moderate pressures, high airway pressures alter their behavior. Specifically, when a flow-limited ventilator with only a moderate driving pressure encounters high airway pressures, the device behaves more like a pressure generator. Instead of flow remaining constant, it decreases or tapers off throughout inspiration. As shown in Figure 30-15, this change in flow can increase the inspiratory time, and thus alter other time-dependent parameters of ventilation.[11]

Cycle variables

A cycle variable is a parameter that, when reached, ends inspiration by cycling the ventilator off.[2] Either pressure, volume, flow, or time can be the cycle variable. Manual cycling is also available on the most modern ventilators.[7] This control, usually a simple

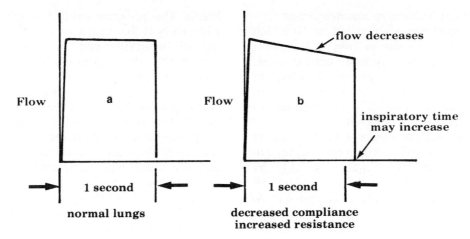

Fig. 30-15 The above inspiratory curves represent the changes in flow that can occur using a constant pressure generator with moderate generating pressures. Under normal conditions, flow is nearly constant (curve on left, *a*). As CL decreases or Raw increases, the flow decreases slightly (curve on right, *b*). If the ventilator is volume limited, the volume will be delivered from the ventilator but inspiratory *(I)* time may increase *(b)*, and this can affect the I:E ratio. (From Pilbeam SP: Mechanical ventilation: physiological and clinical applications, St Louis, 1986, Mosby.)

button, allows the clinician to end inspiration at any time.

Pressure cycling. When a ventilator is set to pressure-cycle, it delivers gas under pressure during inspiration until an adjustable, preselected pressure is reached.[5,6] When the set pressure is achieved, inspiration ends, the machine cycles off, and expiration begins. The volume and flow delivered when pressure-cycling is in effect vary according to other ventilator and patient characteristics. Pressure-cycled ventilators are most commonly used for IPPB therapy (see Chapter 27). However, this approach may also be used for continuous ventilatory support under selected conditions.

The RCP must be careful not to confuse pressure cycling with pressure limiting. Both result in delivery of a preset peak airway pressure. During true pressure cycling, however, inspiration ends when that pressure is reached. During pressure-limited ventilation, the preset peak pressure is often reached early in inspiration, but is held at that level until another parameter (volume, flow, or time) serves to cycle the breath off.

Volume cycling. When a ventilator is set to volume-cycle, it provides gas under pressure during inspiration until an adjustable, preselected volume has been expelled from the device.[5,6] When the set volume is delivered out of the system, inspiration ends, the machine cycles off, and expiration begins. The pressure and flow delivered when volume-cycling is in effect vary according to other ventilator and patient characteristics.

Time cycling. When a ventilator is set to time-cycle, it provides gas under pressure during inspiration for a preselected time interval.[5,6] When the set time interval is over, inspiration ends, the machine cycles off, and expiration begins. During time-cycling, inspiratory time is constant breath to breath. The pressure, volume, and flow delivered when time-cycling may vary according to other ventilator and patient characteristics.

If flow is the controlled variable during inspiration, then time and volume cycling are functionally equivalent. This is because volume is the integral of flow, and flow is the derivative of volume.[2] For example, when using a time-cycled constant flow generator, the delivered volume is simply the product of a constant flow times a constant time:

$$\dot{V}\ (L/sec) \times time\ (sec) = V\ (Liters)$$

Flow cycling. When a ventilator flow-cycles, it provides gas under positive pressure during inspiration until flow drops down to a specified level. When this specified low "terminal" flow is reached, inspiration ends, the machine cycles off, and expiration begins.

Flow cycling can be achieved either mechanically or via electronic control. The Bennett valves found in the Bennett PR and AP series ventilators are examples of a mechanical flow cycling mechanism. These valves close and cycle the device off when a low terminal flow is reached (see Chapter 27).

The more common approach in modern critical care ventilators is to flow-cycle using electronic control. For example, electronic controlled flow-cycling is the usual means for ending inspiration during pressure support ventilation (PSV). PSV is patient-cycled, pressure-limited, flow-cycled ventilation. During PSV, a set level of pressure is applied and maintained at the airway until the patient's inspiratory flow decreases to some minimal level. At this point, inspiration ends and expiration begins. More detail on PSV is provided later in this chapter.

Clinical importance of the cycling mechanism

For decades, arguments have raged as to which ventilator cycling mechanism is best. Given that volume and time-cycled flow-limited ventilation are functionally equivalent, and that pressure-limited and pressure-cycled ventilation are physiologically similar, the argument often boils down to whether to target volume or pressure as our goal.

Targeting volume. Volume-targeted modes include volume and time-cycled, flow-limited ventilation. Advocates of these approaches argue that only by targeting volume can a consistent minute volume be assured, especially under conditions of changing compliance or resistance.[9,30-32] With volume or time-cycled, flow-limited ventilation, the breath-to-breath volume delivered by the ventilator remains relatively constant, while the airway pressure varies according to the patient's lung mechanics. For example, should either compliance decrease or airway resistance in-

crease, the pressure needed to deliver the volume rises. Only if the pressure exceeds a set alarm threshold will inspiration end.

In reality, the volume delivered to a patient during volume or time-cycled, flow-limited ventilation (and, for that matter, with any positive pressure ventilator) is *always* less than that expelled from the machine.[7] Two factors account for this volume loss. First, gases are compressed when delivered under pressure. Thus, the expelled volume (at atmospheric pressure) occupies less space when delivered under pressure. Second, most ventilator circuits are somewhat compliant. Expansion of this tubing under pressure robs some of the volume that would otherwise go to the patient. In combination, these factors contribute to the compressed volume loss during PPV. See the accompanying MiniClini for details.

In general, compressed volume loss is critical only when delivered volumes are small, as in infant, pedi-

---

■ MINI CLINI ■

30-1

Compressed Volume Loss During Positive Pressure Ventilation

A ventilator's compressed volume depends on three factors: (1) the ventilator's internal volume, (2) the compliance of the ventilator circuit, and (3) the applied pressure. Given that the ventilator's internal volume remains fixed, compressed volume loss varies mainly with circuit compliance and applied pressure. By measuring both circuit compliance and applied pressure, the RCP can determine compressed volume loss and thus the corrected volume actually delivered to the patient.

Problem: A patient is receiving ventilatory support via a volume-cycled ventilator set to deliver 800 mL per breath. Initially, the peak pressure is 30 cm H_2O. Over time, the patient's compliance decreases, and the peak pressure rises to 60 cm H_2O. What initial volume was actually received by the patient, and how did the decrease in compliance alter this volume?

Solution: To solve this problem, the RCP would first have to know the circuit compliance factor (also called compression factor). This is determined by occluding the circuit (when off the patient), filling it with a known volume of gas (ΔV), and measuring the resulting statis pressure (ΔP):

$$\text{circuit compliance factor} = \frac{\Delta V}{\Delta P}$$

Typically, the actual measurement is performed by setting the ventilator to deliver a small volume (200 to 300 mL) at minimal flow into a circuit with the patient outlet occluded. ΔP is taken as the end-inspiratory peak pressure.

For example, after setting up a new circuit, you occlude it at the patient connector and set the ventilator to deliver 200 mL. You then observe and record an end-inspiratory peak pressure of 50 cm H_2O. The circuit compliance is:

$$\frac{\text{circuit}}{\text{compliance}} = \frac{200 \text{ mL}}{50 \text{ cm } H_2O}$$
$$= 4 \text{ mL/cm } H_2O$$

This means that for every cm H_2O pressure, about 4 mL of the preset volume will not reach the patient, but be compressed in the ventilator system.

Figure 30-16 applies this factor to our patient. In the first example, the tidal volume is set for 800 mL, and the peak pressure is 30 cm H_2O. Knowing that the compliance factor is 4 mL/cm H_2O, we compute the compressed volume by simply multiplying the airway pressure times the factor:

$$\frac{\text{airway}}{\text{pressure}} \times \frac{\text{compliance}}{\text{factor}} = \frac{\text{compressed}}{\text{volume loss}}$$

$$30 \text{ cm } H_2O \times 4 \text{ mL/cm } H_2O = 120 \text{ mL}$$

Thus, only 680 mL of the set 800 mL actually reaches the patient's airways, while the remaining 120 mL is effectively "lost" by compression in the system.

After the patient's compliance decreases, the peak pressure rises to 60 cm H_2O (second example in Figure 30-16). Using the same factor of 4 mL/cm H_2O we multiply the pressure by the factor again: $60 \times 4 = 240$. Now only 560 mL of the set 800 reaches the patient, while 240 mL is compressed in the system. Of course, this represents a significant drop in actual delivered tidal volume.

Fortunately, many third generation ventilators compute the circuit compliance factor during routine setup or circuit changes, and apply this information to continually correct the delivered tidal volume.

atric, and high frequency applications. As a rule of thumb, the smaller the tidal volume required, the smaller the compression factor needed. To achieve the lowest possible compression factor, the RCP must use: (1) a ventilator with minimal internal volume, (2) low volume, low compliance tubing, and (3) a low volume humidifier.

Compressed volume loss must also be accounted for in certain monitoring functions, such as when performing bedside estimation of compliance and resistance (see Chapter 33).

An additional factor that can cause the patient to receive less volume than the ventilator delivers is a leak. Because the cycle variable during volume-cycle ventilation is the volume expelled from the machine (as opposed to that than actually is received by the patient), a system leak will decrease the volume reaching the patient. For this reason, volume-cycled ventilators are said to compensate poorly for leaks in the system.[13] Because volume cycled ventilators compensate poorly for system leaks, either a low exhaled volume or low inspiratory pressure alarm must be incorporated into their design.[7]

Last, if spontaneous breathing is allowed at all (as during partial ventilatory support), volume-targeted breaths will make up only a portion of the patient's total minute ventilation. Because the level of spontaneous breathing will vary according to patient demand, total minute ventilation will always be changing. Thus the major advantage of the volume-targeted approach, that is a consistent minute volume, simply does not apply during partial ventilatory support.

From these examples we can see that a volume-targeted approach may not provide an absolute constant minute volume under all conditions. In addition, the physiologic changes that require different pressures may also cause changes in gas distribution within the lung, as manifested by alterations in the V/Q ratio. Thus, even if volume-targeting were to provide the same overall ventilation against changing lung mechanics, the resulting arterial blood gases could still vary. All these factors make it important to monitor physiologic parameters as well as exhaled volumes and to make ventilator adjustments accordingly, regardless of cycling mode.

Figure 30-17, page 840, outlines the parameters involved in volume-targeted ventilation. Greyed parameters are those which can be under user control (this will vary by ventilator). Lines connecting parameters show dependency relationships. For example, the cycle time is a function of inspiratory and expiratory time.

Targeting Pressure. Pressure-targeted modes include pressure-cycled and pressure-limited ventilation.[33-36] Pressure-limited ventilation may be either time or flow-cycled. When time-triggered and time-cycled, pressure-limited ventilation is commonly called pressure control ventilation (PCV). When patient-triggered and flow-cycled, pressure-limited ventilation is referred to as pressure support ventilation

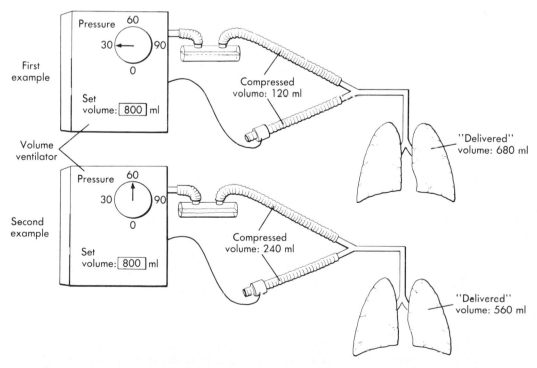

Fig. 30-16 Comparison of volumes delivered to a patient under different end-inspiratory pressures with a volume-cycled ventilator. See text for description of this example.

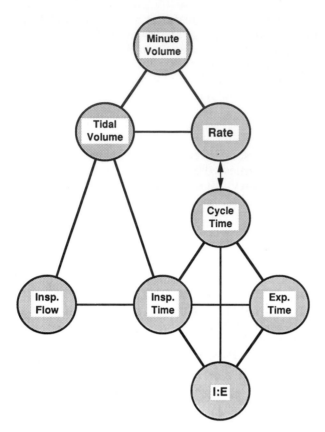

Fig. 30-17 Parameters involved in volume-targeted ventilation. Greyed parameters are those which can be set by the user (varies by ventilator). Lines connecting parameters show dependency relationships. For example, cycle time is a function of inspiratory and expiratory time.

(PSV). Proponents of these modes argue that they can provide greater patient-ventilator synchrony, enhanced gas exchange, and a higher margin of safety than volume-targeted strategies.

The volume delivered during pressure-targeted modes varies with changes in set pressure, patient effort, and lung mechanics. For all pressure-targeted modes, the volume delivered at a given pressure will decrease as compliance falls.[31-36] An increase in resistance will also decrease delivered volume when the cycling variable is pressure, as will active exhalation or muscle tensing by the patient during inspiration.

If pressure serves as the limit variable instead of the cycle variable, changes in airway resistance during pressure-limited ventilation may or may not affect delivered volume. In this case, the key factor is the time available for pressure equilibration. Volume can remain constant even if airway resistance rises, as long as there is sufficient time for alveolar and airway pressures to equilibrate. However, if insufficient time is available for pressure equilibration, delivered volume will decrease as airway resistance increases. The length of time needed for pressure equilibration is usually at least 3 times greater than the time constant for the respiratory system. Figure 30-18 illustrates the

fundamental features of time-cycled, pressure-limited ventilation under different patient conditions.

Since all pressure-targeted modes rely on pressure generation for gas delivery, the flow varies with patient effort and lung mechanics. This tends to enhance patient-ventilator synchrony, as argued by proponents of these modes.

Other proposed advantages of pressure-targeted ventilation are less well-substantiated. Enhanced oxygenation, when it occurs, is probably due to dynamic air trapping or auto-PEEP (see subsequent section on hazards of PPV).[37] In regard to relative safety, proponents cite lower peak airway pressures when using pressure-targeting approaches. Indeed, with all else equal, a pressure generator will deliver a lower peak airway pressure than a flow generator. However, the mean or average airway pressure is typically higher.[38,39] As we shall see, it is mean airway pressure that determines many of the harmful effects of PPV. Moreover, for a given alveolar volume, the peak *alveolar* pressures during pressure-targeted and volume-targeted ventilation must be the same.[40,41] For this reason, pressure-targeted strategies have no intrinsic safety advantage over volume-targeted approaches. As with volume-targeted ventilation, the safety and efficacy of this approach depends on careful and continuous monitoring of the patient's physiologic response to treatment, with appropriate ongoing adjustment.

Figure 30-19 outlines the parameters involved in pressure-targeted ventilation. As previously described for volume-targeted strategies, greyed parameters are those that can be directly adjusted by the clinician. All other parameters are outside direct clinician control.

Baseline variable

The baseline variable is the parameter controlled during expiration. Although either pressure, volume, or flow could theoretically serve as the baseline variable, pressure control is the most practical, being implemented by all commonly used ventilators.

Baseline or expiratory pressure is always measured and set relative to atmospheric pressure. Thus, when we want baseline pressure to equal atmospheric pressure, we set it at zero. This is often called *zero end-expiratory pressure,* or ZEEP. When we want baseline pressure to exceed atmospheric pressure, we set a positive value, called *positive end-expiratory pressure* or PEEP. Although seldom used, we could also set the baseline below atmospheric pressure, a technique called negative end-expiratory pressure, or NEEP.

Zero end-expiratory pressure (ZEEP). ZEEP is the default baseline value during PPV, meaning that it is normally in effect unless purposely changed. Regardless of the mechanism by which gas is delivered to the lungs, it must leave before the next inspiration. Exha-

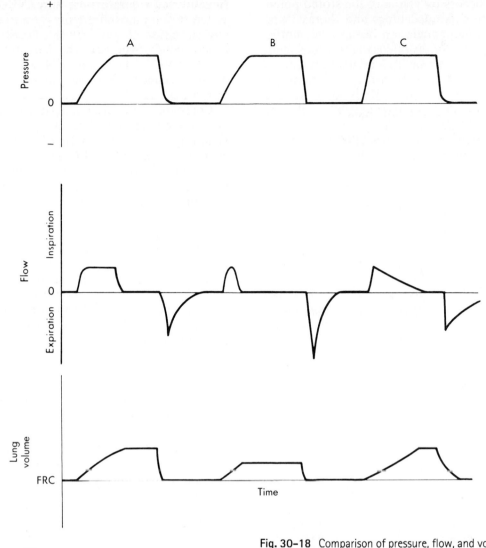

Fig. 30-18 Comparison of pressure, flow, and volume waveforms for time-cycled, pressure-limited ventilation with different patient conditions. *A* shows normal conditions while in *B* there is a decrease in CL and *C* illustrates an increase in Raw. Inspiratory time is equal in *A, B,* and *C.* Note that *B* shows a decrease in volume due to a decrease in CL. *C* shows the same volume as *A*, but more time is required during inspiration to reach that volume in the lung because of the increased Raw.

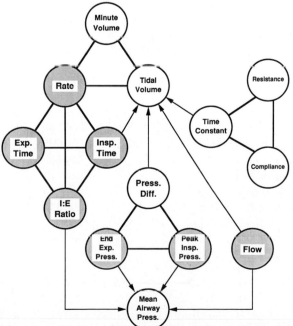

Fig. 30-19 Parameters involved in pressure-targeted ventilation. Greyed parameters are those which can be set by the user (varies by ventilator). Lines connecting parameters show dependency relationships. For example, tidal volume depends on the pressure differential (Peak-PEEP), inspiratory time, inspiratory flow, and time constant of the lung.

lation normally occurs by virtue of the stored potential energy in the expanded lungs and thorax. With ZEEP in effect, when exhalation begins, the ventilator's expiratory valve simply opens to the atmosphere, exposing the patient's airway to a relative pressure of zero. At this point, alveolar pressure exceeds airway pressure, gas moves from alveoli out to the atmosphere, and the lungs and thorax passively recoil down to their resting volume, or FRC.

Positive end-expiratory pressure (PEEP). PEEP is the application and maintenance of pressure above atmospheric at the airway throughout expiration.[42,43] Although PEEP is often referred to as a ventilatory support mode, this is incorrect. PEEP is simply an alteration in the baseline variable and thus can be added to any support mode. When PEEP is combined with mandatory or machine breaths only, we use the term CMV with PEEP. When PEEP is combined with machine *and* spontaneous breaths, we use the term IMV with PEEP.[44] When pressure above atmospheric is maintained at the airway during spontaneous breaths, the term continuous positive airway pressure (CPAP) is used.[45] Figure 30-20 illustrates the various airway pressure waveforms created when the baseline variable is set to deliver PEEP.

Negative end-expiratory pressure (NEEP), is the application of subatmospheric pressure to the airway during expiration (Figure 30-21). NEEP was originally developed to overcome the harmful cardiovascular effects of PPV. The assumption was that NEEP could offset the **impedance** to venous return created by the positive pressure during inspiration.

Compared to positive pressure alone, NEEP does lower airway and pleural pressures, and enhances venous return.[3] However, NEEP can also cause airway collapse, decrease the FRC, and worsen V/Q relationships. Because other, safer approaches to minimizing the harmful effects of PPV are available, there is presently no good indication for using NEEP during continuous ventilatory support.

Inspiratory–expiratory time ratios

The relationship between the inspiratory and expiratory time provided during PPV is called the inspiratory-expiratory time ratio, abbreviated as I:E. In general, I:E ratios are most important in the control and assist-control modes of CMV.[26] In these modes, the I:E ratio, in combination with the rate and delivered volume or pressure, determines the net effect of PPV on both ventilation circulation. When inspiration is ended by volume or time cycling, both the inspiratory and expiratory times can be manipulated to achieve an acceptable balance between efficient ventilation and the least cardiovascular effect. In addition, extending the inspiratory time so that it is longer than expiration (an inverse I:E ratio or I:E > 1.0) has been used to improve oxygenation in patients with acute lung injury.[46]

Table 30-1 summarizes the major terms, symbols and formulas used in calculating the time variables that may be manipulated during the control and assist-control modes of mechanical ventilation.

MODES OF VENTILATION

A mode of ventilation is a particular set of control and phase variables applied to either a mandatory or spontaneous breath.[2] Currently, there are nearly two dozen ventilatory support modes described in the literature. All represent variations within one of three

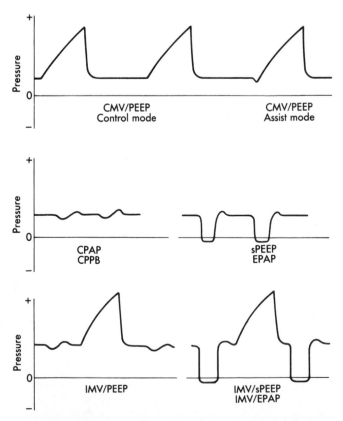

Fig. 30-20 Pressure waveforms for various forms of ventilatory support with end-expiratory pressure at a positive level. See text for description.

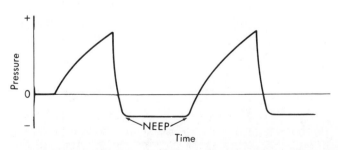

Fig. 30-21 Pressure waveform during CMV with NEEP added.

Table 30-1 Time variables in mechanical ventilation

Term	Symbol	Formula for Calculation
Frequency (rate)	f	Count breaths/minute or $\dfrac{60}{T_I + T_E}$
Cycle time	$T_I + T_E$	Add $T_I + T_E$ or $\dfrac{60}{f}$
Inspiratory time	T_I	$T_I = \dfrac{60}{f} - T_E$ or $T_I = \%T_I \times (T_I + T_E)$
Expiratory time	T_E	$T_E = \dfrac{60}{f} - T_I$
Inspiratory-expiratory time ratio	I:E or T_I:T_E	$I{:}E = \dfrac{T_I}{T_E}$
Percentage inspiratory time (duty cycle)	$\%T_I$	$\%T_I = \dfrac{T_I}{T_I + T_E} \times 100$

major categories: (1) continuous mandatory ventilation (CMV), in which all breaths are mandatory, (2) intermittent mandatory ventilation (IMV), in which mandatory and spontaneous breaths are mixed, and (3) spontaneous modes, in which all breaths are spontaneous. Of course, with any of these three "meta" modes, we can change the baseline variable by adding PEEP.

Continuous mandatory ventilation

Time-triggered CMV (controlled ventilation)

Controlled ventilation is a full ventilatory support mode in which mandatory breaths are triggered according to a preset time interval, independent of patient's effort.[47] Controlled ventilation may target either volume or pressure. With the parameters of ventilation entirely in the hands of the clinician, controlled ventilation is the only mode of ventilatory support that can provide precise and predictable physiologic results.

Indications. For this reason, controlled ventilation is the preferred mode of ventilatory support when a precise minute ventilation or $PaCO_2$ has to be maintained, such as in patients with closed head injuries who require hypoventilation. Moreover, controlled ventilation is required when delivering unnatural I:E ratios, as during inverse ratio PCV.

Clinical application. Technically, controlled ventilation is easy to apply, requiring only a ventilator that can be set to prevent patient triggering. Thus, the challenge of controlled ventilation lies not so much in the design of the apparatus as in the management of the patient.

Controlled ventilation is poorly tolerated by most patients, often resulting in asynchronous breathing efforts against the mechanically controlled breaths, or strenuous, but futile attempts to breathe spontaneous-

ly. Both conditions can dramatically increase the work of breathing, and with it, the oxygen consumption of the respiratory muscles. Clearly, these adverse effects can negate any advantages to the use of this mode of ventilatory support, and have been cited by some as a reason for abandoning this approach altogether.[48] However, most clinicians would argue that controlled ventilation still has a proper, albeit limited, place in the support of selected patients in respiratory failure.

Time or patient-triggered CMV (assist–control ventilation)

Assist-control ventilation is a full ventilatory support mode delivery in which mandatory breaths can be triggered either by the patient or the machine. Assist-control ventilation can be volume or pressure-targeted. Regardless of target, the machine provides a base breathing rate, which the patient can exceed. If the patient's rate drops below the preset backup rate, time-triggered mandatory breaths are provided.[47]

Indications. Before IMV, assist-control ventilation was the primary mode of ventilatory support used on adults. Subsequently, assist-control ventilation went out of favor. However, assist-control ventilation is still considered useful in patients with stable ventilatory drives who are unable to generate sufficient spontaneous inspiratory volumes.

Clinical application. Traditional flow-limited assist-control ventilation is available on most modern ventilators, requiring only selection of the mode, and setting of an appropriate trigger level. Unfortunately, traditional flow-limited assist-control ventilation can cause excessive patient work if the flow is inadequate or the trigger level is incorrectly set. In addition, assist-control ventilation may worsen air trapping in COPD patients.[47] Some newer ventilators provide pressure-limited assist-control (usually PSV with a back-up rate) as an option. This approach can help overcome some of the patient interaction problems encountered with flow-limited assist-control ventilation.

Intermittent mandatory ventilation (IMV)

IMV is a partial ventilatory support mode that combines spontaneous breaths with periodic mandatory or machine breaths.[44,47,49,50] These periodic breaths may be time-triggered or patient-triggered. When machine breaths are time-triggered, the term controlled IMV is often used. When machine breaths are patient-triggered, the term *synchronous intermittent mandatory ventilation,* or SIMV, is preferred. A variation of IMV is which the level of mandatory support varies to achieve a given minute volume is called mandatory minute ventilation or MMV. IMV may also be combined with PEEP or pressure support ventilation (PSV), both discussed later.

Intermittent mandatory ventilation

Figure 30-22 depicts the airway pressure events occurring during IMV. Table 30-2 compares IMV with CMV.

Indications. Considerable controversy still exists regarding the appropriate use of IMV. Many advocate its use mainly for weaning,[51] while others claim that IMV should be used as the primary mode of ventilatory support.[44] The fact is that many of the purported advantages of IMV have yet to be studied in a controlled fashion.[52]

As a partial support mode, IMV allows or requires the patient to sustain some of the work of breathing. When the patient is capable of providing more work, the ventilator's rate can be decreased accordingly. This allows for smooth transitions during ventilatory support. In addition, for a given minute ventilation, ventilatory support with IMV results in a lower mean pleural pressure than CMV.[49,50] This is because the spontaneous breaths during IMV decrease pleural pressure. IMV is also useful when combined with PEEP. Most newer generation ventilators incorporate a system for application of the IMV mode;[7] for ventilators not equipped with an IMV mechanism, special circuits can be added.[50]

Despite these proven advantages, IMV must not be viewed as an indispensable ingredient in all ventilator

Table 30-2 Physiologic effects of CMV versus IMV

CMV	IMV
All breaths mandatory (spontaneous breathing prohibited)	Mandatory and spontaneous breaths mixed
Ventilator responsible for minute ventilation (full ventilator support)	Patient contributes to minute ventilation (partial ventilatory support)
Patient may (assist/control mode) or may not (control mode) determine rate of breathing	Above IMV rate patient controls rate and depth of breathing
Higher mean pleural pressure for given minute ventilation	Lower mean pleural pressure for given minute ventilation

management or as a solution to all management problems.[49,52] For example, we must be careful not to burden some patients too early or too frequently with their own breathing. They may have an adequate central drive to breathe spontaneously, but because of their disease, may not possess adequate musculoskeletal power to convert the drive into significant tidal volumes. For such patients, either the assist/control mode[53] or IMV with pressure support[54] should be used

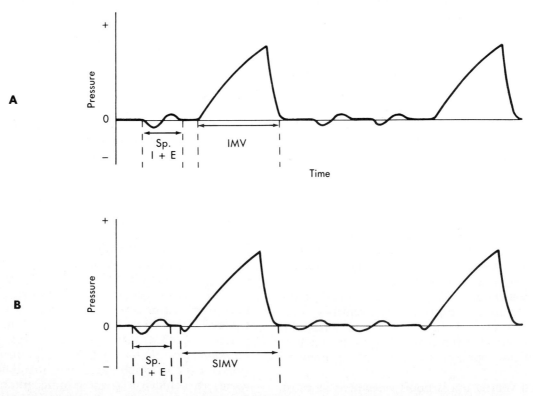

Fig. 30-22 Pressure waveforms for IMV and SIMV. Spontaneous inspiration and expiration *(Sp. I + E)* are shown combined with pressurized (IMV) breaths. **A,** shows the IMV breaths occurring like control mode breaths while **B,** shows IMV breaths triggered by patient (SIMV).

until resolution of the underlying disease process can be achieved.

Clinical application. During IMV, some system must provide fresh gas by which spontaneous breathing can occur at a rate and volume that is patient determined. Currently there are two major categories of IMV systems: continuous flow and demand flow.[55] In general, continuous flow IMV systems are special circuits added to ventilators not equipped with their own IMV mechanism. Built-in demand flow IMV systems are used on most newer generation ventilators.

Continuous flow IMV. As the name implies, a continuous flow IMV system employs a constant flow of fresh gas from which the patient can spontaneously breathe. Figure 30-23 depicts a typical continuous flow IMV system.

A separate blended gas source provides a continuous flow of mixed gases into a 3 to 5 L reservoir bag. This reservoir bag is joined to the inspiratory limb of the circuit proximal to the humidifier via a T connector. A one-way valve separates the reservoir bag from the ventilator circuit. Distension of the bag by continuous gas flow creates a slight pressure difference which normally keeps the one-way valve open, except during mandatory machine breaths.

When a machine breath is provided, the one-way valve is forced closed, and gas under pressure goes to the patient as usual. Simultaneously, the continuous flow fills and distends the reservoir bag, with its pressure limited by a safety relief valve.

Between mandatory breaths, the valve opens, and gas flows from the bag into the ventilator circuit. The patient may then breath spontaneously from this gas flow. During spontaneous exhalation, the patient's expired gases mix with and are flushed out the expiratory port of the ventilator circuit by the continuous flow.

Such a system can easily be used with PEEP. This is because the bag pressure always equals the ventilator circuit pressure between mandatory breaths. With little or no pressure differential across the valve, minimal patient effort is required to draw gas from the reservoir bag.

Nonetheless, in order to ensure minimal patient effort, flows through the system generally must be sufficient to meet the peak inspiratory demands of the patient. Alternatively, using a larger bag (12 to 18 L) or an elastic one may help minimize patient effort during spontaneous breathing.[56-57]

Unfortunately, conventional continuous flow IMV is effective only when the mandatory breaths are time-triggered (control mode). In addition, since the patient's expired gases mix with the continuous flow within the ventilator circuit, expired volume monitoring is difficult. This problem can be overcome, in part, by using a specialized continuous flow circuit, as shown in Figure 30-24, page 846.[58,59] Such a circuit makes expired volume monitoring possible by diverting the excess flow out the exhalation valve, without passing through the monitoring device.

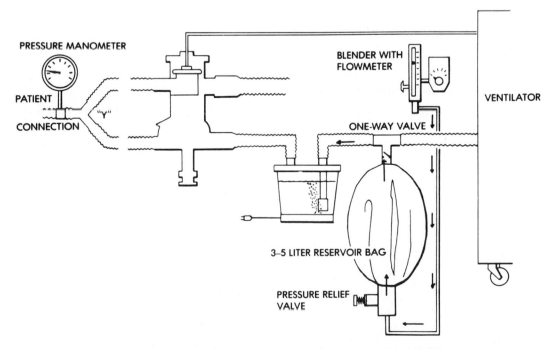

Fig. 30-23 Pressure reservoir IMV system. Continuous gas flow from the blender fills the bag and flows through the circuit to allow spontaneous breathing. The pressure relief valve on the bag is used to vent excess flow during a mechanical breath. See text for description. (From Kirby RR, Smith RA, Desautels DD, editors: Mechanical ventilation, New York, 1985, Churchill Livingstone.)

Another limitation of this approach is the potential for increased pressure in the circuit during exhalation. Not only must the patient's expired gases escape through the expiratory port, but also the excess flow from the reservoir bag. This increase in downstream pressure during exhalation can increase the patient's work of breathing.

Continuous flow IMV may also increase the work of breathing during inspiration, especially if the patient must "pull" gas through a cascade or bubble type humidifier.[60] At inspiratory flows of 120 L/min (mimicking a tachypneic patient), pressure drops as high as 11 cm H_2O have been recorded across some humidifiers.[61] Although higher inspiratory flows through the system can help overcome the increased inspiratory impedance, this effect is negated, in part, by the increase in downstream pressure during exhalation, as previously described. The use of low resistance, wick-type, blow-over humidifers can help resolve this problem.

Demand flow IMV. In lieu of providing fresh gas for spontaneous breathing by continuous flow, most 3rd generation ventilators incorporate a demand valve system.

In concept, a demand valve provides flow to the patient in proportion to inspiratory needs. Early versions of these demand valves were simple pneumatic devices consisting of a diaphragm in a chamber (Figure 30-25). One side of the diaphragm (*A*) is exposed to a reference pressure, with the other side exposed to the patient circuit (*B*). Attached to the diaphragm is a valve (*C*), which controls flow from a high pressure gas source. During spontaneous breathing, a small drop in pressure on the patient side of the valve (*B*) causes it to open. Because the valve attempts to maintain a constant pressure differential across the diaphragm, blended gas will enter the system through (*C*) at a rate proportional to the patient's inspiratory

effort. Typically, such valves can provide flows between 0 and 180 L/min.[7]

Unfortunately, many of these demand valves do not perform as expected. First, ventilator manometers measuring internal or machine (as opposed to airway) pressure underestimate the negative pressure required to open such demand valves.[62] Second, tests of such devices under conditions of a short inspiratory time have indicated that pressure drops as high as 23 cm H_2O may be needed to initiate gas flow, with 4 cm to 10 cm H_2O differentials being the rule.[62,63] As expected, such pressure drops increase the patient's spontaneous work of breathing.[64-66]

Although some of this imposed work of breathing may be associated with pressure drops across high resistance humidifiers, most is probably due to limitations inherent in the design of these valve systems.[47] Of particular concern is the substantial delay time between the initiation of patient inspiratory effort and demand valve opening, ranging between 180 and 250 msec.[66] A continuous flow pressure reservoir system, on the other hand, can respond in as little as one-eighth this time, or about 33 msec.[54]

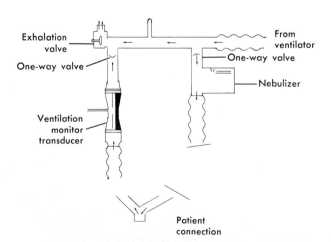

Fig. 30-24 Circuit used for continuous-flow ventilation. (From McPherson SP: Respiratory therapy equipment, ed 4, St Louis, 1989, Mosby.)

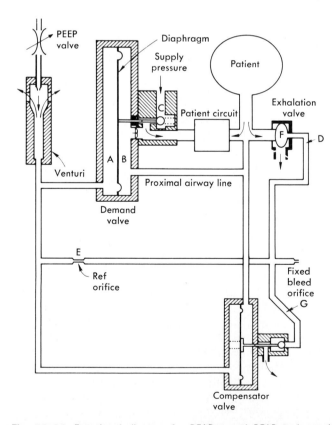

Fig. 30-25 Functional diagram for BEAR-1 and BEAR-2 demand valve, PEEP, and compensator valve systems. (Courtesy Bear Medical Systems, Inc. Riverside, Calif; from McPherson SP: Respiratory therapy equipment, ed 4, St Louis, 1989, Mosby.)

These simple pneumatic systems have given way to microprocessor controlled electromechanical valves.[67] These valves tend to be more sensitive than the typical pneumatic system. In addition, microprocessor control now allows flow-triggering of spontaneous breaths. As previously described, flow-triggering can significantly lower the work of breathing imposed on patients during spontaneous breathing through mechanical ventilation circuits.[8,9]

Mandatory minute ventilation (MMV)

The technique called Mandatory Minute Ventilation, or MMV, first appeared in the medical literature in 1977.[68]

Indications. As originally described, MMV was conceived as a technique designed to aid weaning from ventilatory support. According to its originators, the MMV mode ensures delivery of a preset minimum minute volume, with the patient allowed to breathe spontaneously. Should the patient meet this preset $\dot{V}_E$ entirely by spontaneous effort, a ventilator in the MMV mode will remain passive, delivering no positive pressure breaths. On the other hand, should the patient's spontaneous $\dot{V}_E$ fall below the preset MMV minimum, a ventilator operating in this mode will provide the mechanical support necessary to ensure that the minimum minute ventilation goal is achieved.[47,69-71]

Clinical application. Currently, MMV represents the only commercially available example of true "closed-loop" ventilatory support system.[72] A closed-loop system incorporates both a computerized control process that constantly monitors a given parameter (in this case the $\dot{V}_E$), and a means to *automatically* adjust that parameter to the value previously set by the user. For this reason, only the newer generation microprocessor ventilators have the capacity to operate in the MMV mode. Currently, MMV is available on the Bear 5, Bear 1000, Engstrom Erica, Hamilton Veolar, Ohmeda CPU-1, Ohmeda Advent, and PPG Irisa ventilators.

At present, two different approaches are used to implement MMV. On the Engstrom Erica, and BEAR 1000, for example, the clinician presets both an SIMV frequency and tidal volume, and the minimum MMV level desired. Should the total $\dot{V}_E$ (patient plus IMV breaths) fall below the MMV minimum, then these ventilators will increase the SIMV frequency to maintain the preset $\dot{V}_E$. If, on the other hand, the patient's $\dot{V}_E$ meets or exceeds the minimum MMV level, these devices will not deliver *any* mechanical breaths. However, the BEAR 1000 lets the clinician set a minimum SIMV frequency that is provided regardless of the total minute volume, thereby assuring the delivery of a preset number of periodic mandatory breaths.

The Hamilton Veolar ventilator employs a slightly different approach. When using this device in the MMV mode, the clinician sets both a minimum minute ventilation and an initial level of pressure support (Ppsv). In turn, the ventilator varies the Ppsv to maintain the desired $\dot{V}_E$. A backup SIMV mode is available should the patient become apneic.

In principle then, the application of the MMV mode ensures that a constant minute volume of fresh gas is breathed by a patient, despite minute-to-minute changes in his or her ability to breathe spontaneously. Moreover, MMV should allow simpler and more direct control over a patient's $PaCO_2$ than that provided by comparable weaning methods.[68] Successful use of this mode has been described in the perioperative management of a patient with myasthenia gravis.[74] In addition, favorable results have been reported in one clinical trial comparing MMV to SIMV.[75]

Moreover, most current MMV systems cannot assure an efficient pattern of ventilation. For example, on current ventilators employing this mode, an MMV setting of 8.0 L/min (8,000 mL) could be met by either of the following patterns:

Pattern	Frequency	Tidal volume	Minute ventilation
A	20	400 mL	8,000 mL
B	40	200 mL	8,000 mL

Assuming equivalent deadspace, pattern A clearly has a more efficient combination of rate and tidal volume, resulting in both less deadspace ventilation and more alveolar ventilation per minute. Pattern B, on the other hand, has a grossly inefficient combination of rate and tidal volume, with a large proportion of deadspace ventilation. Yet, with current MMV-capable ventilators, both patterns achieve the desired goal of 8.0 L/min, and would thus be acceptable to the machine.

Ideally, this problem would be avoided by letting the clinician set both a minimum $\dot{V}_E$ *and* a maximum allowable spontaneous breathing rate. In this case, should the spontaneous breathing rate exceed the preset maximum, either a ventilator alarm would activate (signalling the practitioner to respond), or the ventilator would automatically increase the tidal volume (or pressure support level) until the spontaneous breathing frequency returned to the desired range.

Given its present technical limitations, the use of MMV as a primary mode of ventilatory support should be done with extreme caution. Moreover, contrary to those who claim this mode allows patients to "wean themselves," MMV—like any mode of ventilatory support—is no substitute for careful and continuous bedside monitoring by astute clinicians.

Positive end-expiratory pressure (PEEP)

As previously described, PEEP is not a mode of ventilation per se, but simply the application of positive pressure to change the baseline variable during either CMV or IMV.

Indications

PEEP is primarily used to improve oxygenation in patients with severe hypoxemia. As a rule of thumb, severe hypoxemia exists when a patient's PaO_2 cannot be maintained above 50 mm Hg with an FIO_2 above 0.50.

PEEP improves oxygenation in these patients by increasing the FRC, and decreasing physiologic shunting. As a side benefit, the improved oxygenation provided by PEEP allows use of lower FIO_2s.[76-80] Other parameters such a lung compliance and V_D/V_T ratio may also improve when PEEP is applied to some patients.[79,80] PEEP is also indicated in patients with COPD who develop dynamic hyperinflation or auto-PEEP during mechanical ventilatory support.[81]

Hazards

There are several harmful effects associated with the use of PEEP. Table 30-3 summarizes the beneficial and harmful effects of positive end-expiratory pressure.[47] More detail on these effects is provided in the subsequent section on the physiologic effects of PPV.

Contraindications

PEEP is contraindicated in the presence of an untreated bronchopleural fistula or pneumothorax. Application of PEEP to both lungs is contraindicated in severe unilateral lung disease. In these cases, independent lung ventilation (ILV) can be used to apply separate inspiratory and baseline pressures to the right and left lung.[82,83]

Clinical application

Up to 15 cm H_2O PEEP is commonly used, although some patients may require PEEP levels as high as 40 cm H_2O to maintain adequate oxygenation.[80]

Table 30-3 Physiologic effects of positive end-expiratory pressure (PEEP)

Beneficial	Detrimental
Increased FRC	Increased incidence of pulmonary barotrauma
Decreased shunt fraction	Potential decrease in venous return and cardiac output
Increased lung compliance/ decreased work of breathing	Increased work of breathing (with overdistention)
Increase PaO_2 for given FIO_2	Increased pulmonary vascular resistance
	Increased intracranial pressure
	Decreased renal and portal blood flow
	Increased dead space

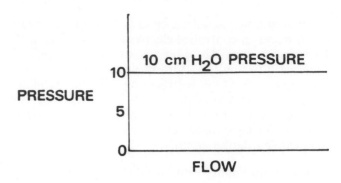

Fig. 30-26 Characteristics of a true threshold resistor.

When infants are receiving PEEP or CPAP, 15 cm H_2O pressure or less normally is applied, though, as with adults, higher pressures have been used.[84]

There are several ways to apply PEEP during mechanical ventilation.[85] We will look first at the mechanisms used to generate PEEP, followed by an analysis of differences in the use of PEEP during various support modes. As we shall see later, most of the methods used to generate PEEP in a ventilator circuit can also be used to apply CPAP during spontaneous breathing.

Generating PEEP. Ideally, a true PEEP mechanism should be capable of maintaining a given pressure level in a ventilator circuit independent of flow, thus acting as a *threshold resistor*.[85,86] As shown in Figure 30-26, a true threshold resistor maintains a given pressure independent of flow. Common devices used to provide PEEP are listed in the accompanying box.

Underwater columns. Figure 30-27 depicts a simple water column PEEP device connected to the expiratory port of a ventilator circuit. By diverting exhaled gases to a diaphragm placed *under* a water column, further exhalation of gas below a certain pressure level is impossible. In this case, the PEEP level is adjusted simply by varying the water level, with each centimeter of column height equal to 1 cm H_2O PEEP.

Spring-loaded diaphragms or disks. Figure 30-28 depicts a simple spring-loaded disk PEEP device, also connected to the expiratory port of a ventilator circuit. With this device, PEEP is adjusted by altering

---

Devices used to generate PEEP

- Underwater columns
- Spring-loaded diaphragms or disks
- Balloon valves
- Electromechanical valves

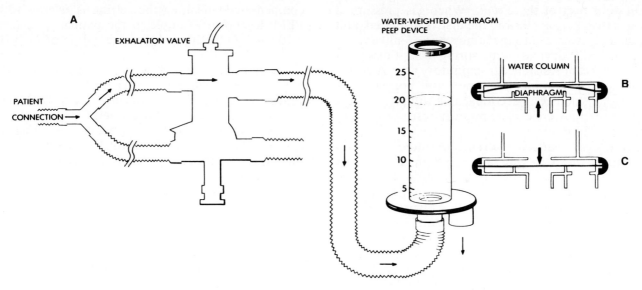

Fig. 30-27 Water-weighted diaphragm PEEP device. **A,** Typical ventilator circuit. **B,** Detail of diaphragm mechanism. When airway pressure is higher than that of the water column, the diaphragm is displaced upward and exhaled gas passes out of the circuit. **C,** When pressures equalize, the diaphragm "seats" and expiratory flow ceases. (From Kirby RR, Smith RA, Desautels DD, editors: Mechanical ventilation, New York, 1989, Churchill Livingstone.)

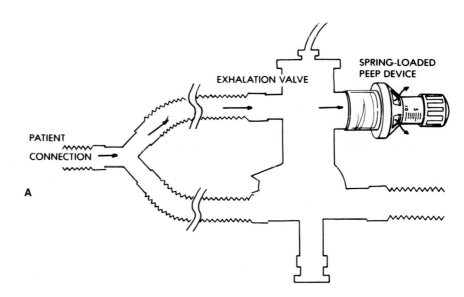

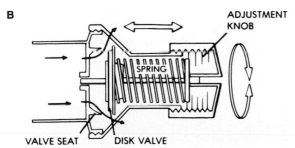

Fig. 30-28 Spring-loaded disk valve. **A,** Typical ventilator circuit. Arrows show direction of expiratory flow. **B,** Detail of spring-loaded valve. See text for description. (From Kirby RR, Smith RA, Desautels DD, editors: Mechanical ventilation. New York, 1985, Churchill Livingstone.)

spring tension on the disk, which seats against the expiratory port of the circuit. When gas pressure is greater than spring tension, the disk is displaced, and exhaled air is vented to the atmosphere. Unlike water column PEEP devices, some spring-loaded disks can offer significant resistance to expiratory flow. A device characterized by a highly elastic "stiff" spring and a seat with a small cross-sectional area will act as a flow resistor, thereby creating expiratory resistance in addition to PEEP.

Pressurized balloon valves. The most common mechanism used to generate PEEP in a ventilator circuit is by pressurization of the expiratory balloon valve. As shown in Figure 30-29, this may be accomplished using either a small venturi (Figure 30-29, *A*), an adjustable pressure regulator (Figure 30-29, *B*), or flow through a fixed orifice (Figure 30-29, *C*).[87] Like some spring-loaded disks, pressurized balloon valves can offer significant resistance to expiratory flow. A balloon valves PEEP mechanism will offer high resistance if the balloon cannot empty readily, or if the cross-sectional area under the valve is small.[87]

Electromechanical valves. More recently, ventilators have begun using electromechanical valves to generate PEEP (Figure 30-30). In this application, a electromechanical valve is linked to a pressure transducer and an electronic processing circuit. Once a PEEP pressure is set by the operator, the processor uses input from the pressure transducer to maintain the desired pressure level, either by closing or opening the valve.

Applying PEEP. PEEP may be applied in the CMV-control, CMV-assist/control, and IMV modes of ventilatory support. PEEP also may be used in conjunction with pressure support ventilation (PSV).

In order for PEEP to work well with any patient-triggered mode, great care must be taken to properly adjust the ventilator's sensitivity setting. Most ventilator sensitivity mechanisms are automatically PEEP-compensated, meaning the setting is *relative* to the PEEP level. For example, if the patient is receiving +10 cm H_2O PEEP, and a pressure drop of 2 cm H_2O was the desired sensitivity, a setting of "−2" would cause the ventilator to trigger at +8 cm H_2O PEEP.

On the other hand, a setting of "−2" on some ventilators may, in fact, mean −2 cm H_2O below atmospheric pressure. This is referred to as a *absolute* "trigger" level. In this case, a patient receiving +10 cm H_2O PEEP would have to decrease the airway pressure by 12 cm H_2O (+10−(−2)) just to trigger the machine on. Clearly, the RCP must know which of these approaches is used on the equipment used to deliver PEEP.

An additional problem when using PEEP with patient-triggered modes is the potential for ventilator self-triggering with system leaks. In these cases, a drop in system pressure due to a leak can trigger the ventilator to begin inspiration. If the leak is large, the ventilator will tend to cycle to inspiration as soon as exhalation is completed, resulting in a undesirably fast rate, and potential hyperventilation of the patient. Systems incorporating PEEP compensated demand valves overcome this problem, in part, by providing additional flow to the system to "feed" the leak, thereby maintaining PEEP pressure. However, this approach only compensates for, but does not correct the leak. Obviously, once identified, such a problem should be corrected.

Details on the management and monitoring of patients receiving PEEP, including how to establish appropriate PEEP levels, are provided in Chapter 33.

Spontaneous breath modes

Spontaneous breath modes include those in which *all* breaths are initiated and ended by the patient. Spon-

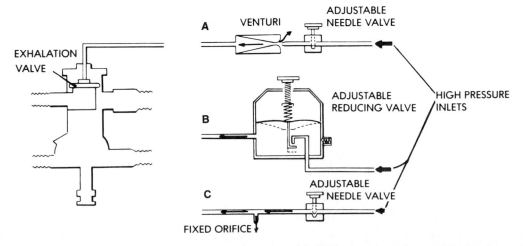

Fig. 30-29 "Trapped" pressure in exhalation valve balloon can be used to generate PEEP in the patient circuit. *A* to *C*, Three ways gas pressure within the balloon is controlled. See text for descriptions. (From Kirby RR, Smith RA, Desautels DD, editors: Mechanical ventilation. New York, 1985, Churchill Livingstone.)

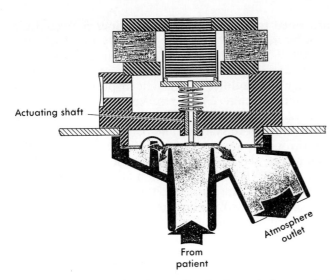

Actuating shaft

Atmosphere outlet

From patient

Fig. 30-30 Diagram of veolar ventilator's electronically controlled exhalation valve. (Courtesy Hamilton Medical, Reno, Nev.)

taneous breath modes include pressure support ventilation (PSV), continuous positive airway pressure (CPAP), bi-level CPAP or BiPAP®, and airway pressure release ventilation (ARPV).

Pressure support ventilation (PSV)

PSV is a spontaneous breathing mode consisting of patient-triggered, pressure-limited, flow-cycled breaths.[54] In this mode, each patient breath is augmented with a set amount of positive pressure.[54] At low support levels, such as 5 cm H_2O, PSV can help unload the respiratory muscles from the imposed work of breathing caused by artificial airways and/or ventilator circuitry.[88-91] At higher levels, pressure support progressively unloads the respiratory muscles from ventilatory work.[92] At pressure support levels resulting in tidal volumes of 10 to 12 mL/kg, essentially all the work of breathing is being assumed by the ventilator.[93]

Regardless of the pressure support level provided, the patient has primary control over the frequency of breathing, and the inspiratory time and flow.[54] Thus, the tidal volume resulting from a PSV breath depends on pressure level set, the patient effort, and mechanical forces opposing ventilation.

As compared to spontaneous breathing (including that occurring during IMV), clinical studies have shown that PSV can result in a decreased respiratory rate, increased VT, reduced respiratory muscle activity, and decreased oxygen consumption.[94-98] Moreover, heart rate, blood pressure, hemoglobin saturation and end-tidal CO_2 levels achieved with PSV are comparable to those realized with SIMV.[95] PSV may also change the nature of patient work during ventilatory support, improving the endurance conditioning of the respiratory muscles, and thereby facilitating weaning.[93] Lastly, PSV apparently is preferred by patients over more traditional modes of ventilatory support.[93,99]

Indications. Although research on PSV is still in progress, there are several specific clinical situations in which this mode of ventilatory support may be indicated. Situations in which PSV may represent the preferred mode of ventilatory support include the following:[54]

- Spontaneously breathing patients who require ventilatory support, and have smaller than optimal artificial airways, especially when breathing at frequencies greater than 20/min and with minute ventilations (VE) in excess of 10 L/min;

- Spontaneously breathing patients with a history of COPD or evidence of muscle weakness who requires long-term mechanical ventilation (greater than 24 to 48 hrs), and are being supported on demand flow systems in the SIMV or CPAP mode;

- Spontaneously breathing patients who exhibit clinical evidence of muscle weakness or COPD patients who experience difficulty on continuous flow IMV systems at low frequencies or CPAP.

Clinical application. PSV is a form of pressure-limited mechanical ventilation, similar in concept to IPPB.[54] PSV may be used as the sole mode of ventilatory support, or incorporated with either IMV, IMV with PEEP, or CPAP. Figure 30-31, page 852, shows the pressure, flow, and volume changes occurring during two different levels of PSV, as compared to those occurring during spontaneous breathing.

As depicted in Figure 30-31, when the patient activates a ventilator in the PSV mode, a ventilatory assist is provided at a preset pressure limit. Normally, the pressure limit is achieved and maintained until the patient's inspiratory flow decreases to some minimal level, usually 25% of the initial peak flow value.[100] At this point, inspiration ends, and the ventilator's exhalation valve opens.

Although similar in concept to IPPB, PSV is technically much more complex, requiring sophisticated, microprocessor-based electromechanical control mechanisms. Only in this manner can the flow be instantaneously adjusted according to both the preset pressure support level and the patient's changing inspiratory demands.

Continuous positive airway pressure (CPAP)

CPAP is simply a spontaneous breath mode, with the baseline pressure elevated above zero.

Indications. CPAP is an appropriate mode of ventilatory support for patients who have adequate spontaneous ventilation, but persistent hypoxemia due to physiologic shunting. However, great care must be taken in judging a patient's adequacy of ventilation. Of and by itself, a normal or low $PaCO_2$ is not

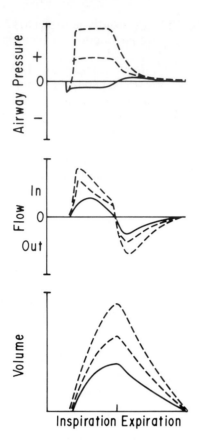

Fig. 30-31 Schema of airway pressure in the distal endotracheal tube (top panel), airflow (middle panel), and lung-volume changes (lower panel), in a spontaneously breathing patient on a mechanical ventilator. Solid lines depict an unassisted breath. Dashed lines depict two levels of pressure-assisted breaths with PSV. Note patient's continued negative-pressure effort when unassisted, compared with the brief period of such patient effort when PSV is used. (From MacIntyre NR: *Respir Care* 32(6):448, 1987)

sufficient evidence that a patient can maintain adequate spontaneous ventilation.

First, there must be evidence that the patient's ventilation is efficient, without unnecessary wasted effort. In general, ventilation is efficient if an adult patient can maintain a normal or low arterial PCO_2 with a minute ventilation less than 10 L/min. Second, there should be no clinical signs or symptoms of respiratory muscle fatigue present. Such signs and symptoms, including dyspnea, tachypnea, asynchronous or paradoxical breathing, and respiratory alternans, are discussed more fully in Chapter 33.

In the presence of refractory hypoxemia, if either or both of these conditions are not met, CMV or IMV with PEEP should be considered the ventilatory support mode of choice. The exception to these rules of thumb is the use of CPAP in infants, as discussed in Chapter 35.

Clinical application. The methods used to generate CPAP are basically the same as those previously described for PEEP. Since CPAP does not require a ventilator, a CPAP system can be very simple (Figure 30-32).[101,102] In this system, a breathing gas mixture from an oxygen blender (A) flows continuously through a humidifier (B) into the inspiratory limb of a breathing circuit (C). A reservoir bag (D) provides reserve volume if the patient's inspiratory flow exceeds that of the system. The patient breathes in and out through a simple valveless T-piece connector (E). A pressure alarm system with manometer (F) monitors the CPAP pressure at the patient's airway. The alarm system can warn of either low or high system pressure. The expiratory limb of the circuit (G) is connected to a threshold resistor, in this case a water column (H).

However, since the work of breathing increases as system pressure decreases from baseline, an ideal CPAP system should be capable of maintaining a near constant (+/− 2 cm H_2O) baseline pressure.[103,104] In order to minimize pressure fluctuations, flows through the system generally will need to be in the 60 to 90 L/min range.[105] Moreover, to accommodate inspiratory flow demands in excess of this range, a reservoir system, preferably one which is elastically loaded, should be incorporated into the system. Alternatively, lower flows—in the 20 to 30 L/min range—may be used, but only if a reservoir of 12 to 18 liters capacity is employed.[56,57] Last, the device used to develop the CPAP pressure must behave as a true threshold resistor, ideally generating *no flow resistance whatsoever* over the full range of available flows.[48]

Many newer ventilators incorporate a demand flow CPAP mode. However, all of the reservations previously cited regarding demand flow IMV apply to their use with CPAP.[62-66] Indeed, the use of these devices may be responsible for many of the reported failures of IMV or CPAP.[48,65] Of course, pressure support ventilation overcomes some of these inherent shortcomings. However, this approach merely compen-

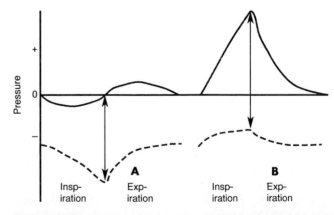

Fig. 30-32 Alveolar (solid lines) and pleural (dotted lines) pressure changes during (A) spontaneous breathing and (B) IPPB. Note the difference in transpulmonary pressure gradients (arrowed lines).

sates for the problem, rather than solving it. A better approach is flow-triggering the spontaneous breaths, which does overcome the basic problem with pressure-triggered demand valves.

Although the application CPAP to adults was originally based on the presence of an endotracheal tube, recent clinical reports have demonstrated its short-term effectiveness with a tightly fitted face mask.[106-108] Problems with administering CPAP by mask include pressure necrosis on the face, increased dead space in the mask, and gastric rupture. Aspiration of gastric contents can occur if the patient vomits when the mask is strapped to the face, but the use of a nasogastric tube and careful selection of patients can help avoid this problem. In one study, 44 awake, cooperative, spontaneously breathing adult patients with evidence of increased physiologic shunting and a normal or low $PaCO_2$ were treated with CPAP by mask, with tracheal intubation avoided in all but one.[108] In this series, no problems with gastric distension or vomiting were reported.

Bi-level CPAP or BIPAP®

Like CPAP, BiPAP® is a spontaneous breath mode, with the baseline pressure elevated above zero. Unlike CPAP, however, BiPAP® allows separate regulation of the inspiratory and expiratory pressures (Figure 30-33).[109,110]

Indications. BiPAP® was originally developed to enhance the capabilities of home CPAP systems used for treatment of obstructive sleep apnea.[110] Subsequently, BiPAP® has been successfully applied in the home for nocturnal ventilatory support to patients with both chronic restrictive and obstructive disorders.[111,112] Although these case reports show promise, as of this writing, BiPAP® has not undergone any comparative clinical trials in either the acute or long-term care settings.

Clinical application. BiPAP® is essentially a mixture of pressure support ventilation with CPAP. The BiPAP® circuit is adjusted to switch between a high inspiratory positive airway pressure (IPAP), and a low expiratory positive airway pressure (EPAP). The volume displacement caused by the difference between IPAP and EPAP contributes to the total ventilation. The duration of IPAP and EPAP can be independently adjusted, yielding a BiPAP® phase ratio, much like an I:E ratio.

Airway pressure release ventilation (APRV)

APRV represents a simple modification of CPAP.[113] Instead of the baseline pressure being maintained at a constant level, however, APRV intermittently decreases or "releases" the airway pressure from the CPAP baseline to a lower pressure level (Figure 30-34). The pressure release usually lasts 1.5 sec or less.

This intermittent pressure release allows gas to passively leave the lungs, thus helping eliminating CO_2. Thus APRV provides all the physiologic benefits of CPAP, with the additional advantage of enhanced ventilation.

Indications. Specific indications for APRV are not clear.[47] APRV was originally proposed as a treatment for severe hypoxemia; however, it has not been shown to significantly improve oxygenation in humans with acute lung injury.[114] APRV appears more effective in improving alveolar ventilation rather than oxygenation.[115,116] For this reason, APRV may be better suited as a treatment for patients with airflow obstruction and alveolar hypoventilation.[47] As with BiPAP®, controlled studies of APRV are still needed.

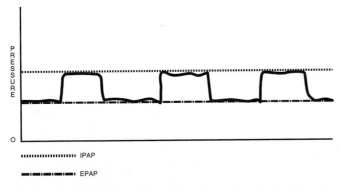

Fig. 30-33 Bi-level continuous positive airway pressure, or BiPAP®. As with CPAP, BiPAP® is a spontaneous breathing mode in which the baseline airway pressure is elevated above zero. However, BiPAP provides *separate* levels of inspiratory and expiratory positive airway pressure, referred to as IPAP and EPAP, respectively. This difference in inspiratory and expiratory pressures during BiPAP® causes gas to flow into and out of the lungs. Thus, unlike CPAP, BiPAP® provides some ventilation.

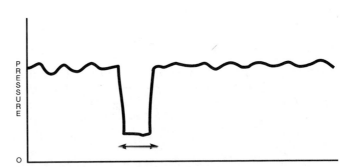

Fig. 30-34 Airway pressure release ventilation (APRV). APRV is a simple modification of CPAP. During APRV, the CPAP pressure is intermittently released or lowered for a short period, usually less than 1.5 sec (bidirectional arrow). This intermittent pressure release helps eliminate CO_2.

PHYSIOLOGIC EFFECTS OF PPV

Safe and effective application of positive pressure ventilation requires knowledge of both its beneficial and harmful effects. When artificially ventilating a patient, we deliberately attempt to change a physiologic condition, ideally from a poor to an improved status. Nonetheless, we are interfering with a level of function, even if that function is abnormal. It is thus vital that RCPs be fully knowledgeable of not only the objectives of treatment, but also the effect of intervention, including its unwanted or harmful consequences.

Generally, the effects of PPV are most apparent as they apply to the lung itself, and to the circulatory and renal systems. Effects of PPV on other elements of physiologic function are evident, though less pronounced.

Pulmonary effects of PPV

The beneficial effects of PPV on the lungs provide the basis for its use. Harmful effects, on the other hand, represent the potentially adverse consequences of applying PPV to a critically ill patient. Obviously, when PPV is indicated, it must never be withheld from a patient. However, knowledge of the harmful effects of PPV must be part of the clinical decision making process. Moreover, once PPV is started, the clinician must continuously be on guard for the many potentially harmful effects of this mode of ventilatory support.

Beneficial effects

Properly applied PPV can maintain or improve alveolar ventilation, help restore normal acid-base balance, and reduce a patient's work of breathing. Further, when used in conjunction with oxygen and supplementary manipulation of expiratory pressures, PPV can assist the clinician in normalizing or improving oxygenation. Of course, these desirable effects can be realized only when the parameters of ventilation are properly chosen and adjusted, as detailed in Chapter 32.

The relationship between improved alveolar ventilation and the correction of abnormal acid-base balance is apparent, and in these areas PPV performs some of its most important functions. More effective alveolar ventilation lowers the $PaCO_2$ and elevates the arterial pH.

PPV can also significantly reduce the work energy expended by patients with actual or impending respiratory muscle fatigue.[93,95,97,98,117] The RCP will frequently see the gratifying physical relaxation enjoyed by patients as a mechanical ventilator assumes a major portion of their work of breathing.

Obviously, to lessen the work of breathing, ventilation must be sufficient to meet the patient's needs. Otherwise, the spontaneously breathing patient will tend to "fight" the ventilator. Early studies demonstrated that inappropriately applied PPV actually resulted in alveolar *hypoventilation* and, as a result of patient struggling, an *increase* in the work of breathing of as much as 250%.[118]

In terms of improving oxygenation, early studies on the effects of simple positive pressure breathing demonstrated an elevation in arterial blood oxygen tension, even with ambient air as the source gas.[119,120] Although these findings were taken as evidence of an increased uniformity of alveolar ventilation and an improved V/Q ratio, more recent analysis suggests that this is not the case. More likely, the improved oxygenation observed in these early studies was probably the result of increased alveolar ventilation or decreased work of breathing. Indeed, as discussed in the next section, PPV can actually worsen the V/Q ratio!

On the other hand, when PEEP (with CMV, IMV, or as simple CPAP) is applied to patients with refractory hypoxemia due to physiologic shunting, dramatic improvements in oxygenation can occur. This is attributable to the recruitment of collapsed alveoli and their associated capillary beds, resulting in a decrease in the portion of pulmonary blood flow perfusing unventilated alveoli, that is a decrease in alveolar shunting.

Detrimental effects

PPV represents an abnormal means of moving gas into and out of the lungs. As such, we should expect this treatment to have harmful effects. The potentially harmful pulmonary effects of PPV include alteration in V/Q ratios, hyperventilation and respiratory alkalosis, lung tissue damage (including barotrauma), air trapping, and increased work of breathing. Other pulmonary problems, not directly associated with PPV per se, include airway complications (Chapter 22), the harmful effects of oxygen (Chapter 26), and nosocomial pulmonary infections (Chapter 4).[121-122]

V/Q imbalances. Early studies with COPD patients reported increases in the $P(A-a)O_2$ during positive pressure breathing.[118] These findings suggested that the inspired gas was not being normally distributed throughout the lung.

The early notion that PPV might alter the distribution of gases in the lungs has subsequently been confirmed with normal subjects. The reasons for this alteration in gas distribution are apparent when one compares spontaneous ventilation with positive pressure breathing.

As discussed in Chapter 11, spontaneous ventilation results in gas distribution mainly to the dependent and peripheral zones of the lungs. PPV, on the other hand, tends to reverse this normal pattern of gas distribution, directing the majority of delivered volume to nondependent lung zones (Figure 30-35,).[123] This phenomenon is due, in part, to the inactivity of the diaphragm and chest wall. While these structures actively facilitate gas movement during spontaneous breathing, their inactivity during PPV serves to impede ventilation to dependent lung zones.[48,124]

An increase in ventilation to the nondependent zones of the lung, where there is less perfusion, increases the V/Q ratio, effectively increasing physiologic deadspace. Indeed, PPV does increase deadspace by this mechanism.[125] However, the increase in P(A-a)O$_2$ that is often observed with PPV must be due to areas of *low* V/Q in the lung.

PPV lowers the V/Q ratio mainly by its effect on the pulmonary circulation. PPV can compress the pulmonary capillaries. This increases pulmonary vascular resistance and decreases perfusion volume.[126] Since the greater the pressure, the worse the effect, the least blood flow will go to the areas with the greatest pressure, contributing to a further increase in deadspace. Conversely, blood from these areas will be diverted to regions with lower vascular resistance, which happen to be those receiving the least pressure and ventilation. Thus the majority of pulmonary blood flow during PPV tends to perfuse the least well ventilated lung regions. This lowers the V/Q ratio in these areas, thereby increasing the alveolar-arterial oxygen tension gradient.[127]

A good clinical example of the effect of PPV on V/Q relationships are the changes in oxygenation that occur in patients with unilateral lung disease as their positions are shifted. In most cases, oxygenation improves significantly when the affected lung is kept up. This phenomenon is easily explained by the fact that PPV preferentially distributes gas to the nondependent areas, in this case, the superior lung.

Hyperventilation and respiratory alkalosis. PPV can result in hyperventilation, a decreased PaCO$_2$, and respiratory alkalosis.[48,128,129] As described in Chapter 12, a high pH (alkalosis) impairs oxygen unloading at the tissue level. Moreover, a high pH can cause hypokalemia. Hypokalemia can disturb electrical conduction in both the heart and skeletal muscles, resulting in cardiac arrhythmias and/or **tetany.** Low PaCO$_2$ levels also cause cerebral vasoconstriction, which, if severe, can impair perfusion to the brain.

For these reasons, mechanical hyperventilation generally should be avoided. Exceptions to this rule are conditions in which the physician desires to decrease cerebral perfusion pressures, such as may occur with closed head trauma.

Lung tissue damage and barotrauma. Over the last decade it has become apparent that PPV does direct damage to the lung. Specifically, we now know that the tidal volumes and airway pressure traditionally

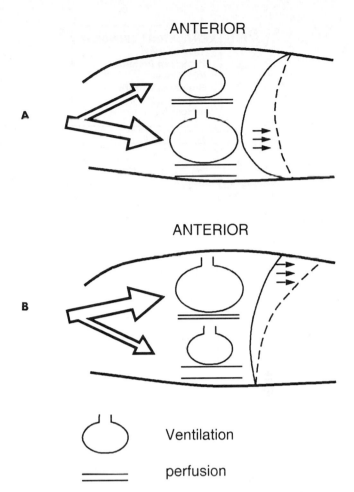

Fig. 30-35 Effect of spontaneous and positive pressure ventilation (PPV) on gas distribution in the prone subject. During spontaneous ventilation (**A**) diaphragmatic action distributes most ventilation to the dependent zones of the lungs, where perfusion is also greatest. The result is a near normal V/Q ratio. Due, in part, to diaphragmatic inactivity, PPV reverses this normal pattern of gas distribution, directing most delivered volume to the upper lung zones (**B**). An increase in ventilation to the upper lung zones, where there is less perfusion, increases the V/Q ratio, effectively increasing physiologic deadspace. At the same time, higher alveolar pressures in the better ventilated upper lung zones divert blood flow away from these areas to those receiving the least ventilation. This results in areas of low V/Q and impaired oxygenation. (Adapted from Kirby RR, Banner MJ, Downs JB, eds.: Clinical Application of Ventilatory Support, New York, 1990, Churchill Livingston.)

used to maintain adequate gas exchange in critically ill patients contributes to lung patholoy.[130,131]

Figure 30-36, page 856, outlines both the factors involved and types of injuries caused. Ventilator factors include large tidal volumes, high airway and PEEP pressures, long inspiratory times, high FiO$_2$s, and nosocomial infection. Patient factors include variations in pulmonary mechanics (compliance, resistance), pre-existing disease, surfactant defects, and host immunity.

In combination, these factors cause inflammation, increased pulmonary vascular filtration pressure, and

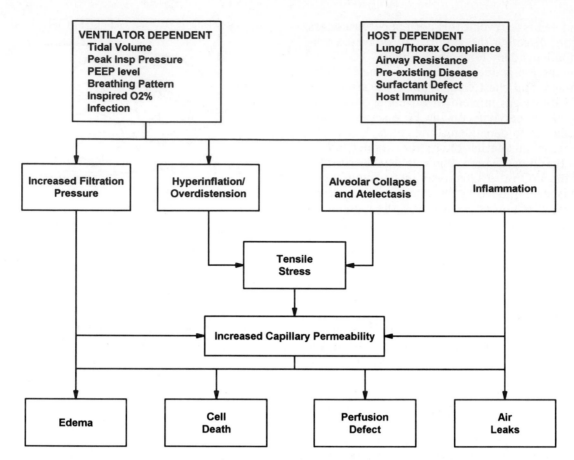

VENTILATOR DEPENDENT	HOST DEPENDENT
Tidal Volume	Lung/Thorax Compliance
Peak Insp Pressure	Airway Resistance
PEEP level	Pre-existing Disease
Breathing Pattern	Surfactant Defect
Inspired O2%	Host Immunity
Infection	

Fig. 30-36 Ventilator and patient/host-dependent factors involved in causing lung injury during ventilatory support. These factors can cause inflammation, atelectasis, overdistension or increased capillary filtration pressures. In turn, increased tensile stress on lung tissue and increased capillary permeability results in one or more of the following lung injuries: air leak, perfusion defect, edema, or cell death. (From Parker JC, et al: Mechanisms of ventilator induced lung injury, *Crit Care Med* 21(1):141, 1993.)

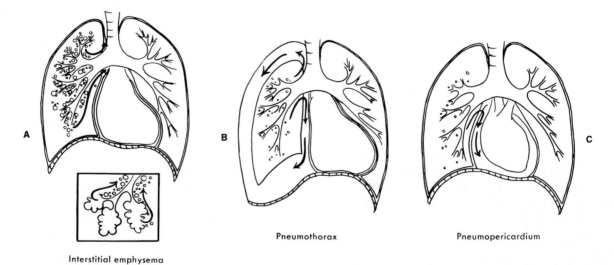

Interstitial emphysema

Pneumothorax

Pneumopericardium

Fig. 30-37 A, Pulmonary barotrauma. Ruptured alveoli are indicated in framed alveoli at bottom. Air dissects from alveoli along vascular sheaths to hilus and thence to pleural space. **B,** Pneumothorax, indicating origin of air in lung tissue and its pathway to inflate pleural space. Heart shifts to left because of high pressure created in right chest. **C,** Course of air from lung to pericardial space. Distended pericardial space causes cardiac tamponade. (From Korones SB: High-risk newborn infants, ed 4, St Louis, 1986, Mosby.)

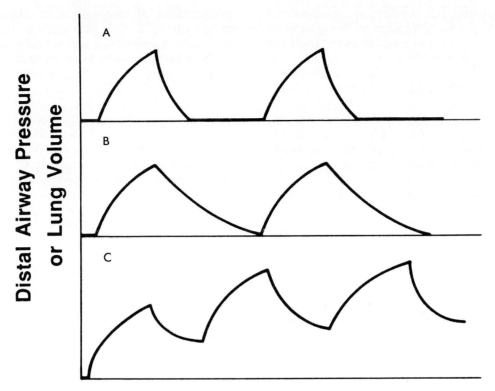

Fig. 30-38 Causes of auto-PEEP. **A,** When airway resistance is normal and expiratory time is long enough, distal airway pressure and lung volume return to normal after a positive pressure breath. **B,** high expiratory resistance prolongs exhalation to the point where air trapping begins, causing auto-PEEP. **C,** shortening the inspiratory time aggravates the problem and worsens auto-PEEP. (From Benson MS, Pierson DJ: Auto-PEEP during mechanical ventilation of adults, *Respir Care* 33(7):557-565, 1988.)

result in heterogeneous changes in lung inflation, with some areas being overdistended while others are collapsed. These inflation changes increase tensile stress on lung tissue, while inflammation and increased filtration pressures increase pulmonary capillary permeability. Fluid moves into the interstitium (edema), cells are damaged or die, and tissues rupture, causing air leaks.

In recent studies, the incidence of pulmonary air leaks was reported to range from 5% to 15% in critically ill patients receiving ventilatory support.[131] Air leaks are associated with specific traumatic injuries which are grouped under the general term *pulmonary barotrauma*. Pulmonary barotrauma include pulmonary interstitial and subcutaneous emphysema, pneumomediastinum, pneumothorax, pneumoperitoneum, and pneumopericardium (Figure 30-37).[132-135] Systemic gas embolism has also been attributed to pulmonary barotrauma.

Methods to avoid or minimize lung tissue damage and barotrauma during PPV are described in Chapter 32.

Air trapping and auto-PEEP. Air trapping represents the incomplete emptying of lung units. As described in Chapter 11, lung units prone to trapping air are those with long time constants, that is, high resistance and/or high compliance.

Air-trapping during PPV is often referred to as auto-PEEP, occult PEEP, or intrinsic PEEP.[136-138] The terms occult and intrinsic are more descriptive, because this form of air trapping can not be discerned by simply observing airway pressures, and thus often go unrecognized.

Figure 30-38, shows the causes of auto-PEEP. As long as airway resistance is normal and expiratory time sufficiently long, distal airway pressure and lung volume return to normal during PPV breaths (Figure 30-38, *A*). Alone or in combination, two factors account for the development of auto-PEEP. First, by effectively increasing the time constant of the lung, high expiratory resistance prolongs exhalation to the point where air trapping begins (Figure 30-38, *B*). Any shortening of the inspiratory time (Figure 30-38, *C*) aggravates the problem, causing a rise in both distal airway pressure and lung volume (auto-PEEP).

By increasing FRC and alveolar pressure, auto-PEEP increases the risk and severity of barotrauma. Auto-PEEP also increases the work of breathing, and decreases venous return and cardiac output. Auto-PEEP may also increase pulmonary vascular resistance.

Patients at greatest risk for developing auto-PEEP are those with high resistance who are being supported by modes which limit expiratory time. High risk patient groups include those with emphysema and asthma. High risk ventilatory support strategies include CMV, especially at high rates or in the assist/control mode, and approaches which purposefully shortens expiratory time, such as inverse ratio ventilation or low inspiratory flows. Means for detecting auto-PEEP are described in Chapter 33; techniques for preventing or minimizing auto-PEEP are discussed in Chapter 32.

Increased work of breathing. As described under beneficial effects, properly applied PPV can decrease the work of breathing. Unfortunately, this ideal is seldom realized. Many modes of ventilatory support can actually increase a patient's work of breathing.

As just discussed, any mode that causes auto-PEEP can increase the work of breathing. This increased work is due to two factors. First, hyperinflation caused by auto-PEEP stretches the diaphragm, which impairs its contractile action. Second, in patient-triggered modes, the high alveolar pressure caused by auto-PEEP must be overcome before any airway pressure change can occur. This effectively reduces machine sensitivity and response time.

Traditional assist-control ventilation (patient-triggered, flow-limited, volume cycled) can also increase a patient's work of breathing. During this mode, the inspiratory flow and trigger level are the primary factors affecting patient work.[139] In general, the less sensitive the trigger level and the lower the flow during assist-control ventilation, the greater the patient's work of breathing.[140]

Modes which include spontaneous breaths can also impose additional work on the patient. When the patient is allowed to breathe spontaneously, as with IMV or CPAP, it is possible to actually *increase* the patient's work of breathing.[48] This seeming paradoxical effect is due mainly to shortcomings in existing equipment function. Increased *inspiratory* work occurs in many IMV or CPAP circuits due to the high resistance to gas flow through some humidifiers, and the slow response time of some demand valve systems.[61-65] Increased *expiratory* work is attributed mainly to high resistance expiratory valves.[141]

The imposed work of breathing created by some IMV or CPAP systems can be avoided by using a continuous high flow of gas through a circuit with minimal flow resistance.[48] Alternatively, pressure support can be used to "unload" the respiratory muscles from the work of breathing during IMV or CPAP.[54]

Cardiovascular effects of PPV

With the close functional relationship between the lungs and heart, it is not surprising that impaired performance of one will affect the other. For this reason, the RCP must fully understand what happens to cardiovascular function when a patient receives positive pressure ventilatory support.

Early studies on the effect of PPV on the cardiovascular system all showed an early, small and transient increase in cardiac output, followed almost immediately by a significant reduction in left ventricular outflow.[142-145] In general, the reduced cardiac output seen in these cases was directly related to the amount of pressure applied. More specifically, the decrease in left ventricular output corresponded to the rise in pleural pressure that occurred with PPV.[146-148]

Spontaneous versus positive pressure ventilation

Figure 30-39 graphically compares the effects of a spontaneous inspiration with that observed during PPV. Normally, negative pleural pressure during inspiration enhances venous return, increases right atrial filling, and improves pulmonary blood flow (Figure 30-39, A). In combination, these factors increase left atrial and left ventricular filling, and left ventricular stroke volume.

When the lung is ventilated with positive pressure, pleural pressure can become positive (Figure 30-39, B). Positive pleural pressure compresses the intrathoracic veins, thereby raising the central venous (CVP) and right atrial filling pressures. As these pressures rise, venous flow back to the heart is impeded, and right ventricular preload and stroke volume decrease, as does pulmonary blood flow.[149] Initially, blood already in the pulmonary circulation is displaced into the left heart, causing a transient increase in its filling pressure and output. However, this initial effect lasts for but a few heart strokes, and, if the positive pressure is continued, flow both to and from the left heart falls.

The high impedance encountered by blood returning to the right heart causes venous pooling, mainly in the capacitance vessels of abdominal viscera.[145] This effectively removes a large volume of blood from the circulation, which can further impair left ventricular output. These interactions are magnified when pleural pressure is further increased or circulating blood volume is low.[150]

The venous impedance caused by PPV is not limited to flow coming from the abdomen. An increase in CVP can also restrict return flow from the brain. Impedance to venous return from the brain can increase the intracranial pressure (ICP), and potentially reduce brain perfusion. In combination with a fall in left ventricular output, an increase in ICP during PPV can significantly impair cerebral perfusion, and potentially result in cerebral ischemia and tissue hypoxia.

In normal subjects, the effects of PPV on cerebral blood flow are minimized by autoregulatory mechanisms that maintain cranial perfusion pressures with-

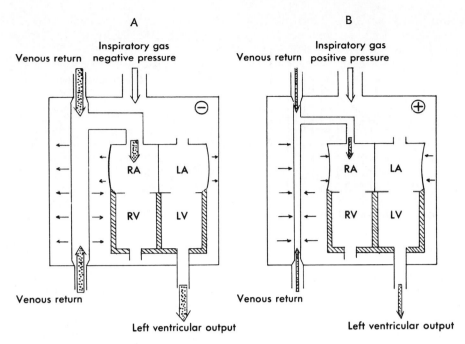

Fig. 30-39 Relationship between Ppl and cardiac output in, **A,** spontaneous and, **B,** positive pressure breathing. (Details are explained in the text.)

in a narrow range. However, patient with pre-existing cerebrovascular problems, and those already exhibiting an elevation in ICP, may be at risk for decreased cerebral perfusion with PPV. Examples include neurosurgical patients, and those with head injuries, intracranial tumors, or cerebral edema of any cause. In these patients, ICP monitoring may be necessary.

Interestingly, PPV can actually improve cardiac output in some patients. Specifically, in patients with left ventricle failure, application of PPV can increase both the left ventricular ejection fraction (EF) and cardiac output.[151] These improvements occur because PPV decreases left ventricular afterload. This phenomenon also explains why the cardiovascular status of some patients deteriorates when they are removed from positive pressure ventilation or they go from full to partial ventilatory support.

Factors affecting the cardiovascular impact of PPV

The impact of PPV on the circulatory system primarily depends on two major factors: (1) the mean pleural pressure, and (2) the subject's cardiovascular status.

Mean pleural pressure

The mean pleural pressure is the average pressure in the pleural "space." At the bedside, pleural pressure is usually measured through an esophageal balloon connected to a pressure transducer.

As an alternative to measuring mean pleural pressure, we can measure mean airway pressure instead. Mean airway pressure is linearly related to mean pleural pressure and can be used clinically to monitor pressure changes.[152]

As shown in Figure 30-40, page 860, mean airway pressure is equivalent to the area under the pressure curve taken over a time span (to include both inspiration and expiration). Because expiratory pressure is always lower than inspiratory pressure, the mean pressure falls somewhere in between. Mathematically, mean airway pressure is computed as the integral of the pressure signal over time. The many variables affecting mean pleural and airway pressures are summarized in the box below.

In terms of ventilatory support mode, the greater the ratio of spontaneous to mandatory breaths, the lower will be the mean airway and pleural pressures.

Factors affecting mean pleural pressure

- Mode of ventilatory support
- Level of positive pressure
- Duration of inspiration
- Duration of expiration
- Nature of the inspiratory waveform
- Level of PEEP
- Lungs/thorax mechanics

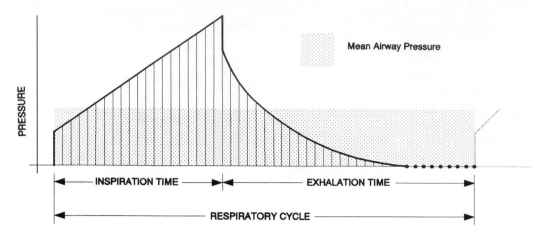

Fig. 30-40 Mean airway pressure is defined as area under pressure curve for duration of respiratory cycle. Area can be approximated by drawing equally spaced vertical lines extending from the pressure curve to line of zero pressure on time axis. When pressure curve reaches zero pressure, equally spaced dots are substituted for vertical lines. When heights of each line (including dots) are measured against corresponding pressure scale, dividing sum of pressure readings by number of readings results in mean airway pressure (shaded area).

Thus, for a given minute volume, partial ventilatory support modes like SIMV will result in a lower mean airway and pleural pressure than full support modes like CMV.

For an individual mandatory breath, the higher the peak pressure, the greater will be the area under the pressure curve, and thus the higher the mean pressures. As seen in Figure 30-41, pressure wave form *E* has the highest applied pressure over a constant time and thus exerts the greatest area and mean pressure.

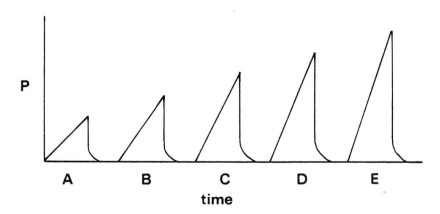

Fig. 30-41 Effect of changes in peak pressure on mean airway pressure.

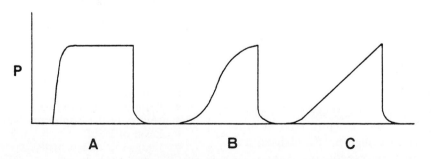

Fig. 30-42 Effect of inspiratory time on mean airway pressure.

Likewise, long inspiratory times increase the area under the pressure curve (Figure 30-42) and, with it, the mean pressures. Expiratory time has an opposite effect on mean pressures. In general, harmful cardiovascular effects of PPV are most likely to occur when the I:E is greater than 1:2.[142]

A mandatory breath's pressure waveform also effects mean pressures.[153] As shown in Figure 30-43, for a given inspiratory time, the constant pressure pattern (curve, *A*) results in the greatest area and thus the highest mean pressure. Of course, a constant pressure pattern is normally produced by a pressure generator that provides decelerating (descending ramp) flow. However, this same pattern can be produced by a nonconstant flow generator.

The effect of PEEP on mean airway pressure is simple to understand; every 1 cm H_2O applied PEEP raises the mean airway pressure by 1 cm H_2O.[154,155] PEEP's effect on mean pleural pressure is more complex, and depends on the patient's lungs and thoracic mechanics.

Of course, some of the pressure generated by a ventilator eventually reaches the alveoli, where it is transmitted across their walls to the pleural space. How much of this alveolar pressure is actually transmitted to the pleural space depends on the patient's lungs and thoracic mechanics.

In general, for a given alveolar pressure, the more compliant the lung, the greater will be the increase in pleural pressure. Thus, a patient with a disease process causing a loss of elastic tissue, such as emphysema, will be more subject to the cardiovascular effects of positive pressure than an individual with normal lungs.

In contrast, a lung with low compliance will transmit less pressure to the pleural space. This explains, in part, why high levels of PEEP may often be used with minimal cardiovascular effects on patients with low lung compliance.

On the other hand, when the compliance of the chest wall is reduced, expansion of the thorax is limited, and more alveolar pressure gets transmitted to the pleural space. Thus, patients who have normal lungs, but suffer from thoracic restriction (such as kyphoscoliosis and spondylitis) will be more subject to the cardiovascular effects of positive pressure than individuals with normal chest wall compliance.

A similar effect can occur in patients with normal thoracic compliance who actively oppose a mandatory breath by contracting their expiratory muscles (as might occur when a patient "fights" a ventilator). Contraction of the expiratory muscles effectively lowers thoracic compliance, also causing more alveolar pressure to be transmitted to the pleural space.

Finally, if resistance to airflow is high, less of the pressure generated at the airway will actually reach the alveoli. Thus, the high airway pressures common in patients with obstructive disorders are not necessarily reflected in high pleural pressures.

Cardiovascular status

The effects of moderate rises in pleural pressure on cardiac output in normal subjects are minimal. In normal subjects, as left ventricular stroke volume decreases, compensatory responses increase both the cardiac rate and the tone of the venous capacitance vessels (refer to Chapter 10). These normal responses ensure adequate blood flow and perfusion pressures.

However, should the subject already be hypovolemic, or have lost peripheral venomotor tone, cardiovascular compensation may be impossible. In these cases, even a small rise in pleural pressure may result in a precipitous fall in cardiac output.

Other effects of PPV

Renal effects

It has long been known that some patients receiving long-term PPV retain salt and water. Among critically ill patients, water retention is usually evident when rapid weight gains occur. In addition, such patients may have a reduced hematocrit, also consistent with hypervolemia due to water retention.[156,157] These early observations are now attributed to both the direct and indirect effect of PPV on renal function.

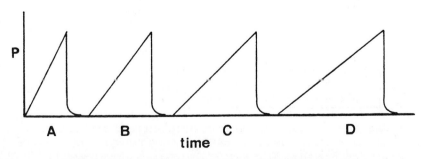

Fig. 30-43 Effect of inspiratory waveform on mean airway pressure.

In terms of direct effect, PPV can reduce urinary output by as much as 30% to 50%.[157-159] This reduced urinary output during PPV is associated with a simultaneous reduction in renal blood flow, glomerular filtration rate, and sodium and potassium excretion.[159]

Indeed, falls in mean arterial blood pressure below 75 mmHg do reduce renal blood flow, glomerular filtration rates, and urinary output. However, mean arterial pressures this low are seldom caused by PPV alone, and kidney **autoregulatory** mechanisms generally can keep renal perfusion pressures within normal limits over a wide range of arterial pressures. Moreover, since restoring cardiac output to normal does not entirely restore urinary output compromised by PPV, other mechanisms must be involved.

Early evidence suggested that the decreased urinary output seen with PPV was due to a redistribution rather than reduction in renal blood flow.[160] More recent analysis tends to refute this explanation, instead showing that impaired renal function during PPV is better associated with a decrease in intravascular volume.[161]

The indirect impact of PPV on renal function may be most important. PPV has a significant effect on the water and sodium-retaining hormonal systems. Specifically, long-term PPV increases plasma renin activity, plasma aldosterone, and **vasopressin** (urinary antidiuretic hormone or ADH).[159,162] In addition, PPV decreases **atrial natriuretic hormone** levels.[163,164]

Decreased right atrial transmural pressure is primarily responsible for the decreases in atrial natriuretic hormone, which leads to sodium retention. Similarly, increased vasopressin secretion may be enhanced by stimulation of the left atrial stretch receptors, which innervate the posterior pituitary. Increased secretion of vasopressin and activation of

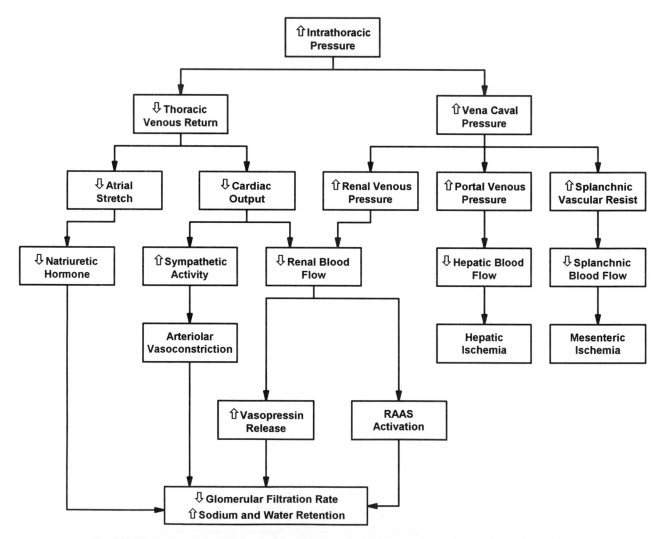

Fig. 30-44 Cardiac, renal, hepatic and splanchnic effects associated with increased intrathoracic pressure due to positive pressure ventilation. **RAAS**=renin-angiotensin-aldosterone system. ↑ =increased; ↓ =decreased. (From: Florete OG, Gammage GW: Complications of ventilatory support. In Kirby RR, Banner MJ, Downs JB: Clinical Applications of Ventilatory Support, New York, 1990, Churchill Livingstone.)

the renin-angiotensin-aldosterone system may also be stimulated by the reduction in renal blood flow associated with PPV.

Hepatic and gastrointestinal effects

Related to its effects on the cardiovascular system, are the impact of PPV on the liver and gut. Hepatic dysfunction with PPV can occur in patients with otherwise normal livers, and is manifested by an increase in serum bilirubin levels.[165] These effects appear directly related to the reduction in hepatic blood flow that occurs with PPV.[166,167] Regardless of cause, these effects are aggravated by PEEP,[168] but reversible by returning cardiac output to pre-PEEP levels with intravascular volume infusions.[169]

An increase in **splanchnic** resistance may also contribute to gastric mucosal ischemia, and helps explain the high incidence of gastrointestinal bleeding and stress ulceration in patients receiving long-term PPV.[84]

Figure 30-44 summarizes the relationship among cardiac, renal, hepatic and other effects of increased pleural pressure caused by PPV.

CHAPTER SUMMARY

Modern modes of ventilatory support cannot be used either safely or effectively unless those responsible for these applications understand both the underlying physical principles *and* physiologic effects.

All modes of ventilatory support cause lung expansion by increasing the transpulmonary pressure gradient. Negative pressure ventilation decreases body surface or chest wall pressure during inspiration. PPV raises alveolar pressure during inspiration, thus reversing normal spontaneous pressure gradients. CPAP also increases the transpulmonary pressure gradient, but solely by keeping airway pressure constant throughout the breathing cycle. Thus gas flow in and out of the lung during CPAP depends on spontaneously generated changes in pleural pressure, as with normal breathing.

The systematic description of breath types and control, phase, and conditional variables can help explain the physical action of ventilatory support devices. Most modern ventilators can provide two major types of breaths: mandatory or spontaneous. When all breaths received by the patient are mandatory, we are providing full ventilatory support. If only some breaths are mandatory, while the rest are spontaneous, the level of ventilatory support is considered partial.

For each breath, we can identify and describe four variables. The variable causing a breath to begin is the trigger variable. To describe what happens during inspiration, we must know whether the breath is pressure or flow–generated, and what limit variable is in effect. The variable causing a breath to end is the cycle variable. To describe what happens during expiration, we must know what baseline variable is in effect.

A mode of ventilation is a particular set of control and phase variables applied to either a mandatory or spontaneous breath. All modes fall within one of three major categories: (1) continuous mandatory ventilation (CMV), in which all breaths are mandatory, (2) intermittent mandatory ventilation (IMV), in which mandatory and spontaneous breaths are mixed, and (3) spontaneous modes, in which all breaths are spontaneous.

PPV is not a normal process, and is thus accompanied by a variety of unwanted or adverse consequences. These potentially detrimental effects include interference with gas exchange itself, and cardiovascular, renal, and gastrointestinal complications.

REFERENCES

1. Kreit JW, Eschenbacher WL: The physiology of spontaneous and mechanical ventilation, *Clin Chest Med* 9(1):11-21, 1988.
2. Chatburn RL: Classification of mechanical ventilators, *Respir Care* 37:1009-1025, 1992.
3. Mushin WW, Rendell-Baker L, Thompson PW, Mapleson WW: *Automatic ventilation of the lungs,* ed 3, Oxford, England, 1980, Blackwell Scientific Publications.
4. Sassoon CSH: Mechanical ventilator design and function: the trigger variable, *Respir Care* 37(9):1056-1069, 1992.
5. Report of the ACCP-ATS Joint Committee on Pulmonary Nomenclature, *Chest* 67:583, 1975.
6. Eros B, Powner D, and Grenvik A: Common ventilatory modes: terminology, *Int Anesthesiol Clin* 18:11-23, 1980.
7. McPherson SP: *Respiratory therapy equipment,* ed 4, St Louis, 1990, Mosby.
8. Sassoon CS, Giron AE, Ely EA, Light RW: Inspiratory work of breathing on flow-by and demand-flow continuous positive airway pressure, *Crit Care Med* 17(11):1108-1114, 1989.
9. Branson RD: Flow-triggering systems, *Respir Care* 39:138-144, 1994.
10. Eros B, Powner D, Grenvik A.: Mechanical ventilators: principles of operation, *Int Anesthesiol Clin* 18:23-37, 1980.
11. Pilbeam SP: *Mechanical ventilation: physiological and clinical applications,* ed 2, St Louis, 1992, Mosby.
12. Scanlan CL: Classification of mechanical ventilators V: Clinical application—inspiratory phase, Dallas, 1978, American Association for Respiratory Therapy.
13. Rattenborg CC, Via-Reque E, editors: *Clinical use of mechanical ventilation,* Chicago, 1981, Mosby.
14. Bone RC: Monitoring respiratory function in the patient with adult respiratory distress syndrome, *Semin Respir Med* 2:140, 1981.
15. Bone RC: Diagnosis of causes for acute respiratory distress by pressure-volume curves, *Chest* 70:740, 1976.
16. Boysen PG, Banner MJ, Jaeger MJ: Inspiratory times and flow wave patterns in relation to distribution of ventilation, *Anesthesiol* 63:A560, 1985.
17. Sullivan M, Saklad M, Demers RR: Relationship between ventilator waveform and tidal-volume distribution, *Respir Care* 22: 386-393, 1977.
18. Dammann JF, McAslan TC: Optimal flow pattern for mechanical ventilation of the lungs—evaluation with a model lung, *Crit Care Med* 5:128-136, 1977.
19. Johansson H: Effects on breathing mechanics and gas exchange of different inspiratory gas flow patterns in patients undergoing respirator treatment, *Acta Anaesth Scand* 19:19-27, 1975.
20. Al Saady N, Bennett ED: Decelerating inspiratory flow waveform improves lung mechanics and gas exchange in patients on intermittent positive-pressure ventilation, *Intensive Care Med* 11(2):68-75, 1985.
21. Modell HI, Cheney FW: Effects of inspiratory flow pattern on gas exchange in normal and abnormal lungs, *J Appl Physiol* 46:1103-1107, 1979.

22. Dammann JF, McAslan TC, Maffeo CJ: Optimal flow pattern for mechanical ventilation of the lungs. 2. The effect of a sine versus square wave flow pattern with and without an end-inspiratory pause on patients, *Crit Care Med* 6(5):293-310, 1978.

23. Lindahl S: Influence of an end inspiratory pause on pulmonary ventilation, gas distribution, and lung perfusion during artificial ventilation, *Crit Care Med* 7:540, 1979.

24. Smith RA, Venus B: Cardiopulmonary effect of various inspiratory flow profiles during controlled mechanical ventilation in a porcine lung model, *Crit Care Med* 16(8):769-772, 1988.

25. Connors AF, McCaffree DR, Gray BA: Effect of inspiratory flow rate on gas exchange during mechanical ventilation, *Am Rev Respir Dis* 124:537-543, 1981.

26. Tuxen DV, Lane S: The effects of ventilatory pattern on hyperinflation, airway pressures, and circulation in mechanical ventilation in patients with severe airflow obstruction, *Am Rev Respir Dis* 136:872-879, 1987.

27. Ayres SM, Kozam RL, Lukas DS: The effects of intermittent positive pressure breathing on intrathoracic pressure, pulmonary mechanics and the work of breathing. *Am Rev Respir Dis* 87:370-379, 1976.

28. Marini JJ, Rodriguez RM, Lamb V: The inspiratory workload of patient-initiated mechanical ventilation, *Am Rev Respir Dis* 134:902-909, 1986.

29. Fulheihan SF, et al: Effect of mechanical ventilation with end-expiratory pause on blood gas exchange, *Anesth Analg* 55:122, 1976.

30. Mapleson WW: The effects of changes of lung characteristics on the functioning of automatic ventilators, *Anaesthesia* 17:300, 1962.

31. Elam JO, Kerr JH, Janney CD: Performance of ventilators: effects of changes in lung-thorax compliance, *Anesthesiology* 19:56, 1958.

32. Fleming WH, Bowen JC: A comparative evaluation of pressure-limited and volume-limited respirators for prolonged post-operative ventilatory support in combat casualties, *Ann Surg* 176:49, 1972.

33. Boysen PG, McGough E: Presure-control and pressure-support ventilation: Flow patterns, inspiratory time, and gas distribution, *Respir Care* 33(2):126-134, 1988.

34. Marini JJ; Crooke PS III: Truwit JD. Determinants and limits of pressure-preset ventilation: a mathematical model of pressure control, *J Appl Physiol* 67(3):1081-1092, 1989.

35. Blanch PB, Jones M, et al: Pressure-preset ventilation (part 1): physiologic and mechanical considerations, *Chest* 104:590-599, 1993.

36. Blanch PB, Jones M, et al: Pressure-preset ventilation (part 2): mechanics and safety, *Chest* 104(3):904-912, 1993.

37. Kacmarek RM, Hess D: Pressure-controlled inverse-ratio ventilation: Panacea or auto-PEEP? [editorial], *Respir Care* 35(10):945-948, 1990.

38. Rau JL, Shelledy DC: The effect of varying inspiratory flow waveforms on peak and mean airway pressures with a time-cycled volume ventilator: A bench study, *Respir Care* 36(5):347-356, 1991.

39. Rau JL: Inspiratory flow patterns: the 'shape' of ventilation, *Respir Care* 38(1):132-140, 1993.

40. Chatburn RL: Some possible misconceptions about peak airway pressures [letter], *Respir Care* 36(8):872-874, 1991.

41. Marini JJ: Paying the piper—the linkage of alveolar ventilation to alveolar pressure [editorial], *Intensive Care Med* 16(2):73-74, 1990.

42. Sugerman HJ, Rogers RM, Miller LD: Positive end-expiratory pressure (PEEP): indications and physiologic considerations, *Chest* 62 (part 2):86s, 1972.

43. Ashbaugh DG, Petty TL: Positive end-expiratory pressure: physiology, indications and contraindications, *J Thorac Cardiovasc Surg* 65:165, 1973.

44. Kirby RR, Graybar GB, editors: Intermittent mandatory ventilation, *Int Anesthesiol Clin* 18:1-189, 1980.

45. Gregory GA, et al: Treatment of the idiopathic respiratory distress syndrome with continuous positive airway pressure, *N Engl J Med* 284:1333, 1971.

46. Lain DC, DiBenedetto R, Morris SL, et al: Pressure control inverse ratio ventilation as a method to reduce peak inspiratory pressure and provide adequate ventilation and oxygenation, *Chest* 95(5):1081-1088, 1989.

47. Sassoon CSH, Mahutte CK, Light RW: Ventilator modes: old and new, *Crit Care Clin* 6(3): 605-634, 1990.

48. Downs JB: Ventilatory patterns and modes of ventilation in acute respiratory failure, *Respir Care* 28:586-591, 1983.

49. Fairley HB: In Kirby RR, Graybar GB, editors: Intermittent mandatory ventilation, *Int Anesthesiol Clin* 18:179, 1980.

50. Weisman JM, Rinaldo JE, et al: Intermittent mandatory ventilation, *Am Rev Respir Dis* 127:641-647, 1983.

51. Harboe S: Weaning from mechanical by means of intermittent assisted ventilation (IAV): case reports, *Acta Anesth Scand* 21:252, 1977.

52. Luce JM, Pierson DJ, Hudson LD: Critical review: intermittent mandatory ventilation, *Chest* 79:678, 1981.

53. Hudson LD: Ventilatory management of patients with adult respiratory distress syndrome, *Sem Respir Med* 2:128, 1981.

54. Kacmarek RM: The role of pressure support ventilation in reducing the work of breathing, *Respir Care* 33:99-120, 1988.

55. DeSautels DA, Bartlett JL: Methods of administering intermittent mandatory ventilation, *Respir Care* 19:187, 1974.

56. Braschi A, Lotti G, Locatelli A, et al: Functional evaluation of a CPAP circuit with a high compliance reservoir bag, *Intens Care Med* 11:85-89, 1985.

57. Bishouty ZH, Roeseler J, Reynaert MS: The importance of the balloon reservoir volume of a CPAP system in reducing the work of breathing, *Intens Care Med* 12:153-156, 1986.

58. McPherson SP, et al: A circuit that combines ventilator weaning methods using continuous flow ventilation, *Respir Care* 20:261, 1975.

59. Weled BJ, Winfrey D, Downs JB: Measuring exhaled volume with continuous positive airway pressure and intermittent mandatory ventilation: techniques and rationale, *Chest* 76:166, 1979.

60. Spearman CB, Sanders HG, Jr: Physical principles and functional design of ventilators. In Kirby RR, Smith RA, Desautels DD, editors: *Mechanical ventilation,* New York, 1985, Churchill Livingstone.

61. Poulton TJ, Downs JB: Humidification of rapidly flowing gas, *Crit Care Med* 9:59-63, 1981.

62. Christopher KL, Neff TA, Bowman JL, et al: Demand and continuous flow intermittent mandatory ventilation systems, *Chest* 87:625-630, 1985.

63. Op't Holt TB, Hall MV, Bass JB, et al: Comparison of changes in airway pressure during continuous positive airway pressure (CPAP) between demand valve and continuous flow devices, *Respir Care* 27:1200-1209, 1982.

64. Henry WC, West GA, Wilson RS: A comparison of the oxygen cost of breathing between a continuous-flow CPAP system and a demand-flow CPAP system, *Respir Care* 28:1273-1281, 1983.

65. Gibney RTN, Wilson RS, Pontoppidan H: Comparison of work of breathing on high gas flow and demand valve continuous positive airway pressure systems, *Chest* 82:692-695, 1982.

66. Viale JP, Annat G, Bertrand O: Additional inspiratory work in intubated patients breathing with continuous positive airway pressure systems, *Anesthesiology* 63:536-539, 1985.

67. Spearman CB, Sanders SG, Jr: The new generation mechanical ventilators, *Respir Care* 32:403-414, 1987.

68. Hewlett AM, Platt AS, Terry VG: Mandatory minute volume. A new concept in weaning from mechanical ventilation, *Anaesthesia* 32(2):163-169, 1977.

69. Shelledy DC, Mikles SP: Newer modes of mechanical ventilation: mandatory minute volume ventilation part 2, *Respir Manage* 18(4):21-2, 24, 26-8, 1988.

70. Quan SF, Parides GC, Knoper SR: Mandatory minute volume (MMV) ventilation: an overview, *Respir Care* 35(9):898-904, 1990.
71. Thompson JD: Mandatory minute ventilation. In Perel A, Stock MC, editors: *Handbook of mechanical ventilatory support*, Baltimore, 1992, Williams & Wilkins.
72. Thompson JD: Computerized control of mechanical ventilation: closing the loop, *Respir Care* 32:440-446, 1987.
74. Higgs BD, Bevan JC: Use of mandatory minute volume ventilation in the perioperative management of a patient with myasthenia, *Br J Anaesth* 51:1181-1184, 1979.
75. Davis S, Potgieter PD, Linton DM: Mandatory minute volume weaning in patients with pulmonary pathology, *Anaesth Intensive Care* 17(2):170-174, 1989.
76. Sugerman HJ, Rogers RM, Miller LD: Positive end-expiratory pressure (PEEP): indications and physiologic considerations, *Chest* 62 (part 2):86s, 1972.
77. Gallagher TJ, Civetta JM: Goal-directed therapy of acute respiratory failure, *Anesth Analg* 59:831, 1980.
78. Ralph D, Robertson HT: Respiratory gas exchange in adult respiratory distress syndrome, *Semin Respir Med* 2:114, 1981.
79. Suter PM, Fairley HB, Isenberg MD: Optimal end-expiratory pressure in patients with acute pulmonary failure, *N Eng J Med* 292:284, 1975.
80. Kirby RR, et al: High-level positive end-expiratory pressure (PEEP) in acute respiratory insufficiency, *Chest* 67:156, 1975.
81. Ranieri VM, Giuliani R, et al: Physiologic effects of positive end-expiratory pressure in patients with chronic obstructive pulmonary disease during acute ventilatory failure and controlled mechanical ventilation. *Am Rev Respir Dis* 147(1):5-13, 1993.
82. Hurst JM, DeHaven CB Jr, Branson RD: Comparison of conventional mechanical ventilation and synchronous independent lung ventilation (SILV) in the treatment of unilateral lung injury, *J Trauma* 25(8):766-770, 1985.
83. Stow PJ, Grant I: Asynchronous independent lung ventilation. Its use in the treatment of acute unilateral lung disease, *Anaesthesia* 40(2):163-166, 1985.
84. Gregory GA: in Thibeault DW, Gregory GA, editors: *Neonatal pulmonary care*, ed 2, Menlo Park, CA, 1986, Addison-Wesley.
85. Kacmarek RM, Dimas S, et al: Technical aspects of positive end-expiratory pressure (PEEP): Part I, II and III, *Respir Care* 27:1478-1517, 1982.
86. Tyler DC: Positive end-expiratory pressure: a review, *Crit Care Med* 11:300-307, 1983.
87. Spearman CB, Sanders HG, Jr: Physical principles and functional design of ventilators. In Kirby RR, Smith RA, Desautels DD, editors: *Mechanical ventilation*, New York, 1985, Churchill Livingstone.
88. Fiastry JF, Quan BF, Habib MP: Pressure support compensation for inspiratory work due to endotracheal tubes and demand CPAP (abstract), *Chest* 89:441S, 1986.
89. Forrette TL, Cook EW, Jones LE: Determining the efficacy of inspiratory assist during mechanical ventilation (abstract), *Respir Care* 30:864, 1985.
90. Nagy RS, MacIntyre NR: Patient work during pressure support ventilation (abstract), *Respir Care* 30:860-861, 1985.
91. Linn CR, Gish GB, Mathewson HS: The effect of pressure support on work of breathing (abstract), *Respir Care* 30:861-862, 1985.
92. Brochard L, Harf A, Lorino H, et al: Pressure support (PS) decreases work of breathing and oxygen consumption during weaning from mechanical ventilation (abstract), *Am Rev Resp Dis* 135:A51, 1987.
93. MacIntyre NR. Pressure support ventilation: effects on ventilatory reflexes and ventilatory muscle workload, *Respir Care* 32:447-457, 1987.
94. Grande CM, Kahn RC: The effect of pressure support ventilation on ventilatory variables and work of breathing (abstract), *Anesthesiology* 65:A84, 1986.
95. MacIntyre NR: Respiratory function during pressure support ventilation, *Chest* 89:677-683, 1986.
96. Ershowsky P, Citres D, Krieger B: Changes in breathing pattern during pressure support ventilation in difficult to wean patients (abstract), *Respir Care* 31:946, 1986.
97. Thalman TA, Holter JF, Chitwood WR: Effects of different types of ventilatory support on total body oxygen consumption (abstract), *Respir Care* 30:859, 1985.
98. Brochard L, Pluskwa F, Lemaire F: Improved efficacy of spontaneous breathing with inspiratory pressure support, *Am Rev Resp Dis* 136:411-415, 1987.
99. Prakash O, Meij S: Cardiopulmonary response to inspiratory pressure support during spontaneous ventilation vs. conventional ventilation, *Chest* 88:403-408, 1985.
100. Campbell RS, Branson RD: Ventilatory support for the 90s: pressure support ventilation, *Respir Care* 38(5):526-537, 1993.
101. Hamilton FN, Singer MM: A breathing circuit for continuous positive airway pressure (CPAP), *Crit Care Med* 2:86, 1974.
102. Gjerde GE: A method for spontaneous breathing with expiratory positive pressure, *Respir Care* 20:839, 1975.
103. Kacmarek RM, Goulet RL: PEEP devices, *Anesth Clin N Am* 5:757-775, 1987.
104. Gherini S, Peters R, Virgilio RW: Mechanical work on the lungs and the work of breathing eith positive end-expiratory pressure and continuous positive airway pressure, *Chest* 76:251-256, 1979.
105. Civetta, J.M., et al: A simple and effective method of employing spontaneous positive pressure ventilation, *J Thorac Cardiovasc Surg* 63:312, 1972.
106. Greenbaum DM, et al: Continuous positive airway pressure without tracheal intubation in spontaneously breathing patients, *Chest* 69:615, 1976.
107. Schmidt GB, et al: EPAP without intubation, *Crit Care Med* 5:207, 1977.
108. Smith RA, et al: Continuous positive airway pressure (CPAP) by face mask, *Crit Care Med* 8:483, 1980.
109. Baum M, Benzer H, Putensen C, et al: Biphasic positive airway pressure (BIPAP)—a new form of augmented ventilation, *Anaesthesist* 38(9):452-458, 1989.
110. Strumpf DA, Carlisle CC, et al: An evaluation of the Respironics BiPAP bi-level CPAP deveice for delivery of assisted ventilation, *Respir Care* 35(5):415-422, 1990.
110. Sanders MH, Kern N: Obstructive sleep apnea treated by independently adjusted inspiratory and expiratory positive airway pressures via nasal mask. Physiologic and clinical implications, *Chest* 98(2):317-324, 1990.
111. Hill NS, Eveloff SE, Carlisle CC, Goff SG: Efficacy of nocturnal nasal ventilation in patients with restrictive thoracic disease, *Am Rev Respir Dis* 145(2 Pt 1):365-371, 1992.
112. Waldhorn RE: Nocturnal nasal intermittent positive pressure ventilation with bi-level positive airway pressure (BiPAP) in respiratory failure, *Chest* 101(2):516-521, 1992.
113. Downs JB, Stock MC: Airway pressure release ventilation: A new concept in ventilatory support, *Crit Care Med* 15:459-461, 1987.
114. Garner W, Downs JB, Stock MC, et al: Airway pressure release ventilation (APRV). A human trial, *Chest* 94:779-781, 1988.
115. Rasanen J, Cane RD, Downs JR, et al: Airway pressure release ventilation: A multicenter trial [abstract], *Anesthesiology* 71:A1078, 1989.
116. Rasanen J, Downs JR, Stock MC: Cardiovascular effect of conventional positive pressure ventilation and airway pressure release ventilation, *Chest* 93:911-915, 1988.
117. Ayres SM, Giannelli S: Oxygen consumption and alveolar ventilation during intermittent positive pressure breathing, *Dis Chest* 50:409, 1966.
118. Sheldon GP: Pressure breathing in chronic obstructive lung disease, *Medicine* 42:197, 1963.
119. Gray FD, MacIver S: The use of inspiratory positive breathing in cardiopulmonary disease, *Br J Tuberc* 52:2, 1958.

120. Motley HL: Intermittent positive pressure breathing therapy, *Inhal Ther* 7:1, 1962.
121. Strieter RM; Lynch JP Complications in the ventilated patient, *Clin Chest Med,* ed 3: 9(1):127-39 1988.
122. Pierson DJ. Complications associated with mechanical ventilation, *Crit Care Clin,* 6(3):711-24 1990.
123. Chevrolet JC, Martin JG, Flood R, et al: Topographical ventilation and perfusion distribution in the lateral posture, *Am Rev Respir Dis* 118(5):847-54, 1978.
124. Froese AB, Bryan AC: Effects of anesthesia and paralysis on diaphragmatic mechanics in man, *Anesthesiology* 41:242-255, 1974.
125. Hedenstierna G: The anatomic and alveolar deadspaces during respiratory treatment: Influence of respiratory frequency, minute volume, and tracheal pressure, *Br J Anesthesiol* 47:993-999, 1975.
126. Hedenstierna G, White FE, Wagner PD: Spacial distribution of pulmonary blood flow in the dog with PEEP ventilation, *J Appl Physiol* 47:938-946, 1979.
127. Campbell EJM, Nunn JF, Peckett BW: A comparison of artificial ventilation and spontaneous respiration with particular reference to ventilation-blood flow relationships, *Br J Anesthesiol* 30:166-172, 1958.
128. Downs JB, Douglas ME, Ruiz BC, Miller NL: Comparison of assisted and controlled mechanical ventilation in anesthetized swine, *Crit Care Med* 7:5-8, 1979.
129. Bone RC: Complications of mechanical ventilation and positive end-expiratory pressure, *Respir Care* 27:402-407, 1982.
130. Tsuno K, Prato P, Kolobow T: Acute lung injury from mechanical ventilation at moderately high airway pressures, *J Appl Physiol* 69(3):956-961, 1990.
131. Parker JC, Hernandez LA, Peevy KJ: Mechanisms of ventilator-induced lung injury, *Crit Care Med* 21(1):131-143, 1993.
132. Bone RC: Mechanical trauma in acute respiratory failure, *Respir Care* 28:618-623, 1983.
133. Bone RC: Pulmonary barotrauma complicating positive end expiratory pressure, *Am Rev Respir Dis* 113:921A, 1976.
134. Marcy TW: Barotrauma: detection, recognition and management, *Chest* 104:578-584, 1993.
135. Haake R, Schlichtig R, et al: Barotrauma. pathophysiology, risk factors, and prevention, *Chest* 91(4):608-613, 1987.
136. Pepe PE, Marini JJ: Occult positive end-expiratory pressure in mechanically ventilated patients with airflow obstruction: the auto-PEEP effect, *Am Rev Respir Dis* 126(1):166-170, 1982.
137. Benson MS, Pierson DJ: Auto-PEEP during mechanical ventilation of adults, *Respir Care* 33(7):557-565, 1988.
138. Milic-Emili J: Dynamic pulmonary hyperinflation and intrinsic PEEP: consequences and management in patients with chronic obstructive pulmonary disease, *Recenti Prog Med* 81(11):733-737, 1990.
139. Marini JJ, Rodriguez RM, Lamb V: The inspiratory workload of patient-initiated mechanical ventilation, *Am Rev Respir Dis* 134:902-909, 1986.
140. Sassoon CSH, Mahutte CK, Te T, et al: Work of breathing and airway occlusion pressure during assist-mode mechanical ventilation, *Chest* 93:571-576, 1988.
141. Hall JR, Rendelman RC, Downs JB: PEEP devices: Flow dependent increases in airway pressure, *Crit Care Med* 6:100, 1978.
142. Cournand A, Motley HL, Werko L: Physiologic studies of the effects of intermittent positive pressure breathing on cardiac output in man, *Am J Physiol* 152:162, 1948.
143. Kilburn KH, Sicker HO: Hemodynamic effects of continuous positive and negative pressure breathing in normal man, *Circ Res* 8:660, 1960.
144. Opie LH, et al: Intrathoracic pressure during intermittent positive-pressure respiration, *Lancet* 1:911, 1961.
145. Bashour FA, et al: Effect of intermittent positive pressure breathing on the cardiac output and the splanchnic blood flow, *Inhal Ther* 13:47, 1968.
146. Coonse GK, Aufrance OE: The relation of the pleural pressure to the mechanics of the circulation, *Am Heart J* 9:347, 1934.
147. Printzmetal M, Kounts WB: Pleural pressure in health and disease and its influence on body function, *Medicine* 14:457, 1935.
148. Christie RV, McIntosh CA: The measurement of pleural pressure in man, and its significance, *J Clin Invest* 13:279, 1934.
149. Rankin JS, Olsen CO, Arentzen CE, et al: The effects of airway pressure on cardiac function in intact dogs and man, *Circulation* 66(1):108-120, 1982.
150. Pinsky MR: The effects of mechanical ventilation on the cardiovascular system, *Crit Care Clin* 6(3):663-678, 1990.
151. Mathru M, Rao TL, et al: Hemodynamic response to changes in ventilatory patterns in patients with normal and poor left ventricular reserve, *Crit Care Med* 10(7):423-426, 1982.
152. Marini JJ, Ravenscraft SA: Mean airway pressure: physiologic determinants and clinical importance—Part 1: Physiologic determinants and measurements, *Crit Care Med* 20(10):1461-1472, 1992.
153. Rau JL, Shelledy DC: The effect of varying inspiratory flow waveforms on peak and mean airway pressures with a time-cycled volume ventilator: A bench study, *Respir Care* 36(5):347-356, 1991.
154. Pick RA, Handler JB, Friedman AS: The cardiovascular effects of positive and expiratory pressure, *Chest* 82:345-350, 1982.
155. Marini JJ, Culver BH, Butler J: Mechanical effects of lung distention with positive pressure on ventricular function, *Am Rev Respir Dis* 124:382-386, 1981.
156. Drury DR, et al: The effects of continuous pressure breathing on kidney function, *J Clin Invest* 26:945, 1947.
157. Sladen A, et al: Pulmonary complications and water retention in prolonged mechanical ventilation, *N Engl J Med* 279:448, 1968.
158. Murdaugh HV, et al: Effect of altered intrathoracic pressure on renal hemodynamics, electolyte excretion, and water clearance, *J Clin Invest* 39:834, 1959.
159. Annat G, Viale JP, et al: Effect of PEEP ventilation on renal function, plasma renin, aldosterone, neurophysins and urinary ADH, and prostaglandins, *Anesthesiology* 58(2):136-141, 1983.
160. Marquez JM, et al: Renal function and cardiovascular responses during positive airway pressure, *Anesthesiology* 50:393, 1979.
161. Priebe HJ, Heimann JC, Hedley-Whyte J: Mechanisms of renal dysfunction during positive end-expiratory pressure ventilation, *J Appl Physiol* 50(3):643-649, 1981.
162. Hemmer M, Viquerat CE, et al: Urinary antidiuretic hormone excretion during mechanical ventilation and weaning in man, *Anesthesiology* 52(5):395-400, 1980.
163. Leithner C, Frass M, et al: Mechanical ventilation with positive end-expiratory pressure decreases release of alpha atrial natriuretic peptide, *Crit Care Med* 15(5):484-488, 1987.
164. Andrivet P, Adnot S, et al: Involvement of ANF in the acute antidiuresis during PEEP ventilation, *J Appl Physiol* 65(5):1967-1974, 1988.
165. Hedley-Whyte J, Burgess GE, Feeley TW, Miller MG: *Applied physiology of respiratory care,* Boston, 1976, Little Brown.
166. Sha M, Saito Y, et al: Effects of continuous positive-pressure ventilation on hepatic blood flow and intrahepatic oxygen delivery in dogs, *Crit Care Med* 15(11):1040-1043, 1987.
167. Bonnet F, Richard C, et al: Changes in hepatic flow induced by continuous positive pressure ventilation in critically ill patients, *Crit Care Med* 10(11):703-705, 1982.
168. Bredenberg CE, Paskanik AM: Relation of portal hemodynamics to cardiac output during mechanical ventilation with PEEP, *Ann Surg* 198(2):218-22, 1983.
169. Matuschak GM, Pinsky MR, Rogers RM: Effects of positive end-expiratory pressure on hepatic blood flow and performance, *J Appl Physiol* 62(4):1377-1383, 1987.

CHAPTER

31

Engineering Principles of Ventilatory Support Devices*

■

Robert L. Chatburn

CHAPTER LEARNING OBJECTIVES

1. Differentiate among the power input, power conversion, control mechanism, and output components of ventilator classification;
2. Distinguish between electrically and pneumatically powered ventilators and its clinical significance;
3. Identify the two major types of drive mechanism used on mechanical ventilators, and its clinical significance;
4. Describe how mechanical ventilators use output control valves to regulate the flow of gas to the patient;
5. Apply the equation of motion for the respiratory system to identify the variables that can be manipulated during mechanical ventilation;
6. Differentiate between open and closed loop control systems;
7. Distinguish among the various types of control circuits used in modern mechanical ventilators (i.e., mechanical, pneumatic, fluidic, electric, or electronic);
8. Apply a knowledge of phase variables to examine how a ventilator starts, sustains and stops an inspiration, and what occurs between mechanical breaths;
9. Demonstrate how conditional variables are used during mechanical ventilation to modify breath types;
10. Given any standard mode of ventilation, define its functional characteristics in terms of breath types (i.e., mandatory, spontaneous), control variables, phase variables, and conditional variables;
11. Recognize the pressure, volume, and flow waveforms generated for each type of control variable;
12. Identify the various alarm functions needed on critical care ventilators and what they indicate;
13. Given any common ventilator, classify it according to the scheme introduced in this chapter.

BASIC CONCEPTS

In order to safely and effectively apply a mechanical ventilator, the respiratory care practitioner (RCP) must understand: (1) the physiologic effects of artificial ventilation, including gas exchange and pulmonary mechanics, (2) ventilator design and operation, and (3) the particular disease processes leading to the need for ventilatory support. In addition, because mechanical ventilatory support is still more of an art than science, the RCP must have experience in working with these devices.

This chapter will focus on the design principles and operating characteristics of mechanical ventilators. It will clarify terminology and outline a framework for understanding current and future ventilatory support devices.

Until recently, most authors used some version of Mushin's classic text to classify mechanical ventilators.[1] However, that system was based on ventilators common in the 1960's. This chapter presents an updated classification scheme designed to accommodate both old and new ventilator designs, including foreseen future innovations.[2-4]

*Sections of this chapter excerpted with permission from *Respir Care* 36:1123–1155, 1991, and *Respir Care* 37:1009–1025, 1992.

To understand ventilator operation, one must have some knowledge of basic mechanics. We begin by recognizing that a ventilator is simply a machine. A machine is a system of related elements designed to alter, transmit, and direct applied energy in a predetermined manner to perform useful work.[5]

We provide ventilators with energy in the form of either electricity (energy = volts × amperes × time) or compressed gas (energy = pressure × volume). That energy is transmitted or transformed (by the ventilator's drive mechanism) in a predetermined manner (by the control circuit) to augment or replace the patient's muscles in performing the work of breathing (the desired output). Thus, to understand mechanical ventilators we must first understand their four basic functions:

I. Power input
II. Power transmission or conversion

III. Control scheme
IV. Output (pressure, volume, and flow waveforms)

This simple outline format can be expanded to add as much detail about a given ventilator as desired, as shown in the accompanying box.

INPUT POWER

Ventilators convert input power from a readily available form to one which is more practical for the exacting task of ventilatory support. The most common forms of input power are electric and pneumatic.

Input power should not be confused with the ventilator's control circuit power. For example, many ventilators use pneumatic input power to drive inspiration, but electric power for the control circuit. This key difference is described in the subsequent section on control circuitry.

Electric power

An electrically-powered ventilator uses voltage from an electrical line outlet to power its drive mechanism. In the US, this line voltage is normally 110 to 115 volts **AC** (60 Hz). In addition to powering the drive mechanism, this AC voltage may be reduced and

---

Outline of ventilator classification system

I. *Input Power*
  A. Electric
    1. AC
    2. DC (Battery)
  B. Pneumatic
II. *Power Conversion and Transmission*
  A. Drive Mechanism
    1. Compressed Gas/Reducing Valve
      a. Direct Application
      b. Stored Potential Energy
      c. Indirect Application
    2. Electrical Motor/Compressor
      a. Rotating Crank and Piston
      b. Rotary Vane Compressor
      c. Linear Drive Motor
  B. Output Control Valves
    1. Pneumatic Diaphragm
    2. Pneumatic Poppet Valve
    3. Electromagnetic Poppet/Plunger Valve
    4. Proportional Valve
III. *Control Scheme*
  A. Control Circuit
    1. Mechanical
    2. Pneumatic
    3. Fluidic
    4. Electric
    5. Electronic
  B. Control Variables
    1. Pressure
    2. Volume
    3. Flow
    4. Time
  C. Phase Variables
    1. Trigger Variable
    2. Limit Variable
    3. Cycle Variable
    4. Baseline Variable
  D. Conditional Variables
  E. Modes
    1. Continuous Mandatory Ventilation
      a. Volume Controlled
      b. Pressure Controlled
      c. Dual Controlled

  2. Synchronized Intermittent Mandatory Ventilation
    a. Volume Controlled
    b. Pressure Controlled
    c. Dual Controlled
  3. Continuous Spontaneous Ventilation
    a. Pressure Controlled
    b. Dual Controlled
IV. *Output*
  A. Pressure
    1. Rectangular
    2. Exponential
    3. Sinusoidal
    4. Oscillating
  B. Volume
    1. Ramp
    2. Sinusoidal
  C. Flow
    1. Rectangular
    2. Ramp
      a. Ascending Ramp
      b. Descending Ramp
    3. Sinusoidal
V. *Alarm Systems*
  A. Input Power Alarms
    1. Loss of Electric Power
    2. Loss of Pneumatic Power
  B. Control Circuit Alarms
    1. General Systems Failure (Vent Inoperative)
    2. Incompatible ventilator settings
    3. Inverse I:E Ratio
  C. Output Alarms
    1. Pressure
    2. Volume
    3. Time
      a. High/low ventilatory frequency
      b. High/low inspiratory time
      c. High/low expiratory time
    4. Inspired Gas
      a. High/low inspired gas temperature
      b. High/low FIO_2

converted to direct current (**DC**). This DC source can then be used to power delicate electronic control circuits.

Some ventilators, notably infant and transport ventilators, have rechargeable batteries, to be used as a back-up source of power if AC current is not available. In the home care setting, battery back-up for electrically-powered ventilators is an essential life-saving feature in the event of a power outage.

Pneumatic power

A pneumatically-powered ventilator uses compressed gas to power its drive mechanism. Because compressed air and oxygen are in abundant supply in most hospitals, most modern intensive care ventilators are pneumatically-powered (Figure 31-1).

Pressure is usually defined as force per unit area, but also has the units of energy density (i.e., energy per unit volume). Thus, the more pressure available, the more useful work that can be generated. Besides being used to inflate the lungs, the input pressure can be used to power the control circuit, as is done with fluidic logic systems (discussed later).

Ventilators powered by compressed gas usually have internal pressure reducing valves, so that the normal operating pressure is lower than the source pressure. This allows uninterrupted operation from hospital piped gas sources, which are usually regulated to 50 psi, but are subject to periodic fluctuations.

The obvious advantage of pneumatically-powered ventilators is their ability to function without electricity. For this reason, pneumatically powered ventilators are ideal in situations where electrical power is unavailable (such as during certain types of patient transport), or as a backup to electrically powered ventilators, in case of power failures. In addition, pneumatically-powered ventilators are useful when electrical power is undesirable, as near magnetic resonance imaging (MRI) equipment.

As we shall see, some pneumatically-powered ventilators are electrically controlled (see following section on control mechanisms). These devices will not function properly without *both* a pneumatic power source and an electrical supply to the control mechanism.

POWER CONVERSION AND TRANSMISSION

The power transmission and conversion system consists of the drive and output control mechanisms. The drive mechanism, generates the actual force needed to deliver gas under pressure. The output control consists of one or more valves that regulate gas flow to the patient.

Drive mechanism

There are two broad types of drive mechanisms: (1) direct application of compressed gas via a pressure reducing valve, and (2) indirect application via an

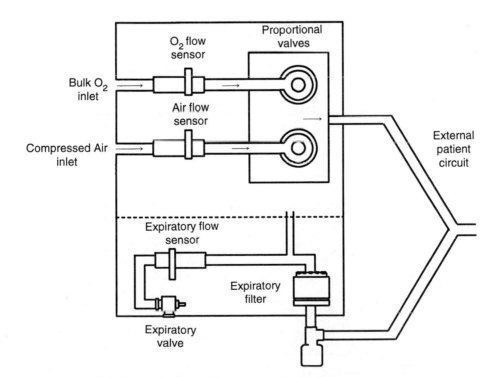

Fig. 31-1 Pneumatic circuit of the Puritian-Bennett 7200ae ventilator. After pressure reduction and flow control, the compressed gas powering the ventilator goes on to directly inflate the lungs

electric motor or compressor. A complete description of all possible drive mechanisms is beyond the scope of this chapter.[6]

Compressed gas/pressure reducing valve

When compressed gas is used as the drive mechanism, its force is usually adjusted via a pressure reducing valve. Delivery of gas to the patient's lungs is then accomplished in one of several different ways. The most common approach is for the compressed gas to directly inflate the lungs, as in the Puritian-Bennett 7200 (see Figure 31-1). Alternatively, the compressed gas may prime a weighted or spring-loaded energy reservoir, as in the Siemens Servo 900C (Figure 31-2). The potential energy that builds up in this reservoir is then used to deliver gas to the lungs. A third approach is for the compressed gas to displace a diaphragm or compress a bag or bellows. This forces the volume *inside* the diaphragm, bag, or bellows into the lungs. A good example of this indirect or "double-circuit" drive scheme is the Engstrom Erica IV ventilator which uses diaphragm displacement to deliver gas to the patient.

Electrical motor/compressor

The drive mechanism in electrically-powered ventilators is an electrical motor that drives a compressor. The compressor may use either a rotating crank and piston, a rotary vane, or a linear drive motor.

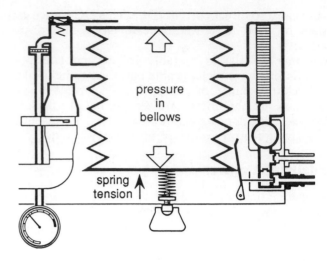

Fig. 31-2 Drive mechanism consisting of a bellows under spring tension (Siemens 900C).

Rotating crank and piston. An electric motor with a rotating crank and piston rod is sometimes referred to as an "**eccentric** wheel." Figure 31-3 shows a schematic of a ventilator using this drive mechanism (Emerson IMV). Air enters the system to the left via a one-way inlet valve, then mixes with oxygen in a reservoir. A pressure relief valve and filter protect against **overpressurization** and contamination. During the downward stroke of the piston, the gas mixture is drawn into the cylinder via a one-way inlet valve.

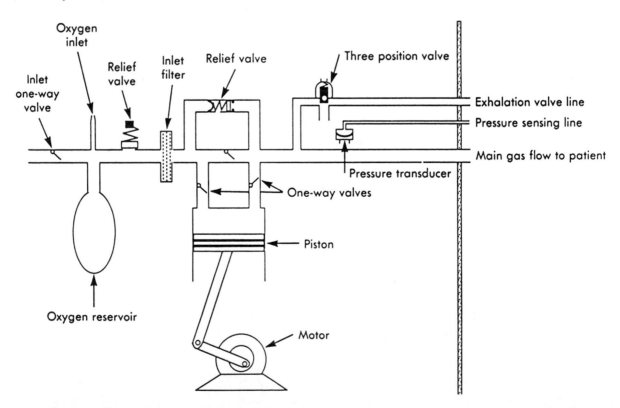

Fig. 31-3 Drive mechanism consisting of eccentric wheel, piston rod, and piston (Emerson IMV). See text for details.

On the upward stroke of the piston, pressurized gas is forced out of the cylinder through a one-way outlet valve, then into the ventilator circuit and patient's lungs.

A ventilator using a rotary driven piston produce characteristic flow and pressure patterns (Figure 31-4). Due to the motion of the eccentric wheel, gas flow out of the cylinder occurs in an accelerating, then decelerating, fashion. This is termed a sinusoidal pattern, meaning "producing a sine wave." We thus refer to this flow pattern as a sine-wave, although it is more precisely one half of a sine wave. Because a sine-wave flow pattern closely resembles that occurring during spontaneously breathing, it theoretically may offer some advantages in selected patients.[7,8]

The resulting airway pressure pattern coincides with the filling rate established by the changes in flow—initially rising slowly, then rapidly, then slowly again. This S-shaped or *sigmoid* pressure pattern is also characteristic of a ventilator using a rotary driven piston.

The Emerson 3-PV, Emerson IMV, and Bennett Companion 2800 are a good example of ventilators using a rotating crank and piston and producing a sine-wave flow pattern. As we shall see, other mechanisms can produce or approximate a sine-wave flow pattern, including microprocessor control.

Rotary Vane Compressor. A rotary vane compressor consists of an electric motor with vanes attached to the motor's shaft. The vanes, acting like blades of a fan, turn rapidly inside a cylinder. The shape and motion of the vanes draws gas into a chamber from which it is expelled under pressure. The Bennett MA-1 drive mechanism is based on a rotary vane compressor, as is the backup air source for the Bear-2.

Linear Drive Motors. A linear drive motor produces linear (as opposed to circular) motion of a piston or diaphragm. For example, an electric motor

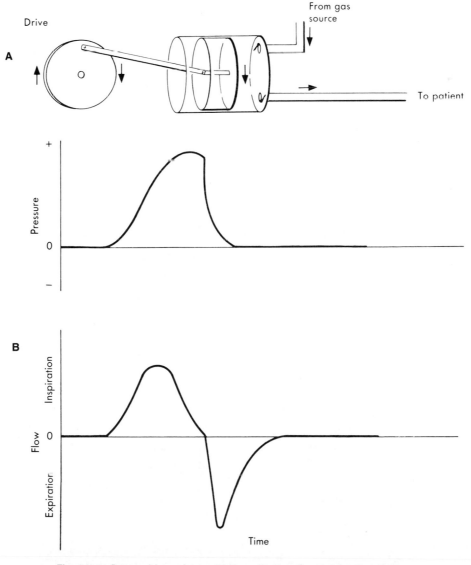

Fig. 31-4 Rotary-driven piston power application. See text for description.

combined with a screw drive produces a linear motion of the piston rod (Figure 31-5). Depending on the control circuit, the piston can be driven forward at either a constant rate (as in the Sechrist 2200) or a variable rate. The linear drive motor is particularly versatile because it can produce a wide variety of easily controllable output waveforms.

Output control valve

The output control valve regulates the flow of gas to the patient. It may be a simple on/off valve (also called an exhalation valve), as in the Bennett MA-1. Alternatively, the output control valve can control the shape of the output waveform, as in the Siemens Servo 300. Commonly used output control valve includes the pneumatic diaphragm, pneumatic poppet valve, **electromagnetic** poppet/plunger valve, and proportional valve.

Pneumatic diaphragm

Usually an on/off type of valve, this device uses a flexible diaphragm or membrane (e.g., a "mushroom" valve) to divert gas from one pathway to another. These are commonly referred to as "exhalation valves." Unfortunately, this is a misnomer, because these valves are primarily responsible for diverting gas into the patient's lungs during inspiration. However, they may also be responsible for slowing exhalation (expiratory retard) or maintaining PEEP. Pneumatic diaphragms are used on many ventilators, such as the Bennett MA-1, MA-2, Bear 2 and 3, and Newport Wave. Figure 31-6 shows the pneumatic diaphragm exhalation valve with PEEP attachment used on the Bennett MA-1.

Pneumatic poppet valve

This type of valve is similar to a solenoid valve except that it uses a small pneumatic pressure (e.g., a fluidic signal) to control a larger pneumatic pressure. They are particularly useful when electronic signals are inconvenient or hazardous (e.g., Omni-Vent MRI).

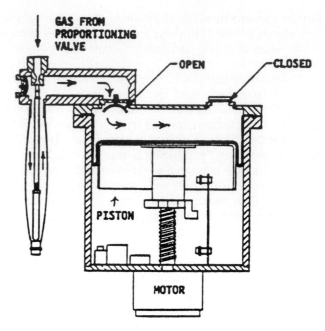

Fig. 31-5 Drive mechanism consisting of a piston rod, and piston driven by a screw mechanism (Sechrist 2200).

Electromagnetic poppet/plunger valves

This device, also called a **solenoid,** uses an electromagnet to open or close a valve, thereby controlling pressure or flow. Examples include the electronic interface valve (e.g., Infrasonics Infant Star, which uses a set of valves to approximate various pressure or flow waveforms), the plunger (e.g., Bear Cub exhalation manifold), and the pinch valve (e.g., Bunnell Life Pulse Jet Ventilator).

Proportional valve

Also known as a mass flow control valve, this device is similar to the solenoid in that it is operated by an electromagnet. The major difference is that rather than simply turning flow on or off, a proportional valve can shape the flow waveform during inspiration by changing the diameter of its outflow port. Thus a proportional valve can control both the magnitude and shape of the flow waveform. Propor-

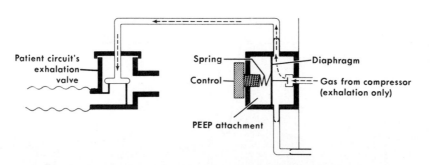

Fig. 31-6 Functional diagram of PEEP attachment for MA-1 ventilator.

tional valves are used in most current model ICU ventilators, including the Puritian-Bennett 7200a, Siemens Servo 900C and 300, Bird 8400 ST, and Hamilton Veolar. Figure 31-7 shows three examples of proportional valves used in modern ventilators.

It should be remembered that many ventilators use more than one output control valve. In particular, one valve is often used to direct flow into the patient's airway (e.g., a mushroom valve) while another may be used to shape the waveform (e.g., a proportional valve).

CONTROL SCHEME

Knowledge of the mechanics of breathing provides a good foundation for understanding how ventilators work. The study of mechanics deals with forces, displacements, and rates of displacement. In physiology, force is measured as pressure (pressure = force ÷ area), displacement is measured as volume (volume = area × displacement) and the relevant rate of displacement is measured as flow (e.g., average flow = volume ÷ time).

Specifically, we are interested in the pressure needed to drive gas into the airway and inflate the lungs. The mathematical expression that relates these variables is known as the equation of motion for the respiratory system:[9,10]

$$\frac{\text{muscle}}{\text{pressure}} + \frac{\text{ventilator}}{\text{pressure}} = \frac{\text{volume}}{\text{compliance}} + (\text{resistance} \times \text{flow}) \quad (1)$$

$$\frac{\text{muscle}}{\text{pressure}} + \frac{\text{ventilator}}{\text{pressure}} = \frac{\text{elastic}}{\text{load}} + \frac{\text{restrictive}}{\text{load}} \quad (1A)$$

In the simplified form (equation 1A), muscle pressure is equivalent to the transrespiratory pressure (airway pressure minus body surface pressure) generated by the muscles during inspiration. Ventilator pressure is the airway pressure generated by the ventilator during inspiration. The combined muscle and ventilator pressure cause gas to flow into the lungs.

Pressure, volume, and flow change with time and hence are variables. Compliance and resistance together constitute the impedance or load against which the muscles and ventilator do work. The elastic load is the pressure needed to overcome the elastance (or compliance) of the lungs and thorax. The resistive load is the pressure needed to overcome frictional resistance, including both airway resistance (anatomic *and* artificial), and tissue viscous resistance.

Note that pressure, volume, and flow are all measured relative to their baseline, or end-expiratory values. This means that the pressure needed to inflate the lungs is measured as the change in airway pressure *above* PEEP. This is the reason, for example, that pressure support levels are measured relative to PEEP. Thinking of ventilator pressure as simply airway pressure limits your understanding of the mechanics involved in breathing.

Volume is measured as the change in lung volume above FRC. The change in lung volume during the inspiratory period is the tidal volume. Flow is measured relative to its end-expiratory value (usually zero). When pressure, volume, and flow are plotted as functions of time, characteristic waveforms for volume controlled ventilation and pressure controlled ventilation are produced (Figure 31-8, page 874).

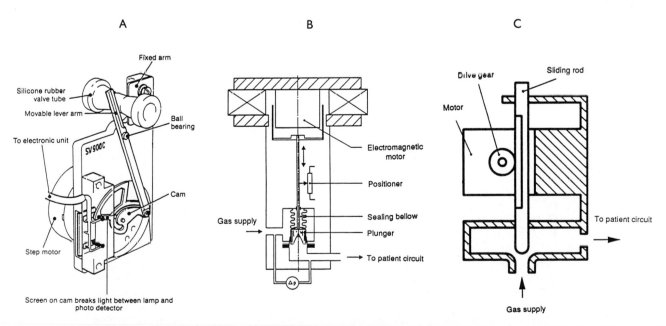

Fig. 31-7 Proportional valves from **A** Siemens 900C, **B** Bennett 7200, **C** Bird 8400 ST.

Notice that if the patient's ventilatory muscles are not working, muscle pressure equals zero. In this case, the ventilator must generate all of the force needed to provide the inspiratory flow and deliver the tidal volume. Under these conditions, we are providing *full ventilatory support*. On the other hand, if ventilator pressure is zero, airway pressure does not rise above baseline during inspiration. In this case, no ventilatory support is provided and the ventilatory muscles must assume all responsibility for breathing (*spontaneous breathing*). In between these two extremes are an infinite number of combinations of some muscle and some ventilator pressure, collectively called *partial ventilatory support.*

The mathematical model of ventilator-patient interaction suggests the proper use of the word "assist", which is another frequently confused concept. Using the equation of motion, whenever ventilator pressure rises above baseline during inspiration, the ventilator is doing some work on the patient. Whenever the

ventilator performs work, the patient is being assisted by the ventilator. Do not confuse this meaning of the word assist with specific names of modes of ventilation (e.g., Assist/Control). Ventilator manufacturers often coin terms for modes without regard to consistency or theoretical relevance.

In the equation of motion, any one of the three primary variables (pressure, volume, or flow) can be predetermined. We call a variable that is determined or set in advance an *independent variable*. When we set one variable as the independent variable, the other two become dependent variables.

This is precisely analogous to the way ventilators operate. For example, during pressure controlled ventilation (PCV), pressure is the independent variable. In this case, the shape of the volume and flow waveforms depend on the shape of the pressure waveform, and the mechanic properties of the respiratory system.

Conversely, during volume controlled ventilation,

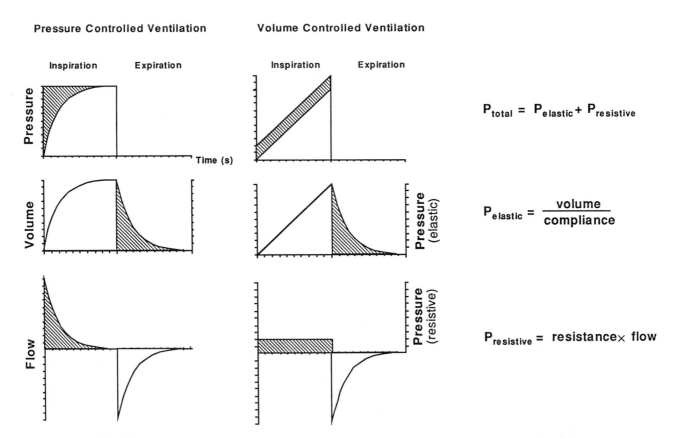

$$P_{total} = P_{elastic} + P_{resistive}$$

$$P_{elastic} = \frac{volume}{compliance}$$

$$P_{resistive} = resistance \times flow$$

Fig. 31–8 Characteristic waveforms for pressure-controlled and volume-controlled ventilation. The order of presentation is pressure, volume, and flow, according to the order specified by the equation of motion. Note that the volume waveform has the same shape as the transthoracic or lung pressure waveform (ie, pressure due to elastic recoil). The flow waveform has the same shape as the transairway pressure waveform (ie, pressure due to airway resistance). The shaded areas represent pressures due to flow resistance, the open areas represent pressure due to elastic recoil.

we specify the shape of the flow waveform. In this case, flow is the independent variable, with the shape of the volume and pressure waveforms being dependent on it. In these cases, the pressure waveform shape also depends on the patient's resistance and compliance.

Control variables

Given that: (1) there are three primary variables in the equation of motion that we can manipulate, and (2) only one of these variables can be controlled at a time, a ventilator must function as either a pressure, volume, or flow controller. In simple terms, then, a ventilator is just a machine that controls either the airway pressure, inspired volume, or inspiratory flow waveform. Time is implicit in the equation of motion and in some cases, will serve as a control variable.

Ventilators can combine control schemes to create complex modes. For example, the Bennett 7200a ventilator can mix flow-controlled breaths with pressure-controlled breaths in the "SIMV+pressure support" mode. The Bear 1000 can mix pressure control with volume control in its pressure augment mode. The Siemens Servo 300 can adjust the level of pressure control automatically to achieve a preset target volume.

The great flexibility of today's ventilators is achieved at the expense of added complexity. Thus, when evaluating ventilator performance, it is important to have simple and clear-cut criteria for deciding which control variables are in effect (Figure 31-9). Note that if the waveforms for all three variables are not predetermined (i.e., none of the variables are independent), then the ventilator controls only the timing of inspiration and expiration phase, and is thus a time controller.

Pressure

The equation of motion (equation 1) tells us that if the ventilator is a pressure controller, then the left side of the equation (i.e., ventilator pressure as a function of time) will be determined by the ventilator settings and will be unaffected by changes in parameter values on the right side (i.e., compliance and resistance).

If the control variable is pressure, the ventilator can control either the airway pressure (causing it to rise above body surface pressure for inspiration) or the pressure on the body surface (causing it to fall below airway opening pressure for inspiration). This is the basis for classifying ventilators as being either positive or negative pressure types.* For example, the Newport Wave would be classified as a positive pressure con-

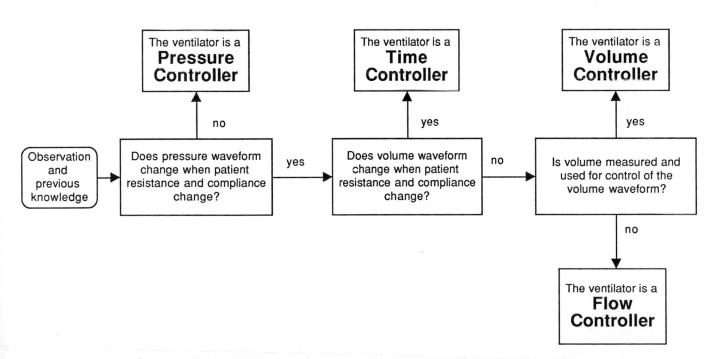

Fig. 31-9 Criteria for determining the control variable during a ventilator assisted inspiration.

troller which generates a rectangular pressure wave-form, while the Emerson Iron Lung is a negative pressure controller which produces a quasi-sinusoidal pressure waveform.

Volume

If the pressure waveform varies as the load imposed by the patient's respiratory system changes, we then examine the volume waveform. If the volume wave-form remains unchanged with changing loads, the device may be either a volume or flow controller (this is because volume and flow waveforms are functions of each other—volume is the integral of flow and flow is the derivative of volume).

To qualify as a true volume controller, a ventilator must: (1) maintain a consistent volume waveform in the face of a varying load, and (2) measure volume and use this signal to control the volume waveform. Volume can be measured directly only by the dis-placement of a piston, bellows, or similar device. With a piston or bellows, controlling the excursion of the device automatically controls the volume wave-form.

Alternatively, the ventilator could electronically convert a flow signal to a volume signal. Note that although some ventilators like the Siemens Servo 900C, the Bennett 7200, the Bear-1000, and the Hamilton Veolar display volume readings, they all actually measure and control flow and calculate vol-ume for displays. Thus, they are all flow controllers unless they are operated in a pressure-control mode (e.g., during pressure support ventilation). An exami-nation of a ventilator's schematic diagrams and oper-ator's manual should provide the information neces-sary to decide whether volume or flow is being measured.

Flow

If the volume change (i.e., tidal volume) remains consistent when compliance and resistance are varied, and if volume change is *not* measured and used for control, the ventilator is classified as a flow controller. The simplest example of open loop flow control in a ventilator consists of a pressure regulator supplying gas to a flowmeter such as found in infant ventilators. An infant ventilator becomes a flow controller rather than a pressure controller if the airway pressure does not reach the set pressure limit.[11] However, the flow-meter is usually not back-pressure compensated

and will vary its output slightly in the face of a changing load. In contrast, the Siemens Servo 900C measures flow and adjusts the output control valve (i.e., the inspiratory scissors valve) accordingly. It can maintain a more consistent inspiratory flow wave-form as the load changes.

Time

Suppose that both pressure and volume are affected by changes in lung mechanics. Then the only form of control is that of defining the ventilatory cycle, or alternating between inspiration and expiration. Therefore, the only variables being controlled are the inspiratory and expiratory times. This situation arises in some forms of high frequency ventilation, where even the designation of an inspiratory and expiratory phase becomes somewhat obscure.

Open versus closed–loop control

Having said what parameters can be controlled, we can now explore how they are controlled. In discuss-ing respiratory mechanics, we have thus far used the term 'system' without definition. A system is a collec-tion of elements that interact according to some particular process or function. Specifically, we are interested in understanding the relation between the input and the output of the system. This understand-ing can help us control system behavior.

We can control a system to achieve a desired output in two different ways:[12]
1. Select an input and wait for an output with no interference during the waiting period. This is known as open-loop control.
2. Select an input, observe the trend in the output, and modify the input accordingly to get as close as possible to the desired output. This is called closed-loop, feedback, or servo-control.

To perform closed-loop control, the output must be measured and compared to a reference value. In ventilators, a transducer and electronic circuitry are needed to perform automatic closed loop control. Closed-loop control provides the advantage of a more consistent output in the face of unanticipated distur-bances. In the case of ventilators, disturbances that might affect function include condensation or leaks in the patient circuit, endotracheal tube obstructions, and changes in respiratory system resistance and compliance.

Control circuit

In order to allow the operator to control pressure, volume, flow, or time, a ventilator must have a control circuit. The control circuit is the subsystem respon-sible for controlling the drive and output control mechanisms. A ventilator control circuit may have

---

*The terms "positive pressure ventilator" and "negative pressure ventilator" obscure the fact that both devices generate a positive transrespiratory pressure. Positive pressure ventilators cause airway pressure to rise above atmospheric pressure (resulting in positive gauge pressure) while negative pressure ventilators cause body surface pressure to fall below atmospheric pressure (resulting in negative gauge pressure). Gauge pressure is defined as pressure measured relative to atmospheric pressure.

mechanical, pneumatic, fluidic, electric, or electronic components. Most modern ventilators combine two or more of these subsystems to provide user control.

Mechanical control

Mechanical control circuits use devices such as levers, pulleys, and cams. These types of circuits were used in the early manually operated ventilators illustrated in history books.[13]

Pneumatic control

Pneumatic control is provided by using pressurized gas itself to regulate the parameters of ventilation. Pneumatically controlled ventilators rely heavily on pressure regulators, needle valves, jet entrainment devices, pressurized gas cartridges, and balloons-valve systems to control ventilator function. The original Bird Mark 7 and 8 and Bennett PR-I and PR-II ventilators depend primarily on pneumatic control.

Fluidic control

Like pneumatically controlled ventilators, fluidically controlled devices use pressurized gas to regulate the parameters of ventilation. However, instead of simple pressurized valves and timers, fluidically-control devices use specialized fluidic "switches" or gates. Several fluid logic components and a simple fluidic ventilator are shown in Figure 31-10, page 878.

Typically, these fluid logic components are combined together into an integrated fluidic logic circuit, which functions like an electronic circuit board.[14] A fluidic logic circuit can provide control over all key ventilator parameters, including pressure, volume, flow, and time. Examples of ventilators using fluidic logic control circuits are the Sechrist IV-100B, Bio-Med MVP-10, and Monaghan 225/SIMV.

The advantage of fluidic control is simple. There are no moving parts to wear out. In addition, since gas flows through the circuit (instead of electrons), fluidic circuits are immune to failure from surrounding electromagnetic interference, as can occur around MRI equipment.

On the other hand, fluidic logic circuits waste a portion of their source gas in controlling ventilator functions. This source gas consumption can be substantial, amounting to as much as 8 to 10 L/min. Although not a key consideration when a bulk supply is available, such gas loss can be critical during patient transport.

Electric control

Electric control circuits use only simple switches, **rheostats** (or **potentiometers**), and magnets to control ventilator operation. One example of a completely electrically controlled ventilator would be the Emerson Iron Lung.

Electronic control

Electronic control circuits use devices such as resistors, capacitors, diodes, and transistors as well as combinations of these components in the form of integrated circuits.

Electronic control, especially that incorporating preprogrammed microprocessors, has quickly become the predominant means of controlling ventilator function. There are two primary reasons for this growth in the use of electronic control mechanisms. First, like fluidic control, electronic control of ventilator parameters can be accomplished with a minimum of moving parts. This increases reliability. Second, electronic control using microprocessors provides functions heretofore unavailable on mechanical ventilators. This increases versatility.

Although there has been a significant evolution in electrical components, the basic concept underlying this type of control mechanism has remained essentially the same over the years. As shown in Figure 31-11 on page 879, an electronic control mechanism consists of three key components: a sensor, a processor, and an effector. The *sensor,* using either electrical or electromechanical means, measures a given parameter, such as pressure or flow. The *processor* receives this signal and interprets it according to either preprogrammed instructions or those provided by operator input. By comparing the sensor signal to the internal or operator provided instructions, the processor determines if an alteration is needed in the *effector* device, usually an electromechanical valve, alarm, or indicator system. If an alteration is needed, the processor sends the appropriate signal to the effector, while continuing to monitor the impact of this change via the sensory loop.

A simple example of this type of electronic control is the pressure limit mechanism on the MA-1 ventilator, as depicted in Figure 31-12, page 879. The sensor, in this case an electromechanical diaphragm, continually monitors airway pressure. The instructions for setting the pressure limited are provided by the operator via a manual adjustment of the diaphragm tension. When the pressure exceeds this diaphragm tension, an electrical circuit is closed, and a signal is sent to the processor, in this case a simple circuit card. Once this input signal is received, the processor immediately sends outputs signals to several effectors, namely the audible and visual alarm indicators, and the main solenoid switch. The main solenoid switch closes, thereby immediately ending the inspiratory phase.

In this example, the processor is simply serving as a "dumb" relay, transferring the input signal from the sensor to the effector. More recently, "smart" processors have been incorporated into mechanical ventilator control systems. Using preprogrammed computer chips, these microprocessors can not only receive and forward signals, but may also interpret and indepen-

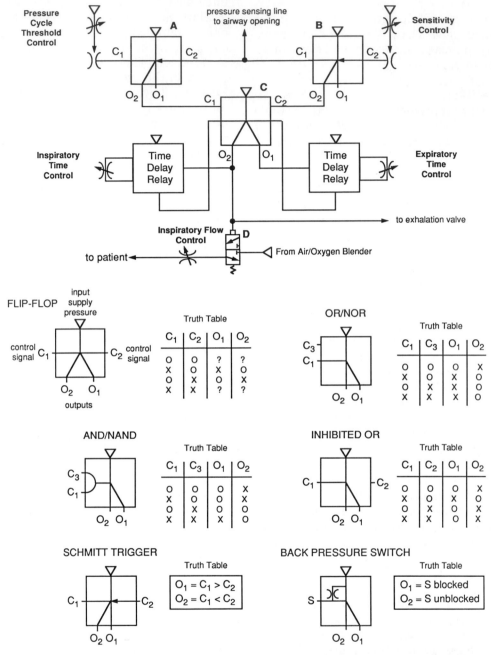

Fig. 31-10 Top A simple time or pressure triggered, pressure cycled ventilator control circuit composed of fluidic components. The circuit consist of two Schmitt triggers *(A and B)*, a flip-flop *(C)*, two timers, a three-way pneumatic valve *(D)*, and needle valves to adjust the sensitivity and peak pressure. The sensitivity valve adjusts a flow of gas through an entrainment device which creates a negative reference pressure. When the patient inspires, airway pressure drops to this threshold, which switches the output from 01 to 02. This signal is input to the flip-flop *(C)* which then outputs a signal to the exhalation valve and the pneumatic valve, causing gas to flow to the patient. When airway pressure rises to the pressure cycling threshold, Schmitt trigger A sends a signal that causes the flip-flop to turn off inspiration and depressurize the exhalation valve. This results in Pressure Controlled Continuous Mandatory Ventilation. If the patient does not trigger inspiration, the inspiratory timer will. If the cycling pressure is set relatively high, inspiration will be time cycled by the expiratory timer, allowing Volume Controlled CMV. Bottom Illustrations of fluidic components used in some ventilator control circuits.

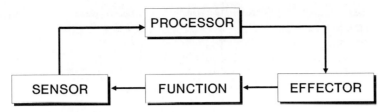

Fig. 31-11 Components of an electronic control mechanism.

dently act on this information, sometimes making *thousands* of minute adjustments in the effector system per second!

Phase variables

Mapleson proposed that a ventilatory cycle be divided into four phases: the changeover from expiration to inspiration, inspiration, the changeover from inspiration to expiration, and expiration.[1] This convention is useful for examining how a ventilator starts, sustains, and stops an inspiration, and what occurs between mechanical breaths.

In each phase, a particular variable, a *phase variable* is measured and used to start, sustain, and end the phases.[15] There are four phase variables: the trigger variable, the limit variable, the cycle variable, and the baseline variable. The criteria for determining phase variables are defined in Figure 31-13, on page 880.

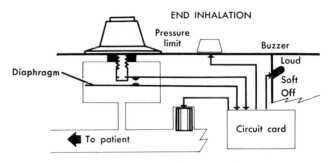

Fig. 31-12 Functional diagram of pressure limit mechanism for MA-1 ventilator. (Courtesy Puritan-Bennett Corp., Los Angeles.) (From McPherson SP: Respiratory therapy equipment, ed 4, St Louis, 1989, Mosby.)

Trigger variable

Inspiration begins when some measured variable reaches a preset value. Thus, the variable of interest is considered an initiating or *trigger variable*. The most common trigger variables are time (when the ventilator starts a breath according to a set rate, independent

---

■ MINI **C**LINI ■

31-1

Problem: A RCP is caring for a critically ill patient who is intubated and requires mechanical ventilatory support. The patient is being ventilated with a Puritan Bennett (PB) 7200 ventilator set in the Intermittent Mandatory Ventilation (IMV) mode. During a routine patient and ventilator assessment, the RCP observes that the patient is making spontaneous efforts which are not being detected by the ventilator. What must the RCP understand about a ventilator's triggering mechanism in order to properly troubleshoot the problem?

Discussion: Failure for a ventilator to trigger in response to a patient's spontaneous effort can be due to multiple causes. The most common variables which control a ventilators ability to activate inspiration are time and pressure. The later variable is

Importance of Setting a Proper Trigger Level

applicable to this current problem since the ventilator should have been able sense the patient's inspiratory effort. The amount of patient work required to trigger a breath is proportional to the volume inspired from the patient ventilator circuit before triggering and the pressure drop from baseline. If the ventilator's sensitivity control is improperly set (that is, less sensitive to patient effort) readjustment of the preset level of inspiratory

triggering effort would be indicated. Should the problem persist despite a properly set sensitivity setting, intervention on the part of the RCP might include examining other methods of decreasing the amount of patient work required to trigger the ventilator. Certain ventilators are capable of providing a flow triggering mechanism versus the traditional pressure triggered variable. The flow triggering feature attempts to avoid excessive respiratory muscle work by allowing for a more sensitive means of detecting spontaneous inspiratory effort. Thus, a change in inspiratory flow is sensed by the ventilator and this information is used as the mechanism which activates inspiration. Since the PB 7200 offers a flow triggering option, the RCP might wish to use this feature and assess patient response.

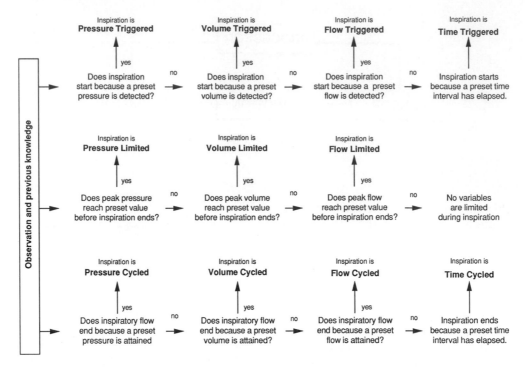

Fig. 31-13 Criteria for determining the phase variables during a ventilator assisted breath

of patient effort) and pressure (when the ventilator senses the patient's inspiratory effort in the form of a drop in baseline pressure and starts inspiration, independent of the set rate). Flow triggering is available on some ventilators, and has been shown to require less patient work than pressure triggering to initiate a breath.[16,17]

The work to trigger a breath is proportional to the volume inspired from the patient circuit before triggering and the pressure drop from baseline. Thus, there is no way to avoid triggering work with a pressure-triggered system. Flow triggering attempts to avoid work by keeping baseline pressure constant and measuring the flow inspired by the patient before triggering. Thus, a perfect flow triggering system would require no work to initiate a breath. A potential problem with flow triggering is noise in the flow signal caused by accumulated condensation in the patient circuit. One way to avoid this is to convert the flow signal to volume and trigger on inspiratory volume. This is the technique used by the Dräger Babylog ventilator.

Any variable that can be measured can potentially be used to trigger inspiration. For example, the Infrasonics Star Sync module allows triggering of the Infant Star ventilator by chest wall movement. Of course most ventilators also allow operators to manually trigger inspiration.

The patient effort required to trigger inspiration is determined by the ventilator's *sensitivity*. Sensitivity is adjusted by changing the preset value of the trigger variable. For example, to make a pressure-triggered ventilator more sensitive, the trigger pressure might be adjusted from 3 to 1 cm H$_2$O below the baseline pressure.

Limit variable

Inspiratory time is defined as the time interval from the start of inspiratory flow to the start of expiratory flow. During inspiration, pressure, volume, and flow increase above their end-expiratory values. If one (or more) of these variables rises no higher than some preset value, the variable is called a *limit variable*.

Limit variables are frequently confused with cycle variables. As we shall see, cycle variables cause inspiration to cease. A limit variable, on the other hand, does not terminate inspiration. In other words, a variable is limited if it increases to a preset value *before* inspiration ends. These criteria are illustrated in Figure 31-13.

Confusion over limit and cycle variables is encouraged by some ventilator manufacturers, who use the term limit to describe what happens when a pressure alarm threshold is met (i.e., inspiration is terminated and an alarm is activated). The term cycle, as defined below, is more appropriate in this situation. Figure 31-14 illustrates the importance of distinguishing between the terms limit and cycle.

Another potentially confusing issue is related to how pressure limits are measured and set. By convention, peak inspiratory and baseline pressures are measured relative to atmospheric pressure. However, a pressure limit can be measured relative to either baseline pressure (as on the Siemens Servo 900C) or atmospheric pressure (as on the Bird VIP).

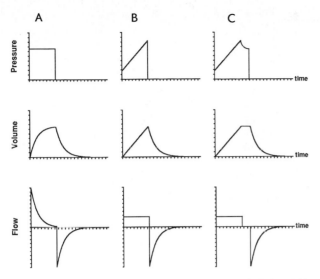

Fig. 31-14 This figure illustrates the importance of distinguishing between the terms "limit" and "cycle". In **A,** inspiration is pressure limited and time cycled. In **B,** flow is limited but volume is not and inspiration is volume cycled. In **C,** both volume and flow are limited (because they reach preset values before end inspiration) and inspiration is time cycled (after the preset inspiratory pause time).

For example, on the Bird VIP, the "High Pressure Limit Control" sets peak inspiratory pressure limit (above ambient pressure) during pressure controlled ventilation, but cycles the breath off and activates a high pressure alarm during volume controlled ventilation. Hence the term "pressure limit" in common usage can indicate several different clinically significant situations, depending on both the mode of ventilation and the manufacturer! Clearly, the lack of standardization among ventilator manufacturers makes it especially important that clinicians understand what they say and say what they mean.

Cycle variable

Inspiration always ends or terminates because some variable has reached a preset value. The variable that is measured and used to end inspiration is called the cycle variable. Pressure, volume, flow, or time can be used as the cycle variable (Figure 31-13).

Deciding whether pressure, volume, flow, or time is the cycle variable on a given ventilator can be confusing. For a variable to be used as a cycle variable, it must first be measured. Most 3rd generation adult ventilators allow the operator to set a tidal volume and inspiratory flow, which would lead one to believe that the ventilator is volume-cycled. However, closer inspection reveals that these ventilators do not measure volume (which is consistent with the fact that all 3rd generation ventilators to date are flow controllers). Rather, they set the inspiratory time needed to achieve the set tidal volume with the set inspiratory flow, making them time-cycled. The tidal volume dial

can be thought of as an inspiratory time dial calibrated in units of volume rather than time.

Baseline variable

The baseline variable is the variable controlled during the expiratory time. Although the baseline value of either pressure, volume, or flow could theoretically be controlled during expiration, pressure control is the most practical, and is implemented by all commonly used ventilators.

Conditional variables

Ventilators may also use pressure, volume, flow, or time (and their derivatives) as conditional variables. A conditional variable is used by a ventilator's control circuit to solve conditional logic formulas. A simple conditional logic formula is an "if-then" statement. That is, if the value of a conditional variable reaches some preset threshold, then some action occurs to change the ventilatory pattern.

A simple example of conditional logic is the Bennett MA-1 sigh function. In the control mode, each breath provided by the MA-1 is time triggered, flow limited, and volume cycled. However, every few minutes, a sigh breath can be introduced with a different set of phase variable values. In this case, the conditional variable is time. *If* a preset time interval has elapsed (i.e., the sigh interval), *then* the ventilator switches to the sigh pattern. Another good example of conditional logic is the switchover between patient-triggered and machine-triggered breaths that occurs during intermittent mandatory ventilation (see below).

Modes of ventilation

A mode of ventilation is a particular set of control variables, phase variables, and conditional variables applied to either a mandatory or spontaneous breath.

The terms "mandatory" and "spontaneous" play a central role in defining and understanding modes of ventilation, so formal definitions must be provided. A spontaneous breath is initiated *and* terminated by the patient. If the ventilator determines *either* the start or end of inspiration, then the breath is considered mandatory. Figure 31-15, page 882, illustrates these definitions with an algorithm.

Figure 31-16, page 882, illustrates that for each breath type (mandatory or spontaneous), the ventilator creates a specific pattern of control and phase variables. The ventilator may either keep this pattern constant for each breath, or it may introduce other patterns (e.g., one for mandatory and one for spontaneous breaths). In essence, the ventilator must decide which pattern of control and phase variables to implement before each breath, depending on the value of some preset conditional variable(s).

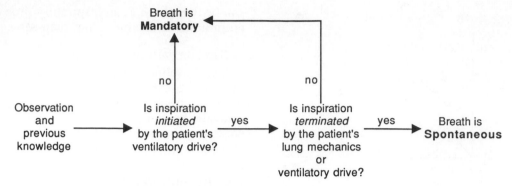

Fig. 31-15 Algorithm defining spontaneous and mandatory breaths. In terms of current technology, if the breath is triggered according to a preset frequency or minimum minute ventilation or cycled according to a preset frequency or tidal volume, the breath is mandatory. All other breaths are spontaneous.

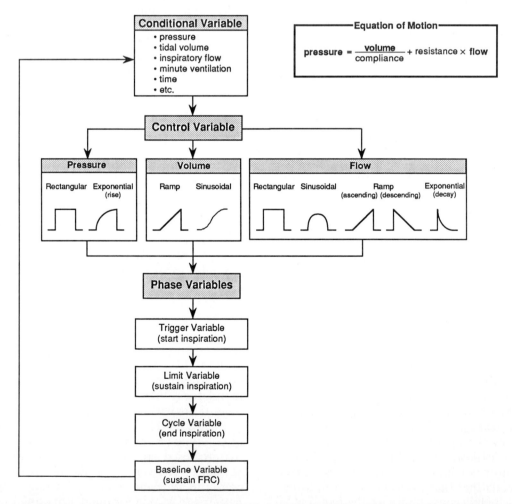

Fig. 31-16 A ventilator classification scheme based on a mathematical model known as the "equation of motion" for the respiratory system. This model indicates that during inspiration, the ventilator is able to directly control one and only one variable at time (ie, pressure, volume, or flow). Some common waveforms provided by current ventilators are shown for each control variable. Pressure, volume, flow, and time are also used as phase variables that determine the parameters of each ventilatory cycle (eg, trigger sensitivity, peak inspiratory flow rate or pressure, inspiratory time, and baseline pressure).

Table 31-1, page 884, applies this scheme to define the most common modes of ventilatory support available on today's ventilators.[4] Note that for each mode the control, phase, and conditional variables are specified for each available breath type.

Using this table, we define CMV (continuous mandatory ventilation) as consisting solely of mandatory breaths which are time-triggered. The control and limit variables during CMV can be pressure, volume, or flow. The CMV breathing cycle can be terminated via either pressure, volume, flow, or time. Likewise, pure PSV pressure support ventilation can be defined as consisting only of spontaneous breaths, which can be triggered by pressure, volume, or flow. The control and limit variables during PSV breaths are pressure. A PSV breath normally cycles-off due to reaching a low terminal flow.

While Table 31-1 defines most ventilatory support modes available on current ventilators, new modes are being created all the time. Unfortunately, manufacturers have not standardized ventilatory support mode nomenclature. Many have even created confusion by applying names that make their products seem unique, hence emphasizing differences rather than similarities.

For these reasons, the individual learning about ventilators is faced with a dilemma. The usual approach to this problem is to try to memorize whatever manufacturers say about their products, and try not to think about the inconsistencies and contradictions. At the time of this writing, there are more than 20 different modes on different types of ventilators, with some individual ventilators offering as many as nine.

A more rational approach is simply to recognize that any mode reduces to one of three general patterns of mandatory and spontaneous breaths: a pattern of all mandatory breaths, all spontaneous breaths, or some combination of the two based on conditional logic. These three groups can be further broken down to eight generic modes based on the control variable for mandatory breaths (i.e., volume control, pressure control, or dual control). For simplicity we will use the term volume control to signify that the inspiratory volume waveform is either directly controlled by the ventilator or indirectly controlled by controlling the flow waveform. Dual control means that both pressure and volume are monitored and used as control signals. As dictated by the equation of motion, however, at any particular moment during inspiration either one or the other is being controlled, but not both. With this system, we need only identify the type of conditional logic that switches between mandatory and spontaneous breaths to account for all current modes of ventilation (Table 31-2, page 885).

By applying these generic modes, any term coined by a manufacturer can be easily understood. Using this system, communication about modes is simplified, yet more precise. An example of more precision is the following: describing a mode as "volume con-

trolled continuous mandatory ventilation" is much more descriptive than saying "assist/control". Depending on the ventilator, the latter term could just as well mean pressure controlled continuous mandatory ventilation, and is also an ambiguous use of the terms assist and control. As mentioned above, any breath is assisted if the ventilator does work on the patient (i.e., if airway pressure rises above baseline during inspiration). To "control" means to regulate, and what is regulated if not the variables of the equation of motion for the respiratory system (i.e., pressure, volume, flow, and time)? Saying "control" without specifying what is being controlled is meaningless.

Additional examples of the simplicity of this scheme can be seen by realizing that synchronized intermittent mandatory ventilation (SIMV) is just IMV with conditional logic that looks at changes in baseline pressure or flow and a time window to synchronize flow delivery with patient effort. Likewise, SIMV with pressure support is just SIMV with the spontaneous breath pressure limit set above 0. Mandatory minute ventilation (MMV) is a form of SIMV with conditional logic that either increases the mandatory rate or the spontaneous assist level. Pressure controlled inverse ratio ventilation (PCIRV), airway pressure release ventilation (APRV), and BiPAP® are similar forms of pressure controlled SIMV.

New modes on the Siemens 300, the Bear 1000, and the Bird 8400ST are described in terms of Dual Control. The unique features of these Dual Control modes are illustrated in Figures 31-17, page 885, and 31-18, page 886.

OUTPUT

To understand heart physiology we study ECGs and blood pressure waveforms. In the same way, to study ventilator operation, we must examine output waveforms. Of course, the output waveforms of interest during ventilatory support are pressure, volume, and flow.

For each control variable, there are a limited number of waveforms produced by current ventilators. Idealized versions of these waveforms are shown in Figure 31-19, page 887.

Output waveforms are ideally graphed in groups of three. The conventional order of presentation is pressure, volume, and flow, respectively, from top to bottom. Convention also dictates that positive flow values (above the horizontal axis) correspond to inspiration and negative flow values (below the horizontal axis) correspond to expiration. The vertical axes are in units of the measured variables (usually cm H_2O for pressure, liters or mL for volume, and L/min or L/sec for flow). The horizontal axis of all graphs is time.

Because the waveforms in Figure 31-19 are idea-

Table 31-1   Classificiation of modes of ventilator operation

Mode	Mandatory Breath				Spontaneous Breath					Control Logic	
	Control	Trigger	Limit	Cycle	Control	Trigger	Limit	Cycle	Supported	Conditional Variable	Action
CMV*	Pressure, volume, or flow	Time	Pressure, volume, or flow	Time, pressure, volume, or flow	—	—	—	—	—	—	—
A/C	Pressure, volume, or flow	Time, pressure, volume, or flow	Pressure, volume, or flow	Time, pressure, volume, or flow	—	—	—	—	—	Time or patient effort	Machine-to-patient triggered
AMV	Pressure, volume, or flow	Pressure, volume, or flow	Pressure, volume, or flow	Time, pressure, volume, or flow	—	—	—	—	—	—	—
IMV	Pressure, volume, or flow	Time	Pressure, volume, or flow	Time, pressure, volume, or flow	Pressure	Pressure, volume, or flow	Pressure	Pressure	No	—	—
SIMV	Pressure, volume, or flow	Time, pressure, volume, or flow	Pressure, volume, or flow	Time, pressure, volume, or flow	Pressure	Pressure, volumn, or flow	Pressure	Pressure	No	Time or patient effort	Machine-to-patient triggered
CPAP	—	—	—	—	Pressure	Pressure, volume, or flow	Pressure	Pressure	No	—	—
PCV	Pressure	Time	Pressure	Time	—	—	—	—	—	—	—
PC-IMV	Pressure	Time	Pressure	Time	Pressure	Pressure, volume, or flow	Pressure	Pressure	No		
PC-SIMV	Pressure	Time, pressure, volume, or flow	Pressure	Time	Pressure	Pressure, volume, or flow	Pressure	Pressure	No	Time or patient effort	Machine-to-patient triggered
PCIRV	Pressure	Time	Pressure	Time	Pressure						
APRV	Pressure	Time or pressure	Pressure	Time	Pressure	Pressure, volume, or flow	Pressure	Pressure	No	Time or patient effort	Machine-to-patient triggered
PSV	—	—	—	—	Pressure	Pressure, volume, or flow	Pressure	flow	Yes		
MMV	Volume or flow	Time	Volume or flow	Time, volume, or flow	Pressure	Pressure, volume, or flow	Pressure	Pressure or volume	Yes*	Minute ventilation, time	Spontan-eous to-mandatory breath
VAPS	—	—	—	—	Pressure, volume, or flow	Pressure, volume, or flow	Pressure	Pressure, volume, or flow	Yes*	Tidal volume	Pressure-to-volume control
BiPAP	Pressure	Time	Pressure	Time	Pressure	Pressure	Pressure	Pressure	No	—	—

*CMV = continuous mandatory ventilation; NA = not applicable; A/C = assist/control; AMV = assisted mechanical ventilation; IMV = intermittent mandatory ventilation; SIMV = synchronized mandatory ventilation; CPAP = continuous positive airway pressure; PCV = pressure-controlled ventilation; PC-IMV = pressure-controlled IMV; PCIRV = PC inverse-ration ventilation; APRV = airway pressure release ventilation; PSV = pressure support ventilation; MMV = mandatory minute ventilation; VAPS = volume-assisted pressure support; BiPAP® = bilevel positive airway pressure.

Table 31-2 "Generic" ventilator modes. All current modes of ventilation can be uniquely described by one of eight basic patterns of mandatory and spontaneous breaths, modified with the appropriate conditional logic.

Pattern	Control	Mandatory Breaths Trigger	Limit	Cycle	Spontaneous Breaths Trigger	Limit	Cycle	Conditional Logic
CMV[1]								
	VC[2]	pt/m[3]	flow[4]	volume/time	—	—	—	• if sigh interval elapsed, increase tidal volume
	PC[5]	pt/m	pressure	time	—	—	—	
	DC[6]	pt/m	pressure	time	—	—	—	• if target espired V_T not met, increase pressure limit[7]
IMV[8]								
	VC	pt/m	flow	volume/time	pt	pressure	flow	• if pt effort in IMV window, synchronize breath (ie, SIMV) • if target minute ventilation not met, increase rate (ie, MMV)[9]
	PC	pt/m	pressure	time	pt	pressure	flow	• if pt effort in SIMV window, synchronize breath (ie, SIMV)
	DC	pt/m	flow	volume	pt	pressure	flow	• if target inspired V_T not met, mandatory, else spontaneous[10]
CSV[11]								
	PC	—	—	—	pt	pressure	flow	
	DC	—	—	—	pt	pressure	flow	• if target expired V_T not met, increase pressure limit[12]

1. Continuous Mandatory Ventilation
2. Volume controlled
3. Patient (pt) or machine (m) triggered
4. An inspiratory hold would create a volume limit
5. Pressure controlled
6. Dual controlled (ie, volume and pressure); either pressure is controlled within a breath and volume controlled over several breaths (ie, Siemens 300) or the ventilator may switch between volume and pressure control within a breath (Bear 1000 or Bird 8400 ST).
7. Pressure Regulated Volume Control (Siemens 300)
8. Intermittent Mandatory Ventilation
9. Mandatory Minute Ventilation; may also be accomplished by increasing spontaneous breath pressure limit instead of mandatory breath rate
10. Pressure Augment (Bear 1000) and Volume Assisted Pressure Support (Bird 8400ST)
11. Continuous Spontaneous Ventilation
12. Pressure Regulated Volume Control (Siemens 300)

lized, they do not show the minor deviations or "noise" often seen during actual ventilator use. Such tions can be caused by many factors, including vibration and turbulence. These waveforms also do not show the impact of expiratory circuit resistance, as this varies depending on the ventilator and type of circuit. Last, one must remember that waveform appearance can be altered by changing the time scale. A faster sweep (shorter time scale) will tend to widen a

given waveform, while a slower sweep speed (longer time scale) will compress the waveform.

Most ventilator waveforms are either rectangular, exponential, ramp, or sinusoidal in shape. Although a variety of subtypes are possible, we will describe only the most common. Waveforms are listed according to the shape of the control variable waveform. Any new waveforms produced by future ventilators can easily be accommodated by this system.

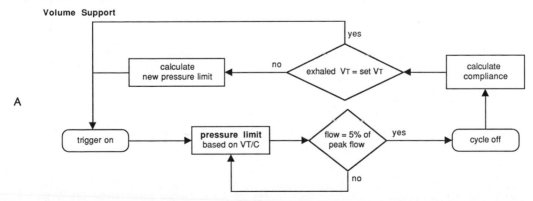

Fig. 31-17 Simplified algorithms for Volume Support (**A**) and Pressure Regulated Volume Control (**B**) modes found on the Siemens 300 ventilator

continued

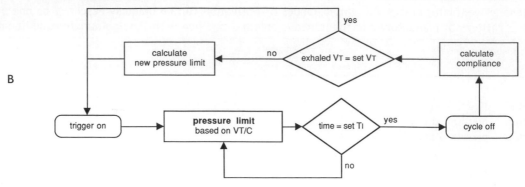

Fig. 31-17 *continued.* For legend see p. 885.

Pressure waveforms

Rectangular

Mathematically, a rectangular waveform is referred to as a step or instantaneous change in transrespiratory pressure from one value to another (Figure 31-19, *A*). In response, volume rises **exponentially** from zero to a steady state value equal to compliance times the change in airway pressure (i.e., PIP-PEEP). Inspiratory flow falls exponentially from a peak value (at the start of inspiration) equal to (PIP-PEEP) ÷ resistance.

Exponential

Exponential pressure waveforms are common during neonatal ventilation, and can also be produced by adjusting the pressure rise control on some newer adult ventilators. The resulting pressure and volume waveforms can take on a variety of shapes ranging from an exponential rise (same shape as the volume waveform in Figure 31-19, *A*) to a linear rise (same shape as the volume waveform in Figure 31-19, *B*). In general, the flow waveform is similar to that seen in Figure 31-19, *A,* except that peak inspiratory flow is reached gradually rather than instantaneously (resulting in a rounded rather than peaked waveform) and peak flow is lower than with a rectangular pressure waveform.

Sinusoidal

As previously described, a sinusoidal pressure waveform can be created by attaching a piston to a rotating crank. In addition, a sine wave pressure pattern can be produced by a linear drive motor driven by an oscillating signal generator. In response, the volume and flow waveforms are also sinusoidal, but they attain their peak values at different times (Figure 31-19, *E*).

Oscillating

Oscillating pressure waveforms can take on a variety of shapes, from sinusoidal (Mira Hummingbird), to

ramp (SensorMedics 3100 Oscillator), to roughly triangular (Infrasonics Star Oscillator). The distinguishing feature of a ventilator classified as an oscillator is that it can generate negative transrespiratory pressure. That is, if the mean airway pressure is set equal to atmospheric pressure, then the airway pressure waveform oscillates above and below zero. If the pressure waveform is sinusoidal, volume and flow will

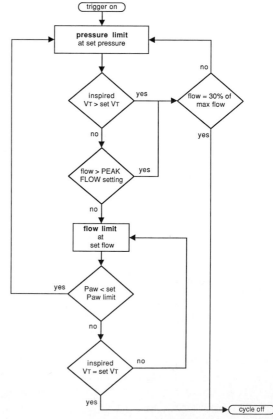

Fig. 31-18 Simplified algorithm for the Pressure Augment mode found on the Bear 1000 ventilator. This is similar to the Volume Assisted Pressure Support algorithm of the Bird 8400 ST ventilator.

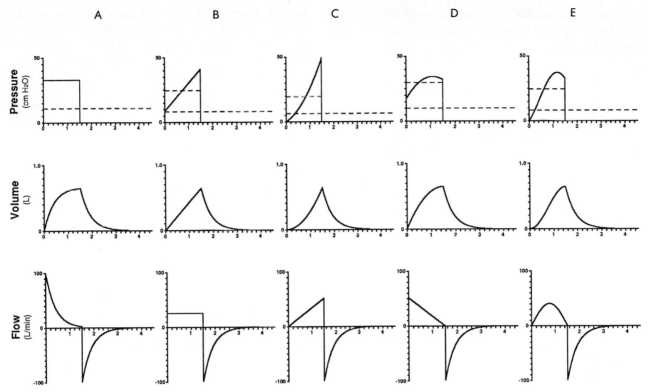

Fig. 31-19 This figure illustrates the theoretical output waveforms for **(A)** pressure controlled inspiration with rectangular pressure waveform. Note that this is identical to flow controlled inspiration with an exponential decay flow waveform; **(B)** flow controlled inspiration with rectangular flow waveform. Note that this is identical to volume controlled inspiration with an ascending ramp volume waveform; **(C)** flow controlled inspiration with an ascending ramp flow waveform; **(D)** flow controlled inspiration with a descending ramp flow waveform, and; **(F)** flow controlled inspiration with a sinusoidal flow waveform. The short dotted lines represent the mean inspiratory pressure while the long dotted lines denote mean airway pressure (assuming zero end expiratory pressure). Note that for the rectangular pressure waveform in A, the mean inspiratory pressure is the same as the peak inspiratory pressure. These output waveforms were created by: (1) defining the control waveform using a mathematical equation (eg, an ascending ramp flow waveform is specified as flow = constant × time) and specifying that the tidal volume equal 644 mL (equivalent to about 9 mL/kg for a normal adult), (2) specifying the desired values for resistance and compliance (for these waveforms, compliance was set at 20 mL/cm H_2O and resistance was set at 20 cm H_2O/L/sec according to ANSI recommendations), (3) substituting the above information into the equation of motion, and (4) using a computer to solve the equations for pressure, volume, and flow and plotting the results against time.

also be sinusoidal, but out of phase with each other (i.e., their peak values occur at different times).

Volume waveforms

Ramp

Volume controllers that produce an ascending ramp waveform (e.g., the Bennett MA-1) produce a linear rise in volume from zero at the start of inspiration to the peak value, or set tidal volume, at end-inspiration (Figure 31-19, *B*). In response, the flow waveform is rectangular. The pressure waveform rises instantaneously from zero to a value equal to (resistance × flow) at the start of inspiration. From here it rises linearly to its peak value (i.e., PIP) equal to (tidal volume/compliance) + (flow × resistance).

Sinusoidal

This volume waveform is most often produced by ventilators whose drive mechanism is a piston attached to a rotating crank (e.g., Engstrom ER-300 and Emerson ventilator). The output waveform of this type of ventilator can be approximated by the first half of a cosine curve, whose shape in this case is referred to as a sigmoidal curve (Figure 31-19, *E*). Because volume is sinusoidal during inspiration, pressure and flow are also sinusoidal.

Flow

Rectangular

A rectangular flow waveform is perhaps the most common output (Figure 31-19, *B*). When the flow waveform is rectangular, volume is a ramp waveform and pressure is a step followed by a ramp as described for the ramp volume waveform.

Ramp

The ramp waveform is what many respiratory care practitioners (and ventilator manufacturers) call an "accelerating" or "decelerating" flow waveform. The term ramp is borrowed from electronic engineering and is preferred for three reasons. First, the name ramp gives a more obvious visual image of actual shape of the waveform. Second, the term ramp has been described mathematically and used universally for much longer than mechanical ventilators have been in existence. Third, the analogy of something accelerating or decelerating is misapplied. For example, when a car is moving we say it has a certain speed (i.e., speed = distance/time). If the speed increases with time we say that the car accelerates (i.e., acceleration = speed/time) not that the speed accelerates. The speed of moving gas is expressed as a flow (i.e., flow = area of tube × distance/time). If the flow increases, we would properly say that the gas accelerates (i.e., acceleration = flow rate/time) not that the flow accelerates. In scientific terms "the acceleration of a particle is the rate of change of its velocity with time."[18]

Ascending ramp. A true ascending ramp waveform starts at zero and increases linearly to the peak value (see Figure 31-19, C). Ventilator flow waveforms are usually truncated. Inspiration starts with an initial instantaneous flow (e.g., the Bear-5 starts inspiration at 50% of the set peak flow). Flow then increases linearly to the set peak flow rate. In response to an ascending ramp flow waveform, the pressure and volume waveforms are exponential with a concave upward shape.

Descending ramp. A true descending ramp waveform starts at the peak value and decreases linearly to zero (Figure 31-19, D). Ventilator flow waveforms are usually truncated; inspiratory flow rate decreases linearly from the set peak flow until it reaches some arbitrary threshold where flow drops immediately to zero (e.g., the Bennett 7200a ends inspiration when the flow rate drops to 5 L/min). In response to a descending ramp flow waveform, the pressure and volume waveforms are exponential with a concave downward shape.

Sinusoidal

Some ventilators offer a mode in which the inspiratory flow waveform approximates the shape of the first half of a sine wave (Figure 31-19, E). As with the ramp waveform, ventilators often truncate the sine waveform by starting and ending flow at some percentage of the set peak flow rather than start and end at zero flow. In response to a sinusoidal flow waveform, the pressure and volume waveforms will also be sinusoidal but out of phase with each other.

Effects of the patient circuit

Pressure, volume, and flow measured at the outlet of a ventilator are never the same as when measured at the patient's airway opening. This is because the patient circuit has its own compliance and resistance. Thus, the pressure measured on the inspiratory side of a ventilator will always be higher than the pressure at the airway opening. In addition, the volume and flow coming out of the ventilator will exceed that delivered to the patient because the effective compliance of the patient circuit.

Patient circuit compliance includes not only the compliance of the material the circuit is made from but the compressibility of the gas within the circuit. This compliance effect absorbs both volume and flow.

■ MINI **C**LINI ■

32-2

Set versus Actual Output of Ventilators

Problem: During patient rounds in the intensive care unit, a RCP is asked by the attending physician if pressure, volume, and flow measured inside a mechanical ventilator are different than pressure, volume, and flow measured at the patient's airway. What would be the correct answer and rationale?

Discussion: This type of question comes up from time to time in clinical practice. In fact, there may be a difference between the "set" values for pressure, volume, and flow and the "output" values from the ventilator once the breath is delivered. The difference could be explained by ventilator transducer calibration error or could be do to the effects of the patient circuit. Patient circuit compliance includes not only the compliance of the material the circuit is made from but the compressibility of the gas within the circuit. Because of the elastic and flow resistive pressure drops created by the ventilator circuit, the compliance effect absorbs both volume and flow. For example, one clinical implication of this effect is that during volume controlled ventilation, the actual delivered tidal volume from the ventilator may, in certain situations, be less than the preset tidal volume.

It can be shown by analogy to electrical circuits that the compliance of the delivery circuit is connected parallel with the compliance of the respiratory system. That is, pneumatic compliance is analogous to electrical capacitance and pneumatic resistance is analogous to electrical resistance.[10] Therefore, the total compliance of the ventilator—patient system is simply the sum of the two compliances. In a similar manner, the resistance of the delivery circuit is shown to be connected in series with the respiratory system resistance so that the total resistance is the sum of the two.

From these assumptions, it can be shown that the relation between the volume input to the patient (at the point of connection to the patient's airway opening) and the volume output from the ventilator (at the point of connection to the patient circuit) is described by:

$$\begin{array}{l} \text{volume} \\ \text{input to} \\ \text{patient} \end{array} = \frac{1}{1 + (Cpc \div Crs)} \times \begin{array}{l} \text{volume} \\ \text{output from} \\ \text{ventilator} \end{array} \quad (2)$$

where Cpc is the compliance of the patient circuit and Crs is the total compliance of the patient's respiratory system.

The equation shows that the larger the patient circuit compliance is compared to the patient's respiratory system, the larger the denominator on the right hand side of the equation and hence the smaller the delivered tidal volume will be compared to the volume coming out of the ventilator's drive mechanism.

Assuming that the volume exiting the ventilator is the set tidal volume, the patient circuit compliance is calculated as:

$$Cpc = \frac{\text{set } V_T}{\text{Pplateau-PEEP}} \quad (3)$$

where Pplateau is the pressure measured during an inspiratory hold maneuver with the wye adapter of the patient circuit occluded (patient is not connected) and PEEP is end expiratory pressure (i.e., baseline pressure). Most authors recommend the use of peak inspiratory pressure, (PIP or Pmax) for Pplateau in the above equation. This is acceptable but it may lead to a slight underestimation of patient circuit compliance. Pplateau is slightly lower than Pmax because of the flow resistive pressure drop of the patient circuit if pressure is not measured at the wye adapter. This difference will be greatest in small bore, corrugated patient circuit tubing, but is probably insignificant.

The effects of patient circuit compliance are most troublesome during volume controlled ventilation. For example, when ventilating neonates, the patient circuit compliance can be as much as three times that of the respiratory system, even with small bore tubing and a small volume humidifier. Thus, when trying to deliver a preset tidal volume, the volume delivered to the patient may be as little as 25% of that coming from

the ventilator, while 75% is compressed in the patient circuit.

Another area where patient circuit compliance causes trouble is in the determination of auto PEEP. The patient's airway opening is occluded at end expiration until static conditions prevail throughout the lungs. The pressure at this time is auto-PEEP (**PEEP$_A$**), and is an index of the volume of gas trapped in the lungs:

$$\text{true PEEP}_A = \frac{Vrs}{Crs} \quad (4)$$

where V_{rs} is the volume of the respiratory system at end expiration and C_{rs} is the respiratory system compliance.

Some ventilators (e.g., Siemens Servo 900C) allow the clinician to perform the maneuver without disconnecting the patient from the ventilator. In this case, however, the end expiratory respiratory system volume is distributed between the lungs and the patient circuit. Thus, the auto-PEEP measured under these conditions will underestimate the true auto-PEEP because the patient circuit compliance is added in parallel with the compliance of the respiratory system:

$$\text{estimated PEEP}_A = \frac{Vrs}{Crs + Cpc} \quad (5)$$

The relation between true and estimated auto-PEEP is derived by solving equation 5 for volume and substituting it into equation 4:

$$\text{true PEEP}_A = \frac{Crs + Cpc}{Crs} \times (\text{estimated PEEP}_A) \quad (6)$$

Thus, true auto-PEEP may be calculated from the estimated auto-PEEP by multiplying by an error factor that is a function of the patient circuit compliance. This error can be substantial for small patients with stiff lungs.

During pressure-controlled ventilation, the compliance of the patient circuit has the effect of rounding the leading edge of a rectangular pressure waveform, which could possibly reduce the volume delivered to the patient. This effect is avoided if the pressure limit is maintained for at least five time constants (i.e., time constants of the respiratory system). The time constant is a measure of the time required for the passive respiratory system to respond to abrupt changes in ventilatory pressure. The time constant is measured in units of seconds and is calculated as resistance times compliance.[10,19]

In summary, the set values for pressure, volume, and flow may be different from the "output (from ventilator)" values due to ventilator transducer calibration errors and different from the "input (to the patient)" due to the effects of the patient circuit. Thus there are two general sources of error that cause discrepancies between the desired and actual patient values.

ALARM SYSTEMS

The ventilator classification scheme described above centers on the basic functions of input, control, and output. If any of these functions fails, a life threatening situation may result. Thus, ventilators are equipped with various types of alarms which may be classified in the same manner as the other major ventilator characteristics.

Day and MacIntyre have stressed that the goal of ventilator alarms is to warn of events.[20,21] They define an event as any condition or occurrence that requires clinician awareness or action. Technical events are those involving an inadvertent change in the ventilator's performance; patient events are those involving a change in the patient's clinical status that can be detected by the ventilator.[20]

Although a ventilator may be equipped with any conceivable vital sign monitor, we will limit the scope here to include only the ventilator's operation, and those variables associated with the mechanics of breathing (i.e., pressure, volume, flow, and time). Because the ventilator is in intimate contact with exhaled gas, we will also include the analysis of exhaled oxygen and CO_2 concentrations as possible variables to monitor.

Alarms may be audible, visual, or both, depending upon the seriousness of the alarm condition. Visual alarms may be as simple as colored lights or may be as complex as alphanumeric messages to the operator indicating the exact nature of the fault condition. Specifications for an alarm event should include: (1) conditions that trigger the alarm, (2) the alarm response in the form of audible and/or visual messages, (3) any associated ventilator response such as termination of inspiration or failure to operate, and, (4) whether the alarm must be manually reset or resets itself when the alarm condition is rectified. Alarm categories include input power alarms, control circuit alarms, and output alarms.

Input power alarms

Loss of electric power
Most ventilators have some sort of battery backup in the case of electrical power failure, even if the batteries only power alarms. Ventilators typically have alarms that are activated if the electrical power is cut off while the machine is still switched on (e.g., if the power cord is accidentally pulled out of the wall socket).

If the ventilator is designed to operate on battery power (e.g., transport ventilators) there is usually an alarm to warn of a low battery condition.

Loss of pneumatic power
Ventilators that use pneumatic power have alarms that are activated if either the oxygen or air supply is cut off or reduced below some specified driving pressure. In some cases, the alarm is activated by an electronic pressure switch (e.g., Bennett 7200) but in others, the alarm is pneumatically operated as a part of the blender (e.g., Siemens Servo 900C).

Control circuit alarms

Control circuit alarms are those that either warn the operator that the set control variable parameters are incompatible (e.g., inverse I:E ratio) or indicate that some aspect of a ventilator self test has failed. In the latter case, there may be something wrong with the ventilator control circuitry itself (e.g., a microprocessor failure) and the ventilator generally responds with some generic message like "Ventilator Inoperative."

Output alarms

Output alarms are those that are triggered by an unacceptable state of the ventilator's output. More specifically, an output alarm is activated when the value of a control variable (pressure, volume, flow, or time) falls outside an expected range. Common output alarms include those for pressure, volume, flow, time, and inspired gas.

Pressure
Pressure alarms may be used to warn of several different types of events, including changes in peak, mean, and baseline airway pressures.

High and low peak airway pressure. These alarms indicate a possible endotracheal tube obstruction, or leak in the patient circuit, respectively.

High and low mean airway pressure. These alarms indicate a possible leak in the patient circuit or a change in ventilatory pattern that might lead to a change in the patient's oxygenation status (i.e., within reasonable limits, oxygenation is roughly proportional to mean airway pressure).

High and low baseline pressure. These alarms indicate a possible patient circuit or exhalation manifold obstruction (or inadvertent PEEP), and disconnection of the patient from the patient circuit, respectively.

Failure to return to baseline pressure. These alarms indicate a possible patient circuit obstruction or exhalation manifold malfunction.

Volume
Volume alarms may be used to warn of several different types of events, the most critical of which are high and low expired volume. These alarms indicate changes in respiratory system time constant during pressure controlled ventilation, leaks around the endotracheal tube or from the lungs, or possible discon-

nection of the patient from the ventilator or circuit. If set to measure cumulative volume over time (minute volume), these alarms can warn of hyperventilation, machine self-triggering, apnea, or disconnection of the patient from the ventilator.

Time

Time-based alarm systems may be used to warn of changes in breathing frequency or an inappropriate inspiratory or expiratory time.

High or low ventilatory frequency. These alarms can indicate hyperventilation, machine self-triggering, and possibly apnea.

Inappropriate inspiratory time. Too long an inspiratory time indicates a possible patient circuit obstruction or exhalation manifold malfunction. Too short an inspiratory time indicates that adequate tidal volume may not be delivered (in a pressure controlled mode) or that gas distribution in the lungs may not be optimal.

Inappropriate expiratory time. Too long an expiratory time may indicate apnea. Too short an expiratory time may warn of alveolar gas trapping (i.e., expiratory time should exceed five time constants).

Inspired gas

Inspired gas alarms require built-in or add-on monitoring systems for temperature and FIO_2.

High/low inspired gas temperature. A high/low inspired gas temperature alarm can warn of overheating or failure of a heated humidifier system. Temperature

Table 31-3 Priorities for mechanical ventilator alarms

Priority	Life-Threatening?	Immediate Response Required?	Redundant	Alarm Type
Level 1	Yes, immediately	Yes	Yes	Loud Audible/visual
Level 2	Yes, potentially	Yes	No	Soft Audible/visual
Level 3	No	No	No	Visual

From AARC: Consensus Statement on the Essentials of Mechanical Ventilators—1992, *Respir Care* 37 (9):1000–1008, 1992.

probe placement can be critical in some applications, especially when using heated enclosures, as with infants (see Chapter 35).

High/low FIO_2. A high/low FIO_2 alarm requires continuous oxygen analysis, usually via a fuel cell or Clark electrode (see Chapter 26). A high/low FIO_2 alarm warns of either source gas failure or oxygen blender failure.

Need for alarm systems

Since not all bedside events are of equal importance, not all alarm systems need have the same status or priority. Table 31-3 describes the priorities for mechanical ventilator alarm systems, as adopted by the American Association for Respiratory Care.[22]

As can be seen, three levels of bedside events are classified:

Table 31-4 Events and monitoring sites for ventilator alarms

Event	Possible Monitoring Site
Level 1	
Power failure (including) when battery in use)	Electrical control system*
Absence of gas delivery (apnea)	Circuit pressures,* circuit flows, timing monitor CO_2 analysis
Loss of gas source	Pneumatic control system*
Excessive gas delivery	Circuit pressures,* circuit flows, timing monitor
Exhalation valve failure	Circuit pressures, circuit flows, timing monitor
Timing failure	Circuit pressures, circuit flows, timing monitor
Level 2	
Battery power loss (not in use)	Electrical control system*
Circuit leak*	Circuit pressures,* circuit flows
Blender failure	FIO_2 sensor
Circuit partially occluded	Circuit pressures, circuit flows
Heater/humidifier failure	Temperature probe in circuit
Loss of/or excessive PEEP	Circuit pressures
Autocycling	Circuit pressures, circuit flows
Other electrical or preventive subsystem out of limits without immediate overt gas delivery effects	Electrical and pneumatic systems monitor
Level 3	
Change in central nervous system drive	Circuit pressures, circuit flows, timing monitor
Change in impedances	Circuit pressures, circuit flows, timing monitor
Intrinsic PEEP (auto) > 5 cm H_2O	Circuit pressures, circuit flows

*Alarms currently defined in the ISO and ASTM standards.
From AARC: Consensus Statement on the Essentials of Mechanical Ventilators—1992, *Respir Care* 37 (9):1000–1008, 1992.

Table 31–5   Application of ventilator classification system

	Bear 1	Bear 2	Bear 5	Bear 1000	Bear Cub	Bird 8400ST	Bird V.I.P.	Dräger Babylog	Emerson 3MV	Hamilton Veolar	Infra. Infant Star	Infra. Adult Star	Newport Breeze	Newport E100I	Newport Wave	PB MA-1	PB 7200	PPG IRISA	Sechrist IV-100B	Sechrist 2200B	Siemens 900C	Siemens 300
I. Drive Power*																						
A. Pneumatic	•	•	•	•	•	•	•	•		•	•	•	•	•	•	•	•	•	•	•	•	•
B. Electric									•												•	•
II. Drive Mechanism																						
A. Compressor																						
1. External			•	•	•	•	•	•		•	•	•	•	•	•		•	•	•		•	•
2. Internal	•	•							•							•				•		
B. Motor and linkage																						
1. Compressed gas/direct	•	•	•	•	•	•	•	•		•	•	•	•	•	•	•	•	•	•		•	•
2. Electric motor/rotating crank									•													
3. Electric motor/threaded rod																				•		
C. Output control valves																						
1. Pneumatic diaphragm	•	•	•	•	•				•			•	•	•		•	•	•				
2. Pneumatic poppet valve									•				•	•	•							
3. Electric poppet valve	•	•		•	•		•			•		•		•		•	•	•		•		
4. Electric proportional valve			•	•		•	•			•		•			•		•	•		•	•	•
III. Control Scheme																						
A. Control circuit																						
1. Mechanical									•						•							
2. Pneumatic	•	•	•	•	•			•		•	•	•	•	•	•	•	•	•	•	•		
3. Fluidic																			•			
4. Electronic	•	•	•	•	•	•	•	•		•	•	•	•	•	•	•	•	•		•	•	•
B. Control Variables																						
1. Pressure	•	•	•	•	•	•	•	•		•	•	•	•	•	•	•	•	•	•	•	•	•
2. Volume	•	•	•						•							•		•			•	
3. Flow			•	•	•	•	•	•		•	•	•	•	•	•		•	•		•	•	•
C. Phase Variables																						
1. Trigger																						
a. pressure	•	•	•	•		•	•		•	•	•	•	•	•	•	•	•	•	•	•	•	•
b. volume									•													
c. flow	•	•				•	1										•					•
d. time	•	•	•	•	•	•	•	•	•	•	•	•	•	•	•	•	•	•	•	•	•	•
e. manual	•	•	•	•	•	•	•	•		•	•	•	•	•	•	•	•	•	•	•	•	•
f. optional external source											•											
2. Limit Variable																						
a. pressure	•	•	•	•	•	•	•	•	•	•	•	•	•	•	•	•	•	•	•	•	•	•
b. volume	•	•	•	•	•		•			•		•			•	•	•	•		•	•	•
c. flow	•	•	•	•	•	•	•	•		•	•	•	•	•	•	•	•	•		•	•	•
3. Cycle Variable																						
a. pressure	•	•	•	•	•	•	•	•		•	•	•	•	•	•		•	•		•	•	•
b. volume				•			•		•							•				•		
c. flow			•	•		•	•			•		•			•		•	•		•	•	•
e. time	•	•	•	•	•	•	•	•		•	•	•	•	•	•	•	•	•	•		•	•
IV. Output																						
A. Pressure																						
1. Rectangular			•	•		•	•	•	•	•	•	•	•	•	•		•	•	•	•	•	•
2. Exponential			•	•													•	•				•
3. Adjustable			•	2		2			2			2		2	2	2		•	2			•
B. Volume																						
1. Ascending Ramp			•											•								
2. Sinusoidal									•													
C. Flow																						
1. Rectangular	•	•	•	•	•	•	•	•		•	•	•	•	•	•	•		•		•	•	•
2. Ascending Ramp			•								•	•								•		
3. Descending Ramp	•	•	•	•		•				•	•	•			•			•		•	•	•
4. Sinusoidal			•	•						•	•	•			•			•		•	•	•
5. Adjustable	•																					
V. Alarms																						
A. Input Power Alarms																						
1. Loss of electric power	•	•	•	•	•	•	•	•	•	•	•	•	•	•	•	•	•	•	•	•	•	•
2. Loss of pneumatic power	•	•	•	•	•	•	•	•	•	•	•	•	•	•	•	•	•	•	•	•	•	•
B. Control Circuit Alarms																						
1. General Systems Failure	•	•	•	•	•	•	•			•		•			•		•	•	•		•	•
2. Incompatible Settings			•	•	•			•		•		•										
3. Inverse I:E Ratio	•	•	•	•	•		•			•		•			•	•	•	•				
C. Output Alarms																						
1. Pressure																						
a. high peak	•	•	•	•	•	•	•	•	1	•	•	•	•	•	•	•	•	•	•	•	•	•
b. low peak	•	•	•	•	•	•	•	•	1	•	•	•	•	•		•	•	•	•	•	•	•
c. high baseline			•	•				•			•	•										
d. low baseline	•	•	•	•	•					•		•			•		•					
e. high/low mean			•																			
2. Volume																						
a. low tidal volume	•	•	•							•		•				•		•		•		
3. Flow																						
a. High minute ventilation			•	•				•		•		•			•		•			•	•	•
b. Low minute ventilation			•	•		•	1	•		•		•			•		•	•		•	•	•
4. Time																						
a. High/low ventilatory rate			•	•	•		•	1		•		•			•		•			•	•	•
b. Apnea	•	•			•	•	•		•		•	•	•		•	•	•				•	•
5. Inspired Gas																						
a. High/low FiO2								•	1	•		•							•	•	•	•

* Power source for generating breath; electricity is usually required for control system.
1 Requires optional monitor.
2 Pressure waveform adjustable as a function of pressure and flow settings.

Level 1—immediately life-threatening if left unattended for even short periods of time; Level 2—potentially life-threatening if left unattended for longer periods of time; and Level 3—nonventilator events that are not likely to be life-threatening but a possible source of patient harm if not addressed.

Based on this priority scheme, Table 31-4, page 891, lists the key events coinciding with each priority level, and possible monitoring sites for detecting each event.[22] In general, critical care ventilators must have alarm systems for all Level I and II events. In this setting, alarm systems for Level III events are recommended, but not required. In addition, alarm system should conform to **ASTM** and **ISO** standards.[23,24]

VENTILATOR CLASSIFICATION

Table 31-5 describes most of the ventilators currently available in the United States according to the classification system described in this chapter.

CHAPTER SUMMARY

The safe and effective use of mechanical ventilators requires in-depth knowledge of ventilator design and operation. To understand mechanical ventilators the RCP must first understand their four basic functions: power input, power conversion, control mechanism, and output.

Knowledge of the mechanics of breathing provides a good foundation for understanding ventilator control mechanisms and output. Using the equation of motion for the respiratory system, we can interrelate all key variables involved in mechanical ventilation, specifically, pressure, volume, flow, and time. Given that only one of these variables can be controlled at a time, all ventilators must function as either pressure, volume, or flow controllers.

Control over the parameters of ventilation is provided by the ventilator's mechanical, pneumatic, fluidic, electric, or electronic control circuits. The control circuits determine when a ventilator starts, how its sustains and stops an inspiration, and what occurs between mechanical breaths. Ventilators may also use pressure, volume, flow, or time (or their derivatives) as conditional variables.

A mode of ventilation is a particular set of control, phase, and conditional variables applied to either a mandatory or spontaneous breath. For each breath type (mandatory or spontaneous), a ventilator creates a specific pattern of control and phase variables. The ventilator may either keep this pattern constant for each breath, or it may introduce other patterns. In essence, the ventilator decides which pattern of control and phase variables to implement before each breath, depending on the value of some preset conditional variable(s).

To understand ventilator operation, we must also examine output waveforms. The output waveforms of interest during ventilatory support are pressure, volume, and flow. For each control variable there are a limited number of waveforms produced by current ventilators.

If any input, control, or output functions fails, a life threatening situation may result. Thus, ventilators are equipped with various types of alarms, which may be classified in the same manner as the other major ventilator characteristics.

REFERENCES

1. Mushin M, Rendell-Baker W, Thompson PW, Mapelson WW: *Automatic ventilation of the lungs,* Oxford: 1980, Blackwell.
2. Consensus statement on the essentials of mechanical ventilators—1992, *Respir Care* 37:1000–1008, 1992.
3. Chatburn RL: Classification of mechanical ventilators, *Respir Care* 37:1009–1025, 1992.
4. Branson RD, Chatburn RL: Technical description and classification of modes of ventilator operation, *Respir Care* 37:1026–1044, 1992.
5. Morris W: *The American heritage dictionary of the English language,* Boston: 1975, American Heritage and Houghton Mifflin.
6. Dupuis YG: *Ventilators: theory and application,* St Louis, 1986, Mosby.
7. Dammann JF, McAslan TC, Maffeo CJ: Optimal flow pattern for mechanical ventilation of the lungs. 2. The effect of a sine versus square wave flow pattern with and without an end-inspiratory pause on patients, *Crit Care Med* 6(5):293–310, 1978.
8. Rau JL: Inspiratory flow patterns: the 'shape' of ventilation, *Respir Care* 38(1):132–140, 1993.
9. Otis AB, McKerrow CB, Bartlett RA, et al: Mechanical factors in distribution of pulmonary ventilation, *J Appl Physiol* 8:427–443, 1956.
10. Chatburn RL, Primiano FP Jr: Mathematical models of respiratory mechanics. In: Chatburn RL, Craig KC: Fundamentals of respiratory care research, Norwalk, 1988, Appleton & Lange.
11. Hess D, Lind L: Nomograms for the application of the Bourns Model BP200 as a volume-constant ventilator, *Respir Care* 25:248–250, 1980.
12. Rubinstein MF: *Patterns of problem solving,* Englewood Cliffs, 409–473, 1975, Prentice-Hall.
13. Morch ET: History of mechanical ventilation. In Kirby RR, Smith RA, Desautels DA: *Mechanical ventilation,* New York, 1985, Churchill Livingstone.
14. Russell DF, Ross DG, Manson HJ: Fluidic cycling devices for inspiratory and expiratory timing in automatic ventilators, *J Biomed Eng* 5:227–234, 1983.
15. Desautels DA: Ventilator performance evaluation. In Kirby RR, Smith RA, Desautels DA: *Mechanical ventilation,* New York, 1985, Churchill Livingstone.
16. Sassoon CSH, Giron AE, et al: Inspiratory work of breathing on flow-by and demand-flow continuous positive airway pressure, *Crit Care Med* 17:1108–1114, 1989.
17. Sassoon CSH, Lodia R, et al: Inspiratory muscle work of breathing during flow-by, demand flow, and continuous-flow systems in patients with chronic obstructive pulmonary disease. *Am Rev Respir Dis* 145(5):1219–1222, 1992.
18. Halliday D, Resnick R: *Fundamentals of physics,* ed 2, New York, 1981, John Wiley & Sons.
19. Chatburn RL, Lough MD, Primiano FP Jr.: Mechanical ventilation, In: Chatburn RL, Lough MD. *Handbook of respiratory care,* ed 2, Chicago, 1990, Mosby.
20. Day S, MacIntyre NR: Ventilator alarm systems. In Fulkerson WJ, MacIntyre NR, *Prob Respir Care* 4:118–126, 1991.
21. MacIntyre NR, Day S: Essentials for ventilator-alarm systems, *Respir Care* 37:1108–1112, 1992.
22. American Association for Respiratory Care: Consensus Statement on the Essentials of Mechanical Ventilators—1992, *Respir Care* 37(9):1000–1008, 1992.
23. American Society for Testing and Materials, ASTM Committee F-29.03.0: Standard specification for ventilators intended for use in critical care; F1 100–90. In Annual Book for ASTM Standards. Philadelphia PA: 1990, American Society for Testing and Materials.
24. International Organization for Standardization, Technical Committee ISO/TC 121: Breathing machines for medical use—lung ventilators (ISO 5369:1987 E). Switzerland: International Organization for Standardization, 1987;1–18; Vol ISO 5369.

CHAPTER

32

Initiating and Adjusting Ventilatory Support

■

Craig L. Scanlan

CHAPTER LEARNING OBJECTIVES

1. Outline the general principles of critical care management for patients in respiratory failure;
2. Given relevant patient data, select the appropriate settings for initiating ventilatory support;
3. Specify the modifications in ventilatory support needed for patients with the following disorders:
   Adult respiratory distress syndrome
   Airway obstruction
   Postoperative complications
   Neuromuscular disease
   Head trauma
   Congestive heart failure
   Unilateral lung disease
   Bronchopleural fistula
4. Identify the key steps in conducting a preliminary assessment of the patient-ventilator system;
5. List all supplementary equipment needed to provide ventilatory support;
6. Identify the major goals and objectives of ventilatory support;
7. Given relevant patient data, recommend appropriate adjustments in ventilatory support settings;
8. Identify and describe how to optimize the key factors affecting patient-ventilator interaction.

The acutely ill patient receiving ventilatory support requires close attention by skilled professionals who are knowledgeable in the clinical aspects of ventilatory support and critical care. These patients should be placed in a specialized critical care unit which is staffed on a 24 hour basis by appropriately trained personnel. In addition, such a unit should be equipped to provide a full range of standard and emergency life support measures, including the ability to continuously monitor key physiologic parameters.[1] Only in such a context can a successful outcome be realized.

THE MANAGEMENT PROCESS

The successful care of patients with respiratory failure involves a systematic management process (Figure 32-1).[2] Key elements in this management process include the following:

1. Selecting initial ventilator settings based on the patient's size and clinical condition. Settings are entered and proper function of the ventilator is verified before connection to the patient.
2. Thorough preliminary assessment of both the patient and ventilator system to assure that all parameters are well tolerated. To assure that the patient is stabilized, including assurance of a patent airway, followed by initial data gathering, to include sampling and analysis of arterial blood gases within 20 to 30 minutes after stabilization.

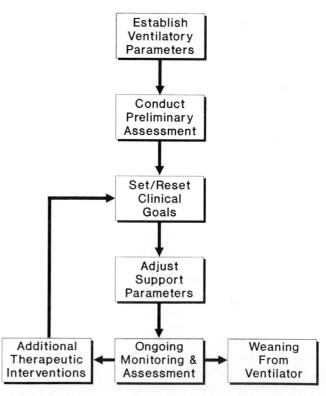

Fig. 32-1 Systematic approach to managing patients in respiratory failure.

3. Setting clinical goals for ventilatory support, in conjunction with the physician and based on the patient's history, physical assessment, and pulmonary status. These goals, along with the length of time the patient is expected to need support, will depend upon the severity of disease and the events leading to the initiation of ventilatory support.

4. Adjustment of support parameters, as indicated by arterial blood gas results and the patient's clinical condition. Several adjustments may be necessary before satisfactory results are achieved. However, in order to evaluate the effect of a parameter change on the patient, it generally is wise to make only a single change at a time. Simultaneous changes in support parameters should be reserved for emergency situations.

5. Ongoing monitoring and assessment of the patient and ventilatory system, as often as indicated. The patient's spontaneous ventilatory effort and capabilities also should be assessed regularly, ideally no less than once per shift. Overall cardiopulmonary function and the relative status of other major body systems should be reviewed and discussed with the patient's nurse and attending physician, as appropriate.

6. Additional therapeutic intervention to treat the cause(s) and complications of respiratory failure, keeping in mind that ventilatory support is a interim measure and does not in itself reverse the initial cause of respiratory failure.

7. Discontinuing ventilatory support (weaning) once the problems resulting in respiratory failure have been corrected. The physiologic and clinical data collected during the course of ventilation are used by the physician, RCP, and nurse to determine patient readiness for weaning.

INITIAL VENTILATORY SUPPORT SETTINGS

When first selecting ventilator settings, the primary aim is to stabilize the patient by assuring adequate oxygenation and ventilation. To do so, one must first select the support mode, FiO_2, and minute ventilation.[2] After selecting these primary settings, one must then adjust the trigger level and inspiratory flow (or time), set all applicable alarms, and assure adequate humidification. After initial stabilization, settings are readjusted according to the specific problem at hand. Table 32-1 provides general guidelines for initial ventilatory support settings.

Mode of ventilatory support

All ventilatory support modes can be classified into one of two broad categories: those that provide full ventilatory support and those that provide only partial support.[3] In full ventilatory support modes, the

Table 32-1 Guidelines for initial ventilatory support settings

Parameter	Setting
Ventilator Mode	If hypercapnia present, start patient on full ventilatory support (CMV or normal rate SIMV)
	If sole problem is hypoxemia, partial ventilatory support with continuous distending pressure (CPAP, APRV, BiPAP) can be used
Target: Volume or Pressure?	Base choice on physiologic considerations, clinical assessment and experience. Use volume as target if lung mechanics unstable; Consider pressure-targeting if patient-ventilator synchrony a potential problem
FiO_2	Set to assure $PaO_2 > 60$ torr or $SaO_2 \geq 90\%$; Decrease to < 0.50 as soon as possible
V_T or Pressure Limit	Start with 8–15 mL/kg according to patient; adjust to keep peak Palv below 35 cm H_2O; may need to accept V_{TS} as low as 5 mL/kg and hypercapnia
Trigger Sensitivity	Set 0.5 to 1.5 cm H_2O below baseline for pressure triggering; 1–3 L/min below baseline for flow triggering
Inspiratory Flow/Time	For flow-limited breaths, set flow ≥ 60 L/min to begin; I:E ratio of 1:3 or less
Inspiratory Flow Pattern	Rectangular or sine acceptable initially; adjust according to patient response
Humidity and Airway Temperature	Provide 30 mg/L water vapor at 30°C; start with HME unless contraindicated; reevaluate patient needs regularly
Sigh breaths	Use only when indicated

machine is responsible for the patient's full minute ventilation. During partial ventilatory support, the patient is responsible for some or all of the minute ventilation. Full ventilatory support modes include CMV (control or assist/control), SIMV set to deliver a normal breathing rate, and **PSVmax**. Partial ventilatory support modes include low rate SIMV (with or without PSV), low-level PSV, **APRV, BiPAP®**, and CPAP.

Whether full or partial ventilatory support is used as the initial mode depends mainly upon the patient's underlying pathophysiologic problem. In general, if the patient's primary problem is inadequate alveolar ventilation (hypercapnic respiratory failure), a full ventilatory support mode, such as CMV or normal rate SIMV, should be chosen. Likewise, if the primary problem is ventilatory muscle weakness or fatigue, the patient should be started on full ventilatory support.

On the other hand, if the problem is a pure hypoxemic respiratory failure, a partial ventilatory support mode that provides continuous distending pressure is usually satisfactory. Partial ventilatory support modes that provides continuous distending pressure include low rate SIMV with PEEP, APRV, BiPAP®, and CPAP. Patients with a combined hypercapnic and hypoxemic respiratory failure are candidates for full ventilatory support (CMV or normal rate IMV) with PEEP.

In selecting the mode, many new generation ventilators also allow the clinician to choose either a volume-targeted or pressure-targeted approach. Table 32-2 compares and contrasts these two different strategies.[3] The primary advantage of the volume-targeted strategy is its ability to guarantee a minimum minute volume, even with changing compliance and resistance. The primary advantage of pressure-targeted ventilation is its ability to limit and control peak airway pressures. In addition, most pressure-targeted modes provide a decelerating inspiratory flow pattern, which may improve patient-ventilator synchrony and gas distribution in some patients.

In fact, both safe pressure limits and decelerating inspiratory flows can be achieved with most newer volume-cycled ventilators.[4,5] In addition, there currently is no firm evidence indicating that either the pressure-targeted or volume-targeted approach results in better clinical outcomes. Thus, the decision as to which strategy to use should be based on physiologic considerations, clinical assessment, and experience.[6]

In terms of physiologic considerations and clinical assessment, patient stability should be the key consideration. If the patient's compliance or resistance is likely to change rapidly, the volume-targeted strategy

is the best place to start. On the other hand, if the clinical assessment indicates that patient-ventilator synchrony is a potential limiting factor in applying ventilatory support, a pressure-targeted strategy can be considered.

Oxygen concentration/FIO_2

The initial FIO_2 setting should provide a PaO_2 of at least 60 torr ($SaO_2 \geq 90\%$) with a wide margin of safety. If the PaO_2 or SaO_2 is known *before* starting ventilatory support, one should use this information to select the initial FIO_2. For example, the initial ventilator FIO_2 setting for a patient who has a PaO_2 of 75 torr while receiving 40% O_2 via T-tube should be at least 0.40.

If the patient's level of arterial oxygenation is unknown and signs of hypoxemia or circulatory failure exist, an initial FIO_2 of 1.0 can be provided. However, to avoid oxygen toxicity and absorption atelectasis, the FIO_2 should be decreased to below 0.50 as soon as possible.[1,7]

Minute ventilation

Whether using full or partial ventilatory support, the general goal in setting the initial minute volume is to assure adequate CO_2 removal, as judged by the normalization of the arterial pH. In addition, one must try to assure that the resulting volumes and alveolar pressures do not cause lung injury.

On volume-cycled ventilators, the base minute ventilation is set in one of two ways. Commonly, the ventilator provides separate tidal volume and rate setting. Minute ventilation ($\dot{V}E$) is thus the product of rate (f) times tidal volume:

$$\dot{V}E = f \times V_T$$

Alternatively, some ventilators have separate minute ventilation and rate settings, with the tidal volume being a derived value:

$$V_T = \frac{\dot{V}E}{f}$$

During full ventilatory support, the total minute ventilation determines the patient's $PaCO_2$. Thus changes in any variable that alters the total minute ventilation will effect the $PaCO_2$. During partial ventilatory support, the total minute ventilation is the sum of that provided by the ventilator plus that generated spontaneously by the patient:

$$\dot{V}E \text{ total} = \dot{V}E \text{ machine} + \dot{V}E \text{ spon}$$

Since the spontaneous contribution ($\dot{V}E$ spon) varies according to the patient's ventilatory drive, only the machine $\dot{V}E$ can be set. However, clinicians should

Table 32-2   Pressure vs volume-targeted ventilation

	Pressure	Volume
Rate	Set or variable	Set or variable
Tidal volume	Variable	Set
Peak pressure	Set	Variable
Peak flow	Variable	Set
Flow waveform	Set	Set
Assist/Control	Yes	Yes
Control	Yes	Yes
Inspiratory time	Variable	Variable
I:E ratio	Variable	Variable

From Kacmarek RM: Methods of providing mechanical ventilatory support. In Pierson DJ, Kacmarek RM, editors: *Foundations of Respiratory Care,* New York, 1992, Churchill Livingston.

still estimate the total minute ventilation requirements for patients receiving partial ventilatory support. This information is useful in setting monitoring and alarm parameters, and in assessing the efficiency of ventilation (as described in subsequent sections).

When using a pressure-targeted strategy, the clinician sets a pressure limit instead of a tidal volume. Tidal volume thus becomes a dependent variable, based on patient effort and pulmonary mechanics. Should this strategy be used to provide initial support, a pressure limit of 30 to 40 cm H_2O is a good starting point.

Nomograms

Patient tidal volume and minute ventilation needs can be estimated with nomograms. The Radford nomogram (Figure 32-2) is the most common tool used for this purpose.[8] To use the nomogram, align the patient's body weight with the desired breathing frequency using a straight edge. The resulting line crosses the predicted male or female tidal volume.

Although correction factors are provided for various conditions, the Radford nomogram tends to underestimate the ventilatory support needs of most critically ill patients. This is because the nomogram is based on healthy subjects and normal resting metabolic requirements.

Estimating formulas

Instead of using a nomogram, initial tidal volumes and breathing rates can be determined by simple formulas. These formulas are based on the patient's age, weight, clinical condition, and mode of ventilatory support (Table 32-3, page 898).[9] Based on these formulas, adult tidal volumes commonly are set be-

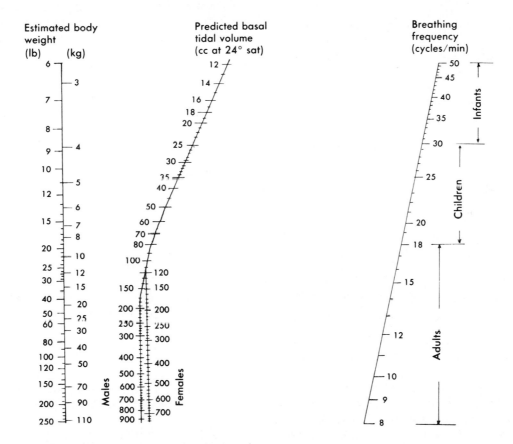

Corrections of predicted basal tidal volumes.

    For patients not in coma: add 10%

    Fever: add 5% for each °F above 99 (rectal)

        add 9% for each °C above 37 (rectal)

    Altitude: add 5% for each 2000 feet above sea level

        add 8% for each 1000 meters above sea level

    Intubation: subtract volume equal to one-half body weight in pounds

        subtract 1 cc/kg of body weight

    Dead space: add equipment dead space

Fig. 32-2 Radford nomogram. (Modified from Radford EP Jr: *J Appl Physiol* 7:451, 1955.)

Table 32–3 Recommended tidal volumes and frequencies*

Patient type	Frequency	Tidal volume
ADULTS		
Normal lungs	8–12	12–15mL/kg
Chronic obstructive disease	8–10 or less	10–12 mL/kg
Chronic restrictive disease	12–20 or more	10 mL/kg or less
Acute lung injury (ARDS)	12–20 or more	10 mL/kg or less
CHILDREN		
Age 8–16	20–30	8–10 mL/kg
Age 0–8	30–40	6–8 mL/kg

*For control and assist/control modes: for IMV mode, rates below these minimums are common, with volumes set at the high end of the prescribed ranges. (From Kacmarek RM, Venegar JV: Mechanical ventilatory rates and tidal volumes, *Respir Care* 32:466–474, 1987.)

tween 10 to 15 mL per kilogram of *ideal* body weight, with rates between 8 to 20/min. For adolescents between 8 to 16 years old, tidal volumes of 8 to 10 mL per kilogram, at rates between 20 to 30/min are usually sufficient. Infants and children (1 month to 8 years old) normally are managed with tidal volumes between 6 to 8 mL/kg and rates between 30 to 40 per minute.

These formulas are adjusted to account for differences in pulmonary mechanics. In adult patients with normal lungs, tidal volumes of 12 to 15 mL/kg are used, with rates of 8 to 12/min. Patients with chronic obstructive airway disorders tend to do better at lower rates of breathing, due to the high expiratory resistance to gas flow. Initial rates in the range of 8 to 10/min are frequently recommended for these patients, with tidal volumes initially set at 10 to 12 mL/kg, and adjusted to maintain an appropriate pH and $PaCO_2$. On the other hand, patients with restrictive pulmonary disease may require rates between 12 to 20/min, sometimes with tidal volumes less than 10 mL/kg.

The set rate of breathing also depends on the mode of ventilatory support. In general, higher base rates are used during full ventilatory support, with lower machine rates used when providing partial support. In the IMV mode, it is probably best to set the initial rate close to that of the patient. The IMV rate can then be adjusted based on subsequent clinical and laboratory assessment. In the CMV-control or CMV-assist/control modes, the machine rate is chosen to assure adequate CO_2 removal and an acceptable pH. In the CMV-assist/control mode, the backup rate should be set at 2 to 4 breaths below the patient's spontaneous

rate. This will help prevent hypoventilation should the patient stop breathing.

Tidal volumes and alveolar pressures

Recently, concern over ventilator-induced lung injuries has increased. Besides causing air-leaks, positive pressure ventilation is now associated with several other lung injuries.[10] These injuries include pulmonary edema, hemorrhage, disruption of the alveolar-capillary membrane, and neutrophil and macrophage infiltration.[11]

Both patient and ventilator factors contribute to these injuries.[10] Key patient factors include pulmonary mechanics (resistance and compliance), and the nature of the disease being treated. Key ventilator factors include the tidal volume and peak alveolar pressure.

In order to avoid the damaging effect of alveolar overdistention, many clinicians are now recommending lower tidal volumes and pressures. Kacmarek and Hickling[11] suggest keeping the peak airway pressure below 35 cm H_2O, while the American College of Chest Physicians recommends maintaining *plateau* pressures below 35 cm H_2O.[12]

To achieve these pressures, tidal volumes as low as 5 mL per kilogram may be required, especially in patients with low compliance or high resistance. Although close to those predicted by the Radford nomogram, such low tidal volumes will typically cause hypercapnia in critically ill patients.

Although contrary to conventional wisdom, allowing a patient's $PaCO_2$ to rise can be beneficial. For example, in some patients it may be safer to allow a high $PaCO_2$ than to risk frank lung damage due to excessive volumes or pressures.[12] This strategy, called *permissive hypercapnia,* has been shown to improve outcomes in selected patient groups, including those with status asthmaticus and ARDS.[11]

However, rapid changes in $PaCO_2$ and pH generally should be avoided. To avoid a rapid fall in pH, the tidal volume should be reduced slowly until the low pressure goal ($\leq$ 35 cm H_2O) is achieved. This will give the kidneys time to compensate for the elevated $PaCO_2$. Should this not be possible (as in acute status asthmaticus), IV bicarbonate may be needed to keep the pH above 7.25 during the acute phase of treatment.[13]

Sensitivity/trigger level

In all modes except CMV-control, the patient can initiate machine-assisted or spontaneous breaths. These breaths may be either pressure or flow-triggered. Where available, flow-triggering is the preferred means for initiating these breaths.[14,15] This is because flow-triggering lessens the work of breathing and results in better patient-ventilator synchrony than pressure-triggering.[15] However, flow-triggering cannot reduce the work of breathing due to small ET tubes or **auto-PEEP**.[15]

Regardless of trigger method, the ventilator delivering assisted or spontaneous breaths should always be set to ensure minimal patient effort. For pressure-triggered systems, this means setting the trigger level 0.5 to 1.5 cm H_2O below the baseline pressure; for flow triggering, the trigger flow should be set 1 to 3 L/min below baseline flow. In either case, system leaks must be avoids as they can result in auto-triggering.[15]

Inspiratory flow and time

During flow-limited mandatory or assisted breaths, the clinician can set both the magnitude and pattern of inspiratory flow. Under these conditions, inspiratory flow also determines inspiratory time. Thus the inspiratory flow setting affects all time parameters, including the I:E ratio. During pressure-limited breaths, the magnitude and pattern of inspiratory flow are usually not under clinician control.

During flow-limited, patient-triggered breaths, the inspiratory flow and trigger level are the primary factors affecting the patient's inspiratory work of breathing.[16-18] In general, the less sensitive the trigger level and the lower the flow, the greater will be the patient's work of breathing.[19] In fact, improper ventilator settings during flow-limited machine breaths may actually increase the work of breathing above that occurring spontaneously (Figure 32-3).[16,20] This can lead to muscle fatigue and hypercapnia.[18]

For these reasons, one should begin flow-limited ventilatory support with relatively high inspiratory flows ($\geq$ 60 L/min). High inspiratory flows minimize the work of breathing,[16-18] decrease auto-PEEP,[21] and improve gas exchange,[22] especially in patients with chronic airflow obstruction. The decrease in auto-PEEP and improved gas exchange is due mainly to the lengthened expiratory time and the lower I:E ratio that occurs with high inspiratory flows.

With high inspiratory flows at normal breathing rates, the resulting I:E ratio will be 1:3 or less. In patients with COPD or asthma I:E ratios of 1:4 or lower may be needed to provide sufficient time for exhalation and prevent auto-PEEP. Obviously, use of low-rate IMV in these patients can help insure sufficient exhalation time.

During pressure-limited breaths, the peak inspiratory flow available from most ventilators is either preset by the manufacturer or limited by the flow capabilities of the device. However, a few ventilators, such as the BEAR 1000 and Siemens 300, allow adjustment of the initial flow delivered during pressure support breaths.[23] Use of this control, typically called the **rise-time** or *pressure slope,* can help tailor pressure support breaths to better meet patient needs

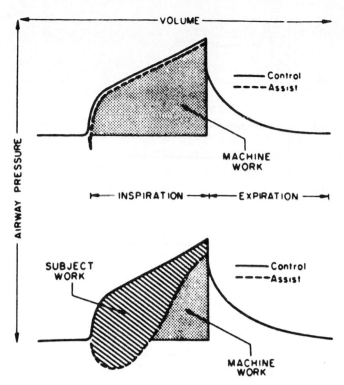

Fig. 32-3 *Above,* plot of an ideal pressure-time waveform during volume-targeted ventilation. *Below,* plot of actual pressure-time curve *(dotted line)* superimposed on the ideal curve. Note the scooped-out actual pressure waveform. The *hatched area* reflects the work performed by the patient during assisted volume-targeted ventilation. This type of actual pressure waveform is indicative of inadequate peak inspiratory flow, or too lengthy an inspiratory time. The peak flow should be increased, normally to between 60 to 90 l/min, to minimize patient effort during volume-limited ventilation. (From Marini JJ, Rodriguez M, Lamb V: *Am Rev Respir Dis* 134:902-909, 1986. Used by permission.)

(Figure 32-4, page 900). Proper adjustment of the initial flow delivered during pressure support breaths can decrease the inspiratory work of breathing and enhance patient-ventilator synchrony.[24]

During pressure control ventilation (PCV), for a given pressure limit and rate of breathing, the ratio of inspiratory time to total cycle time (t_I/t_{total}) has a major impact on minute ventilation, especially in patients with airflow obstruction. As seen in Figure 32-5, page 900, the optimum t_I/t_{total} or "duty cycle" for these patients is about 0.37, meaning 37% inspiratory time.[25] For patients with purely restrictive disorders, alveolar and airway pressures **equilibrate** rapidly for all duty cycles except those that are extremely short or long, and there is no single optimum value for t_I/t_{total}.[26]

In regard to the pattern of inspiratory flow, most ventilators operating in the flow-limited mode offer a choice of several different flow patterns (Figure 32-6, page 901 flow patterns). Unfortunately, the current literature provides conflicting perspectives on the relative benefits of these various flow waveforms.[19,27-29] However, general guidelines have been developed and are summarized in the box, page 900.[30,31]

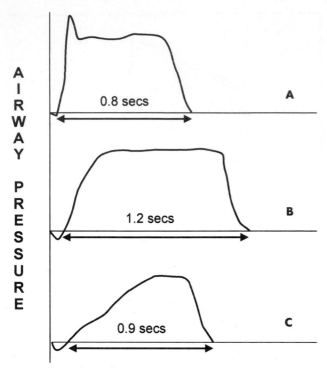

Fig. 32-4 Effect of changing inspiratory rise-time during pressure-limited breaths with a patient preferring a moderate flow. In **A**, flow exceeds patient demand, resulting in a pressure spike and short inspiratory time. In **B**, as flow is decreased, inspiratory time lengthens and the pressure spike disappears. Machine output matches patient demand. When flow is further reduced **C**, patient demand exceeds machine flow, causing deformation of the pressure waveform and a fall in inspiratory time. (From Branson RD, Campbell RS, et al: Altering flowrate during maximum pressure support ventilation (PSVmax): effects on cardiorespiratory function, *Respir Care* 35:1056-1064, 1990.)

Humidification and airway temperature

Humidification must be provided to patients with artificial tracheal airways receiving ventilatory support. Humidification is needed to prevent hypothermia, **inspissation** of airway secretions, destruction of airway epithelium, and atelectasis.[32] Humidification can be provided using either a heated humidifier or a heat and moisture exchanger (HME) (see Chap-

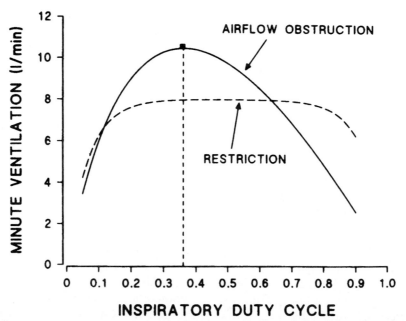

Fig. 32-5 Relationship of minute ventilation to inspiratory duty-cycle (t_I/t_{total}) for pressure control ventilation in patients with severe airflow obstruction and restriction (computer simulation). Note distinct optimum duty cycle for the obstructive case. (From Marini JJ: Patient-ventilator interaction: rational strategies for acute ventilatory management, *Respir Care* 38:482-493, 1993.)

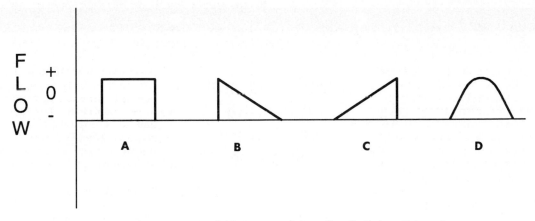

Fig. 32–6 Inspiratory flow patterns available on most moderns flow-limited ventilators. **A,** square wave (or constant flow); **B,** descending ramp (or decelerating flow); **C,** ascending ramp (or accelerating flow); **D,** sine wave.

ter 25). Heated humidifiers should provide at least 30 mg/L water vapor at 30° C; HMEs should be appropriate to the patient's size and tidal[5] volume.[32] HMEs that also provide high-efficiency bacterial filtration may provide added safety and benefit.[33]

When using a heated humidifier, the proximal airway temperature should be set to between 32° and 34° C. Ideally, the airway temperature should be servo-controlled with appropriate high and low alarms.

Once an approach is selected, patients should be reevaluated on a regular basis for their humidification needs (Figure 32-7).[34]

> **Contraindications to use of heat and moisture exchangers**
>
> - Patients with thick, copious, or bloody secretions
> - Patients with an expired V_T < 70% of the delivered V_T
> - Patients with body temperatures less than 32° C
> - Patients with high spontaneous minute volumes (> 10 L/min)
> - During aerosol treatments given via the patient circuit

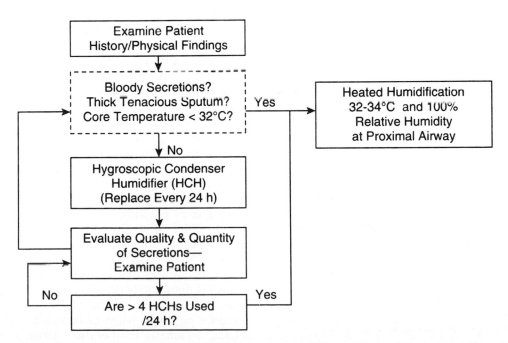

Fig. 32–7 Algorithm for selecting humidification system for patients receiving ventilatory support. (From Branson RD, Chatburn RL: Humidification during mechanical ventilation [editorial], *Respir Care* 38:461-468, 1993.)

■ MINI **C**LINI ■

32–1

Initiating and Adjusting Ventilatory Support

Problem: A mechanically ventilated patient is in the medical intensive care unit recovering from acute respiratory failure secondary to aspiration pneumonia. The patient currently requires airway suctioning every 30 to 60 minutes according to the RCP and staff nurse caring for the patient. In addition, they both note that the secretions are copious and thick in nature. Current ventilator settings are as follows:

Mode	– A/C
V_T	– 900 mL
Preset Rate	– 16/min
Total Rate	– 20/min
FIO_2	– 0.50
PIP	– 45cm H_2O
V_E	– 14-18L/min

The RCP is asked to place a heat and moisture exchanger (HME) unit with high-efficiency bacterial filtration on the ventilator circuit so that the tubing will not need to be changed as frequently. As a RCP who is familiar with HMEs, would this be an appropriate action on this patient?

Discussion: Although useful in many instances, placement of a heat and moisture exchanger (HME) would likely be contraindicated in this patient for multiple reasons. Adequate humidification in a patient with an artificial airway is critical in preventing inspissation of airway secretions, injury, and destruction of the airway epithelium, atelectasis and possible hypothermia. Humidification can be provided by using either a heated humidifier or HME unit. The patient information in this clinical scenario points to several potential problems of using an HME. The most obvious one being copious, thick airway secretions. The HME may not provide sufficient water vapor and heat output relative to consistency which could lead to retained secretions. Furthermore, the airway secretions could be coughed into the HME causing increased resistance to flow and possible obstruction. Since the patient has high ventilatory requirements as evidenced by an elevated exhaled minute volume, it is important that the humidification system be able to maintain adequate heat and moisture output when demands dictate. Other patient situations where an HME should not be used include during aerosol treatments given via the ventilator tubing circuit, high spontaneous minute volumes (>10 L/min), and when body temperature is less than 32° C.

Periodic sighs

Traditionally, ventilators routinely have been set to deliver sigh volumes 1½ to 2 times greater than the tidal volume, at rates between 5 and 20/hour. However, the routine use of sigh breaths during ventilatory support is no longer recommended.[35] Instead, sigh breaths should be applied only when indicated and should probably incorporate a long-duration inspiratory hold. Indications for sigh breaths are provided in the box below.[3]

Limits and alarms

As a component of the initial ventilator set-up, the clinician must activate all appropriate alarms and

verify and document their settings.[36] Details on mechanical ventilator alarms and alarm levels are provided in Chapter 31; here we emphasize initial alarm settings.

There are two basic types of ventilator alarms: (1) those that warn of device malfunction, and (2) those that alert the clinician to changes in patient status.[37,38] In terms of device malfunction alarms, microprocessor ventilators continuously monitor themselves and warn clinicians if power is lost, gas supply is insufficient, or an electronic/pneumatic malfunction has occurred. Typically, these device malfunction alarms are preset by the manufacturer.[38]

In general, only patient status alarms are set by the clinician. Essential patient status alarms include high/low minute ventilation, high/low tidal volume, high/low airway pressure, low PEEP/CPAP, and high/low FIO_2. Table 32-4 provides general guidelines for setting these alarms when initiating ventilatory support.[39,40]

A disconnect alarm (usually warning of low pressure) is mandatory on all ventilatory support apparatus.[41] If available in the CMV mode, an I:E alarm should be set to warn of changes in this parameter. Last, an airway temperature alarm should be set to warn of unexpected changes in the temperature of inspired gas.

Indications for sigh breaths[3]

- Before and after suctioning
- During chest physical therapy
- During and after bronchoscopy
- Before and during extubation
- If small V_Ts are used during controlled ventilation
- During re-expansion of lung collapse

Ventilatory support for specific disorders

The clinician should vary the initial ventilatory support settings based on the specific pathophysiologic problem causing respiratory failure. The most common specific problems the RCP will encounter include ARDS, airway obstruction, postoperative complications, neuromuscular disease, head trauma, and congestive heart failure. Less common special problems include the management of unilateral lung disease and bronchopleural fistula.

ARDS

Ventilatory support modes that have been reported to increase the survival of ARDS patients include pressure-controlled inverse ratio ventilation **(PCIRV)**,[42,43] intentional hypoventilation (permissive hypercapnia),[44] airway pressure release ventilation **(APRV)**,[45,46] and low-frequency positive pressure ventilation with extracorporeal CO_2 removal **(LFPPV-ECCO$_2$R)**.[47,48] The potential benefit of these strategies is linked with the comparatively lower pressures or volumes they deliver. Currently, however, there is no firm evidence that any one mode of ventilatory support (including traditional CMV/SIMV with PEEP) is best for patients with ARDS.[12]

The problem with ARDS is that the lung is not uniformly affected. While large portions of affected lung tissue have low compliance, other regions may retain normal compliance. Unfortunately, most of the V_T delivered by a ventilator goes to these regions with normal compliance. Thus, when using high tidal volumes (10 to 15 mL/kg) in ARDS, large volumes of gas end up overdistending small areas of normal lung tissue. In concept, this **overdistention** is the primary factor in high incidence of ventilator-associated lung injuries seen in ARDS.[12]

In animal models, the best correlate of this type of injury is the plateau pressure. For this reason, a primary emphasis in the ventilatory support of patients with ARDS should be to keep plateau pressures low. Other strategies appropriate to the ventilatory management of ARDS patients are listed in the box below.[12]

Airway obstruction

Patients with asthma and COPD who suffer acute respiratory failure have significant expiratory obstruction and hyperinflation.[12] Patients with asthma may also have high inspiratory resistance. In both groups, efforts should be made to maximize the expiratory time. In obstructive disorders, long expiratory times decrease end-expiratory lung volume, lower auto-PEEP, minimize the hemodynamic impact of positive pressure, and help avoid barotrauma.[49,50]

To lengthen expiration, one shortens inspiration. To shorten inspiration, inspiratory flows must be increased.[51] Unfortunately, high inspiratory flows also increase peak airway pressures. Remember, however,

---

Table 32-4 Initial setting of ventilator alarms

Alarm	Setting
High minute ventilation	10%–15% > set or targeted minute volume
Low minute ventilation	10%–15% < set or targeted minute volume
High V_T	10%–15% > set or targeted tidal volume
Low V_T	10%–15% < set or targeted tidal volume
High pressure Limit	About 10 cm H_2O > average peak airway pressure
Low pressure Limit	5–10 cm H_2O < average peak airway pressure
Low PEEP/CPAP	3–5 cm H_2O < PEEP or CPAP setting
FIO_2	± 5% of setting

From Kacmarek RM: Management of the patient-mechanical ventilator system. In Pierson DJ, Kacmarek RM, editors: *Foundations of Respiratory Care*, New York, 1992, Churchill Livingstone.

Guidelines for ventilatory support of ARDS patients[12]

- Clinician should choose a ventilator mode that can support oxygenation and ventilation in patients with ARDS and with which they have experience;
- An acceptable SaO_2 (usually >90%) should be targeted;
- When plateau pressure equals or exceeds 35 cm H_2O, the tidal volume (V_T) should be decreased (to as low as 5 mL/kg, or lower, if necessary); In conditions where chest wall compliance is low, plateau pressures somewhat greater than 35 cm H_2O may be acceptable;
- To limit plateau pressure (unless contraindicated), the $PaCO_2$ should be permitted to rise; rapid rises in $PaCO_2$ should be avoided, with normal kidney function, a slow reduction in V_T allows renal compensation;
- PEEP helps support oxygenation but is associated with harmful effects; the PEEP level should be set by empirical trial to the minimum needed to provide adequate oxygenation and reassessed regularly;
- Current opinion is that FIO_2 should be kept as low as possible. However, to maintain oxygenation at lower FIO_2s, higher alveolar pressures may be needed. When both high alveolar pressures and high FIO_2s are required to maintain oxygenation, it is reasonable to accept a SaO_2 slightly less than 90%;
- When oxygenation is inadequate, sedation, paralysis, and position change are possible corrective measures. Other factors in oxygen delivery, such as cardiac output and hemoglobin, should also be considered.

that the peak airway pressure is *always* somewhat higher than alveolar pressure when using flow-limited ventilation. In fact, in patients with airway obstruction, the peak airway pressure is usually much higher than the alveolar pressure at end-inspiration. Since it is high alveolar or plateau pressures that cause lung injury, the high flows and peak airway pressures needed in patients with obstructive disorders are not a major concern.

General guidelines for mechanical ventilation of patients with obstructive disorders are provided in the box below. In managing these patients, the RCP should remember to always adjust ventilation to the pH, not $PaCO_2$.[12] In addition, the clinician must recognize that high airway pressures and problems with CO_2 removal are more often seen in the severe asthmatic than in patients with COPD (emphysema and/or chronic bronchitis). If the RCP observes high airway pressures or problems in CO_2 removal in patients with COPD, complicating factors such as pneumothorax, pulmonary edema, mucus plugging, or bronchospasm should be considered.[12]

In managing patients in acute respiratory failure due to asthma, high pressures are predictive of pulmonary hyperinflation.[12] For this reason, both plateau and peak pressures should be minimized in these patients. This often requires a reduction in minute ventilation, with a resulting increase in $PaCO_2$. An elevated $PaCO_2$ is acceptable, as long as pH can be kept at an acceptable level.[13,52]

Some patients with acute severe asthma may "fight" and thus require sedation or paralysis. Sedation or paralysis can decrease active expiratory effort, lower CO_2 production, and help lessen airway collapse.[12] However, muscle paralysis is associated with both acute and long-term complications.

Postoperative patients

It is common practice in some centers to place all postoperative thoracic or abdominal surgery patients on ventilatory support. This is done with the intent of reducing or preventing pulmonary complications.

The fact is that few patients require ventilatory support outside the recovery room. Residual anesthetic effects may require short-term ventilatory support.[12] In addition, some patients who undergo thoracic or upper abdominal surgery show a large drop in FRC after surgery, which predisposes to atelectasis.[53,54] Although lung expansion therapy is usually sufficient to reverse this effect (see Chapter 27), some patients may need a short course of mechanical ventilation.[55] In these cases, the first priority should always be to avoid the common complications associated with ventilatory support.[56,57]

Neuromuscular disorders

Patients with neuromuscular disorders typically retain a normal ventilatory drive and have normal or nearly normal lung function.[58] In these patients, the primary problem is weakness of the ventilatory muscles.[12] Ventilatory muscle weakness can lead to atelectasis (from poor lung inflation) and pneumonia (from impaired cough and mucociliary clearance).[59,60] Atelectasis and pneumonia ultimately lead to respiratory failure. Thus, the main needs of patients with neuromuscular disorders who require ventilatory support are provision of adequate lung inflation and aggressive airway management.[61]

General guidelines for mechanical ventilation of patients with neuromuscular disorders are provided in the box, page 903. These patients are at lower risk for barotrauma than patients with interstitial restrictive problems or COPD. In addition, patients with neuromuscular disorders often prefer large tidal volumes and high inspiratory flows.[12]

The decision as to whether to use full or partial ventilatory support when managing a patient with a neuromuscular disorder requires assessment of the individual's muscle strength and disease process.[12] For example, a patient with a high cervical spine injury will likely need full ventilatory support, while a patient with some ventilatory capability (e.g., Guillian-Barre syndrome) may be adequately managed with a partial ventilatory support mode.

Guidelines for ventilatory support of patients with obstructive disorders[12]

- Volume-targeted, patient- or machine-cycled CMV (assist/control mode) may cause hyperinflation in awake patients with obstructive disorders, and should *not* be used as the initial support mode; clinicians should select an approach other than assist/control that they are familiar with and have used successfully;
- Peak inspiratory flow should be set high enough to meet the patient's inspiratory demands and allow sufficient expiratory time to avoid auto-PEEP;
- Clinicians should monitor for and minimize auto-PEEP:
  Use the lowest minute ventilation and longest expiratory time that produces acceptable gas exchange; this may require the clinician to accept hypercapnia;
  When auto-PEEP occurs in these patients, low levels of externally-applied PEEP may help reduce the work of breathing; Use of PEEP pressures higher than the auto-PEEP level can cause further hyperinflation and should be avoided;
- Wherever possible, the plateau pressure should be kept below 35 cm H_2O; in acutely ill patients with obstructive disorders, sedation or paralysis may be needed to accurately measure plateau pressures.

Guidelines for ventilatory support of patients with neuromuscular disorders[12]

- Large V_Ts (12 to 15 mL/kg) with or without PEEP (5 to 10 cm H_2O) may be needed to relieve dyspnea. High peak flows (>60 L/min) will typically be needed to satisfy patient inspiration demands;
- Use total or partial ventilatory support based on the patient's inherent ventilatory muscle strength.

Head trauma

The goal in providing ventilatory support to stable patients with closed-head injuries who have normal intracranial pressures (ICP) should be to maintain normal arterial blood gases.[62,63] Mechanical hyperventilation (lowering the $PaCO_2$ to 25 to 30 torr) can lower ICP, but should be used only when the ICP is abnormally high.[12] When hyperventilation is used to decrease ICP, the clinical should gradually return the patient's PCO_2 to normal levels over 24 to 48 hours.

Myocardial ischemia and congestive heart failure

General guidelines for mechanical ventilation of patients with myocardial ischemia and congestive heart failure are provided in the box below.

Inappropriately applied mechanical ventilation can increase work of breathing. An increased work of breathing increases oxygen consumption and may impair myocardial oxygenation.[64,65] Thus, in patients with acute myocardial ischemia requiring ventilatory support, it is essential to select a support mode that minimizes the work of breathing.[12]

Conventional wisdom dictates that positive pressure ventilation decreases venous return and cardiac output. In severe congestive heart failure, however, the decrease in afterload caused by positive pressure may actually increase left ventricular stroke volume and cardiac output.[66] In addition, positive pressure ventilation can increase the PaO_2 in patients with congestive heart failure, mainly by increasing lung volume and reducing shunting.[12]

Unilateral lung disease

When traditional positive pressure ventilation is applied to a patient with unilateral lung disease, most of the ventilation goes to the healthy lung. Several strategies have been used to overcome this problem. These approaches include independent lung ventilation (ILV),[67,68] differential CPAP,[69,70] positional changes,[71,72] bronchial blockers, and low inspiratory flows (to even gas distribution).[12] Unfortunately, no single strategy has emerged with proven efficacy in these patients. For this reason, only general guidelines can be offered at this time (see box below).[12] Should these methods not resolve the problem, more aggressive means of ventilatory support must be considered, such as LFPPV-ECCO$_2$R or **ECMO**.[12]

Bronchopleural fistula

There are two common sources of air leakage through a bronchopleural fistula **(BPF)** during positive pressure ventilation. In the first case, air leaks through a rupture in lung tissue caused by trauma, surgery, or other invasive procedures (e.g., central line placement). Alternatively, BPF may develop as a complication of diffuse lung disease like ARDS or *Pneumocystis carinii* pneumonia.[12] Most air leaks are minor; however, large BPFs can cause atelectasis, impair gas exchange, and prolong the need for mechanical ventilation.[12] In some cases, a BPF can be corrected surgically. For example, a bronchial tear can be sutured closed and an irreversibly damaged lung segment causing BPF can be removed. In most cases, however, correction of the BPF requires that the primary disease process be resolved.

Guidelines for ventilatory support of patients with myocardial ischemia or congestive heart failure[12]

- In the patients with acute myocardial ischemia, the clinician should select a mode of ventilatory support that minimizes the work of breathing;
- When severe hypoxemia accompanies congestive heart failure, positive pressure ventilation can decrease venous return and improve oxygenation;
- To assess the effect of positive pressure ventilation on the cardiovascular system, hemodynamic monitoring should be used.

Guidelines for ventilatory support of patients with unilateral lung disease[12]

- Begin with conventional ventilatory support techniques;
- If severe hypoxemia persists, apply a trial of ventilation with the least involved lung in the dependent (down) position;
- If PEEP is used, start with a standard single-lumen ET tube;
- If traditional PEEP does not provide adequate oxygenation, ILV may be tried; ILV need not be synchronous.[73]

All patients with BPF undergoing ventilatory support require chest tube suction to evacuate leaking gas. Ideally, the support mode used should assure adequate gas exchange by inflating the healthy lung areas.[74] Yet, no single ventilatory support mode has proved best in treating patients with BPF.

When the air leak is large and adequate ventilation cannot be maintained, high inspiratory flows and large tidal volumes may be needed at first. If this approach does not work, independent lung ventilation (ILV)[75], or high frequency jet ventilation (HFJV),[76] should be tried.

Once the leak lessens in severity, the ventilatory support strategy should change. In general, manipulations which reduce transpulmonary pressure will help decrease BPF flow and aid in closure.[77] To help close a bronchopleural fistula, the clinician should use a ventilatory support mode and settings that minimize airway and alveolar pressures.[12] Generally, this will require using the lowest possible VT, even to the extent of allowing the $PaCO_2$ top rise. PEEP levels also should be kept as low as possible.

PRELIMINARY ASSESSMENT AND DATA GATHERING

Once the initial ventilatory settings are established, the RCP should conduct a preliminary assessment of the patient and patient-ventilator system to assure that all parameters are well tolerated and the patient is stable and as comfortable as possible. Also during this phase, the RCP must assure that all necessary supplementary equipment necessary to provide patient support is available.

After the patient is stabilized, and the patient-ventilator system is verified in proper working order, initial arterial blood gases are obtained for analysis.

Initial patient assessment and support

Initial evaluation of the patient should include assessment of the patient's appearance and level of consciousness, measurement of vital signs, including heart rate and blood pressure, simple auscultation to verify bilateral ventilation, measurements of key ventilatory parameters (as provided by the support system), and a preliminary assessment of the airway. Other significant observations, such as cardiac arrhythmias, should also be noted. If the patient is conscious during this period of initial assessment, every effort must be made to attend to his or her psychological needs.

Details about the patient's airway should include verification of its position, patency, and cuff pressure. Endotracheal tube placement should be confirmed by either a chest radiograph or fiberoptic laryngoscopy. The initial cuff pressure should be set using either the minimal leak (MLT) or minimal occluding volume

(MOV) technique. In either case, cuff pressure at peak airway pressure should ideally be maintained below 25 mm Hg. An extra endotracheal or tracheostomy tube should be kept at the bedside in case of accidental extubation or rupture of the cuff. The necessary equipment for changing each type of airway must be available and easily accessible (refer to Chapter 22).

A clean, functioning manual resuscitator, connected to oxygen and ready for use, must be available at the bedside in the event of mechanical or electrical failure. A suction source, supply of catheters and sterile water or saline for instillation must also be available, as frequent suctioning may be required and all patients are at risk of airway occlusion by secretions at any time.

Arterial blood gas analysis

Early arterial blood gas analysis is a critical component of initial patient assessment. However, sampling of the arterial blood should be undertaken only after sufficient time has passed to ensure equilibration between the alveolar and arterial gas tensions.

The time necessary for equilibration between the alveolar and arterial gas tensions depends on the underlying disease process. In patients with normal lung function, equilibration between the alveolar and arterial gas tensions can be expected in less than 5 minutes, and arterial blood gases evaluated accordingly. As alveolar ventilation increases and FRC decreases, less time is needed for equilibration of gas tensions. However, in patients with lower than normal alveolar ventilation and larger than normal FRCs, such as those with COPD, equilibration times may be significantly longer than normal. In such patients, it is advisable to wait for 30 minutes after initiation of ventilatory support (or changing support parameters) before sampling the arterial blood.

GOAL SETTING FOR VENTILATORY SUPPORT

The effective application of ventilatory support should be based on clinical goals or objectives.[78,79] Of course, the ultimate end-goal is supporting the patient until the underlying problem is resolved and mechanical ventilation is no longer needed.

In consultation with the patient's physician, the RCP should establish measurable clinical objectives to guide the course of ventilatory support toward discontinuation. Such objectives should provide clear and consistent direction to those involved in the patient's management, yet allow for tailoring the plan according to the patient's condition and individual needs.

The accompanying box outlines the three primary physiologic goals toward which ventilatory support is directed.[12]

Physiologic goals of artificial ventilatory support[12]

- To support or manipulate gas exchange
  alveolar ventilation (eg, arterial PCO_2 and pH)
  arterial oxygenation (eg, PaO_2, SaO_2)
- To increase lung volume
  end inspiratory lung inflation
  functional residual capacity (FRC)
- To reduce or manipulate the work of breathing

Associated with each goal should be tangible interim and end-stage clinical objectives used to determine goal achievement. As an example, if the primary goal is to ensure adequate patient oxygenation, the interim objectives might be to reverse hypoxemia by providing adequate arterial oxygenation (a PaO_2 above 60 torr). On the other hand, the end-stage objective, associated with discontinuance of the support modality, might be the ability of the patient to maintain a PO_2 above 80 torr on an FIO_2 of less than 0.40 without PEEP or CPAP. Clearly, multiple objectives may need to be established for some patients. Specific clinical objectives for ventilatory support are listed in the box below.[12]

ADJUSTING VENTILATORY SUPPORT SETTINGS

As with the management process in general, adjusting ventilator settings should proceed in a systematic manner. Basic physiologic models provide good guidance in this regard. However, the clinician must always keep in mind two basic principles:[12]

1. Although the qualitative response of patients to changes in ventilator settings is usually predictable, the quantitative response is not. For example, raising PEEP usually improves the PaO_2. However, *how much* the PaO_2 increases in any given patient is hard to predict;

Specific clinical objectives of ventilatory support[12]

- To reverse hypoxemia
- To reverse acute respiratory acidosis
- To relieve respiratory distress
- To prevent or reverse atelectasis
- To reverse ventilatory muscle fatigue
- To permit sedation and/or neuromuscular blockade
- To decrease systemic or myocardial oxygen consumption
- To reduce intracranial pressure (ICP)
- To stabilize the chest

---

2. A change in settings designed to improve one physiologic parameter may have adverse effects on others. For example, when one increases PEEP, the PaO_2 may rise but the cardiac output may fall, causing an actual decrease in O_2 delivery. The extent of harmful side effects due to ventilator changes also varies greatly among individual patients.

There are three key categories of adjustments to be made after starting ventilatory support. These include adjustments in ventilation and delivered volume, adjustments in FIO_2 and PEEP/CPAP, and adjustments in patient-ventilator interaction.

Adjusting ventilation and delivered volume

The goal in adjusting ventilatory parameters is to maintain adequate ventilation at safe pressures. You judge the adequacy of ventilation by assessing the patient's $PaCO_2$, as related to the pH. In most cases you will adjust ventilatory parameters to achieve a $PaCO_2$ which normalizes the pH.

You change the patient's $PaCO_2$ by altering the minute ventilation. The following formula estimates of the change in minute ventilation needed to achieve a desired $PaCO_2$:

$$\text{New } \dot{V}_E = \text{Current } \dot{V}_E \times \frac{\text{current } PaCO_2}{\text{desired } PaCO_2}$$

For example, assume a patient being ventilated in the CMV-control mode with a $\dot{V}_E$ of 6.5 L/min has a $PaCO_2$ of 55 torr. If you wish to bring the $PaCO_2$ down 40 torr, the new $\dot{V}_E$ would be calculated as follows:

$$\text{New } \dot{V}_E = 6.50 \text{ L/min} \times \frac{55 \text{ torr}}{40 \text{ torr}}$$
$$\text{New } \dot{V}_E = 8.94 \text{ L/min}$$

Once you know what the new $\dot{V}_E$ should be, you must decide how to achieve it. How you change a patient's minute ventilation depends on the ventilatory support mode being used.

As shown in Table 32-5, page 908, in volume-targeted modes we can change $\dot{V}_E$ by changing either the rate or tidal volume. When our goal is to increase $\dot{V}_E$ while using a volume-targeted CMV mode, we generally increase the tidal volume rather than the rate. This is because raising the tidal volume is a more efficient way to increase $\dot{V}_E$ than increasing the rate (raising V_T decreases deadspace ventilation per minute).

To decrease $\dot{V}_E$ in volume-targeted CMV modes, we generally lower the rate (if tolerable) rather than V_T. The exception is when we want to decrease V_T to avoid lung injury due to excessive pressure. In these cases, we may decrease V_T to as low as 5 mL/kg.

In the CMV-assist/control mode, a simple decrease in $\dot{V}_E$ may not result in the desired rise in $PaCO_2$. In these cases, the clinician can add mechanical dead-

Table 32–5 Changing the minute ventilation

Mode	To Increase $\dot{V}_E$	To Decrease $\dot{V}_E$
VOLUME-TARGETED:		
CMV-Control	- increase V_T	- decrease rate
CMV-Assist/Control	- increase V_T	- decrease rate
		- add deadspace
SIMV	- increase rate	- decrease rate
	- add pressure support	
PRESSURE-TARGETED:		
PCV	- increase ΔP	- decrease ΔP
	- increase rate	- decrease rate
PSV	- increase ΔP	- decrease ΔP
BiPAP(c)	- increase ΔP (IPAP-EPAP)	- decrease ΔP (IPAP-EPAP)
APRV	- increase ΔP	- decrease ΔP
	- increase release frequency	- decrease release frequency

space to the ventilator circuit. To add mechanical deadspace to a ventilator circuit, you place a section of large-bore tubing between the circuit Y and the airway connector.

As rebreathed volume, mechanical deadspace increases the inspired PCO_2. An increase in inspired PCO_2 raises the alveolar and arterial CO_2 tensions. Although nomograms exist to estimate the amount of deadspace needed for a given $PaCO_2$,[80] most clinicians simply add 50 to 100 mL increments until the desired $PaCO_2$ is achieved. Adding mechanical deadspace in the IMV mode is contraindicated, due to the smaller patient tidal volumes.

During volume-targeted SIMV, the total minute ventilation has two components: (1) the machine or ventilator $\dot{V}_E$, plus (2) the spontaneous or patient $\dot{V}_E$:

$$\dot{V}_E \text{ total} = \dot{V}_E \text{ machine} + \dot{V}_E \text{ spon}$$

Since we only can change the ventilator component, we only have partial control over the total minute ventilation during SIMV. To change the minute ventilation during SIMV, we usually increase or decrease the SIMV (machine) rate. In addition to assessing the patient's $PaCO_2$ and pH, however, we also must closely follow the spontaneous breathing rate. This is particularly important when decreasing the $\dot{V}_E$ by lowering the SIMV rate. Should the patient's spontaneous breathing rate rise above 25 to 30/min while lowering the SIMV rate, a higher SIMV rate with lower V_T should be tried.

In pressure-targeted modes, we usually alter minute ventilation by changing the pressure differential.

The *pressure differential* (ΔP) is the difference between the peak and baseline or PEEP pressure:

$$\Delta P = (P_{peak} - PEEP)$$

For a given set of lung characteristics, ΔP determines the transpulmonary pressure gradient and thus the delivered V_T. Any change which increases ΔP thus increases V_T. Conversely, any change which lowers ΔP decreases V_T. Unfortunately, how much V_T will change for a given change in ΔP cannot be predicted in advance. For this reason, changing the minute ventilation in pressure-targeted modes is very much a trial and error process.

During pressure control and pressure support ventilation, we normally increase or decrease ΔP by increasing or decreasing P_{peak} (the pressure limit). Of course, the same results could be achieved by holding the peak pressure constant while altering the PEEP level, but this is seldom done. Changing the rate of breathing will also alter $\dot{V}_E$ in the pressure control mode, but this is generally less effective than altering P_{peak}.

When using BiPAP®, the clinician sets two pressure levels: the inspiratory positive airway pressure (IPAP) and the expiratory positive airway pressure (EPAP). In this case, the pressure differential is simply the difference between the two:

$$\Delta P = (IPAP - EPAP)$$

Any change that increases this pressure differential will tend to raise the delivered V_T. Conversely, any change that decreases the difference between IPAP and EPAP will tend to lower V_T. However, since changes in spontaneous patient effort and rate of breathing also affect $\dot{V}_E$ during BiPAP®, changing the pressure differential alone may not alter the $PaCO_2$ as much as expected.

During APRV, the clinician has control over four parameters: (1) the baseline pressure, (2) the release pressure, (3) the release frequency, and (4) the release time. The baseline pressure, release pressure, and release frequency all affect ventilation.

To increase CO_2 excretion during ARPV, one can raise the baseline pressure, lower the release pressure, or increase the release frequency. Conversely, one can decrease CO_2 removal during ARPV by lowering the baseline pressure, raising the release pressure, or decreasing the release frequency.

In most patients, you will adjust ventilator settings to keep the $PaCO_2$ between 35 and 45 torr, with the pH in the normal range (7.35 to 7.45). There are several situations, however, in which this PCO_2 target is not appropriate. First, in patients with chronic CO_2 retention, 'normal' $PaCO_2$s can be as high as 55 to 65 torr. In these patients, adjusting the $PaCO_2$ to 35 to 45 torr will cause alkalosis. Second, these will be cases in which deliberate hyperventilation is one of the goals of ventilatory support, as when trying to decrease the

ICP in closed head injuries. Last, to limit dangerously high plateau pressures (> 35 cm H_2O), we may purposefully use a low V_T or pressure limit and allow the $PaCO_2$ to rise.[11]

Adjusting oxygenation

In adjusting oxygenation, the ultimate goal is to maintain adequate oxygen delivery to the tissues, while keeping the FIO_2 at a safe, nontoxic level. To this end, each patient must be evaluated individually, taking into account their history, age, and normal PaO_2.

You can adjust oxygenation by changing either the FIO_2 or the PEEP/CPAP level. In general, FIO_2 adjustments alone are satisfactory when hypoxemia is due to a low V/Q ratio. However, PEEP/CPAP usually will be needed to improve oxygenation when physiologic shunting is present.

Adjusting the FIO_2

For patients with normal oxygen carrying capacities and cardiovascular performance, we adjust the FIO_2 to achieve PaO_2s between 60 and 100 torr or SaO_2s $\geq$ 90%. For patients with chronic lung disease and acute-on-chronic hypoxemia, PaO_2s slightly below 60 torr are satisfactory, as long as the SaO_2 exceeds 85%.[81]

The response to changes in FIO_2 depends on the underlying disease process. Patients with normal lungs will have adequate PaO_2s at low FIO_2s. Patients who are hypoventilating or have a minor V/Q mismatch will also respond well to small changes in FIO_2. In contrast, patients with large physiologic shunts will not show much improvement in oxygenation, even when high FIO_2s are applied.

Because the response to changing the FIO_2 varies, simple predicting formulas that do not account for the severity of the disease process are unreliable. However, by using an index of oxygenation that reflects the severity of hypoxemia, we can accurately predict FIO_2 needs.

Among the most reliable indices of oxygenation is the ratio of PaO_2 to PAO_2, also called the a/A ratio.[82,83] To compute the a/A ratio, one must first compute the alveolar oxygen tension (PAO_2), using the alveolar air equation (see Chapter 12). Then one simply divides the arterial PO_2 by the computed PAO_2. The result is a decimal value between 0 and 1.0.

For example, take a patient receiving ventilatory support with 35% oxygen at sea level who has a $PaCO_2$ of 48 torr and a PaO_2 of 50 torr. We calculate the alveolar PO_2 as follows:

$$PAO_2 = FIO_2(PB - PH_2O) - \frac{PaCO_2}{R}$$

$$PAO_2 = .35(760 \text{ torr} - 47 \text{ torr}) - \frac{48 \text{ torr}}{0.8}$$

$$= 250 \text{ torr} - 60 \text{ torr}$$

$$= 190 \text{ torr}$$

To compute the a/A ratio, simply divide the arterial PO_2 (50 torr) by the alveolar PO_2 (190 torr):

$$\text{a/A ratio} = \frac{PaO_2}{PAO_2}$$

$$\text{a/A ratio} = \frac{50}{190}$$

$$\text{a/A ratio} = 0.26$$

The a/A ratio is useful for interpreting the cause and severity of hypoxemia, especially when mixed venous oxygen measures are not available.[84] In simple terms, this value represents the proportion of alveolar oxygen that actually gets into the blood. Normally, the a/A ratio ranges from 0.9 in healthy young subjects to 0.74 in the elderly. a/A values below 0.6 indicate V/Q imbalances requiring simple oxygen therapy. a/A values below 0.15 indicate refractory hypoxemia caused by significant intrapulmonary shunting.

The a/A ratio also can be used to predict the FIO_2 needed for a desired arterial oxygen tension.[85,86] The predicting formula is:

$$FIO_2 \text{ needed} = \frac{(\text{desired } PaO_2 \div \text{a/A ratio}) + PaCO_2}{(PB - 47)}$$

Using our prior patient as an example (PaO_2 = 50 torr, $PaCO_2$ = 48 torr, a/A = 0.26), we will try to raise the PaO_2 to 90 mm Hg (the desired PaO_2). For this patient, the FIO_2 needed for a PaO_2 of 90 torr is estimated as follows:

$$FIO_2 \text{ needed} = \frac{(\text{desired } PaO_2 \div \text{a/A ratio}) + PaCO_2}{(PB - 47)}$$

$$FIO_2 \text{ needed} = \frac{(90 \div 0.26) + 48}{(760 - 47)}$$

$$FIO_2 \text{ needed} = 0.55$$

Instead of using the formula method, you can use a nomogram to predict a patient's needed FIO_2 (Figure 32-8, page 910). To use this nomogram, first align the patient's current FIO_2 and $PaCO_2$ (on the left) with a straightedge. This line will intersect the vertical lines corresponding to the patient's current PAO_2 and PaO_2. Intersecting the PaO_2 vertical at this point will be a diagonal line corresponding to the patient's a/A ratio. Next, move along this diagonal line to a point above the desired PaO_2. From this point (the patient's a/A ratio and desired PaO_2), draw a horizontal line to the left until you intersect the PAO_2 vertical. Last, connect this point (the needed PAO_2) to the patient's $PaCO_2$. Where this line intersects the FIO_2 vertical is the needed FIO_2.

For example, take a patient with a $PaCO_2$ of 40 torr and a PaO_2 of 50 torr breathing 40% oxygen (FIO_2 = 0.40). Assume we want to raise the PaO_2 to 80 torr. First, align the $PaCO_2$ of 40 with the FIO_2 of 0.40. Following this line to right, we read a PAO_2 of 240 torr from its vertical. Next, the patient's line intersects the

PaO$_2$ = 50 vertical on the a/A ratio diagonal of 0.2. Go up this diagonal to a point above desired PaO$_2$ of 80 torr. From here, follow a horizontal line back to the left to intersect the PaO$_2$ vertical at about 400 torr. Connect this point with the PaCO$_2$ of 40. This new line intersects the FIO$_2$ at about 0.63, the FIO$_2$ needed to obtain a PaO$_2$ of 80 torr.

Adjusting PEEP or CPAP

Positive end expiratory pressure (PEEP) or continuous positive airway pressure (CPAP) are indicated for patients with arterial hypoxemia that do not respond to high FIO$_2$s. Clinically, this is known as *refractory hypoxemia.* A patient has refractory hypoxemia when the PaO$_2$ cannot be maintained above 60 torr while breathing 60% or more oxygen.

Because both PEEP and CPAP can impair cardiovascular function and cause barotrauma, it is important to carefully monitor the levels being used and the effect on the patient.[87,88] When you initiate PEEP or CPAP, the goal should be to achieve adequate oxygenation, with an acceptable FIO$_2$, without impairing cardiovascular function. In principle, this optimum level of PEEP or CPAP is indicated when oxygen delivery to the tissues is maximized. Thus precise determination of the optimum level of PEEP or CPAP level can be accomplished only when hemodynamic data—specifically cardiac output and mixed venous PO$_2$ measures—are available.

This approach to optimizing PEEP or CPAP involves applying incremental levels of distending pressure, while monitoring the patient's cardiopulmonary response. Figure 32-9, provides an example of a PEEP study using this empirical method. As distending pressures are raised, careful attention is given to changes in arterial and mixed venous oxygenation as related to cardiac output and blood pressure. Total oxygen delivery is calculated at each incremental level of pressure, with the optimum pressure level corresponding to the point at which these parameters indicate the best effect. In the example provided, PEEP levels of 20 and 25 appear equally effective. However, in this case, the lower level (20 cm H$_2$O) is chosen to minimize the potential for barotrauma.

Obviously, this approach can only be used when the patient has a pulmonary artery catheter in place (see Chapter 33). As an alternative, one can adjust PEEP/CPAP without pulmonary artery monitoring by assessing PaO$_2$ levels as related to effective compliance and arterial blood pressure. As depicted in Figure 32-10, page 912, increasing levels of PEEP/CPAP are normally associated with an increase in both the FRC and the compliance of the lung, as well as an increase in PaO$_2$. This phenomenon is due to both recruitment of additional alveoli and the characteristic steepening of the pressure-volume curve that occurs at higher lung volumes.

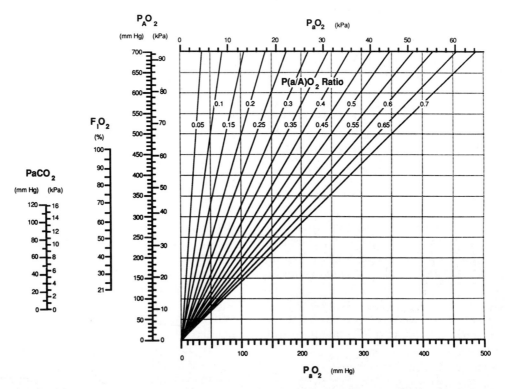

Fig. 32-8 Nomogram for computing a/A ratio and predicting the FIO$_2$ needs of patients. See text for description. (From Chatburn RL: Principles and practice of neonatal and pediatric mechanical ventilation, *Respir Care,* 36:569-593, 1991.)

	0	5	10	15	20	25	30
Minutes/time	15	30	45	60	75	90	105
Blood Pressure (mm Hg)	117/80	120/85	120/80	110/70	115/75	115/75	90/65
P_{Peak} (cm H_2O)	33	39	43	51	51	53	60
P_{PL} (cm H_2O) (plateau)	28	33	37	48	45	47	58
$V_{t\ spontaneous}/V_{t\ ventilator}$	200/1000	200/1000	250/1000	250/1000	250/1000	250/1000	250/1000
$f_{spontaneous}/f_{ventilator}$	4/10	4/10	3/10	4/10	3/10	5/10	6/10
$\dot{V}_E$ Total (l/min)	10.8	10.8	10.8	11.0	10.8	11.3	11.5
C_s (ml/cm H_2O)	36	36	37	35	40	45	36
PaO_2 (F_IO_2 = 1.0)	43	59	65	73	103	152	167
CaO_2 (vol %)	15.3	17.8	18.3	18.9	19.2	19.4	19.6
$PaCO_2$ (mm Hg)	37	37	38	37	39	37	38
pH	7.41	7.42	7.42	7.42	7.40	7.41	7.41
$P(A-a)O_2$ (mm Hg)	607	591	585	577	547	498	483
$PaCO_2 \cdot P_{ET}CO_2$ (mm Hg)	16	15	13	10	9	8	15
$P\bar{v}O_2$ (or $S\bar{v}O_2$) (mm Hg or %)	27	37	38	38	39	40	34
C.O. L/min	4.1	4.2	4.0	4.5	4.4	4.4	3.3
$C(A-\bar{V})O_2$ (vol %)	5.3	5.2	5.4	5.0	4.9	4.9	6.7
PCWP (mm Hg)	3	5	8	11	12	13	18
PAP (mm Hg)	37/21	39/25	41/24	43/25	40/21	38/24	45/30
C.O. x CaO_2 Oxygen transport	790	811	772	869	854	854	776

Comments: Bilateral scattered crackles present in both lungs.

Fig. 32-9 Example of a PEEP study flow sheet including ventilation, oxygenation, and hemodynamic data. Key points to observe when first reviewing a PEEP study are: (1) blood pressure, (2) mixed venous oxygen, and (3) oxygen transport. Notice that these three values decline at a PEEP of 30 cm H_2O. Blood pressure drops to 90/65, PvO_2 drops to 34 mmHg, and oxygen transport drops to 776 mL/min. A more optimum PEEP level is +20 cm H_2O where these parameters and others indicate that oxygen transport is improving without significant cardiovascular side effects. (From Pilbeam SP: Mechanical ventilation: physiological and clinical applications, St Louis, 1986, Mosby.)

In principle, a point is reached at which lung compliance is maximized, beyond which alveoli become overdistended and compliance falls.[89] As long as the blood pressure remains stable, this point represents a rough estimate of the optimum PEEP level.[90] This level should be confirmed by bedside assessment of the adequacy of circulation and oxygenation.

Adjusting patient-ventilator interaction

Patient-ventilator interaction refers to how the machine setup influences patient work, comfort, and synchrony during ventilator-assisted breaths.[26] Key factors affecting patient-ventilator interaction are listed in the accompanying box.[91,92]

Level/type of ventilatory support

The level and type of ventilatory support has a major impact on patient-ventilator interaction. Un-

---

Key factors affecting patient-ventilator interaction[91,92]

Level of ventilatory support
Artificial airway
Inspiratory flow
Trigger sensitivity
Humidification systems
Demand valve function
Flow-triggered system function
PEEP valve function
Presence of auto-PEEP

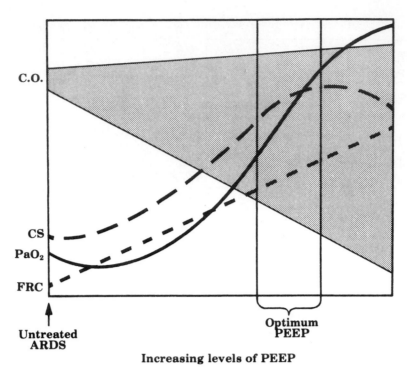

Fig. 32-10 The curves above represent the physiologic factors that change during the application of PEEP or CPAP. As the PEEP level is increased PaO$_2$, FRC, and static compliance (Cs) normally increase. Cardiac output (CO), represented by the shaded area, can increase slightly, stay the same, or decrease. The optimum PEEP level can be expected to occur where PaO$_2$, FRC, and Cs are high. Cardiac output should be maintained near normal so that oxygen transport to the tissues remains high. (From Pilbeam SP: Mechanical ventilation: physiological and clinical applications, St Louis, 1986, Mosby.)

■ MINI **C** LINI ■

32-2

Initiating and Adjusting Ventilatory Support

Problem: A RCP is involved in the clinical management of an 30 year old man who is in the critical care unit for blunt trauma to the chest following a motor vehicle accident. The patient is currently receiving mechanical ventilatory support with machine settings as follows;

    Mode – Volume A/C
    V$_T$ – 900 mL
    Rate – 20/min
    FIO$_2$ – 0.70

Arterial blood gases are drawn with the following results: pH—7.38, PaCO$_2$—36 torr, PaO$_2$—48torr, oxygen saturation—81%. The RCP considers a recommendation that positive end-expiratory pressure (PEEP) be instituted. What are the goals of this type of adjunctive therapy and what are some of the potential adverse effects of PEEP that the RCP should be alert for?

Discussion: The general goals of PEEP are to recruit and stabilize closed alveolar units to achieve adequate oxygenation and to avoid potentially unsafe levels of FIO$_2$ and impairment of systemic oxygen transport. Improvement is most commonly assessed by arterial blood gas analysis; in particular oxygen tension and oxyhemoglobin saturation. The use of PEEP in this situation may be appropriate since the PaO$_2$ and SaO$_2$ values suggest poor arterial oxygenation despite and elevated FIO$_2$ level. When the PaO$_2$ fails to respond to a high FIO$_2$, this condition is referred to as refractory hypoxemia. The precise determination of an "optimum" level of PEEP can be problematic unless measures of oxygen transport and utilization are available. This however, would require placement of a pulmonary artery catheter with measurement of cardiac output and acquisition of mixed venous blood. As the level of PEEP is increased, the RCP must be alert for signs of potential complications such as but not limited to: barotrauma from high peak and mean airway pressures, decreased cardiac output and oxygen transport (despite an improvement in PaO$_2$ and SaO$_2$) from decreased venous return, and increased pulmonary vascular resistance from intrathoracic pressure. In the absence of a pulmonary artery catheter, assessment of arterial blood pressure and heart rate would be helpful. Lastly, measurement of effective compliance may be useful in certain situations where higher levels of PEEP are indicated and concern of alveolar overdistention is possible.

fortunately, the optimum amount and type of support is not known, and surely varies between patients.[91] Too much support may produce respiratory muscle weakness or atrophy; too little support may lead to fatigue. Thus, the primary objective in adjusting the level and type of support is to have the ventilator perform sufficient work to prevent patient fatigue, while allowing the patient to perform enough work to prevent atrophy.[93]

Thus, soon after initiating ventilatory support, and once the patient is adequately stabilized, the clinician should allow the patient to take on some of the breathing workload. By definition, this means switching to a partial ventilatory support mode, such as SIMV (with or without PSV), low-level PSV, BiPAP®, or APRV.

Unfortunately, the partial support provided by some of these modes does not always relieve the patient's breathing workload as intended.[94] For example, during flow-limited volume-cycled SIMV, dyspneic patients often fail to take full advantage of the power assist available from the machine. Specifically, the inspiratory pressure-time product for the patient-triggered SIMV breaths is often the same as for spontaneous breaths. This makes one breathing effort look very much like the next—machine aided or not.[94]

This contradicts the common assumption that the patient need only trigger the machine, after which the ventilator will take over the breathing workload. In reality, patients seldom stop their breathing efforts once the machine triggers on. In this respect, the ventilator and patient act together to accomplish the work associated with a given breath.[26] Thus, for a given patient-triggered machine breath, the harder the patient pulls, the less effectively is work off-loaded to the ventilator.[16,17]

With the patient required to take on a portion of the work of breathing during partial ventilatory support, we must make every effort not to impose any unnecessary workload. Airway and machine factors that can impose additional work on the patient are discussed subsequently. In terms of the level of partial support, we should off-load sufficient work to the ventilator to allow the patient to breathe comfortably at spontaneous rates less than 20/min.[92] To do so, we should: (1) provide a sufficient number of machine-assisted breaths to prevent tachypnea, (2) assure adequate inspiratory flows during these machine-assisted breaths,[92] and (3) use pressure support ventilation, when necessary, to help augment spontaneous tidal volumes.[95-97]

Artificial airway

Next to the level and type of support, the artificial airway is the most important factor affecting work of breathing during ventilatory support.[96,98] This is because artificial airways, especially nasotracheal tubes,

offer the greatest resistance to gas flow of all circuit components.[98]

As a rule of thumb, the smaller the tube and the greater the minute ventilation, the greater the imposed work of breathing.[99] Bends and kinks in ET tubes, and adherence of secretion to their inner walls, further increase flow resistance and thus the breathing workload imposed on patients.[100] Small ET tubes can also worsen the auto-PEEP effect, thereby further elevating workload and contributing to patient-ventilator **asynchrony.**

The ideal solution is to use the largest possible ET tube. Generally, this means ≥ 7.5 mm for women and ≥ 8.0 mm for men.[102] If this is not possible, one can add a low level of pressure support ventilation to overcome the work of breathing imposed by a small airway.[92,96,97]

Inspiratory flow and time

As previously described, the inspiratory flow, together with the trigger level, is a key factor affecting the patient's inspiratory workload.[16-18] Once the initial flow is set, the clinician should reassess its adequacy, and, where necessary, make appropriate changes.

To determine the adequacy of machine flow, one assesses the airway *pressure* waveform. Deviation of the pressure waveform from normal usually indicates that the inspiratory flow is not properly adjusted (Figure 32-11, page 914).[103] The clinician then increases or decreases the flow until the pressure waveform is restored to its normal configuration.

In addition to flow **dysynchrony** during inspiration, some patients may experience timing dysynchrony.[26] For example, during volume-cycled modes, the patient may try to begin exhalation before the ventilator has completed its inspiratory cycle. Although this problem is diminished with pressure-limited modes, it is not eliminated. During pressure-limited ventilation of patients with obstructive disorders, flow may simply decelerate too slowly to cycle the machine off in time for exhalation to begin synchronously with the patient's own rhythm (Figure 32-12, page 914).[26] Under such conditions, exhalation must be initiated by active expiratory muscle action. This adds to the total breathing workload, and can even increase the severity of obstruction.[26]

Trigger sensitivity

After initiating ventilatory support, the clinician should "fine-tune" the trigger sensitivity setting. Fine-tuning is necessary because too sensitive a setting can cause some ventilators to auto-trigger, while an unresponsive trigger level can add to the breathing workload and cause patient-ventilator asynchrony.[91] For example, clinical studies have shown that decreas-

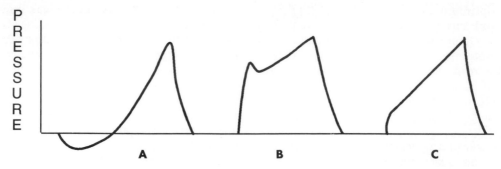

Fig. 32-11 Using the airway pressure waveform to determine the adequacy of machine flow (applies only when ventilator is set to deliver a constant flow). **A**, when the pressure rise lags, inspiratory flow is too low and should be increased. **B**, when the pressure spikes early on, inspiratory flow is too high and should be decreased. **C**, when the flow is adequate to meet patient needs, a small early rise in pressure (equivalent to that needed to overcome airway resistance) is followed by a more gradual ascent to the peak level.

ing the trigger level from 2 to 5 cm H_2O can increase the patient's work of breathing by as much as 34%.[16]

In addition, the less sensitive the trigger setting, the greater the "lag time" between the onset of muscle contraction and the initiation of ventilator flow.[104] This prolonged response time impairs patient-ventilator synchrony and adds to the total breathing workload.

Rather than relying strictly on a trigger setting, the clinician should always observe the effect by reference to the appropriate display. For pressure-triggered systems, the clinician should use either the pressure manometer or graphics display to confirm that airway pressure deflections of no more than 0.5 to 1.5 cm H_2O below baseline actually initiate a machine-assisted breath. Appropriate flow-triggering is more difficult to confirm, since not all systems display the baseline flow. Lacking this information, one should carefully observe the patient's inspiratory efforts, while tallying machine responses. If several patient efforts occur without an expected machine breath, chances are the sensitivity needs to be increased.

Other factors that can prolong ventilator response time other than an incorrect trigger sensitivity setting are listed in the accompanying box.[91,104] The use of unresponsive demand valves is discussed separately.

Humidification systems

The classic bubble-through humidifier presents a special problem in assuring patient-ventilator synchrony. If a bubble-through humidifier is used on a ventilator that senses inspiratory effort proximal to the humidifier, the patient effort needed to trigger the machine on will markedly increase.[92,105]

Heat and moisture exchanges are less of a problem, but can increase flow resistance and work of breath-

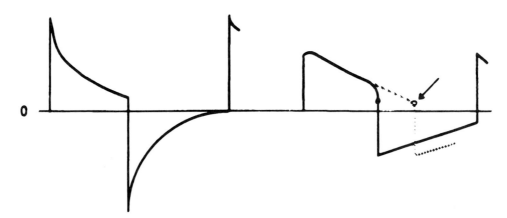

Fig. 32-12 Off-switch triggering during pressure controlled ventilation for normal (*left*) and for severely obstructed patient (*right*). Flow profile during airflow obstruction may require patient to use expiratory effort to lower flow enough to cycle machine off. Passive exhalation (*dashed line*) would require excessive inspiratory time. (From Marini JJ: Patient-ventilator interaction: rational strategies for acute ventilatory management, *Respir Care* 38:482-493, 1993.)

<table>
<tr><td>

**Factors that can prolong
ventilator response time[91,104]**

- Low trigger sensitivity
- Abdominal/rib cage paradox
- Auto-PEEP (dynamic hyperinflation)
- High tubing compliance
- High circuit deadspace
- Transducer variability
- High bias flow in the circuit
- Unresponsive demand valves

</td></tr>
</table>

ing, especially when water-laden.[106] The solution is to always use a pass-over or wick-type humidifier whenever applying partial ventilatory support to patients with high spontaneous minute ventilations.

Demand valve function

Unfortunately, many ventilators which provide spontaneous breaths via mechanical demand valves do not perform as expected. First, on ventilators measuring *internal or machine* pressure, the amount of pressure needed to open the demand valves is significantly more than the pressure change observed on the manometer.[107] Second, when the patient's inspiratory time is short, pressure drops as high as 23 cm H_2O may be needed to start gas flow, with 4 to 10 cm H_2O differentials being the rule.[107,108] As expected, such pressure drops can increase both the mechanical work and oxygen cost of breathing.[109-111]

Although some of this imposed work is due to pressure drops across high resistance humidifiers, most is caused by design flaws in these valve systems.[96] For example, the response time of some demand valves is as slow as 180 to 250 msec.[111] A continuous flow pressure reservoir system, on the other hand, can respond in as little as one-eighth this time, or about 33 msec.[111]

The ideal solution to this problem is to avoid using mechanical demand valves altogether and switch to a flow-triggered system. A flow-triggered system provides a continuous low bias flow of 3 to 20 L/min through the patient circuit while responding to patient needs via changes in flow, rather than pressure.[112,113] The work of breathing through most flow-triggered systems is comparable to that observed during unrestricted T-tube breathing.[113]

If a flow-triggered system is not available, the addition of 5 cm H_2O pressure support to a demand-flow system reduces the inspiratory work to a level comparable with that of a continuous flow system.[113]

Flow-triggered system function

Not all flow-triggered systems are equal. Although most minimize the effort needed for a patient to start a spontaneous breath, not all provide sufficient flow

during inspiration.[92,105] Peak flows available for spontaneous breathing should be at least 60 to 90 L/min. What the available *base flow* is seems less important, since variations in base flow apparently have no effect on the patient's work of breathing.[114]

PEEP valve function

The ideal PEEP/CPAP valve is a true threshold resistor, offering zero flow resistance and generating a pressure totally independent of flow. No PEEP valve meets this ideal. All PEEP valves offer some flow resistance and can therefore impose additional *expiratory* workload on the patient.[115]

Ideally, clinicians should be familiar with the flow resistive properties of the PEEP/CPAP valves used on their patients. One should always select and use those valves which offer minimal flow resistance. Decreased expiratory flow, prolongation of expiratory time, or active expiratory muscle effort during ventilatory support are all signs of increased expiratory flow resistance that might be due to PEEP/CPAP valve resistance.

Presence of auto-PEEP

Auto-PEEP or air-trapping occurs in as many as half of all patients undergoing ventilatory support.[116] The incidence of auto-PEEP is greatest in patients with high minute volumes or respiratory rates, and when 10 or more cm H_2O PEEP is being used.[116] Methods for detecting auto-PEEP are described in the next chapter; here we focus on the impact of auto-PEEP and how best to minimize or avoid its effects.

Air-trapping caused by auto-PEEP flattens the diaphragm and impairs respiratory muscle function, thereby reducing a patient's ability to assume the ventilatory workload.[117,118] In addition, when auto-PEEP exists, the patient must generate a larger than normal pressure gradient to initiate spontaneous flow or trigger a ventilator.[119] This impairs patient-ventilator synchrony and further adds to the work of breathing.[120]

Technique for minimizing these auto-PEEP effects in patients receiving ventilatory support are summarized in the box, page 916.[92] As can be seen, there are three general approaches used: decreasing airflow obstruction, modifying the ventilatory pattern, and applying PEEP/CPAP. Depending on the clinical situation, these approaches may be used alone or in combination.

Methods designed to decrease airflow obstruction are appropriate when there is a reversible component to the obstruction disorder, and should always be implemented in these cases. Most efforts to modify the ventilatory pattern focus on increasing the expiratory time, which ideally will allow trapped gas to be fully exhaled. The last strategy for minimizing auto-PEEP, by applying PEEP/CPAP, requires explanation.

Techniques for minimizing auto-PEEP effects

■ Decrease airflow obstruction
    Aggressive bronchodilation
    Secretion removal
    Use larger size ET tube
■ Modify ventilatory pattern by
    Minimizing inspiratory time vs. total time
    Decrease rate/increase tidal volume
    Increase peak inspiratory flow
    Use low-compressed volume circuit
    Use low rate SIMV
    Decrease tidal volume, allow $PaCO_2$ to rise
      (permissive hypercapnea)
■ Apply PEEP/CPAP

Adapted from Kacmarek RM: Optimizing Ventilatory Muscle Function during Mechanical Ventilation. In Pierson DJ, Kacmarek RM, Eds.: *Foundations of respiratory care*, New York, Churchill Livingston, 1992.

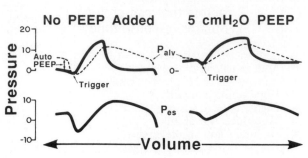

Fig. 32-13 Effect on trigger sensitivity of adding PEEP to auto-PEEP during an assisted machine cycle. To initiate the cycle, the patient must reverse auto-PEEP plus overcome the trigger level (left). Adding PEEP helps equilibrate alveolar and airway pressures, thereby improving trigger sensitivity and decreasing breathing effort. (From Marini JJ: Patient-ventilator interaction: rational strategies for acute ventilatory management, *Respir Care* 38:482-493, 1993.)

The use of externally applied PEEP/CPAP to overcome auto-PEEP is most effective in patients with chronic airflow obstruction due to airway closure.[121] Externally applied PEEP/CPAP helps support these airways during exhalation. By preventing airway closure, applied PEEP/CPAP allows central airway and alveolar pressures to equilibrate. As a result, the pressure gradient needed to initiate spontaneous flow or trigger a ventilator decreases, and with it the work of breathing (Figure 32-13).[122-124]

One must be very careful when using PEEP/CPAP to overcome auto-PEEP. Too much PEEP/CPAP can cause further hyperinflation and compromised hemodynamics and gas exchange. As a general guide, the applied PEEP/CPAP level should be no more than about 85% of the measured auto-PEEP pressure.[125] PEEP/CPAP levels greater than this can worsen auto-PEEP and cause further hyperinflation.

Alternatively, one can gauge the required level of PEEP/CPAP by monitoring the end-expiratory lung volume using inductive plethysmography (see Chapter 33). With a graphics display, the clinician can also inspect the flow/volume curves during application of increasing levels of PEEP. The shape of the expiratory limb of these curves can reveal the presence of and changes in the auto-PEEP effect.[126]

CHAPTER SUMMARY

The successful care of patients requiring ventilatory support involves a systematic management process. Key elements in this management process include: (1) selecting the initial ventilator, (2) conducting a thorough preliminary assessment of the patient-ventilator system, (3) setting clinical goals for ventilatory support, and (4) adjusting support parameters.

When selecting initial ventilator settings, the primary aim is to stabilize the patient by assuring adequate oxygenation and ventilation. To do so, one must first select the support mode, FiO_2, and minute ventilation. After selecting these primary settings, one must then adjust the trigger level and inspiratory flow (or time), set all applicable alarms, and assure adequate humidification. After initial stabilization, settings are readjusted according to the specific problem at hand and the objectives of ventilatory support. Ultimately, our aim should be to provide the patient with needed ventilatory support until it can be safely withdrawn.

REFERENCES

1. Society of Critical Care Medicine, Task Force on Guidelines: Guidelines for standards of care for patients with acute respiratory failure on mechanical ventilatory support, *Crit Care Med* 19(2):275-278, 1991.
2. Kacmarek RM: Systematic modification of ventilatory support. In Barnes, TA, editor: *Respiratory care practice,* Chicago, 1988, Mosby.
3. Kacmarek RM: Methods of providing mechanical ventilatory support, in Pierson DJ, Kacmarek RM, editors: *Foundations of Respiratory Care,* New York, 1992, Churchill Livingston.
4. Ravenscraft SA, Burke WC, Marini JJ: Volume-cycled decelerating flow, *Chest* 101(5):1342-1351, 1992.
5. Kacmarek RM: Essential gas delivery features of mechanical ventilators, *Respir Care* 37(9):1045-1055, 1992.
6. MacIntyre NR: Clinically available new strategies for mechanical ventilatory support, *Chest* 104(2):560-565, 1993.
7. Register SD, Downs JB, Stock MC: Is 50% oxygen harmful? *Crit Care Med* 15:598, 1987.
8. Radford EP: Ventilation standards for use in artificial respiration, *J Appl Physiol* 7:451, 1955.
9. Kacmarek RM, Venegar JV: Mechanical ventilatory rates and tidal volumes, *Respir Care* 32:466-474, 1987.
10. Parker JC, Hernandez LA, Peevy KJ: Mechanisms of ventilator-induced lung injury, *Crit Care Med* 21(1):131-143, 1993.
11. Kacmarek RM, Hickling KG: Permissive hypercapnia, *Respir Care* 38(4):373-387, 1993.
12. Slutsky AS (Chair): ACCP Consensus Conference: mechanical ventilation, *Chest* 104:1833-1859, 1993.
13. Menitove SM, Goldring RM: Combined ventilator and bicarbonate strategy in the management of status asthmaticus, *Am J Med* 74:898-890, 1983.
14. Sassoon CSH: Mechanical ventilator design and function: the trigger variable, *Respir Care* 37(9):1056-1069, 1992.
15. Branson RD: Flow-triggering systems, *Respir Care* 39(2):138-144, 1994.
16. Marini JJ, Capps JS, Culver BH: The inspiratory work of breathing during assisted mechanical ventilation, *Chest* 87:612-618, 1985.
17. Marini JJ, Rodriguez RM, Lamb V: The inspiratory workload of patient-initiated mechanical ventilation, *Am Rev Respir Dis* 134:902-909, 1986.
18. Sassoon CSH, Mahutte CK, Te T, et al: Work of breathing and airway occlusion pressure during assist-mode mechanical ventilation, *Chest* 93:571-576, 1988.
19. Sassoon CSH, Mahutte CK, Light RW: Ventilator modes: old and new, *Crit Care Clin* 6(3):605-634, 1990.
20. Ayres SM, Kozam RL, Lukas DS: The effects of intermittent positive pressure breathing on intrathoracic pressure, pulmonary mechanics and the work of breathing, *Am Rev Respir Dis* 87:370-379, 1976.
21. Tuxen DV, Lane S: The effects of ventilatory pattern on hyperinflation, airway pressures, and circulation in mechanical ventilation in patients with severe airflow obstruction, *Am Rev Respir Dis* 136:872-879, 1987.
22. Connors AF, McCaffree DR, Gray BA: Effect of inspiratory flow rate on gas exchange during mechanical ventilation, *Am Rev Respir Dis* 124:537-543, 1981.
23. Campbell RS, Branson RD: Ventilatory support for the 90s: pressure support ventilation, *Respir Care* 38(5):526-537, 1993.
24. Branson RD, Campbell RS, et al: Altering flowrate during maximum pressure support ventilation (PSVmax): Effects on cardiorespiratory function, *Respir Care* 35(11):1056-1064, 1990.
25. Marini JJ, Crooke PS: A general mathematical model for respiratory dynamics relevant to the clinical setting, *Am Rev Respir Dis* 147(1):14-24, 1993.
26. Marini JJ: Patient-ventilator interaction: rational strategies for acute ventilatory management, *Respir Care* 38(5):482-493, 1993.
27. Johansson H: Effects on breathing mechanics and gas exchange of different inspiratory gas flow patterns in patients undergoing respirator treatment, *Acta Anaesth Scand* 19:19-27, 1975.
28. Modell HI, Cheney FW: Effects of inspiratory flow pattern on gas exchange in normal and abnormal lungs, *J Appl Physiol* 46:1103-1107, 1979.
29. Al-Saady N, Bennett ED: Decelerating inspiratory flow waveform improves lung mechanics and gas exchange in patients on intermittent positive pressure ventilation, *Intensive Care Med* 11:68-75, 1985.
30. Rau JL: Inspiratory flow patterns: the 'shape' of ventilation, *Respir Care* 38(1):132-140, 1993.
31. Rau JL, Shelledy DC: The effect of varying inspiratory flow waveforms on pcak and mean airway pressures with a time-cycled volume ventilator: A bench study, *Respir Care* 36(5):347-356, 1991.
32. American Association for Respiratory Care. Clinical practice guideline. Humidification during mechanical ventilation, *Respir Care* 37(8):887-890, 1992.
33. Shelly MP: Inspired gas conditioning, *Respir Care* 37(9):1070-1080, 1992.
34. Branson RD, Chatburn RL: Humidification during mechanical ventilation [editorial], *Respir Care* 38(5):461-468, 1993.
35. Branson RD, Campbell RS: Sighs: wasted breath or breath of fresh air? *Respir Care* 37(5):462-468, 1992.
36. American Association for Respiratory Care. Clinical practice guideline. Patient-ventilator system checks, *Respir Care* 37(8):882-886, 1992.
37. MacIntyre NM, Day SD: Essentials for ventilator alarm systems, *Respir Care* 37(9):1108-1112, 1992.
38. Campbell RS: Managing the patient-ventilator system: system checks and circuit changes, *Respir Care* 39(3):227-236, 1994.
39. Martz K, Joiner JW, Shepherd RM: *Management of the patient-ventilator system, A team approach,* ed 2, St Louis, 1984, Mosby.
40. Kacmarek RM: Management of the patient-mechanical ventilator system. In Pierson DJ, Kacmarek RM, editors: *Foundations of Respiratory Care,* New York, 1992, Churchill Livingston.
41. US Food and Drug Administration: Accidental breathing circuit disconnections in the critical care setting [HHS publication No. FDA 90-4233], Rockville, MD, 1990, Department of Health and Human Services.
42. Lain DC, DiBenedetto R, Morris SL, et al: Pressure control inverse ratio ventilation as a method to reduce peak inspiratory pressure and provide adequate ventilation and oxygenation, *Chest* 95(5):1081-1088, 1989.
43. Marcy TW, Marini JJ: Inverse ratio ventilation in ARDS, Rationale and implementation, *Chest* 100(2):494-504, 1991.
44. Hickling K: Low volume ventilation with permissive hypercapnia in the adult respiratory distress syndrome, *Clin Intensive Care* 3:67-78, 1992.
45. Cane RD, Peruzzi WT, Shapiro BA: Airway pressure release ventilation in severe acute respiratory failure, *Chest* 100(2):460-463, 1991.
46. Rasanen J, Cane RD, Downs JB, et al: Airway pressure release ventilation during acute lung injury: a prospective multicenter trial, *Crit Care Med* 1991 19(10):1234-1241, 1991.
47. Morris AH, Wallace CJ, Clemmer TP, et al: Extracorporeal CO_2 removal therapy for adult respiratory distress syndrome patients, *Respir Care* 35:224-31, 1990.
48. Morris AH, Wallace CJ, Clemmer TP, et al: Final report: computerized protocol controlled clinical trial of new therapy which includes $ECCO_2R$ for ARDS (abstract), *Am Rev Respir Dis* 145(2):A184, 1992.
49. Pepe PE, Marini JJ: Occult positive end-expiratory pressure in mechanically ventilated patients with airflow obstruction: the anto-PEEP effect, *Am Rev Respir Dis* 126:166-170, 1982.

50. Williams TJ, Tuxen DV, Scheinkestel CD, et al: Risk factors for morbidity in mechanically ventilated patients with acute severe asthma, *Am Rev Respir Dis* 146:607–615, 1992.
51. Scott LR, Benson MS, Pierson DJ: Effect of inspiratory flow-rate and circuit compressible volume on auto-PEEP during mechanical ventilation, *Respir Care* 31:1075–1079, 1986.
52. Darioli R, Perret C: Mechanical controlled hypoventilation in status asthmaticus, *Am Rev Respir Dis* 129:385–387, 1984.
53. Meyers JR, Lembeck L, O'Kane H et al: Changes in functional residual capacity of the lungs after operation, *Arch Surg* 110:576–83, 1975.
54. Ali J, Weisel RD, Layug AB, et al: Consequences of postoperative alterations in respiratory mechanics, *Am J Surg* 128:376–382, 1974.
55. Pierson DJ, Lakshminarayan S: Postoperative ventilatory management, *Respir Care* 29:603–609, 1984.
56. Cullen DJ, Cullen BL: Postanesthetic complications, *Surg Clin North Am* 55:987–98, 1975.
57. Zwillich CW, Pierson DJ, Creagh CE, et al: Complications of assisted ventilation. A preospective study of 354 consecutive episodes, *Am J Med* 57:161–169, 1974.
58. O'Donohue WJ Jr, Baker JP, Bell GM, et al: Respiratory failure in neuromuscular disease, *JAMA* 235:733, 1975.
59. Gibson GJ, Pride NB, Davis JN, et al: Pulmonary mechanics in patients with respiratory muscle weakness, *Am Rev Respir Dis* 115:389–395, 1977.
60. Tobin MJ: Respiratory muscles in disease, *Clin Chest Med* 9:263–286, 1988.
61. Mansel JK, Norman JR: Respiratory complications and management of spinal cord injuries, *Chest* 97:1446–1452, 1990.
62. Muizelaar JP, Marmarou A, et al: Adverse effects of prolonged hyperventilation in patients with severe head injury: a randomized clinical trial, *J Neurosurg* 75:731–39, 1991.
63. Cooper KR: Respiratory complications in patients with serious head injuries. In: Becker DP Gudeurar SK, editors: Textbook of head injury, Philadelphia, 1989, WB Saunders.
64. Aubier M, Trippenbach T, Roussos C: Respiratory muscle fatigue during cardiogenic shock, *J Appl Physiol* 51:499–508, 1981.
65. Rasanen J, Nikki P, Heikkila J: Acute myocardial infarction complicated by respiratory failure: the effects of mechanical ventilation, *Chest* 85:21–28, 1984.
66. Mathru M, Rao TL, El-Etr AA, et al: Hemodynamic response to changes in ventilatory patterns in patients with normal and poor left ventricular reserve, *Crit Care Med* 10:423–426, 1982.
67. Parish JM, Gracey DR, Southern PA, et al: Differential mechanical ventilation in respiratory failure due to severe unilateral lung disease, *Mayo Clin Proc* 59:822–828, 1984.
68. Adoumie R, Shennib H, Brown R, et al: Differential lung ventilation. Applications beyond the operating room, *J Thorac Cardiovasc Surg* 105:229–233.
69. Venus B, Pratap KS, Op't Holt T: Treatment of unilateral pulmonary insufficiency by selective administration of continuous positive airway pressure through a double-lumen tube, *Anesthesiology* 53(1):74–77, 1980.
70. Wendt M, Hachenberg T, Winde G, Lawin P: Differential ventilation with low-flow CPAP and CPPV in the treatment of unilateral chest trauma, *Intensive Care Med* 15(3):209–211, 1989.
71. Baraka A, Serhal A: Lateral decubitus improves oxygenation during conventional ventilation in unilateral lung injury, *Middle East J Anesthesiol* 10(3):329–332, 1989.
72. Dhainaut JF, Bons J, et al: Improved oxygenation in patients with extensive unilateral pneumonia using the lateral decubitus position, *Thorax* 35(10):792–793, 1980.
73. East TD, Pace NL, Westenskow DR: Synchronous versus asynchronous differential lung ventilation with PEEP after unilateral acid aspiration in the dog, *Crit Care Med* 11(6):441–444, 1983.
74. Pierson DJ: Persistent bronchopleural air leak during mechanical ventilation, *Respir Care* 27:408, 1982.
75. Feeley TW, Keating D, Nishimura T: Independent lung ventilation using high-frequency ventilation in the management of a bronchopleural fistula, *Anesthesiology* 69(3):420–422, 1988.
76. Bishop MJ, Benson MS, Sato P, Pierson DJ: Comparison of high-frequency jet ventilation with conventional mechanical ventilation for bronchopleural fistula, *Anesth Analg* 66(9):833–838, 1987.
77. Walsh MC, Carlo WA: Determinants of gas flow through a bronchopleural fistula, *J Appl Physiol* 67(4):1591–1596, 1989.
78. Gallagher TJ, Civetta JM: Goal-directed therapy of acute respiratory failure, *Anesth Analg* 59:831, 1980.
79. Pierson DJ: Indications for mechanical ventilation in acute respiratory failure, *Respir Care* 28:570–577, 1983.
80. Selecky PA, Wasserman K, Klein M, Ziment I: A graphic approach to assessing interrelationships among minute ventilation, arterial carbon dioxide tension, and ratio of physiologic deadspace to tidal volume in patients on respirators, *Am Rev Respir Dis* 117:181, 1978.
81. Bone RC, Pierce AK, Johnson RL: Controlled oxygen administration in acute respiratory failure in chronic obstructive pulmonary disease: A reappraisal, *Am J Med* 65:896, 1978.
82. Gilbert R, Keighley JF: The arterial-alveolar oxygen tension ratio. An index of gas exchange applicable to varying inspired oxygen concentrations, *Am Rev Respir Dis* 109:142–145, 1974.
83. Nelson LD: Assessment of oxygenation: oxygenation indices, *Respir Care* 38(6):631–640, 1993.
84. Peris LV, Boix JH: Clinical use of the arterial/alveolar oxygen tension ratio, *Crit Care Med* 11:888–891, 1983.
85. Gross R, Israel RH: A graphic approach for prediction of arterial oxygen tension at different concentrations of inspired oxygen, *Chest* 79:311–315, 1981.
86. Maxwell C, Hess D, Shefet D: Use of the arterial/alveolar oxygen tension ratio to predict the inspired oxygen concentration needed for a desired arterial oxygen tension, *Respir Care* 29:1135–1139, 1984.
87. Craig KC, Pierson DJ, Carrico CJ: The clinical application of PEEP in ARDS, *Respir Care* 30:184–201, 1985.
88. Maunder RJ, Rice CL, Benson MS, Hudson LD: Managing PEEP: the Harborview approach, *Respir Care* 31:1059–1068, 1986.
89. Suter PM, Fairley HB, Isenberg MD: Effect of tidal volume and positive end-expiratory pressure on compliance during mechanical ventilation, *Chest* 73(2):158–162, 1978.
90. Suter PM, Fairley B, Isenberg MD: Optimum end-expiratory airway pressure in patients with acute pulmonary failure, *N Engl J Med* 292(6):284–289, 1975.
91. Tobin MJ: What should the clinician do when a patient "fights the ventilator"? *Respir Care* 36(5):395–406, 1991.
92. Kacmarek RM: Optimizing Ventilatory Muscle Function during Mechanical Ventilation. In Pierson DJ, Kacmarek RM, editors: *Foundations of respiratory care*, New York, 1992, Churchill Livingston.
93. Marini JJ: Strategies to minimize breathing effort during mechanical ventilation, *Crit Care Clin* 6(3):635–661, 1990.
94. Marini JJ, Smith TC, Lamb VJ: External work output and force generation during synchronized intermittent mechanical ventilation. Effect of machine assistance on breathing effort, *Am Rev Respir Dis* 138(5):1169–1179, 1988.
95. MacIntyre NR: Respiratory function during pressure support ventilation, *Chest* 89(5):677–683, 1986.
96. Kacmarek RM: The role of pressure support in reducing the work of breathing, *Respir Care* 33:99–120, 1988.
97. Brochard L, Pluskwa F, Lemaire F: Improved efficacy of spontaneous breathing with inspiratory pressure support, *Am Rev Respir Dis* 136(2):411–415, 1987.
98. Bolder M, Healey TEJ, Bolder AR, et al: The extra work of breathing through endotracheal tubes, *Anesth Analg* 65:853–859, 1986.
99. Shapiro W, Wilson RK, Casar G, et al: Work of breathing through different sized endotracheal tubes, *Crit Care Med* 14:1028–1031, 1986.

100. Wright PE, Marini JJ, Bernard GR: In vitro versus in vivo comparison of endotracheal tube airflow resistance, *Am Rev Respir Dis* 140:10–16, 1989.
101. Kacmarek RM: The role of pressure support in reducing the work of breathing, *Respir Care* 33:99–120, 1988.
102. Kacmarek RM: Interactions between patients and mechanical ventilators, *Curr Opinion Anesthesiol* 3:228–234, 1990.
103. Marini JJ: Minimizing breathing effort during mechanical ventilation. In: LeMaire F, Zapol WM, editors: *Acute respiratory failure,* New York, 1990, Marcel Dekker.
104. Gurevitch MJ, Gelmont D: Importance of trigger sensitivity to ventilator response delay in advanced chronic obstructive pulmonary disease with respiratory failure, *Crit Care Med* 17:354–359, 1989.
105. Hirsch C, Kacmarek RM, Stanek K: Work of breathing during CPAP and IPS imposed by the new generation mechanical ventilators, *Respir Care* 36:815–828, 1991.
106. Ploysongsang Y, Branson R, et al: Pressure flow characteristics of commonly used heat-moisture exchangers, *Am Rev Respir Dis* 138(3):675–678, 1988.
107. Christopher KL, Neff TA, Bowman JL, et al: Demand and continuous flow intermittent mandatory ventilation systems, *Chest* 87:625–630, 1985.
108. Op't Holt TB, Hall MV, Bass JB, et al: Comparison of changes in airway pressure during continuous positive airway pressure (CPAP) between demand valve and continuous flow devices, *Respir Care* 27:1200–1209, 1982.
109. Henry WC, West GA, Wilson RS: A comparison of the oxygen cost of breathing between a continuous-flow CPAP system and a demand-flow CPAP system, *Respir Care* 28:1273–1281, 1983.
110. Gibney RTN, Wilson RS, Pontoppidan H.: Comparison of work of breathing on high gas flow and demand valve continuous positive airway pressure systems, *Chest* 82:692–695, 1982.
111. Viale JP, Annat G, Bertrand O: Additional inspiratory work in intubated patients breathing with continuous positive airway pressure systems, *Anesthesiology* 63:536–539, 1985.
112. Saito S, Tokioka H, Kosaka F: Efficacy of flow-by during continuous positive airway pressure ventilation, *Crit Care Med* 18(6):654–656, 1990.
113. Sassoon CS, Lodia R, et al: Inspiratory muscle work of breathing during flow-by, demand-flow, and continuous-flow systems in patients with chronic obstructive pulmonary disease, *Am Rev Respir Dis* 145(5):1219–1222, 1992.
114. Sassoon CS, Giron AE, Ely EA, Light RW: Inspiratory work of breathing on flow-by and demand-flow continuous positive airway pressure, *Crit Care Med* 17(11):1108–1114, 1989.
115. Marini JJ, Culver BH, Kirk W: Flow resistance of exhalation valves and positive end-expiratory pressure devices used in mechanical ventilation, *Am Rev Respir Dis* 131(6):850–854, 1985.
116. Wright J, Gong H Jr: "Auto-PEEP": incidence, magnitude, and contributing factors, *Heart Lung* 19(4):352–357, 1990.
117. Kimball WR, Leith DE, Robins AG: Dynamic hyperinflation and ventilator dependence in chronic obstructive pulmonary disease, *Am Rev Respir Dis* 126:991–995, 1982.
118. Macklem PT: Hyperinflation (editorial), *Am Rev Respir Dis* 129:1–2, 1984.
119. Pepe PE, Marini JJ: Occult positive end-expiratory pressure in mechanically ventilated patients with airflow obstruction: the auto-PEEP effect, *Am Rev Respir Dis* 126:166–170, 1982.
120. Benson MS, Pierson DJ: Auto-PEEP during mechanical ventilation of adults, *Respir Care* 33(7):557–565, 1988.
121. Marini JJ: Should PEEP be used in airflow obstruction? [editorial], *Am Rev Respir Dis* 140(1):1–3, 1989.
122. Ranieri VM, Giuliani R, et al: Physiologic effects of positive end-expiratory pressure in patients with chronic obstructive pulmonary disease during acute ventilatory failure and controlled mechanical ventilation, *Am Rev Respir Dis* 147(1):5–13, 1993.
123. Petrof BJ, Legare M, Goldberg P, et al: Continuous positive airway pressure reduces work of breathing and dyspnea during weaning from mechanical ventilation in severe chronic obstructive pulmonary disease, *Am Rev Respir Dis* 141(2):281–289, 1990.
124. Smith TC, Marini JJ: Impact of PEEP on lung mechanics and work of breathing in severe airflow obstruction, *J Appl Physiol* 65(4):1488–1499, 1988.
125. Munoz J, Guerrero JE, et al: Interaction between intrinsic positive end-expiratory pressure and externally applied positive end-expiratory pressure during controlled mechanical ventilation. *Crit Care Med* 21(3):348–356, 1993.
126. Rossi A, Brandolese R, Milic-Emili J, et al: The role of PEEP in patients with chronic obstructive pulmonary disease during assisted ventilation, *Eur Respir J* 3(7):818–822, 1990.

Patient Monitoring and Management

■

Craig L. Scanlan

No aspect of clinical practice is more complex or demanding than the management of critically ill patients who require ventilatory support. Over the past several decades, the specialized knowledge and skills of the respiratory care practitioner (RCP) have become recognized as an essential ingredient in the effective management and monitoring of these patients.

To fulfill this important role, RCPs must be able to accurately gather, interpret, and act on a wide array of patient data, gathered via both direct observation and physiologic monitoring. Such data includes both invasive and noninvasive measures of patient oxygenation, ventilation, and respiratory mechanics. In addition, RCPs must have general knowledge of other elements of patient assessment related to the care of patients receiving ventilatory support, especially hemodynamic monitoring. Last, RCPs are *the* members of the critically care team most responsible for direct oversight of the patient–ventilator system. Competence, care, and diligence in managing and troubleshooting the patient–ventilator system are central to the role of the RCP in critical care.

GENERAL PRINCIPLES IN MANAGING AND MONITORING PATIENTS IN RESPIRATORY FAILURE

The management of critically ill patients is among the most complex and demanding aspects of respiratory care.[1,2] Patient management is an ongoing process involving three major components: data collection, data analysis and interpretation, and decision-making.

Data collection involves gathering information by either repeated or continuous observations. Pertinent information is obtained via traditional physical assessment procedures, in conjunction with standard diagnostic testing, including laboratory and radiologic evaluation. Observations made by physiologic monitoring of the patient's cardiopulmonary status supplement these data in critical care.

The supplementary information provided by physiologic monitoring serves two major purposes. First, monitoring helps define the nature of the problem, its progression, and (ideally) its resolution. Such information provides valuable assistance to clinicians in choosing and evaluating appropriate treatments, thus increasing the likelihood of successful outcomes.

Second, physiologic monitoring also increases our ability to detect complications, hopefully before they become life-threatening.[3] Given the inherent instability of the critically ill, and the high risks involved with their management, it should come as no surprise that complications are common in the intensive care setting. As an example, Table 33-1 summarizes the major complications found over a five year period in the management of 350 patients receiving continuous ventilatory support.[4] As many as half of such incidents can result in actual harm to the patient.[5]

Data collection alone is of little value unless it is used to affect patient management. Indeed, clinicians today are often overwhelmed with patient information, some of which is of questionable help in patient care. As a general rule of thumb, only information that will be used in clinical decision-making should be gathered. This rule minimizes the cost and

Table 33-1 Potential complications of mechanical ventilation

	No. of cases	Percent incidence
COMPLICATIONS ATTRIBUTED TO INTUBATION, EXTUBATION OR TUBE MALFUNCTION		
Prolonged intubation attempts	46	30
Intubation of the right main-stem bronchus	34	10
Premature extubation	21	7
Self extubation	30	9
Tube malfunction	21	6
Nasal necrosis	6	2
COMPLICATIONS ATTRIBUTED TO OPERATION OF THE VENTILATOR		
Machine failure	6	2
Alarm failure	12	4
Alarm found off	32	9
Inadequate nebulization or humidification	45	13
Overheating of inspired air	7	2
MEDICAL COMPLICATIONS OCCURRING WITH MECHANICAL VENTILATION		
Alveolar hypoventilation	35	10
Alveolar hyperventilation	39	11
Massive gastric distention	5	2
Pneumothorax	15	4
Atelectasis	16	5
Pneumonia	13	4
Hypotension	16	5

From Zwillich CW, Pierson DJ, Creagh CE, et al: Complications of assisted ventilation. A prospective study of 354 consecutive episodes, *Am J Med* 57:161–169, 1974.

potential patient hazards associated with needless information gathering.

Once necessary data has been gathered, it must be analyzed and interpreted. Interpretation of patient data requires extensive knowledge of both normal and abnormal parameters, including their significance in various disease states. The respiratory care practitioner (RCP) must be able to gather and interpret physiologic data pertinent to assessing patient oxygenation, ventilation, and respiratory mechanics.[6] In addition, the RCP must possess general knowledge of other elements of patient assessment related to the care of patients in respiratory failure, especially hemodynamic monitoring.[7]

Sound clinical decision-making follows data collection and interpretation. Decision-making involves assessing the potential benefits and risks associated with available management options, and choosing the approach most likely to help and least likely to harm the patient.

Of course, the management process does not end with the initial selection and implementation of a course of action. As described in Chapter 32, patient management is a cyclical and ongoing process.[8] Interventions, once taken, are assessed for their effect. New data is analyzed and interpreted, and refinements or changes are made in the approach used. This process continues until the goals of intervention are achieved, or, as is too often the case in the care of the critically ill, the patient succumbs to the disease process.

Due to the complexities of ventilatory support and its use as a life sustaining measure, careful ongoing monitoring of the patient and patient-ventilator system is essential. Both the patient and patient-ventilator system should be thoroughly assessed at least every two hours, or whenever changes in parameters are made. With unstable patients, continuous monitoring and assessment may be indicated.

For convenience, the process of ongoing monitoring and assessment can be divided into three major components: general patient assessment, physiologic monitoring, and evaluation of the patient-ventilator system.

GENERAL PATIENT ASSESSMENT

General patient information is obtained through observation and assessment techniques.[9] Some of these procedures are performed by the RCP. Other information is secured from the chart or by discussion with the attending physician or nurse. Communication of patient status should also occur through participation in bedside rounds and shift reports. The following assessments are particularly appropriate in monitoring patients receiving ventilatory support.

Vital signs

Vital signs inform the RCP about the overall status of the patient. The most basic signs include temperature, pulse, blood pressure, and respiratory rate. Details on the measurement of vital signs are provided in Chapter 16. Table 33-2, page 922, provides guidance in interpreting changes in vital signs occurring with patients receiving ventilatory support.

Temperature normally is measured by nursing personnel and found on the nursing flow sheet. An elevated temperature might indicate infection and may warrant further investigation, such as culture and sensitivity tests on sputum, blood, or urine. Elevation of the patient's temperature can also occur when the airway temperature is set too high, or the humidifier control mechanism fails.

Pulse rate can and should be obtained and recorded by the RCP. Pulse rates over 120 or under 70/min are a bad sign.[10] The strength of the pulse in various parts of the respiratory cycle must also be noted. Weakening of the pulse during inspiration (pulsus paradoxus) may indicate variations in output due to positive

Table 33-2 Troubleshooting changes in vital signs

Clue	Possible problem	Advice
Hypotension	Decreased venous return (caused by changes in intrathoracic pressure)	Evaluate fluid balance and possible need for filling of vascular bed
Hypertension	Anxiety response to decreased PaO_2, decreased $PaCO_2$	Reassure, alleviate fear
		Check patient-ventilator system; if not easily correctable obtain and evaluate ABG value
Respiratory swing of blood pressure	Decreased venous return (caused by changes in intrathoracic pressure)	If systolic/diastolic pressures below levels for adequate perfusion, evaluate fluid balance consider filling vascular bed
New arrhythmias, tachycardia, bradycardia	Anxiety	Reassure, alleviate fear
	Decreased PaO_2, decreased $PaCO_2$, increased $PaCO_2$	Check patient-ventilator system; if not quickly correctable, obtain and evaluate ABG values
	Decreased venous return	Check for other hemodynamics parameters for adequacy of perfusion
Large swings in CVP or PAWP	Decreased venous return	Evaluate other hemodynamics parameters for adequacy of perfusion
Decreased urinary output	Decreased cardiac output owing to decrease	Evaluate other hemodynamics parameters for adequacy of perfusion
Fever	Increased metabolic rate caused by inspiratory effort or patient-ventilator asynchrony	Check sensitivity and patient triggering effort settings
	Infection	Treat infection; review preventive measures
	Atelectasis	Check patient-ventilator system for secretions, plugs, slippage of tube into right mainstem bronchus
	Overheated humidifier	Check temperature of humidifier heater
Weight gain	Fluid retention caused by decreased venous return	Evaluate other hemodynamic parameters for adequacy of perfusion; consider diuresis
Changes in respiratory rate	Altered settings	Check patient-ventilator setting
	Change in metabolic needs	Evaluate patient's metabolic rate
	Anxiety	Reassure, alleviate fears
	Sleep	Normal-metabolic rate is decreased
Use of accessory muscles or paradoxic breathing	Increased work of breathing	Increase support level
	Patient-ventilator dyssynchrony	Provide pressure support ventilation
		Increase sensitivity
	Auto-PEEP	Eliminate auto-PEEP

pressure, cardiac tamponade, or severe broncho-spasm. The pulse can also help indicate the adequacy of circulation (necessary for arterial blood sampling) and provide corroborating information regarding blood pressure (weak or thready in hypotension).

Patient heart rate can normally be observed continuously using the ECG monitor. This index is particularly important during suctioning, which can cause arrhythmias. Abnormal rhythms may also indicate hypoxemia, ischemic heart disease, an acute cardiopulmonary process such as pulmonary embolism, or the development of congestive heart failure. The RCP should have a basic understanding of ECG interpretation and should be able to recognize changes from the patient's baseline heart rate and rhythm. Interpreting skills should also include the immediate recognition of life threatening arrhythmias such as complete heart block, ventricular tachycardia, and ventricular fibrillation (refer to Chapter 23).

Although a nonspecific indicator, the respiratory rate is a helpful sign. Tachypnea tends to occur early

in respiratory distress.[11] In adults, spontaneous respiratory rates over 30/min are a bad sign.[10] In general, the greater the respiratory rate, the more severe the underlying disease.[12]

Physical assessment

As discussed in Chapter 16, physical assessment includes inspection, palpation, percussion, and auscultation.[13] Although it is more difficult to perform a thorough physical exam on a critically ill patient, the basic principles still apply, but they may need modification. Astute observation can often spot a potential problem before diagnostic test results are available.[9] Moreover, simple physical assessment, in combination with the measurement of vital signs, can help determine the severity of respiratory failure and the potential outcomes of patient management.[10]

Key aspects of bedside assessment involve observation of respiratory muscle activity. Use of the accessory muscles of ventilation almost always signals an increased work of breathing.[14] Specifically, the presence of scalene or sternocleidomastoid muscle activity during inspiration is a bad sign, indicating a ventilatory load in excess of capacity.

In addition to observing the activity of the accessory muscles, the RCP should assess and compare diaphragmatic and chest wall excursion. To enhance accuracy, the patient should be placed in either the supine or semi-Fowler's position, with the RCP observing at a level parallel to the abdomen.

Figure 33-1 schematically illustrates the three major patterns of diaphragmatic and chest wall excursion that can be observed.[15,16] In normal patients in the supine position, the descent of the diaphragm causes outward movement of the abdomen (Ab), with the intercostals causing outward movement of the rib cage (RC). As evident in Figure 33-1, these normal events are coordinated and occur simultaneously with the increment in inspired tidal volume (VT). It is important to note that normal abdominal activity tends to be greater in males than in females.

If the rib cage and abdomen do not move outward at the same time, the breathing pattern is described as *asynchronous*. For example, if the abdomen moves outward noticeably faster than the rib cage, this indicates that the respiratory muscles are not working in synchrony. This pattern often serves as an early indicator of an excessive respiratory muscle load.[17]

Asynchronous breathing may sometimes progress to a more severe pattern called *paradoxical breathing*. In this pattern, the abdomen moves outward while the lower rib cage moves inward during inspiration. As with asynchrony, paradoxical breathing indicates an excessive respiratory muscle load and may be an early signal of fatigue.[18-20]

Not shown in Figure 33-1, but also indicative of excessive muscle loads, is a breathing pattern called *respiratory alternans*. Respiratory alternans occurs when the patient switches back and forth between mainly abdominal and mainly rib cage activity. This pattern may be an effort to alternately rest each muscle group.

Newer quantitative approaches to assessing respiratory muscle function are described later in this chapter.

Chest X-rays

In critical care, chest X-rays are commonly used by the RCP to evaluate endotracheal tube placement. In consultation with the attending physician and/or consulting radiologist, the RCP can also use the chest film to help determine if the lungs are being properly aerated, and to detect major pathological changes such as hyperinflation, atelectasis, consolidation, pneumothorax, pleural effusion, and congestion from pneumonia or heart failure (refer to Chapter 19). A chest film should be obtained immediately after intubation, and daily during the critical period of the patient's illness.[21-24] More advanced techniques, including digital radiography, CT and MRI scans, are playing an increasingly important role in the evaluation of the critically ill patient.[25]

Medications

In order to make informed judgments regarding the patient's stability, need for therapy, and readiness for weaning, the RCP should be familiar with all drugs being administered to the patient. Drugs most likely to affect the patient's respiratory status include those given for pain, sedation, muscle relaxation, arrhythmia, and blood pressure control.

Clinical laboratory studies

The major clinical laboratory studies of use in monitoring the patient in respiratory failure are summa-

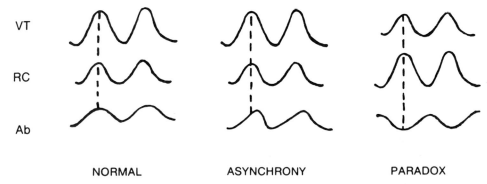

VT

RC

Ab

NORMAL   ASYNCHRONY   PARADOX

Fig. 33-1 Schema of motion of the rib cage *(RC)* and abdomen *(Ab)*, and the calibrated sum of these signals, which is tidal volume *(VT)*. In normal subjects the RC and Ab signals increase and decrease in synchrony. The rate of motion of the two compartments differs during asynchronous breathing, while during paradoxical breathing one compartment moves in an opposite direction to the VT signal. (From Dantzker DR, Tobin MJ: *Respir Care* 30(6):423, 1985.)

rized in Table 33-3. Hematology data are useful in assessing the oxygen carrying capacity of the blood, the response to infection, and the potential for bleeding. Clinical chemistry data help in assessing acid-base imbalances, particularly metabolic or renal problems. For these reasons, RCPs must be familiar with the use, application, and interpretation of these major clinical laboratory studies.[26,27]

Fluid balance

In most critical care units, nursing personnel assume primary responsibility for monitoring a patient's fluid balance. This is done by evaluating fluid intake and output (I/O), often in conjunction with patient weight. Central venous and pulmonary arterial pressures are also used to assess and guide fluid balance.

Fluid balance is particularly relevant to the RCP as it relates to renal function. In addition, careful management of fluid balance is essential in congestive heart failure (CHF), pulmonary edema, and shock of any origin. Moreover, given the sensitivity of the kidneys to changes in O_2 delivery, renal function may be an indicator of disturbances in overall oxygen transport.

Insensible water loss through the lungs is eliminated when providing saturated gas at body temperature to the airway. Since this elimination of water loss is equivalent to water gain, it must be accounted for, especially in patients on fluid restrictions. Moreover, any significant water delivery above body humidity levels, such as occurs with supplementary heated aerosol therapy, should be estimated and reported as fluid intake.

Nutrition

The ability to discontinue ventilatory support can be impacted by a patient's nutritional status (see Chapter 34).[28] Oxygen consumption and carbon dioxide production are affected by the relative balance among the intake and metabolism of carbohydrates, proteins, and fats. Malnutrition may occur in the critically ill patient as a consequence of decreased nutrient intake and the increased metabolic demands of the body.[29]

Careful evaluation should be done by a clinical

Table 33-3   Useful clinical laboratory data

Test	Normal Value	Significance
HEMATOLOGY TESTS		
Red blood cells	M 4.6–6.2 × 10–6/mm³	Oxygen transport
	F 4.2–5.4 × 10–6/mm³	Response to hypoxemia
		Degree of cyanosis
Hemoglobin	M 14.5–16.5 g/dL	Oxygen transport
	F 12.0–15.0 g/dL	Response to hypoxemia
		Degree of cyanosis
Hematocrit	M 40–50%	Hemoconcentration (high)
	F 38–47%	Hemodilution (low)
White blood cells	4500–10,000/mm³	Infection (high)
		Decreased immunity (low)
Platelets	150,000–4000,000/mm³	Slow blood-clotting (low)
		Check before ABG
Prothrombin Time (PT)	12–14 seconds	Slow clotting (high)
		Check before ABG
Partial thromboplastin Time (PTT)	25–37 seconds	Slow clotting (high)
		Check before ABG
CLINICAL CHEMISTRY TESTS		
Sodium	137–147 mEq/L	Acid-base/fluid balance
Potassium	3.5–4.8 mEq/L	Metabolic acidosis (high)
		Metabolic alkalosis (low)
		Cardiac arrhythmias (low)
Chloride	98–105 mEq/L	Metabolic alkalosis (low)
CO_2 content	25–33 mEq/L	Equivalent to $HCO_3 + H_2CO_3$
Blood urea Nitrogen (BUN)	7–20 mg/dL	Renal failure (high) nonvolatile acid
Creatinine	0.7–1.3 mg/dL	Renal disease (high)
Glucose	70–105 mg/dL	Ketoacidosis (high)

From Tilkian SM, Conover MB, Tilkian AG: Clinical implications of laboratory tests, St Louis, 1983, Mosby.

dietician for all patients receiving long-term ventilatory support.[30,31] This topic will be discussed later as it relates to patients' ventilatory requirements.

PHYSIOLOGIC MONITORING

Physiologic data useful in managing patients receiving ventilatory support includes information on oxygenation, ventilation, ventilatory mechanics, and hemodynamics.[32] Table 33-4 provides a summary of the key respiratory parameters, including the minimally acceptable threshold values. A similar summary of hemodynamic parameters is provided later in Table 33-12.

Not all such data need be gathered on all patients. In selecting relevant monitoring parameters, the clinician should be guided by the nature of the underlying cause of respiratory failure, as balanced against the potential risks and benefits associated with the data gathering procedure.

Monitoring may be either invasive or noninvasive.[33] Invasive procedures require insertion of a sensor or collection device into the body, while noninvasive monitoring gather data externally. Generally,

Table 33-4 Physiologic monitoring data (respiratory parameters)

Function Assessed	Parameter Description	Symbol/Formula	Acceptable Value(s)
OXYGENATION			
Lung exchange (external)			
Adequacy	Arterial oxygen partial pressure	PaO_2	60–100 torr
	Arterial oxygen saturation	SaO_2	> 90%
	Transcutaneous oxygen partial pressure	$PtcO_2$	60–100 torr
Efficiency	Alveolar to arterial O_2 tension gradient	$P(A-a)O_2$	< 350 torr (100% O_2)
	a/A ratio	$PaO_2 \div PAO_2$	> 0.6
	Respiratory index	$P(A-a)O_2 \div PaO_2$	< 5.0
	P/F ratio	$PaO_2 \div FiO_2$	> 200
	Percent shunt	$\dot{Q}_s \div \dot{Q}_t$	< 20%
Tissue exchange (internal)	Mixed venous oxygen content	$C\bar{v}O_2$	> 10.0 mL/dL
	Mixed venous oxygen partial pressure	$P\bar{v}O_2$	> 30 torr
	Mixed venous oxygen saturation	$S\bar{v}O_2$	> 65%
	Arterial-venous oxygen content difference	$C(a-\bar{v})O_2$	< 7.0 mL/dL
	Oxygen extraction	$S(a-\bar{v})O_2 \div SaO_2$	< 0.35
VENTILATION			
Adequacy	Minute ventilation	$\dot{V}_E$	5–10 L/min
	Arterial carbon dioxide partial pressure	$PaCO_2$	35–45 torr (normal pH)
	Transcutaneous CO_2 partial pressure	$PtcCO_2$	35–45 torr (normal pH)
	End-tidal CO_2 partial pressure	$PetCO_2$	35–43 torr (4.6-5.6%)
Efficiency	Physiologic deadspace	V_{DS} phy	see V_{DS} phy below
	Deadspace to tidal volume ratio	$V_{DS} \div V_T$	< 0.6
	Minute ventilation vs CO_2 partial pressure	$\dot{V}_E$ vs $PaCO_2$	$\dot{V}_E$ < 10 L/min wth $PaCO_2$ < 40 torr
VENTILATORY LOAD			
Total impedance	Dynamic characteristic	$\dfrac{(V_T-V_C)}{(PIP-PEEP)}$	35–50 mL/cm H_2O
Compliance	Effective compliance (C_{eff})	$\dfrac{(V_T-V_C)}{(Pplat-PEEP)}$	60–100 mL/cm H_2O
Work of breathing	Work kg · m/L or j/L	Work = P × V	< 0.15 kg · m/L < 1.5 j/L
VENTILATORY CAPACITY			
Drive	Occlusion pressure	$P_{0.1}$	< 6 cm H_2O
	Mean inspiratory flow	V_t/t_i	not established
Strength	Vital capacity	VC	> 15 mL/kg
	Negative inspiratory force	NIF; $Pimax$	> −30 cm H_2O
Endurance	Maximum voluntary ventilation	MVV	> 20 L/min
	Ratio of minute volume to MVV	$\dot{V}_E$:MVV	< 1:2
	Pressure-time index	$(Pdi/P_{max}) \times t_i/t_{tot}$	< 0.15

invasive procedures tend to provide more accurate data than noninvasive methods, but carry greater risk.

When both approaches are available, choosing between an invasive or noninvasive approach should depend on the need for measurement precision. On the other hand, it is often useful to combine the two approaches, using the invasive approach to establish accurate baseline information, while applying the noninvasive method for ongoing monitoring.

Physiologic data may also be gathered intermittently or continuously. Generally, the less stable the patient, the greater the need for continuous data gathering.

For each major category of data collection discussed, we will emphasize, where applicable, the variety of options currently available. The final decision on what parameters to monitor and how to collect the data should be made by the care team as a whole, as guided by the above considerations.

Assessing oxygenation

We can assess oxygenation either at the lungs or tissue level. At the lungs, we assess oxygen movement between the alveoli and the blood (external respiration).[34] Oxygen exchange at the lungs should be assessed in terms of both its adequacy and efficiency. At the tissue level, we evaluate oxygen transfer between blood and tissue cells (internal respiration).[35] A full evaluation should consider each in careful detail. As the RCP is most directly responsible for pulmonary gas exchange, we discuss this aspect first, followed by an analysis of the methods used to determine tissue oxygenation.

Adequacy of pulmonary oxygenation

The adequacy of pulmonary O_2 exchange is generally assessed by measuring either the PaO_2 or SaO_2. Both invasive and noninvasive, and continuous and intermittent approaches can be used.

Arterial PO_2. The arterial PO_2 is the most frequently obtained measure of the adequacy of oxygen exchange at the lung. In general, oxygen exchange at the lung is adequate if the arterial PO_2 can be maintained in the 60 to 100 torr range.

The PaO_2 is obtained intermittently by invasive sampling of arterial blood, either percutaneously or by an indwelling arterial line (see the subsequent section on hemodynamic monitoring). Miniaturized intravascular Clark electrodes have been used to provide direct and continuous monitoring of PaO_2.[36,37] However, technical difficulties with these devices have generally precluded their widespread use.[38]

More recently, fluorescence-based sensors called *optodes* have shown promise for invasive blood-gas analysis.[39] Optodes located at the tip of a flexible fiberoptic strand can provide continuous measurement of intravascular PO_2, PCO_2, and pH.[40-42] Clinical

performance of these optode-based blood gas monitoring systems indicates a high degree of stability, consistency, and accuracy when compared to *in-vitro* blood gas analysis.[43]

Transcutaneous PO_2. Noninvasive, continuous estimation of PaO_2 can be provided with the transcutaneous Clark electrode.[44,45] Monitoring the transcutaneous PO_2 ($PtcO_2$) provides a reasonable estimate of oxygen tension, particularly in infants. A modified, heated Clark electrode is used (Figure 33-2). Skin temperatures between 43 and 45° C cause dilation of capillaries under the probe and arterialization of the blood. Oxygen diffuses from the capillaries, across the dermal and epidermal cell layers, and into the electrode. This diffusion cascade may reduce the PO_2 measured at the electrode, particularly as skin thickness increases with patient age. In neonates, the PO_2 diffusion gradient between the capillaries and epidermis is largely offset by the heating effect.

In the stable patient with good cardiac output and fluid balance, the PaO_2 and $PtcO_2$ are highly correlated, with a relatively constant difference between the two values. In such patients, the PaO_2 can be "calibrated" against the $PtcO_2$, thus decreasing the need for repeated arterial samples. In shock or low flow states, however, peripheral vasoconstriction lowers cutaneous blood flow and makes accurate estimations of PaO_2 difficult.[45,46] For this reason, $PtcO_2$ monitoring should generally be used only on patients with stable hemodynamics.

The accompanying box outlines the basic procedure used to set-up a transcutaneous PO_2/PCO_2 system.[45] In terms of electrode placement, the abdomen, chest, or lower back are the most common sites for infants, children and adults.

Procedure for use of transcutaneous monitor

- Place unit at bedside and provide manufacturer-specified warm-up time
- Check membrane to make sure it is free of bubbles or scratches; change membrane if needed
- Select monitoring site by evaluating perfusion, skin thickness, absence of bones
- Prepare the sensor with adhesive ring and contact solution
- Set appropriate probe temperature (based on patient's age, skin and skin manufacturer's recommendations)
- Prepare the site (remove excess hair, clean skin)
- Attach probe to patient, assuring that it is secure
- Allow stabilization time of 10 to 20 min
- Schedule site change time (2 to 6 hrs, depending on patient)
- Set high and low alarms
- Monitor and document results as per institutional protocol
- Change site at appropriate intervals

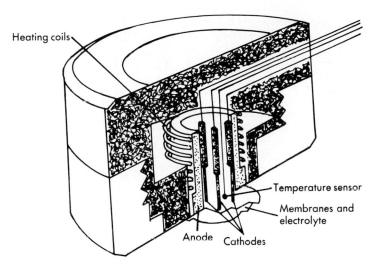

Heating coils

Temperature sensor

Membranes and electrolyte

Anode   Cathodes

Fig. 33-2 Transcutaneous PO_2 electrode. A cross-sectional diagram of the components of the $PtcO_2$ electrode shows a circular anode around a series of cathodes and a temperature sensor. A heating coil causes local hypermia so that surface PO_2 more closely resembles PaO_2. A double membrane separates the electrode proper from the skin. (From Ruppel G: Manual of pulmonary function testing. In McPherson SP: Respiratory therapy equipment, ed 4, St Louis, 1989, Mosby.)

Arterial hemoglobin saturation. The arterial hemoglobin saturation (SaO_2) is also a good indicator of the adequacy of pulmonary oxygen exchange. As with PaO_2 measurements, both invasive and noninvasive, and continuous and intermittent approaches may be used to measure SaO_2.

Estimates of hemoglobin saturation. SaO_2 estimates are normally provided with arterial blood gas reports. Using the obtained PaO_2, temperature, and pH, the SaO_2 is derived by nomogram or computer algorithm. Of course, this derivation assumes that all other parameters are normal, including the type of hemoglobin present.

Oximetry. Actual measurement of the SaO_2 is obtained by spectrophotometric analysis of an arterial blood sample, a procedure called oximetry (see Chapter 17 for details). There are two types of oximeters used in clinical practice: the laboratory CO-oximeter and the bedside pulse oximeter.

Only the laboratory CO-oximeter actually measures SaO_2. CO-oximeters analyze blood samples using three different wavelengths of light (Figure 33-3, page 928). By comparing the differences in light absorbance among these different wavelengths, the CO-oximeter can measure the relative proportion of Hb, HbO_2, and HbCO.

The bedside pulse oximeter uses a transcutaneous probe to estimate arterial saturation.[47-49] This probe transmits two wavelengths of light (red and infrared) through a capillary bed, such as those in the finger. Because only two wavelengths of light are used, the pulse oximeter can only detect the amount of unsaturated hemoglobin present. Results, however, are reported as saturation values, abbreviated as the SpO_2 (pulse saturation). Unfortunately, the SpO_2 includes not only oxyhemoglobin, but also other "saturated" hemoglobins, such as carboxyhemoglobin. The result is an overestimation of SaO_2 in the presence of these abnormal hemoglobins. Other technical limitations of pulse oximetry are described in Chapter 17.

Of course, the relationship between PaO_2 and SaO_2 is described by the oxyhemoglobin dissociation curve. On the middle portion of the curve, where the slope is steep and changes in the PaO_2 result in larger changes in saturation, oximetry provides a sensitive indication of changes in oxygenation status. However, when operating on the flat upper portion of the curve, where large changes in PaO_2 can occur with minor alterations in saturation, oximetry becomes less useful. For this reason, an understanding of the oxyhemoglobin dissociation curve is essential for appropriate interpretation of oximetry data.

Pulse oximetry is considered a safe procedure. However, given its limited accuracy, both false-negative and false-positive results are common. Combined with the need for careful interpretation of results, this limited accuracy can lead to inappropriate treatment decisions.[50]

To avoid these problems, pulse oximeter readings initially should be validated by comparison to direct measures of SaO_2.[50] Thereafter, periodical re-evaluation should occur as the patient's clinical state changes.

In addition to problems of accuracy and interpretation, pulse oximetry can cause tissue injury. Tissue injury occurs at the measuring site and is most commonly due to probe misuse. Examples include pressure sores from prolonged application, and burns from using incompatible probes between instruments.[50]

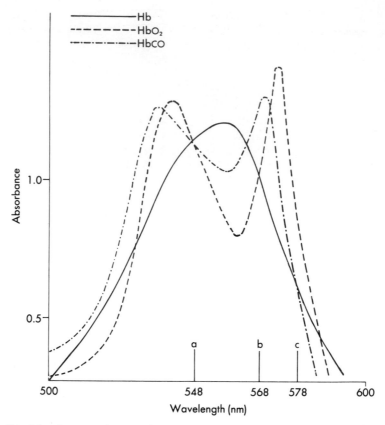

Fig. 33-3 Principle of spectrophotometric oximetry. Absorbance measurements are made at three distinct wavelengths (548, 568, and 578 nm) as light passes through a blood sample. At 548 nm all three forms of HB (Hb, HbO$_2$, and HBCO) have identical absorbances. At 568 nm only Hb and HbO$_2$ coincide, whereas at 578 nm Hb and HbCO coincide. The solution of three simultaneous equations provides the relative proportions of each species as well as the total Hb. (From Ruppel G: Manual of pulmonary function testing. Mosby. In McPherson SP: Respiratory therapy equipment, ed 4, St Louis, 1989, Mosby.)

Efficiency of pulmonary oxygenation

Unfortunately, neither the PaO$_2$ or SaO$_2$ reveals how efficient the lung is in exchanging oxygen. In order to assess the lung's efficiency in oxygenating the blood, we must compare the amount of O$_2$ being delivered to the alveoli with that actually entering the pulmonary capillaries. Measures of oxygenation efficiency at the lung include the alveolar-arterial oxygen tension gradient, various oxygenation ratios, and the physiologic shunt.

Alveolar-arterial oxygen tension gradient. Historically, the efficiency of pulmonary oxygen exchange has been assessed by computing the alveolar-arterial oxygen tension gradient, or P(A−a)O$_2$ (see Chapter 12).

For consistency, this measure is performed with the subject breathing 100% oxygen. Pulmonary oxygen exchange is normal and efficient when the P(A−a)O$_2$ breathing 100% oxygen is between 25 to 65 torr. This small normal difference in PO$_2$ is due mainly to anatomic shunting within the lungs and heart. Higher P(A−a)O$_2$s indicates abnormal inefficiencies in oxygen exchange.

As a rule of thumb, when breathing 100% oxygen, every 100 torr P(A−a)O$_2$ equals about a 5% shunt. Unfortunately, when the PaO$_2$ is below 100 torr, this rule of thumb becomes grossly inaccurate. Alternatively, assuming a normal C(a−$\overline{v}$)O$_2$, one may estimate the percent shunt ($\dot{Q}_s/\dot{Q}_t$) of a patient breathing 100% oxygen as follows:[51]

$$\dot{Q}_s/\dot{Q}_t \approx \frac{P(A−a)O_2 \times 0.003}{[P(A−a)O_2 \times 0.003] + 5}$$

where 5 represents the normal C(a−$\overline{v}$)O$_2$ in mL/dL.

As long as the inspired oxygen concentration is kept constant, changes in P(A−a)O$_2$ provide a valuable index of changes in the efficiency of gas exchange over time. However, the P(A−a)O$_2$ does not change linearly with changes in FiO$_2$.[12] In addition, administration of 100% oxygen actually increases the percent shunt in many patients, probably by causing absorption atelectasis.[52] For this reason, various oxygen tension indices have been used to assess the efficiency of oxygenation. Unlike the P(A−a)O$_2$, these indices yield a constant value for a given degree of shunting, regardless of FiO$_2$.

Oxygen tension indices. There are three oxygen tension indices common in clinical practice (Table 33-5).[53,54] These include the ratio of arterial to alveolar oxygen partial pressures (PaO_2/PAO_2), or a/A ratio; the ratio of the arterial partial pressure of oxygen to the inspired fractional concentration of oxygen (PaO_2/FiO_2), or P/F ratio; and the ratio of the alveolar-arterial oxygen tension gradient to the arterial partial pressure of oxygen ($P(A-a)O_2/PaO_2$), or Respiratory Index (RI).

Normally, a/A ratio ranges from 0.74 in the elderly, to 0.9 in healthy young subjects. a/A values below 0.6 indicate inefficiencies in oxygenation requiring O_2 therapy. a/A values below 0.15 indicate refractory hypoxemia due to significant physiologic shunting.[55,56]

Unlike the a/A ratio, the P/F ratio (PaO_2/FiO_2) does not require the calculation of the PAO_2, and is thus simpler to compute.[12,54] In normal subjects, the P/F ratio should exceed 200, regardless of FiO_2. A P/F ratio below 200 indicates hypoxemia due to significant V/Q inequalities, while a P/F ratio less than 150 signifies the presence of a large physiologic shunt.[57]

With the PaO_2 in its denominator, a low RI is a good sign. Specifically, an RI less than 1.0 indicates normal oxygen exchange, while higher values indicate increasing inefficiency in pulmonary oxygenation. For example, RI values between 1.0 and 5.0 suggest V/Q imbalances treatable with oxygen therapy, while an RI above 5.0 indicates the presence of refractory hypoxemia caused by physiologic shunting.[58,59]

In general, these indices are most accurate for estimating oxygenation efficiency when oxygenation function is good. They become less accurate when lung function is severely impaired.[60]

Physiologic shunt. The most accurate and reliable measure of pulmonary oxygenation efficiency is direct computation of the physiologic shunt ($\dot{Q}_s/\dot{Q}_t$). The physiologic shunt in the lungs is computed using the following equation:

$$\dot{Q}_s/\dot{Q}_t = \frac{Cc'O_2 - CaO_2}{Cc'O_2 - C\bar{v}O_2}$$

where $\dot{Q}_s$ equals the volume of blood bypassing ventilated alveoli, $\dot{Q}_t$ equals the total cardiac output, $Cc'O_2$

equals the "ideal" pulmonary end-capillary oxygen content, CaO_2 equals the arterial oxygen content, and $C\bar{v}O_2$ equals the oxygen content of the mixed venous blood.

In order to measure the physiologic shunt, both an arterial and mixed venous blood sample must be obtained. Arterial blood is obtained for analysis in the usual manner, with its total oxygen content calculated according to the formulas provided in Chapter 12. A true mixed venous blood sample can be obtained only via the distal sample port of an indwelling pulmonary artery catheter. The total oxygen content of the mixed venous blood is calculated in the same manner as the arterial sample.

True end-capillary pulmonary blood cannot be sampled. However, the oxygen content of "ideal" end-capillary pulmonary blood is assumed to equal that which would be obtained if the end-capillary PO_2 were equal to the alveolar PO_2. Thus, to determine the "ideal" end-capillary pulmonary blood content, one simply substitutes the PAO_2 into the formula for calculating total O_2 content.

When only arterial blood is available, an estimated shunt equation may be used.[60] The estimated shunt equation is derived from the physiologic shunt equation, above. An assumed $C(a-\bar{v})O_2$ of 3.5 mL/dL is inserted in the denominator of equation:

$$\dot{Q}_s/\dot{Q}_t = \frac{Cc'O_2 - CaO_2}{Cc'O_2 - (CaO_2 - 3.5)}$$

Using this method, the correlation between actual $\dot{Q}_s/\dot{Q}_t$ and estimated shunt (r= 0.94) has been found higher than the correlations observed using oxygen tension indices.[60]

Adequacy of tissue oxygenation

Oxygen delivery to the tissues per minute (DO_2) is a function of both the arterial oxygen content and the cardiac output:[61]

$$DO_2 \text{ (mL/min)} = \dot{Q}_t \text{ (dL/min)} \times CaO_2 \text{ (mL/dL)}$$

Thus, assuring adequate arterial oxygen content satisfies only half of our concern in providing oxygen to the tissues. In order to meet cellular needs for oxygen, a sufficient volume of arterialized blood must perfuse the tissues each minute.

Classically, whole body perfusion per minute, or cardiac output, can be measured according to the Fick equation:

$$\dot{Q}_t \text{ (L/min)} = \frac{\dot{V}O_2}{C(a-\bar{v})O_2 \times 10}$$

where $\dot{Q}_t$ is the cardiac output in liters per minute, $\dot{V}O_2$ is the whole body oxygen consumption (uptake) in L/min, and $C(a-\bar{v})O_2$ in the arterial-mixed venous oxygen content difference in mL/dL.

Table 33-5   Oxygen tension indices

Index	Formula	Correlation with $\dot{Q}_s/\dot{Q}_t$	Normal	Moderate Hypoxemia	Severe Hypoxemia
a/A	$PaO_2 \div PAO_2$	−0.72	>0.74	<0.74 >0.15	<0.15
P/F	$PaO_2 \div FiO_2$	−0.71	>200	<200 >100	<100
RI	$P(A-a)O_2 \div PaO_2$	+0.74	<1.0	>1.0 <5.0	>5.0

Rearranging the equation to solve for oxygen uptake, we derive:

$$\dot{V}O_2 = Q_t \times C(a\text{-}\bar{v})O_2$$

According to this formula, in order to assess the adequacy of tissue oxygenation, we must not only know how much oxygen is delivered ($\dot{Q}_t \times CaO_2$), but also how much oxygen is left over after tissue exchange.

Mixed venous oxygen content. The amount of oxygen remaining after tissue exchange is the mixed venous oxygen content, or $C\bar{v}O_2$. With a normal hemoglobin level, PaO_2, and cardiac output, the $C\bar{v}O_2$ averages about 14 to 16 mL/dL.

Rearranging the Fick equation once again to solve for $C\bar{v}O_2$, we obtain the following formula:

$$C\bar{v}O_2 = CaO_2 - \frac{\dot{V}O_2}{\dot{Q}_t}$$

As indicated in this formula, the $C\bar{v}O_2$ will fall if either: (1) the arterial oxygen content (CaO_2) falls, (2) tissue oxygen uptake ($\dot{V}O_2$) increases, or (3) cardiac output (Q_t) decreases. Thus the $C\bar{v}O_2$ is a key indicator of the adequacy of both oxygen delivery and uptake at the tissue level.[62] The accompanying box summarizes the clinical conditions associated with changes in mixed venous oxygen content.[12]

$P\bar{v}O_2$ and $S\bar{v}O_2$. In clinical practice, either the mixed venous PO_2 or hemoglobin saturation ($S\bar{v}O_2$) may be used in lieu of the actual oxygen content. Oxygen delivery and tissue uptake are considered normal if the $P\bar{v}O_2$ is between 38 and 42 torr, or the $S\bar{v}O_2$ is between 68% to 77%.[13] Patient values below these normals indicate inadequate oxygen delivery to the tissues. A drop in $S\bar{v}O_2$ below 50% indicates impaired tissue oxygenation, while $S\bar{v}O_2$ values less than 30% can cause unconsciousness due to hypoxemia. Likewise, $P\bar{v}O_2$ values less than 30 torr indicate severe hypoxia.

Normally, blood samples are obtained intermittently from the distal port of a pulmonary artery catheter. The blood sample must be withdrawn slowly and with the balloon deflated. Incorrect technique could cause oxygenated blood to be drawn from the pulmonary capillaries to the catheter, thus contaminating the sample and increasing its measured oxygen values.

Alternatively, $S\bar{v}O_2$ may be measured continuously using *venous oximetry*.[63,64] Venous oximetry is of potential value in certain conditions of decreased O_2 transport, especially in low cardiac output states.

Continuous venous oximetry employs the same general principles of oximetry previously discussed, with two major differences (Figure 33-4). The first difference is that light transmission occurs through a special fiberoptic pulmonary artery catheter. The second difference is that the device measures the magnitude of reflected, as opposed to absorbed light.

Studies of continuous venous oximetry in patients with acute myocardial infarction indicate that high $S\bar{v}O_2$ levels do consistently correspond to increases in cardiac output. On the other hand, decreases in $S\bar{v}O_2$ are not as reliably associated with decreases in cardiac output. In addition, changes in cardiac output of ±20% were only associated with corresponding changes in $S\bar{v}O_2$ in about 1/3 of the measurement.[65]

A unique approach is to combine arterial pulse oximetry with venous oximetry, a method called *dual oximetry*. Studies indicate that this technique is a reliable and accurate method for real-time assessment of gas exchange at both the lung and tissues in patients with acute respiratory failure.[66,67]

Two key oxygenation indices are provided from data obtained via dual oximetry: the ventilation-perfusion index **(VQI),** and an estimate of the oxygen extraction ratio **(O_2ER).**[66-68] The VQI is computed as follows:

$$VQI = \frac{1 - SaO_2}{1 - S\bar{v}O_2}$$

The VQI provides an estimate of the venous admixture which correlates well with $\dot{Q}s/\dot{Q}_t$ (r = 0.78).

The oxygen extraction ratio is the ratio between tissue oxygen consumption and oxygen delivery:

$$O_2ER = \frac{\dot{V}O_2}{DO_2}$$

Accurate measurement of the O_2ER requires careful analysis of whole body O_2 consumption using indirect calorimetry. Dual oximetry provides a close estimate of the O_2ER, using the following formula:

$$O_2ER = \frac{SaO_2 - S\bar{v}O_2}{SaO_2}$$

Clinical conditions associated with changes in $C\bar{v}O_2$

Decreased $C\bar{v}O_2$
  Decreased cardiac output
  Decreased arterial O_2 saturation
  Decreased hemoglobin concentration
  Increased O_2 consumption

Increased $C\bar{v}O_2$
  Increased O_2 delivery to tissues
  Decreased O_2 consumption
  Decreased O_2 extraction by tissues
  Left-to-right intracardiac shunt
  Severe mitral **regurgitation**
  Wedged pulmonary artery catheter
    (false increase in $S\bar{v}O_2$)

From Tobin MJ: Respiratory monitoring during mechanical ventilation, *Crit Care Clin* 6(3):679–709, 1990.

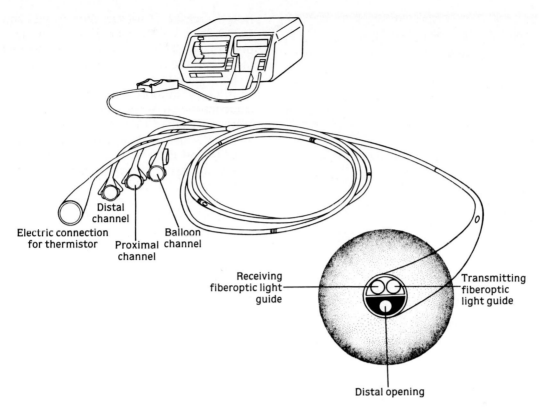

Fig. 33-4 Fiberoptic pulmonary artery catheter system used for continuous monitoring of venous oxygen saturation. (Courtesy Oximetrix, Inc, Mountain View, Calif. From Wilkins RL, Sheldon RL, Krider SJ: *Clinical assessment in respiratory care*, St Louis, 1985, Mosby.)

Normally, the O_2ER is 0.25 or less, indicating that only about a quarter of the oxygen delivered to the tissues is consumed. If either delivery decreases or consumption increases, the O_2ER will rise. An O_2ER greater than 0.35 suggests an excessively high oxygen extraction to meet metabolic needs.[53]

In evaluating the $P\bar{v}O_2$ or $S\bar{v}O_2$, the clinician must taken into account the fact that different organ systems have different oxygen needs. For example, whereas the total body $C(a-\bar{v})O_2$ ranges from 4 to 6 mL/dL, the difference between the arterial and venous oxygen content of the heart is about 11 to 12 mL/dL. Thus a venous oxygen level (representing an average for the body as a whole) does not necessarily indicate that tissue oxygenation is adequate for all body systems.

In addition to these considerations, there are several clinical circumstances in which mixed venous oxygen levels can be misleading. Collectively, these conditions are all forms of *dysoxia* (refer to Chapter 15).[69] Dysoxia is a form of hypoxia in which the cellular use of O_2 is abnormally decreased. The best example of dysoxia is cyanide poisoning. Cyanide disrupts the intracellular cytochrome oxidase system, thereby preventing cellular use of O_2. When cells cannot extract the oxygen delivered to them, the $C\bar{v}O_2$ rises and become *higher* than normal—this despite the presence of tissue hypoxia.

Similar conditions may exist in clinical states such as sepsis, ARDS and multiple organ failure.[70 73] In these cases, tissue oxygen consumption ($\dot{V}O_2$) appears limited by the rate of oxygen delivery; as cardiac output decreases so too does the $\dot{V}O_2$. According to the Fick principle, if both the cardiac output ($\dot{Q}_t$) and tissue $\dot{V}O_2$ decrease, the $C\bar{v}O_2$ and $S\bar{v}O_2$ may remain unchanged, even in the presence of tissue hypoxia. For this reason, some investigators have suggested using mixed venous levels of lactate and pyruvate (by-products of anaerobic metabolism) as the basis for assessing the state of tissue oxygenation in patients with compromised oxygen delivery.[74]

Assessing ventilation

In order to properly assess ventilation, the RCP must understand what factors determine ventilatory demand. Key factors determining ventilatory demand include the following:

- Metabolic rate (carbon dioxide production)
- Acid-base status
- Central respiratory drive
- Physiologic deadspace
- Lung and thoracic mechanics

The box on page 932 differentiates between the primary causes of increased and decreased ventilatory demand.

Factors altering ventilatory demand

Factors increasing ventilatory demand:

Arterial hypoxemia
Increased metabolic rate
Increased physiologic deadspace
Metabolic acidosis
J-receptor stimulation (e.g., pulmonary edema)
Increased work of breathing
Singultus (hiccup)
Confusion/irritation
CNS stimulation
Early salicylate poisoning

Factors decreasing ventilatory demand:

Severe metabolic alkalosis
Decreased metabolic rate
Hyperoxia in chronic respiratory acidosis
Narcotic CNS depression
Neurologic disease
Neuromuscular disease

In assessing metabolism, one also must take into account the type of nutrients being metabolized. Carbohydrates produce the most CO_2 relative to oxygen consumption, one CO_2 for each O_2. Metabolism of pure fat protein produces 30% less CO_2 than pure carbohydrate metabolism, while protein metabolism producing 20% less CO_2.[75]

For this reason, patients who receive only dextrose IVs may have a comparably higher CO_2 production than those metabolizing proteins or fats, and may thus have a greater ventilatory demand.[76] Moreover, as shown in Table 33-6, fever, injury, and burns all increase metabolic rate substantially.

As described in Chapter 11, the relationship between carbon dioxide production ($\dot{V}CO_2$) and alveolar ventilation ($\dot{V}A$) is defined by the following relationship:[77]

$$PACO_2 \approx \frac{\dot{V}CO_2}{\dot{V}A}$$

This formula states that the alveolar PCO_2 is directly proportional to carbon dioxide production and inversely proportional to alveolar ventilation. Of course, we know that the $PACO_2$ rises when ventilation decreases. However, the formula shows that the $PACO_2$ can climb even if the ventilation remains unchanged. This could occur if the metabolic rate increased and alveolar ventilation stayed constant.

For example, if a patient receiving control mode ventilatory support developed an infection and became febrile, his or her metabolic rate would increase. With no change in ventilator rate or tidal volume, alveolar ventilation would remain constant and the $PACO_2$ (and $PaCO_2$) would rise. Of course, the opposite would occur if metabolism were too slow.

In terms of acid-base status, ventilation must always be judged according to its effect on pH. For example, increased ventilatory demands will occur during compensation for metabolic acidosis, yet low levels of alveolar ventilation may be "normal" in compensated respiratory acidosis.

Associated with acid-base balance is the patient's central respiratory drive. However, respiratory drive may be increased or decreased independent of alteration in acid-base balance.

The physiologic deadspace will also affect a patient's ventilatory demands. In patients with normal respiratory drive, an increase in deadspace always increases ventilatory demand.

Last, the mechanics of the lungs and thorax will affect ventilatory demand, both directly and indirectly. Changes in compliance and resistance directly affect ventilatory demand via their influence on the rate and depth of breathing (refer to Chapter 11). Decreased compliance or increased resistance indirectly affect ventilatory demand by increasing the work of breathing, thereby increasing metabolic rate and CO_2 production.

In combination then, the assessment of ventilation must take into account the relationship among multiple factors. As with oxygenation, we can assess ventilation in terms of both its adequacy and efficiency.

Adequacy of ventilation

As with oxygenation, we can measure both the adequacy and efficiency of ventilation. Common techniques for assessing the adequacy of ventilation include the minute volume, arterial PCO_2, transcutaneous PCO_2, and end-tidal PCO_2.[78]

Minute volume. Although fraught with limitations, a patient's minute volume can be used as a rough estimate of the adequacy of ventilation. Indeed, before ABG analysis was available, the adequacy of ventilation was judged mainly by observing the patient and measuring the minute volume. The measured minute volume was then compared to established norms (such as the Radford nomogram). Although this approach has given way to more precise indices of ventilatory adequacy, it still has a place in bedside assessment.

The minute ventilation is normally measured with a mechanical (vane-type) or electronic respirometer

Table 33-6 Factors affecting metabolic rate

Condition	Metabolic Rate
Basal	25 kcal/kg/day
Fever	Basal + 3.0 kcal/kg/day/° C
Injury	50–60 kcal/kg/day
Burns	40 kcal/kg × percent body surface area burned

attached to the ET tube (Figure 33-5).[79] While the patient breathes through the device, the RCP counts the rate and times the procedure for exactly one minute. With this information, minute ventilation ($\dot{V}E$), respiratory rate (f), and average tidal volume (V_T = $\dot{V}E/f$) can be documented. If the respirometer is placed after the exhalation valve in a ventilator circuit, the tidal volume must be corrected for the additional compressed volume collected with the patient's expired gas.

Unfortunately, problems arise when trying to make these measurements in non-intubated patients.[12] Critically ill patients have a low tolerance for devices using mouthpieces or masks. Furthermore, these devices themselves tend to alter the breathing pattern, resulting in a larger tidal volume and lower respiratory rate.[80] Use of the electronic volume accumulators on some third generation ventilators can help overcome this effect, but only on intubated patients.

A normal adult minute volume ranges between 5 and 7 L/min. Of and by itself, a normal minute ventilation does not necessarily indicate adequate ventilation. However, the use of the minute ventilation in conjunction with other measures can be helpful in assessing the efficiency of ventilation and certain elements of respiratory mechanics (discussed subsequently).

Arterial PCO_2. The arterial partial pressure of carbon dioxide, or $PaCO_2$, is the "gold standard" for assessing the adequacy of ventilation. The $PaCO_2$ is usually obtained invasively by arterial puncture or, alternatively, through an indwelling arterial line. In general, ventilation is deemed adequate if the arterial PCO_2 level results in a normal arterial pH. For normal subjects, this means a $PaCO_2$ between 35 and 45 torr.

Continuous, noninvasive monitoring of ventilation can be a useful addition to the standard practice of sampling arterial blood for the PCO_2. Noninvasive monitoring of ventilation can be performed using either a transcutaneous CO_2 electrode or a capnometer.

Transcutaneous PCO_2. Transcutaneous CO_2 monitoring ($PtcCO_2$) is similar to $PtcO_2$ monitoring.[45] Many devices combine O_2 and CO_2 electrodes into a single sensor. A transcutaneous CO_2 probe is a miniaturized Severinghaus pH electrode, combined with a heating element for warming the skin. This probe is attached to the skin surface. The heating from the probe causes a localized increase in CO_2 production which causes the probe to overestimate $PaCO_2$. This error is accounted for by comparing the $PtcCO_2$ to a baseline $PaCO_2$. As with measurement of $PtcO_2$, transcutaneous CO_2 monitoring is affected by low perfusion states. However, transcutaneous CO_2 moni-

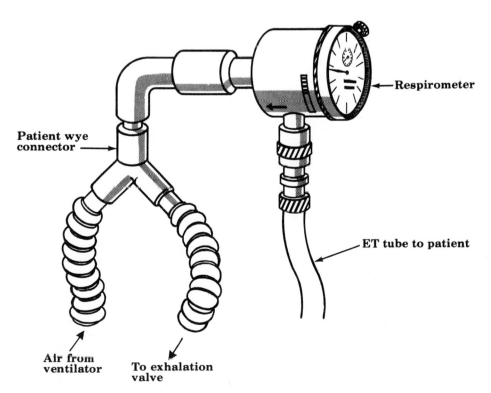

Patient wye connector

Respirometer

ET tube to patient

Air from ventilator

To exhalation valve

Fig. 33-5 Minute volume measurement at the endotracheal tube. The respirometer is attached to the endotracheal tube so that the patient's actual exhaled air can be measured. The respirometer can also be attached at the exhalation valve. Some respirometers read both inspiration and expiration by measuring flow in both directions. (From Pilbeam SP: Mechanical ventilation: physiological and clinical applications, St Louis, 1986, Mosby.)

toring can be a useful technique for analyzing changes in ventilation, especially when used in conjunction with intermittent arterial PCO_2 analysis and minute ventilation measurements.

Capnometry/capnography. *Capnometry* is the clinical measurement of exhaled gas for its CO_2 content.[81] The device making such measurements is called a *capnometer*. A capnometer may offer readings in either %CO_2 or torr. A device which can measure and graphically display changes in CO_2 levels over time (while the patient breathes) is called a *capnograph*. The graphic display provided by a capnograph is called a *capnogram*.

The technical aspects of capnometry were reviewed in Chapter 17.[82] Here we emphasize the interpretation and use of the data so obtained. Figure 33-6 shows a typical normal single breath capnograph tracing. During the first portion of exhalation (Phase I), the expired partial pressure of carbon dioxide, or $P\text{E}CO_2$ is normally 0 torr, indicating exhalation of pure deadspace gas. In Phase II, alveolar gas begins mixing with deadspace gas, causing an increase in the $P\text{E}CO_2$. During Phase III, gas entering the capnometer comes mainly from the alveoli. This results in a leveling of the CO_2 concentration, see visually as the *alveolar plateau*. Gas gathered toward the end of the alveolar plateau is called end-tidal gas, with its carbon dioxide partial pressure abbreviated as $P\text{ET}CO_2$.

The normal $P\text{ET}CO_2$ averages 1 to 5 torr less than the normal $PaCO_2$, ranging between 35 and 43 torr.[12] Expressed as a percentage, this normal value equates to an end-tidal CO_2 concentration of about 4.6% to 5.6%. Since the $P\text{ET}CO_2$ in normal subjects closely approximates the $PaCO_2$, this measure is a potentially

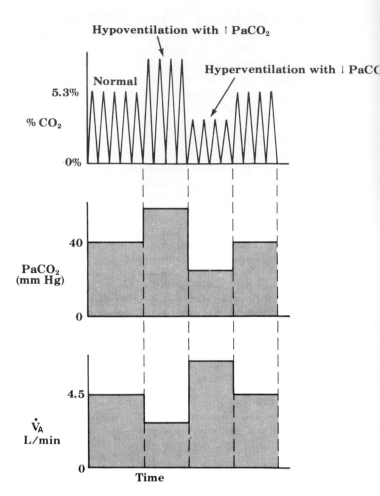

Fig. 33-7 Shows the changes in end-tidal CO_2 with changes in ventilation. During normal alveolar ventilation ($\dot{V}A$), $PaCO_2$ and end-tidal CO_2 are normal. During hypoventilation, $PaCO_2$ and end-tidal CO_2 increase. During hyperventilation, $PaCO_2$ and end-tidal CO_2 decrease. (From Pilbeam SP: Mechanical ventilation: physiological and clinical applications, St Louis, 1986, Mosby.)

useful noninvasive index of the adequacy of ventilation.[83] Using trend analysis, Figure 33-7 demonstrates the close relationship between end-expired CO_2 concentrations, and $PaCO_2$ levels as related to changes in alveolar ventilation in normal subjects.

However, in patients with abnormal V/Q ratios, visible changes in the expired CO_2 tracing are observed, particularly in Phases II and III (Figure 33-8).

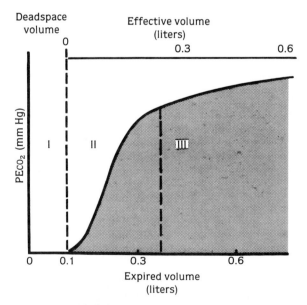

Fig. 33-6 Single-breath tracing for exhaled carbon dioxide. (From Wilkins RL, Sheldon RL, Krider SJ: *Clinical assessment in respiratory care*, St Louis, 1985, Mosby.)

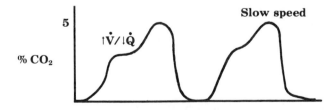

Fig. 33-8 With a slow tracing it is possible to pick up abnormalities in the CO_2 curve. A sloping expiratory curve may indicate a V/Q abnormality. (From Pilbeam SP: Mechanical ventilation: physiological and clinical applications, St Louis, 1986, Mosby.)

Typically, these changes include a slower and more irregular rise in CO_2 levels during phase II, and/or a lower than normal end-tidal CO_2 levels during Phase III. The irregular rise in CO_2 levels during phase II indicates a V/Q imbalance, specifically a high V/Q. In addition, lower than normal Phase III CO_2 levels suggests the presence of a abnormally high P(a-ET)CO_2 gradient, also indicative of a high V/Q.

Conditions such as COPD, pulmonary embolism, and low perfusion states caused by shock or left ventricular failure may all decrease perfusion to ventilated areas of the lung, thereby raising the V/Q ratio and altering the expired CO_2 waveform. As shown in Figure 33-9, these conditions cannot be easily distinguished unless the patient exhales maximally below the resting FRC. Such patterns, while not diagnostic in themselves, provide a useful indication of the severity of the V/Q disturbance, and can warn of developing problems, such as acute pulmonary embolization.

As with electrocardiography, it is probably best to use a systematic approach when assessing the capnogram. To do so, you should always evaluate the CO_2 waveform for the following:

- Height
- Contour
- Baseline
- Frequency
- Rhythm

The height of the capnogram (its peak value) indicates the end-tidal CO_2 value. For a given display setting, changes in height correspond directly to $PetCO_2$ levels.

As previously described, the overall contour of a normal capnogram should consist of a sharp upstroke, a plateau, and a rapid downstroke. Physiologically, changes in waveform contour can indicate changes in the distribution of ventilation and perfusion, or airway obstruction. Waveform changes may also occur with equipment malfunction.

The capnogram baseline indicates the *inspired* CO_2 level. Normally, *inspired* CO_2 level is 0 torr, so the baseline should also be at zero. An elevated baseline (above 0 torr) indicates rebreathing, either intentional or accidental. An elevated baseline during capnography looks much like the airway pressure waveform with PEEP.

The frequency and rhythm of the capnogram breaths correspond to the frequency and rhythm established by either the patient (spontaneous breathing) or ventilator.

Once the capnogram waveform is assessed, the RCP should compare the patient's $PetCO_2$ to the measured $PaCO_2$. As indicated previously, this P(a-ET)CO_2 gradient is usually between 1 and 5 torr. A P(a-ET)CO_2 higher than 5 to 6 torr is abnormal and represents another key finding. For example, mechanical ventilation increases the V/Q ratio.[84] This typically causes an increase in P(a-ET)CO_2, often to as high as 10 to 15 torr. Most pulmonary and cardiovascular problems also cause a rise in P(a-ET)CO_2. A few clinical conditions, however, can actually result in the $PetCO_2$ exceeding the $PaCO_2$.[85] Exercise and large tidal volumes are two examples.[82]

When combined, knowledge of the capnogram waveform, the measured $PaCO_2$ and the P(a-ET)CO_2, can help clinicians identify a number of important clinical problems. These problems include metabolic,

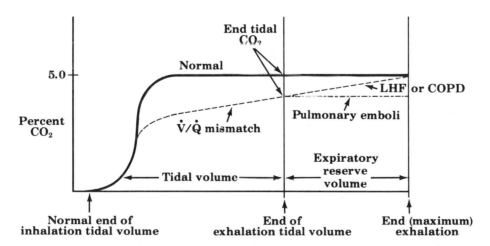

Fig. 33-9 This graph represents the percentage of CO_2 at varying exhaled lung volumes. For a normal individual (solid line) the end-tidal CO_2 at the end of normal tidal exhalation is equal to that at maximum exhalation. With left ventricular failure (LVF) and chronic obstructive pulmonary disease (COPD), the end-tidal CO_2 is less than normal at the end of a normal exhalation and may rise slightly at the end of a maximum exhalation. With pulmonary emboli present, a low end-tidal CO_2 will not rise in value at the end of a maximum exhalation. (From Pilbeam SP: Mechanical ventilation: physiological and clinical applications, St Louis, 1986, Mosby.)

respiratory, and cardiovascular changes; and equipment malfunction. Table 33-7 summarizes the capnographic findings associated with the most common of these clinical problems. Figure 33-10 shows several examples of abnormal capnograms.

Although the $P_{ET}CO_2$ and $PaCO_2$ tend to show a high correlation at single points in time, correlation between changes in $P_{ET}CO_2$ and changes in $PaCO_2$ tend to be much weaker.[12] Indeed, in one study, only 18% of the changes in $P_{ET}CO_2$ corresponded closely with changes in $PaCO_2$, and 1 in 5 cases, the directional trends in $P_{ET}CO_2$ were opposite of those occurring with $PaCO_2$.[86] This has lead some clinicians to recommend against using capnometry as a routine bedside monitoring tool, at least as related to weaning.[87]

As with pulse oximetry, however, capnometry has a place in the monitoring "tool-box." Patients for whom capnometry may be a useful monitoring tool include those with unstable ventilatory drives who are breathing spontaneously or receiving low-level ventilatory support. In these patients, capnometry readings should initially be validated by comparison to the measured $PaCO_2$. Changes in $P_{ET}CO_2$ can then be used to alert the clinician to potential changes in patient ventilation. Thereafter, periodical reevaluation should occur as the patient's clinical state changes.

Table 33-7   Changes in the exhaled capnogram with changes in metabolism, respiration, circulation and equipment function

Condition	Waveform	$P_{ET}CO_2$	$PaCO_2$	$PaCO_2$-$P_{ET}CO_2$	Insp CO_2%
METABOLISM					
Hyperthermia	Normal	↑	↑	Normal	0
Sepsis	Normal	↑	↑	Normal	0
Pain, shivering convulsions	Normal	↑	↑	Normal	0
Hypothermia	Normal	↓	↓	Normal	0
Miscellaneous					
NaHCO3 injection	Normal	↑	↑	Normal	0
Increased depth of anethesia	Normal	↓	↓	Normal	0
Use of muscle relaxants	May see cleft	↓	↓	Normal	0
RESPIRATORY					
Ventilator disconnection	Absent	↓	↑	Widened	0
Apneic patient	Absent	↓	↑	Widened	0
Esophageal intubation	Absent	↓	↑	Widened	0
Hypoventilation, mild	Normal	↑	↑	Normal	0
Hypoventilation, moderate to extreme	Abnormal	↓	↑	Widened	0
Hyperventilation	Normal	↓	↓	Normal	0
Airway obstruct, mild	Abnormal	↑	↑	Normal	0
Airway obstruct, moderate to extreme	Abnormal	↓	↑	Widened	0
Rebreathing	Baseline elevated	↑	↑	Normal	↑
Increased physiologic deadspace	Normal	↓	↑	Widened	0
PEEP (positive end-expiratory pressure)	Normal	↓	↑	Widened	0
High-rate, low tidal volume ventilation	Normal	↓	↑	Widened	0
CARDIOVASCULAR					
Increased CO_2 delivery to lungs (e.g., tourniquet release)	Normal	↑	↑↓	Normal	0
Decreased CO_2 to lungs (pulmonary embolus)	Normal	↓	↑	Widened	0
Right to left shunt	Normal	↓	↑	Widened	0
Decreased blood volume	Normal	↓	↑	Widened	0
Cardiac arrest	Normal	↓	↓	Widened	0
EQUIPMENT					
Increased apparatus dead space	Baseline elevated	↑	↑	Normal	↑
Malfunctioning non-rebreathing valve	Baseline elevated	↑	↑	Normal	↑
Mucus in sampling cell (mainstream)	Abnormal	↑	↑↓	Widened	↑
Leakage in breathing system (sidestream)	Abnormal	↓	↑↓	Widened	0
Water blocking sampling line	Absent	—	—	—	—
Leakage in sampling system	Abnormal	↓	↑↓	Widened	0
Leak around ET tube	Abnormal	↓	↑↓	Widened	0

↑ = increased; ↓ = decreased; ↑↓ = variable (independent) change. (Adapted from Shelly EJ: Capnography training manual, Criticare System, 1989.)

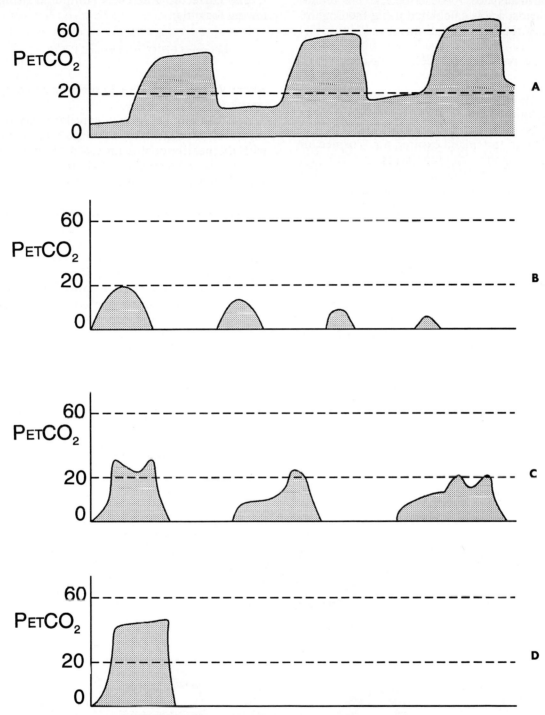

Fig. 33-10 Examples of abnormal capnograms. **A,** progressive rebreathing causing a rise in baseline PETCO$_2$. **B,** Placement of endotracheal tube in esophagus, causing a drop in PETCO$_2$ to zero. **C,** Leak in sample line or around ET tube cuff, resulting in low and variable PETCO$_2$ levels. **D,** ventilator disconnect, causing an abrupt drop in PETCO$_2$ to zero.

Capnometry also has been used for special applications, including detection of esophageal intubation, assessment of blood flow during cardiac arrest, and for determination of PEEP levels.[82] A capnometer may also be used to measure mixed expired CO$_2$ levels when measuring physiologic deadspace.

Efficiency of ventilation

The efficiency of ventilation is assessed by measuring the patient's physiologic deadspace. Alternatively, less precise estimates of the efficiency of ventilation can be obtained using clinical rules of thumb or assessment nomograms.

Physiologic deadspace. As described in Chapter 11, physiologic deadspace is calculated using the Enghoff modification of the Bohr equation:

$$V_{DSphy} = [V_T \times \frac{PaCO_2 - P\overline{E}CO_2}{PaCO_2}] - V_{DSmec}$$

where V_{DSphy} is the physiologic deadspace, V_T is the average tidal volume, $PaCO_2$ is the partial pressure of CO_2 in the arterial blood, $P\overline{E}CO_2$ is the average partial pressure of CO_2 in the mixed expired air. V_{DSmec}, or the mechanical deadspace, represents a correction factor for that portion of the patient's expired air that is rebreathed through the connecting apparatus.

Rearranging the equation to calculate the physiologic deadspace to tidal volume ratio, or V_{DS}/V_T, we derive the following formula:

$$V_{DS}/V_T = \frac{PaCO_2 - P\overline{E}CO_2}{PaCO_2} - \frac{V_{DSmec}}{V_T}$$

If the patient is being supported by positive pressure ventilation, an additional correction is required. This is because the compressed volume of the ventilator contributes to the expired gas, without raising its CO_2 content. Thus, the partial pressure of CO_2 collected from a patient receiving positive pressure ventilation will be lowered by an amount equivalent to the size of the compressed volume.

The corrected $PECO_2$ is computed using the following formula:

$$\text{Corrected } P\overline{E}CO_2 = \text{Measured } P\overline{E}CO_2 \times \frac{V_T}{(V_T - V_c)}$$

where V_c is the calculated compressed volume of the ventilator system.

Alternatively, a special ventilator circuit can be used to eliminate mixing of the patient's expired gases with the ventilator's compressed volume (Figure 33-11). By placing a second exhalation port and one-way valve at the airway connection, this circuit diverts the patient's expired gas to the collection system. The compressed volume then escapes through the normal exhalation port.[88]

Exhaled gas is collected in a large air-tight collection bag, traditionally called a "Douglas" bag (Figure 33-11). Total exhaled volume is measured by an inline mechanical or electronic respirometer. Exhaled gas should be collected for a period of at least three minutes, with an ABG drawn *during* collection. The gas and blood samples are analyzed, and the respective PCO_2 values applied in the above formula.

In lieu of measuring the V_{DS}/V_T ratio by intermittent collection of expired gases and arterial blood gas sampling, a capnometer can be used to estimate physiologic deadspace. In this approach, the $P_{ET}CO_2$ is

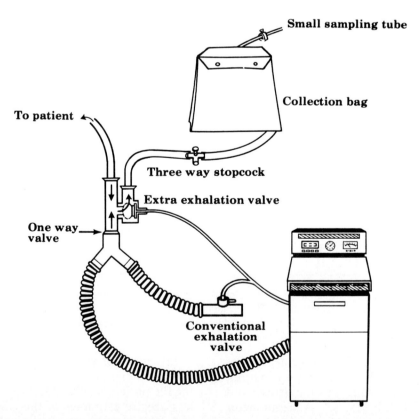

Fig. 33-11 Equipment used for collecting mixed gases from a patient on mechanical ventilation. (From Pilbeam SP: Mechanical ventilation: physiological and clinical applications, St Louis, 1986, Mosby.)

substituted for the PaCO$_2$. The mean expired CO$_2$ is either computed by the capnometer from the waveforms or obtained directly via collection bag. As with the intermittent method, correction must be made for both mechanical deadspace and compressed gas volume.

In healthy subjects, the VDS/VT ratio is between 0.33 and 0.45, indicating efficient ventilation.[12] Ventilation is efficient when the VDS/VT falls within this range. However, since positive pressure ventilation increases deadspace, this normal range will seldom be observed in patients receiving ventilatory support. For this reason, VDS/VT ratios in the 0.4 to 0.6 range are clinically acceptable. VDS/VT ratios above 0.6 indicate grossly inefficient ventilation that may impair a patient's ability to maintain normal CO$_2$ levels.

Estimates of ventilation efficiency. Although the efficiency of ventilation is best assessed by measuring VDS/VT, this approach is not always feasible or necessary. Instead, the RCP may estimate the efficiency of ventilation using clinical rules of thumb, nomograms, or computed indices.

As a rule of thumb for adult patients, ventilation is inefficient if the minute volume exceeds 10 L/min and the PCO$_2$ is normal or high. Exceptions to this rule are patients with increased ventilatory demands due to high metabolic rates, as described earlier.

This clinical rule of thumb is based on assessment nomograms like that shown in Figure 33-12.[89] On this nomogram, the VDS/VT is estimated as the point of intersection between the minute ventilation (Y axis) and the PaCO$_2$ (X axis) lines. Alternatively, this nomogram can be used to determine the $\dot{V}$E required to maintain a desired PaCO$_2$ when deadspace is known. The reader should note that this nomogram assumes a normal CO$_2$ production, and is thus not appropriate for use on patients with high metabolic rates.

Assessing ventilatory mechanics

Early emphasis on monitoring patients in respiratory failure was on gas exchange parameters. This perspective has recently been supplemented with increasingly sophisticated assessment of ventilatory mechanics.[90-92] The importance of monitoring ventilatory mechanics

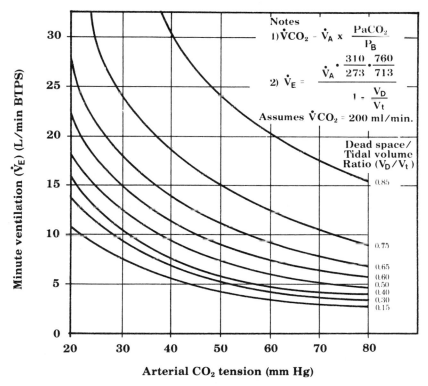

Fig. 33-12 This graph shows the relationship between minute ventilation and PaCO$_2$ for various isopleths of the ratio of dead space to tidal volume (VDS/VT). The upper right hand corner contains the basic assumptions for this relationship. $\dot{V}$CO$_2$ = CO$_2$ output. $\dot{V}$A = alveolar ventilation, PB = barometric pressure. To obtain the VDS/VT, measure the $\dot{V}$E and the PaCO$_2$ and plot these points on the graph. The VD/VT is obtained by noting the isopleth that coincides with this point. To obtain the $\dot{V}$E required to achieve a desired PaCO$_2$, draw a vertical line from the desired PaCO$_2$ on the abscissa to the VDS/VT isopleth obtained in the first step above. Draw a horizontal line from this point to the ordinate to obtain the required $\dot{V}$E. (Reproduced with permission from Selecky PA, et al: *Am Rev Respir Dis* 117:181, 1978. In Pilbeam SP: Mechanical ventilation: physiological and clinical applications, St Louis, 1986, Mosby.)

is based on the relationship between increased work of breathing and respiratory failure.

A complete assessment of ventilatory mechanics must include measures of both the mechanical demands or *load* placed on the respiratory system, and the *capacity* of the system to handle this load.[93]

Assessing ventilatory load

Measures useful in assessing the mechanical load imposed on the respiratory system include total impedance and its components (compliance and resistance), total mechanical work, and the pressure-time product.

Total impedance. The total impedance to inflation represents the sum of all forces opposing movement of gas into the lung. Under conditions of passive inflation, the pressure change needed to inflate a patient's lungs (PIP-PEEP) is a measure of the force needed to overcome total impedance.[93]

To compute total impedance while a patient is on a ventilator, you simply divide the corrected tidal volume by the change in airway pressure:

$$\text{Total impedance} = \frac{(V_T - \text{Compressed volume})}{(\text{PIP} - \text{PEEP})}$$

Normal total impedance values for an intubated adult are between 35 and 50 mL/cm H_2O. Since the units of measure are the same as those used for compliance, some authors refer to this measure as "dynamic" compliance. However, this label is misleading, since, unlike compliance, total impedance includes elastic, frictional, and tissue viscous resistance.

Effective compliance. In order to partition, or separate out the elastic and frictional components of total impedance, the RCP can institute an inflation hold.[94]

As shown in Figure 33-13, the inflation hold momentarily holds the delivered volume in the lungs under static conditions. If the time is sufficient to ensure equilibration of airway and alveolar pressures, a pressure plateau results. The difference between this

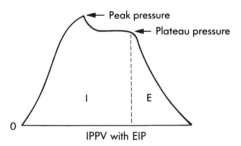

Fig. 33-13 Effect of inflation hold. The difference between peak pressure and plateau pressure is caused by airways resistance. The difference between plateau pressure and end-expiratory pressure is that amount of pressure needed to distend the system (tubing, lungs, chest wall), and the difference can be used to calculate system compliance. See text for further discussion. (From Martin L: Pulmonary physiology in clinical practice, St Louis, 1987, Mosby.)

plateau pressure (P_{plat}) and the baseline or PEEP pressure is the force needed to maintain the lungs and thorax at the delivered volume under static conditions.[95]

By dividing the corrected tidal volume by the plateau pressure, we derive a close estimate of total lung and chest wall compliance, called *effective compliance,* or C_{eff}:

$$\text{effective compliance } (C_{eff}) = \frac{(V_T - \text{Compressed volume})}{(P_{plat} - \text{PEEP})}$$

If auto-PEEP (aPEEP) is present, it must be accounted for, otherwise the computed C_{eff} will be erroneously high. To account for auto-PEEP, simply subtract both it *and* the externally applied PEEP from the plateau pressure:[96]

$$\text{effective compliance } (C_{eff}) = \frac{(V_T - \text{Compressed volume})}{(P_{plat} - \text{PEEP} - \text{aPEEP})}$$

Normal C_{eff} ranges between 60 and 100 mL/cm H_2O. Diseases of the lung parenchyma such as pneumonia, pulmonary edema, and any chronic diseases causing fibrosis are all associated with decreased effective compliance. Acute changes, such as atelectasis, pulmonary edema, ARDS, or lung compression due to a tension pneumothorax cause a rapid drop in C_{eff}.[97,98] When C_{eff} is less than 25 to 30 mL/cm H_2O, as may occur in severe ARDS, the amount of work needed to maintain adequate ventilation is inordinately high, and can quickly lead to muscle fatigue. C_{eff} values less than 25 to 30 mL/cm H_2O thus making weaning from ventilatory support difficult.

Measured on a regular basis, C_{eff} can help establish trends in pulmonary status, and guide the application of PEEP or CPAP therapy. The use of C_{eff} to guide selection of PEEP levels will be discussed in a subsequent section.

Airway resistance. An estimate of expiratory airway resistance can also be obtained using an inflation hold. Since the peak inspiratory pressure reflects total impedance, and P_{plat}-PEEP corresponds to its elastic component, then the difference between PIP and P_{plat} must be due to airway resistance (Raw).

If the inspiratory flow is constant and known with accuracy, then the airway resistance may be estimated according to the following formula:[93]

$$\text{Estimated Raw (cm } H_2O/L/\text{sec}) = \frac{\text{PIP} - P_{plat}}{\dot{V} \text{ (L/min)} \div 60}$$

Normal adult airway resistance ranges from about 0.5 to 2.5 cm H_2O/L/sec. In a normal adult intubated with an 8.0 mm ET tube in place, we would expect airway resistance to be 4 to 6 cm H_2O higher than this normal range, due to the additional resistance imposed by the tube.[99] An increase in Raw above 10 to 15 cm H_2O/L/sec in an intubated patient with otherwise normal lungs signals abnormal airway narrowing due to such factors as increased secretions, bronchospasm, pulmonary vascular congestion, or partial occlusion of the artificial airway.

Some third generation ventilators, such as the Bear 1000, Puritan-Bennett 7200a, and the Hamilton Veolar provide an automated routine to compute both C_{eff} and Raw. These automated computations are valid only if the inflation hold is long enough to allow complete pressure equilibration throughout the lung, and the device is set in the constant flow mode. Most clinicians suggest that an inflation hold of at least 1 to 2 seconds may be needed to ensure pressure equilibration throughout the lung. Even longer time intervals may be required when taking these measures on some COPD patients.

Whether using manual or automated methods, the RCP should simultaneously observe the patient's breathing pattern to be certain that a normal exhalation precedes the pressure measurements. Failure to do so will cause inaccurate measurements of pressure and cause errors. Plateau pressure readings are particularly susceptible to fluctuations caused by spontaneous breathing.

Curve analysis. Instead of single-point computation of C_{eff} and Raw, some clinicians suggest multipoint curve analysis.[100] This approach involves calculating and plotting total impedance and effective compliance points over a series of standardized tidal volumes, such as 7, 10, 13, and 16 mL/kg. As depicted in Figure 33-14, this results in two curves: the effective static compliance curve (ESCC), and the effective dynamic characteristics curve (EDCC).

Comparison of these curves over time provides a graphic portrayal of changing pulmonary mechanics.[101,102] As shown in Figure 33-15, page 942, conditions causing increased airway resistance cause a shift in the EDCC downward and to the right. On the other hand, conditions causing decreased lung or chest wall compliance shift both the EDCC and ESCC downward and to the right. If the condition of the patient acutely worsens without a change in either EDCC or ESCC, the clinician should suspect a problem not directly affecting the lung parenchyma or airways, such as a pulmonary embolism.

Work of breathing. A patient's work of breathing is directly measured as the area of the pleural pressure-volume curve (see Chapter 11). If pressure is measured in kg · m, and volume in liters, then the work of breathing is expressed in kg · m/L. Alternatively, the work of breathing can be expressed in joules per liter (j/L), with one kg · m equal to about 10 joules.

The total work of breathing normally has two components: work done on the lung and work done on the thorax. Additional work will be imposed on a patient who must breathe through an ET tube or ventilator circuit.

A patient's total work of breathing (lung+thorax +imposed) can be measured during ventilatory support only when all the work is being done by the ventilator (controlled breath with passive inflation).

To measure work during controlled ventilatory

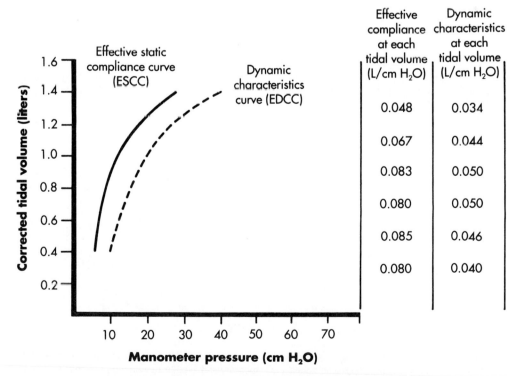

	Effective compliance at each tidal volume (L/cm H₂O)	Dynamic characteristics at each tidal volume (L/cm H₂O)
	0.048	0.034
	0.067	0.044
	0.083	0.050
	0.080	0.050
	0.085	0.046
	0.080	0.040

Fig. 33-14 Effective and dynamic compliance curves and values.

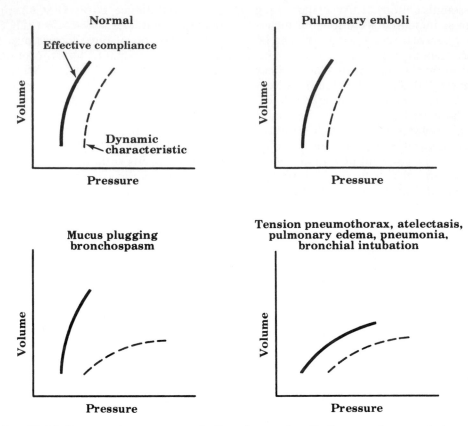

Fig. 33-15 Pressure-volume curves reflecting changes in effective compliance and dynamic characteristics (dynamic compliance) during mechanical ventilation. Under normal conditions the effective and dynamic characteristic curves will be similar. Since pulmonary emboli does not affect resistance or compliance, neither curve will change in this condition. With mucus plugging, airway resistance increases and the dynamic curve shifts to the right and flattens (more pressure is required) while the static compliance curve does not change. In conditions which reduce lung compliance, both curves will shift to the right and flatten. (From Pilbeam SP: Mechanical ventilation: physiological and clinical applications, St Louis, 1986, Mosby.)

support, one must simultaneously measure changes in airway pressure and delivered volume. Typically these measurements are made with a differential pressure pneumotachometer attached between the ventilator and patient at the proximal airway. Total work is then computed as the integral of change in pressure times change in volume:[93]

$$\text{total work} = \int_0^{ti} (\text{Paw} - \text{Patm})\text{Vdt}$$

Figure 33-16 show a pressure-volume loop with computation of the work of breathing in joules/L.

Because inspiratory time is an analog of delivered volume when constant flow is applied, one can estimate the inspiratory work of breathing during mechanical ventilation using the area beneath the airway pressure curve. Of course, this accurately reflects inspiratory work only for controlled breaths.

To compute the spontaneous work of breathing,

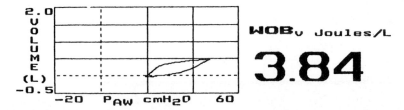

Fig. 33-16 Airway pressure-volume loop recorded on a patient with ARDS during controlled ventilation. Note the decrease in area representing nonelastic inspiratory and expiratory work and the shifting of the curve to right. Compliance is about 10 to 15 mL/cm H_2O.

changes in transpulmonary pressure must be measured. This requires measurement of pleural pressure, normally estimated by placement of an esophageal balloon. Details on the use of esophageal pressure (P_{es}) are provided later in our discussion of pressure, volume, and flow waveforms.

For normal individuals, the average total work of breathing ranges between 0.030 and 0.050 kg · m/L (0.3 and 0.5 j/L).[104] Patients with severe obstructive or restrictive lung disease may have work levels 2 to 3 times this normal value at rest, with marked increases in work at higher minute ventilations.

How much work a patient can tolerate before the ventilatory muscles fatigue is not entirely clear. Maintaining adequate spontaneous ventilation over a long term is probably not possible when work loads exceed 0.15 kg · m/L, or 1.5 j/L. This threshold level surely varies according to patient condition.[105,106] For this reason, and because bedside measurement of the work of breathing is currently a relatively complex and expensive procedure, other indirect measures of work, such as compliance and resistance estimates, are more commonly used.

Assessing ventilatory capacity

While compliance, resistance, and work of breathing measures tell us what load the ventilatory muscles are carrying, they do not indicate how well the respiratory system is responding to that load. To assess the respiratory system's capacity to respond to a load, we must measure its output (drive), and its strength and endurance.

Respiratory drive. There are two common measures used to assess respiratory drive: $P_{0.1}$ and V_T/t_i.[12] $P_{0.1}$ is the pressure recorded 100 msec after initiating an inspiratory effort against an occluded airway.[107,108] V_T/t_i is the spontaneous tidal volume by the inspiratory time, or mean inspiratory flow.[108,109] $P_{0.1}$ is the best studied of the two measures, and has been shown helpful in predicting weaning success.[110,111] $P_{0.1}$ can be measured using digitized signals generated directly from new generation ventilators.[112]

Respiratory muscle strength. The two most common methods used for bedside assessment of respiratory muscle strength are the forced vital capacity (VC) and the negative inspiratory force (NIF).

Vital capacity (VC). The VC maneuver can be performed at the bedside using a mechanical or electronic spirometer attached directly to the patient's airway. Since the VC maneuver is effort dependent, accurate measurements can be obtained only with conscious and cooperative patients. Given the inherent variability in bedside results, 2 to 3 measures should be taken, with the best as the final result.

The VC maneuver represents an integrated measure of coordinated inspiratory and expiratory muscle function as related to the compliance of the lungs and chest wall. Normal individuals are able to generate a VC of about 65 to 75 mL/kg. Values below 65 to 75 mL/kg indicate a generalized restrictive process, which may be due to neuromuscular weakness, acutely decreased lung volumes, or chronic parenchymal disease. A VC below 10 to 15 mL/kg indicates significant muscle weakness, which may impair spontaneous ventilatory capacity.

Negative inspiratory force (NIF). The negative inspiratory force, also known as the maximum inspiratory force (MIF) or maximum inspiratory pressure (P_{Imax}), is a more specific measure than the VC, providing information solely on the output of the inspiratory muscles against a maximum stimulus. The maximum stimulus is provided either by total occlusion of the airway, or by preventing inspiratory gas flow. Unlike the VC maneuver, the NIF can be performed on unconscious or uncooperative patients.

Measurement of NIF at the bedside is normally done with using an aneroid manometer equipped with a maximum value indicator (Figure 33-17). In order to assure maximum stimulation, one of two methods is used (Figure 33-18, page 944). In the first, the RCP completely occludes the airway for a full 20 seconds, observing and recording the maximum deflection of the manometer. Alternatively, the RCP uses a one-way valve that allows exhalation but not inspiration. With this device, the patient will "buck down" toward residual volume on each successive breath, at which point a maximum inspiratory effort is assured (Figure 33-18, Method II).

Both techniques can cause extreme anxiety in alert patients, and should be preceded by a careful and reassuring explanation. Moreover, if using the one-

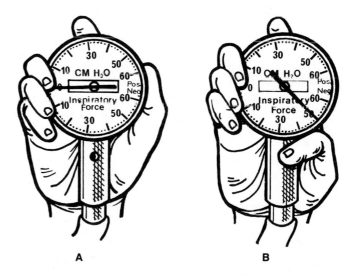

Fig. 33-17 An inspiratory force measurement. The gauge is attached to the patient's endotracheal tube, **A.** The patient is instructed to take in a deep breath while the clinician obstructs the airway by closing the open port on the gauge, **B.** The negative pressure detection, measured here as −50 cm H_2O, is the patient's inspiratory force or peak inspiratory pressure. (From Pilbeam SP: Mechanical ventilation: physiological and clinical applications, St Louis, 1986, Mosby.)

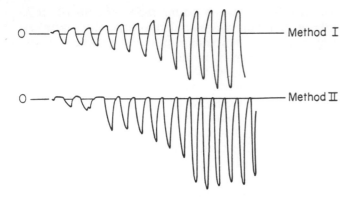

Fig. 33-18 Time course for NIF during the first 25 seconds of airway occlusion in a poorly cooperative intubated patient. Method I uses simple occlusion, while Method II uses one-valve in the expiratory pathway which prevents inspiration. Both methods require 15-25 seconds to reach maximum values. Method II (with the one-way valve) produces largest negative pressure. (From Marini JJ: Mechanical ventilation: taking the work out of breathing?, *Respir Care* 31(8): 695-702, 1986.)

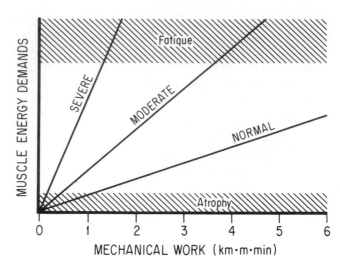

Fig. 33-19 Schematic relationship between ventilatory muscle loads (horizontal axis) and energy demands (vertical axis). As loads increase (either from impedance changes or ventilation requirements), energy demands increase, and when energy demands exceed muscle capabilities, fatigue develops. Disease states steepen the relationship between loads and energy (ie, the muscles become less efficient), and fatigue occurs at a lower load. If a muscle is totally unloaded with mechanical ventilatory support for an excessive period of time, atrophy develops. (From MacIntyre NR: *Respir Care* 33(2):121, 1988.)

way valve method, the RCP should ensure restoration of lung volume after the test by providing several large tidal volumes, either via the ventilator sigh mechanism or with a manual resuscitator.

As indicated in Table 33-8, normal NIF values vary by patient age and sex. Values less than these norms indicate either inspiratory neuromuscular weakness or an abnormal ventilatory drive. When the NIF drops below −20 to −30 cm H₂O, it is unlikely that the patient has sufficient muscle strength to support adequate spontaneous ventilation.

Respiratory muscle endurance and fatigue. Endurance is the capacity of a muscle to sustain a contractile force. Fatigue is the opposite of endurance. Fatigue is the inability of a muscle to generate and sustain a required contractile force.[113,114]

Respiratory muscles fatigue when the workload imposed on them exceeds their energy utilization capabilities. As shown in Figure 33-19, diseased states steepen the relationship between imposed loads and energy demands, causing fatigue to develop faster and at a lower load.[115,116]

Respiratory muscle fatigue may be either a cause or effect of respiratory failure. As cause, muscle fatigue

Table 33-8 Normal negative inspiratory force (cm H₂O) by age/sex

	Mean (± SD) PImax From Residual Volume	
Age Group	**Male**	**Female**
9–18	−96 ±35	−90 ±25
19–50	−127 ±28	−91 ±25
51–70	−112 ±20	−77 ±18
>70	−76 ±27	−66 ±18

From Rochester DF, Hyatte RE: Respiratory muscle failure, *Med Clin N Am*, 67:573–579, 1983.

itself can lead to a decreased minute ventilation, respiratory acidosis, and ultimately, respiratory and cardiac arrest. As an effect, respiratory muscle fatigue is simply a manifestation of other primary problems causing either increased impedance or increased ventilatory demand. Whether cause or effect, fatigued respiratory muscles may take anywhere from 24 to 48 hours to fully recover. The need for this recovery period should be considered by the RCP when selecting the type and length of ventilatory support needed by a given patient.

Common measures used to assess respiratory muscle endurance or fatigue include the maximum voluntary ventilation (MVV), ratio of minute volume to MVV (V̇E:MVV), the **pressure-time index,** and breathing pattern analysis.

Maximum voluntary ventilation (MVV). Whereas the VC assesses the patient's coordinated muscle function on a single breath, the MVV determines the ability of a patient to sustain an increased respiratory load over a period of time. As with the VC maneuver, the MVV procedure can be performed at the bedside using a hand-held spirometer attached to the patient's airway. Similar to its performance in the PFT laboratory, the patient is encouraged to breath as deep and as fast as possible over a predefined time interval, such as 15 or 30 seconds. The value is then extrapolated to a full minute.

Normal MVV values for adults range from 120 to 180 L/min. MVV values below 20 L/min indicate inadequate endurance and are associated with difficulty maintaining spontaneous ventilation without mechanical assistance. Unfortunately, most critically ill patients may not be able to perform this procedure.

Ratio of minute volume to MVV ($\dot{V}E$:MVV). A ratio of minute volume to MVV less than 1:2 reliably indicates that spontaneous ventilation can be sustained without machine support.[12] Conversely, if the MVV is less than twice the resting minute volume, the patient has inadequate muscle endurance and will have difficulty sustaining adequate spontaneous ventilation.

Pressure-time index. The pressure-time index (**PTI**) is a measure of load that correlates highly with oxygen consumption of the ventilatory muscles.[117]

To compute the PTI, one has to measure the pressure changes across the diaphragm during a tidal breath (transdiaphragmatic pressure or P_{di}) and the ratio of inspiratory time to total breath cycle duration, or *duty cycle* (t_i/t_{tot}):

$$PTI = (P_{di}/P_{max}) \times t_i/t_{tot}$$

In studies of normal subjects, high PTI values are strongly correlated with development of diaphragmatic fatigue, with a PTI exceeding 0.15 predicting inability to sustained targeted pressures for more than 45 min.[93]

Breathing pattern analysis. Breathing pattern analysis provides a quantitative way to analyze the interaction of abdomen and rib cage activity previously described under physical assessment. Breathing pattern analysis can be performed at the bedside using respiratory inductance plethysmography (RIP).[118-120]

RIP uses a series LC electrical circuit to measure relative displacement of the abdomen and rib cage. Two separate bands, each containing an electrical coil through which a small current is passed, are wrapped around the abdomen and rib cage (Figure 33-20). Expansion of the bands stretches the electrical coils and changes circuit inductance. Changes in circuit inductance cause a reciprocal change in current flow, proportional to the magnitude of stretch or expansion.[118]

The RIP device can display relative motion of the abdomen and rib cage simultaneously against a time axis, as previously depicted in Figure 33-1. Alternatively, abdominal and rib cage motion may be plotted against each other on an X-Y recorder or oscilloscope. Data from this X-Y plot, when combined with tidal volume information, is used to derive measures such as the percent abdominal paradox, and the average asynchrony index. Figure 33-21, page 946, shows the close relationship between these newer measures of respiratory muscle function and the deterioration in minute ventilation and pH observed after removal of a patient from a ventilator.[121-122]

Assessment of hemodynamics

Hemodynamic monitoring is used to obtain information on various pressure and flow parameters in both the systemic and pulmonary circulations.[123-125] This data can serve both diagnostic and therapeutic purposes. Diagnostically, hemodynamic data can help the clinician distinguish among various cardiovascular and pulmonary problems. Therapeutically, pressure and flow data can guide the selection and modification of treatment protocols.

As with previous methods of assessment, hemodynamic monitoring can be invasive or noninvasive. Simple noninvasive methods, such as the physical examination, vital signs, and the ECG have already been discussed in detail in prior chapters. Noninvasive cardiac output via thoracic electrical impedance, Doppler flow, and CO_2 rebreathing show promise but await confirmation of clinical usefulness.[126,127]

Our focus here will be on invasive hemodynamic monitoring techniques, in particular the use of systemic and pulmonary arterial catheterization to obtain measurements of blood pressures and flow.

Arterial pressure monitoring

Systemic arterial blood pressure is the most commonly measured hemodynamic parameter. As with ABGs, blood pressure can be measured either invasively by arterial cannulation, or noninvasively using traditional cuff occlusion, **oscillometric** measurements, or servo-controlled plethysmography.[126]

Each method has its advantages, but the invasive approach is most accurate. In addition, invasive monitoring allows for display of the arterial pressure waveform on a bedside station, usually in conjunction

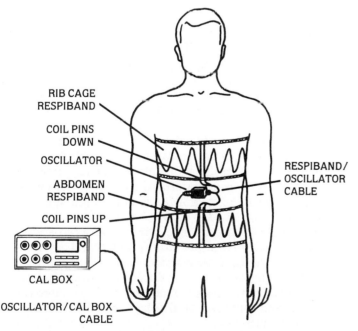

RIB CAGE RESPIBAND

COIL PINS DOWN

OSCILLATOR

ABDOMEN RESPIBAND

COIL PINS UP

RESPIBAND/ OSCILLATOR CABLE

CAL BOX

OSCILLATOR/CAL BOX CABLE

Fig. 33-20 Inductive plethysmograph using chest and abdominal band (Respitrace Corporation, Courtesy of Ambulatory Monitoring, Ardsley, NY).

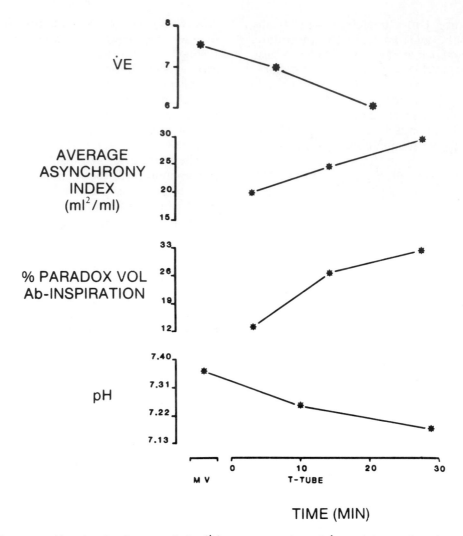

Fig. 33-21 Alterations in minute ventilation ($\dot{V}E$), average asynchrony index, percent paradox volume of the abdomen (*Ab*) during inspiration, and arterial blood pH in a patient who failed a T-tube trial of weaning from mechanical ventilation (MV). (From Dantzker DR, Tobin MJ: *Respir Care* 30(6):428, 1985.)

with the ECG. In combination, these two parameters provide the clinician with considerable information regarding the electrical and mechanical functions of the heart, as related to the status of the peripheral circulation.

Sites for systemic arterial cannulation are the radial, brachial, and femoral arteries. As with arterial puncture, collateral circulation through the ulnar artery makes the radial site first choice. Patency of this artery is always determined by performing the Allen test before catheter placement. Placement of a catheter is by percutaneous puncture or surgical cutdown. In addition to providing hemodynamic monitoring data, an arterial catheter, or "A-line" provides a direct source for obtaining ABG samples without the discomfort associated with **percutaneous** puncture.

Equipment. Figure 33-22 depicts the typical equipment setup for invasive monitoring of arterial blood pressure. The catheter is connected to a disposable continuous flush device (Intraflow) that maintains patency of the system by providing a small, but continuous flow of IV fluid through the system (2 to 4 mL/hr). Because arterial pressures are much higher than venous pressures, gravity infusion is insufficient to drive the IV fluid into the artery. For this reason, the IV bag containing the infusion fluid must be pressurized, usually with a hand bulb pressure pump.

Normally, stopcocks placed in line with the continuous flush device allow calibration of the systems against atmospheric pressure and arterial sampling. A strain gauge pressure transducer, connected to the flush device, provides an analog electrical signal to the amplifier/monitor, which displays the corresponding pressure waveform.

Waveform analysis. Figure 33-23 depicts a typical normal arterial pressure waveform for a single cardiac cycle, with time on the x-axis and pressure on the

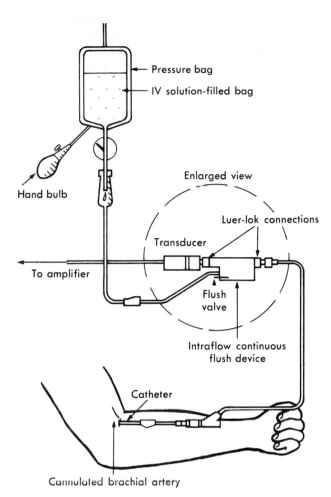

Fig. 33-22 Use of pressurized IV fluid bag and Intraflow flush device for optimal maintenance of arterial catheter patency. Stop-cocks may be placed on each side of the flush device for room air reference and blood sampling. (From Schroeder JS, Daily EK: Techniques in bedside hemodynamic monitoring, St Louis, 1976, Mosby.)

y-axis. For clarity, this waveform is wider than that normally observed on a pressure monitor, which generally operates at a slower "sweep" speed.

As with the cardiac cycle, the arterial pressure waveform is divided into two phases: systole and diastole. In terms of pressure events, systole begins with the opening of the **aortic** valve. Arterial pressure then rises to its peak systolic level, then begins to taper off as the stroke volume is fully ejected into the aorta. Once ventricular pressure drops sufficiently below that in the aorta, ventricular systole ends and the aortic valve closes, as indicated on the waveform by the dichrotic notch. Thereafter, arterial pressure gradually declines until the next systole. The potential energy stored as a result of the elastic expansion of the aorta and large arteries provides for continuous blood flow during diastole.

The pressure components of this normal arterial waveform include the systolic pressure, diastolic pressure, pulse pressure, and mean arterial pressure (Figure 33-23). The systolic pressure (SP) is the peak of the arterial pressure waveform, normally ranging between 90 and 140 mmHg (brachial). The diastolic pressure (DP), is the low point of the waveform, normally ranging between 60 and 90 mmHg. The pulse pressure represents the difference between systolic and diastolic pressures, averaging about 40 mm Hg in healthy adults. The mean arterial pressure (MAP) is the average pressure throughout the cardiac cycle, and averages between 70 and 105 mmHg in adults. MAP is calculated by integration of the arterial pressure waveform over time. Without fancy equipment, the MAP can be estimated by the following formula:

$$MAP = \frac{SP + (DP \times 2)}{3}$$

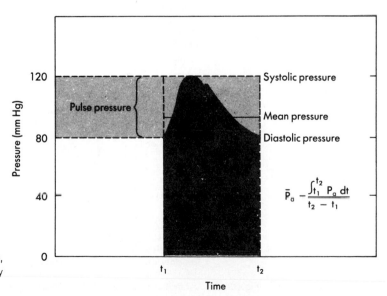

Fig. 33-23 Arterial pressure wave form showing anacrotic limb, systolic peak, dicrotic notch, and diastolic pressure. (From Berne RM, Levy MN: Cardiovascular physiology, ed 5, St Louis, 1986, Mosby.)

Normal values for arterial pressures obtained by arterial cannulation are summarized in the accompanying box.

Normal adult systemic arterial blood pressures	
Pressure	Normal Range
Systolic	100 - 140 mmHg
Diastolic	60 - 90 mmHg
Mean	70 - 105 mmHg

Most modern arterial pressure monitors provide continuous digital display of these pressures, also allowing output to be diverted to a strip-chart recorder for permanent record keeping. Figure 33-24 compares and contrasts strip-chart recordings of a normal arterial waveform *(A)* with those observed in patients with aortic insufficiency *(B)*, cardiogenic shock *(C)*, pulsus alternans due to CHF *(D)*, a bigeminal arrhythmia *(E)*, and pulsus paradoxus due to pericardial tamponade *(F)*.

Maintenance and troubleshooting. In many settings, RCPs are responsible for arterial pressure lines. This responsibility includes ensuring optimum on-

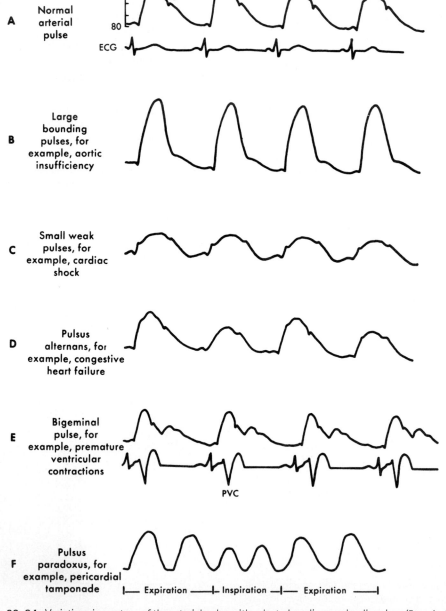

Fig. 33-24 Variations in contour of the arterial pulse with selected cardiovascular disorders. (From Andreoli KG et al: Comprehensive cardiac care, ed 6, St Louis, 1987, Mosby.)

going function of the system and troubleshooting problems. Table 33-9 provides common-sense guidelines to optimize arterial pressure monitoring. Table 33-10, page 950, outlines the cause, prevention and corrective action for several of the most common causes for inaccurate measurements.

Complications. Invasive arterial pressure monitoring carries significant risks. Hemorrhage is always a possibility with arterial cannulation. It can be avoided only by careful equipment setup and scrupulous monitoring. Infection is another major risk, as this may lead to systemic sepsis. Thrombi may form on the catheter and lead to embolization of peripheral arteries. In the worst case, tissue necrosis may develop distal to the insertion site, requiring amputation of the involved area. This latter complication is of particular concern when large artery sites are used with small infants. Care must also be taken on insertion to prevent nerve damage, which may lead to paralysis or chronic pain syndromes.

Pulmonary artery (PA) monitoring

In order to obtain a complete bedside picture of a patient's hemodynamic status, arterial measurements need to be supplemented with data obtained from the pulmonary artery.

Table 33-9 Guide for optimal arterial monitoring

Procedure	Reason
Label IV tubing of arterial line as "artery" or "arterial line."	Visual aid may help to avoid confusion with venous lines
Keep pressure bag inflated to pressure greater than patient's arterial pressure.	Slow deflation of bag will result in blood flow back into tubing
Maintain constant fluid flow with continuous flush device (2 to 4 mL/hr).	Constant fluid flow maintains patency and prevents clotting
Check all connections.	Loose connections can introduce air or allow blood loss
Immobilize extremity.	Extremity movement can result in needle or catheter displacement
Keep all connectors and puncture sites visible.	Possible bleeding may be observed
Frequently check pulse distal to puncture site.	Weakening or loss of pulse may indicate thrombosis
Check circulation, movement, and sensation of extremity distal to puncture site.	Any changes in circulation, movement, or sensation may indicate hematoma formation
Label date of catheter insertion on dressing.	Removal of catheter after 72 to 96 hr may reduce risk of infection

From Daily EK, Schroeder JS: *Techniques in bedside hemodynamic monitoring*, ed 4, St Louis, 1989, Mosby.

Equipment. Equipment needed to obtain data via pulmonary artery catheterization include a specialized, flow-directed balloon-tipped catheter (also called a Swan-Ganz catheter), a continuous flush pressure transducer system like that used for arterial monitoring, a pressure amplifier/monitor with continuous display capabilities, and a bedside cardiac output computer.

Pressures measured with a PA catheter provide information useful in distinguishing between right and left ventricular failure and other cardiopulmonary disorders. These pressure measurements also are helpful in guiding fluid management and drug therapy. In addition, the PA catheter provides a mechanism for direct measurement of cardiac output. Last, as previously discussed, the PA catheter provides a sampling route for mixed venous blood, and thus is a crucial tool in assessing tissue oxygenation.

A typical PA catheter is made of pliable, radiopaque polyvinyl chloride (Figure 33-25, page 951). Most models have four channels: (1) a distal channel, terminating at the tip of the catheter, which allows measurement of PA pressures and the withdrawal of mixed venous blood, (2) a balloon inflation channel, used to inflate or deflate a small balloon located about 1 cm from the catheter tip, thus allowing determination of pulmonary capillary "wedge" pressures, (3) a proximal channel located 30 cm from the catheter tip, which permits measurement of right **atrial** or central venous pressures and allows injection of solutions for cardiac output determination, and (4) an extra injection port to provide continuous infusion capabilities. Also running the length of the catheter is a wire connected to a thermistor bead, located approximately 4 cm from the catheter tip. Connection of this thermistor sensor system to a cardiac output computer allows bedside measurement of cardiac output using the thermal dilution technique.

Indications. Given the numerous risks and complications associated with its use, a PA catheter should be inserted only when the information it can provide is required for effective patient management. Conditions for which effective patient management depends on data obtainable only via a PA catheter are listed in the accompanying box.

Indications for pulmonary artery catheter insertion

- Shock states (cardiogenic, hypovolemic, septic, etc.)
- Myocardial infarction causing cardiovascular instability
- Pulmonary vascular disease
- Pulmonary edema (cardiogenic and noncardiogenic)
- Adult respiratory distress syndrome

Table 33-10 Inaccurate arterial pressure measurements

Problem	Cause	Prevention	Treatment
Damped pressure tracing	Catheter tip against vessel wall	Usually cannot be avoided	Pull back, rotate, or reposition catheter while observing pressure waveform
	Partial occlusion of catheter tip by clot	Use continuous drip under pressure Briefly "fast flush" after blood withdrawal (<2 to 4 mL) Adding 1 unit heparin/1 mL IV fluid may help	Aspirate cloth with syringe and flush with heparinized saline (<2 to 4 mL)
	Clot in stopcock or transducer	Carefully flush catheter after blood withdrawal and reestablish IV drip Use continuous flush device	Flush stopcock and transducer; if no improvement, change stopcock and transducer
Abnormally high or low readings	Change in transducer reference level	Maintain air-reference port of transducer at midchest and/or catheter tip level for serial pressure measurements	Recheck patient and transducer positions
Damped pressure without improvement after flushing	Air bubbles in transducer or connector tubing	Carefully flush transducer and tubing when setting up system and attaching to catheter	Check system; flush rapidly; disconnect transducer and flush out air bubbles
	Compliant tubing	Use stiff, short tubing	Shorten tubing or replace softer tubing with stiffer tubing
No pressure available	Transducer not open to catheter Settings on monitor amplifiers incorrect—still on *zero, cal,* or *off*	Follow routine, systematic steps for setting up system and turning stopcocks	Check system—stopcocks, monitor, and amplifier setup
	Incorrect scale selection	Select scale appropriate to expected range of physiologic signal	Select appropriate scale

From Daily EK, Schroeder JS: *Techniques in bedside hemodynamic monitoring,* ed 4, St Louis, 1989, Mosby.

Insertion. Assuming ECG and pressure monitoring is available, PA catheterization can be performed by a physician at the bedside. The distal port of the catheter is attached to a pressure transducer connected to a bedside display monitor. The basilic, brachial, femoral, subclavian, or internal jugular veins may be used for insertion, with the latter two being the most common.

After entry into the selected vein, the catheter is advanced until the tip is in the right atrium. At this time the balloon is inflated to the recommended volume (usually 1.5 cc), and the catheter is advanced further. As shown in Figure 33-26, the catheter pressure reading and waveform is continuously observed as the catheter proceeds from the right atrium (RA), through the tricuspid valve, into the right ventricle (RV), through the pulmonary semilunar valve, into the pulmonary artery (PA), and finally into a "wedge" position (PAWP). After insertion and stabilization, the catheter position in the pulmonary circulation is confirmed with a chest X-ray.

Immediately after the pulmonary capillary wedge pressure is obtained, the balloon is deflated, allowing blood to flow past the catheter and exposing the tip to pulmonary artery pressures for continuous monitoring. It is important to note that the wedge position should not be maintained for longer than 15 consecutive seconds to prevent pulmonary infarction.

Pressure measurements. Table 33-11 summarizes the pressures that can be measured with the four channel pulmonary artery catheter, including their normal ranges.

Table 33-11 Basic pressure measurements from pulmonary artery catheter

Measurement	Normal range
Central venous pressure	< 6 mmHg
Right atrial pressure	2–6 mmHg
Right ventricular pressure, systolic	20–30 mmHg
Right ventricular pressure, diastolic	2–6 mmHg
Pulmonary artery pressure, systolic	20–30 mmHg
Pulmonary artery pressure, diastolic	6–15 mmHg
Pulmonary artery pressure, mean	10–20 mmHg
Pulmonary artery wedge pressure, mean	4–12 mmHg

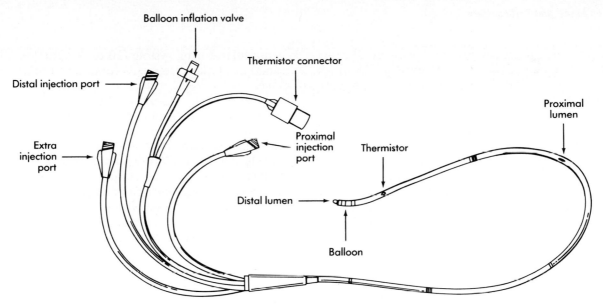

Fig. 33-25 The quadruple-channel pulmonary artery catheter. The most distal channel (distal injection port) is for pulmonary artery pressure measurement; blood can also be aspirated from this channel for mixed venous oxygen measurements. A second channel (balloon inflation valve) is used to inflate-deflate the distal balloon. A third channel (proximal injection port), which exits 30 cm from the catheter tip, is used for central venous (right atrial) pressure monitoring and fluid infusion. The fourth channel (extra injection port), which is not present on all catheters, can be used for continuous infusion of hyperalimentation fluids. The thermistor connector plugs into a bedside cardiac output computer. (From Martin L: Pulmonary physiology in clinical practice, St. Louis, 1987, Mosby.)

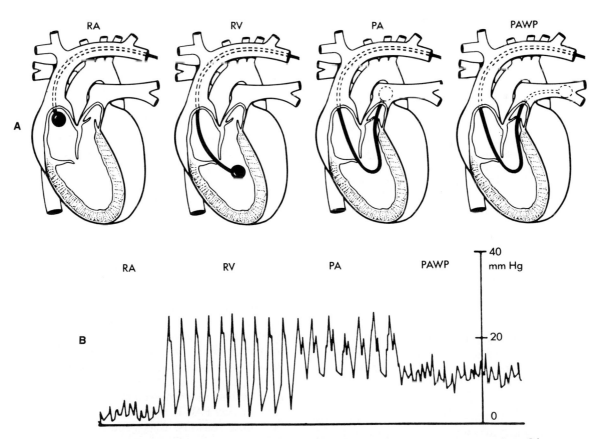

Fig. 33-26 A, Pulmonary artery catheter position in heart. **B,** As monitored by pressure tracings. *RA,* Pressure tracing from right atrium; *RV,* pressure tracing from right ventricle; *PA,* pressure tracing from pulmonary artery; *PAWP,* pulmonary artery wedge pressure tracing.) (From Martin L: Pulmonary physiology in clinical practice, St Louis, 1987, Mosby.)

RA pressures normally are the lowest in all heart chambers, ranging from 2 to 6 mmHg. Although difficult to see in real time, the normal RA pressure waveform includes three distinct waves: the a, c, and v waves. The a wave represents atrial contraction, the c wave ventricular contraction, and the v wave atrial filling against a closed tricuspid valve. Mean RA pressure is the same as central venous pressure (CVP). CVP is a measure of atrial preload. Atrial preload is determined by the balance between the capacity of the cardiovascular system, its circulating volume, and the amount venous return to the heart (refer to Chapter 10). Causes of abnormal RA/CVP pressures are summarized in the accompanying box.

The PA pressure waveform is similar to that seen in the systemic arterial circulation, but with pressures averaging one-sixth those observed in the aorta. PA systolic pressure normally equals that in the right ventricular during systole (20 to 30 mmHg), and is a function of the ejection volume and outflow resistance.

With diastole, closure of the pulmonic valve (also marked by a dichrotic notch) keeps PA diastolic pressures above those of right ventricular diastole. PA diastolic pressures normally range between 6 and 15 mmHg. The mean PA pressure, abbreviated as MPAP or $\overline{PAP}$, ranges between 10 and 20 mmHg. $\overline{PAP}$ is an indicator of right ventricular afterload.

PA pressures increase with increased right ventricular stroke volumes, increased pulmonary vascular resistance, or with elevated left atrial pressures (as occurs in mitral stenosis, or left ventricular failure). PA pressures decrease when blood volume decreases, or pulmonary vascular resistance decreases, as with vasodilation.

The pulmonary artery wedge pressure, abbreviated by various authors as PAWP, PCWP (pulmonary capillary wedge pressure), or PAo (pulmonary artery occluded pressure), normally ranges between 4 and 12 mmHg. When properly measured, the PAWP reflects the downstream pressure in the pulmonary circulation, or pulmonary venous pressure. Pulmonary venous pressure, in turn, reflects left atrial pressure. Under optimum conditions, left atrial pressure equals left ventricular end-diastolic pressure (**LVEDP**), or left ventricular preload. Thus the pulmonary artery wedge pressure provides a "window" on the events occurring in the left side of the heart.

There are, however, several situations in which the PAWP does not accurately reflect left ventricular preload. As summarized in the box on page 953, these may be categorized into those situations in which: (1) PAWP is less than LVEDP, (2) PAWP is greater than LVEDP, and (3) PAWP equals LVEDP, but the LVEDP does not correlate with the left ventricular end-diastolic volume.[128]

Of special importance to the RCP involved in making PAWP measurements is the effect positive pressure has on the accuracy of the data obtained. Whether positive pressure ventilation will affect PAWP accuracy depends on several factors, including the fluid status of the patient, the level of airway pressure, and the position of the catheter in the lungs. As long as the patient has a normal circulating blood volume, and the catheter tip is located in an area of the lung where pulmonary blood flow is uninterrupted by changes in alveolar pressure ("Zone 3"), and the measurement is made at end-exhalation, then the PAWP will provide a close approximation of left ventricular preload. Moreover, PEEP levels of 10 cm H_2O or less in **normovolemic** patients do not significantly affect PAWP, as measured in Zone 3 of the lung. For these reasons, it is generally unnecessary to remove the patient from positive pressure ventilation to measure the PAWP.[129,130]

Cardiac output determinations. The pulmonary ar-

Alterations in right atrial/CVP pressures

Increased right atrial/CVP pressures

1. Right ventricular failure (myocardial infarction, cardiomyopathy)
2. Pulmonary valvular stenosis
3. Tricuspid stenosis and regurgitation
4. Pulmonary hypertension
5. Pulmonary embolism
6. Volume overload
7. Compressions around the heart; constrictive pericarditis, cardiac tamponade
8. Increased large vessel tone throughout the body, resulting in venoconstriction
9. Arteriolar vasodilation that increases the blood supply to the venous system
10. Increased intrathoracic pressure (positive pressure breath or pneumothorax)
11. Placement of the transducer below the patient's right atrial level; raising the patient above the transducer
12. Infusion of solution (especially by pressure infusion pumps) into the central venous pressure line
13. Left heart failure

Decreased right atrial/CVP pressures

1. Vasodilation (by drug or increase in body temperature)
2. Inadequate circulating blood volume (hypovolemia) caused by dehydration; actual blood loss; and large amounts of gastrointestinal loss, wound drainage, perspiration, urine output (diuresis), insensible losses (high temperature, low humidity), and losses to the interstitial space (edema, "third spacing")
3. Spontaneous inspiration
4. Placement of the transducer above the patient's right atrial level
5. Air bubbles or leaks in the pressure line

Clinical conditions when pulmonary artery wedge pressure (PAWP) may not accurately reflect left ventricular preload

1. If PAWP is less than LVEDP:
   Aortic reguritation
   Reduced left ventricular compliance (see number 3)
2. PAWP is greater than LVEDP:
   When catheter tip is in zone 1 or 2; may occur from artificial ventilation, with or without PEEP, or from volume depletion
   Atrial **myxoma**
   Thoracic tumors pressing on pulmonary veins
   Mitral stenosis or regurgitation
   Increased left ventricular compliance (see number 3)
3. PAWP equals LVEDP, but LVEDP does not correlate with LVEDV:

Decreased left ventricular compliance	Increased left ventricular compliance
Increased right ventricular volume	Decreased right ventricular volume
Pericardial tamponade	Removal of pericardium
Some drugs, eg, isoproterenol	Some drugs, eg, nitroglycerin
High LVEDV	Low LVEDV
Tachycardia	Bradycardia
PEEP	Myocardial ischemia/infarction
Myocardial hypertrophy	

From Martin L: Pulmonary physiology in clinical practice, the essentials for patient care and evaluation, St Louis, 1987, Mosby.

tery catheter also can be used to measure cardiac output (CO). Although the Fick method (previously described) can be used, thermodilution measurement is more common. As shown in Figure 33-27, cardiac output is obtained by injecting either a dextrose or saline solution at 0° C (or room temperature) into the proximal port (RA lumen) of the pulmonary artery catheter. On injection, the solution loses heat as it moves from the proximal port to the thermistor bead near the tip of the catheter. How much heat is lost depends on the rate of blood flow, which is computed by a microprocessor.

Hemodynamic profiles. In combination with the pressure measurements previously described, knowledge of the patient's cardiac output allows the clinician to calculate a variety of important hemodynamic parameters. These include the cardiac index, stroke volume, left and right ventricular stroke work indices, and systemic and pulmonary vascular resistances. Formulas and normal values for these important hemodynamic parameters are summarized in Table 33-12, page 954.

Based on this derived information, it is possible to differentiate among a variety of common conditions encountered in critical care, as delineated in Table 33-13, page 954. As always, such quantitative analysis can serve to complement and refine—but never replace—traditional methods of patient assessment.

Pitfalls and complications. Pulmonary artery catheterization is among the most hazardous forms of monitoring used in critical care.[131] These hazards are due to both the many technical complications that can occur when inserting or using a pulmonary artery catheter, and the errors in judgment or management associated with the data it provides. The most common pitfalls and complications of pulmonary artery

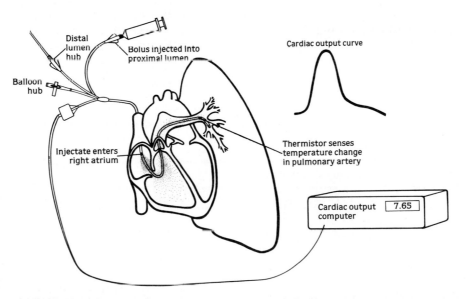

Fig. 33-27 Thermodilution cardiac output measurement. (From Wilkins RL, Sheldon RL, Kirder SJ: Clinical assessment in respiratory care, St Louis, 1985, Mosby.)

Table 33-12   Common values calculated for hemodynamic measurements

Value	Formula*	Normal range
Cardiac output	Heart rate × stroke volume	4.0–8.0 L/min
Cardiac index (CI)	$\dfrac{\dot{Q}_t \text{ (L/min)}}{\text{Body surface area (m}^2)}$	2.5–4.0 L/min/m²
Stroke volume (SV)	$\dfrac{\dot{Q}_t \text{ (mL/min)}}{\text{Heart rate (beats/min)}}$	60–130 mL/beat
Stroke index (SI)	$\dfrac{\text{Stroke volume (mL/beat)}}{\text{m}^2}$	30–50 mL/beat/m²
Left ventricular stroke work	SI × (MSAP − PAWP) × 0.0136	50–62 gm · meters/m²
Right ventricular stroke work	SI × (MPAP − CVP) × 0.0136	8–10 gm · meters/m²
Systemic vascular resistance (SVR)+	$\dfrac{\text{MSAP − CVP (mmHg)}}{\dot{Q}_t \text{ (L/min)}}$	15–20 mmHg/L/min
Pulmonary vascular resistance+	$\dfrac{\text{MPAP − PAWP (mmHg)}}{\dot{Q}_t \text{ (L/min)}}$	1.5–3.0 mmHg/L/min

*MSAP, mean systemic arterial pressure; CVP, central venous pressure; MPAP, mean pulmonary artery pressure; PAWP, pulmonary artery wedge pressure; m², square meters of body surface area; $\dot{Q}_t$ cardiac output; +To convert resistance units to dynes/sec/cm⁻⁵, multiply by a factor of 80.

catheterization are summarized in the accompanying box.

Most of these problems are the responsibility of the attending physician. However, RCPs involved in pulmonary artery monitoring procedures can take an active role in minimizing patient risk by recognizing common problems and taking appropriate corrective action, as specified by institutional protocols.

Pitfalls and complications in hemodynamic monitoring

Pitfalls (errors in judgement or management)

1. Inappropriate indications (when less invasive methods are just as good and when data will not change therapy)
2. Obtaining data incorrectly (inaccurate machine calibration and incorrect transducer placement)
3. Misusing data (improper interpretation of data obtained)
4. Not checking all relevant or related data before making therapeutic decisions (data such as chest X-ray, serum albumin, and urine output)
5. Not removing catheter when hemodynamic data are no longer used or are no longer useful in patient management

Complications from the technique

1. Ruptured or torn pulmonary or tricuspid valve
2. Pneumothorax (usually from subclavian insertion)
3. Pulmonary thrombosis and hemorrhage, including rupture of pulmonary artery
4. Right-sided endocardial damage (including hemorrhage, thrombus, and infection)
5. Knotting or kinking of catheter
6. Thrombosis in venous site of insertion
7. Cardiac arrhythmias, including heart block
8. Infection at site of insertion or at catheter tip
9. Balloon rupture
10. Loss of guide wire or portion of catheter within the venous system

From Martin L: Pulmonary physiology in clinical practice, the essentials for patient care and evaluation, St Louis, 1987, Mosby.

Table 33-13   Some hemodynamic changes in common clinical conditions

Condition	Infiltrate on Chest X-ray	SAP	SVR	Q_t	PAP	PAWP
ARDS	Both sides	↑↓	↑↓	↑↓	↑↓	N to ↓
Left-sided heart failure	1 or both sides	N to ↓	↑	↓	↑	↑
Septic shock	None, 1 or both sides	↓	↓	↑	N to ↓	N to ↓
Dehydration	None	↓	↑	N to ↓	N to ↓	↓
Pulmonary hypertension	None	N	N	N	↑	N

N = Normal; ↑ = increased; ↓ = decreased; ↑↓ = variable; SAP, systemic arterial pressure; SVR, systemic vascular resistance; Q_t, cardiac output; PAP, pulmonary artery pressure; PAWP, pulmonary artery wedge pressure.
From Martin L: Pulmonary physiology in clinical practice, the essentials for patient care and evaluation, St Louis, 1987, Mosby.

MANAGEMENT OF THE PATIENT-VENTILATOR SYSTEM

General patient assessment and physiologic data gathering provide the basis for managing the patient-ventilator system. Chapter 32 provided details on management aspects related to initiating and adjusting ventilatory support. Chapter 34 discusses management of the weaning process. Emphasis here is on routine checks of the patient-ventilator system; assessment of airway pressure, flow and volume waveforms; and troubleshooting common problems.

Routine patient-ventilator system checks

Patients receiving life-support measures must be assessed frequently to assure their safety and comfort and their continued need for and response to support.[132] To do so, we conduct patient-ventilator (P-V) system checks. A P-V system check is a documented evaluation of both the mechanical ventilator system and the patient's response to ventilatory support.[133] Properly conducted, these "vent checks" can prevent untoward incidents, warn of impending events, and assure that proper ventilator settings are maintained.[133] Specific objectives for performing regular P-V system checks are described in the box below.[133]

When to conduct P-V system checks

P-V system checks are performed on a regular schedule, according to institutional protocol. In addition, a P-V system check should be performed prior to obtaining an ABG sample or gathering hemodynamic or bedside PFT data. P-V system checks should also be conducted following any change in ventilator settings, and as soon as possible following an acute change in patient condition. Last, a P-V system check is required any time ventilator performance is questionable.[133]

Components of a P-V system check.

There are four key components to a P-V system check: (1) verification of patient data and ventilator settings, (2) documentation of physician's orders, (3) verification of proper ventilator operation, and (4) clinical observations describing the patient's response to ventilatory support.

Verification of patient data and ventilator settings. P-V system checks must include pertinent patient data and observations indicating the ventilator's settings when checked. The box below outlines the essential information needed in this component of a P-V system check.[132,133] Several third generation ventilators have the capacity to output much of this

---

Objectives for patient-ventilator system checks

- To evaluate and document the patient's response to ventilatory support;
- To assure and document the proper operation of the ventilator;
- To verify and document that the ventilator is functioning and is properly connected to the patient;
- To verify and document that all necessary alarms are activated;
- To verify and document that inspired gas is properly heated and humidified;
- To verify and document that FIO_2 is measured with every change or, at least, every 24 hours (continuous measurement of FIO_2 for infants at risk is warranted);
- To verify and document that ventilator settings comply with physician orders.

Patient data and ventilator settings

- Patient name
- Patient ID number
- Diagnosis
- ET or tracheostomy tube size and position
- Documentation of time of last patient circuit change
- Date of patient-ventilator system check
- Time of patient-ventilator system check
- Current ventilator settings (+indicates where applicable):
  - FDO_2 setting
  - Humidifier temperature setting (when applicable)
  - Mode of support
  - Set ventilator frequency
  - Peak, mean, and baseline airway pressures
  - Presence of auto-PEEP+
  - Set peak inspiratory pressure limit/pressure support level+
  - Set tidal volume+
  - Delivered tidal volume (measured or calculated)
  - Set sigh variables+
  - Set minute ventilation+
  - Set minimum mandatory minute ventilation+
  - Set inspiratory flow and waveform+
  - Set continuous flow (for IMV mode+)
  - Set I:E ratio, % inspiration, or insp/exp times
  - Set sensitivity threshold+
- Documentation of alarm settings/activation of alarms
- A description of any instance of equipment failure
- Signature or initials of person performing check, including credentials (depends on state law and/or hospital policy)

this data to a printer. Although such computerized output can save recording time, the RCP always must verify the accuracy of these data by checking each parameter manually.

Unfortunately, the presence of auto-PEEP cannot be identified by standard observation of airway pressures (this is why some call it *occult* PEEP). Given the high incidence of auto-PEEP among patients receiving ventilatory support, methods to detect its presence should be incorporated as a regular component of all P-V system checks.[134,135]

Two general approaches can be used to detect auto-PEEP. The first is by visual inspection of the expiratory flow and pressure tracings obtained during mechanical ventilation (Figure 33-28). As seen in the bottom Paw tracing, the airway pressure during exhalation falls slowly and barely returns to baseline before the next machine breath begins (arrows). Although these observations confirm that the conditions are prime for developing auto-PEEP, they cannot confirm its presence.

To confirm the presence of auto-PEEP, we must also look at the expiratory flow tracings. Careful inspection of this tracing indicates that expiratory flow does *not* return to zero before the next machine breath begins (arrows). This confirms that auto-PEEP is present.

Since auto-PEEP represents a difference in pressure between alveoli and airway under *dynamic* conditions (with flow still present), we should be able to detect its presence by creating a static state (no flow). Just as we were able to use an inflation hold to measure alveolar pressure during inspiration (to measure compliance), we should be able to use a deflation (or expiratory) hold to measure alveolar pressures at end-expiration.

Figure 33-29 shows how an end-expiratory hold

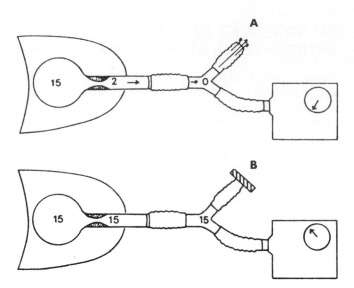

Fig. 33-29 Detection of auto-PEEP during mechanical ventilation. **(A)** auto-PEEP is present (15 cm H_2O at alveoli) but not detected at ventilator manometer because exhalation circuit is open to atmosphere. **(B)** Occlusion of exhalation port just before next machine breath permits pressure to equilibrate throughout the system and auto-PEEP to be detected and measured on pressure manometer. (From O'Quin R, Marini JJ: Pulmonary artery occlusion pressure: clinical physiology, measurement and interpretation, *Am Rev Respir Dis* 128:319-326, 1983.)

can be used to identify *and* measure auto-PEEP. In Figure 33-29, *A*, with the ventilator's expiratory valve open, end-expiratory pressure returns to 0 cm H_2O, despite the presence of an alveolar pressure of 15 cm H_2O (auto-PEEP). In Figure 33-29, *B*, we create an expiratory hold by occluding the expiratory valve of the ventilator, just after the airway pressure returns to baseline. As with an inflation hold, this allows equilibration between alveolar and airway pressure, and we now obtain a reading of 15 cm H_2O on the pressure manometer, equivalent to the auto-PEEP level.

Figure 33-30 shows the same technique being used, but as viewed via an airway pressure tracing. At the point indicated by the arrow, an expiratory hold is activated. Immediately following this maneuver, the airway pressure rises to a level equal to the auto-PEEP pressure.

Documentation of physician's orders. Orders for ventilatory support settings from the attending or consulting physician (or other authorized person) must be documented. Ideally, ventilatory support orders should include both of the following:[136]

- Desired range for $PaCO_2$, $PtcCO_2$, and/or desired range for PaO_2, SpO_2, $PtcO_2$, or SaO_2;
- Ventilator variables to initiate or manipulate in order to achieve desired blood gas results (e.g., mode, tidal volume, airway pressures, ventilatory frequency, or FDO_2).

Any discrepancies between actual ventilator settings and physician orders must be investigated and

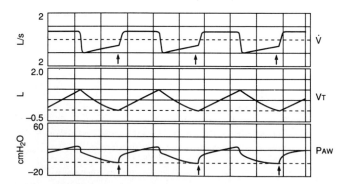

Fig. 33-28 Flow, volume and pressure tracings during time-triggered, volume-cycled ventilation in the presence of auto-PEEP. Expiratory gas flow does not return to zero *(arrow)* in the presence of auto-PEEP. In addition, airway pressure during exhalation falls slowly and barely returns to baseline before the next machine breath begins *(arrow)*. (From Kacmarek RM: Positive end-expiratory pressure. In Kacmarek RM, Hess D, Stoller JK, editors: *Monitoring in Respiratory Care*, St. Louis, 1993 Mosby.)

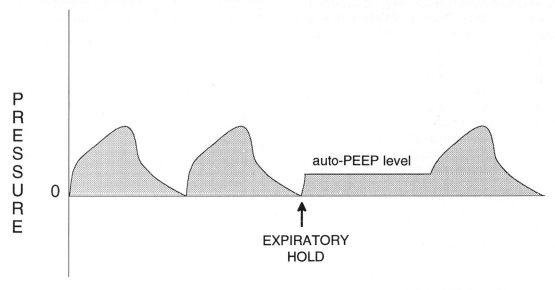

Fig. 33-30 Measurement of auto-PEEP using end-expiratory hold method. Upon initiation of an end-expiratory hold (arrow), airway pressure rises to a level equal to auto-PEEP.

resolved. Some clinicians suggest that parameters should always be returned to those indicated on the last valid order. However, careful investigation may reveal extenuating circumstances which justify the changes made. Nonetheless, if in the judgment of the RCP undocumented changes endanger the patient, parameters should be restored to their previously values while the matter is resolved.

Verification of proper ventilator operation. A P-V system check must include observations that verify proper ventilator operation. Such observations must include confirmation that the ventilator is turned on, the patient circuit is securely attached, and an airway disconnection alarm is functional and properly set.[133,137] In addition, the RCP should verify the FDO_2 with a calibrated analyzer and document inspired gas temperature. Last, prior to connecting a patient to a ventilator and whenever the breathing circuit is changed or disassembled, the RCP must conduct an operational verification procedure, or **OVP.**[133]

At a minimum, an OVP includes a test of circuit integrity and computation of compressed volume. This can be done by manually occluding the patient connection and observing airway pressure rise on a pressure gauge. Alternatively, many third generation ventilators provide various levels of self-testing designed to verify proper function. These self-tests are equivalent to an OVP, and should be conducted as per manufacturer specifications.

Clinical observations of the patient. The RCP must always place emphasis on the assessment of the patient, rather than simply checking the function of the ventilator and documenting the settings.[132] The accompanying box outlines the key patient observations that should be conducted in this component of a P-V system check.[133]

In assessing the frequency of breathing, the RCP should determine both the rate at which the ventilator is set to deliver breaths, as well as the rate of patient-triggered and spontaneous breaths. The machine rate must be verified by actually counting the number of breaths delivered per minute. Analog and digital read-outs, while generally accurate, should not be depended on to verify these values. If in the assist/control mode, the ventilator will generally have an indicator of patient initiated breaths. In the IMV mode, the spontaneous breaths may be indicated, but

---

Clinical observations of the patient during P-V system checks

- Breath sounds
- Spontaneous respiratory rate, volume, and pattern
- Chest and abdominal motion/synchrony
- Pallor, skin color
- Patient's level of consciousness or remarks
- ET tube stability/position
- ET tube cuff pressure
- Volume/character of secretions
- Condition of ancillary equipment (e.g., manual resuscitator)
- Results of bedside pulmonary function evaluations
- Response to ventilator disconnection during bedside procedures
- Documentation of oxygenation and ventilation status (e.g., ABG results, $PETCO_2$ measurements, and SpO_2, etc)
- Documentation of patient-ventilator synchrony during assisted or supported breaths

should be observed and verified by observing the patient's chest expansion, in conjunction with either the negative deflections occurring on the pressure manometer, or actual graphic display of spontaneous breaths (see subsequent section).

Hazards and complications.

Routine P-V system checks generally present minimal risk to patients. However, some critically ill patients may rapidly develop hypoventilation, hypoxemia, bradycardia, and/or hypotension when disconnected from a ventilator during a system check.[133] These potential complications can be minimized by preoxygenating and hyperventilating the patient prior to disconnection. In addition, some ventilators generate a high circuit flow when the patient is disconnected; this high flow may aerosolize contaminated tubing condensate, and increase the risk of nosocomial infection.[133] Obviously, the RCP can minimize this risk by adhering to appropriate CDC precautions during the P-V system checks (see Chapter 4).

Assessing flow, volume, and pressure waveforms

Until recently, analog display of pressure via an aneroid manometer was the only real-time monitoring data provided by ventilator systems. Recent technologic developments have dramatically enhanced the scope and quality of real-time data acquisition and display. Nowhere is this more evident than in the availability of continuous flow, volume, and pressure waveform displays.[138,139]

Typically, these displays are either provided as part of the ventilator's regular monitoring functions, or via

---

> ### Uses of flow, volume and pressure waveform data
>
> - To confirm mode functions
> - To detect auto-PEEP
> - To determine patient-ventilator synchrony
> - To assess and adjust trigger levels
> - To measure the work of breathing
> - To adjust tidal volume and minimize overdistention
> - To assess the effect of bronchodilator administration
> - To help detect equipment malfunctions

---

a separate external monitoring system. In the prior section, we saw how useful such output was in helping detect auto-PEEP. Here we look at other concrete examples of how this data can be used by the RCP, as summarized in the preceding box.[140]

The following flow, volume and pressure waveforms were provided courtesy of BICORE Monitoring Systems, Irvine, CA. Each graph represents a 10 second interval, with vertical 1.0 second time markers. Y-axis parameters and ranges are as labeled. Note that in addition to airway pressure, esophageal pressure (Pes) is being measured and displayed.

To recognize mode, determine patient–ventilator synchrony

Figure 33-31 shows the flow, volume, and pressure tracings typical for a patient receiving machine or patient-triggered (assist-control), volume-targeted ventilation. The upper flow tracing clearly shows a square wave flow pattern being delivered to the

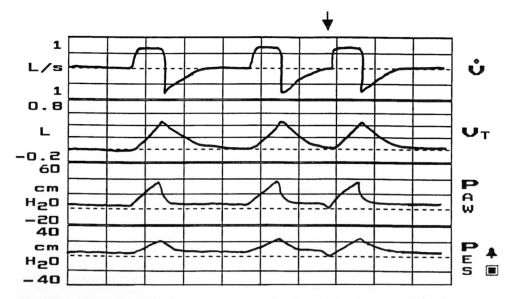

Fig. 33-31 Normal flow, volume, and pressure tracings for a patient receiving machine or patient-triggered (assist-control), volume-targeted ventilation. (Tracing courtesy of BICORE Monitoring Systems, Irvine, CA.)

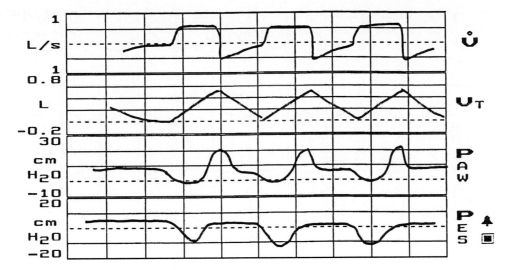

Fig. 33-32 Flow, volume, and pressure tracings for a patient receiving volume-targeted assist-control ventilation. Paw changes and Pes changes indicate flow-starvation. See text for details. (Tracing courtesy of BICORE Monitoring Systems, Irvine, CA.)

airway, typical of a constant flow generator. The linear increase in airway pressure (Paw) is consistent with provision of constant flow, as is the linear change in volume. The arrow marks the beginning of a patient-triggered breath. This event is confirmed by the simultaneous pressure drop in both Paw and esophageal pressure (Pes). After triggering, Paw and Pes changes resemble those during machine-triggered breaths, indicating good patient-ventilator synchrony.

Compare these tracing to those in Figure 33-32. Again, the patient is receiving volume-targeted assist-control ventilation. Flow and volume waveforms appear normal. However, rather than increasing linear-

ly, as expected, Paw changes are erratic, sinking throughout most of inspiration, and then rising rapidly at end-inspiration. A look at the Pes explains the erratic Paw tracing; the large inspiratory decrease in Pes indicates that the patient is being flow-starved, pulling with the respiratory muscles to get more flow than the ventilator is providing. The solution is to either increase the flow or switch to a pressure generation mode, where flow will vary with patient demand.

To recognize, adjust trigger levels

Figure 33-33 shows a patient spontaneously breathing on a demand valve CPAP system at a rate of about

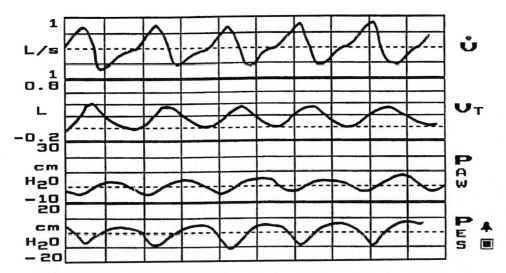

Fig. 33-33 Flow, volume, and pressure tracings for a patient breathing spontaneously breathing on a demand valve CPAP system at a rate of about 30/min. Wide swings in Paw and Pes indicates that excessive effort trigger the demand valve. See text for details. (Tracing courtesy of BICORE Monitoring Systems, Irvine, CA.)

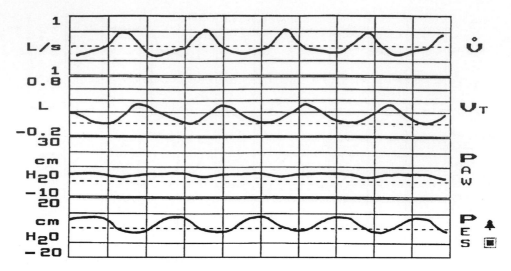

Fig. 33-34 Same patient as in Figure 33-33 after readjusting demand valve sensitivity. See text for details. (Tracing courtesy of BICORE Monitoring Systems, Irvine, CA.)

30/min. Peak inspiratory flows are about 0.6 L/sec (36 L/min), with spontaneous tidal volumes of 350 to 400 mL. Most evident are the wide swings in both Paw and Pes. Breath to breath, Paw varies about ± 4 cm H_2O, with correspondingly large drops in Pes. Tracing indicates that an excessive inspiratory effort is being required to trigger the demand valve.

Figure 33-34 shows the flow, volume, and pressure tracings from the same patient after readjusting demand valve sensitivity to −0.1 cm H_2O. Note especially the effect on pressures. Changes in Paw have been minimized, and Pes swings have become more reasonable.

To adjust tidal volume and minimize overdistention

The pressure-volume loop obtained during a volume-cycled breath provides valuable information regarding patient mechanics. Total compliance can easi-

ly be computed from the slope of the pressure-volume loop, with total machine work equaling its area. Also, inspection of the loop's shape can yield significant information.

In Figure 33-35, Paw is plotted on the x-axis with tidal volume on the y-axis. Delivered tidal volume is 1.2 L, resulting in a peak inspiratory pressure of about 30 cm H_2O. The slope of the pressure-volume loop indicated near normal total compliance. At end-inspiration, however, there is a rapid rise in Paw with little corresponding change in volume (marked by the arrow), giving the loop a bird-like "beaked" appearance. When an extended upper flat portion of the pressure-volume curve is observed, portions of the lung are being overdistended.

Figure 33-36 shows the flow, volume, and pressure tracings from the same patient after decreasing the tidal volume to 900 mL. Note that the pressure-volume loop "beak" is gone, indicating a reduction in unnecessary pressure.

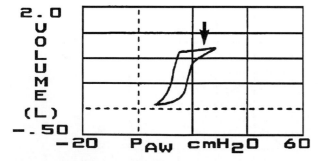

Fig. 33-35 Pressure-volume loop for a patient receiving volume-targeted breath of 1.2 L, with a peak inspiratory pressure of about 30 cm H_2O. Note extended upper flat portion or "beaked" appearance of the curve, indicating overdistention. See text for details. (Tracing courtesy of BICORE Monitoring Systems, Irvine, CA.)

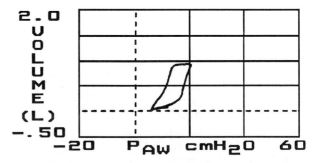

Fig. 33-36 Same patient as in Figure 33-33 after decreasing the tidal volume to 900 mL. Note that the pressure-volume loop "beak" is gone, indicating reduction in unnecessary pressure. See text for details. (Tracing courtesy of BICORE Monitoring Systems, Irvine, CA.)

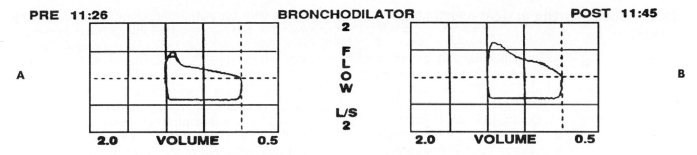

PRE 11:26   **BRONCHODILATOR**   **POST 11:45**

A   **B**

Fig. 33-37 Flow-volume loops taken on a patient before (33-37, *A*) and after (33-37, *B*) administration of albuterol via MDI through the ventilator. Note change in expiratory peak flow and shape of flow-volume curve. See text for details. Tracing courtesy of BICORE Monitoring Systems, Irvine, CA.

To assess the effect of bronchodilator administration

Switching channels and displaying flow versus volume (a flow-volume loop) provides additional information regarding patient mechanics, especially dynamic characteristics like airway resistance.

In Figure 33-37, *A*, volume is plotted on the x-axis with flow on the y-axis. The bottom half of the loop shows constant inspiratory flow delivery to a volume of 1.0 L. The upper half of the loop portrays expiratory events. Here, the peak expiratory flow rate (PEFR) is 0.82 L/sec, with a rapid and early decline.

After administration of albuterol via MDI through the ventilator (Figure 33-37, *B*), both the peak flow and loop shape have changed. PEFR is now 1.26 L/sec, and the early decline in expiratory flow has been eliminated. In combination, these observations indicate a good response to the bronchodilator treatment.

Detecting equipment malfunction

Figure 33-38 shows the flow, volume, and pressure tracings for a patient receiving pressure-limited IMV at a machine rate of 10/min. The most obvious abnormality is the discrepancy between the patient's inspired and expired volumes—the expired volume tracing does not return to its baseline. This indicates volume loss (a leak) during inspiration. Gas leakage during inspiration is confirmed by inspecting the inspiratory flow tracing. With pressure-limited ventilation in effect, we would expect a decelerating flow pattern. Instead, flow remains elevated throughout inspiration, as the system tries to maintain the targeted pressure despite the leak. In this case, inspection of the patient and assessment of the airway revealed a blown ET tube cuff.

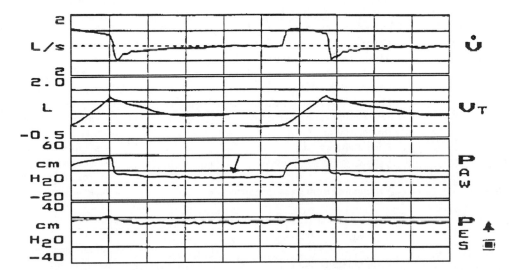

Fig. 33-38 Flow, volume, pressure tracings for a patient receiving pressure-limited IMV at a machine rate of 10/min. Note discrepancy between inspired and expired volume, indicating an inspiratory leak. See text for details. (Tracing courtesy of BICORE Monitoring Systems, Irvine, CA.)

Troubleshooting the patient–ventilator system

Troubleshooting is the identification and correction of mechanical and patient-related problems occurring during ventilatory support.[141,142] The ultimate goal of troubleshooting is to detect potential problems *before* they occur, or before they can cause any stress or harm to the patient. Thus troubleshooting is an ongoing process that requires foreknowledge of what problems can occur and how best to solve them.

Potential problems which may occur during ventilatory support include leaks or malfunctions in the ventilator system, and changes in the clinical condition of the patient. Table 33-14 lists clues to common problems with the patient-ventilator system, possible reasons for the observed problems, and corrective actions. The reader is encouraged to become familiar with these situations by replicating them in a simulated laboratory setting.

There are times when the ventilator may be performing as expected, but the patient exhibits progressive signs of acute respiratory distress. These signs include dyspnea, tachypnea, tachycardia, hypotension, diaphoresis, use of the accessory muscles, and a paradoxical breathing pattern.[143] In addition, the patient's erratic spontaneous breathing efforts cause severe dysynchrony with the ventilator, a phenomenon referred to as 'bucking' or 'fighting' the machine.[143]

Table 33-14 Trouble shooting the patient-ventilator system

Clue	Possible Reason	Corrective Action
VENTILATOR		
Decreased minute or tidal volume	Leak around endotracheal tube, from the system, or the chest tube	Check all connections for leaks
	Decreased patient-triggered respiratory rate	Check respiratory rate
	Decreased lung compliance	Evaluate patient
	Airway secretions	Clear airway of secretions
	Altered settings	Check patient-ventilator system
	Malfunctioning spirometer	Calibrate spirometer
Increased minute or tidal volume	Increased patient-triggered respiratory rate	Check respiratory rate
	Altered settings	Check patient-ventilator system
	Hypoxia	Evaluate patient; consider ABG findings
	Increased lung compliance	Good news
	Malfunctioning spirometer	Calibrate spirometer
Change in respiratory rate	Altered setting	Check patient-ventilator system
	Increased metabolic demand	Evaluate patient
	Hypoxia	Evaluate patient; consider ABG findings
Sudden increase in peak airway pressure	Coughing	Alleviate uncontrolled coughing
	Airway secretions or plugs	Clear airway secretions
	Ventilator tubing kinked or filled with water	Check for kinks and water
	Changes in patient position	Consider repositioning
	Endotracheal tube in right mainstem bronchus	Verify position
	Patient-ventilator asynchrony	Correct asynchrony
	Bronchospasm	Identify cause and treat
	Pneumothorax	Chest tubes
Gradual increase in peak airway pressure	Diffuse obstructive process	Evaluate for problems: atelectasis increased lung water bronchospasm
Sudden decrease in peak airway pressure	Volume loss from leaks in system	Check patient-ventilator system for leaks
	Clearing of secretions, relief of bronchospasm, increase in compliance	Good news
FIO_2 drift	O_2 analyzer error	Calibrate analyzer
	Blender piping failure	Correct failure
	O_2 source failure	Correct failure
	O_2 reservoir leak	Check ventilator reservoir

continued

Table 33-14 Trouble shooting the patient-ventilator system—*cont'd*

Clue	Possible Reason	Corrective Action
VENTILATOR		
I:E ratio too high or too low	Altered inspiratory flow	Check flow setting and correct
	Alteration in other settings that control I:E ratio	Check settings and correct
	Alteration in sensitivity setting	Check settings and correct
	Airway secretion (pressure ventilator)	Clear airway of secretions
	Subtle leaks	Measure minute ventilation
Inspired gas temp too high	Addition of cool water to humidifier	Wait
	Altered settings	Correct temperature control setting
	Thermostat failure	Replace heater
Changes in PEEP level	Change in tidal volume	Adjust PEEP level
	Change in compliance	Adjust PEEP level
	Altered settings	Check settings and correct
Changes in static pressure	Changes in lung compliance	Evaluate patient and correct if possible
Changes in ventilator settings	Changes in these setting resulting from deliberate or accidental adjustment of dials or knobs	Check to determine whether current settings are the intended ones

From Martz K, Joiner JW, Shepherd RM: Management of the patient-ventilator system, A team approach, ed 2, St Louis 1984, Mosby.

Both patient and ventilator-related problem can cause these acute incidents (Table 33-15).[143] Airway-related problems are discussed in detail in Chapter 22. Corrective actions for inadequate ventilatory support, improper trigger sensitivity, dynamic hyperinflation, improper inspiratory flow setting, and patient-ventilator asynchrony are described in Chapter 32.

Regardless of the problem source, the first priority is always to assure that the patient is adequately ventilated and oxygenated.[144] If there is any doubt as to cause or solution of the problem at hand, the patient should be disconnected from the ventilator device and ventilated with 100% oxygen via a manual resuscitator until the problem is resolved.[143] If the distress resolves, it indicates a ventilator problem. If the distress continues, it indicates a patient-based problem.[143] Additional steps to be taken in this situation are listed in the accompanying box.

If medical and mechanical problems have been excluded and the patient continues to show agitation and distress, the patient may have to be sedated or paralyzed.[143] Drug categories and agents used for these purposes in patients receiving ventilatory support are listed in the box on page 964.[145] Unfortunately, the use of neuromuscular blocking agents can mask a patient's problems, impair physical diagnosis, and lead to life-threatening incidents with accidental ventilator disconnection.[143] For these reasons, paralytic agents should be given only as a last resort.

Table 33-15 Causes of sudden respiratory distress in a patient receiving ventilatory support

Patient-Related Causes	Ventilator-Related Causes
Artificial airway problems	System leak
Pneumothorax	Circuit malfunction
Bronchospasm	Inadequate FIO_2
Secretions	Inadequate ventilatory support
Pulmonary edema	Improper trigger sensitivity
Dynamic hyperinflation	Improper inspiratory flow setting
Abnormal resp drive	Patient-ventilator asynchrony
Alteration in body posture	
Drug-induced problems	
Abdominal distension	
Anxiety	
Patient-ventilator asynchrony	

From Tobin MJ: What should the clinician do when a patient "fights the ventilator"? *Respir Care* 36(5):395–406, 1991.

Steps to be taken in managing sudden distress in a patient receiving ventilatory support

1. Remove the patient from the ventilator;
2. Initiate manual ventilation with 100% oxygen using a self-inflating bag;
3. Perform a rapid physical examination and assess monitored indices;
4. Check patency of the airway and try to pass a suction catheter;
5. If death appears imminent, consider and treat most likely causes, i.e., airway obstruction or pneumothorax;
6. Wait until the patient is stabilized to perform more detailed assessment and management.

From Tobin MJ: What should the clinician do when a patient "fights the ventilator"? *Respir Care* 36(5):395–406, 1991.

Pharmacologic agents used to produce sedation or paralysis

Tranquilizing agents

   Diazapam (Valium)
   Chlordiazepoxide HCL (Librium)
   Midazolam (Versed)

Sedative-hypnotics

   Sodium thiopental (Pentothal)
   Etomidate (Amidate)

Narcotic-analgesics

   Morphine
   Fentanyl (Sublimaze)

Neuromuscular blocking agents

   Competitive (nondepolarizing):
     d-tubocurarine
     Pancuronium Bromide (Pavulon)
   Depolarizing:
     Succinylcholine (Anectine)

CHAPTER SUMMARY

The management of critically ill patients is an ongoing process involving three major components: data collection, data analysis and interpretation, and decision-making. Pertinent information is obtained via traditional physical assessment procedures, in conjunction with standard diagnostic testing, including laboratory and radiologic evaluation. Supplementing these data in critical care are observations made via physiologic monitoring of the patient's cardiopulmonary status.

Physiologic monitoring serves two major purposes. First, it helps define the nature of the problem, its progression, and (ideally) its resolution. In addition, physiologic monitoring increases our ability to detect complications, hopefully before they become life-threatening.

RCPs must be able to gather and interpret physiologic data pertinent to assessing patient oxygenation, ventilation, and respiratory mechanics. Moreover, RCPs must possess general knowledge of other elements of patient assessment related to the care of patients in respiratory failure, especially hemodynamic monitoring.

General patient assessment and physiologic data gathering provide the basis for managing the patient-ventilator system. Key aspects involved in managing the patient-ventilator system include routine patient-ventilator checks, assessment of airway pressure, flow and volume waveforms; and system troubleshooting.

REFERENCES

1. Bone RC: Monitoring patients in acute respiratory failure, *Respir Care* 27:700-701, 1982.
2. Vaz Fragoso CA: Monitoring in adult critical care. In Kacmarek RM, Hess D, Stoller JK, editors: *Monitoring in Respiratory Care,* St Louis, 1993, Mosby.
3. Tobin MJ: Respiratory monitoring in the intensive care unit, *Am Rev Respir Dis* 138(6):1625-1642, 1988.
4. Zwillich CW, Pierson DJ, Creagh CE, et al: Complications of assisted ventilation. A prospective study of 354 consecutive episodes, *Am J Med* 57:161-169, 1974.
5. Abramson RS, Wald RS, Grenvik ANA, et al: Adverse occurrences in intensive care units, *JAMA* 244:1582-1588, 1980.
6. Spearman CB: The respiratory therapist's role in intensive care monitoring, *Respir Care* 30(7):602-609, 1985.
7. Kacmarek RM, Hess D, Stoller JK: Perspectives on monitoring in respiratory care. In Kacmarek RM, Hess D, Stoller JK, editors: *Monitoring in Respiratory Care,* St Louis, 1993, Mosby.
8. Low GGJ: Ongoing patient assessment. In Barnes TA, editor: *Respiratory care practice,* Chicago, 1988, Mosby.
9. MacIntyre NR: Respiratory monitoring without machinery, *Respir Care* 35(6):546-553, 1990.
10. Pardee NE, Winterbauer R, Allen J: Bedside evaluation of respiratory distress, *Chest* 85:203-206, 1984.
11. Gravelyn TR, Weg JR: Respiratory rate as an indicator of acute respiratory dysfunction, *JAMA* 244:1123-1125, 1980.
12. Tobin, MJ: Respiratory monitoring during mechanical ventilation, *Crit Care Clin* 6(3):679-709, 1990.
13. Wilkins RL, Sheldon RL, and Krider SJ: *Clinical assessment in respiratory care,* ed 2, St Louis, 1990, Mosby.
14. Tobin MJ: Respiratory muscles in disease, *Clin Chest Med* 9:263-286, 1988.
15. Tobin MJ, Chadha TS, Jenouri G, et al: Breathing patterns, *Chest* 84:202-205, 1983.
16. Sackner MA, Gonzalez H, Rodriguez M, et al: Assessment of asynchronous and paradoxic motion between rib cage and abdomen in normal subjects and in patients with chronic obstructive pulmonary disease, *Am Rev Respir Dis* 130:588-593, 1984.
17. Ashutosh K, Gilbert R, Auchincloss JH, Jr, et al: Asynchronous breathing movements in patients with chronic obstructive pulmonary disease, *Chest* 67:553-567, 1975.
18. Cohen CA, Zagelbaum G, Gross D, et al: Clinical manifestations of inspiratory muscle fatigue, *Am J Med* 73:308-316, 1982.
19. Gallagher CG, Hof VIM, Younes M: Effect of inspiratory muscle fatigue on breathing pattern, *J Appl Physiol* 59:1152-1158, 1985.
20. Grassino A, Bellemare F, Laporte D: Diaphragm fatigue and the strategy of breathing in COPD, *Chest* (suppl) 83:85-89, 1984.
21. Calhoon S, Crapo RO, Ostler DB, et al: Efficacy of chest radiographs in a respiratory intensive care unit, *Chest* 80:379, 1981.
22. Greenbaum DM, Marschall KE: The value of routine daily chest X-rays in intubated patients in the medical intensive care unit, *Crit Care Med* 10(1):29-30, 1981.
23. Henschke CI, Pasternack GS, et al: Bedside chest radiography: diagnostic efficacy, *Radiology* 149(1):23-26, 1983.
24. Bekemeyer WB, Crapo RO, et al: Efficacy of chest radiography in a respiratory intensive care unit. A prospective study, *Chest* 88(5):691-696, 1985.
25. Wiener MD, Garay SM, et al: Imaging of the intensive care unit patient, *Clin Chest Med* 12(1):169-198, 1991.
26. Tilkian SM, Conover MB, Tilkian AG: *Clinical implications of laboratory tests,* St Louis, 1983, Mosby.
27. Pagana KD, Pagana TJ: *Mosby's diagnostic and laboratory test reference,* St Louis, 1992, Mosby.
28. Bassili HR, Deitel M: Effect of nutritional support on weaning patients off mechanical ventilators, *JPEN* 5:161, 1981.
29. Barrocas A, Tretola R, Alonso A: Nutrition and the critically ill patient, *Respir Care* 28:50-59, 1983.
30. Grossman GD: Nutritional assessment of critically ill patients, *Respir Care* 30:463-468, 1985.
31. Peters JA, Burke KI: Nutritional assessment of the patient with respiratory disease. In Wilkins RL, Sheldon RL, Krider SJ, editors: *Clinical assessment in respiratory care,* ed 2, St Louis, 1990, Mosby.
32. Bone RC, Gravenstein N, Kirby RR: Monitoring respiratory and hemodynamic function in the patient with respiratory failure. In Kirby RR, Banner MJ, Downs JB, editors: *Clini-*

cal Application of Ventilatory Support, New York, Churchill Livingston. 1990.

33. Hess D: Noninvasive monitoring in respiratory care—present, past and future: An overview, *Respir Care* 35(6):482-496, 1990.

34. Teplick R: Oxygen transport from lung to tissue. In Kacmarek RM, Hess D, Stoller JK, editors: *Monitoring in Respiratory Care,* St Louis, 1993 Mosby.

35. Dantzker DR, Gutierrez G: The assessment of tissue oxygenation, *Respir Care* 30:456-461, 1985.

36. Carlon, GC, Kahn, RC, Ray C, Howland, WS: Evaluation of an "in vivo" PaO_2 and $PaCO_2$ monitor in the management of respiratory failure, *Crit Care Med* 8(7):410-413, 1980.

37. Goeckenjan, G: Continuous measurement of arterial PO_2: significance and indications in intensive care, *Biotel Patient Montitg* 6:51, 1979.

38. Tobin MJ: *Essentials of Critical Care Medicine,* New York, 1989, Churchill Livingstone.

39. Opitz N, Lubbers DW: Theory and development of fluorescence based optical sensors: Oxygen optodes, *Int Anes Clin* 25:177-197, 1987.

40. Barker SJ, Tremper KK: Intra-arterial oxygen tension monitoring, *Int Anes Clin* 25:199-208, 1987.

41. Green GE, Hassell KT, Mahutte CK: Comparison of arterial blood gas with continuous intra-arterial and transcutaneous PO_2 sensor in adult critically ill patients, *Crit Care Med* 15:491-494, 1987.

42. Shapiro BA, Cane BD, Chomka CM, et al: Preliminary evaluation of an intra-arterial blood gas system in dogs and humans, *Crit Care Med* 17:455-460, 1989.

43. Shapiro BA, Mahutte CK, Cane RD, Gilmour IJ: Clinical performance of a blood gas monitor: a prospective, multicenter trial, *Crit Care Med* 21(4):487-494, 1993.

44. Martin RJ: Transcutaneous monitoring: instrumentation and clinical applications, *Respir Care* 35(6):577-583, 1990.

45. Koff PB, Hess D: Transcutaneous oxygen and carbon dioxide measurements. In Kacmarek RM, Hess D, Stoller JK, editors: *Monitoring in Respiratory Care,* St Louis, 1993, Mosby.

46. Tremper, KK, and Shemaker, W: Transcutaneous oxygen monitoring of critically ill adults, with and without low flow shock, *Crit Care Med* 9:709, 1981.

47. Thys D, Cohen E, Girard D: The pulse oximeter, a noninvasive monitor of oxygenation during thoracic surgery, *Thorac Cardiovasc Surg* 34(6):380-383, 1986.

48. Welch JP, DeCesare R, Hess D: Pulse oximetry: instrumentation and clinical applications, *Respir Care* 35(6):584-596, 1990.

49. McCarthy K, Decker MJ, et al: Pulse oximetry. In Kacmarek RM, Hess D, Stoller JK, editors: *Monitoring in Respiratory Care,* St Louis, 1993, Mosby.

50. American Association for Respiratory Care. Clinical practice guideline. Pulse oximetry, *Respir Care* 36(12):1406-1409, 1991.

51. Hess D, Maxwell C, Dganit S: Determination of intrapulmonary shunt: comparison of an estimated shunt equation and a modified equation with the classic equation, *Respir Care* 32:268-273, 1987.

52. Shapiro BA, Cane R, Harrison R, et al: Changes in intrapulmonary shunting with administration of 100% oxygen, *Chest* 77:138, 1980.

53. Nelson LD: Assessment of oxygenation: oxygenation indices, *Respir Care* 38(6):631-640, 1993.

54. Covelli HD, Nessan VJ, Turtle WK: Oxygen derived variables in acute respiratory failure, *Crit Care Med* 11:646-649, 1983.

55. Gilbert R, Keighley JF: The arterial-alveolar oxygen tension ratio, an index of gas exchange applicable to varying inspired oxygen concentrations, *Am Rev Respir Dis* 109:142-145, 1974.

56. Gilbert R, Auchincloss JH Jr, Kuppinger M, et al: Stability of the arterial/alveolar oxygen partial pressure ratio: Effects of low ventilation/perfusion regions, *Crit Care Med* 7:267-272, 1979.

57. Horovitz JH, et al: Pulmonary response to major injury, *Arch Surg* 108:349-355, 1974.

58. Goldfarb M, Ciurej T, McAslan T, et al: Tracking respiratory therapy in the trauma patient, *Am J Surg* 129:255-258, 1975.

59. Sganga G, Siegel JH, Coleman B, et al: The physiologic meaning of the respiratory index in various types of critical illness, *Clrc Shock* 17:179-193, 1985.

60. Cane RD, Shapiro BA, Templin R, et al: Unreliability of oxygen tension-based indices in reflecting intrapulmonary shunting in critically ill patients, *Crit Care Med* 16:1243-1245, 1988.

61. Snyder JV: Assessment of systemic oxygen transport. In Snyder JV, Pinsky MR, editors: *Oxygen Transport in the Critically Ill,* Chicago, 1987, Mosby.

62. Mithoefer, JC: Assessment of tissue oxygenation, in Simmons, DH, editor: *Current pulmonology,* vol. 4, New York, 1982, John Wiley & Sons.

63. Fahey PJ, Harris K, Vanderwarf C: Clinical experience with continuous monitoring of mixed venous oxygen saturation in respiratory failure, *Chest* 86(5):748-752, 1984.

64. Paulus, DA: Invasive monitoring of gas exchange: continuous measurement of mixed venous oxygen saturation, *Respir Care* 32:535-541, 1987.

65. Kuff JV, Vaughn S, Yang SC, et al: Continuous monitoring of mixed venous oxygen saturation in patients with acute myocardial infarction, *Chest* 95:607-611, 1989.

66. Rasanen J, Downs JB, Hodges MR: Continuous monitoring of gas exchange and oxygen use with dual oximetry, *J Clin Anesth* 1(1):3-8, 1988.

67. Rasanen J, Downs JB, Malec DJ, et al: Real-time continuous estimation of gas exchange by dual oximetry, *Intensive Care Med* 14(2):118-122, 1988.

68. Rasanen J, Downs JB, Malec DJ, et al: Estimation of oxygen utilization by dual oximetry, *Ann Surg* 206(5):621-623, 1987.

69. Robin ED: Dysoxia: abnormal tissue oxygen utilization, *Arch Int Med* 137:905, 1977.

70. Danck SJ, Lynch JP, Dantzker DR: The dependence of oxygen uptake on oxygen delivery in the adult respiratory distress syndrome, *Am Rev Respir Dis* 122:387, 1980.

71. Mohsenifar Z, et al: Relationship between O_2 delivery and O_2 consumption in the adult respiratory distress syndrome, *Chest* 83:267, 1983.

72. Pierson DJ: Normal and abnormal oxygenation: physiology and clinical syndromes, *Respir Care* 38(6):587-599, 1993.

73. Phang PT, Russell JA: When does VO_2 depend on DO_2? *Respir Care* 38(6):618-626, 1993.

74. Weil MH, Afifi AA: Experimental and clinical studies on lactate and pyruvate as indicators of the severity of acute circulatory failure (shock), *Circulation* 41:989, 1970.

75. Benotti P, Blackburn GL: Protein and caloric or macronutrient metabolic management of the critically ill patient, *Crit Care Med* 7:520, 1979.

76. Bassili HR, Deitel M: Nutritional support in long term intensive care with special reference to ventilator patients: a review, *Can Anaesth Soc J* 28:17, 1981.

77. Neff TA: Monitoring alveolar ventilation and respiratory gas exchange, *Respir Care* 30(6):413-421, 1985.

78. Ledingham IM, MacDonald AM, Douglas HS: Monitoring of ventilation, in Shoemaker WC, Thompson WL, Holbrook PR, editors: *Textbook of critical care,* Philadelphia, 1984, WB Saunders.

79. Tobin MJ: Assessment of pulmonary function in critically-ill patients, in Shoemaker WC, Ayres SM, Grenvik A, editors: et al: *The Society of Critical Care Medicine Textbook of Critical Care Medicine,* ed 2, Philadelphia, WB Saunders, 1989.

80. Perez W, Tobin MJ: Separation of factors responsible for change in breathing pattern induced by instrumentation, *J Appl Physiol* 59:1515-1520, 1985.

81. Hess D: Capnometry and capnography: Technical aspects, physiologic aspects, and clinical applications, *Respir Care* 35(6):557-573, 1990.

82. Hess D: Capnography: technical aspects and clinical applica-

tions. In Kacmarek RM, Hess D, Stoller JK, editors: *Monitoring in Respiratory Care,* St Louis, Mosby, 1993.

83. Harris K: Noninvasive monitoring of gas exchange, *Respir Care* 32:544-552, 1987.
84. Carlon GC, Ray C, Mee SM, et al: Capnography in mechanically ventilated patients, *Crit Care Med* 16:550-556, 1988.
85. Moorthy SS, Losasso AM, Wilcox J: End-tidal PCO_2 greater than $PaCO_2$, *Crit Care Med* 12:534-535, 1984.
86. Hoffman IRA, Krieger BP, Kramer MR, et al: End-tidal carbon dioxide in critically ill patients during changes in mechanical ventilation, *Am Rev Respir Dis* 140:1265-1268, 1989.
87. Hess D, Schlottag A, et al: An evaluation of the usefulness of end-tidal PCO_2 to aid weaning from mechanical ventilation following cardiac surgery, *Respir Care* 36(8):837-842, 1991.
88. Pilbeam SP: Mechanical ventilation: physiological and clinical applications, ed 2, St Louis, 1992, Mosby.
89. Selecky PA, Wasserman K, et al: A graphic approach to assessing interrelationships among minute ventilation, arterial carbon dioxide tension, and ratio of physiologic deadspace to tidal volume in patients on respirators, *Am Rev Respir Dis* 117:181, 1978.
90. Bone RC: Monitoring ventilatory mechanics in acute respiratory failure, *Respir Care* 28:597-607, 1983.
91. Fairley HB: Monitoring respiratory mechanics, *Respir Care* 30:406-410, 1985.
92. Chatburn RL: Dynamic respiratory mechanics, *Respir Care* 31:703-711, 1986.
93. Marini JJ: Lung mechanics determinations at the bedside: Instrumentation and clinical application, *Respir Care* 35(7):669-693, 1990.
94. Hubmayr RD, Gay PC, Tayyab M: Respiratory system mechanics in ventilated patients: techniques and indications, *Mayo Clin Proc* 62(5):358-368, 1987.
95. Rossi A, Gottfried SB, Zocchi L, et al: Measurement of static compliance of the total respiratory system in patients with acute respiratory failure during mechanical ventilation, *Am Rev Respir Dis* 131:672-677, 1985.
96. Kacmarek RM, Hess D: Airway pressure, flow and volume waveforms, and lung mechanics during mechanical ventilation, in Kacmarek RM, Hess D, Stoller JK, editors: *Monitoring in Respiratory Care,* St Louis, 1993, Mosby.
97. Mancebo J, Calaf NN, Benito S: Pulmonary compliance measurement in acute respiratory failure, *Crit Care Med* 13:589-594, 1985.
98. Milic EJ, Ploysongsang Y: Respiratory mechanics in the adult respiratory distress syndrome, *Crit Care Clin* 2:573, 1986.
99. Demers RR, Sullivan MJ, Paliotta J: Airflow resistances of endotracheal tubes, *JAMA* 237:1362, 1977.
100. Bone RC: Compliance and dynamic characteristics curves in acute respiratory failure, *Crit Care Med* 4(4):173-9, 1976.
101. Bone RC: Diagnosis of causes for acute respiratory distress by pressure-volume curves, *Chest* 70(6):740-746, 1976.
102. Hylkema BS, Barkmeyer-Degenhart P, Grevick RG, et al: Lung mechanical profiles in acute respiratory failure: diagnostic and prognostic value of compliance at different tidal volumes, *Crit Care Med* 13:637-640, 1985.
103. Marini JJ, Rodriguez RM, Lamb V: Bedside estimation of the inspiratory work of breathing during mechanical ventilation, *Chest* 89(1):56-63, 1986.
104. Peters RM: Work of breathing and abnormal mechanics, *Surg Clin N Am* 54:955-966, 1974.
105. Proctor HJ, Woolson R: Prediction of respiratory muscle fatigue by measurement of the work of breathing, *Surg Gynecol Obstet* 136:367-370, 1973.
106. Sharp JT, Henry JP, Sweany SK, et al: The total work of breathing in normal and obese men, *J Clin Invest* 43:728-739, 1964.
107. Whitelaw WA, Derenne JP, Milic-Emili J: Occlusion pressure as a measure of respiratory center output in conscious man, *Respir Physiol* 23(2):181-199, 1975.

108. Milic-Emili J: Recent advances in clinical assessment of control of breathing, *Lung* 160:1-17, 1982.
109. Tobin MJ, Mador MJ. Guenther SM, et al: Variability of resting respiratory drive and timing in healthy subjects, *J Appl Physiol* 65:309-317, 1988.
110. Herrera M, Blasco J, et al: Mouth occlusion pressure ($P_{0.1}$) in acute respiratory failure, *Intensive Care Med* 11(3):134-139, 1985.
111. Sassoon CS, Te TT, et al: Airway occlusion pressure. An important indicator for successful weaning in patients with chronic obstructive pulmonary disease, *Am Rev Respir Dis* 135(1):107-113, 1987.
112. Brenner M, Mukai DS, et al: A new method for measurement of airway occlusion pressure, *Chest* 98(2):421-427, 1990.
113. Sharp J: Respiratory muscles: a review of old and newer concepts, *Lung* 157:185, 1980.
114. Roussos C, Macklem PT: Inspiratory muscle fatigue, in *Handbook of physiology,* Section 3, Respiration, 1986, American Physiologic Society.
115. Macklem P: The clinical relevance of respiratory muscle research, *Am Rev Respir Dis* 134:812-815, 1986.
116. Rochester DF, Hyatt RE: Respiratory muscle failure, *Med Clin N Am* 67:573-579, 1983.
117. Field S, Sanci S, Grassino A: Respiratory muscle oxygen consumption estimated by the diaphragm pressure-time index, *J Appl Physiol* 57:44-51, 1984.
118. Krieger BP: Ventilatory pattern monitoring: Instrumentation and applications, *Respir Care* 35(7):697-706, 1990.
119. Tobin M, Jenouri G, Lind B, et al: Validation of respiratory inductive plethysmography in patients with pulmonary disease, *Chest* 83:615-620, 1983.
120. Warren RH, Alderson SH: The accuracy of inductance plethysmography in measuring breathing patterns of sedated piglets receiving controlled mechanical ventilation, *Respir Care* 33(10):846-851, 1988.
121. Gallagher CG, Hof VIM, Younes M: Effect of inspiratory muscle fatigue on breathing pattern, *J Appl Physiol* 59:1152-1158, 1985.
122. Grassino A, Bellemare F, Laporte D: Diaphragm fatigue and the strategy of breathing in COPD, *Chest* (suppl.) 83:85-89, 1984.
123. Osgood CF, Watson MH, et al: Hemodynamic monitoring in respiratory care, *Respir Care* 29:25-34, 1984.
124. Matthay RA, Weidman HP, Matthay MA: Cardiovascular function in the intensive care unit: invasive and noninvasive monitoring, *Respir Care* 30:432-449, 1985.
125. Connors AF: Hemodynamic monitoring. In Kacmarek RM, Hess D, Stoller JK, editors: *Monitoring in Respiratory Care,* St Louis, 1993, Mosby.
126. Durbin CG: Noninvasive hemodynamic monitoring, *Respir Care* 35(7):709-716, 1990.
127. Meeker DP, Wiedemann HP: Cardiovascular function, in Kacmarek RM, Hess D, Stoller JK, editors: *Monitoring in Respiratory Care,* St Louis, 1993, Mosby.
128. Martin L: *Pulmonary physiology in clinical practice, the essentials for patient care and evaluation,* St Louis, 1987, Mosby.
129. Collee, GG, Lynch, KE, Hill, RD, Zapol, WM: Bedside measurement of pulmonary capillary pressure in patients with acute respiratory failure, *Anesthesiol* 66:614-620, 1987.
130. Marini JJ: Obtaining meaningful data from the Swan-Ganz catheter, *Respir Care* 30:572-581, 1987.
131. Puri VK, Carlson RW, Bander JJ, Weil MH: Complications of vascular catheterization in the critically ill: a prospective study, *Crit Care Med* 8:495, 1980.
132. Campbell RS: Managing the patient-ventilator system: system checks and circuit changes, *Respir Care* 39(3):227-236, 1994.
133. American Association for Respiratory Care: Clinical practice guideline. Patient-ventilator system checks, *Respir Care* 37(8):882-886, 1992.
134. Benson MS, Pierson DJ: Auto-PEEP during mechanical ventilation of adults, *Respir Care* 33(7):557-565, 1988.

135. Wright J, Gong H Jr: "Auto-PEEP": incidence, magnitude, and contributing factors, *Heart Lung* 19(4):352-357, 1990.

136. Pierson DJ: What constitutes an order for mechanical ventilation, and who should give the order? *Respir Care* 37(9):1124-1130, 1992.

137. US Department of Health and Human Services: Accidental breathing circuit disconnections in the critical care setting, Rockville, MD, 1990, IIIIS publication No. FDA 90-4233.

138. Kacmarek RM, Hess D: Airway pressure, flow and volume waveforms, and lung mechanics during mechanical ventilation. In Kacmarek RM, Hess D, Stoller JK, editors: *Monitoring in Respiratory Care,* St Louis, 1993, Mosby.

139. Tobin MJ: Monitoring of pressure, flow, and volume during mechanical ventilation, *Respir Care* 37(9):1081-1096, 1992.

140. MacIntyre N, Branson R: *Ventilator patient management with pulmonary mechanics monitoring: a casebook,* Irvine, CA, 1993, BICORE Monitoring Systems.

141. Martz K, Joiner JW, Shepherd RM: *Management of the patient-ventilator system, A team approach,* ed 2, St Louis, 1984, Mosby.

142. Grossbach I: Troubleshooting ventilator and patient-related problems, *Crit Care Nurse* 6(5):64-79, 1986.

143. Tobin MJ: What should the clinician do when a patient "fights the ventilator"? *Respir Care* 36(5):395-406, 1991.

144. Hudson LD: Diagnosis and management of acute respiratory distress in patients on mechanical ventilators. In Moser KM, Spragg RG, editors: *Respiratory emergencies,* ed 2, St Louis, 1982, Mosby.

145. Miyagawa CI: Sedation of the mechanically ventilated patient in the intensive care unit, *Respir Care* 32:792-805, 1987.

34

Discontinuing Ventilatory Support

■

Craig L. Scanlan

Ventilatory support can sustain life, but cannot cure disease. Thus, ventilatory support is usually a temporary measure that allows clinicians to "buy time" and treat the underlying problems leading to respiratory failure. For this reason, the end goal for most patients receiving ventilatory support is successful removal or discontinuation.

Removing most patients from ventilatory support is a relatively quick and easy process.[1-3] For some patients, including those with severe lung disease, neuromuscular disorders, or multisystem failure, withdrawing ventilatory support is more difficult.[1] These patients require a slower, more deliberate reduction of ventilatory support.[2,3] The process of slowly reducing ventilatory support is commonly referred to as *weaning*.

Last, there are a small number of patients who become "ventilator-dependent." For these patients, weaning is extremely difficult, and sometimes impossible. This last group poses significant clinical, economic and ethical problems.[1]

Ideally, we should be able to objectively determine who can be successfully removed from ventilatory support, and then simply proceed with the best weaning method. However, because weaning is as much art as science, this ideal scenario is uncommon.

Two key factors hinder the 'science' of weaning. First, our ability to accurately predict who can or cannot be successfully weaned is limited, especially among the chronically ill. In addition, although several weaning techniques are available, none has yet emerged as superior to all others.[1,4]

For these reasons, weaning must be tailored to each individual patient. From this perspective, the key questions underlying the weaning process are WHEN? and HOW? Success cannot be expected unless or until the common problems leading to the patient's ventilator dependency are first resolved (the *when*).[1-4] Once these problems are resolved, an organized plan or protocol should be developed and followed, with variations based on each patient's individual response (the *how*).[1,3,5-7]

SCOPE AND NATURE OF THE PROBLEM

Reported success rates in withdrawing patients from ventilatory support are extremely variable. Several studies of general medical and surgical patients, including the elderly, indicate that better than 9 out of 10 are easily removed from ventilatory support.[8-11] On the other hand, weaning success among patients with chronic lung disease, or those receiving long-term mechanical ventilation (> 1 to 2 weeks), is less common. Between 20% and 40% of these patients are difficult to remove from ventilatory support, with many becoming ventilator-dependent.[12-15]

Data from these studies indicates that patients being considered for removal from ventilatory support fall into three primary categories: (1) those for whom removal is quick and routine, (2) those requiring a slower, more deliberate reduction of support (weaning), and (3) ventilator-dependent or "unweanable" patients who require special strategies if discontinuation is to succeed.

To understand which patients fall into what categories, the clinician must first understand the causes of ventilator dependence.

CAUSE OF VENTILATOR DEPENDENCE

The primary reason why patients cannot be removed from ventilatory support is an imbalance between ventilatory demand and ventilatory capacity (Figure

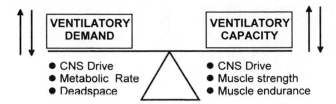

Fig. 34-1 The relationship between ventilatory demand and ventilatory capacity. Normally the two are in balance. In patient who are ventilator-dependent, demand chronically exceeds capacity. See text for details.

Table 34-1   Factors affecting ventilatory drive

CO₂ Production	Deadspace	CNS Drive
Fever	Lung disease	Neurogenic
Shivering	Hypovolemia	Psychogenic
Pain/agitation	Vascular occlusion	Metabolic
Trauma	External apparatus	Acidosis
Sepsis		Sepsis
Overfeeding		Hypoxemia
		Hypotension

Adapted from Marini JJ: The physiologic determinants of ventilator dependence, *Respir Care* 31(4):271–282, 1986.

34-1).[16] Other contributing factors are listed in the accompanying box.

A patient's ventilatory demand is primarily determined by three factors: (1) metabolic rate (CO_2 production), (2) CNS drive, and (3) ventilatory deadspace. Table 34-1, page 968, summarizes how various clinical conditions affect patients' ventilatory demands.[16]

A patient's ventilatory capacity is determined by two key components: CNS drive and muscle performance (Figure 34-1).[16] In terms of neurologic stimulation, most patients undergoing withdrawal of ventilatory support have a normal or increased drive to breathe. On the other hand, patients with certain neuromuscular disorders, and those receiving sedatives, narcotic-analgesics or neuromuscular blocking agents, may have a reduced CNS drive.[16-19] Other factors that can decrease ventilatory drive include neuromuscular fatigue, malnutrition, starvation, metabolic alkalosis, **hypothyroidism,** and sleep deprivation.[16]

Two aspects of muscle performance affect ventilatory capacity: strength and endurance. Overall muscle strength is mainly influenced by age, sex, and muscle bulk. Clinically, respiratory muscle strength is impaired by disuse, malnutrition, starvation, and electrolyte imbalances—especially calcium, magnesium, potassium, and phosphate.[16,20]

A muscle's endurance is best described as its ability to sustain work load over time. Endurance is a function of the muscle's energy supply versus its demand. Energy supply, in turn, is affected by nutritional status, perfusion, and cellular utilization.

Energy demands on a muscle are dictated by the amount of work performed. Respiratory muscle work load is determined by the interaction between lung-thorax mechanical properties (frictional and elastic resistance) and the needed minute ventilation. Additional factors impacting on respiratory work include the added impedance of the breathing apparatus (airway and ventilator circuit), inappropriate ventilator settings, and the presence of **auto-PEEP.**[4,21,22]

In terms of respiratory muscle endurance, normal individuals can sustain about 40% of their maximum voluntary ventilation (MVV) for extended periods of time. For some critically ill patients, however, spontaneously maintaining even a normal minute ventilation can cause muscle energy demands to exceed supply. The result is muscle fatigue and an inability to withdraw ventilatory support.

THE WEANING PROCESS

The process of withdrawing a patient from ventilatory support is best viewed as consisting of several key phases, each with defined endpoints. Three key stages include the preweaning phase, the weaning phase, and the extubation phase.[23] During the preweaning phase, the decision is made whether or not to begin withdrawing ventilatory support. During the weaning phase, withdrawal methods are chosen and applied until the patient is able to maintain adequate spontaneous ventilation. During the extubation phase, the artificial airway is removed and the patient is restored to normal full physiologic function.

Preweaning phase

During the preweaning phase, clinicians must decide whether or not to begin withdrawing ventilatory support.[23] Typically, this decision is based on assessment of the patient's physiologic and psychologic readiness. A quick preliminary patient screening can help identify patients not ready to be weaned.

With the advent of newer ventilator modes, it has become increasingly difficult to define the exact time at which weaning begins.[4,7] As shown in Figure 34-2, *A* and *B*, page 970, traditional weaning approaches involved switching the patient from full ventilatory support (usually volume-cycled assist/control) to no

---

Major factors contributing to ventilator dependence

- Ventilatory demand in excess of capacity
- Arterial hypoxemia
- Cardiovascular instability
- Malnutrition
- Psychologic dependence
- Equipment shortcomings

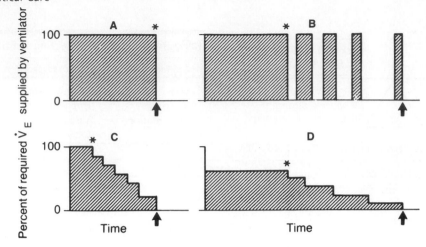

Fig. 34-2 Traditional weaning approaches involved removing the patient from full ventilatory support either abruptly (**A**) or using progressively longer T-tube trials (**B**). Using partial support modes such as SIMV or pressure support, ventilatory support is progressively decreased, from either initial full support (**C**), or initial partial support (**D**). *Asterisks* indicate the points at which weaning is begun; *arrows* indicate successful withdrawal of ventilatory support. (From Pierson OJ: Weaning from mechanical ventilation in acute respiratory failure: concepts, indications, and techiques, *Respir Care* 28:646-660, 1983.)

support (T-tube trials). Although this method is still used, most patients today receive only partial ventilatory support (IMV, pressure support, etc.) (Figure 34-2, *C* and *D*). During partial support, the traditional distinction between being on or off the ventilator no longer applies. In fact, with these modes, the withdrawal process often begins as soon as the patient starts receiving support.

Nonetheless, the decision as to when to begin withdrawing ventilatory support is critical. Premature efforts to remove a patient from a ventilator or decrease the support level typically results in excessive fatigue and leads to weaning failure. On the other hand, waiting too long to begin the withdrawal process can result in greater morbidity (pulmonary and airway injuries, infection, etc.) and psychologic stress, not to mention increased cost.[23,24]

Screening patients for weaning

Before going ahead with complex assessments of physiologic and psychologic readiness, clinicians should conduct a simple patient screening. The purpose of this screening is to identify patients who are clearly not ready to be weaned. To conduct the screening review, the clinician need only answer three simple questions:[25]

1. Is the patient getting better?
2. Is the initial reason for providing ventilatory support being resolved?
3. Is the patient clinically stable?

If the answer to any one or more of these questions is negative, the likelihood of successful weaning is poor. In these cases, ventilatory support should be continued and the patient reevaluated as treatment of the underlying problems progresses. Positive responses to all three preliminary questions support further

consideration of whether or not to begin weaning.

A quick review of six simple physical signs can help answer these questions.[10] These signs include: (1) a pulse rate over 120 or under 70/min, (2) a respiratory rate of over 30/min, (3) the presence of palpable scalene muscle use during inspiration, (4) the presence of palpable abdominal tensing during expiration, (5) the presence of an irregular breathing pattern, and (6) the inability of the patient to alter his/her ventilatory pattern on command. Patients exhibiting none of these signs are clinically stable and have a 90% chance of recovery. Patients exhibiting 1 or 2 of these signs usually require further ventilatory support. When three or more of the signs are present at the same time, the patient is unstable and has a poor prognosis.

After the preliminary screening, the clinician should conduct a more comprehensive assessment. To determine a patient's physiologic readiness to wean, one must conduct a thorough review of all CNS, metabolic, cardiovascular, pulmonary, and renal factors contributing to ventilator dependence. To determine psychologic readiness, the feelings and emotions of the patient should be assessed.[23]

To assist the clinician in conducting this preweaning assessment, a form like that shown in Figure 34-3, can be used.[26] Based on this method, whenever a potential obstacle to weaning is identified, efforts must first be made to correct the problem before the withdrawal process begins.

Physiologic readiness

After conducting the preliminary screening, the clinician should: (1) confirm that the major factors precipitating respiratory failure are being reversed, and (2) perform a more in-depth review of systems. The intent here is to identify and correct any clinical

PREWEANING ASSESSMENT

GENERAL QUESTIONS

Is the patient:	YES	NO
Not impeded by the ET tube?		
Not compromised by bronchospasm?		
Receiving adequate secretion clearance?		
Without dyspnea?		
Optimally positioned?		
Without respiratory muscle fatigue?		
Hemodynamically stable?		
Adequately hydrated?		
Without fever or infection?		
Adequately nourished?		
Without constipation, diarrhea or ileus?		
Improving in general body strength/endurance?		
Calm, relaxed and motivated to wean?		
Getting adequate sleep?		
Free of pain?		

DRUGS

Have drugs been discontinued that:	YES	NO
Decrease respiratory drive?		
Increase muscle weakness?		
Increase anxiety?		

LABORATORY VALUES

K^+		Albumin
Cl^-		T3-T4
$PO4^{--}$		Hct/Hb
Ca^{++}		theophylline
Mg^{++}		pH

PROBLEMS/ACTION PLAN

1.
2.
3.
4.

Fig. 34-3 Example of a preweaning assessment form used to assist in determining patients' readiness to wean. (Adapted from Norton C, Nureuter A: Weaning the long-term ventilator-dependent patient: common problems and management, *Crit Care Nurs* 9(1):42–52, 1989.)

conditions that can hinder weaning (see box on page 972).

Reversal of precipitating factors. Ventilator support is typically started due to an episode of acute respiratory failure. Most clinicians would consider it unwise to begin withdrawing support until the factors precipitating the original illness are being resolved.[4] Unfortunately, objective clinical indices have never been proposed to help to define this point.

CNS assessment. Adequate CNS function is needed in order to assure a stable ventilatory drive and provide secretion clearance and airway protection. Ideally, the patient should be awake and alert, free of seizures, and able to follow instructions.

At a minimum, obtunded patients should possess a gag reflex and good cough response.[23] Any drugs

---

Common clinical conditions that can hinder weaning

Anemia
Atelectasis
Abdominal distention
Acid-base imbalance
Bronchospasm
Drugs-sedatives or analgesics
GI/bowel problems
Cardiovascular collapse (shock, heart failure)
CNS depression
Electrolyte imbalance
Equipment malfunction
Fluid overload
Hypoxemia
Improper weaning procedure
Increased work of breathing
Infection/sepsis
Malnutrition
Malpositioning
Metabolic derangements
Respiratory muscle atrophy
Respiratory muscle weakness/fatigue
Pain
Psychologic impairment
Renal failure
Secretions (excessive)
Sleep disturbances
Starvation

Basic criteria for confirming cardiovascular stability[23]

- Heart rate is less than 120/min
- Systolic blood pressure 80-180 mm Hg
- No major arrhythmias present
- Hemoglobin 12-15 mg/dL
- Hematocrit 40-50%
- No angina present

---

with depressant effects should be discontinued before the withdrawal process begins, and normal acid-base balance should be confirmed. Further, the patient should be rested and not fatigued and sleep deprived as is commonly seen in the intensive care unit.

Cardiovascular assessment. Adequate cardiovascular function is needed in order to provide sufficient tissue perfusion and cellular gas exchange. Although more sophisticated approaches are available for assessing cardiovascular function, basic information should not be overlooked. The accompanying box provides basic criteria for confirming cardiovascular stability.[23]

Based on medical history and/or bedside assessment of hemodynamic performance, clinicians should also identify patients with poor left ventricular reserve who are being considered for withdrawal from ventilatory support. Among these patients, an abrupt transition to spontaneous breathing can actually worsen cardiovascular function.[27-29] This is due to the increases left ventricular afterload that occurs with restoration of normal venous return.

Metabolic and acid-base assessment. The metabolic assessment should focus on the adequacy and appropriateness of patient nutrition. Appropriate nutrition maintains respiratory muscle mass and contractile force, which enhances the likelihood of successful weaning.[30,31]

Feeding formulas should be adjusted according to the nutrient requirements and efficiency of gas exchange in the individual patient.[32] Most patients should receive a daily caloric intake between 1.5-2.0 times their resting energy expenditure (**REE**).[23] In addition, protein intake should be between 1-1.5 gm/kg/day.

Too high a carbohydrate load can increase the respiratory quotient, raise CO_2 production and precipitate acute hypercapnic respiratory failure.[33] Parenteral nutrition solutions containing amino acid-chloride formulas (arginine/lysine) can cause metabolic acidosis and can also increase ventilatory demand.

In terms of acid-base status, the patient should ideally have normal metabolic balance. Metabolic imbalances can impair weaning in one of two ways. As just indicated, metabolic acidosis tends to increase ventilatory demand and thus muscle load. On the other hand, metabolic alkalosis tends to decrease ventilatory drive.

Renal assessment. Adequate renal function is required to maintain proper acid-base equilibrium, electrolyte concentrations, and fluid balance. Disruptions in acid-base balance can affect either ventilatory drive or load, electrolyte imbalances can impair muscle function, and fluid overload can disrupt pulmonary gas exchange.

Ideally, the patient being considered for withdrawal of ventilatory support should have an adequate renal output (equal to intake and exceeding 1000 mL/day). There should be no inappropriate weight gain or edema present. Key electrolyte concentrations should be within normal limits (Mg^{+++} = 1.8-3.0 mEq/L; PO_4^{--} = 2.5-4.8 mg/dL; K^+ = 3.5-5.0 mEq/L), and the arterial pH should be between 7.35-7.45.[23]

Respiratory assessment. Numerous respiratory indicators have been proposed to help assess readiness for weaning.[4] Traditional indicators include measures of oxygenation, ventilation, and mechanics (Table 34-2).[7,34-50] As evident, these indicators are similar to those used to determine the need for mechanical ventilation (Chapter 29).

Traditional indicators. Among these indicators, the most commonly used are the vital capacity (VC), maximum inspiratory pressure (MIP or Pi max), minute ventilation ($\dot{V}$E), and maximum voluntary ventilation (MVV) (see Chapter 33 for details). In general, these parameters have proved useful as predictors of successful withdrawal only among patients receiving short-term ventilatory support or those with no major pulmonary disease.[3,51] These measures do not correlate well with weaning ability in patients on long-term ventilatory support,[3] the elderly,[11] or those with major pulmonary pathology.[1,13,24,36,50-52] Moreover, these traditional indicators have never proved useful in helping clinicians select a particular weaning method.[4]

Notwithstanding their limitations, measurement of these parameters—as part of a comprehensive pre-weaning assessment—can assist clinicians in the decision-making process. For example, a patient with strong performance on bedside ventilatory parameter tests may be considered for weaning sooner than might otherwise have been thought possible.[4] On the other hand, when an indicator suggests that successful weaning is unlikely, it may provide useful information on the patient's underlying pathophysiologic state.[4]

Obviously, to support decision-making, these measures must be accurate, reliable and current.[53] Fortunately, with the exception of vital capacity, most spontaneous ventilatory parameters can be measured reliably with bedside instruments using a standard technique.[54] However, variation in method or differences between evaluators can result in erroneous data and thus misguided decisions.[55,56] In addition, clinicians must remember that the status of patients receiving ventilatory support can vary from day-to-day. Thus, a patient's ability to successfully resume spontaneous ventilation should be evaluated on a recurrent basis.[4]

Newer indicators. The shortcomings of traditional indicators have led investigators to pursue other measures to predict weaning success. These newer indices include the airway occlusion pressure ($P_{0.1}$),[57,58] the rapid-shallow breathing index (f/V_T ratio),[36] the work of breathing (both mechanical and oxygen cost),[51,59-62] and breathing pattern analysis.[63-65]

An airway occlusion pressure, or $P_{0.1}$, is the inspiratory pressure measured 100 milliseconds after airway occlusion.[57,58] $P_{0.1}$ correlates with central respiratory drive and is **effort-independent**. $P_{0.1}$ can be measured using a standard analog recorder or via computer analysis of digitized signals from a ventilator.[66]

Among patients with COPD receiving ventilatory support, those who fail to wean tend to have $P_{0.1}$ values greater than 6 cm H_2O; those successfully weaned have lower values on this criterion.[57] Both the sensitivity (ability to predict successful weaning) and specificity (ability to predict unweanability) of the $P_{0.1}$ can be enhanced by measurement before and during a brief hypercapnic challenge. Successfully weaned patients show a greater increase in $P_{0.1}$ during hypercapnia than those who fail weaning.[67]

Table 34-2 Traditional measurements used to predict weaning success

Measurement	Criterion	Text References
OXYGENATION		
PaO_2 (torr) ($\leq 40\% O_2$)	> 60	34
SaO_2 (%) ($\leq 40\% O_2$)	> 90%	35
PaO_2/PaO_2 ratio	> 0.35	36
PaO_2/FiO_2 ratio	> 200	34,37
Qs/Qt (% shunt)	< 20%	38
VENTILATION		
$PaCO_2$ (torr)	< 50	34
pH	> 7.35	39
VENTILATORY MECHANICS		
Respiratory rate (f) (breaths/min)	< 30	40,41
Tidal volume (V_T) (mL/kg)	> 5	7
Vital capacity (VC) (mL/kg)	> 10–15	35,37,38,41–46
Static compliance (mL/cm H_2O)	> 30–33	37
RESPIRATORY MUSCLE STRENGTH		
Maximum inspiratory force (MIF) (−cm H_2O)	> 20–30	35,37,38,41,43–46
VENTILATORY DEMAND		
Minute volume ($\dot{V}$E) for normal PCO_2 (L/min)	< 10	35,37,38,41,44,47,48
V_{DS}/V_T (dead space fraction) %	< 0.60	37,38,41,47,48
VENTILATORY RESERVE		
Maximum voluntary ventilation (MVV) (L/min)	> 20 > twice $\dot{V}$E	35,37,38,41,44,45,49,50

An extremely simple but apparently powerful weaning index is the ratio of spontaneous breathing frequency to tidal volume (f/V_T), commonly called the rapid-shallow breathing index.[36] f/V_T is calculated by dividing the spontaneous rate of breathing (breaths/min) by the average tidal volume, *in liters* (see accompanying MiniClini). Using a threshold criterion of 100 breaths/min/L, f/V_T has a sensitivity of 0.97 and a specificity of 0.64. This index loses some predictive power in patients receiving ventilatory support for more than 8 days, and may not be as useful in predicting weaning success among the elderly.[36,53,68]

As described in Chapter 11, we can measure either the mechanical or physiologic work of breathing. Studies of the mechanical work of breathing in patients receiving ventilatory support indicate successful weaning is unlikely unless spontaneous work levels are below 1.6 Kg · m/min (or 0.14 Kg · m/L).[51,59]

Instead of measuring mechanical work, several investigators have assessed its physiologic equivalent, the oxygen cost of breathing (OCB). OCB is measured as the difference between the whole body oxygen consumption ($\dot{V}O_2$) during spontaneous breathing versus that obtained during controlled ventilation:

$$OCB = \dot{V}O_2 \text{ (spontaneous)} - \dot{V}O_2 \text{ (controlled ventilation)}$$

Once you measure the OCB, you can easily estimate the relative proportion of oxygen consumed by the respiratory muscles, as compared to the body as a whole:

$$\% \dot{V}O_2 \text{ (resp)} = \frac{OCB}{\dot{V}O_2 \text{ (spon)}}$$

Both the OCB and $\dot{V}O_2$ are directly correlated with the number of days required to wean patients.[60,61] In addition, patients successfully weaned tend to exhibit lower OCB values than those who fail attempts at ventilator withdrawal.[62] A threshold OCB of 15% appears to have the best sensitivity and specificity (ability to predict unweanability).[62]

Enthusiasm for using work of breathing measures to predict "weanability" must be tempered with the knowledge that most cited studies have significant methodologic flaws.[1] Even allowing for these limitations, it is doubtful that a single threshold value of work can, by itself, predict weaning success.[4] After all, work represents only one side of ventilatory demand vs. capacity equation. Thus, measuring work without simultaneously considering muscle strength or endurance provides only partial information.

Breathing pattern analysis is also being proposed as a method to predict weanability. As described in Chapter 33, breathing patterns are assessed using respiratory inductance plethysmography (RIP). Using an RIP monitor, abdominal and rib cage motion can be plotted against each other on an x-y recorder or graphics display. Data from this x-y plot, when combined with tidal volume information, is used to derive measures such as the percent abdominal paradox, and the average asynchrony index. Figure 34-4 shows the relationship between these breathing pattern measures and the deterioration in minute ventilation and pH observed in a patient who failed a spontaneous breathing trial after mechanical ventilation.

Patients who fail spontaneous breathing trials tend to exhibit significantly greater asynchrony and paradox than those having a successful outcome.[63] Unsuccessful weaning outcomes are also associated with an increase in the rib cage, as opposed to abdominal, component of breathing.[64] This transition to greater rib cage breathing among unsuccessfully weaned patients is probably due to an early fall in diaphragmatic power that occurs in this group.[65] Whether these changes are due to muscle fatigue or increased load is not entirely clear; the fact that they occur almost immediately after discontinuing mechanical ventilation suggests, however, that increased load is the primary cause.[1]

No longer restricted to the research laboratory, breathing pattern analysis is adding to our knowledge of the factors affecting withdrawal from ventilatory support. Although apparently helpful in predicting weaning outcomes, this approach should still be considered investigational.

Multivariate indices. Given the multitude of factors affecting patients' responses to withdrawal from ventilatory support, and the knowledge that no single indicators provides sure answers, it is not surprising that investigators have developed and studied several **multivariate** indices. Currently, these include the CROP[36] and adverse factor/ventilator scores,[13] and the weaning index (WI).[69]

The CROP score combines measures of respiratory load, respiratory muscle strength, and gas exchange.[36]

■ MINI **C**LINI ■

34-1

Calculating and Interpreting the Rapid-Shallow Breathing Index

Problem: You measure the following spontaneous breathing parameters on two patients being considered for weaning from mechanical ventilation:

Patient	Rate (f)	V_T
A	32	0.30
B	28	0.40

For which patient is successful weaning *least* likely?

Discussion: First, compute the rapid-shallow breathing index for each patient:

Patient	Rate (f)	V_T	f/V_T
A	32	0.30	107
B	28	0.40	70

Patient A clearly exceeds the threshold criterion of 100 breaths/min/L, while Patient B falls well below this criterion. Thus, all else being equal, patient A is least likely to be successfully weaned.

As a rule of thumb, patients with rates in excess of 30 and tidal volumes below 350mL will be hard to wean.

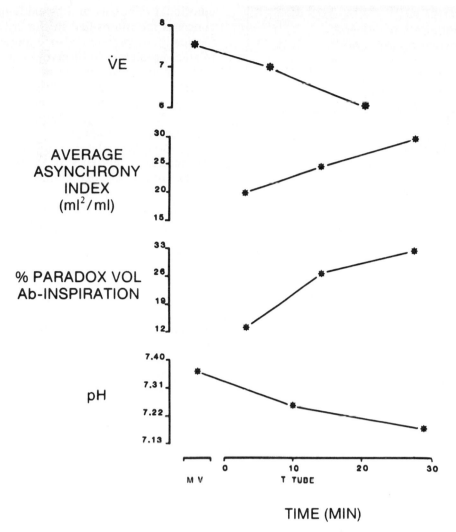

Fig. 34-4 Alterations in minute ventilation ($\dot{V}E$), average asynchrony index, percent paradox volume of the abdomen *(Ab)* during inspiration, and arterial blood pH in a patient who failed a T-tube trial of weaning from mechanical ventilation (MV). (From Dantzker DR, Tobin MJ: *Respir Care* 30(6):428, 1985.)

CROP stands for *c*ompliance, *r*ate, *o*xygenation, and *P*Imax. The actual formula for computing the CROP score is:[36]

$$CROP = \frac{(C_{dyn} \times PImax \times a/A)}{f}$$

where C_{dyn} is the patient's dynamic compliance in mL/cm H_2O, PImax is the maximum inspiratory pressure (or MIP) in cm H_2O, a/A is the arterial-to-alveolar oxygen tension ratio, and f is the patient's spontaneous breathing frequency. In preliminary studies of this multivariate index, patients with CROP scores > 18 had an 87% likelihood of a successful weaning outcome.[36] In comparison, the likelihood of successful outcomes using the traditional **univariate** measures of $\dot{V}E \leq 10$ L/min and PImax ≥ 30 cm H_2O were only 55% and 61%, respectively.

The Adverse Factor/Ventilator Score combines ratings of several "adverse factors" and six ventilatory support parameters into a single measure designed to predict weanability (see box on page 976).[13] Ratings for each parameter are summed to derive a composite score. Based on preliminary analysis of a small sample of patients receiving long-term ventilatory support (≥ 30 days), an Adverse Factor/Ventilator Score exceeding 55 accurately predicted failure to wean in 97% of cases.[13] Whether this strong negative relationship will be replicated in larger prospective studies awaits determination. Also of concern is the relative cumbersomeness of using this scoring system.[22]

Another multivariate weaning predictor under investigation is the weaning index (WI).[69] The WI combines measures of ventilatory endurance and the efficiency of gas exchange. WI is computed as:

$$WI \text{ (weaning index)} = PTI \times \frac{\dot{V}E40}{V_{Tsb}}$$

where PTI is a modified pressure-time index (based on data readily available at the bedside), $\dot{V}E40$ is the

---

Components of adverse factor/ventilator score[13]

Adverse factor score

Hemodynamics and vital signs
　Heart rate
　Blood pressure
　Temperature
　Central venous pressure
　Arrhythmias
　Vasopressors needed?
Presence of Infection
　Oral antibiotics needed?
　Parenteral antibiotics needed?
Nutrition
　Calories/24 h
Neurologic/psychiatric state
　Level of consciousness
　Communication
　Mobility
　Emotional state
　Sedatives needed?
　Pain medication needed?

Ventilator score

Fraction inspired oxygen
Level of PEEP
Static compliance
Dynamic compliance
Minute volume
Triggered respiratory rate

---

minute ventilation needed to achieve a $PaCO_2$ of 40 torr, and V_{TSB} is the spontaneous tidal volume.

Patients who fail weaning trials exhibit higher PTI and $V_{E}40/V_{TSB}$ values than those who are successfully removed from ventilatory support.[69] Although neither variable alone can accurately predict weaning outcome, the composite index does show promise and bears further study.

Limitations of purely quantitative approaches. The emphasis on objective physiologic criteria as a basis for determining patient readiness for weaning is not shared by all clinicians.[7] Some even argue that reliance on these measures only delay the weaning process. Clearly, a middle ground exists. This combined approach, emphasizing both objective data analysis and astute clinical observational skills, is probably the most useful.

Psychologic readiness

Psychologic factors are a major determinant of outcome in some patients, especially those requiring prolonged ventilatory support.[4] However, because minimal research exists in this important area, the relative importance of psychologic factors in determining weaning outcomes is currently unknown.

We do know that any illness creates anxiety and emotional concerns among patients, and that these concerns are intensified in the critical care setting.[26] Critically ill patients also experience dependence-related problems. Subjected to depersonalized routines, many develop **regressive behavior** and self-centeredness. Symptoms of this behavior include preoccupation with bodily functions, interest in the present moment only, and unwarranted concern with surrounding equipment.[26]

Compounding these problems is the inability to communicate. Patients' inability to communicate causes problems in expressing fears, frustrations, and needs, and is a primary cause of emotional stress.[26,70] Indeed, patients perceive the isolation caused by communication difficulties as a greater problem than most other discomforts experienced during ventilatory support (Table 34-3).[71] Other important stressors affecting these patients include disorientation, loss of memory, emotional instability, and physical discomfort.[70]

Physical signs associated with stress and anxiety include diaphoresis, hypertension, increased heart rate, increased respiratory rate, and dilated pupils.[72] Obviously, these signs are nonspecific, being caused by many physiologic as well as psychologic problems. In the absence of an identifiable physiologic cause, however, the presence of these signs should direct the clinician to explore underlying psychologic or emotional determinants.

A related psychologic factor impacting on weaning success is sleep deprivation.[73] Sleep deprivation is an all too common finding among intensive care patients. Progressive sleep deprivation results in patient anxiety, irritability, and sluggish thought processes. Taken to the extreme, sleep deprivation also contributes to a form of **psychosis** that often develops among ICU patients.[73] Given that resuming spontaneous breath-

Table 34-3 Discomforts experienced during ventilatory support as perceived by patients

Discomforts	% Reporting
Anxiety/fear	47%
Not able to talk	46%
Secretions	39%
Pain	36%
Difficulties in sleeping	35%
Panic	30%
Suctioning	30%
Insecurity	29%
Nightmares	26%
Extubation	20%
Ventilator synchronization problems	18%
Problems in resuming spontaneous breathing	11%

From Bergbom-Engberg I, Haljamae H: Assessment of patients' experience of discomforts during respirator therapy, *Crit Care Med* 17(10):1068–1072, 1989.

ing is itself a perceived cause of discomfort (Table 34-3), patients who are already anxious, irritable, or psychotic from sleep deprivation are poor candidates for withdrawal from ventilatory support.

Resolving problems

Whenever a potential obstacle to weaning is identified, efforts must first be made to correct the problem before the withdrawal process begins. Table 34-4, page 978, 979, outlines several management strategies useful in resolving the most common impediments to successful weaning. Although not every obstacle has to be completely resolved, neglecting these major problem areas will surely result in failed weaning efforts.

Weaning phase

Upon completion of the preweaning phase (including resolution of major problems), the patient is considered ready for weaning. At this point, the actual weaning phase begins. During the weaning phase, a withdrawal method is selected and applied, and the patient is carefully monitored for response.

The weaning phase is considered successful if the patient can sustain adequate spontaneous ventilation over time without major adverse effects. If this end is not achieved on first attempt, additional trials may be conducted, or a different weaning method may be tried. Continued failure to wean, however, usually requires reconsideration of the underlying causes of ventilator dependence and return of the patient to the preweaning phase.

Weaning methods

The primary methods available for withdrawing patients from ventilatory support are T-tube trials, intermittent mandatory ventilation (IMV), pressure support ventilation (PSV), and mandatory minute ventilation (MMV). In addition to these common strategies, several computer-based expert systems are being tested and applied as weaning tools. Table 34-5, page 980, compares the advantages and disadvantages of these various approaches to discontinuing ventilatory support.

T-tube trials. When full ventilatory support was the only option, the T-tube trial was the only method available for weaning. With the development of IMV, the T-tube trial became less favored and little used. Today, the T-tube trial has regained legitimacy as one of many tools used for discontinuing ventilatory support.

There are two common variations used in applying T-tube trials for withdrawing ventilatory support: (1) the abrupt or rapid withdrawal, and (2) the gradual transition.[1,4] Both methods usually involve actual transition to a T-tube oxygen delivery system. More recently, patients are being kept on ventilators and provided with the equivalent of T-tube breathing, flow-triggered spontaneous ventilation.

Using the rapid withdrawal method, full ventilatory support is provided up until the patient is deemed ready for removal from mechanical ventilation, as determined by assessment of physiologic indices. At this point, the ventilator is removed, and the patient placed on a T-tube and carefully observed.

The typical trial may last anywhere from 30 minutes to several hours. If the patient remains stable during the trial and upper airway protection is assured, the patient is extubated.[4] If, on the other hand, deterioration in gas exchange occurs, ventilatory support is reinstated.[4] Some clinicians wait at least 24 hours after a failed attempt before trying another trial. An example of a rapid weaning protocol is provided in the box on page 980.

Use of rapid weaning protocols is common among postoperative patients receiving ventilatory support, such as those undergoing thoracic or cardiac surgery.[9] This procedure is also common when ventilatory support is applied for short periods of time solely to maintain alveolar ventilation, such as may occur after heavy anesthesia or in uncomplicated cases of narcotic drug overdose.

Rather than abruptly switching from mechanical to spontaneous ventilation, the clinician may choose a more gradual transition. In this approach, intermittent T-tube trials are applied. Either the duration or frequency of the trial is increased gradually over time. For example, if duration is varied, the clinician may begin with 5 minute trials and, based on patient response, progress to 60 minutes or more, every 2 to 3 hours. If frequency is varied, the clinician might set up a schedule whereby the patient breathes unassisted for 5 minutes every hour, then 5 minutes each half hour, quarter hour, and so on, until mechanical support is discontinued. The decision to continue such trials is always **empirical.**

This gradual approach is more common when ventilatory support is prolonged, as in the management of acute exacerbations of COPD, or with neuromuscular disorders resulting in respiratory failure.

Instead of using a T-tube for weaning trials, the RCP can switch the ventilator to a spontaneous breathing mode (usually CPAP). Before considering this option, however, the RCP must take into account the work of breathing imposed by the particular ventilator being used. The work imposed by most older ventilators that use mechanical demand valves (such as the Bear 1 and 2) is prohibitively high.[74-79] On the other hand, the work imposed by microprocessor-controlled ventilators that use flow-triggering to initiate spontaneous breaths ("flow-by" ventilation) is no more than that occurring with a properly functioning T-tube system.[80-82] In addition, these ventilators have

Table 34–4 Management of common problems in the difficult-to-wean patient

Problem	Management Strategy
Anemia	1. Transfuse when Hb $\leq$ 10 and Hct $\leq$ 30% if thought to be a factor in decreased tissue oxygenation

Increased work of breathing	1. Tube-related
	  a. Apply pressure support
	  b. Change size of small ET tube
	  c. Cut length of ET tube if 2 inches past mouth
	  d. Deflate cuff if all breathing is spontaneous and risk of aspiration is minimal
	2. Secretion-related (see below)
	3. Bronchospasm-related
	  a. Administer bronhodilators
	    - methylxanthines
	    - B_2-agonists via nebulizer
	    - steroids
	    - anticholinergics
	  b. Apply CPAP to reduce auto-PEEP
	  c. Treat cause
	4. Ventilator-related
	  a. Assure synchrony for machine breaths
	  b. Eliminate auto-PEEP

Secretions, atelectasis plugging	1. Systemically hydrate 2. Provide extra humidity 3. Maximally bronchodilate when necessary 4. Perform coughing exercises 5. Perform chest physiotherapy 6. Suction

Dyspnea	1. Use positioning (OOB, dangling, leaning forward)
	2. Decrease tidal volume on ventilator slowly
	3. Provide periodic bag insufflation while off ventilator
	4. Increase endurance
	  a. Alternate weaning with rest to promote endurance
	  b. Provide inspiratory resistive training
	5. Administer codeine to block dyspnea sensation
	6. Provide distraction

Malposition	1. Position to maximize diaphragm excursion, improve lung volume and gas exchange (sitting or dangling) 2. Use rocking chair 3. Follow $\dot{V}_E$, V_T, rate, MIP, MVV, ABGs for optimum position

Respiratory muscle fatigue	1. Direct at cause
	2. Assure adequate O_2 transport/cardiac output
	3. Nourish patient
	4. Replace depleted electrolytes
	5. Decrease work of breathing
	  a. Supplemental oxygen
	  b. Secretion clearance
	  c. Decrease airway resistance
	  d. Mechanical ventilation to rest fatigued muscles, then rotating weaning and rest
	  e. T-piece weaning

Hemodynamic and fluid problems	1. Volume replacement and drugs to increase contractility, increase or decrease preload, and decrease afterload 2. Delay weaning until cardiovascular stability 3. With left ventricular dysfunction, wean with IMV with PEEP or CMV
Infection	1. Identity potential infection sites 2. Remove lines early or replace periodically 3. Treat infection 4. Wash hands 5. Nourish patient

Continued

Table 34-4   Management of common problems in the difficult-to-wean patient—*cont'd*

Problem	Management Strategy
Metabolic problems	1. Treat cause and postpone weaning with acidosis
	2. Keep CO_2 at baseline level in COPD or allow progressive renal compensation during longterm weaning
	3. Provide moderate carbohydrate loading with total parenteral nutrition
Low Mg	4. Give supplements
High Mg	5. Provide dialysis or calcium chloride
Low Ca	6. Treat cause before weaning
Low PO_4	7. Replace PO_4 before weaning
Nutrition	1. Assess weight, albumin, and total lymphocyte count on admission
	2. Label degree of malnutrition and calculate protein needs
	3. Nourish
Exercise	1. Exercise to increase muscle function, prevent contracture, and maintain joint integrity (passive to active range of motion and sitting to ambulating)
	2. Increase strength during activities of daily living
	3. Secure physiotherapy consult
	4. Use exercise bicycle
	5. Encourage wheelchair rides to walks with portable ventilator
	6. Provide breathing retraining
Psychologic problems	1. Secure early psychiatric consult
	2. Allow patient control
	3. Demonstrate staff accountability/honesty
	4. Provide communication method
	5. Decrease environmental stress
	6. Teach relaxation method
	7. Provide mental stimulation
	8. Provide recreation
	9. Provide rewards for short-term goals
	10. Encourage self care
	11. Allow other patients to visit
	12. Provide flexible visiting hours
	13. Take patient out of ICU environment
Sleep disturbances	1. Provide quiet environment (dim lights), reposition patient, backrub, and sedation
	2. Provide for uninterrupted sleep
	3. Avoid weaning at night
	4. Provide relaxation method (hypnosis, biofeedback, progressive muscle relaxation)
	5. Prescribe short-acting sedative hypnotics
Pain	1. Administer minimal analgesia
	2. Provide relaxation methods
	3. Provide alternative method of pain control (accupressure, nerve block, TENS, etc)

Adapted from Norton LC, Neureuter A: Weaning the long-term ventilator-dependent patient: common problems and management, *Crit Care Nurse* 9(1):42-52, 1989.

alarm and monitoring capabilities that are difficult to provide with a simple T-tube system.[83] For these reasons, the use of flow-triggered spontaneous ventilation is a reasonable alternative to traditional T-tube trials.

The last consideration in using T-tube trials is whether or not to apply CPAP. At least three reasons have been proposed to apply CPAP during T-tube weaning.

First, some claim that CPAP may prevent the deterioration in oxygenation that often occurs when patients are switched from mechanical ventilation to spontaneous breathing. A recent study tends to refute this assumption, providing evidence that the T-piece method does not impair arterial oxygenation, and may in fact be superior to CPAP.[84]

The second argument in favor of CPAP during T-tube weaning trials is based on the use of this approach in infants with RDS. In theory, use of an artificial tracheal airway prevents glottic closure. Glottic closure during expiration in infants (as manifested by grunting) is thought to be a normal protective reflex that helps prevent airway collapse and maintains the FRC. In concept, CPAP replaces this normal mechanism while the artificial airway is in place. Although this line of reasoning is compelling,

Table 34–5 Comparison of available weaning methods

Method	Advantages	Disadvantages
T-Tube	Tests patient's true spontaneous ability Allows periods of work and rest Minimal imposed work of breathing	More staff time Abrupt transition difficult for some patients
IMV	Less staff time Gradual transition	Patient-ventilator dysynchrony Potentially high work of breathing May prolong weaning May worsen fatigue
PSV	Less staff time Gradual transition Reduced work of breathing (vs IMV) Prevents fatigue Maintains activity of diaphragm Increased patient comfort/synchrony	Backup ventilation uncertain Large change in minute volume can occur
MMV	Less staff time Maintains activity of diaphragm	Backup ventilation assured May not assure efficient pattern of breathing

there is no evidence to support this generalization to adults.

The last and perhaps best-supported reason for using CPAP during T-tube weaning trials is in patients

---

Rapid weaning protocol using T-tube trial

1. Fulfill physiologic criteria for initiating weaning
   a. Primary respiratory process improved
   b. $PaO_2 \geq 60$ torr on $FiO_2 \leq 0.4$ with PEEP ≤ 5 cm H_2O
   c. Acceptable ventilatory demand:
      $\dot{V}E < 10$ L/min for $PaCO_2$ 40 torr
   d. Adequate ventilatory mechanics:
      – VC > 10–15 mL/kg
      – MIF > 20 cm H_2O
      – MVV > 2 × resting $\dot{V}E$ requirement
2. Choose appropriate time for attempt
   a. Adequate personnel available
   b. No other ongoing procedures or other major activities
3. Eliminate or minimize respiratory depressants
   a. Narcotics, other analgesics
   b. Sedatives
4. Suction airway as needed
5. Place patient in semi-Fowler's or head elevated position
6. Switch to spontaneous ventilation at same or slightly higher FiO_2
   a. T-piece circuit
   b. Via ventilator if applicable
7. Observe patient continuously
8. Measure arterial blood gases in 20 to 30 min; continue trial if:
   a. PaO_2 acceptable (>80% of preweaning value)
   b. pH > 7.30 and stable

Adapted from Pierson DJ: Weaning from mechanical ventilation in acute respiratory failure: concepts, indications and techniques, *Respir Care* 28(5):646–660, 1983.

---

with severe COPD. In these patients, dynamic hyperinflation and auto-PEEP are common, even during spontaneous breathing. Because auto-PEEP increases the work of breathing, it can contribute to weaning failure. In these patients, CPAP reduces the inspiratory work of breathing without further increasing end-expiratory lung volume.[85] In addition, the use of CPAP can reduce the sensation of dyspnea in these patients, thereby minimizing another factor responsible for weaning failures.[85] For these reasons, patients with dynamic hyperinflation and auto-PEEP being considered for T-tube trials via an artificial airway should probably be placed on at least a 5 cm H_2O CPAP.

Intermittent mandatory ventilation (IMV). In prior chapters we looked at the physiologic and technical aspects of IMV, and only touched on its role in weaning. IMV was originally developed over two decades ago as a weaning method.[86] Today, IMV is not only the most widely used weaning technique, but also the most common primary mode of ventilation.[87,88]

As a weaning tool, IMV involves a gradual reduction in the amount of machine support, with a progressive increase in the amount of respiratory work performed by the patient (Figure 34-5).[4] Typically, the level of ventilatory support is reduced by decreasing the IMV rate. The pace of rate reduction is usually based on clinical assessment and measurement of blood gas values. However, precise guidelines do not exist.[4]

Proponents of IMV as a weaning tool argue that this approach helps prevent asynchronous breathing,[89] prevents respiratory alkalosis,[90] improves intrapulmonary gas distribution,[91] shortens weaning time,[86] maintains respiratory muscle function,[92] lowers mean airway pressure and reduces the cardiovascular effects of PEEP,[93] and has psychological benefits for the patient.

On the other hand, those opposed to this method argue that, by definition, the IMV mode cannot respond to changes in patient status and thus requires more careful monitoring. Moreover, they suggest that IMV can increase the work of breathing[94] and may not shorten weaning time.[95]

Of course, no technique is foolproof, and IMV is no exception. IMV is probably the best approach with which to start weaning stable patients who cannot tolerate a rapid withdrawal of mechanical ventilation. IMV should probably not be used to wean patients who are unstable and cannot be monitored closely, or those with CNS depression or impaired respiratory drive.

Even under the best of circumstances, IMV weaning often "stalls" at rates of 2 to 4/min, with further reductions resulting in unacceptable respiratory acidosis or fatigue. This common clinical problem is probably due to the high work of breathing imposed by the artificial airway, the ventilator, or both. If a small artificial airway is at fault, it should ideally be replaced with a larger tube. If this is impossible, pressure support should be applied (see next section). If the ventilator is adding to the patient's spontaneous breathing load, one of three options should be considered: (1) a T-tube trial off the ventilator, (2) a switchover to flow-triggered spontaneous ventilation, or (3) the addition of pressure support.

In summary, IMV is a satisfactory weaning approach, but only when used on appropriately selected patients, and with properly set equipment and bedside personnel support.[88]

Pressure support ventilation. As discussed in Chapter 30, pressure support ventilation (PSV) augments spontaneous breathing with a set amount of positive pressure. At low levels, PSV helps unload the respiratory muscles from the imposed work of breathing caused by artificial airways and/or machine circuitry, a problem common with some ventilators in the IMV mode.[96,97] At higher pressures, essentially all the work of breathing can be assumed by the ventilator.[98]

To assist in withdrawing ventilatory support, low level PSV (usually 5 to 15 cm H_2O) is typically combined with SIMV.[96] Even at these low levels, PSV improves the efficiency of spontaneous breathing. Typically, as PSV is applied, the patient's spontaneous respiratory rate decreases, the tidal volume increases, dead space ventilation decreases, muscle activity becomes more efficient, and oxygen consumption falls.[99-105]

Heart rate, blood pressure, hemoglobin saturation and end-tidal CO_2 levels achieved with PSV are comparable to those seen with SIMV.[100] PSV may also change the nature of patient work during ventilatory support, helping avoid fatigue and improving the endurance conditioning of respiratory muscles.[106,107] Last, PSV is preferred by patients over more tradtional modes of ventilatory support.[106,108]

Patients most likely to benefit from adding low level PSV to IMV during weaning are those for whom IMV alone is not working. These include patients on IMV who have $PaCO_2$s > 45 torr, spontaneous rates > 30/min, spontaneous minute volumes > 10 L/min, and spontaneous tidal volumes < 2 mL/kg.[105]

There are several ways to determine how much pressure support to apply during IMV weaning. The simplest approach is to increase the PSV level until the patient's spontaneous V_T equals or exceeds 4 mL/kg.[105] Alternatively, one can use the patient's spontaneous rate as a gauge. Using this method, the clinician raises the support pressure until the patient's spontaneous rate of breathing falls to an acceptable level (usually 20/min or less).

In patients exhibiting signs of muscle dysfunction while on IMV (tachypnea, use of accessory muscles, paradoxical breathing), the clinician should raise the PSV level until a reasonable ventilatory pattern is observed. Particularly useful in this regard is clinical monitoring of sternocleidomastoid muscle activity. In one clinical study, optimum pressure support coincided with a marked decrease in the activity of this accessory muscle of ventilation.[107]

When pressure support is used specifically to overcome the imposed work of breathing during IMV weaning, an estimating formula can be helpful. To determine the PSV level under these conditions, the clinician multiplies the total flow resistance of the patient-ventilator system times the patient's peak inspiratory flow.[108] Mathematically:

$$P_{psv} = \frac{P_{peak} - P_{plateau} \times \dot{V}_{Imax}}{V_{mech}}$$

where P_{psv} is the needed PSV level in cm H_2O, P_{peak} is the peak airway pressure in cm H_2O during a machine

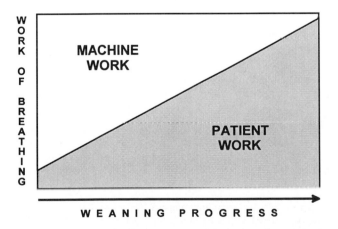

Fig. 34-5 Machine and patient work of breathing during weaning with IMV. The goal is to gradually reduce the amount of work done by the machine, while progressively increasing that done by the patient.

provided volume-cycled breath, $P_{plateau}$ is the plateau pressure in cm H_2O achieved during a mechanical inspiratory volume hold, V_{mech} is the flow in L/sec provided during the mechanical breath, and $\dot{V}Imax$ is the patient's spontaneous peak inspiratory flow in L/sec.

For example, given respective values of 50 cm and 40 cm H_2O for the peak and plateau pressure during a mechanical breath delivered at 60 L/min (1.0 L/sec), and a patient peak inspiratory flow of 30 L/min (0.5 L/sec), you could estimate the needed PSV level as follows:

$$P_{psv} = \frac{50 \text{ cm } H_2O - 40 \text{ cm } H_2O}{1.0 \text{ L/sec}} \times 0.5 \text{ L/sec}$$
$$= 5 \text{ cm } H_2O$$

Alternatively, direct measurement of imposed work of breathing can be used to adjust the PSV level.[109] By measuring pressure changes at the endotracheal tube and volume changes at the airway, pressure-volume loops can be generated and used to compute the imposed work of breathing. Figure 34-6 shows how these loops can be used to help adjust the PSV level and lower the imposed work of breathing to zero.

Rather than using pressure support to supplement IMV, it may be used as the sole weaning mode (see the example protocol in the accompanying box). In this case, the initial PSV level is set to achieve a tidal volume of 10 to 12 mL/kg, referred to as PSV_{max}. In contrast to IMV weaning (where you reduce the rate), you decrease the level of machine assist by reducing the pressure level. Over time, the PSV level is progressively reduced, with an increased rate of breathing being the primary indicator of patient intolerance.

Pressure support weaning protocol

1. Patient selection: Resolving pulmonary process, reliable respiratory drive (similar to point at which traditional IMV weaning begins);
2. Initial settings: Start at PSV_{max} ($VT = 10-12$ mL/kg, work = 0);
3. Reduce PSV as tolerated (rate of breathing reflects tolerance);
4. Extubate at 5 cm H_2O PSV.

Consideration: $PSV_{max} > 50$ cm H_2O is rarely needed. Higher pressures indicate an unstable patient.

Consideration: Backup controlled ventilation can be used as "safety net."

From MacIntyre NR: Weaning from mechanical ventilatory support: volume-assisting intermittent breaths versus pressure-assisting every breath, *Respir Care,* 33:121–125, 1988.

Extubation is indicated when the PSV level can be maintained at 5 cm H_2O with an acceptable ventilatory pattern.[98]

Clearly, pressure support ventilation represents a major addition to the weaning "toolbox." This method appears best suited for patients who are difficult to wean using traditional T-tube trials or IMV. However, no clinical practice guidelines on the use of pressure support during weaning have been developed. Furthermore, although pressure support appears to aid the weaning *process,* there is currently no evidence that its use affects weaning *outcomes.*[88]

Mandatory minute ventilation (MMV). MMV is a ventilatory support mode that ensures delivery of a preset minute volume, with the patient allowed to

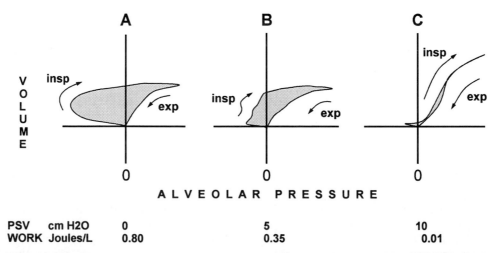

PSV cm H2O	0	5	10
WORK Joules/L	0.80	0.35	0.01

Fig. 34-6 Impact of progressive increase in pressure support level on a patient's imposed work of breathing. Area of loop indicate amount of work. In this example, the imposed work of breathing without pressure support is 0.80 Joules/L (**A**). As the level of pressure support is raised from 5 cm H_2O (**B**) to 10 H_2O (**C**), the imposed work of breathing drops to near zero. (Adapted from Banner MJ, Kirby RR, et al: Decreasing imposed work of the breathing apparatus to zero using pressure support ventilation, *Crit Care Med* 21(9):1333–1338, 1993.)

breathe spontaneously.[88,110] Should the patient meet this preset V̇E on their own, a ventilator providing MMV will remain passive and deliver no machine breaths. On the other hand, should the patient's spontaneous V̇E drop below the preset minute volume, the machine will automatically "kick in" and provide the support needed to achieve the minute ventilation goal (Figure 34-7).[111-113] Currently, MMV is available on the Bear 5, Bear 1000, Engstrom Erica, Hamilton Veolar, Ohmeda CPU-1, Ohmeda Advent, and PPG Irisa ventilators.[112]

Because MMV guarantees a constant minute volume, despite minute-to-minute changes in the patient's spontaneous breathing ability, many consider it an ideal weaning tool.[112] Moreover, MMV should allow simpler and more direct control over a patient's $PaCO_2$ than that provided by comparable weaning methods.[110] Unfortunately, changes in minute volume do not always coincide with changes in $PaCO_2$. Thus, as long as MMV algorithms use minute volume as the goal (as opposed to $PaCO_2$ or, better, pH), the utility of this support mode will be limited.

Of the different MMV algorithms available, that used by the Hamilton Veolar is perhaps the most useful for weaning.[88] When using this device in the MMV mode, the practitioner sets both a minute volume goal *and* an initial pressure support level. In turn, the ventilator varies the pressure support level (P_{psv}) to maintain the desired V̇E. This ensures adequate VT in patients with shallow rapid breathing, which other MMV algorithms neither detect nor

correct.[88] A backup SIMV mode is available should the patient become apneic.

Computer-controlled weaning. MMV is a crude example of computer-controlled mechanical ventilation. Several more complex systems have been developed and are currently being studied in specialized centers.[114-117] At present, none of these systems is available commercially.[4]

The desire to develop computer-based weaning protocols is based on two factors.[116] First, weaning is a time-consuming, labor-intensive process. If computer control can expedite or simplify this process, considerable time and money could be saved. Second, since most weaning decisions are based on objective data, computer-based weaning protocols are relatively easy to develop.

As an example, Strickland and Hasson developed an automatic, computer-controlled ventilator weaning system which interfaces a laptop computer to a ventilator and pulse oximeter.[116] The computer program monitors respiratory rate, minute ventilation and SpO_2, and uses these data to control the ventilator.

The computer begins weaning by decreasing the SIMV rate by 2 breaths/min every 5 min. As long as the patient's breathing rate stays between 8 and 25 breaths/min, the V̇E remains between 6 and 14 L/min, and the SpO_2 equals or exceeds 90%, the computer continues to decrease the SIMV rate until it reaches 2 breaths/min. At this point, the algorithm begins decreasing the pressure support level by 4 cm H_2O every

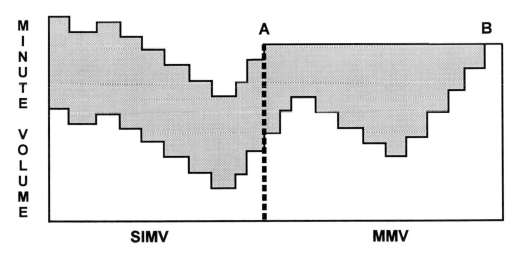

Fig. 34-7 Comparison of mandatory minute ventilation (MMV) with SIMV. Grey area indicates machine-provided minute volume, white area is patient's spontaneous ventilation. Sum of grey plus white is total minute volume. During SIMV, the machine minute volume remains constant. Thus, changes in the patient's spontaneous ventilation cause variations in the total minute ventilation. At point *A*, the patient is switched over to MMV. After this point the total minute ventilation remains constant. However, as the patient's spontaneous ventilation decreases, the machine-provided minute volume increases. Likewise, if the patient's spontaneous ventilation rises, the machine provides less and less of the total. At point *B*, the patient is meeting the total minute ventilation goal entirely with spontaneous breaths; the machine provides no additional ventilation.

5 min, using the same patient monitoring thresholds. Should any one of the monitored parameters fall outside their threshold, the system automatically returns the patient to the previous weaning level.

The primary advantage cited for computer-based weaning protocols are their ability to adapt the nature and level of ventilatory support to the needs of the patient.[4] Potential disadvantages include the following: (1) the algorithm may induce nonphysiologic breathing patterns, (2) the adequate target value can be difficult to adjust, and (3) measurement of the target variable may give false information if other data is not considered. In addition, published data and clinical experience with computer-based weaning protocols are minimal.[4]

Selecting a weaning approach. Ultimately, clinicians want to know which weaning method is best. At present, this question cannot be answered conclusively. The existing literature provides some direction, but there currently are no definitive studies that compare weaning outcomes among the major approaches just described.[4]

Perhaps the best researched area is the use of T-tube trials versus IMV. Both retrospective records analyses[118] and prospective clinical comparisons[119,120] fail to show any major benefit of IMV over T-tube trials. Indeed, in one study, the investigators showed that abrupt T-tube trials resulted in both a shorter duration of weaning and higher success rate than IMV.[120] Based on these findings, it is safe to conclude that—as long as all adverse factors are corrected and the process is carefully monitored—either weaning technique can be used successfully.[3]

In regard to the use of T-tube (zero airway pressure), CPAP, or pressure support for spontaneous breathing, current research provides a conflicting perspective. Initial studies showed that the work associated with T-tube breathing was comparable to that with CPAP.[121] More recently, both CPAP and pressure support (both at 5 cm H_2O) have been shown to decrease mechanical energy expenditure by as much as 43% over simple T-tube breathing.[122] Based on these more recent findings, it is safe to conclude that low levels of either CPAP or pressure support should be used when conducting initial spontaneous breathing trials, especially with COPD patients.[85]

An important, but poorly researched area is that of patient comfort during weaning. Given that weaning success probably depends heavily on the individual patient's subjective response to the experience, relative patient comfort is a key consideration. In terms of patients' sensations of dyspnea or anxiety, there appears to be no major difference among T-tube, SIMV, or pressure support weaning strategies.[123,124] However, dyspnea and anxiety tend to be greater than expected among patients receiving *full* ventilator support.[124] This last finding supports the conventional wisdom that partial support modes are better accepted by patients than full ventilatory support.

Last, a recent prospective comparison of SIMV and MMV provides some interesting results and possible future directions.[125] Among patients with pulmonary pathology who fulfilled traditional weaning criteria, these investigators found comparable success rates for both IMV (86%) and MMV (89%). However, MMV weaning was more rapid and proved less demanding on the ICU staff. Clearly, more research is needed on automated approaches to weaning. Nonetheless, the reported success of MMV in this study raises the possibility that computerized weaning protocols may play an increasingly important role in future approaches to discontinuing ventilatory support.

Obviously, more clinical research is needed before any definitive conclusions as to which of the currently available modes for discontinuing ventilatory support are best. Indeed, with experience as our guide, we should probably not be asking which mode is best, but under what conditions a given mode produces the best results.

Until such answers are available, selection of a weaning approach should be guided by sound knowledge of the relative advantages and disadvantages of each method, as related to the patient's underlying pathology and individual needs. Slavish adherence to uniform protocols on patients as different as those regularly encountered by the RCP should be avoided. Ultimately, the choice of weaning mode is probably less important than providing careful preliminary evaluation to determine patient readiness, and conducting astute observation once the withdrawal process has begun.[126,127]

Patient monitoring during ventilator withdrawal

As just indicated, astute patient observation and monitoring are critical components of the weaning process. The key to success is knowing what to monitor (the parameters) and how to monitor (the technique).

In terms of the parameters that one should monitor, there is a large body of knowledge describing the typical physiologic changes that occur during weaning (Table 34-6). Knowing what changes to expect can aid the decision-making process by helping the clinician determine whether to continue weaning or reinstitute ventilatory support.

Respiratory changes. When ventilatory support is reduced or removed, several physiologic changes are common to most patients and should be expected. Typically, minute volume ($\dot{V}E$) remains about the same when switching to spontaneous ventilation; however, tidal volume usually decreases and respiratory rate increases.[128-130] Respiratory rate increases of more than 14/min, combined with low tidal volumes and high inspiratory flows (VT/TI) are bad signs, as are either a large decrease or increase in $\dot{V}E$.[128-129]

In terms of blood gases, 5 to 10 torr "swings" in $PaCO_2$ and PaO_2 are common. Since ventilation of high $\dot{V}/\dot{Q}$ ratio units remains unchanged during weaning,[130] higher $PaCO_2$s are probably due to the lower V_Ts and resultant decrease in alveolar ventilation. An increased metabolic rate (increased $\dot{V}CO_2$) may also play a role in raising the $PaCO_2$.[131] Increases in $PaCO_2$ greater than 10 torr indicate a failed weaning attempt.[129,131]

Drops in PaO_2 are probably due to redistribution of blood flow to areas of low $\dot{V}/\dot{Q}$ combined with an increase in $\dot{V}O_2$; physiologic shunting tends not to increase.[130-133] For this reason, decreases in PaO_2 during weaning can usually be offset simply by increasing the FiO_2.

Cardiovascular changes. In terms of patients' cardiovascular response to withdrawal of ventilatory support, heart rate increases of 15 to 20/min are common, and usually occur without harmful effect.[128] Most patients also exhibit a moderate increase in arterial blood pressure when switched to spontaneous breathing.[134-135] This is due to both an increase in plasma epinephrine and norepinephrine levels,[135] and a rise in stroke volume and **cardiac index**.[28] The increase in cardiac output occurs secondary to an abrupt increase in venous return to the lungs.[133]

Patients with poor ventricular function (as exhibited by a pre-existing high LVEDP or low **ejection fraction**) respond differently to withdrawal of ventilatory support. In these patients, the fall in pleural pressure that occurs with the return of spontaneous breathing increases left ventricular afterload.[27] This causes an increase in left ventricular end-diastolic volume and a fall in stroke volume, cardiac index, and mean arterial pressure.[28,29]

Another cardiovascular problem, although rare, bears mentioning. A severe bradycardia has been observed among some patients when removed from ventilatory support.[136] The precise mechanism of these episodes remains unclear, but apparently is not due to either hypoxemia or an acid-base imbalance.

Monitoring techniques. In general, simple vital signs and observational assessment remain the best indicators of weaning success or failure.[127] Signs suggesting failure include agitation, tachypnea, tachycardia, bradycardia, hypotension, cyanosis, asynchronous or paradoxical breathing, angina, and cardiac arrhythmias. Generally, the appearance of these signs indicates that the patient is not tolerating the procedure and that ventilatory support should be reinstituted.

For patients remaining attached to a ventilator for weaning via CPAP or flow-by ventilation, continuous monitoring of spontaneous respiratory rate, V_T and $\dot{V}E$ is provided and should be used. For patients on a T-tube, direct continuous measurement of these parameters is less feasible. If V_T and $\dot{V}E$ must be monitored on these patients during weaning, respiratory inductance plethysmography is a good alternative.

A more sophisticated approach is to combine vital signs and observational assessment with noninvasive monitoring of gas exchange. The addition of pulse oximetry to the monitoring regimen can reduce the need for serial ABGs and aid the weaning process.[137] Capnometry also has been applied successfully as a monitoring tool during weaning.[138] However, unlike pulse oximetry (where the SpO_2 and SaO_2 are highly correlated), changes in end-tidal PCO_2 do not always reflect changes in arterial PCO_2 during weaning. For this reason, some clinicians recommend against using capnometry as a routine monitoring tool during weaning from ventilatory support.[139]

For patients with congestive heart failure, additional information on left ventricular performance will usually be needed in order to assess the response to withdrawal of ventilatory support. Typically, this information (including cardiac output and pulmonary capillary wedge pressure) will be provided by a pulmonary artery catheter.

Table 34-6   Changes occurring during withdrawal of ventilatory support

Expected changes	Deleterious changes
Respiratory:	
↑ Resp rate up to 14/min	Resp rate ≥ 30/min
Stable minute volume	Large rise/fall in $\dot{V}E$
5–10 torr swing in PaO_2	$PaO2 < 60$ torr
5–10 torr swing in $PaCO_2$	$PaCO2 > 50$ torr
pH > 7.30 and < 7.50	ph < 7.30
Minimal use of accessory muscles	Increased use of accessory muscles
No paradoxical breathing	Paradoxical breathing
Cardiovascular:	
↑ Heart rate 15–20/min	Persistent tachycardia
↑ Blood pressure 10–15 mm Hg	Hypotension
↑ Stroke volume	New arrhythmias
↑ Cardiac index	↑ PAWP
	↓ Cardiac index
	↓ Stroke volume
	Diaphoresis
	Angina

Extubation phase

The weaning phase ends when the patient is able to sustain adequate spontaneous ventilation without mechanical assistance. After successfully withdrawing ventilatory support, the goal should be to remove the artificial airway. Details on extubation technique are covered in Chapter 22; here we consider only determining when to extubate.

In general, patients should be extubated as soon as adequate airway function is restored. Early extubation is particularly important among patients with endotracheal tubes due to the high work of breathing typically imposed by these devices.[23,140] Due to their larger diameter and shorter length, tracheostomy tubes pose less of a problem; thus extubation of patients with these airways is less urgent.

In general, weaning indicators are helpful only in evaluating a patient's ability to sustain spontaneous ventilation. These same measures, however, are of little use in assessing a patient's ability to protect the upper airway.

Indicators of upper airway function have been developed for treating postoperative patients, but have not been evaluated in critically ill patients (see accompanying box).[1,4,23]

In addition, the ability of a patient to sustain a head lift is associated with recovery of protective airway reflexes in patients previously paralyzed.[141] Last, a negative indicator is the absence of a gag reflex when a tongue depressor is rubbed against the rear of the throat. Unfortunately, this test can be misleading, since as many as 1 out of 5 healthy subjects do not exhibit a gag reflex. Moreover, aspiration can still occur, even in the presence of a gag reflex.[1]

Immediately after extubation, the clinician should expect to see a moderate increase in the patient's respiratory rate, tidal volume, and minute ventilation.[1] With successful extubation, these parameters return back to pre-extubation values within 30 minutes.[142] Signs of unsuccessful extubation include all those identified as occurring during unsuccessful weaning (see Table 34-6). In addition, the RCP should always be on the lookout for postextubation stridor.

STRATEGIES FOR THE CHRONICALLY VENTILATOR–DEPENDENT PATIENT

The chronically ventilator-dependent patient presents a special challenge to caregivers. Although no precise definition exists, patients are considered chronically ventilator-dependent when they cannot be withdrawn from ventilatory support after repeated attempts using standard weaning strategies. In simple terms, the chronically ventilator-dependent individual is considered "unweanable."

Indicators of adequate upper airway function (postoperative patients)

- Deep cough on suctioning
- $VC > 20$ mL/kg
- $MIP > -40$, cm H_2O
- $MEP > 60$, cm H_2O

Scope of the problem

There are probably at least 10,000 ventilator-dependent patients in the United States today.[143] The single most important cause of ventilator-dependency is COPD, although—taken together—neuromuscular conditions predominate. Interestingly, most of these patients are still cared for in acute care facilities.

Given both the high cost of care and marginal quality of life experienced by many of these patients, every effort must be made to restore them to as normal a functional capacity as possible. Ideally, this means weaning the unweanable.

Strategies to aid weaning

Obviously, the first step in withdrawing ventilatory support from a ventilator-dependent patient is to assure that all physiologic and psychologic barriers to weaning have been corrected or abated (see Table 34-4). In considering selected strategies, first on the list should be nutritional repletion.[22,144,145]

Other physiologic approaches that are showing some promise in the management of chronically ventilator-dependent patients include pharmacologic therapy, periodic ventilatory support, and inspiratory muscle training.[22,146]

In terms of pharmacologic therapy, both methylxanthines and **sympathomimetic** agents have shown some promise in enhancing respiratory muscle strength and endurance.[147-150] Although controlled trials are lacking, favorable experience suggests that a trial of aminophylline may occasionally be warranted before a patient is deemed unweanable.[22]

Providing periodic (as opposed to continuous) ventilatory support has proven particularly useful in the management of ventilator-dependent patients with neuromuscular disorders. Although not fully withdrawn from mechanical ventilation, these patients can usually tolerate prolonged periods of spontaneous ventilation as long as recurrent (usually nightly) rest periods are provided. Typically, this approach involves noninvasive positive pressure ventilation (NIPPV) provided via a nasal appliance.[151] For more details, see the section on NIPPV in Chapter 38.

In select instances, exercise conditioning of the inspiratory muscles also appears to be helpful in weaning some ventilator-dependent patients.[14,152-154] Combining conditioning exercises with nutritional support is a particularly appealing strategy.[155] However, the benefit of exercise conditioning in weaning ventilator-dependent patients has yet to be evaluated prospectively.[4,22] Nonetheless, as with drug therapy, a trial of inspiratory muscle conditioning should probably be considered in ventilator-dependent patients for whom other methods fail.[22]

Given the importance of psychologic readiness in weaning, one would expect to find relevant strategies in this area to help withdraw the ventilator-dependent from mechanical support. The two most promising approaches are **biofeedback** and hypnosis. Case reports of hypnosis and biofeedback,[156-158] and a randomized trial of biofeedback[159] suggests that these methods may help the withdrawal of difficult-to-wean patients from ventilatory support.

Successful weaning of most chronically ventilator-dependent patients is possible. However, the use of these specialized methods and the need for specialized personnel are beyond the scope of most facilities. Selection and training of a specialized weaning team can enhance success;[160] however, this approach is not always feasible. Alternatively, good success in withdrawing chronically ventilator-dependent patients from ventilatory support has been achieved in specialized centers designed for this purpose.[161]

Last, one must recognize that some patients will remain ventilator-dependent throughout their lives. For these patients, two considerations are paramount: cost, and quality of life. In terms of cost, many satisfactory and lower cost alternatives exist for ventilator-dependent patients outside the acute care setting.[162] Increasingly, the most cost-effective alternative setting for these patients is the home. Of course, simple transfer to the home can decrease cost, but does little to improve the patient's quality of life. To improve a ventilator-dependent patient's quality of life, a comprehensive rehabilitation program is needed. The goal of such rehabilitation should be to assist the patient in achieving independent self-care.[163]

CHAPTER SUMMARY

The end goal for most patients receiving ventilatory support is successful removal or discontinuation. Although most patients can be removed from ventilatory support quickly and easily, this is not always the case. These patients require a slower, more deliberate process called weaning.

The process of weaning consists of several key phases, each with defined endpoints. Three key stages include the preweaning phase, the weaning phase, and the extubation phase.

During the preweaning phase, clinicians must decide whether or not to begin withdrawing ventilatory support. Typically, this decision is based on assessment of the patient's physiologic and psychologic readiness.

Upon completion of the preweaning phase (including resolution of major problems), the patient is considered ready for weaning. During the weaning phase, a withdrawal method is selected and applied, and the patient is carefully monitored for response.

The weaning phase ends when the patient is able to sustain adequate spontaneous ventilation without mechanical assistance. After successfully withdrawing ventilatory support, the goal should be to remove the artificial airway.

A small number of patients become chronically ventilator-dependent. For these patients, weaning is extremely difficult, and sometimes impossible. Special strategies exist to help wean these patients, but some will remain ventilator-dependent for the remainder of their lives.

REFERENCES

1. Tobin MJ, Yang K: Weaning from mechanical ventilation, *Crit Care Clin* 6(3):725-47, 1990.
2. Stone AM, Bone RC: Successful weaning from mechanical ventilation. Strategies to avoid failure, *Postgrad Med* 86(5):315-9, 1989.
3. Sporn PH, Morganroth ML: Discontinuation of mechanical ventilation, *Clin Chest Med* 9(1):113-26, 1988.
4. American College of Chest Physicians: ACCP Consensus Conference: mechanical ventilation, *Chest* 104:1833-1859, 1993.
5. Bowser MA, et al: A systematic approach to ventilator weaning, *Respir Care* 20:959, 1975.
6. Modell JH: Weaning patients from mechanical ventilation, *Respir Care* 20:373, 1975.
7. Pierson DJ: Weaning from mechanical ventilation in acute respiratory failure: concepts, indications and techniques, *Respir Care* 28(5):646-660, 1983.
8. Larca L, Greenbaum DM: Effectiveness of intensive nutritional regimes in patients who fail to wean from mechanical ventilation, *Crit Care Med* 10:297-300, 1982.
9. Gorback MS, Kantor KK: Extubation without a trial of spontaneous ventilation in the general surgical population, *Respir Care* 32(3):178-182, 1987.
10. Pardee NE, Winterbauer RH, Allen JD: Bedside evaluation of respiratory distress, *Chest* 85:203-206, 1984.
11. Krieger BP, Ershowsky PF, et al: Evaluation of conventional criteria for predicting successful weaning from mechanical ventilatory support in elderly patients, *Crit Care Med* 17(9):858-861, 1989.
12. Sivak ED: Prolonged mechanical ventilation: An approach to weaning, *Cleve Clin Q* 47(2):89-96, 1980.
13. Morganroth ML, Morganroth JL, Nett LM, Petty TE: Criteria for weaning from prolonged mechanical ventilation, *Arch Intern Med* 144:1012-1016, 1984.
14. Aldrich TK, Karpel JP, Uhrlass RM, et al: Weaning from mechanical ventilation: Adjunctive use of inspiratory muscle resistive training, *Crit Care Med* 17:143-147, 1989.
15. Menzies R, Gibbons W, Goldberg P: Determinants of weaning and survival among patients with COPD who require mechanical ventilation for acute respiratory failure, *Chest* 95(2):398-405, 1989.
16. Marini JJ: The physiologic determinants of ventilator dependence, *Respir Care* 31(4):271-282, 1986.
17. Spitzer AR, Giancarlo T, et al: Neuromuscular causes of prolonged ventilator dependency, *Muscle Nerve* 15(6):682-686, 1992.
18. Haake RE, Saxon LA, et al: Depressed central respiratory drive causing weaning failure. Its reversal with doxapram, *Chest* 95(3):695-697, 1989.
19. Bolton CF: Polyneuropathy as a cause of respiratory failure in critical illness, *Intensive Crit Care Dig* 7:7-9, 1988.
20. Knochel JP: Neuromuscular manifestations of electrolyte disorders, *Am J Med* 72:521-535, 1982.
21. Geisman LK, Ahrens T: Auto-PEEP: an impediment to weaning in the chronically ventilated patient, *AACN Clin Issues Crit Care Nurs* 2(3):391-397, 1991.
22. Stoller JK: Establishing clinical unweanability, *Respir Care* 36(3):186-198, 1991.
23. Knebel AR: Weaning from mechanical ventilation: current controversies, *Heart Lung* 20(4):321-31, 1991.
24. Bridges EJ: Transition from ventilatory support: knowing when the patient is ready to wean, *Crit Care Nurs Q* 15(1):14-20, 1992.

25. Scoggin CH: Weaning respiratory patients from mechanical support, *J Respir Dis* 1:13-23, 1980.
26. Norton C, Nureuter A: Weaning the long-term ventilator-dependent patient: common problems and management, *Crit Care Nurs* 9(1):42-52, 1989.
27. Beach T, Millen E, Grenvik A: Hemodynamic response to discontinuation of mechanical ventilation, *Crit Care Med* 1:85-90, 1973.
28. Mathru M, Rao TL, et al: Hemodynamic response to changes in ventilatory patterns in patients with normal and poor left ventricular reserve, *Crit Care Med* 10(7):423-426, 1982.
29. Lemaire F, Teboul JL, et al: Acute left ventricular dysfunction during unsuccessful weaning from mechanical ventilation, *Anesthesiology* 69(2):171-179, 1988.
30. Bassili HR, Deitel M: Effect of nutritional support on weaning patients off mechanical ventilators, *J Parenter Enteral Nutr* 5(2):161-163, 1981.
31. Rochester DF: Malnutrition and the respiratory muscles, *Clin Chest Med* 7(1):91-99, 1986.
32. Benotti PN, Bistrian B: Metabolic and nutritional aspects of weaning from mechanical ventilation, *Crit Care Med* 17(2):181-185, 1989.
33. Dark DS, Pingleton SK, Kerby GR: Hypercapnia during weaning. A complication of nutritional support, *Chest* 88(1):141-143, 1985.
34. Higgins TL, Stoller JK: Discontinuing ventilatory support. In Pierson DJ, Kacmarek RM (editors): *Foundations of Respiratory Care,* New York, Churchill-Livingstone, 1992.
35. Hudson LD: Ventilator management, In Shires GT: *Care of the trauma patient,* ed 2, New York, 1979, McGraw-Hill.
36. Yang KL, Tobin MJ: A prospective study of indexes predicting the outcome of trials of weaning from mechanical ventilation, *N Engl J Med* 324(21):1445-1450, 1991.
37. Jung RC: Weaning criteria for patients on mechanical respiratory assistance, *West J Med* 131:49, 1979.
38. Lanken PN: Weaning from mechanical ventilation. In Fishman AP, editor: Update: Pulmonary diseases and disorders. New York, 1982, McGraw-Hill.
39. Millbern SM, Downs JB, et al: Evaluation of criteria for discontinuing mechanical ventilatory support, *Arch Surg* 113(12):1441-1443, 1978.
40. Meek PM, Tyler ML: Respiratory rate and discontinuation of mechanical ventilation [abstract], *Am Rev Respir Dis* 131:A166, 1985.
41. Pierson DJ: Acute respiratory failure. In Sahn SA, editor: *Pulmonary emergencies,* New York, 1982, Churchill Livingstone.
42. Bendixen HH, Egbert LD, Hedley-Whyte J, et al: *Respiratory care* St Louis, 1965, Mosby.
43. Feeley TW, Hedley-Whyte J: Weaning from intermittent positive-pressure ventilation, *N Engl J Med* 292:903-906, 1975.
44. Marini JJ: Respiratory medicine and intensive care for the house officer, Baltimore, 1981, Williams and Wilkins.
45. Sahn SA, Lakshminarayan S: Bedside criteria for discontinuation of mechanical ventilation, *Chest* 63:1002-1005, 1973.
46. Hilberman M, Dietrich HP, et al: An analysis of potential physiological predictors of respiratory adequacy following cardiac surgery, *J Thorac Cardiovasc Surg* 71(5):711-720, 1976.
47. Pontoppidan H, Laver MB, Gelfin B: Acute respiratory failure in the surgical patient. In Welch CE, editor: *Advances in surgery,* Chicago, 1970, Mosby.
48. Skillman JJ, Malhotra IV, Pallotta JA, et al: Determinants of weaning from controlled ventilation, *Surg Forum* 22:198-200, 1971.
49. Stetson JB, editor: *Prolonged tracheal intubation,* Boston, 1970, Little, Brown.
50. Tahvanainen J, Salmenpera M, Nikki P: Extubation criteria after weaning from intermittent mandatory ventilation and continuous positive airway pressure, *Crit Care Med* 11(9):702-707, 1983.
51. Fiastro JF, Habib MP, et al: Comparison of standard weaning parameters and the mechanical work of breathing in mechanically ventilated patients, *Chest* 94(2):232-238, 1988.
52. DeHaven DB, Hurst JM, Branson RD: Evaluation of two different extubation criteria: attributes contributing to success, *Crit Care Med* 14:92-94, 1986.
53. Mador MJ: Weaning parameters, Are they clinically useful? *Chest* 102(6):1642-3, 1992.
54. Yang KL: Reproducibility of weaning parameters. A need for standardization, *Chest* 102(6):1829-32, 1992.
55. Yang KL, Tobin MJ: Measurement of minute ventilation in ventilator-dependent patients: need for standardization, *Crit Care Med* 19(1):49-53, 1991.
56. Multz AS, Aldrich TK, et al: Maximum inspiratory pressure is not a reliable test of inspiratory muscle strength in mechanical ventilation patients, *Am Rev Respir Dis* 142:529-532, 1990.
57. Sassoon CS, Te TT, et al: Airway occlusion pressure. An important indicator for successful weaning in patients with chronic obstructive pulmonary disease, *Am Rev Respir Dis* 135(1):107-113, 1987.
58. Conti G, De Blasi R, et al: Early prediction of successful weaning during pressure support ventilation in chronic obstructive pulmonary disease patients, *Crit Care Med* 20(3):366-371, 1992.
59. Henning RJ, Shubin H, Weil MH: The measurement of the work of breathing for the clinical assessment of ventilator dependence, *Crit Care Med* 5(6):264-268, 1977.
60. Harpin RP, Baker JP, et al: Correlation of the oxygen cost of breathing and length of weaning from mechanical ventilation, *Crit Care Med* 15(9):807-812, 1987.
61. McDonald NJ, Lavelle P, et al: Use of the oxygen cost of breathing as an index of weaning ability from mechanical ventilation, *Intensive Care Med* 14(1):50-54, 1988.
62. Shikora SA, Bistrian BR, et al: Work of breathing: reliable predictor of weaning and extubation, *Crit Care Med* 18(2):157-162, 1990.
63. Tobin MJ, Guenther SM, et al: Konno-Mead analysis of ribcage-abdominal motion during successful and unsuccessful trials of weaning from mechanical ventilation, *Am Rev Respir Dis* 135(6):1320-1328, 1987.
64. Ochiai R, Shimada M, et al: Contribution of rib cage and abdominal movement to ventilation for successful weaning from mechanical ventilation. *Acta Anaesthesiol Scand* 37(2):131-136, 1993.
65. Pourriat JL, Lamberto C, et al: Diaphragmatic fatigue and breathing pattern during weaning from mechanical ventilation in COPD patients, *Chest* 90(5):703-707, 1986.
66. Brenner M, Mukai DS, et al: A new method for measurement of airway occlusion pressure, *Chest* 98(2):421-427, 1990.
67. Montgomery AB, Holle RH, et al: Prediction of successful ventilator weaning using airway occlusion pressure and hypercapnic challenge, *Chest* 91(4):496-499, 1987.
68. Breitenbucher A, Ershowski PF, Krieger BP: Rapid shallow breathing index as a predictor of weaning outcome in the elderly, *Am Rev Respir Dis* 145:A520, 1992.
69. Jabour ER, Rabil DM, et al: Evaluation of a new weaning index based on ventilatory endurance and the efficiency of gas exchange, *Am Rev Respir Dis* 144:531-537, 1991.
70. Riggio RE, Singer RD, et al: Psychological issues in the care of critically-ill respirator patients: differential perceptions of patients, relatives, and staff, *Psychol Rep* 51(2):363-369, 1982.
71. Bergbom-Engberg I, Haljamae H: Assessment of patients' experience of discomforts during respirator therapy, *Crit Care Med* 17(10):1068-1072, 1989.
72. Grossbach-Landis I: Weaning from mechanical ventilation, *Crit Care Update* 10(3):7-27, 1983.
73. Helton MC, Gordon SH, Nunnery SL: The correlation between sleep deprivation and the intensive care unit syndrome, *Heart Lung* 9(3):464-468, 1980.
74. Gibney RTN, Wilson RS, Pontoppidan H: Comparison of work of breathing on high gas flow and demand valve continuous positive airway pressure systems, *Chest* 82:692-695, 1982.

75. Op't Holt TB, Hall MV, Bass JB, et al: Comparison of changes in airway pressure during continuous positive airway pressure (CPAP) between demand valve and continuous flow devices, *Respir Care* 27:1200-1209, 1982.

76. Henry WC, West GA, Wilson RS: A comparison of the oxygen cost of breathing between a continuous-flow CPAP system and a demand-flow CPAP system, *Respir Care* 28:1273-1281, 1983.

77. Christopher KL, Neff TA, Bowman JL, et al: Demand and continuous flow intermittent mandatory ventilation systems, *Chest* 87:625-630, 1985.

78. Viale JP, Annat G, Bertrand O: Additional inspiratory work in intubated patients breathing with continuous positive airway pressure systems, *Anesthesiology* 63:536-539, 1985.

79. Samodelov LF Falke KJ: Total inspiratory work with modern demand valve devices compared to continuous flow CPAP, *Intensive Care Med* 14(6):632-639, 1988.

80. Sassoon CS, Giron AE, et al: Inspiratory work of breathing on flow-by and demand-flow continuous positive airway pressure, *Crit Care Med* 17(11):1108-1114, 1989.

81. Saito S, Tokioka H, Kosaka F: Efficacy of flow-by during continuous positive airway pressure ventilation, *Crit Care Med* 18(6):654-656, 1990.

82. Sassoon CS, Lodia R, et al: Inspiratory muscle work of breathing during flow-by, demand-flow, and continuous-flow systems in patients with chronic obstructive pulmonary disease, *Am Rev Respir Dis* 145(5):1219-1222, 1992.

83. Herschman Z, Sonnenklar N, et al: A comparison of the Puritan-Bennett 7200a ventilator's flow-by mode to the T-piece mode prior to extubation in postsurgical patients, *Respir Care* 36(10):1119-1122, 1991.

84. Jones DP, Byrne P, et al: Positive end-expiratory pressure vs T-piece. Extubation after mechanical ventilation, *Chest* 100(6):1655-1659, 1991.

85. Petrof BJ, Legare M, et al: Continuous positive airway pressure reduces work of breathing and dyspnea during weaning from mechanical ventilation in severe chronic obstructive pulmonary disease, *Am Rev Respir Dis* 141(2):281-289, 1990.

86. Downs, JB, et al: Intermittent mandatory ventilation: a new approach to weaning patients from mechanical ventilators, *Chest* 64:331-335, 1973.

87. Venus B, Smith RA, Mathru M: National survey of methods and criteria used for weaning from mechanical ventilation, *Crit Care Med* 15(5):530-533, 1987.

88. Sassoon CSH, Mahutte CK, Light RW: Ventilator modes: old and new, *Crit Care Clin* 6(3):605-634, 1990.

89. Petty TL: Intermittent mandatory ventilation reconsidered, *Crit Care Med* 9:620-621, 1981.

90. Downs JB, Block AJ, et al: Intermittent mandatory ventilation in the treatment of patients with chronic obstructive pulmonary disease, *Anesth Analg* 55:437-443, 1974.

91. Downs JB: Ventilatory patterns and modes of ventilation in acute respiratory failure, *Respir Care* 28:586-591, 1983.

92. Andersen JB, Kann T, Rasmussen JP, et al: Intermittent mandatory ventilation assists the diaphragm in weaning patients from mechanical ventilation, *Danish Med Bull* 26:363, 1979.

93. Kirby RR, Downs JB, Civetta JM, et al: High level positive end-expiratory pressure (PEEP) in acute respiratory insufficiency, *Chest* 67:156-163, 1975.

94. Gibbons WJ, Rotaple MJ, Newman SL: Effect of intermittent mandatory ventilation on inspiratory coordination in prolonged mechanically-ventilated patients, *Am Rev Respir Dis* 133:A123, 1986.

95. Schachter EN, Tucker D, Beck GJ: Does intermittent mandatory ventilation accelerate weaning? *JAMA* 246:1210-1214, 1981.

96. Kacmarek RM: The role of pressure support in reducing the work of breathing, *Respir Care* 33:99-120, 1988.

97. Brochard L, Rua F, Lorino H, et al: Inspiratory pressure support compensates for the additional work of breathing caused by the endotracheal tube, *Anesthesiology* 75:739-45, 1991.

98. MacIntyre NR: Weaning from mechanical ventilatory support: volume-assisting intermittent breaths versus pressure-assisting every breath, *Respir Care* 33:121-125, 1988.

99. Grande CM, Kahn RC: The effect of pressure support ventilation on ventilatory variables and work of breathing (abstract), *Anesthesiology* 65:A84, 1986.

100. MacIntyre NR: Respiratory function during pressure support ventilation, *Chest* 89:677-683, 1986.

101. Ershowsky P, Citres D, Krieger B: Changes in breathing pattern during pressure support ventilation in difficult to wean patients (abstract), *Respir Care* 31:946, 1986.

102. Thalman TA, Holter JF, Chitwood WR: Effects of different types of ventilatory support on total body oxygen consumption (abstract), *Respir Care* 30:859, 1985.

103. Brochard L, Pluskwa F, Lemaire F: Improved efficacy of spontaneous breathing with inspiratory pressure support, *Am Rev Resp Dis* 136:411-415, 1987.

104. Annat GJ, Viale JP, et al: Oxygen cost of breathing and diaphragmatic pressure-time index. Measurement in patients with COPD during weaning with pressure support ventilation, *Chest* 98(2):411-414, 1990.

105. Hurst JM, Branson RD, et al: Cardiopulmonary effects of pressure support ventilation, *Arch Surg* 124(9):1067-1070, 1989.

106. MacIntyre NR: Pressure support ventilation: effects on ventilatory reflexes and ventilatory muscle workload, *Respir Care* 32:447-457, 1987.

107. Brochard L, Harf A, et al: Inspiratory pressure support prevents diaphragmatic fatigue during weaning from mechanical ventilation, *Am Rev Respir Dis* 139(2):513-521, 1989.

108. Prakash O, Meij S: Cardiopulmonary response to inspiratory pressure support during spontaneous ventilation vs. conventional ventilation, *Chest* 88:403-408, 1985.

108. Chatburn RL: Estimating appropriate pressure support levels (letter), *Respir Care* 30:925-926, 1985.

109. Banner MJ, Kirby RR, et al: Decreasing imposed work of the breathing apparatus to zero using pressure support ventilation, *Crit Care Med* 21(9):1333-1338, 1993.

110. Hewlett AM, Platt AS, Terry VG: Mandatory minute volume. A new concept in weaning from mechanical ventilation, *Anaesthesia* 32(2):163-169, 1977.

111. Shelledy DC, Mikles SP: Newer modes of mechanical ventilation: mandatory minute volume ventilation part 2, *Respir Manage* 18(4):21-2, 24, 26-8, 1988.

112. Quan SF, Parides GC, Knoper SR: Mandatory minute volume (MMV) ventilation: an overview, *Respir Care* 35(9):898-904, 1990.

113. Thompson JD: Mandatory minute ventilation, in Perel A, Stock MC, editors: *Handbook of mechanical ventilatory support*, Baltimore, 1992, Williams & Wilkins.

114. Hernandez-Sande C, Moret-Bonillo V, Alonso-Betanzos A: ESTER: an expert system for management of respiratory weaning therapy, *IEEE Trans Biomed Eng* 36(5):559-564, 1989.

115. Sitting DF, Gardner RM, Morris AH, et al: Clinical evaluation of computer-based respiratory care algorithms, *Int J Clin Monit Comput* 7:177-185, 1990.

116. Strickland JH Jr, Hasson JH: A computer-controlled ventilator weaning system, *Chest* 100(4):1096-1099, 1991.

117. Dojat M, Brochard L, Lemaire F, et al: A knowledge-based system for assisted ventilation of patients in intensive care units, *Int J Clin Monit Comput* 9:239-250, 1992.

118. Schachter EN, Tucker D, Beck GJ: Does intermittent mandatory ventilation accelerate weaning? *JAMA* 246(11):1210-1214, 1981.

119. Tomlinson JR, Miller KS, et al: A prospective comparison of IMV and T-piece weaning from mechanical ventilation, *Chest* 96(2):348-352, 1989.

120. Ashutosh K: Gradual versus abrupt weaning from respiratory support in acute respiratory failure and advanced chronic obstructive lung disease, *South Med J* 76(10):1244-1248, 1983.

121. Swinamer DL, Fedoruk LM, et al: Energy expenditure associated with CPAP and T-piece spontaneous ventilatory trials. Changes following prolonged mechanical ventilation, *Chest* 96(4):867–872, 1989.

122. Sassoon CS, Light RW, et al: Pressure-time product during continuous positive airway pressure, pressure support ventilation, and T-piece during weaning from mechanical ventilation, *Am Rev Respir Dis* 143(3):469–475, 1991.

123. Bouley GH, Froman R, Shah H: The experience of dyspnea during weaning, *Heart Lung* 21(5):471–476, 1992.

124. Knebel AR, Janson-Bjerklie SL, et al: Comparison of breathing comfort during weaning with two ventilatory modes, *Am J Respir Crit Care Med* 149(1):14–18, 1994.

125. Davis S, Potgieter PD, Linton DM: Mandatory minute volume weaning in patients with pulmonary pathology, *Anaesth Intensive Care* 17(2):170–174, 1989.

126. Coates NE, Weigelt JA: Weaning from mechanical ventilation, *Surg Clin North Am* 71(4):859–876, 1991.

127. Boysen PG: Weaning from mechanical ventilation: Does technique make a difference? *Respir Care* 36(5):407–416, 1991.

128. Gilbert R, et al: The first few hours off a respirator, *Chest* 65:152, 1974.

129. Tobin MJ, Perez W, Guenther SM, et al: The pattern of breathing during successful and unsuccessful trials of weaning from mechanical ventilation, *Am Rev Respir Dis* 134:1111–1118, 1986.

130. Torres A, Reyes A, et al: Ventilation-perfusion mismatching in chronic obstructive pulmonary disease during ventilator weaning, *Am Rev Respir Dis* 140(5):1246–1250, 1989.

131. Kemper M, Weissman C, et al: Metabolic and respiratory changes during weaning from mechanical ventilation, *Chest* 92(6):979–983, 1987.

132. Dantzker DR, Cowenhaven WM, et al: Gas exchange alterations associated with weaning from mechanical ventilation following coronary artery bypass grafting, *Chest* 82(6):674–677, 1982.

133. Rodriguez-Roisin R: Gas exchange during weaning in patients with chronic obstructive pulmonary disease, *Schweiz Med Wochenschr* 124(6):221–226, 1994.

134. Westendorp RG, Roos AN, et al: Plasma atrial natriuretic peptide concentrations in patients weaning from positive-pressure ventilation, *Neth J Med* 38(5–6):249–253, 1991.

135. Oh TE, Bhatt S, et al: Plasma catecholamines and oxygen consumption during weaning from mechanical ventilation, *Intensive Care Med* 17(4):199–203, 1991.

136. Robert R, Malin F, et al: Severe non-hypoxic bradycardia during disconnection from the ventilator during the recovery phase of ARDS, *Intensive Care Med* 17(8):494–496, 1991.

137. Rotello LC, Warren J, et al: A nurse-directed protocol using pulse oximetry to wean mechanically ventilated patients from toxic oxygen concentrations, *Chest* 102(6):1833–1835, 1992.

138. Thrush DN, Mentis SW, Downs JB: Weaning with end-tidal CO2 and pulse oximetry, *J Clin Anesth* 3(6):456–460, 1991.

139. Hess D, Schlottag A, et al: An evaluation of the usefulness of end-tidal PCO2 to aid weaning from mechanical ventilation following cardiac surgery, *Respir Care* 36(8):837–842, 1991.

140. Hess D: Perspective on weaning from mechanical ventilation—with a note on extubation, *Respir Care* 32(3):167–171, 1987.

141. Pavlin EG, Holle RH, Schoene RB: Recovery of airway protection compared with ventilation in humans after paralysis with curare, *Anesthesiology* 70(3):381–385, 1989.

142. Krieger BP, Chediak A, et al: Variability of the breathing pattern before and after extubation, *Chest* 93(4):767–771, 1988.

143. Make B, Bayno S, Gertman P: Prevalence of chronic ventilator-dependency, *Am Rev Respir Dis* 133(4, Part 2):A167, 1986.

144. Larca L, Greenbaum DM: Effectiveness of intensive nutritional regimes in patients who fail to wean from mechanical ventilation, *Crit Care Med* 10:297–300, 1982.

145. Whittaker JS, Ryan CF, et al: The effects of refeeding on peripheral and respiratory muscle function in malnourished chronic obstructive pulmonary disease patients, *Am Rev Respir Dis* 142:283–288, 1990.

146. Aldrich TK: The patient at risk of ventilator dependency, *Eur Respir J Suppl* 7:645s–650s, 1989.

147. Aubier M: Pharmacotherapy of respiratory muscles, *Clin Chest Med* 9:311–324, 1988.

148. Viires N, Aubier M, et al: Effects of aminophylline on diaphragmatic fatigue during acute respiratory failure, *Am Rev Respir Dis* 129:396–402, 1984.

149. Stoller JK, Wiedemann HP, et al: Terbutaline and diaphragm function in chronic obstructive pulmonary disease: A double-blind randomized clinical trial, *Br J Dis Chest* 82:242–250, 1988.

150. Aubier M, Murciano D, et al: Dopamine effects on diaphragmatic strength during acute respiratory failure in chronic obstructive pulmonary disease, *Ann Intern Med* 110:17–23, 1989.

151. Udwadia ZF, Santis GK, et al: Nasal ventilation to facilitate weaning in patients with chronic respiratory insufficiency, *Thorax* 47(9):715–718, 1992.

152. Shekleton ME: Respiratory muscle conditioning and the work of breathing: a critical balance in the weaning patient, AACN *Clin Issues Crit Care Nurs* 2(3):405–414, 1991.

153. Aldrich TK, Karpel JP: Inspiratory muscle resistive training in respiratory failure, *Am Rev Respir Dis* 131:461–462, 1985.

154. Lerman RM, Weiss MS: Progressive resistive exercise in weaning high quadriplegics from the ventilator, *Paraplegia* 25(2):130–135, 1987.

155. McMahon MM, Benotti PN, Bistrian BR: A clinical application of exercise physiology and nutritional support for the mechanically ventilated patient, *J Parenter Enteral Nutr* 14(5):538–542, 1990.

156. Bowen DE: Ventilator weaning through hypnosis, *Psychosomatics* 30(4):449–450, 1989.

157. Corson JA, Grant JL, et al: Use of biofeedback in weaning paralyzed patients from respirators, *Chest* 543–545, 1979.

158. LaRiccia PJ, Katz RH, et al: Biofeedback and hypnosis in weaning from mechanical ventilators, *Chest* 87(2):267–269, 1985.

159. Holliday JE, Hyers TM: The reduction of weaning time from mechanical ventilation using tidal volume and relaxation biofeedback, *Am Rev Respir Dis* 141:1214–1220, 1990.

160. Cohen IL, Bari N, Strosberg MA, et al: Reduction of duration and cost of mechanical ventilation in an intensive care unit by use of a ventilatory management team, *Crit Care Med* 19:1278–1284, 1991.

161. Scheinhorn DJ, Artinian BM, Catlin JL: Weaning from prolonged mechanical ventilation. The experience at a regional weaning center, *Chest* 105(2):534–539, 1994.

162. Nochomovitz ML, Montenegro HD, et al: Placement alternatives for ventilator-dependent patients outside the intensive care unit, *Respir Care* 36(3):199–204, 1991.

163. Make B, Gilmartin M, et al: Rehabilitation of ventilator-dependent subjects with lung diseases. The concept and initial experience, *Chest* 86(3):358–365, 1984.

Neonatal and Pediatric Respiratory Care*

■

Kathleen Smith-Wenning

Catherine C. Smith

Robert L. Zanni

Craig L. Scanlan

CHAPTER LEARNING OBJECTIVES

1. Differentiate between the major events characterizing the prenatal, perinatal, and postnatal periods of lung growth and development;
2. Describe the key elements of functional anatomy and normal fetal circulation;
3. Describe the anatomic and physiologic events associated with the normal transition of the fetus from uterine to extra uterine life;
4. List and describe the key anatomic and physiologic differences between the neonate, child, and adult;
5. Differentiate among the various methods of assessing the newborn infant, including maternal and fetal factors;
6. Describe the indications, hazards, and special tool and techniques involved in applying respiratory care modalities to infants and children, with a special emphasis on ventilatory support;
7. Describe the etiology, pathophysiology, clinical manifestations, and treatment for the following neonatal disease processes:
   Meconium aspiration syndrome
   Respiratory distress syndrome
   Transient tachypnea of the newborn
   Apnea of prematurity
   Persistent pulmonary hypertension
   Congenital abnormalities
   Bronchopulmonary dysplasia
8. Describe the etiology, pathophysiology, clinical manifestations and treatment regimens for the following common pediatric disorders.
   Sudden infant death syndrome
   Gastroesophageal reflux
   Bronchiolitis
   Croup
   Epiglottitis
   Cystic fibrosis

Caring for infants and children is one of the most challenging and rewarding aspects of respiratory care. Neonatal and pediatric respiratory care has evolved into one of the most exciting specialties in the field, demanding from practitioners the utmost in skill and knowledge.

Competent practice in this area requires knowledge of the many differences between infants, children, and adults. In addition, one must understand the unique pathophysiology involved in common neonatal and pediatric respiratory disorders. Only with such knowledge can the respiratory care practitioner (RCP) provide quality of care to this special category of patients.

---

*We thank Ken Watson of Childrens' Hospital, Boston, for his technical assistance, especially in the areas of ECMO and HFOV.

DEVELOPMENT OF THE RESPIRATORY SYSTEM

Unlike the other major organs that begin working early in fetal life, the lung is not afforded any "practice" for its role. Hence, embryonic development must prepare the respiratory system to take on its new role immediately at birth.

Respiratory system development is an ongoing process that begins in the early embryo and extends for years after birth. Table 35-1, page 992, summarizes the major developmental events. Table 35-2, page 992, compares lung structure and function of the newborn, 8 to 10 year old child, and the fully developed adult. As seen in Table 35-2, major changes in both lung structure and function occur after birth.

Respiratory system development is divided into

Table 35-1   Summary of respiratory tract development

Approximate time of occurrence	Developmental event
24 days	Laryngotracheal groove develops
26-28 days	Bronchial buds form
2 weeks	Intraembryonic coelom forms
3 weeks	Diaphragm development begins
4 weeks	Primitive nasal cavities
	Tongue development
	Pharynx formation begins
	Pulmonary artery development
	Pulmonary vein development
	Phrenic nerves originate
6 weeks	Pseudoglandular phase begins
6 weeks	Arytenoid swellings (lead to formation of larynx)
	Lung bud migration into pleural canals
7 weeks	Oropharynx
	Tracheal cartilage development begins
	Smooth muscle cells of bronchi develop
8 weeks	Bronchial arteries develop
10 weeks	Secondary palate
	Vocal cords
	Ciliary development
	Cartilaginous rings of trachea
11 weeks	Lymphatic tissue appears
12 weeks	Mucous glands appear
13 weeks	Goblet cells appear
17 weeks	Canalicular phase begins
22 weeks	Methyltransferase system for lecithin synthesis
	Lecithin appears
24 weeks	Alveolar phase begins
	Respiratory bronchioles
	Alveoli develop
26-28 weeks	Alveolar-capillary surface area of respiratory system developed sufficiently to support extrauterine life
35 weeks	Phosphocholine transferase system for lecithin synthesis

Reproduced with permission from Richmond B and Galgoczy M; Development of the Cardiorespiratory System. In Lough MD et al: editors: *Newborn Respiratory Care.* Copyright © 1979 by Year Book Medical Publishers, Inc, Chicago.

Table 35-2   Postnatal development of lung structure and function

	Newborn	8–10 yrs	Adult
Lung weight, g	50	350	800
Lung tissue, % total	28	15	9
Number of alveoli, $\times 10^6$	20	300	300
Diameter of alveoli, μm	50	150	300
Surface area, m^2	3	32	70
Generations of airways	23	23	23
Number of respiratory airways, $\times 10^6$	1.5	14	14
Total lung capacity, L	0.2	3.0	6.0
Vital capacity, L	0.15	2.2	4.5
P_{tp} at 80% TLC, cm H_2O	8	10	15
Anatomic dead space, ml	7	50	150
$\dot{V}_{max50\%}$, FVC/s ↑	1.5-2.2	0.8-1.2	0.8-1.2

Data courtesy of EK Motoyama. From Fishman AP: *Assessment of pulmonary function,* New York, 1980. McGraw-Hill.
Note: P_{tp} = transpulmonary pressure at 80% of total lung capacity (TLC); $\dot{V}_{max50\%}$ = maximum expiratory flow rate at 50% of forced vital capacity (FVC).

structures increase in both number (hyperplastic growth) and size (hypertrophic growth). Like growth of the body as a whole, postnatal lung development is influenced by a variety of physiologic, anatomic, and environmental factors. Any one of these factors can hinder development and thus impair normal adult lung function.

Prenatal development

Development of the respiratory system in utero traditionally is divided into four stages. These stages are called the embryonic, pseudoglandular, canalicular, and alveolar (or terminal sac).[5] Figure 35-1 shows the major changes occurring in each stage.

Embryonic stage

The embryonic stage begins with fertilization and lasts 5-6 weeks. During this stage one central tube is formed from an inpouching of the embryo's surface. This tube develops into the gastrointestinal tract and its derivatives. At about 21 days, the diaphragm begins to form. At about 24 days, a laryngotracheal groove develops, followed by the formation of a lung bud at 28 days. At about the same time, the palate begins development, separating the nasal and oral cavities. At the end of 4 weeks, the tongue and pharynx have formed, as has the primitive pulmonary circulation.

Pseudoglandular stage

The pseudoglandular stage lasts from weeks 7 to 16. During this stage, the lung bud divides, grows distally, and evolves into the major airways, blood vessels and nerves. By week 7, development of the

three major periods.[1-4] During the first, or *prenatal period* the major airway and lung structures develop. Abnormalities during this period often result in congenital anatomical anomalies. The second phase of development is the *perinatal period.* During the perinatal period, the respiratory system must prepare to take over the role of gas exchange from the placenta. Many of the respiratory problems seen in premature infants are due to incomplete perinatal development. The third or *postnatal period* occurs after birth. During the postnatal period, important respiratory

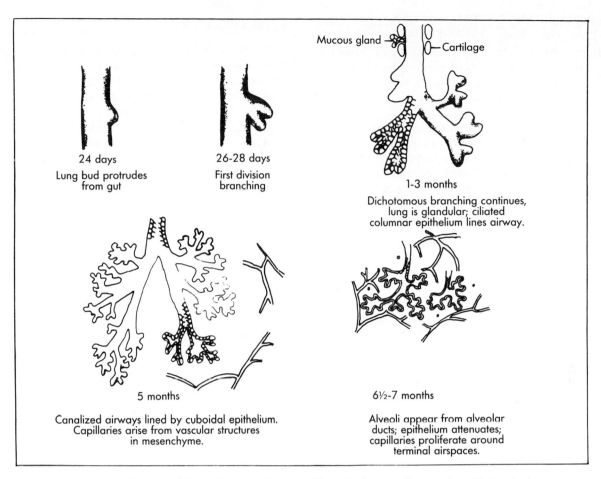

Fig. 35-1 Diagram of the major prenatal stages of lung development. (Redrawn from WB Saunders.)

diaphragm is complete.[5] By week 12, cartilage, glandular, and lymphatic tissues have developed, and lung lobes are identifiable. By the end of the 15th week, all upper airway structures are recognizable and formation of the bronchial tree is complete.

Common developmental abnormalities that occur during the pseudoglandular phase include **congenital** diaphragmatic hernia and trachcocsophageal (T-E) fistula. A congenital diaphragmatic hernia is a abnormal opening between the abdominal and thoracic cavities. Because abdominal viscera are usually displaced through the hernia into the thorax, lung growth on the affected side can be retarded. A T-E fistula is a developmental abnormality in which the early embryonic connection between these two tubes fails to close. Although many variations exist, all can lead to aspiration of stomach contents and severe respiratory complications.

Canalicular stage

The canalicular stage begins at week 17 and runs through week 24. During this stage, development of pulmonary blood vessels progresses rapidly, and respiratory bronchioles begin forming. At the cellular level, the respiratory epithelial and capillary endothelium fuse into a primitive gas exchange surface. Toward the end of the canalicular stage, immature type II cells begin to develop and produce surfactant, a surface-active substance which helps maintain alveolar stability.

Alveolar stage

At 24 to 26 weeks gestation, the fetal lung begins its final alveolar stage of prenatal development. During this stage, alveolar formation progresses, and the surfactant-producing type II cells fully develop. At about 35 weeks, these cells become capable of stable surfactant production. At this point, the fetal lung is mature enough to begin air breathing without major complications.

Perinatal development

During the perinatal period, the lung makes a rapid transition from a nonaerated, fluid-filled, and poorly perfused structure to an efficient organ of extrauterine gas exchange. A successful transition to air breathing involves many complex factors, the most important of which are the maturation of the lung and central nervous system.

Toward the end of **gestation,** the respiratory units of the normal fetal lung consist of three generations of respiratory bronchioles, a generation of alveolar ducts, and terminal clusters of alveolar saccules and primitive alveoli. Thinning of the alveolar-capillary membrane is by now sufficient to provide adequate gas exchange.

Also near the end of gestation, the fetus begins making respiratory movements. These include gasps or deep breaths, small rapid breaths, and coughing. Prior to birth, the normal fetal nervous system also becomes sensitive to maternal changes in blood O_2 and CO_2. In combination, these changes help ensure that the transition to air breathing proceeds quickly and uneventfully.

Postnatal growth

In the newborn infant, airway branching is complete, but alveolar formation is not. The gas exchange portions of the newborn lung mainly consist of thick-walled saccules or pouches. True alveoli are small in size and number, and the ratio of the lung's surface area to its weight is low (see Table 35-2).

Postnatal growth of the respiratory system involves two major stages: hyperplastic and hypertrophic.[1] During the first 8 to 10 years of life, lung growth is mainly hyperplastic, with the number of alveoli increasing by 10 fold to 15 fold (see Table 35-2).

Alveolarization occurs via two related mechanisms. First, additional alveolar buds form from the large saccules, dividing these pouches into many smaller compartments. Second, alveoli form off the walls of the terminal bronchioles. This increases the number of alveolar ducts and respiratory bronchioles.

The second, or hypertrophic period of postnatal growth begins at 8 to 10 years, and continues through adolescence and young adulthood. Development during this final period involves enlargement of lung structures, with little new alveolar formation. Connective tissue synthesis also continues, and the collagen content of the lung increases. However, tissue mass increases less than total volume. The overall size of the lung increases some threefold, and the average size of alveoli double.[6] By the end of adolescence, all respiratory structures are fully mature.

TRANSITION FROM UTERINE TO EXTRAUTERINE LIFE

Many of the problems that occur in the perinatal period are due to difficulties in making the transition to air breathing. In order to understand these problems, one must know both how the fetus survives in utero, and how the changeover to air breathing is made.

Fetal circulation

Survival of the fetus in utero requires a circulatory link between the mother and embryo. Within a week of uterine implantation, finger-like projections called *chorionic villi* arise from the embryo's aorta and invade the uterine endometrium.[7-9] These villi consist of an outer epithelial layer and a connective tissue center containing the fetal capillaries. As the villi increase in size and number, they further erode the endometrium, creating irregular pockets called *intervillous spaces.* Ultimately, maternal blood fills these spaces, continually bathing the fetal capillaries in an oxygen and nutrient-rich environment (Figure 35-2).

As gestation progresses, the villi decrease in size but increase in number. This increases the surface area for maternal-fetal exchange, up to about 14 m² at term. Thinning of the villous connective tissue also improves exchange by decreasing the distance between the maternal blood and fetal capillaries.

The placental circulation

In combination, the maternal uterine tissues and blood vessels of the fetal chorionic villi make up the *placenta.* Figure 35-3 shows a well-developed placenta in cross-sectional. Maternal blood flows into the intervillous space through the spiral arteries. In the intervillous space, maternal and fetal blood come into close proximity, aiding diffusion of O_2, CO_2, and metabolic products. After exchange takes place, maternal blood exits through venous channels, and returns to the maternal circulation. Freshly oxygenated fetal blood leaves the chorionic villi capillaries to join placental venules, which eventually merge to form a single umbilical vein.

On the fetal side of the placenta, the chorionic and amnionic layers give rise to the umbilical cord. As seen in cross-section (Figure 35-4), the umbilical cord contains a single umbilical vein (returning to the

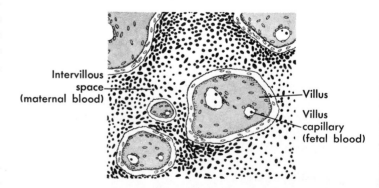

Fig. 35-2 Microscopic appearance of the villi in an intervillous space. Fetal capillaries permeate the villi, which are immersed in maternal blood within the intervillous spaces. (From Korones SB: *High-risk newborn infants:* the basis for intensive nursing care, St Louis, 1986, Mosby.)

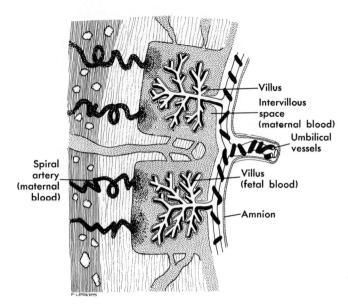

Fig. 35-3 Section through the placenta showing the spiral arteries that supply maternal blood to the intervillous space, the branching villi immersed in the intervillous space, and the umbilical vessels that branch repeatedly to terminate as villous capillaries. (Modified from Netter. In Oppenheim E, editor: Ciba collection of medical illustrations, vol 2, Reproductive system, 1965, From Korones SB: *High-risk newborn infants: the basis for intensive nursing care*, ed 4, St Louis, 1986, Mosby.)

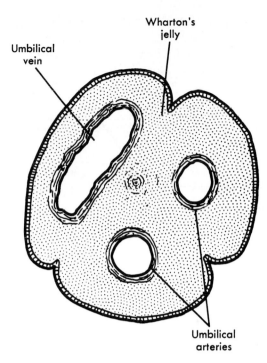

Fig. 35-4 Cross-section of umbilical cord. The arteries have thick walls; the lumen of the vein is larger than those of the arteries, and its wall is thin. (From Korones SB: *High-risk newborn infants: the basis for intensive nursing care*, ed 4, St Louis, 1986, Mosby.)

fetus) and two umbilical arteries (coursing toward the placenta). Generally, the umbilical vein is larger than the arteries, but thinner-walled. Surrounding all three blood vessels is a white gelatinous material called Wharton's jelly. For a short time after birth (up to 24 hours in some infants), the umbilical arteries remain open and can be used for infusion or blood sampling.

Abnormal implantation of the placenta (**placenta abruptio, placenta previa**) or decreased placental blood flow (**uteroplacental insufficiency**) can cause intrauterine growth retardation or fetal asphyxia. The detrimental affects of such conditions can result in respiratory distress in the immediate postnatal period.

Factors affecting placental exchange

Although in close proximity, maternal blood and fetal blood never physically mix. Nonetheless, certain drugs, bacteria, and viruses can cross the intervillous space and cause a variety of problems.

In the intervillous space, various factors favor diffusion of oxygen to the fetus.[8] Maternal oxygen, with its PaO_2 of 80 to 100 torr, readily diffuses to fetal blood, with its PaO_2 of about 16 torr. The Bohr effect also aids oxygen uptake by the fetus (see Chapter 12). In addition, fetal blood usually has more Hb than adult blood, thus increasing O_2 carrying capacity. However, the major factor responsible for fetal survival in this hypoxic environment is fetal hemoglobin (HbF).[8-11]

As compared to adult hemoglobin, HbF combine less readily with 2,3 DPG. This increases HbF affinity for oxygen. As seen in Figure 35-5 on page 996, this increased oxygen affinity is manifested by a left shift of the HbF dissociation curve, with a P_{50} about 6 to 8 torr less than adult hemoglobin (HbA). For example, at a PO_2 of 30 torr, HbF is over 75% saturated with oxygen, as compared to about 60% for HbA.

HbF is replaced by adult hemoglobin after the first four to six months of life. During this time, the RCP must be aware that cyanosis will appear later and at lower PO_2 values than in the adult. As indicated in Chapter 15, cyanosis generally becomes apparent only when the SaO_2 drops to around 75%. In the infant with a high proportion of HbF, a SaO_2 of 75% does not occur until the PaO_2 drops below 30 torr.

Despite these factors, the PO_2 in blood returning to the fetus through the umbilical vein is only about 30 torr.[8,9] This high maternal-fetal diffusion gradient is due to local variations in placental diffusing capacity, the uneven distribution of maternal blood flow, shunting on both sides of the placenta, and the placenta's high O_2 consumption. The accompanying box summarizes the normal blood gas values of a term fetus in both the umbilical arteries and vein.

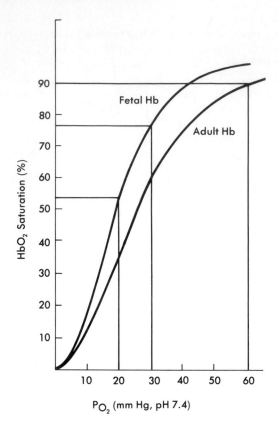

Fig. 35-5 Fetal hemoglobin produces left shift of oxyhemoglobin curve. (From Koff PB, Eitzman DV, and Neu J: *Neonatal and pediatric respiratory care,* St Louis, 1988, The CV Mosby Co.)

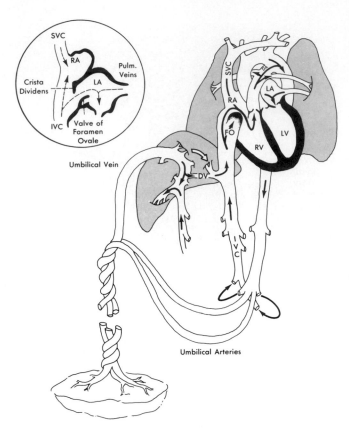

Fig. 35-6 Fetal circulation. SVC, Superior vena cava; IVC, inferior vena cava; RA, right atrium; FO, foramen ovale; LA, left atrium; DV ductus venosus; RV right ventricle; LV, left ventricle; DA, ductus arteriosus. (From Clinical education aid 7, Ross Laboratories. Reprinted with permission from Ross Laboratories, Columbus, Ohio.)

Fetal circulation

Oxygenated blood from the placenta is carried in the umbilical vein to the fetal circulation via the hepatic system (Figure 35-6). About one-third of this blood flows to the lower trunk and extremities. The other two-thirds is shunted past the liver through the *ductus venosus* into the inferior vena cava. This freshly oxygenated blood mixes with the venous blood returning from the lower trunk and extremities, and enters the right atrium.

About 50% of this blood is shunted from the right atrium into the left atrium through the *foramen ovale.* This blood then goes to the left ventricle, and ascending aorta, where it continues on to the brain, brachiocephalic trunk, and descending aorta.

Blood gas values of term fetus	
Umbilical arteries	Umbilical vein
PO$_2$ 16 torr	PO$_2$ 29 torr
PCO$_2$ 46 torr	PCO$_2$ 42 torr
pH 7.33 torr	pH 7.35

Adapted from Seeds AE: *Pediatr Clin North Am* 17:811, 1970. From Koff PB, Eitzman DV, Neu J: *Neonatal and pediatric respiratory care,* St Louis, 1988, Mosby,

Venous blood from the superior vena cava is directed downward into the right ventricle, then into the main pulmonary artery. Due to the low PO$_2$ in the fetal environment, pulmonary vascular resistance is high. For this reason, the mean pulmonary artery pressure in the fetus is higher than in the aorta. Since blood follows the path of least resistance, less than 10% of the blood entering the pulmonary artery actually flows into the lungs.[8,9] The rest is shunted from the main pulmonary artery to the descending aorta via the *ductus arteriosus.* This shunted flow then mixes with the blood ejected from the left ventricle. A portion of this less oxygenated blood circulates to the gut and lower extremities, with the rest returning to the placenta for reoxygenation via the two umbilical arteries.

Cardiopulmonary events at birth

Before birth, the placenta acts as the fetus' nutritive, respiratory, digestive, and renal organs. When the fetus and placenta separate at birth, rapid and dramatic changes must occur before air breathing can begin.

First, the lung liquid must be cleared, and the lungs inflated with air. The fetal lung is normally filled with a liquid ultrafiltrate of the plasma to a volume equal to the FRC, or about 30 mL/kg. During normal vaginal delivery, about one-third of this fluid is cleared by compression of the thorax in passage through the birth canal. The rest of the fluid is cleared by the pulmonary capillaries and lymphatics during the first few breaths.

In order to replace the remaining lung fluid with air and establish a stable FRC, the newborn must develop very high transpulmonary pressure gradients during the first few breaths. These high pressure gradients are needed to overcome the opposing forces of fluid viscosity in the airways and surface tension in the alveoli.

The stimulus for these initial efforts is both peripheral and central in origin. First, the newborn infant is bombarded by new tactile and thermal stimuli, all of which stimulate breathing. In addition, as placental gas transfer is suddenly interrupted, the newborn quickly becomes hypoxemic, hypercapnic, and acidotic.

As shown Figure 35-7, essentially no air enters the newborn lung until the transpulmonary pressure gradient exceeds 40 cm H_2O. As lung volume increases in a stepwise fashion with each breath, less and less pressure is needed to overcome the opposing forces. Normally, the resting FRC is achieved within 3 to 4 breaths. Two factors help the newborn achieve a normal FRC: Head's reflex (Chapter 14), and expiration against a partially closed glottis.[10]

As shown in Figure 35-8, on page 998, when the lung expands and breathing begins, the PaO_2 increases, the $PaCO_2$ decreases, and the pH rises back toward normal. These factors decrease pulmonary vascular resistance and constrict the ductus arteriosus. In combination, the fall in pulmonary vascular resistance and constriction of the ductus increase blood flow through the lungs. The decrease in pulmonary vascular resistance also lowers pulmonary artery pressures, which helps reabsorb any remaining lung fluid back into the pulmonary capillaries.

At about the same time, cessation of umbilical flow causes a rapid rise in systemic vascular resistance. As systemic vascular resistance increases, left sided heart pressures rise. With left sided heart pressures now higher than those on the right, the foramen ovale closes.

When this last right-to-left shunt closes, the transition between the fetal and normal extrauterine circulations is functionally complete. Full transition occurs later, as the ductus arteriosus and foramen ovale

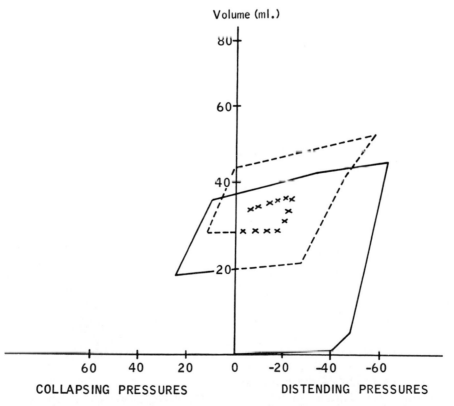

Fig. 35-7 Transpulmonary pressures developed in the human neonate during the first three breaths after birth. (From Avery ME: *The lung and its disorders in the newborn infant*, ed 2, Philadelphia, 1964, WB Saunders.)

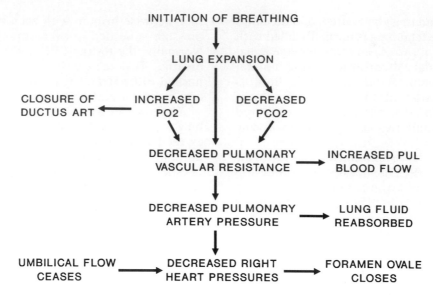

INITIATION OF BREATHING

↓

LUNG EXPANSION

CLOSURE OF ← INCREASED   DECREASED
DUCTUS ART   PO2   PCO2

DECREASED PULMONARY → INCREASED PUL
VASCULAR RESISTANCE   BLOOD FLOW

DECREASED PULMONARY → LUNG FLUID
ARTERY PRESSURE   REABSORBED

UMBILICAL FLOW → DECREASED RIGHT → FORAMEN OVALE
CEASES   HEART PRESSURES   CLOSES

Fig. 35-8 Newborn respiratory and circulatory changes. (From Kirby RR, Smith RA, Desautels DD, editors: *Mechanical ventilation*, New York, 1985, Churchill Livingstone.)

anatomically close. Anatomic closure of the ductus, through fibrosis, normally occurs within three weeks. Permanent adherence of the tissue flap covering the foramen ovale may take several months.

All these changes normally occur during the first few minutes after birth, and allow the newborn infant to achieve essentially normal gas exchange within the first 12 to 24 hours of life. However, a number of abnormal conditions can interfere with these transition events and lead to failure of the respiratory or cardiovascular systems.

ANATOMIC AND PHYSIOLOGIC DIFFERENCES

There are many anatomic and physiologic differences between infants, children, and adults. Of course, these differences are most pronounced between the newborn and adult, with a gradual development toward adult features over time.

Anatomic differences

The key respiratory structures of infants, children and adults differ not only in size, but also in the position and function.[11-13]

Head and upper airway

As shown in Figure 35-9, relative to its body, the head of the infant is larger than in adults. In infants with poor muscle tone, the weight of the head can cause acute flexion of the cervical spine. Infant neck flexion causes airway obstruction, probably in the pharynx.[14]

Although its head is larger, an infant's nasal passages are proportionately smaller than an adult's. Combined with large and highly vascular adenoid tissue, these small nasal passages makes nasal intubation more difficult and risky in infants. In addition, the infant's jaw is much rounder and the tongue much larger relative to the oral cavity. This increases the likelihood of airway obstruction with loss of muscle tone.

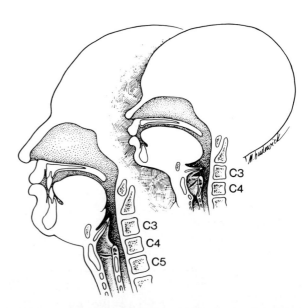

Fig. 35-9 Comparison of adult and pediatric airways. (From Finucane BT, Santora AH: *Principles of airway management*, Philadelphia, 1988, FA Davis.)

Traditionally, infants have been considered obligate nose breathers, hence dependent upon a patent nasal airway for ventilation. In fact, most infants do breathe exclusively through the nose. However, 30% to 40% of newborn infants will sometimes breathe through the mouth, both spontaneously and in response to nasal occlusion.[15] Unfortunately, oral breathing in preterm infants can lead airway obstruction.[16] As normal infants mature, they to do more oral breathing, especially when faced with nasal obstruction.[16] At about 4 to 5 months of age, most infants are capable of full oral ventilation.[13]

Larynx and epiglottis

The infant larynx lie higher in the neck than in later years, with the glottis being located between C3 and C4. In addition, the larynx of the infant is more funnel-shaped than the adult's. For this reason, the narrowest passage is through the cricoid cartilage, rather than the glottis, as in adults.[12,13]

The infant epiglottis is longer, and less flexible than the adult's and lies higher and in a more horizontal position. During swallowing, the infant's larynx provides a direct connection to the nasopharynx above. This creates two nearly separate pathways, one for breathing and one for swallowing. It also helps explain why infants can breath and suckle at the same time. Anatomic descent of the epiglottis begins between 2 1/2 and 3 months of age.

The mucosa of the infant's upper airway, especially the larynx, is thin and easily traumatized. For this reason, continuous attempts at intubation and/or suctioning can easily cause swelling and obstruction in these areas. In addition, mechanical stimulation of the neonatal larynx may result in prolonged apnea.[17]

Conducting airways

The large conducting airways of the infant are shorter and narrower than an adult's. The normal newborn trachea is about 5 to 6 cm long and 4 mm in diameter, while that in small preterm infants may be only 2 cm long and 2 to 3 mm wide. With smaller airways, a newborn's anatomic dead space is proportionately smaller than an adult's, being about 0.75 mL/lb of body weight.

As shown in Figure 35-10, the mainstem bronchi branch off the infant trachea at less acute angles than in the adult, particularly on the right. As with adults, however, the right mainstem bronchi of the infant is still more in line with the trachea than the left.[18]

The tracheobronchial tree of the newborn is more compliant than its adult counterpart. In children under 5 months of age, the bronchiolar structure has few elastic fibers. Lacking the normal supportive structures found in the adult, the infant airway is more prone to collapse, both during inspiration and

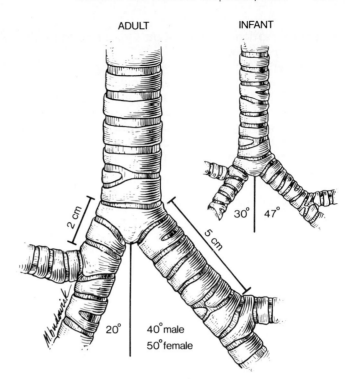

Fig. 35-10 Comparison of adult and pediatric tracheas. (From Finucane BT, Santora AH: Principles of airway management, Philadelphia, 1988, FA Davis.)

expiration. Airway collapse can result in air trapping, overdistention, and atelectasis.[11,12]

Respiratory zone

Although the infant's airway is smaller than the adult's, the respiratory bronchioles, alveolar ducts and alveolar sacs have the same volume. Respiratory units increase in number, whereas airways increase in size as infants age. However, by 8 to 10 years of age, the number of alveoli in the child's lung is about the same as in the adult. Thereafter, increased gas exchange ability occurs by virtue of a growth in the size, rather than number of alveoli.[1,3,4]

Chest wall and musculature

Because it consists mainly of cartilage, the chest cage of the newborn is highly compliant. For this reason, during periods of respiratory distress, the infant chest wall is more readily drawn inward.[19] Indrawing of the chest wall can be observed above and below the sternum, or between the ribs (suprasternal, substernal, and intercostal retractions).

Also unlike that of the adult, an infant's thoracic muscles are immature, providing little structural support and minimally supporting ventilation.[19] In addition, the infant thoracic cage is more rounded than an adult's, with the ribs being horizontally orientated.[11,12] For these reasons, the A-P diameter of the infant thorax changes little during inspiration. This places a greater burden on the infant's diaphragm as the primary inspiratory muscle.

The diaphragm of the newborn infant lies at about T8-T9 posteriorly, higher than the position in adults. In addition, the infant diaphragm moves mainly up and down, having little effect on lateral chest dimensions. Even its vertical motion is restricted by proportionately larger abdominal viscera. Gastric insufflation, common in infants, can further limit diaphragmatic motion.

Physiologic differences

The key physiologic differences between the infants and adults are listed in Table 35-3.[6] We will highlight the clinical significance of these differences, particularly those related to the control of breathing, metabolic and ventilatory requirements, and the mechanics of ventilation.

Control of breathing

Neonates, especially preterm infants, have frequent short periods of apnea and periodic breathing. Apneic spells occur most often during sleep or oral feeding, and may be accompanied by bradycardia. Apnea and periodic breathing are probably due to a decreased responsiveness to CO_2.[20]

Although peripheral chemoreceptors are active in the neonate, both premature infants and full term babies exhibit a paradoxical response to hypoxemia. Unlike adults, a newborn exposed to severe hypoxemia (a PaO_2 below 30 to 40 torr), responds with either hypopnea or apnea. CNS depression is the best explanation for this phenomenon.[21,22]

As already described, the full-term infant has an active inflation reflex, which helps establish the initial FRC. Although it lessens after birth, this reflex contributes to the increased inspiratory efforts that occur with airway obstruction or atelectasis. On the other hand, infants less than 32 weeks gestation often become apneic when faced with increased respiratory work loads, suggesting that this reflex is not fully developed.

Metabolism and ventilatory requirements

The basal metabolic rate of a full-term 3 kg infant is about 2 cal/kg/hr, nearly twice that of an adult. This means that the infant's O_2 consumption and CO_2 production (per kilogram) are also double an adult's. This high metabolic rate demands twice as much ventilation per minute, ($\dot{V}E$) per kilogram, as compared to adults.

When adjusted for body weight, infant tidal volumes are about the same as in the adult (6 to 7 mL/kg). To meet its greater ventilatory demand, the infant must therefore increase its breathing rate, to an average of 30 to 40 breaths/min. This high rate of breathing, in turn, wastes more ventilation per minute than in the adult. This occurs despite the fact that the anatomic dead space of an infant is proportionately smaller than the adult's.

Mechanics of breathing

The absolute compliance of the neonatal lung is less than an adult's. However, if you correct the compliance value for lung volume at FRC (a measure called *specific compliance*), the newborn infant's lung compliance is about the same as an adult's, or about 60 mL/cm H_2O/L.

However, because the infant's chest wall is so compliant, the recoil tendency of the lungs goes mainly unopposed. This results in a smaller FRC of about 30 mL/kg (as compared to an adult's 35 ml/kg).[23] With a smaller FRC, airway closure and atelectasis can occur more easily, resulting in lowered V/Q ratios and increased shunting. Moreover, a small FRC means that changes in ventilation will cause more rapid changes in blood gas values.[24-26] Last, with a small FRC providing less O_2 reserves, and with double the adult metabolic rate, an infant deprived of oxygen can become severely hypoxemic within seconds.

ASSESSMENT OF THE NEWBORN INFANT

Detailed analysis of pediatric and neonatal assessment is beyond the scope of this chapter. Instead, we will highlight the basic assessment methods needed to recognize common perinatal problems. More comprehensive reviews detailing clinical assessment of both the neonate and child can be found in other sources.[27-29]

Table 35-3   Physiologic differences between neonate and adult

Variable	Newborn	Adult
Body weight (kg)	3	70
Tidal volume (V_T) (mL/kg)	6	6
Respiratory rate (breaths/min)	35	15
Volume expired (mL/kg/min)	210	90
Physiologic dead space/V_T ratio	0.30	0.33
O_2 consumption (mL/kg/min)	6.4	3.5
CO_2 consumption (mL/kg/min)	6.0	3.0
Calories (kg/hr)	2	1
Total lung capacity (TLC) (mL/kg)	63	86
Functional residual capacity (FRC) (mL/kg)	30	35
Vital capacity (VC) (mL/kg)	35	70

Modified from Godinez RI: Special problems in pediatric anesthesia, *International Anesthesiology Clinics,* Boston, 1985, Little, Brown, p 88.

General assessment

Ideally, assessment of the newborn infant begins prior to birth. Due consideration should be given to both the maternal history and condition, and the fetal and newborn status.

Maternal factors

The most important maternal factors related to the health of the fetus and the outcomes of pregnancy are listed in the accompanying box.

In terms of maternal history, risk is highest with either very young mothers (less than 16 years old) or older women (over 40). In addition, first pregnancies (primagravida) grand multiparity (more than five prior pregnancies), or a recurrent history of difficult pregnancies increase the risk of a poor outcome.

Prior or existing maternal disease all increase risk to the fetus. Common examples include hypertensive disorders, diabetes mellitus, and viral or bacterial infections during pregnancy. For example, diabetes increases the risk of both congenital heart defects and hyaline membrane disease. On the other hand, renal disease, toxemia of pregnancy, and primary hypertension can all lead to placental insufficiency, and the associated risk of fetal distress during labor and delivery.[29]

Infections can be passed to the fetus across the placenta, although transmission during labor and delivery is more common. Unfortunately, some maternal infections passed to the fetus early on, such as rubella, can cause severe developmental abnormalities.

Recently, the effect of various drugs has gained attention as a factor affecting fetal and newborn health. We have known for years that use of maternal analgesic or anesthetic agents during labor and delivery increases the risk of newborn respiratory distress. More recently, we have learned that maternal addiction to narcotics can cause growth retardation and severe neonatal withdrawal symptoms after birth. Excessive use of alcohol during pregnancy causes the fetal alcohol syndrome (FAS). Last, we now know that mothers who smoke tend to give birth to low birth weight babies.

Fetal assessment

In years gone by, evaluation of the fetus was limited to simple physical assessment methods, including palpation and auscultation. Modern technology has made available several sophisticated approaches for assessing the fetus before birth. These methods include **ultrasonography,** amniocentesis, fetal heart rate monitoring, and fetal blood gas analysis.[31,32]

Ultrasonography. Ultrasonography uses high frequency sound waves to obtain a picture of the infant in utero. This allows the physician to: (1) view the position of the fetus and placenta, (2) measure fetal growth (to help set gestational age), (3) see whether

---

Maternal factors affecting outcomes of pregnancy
■ Mother's age and parity
■ History of previous births
■ Prior or existing maternal disease
■ Use of drugs, alcohol or tobacco during pregnancy

---

anatomic anomalies exist, and (4) qualitatively assess the amniotic fluid.

Amniocentesis. Amniocentesis involves direct sampling and quantitative assessment of amniotic fluid. Amniotic fluid may be inspected for meconium (fetal bowel contents) or blood. In addition, sloughed fetal cells can be analyzed for genetic normality.

Of critical importance to the RCP is the ability to assess lung maturation via amniocentesis. This test, called the L/S ratio, involves measurement of two phospholipids, lethicin and sphingomyelin, synthesized by the fetus in utero. As shown in Figure 35-11 on page 1002, the lethicin to sphingomyelin ratio rises with increasing gestational age. At about 34 to 35 weeks gestation, this ratio abruptly rises above 2:1. An L/S ratio greater than 2:1 indicates stable surfactant production and a mature lung.

Phosphatidylglycerol (PG) is another lipid found in the amniotic fluid that is used to assess fetal lung maturity. PG first appears when a stable pathway for surfactant exits, at about 35 to 36 gestation.[33]

Fetal heart rate monitoring. Fetal heart rate monitoring involves concurrent measurement of fetal heart rate and uterine contractions during labor and delivery. A normal fetal heart rate ranges between 120 to 160/min. By itself, a drop in fetal heart rates of 20 beats/min below baseline, or an absolute fall below 120/min, is a bad sign.

Knowledge of heart rate changes as related to contractions provides additional information. As shown in Figure 35-12 on page 1002 there are three major patterns of fetal heart rate changes during labor: early deceleration, late deceleration, and variable deceleration.

In early deceleration (type I), the heart rate drops below 100/min soon after a contraction begins. Following the onset of contraction, the heart rate quickly returns to normal. An early deceleration pattern is believed to be due to vagal stimulation caused by head compression. Early deceleration is harmless.

Late deceleration (type II) occurs 10 to 30 seconds after onset of contractions. The heart rate returns to baseline only after the contraction ends. A late deceleration pattern indicates impaired maternal-placental blood flow, or uteroplacental insufficiency. Uteroplacental insufficiency is a primary cause of fetal asphyxia.

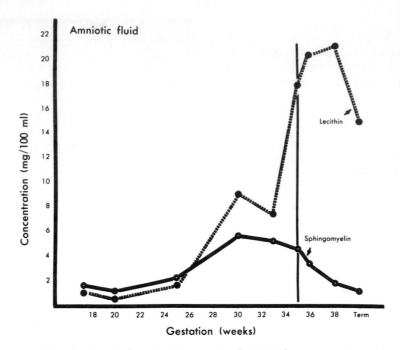

Fig. 35-11 Lecithin *(broken line)* and sphingomyelin *(solid line)* concentrations plotted against gestational age. L/S ratio rises to 1.2 at 28 weeks and to 2 or more at 35 weeks, indicating maturation of the fetal lung. (From Gluck L et al: *Am J Obstet Gynecol* 109:440, 1971.)

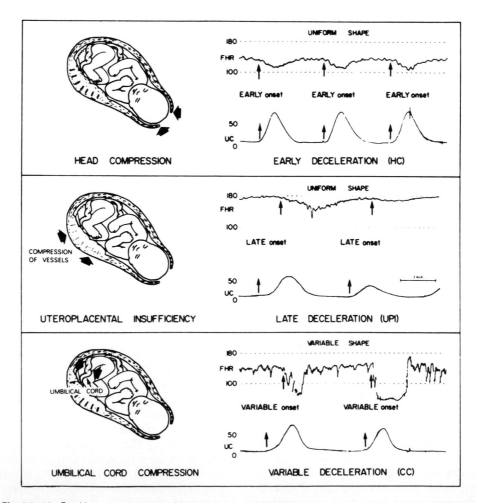

Fig. 35-12 Fetal heart rate patterns. (From Avery GB, editor: *Neonatology: pathophysiology and management of the newborn*, ed 2, Philadelphia, 1981, JB Lippincott.)

With variable deceleration (type III), there is no clear relationship between contractions and heart rate. This pattern is the most common of the three, and is probably due to umbilical cord compression. Short periods of cord compression are harmless. Longer period of imparied umbilical blood flow, however, can lead to hypoxic fetal distress. Cord compression often can be relieved by repositioning the mother.

Fetal blood gas analysis. When other factors indicate potential problems during labor and delivery, fetal blood gases can help determine their severity. Normally, fetal blood is obtained from a capillary sample taken from the presenting part, usually the scalp. Blood is analyzed mainly for the pH.

The normal fetal capillary pH ranges from 7.35 to 7.25, with the lower values occurring late in labor. A pH below 7.20 indicates a combined respiratory and metabolic acidosis. Metabolic acidosis indicates tissue hypoxia, anaerobic metabolism, and lactic acid accumulation.

Assessment of the newborn

Neonate assessment begins immediately upon delivery. There are two basic aspects of neonatal assessment that the RCP must understand. These include the Apgar score and assessment of gestation age.[31]

Apgar score. The Apgar score is a objective scoring system used to rapidly evaluate neonates. As shown in Table 35-4, the system has five components: heart rate, respiratory effort, muscle tone, reflex irritability, and skin color. Each component is rated according to set definitions, resulting in a composite score. To establish a trend, infants normally are scored at 1 and 5 minutes after birth. Additional scoring may occur thereafter to assess how an infant is responding to resuscitation. The need for resuscitation, however, is established right after delivery and never postponed for Apgar scoring.

In general, infants scoring 7 or higher at 1 minute are considered normal, requiring only routine care and observation. Infants with a 1 minute Apgar score of 3 to 6 usually need stimulation and supplemental oxygen. An infant with an Apgar score of 6 or less at

five minutes is still severely depressed and at risk of developing major complications. Such infants are normally placed in intensive care.

When combined with birth weight, the 5 minute Apgar score is a good predictor of subsequent neurologic status. On an average, less than 2% of normal birth weight infants with 5 minute Apgar scores between 7 to 10 will have a neurological problem at 1 year of age. Similar size infants with 5 minute Apgar scores of 3 or less have three times the incidence of neurological problems. The incidence of these problems increases to nearly 20% among smaller infants with low Apgar scores.

Assessment of gestational age. Determination of gestational age involves assessment of multiple physical characteristics and neurologic signs. Two common systems are used to determination gestational age: the Dubowitz scales and the Ballard scales.

The Dubowitz scales involves assessment of 11 physical and 10 neurologic signs (see accompanying box).[34] Each sign is given a score of 0 to 5. All scores for all signs are then totaled. When used within the first five days of life, the total Dubowitz score predicts gestational age with an accuracy of about 2 weeks.

The Ballard scales are a simplified version of the Dubowitz method. The Ballard scale includes 6 physical and 6 neurologic signs (Figure 35-13, page 1004).[35]

Dubowitz gestational age assessment criteria

Physical criteria:	Neurologic criteria:
Edema	Posture
Skin texture	Square window
Skin color	Ankle dorsiflexion
Skin capacity	Arm recoil
Lanugo	Leg recoil
Plantar creases	Popliteal angle
Nipple formation	Heal to ear
Breast size	Scarf sign
Ear form	Head lag
Ear firmness	Ventral suspension
Genitalia	

Table 35-4   Apgar scoring system for newborn assessment

Sign	Score		
	0	1	2
Heart rate	Absent	Slow (<100/min)	>100/min
Respirations	Absent	Slow, irregular	Good, crying
Muscle tone	Limp	Some flexion	Active motion
Reflex irritability (catheter in nares, tactile stimulation)	No response	Grimace	Cough, sneeze, cry
Color	Blue or pale	Pink body with blue extremities	Completely pink

From Koff PB, Eitzman DV, Neu J: *Neonatal and pediatric respiratory care*, St Louis, 1988. Mosby.

Neuromuscular maturity

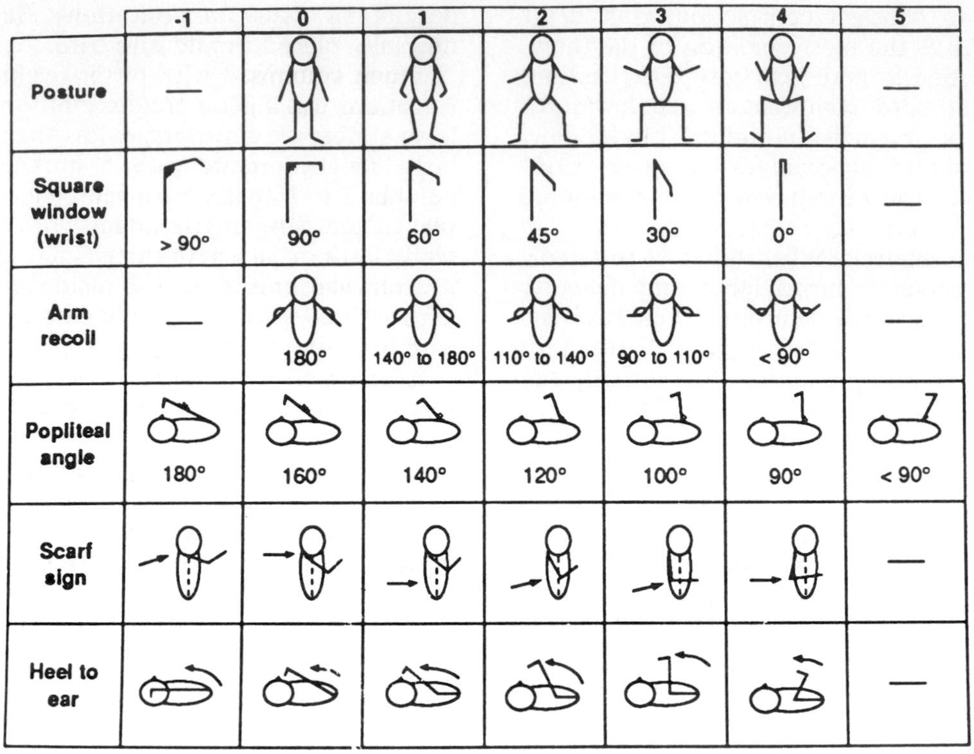

	-1	0	1	2	3	4	5
Posture	—						—
Square window (wrist)	> 90°	90°	60°	45°	30°	0°	
Arm recoil	—	180°	140° to 180°	110° to 140°	90° to 110°	< 90°	—
Popliteal angle	180°	160°	140°	120°	100°	90°	< 90°
Scarf sign							—
Heel to ear							—

Physical Maturity

	-1	0	1	2	3	4	5
Skin	Sticky, friable, transparent	Gelatinous, red, translucent	Smooth, pink; visible vessels	Superficial peeling or rash; few visible vessels	Cracking; pale areas; rare visible vessels	Parchment-like; deep cracking; no visible vessels	Leathery, cracked, wrinkled
Lanugo	None	Sparse	Abundant	Thinning	Bald areas	Mostly bald	——
Plantar surface	Heel-toe 40 to 50 mm: −1; <40 mm: −2	> 50 mm; no crease	Faint red marks	Anterior transverse crease only	Creases over anterior two-thirds	Creases over entire sole	——
Breast	Imperceptible	Barely perceptible	Flat areola, no bud	Stippled areola; 1- to 2-mm bud	Raised areola; 3- to 4-mm bud	Full areola; 5- to 10-mm bud	——
Eye and ear	Lids fused, loosely: −1; tightly: −2	Lids open; pinna flat, stays folded	Slightly curved pinna; soft, slow recoil	Well-curved pinna; soft but ready recoil	Formed and firm; instant recoil	Thick cartilage; ear stiff	——
Genitalia, male	Scrotum flat, smooth	Scrotum empty; faint rugae	Testes in upper canal; rare rugae	Testes descending; few rugae	Testes down; good rugae	Testes pendulous; deep rugae	——
Genitialia, female	Clitoris prominent; labia flat	Prominent clitoris; small labia minora	Prominent clitoris; enlarging minora	Majora and minora equally prominent	Majora large; minora small	Majora cover clitoris and minora	——

Maturity rating

Score	-10	-5	0	5	10	15	20	25	30	35	40	45	50
Weeks	20	22	24	26	28	30	32	34	36	38	40	42	44

Fig. 35-13 The Ballard Gestational Age Assessment. (From: Ballard JL, et al: A simplified score for assessment of newly born infants, *J Pediatrics* 95(5)769-774, 1979.)

Ideally, assessment of the neonate using the Ballard method should be conducted between 30 and 42 hours after birth.

As shown in Figure 35-14, by plotting the infant's gestational age against weight, one can classify the newborn's relative developmental status.[36] In terms of age, *term* infants are born between 38 to 42 weeks gestation. Infants born prior to 38 weeks are *preterm,* while those born after 42 weeks are *post-term.* In terms of weight, infants between the 10th and 90th percentiles are appropriate for gestational age, or *AGA.* Those above the 90th percentile are large for gestational age (*LGA*), while those below the 10th percentile are small for gestational age (*SGA*). By classifying infants into one of the resulting nine categories—such as "preterm, AGA"—the clinician can help identify those at highest risk, and predict both the nature of the risks involved and the likely mortality rate.

Small, preterm infants are at highest risk. Com-pared to term babies, the lungs of these infants are not yet fully prepared for gas exchange. In addition, their digestive tracts cannot absorb fat as well, and their immune systems are not yet capable of warding off infection. Small, preterm infants also have a very large surface area to body weight ratio. This increases heat loss and impairs thermoregulation. Last, the vasculature of these small infants is less well developed, increasing the likelihood of hemorrhage (especially in the ventricles of the brain).

Years ago, over 2 out of 3 infants weighing less than 1500 g died after birth. Improvements in neonatal care have dramatically changed the outlook for these patients. Today, an infant born past 28 weeks gestation and weighing over 1200 g has about an 80% chance of survival.

Unfortunately, this increase in survival has created a new set of problems. We now see extended morbidity and poor physical growth among some of these infants, often requiring many rehospitalizations. In

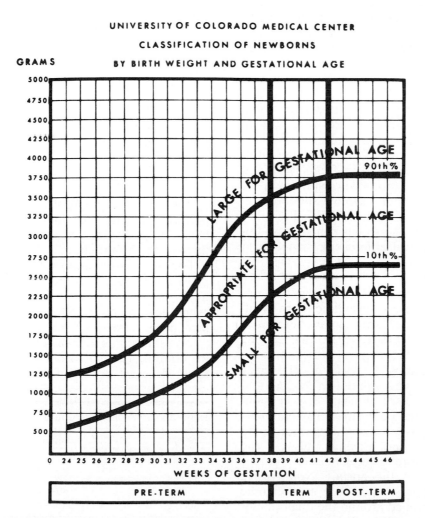

Fig. 35-14 Colorado intrauterine growth chart. (From Avery GB, editor: Neonatology: pathophysiology and management of the newborn, ed 2, Philadelphia, 1981, JB Lippincott.)

addition, serious medical complications of treatment have increased, including chronic pulmonary disease, and increased infection rates.

One might expect LGA infants (those weighing over 4000 g at birth) to be problem-free. In fact, LGA infants also have higher mortality rates than normal term babies. This higher death rate is due to several factors, including the obvious mechanical problems occurring during labor and delivery. Labor and delivery problems may help explain why LGA infants tend to have lower Apgar scores than normal term babies.

LGA infants are more common among diabetic mothers (except those with advanced disease), but this population is only a small proportion of all LGA births. In many cases, high birth weight may simply be based on genetic factors. In addition, many infants may be classified as LGA due to underestimation of actual gestational age.

Respiratory assessment of the infant

Of course not all respiratory problems occur at birth. As shown in Table 35-5, only a small number of the many infant respiratory disorders are seen at this time.[32] Most respiratory disorders show up after birth, developing either slowly or suddenly. Knowledge of when and how a problem begins can help determine its cause.

Although some RCPs are involved in delivery room care, they are more commonly called upon to help assess and treat infants who develop respiratory problems after birth. In this regard, many of the adult assessment techniques discussed in Chapter 16 and Chapter 18 either must be modified or simply do not apply. In addition, both ABG sampling and interpretation differ substantially from that applied to adult patients.[37] Proper infant assessment demands an understanding of these critical differences.

Physical assessment

As with adults, infant physical assessment includes measurement of vital signs. A normal newborn respiratory rate is 40 to 60/min. Normal infant heart rates vary between 100 to 160/min. Heart rate can be assessed by auscultation of the apical pulse, normally located at the 5th intercostal space, midclavicular line. Alternatively, one can palpate the brachial and femoral pulse. Weak pulses indicate hypotension, shock, or vasoconstriction. Bounding peripheral pulses occur with major right-to-left shunting through the ductus arteriosus. A strong brachial pulse in the presence of a weak femoral suggests either a patent ductus or coarctation of the aorta.[33] Noninvasive blood pressure assessment is made using an electronic cuff system, usually wrapped around the thigh (femoral artery). Normal ranges of blood pressure are listed for various sized neonates in Table 35-6.[33]

Table 35-5 Causes of respiratory distress grouped by characteristics of onset

Onset	Sudden	Gradual or progressive
At birth	Pneumothorax	HMD
	Apnea	TTNB
	Asphyxia	Pneumonia (eg, group B
	Maternal drugs	streptococci)
	Choanal atresia	Meconium aspiration
	Diaphragmatic hernia	Congenital heart disease
		Hypoplastic left heart
		syndrome
		Transposition
		Pulmonary atresia
0 to 7 days	Pneumothorax	Pneumonia
	Pneumomediastinum	T-E fistula
	Apnea	Congenital intrathoracic
	Prematurity	lesions
	CNS hemorrhage	Congenital heart disease
	Sepsis	Hypoplastic left heart
	Hypoglycemia	syndrome
	Pulmonary hemorrhage	Coarctation
	Aspiration	Ventricular defect
		Tetralogy of Fallot
		Patent ductus arteriosus
		Endocardial cushion
		defect
		Malposition
		Distended abdomen

From Guthrie R, Hodson WP: Clinical diagnosis of pulmonary insufficiency. In Thibeault DW, Gregory GA: *Neonatal pulmonary care,* Norwalk Conn, 1986, Appleton Century-Crofts.
HMD, Hyaline membrane disease; *TTNB,* transient tachypnea of the newborn; *T-E,* tracheoesophageal; *CNS,* central nervous system.

Thoracic assessment of infants is more difficult to perform and interpret than in adults. This is due to both the small size and ease of sound transmission through the infant chest.

For this reason, observational assessment is emphasized. Infants in respiratory distress typically exhibit one or more of six key signs: nasal flaring, cyanosis, or blueness of the skin, expiratory grunting, tachypnea, retractions, and paradoxical breathing.

Nasal flaring is seen as dilation of the alar nasi on inspiration. The extent of flaring varies according to facial structure of the infant. Nasal flaring coincides

Table 35-6 Normal neonatal blood pressures (mm Hg)

Weight	Systolic	Diastolic
750 g	34–54	14–34
1000 g	39–59	16–36
1500 g	40–61	19–39
3000 g	51–72	27–46

Source: Whitaker K: *Comprehensive perinatal and pediatric respiratory care,* Albany, NY, Delmar, 1992.

with an increase in ventilatory demand and the work of breathing. In concept, nasal flaring decreases the resistance to air flow. It also may help stabilize the upper airway by minimizing negative pharyngeal pressure during inspiration.[38]

Chapter 15 described the limits of cyanosis as a physical sign in adults. As with adults, cyanosis may be absent in infants with anemia, even when PaO_2s are low. In addition, infants with high HbF levels may not become cyanotic until the PaO_2 falls below 30 torr. Last, hyperbilirubinemia can mask cyanosis. Hyperbilirubinemia is a hepatic condition causing increased blood and tissue levels of the bile pigment, **bilirubin.** Bilirubin causes jaundice, a yellow discoloration of the skin. It is this discoloration that may mask the presence of cyanosis.

Grunting occurs when infants exhale against a partially closed glottis. By increasing airway pressure during expiration, grunting helps prevent airway closure and alveolar collapse. Grunting can vary from mild (audible only by stethoscope) to severe (audible with the naked ear). Grunting is most common in hyaline membrane disease, but is also seen in other respiratory disorders associated with alveolar collapse.

For infants, tachypnea exists when the breathing rate rises above 60/min. Since it is the most common of all signs of infant respiratory distress, tachypnea is not a very specific indicator. Periods of apnea lasting 20 seconds or more are a more ominous sign of newborn distress.

Retractions represent the indrawing of chest wall muscle and tissue between bony structures. Retractions can occur in the suprasternal, substernal, and intercostal regions. Retractions indicate an increase in

work of breathing, especially due to decreased pulmonary compliance.

As a sign of respiratory distress, paradoxical breathing in infants differs from the adult form. Instead of drawing the abdomen in during inspiration, the infant with paradoxical breathing tends to draw in the chest wall. This inward movement of the chest wall may range in severity from a simple time lag during inspiration, to a full blown see-saw motion, in which the chest caves inward while the abdomen moves out. As with retractions, paradoxical breathing indicates an increase in ventilatory work.

Several of these signs of respiratory distress have been combined into an assessment system called the Silverman Index (Figure 35-15). The Silverman Index can be used by the RCP to help grade and track the severity of respiratory distress.[39] Low composite scores (0 to 3) indicate minimal distress. Higher Silverman scores indicate significant respiratory impairment.

Arterial blood gas analysis

As with adults, arterial blood gas (ABG) analysis is among the most important and reliable tool for assessing infant respiratory distress. Also as with adults, many noninvasive techniques—such as transcutaneous PO_2 and PCO_2 electrodes, and pulse oximeters—are used to obtain comparable data.[37] Nonetheless, ABG analysis remains the principle approach when precise results are critical.

Methods. As with adults, infant ABG samples can be obtained by either arterial puncture or peripheral arterial line. However, these procedures are technically difficult in neonates. Alternate means for obtaining infant arterial blood samples are: (1) umbilical artery

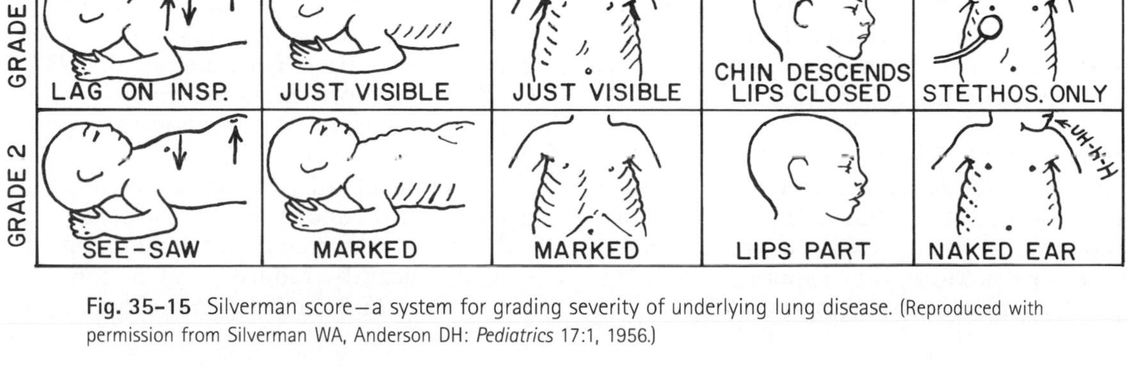

	UPPER CHEST	LOWER CHEST	XIPHOID RETRACTION	CHIN MOVEMENT	EXPIRATORY GRUNT
GRADE 0	SYNCHRONIZED	NO RETRACTION	NONE	NO MOVEMENT OF CHIN	NONE
GRADE 1	LAG ON INSP.	JUST VISIBLE	JUST VISIBLE	CHIN DESCENDS LIPS CLOSED	STETHOS. ONLY
GRADE 2	SEE-SAW	MARKED	MARKED	LIPS PART	NAKED EAR

Fig. 35-15 Silverman score—a system for grading severity of underlying lung disease. (Reproduced with permission from Silverman WA, Anderson DH: *Pediatrics* 17:1, 1956.)

catheterization, and (2) capillary sampling or heel sticks. Table 35-7 summarizes the advantages, disadvantages, and complications of these sampling methods.[37]

Care must be taken in assessing the results of capillary sampling. First, differences in method make this the least reliable of all sampling procedures. Second, even when properly obtained, capillary samples do not accurately predict arterial values in neonates.[40] At best, a capillary sample can only be used to assess pH. As with transcutaneous monitoring, peripheral vasoconstriction or hypoperfusion makes capillary O_2 tensions unreliable.

Regardless of method, the RCP must remember that the total blood volume of the infant is very small. Too frequent sampling, or too large a sample, can critically deplete an infant's blood volume. For this reason, an ongoing record of all blood-outs must be maintained.

Assessment. To properly assess ABG results in the immediate postnatal period, the RCP must know infant normals. As shown in Table 35-8, page 1010, soon after delivery, normal term infants tend toward a mild metabolic acidosis. Normal preterm infants have a slightly greater acidemia (due mainly to an additional respiratory component) with a moderate hypoxemia.[41] This hypoxemia is probably due to both impaired gas exchange in the immature lung and some persistent right-to-left anatomic shunting, especially through the ductus arteriosus.

These differences from adult values reflect both the stressful events of birth and a lower buffering capacity of fetal blood, neither of which require treatment. Five days after birth, a normal infant's blood gases are basically the same as an adult's, with a slightly lower PO_2.

Also important in assessing neonatal blood gases is the impact of right-to-left shunting through a patent ductus arteriosus **(PDA)**. The result is an umbilical artery PaO_2 that is lower than that in the right radial and temporal arteries.[42] This is because blood flowing through a PDA normally enters the aorta distal to both the brachiocephalic and left common carotid arteries, but proximal to the left subclavian. Thus umbilical artery blood (and that from the left arm) is postductal, being lower in O_2 content than the preductal flow going to the brain and right arm. This is why right arm samples are preferred when an infant's oxygenation status is marginal. Samples from this location best reflect O_2 delivery to the brain.

Pulmonary function testing

In adults and older children, a voluntary forced exhalation is needed to produce maximum flow. Because infants and young children are unable to cooperate with instructions, they cannot perform the forced expiratory maneuver on command.[43]

In order to overcome this problem, a partial expiratory flow volume (PEFV) technique was developed and applied to young children.[44] The same method has been used to produce the PEFV curves in infants.[45]

The maneuver is performed using a compressive cuff placed around the chest and abdomen of a sedated infant.[43] The cuff is rapidly inflated to various pressures. This rapid external compression forces air out of the lungs, with the flow measured via a pneumotach attached to a mask. Volumes are integrated from the flow signal.

Figure 35-16, on page 1010 depicts an ideal PEFV curve. Results are used to study normal lung growth and development, pathophysiology, and airway responsiveness.[43] Although these tests of infant pulmonary function are being widely used, procedural guidelines or equipment standards do not yet exist.[46]

GENERAL MANAGEMENT OF THE CRITICALLY ILL NEONATE

Many of the principles underlying care of the critically ill infants are similar to those for adults. However, neonatal intensive care involves several treatment differences. Key considerations in neonatal intensive are temperature regulation, fluid and electrolyte balance, nutrition, and infection control.[27,28,47]

Temperature regulation

Due to their large surface area-to-weight ratio, newborn babies loose body heat faster than adults. In addition, infants' temperature regulation mechanisms may not be fully developed. Thus small infants cannot readily adapt to changing environmental temperatures, especially cold. Hypothermia in neonates increases oxygen consumption and can cause hypoglycemia, metabolic acidosis, pulmonary vascular hypertension, increased right-to-left shunting, and apnea (Figure 35-17, page 1010).

Infants' external body temperatures must be kept between 36.5 and 36.8° C.[48] To maintain this temperature, a *neutral thermal environment* must be established. The ambient temperature needed to maintain an NTE varies between 32° C and 35° C, depending on the infant's size. In general, the smaller the infant, the higher the NTE within this range. The NTE also decreases over time. For example, the NTE for a 1500 to 2500 g newborn infant is between 32.8 and 33.8° C. Six weeks later, the same infant can be kept between 29.0° C and 31.8° C.

Either incubators or radiant warmers are used to achieve NTE conditions. In addition to these methods, placing a layered thermal hat on the infant's head can significantly reduce oxygen consumption and extend the NTE range by as much as 1° C.

Table 35-7 Advantages, disadvantages, and complications of invasive blood gas-sampling techniques

Peripheral artery catheterization	Umbilical artery catheterization	Peripheral artery puncture	Capillary sampling
ADVANTAGES			
Provides frequent blood gas sampling with minimum discomfort; provides accurate ABG values; is rapid to perform (if arterial puncture is easy); provides continuous blood pressure monitoring; artery may be identified with cutaneous transillumination or by Doppler ultrasound techniques.	Provides frequent blood gas sampling with minimum discomfort; is usually simple and rapid to perform; provides large vessel for access in small infants; may be used for certain infusions; provides continuous blood pressure monitoring	Provides accurate ABG values; is rapid to perform on older child; has less risk of infection or embolism; provides sampling from different sites to diagnose heart anomalies; artery may be identified with cutaneous transillumination or by Doppler ultrasound techniques	Provides least invasive sampling technique; provides least risk of infection or embolism; is able to be repeated frequently; is suitable for long-term follow-up care of chronic respiratory infant
DISADVANTAGES			
Often is technically difficult to place catheter without surgical "cutdown;" fluid overload can occur from infusion fluid; volume depletion can occur from frequent blood sampling; requires collateral circulation	Fluid overload can occur from infusion fluid; volume depletion can occur from frequent blood sampling; postductal admixture results in lower PO_2 values than are delivered to retina	Often is technically difficult to obtain (especially with frequent sampling or from patient in shock); crying or pain alters reported values; requires collateral circulation	Is not reliable for older infant or child; is usually imprecise and not used for critically ill infant; PO_2 may not reflect arterial trends; crying or pain alters reported values
COMPLICATIONS			
Infection; embolism (thromboembolism or air embolism); infiltration of infusion fluid; nerve damage; severe bleeding around catheter or around tubing connections; vasospasm	Infection; embolism (thromboembolism or air embolism); abdominal organ necrosis can occur from hypertonic infusion; severe bleeding around catheter or around tubing connection; vasospasm	Risk of infection can occur without aseptic technique; severe bleeding; risk of embolism; nerve damage; hematoma	Increased work of breathing and possibly fatigue; cutaneous fibrosis of heel; bone spurs from deep punctures; puncture of posterial tibial artery

Adapted from Burton GG, Hodgkin JE: *Respiratory care: a guide to clinical practice*, ed 2, Philadelphia, 1984, JB Lippincott, p. 264; Fletcher MA, MacDonald MG, Avery GB: *Atlas of procedures in neonatology*, Philadelphia, 1983, JB Lippincott Co, p. 146; Merenstein GB, Gardner SL: *Handbook of neonatal intensive care*, St Louis, 1985, Mosby, p 99. From Koff PB, Eitzman DV, Neu J: *Neonatal and pediatric respiratory care*, St Louis, 1988, The CV Mosby Co.
ABG, arterial blood gas.

Table 35-8   Age-related values commonly reported for normal arterial blood gases

	Normal preterm infants (at 1 to 5 hours)	Normal term infants (at 5 hours)	Normal preterm infants and term infants (at 5 days)	Children, adolescents, and adults
pH	7.33	7.34	7.38	7.40
range	7.29 to 7.37	7.31 to 7.37	7.34 to 7.42	7.35 to 7.45
PCO$_2$	47	35	36	40
range	39 to 56	32 to 39	32 to 41	35 to 45
PO$_2$	60	74	76	95
range	52 to 67	62 to 86	62 to 92	85 to 100
HCO$_3^-$	25	19	21	24
range	22 to 23	18 to 21	19 to 23	22 to 26
BE	−4	−5	−3	0
range	−5 to −2.2	−6 to −2	−5.8 to −1.2	−2 to +2

Adapted from Orzalesi MM, et al: *Arch Dis Child* 42:174, 1967; Koch G, Wendel H: *Biol Neonate* 12:136, 1968. From Koff PB, Eitzman DV, Neu J: *Neonatal and pediatric respiratory care,* St Louis, 1988, Mosby.
HCO$_3^-$ bicarbonate; *BE,* base excess.

Fluid and electrolyte balance

It is more difficult to maintain fluid balance in newborn infants than in adults. Factors contributing to this problem are the newborn's small total body fluid volume, larger body surface area to weight ratio, increased skin permeability, and immature renal function. For these reasons, fluid balance must take into account gestational age, postpartum age, environmental temperature and humidity, and underlying pathology.

In terms of acid-base balance, the kidneys are not fully functional until about one month of age. Thus the newborn infant has difficulty compensating for ventilatory acid-base problems. In addition, a neonate's extracellular fluid compartment is proportionately about twice as large as an adult's. Given the large extracellular volume, fluid and electrolyte shifts from one body compartment to another can occur readily, and the acid-base status of the blood can quickly fluctuate.

Nutrition

Due to their high metabolic rates, infants require twice as many calories per kilogram as adults. As with adults, illnesses causing tissue damage and repair, infection, and fever greatly increase metabolic rates.

Since sick infants generally cannot be fed orally, nutrition must be supplied parenterally. In most centers, 10% dextrose at the rate of 150 mL/kg/day is used initially to meet basic caloric needs. If oral feedings cannot start within 3 to 5 days, amino acids and fats must be given either orally or parenterally.[47]

Infection control

Due to their immature immune systems, critically ill newborn infants are highly susceptible to nosocomial infections.[49] Many of these begin as localized infections of areas such as the skin and conjunctiva.

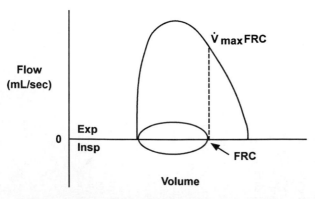

Fig. 35-16 Ideal infant peak expiratory flow-volume (PEFV) curve obtained by thoracic compression. Note identification of V̇$_{max}$FRC, the maximum flow at functional residual capacity.

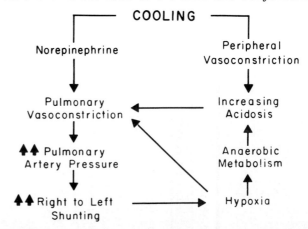

Fig. 35-17 The vicious circle resulting from cooling in the neonate. (From WB Saunders.)

However, any infection in a critically ill neonate can rapidly progress to more serious and life-threatening systemic infections.

Staphylococcus aureus, and group B beta hemolytic *Streptococcus* are the major gram positive offenders. Colonization with these organisms occurs mainly through contaminated hands. Gram negative infections, such as those caused by *Pseudomonas aeruginosa,* are more likely caused by contaminated equipment, particularly that used in respiratory care. Only strict adherence to infection control procedures can minimize the likelihood of hospital-acquired newborn infections (see Chapter 4).

BASIC RESPIRATORY CARE

Respiratory care of the infant and child involves most of the approaches used with adults. However, there are many differences between adults and infants, and several neonatal and pediatric respiratory disorders are unique to these age groups. For these reasons, some variations in therapy are required. We will focus primarily on the special tools and techniques used in oxygen therapy, bronchial hygiene, humidity and aerosol therapy, airway management, and resuscitation. CPAP and ventilatory support will be discussed separately.

Oxygen therapy

There are several unique aspects of oxygen therapy in infants and children.[50] These include special indications, hazards and precautions, methods of administration and monitoring techniques.

Indications

As in adults, the primary indication for O_2 therapy in infants and children is documented hypoxemia. In children and infants older than 28 days, hypoxemia exists when the PaO_2 is less than 60 torr or SaO_2 is below 90%. In neonates, a PaO_2 less than 50 torr or a SaO_2 less than 88% indicates hypoxemia.[51]

Oxygen therapy also is indicated in infants with pulmonary hypertension due to bronchopulmonary **dysplasia.**[52] Supplemental oxygen lowers pulmonary vascular resistance in these patients, and thus decreases right ventricular workload.

Supplemental oxygen should likewise be used during any procedure known to cause arterial desaturation. Intubation and fiberoptic bronchoscopy are good examples of procedures known to cause hypoxemia in infants and children.[53]

Hazards and precautions

The goal of O_2 therapy is to provide adequate tissue oxygenation at a safe FIO_2. A safe FIO_2 is one which causes neither pulmonary nor retinal damage.[54]

In terms of pulmonary toxicity, some evidence suggests that the growing lung is more sensitive to O_2 than the adult lung.[54] High PO_2s may also contribute to the development of bronchopulmonary dysplasia (to be discussed subsequently).

In addition to its pulmonary effects, hyperoxia can cause **retinopathy** in premature infants. Retinopathy of prematurity (ROP) affects neonates up to about one month of age, by which time the retinal arteries have sufficiently matured. There is evidence that retinal damage is most likely in infants weighing less than 1500 g.[55]

Oxygen is not the only factor associated with ROP. Other factors linked with ROP are listed in the accompanying box.[56-58]

Hyperoxia may also have harmful cardiovascular effects. First, increased PaO_2s in newborn infants constrict the ductus arteriosus. Although this is normally a desired response, it can cause problems in infants with ductus-dependent heart lesions.[59] In addition, in children with acyanotic congenital heart disease, hyperoxia can increase aortic pressures and systemic vascular resistance, and decrease cardiac index and oxygen transport.[60]

Another precaution in newborn O_2 therapy is the flip-flop phenomenon. Flip-flop refers to a larger than expected drop in the PaO_2 when the FIO_2 is lowered. Then, when the FIO_2 is raised back up, the PaO_2 fails to return to its original level.

The cause for this phenomenon is not known. In some infants, the pulmonary vessels are particularly sensitive to changes in PO_2. In these infants, lowering

---

Factors other than oxygen associated with retinopathy of prematurity[56-58]

Immaturity
Multiple episodes of bradycardia apnea
Prolonged parenteral nutrition
Number of blood transfusions
Hypoxemia
Hypercapnia
Hypocapnia
Hyperoxia
Blood transfusions
Intraventricular hemorrhage
Infection
Patent ductus arteriosus
Prostaglandin synthetase inhibitors
Vitamin E deficiency
Lactic acidosis
Respiratory distress syndrome
Hyaline membrane disease
Anemia of prematurity
Hyperbilirubinemia
Cardiovascular defects
Hypocalcemia
Hypothermia

the FIO_2 causes severe pulmonary vasoconstriction. This may alter regional V/Q ratios or increase right-to-left shunting. Under these conditions, the PaO_2 would drop out of proportion to the reduction in FIO_2. Flip-flop can usually be prevented by changing the FIO_2s in small, as opposed to large, increments.

Despite these hazards, O_2 must never be kept from an infant in need. In order to maintain an acceptable PaO_2 in some sick babies, a dangerously high FIO_2 may at times be needed.

Safe levels

Unfortunately, there is no firm agreement as to the safe upper limit for either FIO_2 or PaO_2. In general, most clinicians aim to keep the FIO_2 below 0.50 when possible. In terms of blood levels, keeping the PaO_2 between 60 and 80 torr or the SaO_2 between 87% and 92% appears to minimize risk.[61-63] Conditions such as persistent fetal circulation may require higher PO_2s.

Methods of administration

Oxygen can be given to infants via mask, cannula, catheter, isolette, or oxyhood. Table 35-9 compares the advantages and disadvantages of these standard delivery methods.[30]

Alternative O_2 delivery systems for special situations have also been developed. These include systems for post-anesthesia recovery[64] and home care of tracheostomized infants.[65]

As with adults, the mask is the device of choice in emergencies. Masks are also useful during infant transport or when a baby must be removed from an O_2 enclosure for special procedures. However, masks are poorly tolerated by infants and toddlers. In addition, masks can easily cause pressure necrosis when applied to delicate neonatal skin.

The oxyhood is better tolerated by infants, and is the only method capable of delivering a precise FIO_2. This makes it the device of choice for controlled O_2 therapy to infants. An oxyhood can be set-up either with or without an O_2 blender. Table 35-10 compares the equipment needs and procedures for these two methods.[61]

Gas in an oxyhood system is delivered through either a heated humidifier or nebulizer. In either case, in order to ensure removal of exhaled CO_2, system flow must be at least 7 L/min.[66] Delivery of dry gas must be avoided. Dry gas damages the respiratory mucosa and increases insensible water loss. Unheated gas delivery is also contraindicated, since it causes hypothermia, with its associated problems.

If a heated jet nebulizer is used without a blending system, care must be taken to reduce tubing rainout. Excess water in the tubing increases flow resistance and FDO_2. Excessive noise levels in the hood also must be avoided, as subsequent hearing loss can occur.[67,68] In addition, oxyhoods should be changed on a regular basis to avoid nosocomial infection.[69]

Recently, microprocessor-based control of oxyhood FDO_2 has been demonstrated.[70,71] These systems adjust the FDO_2 delivered by a blender to achieve a user-set target SpO_2, usually between 92% to 95%. Alarms are actuated if the neonate's SpO_2 falls outside these predefined limits. These systems are able to achieve and maintain the targeted SpO_2 for most infants in an acceptable range. In addition, fluctuations in SpO_2 and overshoots are less common with these systems than with manual control of FDO_2.

When an infant or child needs low to moderate O_2 concentrations, either a nasal cannula or catheter can be used. Modified infant cannulas have been developed to enhance tolerance and reduce complications.[72,73]

In general, the catheter is preferred for long-term therapy, including home care.[74-76] As in adults, these nasal devices perform as low-flow systems. The FIO_2 varies with the rate and depth of breathing and the input flow.

Table 35-9   Oxygen delivery devices

Device	Advantages	Disadvantages
Mask	Ease of application	CO_2 buildup with inadequate flow; pressure necrosis; inaccurate FIO_2, difficult to fit and maintain on infant
Cannula/catheter	Good for long-term care in chronic disease; usually tolerated well	Inaccurate FIO_2; insufficient humidity; insertion difficulties with catheter
Isolette	Warmed and humidified gas; good for low oxygen levels in stable infants	Varying FIO_2; long stabilization time; risk of bacterial contamination
Oxyhood	Warmed and humidified gas at any FIO_2 when used with oxygen blender. Stable FIO_2 not interrupted by routine care of infant	Overheating can cause apnea and dehydration; underheating will cause increased oxygen consumption; inadequate flow will cause CO_2 buildup; noise may lead to hearing loss

From Aloan CA: *Respiratory care of the newborn: a clinical manual*, Philadelphia, 1987, JB Lippincott.

Table 35-10 Setup procedure for oxyhood administration

Equipment needed	Procedure
With blender	
1. Air/oxygen blender with flowmeter and nebulizer (heater if indicated)	1. Connect nebulizer to blender and set nebulizer collar at 100%. Dial blender to desired FIO_2
2. Large-bore tubing and water trap	2. Attach large-bore tubing to water trap and nebulizer and attach more tubing from the water trap to oxyhood
3. Oxyhood of appropriate size	3. Place oxyhood in Isolette or radiant warmer
4. Nebulizer	4. Turn on flow to minimum of 7 L/min (check for aerosol production—should see a mist)
	5. Analyze FIO_2
	6. Monitor temperature if nebulizer is heated.
	7. Chart on appropriate respiratory progress notes
Without blender	
5. Air and oxygen flowmeters and nebulizer	1. Connect nebulizer to air flowmeter. Set nebulize collar at 100%.
6. Bleed-in adapter and oxygen connective tubing	2. Connect oxygen connective tubing to bleed-in adapter and to nipple on oxygen/air flowmeter
7. Oxygen flowmeter nipple adapter	3. Connect bleed-in adapter to nebulizer port
8. Large bore tubing and water traps	4. Adjust air and oxygen flowmeters to desired FIO_2 ensuring that combined flow is greater than 7 L/min
	5. Attach large bore tubing to bleed-in adapter and water trap. Attach second piece from water trap to oxygen hood.
	6. Analyze FIO_2 as above; note: it will take a few minutes for desired FIO_2 concentration to stabilize
	7. Chart as above

From Koff PB, Eitzman DV, Neu J: *Neonatal and pediatric respiratory care,* St Louis, 1988, Mosby.

Nasal flows in smaller infants usually range from .25 to 1.0 L/min. Normally, this requires a calibrated low-flow metering device. When using a catheter, flow of 150 mL/kg/min provide an FIO_2 of about 0.50.[77] However, even minor changes in flow can cause large changes in delivered FIO_2.[78] In addition, high flows may irritate the nasal mucosa, cause gastric distension, and unknowingly create CPAP.[79] A rare but more serious complication of infant O_2 therapy by catheter is pneumocephalus.[80]

More precise control of nasal O_2 therapy for infants can be achieved by using a blender. With this setup, the clinician can alter both the flow and FDO_2. In addition, this approach helps avoid the excessive and abrupt changes in FIO_2 that are so poorly tolerated by infants with chronic lung disease.[78]

Monitoring

Due to the unique hazards of O_2 therapy in infants and children, both FDO_2 and oxygen blood levels must be carefully monitored.[81]

FDO_2. In infants, FDO_2 should be analyzed continuously, with a system check at least every 4 hours.[51] If continuous monitoring is not feasible, the FDO_2 must be sampled and confirmed at least every 2 hours with a properly calibrated O_2 analyzer.[63] It is especially important to analyze the FDO_2 when using a blender, since these devices are notoriously inaccurate.[82,83]

PaO_2, $PTCO_2$, and SpO_2. Blood oxygen levels can be assessed via both invasive and noninvasive methods. Invasive measurement of actual blood PO_2 is still the standard for comparison. Invasive methods include intermittent sampling via arterial puncture or arterial/umbilical lines.

Unfortunately, vascular puncture in newborns affects the accuracy of results, causing a fall in both $PaCO_2$ and PaO_2.[84] Although use of indwelling arterial/umbilical lines overcomes this problem, these approaches are fraught with serious complications.[85] In addition, intermittent sampling fails to identify many critical events, making evaluation of an infant's course incomplete and, at times, incorrect.[86,87] Continuous assessment by intravascular optodes is now being used in children, but not yet with infants (see Chapter 17).

Noninvasive methods include transcutaneous PO_2 electrodes and pulse oximetry (see Chapter 17 for technical details). Both these methods provide continuous data.

Measurement of transcutaneous PO_2 ($PTCO_2$) via PO_2 electrode is a reliable method for assessing blood oxygenation in infants and children with good tissue perfusion.[88,89] When tissue perfusion is low, the $PTCO_2$ tends to underestimate the actual PaO_2s (see the box on page 1014).[33,87]

Continuous $PTCO_2$ monitoring can also help avoid

Conditions causing inaccurately low PtcO$_2$ readings in neonates

- Shock
- Hypothermia
- Anemia
- Peripheral edema
- Pulmonary vasodilators (e.g., tolazoline)
- Hyperoxia (PaO$_2$ > 100 torr)
- Severe acidosis
- Chronic lung disease (e.g., BPD)

Situations in which continuous pulse oximetry is indicated

- Mechanical ventilation
- Artificial airways
- Continuous oxygen therapy
- Invasive procedures
- Signs or symptoms of respiratory distress
- Transport of critically ill
- Central or obstructive apnea
- Delivery room resuscitation

---

retinopathy in neonates weighing 1,000 g or more.[90] In addition, dual PtcO$_2$ monitoring (right shoulder, abdomen) can help detect and quantify ductal shunting.[91] With significant shunting through the ductus arteriosus, the right shoulder (preductal) PtcO$_2$ is higher than the post-ductal measure (abdomen). Continuous PtcO$_2$ monitoring can also be used to assess changes in perfusion.[33] Last, if it reduces the frequency of invasive sampling, PtcO$_2$ monitoring can lower intensive care costs.[92]

The calibrated PO$_2$ electrode is usually placed on a fleshy portion of the chest, abdomen, inner thigh, or lower back using an adhesive ring. Inaccurate results may occur if the electrode is placed over poorly perfused sites, such as distal extremities, pressure points, or boney prominences.[93] The electrode is heated to 43°C to 44°C. Heating aids gaseous diffusion through the skin and causes vasodilation. Vasodilation speeds blood flow through the capillaries (arterialization).

An improper electrode temperature may cause false readings. However, even normal heating can cause skin blistering, especially in low birth weight infants.[93] For this reason, electrode position should be changed every 2 to 4 hours.

After temperature equilibration (10 to 20 minutes), the initial PtcO$_2$ reading should be compared to a concurrent measure of PaO$_2$. Thereafter, agreement between the PtcO$_2$ and PaO$_2$ should be reevaluated whenever a major change in the patient's clinical state occurs.[93]

Hemoglobin saturations measured by pulse oximetry (SpO$_2$) correlate well with measured SaO$_2$ and PaO$_2$ values in neonates with chronic lung disease and prolonged oxygen dependence. However, in infants with acute cardiorespiratory problems, pulse oximetry is less useful in reflecting changes in the arterial blood.[94] Specifically, the SpO$_2$ tends to overestimate SaO$_2$ when SaO$_2$ decreases.[95] Nonetheless, continuous pulse oximetry can warn of clinical deterioration.[94] In addition, continuous pulse oximetry can be used to detect hyperoxemia and thus help avoid ROP.[96] The accompanying box lists situations in which continuous pulse oximetry may be indicated.[87,97]

As with transcutaneous monitoring, pulse oximeter readings initially should be validated by comparison to actual invasive SaO$_2$ measures. Reevaluation should occur whenever the patient's clinical status changes.[98]

Positioning and bronchial hygiene therapy

As with adults, therapeutic positioning and bronchial hygiene therapy can be applied to infants and children.[30,99] However, variations in method are required to account for differences in anatomy, physiology, and pathophysiology.[100]

Therapeutic positioning

As in adults, the body position assumed by sick infants and children affects both gas exchange and the mechanics of breathing. Positioning is a simple and safe therapeutic maneuver that has prompt and proven benefits.

In premature infants, elevated respiratory workloads and musculoskeletal immaturity may predispose to respiratory failure. Likewise, in infants with respiratory insufficiency due to conditions like respiratory distress syndrome or bronchopulmonary dysplasia, mechanical changes in the lung increase the work of breathing. Placement of these patients in prone and elevated positions can improve oxygenation, decrease respiratory rate, and decreased asynchronous breathing.[101-105]

Improved oxygenation in the prone and elevated positions is probably due to enhanced V/Q ratios. Decreases in respiratory rate most likely occur because the FRC increases when abdominal stress on the diaphragm is reduced. Likewise, improvements in thoracoabdominal synchrony in the prone position are probably due to changes in the diaphragm's position against the anterior rib cage wall, and an increase in passive tension of the rib cage muscles.[105] Although these positional changes affect oxygenation, there is no impact on carbon dioxide removal.[106] The effect of positioning on older infants and children is less consistent and probably should be evaluated on an individual basis.[107] In addition, prone positioning is associated with a higher risk of sudden infant death syndrome (SIDS) in nonhospitalized infants during the first 6 months of life.[108]

Lateral or side-lying positions have no major impact on gas exchange in infants with bilateral lung disease.[109,110] However, use of the side-lying position is an important therapy for unilateral lung disorders in infants, especially pulmonary interstitial emphysema.[111-115] In these cases, oxygenation improves when the good lung is uppermost—the reverse of the situation in adults. This reversal of the adult pattern is most likely due to differences between infants and adults in lung mechanics and diaphragmatic function.[113]

Bronchial hygiene therapy

Bronchial hygiene methods applicable to infants and children include postural drainage, percussion and vibration, directed coughing, and positive expiratory pressure (PEP) therapy.

Indications. Bronchial hygiene therapy is indicated when excessive secretions impair pulmonary function.[116] Due to their smaller airways, increased secretions are a major problem for infants and small children.[100]

Among infants, increased secretions are common in meconium aspiration, pneumonia, bronchopulmonary dysplasia, and atelectasis.[117] In addition, many infants have impaired cough reflexes due to muscle weakness or endotracheal intubation.[118] In these patients, properly performed bronchial hygiene therapy can help remove secretions and improve oxygenation.[119-121]

In children, increased secretions occur in cystic fibrosis, bronchiectasis, and pneumonia. Bronchial hygiene therapy can also be valuable in the initial management of aspirated foreign bodies.[122] Bronchial hygiene therapy is probably not of value in bronchiolitis,[118,123] or in *preventing* postoperative atelectasis.[124]

Methods. For postural drainage and percussion, infants and small children are best managed by holding them on one's lap or shoulder. This provides more comfort and security for the child, and helps achieve the treatment objectives.

As shown in Figure 35-18, on page 1016 anatomic differences in the structure of the tracheobronchial tree in infants and children require minor modifications in both positioning and percussion sites.[125]

Because even minor impact below the rib margins can damage abdominal viscera, the RCP must be extremely careful when percussion and vibration is applied. This potential problem is greatest in small infants, due to the relative size of the abdominal contents. Also for this reason, cupped hands or adult mechanical percussors cannot be used in infants. Tenting of the middle three fingers of the hand may suffice for larger infants and small children. For tiny infants and neonates, small percussion cups can be purchased. Likewise, special downsized mechanical vibrators are available for small infants.

Unlike adults, infants and small children cannot cough on command. For this reason, secretions mobilized with postural drainage and percussion must be cleared by suctioning. In some situations, these techniques will not be effective, and therapeutic bronchoscopy may be needed.

For larger children with excessive secretions, combining directed coughing with postural drainage and percussion may help improve clearance.[126] As an alternative to traditional percussion and vibration, high frequency oscillations, applied either externally[127] or internally,[128] may help mobilize mucous. Likewise, positive expiratory pressure (PEP) therapy by mask has shown promise as an aid to secretion clearance, especially in cystic fibrosis patients.[129,130] Last, the beneficial effects of postural drainage and percussion can probably be enhanced if preceded by aerosol inhalation of an adrenergic bronchodilator and a mucolytic.[131] Chapter 28 provided more details on these bronchial hygiene methods.

Complications. Complications of bronchial hygiene therapy in infants and children are similar to those in adults (see Chapter 28). Infants are more prone to regurgitation (and possible aspiration), especially if postural drainage is done soon after feeding. This problem can be avoided if a nasogastric tube is already in place.

Other potential complications of percussion and drainage in infants include rib fractures,[132] subperiosteal hemorrhages,[133] and an increased risk of severe (grade III/IV) intraventricular hemorrhage.[134]

Of additional concern is the rise in intracranial pressure (ICP) caused by any head-down position.[135,136] Increases in ICP due to head-down positions are especially harmful to infants at risk for intraventricular hemorrhage or cerebral edema. For this reason, head-down positions are contraindicated in infants and any child for whom ICP levels are a concern. Head-down positions also are poorly tolerated by children with status asthmaticus or congestive heart failure.

Monitoring. Given the instability of most critically ill infants and children, both a thorough initial assessment and ongoing patient evaluation during and after treatment are mandatory. Traditional assessment of the vital signs, blood pressure, color, and breath sounds before, during, and after treatment should be supplemented with pulse oximetry monitoring, especially if hypoxemia is suspected.[116] If an ICP monitoring system is in use, ICP also should be assessed.

Of particular concern is the fact that head-down positions cause hypoxemia in many critically ill infants and children.[104,137,138] To offset hypoxemia in such patients, the FIO_2 may need to be raised during therapy. The RCP must always assure that the SpO_2 is restored to pretreatment levels before ending therapy and leaving the patient.

Humidity and aerosol therapy

Humidity and aerosol therapy techniques for infants and children are generally similar to those used with adults. Key differences in humidity therapy involve both physiology and equipment application.[139] Aerosol therapy differs from adult approaches mainly in regard to drug dosing and delivery methods.[140]

Humidity therapy

Humidification of inspired gases delivered to infants and children is based on the same basic principles as in adults (Chapter 25). In addition, high ambient humidity levels decrease evaporative heat and water loss, which is especially important in managing premature infants.[141] High ambient humidity can be provided to the entire nursery room, or just inside infant enclosures or incubators. High ambient humidity is not as critical for infants born after 30 weeks gestation.[142]

Due to problems with thermoregulation in newborn infants, adjustment and monitoring of inspired gas temperature is more critical, especially in enclosures. Too high a gas temperature can result in hyperpyrexia and overhydration. Too low a temperature can cause hypothermia and increased oxygen consumption. In addition, low airway temperatures in mechanically ventilated low-birth-weight infants have been associated with an increased incidence of pneumothorax and chronic lung disease.[143]

Because nasal oxygen flows used in older infants and children are usually low, humidification is generally not needed when this approach is used. When the upper airway is bypassed, however, supplemental

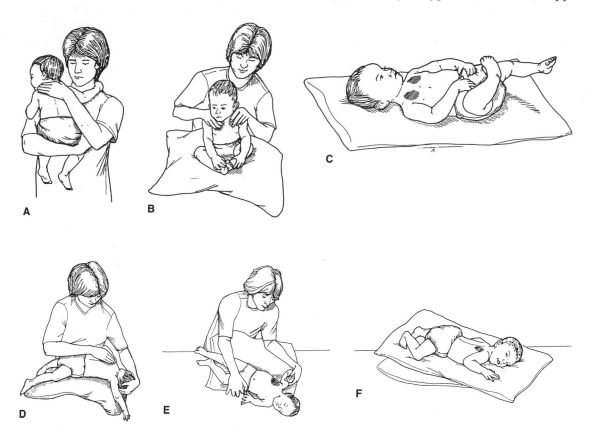

Fig. 35–18 Postural drainage and percussion positions for infant and child. Angles of drainage for infant are not as obtuse as those for child. **A,** Posterior segments of right and left upper lobes are drained with patient in upright position at 30-degree angle forward. Percuss over upper posterior thorax. **B,** Apical segments of right and left upper lobes are drained with patient in upright position, leaning forward 30 degrees. Percuss over area between clavicle and tip of scapula on each side. **C,** Anterior segments of right and left upper lobes are drained with patient in flat, supine position. Percuss anterior side of chest directly under clavicles to around nipple area (shaded). Avoid direct pressure on sternum. **D,** Right and left lateral basal segments of lower lobes are drained at 30 degrees Trendelenburg. Patient lies on appropriate side, rotated 30 degrees forward. Percuss over uppermost portions of lower ribs. **E,** Right and left anterior basal segments of lower lobes are drained at 30 degrees Trendelenburg. Patient lies on appropriate side with 20 degree turn backward. Percuss above anterior lower margin of ribs. **F,** Right and left superior segments of lower lobes are drained at 15 degrees Trendelenburg, with patient in prone position. Percuss below scapula in midback area. (From Levin DL, Morriss FC, Moore GC, editors: *A practical guide to pediatric intensive care*, ed 2, St Louis, 1984, Mosby.)

humidification must be provided. In these cases, the ANSI minimum of 30 mg/L also is applied to infants and children. This usually means using either a heated humidifier or nebulizer. Due to potential problems with infection and water balance, continuous nebulization is usually avoided in infants.

Humidification of inspired gases for infants and children receiving mechanical ventilation is usually provided by a servo-controlled heated wick humidifier. Ideal design features for these systems include: (1) minimal internal volume and constant water level (to decrease compressed volume loss), (2) closed, continuous feed water supply (to avoid contamination), (3) detachable hot plate heating (to make changes easily), and (4) distal airway temperature sensor and high/low alarms (for safety).

Newer membrane humidification systems perform as well or better than traditional wick humidifiers.[144] In membrane humidifiers, a hydrophobic membrane covers a heated water chamber. When dry gas enters the humidifier, molecular water readily diffuses across the membrane, while the liquid water stays behind.

Common problems with humidifier systems include condensation, inadequate humidification,[145] and variable humidification.[146] Condensation can be prevented by using heated wire circuits.[147] However, heated wire circuits can malfunction, especially when the temperature sensor is improperly placed.[148,149] As an alternative, the inspiratory side of the circuit can be insulated, but this only reduces condensation by about 15%.[146]

Inadequate and variable humidification are usually the result of improper placement of the temperature sensors. Inadequate humidification can occur in nonheated circuits when the humidifier temperature probe is placed too far upstream from the airway connector. This causes the humidifier servocontroller to cycle off prematurely, resulting in a lower than desired airway temperature.

Variable humidification problems occur mainly when ventilator circuits must pass through a room, then into a warmed enclosure. As a general rule, in incubators set to high temperatures (33° C to 35° C), inspired gas humidity is linearly related to humidifier temperature. In cooler incubators (31° C to 33° C), inspired humidity levels tends to vary inversely with humidifier temperature. This latter observation is due to the increased circuit condensation seen in cooler incubators.[146]

Use of heated wire circuits in conjunction with warmed enclosures presents a slightly different problem. As shown in Figure 35-19, the temperature of the humidifier, heated circuit, room, and incubator all influence the relative humidity of the gas delivered to the infant's airway. Proper placement of the heated circuit temperature probe immediately outside the incubator (with proper settings for the humidifier and circuit) provides the desired results.[147]

As an alternative to heated humidification systems, hygroscopic condenser humidifiers (HCH) have been developed and tested with neonates receiving mechanical ventilation.[150] With tidal volumes between 10 and 50 mL, and at ambient temperatures of 24° C and 38° C, these units meet or exceed the ANSI minimum of 30 mg/L, even with airway leaks up to 15% of the delivered volume. Unlike their use in adults, however, no guidelines exist for HCH application to infants. Until guidelines are developed, due caution should be used in applying HCH or HME devices to infants.

High-frequency jet ventilation (HFJV) presents a unique problem. Early reports in the literature indicated a high incidence of tracheal obstruction from thickened secretions with prolonged HFJV. Subsequently, actual tissue damage, called *necrotizing tracheobronchitis,* also was observed. These findings have been attributed to both inadequate humidification and shear force damage to tracheal tissues. Recent research indicates both factors are involved. Based on this research, tracheal erosion can be minimized if the HFJV device delivers heated, humidified gases through a jet centered in and located proximal to the endotracheal tube tip.[151]

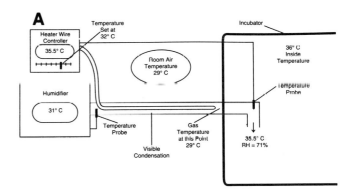

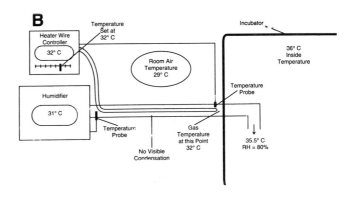

Fig. 35-19 Illustration of the problem encountered with heated wire circuit inside incubator. **(A),** When temperature probe is inside incubator with set temperature higher than humidifier, condensation forms in circuit and relative humidity of inspired gas drops. **(B),** Placing probe just outside incubator resolves problem. From: Chatburn RL: Principles and practice of neonatal and pediatric mechanical ventilation, *Respircare* 36(6):569-593, 1991.

Aerosol drug therapy

Drug action in infants and children differs significantly from that in adults. Differences include missing enzyme systems, immature receptors, variable GI absorption, and altered volume of distribution.[140] Dosing is thus imprecise and systemic effects hard to predict. For these reasons, topical administration via aerosol is a good alternative to systemic routes, especially for pulmonary disorders. The aerosol route is also safer and more comfortable than oral and parenteral approaches.

Table 35-11   Dosage guidelines for nebulized solutions for neonates, infants and children

Drug	Dosage
Sympathomimetic bronchodilators	
Racemic epinephrine	0.05 mL/kg of 2.25% solution; not more frequently than q2 maximum dose 0.5 mL
Isoproterenol	0.025 mL of 1:200 solution or 0.01 mL/kg maximum = 0.05 mL; tid, qid
Isoetharine	0.25–0.5 mL of 1% solution; q4h
Metaproterenol	0.2–0.3 mL of 5% solution; q4h 0.01 mL/kg of 5% solution for 3–6 year olds
Albuterol	0.01–0.03 mL/kg of 0.5% solution maximum = 0.5 mL; tid, qid
Bitolterol	MDI only
Pirbuterol	MDI only
Anticholinergic bronchodilators	
Atropine sulfate	0.05 mg/kg, maximum = 1 mg
Ipratropium	MDI only
Mucolytic agents	
Acetylcysteine	3–5 mL of 10 or 20% solution; tid, qid
Corticosteroids	
Dexamethasone	MDI only
Beclomethasone	MDI only
Flunisolide	MDI only
Triamcinolone	MDI only
Antiasthmatics	
Cromolyn sodium	< 2 years, 20 mg qid
Nedocromil	MDI only
Antiinfectives	
Ribavirin	6 g/300 mL (2%), 12–18 h/day
Pentamidine	< 5 years, 300 mg/month by Respirgard*

*JAMA 1991; 265:1637–1644.

From Rau JL: Delivery of aerosolized drugs to neonatal and pediatric patients, *Respir Care* 36(6):514–542, 1991.

Drug dosages. Table 35-11 lists dosage guidelines for administration of aerosolized drugs to infants and children.[140] With the exception of ribavirin and metaproteronol, no actual infant or child doses have been set by clinical studies. Instead, these doses are based on manufacturers' recommendations.

Delivery systems. Small volume jet nebulizers (SVN), metered dose inhalers (MDI), and dry powder inhalers (DPI) can be used to deliver aerosolized drugs to infants and children. Table 35-12 lists guidelines for using these devices among these age groups.[140]

A particular problem is aerosol drug administration to intubated infants and children. Baffling caused by the small ET tubes in these patients prevents most of the drug from entering the lungs. In fact, less than 1% pulmonary deposition occurs in these patients, regardless of delivery system.[140] In addition, unless proper adjustments are made, nebulizer flows can alter both the volumes and pressures delivered to patients. Guidelines to assure safe and effective aerosol drug delivery to intubated infants and children receiving ventilatory support using a small volume nebulizer (SVN) appears in the accompanying box.[152]

Airway management

Due to the significant anatomical differences between the neonate and adult, the airway management methods in infants are somewhat unique. Specifically, both equipment and technique must be individually tailored to each infant, according to his or her size, weight, and postpartum age.[153-155]

Equipment

A wide selection of infant and pediatric sized masks, oral airways, suction catheters, laryngoscope blades, and endotracheal tubes is needed to account for variations in patient age and weight. Table 35-13 provides recommendations regarding endotracheal tube and suction catheter sizes for infants and children.[153,156]

Table 35-12   Age guidelines for modes of aerosol drug delivery

Mode*	Minimum age
SVN	Neonate (0-1 month)
MDI	7 years
—with spacer	3 years
—with spacer and mask	Infant (1-12 months)
—with ETT	Neonate
DPI	3-4 years

From Rau JL: Delivery of aerosolized drugs to neonatal and pediatric patients, *Respir Care* 36(6):514–542, 1991.
SVN = small volume nebulizer; MDI = metered dose inhaler; ETT = endotracheal tube; DPI = dry powder inhaler.

<table>
<tr><td colspan="2">

Guidelines for aerosol drug
delivery via small volume
nebulizer to intubated infants
and children receiving
ventilatory support
</td></tr>
</table>

- Position SVN in inspiratory limb of ventilator circuit 18 inches upstream from the patient Y-piece
- Dilute drug with 4 mL physiologic saline (0.9%)
- Set nebulizer flow to 6 to 8 L/min
- Adjust ventilator flow to maintain pretreatment setting
- Tap sides of nebulizer to minimize dead volume
- Continue treatment until no aerosol is produced
- Remove equipment and be sure to return ventilator to pretreatment setting
- Monitor patient for side effects

From: Kacmarek RM, Hess D: The interface between patient and aerosol generator, *Respir Care* 36(9):952-976, 1991.

Using oral airways and masks

When using an oral airway in infants, a Guedel type, with a central passageway, is probably the best choice. This is because the infant tongue can easily occlude the lateral slots of other designs, thereby worsening the obstruction. When using a mask on an infant, the RCP should be careful not to overextend the neck, as this may worsen airway obstruction.

Furthermore, one should never raise the mandible forcefully to close the mouth, as sometimes done with adults. In infants, this maneuver will press the tongue up against the soft palate and occlude the nasopharynx. To establish a good airway in neonates, one must often gently advance the jaw and kept the mouth open beneath the mask.

Endotracheal intubation

Endotracheal intubation is a generally safe method of airway management in infants and children, even when used for extended periods.[157] Unique complications and hazards associated with intubation in these age groups are listed in the box on page 1020. The overall complication rate for endotracheal intubation is about 8%, with accidental extubation and tube blockage being the most frequent problems.[159]

As listed in Table 35-13, proper ET tube size and depth of insertion can be estimated by the infant's age or height. If the tube is too small, a large leak may result, making positive pressure ventilation ineffective. Small tubes also have high flow resistance, increasing the spontaneous work of breathing.[165]

On the other hand, too large a tube can cause mucosal and laryngeal damage. Too large a tube may cause inward sloughing of the laryngeal membranes after extubation, resulting in severe upper airway obstruction. To avoid these problems in infants, the ratio of tube size (in mm) divided by the patient's gestational age in weeks should be less than 0.1.[162] As

Table 35-13   Endotracheal tube and suction catheter sizes for infants and children

Age or weight	ET tube ID (mm)	Tube length (cm) oral	Tube length (cm) nasal	Suction cath (F)
NEWBORN				
Less than 1000 g	2.5	9-11	11-12	5
1000 to 2000 g	3.0	9-11	11-12	6
2000 to 3000 g	3.5	10-12	12-14	6
More than 3000 g	4.0	11-12	13-14	8
CHILDREN				
6 months	3.0-4.0	11-12	12-14	6-8
18 months	3.5-4.5	11-13	13-15	8
2 years	4.0-5.0	12-14	14-16	8-10
3 years	4.5-5.0	12-14	14-16	8-10
4 years	4.5-5.5	13-15	15-17	8-10
5 years	4.5-5.5	13-15	15-17	8-10
6 years	5.5-6.0	14-16	16-18	10
8 years	6.0-6.5	15-17	17-19	10
12 years	6.0-7.0	17-19	19-21	10
16 years	6.5-7.5	19-21	21-23	10-12

Estimating formula for tube internal diameter (ID) in mm:
(1) Tube ID = (Age + 16)/4
(2) Tube ID = Height(cm)/20
Estimating formula for tube length (cm):
(1) Oral: 12 + (Age/2)
(2) Nasal: 15 + (Age/2)

**Complications and hazards of
endotracheal intubation in
infants and children**

- Palatal grooving (neonates)[158]
- Incisal enamel hypoplasia (neonates)[158]
- Accidental extubation[159,160]
- Tube blockage[159]
- Tracheal stenosis[161,162]
- Esophageal perforation[163]
- Tracheal perforation[164]

---

an example, for an infant born at 35 weeks gestation, the ET tube should be smaller than 35 × 0.1, or 3.5 mm (internal diameter).

Most infant ET tubes are uncuffed. Cuffless tubes are used because cuffs can quickly erode the soft tracheal walls of infants. However, without a cuff, the incidence of aspiration in intubated infants is high.[166]

Even without cuffs, infant ET tubes are very small, and can be very easily kinked or obstructed. For these reasons, proper head positioning, avoidance of cumbersome connecting apparatus, and extreme care in suctioning to avoid mucous plugs becomes very important.[167]

Due to the relative ease and safety of oral insertion, oral intubation is the preferred route for neonates requiring prolonged ventilatory support.[168] Postintubation problems with tube position, infection, and extubation (including atelectasis and stridor) are about the same for the oral and nasal routes.[168]

Because the tongue is large and the epiglottis high, most RCPs find the Miller (straight) laryngoscope blade best for intubating infants. Since even small amounts of edema can cause serious airway obstruction in infants, great care must be taken to avoid mucosal trauma during intubation. The distance between the cords and carina is much smaller in infants, making endobronchial intubation more likely.[169] In addition, because small tube movement can result in either bronchial insertion or extubation,[170,171] the RCP must confirm tube placement after intubation.

Because breath sounds are so difficult to assess in infants and small children, other methods to initially determine proper tube position must be used. Disposable colorimetric end-tidal CO_2 detectors can accurately identify proper tube position in children and infants with spontaneous circulation who weigh more than 2 kg, even with uncuffed tubes.[172,173] Once positioning in the lungs is established, ET tube placement should be confirmed by X-ray. Alternatively, tube position in neonates can be confirmed by ultrasonography.[174] Optimal ET tube tip position by sonography is 1 cm above the aortic arch.[175]

Once proper ET tube position is assured, the tube must be carefully stabilized. Factors associated with accidental extubation of infants include patient agita-

tion, suctioning, head-turning, chest physiotherapy, loose tape, too short a tube between lip and adapter, weighing, and endotracheal tube taping.[176] Figure 35-20 demonstrates a traditional approach to stabilization of an oral endotracheal tube using tape and tincture of Benzoin.

Suctioning

Properly performed nasopharyngeal and tracheal suctioning can help minimize aspiration, prevent ET tube occlusion, and lower airway resistance in infants and children.[33,177] Suctioning, however, is a hazardous procedure. As with adults, complications are many and frequent. The accompanying box lists the common complications and hazards associated with tracheal suctioning of infants and children.[33,178-186]

Of special concern in small infants are the cardiovascular and cerebrovascular changes that occur with suctioning. Many of these effects are independent of changes in oxygenation and ventilation.[178] In addition, these vascular effects may be especially harmful for the preterm infant at risk for intraventricular hemorrhage.[180]

For these reasons, tracheal suctioning of preterm infants and neonates should only be performed when clinical signs indicate a need.[180] Clinical signs indicating a need for suctioning of infants and children

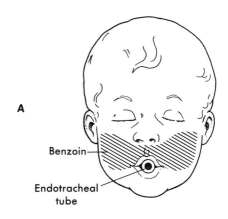

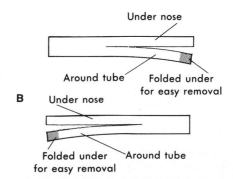

Fig. 35-20 Method for taping endotracheal tube. **A,** Benzoin is applied to cheeks and upper lip. Skin bond cement may also be used. **B,** Split tape is applied. (From Koff PB, Eitzman DV, Neu J: *Neonatal and pediatric respiratory care,* St Louis, 1988, Mosby.)

Complications and hazards of tracheal suctioning in infants and small children

- Infection[33]
- Accidental extubation[176]
- Atelectasis[33]
- Increased blood pressure[178-181]
- Increased intracranial pressure[178,180]
- Cerebral vasodilation/increased blood volume[182]
- Arterial hypoxemia[178,181,183]
- Cerebral hypoxemia[182,184]
- Hypercapnia[178]
- Bradycardia[179,181]
- Pneumothorax[185,186]
- Mucosal damage[33]

---

include abnormal breath sounds (course crackles or rhonchi), visible secretions at the ET tube, and evidence of respiratory distress.[33]

Equipment. Oral and pharyngeal suctioning of infants is best done with a bulb syringe. Either a DeLee trap or a mechanical vacuum source with catheter may be used for nasopharyngeal and nasotracheal suctioning of neonates. Equipment for suctioning larger infants and children is the same as for adults (refer to Chapter 22), with appropriate modifications in vacuum pressure and catheter size.[99] Recommended suction pressures for neonates range from -60 to -80 mmHg although copious, and thick secretions may require lower pressures. With large infants and children, pressures in the 80 to 100 mmHg range are generally safe and effective. Catheter sizes are chosen according to the age of the patient and, where applicable, the size of the tracheal airway (refer to Table 35-13).

Procedure like

Nasopharyngeal and nasotracheal suctioning in infants and children is similar to the adult procedure. Key exceptions are outlined below.

To avoid hypoxemia, infants and children should be preoxygenated and hyperinflated prior to suctioning. In infants less than 6 months old, preoxygenation with 100% oxygen should be avoided, due to the risk of retinopathies.[33,99] Instead, most clinicians recommend raising the FIO_2 by 10% to 15% for at least 1 minute prior to suctioning.[33] This increase in FIO_2 is usually sufficient to prevent arterial and cerebral hypoxemia in these patients.[182] Older children can receive 100% oxygen.[183]

Hyperinflation of infants should always be done with an appropriate sized bag-valve-mask device with airway pressure manometer.[187] The pressure used should be carefully monitored and never exceed that used for mechanical ventilation by more than 25%.

Since desaturation in the arterial and cerebral circulations begins within 5 seconds of the onset of suctioning,[182] hypoxemia also can be minimized by limiting the duration of suctioning to 5 seconds or less. Other techniques for averting hypoxemia include use of endotracheal tube adaptors that allow preoxygenation and suctioning without disconnection of the ventilator,[188-190] catheters that alternately deliver oxygen or suction,[191] and closed tracheal suction systems.[192]

Given an infant's small lung volume and airway size, suctioning can quickly cause atelectasis unless close attention is paid to detail. Catheter insertion to the point of resistance without partial withdrawal can obstruct a distal airway and quickly collapse that lobe or segment. Although rare, deep endotracheal suction in infants and children can also cause pneumothorax.[186] For these reasons, the RCP should limit catheter insertion in infants and children to just beyond the tip of the ET tube.[30,33] To do so, one first must measure the ET tube length (including adapter). This length is then recorded for the patient and used as the maximum catheter insertion distance ($\pm$ 1 cm).

If deep suctioning is deemed necessary in neonates, turning the head aids passage of the catheter into the contralateral bronchus.[193-195] Thus, to increase the likelihood of left bronchial insertion, the head should be turned to the right. Curved tip catheters also can help assure selective bronchial insertion in infants.[194]

Saline irrigation or lavage prior to suctioning is well tolerated by infants and children, and may actually improve airway resistance in neonates with meconium aspiration.[196,197] For infants, lavage volume should be no more than 0.25 to 0.5 mL.[196] In larger infants and children, 0.5 to 3.0 ml of saline may be used.

Because the cardiovascular and cerebrovascular effects of suctioning occur separate from changes in oxygenation, none of the methods just described will limit these serious hazards. Instead, sedation and muscle paralysis (with pancuronium) can be used to lessen the vascular response to suctioning that occurs in infants.[198,199]

Perhaps the simplest and best way to minimize the harmful effects of suctioning is to decrease its frequency. A study conducted among low birthweight infants requiring ventilatory support for RDS showed no significant differences in respiratory outcomes when comparing 12-hourly and 6-hourly suction regimens.[200] Based on these results, infrequent suctioning is probably the safest approach to airway management of the intubated RDS infant.

Monitoring

Given the many hazards of suctioning, careful monitoring is a must. Assessment of the patient's respiratory rate, color, pulse, and blood pressure should be supplemented with either continuous transcutaneous PO_2 or SpO_2 monitoring, especially if the patient's oxygenation status is marginal or unstable.[201] Where available, the RCP should also observe the ECG on the bedside monitor, as cardiac arrhythmias—particularly bradycardia—represent common complications of suctioning neonates.[202]

Upon completion of the suctioning procedure, the RCP must assure that the patient is stable and adequately ventilated. Last, careful auscultation should be conducted to verify proper ET tube placement, since accidental extubation or endobronchial intubation are so common when suctioning small infants.

Neonatal resuscitation

Resuscitation procedures for infants and children were detailed in Chapter 23. Given the increasing frequency of RCP involvement in the delivery room, a separate discussion of newborn resuscitation is in order.

Procedures for resuscitation of the newborn have been established by the American Academy of Pediatrics.[203] Figure 35-21 outlines the basic protocol. As with adult crash carts, neonatal resuscitation equipment should be checked at least every shift.[33,203]

Immediately after delivery, efforts must be made to keep the infant warm. Failure to ensure proper body temperature may impair all subsequent resuscitation efforts.[203] Once the infant is warmed, the mouth and nose are suctioned with either a bulb syringe or De Lee catheter. If meconium is visible in the larynx, the tracheal should also be suctioned, ideally through an endotracheal tube. Also at this time, tactile stimulation is provided.

If the infant is not breathing or the heart rate is below 100/min, positive pressure ventilation (PPV) with 100% oxygen is provided with a bag-valve-mask device. After application of PPV, the heart rate is reassessed. If the heart rate is below 60/min, chest compressions are begun and PPV maintained. If after 30 seconds the heart rate is still below 80/min, appropriate medications are given. If the heart rate is rising and exceeds 80/min, PPV continues without compressions. When the heart exceeds 100/min, one looks for spontaneous respiratory efforts. If spontaneous respirations appear, PPV is stopped and the infant evaluated for color. If central cyanosis is present, supplemental oxygen is given. Otherwise the patient is carefully observed and monitored.

CONTINUOUS POSITIVE AIRWAY PRESSURE (CPAP)

The primary indication for CPAP in infants is the same as for adults. Specifically, CPAP is indicated when arterial oxygenation is inadequate despite a high FIO_2.[204-207] For infants, this means a PaO_2 less than 50 torr while breathing an $FIO_2 \geq 0.50$, or an a/A ratio less than 0.2 to 0.4.

As with adults, CPAP increases the FRC and recruits additional alveoli for gas exchange. In infants prone to alveolar collapse, CPAP usually decreases right-to-left shunting. However, unlike the adult response, infant CPAP can decrease lung compliance, especially in patients with respiratory distress syn-

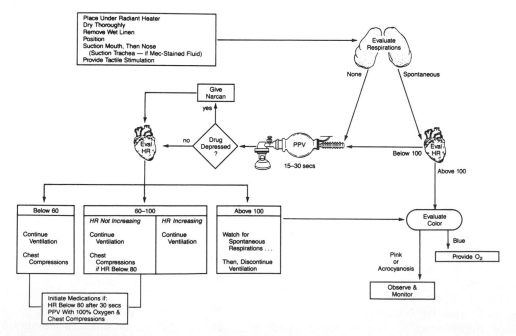

Fig. 35-21 Protocol for resuscitation of the newborn. (Reproduced with permission. Textbook of Neonatal resuscitation,© 1987, 1990, American Heart Association.)

drome. This paradoxical response is probably due to the overdistention of normal lung units.[47]

Since a fall in compliance increases the work of breathing, CPAP should be used cautiously in infants with CO_2 retention. The exception is infants with small airways obstruction, such as meconium aspiration. In these cases, low levels of CPAP can decrease airway resistance and actually improve minute ventilation, thereby lowering the $PaCO_2$.[47] Conversely, too much CPAP applied to infants with meconium aspiration may only worsen hyperinflation and air-trapping.

Since CPAP is most successful when started early in hypoxemic respiratory disorders, many centers begin treatment as soon as an infant shows clear signs of respiratory distress. Earlier prophylactic application is of no value.[208] Signs of respiratory distress indicating a need for CPAP are summarized in the accompanying box.[207,209]

In addition to its therapeutic use, infant CPAP can also be used for supportive purposes. Supportive indications for CPAP include apnea, tracheobronchial malacia, and small airways obstruction.

Methods of administration

Most modern infant CPAP systems consist of a continuous flow "Y" circuit with a threshold resistor on the expiratory limb.[210] Threshold resistors used to create CPAP include spring loaded disks, gravity weighted valves, and electronic solenoids. In addition, most infant ventilators are CPAP-capable. These systems take advantage of the built-in FIO_2 control, humidification, and alarm features of these ventilators. Regardless of design or features, CPAP systems should impose as little additional work of breathing on the infant as possible.[211,212]

The major problem with infant CPAP is not how to create the pressure, but how to apply it to the airway. The four major ways to apply CPAP include: (1) nasal prongs, (2) endotracheal tubes, (3) nasopharyngeal tubes, and (4) face masks. Table 35-14 compares and contrasts these modes of CPAP application in regard to their various design features.[30] Due to the many problems with mask application, this approach is seldom used. Today, most CPAP is applied via either

---

the nasal or tracheal route. Since nasal CPAP can cause gastric distension, a gastric tube is often needed.

Initiating CPAP

When starting infant CPAP, the RCP should carefully check both the circuit pressure and flow before attaching the device to the patient. Once the infant is attached to the circuit, the RCP should check and confirm that the airway pressure equals that prescribed. Generally, CPAP pressures are set between 2 cm and 8 cm H_2O. The flow should be set high enough to meet patient needs, initially about 3 times the infant's estimated minute ventilation. Later, flow should be adjusted to keep airway pressure deflections to 1 cm H_2O or less during inspiration. Too high a flow can create additional, unintended airway pressure.[213]

Monitoring and adjustment

Infant CPAP levels are usually determined on a trial and error basis. The usual routine is to adjust the CPAP level in small increments (2 cm H_2O), while carefully observing changes in both arterial oxygenation and the infant's clinical response.[47,204]

When CPAP is successful, the infant's respiratory rate usually drops toward normal, and grunting and retractions, if present, tend to lessen or cease. Arterial blood gas analysis will show an improved PaO_2, usually sufficient enough to allow a reduction in FIO_2.

Newer methods for determining the best CPAP level in infants include computerized bedside flow-volume analysis[214] and respiratory inductance plethysmography (RIP) assessment of thoracoabdominal motion.[215]

In general, CPAP pressure levels should be raised if severe hypoxemia, grunting, sternal retractions, and cyanosis persists. Worsening hypoxemia or hypercapnia, tachypnea, and active abdominal muscles use during expiration indicate excessive CPAP. Excessive CPAP can also reduce cardiac output. Decreased arterial blood pressure, peripheral vasoconstriction, and metabolic acidosis are all signs of this harmful effect.[216]

Mechanical ventilation is indicated if: (1) adequate oxygenation cannot be maintained with CPAP, (2) prolonged apneic spells continue, or (3) hypercapnia persists or worsens.

Discontinuation

CPAP should be decreased or discontinued when the results of ABG analysis, chest X-rays, and clinical assessment indicate resolution of the underlying disorder. In general, the first step is to decrease the FIO_2 to nontoxic levels, followed by lowering the CPAP pressure. Since simultaneous changes in pressure and FIO_2 make it hard to interpret the infant's

---

Signs of respiratory distress indicating a need for infant CPAP[207,209]
Tachypnea
Severe retractions
grunting
Cyanosis with $FIO_2 \geq 0.50$
Periodic breathing
Recurrent apnea
Chest X-ray indicating RDS

Table 35-14   Comparison of CPAP methods

Method	Advantages	Disadvantages
Endotracheal tube	Patent airway; easy attachment to resuscitator or mechanical ventilator; easily stabilized and controlled	Hazards associated with intubation
Nasal prongs	Eliminates need for intubation; easily applied	Pressure necrosis and trauma; loss of CPAP with crying or leaks; false pressure reading with high flows; positioning difficult to maintain
Nasopharyngeal tube	Eliminates need for intubation; easily inserted	Pressure necrosis and trauma; loss of CPAP with crying or leaks
Mask	Eliminates need for intubation; easily applied	Mouth care difficult; leaks; danger of increasing CO_2 with inadequate flow; pressure necrosis; danger of aspiration

From Aloan CA: *Respiratory care of the newborn: a clinical manual,* Philadelphia, 1987, JB Lippincott.

response, only one parameter should be changed at a time.

The endotracheal or nasal tube should be removed when the infant can maintain adequate oxygenation without signs of respiratory distress on 2 cm to 3 cm H_2O CPAP at an FiO_2 of ≤ 0.40. Once disconnected from the CPAP apparatus, the infant should be placed in an oxyhood at an equivalent or slightly higher FiO_2. The endotracheal tube should never be left in place without CPAP, since it increases the work of breathing and prevents glottic closure. This can decrease the FRC and worsen arterial oxygenation.

Hazards and complications

Most of the hazards and complications of infant CPAP are similar to those in adults.[216] As previously mentioned, infant CPAP can overdistend normal lung units and decrease lung compliance. Overdistension also increases the risk of pulmonary barotrauma, and may increase physiologic dead space. CPAP also increases pleural pressure and can impede venous return to the heart. Decreased venous return can lower cardiac output and increase intracranial pressure (ICP). Increased ICP levels are associated with intraventricular hemorrhage in infants.

As with adults, CPAP can increase pulmonary vascular resistance by compressing pulmonary capillaries. In infants, a rise in pulmonary vascular resistance can worsen hypoxemia by increasing right-to-left shunting through the foramen ovale and ductus arteriosus. This problem becomes evident when increases in CPAP worsen, rather than improve, arterial oxygenation.

Other hazards and complications unique to infant nasal CPAP include pressure necrosis, plugging of the nares with mucus, and loss of pressure through an open mouth.

MECHANICAL VENTILATION

Mechanical ventilation of the infant and small child differs significantly from adult approaches. These differences are most evident in the neonatal period. Over time, these differences become less important. For older children, mechanical ventilation is basically the same as with adults.

General indications

The accompanying box summarizes the major indications for mechanical ventilation of newborn infants. As with adults, acute respiratory failure is the primary indication. Also as with adults, acute respiratory failure falls into two major categories: hypoxemic and hypercapneic.

Indications for mechanical ventilation of neonates

Respiratory failure:

$PaCO_2 > 55$ torr
$PaO_2 < 50$ torr

Depression of respiratory drive:

Apnea of prematurity
Intracranial hemorrhage
Drug depression

Impaired pulmonary function:

RDS
Meconium aspiration
Pneumonia

Hypoxemic respiratory failure exits when the signs of respiratory distress and hypoxemia persist despite treatment with CPAP and supplemental oxygen. In some clinical centers, a trial of CPAP is bypassed. Instead, mechanical ventilation is begun when the infant's PaO_2 drops below 50 torr on an $FiO_2 \geq 0.50$.[47,217]

Newborn hypercapneic respiratory failure is usually due to depression of the central respiratory drive. Common conditions causing CNS depression include neonatal asphyxia, apnea of prematurity, intraventricular hemorrhage, and depressant drugs transmitted from the mother during labor and delivery.

Ventilatory support may also be needed when alterations in lung function create V/Q imbalances or increase the work of breathing. These conditions occur together when the FRC is decreased, as in respiratory distress syndrome and interstitial pneumonia. Conversely, when small airway obstruction is the problem, as in meconium aspiration, portions of the lung may be hyperinflated. However, airway obstruction and hyperinflation also cause V/Q imbalances and increase the work of breathing.[47]

Basic principles

Currently, there are three major approaches to infant ventilatory support: (1) time-cycled, pressure-limited continuous flow IMV, (2) patient-triggered ventilation (SIMV or assist/control), and (3) high frequency ventilation. Another option, negative pressure ventilation, is being used with some success in managing refractory hypoxemia and pulmonary interstitial emphysema.[218,219]

Time-cycled, pressure-limited IMV

Figure 35-22 diagrams the function of a modern time-cycled, pressure-limited continuous flow IMV infant ventilator. In Figure 35-22 *A,* the ventilator is in its expiratory phase. Air and oxygen are blended and delivered continuously at a constant flow via a calibrated flowmeter into the patient circuit (single-circuit system).

A pneumatic, fluidic or electronic timer controls the function of an expiratory valve. The typical expiratory valve is either a gas-powered diaphragm or electronic solenoid. During the ventilator's expiratory phase, this valve stays open, allowing the infant to spontaneously draw fresh gas from the breathing circuit. During spontaneous exhalation, the continuous flow flushes expired gas out the circuit. Most expiratory valves also provide variable CPAP or PEEP.

When the expiratory time interval ends, the expiratory valve closes, and the ventilator begins inspiration (Figure 35-22, *B*). With the expiratory valve closed, gas now must flow into the infant's lungs.

As gas flows into the infant's lungs, the system pressure rises until the preset pressure limit is reached

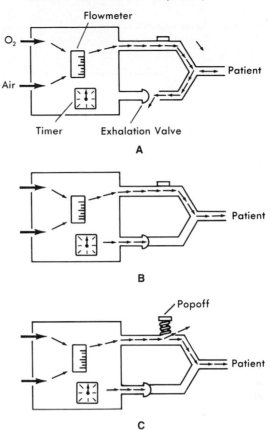

Fig. 35-22 Schema of neonatal ventilator. **A,** Spontaneous phase. **B,** Inspiratory phase. **C,** Pressure-limiting phase. (From Koff PB, Eitzman DV, Neu J: *Neonatal and pediatric respiratory care,* St Louis, 1988, Mosby.)

(Figure 35-22, *C*). At this point, a pressure pop-off or relief valve opens. With the exhalation valve closed, but the pressure pop-off open, gas now escapes out the relief valve, no longer flowing into the infant's lungs. As long as the exhalation valve is closed and the relief open, system pressure remains constant at preset pressure limit.

As shown in Figure 35-23 on page 1026, the length of this pressure hold or plateau is determined by the inspiratory time. Once inspiration ends, the exhalation valve opens and a new expiratory phase begins, allowing the infant to again breathe spontaneously.

Advantages and disadvantages. Time-cycled, pressure-limited ventilatory support provides full user control over mechanical rate, inspiratory and expiratory times, and airway pressure. On the other hand, when using this mode, both tidal volume and minute ventilation can vary with changes in infant lung mechanics. In addition, while some infants tolerate this mode well, other tend to fight the ventilator.[220] This results in active expiration against mechanical breaths, asynchronous breathing, and decreased oxygenation.[221] Fighting the ventilator may also increase the risk of barotrauma[222] and intraventricular hemorrhage.[223]

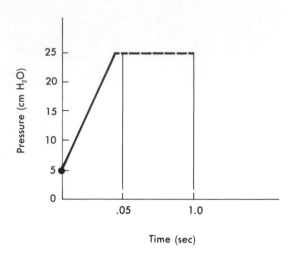

Fig. 35-23 Prolonging inspiration increases plateau period. (From Koff PB, Eitzman DV, Neu J: *Neonatal and pediatric respiratory care,* St Louis, 1988, Mosby.)

Key design considerations. The accompanying box outlines the key features for an ideal time-cycled, pressure-limited infant ventilator.[47] Other than reliability and ease of use, the most important features involve monitoring and limiting of delivered pressure and limiting the breathing circuit.

In terms of pressure monitoring, the manometer readings of many infant ventilators consistently underestimate true peak pressures, and are very unreliable regarding PEEP values.[224] In addition, peak inspiratory pressure overshoots occur with many of these devices, especially during asynchronous expiration.[225] This may contribute to barotrauma in newborn infants who fight positive-pressure ventilation.

Due to the small tidal volumes used in neonatal mechanical ventilation, both circuit deadspace and compressed volume must be minimal.[226] Moreover, changes in the circuit's internal volume, as occur when humidifier water levels change, are unacceptable. Patient circuits are thus relatively noncompliant. The ideal humidifier has a small internal volume and the means to keep the water level constant.

Condensation in infant ventilator circuits is a particularly vexing problem, which can result in grave hazards to the infant if the water finds its way to the airway.[227] See the prior discussion on humidity therapy for technical details on these problems.

As in adults, spontaneous breathing through some ventilator circuits can increase the work of breathing. This is most likely to occur in infant circuits with high

---

Desired characteristics for neonatal ventilators

General characteristics

Designed specifically for neonatal use
Reliable and easy to operate
Simple, inexpensive, and readily accessible calibration and repair
100% Relative humidity of inspired gas
Minimal dead space
Minimal internal compressible and distensible volume; nondistensible ventilator circuit tubing
Minimal noise
Low cost

Functional characteristics

Precisely controlled FIO_2
Cycling rate 0 to 200/min
Continuous flow system for IMV
V_{TS} 5 to 100 mL
CPAP or PEEP, 0 to 15 cm H_2O (independent of flow, peak inspiratory pressures, or rate)
Independently adjusted inspiratory and expiratory times (inspiratory time 0.2 to 1.5 sec)
Adjustable inspiratory flow rate 0 to 20 L/min
Manual cycling device
Adjustable inspiratory time-limiting device
Adjustable pressure-limiting valve
Failsafe valve in case of ventilator malfunction

Alarms

Visual, audible, adjustable, and battery-powered
High and low pressure for PEEP and peak inspiratory pressure (based on proximal airway pressure)
High and low rate
High and low FIO_2
Prolonged inspiratory time
Inspired gas temperature
Electrical or pneumatic power failure

Monitoring capability

FIO_2
Inspiratory and expiratory time
I:E ratio
Proximal airway pressure
Duration of positive pressure
Respiratory rate
Mean airway pressure

From Kirby RR, Smith RA, and Desautels DD, editors: Mechanical ventilation, New York, 1985, Churchill Livingstone.

Table 35-15 Functional comparison of time-cycled, pressure-limited infant ventilators

Ventilator*	Control mechanism	Ventilator rate	Inspiration time	Expiration time	I:E ratio
Babybird	Pneumatic	Resultant	Preset	Preset	Resultant
Babybird 2A	Electronic	Preset	Preset	Resultant	Resultant
Bourns BP-200	Electronic	Preset	Resultant	Resultant	Preset
Bourns Bear Cub	Electronic	Preset	Preset	Resultant	Resultant
Bio-Med MVP-10	Fluidic	Resultant	Preset	Preset	Resultant
Sechrist IV-100B	Fluidic	Resultant	Preset	Preset	Resultant
Healthdyne 102/105	Electronic	Preset	Preset	Resultant	Resultant
Infrasonics Infant Star	Electronic	Preset	Preset	Resultant	Resultant

*Except for the Infrasonics Infant Star, all the above ventilators are based on the continuous-flow IMV principle of operation and are normally used in the pressure-limited time-cycled mode. The Infrasonic Infant Star provides an alternative demand flow mode. Note: a preset parameter is user selectable through a ventilator control; a resultant parameter cannot be set by the user but derives from the interaction of two or more preset values.

resistance exhalation valves.[228] The ideal infant circuit exhalation valve should be a true threshold resistor.

Table 35-15 compares and contrasts the operational features of several time-cycled, pressure-limited infant ventilators. The reader interested in more detail regarding actual operation of these ventilators should consult either the manufacturers' literature or standard equipment reference texts.[47,210,229] Purchase decisions should go beyond product literature and be based on rigorous testing under standardized conditions.[230]

Patient-triggered infant ventilation

To overcome the problems associated with asychronous breathing during time-cycled, pressure-limited IMV, two patient-triggered infant ventilation modes have been introduced. These include assist-control (A/C) and SIMV.[220,231,232]

These modes are similar in concept to their adult counterparts. During infant SIMV, selected spontaneous breaths trigger the ventilator to deliver a mechanical breath, at settings determined by the clinician. If the infant becomes apneic during SIMV, controlled breaths are delivered at the base SIMV rate. During A/C, every spontaneous breath triggers an assisted mechanical breath, resulting in a variable, and usually high, rate. If apnea occurs during A/C breathing, controlled breaths will be delivered at the preset minimum (control) rate.[220]

Advantages and disadvantages. Advantages of patient-triggered infant ventilation over time-cycled IMV are listed in the accompanying box.

There currently are three primary indications for using patient-triggered ventilation with infants. First, the A/C mode is useful for short-term support of unstable infants who need fast ventilator rates, similar to hand bagging.[220] Second, SIMV is a good choice for supporting larger, more mature babies (> 28 weeks gestation) with acute respiratory distress who breath asynchronously on traditional IMV.[232,239-242] Last, SIMV may be preferable to time-cycled IMV for weaning.[235,236]

Patient-triggered ventilation does not offer any major advantages over traditional IMV for infants who are chronically ventilator-dependent.[240] Also, if an infant is apneic or breathing synchronously with IMV, or has minimal lung disease, there is unlikely to be any improvement on changing to SIMV.[220] Failure of patient-triggered ventilation becomes evident when oxygenation does not improve, and the triggering rate remains slow after switchover.[242]

Failure of patient-triggered infant ventilation may be due either the patient's breathing pattern or the equipment.[243] In infants in whom mechanical inflation extends beyond patient inspiration, synchrony may not be properly achieved. In terms of equipment, a slow response time can also result in failure.

Equipment. Table 35-16 on page 1028, describes the characteristics of available patient-triggered infant ventilation systems, including the sensor mechanism, response time, modes and special features.[220] Each of these systems has a visual display that indicates when spontaneous breaths occur, and whether mechanical breaths are patient-triggered or controlled.

Application. The key to successful patient-triggered infant ventilation is proper system triggering. As can be seen, most systems sense patient effort via flow changes, using either a hot-wire anemometer or pneumotachometer.

Advantages of patient-triggered infant ventilation over time-cycled IMV

Improved oxygenation[231,233]
Decreased cerebral vascular effects[234]
Less time on ventilator/faster weaning[235,236]
Decreased duration of oxygen therapy[235]
Decreased progression of IVH[235]
Low incidence of pneumothorax[237]
Less air-trapping (auto-PEEP)[238]

Table 35-16   Characteristics of available patient-triggered systems for neonatal ventilation

PTV system	Sensor	Response time-ms	Modes	Features
InfantStar and Star Sync	Graseby capsule -detects abdominal movement	52±13	SIMV and A/C	*Displays spontaneous TI and RR *Audible signal during inspiration aids capsule placement *No sensitivity setting needed
Bear Cub, NVM–1 TV monitor and Bear CEM	HWA flow sensor	65+15	SIMV and A/C	*NVM–1 displays VT and minute volume data, airway leak size *NVM–1 alarm limits hard to set/disable (minute volume) *C02 retention often evident, requiring an increase in PIP or ventilator rate (VLBW infants)
Drager Babylog 8000	HWA flow sensor	95±24*	SIMV and A/C	*Sensor built into the Y-piece *Fully integrated, easy to use *Graphic display of pressure or flow waveform. Displays tidal and minute ventilation data, airway leak size
Bird VIP and Partner TV monitor	VOP flow sensor	30–70	SIMV and A/C	*Partner displays VT and min volume data, airway leak size *Graphic display optional *Can end positive pressure when inspiration ends *Low rate of autocycling
Sechrist IV HP monitor and SAVI module	Chest leads Impedance	40–80**	A/C	*CR graph aids correct lead placement and sensitivity setting *Terminates positive pressure on active expiration

HWA-Hot-wire anemometer
VOP-Variable-orifice pneumotachometer
* 15% lower in future software versions
** Trigger delay. Additional system delay not reported.
From Bernstein G: Synchronous and patient-triggered ventilation in newborns, *Neonatal Respir Dis,* 3(2):1–4, 9–11, 1993.

System response time is the delay (in milliseconds) from the start of a spontaneous breath to the onset of the triggered breath. To avoid stimulating active expiration, response time on infant ventilators should be less than 100 ms.[220]

Common problems with triggering include missed breaths and inappropriate cycling. Missed breaths occur when the sensor fails to detect spontaneous effort. Clinical signs indicating missed breaths include: (1) a patient breathing rate obviously higher than that displayed by the ventilator, and (2) delivery of many controlled breaths (some being asynchronous).[220]

Reasons why sensors fail to detect spontaneous breaths include insufficient sensitivity, collection of foreign material (secretions, exogenous surfactant, etc) on the sensor, or a large air leak around the ET tube. Detachment of abdominal or chest sensors will also result in missed breaths.

Inappropriate triggering is due to either autocycling or incorrect sensor placement.[220] Autocycling usually occurs at higher sensitivity settings. When the sensitivity is set too high, the ventilator may incorrectly trigger on when it senses artifactual signals. For example, systems with pressure or flow sensors may autocycle when condensed water causes vibrations in the breathing circuit. Autocycling is also common in flow-triggered systems when leaks around the ET tube cause a compensatory rise in flow to maintain PEEP.

In the A/C mode, autocycling results in an abnormally rapid ventilator rate. If this causes hyperventilation, the infant may become apneic.[220] When autocycling occurs during SIMV, the ventilator rate does not change, but asynchrony may occur.

Incorrect sensor placement can also cause triggering errors. For example, improper placement of chest impedance leads on the Sechrist can cause triggering with cardiac impulses.[220] Likewise, placing the Infant-Star Graseby abdominal sensor capsule too close to the ribs may cause the ventilator to trigger on during expiration.

High frequency ventilation

High frequency ventilation (HFV) in infants and children is broadly defined as ventilatory support at mechanical rates greater than 60/min. First developed in the 1970's, the methods and approaches to high frequency ventilation continues to undergo research and development.

Methods. There are four different types of high frequency ventilation used in infants and children (Table 35-17).[217,244]

High-frequency positive-pressure ventilation (HFPPV) is delivered with conventional ventilators using modified low-compliance circuits which allow adequate VTs despite short inspiratory times. Most conventional neonatal ventilators now provide rate adjustment up to 150/min.

High-frequency jet ventilation (HFJV) employs a high pressure source to deliver gas through a small-bore injector cannula at rates between 60 and 600/min. Gas entrainment may occur and delivered VT may be large. However, even when volumes are smaller than the deadspace, adequate CO_2 elimination can occur.[244]

High-frequency flow interrupters (HFFI) provide small volumes at high rates (300 to 1200/min) by interrupting a flow or high-pressure source. In contrast to jet ventilation, no injector is used and no gas entrainment occurs.[244]

Because expiration is active, high-frequency oscillatory ventilation (HFOV) is unique.[244] Delivered volumes are usually very small (even less than dead space) and rates very high (up to 50 Hz or 3,000/min).[217] Either a piston pump or acoustic speaker provides volume delivery and active expiration. Because expiration is active, shorter expiratory times are possible, and gas trapping may be less of a problem.[244]

Despite many differences, these various high-frequency methods have much in common. Regardless of approach, delivered VT tends to decrease with increasing ventilatory rate and decreasing ET tube size. In addition, delivered volumes are relatively unaffected by lung compliance.[245] However, dynamic lung volume (FRC) tends to increase at higher rates.[246] Oxygenation is adjusted mainly by altering mean airway pressure ($\bar{P}aw$) and FiO_2. CO_2 elimination depends mainly on the pressure amplitude or gradient (PIP-PEEP).[244]

Indications. Current research provides a mixed picture on the clinical use of high frequency ventilation in infants and children.

HFPPV provides adequate gas exchange in critically ill neonates with lower PIP and $\bar{P}aw$ levels, and may be associated with a decreased incidence of pneumothorax.[247-249] In addition, higher rates are associated with less asynchronous breathing in the time-cycled IMV mode.[250]

Likewise, HFJV maintains or improves gas exchange in infants with RDS at lower airway pressures than conventional ventilation.[251,252] HFJV also can reduce flow through a bronchopleural fistula and may promote its healing.[253] Early problems with necrotizing tracheobronchitis during HFJV have been eliminated with adequate humidification mechanisms and improved injector designs. However, even though short-term benefits in gas exchange and airway pressure occur, HFJV has little effect on the morbidity, mortality, or complications associated with infant ventilation.[254,255]

HFFI at rate between 300 to 1200/min improves gas exchange, both oxygenation and ventilation, in infants with RDS and **PIE** at a lower PIP levels than conventional mechanical ventilation.[256,257]

HFOV can improve gas exchange while lowering $\bar{P}aw$.[258] As compared to conventional mechanical ventilation, however, HFOV does not affect mortality or support needs in patients at risk for bronchopulmonary dysplasia.[259,260] Furthermore, HFOV may increase the incidence of air leaks, and serious intraventricular hemorrhage.[259] The exception may be for RDS infants started on HFOV, as opposed to switched over from conventional ventilation. For these infants, continuous HFOV is as safe as conventional ventila-

Table 35-17   Techniques for high-frequency ventilation

	HFPPV*	Jet ventilation	Flow interruption	Oscillation
Tidal volume	>VDS+	> or < VDS	> or <VDS	>VDS
Expiration	Passive	Passive	Passive	Active
Pressure waveform	Variable	Triangular	Triangular	Sine wave
Entrainment	None	Possible	None	None
Frequency	60–150/min	60–600/min	300–1200/min	300–3000/min

*HFPPV—high-frequency positive-pressure ventilation

From Coghill CH, Haywood JL, Chatburn RL, Carlo WA: Neonatal and pediatric high-frequency ventilation: principles and practice, *Respir Care* 36(6): 596–609, 1991.

tion and can decrease the incidence of chronic lung disease.[261]

High frequency ventilation also has been combined with IMV in patients with severe respiratory failure.[262-264] As with high frequency ventilation, combined HFV-IMV tends to improve gas exchange at lower $\overline{P}$aws, while allowing a reduction in the IMV rate.[244] The rationale behind the IMV breaths is that they may prevent or resolve atelectasis that sometimes complicates prolonged periods of HFV, especially at small tidal volumes.[244]

In summary, the various HFV modes offer some practical advantages over conventional ventilation, but generally do not improve outcomes in infants suffering from respiratory failure. Current research indicates that the infants most likely to benefit from HFV are the tiny, ventilator-dependent babies at risk for air leaks.[244] Other potential uses for HFV are described in the accompanying box.

Adjusting ventilator parameters

Adjusting settings on modern infant ventilators is easy. Exactly what values to set, however, remains controversial.

All clinicians do agree that settings must be adjusted according to the needs of each individual patient. In addition, ventilator settings depend on the mode being used (time-cycled IMV, A/C, HFV, etc.).

Key settings common to all modes include the rate or frequency (f), inspiratory time (TI), I:E ratio, pressure gradient (PIP-PEEP), and FIO$_2$. In IMV, SIMV and A/C modes, the clinician must also set the flow rate ($\dot{V}$). Another key parameter is the mean airway pressure ($\overline{P}$aw). Although not directly adjustable, $\overline{P}$aw must be carefully monitored. This is because $\overline{P}$aw levels are linked to both the severity of illness and the likelihood of complications during infant ventilatory support.

These parameters are initially set to average values using clinical rules of thumb. Later, settings are adjusted to ensure adequate ventilation and oxygenation, while attempting to minimize complications.

Potential clinical uses of HFV[244]

Air leak syndromes
  Pulmonary interstitial emphysema (PIE)
    Bronchopleural fistula and pneumothorax
    Pneumomediastinum
    Pneumoperitoneum

Impaired cardiac function

Bronchoscopy and airway and thoracic surgery

Rescue therapy for those awaiting ECMO

Conventional ventilation and HFPPV

Over the last decade, the differences between conventional infant ventilation and HFPPV have become minimal. This is especially true in regard to rates and time parameters.

Rate. On most conventional infant ventilators, the rate is a preset parameter. In this case, the RCP simply selects the desired value. On a few ventilators, such as the Sechrist IV-100B and BioMed MVP-10, there is no rate control. Instead, the RCP sets the rate by adjusting separate inspiratory and expiratory time controls. In this case, the rate is a derivative value or resultant. A resultant is a parameter whose value results from two or more preset values.

In either case, the machine rate is the major factor affecting alveolar ventilation and PaCO$_2$ during conventional ventilation. In addition, the machine rate affects the degree of synchrony between spontaneous and IMV breaths.

In the past, IMV rates of 30 to 40 breaths/min were the norm for infants.[217] This is still the case for full-term babies with mild respiratory distress. For premature infants, however, current research indicates that rates between 60 and 120/min are more beneficial. These higher rates provide the best synchrony and highest minute volume.[250,265] In addition, higher rates (with shorter TIs) lower the risk of barotrauma.[266] If an acceptable PaCO$_2$ cannot be achieved using these rates, either the pressure limit or inspiratory time may have to be changed.

Inspiratory time (TI) and I:E ratio. By definition, all conventional infant ventilators provide user control over TI. If the breathing rate is preset, then the expiratory time (TE) simply equals the remainder of the total cycle time. In this case, changes in TI will not affect the rate, but will alter the I:E ratio.

On the other hand, when the breathing rate is set using separate inspiratory and expiratory time controls, changes in TI will alter both the rate and the I:E ratio. For a constant TE, an increase in TI will lower the rate and raise the I:E ratio. Conversely, a decrease in TI will increase the rate and lower the I:E ratio.

Initially, the inspiratory time is set between 0.2 and 0.5 seconds, with an I:E ratio between 1:1 and 1:3. Individual adjustments are made according to both the underlying disorder and the results of clinical assessment. For preterm infants, high rates and short inspiratory times tend to result in the best synchrony with the ventilator and the highest minute volume.[250,265] In addition, animal studies fail to show any advantage to prolonging TI beyond the point where volume ceases to accumulate.[267]

Peak inspiratory pressure (PIP). The peak inspiratory pressure, or PIP, is the preset pressure limit that is set and maintained during inspiration. The PIP, together with the TI and flow, determine the delivered tidal volume.

Although initial PIP settings vary, most centers begin with 20 to 25 cm H_2O.[47,217] Thereafter, the PIP is adjusted accordingly, with the goal being the lowest value needed to obtain satisfactory ventilation and oxygenation.

Gas flow. Conventional infant ventilators operate in the continuous flow IMV mode. In this mode, circuit flow must be sufficient to: (1) meet the infant's spontaneous breathing demands, and (2) provide an adequate mechanical tidal volume at the selected PIP and t_I.

An initial flow of 6 to 8 L/min generally meets these needs.[33] Usually, this range of flow also provides the typical pressure plateau seen in time-cycled, pressure-limited ventilation (Figure 35-24, A).[217]

Lower flows slow the rise in pressure, such that the pressure limit may not be reached until the end of inspiration (Figure 35-24, B). Thus, a change in flow alters both the pressure waveform and the time required to reach the pressure limit. However, if the flow is too low, the infant's spontaneous demands will not be met. The RCP can detect inadequate flow by observing the airway pressure manometer. When the flow is too low, spontaneous inspiration causes a negative deflection on the manometer. If this occurs, the flow should be increased.

In some newer infant ventilators, such as the Bird VIP, a parallel demand system can augment flow as needed. Typically, the clinician sets a system minimum flow. When the infant's spontaneous flow demands exceed the system minimum, the ventilator provides additional flow. When the infant no longer needs the extra flow, it returns to the preset value.[229]

If the pressure limit is set above that needed to deliver the flow during inspiration, the ventilator will

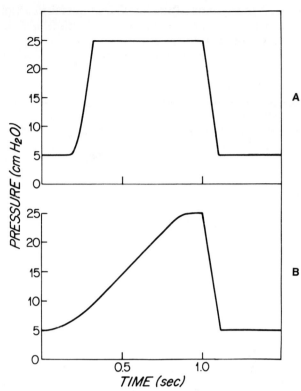

Fig. 35-24 Pressure wave pattern of neonatal ventilator. **A,** High flow rate. **B,** Low flow rate. (From Koff PB, Eitzman DV, Neu J: *Neonatal and pediatric respiratory care,* St Louis, 1988, Mosby.)

function in a volume-limited mode. In this case, increases in either flow or TI will increase the tidal volume. In addition, changes in lung compliance and airway resistance will affect the PIP.[75] See the accompanying MiniClini for a discussion.

■ M I N I C L I N I ■

35-1

Volume-Limiting Inspiration with a Time-Cycled Infant Ventilator

By setting the pressure limit above that required to deliver the gas flow over the duration of inspiration, the constant flow time-cycled infant ventilator may be volume-limited.

As an example, if the gas flow is preset at 6.0 L/min (100 mL/sec) and the inspiratory time is preset to 0.5 seconds, then the tidal volume delivered by the ventilator is calculated as the product of flow ($\dot{V}$) times inspiratory time (TI):

$V_T = \dot{V} \times T_I$
$V_T = 100 \text{ mL/sec} \times 0.5 \text{ sec}$
$\quad = 50 \text{ mL}$

Of course, not all of this volume will actually enter the patient's lungs. As with adult ventilators, a component of the delivered volume will be compressed in the ventilator circuitry, thus effectively lowering that which is actually available to the patient.

Volume-limiting provides more precise control over the infant's minute ventilation than does the time-cycled, pressure-limited mode. However, volume-limiting allows breath stacking. Moreover, with a high pressure limit setting, airway pressures can rise to dangerous levels and lead to pulmonary barotrauma. Last, since volume-limiting with small infants generally requires lower flows than those used in the time-cycled, pressure-limited mode, the imposed work of breathing through the circuit may be increased. For these reasons, the time-cycled, pressure-limited mode is generally preferred for conventional ventilation.

Last, if the system's PEEP or CPAP device has high flow resistance, increases in flow will raise, and decreases in flow will lower system pressure.[210]

FIO_2. To avoid the risk of ROP and oxygen toxicity, the FIO_2 during mechanical ventilation should be kept as low as tolerated. Oxygen may also be a contributing factor in the development of bronchopulmonary dysplasia (BPD).

Positive end-expiratory pressure (PEEP). As in adults, PEEP is indicated in infants with refractory hypoxemia. Typically, refractory hypoxemia in infants is due to alveolar instability and decreased lung volumes.[207] By stabilizing alveoli and increasing the FRC, PEEP improves arterial oxygenation. As the PaO$_2$ rises, pulmonary vascular resistance decreases. If not offset by PEEP, a fall in pulmonary vascular resistance can lessen both pulmonary and cardiac shunting. PEEP may also be helpful in decreasing flow resistance and improving ventilation in infants with small airway obstruction.[47]

PEEP levels are usually set between 4 to 10 cm H$_2$O.[217] In general, moderate levels of PEEP have little effect on the neonatal cardiovascular or cerebral circulations.[268] However, even at low levels, PEEP can have harmful effects on preterm infants. These effects include a decrease in both compliance and minute ventilation.[269] Higher PEEP levels are poorly tolerated by most infants. This is because further overdistension can suppress venous return, increase deadspace ventilation, and cause CO$_2$ retention.[47] High PEEP levels can also increase pulmonary vascular resistance and right-to-left shunting, due to compression of the blood vessels. This is apparent when oxygenation worsens, rather than improves as PEEP is applied.

Mean airway pressure. The mean airway pressure, or P̄aw, is the average pressure applied to the lungs over time. As shown in Figure 35-25, this represents the total area under the curve of pressure over time. Parameters that affect P̄aw include the breathing rate, PIP, inspiratory pressure waveform, TI, I:E ratio, and PEEP level.

Clinical research shows that higher P̄aws are associated with better arterial oxygenation.[24,270] However, the higher the P̄aw, the greater the likelihood of pulmonary barotrauma. Pulmonary air leaks are most common when the P̄aw rises above 12 cm H$_2$O.[47]

The best P̄aw level is that which provides adequate oxygenation and ventilation with minimal risk of barotrauma and cardiovascular depression. P̄aw levels must be individualized.[25] The same P̄aw level can be achieved by a host of different time and pressure settings.

Of course, it is control over these time and pressure parameters that gives the RCP flexibility in patient management. Lumping these parameters together into a single measure can help us understand their combined impact. However, establishing normal or desired P̄aw levels should be discouraged.[47]

Patient-triggered ventilation

Settings used for patient-triggered infant ventilation are similar to those used with conventional ventilation, with a few key exceptions. In unstable infants, the A/C mode is initially applied, usually at base rates of 70 to 100/min.[220] In more stable infants requiring SIMV, initial rates of 50 to 70/min are used, with inspiratory times between 0.2 and 0.4 sec.[271] Flow, PIP, FIO_2 and PEEP adjustments are as described above.

High frequency ventilation

Settings used in high frequency infant ventilation differ considerably from conventional approaches. We will highlight common strategies used with HFJV and HFO.

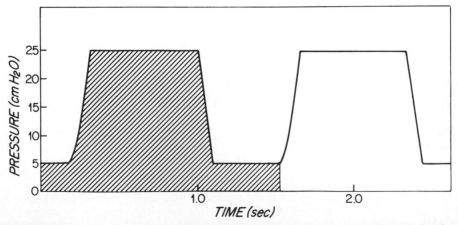

Fig. 35-25 Pressure wave pattern of neonatal ventilator, with shaded area representing calculated mean airway pressure (P̄aw). (From Koff PB, Eitzman DV, Neu J: Neonatal and pediatric respiratory care, St Louis, 1988, Mosby.)

High frequency jet ventilation (HFJV). HFJV usually is used together with conventional ventilation. The main lumen of a special ET tube connects to the conventional ventilator, while the jet ventilator has its own port. A third port is used to monitor distal airway pressure.

A typical HFJV ventilator provides operator control over PIP, inspiratory time, and rate.[244] Depending on the device, available rates vary between 60 to 660/min (1 and 11 Hz). Peak inspiratory pressure can usually be set between 4 and 50 cm H_2O, and inspiratory time is adjustable between 0.020 and 0.050 sec (20 to 50 milliseconds).

HFJV is started with rates between 300 and 500/min, PIPs about 10% to 30% below the conventional PIP, and a jet inspiratory time of about 0.02 seconds.[244] The PIP on the conventional ventilator is then kept about 10 cm H_2O above the HFJV PIP. IMV breaths are rapidly reduced over several minutes to the desired background rate (2 to 10/min).

Oxygenation is adjusted by altering FIO_2 and $\overline{Paw}$.[244] When lung underexpansion is the problem (as in RDS), $\overline{Paw}$ can be raised by increasing either PIP, PEEP, rate, or Ti. PEEP, however, is usually the variable adjusted upward. If oxygenation is poor and the lungs are overexpanded, then excessive pressure or gas trapping should be suspected. In this situation, oxygenation might improve with reduction in $\overline{Paw}$.[244]

CO_2 elimination depends mainly on VT and somewhat on rate.[244] VT is determined by the pressure gradient (PIP-PEEP). Either decreasing PEEP or increasing the PIP increases the pressure gradient and improves CO_2 elimination. If this fails to improve CO_2 elimination, an increase in frequency can be attempted.[244]

High frequency oscillatory ventilation (HFOV). A typical HFOV ventilator provides operator control over rate, I:E ratio, and oscillatory pressure amplitude, (referred to as *power* on some HFOV devices).

There are two basic strategies used with HFOV: low and high volume. In both cases, the initial frequency is set between 600 and 900/min (10 to 15 Hz), with an I:E ration of 1:2. Therapy is begun by adjusting oscillatory amplitude until chest-wall vibrations become visible.[244]

The low volume strategy is used to minimize or prevent problems with air leaks.[272] With this strategy, the mean airway pressure is kept as low as possible. If the initial oscillatory amplitude does not provide adequate CO_2 removal, then the frequency is reduced from 15 to 10 Hz. The lower frequency causes less loss of oscillatory power across the ET tube, thus providing a higher amplitude to the airway and lungs.[244] If hypoventilation persists after lowering the frequency, then inspiratory time can be increased toward 50% (I:E of 1:1).

The high volume strategy is used to treat hypoxemia due to diffuse alveolar disease which does not respond to conventional ventilation. Instead of aiming for a low mean airway pressure, oxygenation is managed by increasing $\overline{Paw}$ to a level 10% above that used with conventional ventilation.[244] This high mean airway pressure is used to achieve maximum alveolar recruitment.

HFOV is also used as a rescue treatment for infants being considered for ECMO.[273,274] The goal in these cases is to improve gas exchange at the lowest possible mean airway pressure and FIO_2 while the patient is being prepared for ECMO.

Monitoring during ventilatory support

Until recently, monitoring of the infant receiving ventilatory support was based almost entirely on observational assessment, combined with blood gas analysis. Advances in technology now allow continuous monitoring of such basic ventilatory parameters as tidal volume and minute ventilation. Direct assessment of ventilation via capnography also is now feasible with infants.[275-276] In addition, bedside testing of pulmonary mechanics can now provide critical data needed to adjust ventilatory parameters.

Recent improvements in computer technology have made available bedside assessment of infant pulmonary function. Table 35-18, on page 1034 summarizes pulmonary function values in well and sick infants.

Particularly important in providing ventilatory support is the ability to measure both the infant's lung compliance and resistance while receiving ventilatory support. This information can be invaluable in adjusting and optimizing ventilator settings. One of the common problems with pressure-limited ventilation is overdistention of the lung, especially when the infant's lung compliance improves. As shown in Figure 35-26, on page 1034 a volume-pressure loop can quickly help identify overdistention and thus help avoid pulmonary barotrauma.[277]

Weaning from ventilatory support

As with adults, mechanical ventilation of infants is supportive in nature. Thus the primary goal always is to resolve the disorder(s) so that ventilatory support can be discontinued as soon as possible. Also as with adults, weaning is not likely to succeed until all major pulmonary, cardiovascular, and metabolic problems are corrected.

Unlike adults, however, few standard protocols have been developed for weaning infants. Thus the process of weaning infants from ventilatory support differs according to mode and varies from center to center.

Weaning from conventional ventilation and HFPPV

Figure 35-27, on page 1035 provides one example of a protocol for weaning infants from conventional

Table 35-18　Pulmonary function in well and sick infants*

Measurement	Well infants	Infants with RDS
Tidal volume (mL/kg)	5–7	4–6
Respiratory rate (breaths/min)	30–40	50–80
Minute ventilation (mL/kg/min)	200–300	250–400
Functional residual capacity (mL/kg)	25–30	20–33
Thoracic gas volume (mL/kg)	30–40	20–35
Dynamic compliance (mL/cm H_2O/kg)	1–2	0.3–0.5
Lung resistance (cm H_2O/L/sec)	25–50	60–150
Work of breathing (g cm/min/kg)	500–1000	800–3,000†
$PaCO_2$ (torr)	30–40	32–50
PaO_2 in air (torr)	105–115	92–108
Alveolar ventilation (mL/kg/min)	110–160	55–90
Physiologic dead space (mL/kg)	2–3	3.0–4.5
Dead space/tidal volume (%)	22–38	60–80
Anatomic dead space (mL/kg)	1.5–2.5	2.5–4.2
Alveolar dead (mL/kg)	0–0.5	0.2–0.7
Pulmonary clearance delay (%)	0–30	7–40
Effective pulmonary capillary perfusion (nitrous oxide) (mL/kg/min)	160–230	75–140
Venous admixture in air (%)	8–22	22–60
$P(a\text{-}A)CO_2$ (torr)	−2 to +4	8–25
$P(A\text{-}a)O_2$ in air (torr)	20–40	25–60
in O_2 (torr)	230–380	270–550
CO_2 response (mL/kg/min/torr CO_2)	25–70	NA

*Adapted from McCann EM, Goldman SL, Brady JP: *Pediatr Res* 21:313, 1987.
RDS = respiratory distress syndrome; NA = not available
†From author's laboratory. Used by permission.

time-cycled, pressure-limited continuous flow IMV. Underlying this approach is early emphasis on removing high-risk interventions. High-risk elements include FIO_2s > 0.7, PIPs > 30 cm H_2O, PEEP levels > 8 cm H_2O, and TI > 0.7 seconds.[47] After these parameters are safely lowered, the breathing rate is

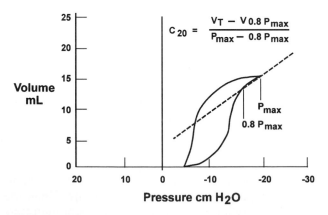

Fig. 35-26　Use of volume-pressure loop to determine presence of overdistention during mechanical ventilation. C_{20} is the compliance over the last 20% of inspiration. In a normal loop, the ratio of C_{20} to overall compliance (C_{20}/C) is close to 2.0. Overdistention exists when C_{20}/C drops below 0.7. (From Fisher JB, Mammel M: Identifying lung overdistention during mechanical ventilation by using volume-pressure loops, *Pediatr Pulmon* 5:10-14, 1988.)

decreased as tolerated. Once the FIO_2s is below 0.5 and the PIP is less than 25 cm H_2O, a switch is made to CPAP. Both CPAP and FIO_2 are then reduced until the infant can maintain satisfactory blood gases on less than 40% oxygen and 2 cm H_2O CPAP. At this point, extubation is indicated.

Recent research indicates that keeping inspiratory times short (0.5 sec or less) can speed the weaning process during both conventional and HFV.[280,281] This is probably due to the better synchrony seen with shorter TIs.

The need for CPAP prior to extubation remains controversial. Many infants tolerate direct extubation from low intermittent mandatory ventilation rates without a trial of CPAP.[282] In fact, a pre-extubation trial of CPAP may cause more frequent apnea in infants when used for more than several hours.[273] However, use of nasal CPAP after extubation may be needed by some low birth weight infants.[284]

Weaning from high frequency ventilation

With HFJV, as ventilation improves and $PaCO_2$ falls, the PIP is reduced. Once the FIO_2 is less than 0.7, PEEP is reduced as oxygenation improves. Once both the HFJV and conventional ventilator PIP are below 15 cm H_2O, only the HFJV PIP is further reduced. Then the frequency is gradually reduced to around

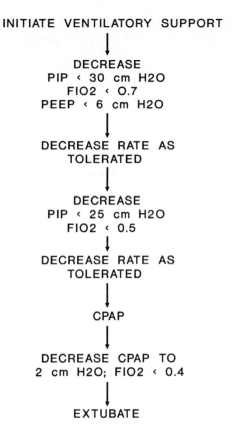

INITIATE VENTILATORY SUPPORT

↓

DECREASE
PIP < 30 cm H2O
FIO2 < 0.7
PEEP < 6 cm H2O

↓

DECREASE RATE AS
TOLERATED

↓

DECREASE
PIP < 25 cm H2O
FIO2 < 0.5

↓

DECREASE RATE AS
TOLERATED

↓

CPAP

↓

DECREASE CPAP TO
2 cm H2O; FIO2 < 0.4

↓

EXTUBATE

Fig. 35-27 General guidelines for weaning infants with acute respiratory failure from conventional mechanical ventilatory support. At each step, try to maintain PaO_2 between 50 and 70 torr and $PaCO_2$ between 35 and 45 torr. If possible, make only one change at a time. (From Kirby RR, Smith RA, Desautels DD, editors. Mechanical ventilation, New York, 1985, Churchill Livingstone.)

360/min, at which point the infant can usually be extubated.[244]

With HFOV, as compliance improves, the FIO_2 is lowered to about 0.7. At this point, $\overline{Paw}$ reduction begins. When $\overline{Paw}$ is down to 10 to 12 cm H_2O and air leaks have resolved, the patient may tolerate weaning to conventional ventilation.[244]

Complications of ventilatory support

Table 35-19 summarizes the most common complications associated with mechanical ventilation of infants.[47,25,217,285-287] Bronchopulmonary dysplasia will be discussed subsequently. Retinopathy of prematurity (ROP) is not a complication of mechanical ventilation itself, but of the accompanying oxygen therapy. Likewise, airway complications can occur separately from mechanical ventilation.[286]

As with adults, positive pressure ventilation can increase pulmonary vascular resistance. However, in infants with certain cardiovascular defects, a rise in pulmonary vascular resistance can worsen extrapulmonary right-to-left shunts.

Table 35-19 Complications of infant mechanical ventilation

Complication	Primary causative factors
Ventilator-induced injuries	
Air leak syndromes:	Peak inspiratory pressure
Pneumothorax	PEEP (set and intrinsic)
Pneumomediastinum	Inspiratory time/asynchrony
Pneumopericardium	
Pneumoperitoneum	
Pulmonary interstitial	
emphysema	
Subcutaneous emphysema	
Parenchymal lung damage	
Bronchopulmonary dysplasia	
Cardiovascular complications:	Peak inspiratory pressure
Decreased venous return	PEEP (set and intrinsic)
Decreased cardiac output	Inspiratory time/asynchrony
Increased pulmonary	
Vascular resistance	
Increased ICP	
Increased incidence of IVH	
Oxygen-induced injuries:	FIO_2 and duration of use
Oxygen toxicity	Inspiratory pressures (BPD only)
Retrolental fibroplasia	
Airway complications:	Mechanical factors
Accidental extubation	Human error
Atelectasis	Inadequate humidification
Endobronchial intubation	Equipment contamination
Postintubation stridor	
Tube plugging/kinking	
Tracheal lesions	
Infection	
General complications:	
Infection	
Acid-base imbalances	

Also as in adults, PPV can overinflate more compliant alveoli and compress the pulmonary capillaries. This can cause redirection of pulmonary blood flow to more poorly ventilated alveoli, further contributing to hypoxemia.[24]

Should increased levels of CPAP or PEEP cause a fall in PaO_2s, it is likely that the pressure level is increasing right-to-left shunting. This situation can be rectified by simply decreasing the CPAP or PEEP.[71,207]

EXTRACORPOREAL MEMBRANE OXYGENATION

Extracorporeal membrane oxygenation (ECMO) is a form of cardiopulmonary bypass used to provide gas exchange. Venous blood is removed from the right atrium, oxygenated by passage by a diffusing membrane, and then returned to the patient (Figure 35-28).

There are two types of ECMO circuits. The most often used is the venoarterial bypass. With this method, a cannula is placed into the right atrium via the right internal jugular vein. The blood is then oxygenated by the ECMO circuit and returned to the aorta through a cannula placed into the right common carotid artery.

The other option is venovenous bypass. In a venovenous bypass circuit, a double lumen catheter is placed into the right atrium, once again via the right internal jugular vein. The large outer lumen allows for venous drainage of blood while the smaller inner lumen permits the return of arterialized blood from the membrane. Venovenous bypass is associated with fewer complications than the venoarterial route and is preferred when cardiac output does not have to be supported.[288,289]

Patients who are selected for ECMO are those who do not respond to conventional mechanical ventilation and maximum pharmacological support. The most common disease states in the neonatal population are persistent pulmonary hypertension (PPHN), meconium aspiration syndrome (MAS), sepsis, perinatal asphyxia, respiratory distress syndrome (RDS),

and congenital diaphragmatic hernia (CDH).[290] Criteria for patient selection are listed in the accompanying box.[291]

ECMO is also being more widely used in the pediatric population, and especially in the treatment of adult respiratory distress syndrome (ARDS) and cardiac defects.[33,289,291]

Stabilization and transport

Treatment of a critically ill infant or child is usually carried out at a tertiary care facility. Such institutions have the trained staff and equipment needed to perform the complicated procedures that sustain life and aid in recovery.[292] Institutions lacking these capabilities must therefore transport their critically ill infants or children to tertiary care facilities.

Modes of transportation include ground ambulance, helicopter, or fixed wing aircraft. Within the vehicle, the transport team sets up an environment that is actually an extension of the receiving intensive care unit.[293]

The transport team should be composed of individuals qualified to care for critically ill or injured children in a transport setting.[294] Typical team members include a physician, registered nurse, RCP, and paramedic.

Training of the transport team is an important issue. Qualifications include at least one year of neonatal/pediatric critical care experience for registered nurses and RCPs. Paramedics should have specific pediatric training and experience, and the RCP should at least be registry eligible.[294] A common prerequisite to becoming a member of the team involves completion of an approved programs in pediatric advanced life support (PALS) and neonatal resuscitation.[294,295]

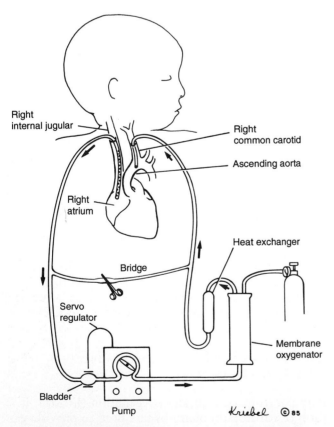

Fig. 35-28 Venoarterial ECMO circuit. (From O'Rourke PP: Ecmo: Where have we been? Where are we going? *Respir Care* 36:7, 1991.)

Inclusion criteria for neonatal ECMO

- Reversible lung disease
- Gestational age > 35 weeks
- No preexisting cerebral hemorrhage
- Significant shunting:

  $$P(A-a)O_2 > 610 \text{ for 2 hours}$$
  $$\text{oxygenation index} > 0.4+$$
  $$\text{oxygenation index} > 0.3 \text{ with air leaks}$$

- Reversible anatomic shunting
- Reversible pulmonary hypertension

$$+\text{Oxygenation index (OI)} = \frac{(FiO_2 \times \overline{Paw})}{PaO_2} \times 100$$

From Thompson JE, Perlman N: Extracorporeal membrane oxygenation In Koff PB, Eitzman DV, *Neu J:* Neonatal and pediatric respiratory care, ed 2, St Louis, 1993, Mosby.

The role of the RCP during transport is to assist in pulmonary stabilization and airway management.[294] This can include patient assessment, monitoring, oxygen therapy, administration of aerosolized medications, ventilator management, and assisting other members of the team. The RCP is also responsible for assuring that the needed equipment and supplies are available to support these responsibilities. The accompanying box lists the basic equipment and supplies needed to provide respiratory care during neonatal and pediatric transport.[295]

COMMON DISORDERS OF THE NEWBORN

There are literally dozens of perinatal disorders affecting the respiratory system. Some of these represent developmental abnormalities of the heart, lungs, or airways. Many conditions are simple due to prematurity itself, while others occur as a result of problems during labor and delivery. Last, some problems occur as a result of treatment.

We will focus mainly on the common disorders in these categories, to include meconium aspiration syndrome, respiratory distress syndrome, transient tachypnea of the newborn, apnea of prematurity, bronchopulmonary dysplasia, persistent pulmonary hypertension, and congenital cardiopulmonary abnormalities.

Meconium aspiration syndrome (MAS)

Toward the end of gestation, the normal fetus exhibits 30 to 70 breathing movements per minute. These movements stop during short incidents of fetal asphyxia. If, however, asphyxia is prolonged, the fetus may take large gasps. This can cause aspiration of surrounding liquid into the lungs.

Pathophysiology

Normally, the liquid around the fetus is pure amniotic fluid. Pure amniotic fluid consists mainly of fetal lung fluid and some fetal urine. Aspiration of this fluid is relatively harmless, since it is easily cleared during the first few breaths.

A greater problem is aspiration of meconium. Meconium is a product of the fetal bowel. Meconium consists of amniotic fluid, mucopolysaccharides, cholesterol, bile acids and salts, intestinal enzymes, and other substances.

Traditionally, the passage of meconium has been associated with fetal asphyxia. Meconium passage is more common when fetal umbilical venous blood oxygen saturation falls below 30%. However, some infants who never experience intrauterine hypoxia also pass meconium. This suggests that other mechanisms may be involved.[296]

Amniotic fluid is stained with meconium in about 12% of all births.[297] The incidence of meconium-stained amniotic fluid is highest when gestation exceeds 37 weeks, in breech deliveries, and with SGA infants. About one third of these infants show evidence of aspiration (meconium present below the vocal cords). However, the actual clinical syndrome develops in only 2 out of every 1000 infants. Ninety-five percent of infants with inhaled meconium clear the lungs spontaneously.[297]

For many years, the aspirated meconium itself was considered the primary cause of the syndrome. Recent evidence suggests that the real culprit is probably the fetal asphyxia that precedes aspiration.[297] Fetal asphyxia causes pulmonary vasospasm and hyperreactivity of the vasculature. Severe asphyxia causes actual lung damage and pulmonary hypertension. In the damaged state, the lungs cannot clear the meconium.

MAS involves two primary problems: pulmonary obstruction and lung tissue damage.[296] As shown in

---

Equipment and supplies needed to provide respiratory care during neonatal and pediatric transport

Equipment

Adequate supply of oxygen and compressed air
Air-oxygen blender
Mechanical ventilator with circuit
Manual resuscitator capable of giving 100% O_2 with PEEP
Noninvasive oxygen monitor (SpO_2 or $PtcO_2$)
Oxygen analyzer
Airway pressure monitor (electronic or mechanical)
Electrocardiograph monitor
Portable suction apparatus
Laryngoscope handle
Laryngoscope blades (sizes newborn to adult)
Extra laryngoscope bulbs and batteries
Stethoscope
Tools

Supplies

Resuscitation masks (sizes 0, 1, 2, 3, 4)
Feeding tubes (size 6, 8, and 10 Fr)
Disposable oxygen hood
Oxygen connecting tubing
Disposable hand-held nebulizer with tubing (for bronchodilators)
Cloth adhesive tape for taping endotracheal tubes (½" & 1")
Tincture of benzoin for taping endotracheal tubes
Pulse oximeter probes (at least two, in case one fails)
Endotracheal tubes (sizes 2.5-7.0)
Stylet
Forceps
Suction apparatus

Figure 35-29, obstruction is due to plugging of the airways with meconium. This obstruction is often of the ball-valve type, allowing gas entry but preventing exit. Ball-valve obstructions cause air-trapping and can lead to barotrauma. The lung tissue injury caused by MAS is like the pneumonitis seen in adult aspiration syndromes. Pulmonary hypertension and persistent fetal circulation, with intracardiac right-to-left shunting, frequently complicate MAS.[297]

Clinical manifestations

Prior to birth, thick meconium, fetal tachycardia, and absent fetal cardiac accelerations during labor identify the fetus at high risk for MAS.[298] If, after delivery, the infant has a low umbilical artery pH, an Apgar score less than 5, and meconium aspirated from the trachea, intensive care and close observation for MAS is warranted.

Infants who develop MAS typically have gasping respirations, tachypnea, grunting, and retractions. The chest X-ray usually shows irregular pulmonary densities, representing areas of atelectasis, combined with hyperlucent areas, representing hyperinflation due to air trapping (Figure 35-30).[299] Arterial blood gases typically show hypoxemia with a mixed respiratory and metabolic acidosis.[296] In the most severe cases there is right-to-left shunting and persistent fetal circulation, with subsequent fetal death.[297]

Treatment

In the presence of thick meconium-stained amniotic fluid, the oropharynx should be suctioned as the head is presented during delivery, before the first breath is taken. Once delivery is complete, the infant should immediately be intubated with the largest ET tube possible.[203] Suction should then be applied directly to the ET tube, not via a catheter.[33] The ET tube is then removed and inspected for meconium. If meconium is present, the procedure is repeated with a new ET tube, until no further meconium is aspirated. To prevent hypoxia, a flow of warmed 100% oxygen

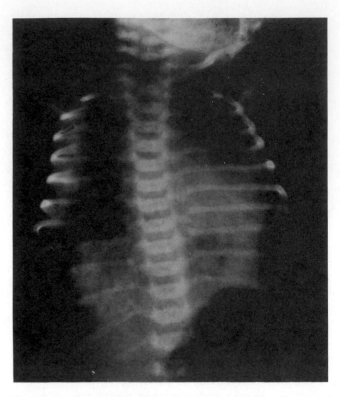

Fig. 35-30 Meconium aspiration is severe in this chest film. Broad areas of density represent atelectasis and interstitial fluid. Regional emphysema is seen in the remaining radiolucent areas. The overall effect of diffuse airway obstruction is over-expansion of the lungs, as indicated by the low position of the diaphragm. (From Korones SB: *High-risk newborn infants: the basis for intensive nursing care,* ed 4, St Louis, 1986, Mosby.)

should be blown across the infant's face during the aspiration efforts. Unfortunately, these interventions at birth may do little to affect the incidence of MAS.[297]

Should the infant worsen, CPAP or mechanical ventilation may be indicated. CPAP is indicated if the primary problem is hypoxemia. By distending the small airways, CPAP can help overcome the ball-valve obstruction, and actually improve both oxygenation

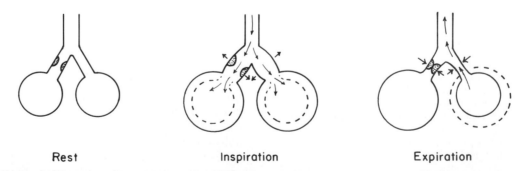

| Rest | Inspiration | Expiration |

Fig. 35-29 Demonstration of ball-valve effect. At rest, airway lumen is partially obstructed; with inspiration, negative intrathoracic pressure opens airway and relieves obstruction. Gas enters and expands alveoli. On expiration, intrathoracic pressure changes to positive force that narrows airway, causing total occlusion. Gas cannot be expelled and is trapped within aveoli. (From Koff PB, Eitzman DV, Neu J: *Neonatal and pediatric care,* St Louis, 1988, Mosby.)

and ventilation.[300] On the other hand, if respiratory acidosis is severe, or clinical assessment indicates an excessive work in breathing, mechanical ventilation should be started.

Infants with severe MAS are very difficult to ventilate. Because they often retain CO_2, high rates and peak pressures are needed.[47] Unfortunately, high rates and pressures increase the threat of barotrauma, especially if air trapping is a major problem. High pressures may also worsen pulmonary hypertension and aggravate any right-to-left cardiac shunting. For these reasons, most clinicians recommend that MAS infants be ventilated with short inspiratory times and low peak pressures, with an I:E ratio long enough to allow complete exhalation from obstructed lung units.[47]

To overcome the problems associated with high pressures, HFJV, alone or in combination with low rate conventional ventilation has been used to treat MAS.[301,302] Results are generally favorable, with HFJV providing better oxygenation and ventilation at a lower mean airway pressure ($\overline{P}aw$).

Since pulmonary infections often complicate MAS, antibiotic therapy may be needed. In addition, vasodilators such as tolazoline may be needed to treat pulmonary hypertension.

Respiratory distress syndrome of the newborn

Neonatal respiratory distress syndrome (RDS) affects 60,000 to 70,000 infants each year in the United States. Although the death rate has decreased dramatically over the last three decades, many infants still die or exhibit chronic effects from the syndrome.

RDS, or hyaline membrane disease, is a disease of prematurity. The major factor in the development of RDS is inadequate surfactant production.[303,304] Not until 34 to 36 weeks gestation is surfactant production stable enough to support extrauterine life.

Surfactant production depends on both the relative maturity of the lung and the adequacy of fetal perfusion. Thus maternal factors that impair fetal blood flow, such as abruptio placenta, **pre-eclampsia,** and maternal diabetes, may also lead to RDS.

Another factor associated with RDS is the persistence of high pulmonary vascular resistance after birth. If the fetus is stressed and develops acidosis and severe hypoxemia, pulmonary vascular resistance rises. This can cause ischemic injury to the lung, and further impair surfactant production.

Pathophysiology

Figure 35-31 outlines the pathophysiologic events associated with RDS.[30] A decrease in surfactant increases alveoli surface tension forces. This causes alveoli to become unstable and collapse, leading to atelectasis and an increased work of breathing. At

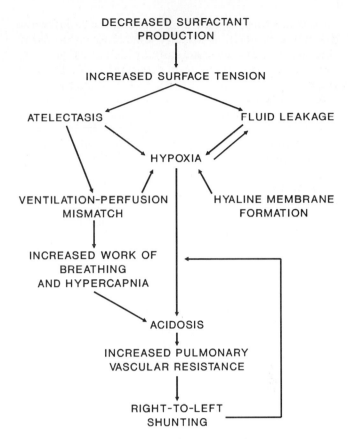

Fig. 35-31 Clinical progression of hyaline membrane disease. (From Aloan CA: *Respiratory care of the newborn: a clinical manual,* Philadelphia, 1987, JB Lippincott.)

the same time, the increased surface tension pulls fluid from the pulmonary capillaries into the alveoli. In combination, these factors impair oxygen exchange and cause severe hypoxemia.

The severe hypoxemia and acidosis increase pulmonary vascular resistance. As pulmonary artery pressures rise, extrapulmonary right-to-left shunting increases, and hypoxemia worsens. Hypoxia and acidosis also impair further surfactant production.

Clinical manifestations

The first signs of respiratory distress in infants with RDS usually occur soon after birth. Tachypnea usually occurs first. Following tachypnea, worsening retractions, paradoxical breathing, and audible grunting are observed. Nasal flaring may also be seen. Chest auscultation often reveals dry, uneven crackling sounds.

Cyanosis may or may not be present. If, however, central cyanosis is observed, it is likely that the infant has severe hypoxemia.

As with ARDS, the hypoxemia caused by infant RDS is refractory to treatment. High FIO_2s do little to improve arterial oxygenation.[304] However, certain other pulmonary conditions, as well as hypotension, hypothermia, and poor perfusion, will mimic this aspect of RDS.

Because these signs are not very specific, definitive diagnosis of RDS is usually made by chest X-ray (Figure 35-32). Reticulogranular densities and the presence of air bronchograms are typical of RDS, and important in staging its severity (see accompanying box). The reticulogranular pattern is caused by the aeration of respiratory bronchioles and the collapse of the alveoli. Air bronchograms appear as aerated, dark, major bronchi surrounded by the collapsed or consolidated lung tissue.

Treatment

CPAP and PEEP are the traditional support modes used to manage RDS. Recently, surfactant replacement therapy, high frequency ventilation, and extracorporeal membrane oxygenation have proved useful as adjuncts or alternatives to these traditional approaches.[305]

CPAP. Unless the infant's condition is severe, a trial with nasal CPAP is indicated. Due to the hazards with ET tubes, nasal prongs are preferred. If signs of respiratory distress persist after CPAP is started, the airway pressure should be raised in small increments (1 cm to 2 cm H_2O). If the infant's clinical condition deteriorates rapidly, a more aggressive approach is required.

Intubation should be performed under controlled conditions as an elective procedure. A trial of endotracheal CPAP with the same settings used with the nasal route should be tried prior to considering mechanical ventilation. Often endotracheal CPAP provides better oxygenation than the nasal route, probably due to less

leakage. If oxygenation does not improve on maximum levels of CPAP and FiO_2, or if the patient is apneic or acidotic, mechanical ventilation with PEEP must be started.

Mechanical ventilation. The aim of mechanical ventilation in RDS is to prevent lung collapse and maintain alveolar inflation. In severe RDS, some alveoli collapse on every breath, requiring very high reinflation pressures. To maintain this pressure for an adequate period of time, a constant pressure pattern is desirable.

Carbon dioxide levels are not normally affected when PEEP is used. Because the time constant of the lungs in RDS is so short, the lung empties very quickly. If, however, alveolar ventilation is inadequate, either the PIP or rate should be increased. To minimize the potential for barotrauma, the PIP should be kept below 30 cm H_2O.[47]

High mean airway pressures do not usually affect blood pressure and cardiac output in infants with hyaline membrane disease.[25] This is because low lung and high chest wall compliance minimize pressure transmission to the pleural space. As the infant with RDS begins to recover, compliance increases, making high mean airway pressures more hazardous.

Surfactant replacement therapy. Currently, two surfactant preparations are being used to treat neonatal RDS in the United States: colfosceril palmitate with cetyl alcohol and tyloxapol (Exosurf Neonatal)[306] and beractant (Survanta).[307] Exosurf Neonatal is a synthetic preparation while Survanta is a natural bovine extract. Both preparations are liquid suspensions that are instilled directly into the trachea.

Prophylactic surfactant replacement therapy is recommended for small infants (< 1,350 g) and for larger infants who show signs of pulmonary immaturity.

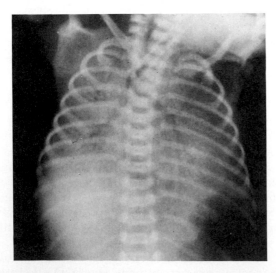

Fig. 35-32 Radiolucent appearance of severe hyaline membrane disease. The lungs are dense. The cardiac shadow is barely disernible in left chest. Prominent black streaks emanating from both hilar areas are air bronchograms. (From Korones SB: *High-risk new born infants: the basis for intensive nursing care*, ed 4, St Louis, 1986, Mosby.)

Staging of RDS by chest X-ray

Stage I is marked by a generalized reticulogranular density over all lung fields. The cardiac shadow is sharp. The hemidiaphragms are located at the level of the eighth rib.

Stage II shows an increase in reticulogranular densities, air bronchograms over the medial two-thirds of the lung fields. The lungs are not as well expanded, and the hemidiaphragms are above the eighth rib.

Stage III shows increasing reticulogranular densities, and more prominent air bronchograms. Inflation of the lungs is only down to the seventh rib. The chest wall may be distorted and have a bell-shape appearance. The cardiac shadow is indistinct.

Stage IV shows the characteristic the white out appearance, with extreme opacification. There is an exaggerated bell-shaping of the chest wall. The cardiac shadow is obliterated, and the hemi diaphragms are above the seventh rib.

Surfactant replacement therapy is also used as rescue treatment for infants who already have RDS.[308-310]

The accompanying box outlines an administration protocol for Exosurf Neonatal. Current protocols for use of this substance demand rigorous respiratory care including either CPAP or mechanical ventilation with PEEP (as indicated). Therapies aimed at decreasing pulmonary edema, improving cardiac output, and weaning from oxygen and high ventilatory pressures are essential in the successful management of infants undergoing surfactant therapy.[311]

Transient tachypnea of the newborn (TTN)

TTN is often referred to as Type II RDS. The cause of TTNB is still unclear, but is most likely due to delayed clearance of fetal lung liquid.[312] During most births, about two-thirds of this fluid is expelled by a thoracic squeeze in the birth canal, with the rest reabsorbed through the lymphatics during initial breathing. However, these mechanisms are impaired in infants born via Cesarean section, or those with incomplete development of the lymphatics (preterm or SGA infants).[312]

Administration protocol—Exosurf Neonatal

1. Prepare the Airway
Five different sized endotracheal tube adapters come with each vial of Exosurf Neonatal. The adapters are clean but not sterile.
   a. Select an adapter corresponding to the ID of the endotracheal tube;
   b. Insert the adapter into the endo tube with a firm push-twist motion;
   c. Connect the breathing circuit wye to the adapter.
2. Prepare the Exosurf Neonatal Suspension
Exosurf Neonatal should be reconstituted immediately before use using only the accompanying 8 mL diluent (preservative-free sterile water). Solutions containing buffers/preservatives should not be used for reconstitution.
   a. Fill a 10 mL or 12 mL syringe with the 8 mL diluent supplied using an 18 or 19 gauge needle;
   b. Allow the vacuum in the vial to draw the water into the vial;
   c. Aspirate as much as possible of the 8 mL out of the vial into the syringe (while maintaining the vacuum), then SUDDENLY release the syringe plunger;
   d. Repeat step c 3 or 4 or four times to assure adequate mixing of the vial contents (if a vacuum is not present, the vial of Exosurf Neonatal should be discarded);
   e. Draw the appropriate dosage volume for the entire dose (5 mL/kg) into the syringe from below the froth in the vial (again assuring a vacuum).
3. Administer the Exosurf Neonatal Suspension
   a. Suction and stabilize the infant prior to Exosurf administration;
   b. Remove the cap from the sideport on the endotracheal tube adapter and attach the syringe containing the Exosurf suspension;
   c. Place the infant in the midline position;
   d. Administer the first 2.5 mL/kg half-dose by instillation slowly over 1 to 2 min (30 to 50 mechanical breaths) in small bursts timed with inspiration
   e. Turn the infant's head and torso 45 degrees to the RIGHT for 30 seconds while mechanical ventilation is continued;
   f. Return the infant to the midline position;
   g. Administer the second 2.5 mL/kg half-dose in an identical manner over another 1 to 2 minutes;
   h. Turn the infant's head and torso 45 degrees to the LEFT for 30 seconds while mechanical ventilation is continued;
   i. Return the infant to the midline position;
   j. Remove the syringe and recap the sideport of the endotracheal tube adapter.
4. Monitor the Response
   a. During dosing, monitor heart rate, color, chest expansion, facial expressions, the oximeter, and the endotracheal tube patency and position;
   b. If heart rate slows, the infant becomes dusky or agitated, transcutaneous SO2 falls more then 15%, or Exosurf backs up the endotracheal tube, dosing should be slowed or halted and, if necessary, the peak inspiratory pressure, ventilator rate, and/or FiO2 turned up;
   c. On the other hand, rapid improvements in lung function may require immediate reductions in peak inspiratory pressure, ventilator rate, and/or FiO2.
5. Follow-up
   a. Confirm the position of the endotracheal tube by listening for equal breath sounds in the axillae;
   b. Continue to carefully monitor chest expansion, color, transcutaneous saturation, and arterial blood gases for at least 30 minutes after dosing;
   c. Avoid suctioning for two hours after Exosurf administration, except when dictated by clinical necessity.

The residual lung fluid causes an increase in airway resistance and an overall decrease in lung compliance. Because compliance is low, the infant must generate more negative pleural pressures to breathe. This can result in hyperinflation of some areas, and air-trapping in others.

Infants who develop TTN are usually born at term without any specific predisposing factors in common. Mothers of neonates who develop TTN tend to have longer labor intervals and a higher incidence of failure to progress in labor, leading to Cesarean delivery.[312] In many cases, however, maternal history and labor and delivery are normal.

Clinical manifestations

During the first few hours of life, infants with TTN breathe rapidly. However, alveolar ventilation, as measured by arterial pH and PCO_2, is usually normal. The chest X-ray, which may initially be confused with true RDS, shows hyperinflation secondary to air-trapping, with perihilar streaking. The perihilar streaking probably represents lymphatic engorgement. Pleural effusions may be evident in the costophrenic angles and interlobar fissues.

Treatment

Infants with TTN usually respond readily to low FIO_2s by oxyhood. Infants requiring higher FIO_2s may benefit from CPAP. Because the retention of lung fluid may be gravity dependent, frequent changes in the infant's position may help speed clearance and minimize V/Q imbalances. Since TTN and neonatal pneumonia have similar clinical signs, IV antibiotics should be considered for at least 3 days after obtaining appropriate cultures. The need for mechanical ventilation is rare and probably indicates a complication. Clearing of the lungs, as evident via both chest X-ray and clinical improvement, usually occurs within 24 to 48 hours.

A small number of infants with TTN go on to develop persistent pulmonary hypertension. This possibility should be considered if the PaO_2 does not increase as expected with supplemental oxygen.

Apnea of prematurity

Apnea is a common, treatable disorder in premature infants, which usually resolves over time.[313] Short apneic spells of 15 seconds or less are normal at all ages. Apneic spells are abnormal if: (1) they last more than 20 seconds, or (2) they are associated with cyanosis, pallor, **hypotonia** or bradycardia.

If no effort to breathe occurs during the spell, the apnea is called *central apnea*. On the other hand, if breathing efforts occur, but obstruction prevents air flow, the apnea is termed *obstructive*. Mixed apnea is a combination of the central and obstructive types.[314]

Etiology

Prematurity is the primary cause of central apnea in newborns. The incidence of apnea of prematurity is inversely proportional to gestational age. Over half of all preterm and SGA infants exhibit one or more apneic episodes, many of which occur with bradycardia. This suggests that apnea of prematurity is associated with an immature respiratory control system.

In addition to prematurity, several other factors can cause apnea in infants. Table 35-20 describes these potential causes, associated signs, and diagnostic indicators.[315]

Treatment

Infants with apnea must be monitored continuously for both heart and respiratory rate. Continuous noninvasive monitoring of oxygenation via transcutaneous electrode or pulse oximetry is also recommended.

Table 35-20 Evaluation of an infant with apnea

Possible causes	Associated signs	Investigation
Infection	Lethargy, respiratory distress, temperature instability	Complete blood count, sepsis evaluation
Metabolic disorder	Poor feeding, lethargy, jittenness	Glucose, calcium, electrolyte levels
Impaired oxygenation	Respiratory distress, tachypnea, cyanosis	Oxygen monitoring, ABGs, chest X-ray
Maternal drugs	Maternal history, hypotonia, CNS depression	Magnesium level, urine drug screen
Intracranial pathology	Abnormal neurologic exam, seizures	Cranial ultrasound
Environmental	Lethargy	Monitor temperature (baby and environment)
Gastroesophageal reflux	Feeding difficulty	Specific observation, barium swallow

From Stark AR: Disorders of respiratory control in infants, *Respir Care* 36(7):673–681, 1991.

Most apneic incidents can be quickly terminated by gentle mechanical stimulation, such as picking the infant up, flicking the sole of the feet, or rubbing the skin.[314] If the cause of apnea is not prematurity, treatment must be directed at resolving the underlying condition. Table 35-21 outlines current treatment strategies for infants with apnea.[315]

Apnea due to prematurity responds well to the methylxanthines, especially theophylline and caffeine.[316] These agents stimulate the central nervous system and increase the infant's responsiveness to carbon dioxide. For infants with apnea that is refractory to treatment with theophylline, doxapram can be used.[317]

CPAP is also used to treat infant apnea. Although its mechanism of action is not clearly established, CPAP probably stimulates vagal receptors in the lung, thereby reflexes increasing the output of the brainstem respiratory centers. Severe or recurrent apnea which is not responsive to these interventions may require mechanical ventilatory support.

As the respiratory response mechanisms mature, apnea of prematurity normally resolves itself. Apneic spells begin to disappear by the 37th to 44th week of postconceptual age, with no apparent long-term effects. Infants who exhibited apnea of prematurity are not at any higher risk for SIDS.[314]

Bronchopulmonary dysplasia (BPD)

Infants with respiratory failure in the first few weeks of life may develop a chronic pulmonary condition called bronchopulmonary dysplasia, or BPD. Immaturity, oxygen toxicity, and positive pressure ventilation have all been implicated in the origin of BPD.[318-320] More recently, malnutrition has been identified as a potential factor.[321]

Pathophysiology

The formation of a hyaline membrane occurs acutely, often complicated by a left-to-right shunt through a PDA or patent foramen ovale. Pulmonary edema occurs next, followed by interstitial fibrosis, and finally by emphysematous changes. A delay in normal lung growth and development is often present, along with episodes of pulmonary insufficiency and chronic lung infections. As with RDS, bronchopulmonary dysplasia develops in stages, both pathologic and radiologic in nature (see box on page 1044). However, BPD develops over a much longer course than RDS.

Clinical manifestations

Initially the infant may have only required a small amount of supplemental oxygen. As the PaO_2 drops, additional O_2 is needed. This cycle progresses until the PaO_2 can no longer be maintained without a toxic FIO_2.

Due to variable obstruction, the lungs have areas of atelectasis and air-trapping. Arterial blood gases reveal varying degrees of hypoxemia and hypercapnia secondary to airway obstruction, air trapping, pulmonary fibrosis, and atelectasis. There is a marked increase in airway resistance with an overall decrease in lung compliance.

Treatment

The best treatment of BPD is prevention. Modern methods of neonatal intensive care apparently are decreasing the incidence of this disorder, but BPD is still too common an outcome in low birth weight infants treated for respiratory distress.

Management of infants with BPD involves steps to minimize further lung damage and prevent pulmonary hypertension and cor pulmonale. These infants may be dependent upon supplemental oxygen or mechanical ventilation for months, and have symptoms of airway obstruction for years.

Therapy is usually supportive throughout the course of the disease, since BPD tends to be self-limiting in surviving infants. The infant with BPD is given respiratory support as needed. Supplemental O_2 can help decrease the pulmonary hypertension that is

---

Table 35-21 Treatment strategies for infants with apnea

Treatment	Rationale
Treat underlying cause if identified	Removes precipitating factor
Tactile stimulation	Increases respiratory drive by sensory stimulation
Continuous positive airway pressure	Reduces mixed and obstructive apnea by splinting the upper airway
Theophylline or caffeine	Increases respiratory center output and CO_2 response, enhances diaphragm strength; adenosine antagonist
Doxapram	Stimulates respiratory center and peripheral chemoreceptors
Transfusion	Decreases hypoxic depression by increasing oxygen carrying capacity
Mechanical ventilation	Provides support when respiratory effort is inadequate

From Stark AR: Disorders of respiratory control in infants, *Respir Care* 36(7):673–681, 1991.

Staging of bronchopulmonary dysplasia

Stage I—Acute Respiratory Distress (days 1 to 3)
This stage may be indistinguishable from severe RDS
Stage II—Regeneration (days 4 to 10)
Necrosis and repair of the alveolar epithelium is evident. Regeneration and proliferation of the bronchial epithelium occurs. Ulceration and membrane formation in bronchioles is also present, but fibrosis is not. X-rays findings are similar to RDS, with opacification of the lungs obscuring the heart border, and air bronchogram (Figure 35-33).
Stage III—Transitional Period to Chronic Disease (days 10 to 20)
As shown in Figure 35-34, the X-ray at this stage shows interstitial edema and focal areas of atelectasis and radiolucency. Radiolucent areas, most prominent in the perihilar region, represent localized emphysema. These areas often increase in size and number for three to four months, until they fill the entire lung fields. Over this time period, the lungs become increasingly hyperexpanded.
Stage IV—Chronic Disease (1 month+)
The pathologic changes show obliterative bronchiolitis, bronchiolar fibrosis, and ulceration. Metaplasia of bronchiolar epithelium with narrowing of the bronchioles may also occur. The X-ray appearance shows that resolution has started in this stage. The cystic areas are replaced by hyperlucency at the bases and streaky infiltrates toward the apices. The hyperlucency and the streaky areas finally resolve over a period of months.

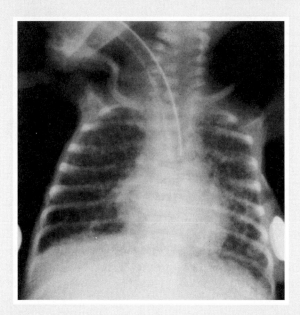

Fig. 35-33 Moderate BPD: interstitial edema and focal atelectasis produce a diffuse density in both lungs. A few small, round radiolucencies represent early regional emphysema. (From Korones SB: *High-risk newborn infants: the basis for intensive nursing care*, ed 4, St Louis, 1986, Mosby Co)

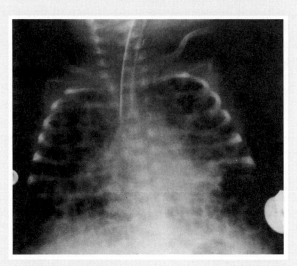

Fig. 35-34 Radiologic appearance of bronchopulmonary dysplasia in advanced stage. White strands are seen throughout both lung fields, representing fibrosis. Lungs are overexpanded in the extreme; diaphragms are at a very low level, and intercostal spaces bulge. (From Korones SB: *High-risk newborn infants: the basis for intensive nursing care*, ed 4, St Louis, 1986, Mosby.)

common with this disorder. Diuretics are given as needed to decrease pulmonary edema, with antibiotics given to treat existing pulmonary infections.[322] Chest physical therapy may help mobilize secretions and prevent further atelectasis. Bronchodilator therapy may be useful in decreasing airway resistance.[323] Steroid therapy with dexamethasone can produce substantial short-term improvement in lung function, often permitting rapid weaning from ventilatory support. However, steroid therapy apparently has little effect on long-term outcomes such as mortality or duration of oxygen therapy.[324-326]

Persistent pulmonary hypertension of the newborn (PPHN)

Persistent pulmonary hypertension of the newborn (PPHN) is a complex syndrome with many causes. The common denominator in PPHN is a return to fetal circulatory pathways, usually due to high pulmonary vascular resistance. In PPHN, blood flow continues to bypass the pulmonary vascular bed through the ductus arteriosus and the foramen ovale. This results in further right-to-left shunting, severe hypoxemia, and metabolic and respiratory acidosis.[33]

Congenital abnormalities affecting respiration

The most common congenital abnormalities affecting respiration are laryngomalacia, tracheomalacia, tracheoesophageal (T-E) fistula, and diaphragmatic hernia. Laryngomalacia and tracheomalacia can cause airway obstruction. T-E fistula can cause aspiration pneumonitis and complicate ventilatory management. Diaphragmatic hernia can cause hypoplasia of both lung tissue and the pulmonary vasculature, and is associated with persistent fetal circulation.[327]

Because they can mimic other problems, all congenital abnormalities affecting respiration require careful differential diagnosis. Most treatment approaches ultimately require surgical intervention. Supportive management of diaphragmatic hernia and T-E fistula often includes high frequency ventilation.[328-330]

Congenital heart disease

A full discussion of congenital heart disease is beyond the scope of this chapter. Basic knowledge of the common defects, however, is essential to good practice in pediatric and neonatal respiratory care.

Figure 35-35, page 1046, diagrams the normal cardiac anatomy and compares it to the five most common congenital defects.

Tetrology of Fallot

Tetrology of Fallot is a cyanotic (right-to-left shunting) defect that includes: (1) obstruction to right ventricular outflow (pulmonary stenosis), (2) ventricular septal defect, (3) dextroposition of the aorta, and (4) right ventricular hypertrophy.

Ventricular septal defect (VSD)

Defects found along the septum separating the right and left ventricles are quite common. VSD can occur alone or in combination with other anomolies. Like Tetrology of Fallot, a VSD normally causes right-to-left shunting, arterial desaturation, and cyanosis.

Atrial septal defect (ASD)

The most common type of ASD is a small, slit-like opening that persists after closure of the foramen ovale. An isolated ASD is of little clinical importance.

Patent ductus arteriosus (PDA)

While in utero the fetus shunts a large percentage of pulmonary blood flow through the ductus arteriosus to the aorta. Closure of the ductus normally occurs at birth (see Cardiopulmonary events at birth, earlier in this chapter). Factors altering pressure gradients or affecting smooth muscle contraction can cause the ductus to open or remain open. Depending on the pressure gradient established, shunting through an open ductus may be either right-to-left (pulmonary pressures greater than aortic) or left-to-right (aortic pressures greater than pulmonary). Treatment is either surgical (by **ligation**) or pharmacologic (indomethacin).

Coarctation of the aorta

Coarctation can be found alone or in combination with other defects. It involves a constriction of the aorta that restricts blood flow. Coarctation is most commonly located near the ductus arteriosus. Coarctation increases afterload on the left ventricle.

PEDIATRIC RESPIRATORY DISORDERS

As compared to the common cardiopulmonary diseases in the neonatal period, the more common conditions in the older infant and child result from airway obstruction due to bacterial or viral infections. Other entities to be discussed are the Sudden Infant Death Syndrome, gastroesophageal reflux, and cystic fibrosis.

Sudden infant death syndrome (SIDS)

SIDS, or crib death, is the leading cause of death in infants less than one year old in the United States. About 2 out of every 1000 infants die of SIDS, accounting for between 5000 and 10,000 deaths per each year in the United States alone.[331]

A presumptive diagnosis is based on the conditions of death, in which a previously healthy baby dies suddenly and unexpectedly, usually during sleep. On autopsy, many infants dying of SIDS show evidence of repeated episodes of hypoxia or ischemia. However, no precise cause of death can be identified.[314,332]

Etiology

The cause of SIDS remains unknown. Apnea of prematurity is not a predisposing factor, and there is no evidence that immaturity of the respiratory centers is a cause. Although infants in families where two or more SIDS deaths have occurred are at slightly higher risk, there is no evidence of a genetic link. Where three or more SIDS deaths have occurred in the same family, the possibility of child abuse (purposeful asphyxia) must be considered.[333]

Epidemiological analysis

Currently, our best knowledge of SIDS comes from population or epidemiological studies.[334] These stud-

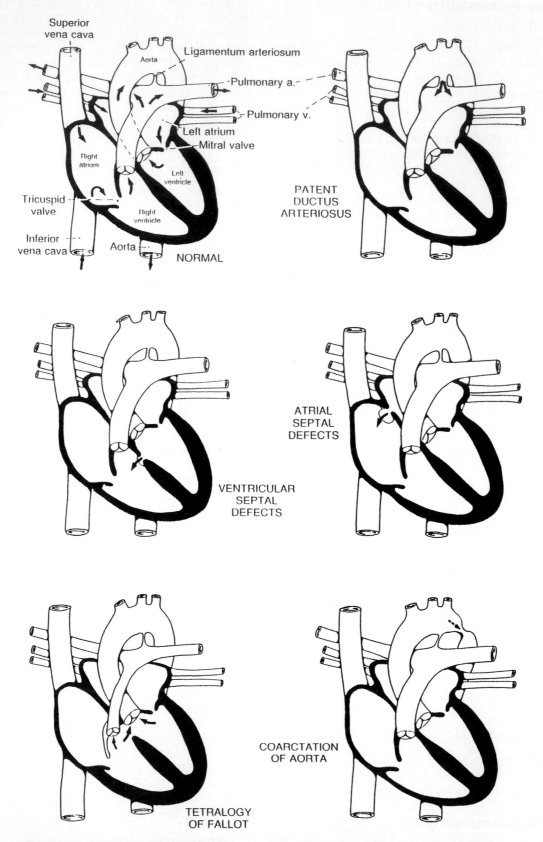

Fig. 35–35 Normal flow of blood through the heart and some congenital defects that cause abnormal flow. (Used with permission from Jabob S, Francone C, Lossow WJ: *Structure and function in man*, ed 5. Philadelphia, 1982, WB Saunders.)

Factors associated with increased frequency of SIDS in victims and their families

Maternal Characteristics

Less than 20 years old
Poor
Black, Native American, or Alaskan native
Previous fetal loss
Cigarette smoking
Narcotic abuse
Ill during pregnancy
Inadequate prenatal care

Infant Characteristics at Birth

Male
Premature birth
Small for gestational age
Low APGAR scores
Resuscitation with oxygen and ventilation
Second or third in birth order or of a multiple birth pregnancy
Previous siblings SIDS victims

Infant Characteristics Near Time of Death

Age less than 6 months (peak between 1 and 3 months)
Winter season
Asleep at night
Mild illness in week before death
History of apparent life-threatening event (ALTE)

From Koff PB, Eitzman DV, Neu J: *Neonatal and pediatric respiratory care,* St Louis, 1988, Mosby.

---

ies reveal statistical risk factors associated with SIDS (see box above). Typically, the infant who dies of SIDS was a preterm black male born to a poor mother less than 20 years old who received inadequate prenatal care. Infants between 1 to 3 months old are most susceptible, and death is most likely to occur at night during the winter months. The risk of SIDS is also higher in infants who previously experienced an apparent life-threatening event (ALTE).[314] An ALTE occurs when a baby becomes apneic, cyanotic, or limp enough to frighten the parent or caregiver. More recently, the prone sleeping position has been strongly associated with an increased risk of SIDS.[335,336]

Prevention

Given its unknown cause and unexpected occurrence, there is no current treatment for SIDS. Instead, prevention is the goal.

Successful prevention requires that high risk infants be identified. Identification of such infants is based on a history of risk factors (above) and documented monitoring or event recording.[337,338] Once the high risk infant is identified, the family is trained in monitoring and CPR. In addition, the American Academy of Pediatrics now recommends that infants be placed in either the supine or side-lying positions throughout the first 6 months of life.[339]

With the potential for parental fear of SIDS extremely high, the possibility for abuse of home monitoring is great. In order to better define the need and appropriate approach for home monitoring of infants, the National Institutes of Health recently developed a consensus statement on infantile apnea and home monitoring. The eight specific NIH recommendations regarding the need for and use of home monitoring are summarized in the box, page 1048.[340]

Gastroesophageal reflux

Gastroesophageal reflux (GER), the regurgitation of stomach contents back up the esophagus, is common in childhood. Some causes of GER are physiologic. There is a general agreement that these are important interactions between GER and a variety of disorders of the respiratory system.[341] Respiratory problems caused by gastroesophageal reflux include reactive airway disease, aspiration pneumonia, laryngospasm, stridor, chronic cough, choking spells, and apnea.

GER should be considered in the infant faced with a sudden life-threatening event, and in the older child or adult presenting with unexplained chronic head and neck complaints.[341]

GER can be diagnosed by testing the esophageal pH. Once GER has been diagnosed, medical therapy can begin. Some cases may require surgical intervention.[342]

Bronchiolitis

Bronchiolitis is an acute infection of the lower respiratory tract, usually caused by the respiratory syncytial virus, or RSV.[343,344] Nearly one in ten infants under the age of two will acquire a bronchiolitis infection, with the greatest incidence in those around six months of age. Outcomes are generally good, although about one percent of infants hospitalized for bronchiolitis die from respiratory failure. Those most prone to develop respiratory failure as a consequence of bronchiolitis are the very young, those who are immunodeficient, and those with congenital heart disease, bronchopulmonary dysplasia, cystic fibrosis, or childhood asthma.

Clinical manifestations

The clinical manifestations of bronchiolitis are those associated with inflammation of the small bron-

---

NIH consensus statement on infantile apnea and home monitoring

1. Home cardiorespiratory monitoring is medically indicated in certain groups of infants at high risk for sudden death including the following:
   a. Infants with one or more severe ALTEs requiring vigorous stimulation, mouth-to-mouth resuscitation, or CPR.
   b. Siblings of two or more victims of SIDS.
   c. Preterm infants with apnea of prematurity who are otherwise ready for discharge.
   d. Infants with conditions such as central hypoventilation or tracheostomy.
2. It is not clear from existing evidence whether the potential benefits of monitoring outweigh the risk for other groups of infants in whom the risk of sudden death is elevated. These groups include the following:
   a. Siblings of one SIDS victim.
   b. Infants with less severe ALTEs.
   c. Infants of opiate-abusing or cocaine-abusing mothers.
3. Cardiorespiratory monitoring is not medically indicated for normal infants or asymptomatic preterm infants.
4. Caregivers must be trained and demonstrate proficiency in infant CPR and must understand that cardiorespiratory monitoring does not guarantee survival.
5. Pneumocardiograms are not useful in screening infants in an attempt to predict SIDS victims or victims of infantile apnea.
6. Decisions for stopping home monitoring should be based on clinical criteria. It is reasonable to discontinue the monitor when the infant has had 2 or 3 months free of events requiring vigorous stimulation, mouth-to-mouth resuscitation, or CPR.
7. Effective home monitoring requires a coordinated, interdisciplinary effort from physicians, nursing and social work services, health care agencies, and medical equipment vendors.
8. In the rare infant with recurrent severe apnea of infancy requiring resuscitation, prolonged hospitalization may be necessary. The vast majority of infants with an ALTE and apnea of infancy have an excellent prognosis without after effects.

---

chi and bronchioles. Bronchiolitis commonly occurs soon after an ordinary upper respiratory infection. The infant may have a slight fever with an intermittent cough. After a few days, signs of respiratory distress develop, particularly dyspnea and tachypnea. Progressive inflammation and narrowing of the airways causes both inspiratory and expiratory wheezing and increased airway resistance. The chest X-ray may show signs of hyperinflation, with areas of consolidation.

The diagnosis of RSV can be established by immunoflourescent assay, or IFA. IFA can confirm the infection the same day and therefore assists in the implementation of a valid treatment plan.

Treatment

As depicted in Figure 35-36, treatment of the patient with bronchiolitis varies with the severity of the infection and the observed clinical picture.[344] Many patients can be treated at home with humidification and oral decongestants. Patients with more severe symptoms are generally hospitalized, with treatment directed at relieving the airway obstruction and associated hypoxemia.

The hospitalized child is frequently treated with systemic hydration and oxygen via oxyhood, croup tent or nasal cannula, and assistance with airway clearance, as needed. Because bronchiolitis and childhood asthma have similar symptoms, a trial course of bronchodilator therapy with a beta$_2$ adrenergic agent may be useful.[345] Antibiotics may be administered to treat secondary bacterial infections.

Severe cases are treated with ribavirin. Ribavirin is a broad spectrum virustatic agent that is active against a wide range viruses. Ribavirin has been shown to be an effective agent in the treatment of bronchiolitis caused by RSV.[346,347] The American Academy of Pediatrics guidelines for the use of ribavirin is summarized in the accompanying box.[348]

Ribavirin is nebulized with a specially designed small particle aerosol generator, or SPAG (refer to Chapter 25). Normally, the aerosol is directed into an oxyhood or croup tent, and given for 12 to 18 hours per day for 3 to 7 days.[346] The treatment can also be given as a high-dose, short-duration therapy for 2-hour periods, 3 times daily for up to 5 days.[347]

Should the child with bronchiolitis progress to true respiratory failure, mechanical ventilation is required.[349] Administration of ribavirin to ventilator-dependent children must be done with caution. Precipitation of the aerosol clogs the expiratory valve and can cause inadvertent PEEP.[350] However, use of a one-way valve on the inspiratory side and a bacterial filter on the expiratory side of the ventilator circuit can prevent these problems.[351]

Due to the obstructive nature of this disorder, low rates and long expiratory times may be needed in order to prevent air trapping. Vigorous bronchial hygiene, including tracheo-bronchial aspiration, is usually needed to maintain a patent airway.

Croup

Common croup is an infectious disorder of the upper airway which normally results in subglottic

BRONCHIOLITIS

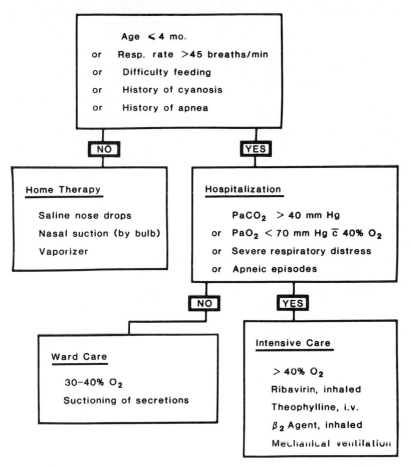

Fig. 35-36 Schema of bronchiolitis therapy shows criteria for and elements of therapy in home versus hospital and hospital ward versus intensive care unit. (From Koff PB, Eitzman DV, Neu J: Neonatal and pediatric respiratory care, St Louis, 1988, Mosby.)

American Academy of Pediatrics
Recommendations for treatment of RSV bronchiolitis

Based on the data currently available, the committee recommends that of the *infants hospitalized* with lower respiratory tract disease caused by RSV, those in the following categories should be considered for treatment with ribavirin aerosol.

1. Infants at high risk for severe or complicated RSV infection. This includes infants with congenital heart disease, bronchopulmonary dysplasia and other chronic lung conditions, and certain premature infants. In addition, children with immunodeficiency, especially those with severe combined immunodeficiency disease, recent transplant recipients, and those undergoing chemotherapy for malignancy, should also be considered to be a high risk for complicated RSV infection.
2. Infants hospitalized with RSV lower respiratory tract disease who are severely ill. Since severity of illness is often difficult to judge clinically in infants with RSV infection, determination of the blood gases is often necessary. Infants with PaO_2 levels of less than 65 torr and those with increasing $PaCO_2$ levels should be considered as candidates for ribavirin therapy. Oximetry may be used as a non-invasive means of determining the arterial oxygen saturation.
3. Infants who might be considered for treatment are those hospitalized with lower respiratory tract disease which is not initially severe, but who may be at some increased risk of progressing to a more complicated course by virtue of young age (<6 weeks), or in whom prolonged illness might be particularly detrimental to an underlying condition, such as those with multiple congenital anomalies, neurologic or metabolic disease.

From *American Academy of Pediatrics:* Policy Statement, Ribavirin therapy of respiratory syncytial virus, AAP News/Dec 1986.

swelling and obstruction.[344] Viral croup, caused by the parainfluenza virus, is the most common form of airway obstruction in children between 6 months to 6 years of age.[352] Less common as causative agents are the respiratory syncytial and influenza viruses.[353-355] Bacterial suprainfections may worsen the disorder. *Staphylococcus aureus*, group A *Streptococcus pyogenes*, or *H. influenzae* are the most common bacterial suprainfections.[344]

Formerly, several different croup syndromes were recognized. The two most common, laryngotracheitis and spasmodic croup, are probably simply two ends of a broad spectrum in the clinical presentation of a single disease.[352]

Clinical manifestations

Signs and symptoms of croup become evident after 2 or 3 days of nasal congestion, fever, and coughing.[344] Typically, the child presents with a slow, progressive inspiratory and expiratory stridor and a croupy barking cough. As the disease progresses, dyspnea, cyanosis, exhaustion, and agitation become evident.

X-ray examination can be helpful in confirming the diagnosis and in ruling out epiglottitis. Classic croup manifests itself on the AP film with a characteristic subglottic narrowing of the trachea, called the steeple sign. Lateral films typically show ballooning of hypopharynx.[356]

Treatment

The evaluation and treatment of the child with croup must focus on the degree of respiratory distress and associated findings. Table 35-22 presents a scoring system for quantifying the severity of croup.

If stridor is mild or occurs only on exertion, and cyanosis is not present (croup "score" of 3 or less), hospitalization is generally not required, and the child is treated at home. If the combined signs total to a score above 4—indicating stridor at rest, accompanied by harsh breath sounds, suprasternal retractions and cyanosis breathing room air—hospitalization is indicated. Although there is little research to support the practice,[352] management of the child with mild to moderate croup traditionally involves cool mist therapy, with or without supplemental oxygen. On the other hand, both aerosolized racemic epinephrine and dexamethasone (> 0.3 mg/kg) are effective in decreasing the length and severity of respiratory symptoms associated with viral croup.[352] Helium-oxygen mixtures may also be useful in the management of refractory viral croup.[357]

Progressive worsening of the patient's clinical signs, combined with arterial blood gas results indicating severe hypercapnia and hypoxemia, indicate the need for intubation and mechanical ventilation. As with bronchiolitis, tracheobronchial aspiration is usually needed to maintain a patent airway.[352]

Epiglottitis

Epiglottitis is an acute and often life-threatening infection of the upper airway which causes severe obstruction secondary to supraglottic swelling.[344,358,359] Although not as common as croup, epiglottitis tends to affect a similar age group, children under the age of 5. The most common cause is *Haemophilus influenzae*, type B.

Clinical manifestations

The child with epiglottitis usually presents with a high fever, cyanosis, and labored breathing.[358,359] The patient does not have a croupy bark, but instead exhibits a muffled voice. Older children may complain of sore throat and difficulty in swallowing. Difficulty in swallowing may cause drooling, which almost always is diagnostic of epiglottitis.

Visual examination of the upper airway should always be performed in a controlled setting. Inadvertent traction of the tongue can cause further and immediate swelling of the epiglottis with an abrupt and total upper airway obstruction. On lateral neck X-ray (Figure 35-37), the epiglottis is markedly thickened and flattened (the *thumb sign*) the aryepiglottic folds are swollen, and the valeculla may not be visualized. As with croup, the hypopharynx may be ballooned out.[344]

Table 35-22   Clinical croup score

	Score		
	0	1	2
Inspiratory breath sounds	Normal	Harsh with rhonchi	Delayed
Stridor	None	Inspiratory	Inspiratory and expiratory
Cough	None	Hoarse cry	Bark
Retractions and flaring	None	Flaring and supersternal retractions	As under 1, plus subcostal, retractions
Cyanosis	None	In air	in 40% O_2

From Downs JJ: Pediatric intensive care: annual refresher course lectures, ASA, 1974.

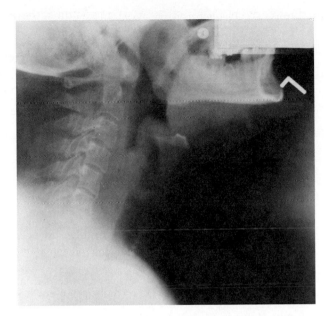

Fig. 35-37 Lateral neck X-ray of patient with epiglottis. Note the prominent "thumb" sign.

Treatment

Once the diagnosis is confirmed, the child should be accompanied by a clinician skilled in airway management who is prepared to intervene in the case of acute airway obstruction. Optimally, children with epiglottitis should be electively intubated under general anesthesia in the operating room. Nasal or orotracheal intubation is commonly performed. A tracheostomy may be needed if the patient's condition warrants it. There should be no attempt to lie the child down, nor attempts to intubate until the patient is sedated, as this may precipitate acute airway obstruction and respiratory arrest. Once an airway is secured, bacterial culture should be taken and antibiotic therapy started.[343,338-360]

Cystic fibrosis (CF)

Cystic fibrosis is an autosomal recessive genetic disorder characterized by pancreatic insufficiency, and abnormally thick secretions from the exocrine glands.[361-362] It affects mainly caucasians, at a rate of about 1 of 2500 births.

The defective gene responsible for cystic fibrosis has recently been identified.[363] This knowledge is already changing the approach to diagnosis and treatment of this disorder.[364]

Clinical manifestations

The clinical features seen in cystic fibrosis are related to pancreatic dysfunction and to a chronic, diffuse, obstructive, and infectious pulmonary process. The earliest defects include secretion of thick mucus which partially obstructs the bronchioles, and infection.[361-362] Infections are persistent, initially from *Staphylococcus aureus,* but later on from *Pseudomonas aeruginosa.* The patient has a frequent cough, tachypnea, and wheezing. There is a progressive thickening of the bronchi, bronchioles, and alveoli. The chest X-ray typically reveals a patchy atelectasis, irregular aeration, and air trapping.[365]

Pulmonary complications include bronchitis and bronchiolitis. Recurrent infections eventually result in the destruction of small airways with a resulting bronchiectasis. In older children, cor pulmonale is evident as an associated cardiac involvement.[361-362]

In addition to pulmonary problems, the highly viscous secretions cause pancreatic duct obstruction. The liver and intestines are also involved. Digestive juices are hindered and the person cannot digest fats or break down nutrients. With fats not being digested, stool becomes fatty (steatorrhea). Because of the inability to absorb fat, patients also have difficulty in absorbing fat soluble vitamins (A, D, E, and K). These patients have difficulty in gaining weight because they cannot digest their food properly. This requires treatment with pancreatic enzymes and vitamin supplements.[361-362]

Treatment

Traditional therapy for cystic fibrosis is a daily and ongoing regimen.[366] A low fat diet, vitamin supplements, and pancreatic enzymes are taken to minimize digestive problems. Antibiotic therapy is based upon culture and sensitivity results. Ribavirin treatment may be of some use since respiratory syncytial virus has been shown to be a contributing factor in the destruction of the pulmonary parenchyma.

Respiratory therapy measures are geared towards decreasing airway obstruction. Humidification, bronchodilators, mucolytic agents, expectorants, and vigorous chest physiotherapy all assist in airway clearance. Measures are usually supportive until the patient progresses to respiratory failure. Patients eventually succumb to chronic and devastating pulmonary infections or cor pulmonale.

A number of promising new treatment approaches are becoming available.[367] Recombinant human DNase, a proteolytic enzyme, is now approved for use by the FDA. In the adults with cystic fibrosis, use of aerosolized DNase results in improvements in both lung function and dyspnea scores.[368] Other drugs are being developed that may correct the basic defect in cellular ion transport that causes the abnormal secretions.[367] Most exciting, however, is the possibility for reversing the actual genetic defect via gene therapy. Currently, human trials of gene therapy for cystic fibrosis are underway, but it is simply too early to know the outcome.

CHAPTER SUMMARY

Neonatal and pediatric respiratory care is among the most sophisticated specialty areas in the field. Competent practice in this area requires a firm understanding of the many anatomic and physiologic differences between the infant, child, and adult, as well as the unique pathophysiology involved in common neonatal and pediatric respiratory disorders.

Many of the cardiopulmonary problems that occur in the perinatal period are associated with difficulties in the fetus' transition from uterine to extrauterine life. Other conditions are related to simple prematurity, while some problems appear to be iatrogenic in origin. On the other hand, pulmonary problems in the older infant and child result mainly from airway obstruction due to bacterial or viral infections, genetic disorders, and preventable accidents.

A critical component in the respiratory care management of infants and children is thorough clinical assessment. Due to the significant anatomic and physiologic differences between adult and infant, many of the assessment techniques useful with older patients simply cannot apply in the young infant. Ideally, general assessment of the infant begins prior to birth, and involves consideration of both the maternal history and condition, and the fetal and newborn status. As the child grows and develops, more of the assessment methods used with adults begin to apply.

Many of the general principles of management of the critically ill newborn infant are similar to those for adults. However, special considerations that apply to neonate care include temperature regulation, fluid and electrolyte balance, nutrition, and infection control. In terms of respiratory care management, substantial variations are required in the tools and techniques applied to the critically ill infant. These special tools and techniques provide the practitioner with the basis for anticipating the unique needs of critically ill infants and children, and planning and implementing their treatment regimens.

REFERENCES

1. Thyurlbeck WM: Postnatal growth and development of the lung, *Am Rev Respir Dis* 111:803–844, 1975.
2. Langston C, Kida K, Reed M, Thurlbeck WM: Human lung growth in late gestation and in the neonate, *Am Rev Resp Dis* 129:607–613, 1984.
3. Dunnill MS: Postnatal growth of the lung, *Thorax* 17:329–333, 1962.
4. Polgar G, Weng TR: The functional development of the respiratory system from the period of gestation to adulthood, *Am Rev Respir Dis* 120:625–695, 1979.
5. Sadler TW: *Langman's medical embryology,* ed 5, Philadelphia, 1985, Williams and Wilkins.
6. Fishman AP: *Assessment of Pulmonary Function,* New York, 1980, McGraw-Hill.
7. Moore KL: *The Developing human–clinically oriented embryology,* ed 3, Philadelphia, 1982, WB Saunders.
8. Koff PB: Development of cardiopulmonary system. In Koff PB, Eitzman DV, Neu J: *Neonatal and pediatric respiratory care,* ed 2, St Louis, 1993, Mosby.
9. Escobedo MB: Fetal and neonatal cardiopulmonary physiology. In Schreiner RL, Kisling JA, editors: *Practical neonatal respiratory care,* New York, 1982, Raven Press.
10. Eitzman DV: Physiologic development. In Koff PB, Eitzman DV, Neu J: *Neonatal and pediatric respiratory care,* ed 2, St Louis, 1993, Mosby.
11. Stave U, editor: *Perinatal physiology,* New York, 1978, Plenum Medical.
12. Crelin ES: *Functional anatomy of the newborn,* New Haven, 1973, Yale University Press.
13. Laitman JT, Crelin ES: Developmental changes in the upper respiratory system of human infants, *Perinatology-Neonatology* 4:15–21, 1980.
14. Reed WR, Roberts JL, Thach BT: Factors influencing regional patency and configuration of the human infant upper airway, *J Appl Physiol* 58(2):635–644, 1985.
15. Miller MJ, Martin RJ, Carlo WA, et al: Oral breathing in newborn infants, *J Pediatr* 107:465–469, 1985.
16. Miller MJ, Carlo WA, Strohl KP, et al: Effect of maturation on oral breathing in sleeping premature infants, *J Pediatr* 109:515–519, 1986.
17. Harding R: Function of the larynx in the fetus and newborn, *Annu Rev Physiol* 46:645–659, 1984.
18. Kubota Y, Toyoda Y, Nagata N, et al: Tracheo-bronchial angles in infants and children, *Anesthesiology* 64(3):374–376, 1986.
19. Muller N, Bryan AC: Chest wall mechanics and respiratory muscles in infants, *Ped Clin N Am* 26:503–516, 1979.
20. Rigatto H, Brady JP, de la Torre Verduzco R: Chemoreceptor reflexes in preterm infants. II. The effect of gestational age on the ventilatory response to inhaled CO2, *Pediatrics* 55:614, 1975.
21. Rigatto H, Brady JP, de la Torre Verduzco R: Chemoreceptor reflexes in preterm infants. I. The effect of gestational age and postnatal age on the ventilatory response to inhalation of 100% and 15% oxygen, *Pediatrics* 55:604, 1975.
22. Brady JP, Ceruti E: Chemoreceptor reflexes in the newborn infant: effect of varying degrees of hypoxia on heart rate and ventilation in a warm environment, *J Physiol* (Brit), 184:631, 1966.
23. Gerhardt T, Bancalari E: Chest wall compliance in full-term and premature infants, *Acta Paediatr Scand* 69:359, 1980.
24. Carlo WA, Martin RJ: Principles of neonatal assisted ventilation, *Ped Clin N Am* 33:221–237, 1985.
25. Greenough A, Roberton NR: Neonatal ventilation, *Early Hum Develop* 13(2):127–136, 1986.
26. Herman S, Reynolds EOR: Methods for improving oxygenation in infants mechanically ventilated for hyaline membrane disease, *Arch Dis Child* 48:612–617, 1973.
27. Klaus MH, Fanaroff AA, editors: *Care of the high-risk neonate,* ed 3, Philadelphia, 1986, WB Saunders.
28. Thibeault DW, Gregory GA, editors: *Neonatal pulmonary care,* ed 2, Norwalk, CT, 1986, Appleton-Centurt-Crofts.
29. Kendig EL, Chernick V, editors: *Disorders of the respiratory tract in children,* ed 4, Philadelphia, 1983, WB Saunders.
30. Aloan, CA: *Respiratory care of the newborn: a clinical manual,* Philadelphia, 1987, JB Lippincott.
31. Korones SB: *High-risk newborn infants,* ed 3, St Louis, 1981, Mosby.
32. Behnke M: Patient assessment. In Koff PB, Eitzman DV, Neu J: *Neonatal and pediatric respiratory care,* ed 2, St Louis, 1993, Mosby.
33. Whitaker K: *Comprehensive perinatal and pediatric respiratory care,* Albany, NY, 1992, Delmar Publishers.
34. Dubowitz LMS, Dubowitz D, Goldberg C: Clinical assessment of gestational age in the newborn infant, *J Pediatr* 77:1–10, 1970.
35. Ballard JL, et al: A simplified score for assessment of fetal maturation of newly born infants, *J Pediatr* 95:769–774, 1979.
36. Yerushalmy JJ: The classification of newborn infants by birth weight and gestational age, *J Pediatr* 71:164, 1967.
37. Czervinske MP: Arterial blood gas analysis and other monitoring. In Koff PB, Eitzman DV, Neu J: *Neonatal and pediatric respiratory care,* ed 2, St Louis, 1993, Mosby.

38. Carlo WA, Martin RJ, Bruce EN, et al: Alae nasi activation (nasal flaring) decreases nasal resistance in preterm infants, *Pediatrics* 72(3):338–343, 1983.
39. Silverman WA, Anderson DH: Evaluation of respiratory status: Silverman and Anderson index, *Pediatrics* 17:1, 1956.
40. Courtney SE, Weber KR, Breakie LA, et al: Capillary blood gases in the neonate. A reassessment and review of the literature, *Am J Dis Child* 144(2):168–172, 1990.
41. Koch G, Wendel H: Adjustment of arterial blood gases and acid base balance in the normal newborn infant during the first week of life, *Biol Neonate* 12:136, 1968.
42. Fan LL, Dellinger KT, Mills AL, et al: Potential errors in neonatal blood gas measurements, *J Pediatr* 97:650, 1980.
43. Morgan WJ, et al: Partial expiratory flow volume curves in infants and young children, *Pediatric Pulmon* 5:232–243, 1988.
44. Taussig LM, Landau LI, Godfrey S, et al: Determinants of forced expiratory flows in newborn infants, *J Appl Physiol* 53(5):1220–1227, 1982.
45. Adler SM, Wohl MEB: Flow-volume relationship at low lung volumes in healthy term newborn infants, *Pediatrics* 6:636–640, 1978.
46. American Thoracic Society: Respiratory mechanics in infants: physiologic evaluation in health and disease, *Am Rev Respir Dis* 147:474–496, 1993.
47. Bancalari E, Eisler E: Neonatal respiratory support. In Kirby RR, Smith RA, Desautels, DD, editors: *Mechanical ventilation,* New York, 1985, Churchill Livingstone.
48. Scopes J, Ahmed I: Ranges of critical temperatures in sick and premature newborn babies, *Arch Dis Child* 41:417, 1966.
49. Quie PG: Lung defense against infection, *J Pediat* 108:813–816, 1986.
50. Bland RD: Special considerations in oxygen therapy of infants and children, *Am Rev Respir Dis* 122(5 Pt 2):45–54, 1980.
51. American Association for Respiratory Care: Clinical practice guideline. Oxygen therapy in the acute care hospital, *Respir Care* 36(12):1410–1413, 1991.
52. Abman SH, Wolfe RR, Accurso FJ, et al: Pulmonary vascular response to oxygen in infants with severe bronchopulmonary dysplasia, *Pediatrics* 75(1):80–84, 1985.
53. Schnapf BM: Oxygen desaturation during fiberoptic bronchoscopy in pediatric patients, *Chest* 99(3):591–594, 1991.
54. Coates AL, Desmond K, Willis D, et al: Oxygen therapy and long-term pulmonary outcome of respiratory distress syndrome in newborns, *Am J Dis Child* 13(10):892–895, 1982.
55. Flynn JT, Bancalari E, Bachynski BN, et al: Retinopathy of prematurity. Diagnosis severity, and natural history, *Opthalmology* 94(6):620–629, 1987.
56. Shohat M, Reisner SH, Krikler R, et al: Retinopathy of prematurity: incidence and risk factors, *Pediatrics* 72(2):159–163, 1983.
57. Luccy JF, Dangman B: A reexamination of the role of oxygen in retrolental fibroplasia, *Pediatrics* 73(1):82–96, 1984.
58. Francois J: Risk factors for retrolental fibroplasia, *Ophthalmologica* 186(4):189–196, 1983.
59. Fay FS: Guinea pig ductus arteriosus. Cellular and metabolic basis for oxygen sensitivity, *Am J Physiol* 221:470–479, 1971.
60. Beekman RH, Rocchini AP, Rosenthal A: Cardiovascular effects of breathing 95 percent oxygen in children with congenital heart disease, *Am J Cardiol* 52(1):106–111, 1983.
61. Bakken E, Desautels DA: Oxygen therapy. In Koff PB, Eitzman DV, Neu J: *Neonatal and pediatric respiratory care,* ed 2, St Louis, 1993, Mosby.
62. Flynn JT, Bancalari E, Snyder ES, et al: A cohort study of transcutaneous oxygen tension and the incidence and severity of retiopathy of prematurity, *N Engl J Med* 326(16):1050–1054, 1992.
63. American Academy of Pediatrics, American College of Obstetricians and Gynecologists: *Guidelines for perinatal care,* ed 2, Evanston, Illinois, 1988.
64. Amar D, Brodman LE, Winikoff SA, et al: An alternative oxygen delivery system for infants and children in the post-anaesthesia care unit, *Can J Anaesth* 38(1):49–53, 1991.
65. Coates AL, Blanchard PW, Vachon F, et al: Simplified oxygen administration in tracheostomized patients with bronchopulmonary dysplasia, *Int J Pedi Otorhinolaryngol* 10(1):87–90, 1985.
66. Gale R, Redner-Carmi R, Gale J: Accumulation of carbon dioxide in oxygen hoods, infant cots, and incubators, *Pediatrics* 60:453, 1977.
67. Dawes GW, Williams TJ: The oxygen hood as a noise factor in infant care (abstract), *Respir Care* 24:12, 1979.
68. Blennow G, Svenningsen NW, Almquist B: Noise levels in infant incubators, *Pediatrics* 53:29, 1974.
69. Lanska MJ, Silverman R, Lanska DJ: Cutaneous fungal infections associated with prolonged treatment in humidified oxygen hoods [letter], *Pediatr Dermatol* 4(4):346, 1987.
70. Bhutani VK, Taube JC, Antunes MJ, et al: Adaptive control of inspired oxygen delivery to the neonate, *Pediatr Pulmonol* 14(2):110–117, 1992.
71. Morozoff PE, Evans RW: Closed-loop control of SaO_2 in the neonate, *Biomed Instrum Technol* 26(2):117–23, 1992.
72. Rotschild A, Schapira D, Kuyek N, Solimano A: Evaluation of nasal prongs of new design for low-flow oxygen delivery to infants, *Respir Care* 34(9):801–804, 1989.
73. Kloor TH Jr, Carbajal D: Infant oxygen administration by modified nasal cannula, *Clin Pediatr* (Phila) 23(9):477–479, 1984.
74. Guilfoile T, Dabe K: Nasal catheter oxygen therapy for infants, *Respir Care* 26:35, 1981.
75. Campbell AN, Zarfin Y, Groenveld M, Bryan MH: Low flow oxygen therapy in infants, *Arch Dis Child* 58(10):795–798, 1983.
76. Coffman JA, McManus KP: Oxygen therapy via nasal catheter for infants with bronchopulmonary dysplasia, *Crit Care Nurse* 4(3):22–23, 1984.
77. Shann F, Gatchalian S, Hutchinson R: Nasopharyngeal oxygen in children, *Lancet* 2(8622):1238–1240, 1988.
78. Vain NE, Prudent LM, Stevens DP, et al: Regulation of oxygen concentration delivered to infants via nasal cannulas, *Am J Dis Child* 143(12):1458–1460, 1989.
79. Locke RG, Wolfson MR, Shaffer TH, et al: Inadvertent administration of positive pressure during nasal cannula flow, *Pediatrics* 91(1):135–138, 1993.
80. Frenckner B, Ehren H, Palmer K, et al: Pneumocephalus caused by a nasopharyngeal oxygen catheter, *Crit Care Med* 18:1287–1288, 1990.
81. Zierler S: Causes of retinopathy of prematurity: an epidemiologic perspective, *Birth Defects* 1:23–33, 1988.
82. Karmann U, Roth F: Prevention of accidents associated with air-oxygen mixers, *Anesthesia* 37(6):680–682, 1982.
83. Emergency Care Research Institute: Inaccurate O_2 concentrations from oxygen-air proportioners, *Health Devices* 18(10):366–367, 1989.
84. Kim EH, Cohen RS, Ramachandran P: Effect of vascular puncture on blood gases in the newborn, *Pediatr Pulmonol* 10(4):287–290, 1991.
85. Guilfoile TD: Bedside monitoring of the acutely ill neonate: the impact of transcutaneous monitoring on neonatal intensive care, *Respir Care* 31(6):507–515, 1986.
86. Cassady G: Transcutaneous monitoring in the newborn infant, *J Pediatr* 103:837–848, 1983.
87. Salyer JW: Respiratory monitoring in the neonatal intensive care unit. In Kacmarek RM, Hess D, Stoller JK, editors: *Monitoring in respiratory care.* St Louis, 1993, Mosby.
88. LeSouef PN, Morgan AK, Soutter LP: Comparison of transcutaneous oxygen tension with arterial oxygen tension in newborn infants with severe respiratory illnesses, *J Pediatr* 92:692–695, 1978.
89. Yahav J, Mindorff C, Levison H: The validity of the trans-

cutaneous oxygen tension method in children with cardio-respiratory problems, *Am Rev Respir Dis* 124:586–587, 1981.

90. Bancalari E, Flynn J, Goldberg RN, et al: Influence of transcutaneous oxygen monitoring on the incidence of retinopathy of prematurity, *Pediatrics* 79(5):663–9, 1987.

91. Heinonen K, Hakulinen A: Transcutaneous PO_2 recording using two sensors in a neonate with preductal coarctation of the aorta, *Crit Care Med* 14(4):298–299, 1986.

92. Peevy KJ, Hall MW: Transcutaneous oxygen monitoring: economic impact on neonatal care, *Pediatrics* 75(6):1065–1067, 1985.

93. American Academy of Pediatrics Task Force on Transcutaneous Oxygen Monitors: Report of consensus meeting, *Pediatrics* 83(1):122–126, 1989.

94. Walsh MC, Noble LM, Carlo WA, Martin RJ: Relationship of pulse oximetry to arterial oxygen tension in infants, *Crit Care Med* 15(12):1102–1105, 1987.

95. Praud JP, Carofilis A, Bridey F, et al: Accuracy of two wavelength pulse oximetry in neonates and infants, *Ped Pulmonol* 6(3):180–182, 1989.

96. Bucher HU, Fanconi S, Baeckert P, Duc G: Hyperoxemia in newborn infants: detection by pulse oximetry, *Pediatrics* 84(2):226–230, 1989.

97. Maxwell LG, Harris AP, Sendak MJ, et al: Monitoring the resuscitation of preterm infants in the delivery room using pulse oximetry, *Clin Pediatr* (Phila) 26(1):18–20, 1987.

98. American Association for Respiratory Care: Clinical practice guideline. Pulse oximetry, *Respir Care* 36(12):1406–1409, 1991.

99. Scott AA, Koff PB: Airway care and chest physiotherapy, in Koff PB, Eitzman DV, Neu J: *Neonatal and pediatric respiratory care,* ed 2, St Louis, 1993, Mosby.

100. Crane L: Physical therapy for neonates with respiratory dysfunction, *Phys Ther* 61(12):1764–1773, 1981.

101. Martin RJ, Herrell N, Rubin D, Fanaroff A: Effect of supine and prone positions on arterial oxygen tension in the preterm infant, *Pediatrics* 63(4):528–531, 1979.

102. Fox MD, Molesky MG: The effects of prone and supine positioning on arterial oxygen pressure, *Neonatal Netw* 8(4):25–29, 1990.

103. Sconyers SM, Ogden BE, Goldberg HS: The effect of body position on the respiratory rate of infants with tachypnea, *J Perinatol* 7(2):118–121, 1987.

104. Thoresen M, Cowan F, Whitelaw A: Effect of tilting on oxygenation in newborn infants. *Arch Dis Child* 63(3):315–317, 1988.

105. Wolfson MR, Greenspan JS, et al: Effect of position on the mechanical interaction between the rib cage and abdomen in preterm infants, *J Appl Physiol* 72(3):1032–8, 1992.

106. Crane LD, Snyder JE, et al: Effects of position changes on transcutaneous carbon dioxide tension in neonates with respiratory distress, *J Perinatol* 10(1):35–37, 1990.

107. Polacek TL, Barth L, et al: The effect of positioning on arterial oxygenation in children with atelectasis after cardiac surgery, *Heart Lung* 21(5):457–462, 1992.

108. Guntheroth WG, Spiers PS: Sleeping prone and the risk of sudden infant death syndrome, *JAMA* 267(17):2359–2362, 1992.

109. Bozynski ME, Naglie RA, et al: Lateral positioning of the stable ventilated very-low-birth-weight infant. Effect on transcutaneous oxygen and carbon dioxide, *Am J Dis Child* 142(2):200–202, 1988.

110. Schlessel JS, Rappa HA, Lesser M, Harper RG: Pulmonary mechanics and gas exchange: effect of lateral positioning during recovery from respiratory distress syndrome. *Pediatr Pulmonol* 15(1):36–40, 1993.

111. Heaf DP, Helms P, et al: Postural effects on gas exchange in infants, *N Engl J Med* 308(25):1505–1508, 1983.

112. Cohen RS, Smith DW, et al: Lateral decubitus position as therapy for persistent focal pulmonary interstitial emphysema in neonates: a preliminary report, *J Pediatr* 104(3):441–443, 1984.

113. Davies H, Kitchman R, et al: Regional ventilation in infancy. Reversal of adult pattern, *N Engl J Med* 313(26):1626–1628, 1985.

114. Swingle HM, Eggert LD, Bucciarelli RL: New approach to management of unilateral tension pulmonary interstitial emphysema in premature infants, *Pediatrics* 74(3):354–357, 1984.

115. Sharp MJ; Goldsmith JP. Ventilatory management casebook. Resolution of pulmonary interstitial emphysema using position therapy, *J Perinatol* 8(2):163–165, 1988.

116. American Association for Respiratory Care: Clinical practice guideline. Postural drainage therapy, *Respir Care* 36(12):1418–1426, 1991.

117. Mellins R: Pulmonary physiotherapy in the pediatric age group, *Am Rev Respir Dis* 1974, 110:137–142.

118. Eid N, Buchheit J, Neuling M, Phelps H: Chest physiotherapy in review, *Respir Care* 36(4):270–282, 1991.

119. Etches PC, Scott B: Chest physiotherapy in the newborn: effect on secretions removed, *Pediatrics* 62(5):713–715, 1978.

120. Finer NN, Boyd J: Chest physiotherapy in the neonate: a controlled study, *Pediatrics* 61(2):282–285, 1978.

121. Curran C, Kachoyeanos M: The effects on neonates of two methods of chest physical therapy, *MCN* 4:309, 1979.

122. Law D, Kosloske AM: Management of tracheobronchial foreign bodies in children: a reevaluation of postural drainage and bronchoscopy, *Pediatrics* 58(3):362–367, 1976.

123. Webb MS, Martin JA, et al: Chest physiotherapy in acute bronchiolitis, *Arch Dis Child* 60(11):1078–1079, 1985.

124. Reines HD, Sade RM, et al: Chest physiotherapy fails to prevent postoperative atelectasis in children after cardiac surgery. *Ann Surg* 195(4):451–455, 1982.

125. Levin D: *Postural drainage and percussion for the infant and child, in Pediatric intensive care,* ed 2, St Louis, 1984, Mosby.

126. American Association for Respiratory Care: Clinical practice guideline. Directed cough, *Respir Care* 38(5):495–499, 1993.

127. Warwick WJ, Hansen LG: The long-term effect of high-frequency chest compression therapy on pulmonary complications of cystic fibrosis, *Pediatr Pulmonol* 11:265–271, 1991.

128. Freitag L, Kim CS, et al: Mobilization of mucous by airway oscillations, *Acta Anaesthesiol Scand Suppl* 90:93–101, 1989.

129. Mahlmeister MJ, Fink JB, et al: Positive expiratory pressure mask therapy: theoretical and practical considerations and a review of the literature, *Respir Care* 36(11):1218–1229, 1991.

130. American Association for Respiratory Care: Clinical practice guideline. Use of positive airway pressure adjuncts to bronchial hygiene therapy, *Respir Care* 38(5):516–521, 1993.

131. Maayan C, Bar-Yishay E, et al: Immediate effect of various treatments on lung function in infants with cystic fibrosis, *Respiration* 55(3):144–151, 1989.

132. Purohit DM, Caldwell C, Levkoff AH: Multiple rib fractures due to physiotherapy in a neonate with hyaline membrane disease, *Am J Dis Child* 129(9):1103–1104, 1975.

133. Wood BP: Infant ribs: generalized periosteal reaction resulting from vibrator chest physiotherapy, *Radiology* 162(3):811–812, 1987.

134. Raval D, Yeh TF, et al: Chest physiotherapy in preterm infants with RDS in the first 24 hours of life, *J Perinatol* 7(4):301–304, 1987.

135. Emery JR, Peabody JL: Head position affects intracranial pressure in newborn infants, *J Pediatr* 103(6):950–953, 1983.

136. Goldberg RN, Joshi A, et al: The effect of head position on intracranial pressure in the neonate, *Crit Care Med* 11(6):428–430, 1983.

137. Raval D, et al: Changes in $tcPO_2$ during tracheobronchial hygiene in neonates, *J Pediatr* 96:1118, 1980.

138. Barnes CA, Asonye UO, Vidyasagar D: Effects of broncho-pulmonary hygiene on PtcO₂ values in critically ill neonates, *Crit Care Med* 9:819, 1981.

139. Chatburn RL: Physiologic and methodologic issues regarding humidity therapy, *J Pediatr* 114:416–420, 1989.

140. Rau JL: Delivery of aerosolized drugs to neonatal and pediatric patients, *Respir Care* 36(6):514–542, 1991.

141. Harpin VA, Rutter N: Humidification of incubators, *Arch Dis Child* 60(3):219–224, 1985.

142. Sauer PJ, Dane HJ, Visser HK: Influence of variations in the ambient humidity on insensible water loss and thermo-neutral environment of low birth weight infants, *Acta Paediatr Scand* 73(5):615–619, 1984.

143. Tarno-Mordi WO, Reid E, et al: Low inspired gas temperature and respiratory complications in very low birth weight infants, *J Pediatr* 114:438–442, 1989.

144. Hanssler L, Tennhoff W, Roll C: Membrane humidification —a new method for humidification of respiratory gases in ventilator treatment of neonates, *Arch Dis Child* 67(10 Spec No):1182–1184, 1992.

145. Tarnow-Mordi WO, Sutton P, Wilkinson AR: Inadequate humidification of respiratory gases during mechanical ventilation of the newborn, *Arch Dis Child* 61(7):698–700, 1986.

146. O'Hagan M, Reid E, Tarnow-Mordi WO: Is neonatal inspired gas humidity accurately controlled by humidifier temperature?, *Crit Care Med* 19(11):1370–1373, 1991.

147. Chatburn RL: Principles and practice of neonatal and pediatric mechanical ventilation, *Respir Care* 36(6):569–593, 1991.

148. Emergency Care Research Institute: Heated wires can melt disposable breathing circuits, *Health Devices* 18(5):174–175, 1989.

149. Levy H, Simpson Q, Duval D: Hazards of humidifiers with heated wires [letter], *Crit Care Med* 21(3):477–478, 1993.

150. Gedeon A, Mebius C, Palmer K: Neonatal hygroscopic condenser humidifier, *Crit Care Med* 15(1):51–54, 1987.

151. Muller WJ, Gerjarusek S, Scherer PW: Studies of wall shear and mass transfer in a large scale model of neonatal high-frequency jet ventilation, *Ann Biomed Eng* 18(1):69–88, 1990.

152. Kacmarek RM, Hess D: The interface between patient and aerosol generator, *Respir Care* 36(9):952–976, 1991.

153. Finucane BT, Santora AH: *Principles of airway management,* Philadelphia, 1988, FA Davis.

154. Barkin RM: Pediatric airway management, *Emerg Med Clin North Am* 6(4):687–692, 1988.

155. Turner BS: Maintaining the artificial airway: current concepts, *Pediatr Nurs* 16(5):487–493, 1990.

156. Keep PJ, Manford ML: Endotracheal tube sizes for children, *Anesth* 29:181, 1974.

157. Dankle SK, Schuller DE, McClead RE: Prolonged intubation of neonates, *Arch Otolaryngol Head Neck Surg* 113(8):841–843, 1987.

158. Angelos GM, Smith DR, et al: Oral complications associated with neonatal oral tracheal intubation: a critical review, *Pediatr Dent* 11(2):133–140, 1989.

159. Black AE, Hatch DJ, Nauth-Misir N: Complications of tracheal intubation in neonates, infants and children: a review of 4 years' experience in a children's hospital, *Br J Anaesth* 65(4):461–467, 1990.

160. Scott PH, Eigen H, et al: Predictability and consequences of spontaneous extubation in a pediatric ICU, *Crit Care Med* 13(4):228–232, 1985.

161. Caldwell CC, Stankiewicz J, et al: Intubation-related tracheal stenosis in very-low-birth-weight infants. Diagnosis and treatment, *Am J Dis Child* 139(6):618–620, 1985.

162. Sherman JM, Lowitt S, et al: Factors influencing acquired subgottic stenosis in infants, *J Pediatr* 109(2):322–327, 1986.

163. Clarke TA, Coen RW, et al: Esophageal perforations in premature infants and comments on the diagnosis, *Am J Dis Child* 134(4):367–368, 1980.

164. McLeod BJ, Sumner E: Neonatal tracheal perforation. A complication of tracheal intubation, *Anaesthesia* 41(1):67–70, 1986.

165. Blom H, Rytlander M, Wisborg T: Resistance of tracheal tubes 3.0 and 3.5 mm internal diameter. A comparison of four commonly used types, *Anaesthesia* 40(9):885–888, 1985.

166. Goodwin SR, Graves SA, Haberkern CM: Aspiration in intubated premature infants, *Pediatrics* 75(1):85–88, 1985.

167. Scott AA, Koff PB: Airway care and chest physiotherapy. In Koff PB, Eitzman DV, Neu J: *Neonatal and pediatric respiratory care,* ed 2, St Louis, 1993, Mosby.

168. McMillan DD, Rademaker AW, et al: Benefits of orotracheal and nasotracheal intubation in neonates requiring ventilatory assistance, *Pediatrics* 77(1):39–44, 1986.

169. Rotschild A, Chitayat D, et al: Optimal positioning of endotracheal tubes for ventilation of preterm infants. *Am J Dis Child* 145(9):1007–1012, 1991.

170. Donn SM, Blane CE: Endotracheal tube movement in the preterm neonate: oral versus nasal intubation, *Ann Otol Rhinol Laryngol* 94(1 Pt 1):18–20, 1985.

171. Roopchand R, Roopnarinesingh S, Ramsewak S: Instability of the tracheal tube in neonates: a postmortem study, *Anaesthesia* 44(2):107–109, 1989.

172. Wee MY, Walker AK: The oesophageal detector device: an assessment with uncuffed tubes in children, *Anaesthesia* 46(10):869–871, 1991.

173. Bhende MS, Thompson AE, et al: Validity of a disposable end-tidal CO2 detector in verifying endotracheal tube placement in infants and children, *Ann Emerg Med* 21(2):142–145, 1992.

174. Lingle PA: Sonographic verification of endotracheal tube position in neonates: a modified technique, *JCU J Clin Ultrasound* 16(8): 605–609, 1988.

175. Slovis TL, Poland RL: Endotracheal tubes in neonates: sonographic positioning, *Radiology* 160(1):262–263, 1986.

176. Brown MS: Prevention of accidental extubation in newborns, *Am J Dis Child* 142(11):1240–1243, 1988.

177. Prendiville A, Thomson A, Silverman M: Effect of tracheobronchial suction on respiratory resistance in intubated preterm babies, *Arch Dis Child* 61(12):1178–1183, 1986.

178. Durand M, Sangha B, et al: Cardiopulmonary and intracranial pressure changes related to endotracheal suctioning in preterm infants, *Crit Care Med* 17(6):506–510, 1989.

179. Fanconi S, Duc G: Intratracheal suctioning in sick preterm infants: prevention of intracranial hypertension and cerebral hypoperfusion by muscle paralysis, *Pediatrics* 79(4):538–543, 1987.

180. Perlman JM, Volpe JJ: Suctioning in the preterm infant: effects on cerebral blood flow velocity, intracranial pressure, and arterial blood pressure, *Pediatrics* 72(3):329–334, 1983.

181. Simbruner G, Coradello H, et al: Effect of tracheal suction on oxygenation, circulation, and lung mechanics in newborn infants, *Arch Dis Child* 56(5):326–330, 1981.

182. Shah AR, Kurth CD, et al: Fluctuations in cerebral oxygenation and blood volume during endotracheal suctioning in premature infants, *J Pediatr* 120(5):769–774, 1992.

183. Kerem E, Yatsiv I, Goitein KJ: Effect of endotracheal suctioning on arterial blood gases in children, *Intensive Care Med* 16(2):95–99, 1990.

184. Skov L, Ryding J, et al: Changes in cerebral oxygenation and cerebral blood volume during endotracheal suctioning in ventilated neonates, *Acta Paediatr* 81(5):389–393, 1992.

185. Alpan G, Glick B, et al: Pneumothorax due to endotracheal tube suction, *Am J Perinatol* 1(4):345–348, 1984.

186. Jaw MC, Soong WJ, et al: Pneumothorax: a complication of deep endotracheal tube suction: report of 3 cases, *Chung Hua I Hsueh Tsa Chih* 48(4):313–317, 1991.

187. Barnes TA: Emergency ventilation techniques and related equipment, *Respir Care* (7):673–90, 1992.

188. Cabal L, Devaskar S, et al: New endotracheal tube adaptor reducing cardiopulmonary effects of suctioning, *Crit Care Med* 7(12):552–555, 1979.

189. Gunderson LP, McPhee AJ, Donovan EF: Partially ventilated endotracheal suction. Use in newborns with respiratory distress syndrome, *Am J Dis Child* 140(5):462–465, 1986.

190. Bodai BI, Briggs SW, et al: Evaluation of the ability of the Neo₂Safe valve to minimize desaturation in neonates during suctioning. *RespirCare* 34(5):355–359, 1989.

191. Graff M, France J, et al: Prevention of hypoxia and hyperoxia during endotracheal suctioning, *Crit Care Med* 15(12):1133–1135, 1987.

192. Monaco FJ, Meredith KS: A bench test evaluation of a neonatal closed tracheal suction system, *Pediatr Pulmonol* 13(2):121–123, 1992.

193. Fewell J, Arrington R, Seibert J: The effect of head position and angle of tracheal bifurcation on bronchus catheterization in the intubated neonate, *Pediatrics* 64(3):318–320, 1979.

194. Placzek M, Silverman M: Selective placement of bronchial suction catheters in intubated neonates. *Arch Dis Child* 58(10):829–831, 1983.

195. Soong WJ, Hwang BT: Selective placement of bronchial suction catheters in intubated full term and premature neonates, *Chung Hua I Hsueh Tsa Chih* 48(1):45–48, 1991.

196. Shorten DR, Byrne PJ, Jones RL: Infant responses to saline instillations and endotracheal suctioning. *J Obstet Gynecol Neonatal Nurs* 20(6):464–9, 1991.

197. Beeram MR, Dhanireddy R: Effects of saline instillation during tracheal suction on lung mechanics in newborn infants, *J Perinatol* 12(2):120–123, 1992.

198. Ninan A, O'Donnell M, et al: Physiologic changes induced by endotracheal instillation and suctioning in critically ill preterm infants with and without sedation. *Am J Perinatol* 3(2):94–97, 1986.

199. Fanconi S, Duc G: Intratracheal suctioning in sick preterm infants: prevention of intracranial hypertension and cerebral hypoperfusion by muscle paralysis, *Pediatrics* 79(4):538–43, 1987.

200. Wilson G, Hughes G, et al: Evaluation of two endotracheal suction regimes in babies ventilated for respiratory distress syndrome, *Early Hum Dev* 25(2):87–90, 1991.

201. Feaster SC, West C, Ferketich S: Hyperinflation, hyperventilation, and hyperoxygenation before tracheal suctioning in children requiring long-term respiratory care, *Heart Lung* 14(4):379–384, 1985.

202. Cordero L, Hon EH: Neonatal bradycardia following nasopharyngeal stimulation, *J Pediatr* 78:441, 1971.

203. Bloom, RS, Cropley C: *Textbook of neonatal resuscitation,* Evanston, IL: American Academy of Pediatrics, 1990.

204. Czervinske MP: Continuous positive airway pressure. In Koff PB, Eitzman DV, Neu J: *Neonatal and pediatric respiratory care,* ed 2, St Louis, 1993, Mosby.

205. Jonzon A: Indications for continuous positive airway pressure and respiratory therapy, *Int J Technol Assess Health Care* 7(Suppl)1:26–30, 1991.

206. Kamper J, Ringsted C: Early treatment of idiopathic respiratory distress syndrome using binasal continuous positive airway pressure, *Acta Paediatr Scand* 79(6–7):581–586, 1990.

207. Duncan, AW, Oh TE, Hillman DR: PEEP and CPAP, *Anaesth Inten Care* 14:236–250, 1986.

208. Han VK, Beverley DW, et al: Randomized controlled trial of very early continuous distending pressure in the management of preterm infants, *Early Hum Dev* 15(1):21–32, 1987.

209. Finer NN, Kelly MA: Optimum ventilation for the neonate. I Continuous positive airway pressure, *Perinatol Neonatal* 7:95–100, 1983.

210. McPherson SP: *Respiratory therapy equipment,* ed 4, St Louis, 1990, Mosby.

211. Weinstein MM, Weinstein MR: Increased airway resistance complicating respiratory distress syndrome, *Crit Care Med* 15:76–77, 1987.

212. Czervinske MP, Durbin CG, Gale TJ: Resistance to gas flow across 14 CPAP devices for newborns, *Resp Care* 31:18, 1986.

213. Simbruner G: Inadvertent positive pressure in mechanical ventilation of the newborn with detection and effects on lung mechanics and gas exchange, *J Pediatr* 168:589–595, 1986.

214. Schulze A, Madler HJ, et al: Titration of continuous positive airway pressure by the pattern of breathing: analysis of flow-volume-time relationships by a noninvasive computerized system, *Pediatr Pulmonol* 8(2):96–103, 1990.

215. Locke R, Greenspan JS, et al: Effect of nasal CPAP on thoracoabdominal motion in neonates with respiratory insufficiency, *Pediatr Pulmonol* 11(3):259–264, 1991.

216. Turney T, et al: Complications of constant positive airway pressure, *Arch Dis Child* 50:128, 1975.

217. Betit P, Thompson JE: Mechanical ventilation. In Koff PB, Eitzman DV, Neu J: *Neonatal and pediatric respiratory care,* ed 2, St Louis, 1993, Mosby.

218. Cvetnic WG, Shoptaugh M, Sills JH: Intermittent mandatory ventilation with continuous negative pressure compared with positive end-expiratory pressure for neonatal hypoxemia, *J Perinatol* 12(4):316–324, 1992.

219. Cvetnic WG, Waffarn F, Martin JM: Continuous negative pressure and intermittent mandatory ventilation in the management of pulmonary interstitial emphysema: a preliminary study, *J Perinatol* 9(1):26–32, 1989.

220. Bernstein G: Synchronous and patient-triggered ventilation in newborns, *Neonatal Respir Dis* 3(2):1–4, 9–11, 1993.

221. Greenough A, Greenall F: Observation of spontaneous respiratory interaction with artificial ventilation, *Arch Dis Child* 63(2):168–171, 1988.

222. Greenough A, Wood S, Morley CJ, et al: Pancuronium prevents pneumothoraces in ventilated premature babies who actively expire against positive pressure ventilation, *Lancet* 1:1–4, 1984.

223. Pertman LM, Goodman S, Kreusser KL, et al: Reduction in intraventricular hemorrhage by elimination of fluctuating cerebral blood flow velocity in preterm infants with respiratory distress syndrome, *N Engl J Med* 312:1353–1357, 1985.

224. Sola A, Farina D, et al: Lack of relationship between the true airway pressure and the pressure displayed with an infant ventilator, *Crit Care Med* 20(6):778–781, 1992.

225. Kirpalani H, Santos-Lyn R, Roberts R: Some infant ventilators do not limit peak inspiratory pressure reliably during active expiration, *Crit Care Med* 16(9):880–883, 1988.

226. Pirie GE, Cain DL: Options for ventilating the pediatric patient-Part 3. circuits and humidification systems, *Perinatol Neonatol* 75–83, 1984.

227. Nelson D, McDonald JS: Heated humidification, temperature control, and "rain-out" in neonatal ventilation, *Respir Therapy* 7:41, 1977.

228. Rasanen J, Leijala M: Breathing circuit respiratory work in infants recovering from respiratory failure, *Crit Care Med* 19(1):31–35, 1991.

229. Desautels DA: Mechanical ventilators. In Koff PB, Eitzman DV, Neu J: *Neonatal and pediatric respiratory care,* ed 2, St Louis, 1993, Mosby.

230. Carr DJ, Rich M, et al: A comparative evaluation of three neonatal ventilators, *Crit Care Med* 14(3):234–236, 1986.

231. Greenough A, Pool J: Neonatal patient triggered ventilation *Arch Dis Child* 63(4):394–397, 1988.

232. Greenough A, Milner AD: Respiratory support using patient triggered ventilation in the neonatal period, *Arch Dis Child* 67(1 Spec No):69–71, 1992.

233. Cleary JP, Bernstein G, Heldt GP, et al: Improved oxygenation during synchronized vs intermittent mandatory ventilation in VLBW infants with respiratory distress: A randomized crossover design, *Pediatr Res* 1993; 33:1226A.

234. Govindaswami B, Heldt GP, Bernstein G, et al: Reduction in cerebral blood flow velocity (CBFV) variability in infants >1500 g during SIMV, *Pediatr Res* 33:1258A, 1993.

235. Vishveshwara N, Freeman B, Peck M, et al: Patient-triggered synchronized assisted ventilation of newborns, *J Perinatol* 4:347–354, 1991.

236. Chan V, Greenough A: Randomised controlled trial of weaning by patient triggered ventilation or conventional ventilation, *Eur J Pediatr* 152(1):51–54, 1993.

237. Hird MF, Greenough A: Randomized trial of patient-triggered ventilation versus high frequency positive pressure ventilation in acute respiratory distress, *J Perinat Med* 19: 379–384, 1991.

238. Greenough A, Hird MF, Chan V: Airway pressure triggered ventilation for preterm neonates, *J Perinat Med* 19(6):471–476, 1991.

239. Hird MF, Greenough A: Gestational age: an important influence on the success of patient triggered ventilation, *Clin Phys Physiol Meas* 11(4):307–12, 1990.

240. Hird MF, Greenough A: Patient triggered ventilation in chronically ventilator-dependent infants, *Eur J Pediatr* 150(10): 732–734, 1991.

241. Hird MF, Greenough A: Patient triggered ventilation using a flow triggered system, *Arch Dis Child* 66(10 Spec No): 1140–1142, 1991.

242. Mitchell A, Greenough A, Hird M: Limitations of patient triggered ventilation in neonates, *Arch Dis Child* 64(7 Spec No):924–929, 1989.

243. Hird MF, Greenough A: Causes of failure of neonatal patient triggered ventilation, *Early Hum Dev* 23(2):101–108, 1990.

244. Coghill CH, Haywood JL, Chatburn RL, Carlo WA: Neonatal and pediatric high-frequency ventilation: principles and practice, *Respir Care* 36(6):596–609, 1991.

245. Fredberg JJ, Glass GM, et al: Factors influencing mechanical performance of neonatal high-frequency ventilators, *J Appl Physiol* 62:2485–2490, 1987.

246. Hoskyns EW, Milner AD, Hopkin IE: Dynamic lung inflation during high frequency oscillation in neonates, *Eur J Pediatr* 151(11):846–850, 1992.

247. Eyal FG, Arad ID, et al: High frequency positive-pressure ventilation in neonates, *Crit Care Med* 12:793–797, 1984.

248. Sedin G: Positive-pressure ventilation at moderately high frequency in newborn infants with respiratory distress syndrome (IRDS), *Acta Anaesthesiol Scand* 30:515–520, 1986.

249. OCTAVE Study Group: Multicentre randomised controlled trial of high against low frequency positive pressure ventilation, *Arch Dis Child* 66(7 Spec No):770–775, 1991.

250. Hird MF, Greenough A: Inflation time in mechanical ventilation of preterm neonates, *Eur J Pediatr* 150(6):440–444, 1991.

251. Pagani G, Rezzonico R, Marini A: Trials of high frequency jet ventilation in preterm infants with severe respiratory disease, *Acta Paediatr Scand* 74:681–686, 1985.

252. Carlo WA, Chatburn RL, Martin RJ: Randomized trial of high-frequency jet ventilation versus conventional ventilation in respiratory distress syndrome, *J Pediatr* 110:275–282, 1986.

253. Gonzalez F, Harris T, et al: Decreased gas flow through pneumothoraces in neonates receiving high-frequency jet versus conventional ventilation, *J Pediatr* 110:464–466, 1987.

254. Carlo WA, Siner B, Chatburn RL, et al: Early randomized intervention with high-frequency jet ventilation in respiratory distress syndrome, *J Pediatr* 117:765–770, 1990.

255. Carlo WA, Beoglos A, Chatburn RL, Walsh MC, Martin RJ: High-frequency jet ventilation in neonatal pulmonary hypertension, *Am J Dis Child* 143:233–238, 1989.

256. Frantz ID, Wethhammer J, Stark AR: High-frequency ventilation in premature infants with lung disease: Adequate gas exchange at low tracheal pressures, *Pediatrics* 71:483–488, 1983.

257. Gaylord MS, Quissell BJ, Lair ME: High frequency ventilation in the treatment of infants weighing less than 1500

258. Kohelet D, Periman M, et al: High-frequency oscillation in the rescue of infants with persistent pulmonary hypertension, *Crit Care Med* 16:510–516, 1988.

259. The HIFI Study Group: High-frequency oscillatory ventilation compared with conventional mechanical ventilation in the treatment of respiratory failure in preterm infants, *N Engl J Med* 320:88–93, 1989.

260. Clark RH, Gertsman DR, Null DM Jr, et al: High-frequency oscillatory ventilation reduces the incidence of severe chronic lung disease in respiratory distress syndrome (abstract), *Am Rev Respir Dis* 141(4, Part 2):A686, 1990.

261. Clark RH, Gerstmann DR, et al: Prospective randomized comparison of high-frequency oscillatory and conventional ventilation in respiratory distress syndrome, *Pediatrics* 89(1): 5–12, 1992.

262. Boynton BR, Mannino FL, et al: Combined high-frequency oscillatory ventilation and intermittent mandatory ventilation in critically ill neonates, *J Pediatr* 105:297–302, 1984.

263. Spitzer AR, Butler S, Fox WW: Ventilatory response to combined high frequency jet ventilation and conventional mechanical ventilation for the rescue treatment of severe neonatal lung disease, *Pediatr Pulmonol* 7:244–250, 1989.

264. Berner ME, Rouge JC, Suter PM: Combined high-frequency ventilation in children with severe adult respiratory distress syndrome, *Intensive Care Med* 17(4):209–214, 1991.

265. Heicher DA, Kasting DS, Harrod JR: Prospective clinical comparison of two methods for mechanical ventilation of neonates: rapid rate and short inspiratory time versus slow rate and long inspiratory time, *J Pediatr* 98(6):957–961, 1981.

266. Pohlandt F, Saule H, et al: Decreased incidence of extra-alveolar air leakage or death prior to air leakage in high versus low rate positive pressure ventilation: results of a randomised seven centre trial in preterm infants, *Eur J Pediatr* 151(12):904–909, 1992.

267. Mammel MC, Boros SJ, et al: Determining optimum inspiratory time during intermittent positive pressure ventilation in surfactant-depleted cats, *Pediatr Pulmonol* 7(4):223–229, 1989.

268. Shortland DB, Field D, et al: Cerebral haemodynamic effects of changes in positive and expiratory pressure in preterm infants, *Arch Dis Child* 64(4):465–469, 1989.

269. Field D, Milner AD, Hopkin IE: Effects of positive end expiratory pressure during ventilation of the preterm infant, *Arch Dis Child* 60(9):843–847, 1985.

270. Boros, SJ, et al: The effect of independent variations in inspiratory-expiratory ratio and end-expiratory pressure during mechanical ventilation in hyaline membrane disease: the significance of mean airway pressure, *J Pediatr* 94:114–117, 1979.

271. Upton CJ, Milner AD, Stokes GM: The effect of changes in inspiratory time on neonatal triggered ventilation, *Eur J Pediatr* 149(9):648–650, 1990.

272. Clark RH, Gerstmann DR, et al: Pulmonary interstitial emphysema treated by high-frequency oscillatory ventilation, *Crit Care Med* 14(11):926–930, 1986.

273. Carter JM, Gerstmann DR, et al: High-frequency oscillatory ventilation and extracorporeal membrane oxygenation for the treatment of acute neonatal respiratory failure, *Pediatrics* 85(2):159–164, 1990.

274. deLemos R, Yoder B, et al: The use of high-frequency oscillatory ventilation (HFOV) and extracorporeal membrane oxygenation (ECMO) in the management of the term/near term infant with respiratory failure, *Early Hum Dev* 29(1–3):299–303, 1992.

275. Badgwell JM, Heavner JE: End-tidal carbon dioxide pressure in neonates and infants measured by aspiration and flow-through capnography, *J Clin Monit* 7(4):285–288, 1991.

276. Sivan Y, Eldadah MK, et al: Estimation of arterial carbon dioxide by end-tidal and transcutaneous PCO_2 measure-

ments in ventilated children, *Pediatr Pulmonol* 12(3):153–157, 1992.

277. Fisher, JB, Mammel M: Identifying lung overdistention during mechanical ventilation by using volume-pressure loops, *Pediatr Pulmon* 5:10–14, 1988.

278. Donahue LA, Thibeault DW: Alveolar gas trapping and ventilator therapy in infants, *Perinatol Neonatol* 3 (June):35–37, 1979.

279. Simbruner G: Inadvertent positive end-expiratory pressure in mechanically ventilated newborn infants: detection and effect on lung mechanics and gas exchange, *J Pediatr* 108(4): 589–595, 1986.

280. Greenough A, Greenall F, Gamsu HR: Inspiratory times when weaning from mechanical ventilation, *Arch Dis Child* 62(12):1269–1270, 1987.

281. Greenough A; Pool J; Gamsu H: Randomised controlled trial of two methods of weaning from high frequency positive pressure ventilation, *Arch Dis Child* 64(6):834–838, 1989.

282. Kim EH, Boutwell WC: Successful direct extubation of very low birth weight infants from low intermittent mandatory ventilation rate, *Pediatrics* 80(3):409–414, 1987.

283. Kim EH: Successful extubation of newborn infants without preextubation trial of continuous positive airway pressure, *J Perinatol* 9(1):72–76, 1989.

284. Higgins RD, Richter SE, Davis JM: Nasal continuous positive airway pressure facilitates extubation of very low birth weight neonates, *Pediatrics* 88(5):999–1003, 1991.

285. Truog WE: Complications of mechanical ventilation and airway control in the neonate, *Respir Care* 31(6):498–506, 1986.

286. Rivera R, Tibballs J: Complications of endotracheal intubation and mechanical ventilation in infants and children, *Crit Care Med* 20(2):193–199, 1992.

287. Chambers HM, van Velzen D: Ventilator-related pathology in the extremely immature lung, *Pathology* 21(2):79–83, 1989.

288. O'Rourke PP: ECMO: where have we been? Where are we going?, *Respir Care* 36(7):683–692, 1991.

289. O'Rourke PP: ECMO: current status, *Neonatal Respir Dis* 3(3):1–4, 9–11, 1993.

290. Null D, Berman LS, Clark R: Neonatal and pediatric ventilatory support. In Kirby RR, Banner MJ, Downs JB, editors: *Clinical application of ventilatory support,* New York: Churchill Livingstone, 1990.

291. Thompson JE, Perlman N: Extracorporeal membrane oxygenation, in Koff PB, Eitzman DV, Neu J: *Neonatal and pediatric respiratory care,* ed 2, St Louis, 1993, Mosby.

292. American Heart Association and American Academy of Pediatrics: *Textbook of advanced pediatric life support,* Dallas, 1990, American Heart Association.

293. Day SE: Intra-transport, stabilization and management of the pediatric patient, *Pediatr Clin N Amer* 40(2):263–274, 1993.

294. American Academy of Pediatrics, Committee on Hospital Care: Guidelines for air and ground transportation of pediatric patients, *Pediatrics* 78(5):943–950, 1986.

295. Sayler JW: Transport of the critically ill and injured, *Respir Care* 36(7):720–733, 1991.

296. Burchfield DJ, Neu J: Neonatal parenchymal diseases. In Koff PB, Eitzman DV, Neu J: *Neonatal and pediatric respiratory care,* St Louis, 1988, Mosby.

297. Katz VL, Bowes WA Jr: Meconium aspiration syndrome: reflections on a murky subject, *Am J Obstet Gynecol* 166 (1 Pt 1):171–83, 1992.

298. Rossi EM, Philipson EH, et al: Meconium aspiration syndrome: intrapartum and neonatal attributes, *Am J Obstet Gynecol* 161(5):1106–10, 1989.

299. Farquhar RC: Roentgenologic changes in meconium aspiration syndrome: review and report of case, *J Am Osteopath Assoc* 80(9):604–608, 1981.

300. Fox WW, Berman LS, et al: The therapeutic application of end-expiratory pressure in the meconium aspiration syndrome, *Pediatrics* 56(2):214–217, 1975.

301. Trindade O; Goldberg RN, et al: Conventional vs high-frequency jet ventilation in a piglet model of meconium aspiration: comparison of pulmonary and hemodynamic effects, *J Pediatr* 107(1):115–120, 1985.

302. Keszler M, Molina B, et al: Combined high-frequency jet ventilation in a meconium aspiration model, *Crit Care Med* 14(1):34–38, 1986.

303. Stahlman, M: Acute respiratory disorders in the newborn, in Avery G, editor: *Neonatology–pathophysiology and management of the newborn,* ed 3, Philadelphia, 1987, JB Lippincott.

304. Stark AR, Frantz ID: Respiratory distress syndrome, *Pediatr Clin North Am* 33(3):533–544, 1986.

305. Wiswell TE, Mendiola J: Respiratory distress syndrome in the newborn: innovative therapies, *Am Fam Physician* 47(2):407–414, 1993.

306. Phibbs RH, Ballard RA, et al: Initial clinical trial of EXOSURF, a protein-free synthetic surfactant, for the prophylaxis and early treatment of hyaline membrane disease, *Pediatrics* 88(1):1–9, 1991.

307. Hoekstra RE, Jackson JC, et al: Improved neonatal survival following multiple doses of bovine surfactant in very premature neonates at risk for respiratory distress syndrome, *Pediatrics* 88(1):10–18, 1991.

308. Jobe AH: Pulmonary surfactant therapy, *N Engl J Med* 328 (12):861–868, 1993.

309. Morley CJ: Surfactant treatment for premature babies—a review of clinical trials, *Arch Dis Child* 66(4 Spec No):445–450, 1991.

310. Yee WF, Scarpelli EM: Surfactant replacement therapy, *Pediatr Pulmonol* 11(1):65–80, 1991.

311. Hallman M, Merritt TA, et al: Factors affecting surfactant responsiveness, *Ann Med* 23(6):693–698, 1991.

312. Rawlings JS, Smith FR: Transient tachypnea of the newborn. An analysis of neonatal and obstetrical risk factors, *Am J Dis Child* 138:869–871, 1984.

313. Miller MJ, Martin RJ: Apnea of prematurity, *Clin Perinatol* 19(4):789–808, 1992.

314. Chesrown SE: Sudden infant death syndrome and apnea disorders. In Koff PB, Eitzman DV, Neu J: *Neonatal and pediatric respiratory care,* ed 2, St Louis, 1993, Mosby.

315. Stark AR: Disorders of respiratory control in infants, *Respir Care* 36(7):673–681, 1991.

316. Kriter KE, Blanchard J: Management of apnea in infants, *Clin Pharm* 8(8):577–587, 1989.

317. Barrington KJ, Finer NN, et al: Physiologic effects of doxapram in idiopathic apnea of prematurity, *J Pediatr* 108(1):124–129, 1986.

318. Nickerman BG: Bronchopulmonary dysplasia: Chronic pulmonary disease following neonatal respiratory failure, *Chest* 87:528–535, 1985.

319. Bancalari E, Gerhardt T: Bronchopulmonary dysplasia, *Pediatr Clin North Am* 33(1):1–23, 1986.

320. Chambers HM, van Velzen D: Ventilator-related pathology in the extremely immature lung, *Pathology* 21(2):79–83, 1989.

321. Frank L, Sosenko IR: Undernutrition as a major contributing factor in the pathogenesis of bronchopulmonary dysplasia, *Am Rev Respir Dis* 138(3):725–729, 1988.

322. Blanchard PW, Brown TM, Coates AL: Pharmacotherapy in bronchopulmonary dysplasia, *Clin Perinatol* 14(4):881–910, 1987.

323. Wilkie RA, Bryan MH: Effects of bronchodilators on airway resistance in ventilator dependent neonates with chronic lung disease, *J Pediatr* 111:278–282, 1987.

324. Benini F, Rubaltelli FF, et al: Dexamethasone in the treatment of bronchopulmonary dysplasia, *Acta Paediatr Scand Suppl* 360:108–112, 1989.

325. Harkavy KL, Scanlon JW, et al: Dexamethasone therapy for chronic lung disease in ventilator- and oxygen-dependent infants: a controlled trial, *J Pediatr* 115(6):979–983, 1989.

326. Avery GB, Fletcher AB, et al: Controlled trial of dexamethasone in respirator-dependent infants with bronchopulmonary dysplasia, *Pediatrics* 75(1):106–111, 1985.

327. Cullen ML, Klein MD. Philippart AI: Congenital diaphragmatic hernia, *Surg Clin North Am* 65(5):1115–1138, 1985.

328. Sawyer SF, Falterman KW, et al: Improving survival in the treatment of congenital diaphragmatic hernia, *Ann Thorac Surg* 41(1):75–78, 1986.

329. Bloom BT, Delmore P, et al: Respiratory distress syndrome and tracheoesophageal fistula: management with high-frequency ventilation, *Crit Care Med* 18(4):447–448, 1990.

330. Goldberg LA, Marmon LM, Keszler M: High-frequency jet ventilation decreases air flow through a tracheoesophageal fistula, *Crit Care Med* 20(4):547–549, 1992.

331. National Institutes of Health, National Institute of Child Health and Human Development: Sudden infant death syndrome (SIDS), 1986, Special Report to Congress.

332. Hunt CE, Brouillette RT: Sudden infant death syndrome, 1987 perspective, *J Pediatr* 110:669, 1987.

333. Rosen CL, Frost JD, Glaze DG: Child abuse and recurrent infant apnea, *J Pediatr* 109:1065, 1986.

334. Kraus JF: Methodologic considerations in the search for risk factors unique to sudden death syndrome. In Tilden, RJ, Roeden, LM, Steinschneider A, editors: *Sudden infant death syndrome,* Proceedings of the 1982 international conference, Baltimore, Md 1983, Academic Press.

335. Dwyer T, Ponsonby AL, et al: Prospective cohort study of prone sleeping position and sudden infant death syndrome, *Lancet* 337(8752):1244–1247, 1991.

336. Guntheroth WG, Spiers PS: Sleeping prone and the risk of sudden infant death syndrome, *JAMA* 267(17):2359–2362, 1992.

337. Weese-Mayer DE, Brouillette RT, Morrow, AS, et al: Assessing the validity of infant monitor alarms with event recording, *J Pediatrics* 115:702, 1989.

338. Weese-Mayer DE, Morrow AS, Conway LP, et al: Assessing the clinical significance of apnea exceeding 15 seconds duration with event recording, *J Pediatrics* 117:568, 1990.

339. American Academy of Pediatrics AAP Task Force on Infant Positioning and SIDS: Positioning and SIDS, *Pediatrics* 89(6 Pt 1): 1120–1126, 1992.

340. Consensus statement: NIH consensus development conference on infantile apnea and home monitoring, *Pediatrics* 79:292, 1987.

341. Bernard F, Dupont C, Viala P: Gastroesophageal reflux and upper airway diseases, *Clin Rev Allergy* 8(4):403–425, 1990.

342. Herbert JJ: Development of gastroesophageal reflux. In Lebenthal: *Textbook of gastroenterology and nutrition in infancy* (ed 2), New York, Raven Press, 1989.

343. Tercier JA: Bronchiolitis: a clinical review, *J Emerg Med* 1:119–123, 1983.

344. Kurth CD, Goodwin SR: Obstructive airway diseases in infants and children. In Koff PB, Eitzman DV, Neu J: *Neonatal and pediatric respiratory care,* St Louis, 1988, Mosby.

345. Schuhs CG, et al: Nebulized albuterol in acute bronchiolitis, *J Pediatr* 117(4):633–637, 1990.

346. Hall CB, McBride JT, et al: Ribavirin treatment of respiratory syncytial viral infection in infants with underlying cardiopulmonary disease, *JAMA* 254:3047–3051, 1985.

347. Englund JA, Piedra PA, Jefferson LS, et al: High-dose, short-duration ribavirn aerosol therapy in children with suspected respiratory syncytial virus infection, *J Pediatr* 117(2 Pt 1):313–320, 1990.

348. American Academy of Pediatrics, Policy Statement, *Ribavirin Therapy of Respiratory Syncytial Virus,* AAP News 1986.

349. Outwater KM, Crone RK: Management of respiratory failure in infants with acute viral bronchiolitis, *Am J Dis Child* 138:1071–1075, 1984.

350. Demers RR, Parker J, et al: Administration of ribavirin to neonatal and pediatric patients during mechanical ventilation. *Respir Care* 31:1188–1196, 1986.

351. Adderley RJ: Safety of ribavirin with mechanical ventilation, *Pediatric Infect Dis J* 9(9 Suppl):ss 112–114, 1990.

352. Skolnick NS: Treatment of croup. A critical review, *Am J Dis Child* 143(9):1045–1049, 1989.

353. Ryckman F, Rodgers SM: Obstructive airway disease in infants and children, *Surg Clin N Am* 65:1663–1687, 1985.

354. McLain LG: Croup syndrome, *Am Fam Physician* 36(4):207–114, 1987.

355. Broniatowski M: Respiratory distress in children, *Ear Nose Throat J* 64:13–19, 1985.

356. Currarino G, Williams B: Lateral inspiration and expiration radiographs of the neck in children with laryngotracheitis (croup), *Radiology* 145(2):365–366, 1982.

357. Nelson DS, McClellan L: Helium-oxygen mixtures as adjunctive support for refractory viral croup, *Ohio State Med J* 78(10):729–30, 1982.

358. Barker GA: Current management of croup and epiglottis, *Ped Clin N Am* 26:565, 1979.

359. Benjamin B: Acute epiglottitis, *Ann Acad Med Singapore* 200(5):696–699, 1991.

360. Faden HS: Treatment of Haemophilus influenzae type B epiglottitis, *Pediatrics* 63(3):402–7, 1979.

361. David TJ: Cystic fibrosis, *Arch Dis Child* 65(1):152–157, 1990.

362. Orenstein DM: Cystic fibrosis, *Respir Care* 36(7):746–752, 1991.

363. Barker PE: Gene mapping and cystic fibrosis, *Am J Med Sci* 299(1):69–72, 1990.

364. Beaudet AL: Genetic testing for cystic fibrosis, *Pediatr Clin North Am* 39(2):213–228, 1992.

365. Carty H: The chest radiograph in cystic fibrosis in children and the role of other radiological techniques, *J R Soc Med* 80 Suppl 15:38–46, 1987.

366. Levison H, Garner D, et al: Living with cystic fibrosis: patient, family, and physician realities, *Compr Ther* 13(10):38–45, 1987.

367. Alton E, Caplen N, et al: New treatments for cystic fibrosis, *Br Med Bull* 48(4):785–804, 1992.

368. Aitken ML, Burke W, et al: Recombinant human DNase inhalation in normal subjects and patients with cystic fibrosis. A phase 1 study, *JAMA* 267(14):1947–1951, 1992.

7

Preventive and Long-Term Care

36

Health Education and Health Promotion

■

Ann W. Tucker

Crystal L. Dunlevy

CHAPTER LEARNING OBJECTIVES

1. Relate lifestyle behaviors to selected indicators of the health status of individuals and groups;
2. Compare and contrast the medical model of health care delivery with alternative approaches to health services;
3. Identify the major priorities and objectives underlying efforts to improve the health status of the Nation;
4. Differentiate between the concepts of health promotion and health education;
5. Compare and contrast the role of the consumer and the health care professional in health education efforts;
6. Describe the components of a systematic model for developing health educational programming;
7. Identify and describe the various settings in which RCPs can assume a role in providing health education activities;
8. Relate the role of the family to the successful provision of health promotion services;
9. Describe specific ways in which RCPs can contribute to improving the health status of the Nation.

As America approaches the twenty-first century, we have many reasons to be proud of our health care system. Although problems of access remain (Chapter 1), our health has never been better. Most of the infectious diseases that ravaged America in the early 1900's have been wiped out. Mortality rates for all ages have declined, and the longevity of the population has improved.[1]

With these important advances has come the recognition that most of our remaining health problems are related to lifestyle behaviors.[2-4] The top five causes of death in the U.S. are heart disease, cancer, accidents and injuries, cerebrovascular disease, and chronic lung disease.[1] In 1990, these problems accounted for nearly 72% of all deaths. Of course, many of these causes of death are linked to individual lifestyles.

As we reach the end of this century, we are beginning to rethink the concepts of health and illness. The result is a growing emphasis on preventing disease, rather than simply treating illness.

In this context, all health professionals, including respiratory care practitioners (RCPs), will have to expand their role beyond that required to simply treat disease. Future RCPs must become experts in cardiopulmonary health promotion, disease prevention, and health education. These new leadership roles will place the RCP in a variety of new and alternative health care settings, including the workplace and community.

CONTEXT FOR HEALTH EDUCATION AND HEALTH PROMOTION

In order to illustrate the importance of this new approach to health care, we will first look at the evidence linking health and lifestyle. We will then explore the shortcomings of the current medical model of health care. Finally, we will examine alternative ways for improving the health status of the population, as developed by the U.S. government.

Relationship between lifestyle behaviors and health status

In the early 1970's, the Canadian government examined the major causes of disease and disability affecting its population. This landmark study clearly demonstrated that the causes of disease and disability fell into four major categories: (1) inadequacies in the existing health care system, (2) **behavioral** factors or unhealthy lifestyles, (3) environmental hazards, and (4) human biological factors. Figure 36-1 depicts these factors and their relative impact on health status.

More recently, a California study found that individual life expectancy could be increased significantly by practicing seven simple behaviors. These behaviors included eating breakfast, eating moderately and regularly, not smoking cigarettes, engaging in exercise, drinking only moderate amounts of alcohol, and obtaining 7 to 8 hours sleep nightly. For males, practicing these behaviors increased life expectancy an average of 11 years. Females following these practices could expect an average increase in lifespan of 7 years.[5]

Such studies have heightened public awareness on the impact that factors like smoking, diet, and exercise have on health. The public is becoming more aware that lifestyle habits affect health and the quality of life. A Harris poll revealed that over 90% of Americans understand the impact of various lifestyle behaviors on their health. Despite this awareness,

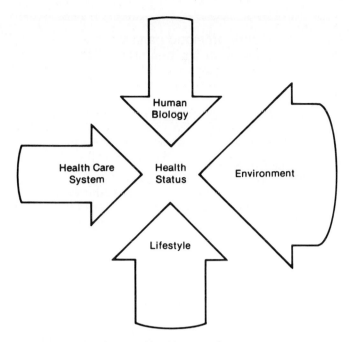

Fig. 36-1 Determinants of health status. (This figure is similar to one developed by Blum HL: Planning for health, development and application of social change theory, New York, 1973, Human Sciences Press, p. 3. Reprinted with permission.)

however, at least one-third of American adults smoke, are overweight, and/or do not exercise regularly.[4] This difference between knowledge and actual behavior stems, in part, from acceptance of the medical model of health care.

Medical model of health care delivery

Throughout this century, the medical model has shaped the organization and delivery of health care. Under this model, primary responsibility for preserving, maintaining, and restoring health rests with the health care system. Consequently, both consumers and health care providers have developed a dependency on this system.

Three assumptions underlying the medical model encourage dependency. First, the medical model asserts that disease and disability arise from outside the individual. Second, because external factors cause illness, victims of disease and disability are not responsible for their conditions. Third, the medical model asserts that these victims must depend on medical care for diagnosis and treatment.[6]

Based on this model, our health care system has evolved to emphasize specialization, high technology, and curative approaches to illness. In addition, the model has promoted high social expectations regarding the importance of the health care system. As a result, many consumers tend to view the health care system as the solution for *all* health-related matters.[6]

Many critics of the medical model argue that this approach has worsened the problems in health care delivery. The system is fragmented, health care resources are unevenly distributed, and health care costs have skyrocketed. Moreover, as the population's reliance on the health care system has grown, individuals have assumed less and less personal responsibility for their own health status. Critics also note that, while the population's health status has improved, it has done so only because vast resources have been devoted to health care.[6]

An alternate approach

As early as 1980, the U.S. government began stressing that the Nation's health strategy had to shift focus from curative treatment of disease to its prevention.[7] That year the Department of Health and Human Services published its landmark report, *Healthy People.* This report established—for the first time in U.S. history—national health goals and objectives and timelines for their achievement (1990).

Recent review of these original goals indicated good achievement in the areas of high blood pressure control, immunization, accident prevention and control, control of infectious diseases, smoking, and alcohol and drug use. On the other hand, progress has been slow in the areas of pregnancy and infant health, nutrition, physical fitness and exercise, family planning, sexually transmitted diseases, and occupational safety and health.[8]

Subsequent to this review, over 300 organizations and 50 state health departments worked together to develop a new set of objectives for the year 2000. The results of that 3-year effort, *Healthy People 2000,* were published in 1990.[9]

Healthy People 2000 sets forth three broad goals for the Nation to achieve by the year 2000. The three goals are: (1) to increase the span of healthy life for Americans, (2) to reduce health disparities among Americans, and (3) to achieve access to preventive services for all Americans.

These goals encompass the essential elements of health promotion and disease prevention: prevention of premature death, disease, and disability, and improvement in the quality of life.

Based on these goals, over 300 specific objectives have been established. The objectives are organized into three major categories and 21 priority areas (see box, page 1064).

Achieving these various goals and objectives requires collaboration among many health professions. By virtue of their numbers, training, and acceptance, allied health professionals such as RCPs are among the best prepared to assume leadership positions in the health promotion movement.[3]

The recognition that allied health professionals have an important role to play in health promotion has changed the way these providers look at them-

Healthy People 2000 priority areas

Health promotion objectives:

- Physical activity and fitness
- Nutrition
- Tobacco
- Alcohol and other drugs
- Family planning
- Mental health and mental disorders
- Violent and abusive behavior
- Educational and community-based programs

Health protection objectives:

- Unintentional injuries
- Occupational safety and health
- Environmental health
- Food and drug safety
- Oral health

Preventive services objectives:

- Maternal and infant health
- Heart disease and stroke
- Cancer
- Diabetes and chronic disabling diseases
- HIV infection
- Sexually transmitted diseases
- Immunization and infectious diseases
- Clinical preventive services

Health promotion and disease prevention position statement American Association for Respiratory Care

The American Association for Respiratory Care (AARC) submits this paper to identify and illustrate the involvement of the respiratory care practitioner in the promotion of health and the prevention of disease and supports these activities.

The AARC realizes that respiratory care practitioners are integral members of the health care team, hospitals, home health care settings, pulmonary laboratories, rehabilitation programs, and all other environments where respiratory care is practiced as outlined in the AARC Statement of Principles.

The AARC recognizes that education and training of the respiratory care practitioner is the best method by which to instill awareness for the opportunity to improve the patient's quality and longevity of life, and that such information should be included in their formal education and training.

The AARC recognizes the respiratory care practitioner's responsibility to participate in pulmonary disease training, smoking cessation programs, pulmonary function studies for the public, air pollution alerts, allergy warnings, and sulfite warnings in restaurants, as well as research in those and other areas where efforts could promote improved health and disease prevention.

Furthermore, the respiratory care practitioner is in a unique position to provide leadership in determining health promotion and disease prevention activities for students, faculty, practitioners, patients, and the general public.

The AARC recognizes the need to provide and promote consumer education related to the prevention and control of pulmonary disease to establish a strong working relationship with other health agencies, educational institutions, Federal and state government, businesses and other community organizations and to monitor such.

Furthermore, the AARC supports efforts to develop personal and professional wellness models and action plans that will inspire and encourage all members and non-members alike to cooperate on health promotion and disease prevention.

Source: American Association for Respiratory Care: Position statements, Dallas, TX: American Association for Respiratory Care, undated.

selves. As a result, in the early 1980's, many health professional organizations changed their standards of education and practice, and developed policy statements regarding health promotion and disease prevention. Organizations that have adopted formal statements include those representing RCPs, occupational therapists, physical therapists, clinical laboratory personnel, registered dieticians, physician assistants, and radiologic technologists.[10] The formal policy statement of the American Association for Respiratory Care on health promotion and disease prevention appears in the accompanying box.

More recently, allied health educators are changing their curricula to include activities directly related to health promotion and disease prevention. For example, the State University of New York at Stony Brook has developed curricular materials designed to introduce students to health promotion and disease prevention practices.[11] Similar curricular changes are now underway in many respiratory care educational programs.

How can RCPs support the goals of *Healthy People 2000?* RCPs can contribute by helping patients and the public develop healthier lifestyles, and by working to effect changes in the environment. Both *Healthy People 2000,* and its follow-up report *Prevention '91/ '92: Federal Programs and Progress* identify several areas that are especially suited for the respira-

tory care profession to either initiate or expand its involvement (see accompanying box).

In addition, RCPs can and should take an active role in developing educational materials to assist other health professionals in counseling and assisting patients with chronic cardiopulmonary disorders. A good example of this type of health promotion activity is the Peak Performance USA Project, developed by the American Association for Respiratory Care.[12] Peak Performance USA is designed to bring better asthma care to the nation's children. The project method uses hospital-based RCPs to teach school

> ## Examples of health promotion activities for respiratory care
>
> - Increasing the span of healthy life by increasing physical activity and the ability to perform self-care;
> - Implementing activities directed at reducing chronic diseases and their modifiable risk factors (pulmonary disease, in particular);
> - Offering smoking cessation programs for various populations including adolescents, geriatric, minority, and pregnant individuals.
> - Identifying specific occupational safety and health hazards in the workplace, and disseminating this information to employees in order to prevent work-related pulmonary disease and injury.

nurses how to develop an effective management program for their asthmatic students. The AARC provides a comprehensive package of materials to participating hospitals, who then work with their local community school districts to implement the program. Everything the school nurse needs to establish the program is provided, including medical forms, action plans for various school personnel, a peak flow meter, and a holding chamber.

Also worthy of attention by RCPs are recent efforts by the **DHHS'** Administration on Aging **(AoA)**. The AoA was developed to support state and local efforts to address the health care, economic, and social concerns of older Americans. The AoA has sponsored several regional conferences designed to facilitate health promotion activities among the elderly. The AoA launched a cooperative initiative in 1991 to let older people know "It's Never Too Late To Quit Smoking." All of these activities could be enhanced by the involvement of RCPs.

HEALTH PROMOTION AND HEALTH EDUCATION CONCEPTS

If health professionals are to help people develop healthier lifestyles, they must begin taking a different approach to health care delivery. Health professionals will be expected to provide services directed toward both preventing disease or disability, and promoting the quality of life through healthier behaviors. In this approach, consumers should assume greater responsibility for their own health. However, people will still turn to health professionals to assist them with assessing their health needs, developing health enhancement strategies, and monitoring progress and achievements.

Clearly, with changing expectations regarding the health care system, health promotion, and health education services are becoming an increasingly important component of our role as health professionals.

Health promotion

Health promotion is a central element in this new strategy. Unfortunately, much confusion exists as to the meaning of this term. Such confusion is made worse when the term is overused or misapplied. According to Duncan and Gold:[13]

> The term health promotion has gained wide popularity in recent years. This widespread usage has been accompanied by a wide diversity of definitions.—In many cases health promotion seems to have become an all-inclusive umbrella term under which any health service may find coverage. Health services have become health promotion services; outpatient clinics have become health promotion centers. In these cases, "health promotion" has become a fad or a gimmick—as meaningless as labeling certain cereals and other foods as natural.

Although still broad in concept, Lawrence Green defines health promotion as that combination of educational, organizational, economical and environmental supports necessary for behavior conducive to health.[13] Breslow applies a similar scope in defining health promotion as "the advancement of well-being and the avoidance of health risks by achieving the optimal levels of behavioral, societal, environmental, and biomedical determinants of health."[14] Mullen proposes that health promotion consists of two components: (1) disease prevention, and (2) wellness.[13]

Assumptions

As discussed earlier, the relationship between lifestyle and health has been well-documented. Health promotion focuses on this relationship. Unlike the traditional medical model, health promotion assumes that an individual's health is highly dependent on factors arising within the individual. In other words, how people live and what lifestyle decisions they make often can predispose them to specific diseases or disabilities.[6] For example, individuals who choose to smoke cigarettes are at a higher risk of contracting diseases such as lung cancer, COPD, respiratory infections, and high blood pressure. Although consumers will be held increasingly accountable for their own health, health professionals will be expected to continue to help individuals pursue healthy lifestyles.

Components

Regardless of definition, health promotion begins with healthy individuals and applies methods designed to maintain or improve their health status. Included are activities that focus on **holistic** health care, high level wellness, and disease prevention.

Holistic health care. The term holistic is derived from the Greek word, *holos,* meaning whole. The phrase holistic health means more than the physical state of being or the absence of disease. Holistic health asserts that health is a dynamic process comprised of many dimensions, each contributing to an individual's quality of life.

Supporters of holistic health care have proposed a multidimensional model of health.[15,16] According to this model, health is composed of six dimensions: physical, social, emotional, mental, spiritual, and vocational (see accompanying box). The model assumes that these dimensions interact with each other, while contributing to the whole.

Within this framework, holistic health care involves promoting health and preventing disease in all six dimensions. Emphasizing one dimension at the expense of the others may result in an imbalance in the health of the individual.

High-level wellness. As first defined in 1961, high-level wellness is oriented toward maximizing individuals' potential.[17] High-level wellness includes all six dimensions of health. When individuals experience high-level wellness, they have achieved and are maintaining a balance in all six dimensions.

Disease prevention. Disease prevention was first emphasized as a component of health promotion by Levall and Clark in 1965.[17] They identified three levels of disease prevention: primary, secondary, and tertiary. Each level is identified by the type of activities used to improve, prevent, or restore health.[18]

Primary prevention focuses on enhancing the well-being of healthy people. Primary responsibility for enhancing health rests with the individual. For instance, choosing not to smoke, to wear seat belts, and to eat a balanced diet are examples of primary prevention behaviors.

Early diagnosis and periodic screening for disease is known as *secondary prevention*. Secondary prevention aims to find and treat disease before it progresses to a permanent disability or results in premature death. Both the consumer and health care provider share responsibility for secondary prevention. Examples of secondary prevention include pulmonary function screening, hypertension screening, breast self-examination, pap smears, oral cancer examinations, and periodic eye testing.

Tertiary prevention includes efforts to rehabilitate and restore individual functioning, while minimizing further consequences of disease or disability. Primary responsibility for tertiary prevention rests with the health care system. Examples of prevention at this level familiar to most RCPs are pulmonary and cardiac rehabilitation programs (Chapter 37).

Health education

At the core of health promotion are the principles of health education. Health education is a process of planned learning designed to enable individuals to make informed decisions and take responsible action regarding their health.[19]

Basic requirements. Understood in this definition are several basic requirements. First, health education is planned. Planning health education programs requires a global assessment of factors and values that predispose or enable people to lead healthy lives. Second, health education programs use various educational and behavioral methods which are reinforced over time. Third, the primary goal of health education is behavioral change. This change must be voluntary and occur with the full knowledge and consent of the participants.[3] Fourth, health education activities can involve both individuals or groups.[19]

Health education strives to promote, maintain, and improve individual and community health.[20] This goal establishes an important link between health and education. It implies that health education covers the continuum between health and disease, as well as the continuum between prevention and treatment. The educational activities suggested in this goal are those relating to the promotion, maintenance, and enhancement of health.[19]

Health education programs address two levels:

Six dimensions of health

Physical. Physical health is the dimension with which most individuals are familiar. Physical health includes the level of physical fitness, the existence of disease or predisposing risk factors, and the level of biological functioning.
Social. Social health is the ability of individuals to function in and interact with society. This dimension of health is concerned with the quality of the interaction and the level of satisfaction with interpersonal relationships.
Mental. Mental health is concerned with the level of intelligence and ability to learn.
Emotional. The level of ability to express feelings when appropriate is indicative of an individual's emotional health.
Spiritual. Spiritual health is a difficult dimension to define. Generally, attributes such as honesty, integrity, purpose, or ambition in life are all considered elements of this dimension. In addition, spiritual health includes the belief in some unifying source.
Vocational. Vocational health expands the conception of health to include the integration between social (community) and personal health components. Vocational health includes financial success and advancement, recognition for contributions, sharing of work experience with others, contribution (sacrifice) to humankind, having an impact on the quality of lives of others, meeting nonrecreational challenges, expanding professional horizons, gaining new perspectives to problem solutions and giving oneself to goals or objectives related to the greater good.

From: Eberst RM: Defining health: A multidimensional model, *J School Health* 54:99–104, 1984, and Greenberg JS: Health and wellness: A conceptual differentiation, *J School Health* 55:403–406, 1985.

individuals and groups. Moreover, health education can occur in several settings, including health care institutions, the community, home, schools, and the workplace. Regardless of setting, health education cannot be effective unless combined with related strategies for health promotion.[2] In addition, effective health education requires active collaboration between health care professionals and consumers.

Role of consumer. Educating for health, rather than treating disease and disability, requires a shift in philosophy regarding responsibility for health. The burden of responsibility is shifted from the health care system to the consumer.[17]

However, health is just one of many factors competing for attention in an individual's life. As discussed earlier, health has many dimensions. The level of wellness achieved in each major dimension is affected by family, cultural, community, and societal norms, as well as economic and politic factors. In addition, the value individuals place on health will determine how well they follow a recommended health strategy.

Both consumers and health professionals must know and understand the variety of forces impacting on an individual's behavior. Once these factors are recognized and accepted, the likelihood of adopting healthy behaviors is high.

Role of the health professional. Although individuals must ultimately assume responsibility for their health, promoting healthy behaviors through education is an important function for health personnel. In this capacity, health professionals must first and foremost serve as role models for the public. Successful health education outcomes cannot be expected unless the professionals involved model healthy behaviors. To this end, the American Association for Respiratory Care has created a role model statement to help RCPs set good examples for the public health (see accompanying box).

Providing a good example alone cannot assure successful health education programming. In order to achieve desired outcomes, health professionals must make sure that certain conditions are met. Key conditions needed for effective health education include the following:[3]

1. Program participants must be actively engaged in the learning process. The educational process is impeded if participants are passive recipients of information.
2. Health education activities must incorporate the values and health beliefs of the learners. Therefore, familial, cultural, societal, and economical barriers must be considered when providing opportunities for individuals to make decisions regarding their health.
3. The role of the health educator is to facilitate behavioral change. Therefore, the learning process should be approached cooperatively.

Role model statement American Association for Respiratory Care

As health professionals engaged in the performance of cardiopulmonary care, the practitioners of this profession must strive to maintain the highest personal and professional standards. A most important standard in the profession is for the practitioner to serve as a role model in matters concerning health.

In addition to upholding the code of ethics of this profession by continually striving to render the highest quality of patient care possible, the respiratory care practitioner shall set himself apart as a leader and advocate of public respiratory health.

The respiratory care practitioner shall participate in activities leading to awareness of the causes and prevention of pulmonary disease and the problems associated with the cardiopulmonary system.

The respiratory care practitioner shall support the development and promotion of pulmonary disease awareness programs, to include smoking cessation programs, pulmonary function screenings, air pollution monitoring, allergy warnings, and other public education programs.

The respiratory care practitioner shall support research in all areas where efforts could promote improved health and could prevent disease.

The respiratory care practitioner shall provide leadership in determining health promotion and disease prevention activities for students, faculty, practitioners, patients, and the general public.

The respiratory care practitioner shall serve as a physical example of cardiopulmonary health by abstaining from tobacco use and shall make a special personal effort to eliminate smoking and the use of other tobacco products from his home and work environment.

The respiratory care practitioner shall uphold himself as a model for all members of the health care team by demonstrating his responsibilities and shall cooperate with other health care professionals to meet the health needs of the public.

Source: American Association for Respiratory Care: Position statements. Dallas, TX: *American Association for Respiratory Care,* undated.

---

4. Developing predisposing, enabling, and reinforcing health attitudes and behaviors requires effort which will only take place over time.
5. The health care professional must be willing to listen **nonjudgmentally** to the concerns of the learners. The health care provider must be empathetic and understanding in order to effectively overcome social, economic, political, and cultural barriers.
6. The level of learners' self-concept and self-esteem may aid or inhibit their ability to make decisions and act on those decisions. Therefore, the health professional should be willing to provide emotional support and assurance when needed.

7. The characteristics of the health educator make a significant difference in the outcome of the education program. Generally, a successful outcome will occur if the educator exudes confidence but is not overly educative and authoritarian.

How health education efforts can be organized to meet these conditions is the subject of the next section of the chapter.

A MODEL FOR HEALTH PROMOTION AND HEALTH EDUCATION PROGRAMMING

There are many approaches to health promotion and health education. Some of these methods are based solely on experience, while others are founded in the behavioral and social sciences. For purposes of illustration, we have chosen the latter type of model.

In 1980, Green and associates developed a systematic approach to health education programming called the PRECEDE Model.[21] The PRECEDE Model (an **acronym** for *P*redisposing, *R*einforcing, and *E*nabling *C*auses in *E*ducational *D*iagnosis and *E*valuation) assumes that health education is used to change behaviors. The model recognizes that behavioral change is complex. In order to affect behavioral change, the model borrows theories from four disciplines: **epidemiology,** social and behavioral sciences, administration, and education.

Consistent with the premises of health education, the model asserts that behavioral change must be voluntary. In other words, change must occur with the full knowledge and consent of the individual. Only when the health of others is threatened should health behaviors be compelled. In addition, the model recognizes that behavioral change must be consistent with the value system of the individual and society. Otherwise, there must be an opportunity to adjust the value system.[21]

As depicted in Figure 36-2, the PRECEDE Model uses a deductive approach to develop health education programs. Using this model, the health educator first diagnoses the intended behavioral outcomes, and then works backward to identify the causes of wanted and unwanted health behaviors.

Green and associates have divided this process into seven phases, with each phase using specific diagnostic strategies from epidemiology, the social and behavioral sciences, education, and administration. A brief description of each phase is provided below.

Phase 1. Quality of life assessment

The first phase assesses the general quality of life in the population. At this level, consideration is given to general problems in the society. These problems

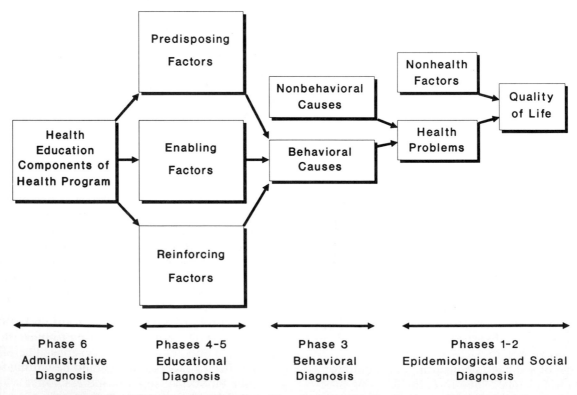

Fig. 36-2 The PRECEDE model. (From Green LW et al: *Health education planning: a diagnostic approach,* Mountain View, Calif, 1980, Mayfield Publishing.)

are defined both subjectively and objectively. The subjective viewpoint comes directly from the community and individuals themselves. Objective data is based on specific social indicators. Social indicators include factors such as population statistics; rates of illegitimacy, unemployment and absenteeism; welfare data; and information on conditions like alienation, hostility, discrimination, voting, riots, crime, and crowding.

Phase 2. Differentiating health and nonhealth problems

The second phase diagnoses specific problems that contribute to the quality of life, as identified in phase one. These specific problems are sorted into health and nonhealth categories. Health problems may involve malnutrition, overpopulation, ill health, alcoholism, cardiovascular diseases, respiratory diseases, various types of cancer, and accidents. Nonhealth factors include unemployment, poor education, lack of industry, race, age, sex, social disintegration, geography, and transportation. Vital indicators such as **morbidity,** mortality, fertility, and disability statistics facilitate the understanding of disease causes and social diagnosis.

Phase 3. Behavioral diagnosis

This phase analyzes behavioral and nonbehavioral causes of the identified health problems. To distinguish between behavioral and nonbehavioral causes, the health care provider should begin by listing all of the known causes of a particular health problem.

For example, if chronic obstructive pulmonary disease (COPD) is identified as a major health problem in a given population, the health care provider would identify all known risk factors:

- Age
- Socioeconomic status
- Occupational exposure (cotton fiber, coal dust, asbestos)
- Air pollution
- Cigarette smoking
- Family history of disease
- Alpha-1 antitrypsin deficiency

Clearly, the behavioral cause of COPD is smoking and associated smoking behaviors. Age, family history, the genetic defect (alpha-1 antitrypsin deficiency), and air pollution are nonbehavioral. Socioeconomic status and occupational exposure are more difficult to categorize, since they have both behavioral and nonbehavioral components. Identifying nonbehavioral factors is important because they provide planners with more realistic expectations regarding program outcomes.

Phases 4 and 5. Educational diagnosis

Phases four and five address the educational diagnosis. Green and associates specify three major categories of factors that impact on health behavior: (1) predisposing, (2) enabling, and (3) reinforcing factors.

Predisposing factors include variables such as an individual's knowledge, attitudes, values and perceptions regarding health behaviors. *Enabling* factors involve the availability and accessibility of resources, and needed skills and knowledge. *Reinforcing* factors, crucial during any change process, include the attitudes and behavior of health personnel or significant others, such as peers, family, and employers.

During phase 4, all factors that may predispose, enable, or reinforce behavioral change are identified. In phase 5, these factors are analyzed, and decisions are made as to which factors will receive intervention.

Phase 6. Administration

Phase 6 is the administrative component. During this phase, the health education program is planned and implemented.

Phase 7. Evaluation

The final phase of the PRECEDE Model is evaluation. Three elements are evaluated. First, the program process (planning and implementation of activities and events) is assessed. Second, the impact of predisposing, enabling, reinforcing, and behavioral factors is determined. Last, program outcomes, such as the health and social benefits, are evaluated. Program planners should be aware that evaluation should be a continuous process throughout all phases of the program.

Ultimately, health education programs are effective only if they influence health behaviors.[19] By providing a systematic approach to diagnosing cause and effect relationships between behavior and health, the PRECEDE Model provides guidance to health education program planners.

IMPLICATIONS FOR RESPIRATORY CARE PRACTITIONERS

Earlier in this chapter we looked at why health professionals' roles are expanding. As a result, health care professionals, including RCPs, are providing services beyond the traditional curing functions. These additional services include health promotion, disease prevention, and health education activities.

In respiratory care, these new services are allowing RCPs to expand the scope and nature of their practice. In addition, RCPs have the opportunity to deliver health care in a variety of new settings, such as the workplace and community. Providing health care in these new settings also has had an impact on the nature of health care practice. RCPs now have the opportunity to offer preventive, as well as rehabilitative, services.

Setting for services

In looking at how health care professionals provide health promotion and education services, it is often useful to identify the various settings of delivery. These settings include traditional health care institutions (hospitals and skilled nursing facilities), worksites, the home, and various community and educational institutions.[10,22]

RCPs provide important health promotion and health education services in all of those settings.[23] The following is a brief summary of the types of services provided by RCPs in each setting.

Health care institutions

Health care institutions where RCPs provide health promotion and health education services include both in-patient facilities (e.g., hospitals and skilled nursing facilities), and ambulatory care centers (e.g., physicians offices, clinics, HMOs, surgical care centers). Within these settings, RCPs perform a variety of vital primary, secondary, and tertiary health promotion services.

In the area of primary prevention, RCPs organize smoking awareness and smoking cessation programs for both staff and patients. In this role, RCPs provide program participants with appropriate information and help them develop the skills needed to stop smoking.[22]

Secondary prevention involves early diagnosis and prevention of the debilitating effects of a disease. RCPs are involved in a variety of diagnostic procedures. This includes early detection of small airway dysfunctions, or other pulmonary disabilities through pulmonary function testing. When pulmonary disease is detected, the RCP assists the patient's physician in providing the patient with relevant information on his or her condition, including how to prevent its progression. This may involve developing a health promotion/education program tailored to the individual patient's needs and values.[22-24]

Tertiary prevention or rehabilitation involves patient education in rehabilitation techniques, exercise conditioning, bronchial hygiene, breathing retraining, and disease education.[22] Chapter 37 provides more detail on pulmonary rehabilitation programs.

Worksite

Health promotion at work has many potential benefits. These include cost-effectiveness, decreased absenteeism, increased job satisfaction, and increased productivity.[10] As a health care team member at the workplace, an RCP's responsibilities could include: (1) performing pulmonary function and blood pressure screening, (2) developing smoking cessation and stress management programs, and (3) consulting on workplace policies related to smoking and occupational exposure to hazards (asbestos, cotton, and other fibers).[22-24] As RCPs become increasingly involved with exercise conditioning, development of workplace exercise programs may also be within their realm of responsibility.

Home

Home health care is one of the fastest growing segments of health care. Home care is defined as the provision of health and related social support services to physically and mentally impaired persons in their places of residence.[25] Advocates of home health care emphasize its cost-effectiveness and humaneness. According to Barhydt-Wezenaar:[25]

> By bringing health care services to people in their own homes, hospitalization can often be prevented and residential health care facility placement can be delayed. Cost savings resulting from the provision of home care services, which can be offered at a cost well below the costs of institutional health care, provide added incentive for the use of home care services—Making available care in one's own home or in an alternative home setting is a realistic and often more humane approach to cultivating the health and well-being of people.

A variety of health care services can be provided in the home. Such services range from chronic care for totally dependent individuals to care for those whose needs are temporary. In the home, RCPs perform traditional functions such as pulmonary function screening, physiologic monitoring, and rehabilitation. RCPs may also help develop patient care plans. In addition to providing therapy, RCPs provide essential education services for smokers, nonsmokers who reside with smokers, asthmatics, and individuals with cystic fibrosis.[22-24] Education relating to respiratory therapy equipment, including operation, troubleshooting, and cleaning is also provided. Chapter 38 provides details on the role of RCPs in the home care setting.

Community

Health promotion and education services performed in health care facilities, at the workplace, and in the home generally focus on individuals. At the community level, health promotion activities are usually directed toward groups. Some community health promotion services that may be performed by RCPs include involvement in smoking cessation programs, family asthma programs, better-breathing clubs, and community group sessions for individuals with COPD. In addition, RCPs may provide important services as volunteers for the American Lung Association, the American Heart Association, and the American Red Cross. They also may serve as educators and exhibitors at community health fairs.[22,23]

Educational institutions

Because many unhealthy behaviors begin in childhood or early adolescence, elementary and secondary schools are an ideal place to begin health education activities. Tobacco education programs are a good example.

Cigarette smoking is the primary risk factor associated with many of today's leading causes of death. Research has proved that most smoking behavior begins in late childhood or adolescence. Thus health education efforts to address this problem must focus on our youth. Educational institutions provide the best setting in which to offer tobacco education programs, and RCPs are among the best equipped health professionals to provide such experiences.

Successful tobacco education programs have several key features. Programs should begin in elementary school, preferably kindergarten or first grade. Even in these early grades, children are aware of cigarettes and have begun to develop beliefs regarding smoking. These factors should be considered in developing any health education program.[26]

Among children, family factors have a strong impact on smoking behaviors, knowledge, and attitudes. With this knowledge, RCPs should plan on reaching parents also. Parents need to learn how they can best promote the development of antismoking values in their children.

Program planners also must recognize that youngsters' beliefs and behaviors are also shaped by influences outside the school and family environment. Consequently, children and adolescents need to understand the impact that their peers and the media have on their health-related behaviors.

The role of the family

Regardless of setting, the family plays a crucial role in maintaining the well-being of its members. Family characteristics affect both the health knowledge and behaviors of its members, and their use of the health care services. These characteristics include **ethnicity**, socioeconomic status, level of education, culture and traditions, and family structure. RCPs intent on developing effective health promotion programs must attend to the needs and values of the family.[27]

Many health care institutions are becoming involved in family health care. Health care facilities are offering disease-specific family support services, family wellness programs, and exercise and health promotion programs. Hospitals, together with community and religious organizations, are forming family support systems. In addition, hospitals are providing referrals to social service agencies.[28]

Home health care providers have long known that a caring family is the key to successful home care. Besides providing emotional support, family members can be trained to perform many of the maintenance functions performed by health care providers. With family support, individuals in need of even complex services such as ventilatory support are able to receive needed health care in the comfort and security of their own home.

In the future, the role of the family will receive even more attention, as the government, health care providers, and public work together to reduce the costs and consequences of the leading causes of premature morbidity and mortality.

SUPPORTING THE HEALTHY PEOPLE 2000 PROCESS

As noted earlier, the U.S. government considers health prevention and promotion services the key to reducing premature morbidity and mortality. Achieving these national health goals requires a concerted effort from all health care providers. Each allied health profession should identify where they can most effectively channel their energies and resources toward achieving these goals.

Data needs

Earlier in this chapter, several areas of health promotion activity applicable to RCPs were identified. In order to set *Healthy People 2000* in motion, states and communities will need help in developing specific objectives. These objectives should be based on objective data that indicates specific health problems.

Healthy People 2000 objectives address this area by calling for more and better data collection, including more state efforts to analyze and distribute relevant information. The Public Health Foundation recently conducted a survey to assess states' ability to measure progress toward the year 2000 objectives. The published study summarizes existing data resources by state, and identifies areas where data needs are greatest.[29] A variety of federal initiatives provide support for data collection.

Health status indicators

A consensus process involving federal, state, and local officials has resulted in a set of 18 Health Status Indicators available to all communities (see box, page 1072). These indicators allow comparison of local and state data with data on similar populations or national norms.[14]

Program planning assistance

Three national programs are designed to help states and communities develop their own objectives. *Healthy Communities 2000: Model Standards* help communities translate the national objectives into specific community-related targets. This program also

---

Health status indicators for the general assessment of community health

Indicators of health status outcome

1. Race/ethnicity–specific infant mortality, as measured by the rate (per 1000 live births) of death among infants less than one year of age.

Death rates (per 100,000 population, age adjusted to the 1940 standard population) for:
2. Motor vehicle crashes
3. Work-related injury
4. Suicide
5. Lung cancer
6. Breast cancer
7. Cardiovascular disease
8. Homicide
9. All causes

Reported incidence (per 100,000 population) of:
10. Acquired immunodeficiency syndrome (AIDS)
11. Measles
12. Tuberculosis
13. Primary and secondary syphilis

Indicators of risk factors

14. Prevalence of low birth weight, as measured by percentage of total number of live-born infants weighing less than 2500 grams at birth
15. Births to adolescents (females aged 10 to 17 years) as a percentage of total live births
16. Prenatal care, as measured by the percentage of mothers delivering live infants who did not receive care during first trimester of pregnancy
17. Childhood poverty, as measured by the proportion of children under 15 years of age living in families at or below the poverty level
18. Proportion of persons living in counties exceeding U.S. Environmental Protection Agency standards for air quality during previous year

Note: Position of indicator does not imply priority.

From US Department of Health and Human Services. *Prevention '91/'92: Federal Programs and Progress,* Washington, DC: US Government Printing Office, 1992.

---

helps communities develop action plans to achieve these objectives.

The most recent edition of Model Standards is organized around the priority areas of *Healthy People 2000,* and includes all national objectives with baseline data and targets.[30] It also allows communities to fill-in-the-blank with data and targets that are more locally relevant.

One example of a Model Standards objective is as follows (numbers in parenthesis refer to national targets):

By _____ (2000), reduce asthma morbidity, as measured by a reduction in asthma hospitalizations, to not more than _____ (160) per 100,000 people.

Model Standards also includes community-orient-ed objectives that go beyond the national goals, suggesting specific implementation approaches. For example:

By _____, the community will be served by codes and regulations to provide control of air pollution problems and by adequate enforcement programs.

The National Healthy Communities Initiative (NCHI) is a cooperative venture between the National City League and Public Health Service. NCHI has begun a two-pronged effort to assist communities in improving their citizens' health and quality of life. The first component is an information network that provides assistance on starting community projects, supplies resources for such projects, and organizes conferences on related topics. The second element involves collaborative training programs with state and local groups on how best to start community health projects. NCHI also encourages communities to critically examine their ability to problem-solve and their health status within the context of the national objectives.

The National Association of County Health Officials, in cooperation with the **CDC,** has developed the Assessment Protocol for Excellence in Public Health (APEX/PH). This protocol is a tool that public health agencies can use to evaluate their strengths and weaknesses in meeting the health needs of their community. It also describes the monitoring and evaluation necessary to ensure that plans are carried out to meet local objectives.

CHAPTER SUMMARY

A revolution in health care has begun. No longer is responsibility for health placed solely on health care providers. There is a growing acceptance that health status is determined mainly by individual behaviors and lifestyle. Based on this recognition of individual responsibility, efforts to improve the health status of the population are beginning to take a new course.

For many years the federal government has asserted that health promotion activities are among the most effective ways to reduce premature morbidity and mortality. To this end, the government has identified national health goals for the year 2000, and defined the steps needed to achieve these goals. Key to this effort are effective health promotion and health education.

Health promotion consists of three interrelated elements: holistic health care, high-level wellness, and disease prevention.

Health education is at the core of health promotion efforts. Ideally, health education should introduce and strengthen healthy behaviors, while eliminating harmful ones. Models like PRECEDE can help health professionals design programs to change undesirable health behaviors.

RCPs deliver health promotion services in a variety of settings, including health care institutions, the workplace, home, community, and educational institutions. In each of these settings, RCPs can provide a variety of educational and therapeutic health care services.

In order to set, implement, and evaluate health objectives, responsibilities must be shared. Because health problems affect so many segments of our population, no single group can undertake such an initiative alone. In order to create a healthier America, collaborative efforts must occur both among the different levels of government, and among lay and professional groups at each level. In this respect, respiratory care is taking a leading role.

REFERENCES

1. US Department of Health and Human Services: *Prevention '91/'92: Federal Programs and Progress.* US Government Printing Office, Washington, DC, 1992.
2. Bunker JF, et al: Curricular implications of health promotion and disease prevention in allied health education, *J Allied Health* 15:329–338, 1986.
3. Hamburg MV: Health education: A tool for preventive care in allied health, *J Allied Health* 15:305–308, 1986.
4. Martin-Peterson J, Cottrell RR: Self-concept, values, and health behavior, *Health Educ* 18:6–9, 1987.
5. Breslow L: A positive strategy for the nation's health, *JAMA* 242:2093–2095, 1979.
6. Du Val MK: Mary Switzer memorial lecture: health education, health promotion, and the allied health professions, *J Allied Health* 11:13–20, 1982.
7. US Department of Health and Human Services: *Promoting health/preventing disease:* Objectives for the Nation. US Government Printing Office: Washington, DC, 1980.
8. Mason JO, McGinnis JM: *"Healthy People 2000":* an overview of the national health promotion and disease prevention objectives, *Public Health Reports* 105:441–446.
9. Public Health Service, Office of Disease Prevention and Health Promotion: *Healthy People 2000,* Washington, DC: US Government Printing Office, 1990. PHS Publication No. (PHS) 90-50212.
10. Douglas PD: Practice implications of health promotion and disease prevention in allied health, *J Allied Health* 15:323–328, 1986.
11. Axton KL, Rice NC: Planning for health promotion in the RC curriculum, *AARC Times* 12(6):20,22,24, 1988.
12. Bunch D: AARC launches nationwide "Peak Performance USA" project, *AARC Times* 17(3):39–41.
13. Duncan DF, Gold RS: Reflections: health promotion—what is it?, *Health Values* 10.47–48, 1986.
14. Breslow L: Health status measurement in the evaluation of health promotion, *Med Care* 27(3 suppl):S205–216, 1989.
15. Eberst RM: Defining health: A multidimensional model, *J School Health* 54:99–104, 1984.
16. Greenberg JS: Health and wellness: A conceptual differentiation, *J School Health* 55:403–406, 1985.
17. Green K: Health promotion: Its terminology, concepts, and modes of practice, *Health Values* 9:8–14, 1985.
18. Alles WF, Rubinson L, Monismith S: Health promotion. In Rubinson L, Alles W, editors: *Health education: foundations for the future,* St Louis, Times Mirror/Mosby College Publishing, 1984.
19. Shirreffs JA: The nature and meaning of health education. In Rubinson L, Alles W, editors: *Health education: foundations for the future,* St Louis, Times Mirror/Mosby College Publishing, 1984.
20. National Task Force on the Preparation and Practice of Health Educators, Inc.: *A Framework for the development of competency-based curricula for entry-level health educators.* New York: National Task Force on the Preparation and Practice of Health Educators, Inc, 1986.
21. Green LW, et al: *Health education planning: A diagnostic approach,* Palo Alto, CA, 1980, Mayfield Publishing.
22. Beckett RG: The respiratory care practitioner role in health promotion. In Kra E, editor: *Proceedings of allied health leadership in health promotion and disease prevention,* University of Connecticut, 1986, Storrs and State University of New York at Stony Brook.
23. Bunch D: RTs take the lead in health promotion, *AARC Times* 12(6):26–33, 66, 1988.
24. Axton KL: Implications of health promotion and disease prevention for the practice of respiratory care. In Kra E, editor: *Proceedings of allied health leadership in health promotion and disease prevention,* University of Connecticut, Storrs and State University of New York at Stony Brook, 1986.
25. Barhydt-Wezenaar N: Home care and hospice. In Jonas S, editor: *Health Care Delivery in the United States,* ed 3, New York, 1986; Springer Publishing.
26. Tucker AW: Elementary school children and cigarette smoking: A review of the literature, *Health Educ* 18(3):18–27, 1987.
27. Crooks CE, Iammarino NK, Weinberg AD: The family's role in health promotion, *Health Values* 11(2):7–12, 1987.
28. Robinson PD, Roe H, Boys LJ: The focus of hospitals on family care, *Health Values* 11(2):19–24, 1987.
29. Public Health Foundation: A report on states' ability to measure progress toward achievement of the year 2000 objectives, submitted to the Office of Disease Prevention and Health Promotion, *Public Health Service* February 1990.
30. American Public Health Association, *Healthy Communities 2000: Model Standards* (Guidelines for community attainment of the year 2000 national health objectives), ed 3, Washington, DC. The American Public Health Association, 1991.

Pulmonary Rehabilitation

■

Kenneth A. Wyka

CHAPTER LEARNING OBJECTIVES

1. Define the concept of pulmonary rehabilitation based on the position statements of the American College of Chest Physicians **(ACCP)** and the American Thoracic Society **(ATS)**;
2. Differentiate between the physical and psychosocial bases of pulmonary rehabilitation;
3. Discuss the importance of goal setting for pulmonary rehabilitation with input from both the patient and members of the multidisciplinary rehabilitation team;
4. Compare and contrast the potential benefits of pulmonary rehabilitation according to their current acceptability and probability;
5. Describe the patient selection process, including criteria for entry, for a pulmonary rehabilitation program;
6. Discuss the importance of cardiopulmonary exercise evaluation in terms of patient selection and pulmonary rehabilitation program evaluation;
7. Describe the process of pulmonary rehabilitation on the basis of format, content, and program implementation;
8. Explain the importance of aerobic exercises and inspiratory muscle resistance training in the physical reconditioning process;
9. Differentiate between pulmonary and cardiac rehabilitation on the basis of focus, procedure, and outcome.

Steady improvements in acute care are presenting new medical and social problems. As more survive the acute phases of various illnesses, there are increasing numbers of individuals with chronic disorders. These chronic disorders are associated with a wide spectrum of physiologic, psychological, and social disabilities.

Foremost among these groups are those with chronic cardiopulmonary disease. Although differences in the original diagnosis can have an impact upon treatment outcomes and long term survival, patients with chronic cardiopulmonary disorders have much in common. All tend to share an inability to cope effectively with the physiologic limitations of their disease. Because of this physiologic disability, they commonly have many **psychosocial** problems. All too often, the end result is lower quality of life.

The high incidence of repeated hospitalizations and the progressive **disability** of these patients require well organized programs of chronic care. Ideally, such programs should address both the physiologic impairment and its psychosocial consequences. This approach requires both a **holistic** and long term perspective for which trained personnel and physical facilities currently are in short supply. Part of the solution to this problem lies in the provision of comprehensive home care (Chapter 38). Many chronically handicapped patients require daily care, some of which can be provided in **ambulatory** centers but the bulk of which must be provided and carried out within the home environment. However, comprehensive home care cannot succeed without efforts to help patients readapt to their physical, mental and social disability. We are in desperate need of both better facilities and a more highly skilled work force that is capable of offering a full spectrum of cardiopulmonary rehabilitation services.

What impact health care reform will have on pulmonary rehabilitation and respiratory home care remains to be seen. Since both these areas focus on reducing hospitalization and overall medical costs, it is hoped that health care reform, as it is phased in, will treat rehabilitation and home care in a favorable light.

Clearly, respiratory care can and should play an important role in the provision of cardiopulmonary rehabilitation services. Until recently, however, respiratory care education has focused almost exclusively on developing the skills necessary to provide acute care services. If respiratory care practitioners (RCPs) are to take a more active role in the long term care and rehabilitation of patients with chronic disorders of the cardiopulmonary system, greater emphasis must be placed on developing the special knowledge and skills needed to assist patients in adapting to and living with their disability.

This chapter will provide foundation knowledge on the goals, methods, and current issues involved in organizing, implementing and evaluating planned programs of rehabilitation for individuals with chronic cardiopulmonary disorders. Because the scope of this text relates primarily to respiratory care, greater emphasis will be given to pulmonary rehabilitation programming.

GOALS OF CARDIOPULMONARY REHABILITATION

Rehabilitation was defined by the Council on Rehabilitation in 1942 as "the restoration of the individual to the fullest medical, mental, emotional, social and vocational potential of which he/she is capable."[1] The overall goal is to maximize the functional ability and to minimize the impact the disability has on the individual, the family, and the community.

In 1974 The American College of Chest Physicians' Committee on Pulmonary Rehabilitation defined pulmonary rehabilitation as:[2]

> an art of medical practice wherein an individually tailored, **multidisciplinary** program is formulated which through accurate diagnosis, therapy, emotional support, and education, stabilizes or reverses both the physio- and psychopathology of pulmonary diseases and attempts to return the patient to the highest possible functional capacity allowed by his/her pulmonary handicap and overall life situation.

In an official statement adopted in 1981, the American Thoracic Society Executive Committee delineated two principal objectives of pulmonary rehabilitation:[3]

1. To control and alleviate as much as possible the symptoms and pathophysiologic complications of respiratory impairment; and
2. To teach the patient how to achieve optimal capability for carrying out his/her activities of daily living (ADL).

Depending on the needs of the specific patient, comprehensive care may include the delivery of a structured, defined program of rehabilitation for the patient's care. In the broadest sense, however, pulmonary rehabilitation represents any method designed to improve the quality of life experienced by patients with a disabling pulmonary disease.[4]

In the same sense, cardiac rehabilitation involves good, comprehensive cardiac care for patients with cardiovascular disease. In many ways, the philosophy, objectives, and methods of both pulmonary and cardiac rehabilitation share much in common. Key differences in the two approaches will be considered later on in this chapter.

HISTORICAL PERSPECTIVE

Pulmonary rehabilitation is not a new concept. In 1951, Alvan Barach and associates commented on the need for training programs for chronic lung patients regarding reconditioning efforts to improve an individual's ability to walk without dyspnea.[5] Our apparent ignorance of the problem persisted into the 1960's as the recommended treatment for patients with chronic lung disease included the administration of oxygen as well as stress avoidance. This produced a vicious cycle in the patient resulting in skeletal muscle deterioration, progressive weakness and fatigue, and increasing levels of dyspnea, even at rest. Patients became home-bound, then room-bound and eventually bed-bound. Improved avenues of therapy and rehabilitation as suggested by Dr. Barach and associates were very much needed.

In 1962, Pierce and associates published results which demonstrated Barach's insight into the value of pulmonary reconditioning.[6] They observed that rehabilitative efforts in patients with chronic obstructive pulmonary disease (COPD) permitted them to perform exercises with lower pulse rates, respiratory rates, minute volumes, and CO_2 production. However, these benefits were achieved without significant changes in pulmonary function.

In 1964, Paez and associates indicated that the efficiency of motion and oxygen utilization were both improved in chronic lung patients as the result of reconditioning techniques.[7] Some 4 years later, Christie demonstrated that these rehabilitative benefits could be acquired on an outpatient basis with minimal supervision.[8]

More recently, Hudson and associates demonstrated a significant reduction in the days of hospitalization of 44 patients after beginning participation in an outpatient pulmonary rehabilitation program.[9] A shorter-term inpatient program conducted by Moser and associates at the University of California (San Diego) School of Medicine shows significant post-program reductions in participants' O_2 consumption, minute ventilation, heart rate, and respiratory rate during exercise.[10] Also, of the 29 patients completing the program, 16 improved in terms of their dyspnea class and 11 demonstrated a significant gain with regard to their activities of daily living or ADL.

Although long-term results of pulmonary rehabilitation are contradictory and often difficult to interpret, recent evidence suggests that program deficiencies may be a contributing factor in cases where no improvements in physical or psychosocial measures are obtained. Specifically, insufficient theoretical and practical training of health professionals in rehabilitation methods, a lack of uniformity in rehabilitation teams, and treatment courses that are too few in number or too short in duration have been implicated as reasons for less than satisfactory outcomes. Early detection of COPD in the asymptomatic stage coupled with smoking cessation also appear to be critical factors which must be considered.[11-12]

These investigations have changed the ways in which patients with chronic lung disease are being managed. With increasing evidence of its efficacy in increasing patients' exercise tolerance, decreasing the frequency and duration of their acute care, and enhancing their quality of life and sense of well-being, well planned and comprehensive programs of pulmonary rehabilitation are being organized in a variety of settings. Regardless of setting or design, such programs must be founded on the sound application of current knowledge in the clinical and social sciences.

SCIENTIFIC BASES

Rehabilitation must focus on the patient as a whole, and not solely on the underlying disease. For this reason, effective programming must combine knowledge from both the clinical and social sciences. Knowledge from the clinical sciences can help quantify the extent of physiologic impairment and help establish outcome expectations for physical reconditioning.[13] Social sciences knowledge is helpful in determining the psychologic, social, and vocational impact of the disability on the patient and family, and in establishing ways to improve the patient's quality of life.

This combined approach is substantiated by recent evidence showing a strong relationship between objective measures of patients' physiologic impairment and their quality of life.[14-15] In these patients, social and psychological indicators better predict both the frequency and length of subsequent acute care rehospitalizations than do traditional measures of pulmonary dysfunction.[16]

Physical reconditioning

At rest, an individual maintains homeostasis by balancing external, internal, and cellular respiration. External respiration is gas exchange effected by the lungs. Internal respiration is gas exchange effected at the tissue level. Cellular respiration represents the oxidative process which occurs in the mitochondria for the production of energy in the form of adenosine triphosphate (ATP).

Physical activity, such as exercise, increases these processes, and in an effort to maintain homeostasis, the cardiorespiratory system must keep pace. As illustrated in Figure 37-1, this is accomplished in a number of ways.[17] Ventilation and circulation increase to supply tissues and cells with necessary oxygen and to eliminate the increased levels of carbon dioxide which result from oxidative metabolism. This production of carbon dioxide ($\dot{V}CO_2$) by the cells and consumption of oxygen ($\dot{V}O_2$) is frequently expressed as a ratio. The ratio is referred to as the respiratory quotient, or RQ. Normally, at rest, an individual consumes about 250 mL of O_2 per minute and, in the process, produces approximately 200 mL of CO_2 per minute. The normal RQ is therefore about 0.8. Although the final pathway for carbohydrate, protein, and fat metabolism is shared, there are differences in the respiratory quotient for each. The RQ of carbohydrate is 1.0, that of protein is 0.8 and that of fat is 0.7.

As depicted in Figure 37-2, $\dot{V}O_2$ and $\dot{V}CO_2$ also increase in linear fashion as exercise levels increase. If

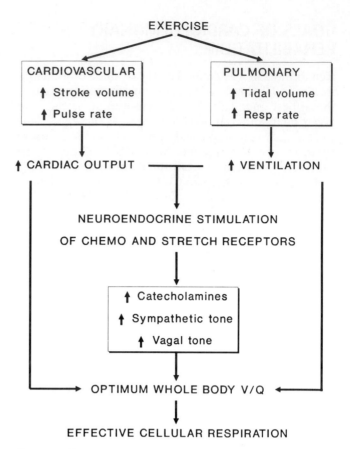

Fig. 37-1 The body's response to increased levels of activity such as exercise.

the body cannot deliver sufficient oxygen to meet the demands of energy metabolism, blood lactate levels increase. The buffering of lactic acid results in increased carbon dioxide production. This provides an added stimulus to ventilation. The point where increased levels of lactic acid result in an increased $\dot{V}CO_2$ and V_E is referred to as the **anaerobic threshold.**[17] The RQ at this point is equal to or greater than 1.0. This indicates that carbon dioxide production has equalled or surpassed oxygen consumption. When the anerobic threshold is exceeded, metabolism becomes anaerobic, thereby decreasing energy production and increasing fatigue.

Increases in physical activity result in increases in ventilation. This, coupled with an increased cardiac output, provides a ventilation to perfusion ratio ideal for adequate gas exchange (refer to Figure 37-1).

The maximum voluntary ventilation (MVV) appears to be a good indicator of the respiratory system's ability to handle increased levels of physical activity. MVV can be measured directly, or it can be estimated by multiplying the forced expiratory volume in one second (FEV_1) by a factor of 35. Normally, an individual can achieve 60% to 70% of their MVV value on maximum exercise. This indicates that sufficient reserve still exists in the respiratory system and

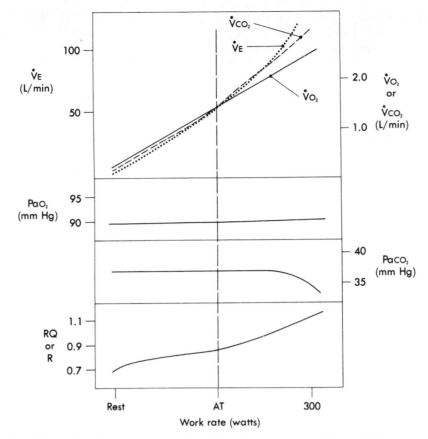

Fig. 37-2 Schematized data representing the relationship between ventilation and O_2 uptake and CO_2 output and the changes in gas tension during incremental exercise. AT, Anaerobic threshold. (From Lane EE, Walker JF: Clinical arterial blood gas analysis, St Louis, 1987, Mosby.)

that ventilation is not the primary limiting factor for the termination of exercise.[17]

Chronic pulmonary patients lacking this reserve will have severe limitations to their exercise capabilities. The high rate of CO_2 production during exercise in these patients results in respiratory acidosis and a shortness of breath out of proportion to the level of activity. In addition, muscles (both skeletal and respiratory) consume higher percentages of the total oxygen consumption as work levels in these patients increase (Figure 37-3, page 1078). Together these factors contribute to a high degree of patient intolerance for any significant increase in physical activity.

Pulmonary rehabilitation must therefore include efforts to physically recondition patients and increase their exercise tolerance. This can be accomplished by strengthening essential muscle groups, improving overall oxygen utilization, and enhancing the body's cardiovascular response to physical activity.

Psychosocial support

If the overall goal of pulmonary rehabilitation is to improve the quality of patients' lives, then physical reconditioning alone is not sufficient. Studies suggest that the success or failure of physical reconditioning plays a lesser role in program retention than meeting patients' psychological and social needs.[18,19]

There is a well-established relationship between patients' physical, mental and social well-being.[20] The term psychosomatic refers to the relationship between the emotional state or outlook of an individual (psyche) and the physical responses of the individual's body (soma). Everyday life is full of such relationships, such as the physical fatigue that follows a period of emotional tension. Many of these associations are considered part of normal human behavior. However, emotional states such as stress can cause or aggravate an existing physical problem. Likewise, physical manifestations of disease, such as recurrent dyspnea, can worsen stress.

Moreover, the progressive nature of COPD can negatively affect patients' overall outlook on their disease and reduce their motivation to adapt to its consequences. RCPs must realize that all their skilled technical services, as well as the best pharmacologic therapy, can be negated, and a patient can be driven on a progressively downhill course because of an unfavorable mental state.

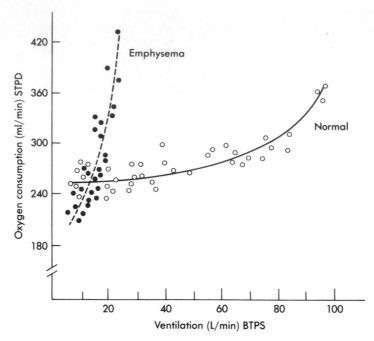

Fig. 37-3   The changes O_2 consumption with increasing ventilation in normal subject (O) and in patient with emphysema (●). BTPS, Body temperature, saturated with water vapor, body pressure; STPD, volume of dry gas at 0° C and 760 mm Hg atmospheric pressure. (From Cherniack RM, Cherniack L, Naimark A: Respiration in health and disease, ed 3, Philadelphia, 1984, WB Saunders.)

Of course, emotional problems are not unique to patients with respiratory disease. Depression and hostility commonly occur with many acute and chronic diseases. In chronic respiratory disease, however, it may be a double-edged sword. Not only can emotional disturbances affect the general well-being of the patient, but they may also directly aggravate the very defects that are responsible for the underlying disability.[21]

The role of emotional and personality problems in the origin of childhood bronchial asthma is well known and has been extensively recorded in medical literature. It is quite probable that certain cases of adult (intrinsic) asthma, for which no specific allergic basis can be found, are attributable, in part, to psychological or emotional disorders. As compared to intrinsic asthma, however, psychological factors in chronic pulmonary disease are more a result of the disease than a cause.[20] Often the patient with progressive emphysema develops severe anxiety, hostility, and stress as a direct consequence of the disability. Because patients are fearful of economic loss and death, they can also develop hostility toward the disease and often toward those people around them.

Unfortunately, proper attention to the psychological component of chronic lung disease has been largely neglected.[20-22] Although the reasons for this neglect are many, a major factor is a disproportionate emphasis on the physical basis of diseases and associated methods of therapy in the education of health professional. Because psychological therapy has been used successfully in the management of bronchial asthma, it is used in nonasthmatic diseases as well.

In regard to the social needs of patients with chronic lung disease, one commonly observes patients spontaneously receiving support and encouragement by simple association with each other. This informal observation suggests that the presence or absence of social support mechanisms may be a factor in determining how well patients adapt to their disability. Recent studies indicate that patients lacking a strong social support structure are at higher risk for rehospitalization than those with such networks.[15] Clearly, well designed pulmonary rehabilitation programming should take advantage of this knowledge and address the social support needs of participating patients.

In terms of social function, the physiologic impairment of chronic lung disease, in combination with other variables, can severely restrict a patient's ability to perform even the most routine tasks requiring physical exertion. Obviously, intolerance for physical exertion lessens the patient's social activity. More importantly, however, are the patients' potential loss of confidence in their ability to care for themselves that can accompany such impairments, and the resultant loss of feelings of dignity and self-worth. These self-perceptions are only worsened when family, friends, or health care professionals label the patient as a pulmonary cripple. Such factors can establish a cycle of further social withdrawal and intensified psychological depression, and an increased frequency of acute exacerbations of the underlying disease. Figure 37-4 presents elements of this cycle and shows how chronic lung disease and other variables can impact on a patient's quality of life.

It is here that the link between the physical reconditioning and psychosocial support components of pulmonary rehabilitation becomes most evident. By reducing exercise intolerance and enhancing the body's cardiovascular response to physical activity, patients can develop a more independent and active lifestyle. For some, simply being able to walk to the market or play with their grandchildren will contribute to a greater feeling of social importance and self-worth. For others, physical conditioning may allow a return to near normal levels of activity, despite the recurrence of periods of dyspnea. Among those for whom physical reconditioning provides a level of normalcy to daily activities, opportunities exist to address vocational needs and expectations.

Many disabled pulmonary patients are in their economically productive years and are anxious to return to economic self-sufficiency. For them, occupational retraining and job placement are necessary ingredients of a purposeful rehabilitation program. Such a program should be based on the individual needs and expectations of each patient.[23] Much study is needed to categorize occupations in terms of their energy requirements on the respiratory system and to derive simple but informative tests of the work of breathing to enable the rehabilitation team to match patients to those jobs in which they would have the greatest chance of success. Not only must the patient's physical status be considered but education, past experience, aptitude, and personality as well.[23-25] Obviously, this requires both the skills of health related professional such as vocational counselors and occu-

pational therapists,[26] and the cooperation of business and industry in the community. Successful vocational rehabilitation efforts have already been made in behalf of disability resulting from such conditions as incapacitating trauma and stroke. Only recently have similar approaches been applied to patients with pulmonary disability.[25,26]

PULMONARY REHABILITATION PROGRAMMING

Program goals and objectives

Pulmonary rehabilitation programs vary in their design and implementation but generally share common goals. Examples of these common goals appear in the accompanying box.[27-33]

Goals common to pulmonary rehabilitation programs

- Control of respiratory infections
- Basic airway management
- Improvement in ventilation and cardiac status
- Improvement in ambulation and other types of physical activity
- Reduction in overall medical costs
- Reduction in hospitalizations
- Psychosocial support
- Occupational retraining and placement (when and where possible)
- Family education, counseling and support
- Patient education, counseling and support

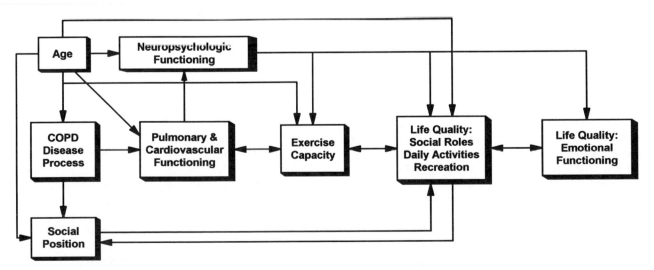

Fig. 37-4 Model describing relationship between physical and psychologic dysfunction in patients with chronic lung disease. (Adapted from McSweeney AJ, et al: Life quality of patients with chronic obstructive pulmonary disease, *Arch Intern Med* 142:473, 1982.)

■ M I N I **C** L I N I ■

37-1

Dimensions of Pulmonary Rehabilitation

Problem: An RCP is asked to consult on a 63-year-old male patient hospitalized with severe chronic obstructive pulmonary disease (COPD) for possible participation in an outpatient pulmonary rehabilitation program. During the patient interview, the RCP is told that if the program will not cure or reverse the disease process, then he sees no reason why going through rehab would be of any benefit. How should the RCP respond to the patient keeping in mind his expectations of what pulmonary rehabilitation should accomplish?

Discussion: It is critical for all RCPs and other caregivers interested in the field of pulmonary rehabilitation to recognize that the focus of any pro- gram should attempt to treat the patient as a whole, and not solely the underlying disease. A well constructed pulmonary rehabilitation program should be able to both quantify the extent of physiologic impairment and assist in establishing outcome expectations for physical reconditioning. Further, regardless of setting or design, such programs must address the psychologic, social, and vocational impact of the disability on the patient and family, and seek ways to improve the patient's quality of life. In this case, the RCP should speak to the benefits of pulmonary rehabilitation outside the traditional measures of pulmonary dysfunction. While pulmonary rehabilitation can not affect the progressive deterioration in lung function that occurs with chronic obstructive pulmonary disease, both education and exercise may improve his ability to perform activities of daily living and exercise tolerance by maximizing the efficiency of muscle use. In addition, effective breathing techniques may lessen the degree of dyspnea sensation. Other important goals of pulmonary rehabilitation are to decrease overall medical costs and reduce the need for hospitalization.

These general goals assist planners in formulating more specific program objectives. When determining objectives, both patients and members of the rehabilitation team should have input. Depending on the specific needs of the participants, program objectives can include the following:

■ Development of diaphragmatic breathing skills
■ Development of stress management and relaxation techniques
■ Involvement in a daily physical exercise regimen to condition both skeletal and respiratory-related muscles
■ Adherence to proper hygiene, diet and nutrition
■ Proper use of medications, oxygen, and breathing equipment (if applicable)
■ Application of postural drainage with chest percussion/vibration (when indicated)
■ Focus on group support
■ Provisions for individual and family counseling

When program objectives are specifically defined and structured in a measurable way, strategies can be tailored to insure the maximum results and benefit. Demonstration of program effectiveness also becomes easier and more acceptable by the medical community.[34] However, benefits realized by participating patients are not always easy to identify and may be controversial.

Benefits and potential hazards

Benefits

An underlying assumption of all pulmonary rehabilitation programs designed for those with chronic lung disorders is that the disease process is progressive and irreversible. Based on this assumption, we cannot expect long term improvements in objective indicators of pulmonary function such as those obtained by spirometry or blood gas analysis. The research literature clearly shows that rehabilitation cannot affect the progressive deterioration in lung function that occurs with chronic pulmonary disorders.[11,35-37]

However, the evidence is just as convincing that properly implemented rehabilitation programs can improve a patient's overall utilization of oxygen by increasing the effectiveness of muscle use and by promoting more effective breathing techniques. We know that exercise ventilation in patients with COPD is inefficient in that the oxygen cost for a given amount of ventilation is excessive.[38] We also know that training of specific skeletal muscle groups alone may not produce an improvement in exercise tolerance, but that training of respiratory-related muscles can improve exercise tolerance.[39-41] Therefore, to maximize rehabilitation outcomes, programs must have activities to recondition and retrain both the respiratory-related and skeletal muscles groups. The accompanying box classifies the benefits of exercise reconditioning for chronic lung patients based on current knowledge of their acceptability and probability.[42]

Reconditioning provides more than just physiologic benefits. However, achieving the related social, psychological, and vocational outcomes requires a complementary and multidisciplinary focus on psychosocial **readaptation.**[43] For this reason, programs that attend solely to physical reconditioning efforts are not truly rehabilitative in nature. Only those that

Benefits from exercise reconditioning[42]

I. Accepted Benefits
- Increased physical endurance
- Increased maximum oxygen consumption
- Increased skill in performance with:
  - Decreased ventilation
  - Decreased oxygen consumption
  - Decreased heart rate
  - Increased anaerobic threshold

II. Potential Benefits
- Increased sense of well-being
- Increased clearance of secretions
- Increased hypoxic drive
- Increased left ventricular function

III. Unlikely or Unknown Benefits
- Prolonged survival
- Improved pulmonary function tests
- Lowered pulmonary artery pressure
- Improved arterial blood gas results
- Improved blood lipids
- Change in muscle oxygen extraction
- Change in step desaturation or apnea

Evaluation of rehabilitation program outcomes[49]

Changes in exercise tolerance
- Pre- and post 6 or 12 minute walking distance
- Pre- and post pulmonary exercise stress test
- Review of patient home exercise logs
- Strength measurement
- Flexibility and posture
- Performance on specific exercise training modalities (e.g., ventilatory muscle, upper extremity)

Changes in symptoms
- Dyspnea measurement comparison
- Frequency of cough, sputum production or wheezing
- Weight loss or gain
- Psychologic test instruments

Other changes
- Activities of daily living changes (ADL)
- Post-program follow-up questionnaires
- Pre- and post-program knowledge tests
- Compliance improvement with pulmonary rehabilitation medical regimen
- Frequency and duration of respiratory exacerbations
- Frequency and duration of hospitalizations
- Frequency of emergency room visits
- Return to productive employment

address both physical and psychosocial needs should be considered true rehabilitation programs.

Naturally, physiologic benefits currently are more acceptable to the medical community and are easier to determine, measure, and document. This can be accomplished by performing a periodic exercise study or evaluation on each patient. Psychosocial benefits, on the other hand, tend to be both more controversial and more difficult to substantiate. Nonetheless, participants in comprehensive rehabilitation programs tend to feel better, experience less dyspnea, have fewer infections and hospitalizations, and are usually able to lead more active and productive lifestyles than those not involved in such services.[44-46] Ultimately, these benefits may be the best indicators of program success.

Another important indicator may be the relationship of pulmonary rehabilitation to patients' survival rates or life expectancy. Although some studies suggest that pulmonary rehabilitation can affect survival rates,[47,48] more research is needed in this area. Results of such studies will help better define and quantify these potential benefits and thus improve the content and delivery of rehabilitation programs.

In combination, these physiologic and psychosocial benefits represent the desired outcomes of pulmonary rehabilitation. As shown in the accompanying box, these outcomes can be categorized and measured using both quantitative and qualitative methods.[49] Results of these assessments can then be used to evaluate patient outcomes and program effectiveness.

Potential hazards

While benefits to physical reconditioning and pulmonary rehabilitation can be expected and realized by most chronic respiratory patients, certain potential hazards do exist. These may be outlined as follows:

a. Cardiovascular abnormalities:
   Arrhythmias (especially life-threatening) can be reduced through the administration of supplemental oxygen during exercise
   Systemic hypotension

b. Blood gas abnormalities:
   Arterial desaturation
   Hypercapnia

c. Muscular abnormalities:
   Functional or structural injuries
   Diaphragmatic fatigue and failure
   Exercise-induced muscle **contracture**

d. Miscellaneous:
   Exercise-induced asthma May be present in young asthmatic patients but is rarely encountered in COPD
   Hypoglycemia
   Dehydration

While short-term and long-term hazards to pulmonary rehabilitation do exist, they can be minimized or eliminated. Proper patient selection, education, supervision, and monitoring are key factors in reducing possible hazards.[47]

Patient evaluation and selection

Before beginning a program of comprehensive pulmonary rehabilitation, criteria for proper patient selection and inclusion into the program need to be defined and established. This should be done through extensive patient testing, evaluation, and assessment.

Patient evaluation

Patient evaluation should begin with a complete patient history—medical, psychological, **vocational,** and social. A well-designed patient questionnaire and interview form will assist with this step. Members of the rehabilitation team should be involved as early as possible with the patient evaluation and selection process. This would include input from each patient's home care company, if applicable, regarding therapeutic regimens and related equipment present in the home environment, compliance with all prescribed therapy, and benefits or problems documented.

The patient's history should be followed by a complete physical examination. A recent chest film, resting electrocardiogram, complete blood count, serum electrolytes, and urinalysis will provide additional information on the patient's current medical status.

To ascertain the patient's cardiopulmonary status, a complete series of pulmonary function and cardiopulmonary stress tests should be performed. The pulmonary function testing should include assessment of pulmonary ventilation, lung volume determinations, diffusing capacity (D_{LCO}), and pre and post bronchodilator spirometry.

The cardiopulmonary stress test should measure blood pressure, heart rate, electrocardiogram, respiratory rate, O_2 saturation, maximum ventilation ($\dot{V}_{E_{max}}$), O_2 consumption (either absolute $\dot{V}O_2$ or **METS,** the multiple equivalents of resting O_2 consumption), CO_2 production ($\dot{V}CO_2$), respiratory quotient (R), and the O_2 pulse during various graded levels of exercise on either an **ergometer** or treadmill. These stages are usually spaced at one to two minute intervals depending upon the program selected and followed. In addition, an arterial line may be inserted in order to allow serial determinations of blood gases during the course of the evaluation. While this will provide the most accurate reflection of oxygenation and ventilation during graded activity, oximetry or transcutaneous membrane measurements are better tolerated and provide acceptable equivalent data.

It should be noted that cardiopulmonary exercise evaluations are also useful in differentiating between primary respiratory or cardiac causes of exercise limitations.[50] Table 37-1 summarizes these key similarities and differences. Obviously, besides helping to differentiate between the underlying cause of exercise

Table 37-1 Exercise parameters distinguishing cardiac and ventilatory (COPD) limitations*

Parameter*	Cardiac†	COPD†
Max $\dot{V}O_2$	↓	↓
Max HR	N or ↓	↓
O_2 pulse	↓	N
Max $\dot{Q}$	↓	↓
$\dot{Q}/\dot{V}O_2$	↓	N
PaO_2	N	↓
$PaCO_2$	↓	↑
$\dot{V}_E/\dot{V}CO_2$	↑	↑
AT	↓	N

From Lane EE, Walker JF: *Clinical arterial blood gas analysis,* St Louis, 1987, Mosby.
*$\dot{V}O_2$, Oxygen consumption; HR, heart rate: $\dot{Q}$, cardiac output: $\dot{V}_E/\dot{V}CO_2$, ratio of ventilation to CO_2 production: AT, anaerobic threshold.
†N, Normal: ↑, increased: ↓, decreased.

intolerance, application of cardiopulmonary exercise evaluation data assists practitioners in the proper placement of qualifying candidates into either pulmonary or cardiac rehabilitation programs.

In order for a cardiopulmonary exercise evaluation to be performed properly and safely, certain measures must be adhered to. A physician must be present during the entire test and a cardiac crash cart with monitor, defibrillator, oxygen, cardiac drugs, suction, and airway equipment must be readily available. Staff conducting and assisting with the procedure must be certified in basic and advanced life support techniques, following either the American Heart Association or American Red Cross standards. The patient should have a physical examination just prior to the test, including a resting electrocardiogram. The test should be terminated promptly if the patient exhibits any major arrhythmias or experiences any angina or severe dyspnea.

With regard to test results, patients should fast 8 hours prior to the procedure and not take any medications which could alter test results. The patient should wear comfortable, loose-fitting clothing and footwear having adequate traction for treadmill or ergometer activity. The mouthpiece or face-mask used during the test should be sized properly and fit comfortably with no leaks. Test conditions should be as standardized as possible to allow for comparison of both pre- and post rehabilitation results, and periodically from year to year as the patient is treated and followed.

Emphasis is being placed on the value of exercise testing because it provides objective criteria for demonstrating the benefits of physical reconditioning and pulmonary rehabilitation in chronic pulmonary patients. While improvement in pulmonary function and arterial blood gases may not be evident, improvement in parameters measured during a cardiopulmonary exercise evaluation are demonstrable. Generally, exercise tolerance is enhanced and the anaerobic threshold is increased along with a reduction in exercise metabolic acidosis. In many individuals, oxygen consumption is increased with an improved METS at all levels of activity, especially at or near the anaerobic threshold. An improved cardiovascular response (heart rate, blood pressure, and cardiac output) has also been identified. Therefore, this type of testing is of definite value and should be included in the patient evaluation process before and after any pulmonary rehabilitation endeavor.[50-52]

All of the procedures and tests identified here are necessary because they evaluate the patient's current cardiopulmonary condition. This will assist in proper patient selection, help to reduce the incidence of any patient injury or cardiopulmonary accident during the course of the rehabilitation program, assure that the patient can exercise and recondition safely, and serve as a basis for post-program evaluation in determining acquired cardiopulmonary benefits and overall patient improvement.

Patient selection and rejection

Patients should be selected into pulmonary rehabilitation programs based on the likelihood of their benefiting from such participation and activity. They should also be ex-smokers. Patients who smoke should be enrolled in a smoking cessation program first before being placed in pulmonary rehabilitation. General indications and contraindications for inclusion in a pulmonary rehabilitation program are listed in the accompanying box.

Indications and contraindications for pulmonary rehabilitation

Indications

- Patients with moderate to severe obstructive lung disease
- Patients with bronchial asthma and associated bronchitis (asthmatic bronchitis)
- Patients with combined obstructive and restrictive ventilatory defects
- Patients with chronic muco-ciliary clearance problems
- Patients having exercise limitations due to severe dyspnea

Contraindications

- Cardiovascular instability requiring cardiac monitoring (consider cardiac rehabilitation)
- Malignant neoplasms involving the respiratory system
- Patients with severe arthritis or neuromuscular abnormalities (consider aquatic exercises for rehabilitation)

Naturally, not all chronic lung patients are candidates for pulmonary rehabilitation. Those pulmonary patients that are end-stage and have little or no cardiopulmonary reserve probably would not be able to participate in the program activities and would therefore not benefit to any meaningful degree. Neither would patients who still smoke (refer to the chapter on health education and health promotion for more information on smoking cessation activities.) Besides the support group format, nicotine gum and patches are available to assist patients in becoming ex-smokers.

Groups or classes for pulmonary rehabilitation should be kept homogeneous. Placing individuals in a program who are at different stages of cardiopulmonary disability can prove to be very defeating. Those with mild to moderate impairment may become discouraged on how severe lung disease can become and those with severe impairment will feel they cannot keep up with or maintain the level of activity exhibited by those with less severe impairment. It is best to group patients together on the basis of severity and overall ability. In this way, patients can participate, compete, and progress together in the program without frustration, fear or a loss of motivation.

Objectively, candidates considered for inclusion into a pulmonary rehabilitation program generally fall into one of the following groups:

- Patients in whom there is a respiratory limitation to exercise resulting in termination at a level less than 75% of the predicted maximum oxygen consumption ($\dot{V}O_2$max)
- Patients in whom there is significant irreversible airway obstruction with a forced expiratory volume in one second (FEV_1) of less than two (2) liters or an FEV_1% (FEV_1/FVC) of less than 60%
- Patients in whom there is a significant restrictive lung disease with a total lung capacity (TLC) of less than 80% of predicted and single breath carbon monoxide diffusing capacity (D_{LCO}) of less than 80% of predicted
- Patients with pulmonary vascular disease in whom the single breath carbon monoxide diffusing capacity (D_{LCO}) is less than 80% of predicted or in whom exercise is limited to less than 75% of maximum predicted oxygen consumption (predicted $\dot{V}O_2$max)

Patients may be excluded from pulmonary reconditioning or rehabilitation programs if they do not fulfill the criteria for inclusion. In addition, patients may also be rejected if there is a significant cardiovascular component to exercise limitation (with exclusion of pulmonary vascular disease) or in whom there is an adverse cardiovascular response to exercise. Cardiac monitoring may be required during their reconditioning. As a result, these patients should be placed in an appropriate cardiac rehabilitation program and followed accordingly.

Program design and implementation

Having identified program objectives in an earlier section of this chapter and having just reviewed the patient selection process, we can now take a serious look at program format, content and implementation.

Format

Essentially, programs can have either an open-ended or closed design, with or without planned followup sessions.[35,53-55] With an open-ended format, patients enter the program and progress through it until certain predetermined objectives are achieved. There is no set time frame. An individual patient can complete the program in weeks or in months, depending upon his/her condition, needs, motivation, and performance. If the clinical objectives are not reached, the patient continues on with the program. This type of format is good for the patient who is self-directed, has scheduling difficulties, and requires certain specific, individual attention. The major drawback is the lack of group support and involvement. This may be minimal at best, or totally lacking. Program content can be presented on an individual basis by the course facilitator or through the use of audio-visual aids.

On the other hand, the closed design is more traditional and uses a set time period in which program content is covered. These pulmonary rehabilitation programs usually run for eight, ten, twelve, or sixteen weeks and classes may meet anywhere from one to three times a week. Class sessions are usually one to three hours long. Presentations are more formal and group support and involvement is encouraged. Patients finish the program when the scheduled sessions are completed—not when predetermined clinical objectives are necessarily met. This can be a drawback. However, patients can enroll again if the anticipated improvements have not been realized. In addition, class size may prevent or reduce the amount of individualized attention a certain patient may receive.

Regardless of the format used, the overall aim of any pulmonary rehabilitation program is to present the essential material to its patients, to have them complete a reconditioning regimen safely, and to demonstrate as much physical and psychosocial improvement as possible. In order for any results to be lasting, these programs must include periodic follow-up sessions and activities for reinforcement. Follow-up must be on-going and available to all patients who complete pulmonary rehabilitation. Frequently, this essential element of the process is difficult, but program coordinators must insure that it is routinely scheduled. Follow-up or reinforcement could be open-ended (available during regular rehabilitation sessions and offering open attendance) or could be scheduled weekly, monthly, bi-monthly, or quarterly. The important thing is to have some type of follow-up available.

Content

The actual content of any pulmonary rehabilitation effort is based on the identified or stated program objectives. However, before patients are admitted to the formal program, they must be non-smokers. Reconditioning and rehabilitation will have little or no value if the patient still smokes.[35] Consequently, as previously stated in this chapter, some form of smoking cessation must be provided as a prerequisite for smokers. This could be achieved through group sessions, individualized counseling, hypnosis, use of nicotine gum or patches, other pharmacological aids, or by using programs conducted through the American Lung Association, American Cancer Society, American Heart Association, or any private concern. Smoking cessation can be conducted at the facility where reconditioning and rehabilitation sessions are held, or patients can be referred to outside programs. However, results are not guaranteed and many patients who are smoking will find it difficult, if not impossible, to quit. Desire and motivation, along with reinforcement, are key elements in eliminating tobacco from one's lifestyle.

Rehabilitation programs can be divided into educational and physical reconditioning components. Table 37-2 outlines a sample session incorporating these two key components. One without the other will result in a less than effective program. Both components are needed in order to rehabilitate the chronic pulmonary patient to improved physical condition and psychosocial outlook.

As shown in Table 37-2, the ideal rehabilitation session should run for about 2 hours. Group size, available equipment and group interaction will dictate whether shorter or longer sessions are needed. Patients should arrive 10 to 15 minutes before a scheduled session in order to allow for informal group interaction and support. Classes should begin on time and conclude promptly as scheduled. Educational presentations should be brief and to the point. The use of audio-visuals or demonstrations should be used to enhance understanding. In order to facilitate patient comprehension, the language should be simple, and unnecessary technical terms or concepts should be avoided. Handouts which enhance certain points made during a presentation are both useful and desirable. A folder or notebook should be maintained by each patient, in which program activities may be recorded and handout materials kept.

The physical reconditioning component of the pulmonary rehabilitation program consists primarily of an exercise prescription with **target heart rate** based on the results of the patient's pre-program cardiopulmonary evaluation. The target heart rate is the heart rate achieved at 65% of the patient's maximum oxygen consumption during the exercise evaluation, and should be maintained during aerobic conditioning.

Table 37-2 Sample pulmonary rehabilitation session

COMPONENT	Focus	Time Frame
EDUCATIONAL	Welcome (group interaction)	5 minutes
	Review of program diaries (past week activities)	20 minutes
	Presentation of educational topic	20 minutes
	Questions, answers and group discussion	15 minutes
PHYSICAL RECONDITIONING	Physical activity and reconditioning	45 minutes
	Individual goal-setting and session summary	15 minutes
	TOTAL	120 min (2 hours)

The exercise prescription should include the following activities:

■ **Aerobic exercises** for the lower extremity involving either walking on a flat, smooth surface for a specified period of time, walking on a treadmill for a specified distance or time, or pedaling a stationary bicycle for a specified distance or period of time. Patients with significant orthopedic deformities or disabilities should participate in aerobic aquatic exercises.

■ Exercises for the upper extremity using either ergometry or a rowing machine. This type of activity increases accessory muscle endurance by progressive exercise. Weights and/or calisthenics (including isometrics) may also be used if upper extremity ergometers and rowing machines are unavailable.

■ Inspiratory resistance exercises to increase exercise capacity by reconditioning the inspiratory muscles. Patients should be trained in the proper use of this or any other inspiratory muscle trainer selected. Resistance will be increased gradually until completion of the pulmonary rehabilitation program.

To ensure success with the physical reconditioning part of the program, patients must actively participate at the facility during each session and at home. While exercising at the facility, patients will have their pulse rates and oxygen saturations monitored through pulse oximetry. This is done before, during and after each activity and represents a form of biofeedback for the patient. Blood pressure and patient temperature measurements may also be made, but these are usually done at the start of each session. In addition, exercise sessions should be upbeat. Lively music helps to maintain a positive atmosphere. Remember, these patients are ill and require a nurturing environment from team members, family and the group itself.

To continue the exercise regimen at home, patients must obtain a treadmill or stationary bicycle (exercycle) and identify a location where daily walking activities can be accomplished. In addition, to help insure compliance with the program, a daily log or diary sheet must be completed. Figure 37-5, page 1086, depicts a sample log sheet which comprises a section of the patient manual. These log or diary forms are reviewed each time the patient attends a session. Based on this information, further individualized reconditioning goals are set.

With the treadmill or stationary bicycle, patients are required to cover a certain distance or duration every day that they are in the program. If distance is the focus, then patients are required to cover greater and greater distances with increasing tension or resistance as they progress through the program. If the focus is on duration, then patients must go for longer periods of time on either the stationary bicycle (exercycle) or the treadmill. Commonly, the duration is set (30 minutes per session BID) and the patients are asked to gradually cover more distance within each 30 minute segment as tension or resistance on the equipment is also gradually increased. Daily results are recorded in each patient's log or manual. The overall result should be a strengthening of the lower extremities with increasing endurance to perform physical activities.

Walking on a flat, smooth surface is another integral part of the reconditioning process. It usually takes the form of a 12 minute walk performed once a day for the duration of pulmonary rehabilitation. The 12 minute walk is a convenient way for a patient to carry out a well-defined amount of activity with increasing vigor and results over a number of weeks. During the 12 minutes, patients are asked to walk on flat ground (zero grade) for as long as they can. When dyspnea becomes uncomfortable, they are instructed to stop and rest (however, the twelve minute interval still continues). After resting briefly, walking should be continued at a pace comfortable to each individual patient.

The objective is for each patient to walk as far as possible during the 12 minutes, stopping as necessary, and quantifying the total distance covered, including number of stops and rest periods. Landmarks such as telephone poles, city blocks or actual measurements in feet or miles may be used in quantifying

Patient Log   **Week #** _____

Day	PFlex	12-min Walk	Exercycle	Remarks
	No. _____ Duration ___	Distance _____ No. Stops _____	Distance _____ Duration _____	
	No. _____ Duration ___	Distance _____ No. Stops _____	Distance _____ Duration _____	
	No. _____ Duration ___	Distance _____ No. Stops _____	Distance _____ Duration _____	
	No. _____ Duration ___	Distance _____ No. Stops _____	Distance _____ Duration _____	
	No. _____ Duration ___	Distance _____ No. Stops _____	Distance _____ Duration _____	
	No. _____ Duration ___	Distance _____ No. Stops _____	Distance _____ Duration _____	
	No. _____ Duration ___	Distance _____ No. Stops _____	Distance _____ Duration _____	

Fig. 37-5 Sample log or diary form on which patient in a pulmonary rehabilitation program records daily physical reconditioning activities and exercises.

distance. This activity can be performed outdoors, weather permitting. However, with adverse weather conditions such as high heat and humidity or rainy days, the activity can be carried out in shopping malls, stores, gyms, hallways, or other indoor areas where walking a measured distance is possible. Patients are encouraged to increase distances covered each time, if possible, and to record their progress in their manuals or diaries. Some patients will double or triple their walking distance from beginning of the program to its end and realize a decrease in the number of stops or rest periods needed.

While outside the scope of this chapter, the RCP should always consider the impact of weather on each patient's condition. This topic may also be informally discussed during rehabilitation education sessions or be included as part of personal care and hygiene. Patients often claim that their condition and ability to breathe relates to the weather conditions of the day. Factors such as barometric pressure, wind velocity and direction, humidity and temperature certainly play a role in one's respiratory condition, including airway resistance and oxygenation. This along with air pollution/ozone alerts and temperature inversions show why a quick lesson in meteorology would be of interest to pulmonary patients.

Upper body strength can be achieved through the use of exercise bicycles, rowing machines, weight-lifting and/or calisthenics with isometrics. These are usually performed during class sessions but may be carried out at home if the necessary equipment is available and if proper supervision exists. Upper body conditioning will help patients perform a number of useful activities at home and will also help to increase their overall physical endurance.

Inspiratory muscle resistance training completes the program of physical reconditioning.[40,56-61] While using inexpensive commercially available devices such as that pictured in Figure 37-6, patients are instructed to breathe at increasing levels of resistance during the course of the program, thus increasing the strength of their inspiratory muscles. Inspiratory resistance breathing exercises may take place once or twice a day for at least 30 minutes per session. Resistance is increased gradually, as tolerated by the patient, usually once a week or once every 2 weeks. Patients are also encouraged to practice their diaphragmatic breathing techniques, another essential component of rehabilitation, during inspiratory muscle training. Once again, the activity with related results and/or problems should be documented in the patient's diary or manual.

To complement the physical reconditioning aspect of the pulmonary rehabilitation effort, the educational portion of the program should cover topics which are both useful and necessary to the patient.[62] The accompanying box provides a sequential listing of topics covered during a 12 week rehabilitation program of the author's design.

Naturally, other topics can be included and covered, but in terms of relative importance, the ones mentioned are generally given the highest priority. The actual content of these sessions includes the following:

- *Respiratory structure, function and pathology, including a discussion of dyspnea.* This presentation lays the groundwork for the program and gives each patient some basic information about the cardiorespiratory system and related disorders. This particular session can be presented by a physician or RCP.

A listing of topics covered during the educational portion of a 12 week pulmonary rehabilitation program

Session 1—Introduction and Welcome Program Orientation

Session 2—Respiratory Structure, Function and Pathology

Session 3—Diaphragmatic and Pursed-Lip Breathing Techniques

Session 4—Methods of Relaxation and Stress Management

Session 5—Proper Exercise Techniques and Personal Routines

Session 6—Aspects of Postural Drainage, Chest Percussion and Vibration

Session 7—Administration of Oxygen and Aerosol Therapy (Respiratory Therapy Procedures and Home Care)

Session 8—Medications—Their Use and Abuse

Session 9—Medications—Use of MDIs and Spacers

Session 10—Dietary Guidelines and Good Nutrition

Session 11—Recreation and Vocational Counselling; Activities of Daily Living

Session 12—Plans for Maintaining Physical Conditioning; Program Conclusion and Evaluation; Graduation

---

- *Diaphragmatic and pursed-lip breathing techniques,* including a section on avoiding or reducing panic breathing. This topic can be given by a physical or RCP and serves as a cornerstone for the physical reconditioning effort. Patients must learn how to control their breathing efforts in order to ensure maximum result (ventilation) at a minimum of effort (energy expenditure). Diaphragmatic breathing with pursed-lips will help to accomplish this, but this technique will require daily practice on the part of the patient and continued reinforcement throughout the entire program by the group facilitator.

- *Methods of relaxation and stress management.* This session is best conducted by a psychologist with experience in lung diseases and breathing disorders. Patients must learn to avoid aggravation and upsetting circumstances and to adopt, instead, a more relaxed attitude about their particular life circumstances. This will help to reduce unnecessary oxygen utilization, help to conserve energy and help to avoid undesirable cardiovascular and nervous responses to stress.

- *Exercise techniques and personal routines.* The rationale for and value of exercise should be covered and discussed along with suggestions for the adoption of personal exercise routines after the rehabilitation program is over. This topic can be

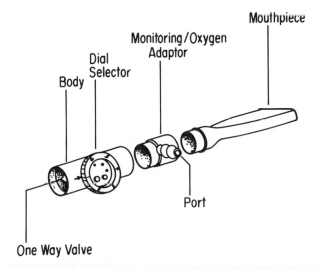

Body
Dial Selector
Monitoring/Oxygen Adaptor
Mouthpiece
Port
One Way Valve

Fig. 37-6 Flow-resistive breathing device.

presented by a physical therapist or an RCP with experience in exercise physiology.

- *Postural drainage, chest percussion and vibration.* This topic is especially helpful to those patients having secretion clearing problems associated with chronic bronchitis and bronchiectasis. Family members and friends may be invited to attend this session in order to acquire some basic skills with these procedures. This area should be taught by either an RCP or physical therapist.

- *Respiratory home care* (oxygen and aerosol therapy). A careful review of home care equipment, procedures, and self-administered therapy should be undertaken by an RCP who has had home care exposure. Safety and equipment cleaning procedures should also be covered for each type of therapy. This topic is essential, especially when patients are using home oxygen, aerosol, or IPPB therapy. Those patients not yet on this type of therapeutic regimen may have questions or fears and be unreceptive to the concept. Presenting the modalities available and having patients discuss their positive experiences with respiratory home care will help alleviate the fears and anxieties of non-users.

- *Medications.* This is another key topic where patients have numerous questions and concerns. It is best presented by a physician or pharmacist but may also be covered by an RCP or respiratory nurse clinician. Proper use of medications should be addressed along with possible abuses and adverse effects. Attention should be focused on adrenergic and anti-cholinergic agents, steroids, metered dose inhalers (MDI), diuretics, theophylline compounds, and pharmaceuticals affecting the cardiovascular system. Sufficient time should also be allotted for questions and answers. Two sessions should be allotted for this topic.

- *Dietary guidelines.* This subject focuses on weight management and good nutrition as it relates to cardiopulmonary health. The topic belongs to the dietitian or nutritionist. Key elements of a good diet, including high protein to build-up atrophied muscles, must be considered. The facilitator should cover proper eating habits, methods of gaining and losing weight, foods to avoid, ways to increase appetite, and daily menu planning. This session will stimulate patients to eat better and thus supply their bodies with the necessary fuel for increased energy production.

- *Recreation and vocational counseling.* This topic can be presented by an occupational therapist or social worker with experience in work counseling. This session should motivate participants to seek-out various types of recreational activities and even part-time work if they are able. The topic is often presented at the end of the pulmonary rehabilitation program when patients should have acquired some physical endurance and should be preparing for a more active and productive lifestyle. The class may brainstorm ideas for recreational or physical activities and from this action plans can be formulated. Changes in attitudes toward physical activity should be perceived by the group facilitator. Patients should no longer feel they cannot walk, exercise, or even be left alone at home. Their overall psychological outlook can definitely change for the better if they have been successful in the program.

These topics need to be presented in an orderly, coherent fashion using supplementary audio-visuals and demonstrations, where appropriate. The program facilitator or leader must insure that rehabilitation sessions are conducted on time and in a way that permits maximum involvement and participation on the part of each patient. This facilitator can be a physician, RCP, physical therapist, or respiratory nurse clinician. However, whoever takes the lead, it is important for that individual to have group facilitating skills, to be able to motivate, to instill confidence, and to have complete knowledge and familiarity with cardiopulmonary diseases and the rehabilitation process.

Motivation on the part of the patient to attend class sessions, to participate both in class and at home, to adhere to program guidelines and to persist with the program's regimen falls on the shoulders of the group facilitator. This individual must constantly encourage, correct, and direct patients toward the achievement of program and personal goals. This task is not an easy one, but with patience and persistence it can be accomplished. The result will be effective pulmonary rehabilitation with patients doing more with less dyspnea and leading more productive lives with decreased hospitalization and overall medical costs.

Implementation

This section will explore various aspects of program implementation. In 1987, the American Association for Respiratory Care (AARC) and the American Association of Cardiovascular and Pulmonary Rehabilitation (AACVPR) jointly conducted the first national survey of pulmonary rehabilitation programs. This National Pulmonary Rehabilitation Survey was published in 1988 and demonstrated the variation existing in program structure, content, staffing, and cost throughout the United States.[63]

With regard to staffing and necessary personnel, pulmonary rehabilitation should be a multidisciplinary endeavor. Team care is enhanced by involving a variety of health care professionals and family members in the planning, implementation, and evaluation components of the program (Figure 37-7). Family will help to provide needed feedback and ensure that

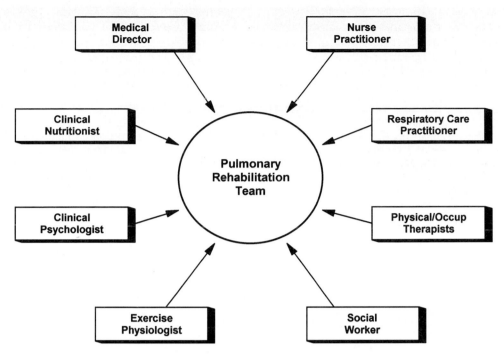

Fig. 37-7 The multidisciplinary nature of pulmonary rehabilitation. Team care is enhanced by involving a variety of health care professionals and family members in program planning, implementation, and evaluation.

instructions and the exercise prescription are carried out at home.[64] The ideal pulmonary rehabilitation program would include the services of a pulmonologist, RCP, physical therapist, occupational therapist, dietitian, social worker, respiratory nurse clinician, pharmacist, and psychologist.

When any of these specialists are not available, then duties or responsibilities for conducting the sessions must be shared. Individuals who are **multi-competent** in a number of disciplines would be an asset and might even function as program facilitators or directors. Institutional policy usually dictates the level of compensation, if any, that professionals receive for participation in the program. Job descriptions and scheduling are other issues that require consideration but are usually handled through effective program administration.

In addition to staffing, facilities are another concern that must be addressed. Patient attendance and participation will be discouraged by having the program in an unreachable facility such as at the top of a hill, inaccessible to public transportation, or with little or no available parking. Arrangements can be made with organizations such as the American Red Cross or community medi-vans to provide transportation to and from the program for elderly patients who do not drive. The facility should also be wheelchair accessible with no barriers present.

In the facility itself, two separate rooms for the

pulmonary rehabilitation program would be ideal—one room for the educational portion of the program, including room for group interaction and support, and one room for physical reconditioning. Rooms should be spacious and comfortable with adequate lighting, ventilation, and temperature control. Chairs should be comfortable with good back support. Restroom facilities should be in or adjacent to the rehabilitation area. A room for individual counseling is desirable but any private office would help meet this need. It is also preferable to have pulmonary function testing and arterial blood gas analysis capabilities on site. If this space is used by other departments for other functions, then proper scheduling of rehabilitation sessions needs to be considered. Adequate time should be allotted for each class session and for necessary setup and breakdown of equipment. Finally, it is important to reemphasize that the area designated for pulmonary rehabilitation should be accessible to the patient, with parking spaces set aside for those who drive to the sessions.

Another aspect of program implementation involves timely scheduling of the rehabilitation sessions. This has already been mentioned in terms of scheduling meeting space and staff participation. The third factor involves patient attendance. With the open-ended format, patients can more or less attend rehabilitation at any time convenient to them as long as the facility is open and staffed accordingly. With

■ MINI CLINI ■

37-2

Problem: An RCP has been asked to assist in the planning process for starting a pulmonary rehabilitation program to support a 350 bed, full service hospital. According to the strategic plan, the physical location of the rehab center is about 3 blocks away from the hospital. The RCP has not seen the proposed site but was asked to approve a recommendation that the facility be used. What factors should the RCP take into account before making a decision on site selection?

Discussion: Since the hospital is currently in the planning process for starting a pulmonary rehabilitation program and has not made final facil-

Importance of Facilities for Pulmonary Rehabilitation

ities selection, the RCP is in a key position to assess, among other areas, issues related to the proposed site. Patient attendance and participation will be adversely affected if the facility is unreachable, such as at the top of a hill. If the location is in an high

crime or unsafe area with little or no security, this too would discourage patients from attending. As true with any program, public transportation which does not permit accessibility to the proposed facility would be a limiting factor, as would little or no available parking. There are numerous other facility considerations outside the actual physical location of the rehab center which would then need to be addressed. For example, the current square footage of available space and room for future expansion would need to be evaluated relative to anticipated needs, as would the facility itself being wheelchair accessible with no barriers present.

the closed format, sessions are scheduled one to three times per week, for 1 to 3 hours, with programs running 8 to 16 weeks. Class times need to be scheduled when the largest number of patients are able to attend. Traffic patterns, bus schedules, and availability of rides are concerns which need to be discussed. The ideal situation involves a separate area set totally aside for pulmonary rehabilitation with a dedicated staff of professionals conducting the program. Then scheduling for either open-ended or closed design programs becomes easier and more manageable. Sessions can be conducted in the morning, afternoon, or evening hours and even on weekends if necessary. Proper scheduling helps to encourage participation and removes potential stumbling blocks which could undermine the rehabilitation process.

Class size is another issue that must be addressed. Theoretically, a rehabilitation program could be conducted with as few as one participant up to fifteen or more, depending on available space, equipment, and staff. However, to foster group identity, interaction, and support, small group discussions are encouraged. The ideal class size should range from three to ten participants. Keeping the class size manageable facilitates vital group interaction processes and allows for more individualized attention. These factors help sustain motivation, thereby reducing the likelihood of participant attrition.

Naturally, economic concerns surface when class size is considered. Although it is clear that program quality must be the first priority, program viability realistically depends on the number of participants. As a general guideline, programs should be conducted

with a class size that is comfortable with regards to space and staffing and one that is also economically feasible. Such an approach will help insure that programs are both economically feasible and capable of producing meaningful patient outcomes.

In addition, equipment is needed for the instruction and reconditioning aspects of the rehabilitation program. To meet the educational needs of the program, a blackboard or flipchart along with a 35 mm slide projector, screen, overhead projector, and cassette tape player are necessary. A videotape player with monitor may also be helpful, especially if individualized instruction or commercially available programs are used. Also, slides, tapes and formal learning packages dealing with the educational topics covered during the rehabilitation program should be available for group and individualized presentation. These can be purchased from outside sources or designed and developed in-house.

For physical reconditioning, stationary bicycles (exercycles), treadmills, rowing machines, upper extremity ergometers, weights, pulse oximeters, and inspiratory resistance breathing devices represent the minimum equipment requirements. The actual quantity of equipment needed depends on class size, scheduling, and available space. Enough equipment should be on hand to keep all patients exercising and to monitor their activity. Emergency oxygen and bronchodilator medications should also be maintained in the rehabilitation area. Equipment guidelines for a class of six to ten participants include the following:

5 exercycles
2 treadmills

2 rowing machines
2 upper extremity ergometers
5 pulse oximeters for monitoring rate and O$_2$ saturation
1 emergency oxygen cylinder (E) and bronchodilator medications

In addition, each patient should be supplied with an inspiratory resistance breathing device.

Because equipment can be expensive, care must be taken in its selection and purchase. Devices and appliances should be durable, easy and safe to use, simple to maintain, and not overly expensive. Initially, basic items are purchased. As a program develops and expands, equipment resources can be enhanced. Finally, other program needs should be reviewed and considered. These include the following:

- Patient manual, including daily log forms or activity diary
- Providing light refreshments for program participants
- Developing a communication network between facility and program participants in the event of schedule changes due to emergencies or cancellation of class sessions due to illness, weather, etc.
- Identification of a home care provider for home oxygen, respiratory therapy equipment, and stationary bicycles. Although this is not absolutely necessary, it is helpful in standardizing the type of equipment used within the program
- Developing a system of charges and mechanism for patient payment. This will be considered further in the next section of this chapter.

By considering all of the factors needed for effective implementation of pulmonary rehabilitation, programs will have lower patient decline and a greater chance for overall success. As programs are conducted, regular evaluations by both patient and staff must be made. Needed changes should be implemented on an ongoing basis. Only in this manner can one expect continued refinement of the process and improvement in patient outcomes.

Cost and reimbursement

Pulmonary rehabilitation program costs are generally based on the average cost per participant. According to regional labor and material prices, costs vary throughout the country. In addition, within a given program, there are several factors to be considered in projecting costs (see accompanying box). Obviously, the larger the class size and the more participants involved in the overall program, the lower the cost will be per patient. The Loma Linda University Medical Center Pulmonary Rehabilitation Program reported for the fiscal year July 1981 to June 1982 that the average cost per patient attending their rehabilitation programs was $452. This was based on total expenses of $519,942 for the year with 1,150 patients participating.[65]

Factors affecting pulmonary rehabilitation program costs

1. Marketing and program promotion
2. Number of personnel involved in program facilitation and administration
3. Space and utility expenses
4. Audio-visual, exercise, and monitoring equipment (purchase and maintenance)
5. Production and duplication of course materials
6. Patient supplies
7. Office supplies
8. Refreshments
9. Miscellaneous expenses

When determining patient charges, consideration must also be given to the type and amount of funding that has been received to offset program expenses and available insurance reimbursement. Pre- and post-program testing and evaluations will naturally generate revenues but should not be included in the formulation of program charges. However, payments for pulmonary function testing, exercise testing, arterial blood gas analysis, and other evaluations may help to keep a pulmonary rehabilitation program financially viable.

Charges for an entire program or for each session must be structured in a way that does not deter patient attendance. Many pulmonary patients are on a fixed income and have other living and medical expenses to account for. A happy medium between a patient's ability to pay and program expenses must be identified. Any scholarships or funding from local charitable organizations, foundations, or agencies, such as the American Lung Association, will help ease the financial burden. The most comprehensive and effective program available will have no impact if patients are unwilling or unable to attend and participate because of financial limitations.

The cost of providing pulmonary rehabilitation has increased over the years, as have health care costs in general. Current nationwide charges for pulmonary rehabilitation range from $50 to $200 per session depending on geographical location of the program, type and level of service provided, and cost of overhead and physician involvement. Depending on total length of the program, charges will range from $400 to $4000 per patient. At three different programs in New Jersey, Lung Diagnostics, The Breathing Center and Better Breathing, program charges range from $100 to $170 per patient per session. With insurance reimbursing 80% after deductible, each patient would be responsible for the remaining 20% or approximately $20 to $35 per session. Additional medical coverage may cover this balance.

Inpatient rehabilitation reimbursement policies vary throughout the country, as do charges for partici-

1092 Preventive and Long-Term Care

pation in these programs. In 1982, the Health Care Financing Administration (HCFA) published the final rules for Medicare reimbursement guidelines for comprehensive outpatient rehabilitative facilities (**CORF**s). Under Part B of Medicare, the scope of services of a CORF now include reimbursement for outpatient activities and one home visit. Reimbursement is dependent on the CORF's meeting the conditions of participation established in section 933 of Public Law 96–499. This also includes provisions for certification of the program. Each CORF must present its program description and anticipated results to local third-party payers to establish both payment and cost-reimbursement policies.[65]

By following these guidelines, Medicare will establish an allowable charge for the program and reimburse 80% of this rate after the patient meets the annual prescribed deductible. Other programs, both inpatient and outpatient in nature, have obtained reimbursement from third-party payers by charging for rehabilitation sessions as physical therapy exercises for COPD, reconditioning exercise sessions, office visits with therapeutic exercises, serial pulse oximetry determinations, and/or physician office visits, intermediate. The goal is to obtain as much insurance reimbursement as possible, thereby decreasing the financial burden on the patient. The accompanying box provides a listing of all possible sources of reimbursement.[66]

Legal issues

In the past, reimbursement for respiratory rehabilitation services provided on an outpatient basis by an RCP was not available. The role of the respiratory practitioner was poorly defined. Efforts at recognition for reimbursement were frustrated by both legislative and regulatory omissions. The creation of the Medicare and Medicaid programs in 1965 under the Social Security Act failed to recognize respiratory therapy, then a growing and emerging health care profession.[67]

In 1980, Medicare proposed creation of comprehensive outpatient rehabilitative facilities (CORFs) which mentioned respiratory care services as reimbursable. This was the first statute to recognize respiratory therapy as such. These regulations were published in 1982. Although the CORF ruling allows for reimbursement for outpatient services provided by an RCP, including one home care visit, more is needed. Respiratory home care has been demonstrated as a cost-saver with regard to health care expenditures.[68] In conjunction with a pulmonary rehabilitation program, even more meaningful patient and economic outcomes are possible. The profession as a whole must continue to seek legal recognition and acceptable reimbursement policies and practices for both rehabilitation and home care activities. With more states achieving legal credentialing, insurance reim-

---

Sources of reimbursement for pulmonary rehabilitation programs[66]

- **Nongovernmental Health Insurance Programs:**
  Private, single or group health insurance plans:
    Health maintenance organizations (HMOs)
    Preferred provider organizations (**PPO**s)
  Medicare supplement
- **Federal and State Health Insurance Programs:**
  Medicare
  Medicaid
  Uncompensated services (Hill-Burton)
  Comprehensive outpatient rehabilitation facility (CORF)
  Veterans administration benefits
  Civilian health and medical programs of the uniformed services (**CHAMPUS**)
  Federal workers insurance
- **Ancillary Liability and Casualty Insurance Programs:**
  Automobile insurance, related to auto accidents
  Worker's compensation, related to accidents on the job
  Business insurance coverage, related to injuries sustained on business premises
  Homeowner's insurance, related to injuries sustained on the owner's premises
  Malpractice insurance on providers of health care
  Product and service liability insurance related to product or service-cased injuries
- **Other Options of Reimbursement:**
  Senior care
  Rehabilitation hospitals
  Grants

---

bursement for RCPs involved in pulmonary rehabilitation will become a reality.

Program results

As previously indicated, pulmonary rehabilitation has not been able to produce any meaningful improvements in the traditional objective measures of lung function. In addition, improved survival, changes in muscle O_2 extraction, enhanced mucociliary clearance, and a more positive psychological outlook are other controversial patient outcomes resulting from participation in pulmonary rehabilitation.[35]

Actual or accepted outcomes include improved exercise tolerance, increased maximum oxygen consumption ($\dot{V}O_2$max), and METS levels plus higher levels of physical activity with positive changes in pulse, ventilation and anaerobic threshold.[10,40,69–71] These improvements can be demonstrated on repeat cardiopulmonary exercise evaluations performed after a pulmonary rehabilitation program. Patients should be able to sustain higher levels of activity for longer periods of time.

Improved physiologic results have been reported in the literature, as well as correlated improvements in patients' functional abilities as measured by their ADL scores and reduction in hospitalization and other medical expenditures.[72,73] Patient and program outcomes must be evaluated at the conclusion of the program and periodically thereafter. Evaluation results must compare pre-program and current patient status and should include physiologic, psychological, and sociological data. Results of pulmonary rehabilitation must be communicated to the patient, family, referring physician, and home care company, if appropriate. From here, further goals and objectives for continued improvement may be established to provide the basis for follow-up and reinforcement activities.

It must be stated that pulmonary rehabilitation cannot eliminate the occurrence of dyspnea in these patients. However, pulmonary rehabilitation can make shortness of breath less debilitating and more manageable. So while patients still become dyspneic, they do so after greater amounts of exercise or other physical activity, and are able to realize more confidence in themselves. They recognize that lack of activity is destructive and that perhaps their only hope for an improved life style is to adhere to program guidelines and to follow through with the prescribed educational and reconditioning regimen.

Rehabilitating the ventilator-dependent patient in an extended care facility or at home requires a different, more labor-intensive approach. Rehabilitation and strengthening of ventilatory muscles allows for improved independence, mobility, and in some cases, ability to wean the individual off the ventilator.[74] This rehabilitative format requires an individualized approach using all available resources and techniques, including the use of variable inspiratory/expiratory positive pressure delivery systems.[74]

CARDIAC REHABILITATION

Before concluding this section of the chapter, some consideration will be given to cardiac rehabilitation. Cardiac rehabilitation is defined as a comprehensive exercise and educational program designed for patients with cardiovascular diseases. Like pulmonary rehabilitation, good cardiac rehabilitation programs are multidisciplinary in approach and focus. Goals include patient education, (which fosters prudent heart living), physical reconditioning, (which can result in improved work capacity), weight loss, and a return to work.

Enrollment is based on a cardiovascular evaluation and related parameters. Because cardiovascular rehabilitation programming has been in existence longer than pulmonary rehabilitation, and because its out-

comes tend to have greater validity and acceptance, reimbursement is more readily available at this time.

The goal of any structured cardiac rehabilitation program is to help patients develop a regular pattern of safe exercise in order to achieve greater cardiovascular performance during activity. Programs are usually divided into monitored and maintenance segments, with home care options available. Exercise prescriptions are individualized for participating patients in an effort to maximize patient outcomes and reduce the chances of adverse effects.

Pulmonary and cardiac rehabilitation share a number of similarities and differences. Some of them have already been briefly discussed. Table 37-3 summarizes these programs by comparing a number of key characteristics. In essence, both programs are similar in many ways, differing only on their rehabilitative focus and type of patient monitoring. It should be added that the average age of patients involved in pulmonary and cardiac rehabilitation programs may differ to some extent. Patients with chronic pulmonary disease, especially COPD, will be in their sixties and seventies. Patients with restrictive diseases will have ages ranging from the teens to the seventies. Patients that are ventilator-dependent present other specialized concerns, including a very broad range in age.[75] On the other hand, cardiac patients will probably range from their late thirties on up to their sixties or seventies. Again, one of the keys to motivation and program success is to keep the programs homogeneous—age, degree of impairment and level of pre-program functional activity and ability. This pertains to either pulmonary or cardiac rehabilitation efforts.

Finally, respiratory care involvement in cardiac

Table 37-3 A comparison of pulmonary and cardiac rehabilitation programs

Characteristic	Pulmonary	Cardiac
Use of an exercise stress test for patient evaluation	Yes (cardiopulmonary)	Yes (cardiac)
Primary focus of cardiovascular program	On breathing techniques and exercise tolerance	On fitness
Use of education and exercise as key program components	Yes	Yes
Patient monitoring pressure during exercise	SaO_2 and pulse	ECG, blood and pulse
Multi-disciplinary approach	Yes	Yes
Reimbursable	Yes	Yes

rehabilitation will probably be significantly less. For the most part, RCPs, unless multicompetent, will be involved with instruction on oxygen use and assisting with patient exercise sessions. Most often, the cardiologist and cardiac nurse specialist or clinician are involved with program facilitation and administration. Other health professionals that may be involved include the dietitian, physical therapist, occupational therapist, pharmacist, social worker, and psychologist.

CHAPTER SUMMARY

Properly planned pulmonary rehabilitation programs can produce certain positive, measurable patient outcomes. The success of such efforts depends upon careful application of current clinical and social science knowledge, and the use of a multidisciplinary approach throughout all phases of program organization, implementation, and evaluation. In this context, RCPs are playing an increasingly important role.

Although these efforts can bring hope to patients for a more active and productive existence, we must remember that the need for pulmonary rehabilitation stems, in part, from the lack of attention currently given to the promotion of healthy lifestyles and the prevention of pulmonary disease (refer to Chapter 36). Ultimately, success in health promotion and disease prevention activities should lessen the need for chronic and rehabilitative care. Until this ideal is achieved, pulmonary rehabilitation will continue to represent a necessary and growing component of respiratory care.

REFERENCES

1. Council on Rehabilitation: *Definition of rehabilitation,* Chicago, 1942, Council on Rehabilitation.
2. Petty TL: Pulmonary rehabilitation, *Basics of RD* 4:1, 1975.
3. American Thoracic Society Executive Committee: Pulmonary rehabilitation—an official statement of the American Thoracic Society, *Am Rev Respir Dis* 124:663–666, 1981.
4. Harris PL: A guide to prescribing pulmonary rehabilitation, *Primary Care* 12:253–66, 1985.
5. Barach AL, Bickerman HA, Beck G: Advances in the treatment of nontuberculous pulmonary disease, *Bull NY Acad Med* 28:353–384, 1952.
6. Pierce AK, Taylor HF, Archer RK, Miller WF: Responses to exercise training in patients with emphysema, *Arch Intern Med* 113:28–36, 1964.
7. Paez PN, Phillipson EA, Masangkay M, Sproule BJ: The physiologic basis of training patients with emphysema, *Am Rev Respir Dis* 95:944–953, 1967.
8. Christie D: Physical training in chronic obstructive lung disease, *Brit Med J* 2:150–151, 1968.
9. Hudson LD, Tyler ML, Petty TL: Hospitalization needs during an outpatient rehabilitation program for severe chronic airway obstruction, *Chest* 70:606–610, 1976.
10. Moser KM, Bokinsky GE, Savage RT, Archibald CJ, Hansen PR: Results of a comprehensive rehabilitation program, *Arch Intern Med* 140:1596–1601, 1980.
11. Gimenez M: Technics and results in respiratory kinesitherapy of chronic obstructive bronchopneumopathies, *Rev Fr Mal Respir* 11:525–43, 1983.
12. Alkalay L, Kaplan AS, Sharma R, Kimbel P: Chronic Obstructive pulmonary disease: rehabilitation program with continuation on an outpatient basis, *J Am Geriatr Soc* 28(2):88–92, 1980.
13. Ries AL: Scientific basis of pulmonary rehabilitation: position paper of the American Association of Cardiovascular and Pulmonary Rehabilitation, *J Cardiopulmonary Rehabil* 10:418, 1990.
14. Daughton D, Fix AJ, Kass I, McDonald T, Stevens C: Relationship between a pulmonary function test (FEV$_1$) and the ADAPT quality-of-life scale, *Percept Mot Skills* 57:359–62, 1983.
15. Bradley BL: Rehabilitation of patients with chronic respiratory disease, *Respir Ther* 13(4):15–16, 19–21, 1983.
16. Jensen PS: Risk, protective factors, and supportive interventions in chronic airway obstruction, *Arch Gen Psychiatry* 40:1203–7, 1983.
17. Zaltzman M, Steinberg H: Normal and abnormal cardiopulmonary responses to exercise, *Appl Cardiol* 14:19–21, 1986.
18. Fix AJ, Daughton D, Kass I, Bell CW, Golden CJ: Emotional, intellectual and physiological predictors of vocational outcome of pulmonary rehabilitation patients, *Psychol Rep* 46:379–82, 1980.
19. Shenkman B: Factors contributing to attrition rates in a pulmonary rehabilitation program, *Heart Lung* 14:53–58, 1985.
20. Dudley DL, Glaser EM, Jorgenson BN, Logan DL: Psychosocial concomitants to rehabilitation in chronic obstructive pulmonary disease. Part 1. Psychosocial and psychological considerations, *Chest* 77:413–20, 1980.
21. Dudley DL, Glaser EM, Jorgenson BN, Logan DL: Psychosocial concomitants to rehabilitation in chronic obstructive pulmonary disease. Part 3. Dealing with psychiatric disease (as distinguished from psychosocial or psychophysiologic problems), *Chest* 77:677–84, 1980.
22. Dudley DL, Glaser EM, Jorgenson BN, Logan DL: Psychosocial concomitants to rehabilitation in chronic obstructive pulmonary disease. Part 2. Psychosocial treatment. *Chest* 77:544–51, 1980.
23. Fix AJ, Daughton D, Kass I, Patil KD, Kass M, Polenz D: Personality traits affecting vocational rehabilitation success in patients with chronic obstructive pulmonary disease, *Psychol Rep* 43:939–944, 1978.
24. Kass I, Dyksterhuis JE, Rubin H, Patil KD: Correlation of psychophysiologic variables with vocational rehabilitation outcome in patients with chronic obstructive pulmonary disease, *Chest* 67:433–40, 1975.
25. Dyksterhuis JE: Vocational rehabilitation of chronic obstructive pulmonary disease patients, *Rehabil Lit* 33:136–138, 1972.
26. Pomerantz P, Flannery EL, Findling PK: Occupational therapy for chronic obstructive lung disease, *Am J Occup Ther* 29:407–11, 1975.
27. Putnam JS, Beechler CR: Comprehensive care in chronic obstructive pulmonary disease. *Prim Care* 3:593–608, 1976.
28. Faling LJ: Pulmonary rehabilitation—physical modalities, *Clin Chest Med* 7:599–618, 1986.
29. Paine R, Make BJ: Pulmonary rehabilitation for the elderly, *Clin Geriatr Med* 2:313–35, 1986.
30. Hodgkin JE, Farrell MJ, Gibson SR, Kanner RE, Kass I, Lampton LM, Nield M, Petty TL: American Thoracic Society. Medical Section of the American Lung Association. Pulmonary rehabilitation, *Am Rev Respir Dis* 124:663–6, 1981.
31. Young A: Rehabilitation of patients with pulmonary disease, *Ann Acad Med Singapore* 12:410–6, 1983.
32. Levi-Valensi P, Palat M, Duwoos H, Hermand H, Nickly N, Muir JF, Ndarurinze S: Rehabilitation of chronic pulmonary patients. Critical study of objectives and methods. Current state of the problem, *Poumon Coeur* 33(1):7–14, 1977.

33. Fergus LC, Cordasco EM: Pulmonary rehabilitation of the patient with COPD, *Postgrad Med* 62:141–144, 1977.

34. MacDonnell RJ: The pulmonary rehabilitation maze, *Respir Care* 28(2):180–190, 1983.

35. Alkalay I, Kaplan AS, Sharma R, Kimbel P: Chronic obstructive pulmonary disease: rehabilitation program with continuation on an outpatient basis, *J Am Geriatr Soc* 28(2):88–92, 1980.

36. Niederman MS, Clemente PH, Fein AM, Feinsilver SH, Robinson DA, Ilowite JS, Berstein MG: Benefits of a multidisciplinary pulmonary rehabilitation program. Improvements are independent of lung function, *Chest* 99(4):798–804, 1991.

37. Zu Wallack RL, Patel K, Reardon JZ, Clark BA 3d, Normandin EA: Predictors of improvement in the 12-minute walking distance following a six-week outpatient pulmonary rehabilitation program, *Chest* 99(4):805–808, 1991.

38. Spiro SG, Hahn HL, Edwards RHT, Pride NB: Cardiorespiratory adaptations at the start of exercise in normal subjects and in patients with chronic obstructive bronchitis, *Clin Sci Molecul Med* 47:165–172, 1974.

39. Casciari RJ, Fairshter RD, Harrison A, Morrison JT, Blackburn C, Wilson AF: Effects of breathing retraining in patients with chronic obstructive pulmonary disease, *Chest* 79:393–398, 1981.

40. Sonne LJ, Davis JA: Increased exercise performances in patients with severe COPD following inspiratory resistive training, *Chest* 81:436–439, 1982.

41. Mohsenifar Z, Horak D, Brown HV, Koerner SK: Sensitive indices of improvement in a pulmonary rehabilitation program, *Chest* 83(2):189–192, 1983.

42. Hughes RL, Davison R: Limitations of exercise reconditioning in COLD, *Chest* 83:241–249, 1983.

43. Kass I, Dyksterhuis JE, Rubin H, Patil KD: Correlation of psychophysiologic variables with vocational rehabilitation outcome in patients with chronic obstructive pulmonary disease, *Chest* 67(4):433–440, 1975.

44. Bebour DE, Hodgkin JE, Zorn EG, Yee AR, Sammer EA: Clinical and physiological outcomes of a university-hospital pulmonary rehabilitation program, *Respir Care* 28(11):1468–1473, 1983.

45. Toshima MT, Kaplan RM, Ries AL: Experimental evaluation of rehabilitation in chronic obstructive pulmonary disease: short-term effects on exercise endurance and health status, *Health Psychol* 9(3):237–252, 1990.

46. Wright RW, Larsen DF, Monie RG, Aldred RA: Benefits of a community-hospital pulmonary rehabilitation program, *Respir Care* 28(11):1474–1479, 1983.

47. Bruce EH, Frederick R, Bruce RA, Fisher LD: Comparison of active participants and dropouts in CAPRI cardiopulmonary rehabilitation programs, *Am J Cardiol* 37(1):53–60, 1976.

48. Daughton DM, James Fix A, Kass I, Patil KD: Three-year survival rates of pulmonary rehabilitation patients with chronic obstructive pulmonary disease, *J Natl Med Assoc* 76(3):265–268, 1984.

49. Reisman-Beytas LJ Connors GL: Organization and management of a pulmonary rehabilitation program. In Hodgkin JE, Connors GL, Bell JE, editors, *Pulmonary Rehabilitation: Guidelines to Success,* ed 2, Philadelphia, JB Lippincott, 1993.

50. Sue D: Exercise testing and the patient with cardiopulmonary disease, *Prob Pulmon Dis* 2:1–8, 1986.

51. Wasserman K, Sue DY, Casaburi R, Moricca RB: Selection criteria for exercise training in pulmonary rehabilitation, *Eur Respir J Suppl* 7:604s–610s, 1989.

52. Casaburi R, Wasserman K, Patessio A, Ioli F, Zanaboni S, Donner CF: A new perspective in pulmonary rehabilitation: anaerobic threshold as a discriminant in training, *Eur Respir J Suppl* 7:618s–623s, 1989.

53. Hodgkin JE: Organization of a pulmonary rehabilitation program, *Clin Chest Med* 7:541–549, 1986.

54. Gilmartin ME: Pulmonary rehabilitation-patient and family education, *Clin Chest Med* 7:619–627, 1986.

55. White B, Andrews JL: Pulmonary rehabilitation in an ambulatory group practice setting, *Med Clin N Am* 63:379, 1979.

56. Ries AL, Moser KM: Comparison of isocapnic hyperventilation and walking exercise training at home in pulmonary rehabilitation, *Chest* 90:285–9, 1986.

57. Levine S, Weiser P, Gillen J: Evaluation of a ventilatory muscle endurance training program in the rehabilitation of patients with chronic obstructive pulmonary disease, *Am Rev Respir Dis* 133:400–6, 1986.

58. Chen H, Dukes R, Martin BJ: Inspiratory muscle training in patients with chronic obstructive pulmonary disease, *Am Rev Respir Dis* 131:251–255, 1985.

59. Belman M, Mittman C: Ventilatory muscle training improves exercise capacity in chronic obstructive pulmonary disease patients, *Am Rev Respir Dis* 121:273:280, 1980.

60. Pardy R: The effects of inspiratory muscle training on exercise performance in chronic airflow limitation, *Am Rev Respir Dis* 123:421–425, 1981.

61. Levine S, Weiser P, Gillen J: Evaluation of a ventilatory muscle endurance training program in the rehabilitation of patients with chronic obstructive pulmonary disease, *Am Rev Respir Dis* 133(3):400–406, 1986.

62. Hanak M: Patient and family education: *Teaching programs for managing chronic disease and disability,* New York, 1986, Springer Publishing Co.

63. Bickford LS, Hodgkin JE: National pulmonary rehabilitation survey, *Respir Care* 33(11):1030–1035, 1988.

64. Gilmartin ME: Pulmonary rehabilitation: patient and family education, *Clin Chest Med* 7(4):619–627, 1986.

65. Nicol J, Hodkin JE, Connors G, Gray L, Tilton D, Zorn E, Dunham J: Strategies for developing a cost effective pulmonary rehabilitation program, *Respir Care* 28:1451–1455, 1983.

66. Connors GL, Hilling L, Grindal S, Wilkison WK: Reimbursement: a determinant of program survival, in Hodgkin JE, Connors GL, Bell JE editors. *Pulmonary Rehabilitation: Guidelines to Success,* ed 2, Philadelphia, 1993, JB Lippincott.

67. Porte P: Legislation and respiratory rehabilitation, *Respir Care* 28:1498–1502, 1983.

68. Roselle S, D'Amico FS: The effect of home respiratory therapy on hospital readmission rates of patients with chronic obstructive pulmonary disease, *Respir Care* 27:1194–1199, 1982.

69. Haas A, Cardon H: Rehabilitation in chronic obstructive pulmonary disease: a five year study of 252 male patients, *Med Clin N Am* 53:593–606, 1969.

70. Mohsenifar KM, Horak D, Brown HV, Koerner SK: Sensitive indices of improvement in a pulmonary rehabilitation program, *Chest* 83:189–192, 1983.

71. Make BJ: Pulmonary rehabilitation: myth or reality?, *Clin Chest Med* 7:519–540, 1986.

72. Hudson LD, Tyler ML, Petty TL: Hospitalization needs during an outpatient rehabilitation program for severe chronic airway obstruction, *Chest* 70(5):606–610, 1976.

73. Olopade CO, Beck KC, Viggiano RW, Staats BA: Exercise limitation and pulmonary rehabilitation in chronic obstructive pulmonary disease, *Mayo Clin Proc* 67(2):144–157, 1992.

74. Make BJ, Gilmartin ME: Rehabilitation and home care for ventilator-assisted individuals, *Clin Chest Med* 7(4):679–691, 1986.

75. Make BJ, Gilmartin M, Brody JS, Snider GL,: Rehabilitation of ventilator-dependent subjects with lung disease, *Chest* 86:358–365, 1984.

Respiratory Home Care

■

Kenneth A. Wyka

Craig L. Scanlan

CHAPTER LEARNING OBJECTIVES

1. Define the concept of respiratory home care;
2. State the standards for respiratory therapy home care as adopted by the American Association for Respiratory Care (AARC);
3. Describe the guidelines for home care of the ventilator-dependent patient as proposed by the American College of Chest Physicians (ACCP);
4. Discuss the delivery of respiratory care in the home on the basis of patient selection, prescribed therapy, factors ensuring success, and potential problems or difficulties;
5. Identify current criteria for home oxygen therapy;
6. Compare and contrast the various home oxygen delivery systems;
7. Describe the appropriate use, advantages, and disadvantages of the various modes of home ventilatory support;
8. Identify and describe other common modes of home respiratory care, with an emphasis on the use of nasal CPAP for treatment of obstructive sleep apnea;
9. Identify and describe the current major issues involved in the delivery of home respiratory care.

Respiratory home care represents one of the fastest growing and most dynamic segments of respiratory care. As the elderly population grows and the health care reform movement strengthens, the need for comprehensive home care has become more keenly felt and recognized.

Since most home care begins after an acute-care hospitalization, a well-designed program must be carefully integrated with the discharge planning process. Moreover, because home care normally involves several disciplines, coordinated teamwork is essential.

Key areas of home care for which respiratory care practitioners (RCPs) are responsible include continuous oxygen therapy, long-term mechanical ventilation, treatment of sleep apnea, and in-home continuation of pulmonary rehabilitation. These and other aspects of respiratory home care are the major focus of this chapter.

HISTORICAL PERSPECTIVE

Provision of respiratory therapy in the home for the management of patients with chronic cardiorespiratory conditions is an accepted and necessary practice today. However, its widespread application, including "high-tech" levels of care, are relatively new. The health care industry is only beginning to realize the positive impact respiratory home care can have on patient management and related health care costs.

Before 1970, respiratory therapy procedures were almost exclusively administered within the hospital. Although there were isolated cases of patients receiving selected therapy in the home, comprehensive respiratory care was simply not available in this setting. The accompanying box lists some of the reasons why.

After 1970, respiratory home care began to emerge as a speciality with its own identity. Electrically driven IPPB units became available, as did small volume liquid oxygen systems, oxygen concentrators, portable ventilators, and disposables supplies. At the same time, the number of accredited respiratory therapy programs grew steadily, producing greater numbers of practitioners who became credentialed through the National Board for Respiratory Care (NBRC). Although Medicare and other insurance carriers did not directly reimburse RCPs for the services they provided, reimbursement for oxygen and other equipment was supported. As a result, the number of companies and organizations providing respiratory home care increased dramatically, as did the competition for patient services.[1]

Federal laws passed in the early 1980's designed to contain health care costs made home care a viable alternative to certain forms of hospitalized care. More recent efforts at health care reform are creating added incentives to use the hospital less and alternative sites, such as the home, more. Essentially all of the necessary elements are now in place to shape the future practice of respiratory home care. And the final key element—direct reimbursement for home respiratory care services—is on the horizon.

GOALS, OBJECTIVES AND STANDARDS

The American Association for Respiratory Care **(AARC)** defines respiratory home care as those specif-

---

Why respiratory home care was not available prior to 1970

Technology: equipment was pneumatic, complicated and cumbersome. Portability needed to be solved. Also, disposables were not readily available.

Personnel: few trained and credentialed RCPs were in existence before 1970. Almost all qualified practitioners were employed by hospitals in supervisory and managerial roles.

Attitudes: many health care professionals did not believe that patients could adhere to prescribed therapeutic routines in the home. They believed that the best place for on-going therapy was in the hospital. As a result, many respiratory therapy departments had outpatient clinics treating patients anywhere from one to five times per week or more.

Home Care Equipment Providers: these were small in number and offered limited services at best.

Reimbursement: was not available for respiratory care delivered by a respiratory technician or therapist. When Medicare and Medicaid came into existence in 1965, respiratory therapy was not mentioned in the reimbursement policies and was thereby excluded. However, oxygen and related equipment became reimbursable under Part B of Medicare in 1967 and this reimbursement would have a significant impact on the growth of home care in the years to come.

Regulatory Standards: Up until 1988, all standards related to provision. Standards of home care were based on federal reimbursement criteria, or state licensing regulations. In 1986, the Joint Commission on Accreditation of Healthcare Organizations (JCAHO) began working on a set of standards for the home health care industry, to include all companies and organizations that provide equipment and/or care for patients outside of the hospital setting. These standards were implemented in 1988.

---

ic forms of respiratory care provided in the patient's place of residence by personnel trained in respiratory therapy working under medical supervision.[2]

Goals and objectives

The primary goal of home care is to provide quality health care services to patients or clients in their home setting, thus minimizing dependence on hospitals as the basis for ongoing treatment.

In regard to respiratory home care, several specific objectives are evident. Respiratory home care can contribute to:

- Supporting and maintaining life
- Improving patients' physical, emotional, and social well-being
- Promoting patient and family self-sufficiency
- Insuring cost-effective delivery of care

Most patients for whom respiratory home care is considered are those with chronic respiratory diseas-

es. Applicable categories of disorders include the following:

- Chronic obstructive pulmonary disease (COPD)
- Cystic fibrosis
- Chronic neuromuscular disorders
- Chronic restrictive conditions
- Carcinomas of the lung

In addition, some acute conditions may best be treated in the home. These disorders include respiratory tract infections not requiring hospitalization and mild forms of asthma.

Although not all aspects of respiratory home care have proven effective, various studies have shown that carefully selected treatment regimens can be of significant benefit to patients. These benefits include increased **longevity,** improved quality of life, increased functional performance, and a reduction in the individual and societal costs associated with hospitalization.[3-10]

Standards for home care

Standards for home care have evolved somewhat haphazardly. Federal regulations have focused mainly on reimbursement criteria for selected home medical equipment and services. State efforts, where applicable, have addressed general licensing requirements for home care providers. Until recently, private sector initiatives have been limited to position statements by relevant professional organizations, such as the AARC. Not until 1988 was a comprehensive effort made to establish national standards for providers of home care.

Federal regulations

Federal regulation of respiratory home care began in 1967 with recognition of oxygen and related equipment as reimbursable under Medicare (Part B). Since then, several changes have occurred. The main change has been a move toward more objective criteria for documenting patient eligibility and much stricter limitations on total costs. Details on these regulations are provided later in this chapter. However, given the frequency of change in this area, the reader should consult sources such as the *Federal Register* for the most current information on federal home care reimbursement regulations.

State efforts

Many states have regulations in effect that govern licensing of home health care providers, such as home health agencies (HHAs) or visiting nurse associations (VNAs). Since these regulations are different in each state, readers should contact their state health department for details.

Private sector initiatives

Like many professional organizations, the American Association for Respiratory Care (AARC) recognized early on the need for home care standards. In fact, the AARC was among the first to be develop a set of home care standards, originally published in 1979.[2] These standards are summarized in the accompanying box.

Subsequently, both the AARC and the American Respiratory Care Foundation AARC have published guidelines dealing with specific aspects of home care, including equipment disinfection[11] and oxygen therapy.[12]

In 1986, the Joint Commission on Accreditation of Healthcare Organizations (JCAHO) initiated a two-year project to develop a comprehensive set of accreditation standards for the home health care providers. This project included field reviews, pilot surveys, and input from organizations representing professional providers, institutions and agencies, third-party payors, and consumers of home health services.

First published in 1988, these standards have since undergone several major revisions and refinements. The current standards are divided into major two sections.[13]

Section 1 contains general standards applicable to *all* home care organizations. These general standards focus on seven major areas: (1) patient/client rights and responsibilities, (2) patient/client care, (3) safety management, (4) infection control, (5) the home care record, (6) quality assessment and improvement, and (7) governance and management.

Section 2 standards are specific to the type of provider. In this section, separate standards are specified for home health services (such as nursing or physical therapy), pharmaceutical services, personal care and support services, equipment management, and clinical respiratory services.

Most agencies providing home respiratory care are responsible for both equipment management and clinical services. Equipment management includes the selection, delivery, setup, and maintenance of equipment. Example of clinical respiratory services provided in the home are chest assessment, monitoring of vital signs, blood pressure testing, pulmonary function testing, drawing blood, suctioning, and chest physical therapy.

Thus, to gain JCAHO accreditation, an agency providing home respiratory care services must meet the seven general standards applicable to all home care providers, and those applicable to equipment management and clinical respiratory services. The current Section 2 standards for equipment management and clinical respiratory services are listed in the accompanying boxes.

With both the AARC and JCAHO standards now providing a sound basis for quality home care, health professionals and consumers alike should now expect providers to comply with these expectations. Of course, the ultimate goal should always be to place the patient needs first in an effort to provide an optimum level of professional service.

HOME CARE PLANNING

Most patients are referred to respiratory home care after an acute care hospitalization. Others are placed in a home care service from a physician's office or an outpatient facility. In almost all these cases, the patient's physician identifies the need for respiratory home care and writes specific orders for implementation.

The home care team

Although the physician normally initiates the home care order, a number of other health care professionals are involved in the discharge process. The box, page 1101, identifies the key home care team members, along with their major duties. As with pulmonary rehabilitation (Chapter 37), a team care approach in home care produces the best patient results. Communication and mutual respect for each team member's talents and abilities are two key elements in making home care work. Any breakdown in the system may delay or affect patient discharge, home care and/or followup.

American Association for Respiratory Care Standards for home respiratory care[2]

Standard I

The need for therapy must be clearly established. There must be criteria and therapeutic objectives for program entry requirements. A unified approach should exist between the physician and therapist for the objectives and modalities of therapy.

Standard II

A medical record that includes the prescription must be established and maintained on all patients receiving any form of respiratory therapy home care.

Standard III

Respiratory therapy equipment used must be safe and appropriate. The patient must demonstrate its effective use, and he/she or the family must demonstrate its proper maintenance, including sterilization or appropriate cleanliness.

Standard IV

There must be evidence that patients are receiving followup evaluations at least once per month, and more often if necessary, by some member of the home care team.

JCAHO standards for home equipment management[13]

EM.1 Organizations providing equipment directly or by contract effectively manage the selection, delivery, setup, and maintenance of equipment.

EM.1.1 Staff providing equipment and related services demonstrate knowledge of and competence in the following:

EM.1.1.1 Specific structural, electrical, and environmental requirements for safe and effective use of equipment in the home setting;

EM.1.1.2 Equipment setup;

EM.1.1.3 Equipment safety checks and troubleshooting;

EM.1.1.4 Routine and emergency response procedures, including backup systems.

EM.1.2 There is a process designed to assure that the equipment provided by the home care organization is safe and is working as intended for the patient's/client's use in the home.

EM.1.2.1 There is documentation of the manufacturer, model, serial number, and maintenance instructions for all appropriate equipment.

EM.1.2.2 There is a process for obtaining timely and accurate information about equipment hazards, defects, and recalls.

EM.1.2.2.1 As appropriate, patients/clients, staff, and the prescribing physician are notified of equipment hazards, defects, and recalls.

EM.1.2.3 Routine and preventive maintenance is performed

EM.1.2.3.1 by qualified individuals and

EM.1.2.3.2 on an ongoing basis.

EM.1.2.3.2.1 The results of the ongoing evaluation of equipment are documented routinely.

EM.1.3 The home care organization has an established procedure for the delivery of equipment and supplies.

EM.1.3.1 The frequency and method of delivery are appropriate to the patient's/client's needs.

EM.1.3.1.1 The method of delivery is designed to assure that equipment and supplies are sanitary and in working order.

EM.1.4 The patient/client receives education appropriate to the equipment or medical supplies.

EM.1.4.1 Patient/client education describes the patient's/client's responsibilities in the care and use of the equipment and/or supplies.

EM.1.4.2 Patients/clients receive written information regarding when and how they can contact the home care organization for equipment maintenance and/or repair.

EM.1.4.2.1 When the equipment becomes the property of the patient/client, he/she is advised of his/her responsibility for maintaining it.

EM.1.4.3 Patient/client education is conducted by a qualified individual.

EM.1.4.3.1 When the equipment is invasive, when an invasive technique is taught, or when the equipment supports life functions, a qualified health care professional conducts patient/client education.

EM.1.5 The home care organization provides for emergency maintenance, replacement, or backup equipment when necessary.

EM.1.5.1 If equipment malfunction may threaten the patient's/client's health, access to 24-hour emergency services is available for equipment maintenance or replacement.

EM.1.5.2 If equipment malfunction may threaten the patient's/client's life, a backup system is provided.

EM.2 Equipment and related medical supplies provided are appropriate to the care delivered and to the home environment.

EM.2.1 As appropriate, the equipment and related medical supplies are provided according to physician order(s).

EM.2.2 Initial and ongoing assessments are designed to assure that equipment or supplies are appropriate for an individual patient's/client's use.

EM.2.2.1 The assessments are conducted by a qualified individual.

EM.2.2.1.1 When equipment is invasive or supports life functions, a qualified health care professional conducts an assessment of its appropriateness for a patient's/client's use.

The discharge decision is usually made by the patient's physician. With difficult cases, family members and the hospital chaplain may also be involved. This decision may also require that specific discharge criteria have been met (education and training, patient status, and home conditions), and that sufficient caregiver support exists at home.[14] Most often, these criteria pertain to home mechanical ventilation. Other forms of respiratory home care require far less planning, and are much easier to provide. Nonetheless, patient and/or caregiver cooperation, acceptance of responsibilities, and education are important aspects of home care delivery, regardless of the type and complexity of equipment and care prescribed.[15,16]

JCAHO standards for clinical respiratory services[13]

RS.1 The number, qualifications, and current competence of the individual(s) providing clinical respiratory services are appropriate to the patient/client needs, the level of care required, and applicable law and regulation.

RS.2 All clinical respiratory services have ongoing supervision.

RS.2.1 Appropriate supervision is available during all hours services are provided.

RS.2.2 The number, qualifications, and current competence of the individuals supervising clinical respiratory staff are appropriate to the scope of clinical respiratory services provided.

RS.2.2.1 When a supervisor does not have appropriate clinical training and experience in clinical respiratory services, the organization provides access to qualified consultation.

RS.3 An individualized plan of treatment is developed for each patient/client receiving clinical respiratory services.

RS.3.1 The patient's/client's physician, or other individual allowed by law and by the organization, establishes the plan of treatment for clinical respiratory services.

RS.3.2 The plan of treatment

RS.3.2.1 is based on a current assessment of the patient/client;

RS.3.2.2 includes information on

RS.3.2.2.1 diagnosis(es),

RS.3.2.2.2 treatment, including procedures and medications, and

RS.3.2.2.3 precautions and limitations that affect the plan of care/service;

RS.3.2.3 is obtained from the patient's/client's physician on a timely basis in accordance with applicable law and regulation;

RS.3.2.4 is periodically reviewed and revised as necessary;

RS.3.2.4.1 The plan of treatment is reviewed by the patient's/client's physician as frequently as required by the patient's/client's condition, the outcome of treatment, or the patient's/client's response to care according to applicable law and regulation.

RS.3.2.4.2 The minimum frequency of the review is specified in organizational policy and procedure.

RS.3.2.5 is included in the home care record.

RS.4 A mechanism is in place to verify that a patient's/client's physician from whom orders are accepted is licensed.

RS.5 There is ongoing communication between the clinical respiratory services staff and the patient's/client's physician.

RS.5.1 Clinical respiratory staff contact the patient's/client's physician whenever warranted by the patient's/client's condition.

RS.5.2 Written reports of the patient's/client's respiratory condition, the outcome of current treat-

ment, and his/her response are periodically provided to his/her physician.

RS.5.2.1 The minimum frequency of the reporting is specified in organizational policy and procedure.

RS.6 On admission and periodically throughout the course of care, individualized assessments of the patient/client are conducted.

RS.6.1 The assessments

RS.6.1.1 are conducted by qualified individuals;

RS.6.1.2 identify the problems, needs, and strengths of the patient/client and the services the family can provide; and

RS.6.1.3 include the patient's/client's family/support system and the home environment.

RS.7 Care provided is

RS.7.1 in accordance with accepted standards of practice;

RS.7.2 in accordance with existing physician orders;

RS.7.3 directed toward the achievement of stated goals; and

RS.7.4 evaluated against established goals to determine achievement of those goals.

RS.8 The organization has written policies and procedures regarding the resuscitation of patients/clients and the forgoing or withdrawal of life-sustaining treatment.

RS.8.1 The policies describe

RS.8.1.1 the documentation required in the home care record, including appropriate orders authenticated by the patient's/client's physician, and

RS.8.1.2 the documentation of any advance directives known to the organization.

RS.9 Organizations providing clinical respiratory services whose staff administers drugs in the home have policies and procedures relating to such drug administration.

RS.9.1 Written policies and procedures address at least the following:

RS.9.1.1 The drugs and/or drug classes that clinical respiratory staff administer, including the route of administration and any exceptions;

RS.9.1.2 Treatment modalities, such as aerosol therapy;

RS.9.1.3 Response to adverse drug reactions; and

RS.9.1.4 Documentation of patient/client education.

RS.9.2 There is a process designed to assure that the drug to be administered by inhalation is

RS.9.2.1 identified as the drug ordered for the patient/client;

RS.9.2.2 stable and within expiration limits; and

RS.9.2.3 not contraindicated for the patient/client.

RS.10 A home care organization that directly provides clinical laboratory services through collection and analysis of specimens promotes the safe and accurate performance of laboratory procedures.

continued

JCAHO standards for clinical respiratory services[13]—*cont'd*

RS.10.1 Current, readily available policies and procedures are in place and address the following, as applicable:
RS.10.1.1 Specimen collection;
RS.10.1.2 Specimen preservation;
RS.10.1.3 Instrument calibration;
RS.10.1.4 Quality control and remedial action;
RS.10.1.5 Equipment performance evaluations; and
RS.10.1.6 Test performance.

RS.10.2 The home care organization performs tests and examines specimens on the written request of individuals authorized by the organization and licensed to engage in the direct treatment of patients/clients.

RS.10.3 Personnel in the organization are designated as responsible for performing tests and for directing or supervising the testing.

RS.10.4 Staff who perform tests have adequate, specific training and orientation to perform the tests.

RS.10.5 Quality control checks are performed for all procedures with suitable positive and, as appropriate, negative reference samples, as recommended by the manufacturer.

RS.10.5.1 Appropriate quality control and test records are maintained.

RS.11 A home care organization whose stated scope of services includes the provision of medical laboratory services through another organization has a written agreement with the laboratory performing the services.

RS.11.1 The written agreement requires that the laboratory is accredited by the Joint Commission on Accreditation of Healthcare Organizations or the College of American Pathologists or demonstrates compliance with applicable federal standards for clinical laboratories.

Members of the respiratory home health care team

Discipline	Responsibilities
Utilization Review	Advises and/or recommends consideration of patient discharge. Documents patient's in-hospital care.
Discharge Planning (Social Service or Community/Public Health)	Brings all the needed home care elements together and insures that a patient can be discharged home. Makes contacts with outside agencies that may assist with patient care.
Physician	Writes order for patient discharge. Evaluates patient's condition and prescribes respiratory home care. Establishes therapeutic objectives.
Respiratory Care	Recommends types of home care modalities. May set-up therapeutic regimen at home and followup accordingly. May suggest home care provider for necessary equipment and supplies.
Nursing	Writes home care plan for patient. Assesses patient's status and provides necessary home care followup.
Dietary	Assesses patient's nutritional needs and writes dietary plan for patient. Makes arrangements for meals as may be necessary.
Physical Therapy	Provides necessary physical therapy and recommends any additional modalities or procedures.
Psychiatry/ Psychology	Assesses patient's emotional status and provides any needed counseling or support.
Durable Medical Equipment (DME) Supplier/Home Care Company	Provides necessary home care equipment and supplies and handles any emergency situations involving delivery or equipment operation.

The discharge plan

The discharge plan should consider the following key points:

- Date of discharge
- Therapeutic goals for home care
- Specific therapies to be given, including frequency
- Necessary equipment for implementation
- Patient instruction and set-up
- Selection of home care agency
- Plans for patient follow-up and evaluation

Therapeutic objectives, as related to patient care, may include any of the following:

- To support ventilation (life support)
- To improve oxygenation (at rest, with activity, or during sleep)
- To reverse bronchospasm
- To promote mucociliary clearance
- To promote bronchial hygiene
- To help maintain upper airway patency
- To promote effective breathing techniques/ avoid panic breathing

By keeping the plan objective, desired patient outcomes will be easier to assess and achieve.

Patient referrals and DMEs

Upon discharge, patients may be referred directly to a visiting nurse service (VNA), home health agency (HHA), or durable medical equipment (DME) supplier.

DME suppliers range in size from multi-million dollar national corporations offering a broad range of services, to small local companies. With the advent of home oxygen reimbursement under Medicare in 1967, the number and diversity of DME companies increased. These companies, both large and small, usually provide the following respiratory home care services:

- 24 hour, 7 day a week service
- Insurance coverage (private, Medicare, and Medicaid)
- Home instruction and follow-up by an RCP
- Most forms of respiratory care

Home care equipment can also be provided through HHAs, VNAs, hospitals, outpatient facilities, charitable organizations, hospice groups, and private concerns (e.g., physician offices, and respiratory practitioners in private practice).

Several factors should be considered when selecting a DME supplier. These factors include accreditation status, cost and scope of services, dependability, location, personnel, past track record, and availability.

To assure a basic level of quality, one should select a DME supplier that is JCAHO accredited. In addition, the service should be problem-free and provided by a reliable, professional and courteous staff. Charges should be reasonable and competitive, and clinical respiratory services by credentialed RCPs should be available.

Due to the profitable nature of DME supply, many agencies and physician groups have set up joint ventures with home care companies. Such partnerships are legal if: (1) all parties are at risk when entering into the agreement, (2) a legal contract is written which identifies responsibilities for all involved parties, and (3) the joint venture is not based on patient referrals alone.

For years, many DME suppliers engaged in highly profitable but dubious practices, such as renting inexpensive equipment that could easily be purchased. To eliminate these practices, Congress wrote laws in 1987 that changed reimbursement policies for home medical equipment. Under these laws (commonly referred to as the "six-point plan") rent payments for inexpensive equipment cannot exceed the purchase price, and payments for expensive equipment are capped at 15 months. Oxygen and O_2 equipment are reimbursed on a monthly basis.

More recently, the home care industry has become the focus for managed care plans. Under these arrangements, third-party payors (excluding Medicare) have designated case managers who oversee reimbursement for home care services. Case managers are responsible for obtaining the best service possible at the lowest possible price. This is commonly done by having DMEs bid on large-volume contracts for equipment and services. Given their decision-making authority over the purchase of services, case managers are becoming integral members of the home care team.

Assessing the home environment

Before beginning any home care regimen, the provider should assess the patient's home. Key considerations include accessibility, equipment, and the general environment (see accompanying box).

The home care provider must also assess the ability of the patient and/or caregiver to understand both equipment use and maintenance, including disinfection, and administration of prescribed therapy. Adequate time must be scheduled for proper instruction and review of all equipment and procedures.

RESPIRATORY HOME CARE SERVICES

The most common home respiratory care services are oxygen therapy and ventilatory support. Other modes of home respiratory care include aerosol therapy, IPPB, airway care, chest physical therapy, **nasal CPAP,** and apnea monitoring.

<table>
<tr><td>

Assessing the home environment

Accessibility

    In and out of home/apartment
    Bathroom
    Kitchen
    Between rooms
    Wheelchair mobility
    Doorway width
    Thresholds
    Stairways
    Carpeting

Equipment

    Available space
    Electrical power supply
      Amperage
      Grounded outlets
    Presence of hazardous appliances

Environment

    Heating/ventilation
    Humidity
    Lighting
    Living space

</td></tr>
</table>

Home oxygen therapy

Oxygen therapy is the most common mode of home respiratory care. Between 500,000 to 800,000 patients are receiving some form of home O_2 therapy in the US.[17,18] This high usage is based, in part, on the fact that O_2 therapy improves survival in selected patient groups, especially those with advanced COPD.[4,19-25] In particular, several studies have shown improved nocturnal oxygen saturation, reduced pulmonary artery pressure, and lower pulmonary vascular resistance with appropriate out-patient O_2 therapy.[26-32]

Goal

There are two major goals of home O_2 therapy: (1) to prevent or alleviate adverse responses to chronic hypoxemia, and (2) to allow the patient to function at the highest possible level of performance.

The accompanying box lists the common adverse responses to chronic hypoxemia. While nocturnal restlessness and morning headache are relatively harmless, conditions such as pulmonary hypertension and chronic cor pulmonale can be life-threatening. In either case, O_2 therapy can help.

In terms of patients' functional performance, the ultimate goal is to restore a normal level of activity. This may include walking or traveling with portable oxygen, both around town and away from home. The psychological uplift is remarkable when patients can venture from their home, even go on vacation, knowing that their O_2 needs will be met. Most home care or

<table>
<tr><td>

Adverse responses to chronic hypoxemia

- Pulmonary hypertension
- Recurring congestive heart failure (CHF)
- Chronic cor pulmonale
- **Erythrocythemia** (Hct > 56%)
- Impaired cognitive processes
- Nocturnal restlessness
- Morning headache

</td></tr>
</table>

DME providers can make arrangements for patients who are planning to travel with oxygen. There is a National Oxygen Travel Service which is available to help with such plans.

Many commercial carriers (airlines, railways) place restrictions on personal O_2 systems.[33,34] For example, only empty portable systems can be taken on airplanes. The airline will provide O_2 for the patient during the flight, with a fee charged for each cylinder used. Specific carriers should be contacted when travel arrangements are being made. Of course, plans must also include supplying oxygen at the patient's destination.

Specific indications and documentation of need

Until recently, O_2 therapy was the most abused forms of home respiratory care. Most of these abuses were eliminated in 1985 when the Health Care Financing Administration (HCFA) published uniform national criteria for home O_2 therapy coverage.[35]

These regulations required that home O_2 prescriptions be based on documented hypoxemia, as determined by either blood gas analysis or oximetry. Prescriptions for O_2 could no longer be based simply on patient diagnosis or signs and symptoms. In addition, "prn" oxygen was no longer acceptable.

Some years later, the AARC developed a clinical practice guideline for oxygen therapy in the home or extended care facility.[17] Indications for home oxygen therapy specified in this guideline are listed in the box, page 1104.

Conditions for which O_2 therapy is *not* indicated or reimbursed include **angina pectoris** without hypoxemia, dyspnea without cor pulmonale or hypoxemia, peripheral vascular disease causing desaturation in one or more extremities, and terminal illnesses that do not affect the lungs.[32]

Once the need for O_2 therapy is established, a prescription is written. A prescription for home O_2 therapy *must* include the following elements:

- Flow rate in liters/minute and/or concentration
- Frequency of use in hours/day and minutes/hour (if applicable)
- Duration of need—a specific number of months up to 12 (lifetime authorization is no longer acceptable)

Indication for O_2 therapy in the home or extended care facility[12]

A. Documented hypoxemia at rest

In adults, children and infants older than 28 days: (1) a $PaO_2 \leq 55$ torr or an $SaO_2 \leq 85\%$ breathing room air, or (2) a PaO_2 of 56–59 torr or an SaO_2 or $SpO_2 \leq 89\%$ in association with specific clinical manifestations of chronic hypoxemia (see "Adverse responses to chronic hypoxemia" box on page 1103 for examples).

B. Desaturation with activity

Some patients may not qualify for O_2 therapy at rest but will qualify for oxygen during ambulation, sleep, or exercise. Oxygen therapy is indicated during these specific activities when the SaO_2 falls to 88% or less.

- Diagnosis—severe primary lung disease, secondary conditions related to lung disease and hypoxia-related conditions or symptoms that may improve with oxygen
- Laboratory evidence—arterial blood gas analysis or oximetry under the appropriate testing conditions. Home care companies cannot provide this testing.
- Additional medical documentation—no acceptable alternatives to home oxygen therapy.

The physician authorizes home O_2 therapy in this fashion, using the **HCFA** Certification of Medical Necessity for Home Oxygen Therapy form (Figure 38-1). When O_2 therapy is begun in the hospital but continues in the home setting, analysis of arterial blood oxygen should be repeated after 1 to 3 months to determine the need for long-term oxygen therapy.[36] Once the need for long-term therapy is documented, repeat ABGs or SaO_2 measurements are not needed.

However, blood oxygen levels may still be measured when the need arises to assess changes in the patient's condition or to adjust the oxygen prescription.[36,37]

Supply methods

Home oxygen is supplied from one of three sources:[38,39]

- Compressed oxygen cylinders
- Liquid oxygen (LOX) systems
- Oxygen concentrators or enrichers

Table 38-1 summarizes the major advantages and disadvantages of each of these systems.

Compressed oxygen cylinders. When home oxygen was first used, large gas cylinders (H or K) were the primary supply source. For the high volume user or the patient receiving mechanical ventilation, these large cylinders were commonly yolked together to provide greater storage capacity.

Advantages of using cylinder oxygen in the home include minimal waste (even when the cylinder is not used), portability (D/E cylinders only), and suitability for small volume users. The primary disadvantage of cylinder gas is the relatively small volume of available oxygen. Other disadvantages include the hazards of high pressure, and the weight, bulkiness and cost of large cylinders. When cylinder use becomes excessive and delivery becomes a problem, other systems, such as liquid oxygen or a concentrator, should be considered.

Safety measures for cylinder oxygen are the same as those covered in Chapter 24. The cylinder should be secured with a stand or "donut" base; the unit should not be placed near extreme heat or cold. Smoking or flames are not permitted in any area where O_2 is being used, and regulator or flowmeter valves and connections should never be lubricated with oil. These safety measures should be thoroughly reviewed by the RCP with both the patient and family. After instruction,

---

Table 38-1 Advantages and disadvantages of the three major home oxygen supply systems

System	Advantages	Disadvantages
Compressed-oxygen cylinder	Good for small-volume user No waste or loss Stores oxygen indefinitely Widespread availability	Large cylinders are heavy and bulky High pressures may represent a safety hazard (2200 psi) Provides limited volume of oxygen Frequent deliveries may be necessary
Liquid oxygen system	Provides large quantities of oxygen Low pressure system (20 to 25 psi) Portable units can be refilled from reservoir (up to 8-hour supply at 2 L/min) Valuable for rehabilitation	Loss of oxygen due to venting when system is not in use LOX must be delivered as needed Low temperature of LOX may represent a safety hazard
Oxygen concentrator	No waste or loss Low-pressure system (15 psi) Cost effective when continual supply of oxygen is needed Eliminates need for oxygen delivery	Disruption in electrical service renders system inoperable Back-up oxygen is necessary Cannot operate ventilators or other high-pressure devices Concentration of oxygen decreases with flow rate Electrical costs for operating system may be substantial

Department of Health and Human Services
Health Care Financing Administration

Form Approved
OMB No. 0938-0534

ATTENDING PHYSICIAN'S CERTIFICATION OF MEDICAL NECESSITY FOR
HOME OXYGEN THERAPY (Legible handwritten entries acceptable)

Public reporting burden for this collection of information is estimated to average 15 minutes per response, including the time for reviewing instructions, searching existing data sources, gathering and maintaining the data needed, and completing and reviewing the collection of information. Send comments regarding this burden estimate or any other aspect of this collection of information, including suggestions for reducing this burden, to HCFA, P.O. Box 26684, Baltimore, MD 21207; and to the Office of Information and Regulatory Affairs, Office of Management and Budget, Washington, DC 20503.

Patient's Name, Address, and HIC No.	Supplier's Name, Address, and Identification No.

Certification: ☐ Initial   ☐ Revised   ☐ Renewed

INFORMATION BELOW TO BE ENTERED ONLY BY PHYSICIAN OR PHYSICIAN'S EMPLOYEE

1. Pertinent Diagnoses, ICD-9-CM Codes, and Findings - CHECK ALL THAT APPLY:

☐ Emphysema (492.8)
☐ COPD (496)
☐ Cor Pulmonale (416.9)
☐ Interstitial Disease (515)
☐ Other _____
    Specify   Code

☐ Chronic Obstructive Bronchitis (491.2)
☐ Chronic Obstructive Asthma (493.20)
☐ Congestive Heart Failure (428.0)
☐ Secondary Polycythemia (289.0)
☐ Hematocrit 57% or more Yes☐ No☐

2.A. I last examined this patient for this condition on:
___/___/___
Month Day Year

2.B. Home oxygen prescribed:
___/___/___
Month Day Year

2.C. Estimated length of need:
☐ 1-3 months ☐ 4-12 months ☐ Lifetime

3.A. Results of Most Recent Arterial Blood Gas and/or Oxygen Saturation Tests (Patient Breathing Room Air)

	PO2	O2 Saturation	Date
(1) At Rest			
(2) Walking..........			
(3) Sleeping.........			
(4) Exercising.......			
(5) Other :			

3.C. Physician/Provider Performing Test(s) (Printed/Typed Name and Address):

3.B. If performed under conditions other than room air, explain:

NOTE: If PO2 Level exceeds 59 mm Hg or the arterial blood saturation exceeds 89% at rest on room air, the claim will be disallowed without compelling medical evidence. Check block ☐ if you have attached a separate statement on your letterhead of additional documentation.

4. Oxygen Flow Rate : _____ Liters per minute   ☐ Continuous (24 hrs/day)

☐ Noncontinuous (Enter hrs/day): _____ Walking _____Sleeping _____Exercise Program _____Other (specify) _____

5. Oxygen Equipment Prescribed If you have prescribed a particular form of delivery, check applicable block(s). Otherwise leave blank.

A. Supply System

(1) Stationary Source
☐ Concentrator   ☐ Liquid Oxygen
☐ Compressed Gas ☐ Other

(2) Portable or Ambulatory Source
☐ Liquid Oxygen
☐ Compressed Gas
☐ Other _____

B. Delivery System

☐ (1) Nasal Cannula
☐ (2) O2 Conserving Device
  ☐ Pulse O2 System
  ☐ Reservoir System
  ☐ Other _____
☐ (3) Transtracheal Catheter
☐ (4) Other _____

6. If you have prescribed a portable or ambulatory system, describe activities/exercise that patient regularly pursues which require this sys in the home and which cannot be met by a stationary system (e.g., amount and frequency of ambulation).

CERTIFICATION

THE PATIENT HAS APPROPRIATELY TRIED OTHER TREATMENT MEASURES WITHOUT SUCCESS. OXYGEN THERAPY AND OXYGEN EQUIPMENT AS PRESCRIBED IS MEDICALLY INDICATED AND IS REASONABLE AND NECESSARY FOR THE TREATMENT OF THIS PATIENT. THIS FORM AND ANY STATEMENT ON MY LETTERHEAD ATTACHED HERETO HAS BEEN COMPLETED BY ME, OR BY MY EMPLOYEE AND REVIEWED BY ME. THE FOREGOING INFORMATION IS TRUE, ACCURATE, AND COMPLETE, AND I UNDERSTAND THAT ANY FALSIFICATION, OMISSION, OR CONCEALMENT OF MATERIAL FACT MAY SUBJECT ME TO CIVIL OR CRIMINAL LIABILITY.

Attending Physician's Signature: (A STAMPED SIGNATURE IS NOT ACCEPTABLE)	Date:

Physician's Name, Address, Telephone No., and Identification No.:

HCFA-484 (5-90)

★ U S GPO 1990 261 114 13580

Fig. 38-1 Form used to certify the medical necessity for home oxygen therapy via the Health Care Financing Administration (HCFA).

the RCP should always confirm and document caregivers' actual ability to safely use the delivery system.

In addition to the cylinder gas, a pressure reducing valve with flowmeter is needed to deliver O_2 at the prescribed flow. Standard clinical flowmeters deliver flows up to 15 L/min; flows used in the home are typically in the 0.25 to 5.0 L/min range. For this reason, specially calibrated low-flow flowmeters may be needed. Alternatively, preset flow restrictors may be used. As described in Chapter 24, flow restrictors provide a fixed flow at a given source pressure. This makes the flow restrictor the device of choice when there are concerns about the patient or caregiver changing O_2 flows on their own.

Although cylinder gas is essentially dry, there is no need to humidify oxygen supplied to adults for nasal administration at flows of 4 L/min or less.[12] If humidification is needed, a simple unheated bubble humidifier is satisfactory for gas administration to the upper airway. Because the mineral content of home tap water may be high (hard water), water used in these humidifiers should be distilled. Otherwise, the porous diffusing element through which the oxygen passes may become occluded. Although complete blockage is unlikely, occlusion of the diffusing element can impair humidification.

Liquid oxygen systems. Because one cubic foot of liquid oxygen equals 860 cubic feet of gas, liquid oxygen systems can store large quantities of oxygen in small spaces. This is ideal for the high volume user who requires a large number of gaseous oxygen cylinders (ten or more per month) to meet therapeutic needs.

As shown in Figure 38-2, a typical home liquid oxygen system is a miniaturized version of that used in hospitals. Like its larger counterpart, the home system consists of a reservoir unit similar in design to a thermos bottle. The inner container of liquid oxygen (LOX) is suspended in an outer container, with a vacuum in between.

The liquid oxygen in the inner reservoir is kept at about $-300°F$. Due to constant vaporization, oxygen exists in the gaseous form above the liquid. When the cylinder is not being used, this vaporization maintains the pressure between 20 to 25 psi. When pressures rise above this level, gas is vented by the primary pressure relief valve.

When flow is turned on, gaseous oxygen leaves the container through a vaporizing coil, where it is warmed by exposure to room temperature. It then leaves the system through a standard oxygen outlet, where it is metered by a flow control valve. With low-flow and oxygen conserving systems being so common in the home care setting, these metering devices are usually calibrated in 0.5 L/min units, and limited to a maximum flow of 5 to 8 L/min.

If the cylinder pressure drops below a preset level during use (usually 20 psig), an economizer valve closes, causing the liquid O_2 to move up the center tube and into the vaporizing coil. When in the vaporizing coil the liquid oxygen is converted to a gas.

Depending on manufacturer and model, small liquid oxygen cylinders hold between 45 to 100 pounds of LOX (18 to 40 liters). In order to calculate the duration of flow available from a liquid O_2 system, one must first convert the weight of liquid oxygen in pounds to the equivalent volume of *gaseous* oxygen in liters. At normal liquid cylinder operating pressures, one pound of stored liquid oxygen equals about 344 liters of gaseous oxygen.

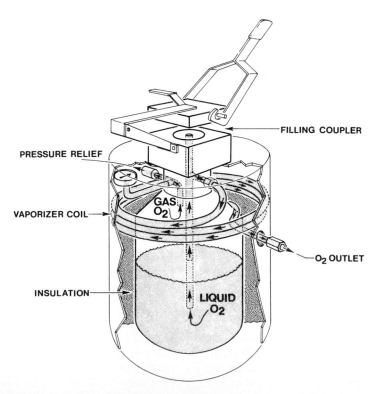

Fig. 38-2 Diagram of a home liquid oxygen supply system. (From Lampton LM: Home and outpatient oxygen therapy. In Brashear RE, Rhodes ML, editors: *Chronic obstructive lung disease,* St Louis, 1978, Mosby.)

For example, given a 100 pound liquid oxygen system with a gauge reading indicating a half-full cylinder, one would compute the available gaseous oxygen (in liters) as follows:

Step 1

$$\text{Available LOX (in pounds)} = 100 \times 0.5$$
$$= 50 \text{ lbs}$$

Step 2

$$\text{Available gaseous oxygen} = \text{Weight (lbs) remaining} \times \text{factor}$$
$$= 50 \text{ lbs} \times 344 \text{ L/lb}$$
$$= 17,200 \text{ L}$$

Finally, in order to compute the actual duration of flow, one simply divides the available volume of gaseous oxygen by the prescribed liter flow. Assuming a prescribed flow of 2 liters per minute, the duration of flow for a half-full 100 pound cylinder would be calculated as follows

Step 3

$$\text{Duration of flow} = \frac{\text{available gaseous oxygen (L)}}{\text{prescribed liter flow (L/min)}}$$

$$\text{Duration of flow} = \frac{17,200 \text{ L}}{2 \text{ L/min}}$$

$$= 8,600 \text{ minutes}$$
$$= 143.3 \text{ hours}$$
$$= 6 \text{ days}$$

To help avoid these computations, many manufacturers provide simple conversion charts for this purpose. Table 38-2 is an example of a conversion chart for a typical 100 pound home liquid oxygen system.

Table 38-2 Conversion chart for computing duration of flow 100 lb (40 L) home liquid O_2 reservoir

Gauge reading	1	2	3	4	5
Weight (lb)	12.5	25	50	75	100
Liquid liters	5	10	20	30	40
Gaseous liters	4303	8606	17,212	25,818	34,424

DURATION OF FLOW (HOURS)

Flow (L/min)					
0.5	143	287	574	861	1147
1	72	143	287	430	574
1.5	48	96	191	287	382
2	36	72	143	215	287
2.5	29	57	115	172	229
3	24	48	96	143	191
3.5	20	41	82	123	164
4	18	36	72	108	143
4.5	16	32	64	96	127
5	14	29	57	86	115
6	12	24	48	72	96
7	10	20	41	61	82
8	9	18	36	54	72

Many home liquid O_2 systems also come with smaller portable units (Figure 38-3). This system is ideal for the ambulatory patient who is capable of exercise or other physical activities conducted outside the home.

Typical portable units weigh between 5 to 14 pounds and can be refilled directly from the stationary reservoir. Although designs vary, most portable units come with a carrying case or small cart, and can

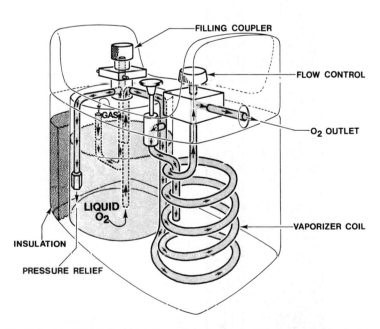

Fig. 38-3 Diagram of a portable liquid oxygen unit. (From Lampton LM: Home and outpatient oxygen therapy. In Brashear RE, Rhodes ML, editors: *Chronic obstructive lung disease*, St Louis, 1978, Mosby.)

provide 5 to 8 hours of O_2 at flow of 2 L/min. Either an adjustable flow restrictor or Bourdon-type gauge is used to meter flow, with a weight gauge used to indicate remaining O_2 contents. The functional use time of portable liquid O_2 units can be extended with oxygen-conserving devices.[12]

Due to the extremely low temperature of liquid O_2, patients and caregivers must be extremely careful when refilling these portable systems. The accompanying box lists the steps needed to fill a portable liquid O_2 unit from a reservoir.[39] The procedure takes about one to two minutes, depending on the size of the portable tank.

Oxygen concentrators. An oxygen concentrator is an electrically-powered device that physically separates the oxygen in room air from nitrogen. Currently, there are two types of O_2 concentrators: (1) the "molecular sieve" concentrator, and (2) the membrane concentrator or oxygen enricher.

The molecular sieve concentrator (Figure 38-4) uses a pump to compress and deliver filtered room air to one of two sets of sieves. These sieves contain **zeolite** pellets (inorganic sodium-aluminum silicate). These pellets absorb nitrogen, carbon dioxide, and water vapor. To remove these unwanted gases from the pellets, an automatic pressure swing cycle switches back and forth between the sieve sets. While one set is pressurized to produce oxygen, the other is depressurized to purge N_2, CO_2, and water vapor.

Gas leaving the sieves is stored in a small accumulator. At flows of 1 to 2 L/min, the typical molecular sieve concentrator provides between 94% and 95% oxygen. However, at higher flows the process becomes less efficient. At 3 to 5 L/min, oxygen concentrations fall to between 85% and 93%. At flows greater than 5 L/min, delivered concentrations are 80% or less.[40]

Membrane concentrators or oxygen enrichers separate oxygen from room air using a thin gas-permeable plastic membrane (Figure 38-5). A vacuum pump

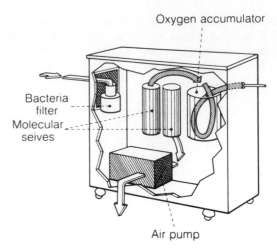

Fig. 38-4 A molecular sieve-type oxygen concentration. (Courtesy DeVilbis, Toledo, Ohio.)

provides a negative pressure gradient across the membrane. The design of the membrane is such that oxygen and water vapor diffuse more rapidly than nitrogen. This provides an enriched mixture of about 40% oxygen at flows up to 10 L/min.[39,41] Although lower than the molecular sieve, the FDO_2 provided by a membrane concentrator is nearly constant throughout the normal range of flow. However, to compensate for the lower FDO_2, higher flows must be used. In general, the flow should be 3 times that used with a 100% source. For example, a patient on 2 L/min nasal oxygen from a 100% O_2 cylinder should receive 6 L/min from the membrane concentrator.

Since water vapor molecules readily diffuse through the membrane, the oxygen mixture delivered by a membrane concentrator need not be humidified. However, excess water vapor is generated in this process and must be removed. This is done using a simple condenser system, with the condensate evaporated into the nitrogen-rich exhaust (refer to Figure 38-5).

Oxygen concentrators are among the most cost-efficient means of supplying oxygen to patients who need continuous low-flow oxygen at home. Depending on local utility rates, a concentrator running 24 hours per day will increase the average monthly electrical bill by only 5% to 10%.

When used with patients receiving low-flow oxygen, O_2 concentrators are just as effective in raising blood oxygen levels as more traditional supply systems (such as 100% cylinder gas with a cannula).[42,43] Moreover, current reimbursement regulations favor use of cost-efficient home oxygen systems. As a result, the use of oxygen concentrators and conserving systems is becoming increasingly popular.

Problem-solving and troubleshooting. Technical problems with home oxygen supply systems are similar to those encountered in the hospital setting (see

---

Steps in filling portable liquid O_2 unit from reservoir[39]

1. Make sure there is enough liquid oxygen in the reservoir to fill the portable unit.
2. Check the connectors on both units to make sure that they are clean and dry. Moisture on these connectors could cause the connectors to freeze together.
3. Connect the portable unit to the reservoir according to the manufacturer's instructions. The flow-rate controller should be turned off.
4. Open the portable unit vent. Allow the portable unit to fill until the vent begins to pass liquid oxygen instead of gas. Close the vent valve.
5. Disengage the portable unit according to the manufacturer's instructions.

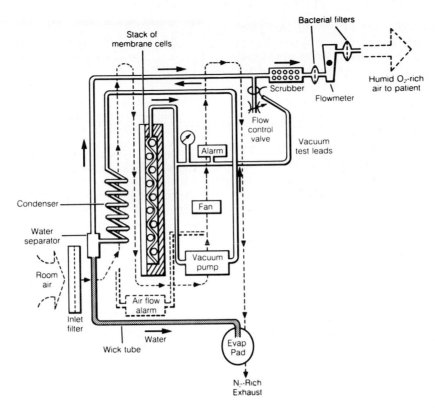

Fig. 38-5 A membrane-type oxygen concentrator. (Courtesy Oxygen Enricher Co, Schenectady, NY.)

Chapter 24). In addition to these technical problems, situations can arise when patients or caregivers fail to properly follow instructions or respond as needed to simple incidents. To help avoid communication problems, the RCP should always reinforce verbal instruction by providing simple written instructions for subsequent reference. In addition, the RCP should always confirm and document caregivers' actual abilities to use the delivery system safely, including how to troubleshoot simple problems.[12]

To help avoid problems before they occur, the patient or caregiver should be instructed to check all O_2 delivery equipment at least once a day.[12] The proper function of all equipment, including liter flow and FDO_2, should be confirmed. In addition, the remaining liquid or compressed gas content of the supply system should be checked. Providing the patient or caregiver with a simple checklist or log diary form can help assure that these important tasks are performed regularly.

Unlike the hospital setting, home oxygen supply problems cannot always be addressed immediately. For this reason, all home oxygen systems must have an emergency back-up supply. This is normally provided by a large H/K cylinder. If the patient's primary O_2 supply is via concentrator, the RCP should also notify the local power company that life support equipment is being used at that home. In the event of an outage, the company will try to restore power to that location first. Alternatively, an emergency gasoline electrical

generator can provide back-up power for a concentrator.

Possible physical hazards to patients and caregivers include unsecured cylinders, ungrounded equipment, mishandling of liquid oxygen (resulting in burns), and fire.[12] Careful preliminary instruction, followed by ongoing assessment of the home environment, can help minimize these problems.

Bacterial contamination associated with certain nebulizers and humidification systems is an additional possibility.[12] Infection control procedures designed to minimize this problem are discussed in detail later in this chapter.

Reports of inaccurate flows or O_2 concentrations with home oxygen supply equipment are another area of concern.[44,45] Accurate flow output of oxygen systems should be confirmed by the supplier (using calibrated laboratory meters) *before* equipment is placed in the home.[46]

On the other hand, the FDO_2s provided by oxygen concentrators should be checked and confirmed as part of a routine monthly maintenance visit.[47] Routine maintenance of these devices should include cleaning and replacing filters, checking the alarm system, and confirming the FDO_2s with a calibrated oxygen analyzer.* If the FDO_2s are lower than the manufacturer's specification at the given flow, the

---

*To help insure the delivery of prescribed concentrations of oxygen, many units are equipped with oxygen sensors for continuous monitoring.

zeolite canisters are probably exhausted and should be replaced.

Since most home liquid oxygen systems operate at pressures below 50 psi, they cannot be used to drive equipment needing this standard pressure, such as pneumatically powered ventilators. Likewise, the pressure generated by oxygen concentrators is not sufficient to operate these devices.

However, since the typical home ventilator is electrically powered and uses a flowmeter to provide supplementary O_2, this limitation is generally not a problem. Nonetheless, when 50 psi oxygen is needed, large gas cylinders are the storage system of choice.

Many home care patients using liquid O_2 express concern when they observe gas venting from their system. It should be explained to patients that venting is a normal feature of liquid O_2 systems. Since liquid O_2 is stored at **cryogenic** temperatures, ambient temperatures speed conversion of the liquid to a gas. When a liquid oxygen system is not in use, pressure builds up and eventually opens the pressure relief or vent valve. This wastes some oxygen. Venting does not occur during continual use, since system pressures never build up to activate the relief valve.

Delivery methods

The most common O_2 delivery system used at home is the nasal cannula. Simple oxygen masks and air entrainment mask (AEMs) may also be used, but are not common. In general, nasal catheters and reservoir masks are not used for home oxygen administration to adults.

Oxygen is not an expensive commodity. However, overuse, inappropriate prescribing practices and other billing abuses have made it an expensive proposition. In addition, the growth in use of home oxygen, the cost of providing this service, and recent changes in reimbursement practices have all helped alter attitudes regarding the economics of this therapy. Medicare and other insurance carriers are taking a closer look at oxygen usage, and related payments.

In an effort to keep oxygen use (and costs) down, a number of oxygen conserving devices have been developed. These include transtracheal oxygen therapy **(TTOT),** the reservoir cannula, and the demand or pulsed-flow oxygen delivery system.[48-52] Since the more traditional methods of oxygen administration are detailed in Chapter 26, we will focus here on the application of these newer conserving devices.

Transtracheal oxygen therapy (TTOT). The transtracheal oxygen catheter was first described by Heimlich in 1982.[53] Transtracheal oxygen therapy (TTOT) involves O_2 delivery directly into the trachea through a thin Teflon catheter inserted by guidewire between the second and third tracheal rings (Figure 38-6). The catheter is secured on the outside by a custom-sized chain necklace, and receives oxygen through standard tubing connected to a flowmeter.[54]

Reported benefits of transtracheal oxygen therapy (TTOT)
Increased patient mobility[54]
Avoidance of nasal and ear irritation[54]
Improved compliance with therapy[50,54]
Improved oxygenation when nasal cannula fails[50]
Enhanced personal image[50]
Better sense of taste, smell, and appetite[50,56]
Reduced oxygen cost of breathing[57]
Increased exercise tolerance[58]
Improved sleep (less hypoxemic)[50]

Not all patients requiring long-term O_2 therapy are candidates for TTOT. TTOT is indicated for only for those patients who meet one or more of the following criteria: (1) they cannot be adequately oxygenated with standard approaches, (2) they do not comply well when using other devices, (3) they exhibit complications from nasal cannula use; (4) they prefer TTOT for cosmetic reasons, and (5) they have need for increased mobility.[54] TTOT may also be an treatment alternative for some patients with sleep apnea when nasal CPAP is not tolerated or when combined oxygen and nasal CPAP are required.[55]

Because O_2 is delivered to the middle of the trachea, oxygen builds up here and in the upper airway during expiration. This effectively expands the anatomic reservoir, thereby increasing the FIO_2 at any given flow. As compared to a nasal cannula, anywhere from 50% to 75% less oxygen flow is needed to achieve a given PaO_2 with TTOT.[18,50] In some patients, adequate oxygenation can be achieved with flows as low as 0.25 L/min.

This can be of great economic benefit to patients who require continuous home oxygen. Currently, the typical cost of home oxygen at 2 L/min is between $400 to $500 per month. In concept, TTOT can cut this cost by $150 or more. Actual cost savings, however, may be significantly less.[50] Other reported benefits of TTOT are listed in the box above.

As with most home care modalities, the success of TTOT depends mainly on good patient education and ongoing self-care with professional followup. Key patient responsibilities include routine catheter cleaning, and recognizing and troubleshooting common problems. The accompanying box describes key self-care guidelines for patients with transtracheal O_2 catheters.[54]

Reservoir cannula. The reservoir cannula (Figure 38-7) represents a hybrid device, combining the concepts of a low-flow and reservoir delivery system.[49-51] The reservoir cannula operates by storing about 20 mL of oxygen in a small reservoir during exhalation.[59] This stored oxygen is then added to the normal flow during early inspiration. This increases the amount of

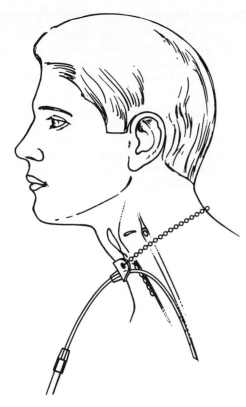

Fig. 38-6   Transtracheal oxygen catheter in position.

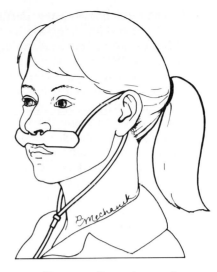

Fig. 38-7   Reservoir cannula.

oxygen available on each breath, and decreases the flow needed for a given FIO_2. Typically, a reservoir cannula can provide SaO_2 levels equal to those achieved with a regular cannula at between 1/3 to 2/5 the flow.[59,60] As with all conserving devices, this gas savings reduces cost and allows longer times away from stationary O_2 sources.

Unfortunately, many patients object to the appearance of the reservoir cannula, often referring to it as a 'mustache.' In addition, patients using a reservoir cannula during exercise show a greater fall in SaO_2 than when using a standard nasal cannula.[61]

To address these concerns, a pendant reservoir system was developed (Figure 38-8). In this design, the reservoir is situated on the anterior chest wall,

---

Self-care guidelines for patients with transtracheal O_2 catheters[61]

1. The catheter should never be out of your tract for more than a few minutes or your tract may close. If you cannot reinsert the catheter, put on a nasal cannula and call your doctor.
2. Always keep the catheter clean to ensure proper function.
3. If you believe the catheter isn't working properly, first clean it. If you still believe that the catheter isn't working, put on a nasal cannula and call your doctor.
4. If your humidifier pop-off is making noise, clear any hose blockage and clean the catheter.
5. The catheter must never be removed or inserted while oxygen is flowing through it.
6. Always keep your tract opening clean and dry. Don't use antibiotics or other ointments.
7. Always keep the oxygen hose under your shirt, blouse, t-shirt, or pajama-top and clipped to the top of your pants, skirt, or pajama bottoms.
8. Don't pull, twist, crush, cut, glue, boil, or abuse the catheter—treat it as your lifeline.
9. Any product which is cracked, broken, develops a permanent kink or a foul odor should be immediately discarded and replaced. Catheters and hoses should be routinely replaced every three months.
10. When traveling, always take catheter cleaning supplies, a nasal cannula, and a spare catheter.

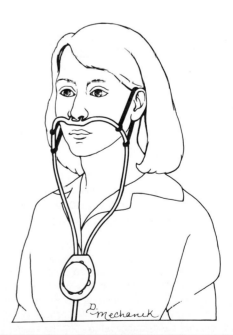

Fig. 38-8   Pendant reservoir oxygen-delivery system.

where it can easily be hidden from view. Performance characteristics of the pendant reservoir system are comparable to those of the reservoir cannula, both at rest and during exercise.[62,63]

For oxygen conserving devices using an external reservoir, the F_{IO_2} varies with the reservoir volume, oxygen input flow and ventilatory pattern. Figure 38-9 shows the relationship among these factors under steady state conditions.[48] As can be seen, for an equivalent input flow, an oxygen reservoir cannula can provide as much as 3% to 7% more O_2 per breath than a simple cannula. Obviously, any change in breathing pattern would change the F_{IO_2} delivered by both types of device. In addition, the amount of oxygen savings varies greatly among individual patients.[64]

Demand flow oxygen delivery systems. Rather than using a reservoir to conserve oxygen during expiration, a demand flow or pulsed oxygen delivery device uses a sensor and valve system to eliminate expiratory oxygen flow altogether.[65-67]

As indicated in Figure 38-10, *A,* with continuous oxygen flow, most of the effective O_2 delivery occurs during the first half of inspiration, with a significant 'precharging' of the anatomic reservoir occurring at the end of each exhalation.[18] All the oxygen delivered during the latter half of inspiration and throughout most of expiration is wasted.

Figure 38-10, *B* shows the effect of a coordinated pulse of oxygen given at the beginning of inspiration. Ideally, this O_2 pulse should occur during the first 25%

of inspiration. Under these conditions, a pulsed oxygen system can produce SaO_2s equal to those seen with continuous flow, while using 60% less oxygen.[18]

Demand flow sensors determine when inspiration begins by either temperature or pressure changes. A thermistor is used to sense temperature changes as inspiratory flow starts, while a fluidic or electromechanical valve senses pressure changes. Immediately after sensing inspiration, the system opens a valve and delivers a quick pulse of oxygen. Closure of the valve prevents oxygen delivery during exhalation.

The amount of oxygen delivered is altered in two different ways. Either the volume of the oxygen pulse is varied, or the O_2 is delivered on a variable breath schedule, such as every 2nd or 3rd inhalation.[50]

In concept, the demand flow delivery system provides the greatest savings in oxygen usage for a given level of arterial saturation. In addition, there is no need for humidification since O_2 is only delivered during inspiration. The drying effects of oxygen on the nasal mucosa during the expiratory phase are eliminated. Demand flow systems also have been successfully adapted for use with transtracheal catheters, resulting in even more efficient oxygen delivery.[68]

Table 38-3 compares and contrasts these oxygen conserving devices according to their principles of operation, performance characteristics, and advantages and disadvantages.[48]

A **CONTINOUS FLOW OXYGEN**

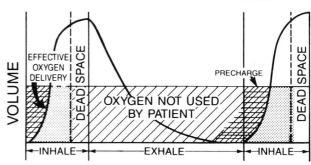

B **PULSE OXYGEN**

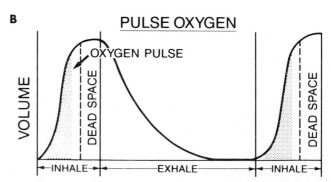

Fig. 38-10 Demand flow oxygen delivery. With continuous flow **(A)** most O_2 is delivered during first half of inhalation, with remainder wasted. With a coordinated pulse during the first 25% of inspiration, no waste occurs. (From O'Donohue WJ: The future of home oxygen therapy, *Respir Care* 33(12): 1125-1130, 1988.)

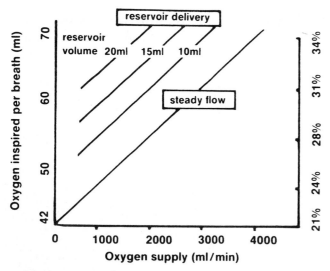

Fig. 38-9 Oxygen-delivery model for reservoir-storage cannulas as compared with steady-flow cannulas. The model is based on the assumptions that the patient is breathing 20 breaths per minute, I:E is 1:2, critical delivery volume is the first 200 mL of inhalation, and the time required to deliver that volume is 0.5 second. The effective inspired oxygen volumes received by the patient are shown for steady-flow conditions and storage reflux conditions using 10, 15, and 20 mL oxygen boluses. (From Tiep BL: *Respir Care* 32(2):109, 1987.)

Table 38-3   Comparison of oxygen-conserving methods

Characteristic	Method		
	Transtracheal catheter	Reservoir cannula	Demand delivery
Conservation mechanism	Reduction of dead space	Storage of oxygen during exhalation	Delivery only during early inhalation
Unique advantages	Unobtrusive; possible improved patient compliance	Disposable. Probably least subject to mechanical failure	Maintains O_2 savings over usual delivery ranges
Oxygen required (expressed as a fraction of continuous-flow requirement)	1/3 to 1/2	1/4 to 1/2	1/2 to 1/3
Need for humidification*	None	None	None
Obtrusiveness	Least obtrusive	Most obtrusive	Comparable to steady flow
Unique disadvantages	Catheter clogging, surgical complications (e.g., infection, subcutaneous emphysema)	Most obtrusive	Theoretically most vulnerable to mechanical failure*

*No incidents reported.

Selecting a home delivery system. As when selecting hospital-based oxygen therapy systems (Chapter 26), the RCP should always remember the 'three Ps:' *Purpose, Patient,* and *Performance.* The goal is always to match the performance of the equipment to both the objectives of therapy (purpose) *and* the patient's special needs.

Because the majority of home care patients who need oxygen are relatively stable, and because their FIO_2 needs are minimal, traditional low-flow therapy via nasal cannula (using either a concentrator or liquid reservoir) is the most common and accepted approach. When combined with a portable gas cylin-der (for backup and limited walking), this combination is ideal for patients with restricted activity.[69]

While conserving devices may lower cost, their primary patient benefit is to extend the usable time of portable O_2 systems. For example, while a portable liquid O_2 unit can provide 5 to 8 hours of O_2 at 2 L/min via standard nasal cannula, use of a conserving device can double or even triple this time frame.

Of course, this benefit is meaningful only to active patients who need or desire increased mobility in, around, and outside the home. For these patients, a conserving device used in conjunction with a portable

---

■ MINI CLINI ■

38-1

Failure to Use Home Portable Oxygen

Problem: An elderly female patient with COPD and rheumatoid arthritis in both hands living alone is being discharged from the hospital with an order that supplemental low-flow oxygen be set up in the home for continuous use at 4 liters per minute. A liquid oxygen system was selected. The week following home discharge, the patient, who had previously been known to regularly take early morning walks and is currently well enough to continue this activity, is no longer doing so according to neighbors close to her. In fact, no one recalls seeing her outside her home since leaving the hospital. This behavior continues despite the fact that she answers the telephone at home and denies there are any problems. In light of these observations, what action(s) might the home care RCP take to further investigate the situation?

Discussion:
There are a number of possible reasons why this individual may have chosen not to leave her home in spite of the fact that she is physically capable. One possible explanation may be related to the psychologic adjustment of having to wear oxygen and feeling self-conscious in public. The RCP can assist the patient by providing reassurance and emotional support. Perhaps the RCP could speak to a close relative or friend about the oxygen system so that they would better understand the types of feelings she might be going through. Another explanation for the patient not leaving her house might be related to an inability to fill her portable liquid system from the reservoir unit. Since the patient is known to have rheumatoid arthritis in both hands, she may be physically unable to perform the filling procedure. Due to the extremely low temperature of liquid oxygen, patients and other caregivers must be extremely careful when refilling these portable systems. If the RCP determines that physical dexterity of her hands limits her from properly and safely operating this type of home oxygen supply system, then another alternative delivery system should be explored.

liquid O_2 system (with the large reservoir used inside the home) is the ideal choice.[69,70]

Which specific conserving device should be used depends on the patient's needs and preferences. Given that reservoir or 'mustache' cannulas are poorly accepted by most patients, and that current demand flow systems are somewhat bulky and unreliable, the choice usually narrows to a transtracheal catheter or pendant reservoir cannula. Patients who meet the criteria for TTOT (see above) *and* can provide meticulous self-care should receive TTOT. Even with good planning, complications or poor acceptance of TTOT are possible and may require catheter removal.[71] When TTOT is not indicated or fails, the pendant reservoir cannula is an acceptable alternative.

An additional consideration in selecting a home O_2 system is whether oxygen desaturation occurs when the active patient exercises while receiving oxygen therapy. If this is the case, either a transtracheal catheter or pendant reservoir cannula should be recommended.[72]

Home care patients with artificial airways who need oxygen present a special problem. Due to both high O_2 usage and infection concerns, an oxygen-powered air entrainment nebulizer is not satisfactory. Instead, a compressor-driven humidifier with supplemental O_2 bled in at low flows from a concentrator should be used.[12] In this case, the RCP must compute the proper flows for air and oxygen (Chapter 26) and confirm the FdO_2 by calibrated analyzer.

Problem-solving and troubleshooting. The most common problems with home oxygen delivery systems are nontechnical in nature. As previously described under supply systems, patients and caregivers often fail to follow instructions or comply with the prescribed therapeutic regimen.[12] As a general rule, caregivers should be allowed to operate and maintain oxygen delivery devices only after they have been instructed by credentialed RCPs and have demonstrated the appropriate level of skill.[12] In no case should the patient or caregiver be allowed or instructed to alter flow settings for a given device. Instead, when in doubt, they should be taught to switch to the backup supply at the same liter flow.

Technical problems are most common with TTOT and demand flow systems. Most problems with TTOT are related to initial catheter insertion or ongoing maintenance. Most problems with demand flow systems are based on the current limits of this technology.

The most common complications of TTOT are listed in the accompanying box.[46,54] Although the incidence of these problems is very low, the RCP responsible for overseeing TTOT must be on constant guard for their occurrence. In particular, any evidence of tract tenderness, fever, excessive cough, increased dyspnea, or subcutaneous emphysema should immediately be reported to the patient's physician.

Complication of transtracheal oxygen therapy[46,54]
Bleeding*
Pneumothorax*
Bronchospasm*
Subcutaneous emphysema
Catheter dislodgement/lost tract
Increased sputum production
Blockage by **inspissated mucous**
Infection/abscess
Cephalad position
Tract tenderness

* complications associated mainly with insertion

To help avoid complications or product failure, catheters and their tubing should be replaced every 3 months, at which time a check-up by the physician is also recommended. Routine cleaning of the catheter should be performed daily by the patient or caregiver, as per the self-care guidelines previously listed. Patients should always be instructed to put on a nasal cannula and call their doctor if any major problem occurs.

Since transtracheal catheters are normally used with humidifiers, the RCP also must be prepared to troubleshoot this equipment. Guidelines for dealing with leaks and obstructions in O_2 delivery systems using humidifiers are provided in Chapter 26. Given the small bore of transtracheal catheters, one should generally use a humidifier with a high pressure (2 psi) relief valve, otherwise, the pop-off will constantly sound. As previously discussed, distilled water is satisfactory for airway humidification in the home. Because nondisposable humidifiers are often used in this setting, patients and caregivers must be taught proper techniques for cleaning and disinfecting this equipment.

Common problems with demand flow oxygen delivery systems are listed in the box on page 1115.[50]

Ventilatory support in the home

For both humane and financial reasons, home ventilatory support is now a recognized and viable form of respiratory care.

Successful home ventilatory support depends on proper patient selection and good discharge planning.[73-76] Key factors include a coordinated team approach, effective family and caregiver education, thorough preparation of the home environment, and careful selection of needed equipment and supplies. Properly planned and carried out, home ventilatory support can provide major benefits for both patient and family, with substantial savings in health care costs.[77-79]

Chronically ill patients have a more positive psychological outlook when they are at home, even while receiving ventilatory support. In addition, there appears to be greater freedom and more motivation to live, including a desire to become involved in productive activities.

Cost savings accrue in two ways. First, on a daily basis, home care is significantly cheaper than hospital care, especially intensive care. Second, when properly planned and implemented, home ventilatory support decreases hospital readmission rates. In fact, home ventilatory support can continue for years without the need for hospitalization.[80-82]

In 1986, over 3,000 ventilator-dependent patients were being successfully cared for at home.[76] Based on current estimates, this number continues to grow. In order to help identify the number and specific needs of this important group, the AARC recently created a national registry for ventilator-dependent patients.

Patient groups

Most patients needing home ventilatory support fall into one of three broad categories:[73]

1. Patients unable to maintain adequate ventilation over prolonged periods of time (nocturnal use in particular);
2. Patients requiring continuous mechanical ventilation for long-term survival;
3. Patients who are terminally ill with short life expectancies.

The accompanying box provides more detailed profiles of these patient groups.[73,76] As can be seen, the primary patient groups best served by home ventilatory support are those with neuromuscular diseases or injuries, chest wall deformities, severe COPD, and malignancies of the lung.

In addition to adults, a growing number of ventilator-assisted children are being managed in the home. The same basic principles of discharge planning and patient care for adult patients should be followed for ventilator-assisted children.[83-90]

Prerequisites

For home ventilatory support to be successful, several prerequisites must be met.[91,92] These include:

- Willingness of family to accept responsibility
- Adequacy of family and professional support
- Overall viability of the home care plan
- Stability of patient
- Adequacy of home setting

Profiles of patient groups requiring mechanical ventilation within the home environment

	Group Description	Diseases Involved
Profile 1	Mainly composed of neuromuscular and thoracic wall disorder; particular stage of disease process allows patient certain periods of spontaneous breathing time during day; generally requires only nocturnal mechanical support	Amyotrophic lateral sclerosis Multiple sclerosis Kyphoscoliosis and related chest wall deformities Diaphragmatic paralysis Myasthenia gravis
Profile 2	Requires continuous mechanical ventilatory support associated with long-term survival rates	High spinal cord injuries Apneic encephalopathies Severe chronic obstructive lung disease Late-stage muscular dystrophy
Profile 3	Usually returns home at request of patient and family; patient's condition is terminal, life expectancy is short, and patient and family wish to spend remaining time at home; patients usually pose management problems in the home because of their rapidly deteriorating conditions	Lung cancer End-stage chronic obstructive pulmonary disease

■ MINI **C**LINI ■

38-2

Considerations in Selecting a Ventilator For Use in the Home

Problem: A ventilator dependent patient who has recently been diagnosed with a neuromuscular disease is to be discharged from the hospital and will require mechanical ventilatory support in the home. What areas of consideration must the RCP take into account when contemplating which type of ventilator will be most appropriate for this setting?

Discussion:
The type of ventilator selected for home mechanical ventilation depends on several factors in this case. The most important issue centers around the severity of the underlying illness which created the need for artificial ventilatory support in the first place. First, the ventilator itself must be able to provide an adequate level of ventilatory support based on the patient's condition. Secondly, the RCP working for the home care provider must perform an assessment of the home environment to determine the amount of available space for the ventilator and supporting equipment, electrical power supply (amperage and grounded outlets), and the presence of hazardous appliances which might be in operation nearby. Much time will be spent by the hospital and home care provider in assessing the ability of the patient and/or caregiver to understand both equipment operation and maintenance. Ideally, the ventilator selected should be placed on the patient while still in the hospital. Of critical importance is that adequate time be scheduled for proper instruction, demonstration, and the opportunity for caregivers to practice newly learned patient care skills prior to home discharge. The RCP plays a key role in evaluating patient tolerance to the home ventilator equipment and caregiver knowledge of procedures, particularly emergency situations such as ventilator or power failure, ventilator circuit problems, airway emergencies, and cardiac arrest.

In regard to the home setting, the same factors listed previously in the box on page 1103, (Assessing the Home Environment) should be evaluated for patients being considered for home ventilatory support.[74]

Planning

Successful home ventilatory support requires extensive planning, education, and followup by all members of the home care team. Basic steps in the discharge process for a ventilator-dependent patient include the following:

1. Family is consulted regarding feasibility;
2. Physician writes appropriate orders;
3. Discharge planner coordinates efforts of team members and discharge plan is formulated;
4. Physician and other team members discuss plan with family and/or care-givers;
5. Education and training are initiated and completed;
6. Patient and family are prepared for discharge;
7. Home layout is assessed with necessary changes made;
8. Equipment and supplies are readied;
9. Discharge planner meets with team and makes final preparations;
10. Patient is discharged (with trial period, if necessary);
11. Local power company is notified regarding the presence of life support equipment. Appropriate back-up power (battery or compressed gas source) is made available;

12. On-going and follow-up care provided by visiting nurse, RCP, and other health care professionals (as necessary).

To properly prepare patients, family, and other caregivers for home discharge, a comprehensive educational program must be undertaken and completed. Essential skills that must be taught include:[74]

■ Simple patient assessment;
■ Airway management, including tracheostomy and stoma care, cuff care, suctioning, changing tubes/ties;
■ Chest physical therapy techniques, including percussion, vibration, coughing;
■ Medication administration, including oral and aerosol;
■ Patient movement and ambulation;
■ Equipment operation and maintenance;
■ Equipment troubleshooting;
■ Cleaning and disinfection;
■ Emergency procedures.

Emergency situations that caregivers must be trained to recognize and properly deal with include ventilator or power failure, ventilator circuit problems, airway emergencies (see Chapter 22), and cardiac arrest.

All caregivers should successfully complete this educational process. This may require 1 to 2 weeks of instruction, demonstration, caregiver practice, and evaluation. Ideally, the patient should be placed on the actual ventilator that will be used in the home setting before discharge. In the early stages after discharge, patient followup by a RCP may need to occur every day. As patient and family become more familiar with the equipment and procedures, follow-up visitations can decrease to weekly or biweekly, as needed.[93,94]

Goals and standards of care

To help assure quality care for ventilator-dependent patients in the home setting, several standards and guidelines have been developed. Both the American College of Chest Physicians (**ACCP**) and AARC have developed and adopted such guidelines.[95-97] The ACCP guidelines specify five major goals for home ventilatory support:[95]
- To extend life
- To enhance the quality of life
- To reduce morbidity
- To improve physical, physiological, social and **psychosocial** function
- To provide cost benefits

These guidelines also indicate that the best candidates for home ventilation are those with neuromuscular or skeletal disorders, such as muscular dystrophy or kyphoscoliosis. Patients with restrictive lung diseases involving the pulmonary parenchyma are poor candidates for home ventilatory support. Most of these patients are acutely ill and unstable. In regard to assessing patient stability, the accompanying box outlines the ACCP criteria.

The standards of care approved by the American Association for Respiratory Care (AARC) for ventilator-assisted individuals in an alternative site are as follows:[97]

Standard I— The provision of care to a ventilator assisted patient located in an alternative site* shall be defined and guided

---

*Alternative site may be defined as any identifiable location outside the acute care hospital setting, such as the home, convalescent center, nursing facility or retirement center where ventilator-assisted patients receive care.

Physiologic stability for home ventilatory support[95]

- Absence of severe dyspnea while on a ventilator
- Acceptable arterial blood gas results
- Inspired oxygen concentrations that are relatively low
- Psychological stability
- Evidence of developmental progress (for pediatric/adolescent candidates)
- Absence of life-limiting cardiac dysfunction and arrhythmias
- If possible, no positive end expiratory pressure (PEEP) or if needed, PEEP should not exceed +10 cm H_2O
- Ability to clear airway secretions—either by cough or suction
- A tracheostomy tube as opposed to an endotracheal tube
- No readmissions expected for more than one month

by established written policies and procedures accepted by both the discharging institution and the alternative care site.

Standard II— The services provided to ventilator-assisted patients shall be dispensed in accordance with a prescription written by the physician responsible for the care of that particular patient.

Standard III—Participants shall be prepared for their responsibilities in the provision of services through appropriate training and education.

Standard IV—The ventilator-assisted patient shall be provided with safe and effective equipment appropriate for that patient's physiologic needs.

Standard V— There shall be established recording and reporting mechanisms for the program.

Standard VI—The quality and appropriateness of care provided under the auspices of the program must be monitored and evaluated by the program's Medical Director and identified problems must be resolved.

Equipment considerations

Essential equipment and supplies needed for ventilator-dependent patients at home include the following:[73,74]

Equipment:
- Ventilator
- Ventilator humidifier/HME with back-up
- Monitoring/alarm devices (e.g., pulse oximeter)
- Stethoscope/sphygmomanometer
- Suction machine with back-up (manual or battery)
- Manual resuscitator (bag-valve-mask unit)
- Compressor/nebulizer (as needed)
- Hospital bed with table
- Patient lift
- Bedside commode, urinal, or bedpan
- Wheelchair

Supplies:
- Oxygen
- Disposable supplies (circuits, catheters, pads)
- Tracheostomy tubes/care kits
- Needed solutions

In addition, a back-up ventilator, battery, battery charger, and cables are required for any patient who cannot maintain spontaneous ventilation for four consecutive hours and who lives in a rural area.[74]

Selecting the appropriate ventilator

In regard to the ventilator itself, both negative-pressure and positive-pressure devices are used in the home setting.[98] Which type is best for a given case depends on several factors. These factors include the patient's underlying disease process (including FIO_2 needs), the status of the patient's airway, the competence of the family and caregivers, the available space, and the need for portability.

In general, if a patient already has a tracheostomy tube in place, a positive-pressure ventilator is selected. For patients with intact upper airways, either negative or positive-pressure ventilation may be considered. Typically, if support must be continuous, a negative-pressure device is used. On the other hand, intermittent support (usually nocturnal) is best provided by noninvasive positive-pressure ventilation **(NIPPV),** usually via nasal mask.

Regardless of power application or patient interface, any ventilator used in the home should be: (1) reliable (operate trouble-free for long periods), (2) simple (have easy to understand controls/circuit), and (3) accident-proof (have stops on dials or a covered control panel to prevent unintended changes in settings).[98,99] More specific characteristics follow.

Positive-pressure ventilators. Common positive-pressure ventilators designed for home use include the Thompson Maxivent, Bear 33 (Figure 38-11), Aequitron LP-6 (Figure 38-12), and Puritan-Bennett C-2801 (Figure 38-13), Table 38-4, page 1119, compares several of the common positive-pressure ventilators designed for home care use.

Key features. A typical home positive-pressure ventilator is time or patient-triggered, flow or pressure-limited and volume-cycled. As shown in Figure 38-14, most home positive-pressure ventilators are electrically powered, and use a rotary-drive piston to generate a sine-wave flow pattern. Depending on the model, available volumes range from 50 to 3000 mL, and rates can be set between 1 to 69 breaths/min (see Table 38-4).[98]

Several home positive-pressure ventilators have an internal battery which can provide up to one hour of use if the electrical power fails. Most of these devices

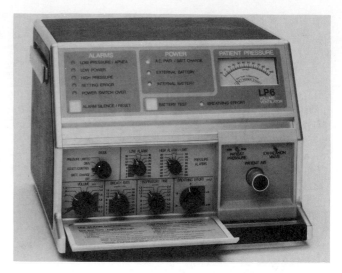

Fig. 38-12 Acquitron LP6. (Courtesy Aequitron Products, Minneapolis, Minn.)

can also be connected to an external power source, such as a marine battery.

Although IMV/SIMV is now available on most of these devices, use of this mode is not recommended for patients with limited inspiratory muscle strength. This is due to the high work of breathing these systems impose on patients in the SIMV mode.[100]

Table 38-5, page 1120, lists the essential, recommended, and optional features that should be available on home positive-pressure ventilators.[101] An *essential* feature is basic to safe and effective operation in most patient care settings. A *recommended* feature helps provide optimal patient management. An *optional* feature is possibly useful in limited situations but not necessary for a majority of patients.

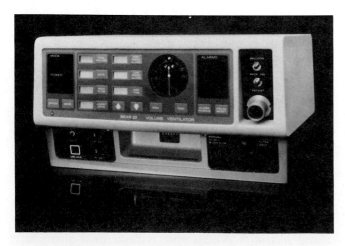

Fig. 38-11 Bear 33 ventilator. (Courtesy Bear Medical Systems, Riverside, Calif.)

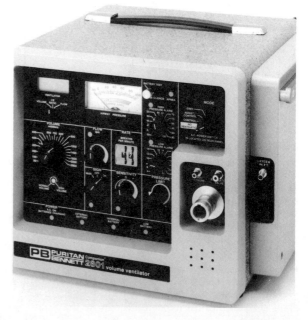

Fig. 38-13 Puritan-Bennett 2801 ventilator. (Courtesy of Bennett Group, Boulder, Colo.)

Table 38-4   Some features of positive-pressure home care ventilators

Features	Aequitron medical LP-5	LP-6	Puritan-Bennett Corp Maxi-Vent	M25B	280	Lifecare PVV	PLV-100	PLV-102	Bear Medical Bear 33
Control	C	C	C	C	C	C	C	C	C
Assist/Control	A/C	A/C	—	A/C	A/C	—	A/C	A/C	A/C
IMV, SIMV	IMV	SIMV	—	—	SIMV	—	SIMV	SIMV	SIMV
Tidal volume range (mL)	100-2,000	100-2,000	Variable	300-2,500	50-2,800	0-3,000	50-3,000	50-3,000	100-2,200
Rate range (per min)	2–28	1–38	8–24	4–23	1–69	8–30	2–40	2–40	2–40
I:E-fixed or variable	Variable	Variable	Fixed 1:1	Variable	Variable	Fixed 1:1	Variable	Variable	Variable
Approximate, maximum pressure (cm H_2O)	80	100	80 (−70 cm H_2O)	65	70	100	100	100	80
Pressure limit——ends inspiration (EI) or holds peak pressure (HPP)	EI	EI	HPP	HPP	HPP	HPP	EI	EI	EI
Typical flow pattern: sine or decelerating (decel)	sine	decel	decel (variable)	sine	sine	sine	sine	sine	sine
Low pressure	yes	yes	yes	yes	yes	yes	yes	yes	yes
High pressure with pressure limit	yes	yes (except in pressure limit mode)	no	no	no	no	yes	yes	yes
High pressure separate from press limit	no	no	no	yes (factory set)	yes	yes	no	no	no
I:E	yes	yes	no	no	yes	no	yes	yes	yes
Insp flow	yes	no	no	no	yes	no	yes	yes	yes
Apnea	yes	yes	no	no	yes	no	yes	yes	yes
Low battery or power loss	yes	yes	yes	yes	yes	yes	yes	yes	yes
Alarm silence	yes	yes	yes	no	yes	no	no	yes	yes
Can provide negative pressure?	no	no	yes	no	no	no	no	no	no
Reservoir for O_2 addition available?	yes	yes	no	yes	yes	no	no	yes	yes

(From Kacmarek RM, Spearman CB: Equipment used for ventilatory support in the home, *Respir Care* 31(4): 310-328, 1986.)

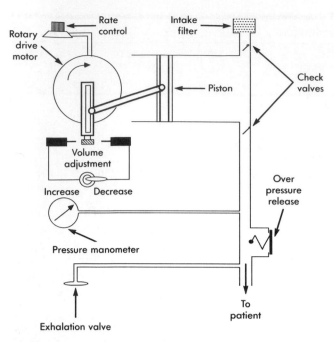

Fig. 38-14 Functional diagram of Life Products LP3. (Courtesy Aequitron Products, Minneapolis, Minn.)

Monitoring and alarms. The only machine parameter considered essential for continuous monitoring when using a home care ventilator is the peak airway pressure.[101] Of course, if the FDO_2 exceeds 0.21 or PEEP is used, these parameters must also be monitored.

On the other hand, home care ventilators should provide a set of alarm systems to warn caregivers of life-threatening events. The box, page 1120, lists the key events that home care ventilator alarms should recognize and indicate.[101] Level 1 events are considered immediately life-threatening, and require an immediate response. These alarms should be redundant and provide a loud audible and visual warning. Level 2 events are considered potentially life-threatening, and also require an immediate response. These alarms need not be redundant and should provide a soft audible and visual warning.

Patient parameters to be monitored during home positive-pressure ventilation are essentially the same as those assessed in the acute care setting, with an emphasis on simplicity.[102] For example, while the caregiver should be assessing the patient's vital signs, lung sounds, and sputum production on a daily basis, ABG analysis (by the RCP) may be conducted only monthly, or only when changes in the care plan are needed. Likewise, compliance and resistance measures will be performed only when other evidence indicates the need.

Negative-pressure ventilators. Seldom used in the acute care setting, negative-pressure ventilation is a popular means of ventilatory support in the home. This mode is most useful for patients with clear, patent airways who require periodic ventilatory support, such as those with chronic neuromuscular disorders.[103-105] Negative-pressure ventilation has also been successfully used to provide intermittent support to patients with COPD.[106]

Types of negative-pressure ventilators used in the home setting include:[107]
- Iron lung (Figure 38-15)
- Chest cuirass
- Raincoat/pneumosuit

A typical iron lung has its own electrical motor and drive system to generate negative pressure. The chest cuirass, raincoat, and pneumosuit systems are simply enclosures that allow negative pressure to be applied to the thorax. Thus, these devices must be powered by a separate negative-pressure generator. Examples of negative-pressure generators used to power a cuirass,

Table 38-5   Essential, recommended, and optional features of a positive pressure ventilator for home care use

Feature	Necessity
Positive pressure tidal breaths	Essential
Mandatory rate	Essential
Flow or 1:E or inspiratory time	Recommended+
Expiratory pressure (PEEP)	Optional
FDO_2 to 1.0	Optional
Patient spontaneous breath (eg, CPAP, IMV)	Optional
Breath-triggering mechanism (flow or pressure sensors to initiate a ventilator breath)	Recommended+
Flow-timing interaction (eg, pressure support)	Optional
Feedback control (eg, mandatory minute ventilation)	Optional

+Essential if patient has intact ventilatory drive and respiratory muscles or possibility of partial or complete ventilator independence is anticipated.

Events for home care ventilator alarms[101]

Level 1 (Essential)
  Power failure (including when battery in use)
  Absence of gas delivery (apnea)
  Loss of gas source
  Excessive gas delivery
  Exhalation valve failure
  Timing failure
Level 2 (Recommended)
  Battery power loss (not in use)
  Circuit leak
  Blender failure
  Circuit partially occluded
  Heater/humidifier failure
  Loss of/or excessive PEEP
  Autocycling

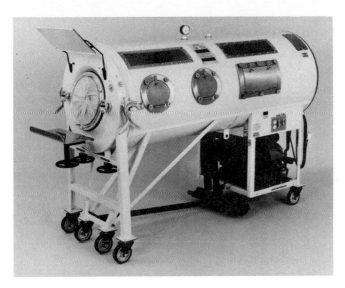

Fig. 38-15 Emerson iron lung negative pressure ventilator (Courtesy J.H. Emerson Co., Cambridge, Mass.)

> ### Problems with home negative-pressure ventilation[108-111]
>
> - Hard to apply
> - Cumbersome
> - Poorly tolerated
> - Limited mobility
> - Poor synchronization
> - Upper airway obstruction and sequelae: Hypoventilation/hypercapnia Hypoxemia/desaturation

Beneficial effects of NIPPV. Although it is simply too soon to draw firm conclusions, both case reports and limited clinical trials are revealing that home NIPPV can provide a number of significant benefits (see the box on page 1122).

raincoat, or pneumosuit include the Emerson 33-CRE, CRX, CRA, the Thompson Maxivent (Puritan-Bennett), and the Lifecare 170C.

In the past, the primary advantage cited for negative-pressure ventilation was its ability to provide support without an artificial airway. While more an indication than an advantage, this distinction no longer pertains. Over a decade' experience with non-invasive positive-pressure ventilation (NIPPV) proves that this alternative approach is safe and feasible. Moreover, comparative experience with NIPPV has clarified many of the problems with home negative-pressure ventilation (see accompanying box).[108-111]

Noninvasive positive-pressure ventilation (NIPPV). NIPPV is not a separate mode of ventilation. It is simply an alternative means for connecting the patient to the ventilator. Specifically, NIPPV is the application of positive pressure to the intact airway via a mouthpiece[112] or mask.[113] Although oro-nasal masks are used,[114] the form-fitting nasal mask is most popular.

Any existing positive-pressure ventilator can be used to provide NIPPV. The current trend, however, is toward use of time or patient-triggered, pressure-limited, flow-cycled devices (pressure support with timed backup).[115,116] Units such as the Respironics BiPAP® S/T-D (Figure 38-16) are specifically designed to provide this type of support.

Indications for NIPPV. Home NIPPV is indicated mainly for intermittent use by patients who cannot maintain adequate ventilation over long periods of time. Most commonly, nocturnal ventilation is provided, although intermittent day use has also been employed. The box on page 1122 summarizes specific patient groups that have been successfully supported in the home with NIPPV.

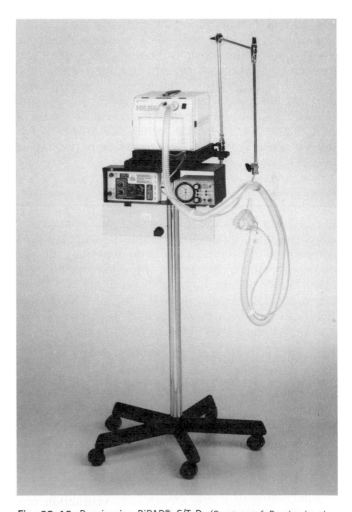

Fig. 38-16 Respironics BiPAP® S/T-D. (Courtesy of Respironics, Inc, Murrysville, PA.)

Indications for non-invasive positive-pressure ventilation

Neuromuscular disorders[110,117-119]

Muscular dystrophy[120,121]
Spinal cord injury/quadraplegia[122,123]
Idiopathic hypoventilation syndrome[124]
Post-polio respiratory insufficiency[125]

Restrictive disorders[117,126]

Chest wall restriction/kyphoscoliosis[115,127]
Severe obesity[116,128]

Obstructive disorders:

Chronic obstructive pulmonary disease[118,126,129,130]
End-stage cystic fibrosis[131,132]

Beneficial effects of noninvasive positive-pressure ventilation (NIPPV)

1. Avoid need for/eliminate use of tracheostomy[112]
2. Decreased inspiratory muscle energy expenditure[126]
3. Decreased incidence of nocturnal desaturation[133]
4. Improved daytime blood gases[108,110,119,133,134]
5. Increased daytime lung volumes[110]
6. Increased respiratory muscle strength/endurance[110,134]
7. Improved nocturnal gas exchange[134]
8. Improved daytime functioning/activity level[119,134]
9. Decreased incidence of daytime headache[108]
10. Decreased daytime insomnia/somnolence[108,116]
11. Improved intellectual capacity[108]

Evaluation and follow-up

Routine follow-up visits by an RCP help ensure the success of patient management within the home. Equipment must be checked and cleaned as necessary. The patient's status should be carefully assessed and appropriate recommendations for change should be made to the primary or prescribing physician. Any prescribed respiratory therapy should be administered during the visit and all necessary supply items left with the patient's caregivers. After each visit, a report form must be completed and kept on record as part of the documentation process. Subsequent follow-up visits should take place regularly (weekly or biweekly), and whenever needed.

Other modes of respiratory home care

In addition to home O_2 therapy and ventilatory support, other modes of respiratory care are now common in the home. These may represent the primary in-home therapy, or may be used to supplement other modes of care. Included for discussion here are bland aerosol therapy, aerosol drug administration, IPPB, chest physical therapy, airway care, nasal CPAP and **BiPAP,** and apnea monitoring.[135-137]

Bland aerosol therapy

Bland (water or saline) aerosol therapy has been a common home care practice for many years. Depending upon patient condition and therapeutic objectives, this therapy may be either continuous or intermittent.

Continuous bland aerosol therapy is indicated for patients with tracheostomies, or children using mist tents for treatment of croup or cystic fibrosis. Either normal saline or sterile distilled water is used. The aerosol is usually produced by jet nebulizers driven by 50 psi air compressors. The major problem is infec-

tion from contaminated equipment.[138] To reduce the incidence of infection, equipment and patient delivery systems must be cleaned and changed every 24 hours. Disinfection procedures are discussed later in this chapter.

Cool or heated bland aerosols also can be given on an intermittent, or treatment basis. Historically, this approach has been used for patients who have difficulty clearing thick secretions. Current knowledge, however, suggests that bland aerosol therapy alone has little effect on the properties of mucous or its clearance.[138] It may, however, be useful as an adjunct to bronchial drainage procedures in patients who regularly produce large amounts of sputum.[139]

Aerosol drug administration

The aerosol route also can be used for self-administration of drugs in the home. Drugs frequently administered via the aerosol route include isoetharine (Bronkosol), metaproterenol (Alupent), albuterol (Proventil or Ventolin), N-acetylcysteine (Mucomyst), and pentamidine (for AIDS patients).

Special precautions must be followed when giving aerosolized pentamidine.[140,141] The delivery system must include one-way valves and a HEPA filter on the expiratory port of the nebulizer. Generally, this nebulizer design requires a 50 psig gas source. All CDC universal precautions should be followed, with proper disposal of contaminated equipment and supplies.[142]

Most other drugs can be given via MDI. Alternatively, a standard small volume nebulizer powered by a low-output diaphragm compressor can be used. As of 1993, Medicare is considering limiting reimbursement for home compressor/nebulizer rentals. These systems will probably require a certificate of medical necessity **(CMN)** completed by the ordering physician. Coverage will depend on: (1) the patient first

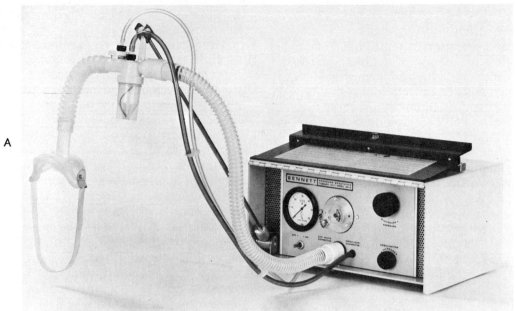

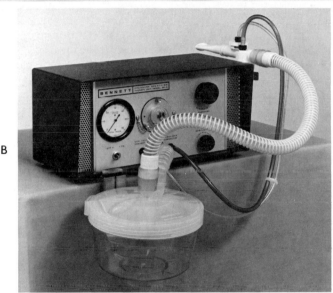

Fig. 38-17 A, Bennett AP-4 **B,** Bennett AP-5 Both units are air compressor-driven ventilators. (Courtesy Puritan-Bennett Corp., Los Angeles, Calif.)

having tried an MDI with a spacer, (2) spirometry showing at least a 12% improvement in either FEV_1 or **peak expiratory flow,** and (3) evidence that nebulizer use can help prevent hospitalization. This medical need would have to be reviewed and recertified after two months.[143]

Intermittent positive pressure breathing (IPPB)

This therapy, although not as widely used as in the past, still has viable home care applications. In the home care setting, IPPB can be used to deliver aerosol drugs to patients with ventilatory muscle weakness (e.g., neuromuscular disease, kyphoscoliosis) or chronic conditions in which intermittent ventilatory support is indicated.[144]

Small electrically-powered units, like the Bennett AP-5, are the most common type of equipment used to deliver home IPPB therapy (Figure 38-17). Older pneumatic devices, such as the Bennett TV-2P, Bennett PR-1 and PR-2, and Bird Mark 7 and 8 are also in use. As with aerosol therapy, the major concerns in providing home IPPB are patient education, ensuring compliance with the prescribed therapy, and equipment disinfection.

Chest physical therapy (postural drainage, percussion and vibration)

Percussion and vibration can be applied manually or mechanically with the aid of a simple percussor/vibrator. Alternatively, a high-frequency chest compression vest can be used for self-administration (see Chapter 28). Medicare reimburses for these items if no one is available or able to provide manual percussion and vibration at home.

Postural drainage, percussion, and vibration should be administered as directed by the physician's prescription, and are best applied *after* any aerosol or IPPB therapy. Patients with cystic fibrosis, bronchiectasis, chronic bronchitis, and any condition resulting in significant sputum production can benefit from this form of therapy. Family members can usually be taught the proper techniques. The presence of any mechanical device will make the therapy session easier for the family member.

Recently, positive airway pressure adjuncts have proven useful as aids in mobilizing secretions in selected patient groups.[145] These methods include positive expiratory pressure (PEP), and expiratory positive airway pressure (EPAP). Since neither technique require a pressurized external gas source, they can easily be used at home. Of course, coughing or other airway clearance techniques (including suctioning) must be used in conjunction with these methods.

Airway care

Small portable suction units have been available for home use since the 1960's. The equipment consists of a suction pump, collection bottle, and suction tubing with catheter.

Patient and family instruction are usually done in the hospital before patient discharge. Home reinforcement and follow-up are also needed. Since pressure is usually measured in inches of mercury (in Hg), care must be taken to properly adjust this suction pressure for each patient. For infants, 5 to 7 in Hg are recommended; for children, 7 to 12 in Hg, and for adults, 12 to 15 in Hg.

Maintenance and cleaning need to be performed on a daily basis. In many cases, suction catheters are used for a day and then discarded. This measure is followed in an effort to control supply costs. Catheters are placed in a disinfecting solution such as hydrogen peroxide or 2.5% acetic acid between suctioning attempts. Tracheostomized patients receive trach care from a trained family member, visiting nurse, or assigned RCP. Trach tube changes are usually performed by the physician, RCP, or home health care nurse.

Nasal CPAP (continuous positive airway pressure)

Nasal CPAP is a relatively new form of home care used to treat **obstructive sleep apnea** (refer to Chapter 20).[146-148] In 1987, Medicare began reimbursing for nasal CPAP equipment for home care patients with a confirmed diagnosis of sleep apnea syndrome. Documentation of this diagnosis must be provided via a sleep study **(polysomnography).**

Equipment. A typical home nasal CPAP apparatus consists of a flow-generator (blower), one-way valve or reservoir bag, nasal mask, and PEEP/CPAP valve (threshold resistor) (Figure 38-18).[149] The pressure

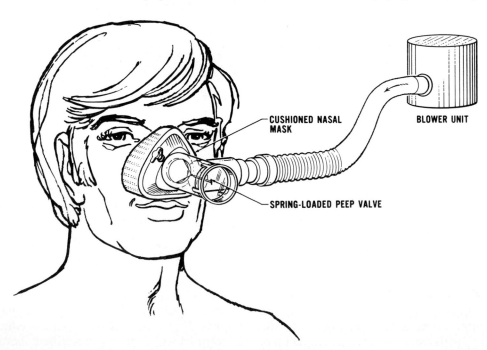

CUSHIONED NASAL MASK

BLOWER UNIT

SPRING-LOADED PEEP VALVE

Fig. 38-18 Home nasal CPAP apparatus.

level can be adjusted, usually between 2.5 to 20 cm H_2O. Newer units have a ramp feature that gradually raises the pressure to the prescribed level over a period of time. This allows the patient to fall asleep and more readily adapt to the therapy.

Determining the proper CPAP level. The proper CPAP level for a given patient is determined by one of several methods. The best method is to repeat the sleep study, using different levels of CPAP. Observed changes in the apnea-hypopnea index **(AHI)** are then correlated with the various CPAP pressures. The prescribed level of CPAP should be the *lowest* pressure at which apneic episodes essentially cease.

Alternatively, CPAP may be titrated against **pulse oximetry** data (Figure 38-19). In this case, the goal is to use the lowest CPAP pressure which prevents episodes of arterial desaturation ($SpO_2 \geq 90\%$).

The last and least objective means for setting the proper CPAP pressure is to have patients assess their response to the therapy. Over a period of several nights, the patient would be instructed to set different levels of pressure (e.g., 4-6-8-10 cm H_2O). Each following morning, the patient would log the severity of key symptoms, such as headache and **hypersomnolence.** Based on a review of this log, the physician would prescribe the lowest CPAP pressure at which these key symptoms resolved.

Use and maintenance. Once the proper CPAP pressure is determined, the patient is fitted for a mask and trained in the proper use, cleaning, and maintenance of the equipment. Typical patient instructions for home nasal CPAP therapy are provided in the accompanying box.

Problem-solving and troubleshooting. Patient problems associated with nasal CPAP include reversible upper airway obstruction,[150] skin irritation,[149] **conjunctivitis,**[151] epistaxis,[152] and nasal discomfort (dryness, burning and congestion).[153] Reversible upper airway obstruction (usually due to a flaccid epiglottis) is a rare problem that contraindicates nasal CPAP. Skin irritation is usually due to tight mask straps or a dirty mask. Persistent redness on the face or about the nose is the primary sign. Adjusting the straps (while maintaining a good mask seal) can help prevent irritation. In addition, the mask should be cleaned daily to remove dirt and facial oils. Even with proper care, most masks hardens over time, causing prob-

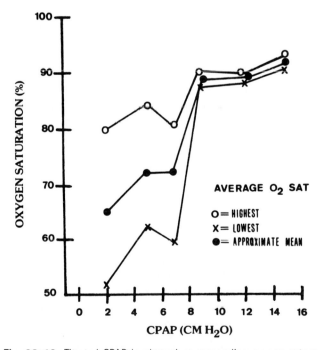

Fig. 38-19 Titrated CPAP levels and corresponding oxygen saturations while patient was asleep and using nasal CPAP. (From Sleeper GP, Strohl KP, Armeni MA: Nasal CPAP for at-home treatment of obstructive sleep apnea: a case report, *Respir Care* 30(2) 90-94,1985.)

Typical patient instructions for home nasal CPAP therapy

Equipment preparation

1. Place blower unit on a level surface (table or nightstand) close to where you sleep.
2. Make sure that the air exhaust and inlet vents are not obstructed.
3. Plug machine into a standard grounded (3 prong) electrical outlet.
4. Check air inlet filter to be sure it is in place and free of dust.
5. Connect one end of the tubing to the airflow outlet on the blower.
6. Connect the other end of the tubing to the mask. Then place the mask over the nose.
7. Adjust strap tightness to seat mask firmly over nose.
8. Turn on the blower and verify a flow of air.
9. Assure proper fit and adjustment of mask and headgear. Air should not be leaking out around the bridge of the nose into the eyes.
10. You are now ready to sleep with mask on.

In the morning

1. Remove mask by slipping strap off of back of head. (You may leave the headstrap connected between cleaning).
2. Turn off blower.
3. Wash the mask every morning with a mild detergent, then rinse with water. This keeps the mask soft and airtight.
4. Store the mask in plastic bag to keep free of dust and dirt.

Weekly

1. Wipe off the blower unit with a clean, damp cloth.
2. Wash the headstrap.
3. Service the filters according to the instructions in your patient manual.

■ MINI **C**LINI ■

38-3

Troubleshooting Home Nasal CPAP

Problem: A 43-year-old obese male with documented obstructive sleep apnea has been advised by his attending physician that home nasal continuous positive airway pressure (CPAP) therapy at night will be necessary. The home care RCP makes an appointment with the patient to assess his tolerance to the CPAP unit. During the visit, the patient notes that he has been experiencing nasal discomfort. How can the RCP assist in problem-solving with this specific complaint and what are some of the other potential patient problems associated with CPAP therapy that the clinician should be alerted to?

Discussion:
Home CPAP devices typically employ some type of nasal mask with supporting headgear. Complaints of nasal discomfort are not uncommon and are most likely due to the effects of dry air generated under continuous positive pressure by the CPAP unit blower. However, there are other contributing factors which may aggravate the sensation of nasal irritation. Nasal mucosa may be prone to dryness depending on the patient's overall hydration status. That is, systemic dehydration in a patient may only worsen a patient's subjective complaints of nasal dryness. In addition, living and breathing in a cold, dry winter climate could potentially aggravate symptoms as well as breathing indoors with a dry forced air heating system. The RCP might suggest the use of saline nasal spray as needed and increasing oral intake of fluids (if no restrictions on fluid intake), an in-line bubble humidifier or heat and moisture exchange unit (HME), and possibly the use of a chin strap to decrease the loss of upper airway moisture. Other patient problems associated with the use of CPAP therapy include conjunctivitis, epistaxis, and skin irritation due to tight mask straps or a dirty mask. The later may be detected by the presence of redness on the face or about the nose. It is important to recognize that skin breakdown on the face and nose can occur from excessive mask pressure, particularly in patients with poor skin turgor. Routine patient assessment should also include checking for a proper fitting mask so that excessive airleak is avoided.

---

lems with irritation and leaks. For this reason, nasal masks should be replaced at least every 3 months, or sooner if leakage or discomfort occur.

Conjunctivitis is probably due to mask leakage around the bridge of the nose, which is easily correct-

Patient instructions for troubleshooting CPAP equipment

Inadequate flow
1. Check to make sure that the unit is plugged into a working electrical outlet.
2. Check and confirm that the unit is turned on.
3. Check to make sure all connections are tight.
4. Check and confirm that airflow is coming from blower.
5. Check to make sure that the intake/exhaust vents are not obstructed.
6. Check the blower inlet filter to confirm that air can easily enter unit. If the filter appears obstructed, wash it.
7. If there is still no flow, contact your home care provider.

Air leaks
1. Check mask fit, and readjust mask or headgear if necessary.
2. Contact your home care provider for a replacement mask if adjustments don't resolve the problem.

ed by assuring a good seal in this area. Epistaxis and nasal discomfort are associated with drying of the nasal mucosa (a particular problem in cold, dry winter climates). Methods used to overcome excessive drying include in-line bubble humidifiers, room vaporizers, heat and moisture exchangers (**HMEs),** chin straps (to decrease loss of upper airway moisture), and saline nasal sprays.[153,154] Since none of these methods have proved satisfactory for all patients, selection should be based on individual patient acceptance and observed improvement in comfort.

The most common problem with the actual CPAP apparatus is an inability to reach or maintain the set pressure. This is usually due to either inadequate flow or system leaks. As part of their initial training, patients and caregivers should be taught how to recognize and correct these common problems. The accompanying box outlines the procedures patients can use to troubleshoot both inadequate flows and system leaks.

BiPAP®. A variation of nasal CPAP is bi-level positive airway pressure, or BiPAP®. While CPAP uses a single pressure level, BiPAP® employs two: IPAP (inspiratory positive airway pressure) and EPAP (expiratory positive airway pressure). In some patients, independent adjustment of IPAP and EPAP achieves the same results as conventional nasal CPAP, but at lower levels of expiratory pressure. This may reduce the adverse effects associated with nasal CPAP therapy and improve long-term therapeutic compliance.[155]

With proper application and patient compliance, nasal CPAP and BiPAP® can dramatically lessen or resolve the many problems associated with sleep apnea (morning headaches, daytime hypersomnolence, cognitive impairment, etc.). This, in turn, can enhance the patient's quality of life and may also lessen the incidence of more severe complications, such as systemic and pulmonary hypertension and cardiac arrhythmias.[146]

Apnea monitoring

Sudden infant death syndrome (**SIDS**) is another disorder with which the home care RCP may become involved. Hospitalized infants at risk for SIDS are frequently set-up on apnea monitors. After extensive family instruction in both equipment use and resuscitation, some of these infants may be discharged to the home with this equipment.

Most apnea monitors detect both respirations and heart rate, and activate audio and visual alarms when pre-set high or low limits are reached. Follow-up visits by an RCP or nurse are usually frequent at first, but become less needed as the family becomes skilled with the equipment and monitoring routine. Apnea monitors are usually discontinued after an infant demonstrates negative **pneumocardiograms.** More details on home apnea monitoring are provided in Chapter 35.[156-159]

Infusion therapy

While not specific to respiratory care, many home care patients receive intravenous or infusion therapy. Of special note are cystic fibrosis and AIDS patients receiving IV antimicrobials, and cancer patients on chemotherapy via infusion. The RCP should be aware of the indications for and problems associated with this type of home care.[160-161]

PATIENT ASSESSMENT AND FOLLOW-UP

As indicated in the AARC's standards for respiratory home care, there must be evidence that patients are receiving follow-up evaluations by a home care team member at least monthly, and more often if needed.[2] This individual could be the attending physician, the visiting nurse, a physical therapist or an RCP. While some DME suppliers may argue against monthly visits by credentialed RCPs, most do provide and cover the cost of such follow-up.

Soon after hospital discharge, patients may require more frequent follow-ups, as in the case of ventilator-dependent patients. However, with time and experience, visits can be less frequent. Nonetheless, some type of follow-up in the home by an RCP is needed periodically. Factors to consider when deciding on the frequency of visits include:

- The patient's condition and therapeutic needs (objectives);
- The level of family or caregiver support available;
- The type and complexity of home care equipment;
- The overall environment the patient lives in;
- The ability of the patient to provide self-care.

When a visit is made by a RCP, a number of functions must be performed. These include:

- Patient assessment (objective and subjective data), including pre- and post-treatment measurements of pulse, respiratory rate, blood pressure, and peak expiratory flow rate (or FVC, FEV_1 and $FEV_1\%$ if appropriate);
- Patient's compliance with prescribed respiratory home care;
- Equipment assessment (operation, cleanliness, and need for related supplies);
- Identification of any problem areas or patient concerns;
- Statement related to patient goals and therapeutic plan.

A standard written report, such as that shown in Figure 38-21, page 1128, should be completed by the visiting RCP. Copies should be sent to the patient's physician, the home care referral source, and any other member of the team requiring this information. The report should be part of the patient's medical record, and should be referred to when following the patient's course and overall progress. Policies and procedures regarding patient set-up and follow-up in the home should be established and kept on file by each DME supplier providing any type of respiratory care in the home setting.

EQUIPMENT DISINFECTION AND MAINTENANCE

With the increase in number of patients receiving home respiratory care, the danger of infection from contaminated equipment has also grown. In order to help minimize home-related infection, the American Respiratory Care Foundation (ARCF) has developed guidelines for disinfecting home respiratory care equipment.[11]

The ARCF guidelines complement the JCAHO home care standards (previously discussed). Emphasis in these guidelines is on the sources of infection, basic principles of infection control, patients at high risk, disinfection methods, equipment processing, and care of solutions and medications.

In regard to the principles of infection control, the ARCF recommends proper handwashing technique by all caregivers. In addition, visits to the patient by friends or relatives with respiratory infections are discouraged.

In regard to DME suppliers, the ARCF guidelines require that all permanent equipment (such as venti-

Home Visitation Report

Name:	Age:
Address:	Telephone:
Physician:	Referral:

Patient Diagnosis/History:

Therapeutic Objectives:

Home Care Prescription:

Patient Evaluation:

Clinical Measurements	Pulse	RR	B/P	PEFR	%PRED
Pre-Treatment					
Post-Treatment					
Predicted PEFR		L/min	% Improvement:		

Therapeutic Plan:

Next Scheduled Visit:

Therapist:	Date:

Fig. 38–21 Example of a form used to document the delivery of home respiratory care.

lator circuits, O_2 delivery equipment, and aerosol systems) be sterilized or receive high-level disinfection before being supplied to another patient. Disposable or single-patient use equipment must be used by one patient only.

In terms of cleaning, the ARCF recommends that all equipment be completely disassembled, and washed first in cool water to soften and loosen dried material. This initial wash should be followed by a soak in warm soapy water for several minutes, with equipment scrubbed as needed to remove any remaining organic material. Following this step, the equipment must be thoroughly rinsed to remove any residual soap, and drained of excess water.

According to the ARCF guidelines, neither quaternary ammonium compounds (quats) or acetic acid should be used to disinfect home care equipment. Instead, high-level disinfection with glutaraldehyde is recommended. In our opinion, this guideline is too stringent for many home care settings. It fails to account for both individual differences in patient risk and the broader bacteriocidal activity exhibited by some new disinfectants. Issues such as infection risk, cost, and safety must be considered by both the provider and patient before selecting the best disinfectant.

In regard to using water for humidification or nebulization, the ARCF recommends that it be boiled, stored in the refrigerator, and discarded after 24 hours. The ARCF also recommends that manufacturers' guidelines for the proper handling of specific medications be strictly followed.

In addition to these general guidelines, the ARCF provides detailed instructions for patients and caregivers on how to clean and disinfect selected home care equipment. The accompanying box provides an example of patient instructions for cleaning and disinfecting a ventilator circuit.[11]

ISSUES IN RESPIRATORY HOME CARE

Reimbursement

Although respiratory care services are fully reimbursed in the hospital, home services are not. Limited reimbursement is available in certain alternative sites such as skilled nursing facilities (**SNF**), and through home health agencies for ventilator-dependent patients. What little reimbursement is available for respiratory home care varies throughout the states. Pending health care reform legislation in Congress may improve home care reimbursement for respiratory services.

While reimbursement for home care equipment is available through Medicare and other insurance carriers, home clinical services performed by RCPs are generally not covered. The reasons for this are political, economical, and clinical. When home care reimbursement for clinical services started, respiratory care was a relatively new profession that was not fully understood or appreciated by the medical community. While the profession has grown and achieved due recognition, the reimbursement picture has not changed. Today, Medicare expenditures are tightly controlled. Other home care providers are not willing to give up their 'piece of the pie.' Thus, any changes in reimbursement for respiratory home care services will have to come about through legislative action.

Patient and caregiver instructions for cleaning and disinfection of ventilator circuits

Before you start to clean and disinfect your equipment, be sure that:
- Your work area is clear and clean;
- You have all of your supplies out and ready for use;
- Your hands are clean;
- Clean gloves are available in case you need them;
- You have a clean apron or a clean old shirt to put over your clothes to protect them from splashes and spills of dirty water that may contain germs.

Considerations

1. The outer surface of the ventilator may be wiped off as necessary with a clean, damp (not wet) cloth. You don't need to worry about cleaning the inside of the machine, but it should be checked and necessary maintenance should be done according to manufacturer's recommendations by someone from the company that supplied the machine.
2. The patient circuit must be taken completely apart and cleaned and disinfected every 24 hours.

Procedure

1. Take the circuit completely apart. Wipe the outer surface of the small tubes with a damp clean cloth. Hang from line with clips or clothes pins. Take large-bore tubings, connectors, nebulizer or humidifier, and exhalation valve apart, wash first in cool water to soften and loosen dried material. Then soak in warm soapy water for several minutes. Scrub with brush to remove any phlegm or secretions or other material that shouldn't be there. Rinse until all soap is gone. Drain off as much water as you can.
2. Place the parts in the disinfectant solution. Be certain that all of the inside and outside surfaces of the parts are covered with the disinfectant. Leave the parts in the disinfectant for at least 15 minutes or the manufacturer's recommended length of time. Check the clock or use a timer.
3. Be sure that your hands or gloves are clean. Rinse all of the parts thoroughly under running water.
4. Drain off as much water as you can and hang tubings to dry. Put small parts on a clean, dry surface.
5. When all parts are completely dry, put the exhalation valve and nebulizer back together, then put the circuit back together ready for use. Be sure that your hands are clean before you start to put the circuit back together. Store the circuit in a clean plastic bag.
6. It is best to have at least 3 complete ventilatory circuits—one in use, one being cleaned or drying, and one in reserve.

Other factors currently impacting on reimbursement for home respiratory care services include:[162]

■ Manpower shortages in related allied health professions;

■ A growing demand for multicompetent practitioners;

■ Legal credentialing (licensure) of RCPs;

■ Changes in education and entry requirements into the field;

■ The development of relevant clinical practice guidelines;

■ A growing public awareness of the respiratory care profession;

■ Proposed federal health care reform measures.

Ethical and legal issues

As respiratory home care has grown, so too has the potential for fraud and abuse. Among the most common areas of potential ethical or legal impropriety are:[163]

"Finders fees"—payment to a practitioner for patients referred to a particular DME supplier.

Hiring hospital staff—RCPs in a particular department are hired or contracted to perform home visits in return for patient referrals from that hospital.

Consultation services—a legal practice so long as neither the service nor payment for services is tied to patient referrals.

Inducements to the patient—offers of "free, noncovered" items to convince a patient to use a particular DME provider.

Free equipment—instead of cash payments, free equipment is offered in return for patient referrals.

Payment of electric bills—another inducement for patient referrals.

Under the Medicare/Medicaid Anti-Fraud and Abuse Amendments of 1977 (PL 95-142) such actions can result in criminal prosecution and very stiff penalties. For example, RCPs found guilty of fraud or abuse under this law can be fined $25,000 and/or imprisoned for up to five years for each offense.

In order to discourage such abuse, the AARC has adopted a statement on the ethical performance of respiratory home care (refer to Chapter 5). In addition, the AARC has taken the position that:[164]

1. Profit or revenue generation must not influence the selection, evaluation or continuation of any respiratory home care services. Fees, kickbacks, or other remunerations paid or offered by DME providers or received or solicited by RCPs for referral of patients are considered unethical and illegal.

2. Individuals who are either employed by or receive remuneration from both health care institutions which may refer patients and by DME suppliers who offer respiratory home care must openly disclose this relationship to both parties.

3. Institutionally-based RCPs who have significant ownership interest in a DME company which provides respiratory home care must openly disclose this relationship to the employing institution, Medicare Part B carriers, and all others who may be involved in the referral process. The practitioner must remove himself from the process of patient referrals to that provider.

Hopefully, these legal and ethical standards will decrease fraud and abuse in respiratory home care. However, only the active involvement of RCPs in supporting and upholding these laws and standards can assure that the occasional unscrupulous provider is exposed and prosecuted. As discussed in Chapter 5, this is the least we can expect from a field that seeks recognition as a true profession.

Finally, we will briefly mention the ethics involved in providing home care to "technology-dependent" children and adults. When home care involves advanced technology, it can strain the traditional concept of caring for a family member who is ill, regardless of age. Support on all levels must be afforded to family and caregivers who provide care outside traditional health care facilities.[165]

CHAPTER SUMMARY

Over the past 25 years, respiratory home care has evolved from an isolated and often neglected responsibility to a key component of comprehensive health care. Much of this rapid growth was associated with poor regulatory control and profiteering. However, with both the government and private sector increasingly seeking ways to lower costs, home care is becoming a viable alternative to hospitalization.

Today, legitimate uses for respiratory home care include long term O_2 therapy and care of ventilator-dependent patients. Other respiratory care modalities may be employed either by themselves or to supplement these forms of care.

The success of home care depends upon careful team planning, effective patient and family education, and coordinated assessment and follow-up. The RCP represents a vital member of the home care team. With other health providers and governmental agencies beginning to appreciate the important role played by RCPs in home care, an increase in their use is assured. RCPs can further this acceptance by continuing to provide highly skilled home care, and by delivering these services ethically and in cost-effective ways.

REFERENCES
1. Wyka KA: A review of respiratory home care, *RX Home Care* 641-49, 1984.
2. American Association for Respiratory Care: Standards for respiratory therapy home care—An official statement by the American Association for Respiratory Care, *Respir Care* 24:1080-1082, 1979.

3. Fischer DA, Prentice WS: Feasibility of home care for certain respiratory-dependent restrictive or obstructive lung disease patients, *Chest* 82:739, 1982.

4. The Medical Research Council Working Party: Long-term domicilliary oxygen therapy in chronic hypoxic cor pulmonale complicating chronic bronchitis and emphysema, *Lancet* 1:681-686, 1981.

5. Sivak ED, Cordasco EM, Gipson WT, Mehta A: Home care ventilation: The Cleveland Clinic experience from 1977 to 1985, *Respir Care* 31:294-302, 1986.

6. Goldberg AJ, Faure EAM: Home care for life-supported persons in England: The Responaut Program, *Chest* 86:910, 1984.

7. Make BJ, et al: Long-term management of ventilator-assisted individuals: The Boston University experience, *Respir Care* 31:303, 1986.

8. Bergner M, Conrad DA, Palmont CM, et al: The cost and efficacy of home care for patients with chronic lung disease, *Med. Care* 26(6):566-579, 1988.

9. Fields AI, Rosenblatt A, Pollack MM, Kaufman J: Home care cost-effectiveness for respiratory technology-dependent children, *Am J Dis Child* 145(7):729-733, 1991.

10. Weimer, HP: Home respiratory therapy for patients with chronic obstructive pulmonary disease, *Respir Care* 28(11):1484-1489, 1983.

11. American Respiratory Care Foundation: Guidelines for disinfection of respiratory care equipment used in the home, *Respir Care* 33:801-808, 1988.

12. American Association for Respiratory Care: Clinical practice guideline: Oxygen therapy in the home or extended care facility, *Respir Care* 37(8):918-922, 1992.

13. Joint Commission on Accreditation of HealthCare Organizations: *1993 Accreditation Manual for Home Care. Volume I: Standards, JCAHO.* Oakbrook Terrace, IL, 1992.

14. O'Ryan J: Discharge planning for the respiratory patient. In Lucas J, Golish JA, Sleeper G, O'Ryan JA, editors: *Home Respiratory Care* Norwalk: Appleton & Lange; 1988.

15. Bagnall P, Heslop A: Chronic respiratory disease: educating patients at home, *Prof Nurse* 2(9):293-296, 1987.

16. Branscomb DV, Weems BP: Home care and COPD patient responsibility, *Respir Ther* 16(5):11-13, 1986.

17. Petty TL: New developments in home oxygen therapy, *Respir Mgmt* 1:724-729, 1987.

18. O'Donohue WJ: The future of home oxygen therapy, *Respir Care* 33(12):1125-1130, 1988.

19. Nocturnal Oxygen Therapy Trial Group: Continuous or nocturnal oxygen therapy in hypoxemic chronic obstructive lung disease, *Ann Intern Med* 93391-398, 1980.

20. Anthonisen NR: Home oxygen therapy in chronic obstructive pulmonary disease, *Clin Chest Med* 7(4):673-678, 1986.

21. Baudouin SV, Waterhouse JC, Tahtamouni T, et al: Long-term domiciliary oxygen treatment for chronic respiratory failure reviewed, *Thorax* 45(3):195-198, 1990.

22. Openbrier DR, Fuoss C, Mall CC: What patients on home oxygen therapy want to know, *Am J Nurs* 88(2):198-201, 1988.

23. Petty TL: Home oxygen—a revolution in the care of advanced COPD, *Med Clin North Am* 74(3):715-729, 1990.

24. Petty TL, Neff TA, Creagh CE, et al: Outpatient oxygen therapy in chronic obstructive pulmonary disease. A review of 13 years' experience and an evaluation of modes of therapy, *Arch Intern Med* 139(1):28-32, 1979.

25. Zinman R, Corey M, Coates AL, et al: Nocturnal home oxygen in the treatment of hypoxemic cystic fibrosis patients, *J Pediatr* 114(3):368-377, 1989.

26. O'Donohue WJ: New concepts in long-term oxygen therapy, *Respir Ther* 5(4):47-53, 1992.

27. Christopher KL: Long-term oxygen therapy. In Pierson DJ and Kacmarek RM editors: *Foundations of respiratory care,* New York, 1992, Churchill Livingstone.

28. Howard P: New thoughts on long-term domiciliary oxygen therapy, *Recenti Prog Med* 81(3):158-161, 1990.

29. Long-term domiciliary oxygen therapy in chronic hypoxic cor pulmonale complicating chronic bronchitis and emphyse-

ma. Report of the Medical Research Council Working Party, *Lancet* 1(8222):681-686, 1981.

30. Long-term oxygen therapy indications and guidelines for use, *Home Healthcare Nurse* 7(3):40-47, 1989.

31. O'Donohue WJ: Home oxygen therapy. Why, when and how to write a proper prescription, *Postgrad Med* 87(2):59-61, 1990.

32. Tiep BL: Long-term home oxygen therapy, *Clin Chest Med* 11(3):505-521, 1990.

33. Christopher KL: Travel for patients with chronic respiratory disease, in Pierson DJ and Kacmarek RM editors: *Foundations of respiratory care,* New York, 1992, Churchill Livingstone.

34. Sleeper G: Traveling with oxygen. In Lucas J, Golish JA, Sleeper G, O'Ryan JA, editors: *Home Respiratory Care,* Norwalk, 1988, Appleton & Lange.

35. Transmittal 702 Final regulations released on home use of oxygen, *AARTimes* 927-30, 1985.

36. Conference Report: New problems in supply, reimbursement and certification of medical necessity for long-term oxygen therapy, *Am Rev Respir Dis* 142:721-724, 1990.

37. O'Donohue WJ: Effect of oxygen therapy on increasing arterial oxygen tension in hypoxemic patients with stable chronic obstructive pulmonary disease while breathing ambient air, *Chest* 100:968-972, 1991.

38. Fleig CP: Evolution of oxygen delivery systems, *Respir Ther* 12(1):79, 81-82, 1982.

39. Sleeper G: Home oxygen therapy equipment. In Lucas J, Golish JA, Sleeper G, O'Ryan JA, editors: *Home Respiratory Care,* Norwalk, 1988, Appleton & Lange.

40. Chusid EL: Oxygen concentrators, Int. Anesthesiol, *Clin* 20:235-247, 1982.

41. McPherson SP: *Respiratory therapy equipment,* ed 4, St Louis, 1990, Mosby.

42. Brown HV, Ziment I: Evaluation of an oxygen concentrator in patients with COPD, *Respir Ther* 5(6):55, 1978.

43. Chusid EL, Librot M, Utzurrum F, et al: Treatment of hypoxemia with an oxygen enricher, *Chest* 76268, 1979.

44. Massey LW, Hussey JD, Albert RK: Inaccurate oxygen delivery in some portable liquid oxygen devices, *Am Rev Respir Dis* 137:204 205, 1988.

45. Bongard JP, Pahud C, DeHaller R: Insufficient oxygen concentration obtained at domiciliary controls of eighteen concentrators, *Eur Resp J* 2(3):280-282, 1989.

46. Lucas J: Selecting the optimum oxygen system. In Lucas J, Golish JA, Sleeper G, O'Ryan JA, editors: *Home Respiratory Care,* Norwalk, 1988, Appleton & Lange.

47. Conference Report: Problems in prescribing and supplying oxygen for Medicare patients. *Am Rev Respir Dis* 1986;134:340-341.

48. Tiep BL: New portable oxygen devices, *Respir Care* 32:106-112, 1987.

49. Myers RJ: Oxygen conservation devices, *RX Home Care* 835 838, 1986.

50. O'Donohue WJ: Oxygen conserving devices, *Respir Care* 32(1):37-42, 1987.

51. Evans TW, Waterhouse JC, Suggett AJ, Howard PA: A conservation device for oxygen therapy in COPD, *Eur Resp J* 1(10):959-961, 1988.

52. Shigeoka JW: Oxygen conservers, home oxygen prescriptions and the role of the respiratory care practitioner, *Respir Care* 36(3): 178-183, 1991.

53. Heimlich HJ: Respiratory rehabilitation with transtracheal oxygen system, *Ann Otol Rhinol Laryngol* 91:643, 1982.

54. Spofford B, Christopher K, McCarty D, et al: Transtracheal oxygen therapy: A guide for the respiratory therapist, *Respir Care* 32(5):345-352, 1987.

55. Farney RJ, Walker JM, Elmer JC, et al: Transtracheal oxygen, nasal CPAP and nasal oxygen in five patients with obstructive sleep apnea. *Chest* 101(5):1228-35, 1992.

56. Wesmiller SW, Hoffman LA, Wiseman, M: Understanding transtracheal oxygen delivery, *Nursing* 19(12):43-47, 1989.

57. Benditt J, Pollock M, Roa J, Celli B: Transtracheal delivery of gas decreases the oxygen cost of breathing, *Am Rev Respir Dis* 147(5):1207-1210, 1993.

58. Wesmiller SW, Hoffman LA, Sciurba FC, et al: Exercise tolerance during nasal cannula and transtracheal oxygen delivery, *Am Rev Respir Dis* 141(3):789-91, 1990.

59. Tiep BL, Nicotra B, Carter R, Phillips R, Otsap B: Evaluation of an oxygen conserving nasal cannula, *Respir Care* 30:19-25, 1985.

60. Soffer M, Tashkin DP, Shapiro BJ, et al: Conservation of oxygen supply using a reservoir nasal cannula in hypoxemic patients at rest and during exercise, *Chest* 88(5):663-668, 1985.

61. Hussey JD, Massey LW, Lakshminarayan S: The efficacy of a reservoir cannula on oxygen saturation during exercise in patients with chronic obstructive pulmonary disease (COPD), *Am Rev Respir Dis* 131:A98, 1985.

62. Tiep BL, Belman MJ, Mittman C, et al: A new pendant storage oxygen-conserving nasal cannula, *Chest* 87:381-383, 1985.

63. Carter R, Williams JS, Berry J, et al: Evaluation of the pendant storage oxygen-conserving nasal cannula during exercise, *Chest* 89:806-810, 1986.

64. Gonzales SC, Huntington D, Romo R, Light RW: Efficacy of the Oxymizer pendant in reducing oxygen requirements of hypoxemic patients, *Respir Care* 31:681-688, 1986.

65. Pflug AE, Cheney FW, Butler J: Evaluation of an intermittent oxygen flow system, *Am Rev Respir Dis* 105:449-452, 1972.

66. Anderson WM, Ryerson G, Block AJ: Evaluation of an intermittent demand nasal oxygen flow system with a fluidic valve, *Chest* 86:313-318, 1984.

67. Franco MA, Liompart MD, Teague R, et al: Pulse dose oxygen delivery system, *Respir Care* 29:1034, 1985.

68. Tiep BL, Christopher KL, Spofford BT, et al: Pulsed nasal and transtracheal oxygen delivery. *Chest* 97(2):364-368, 1990.

69. Nolte D: Indications of different oxygen sources, *Lung* 168 Suppl:809-813, 1990.

70. Moore-Gillon J: The role of oxygen saving devices in patients with chronic hypoxemia, *Lung* 168 Suppl:814-815, 1990.

71. Hoffman LA, Dauber JH, Ferson PF, et al: Patient response to transtracheal oxygen delivery, *Am Rev Respir Dis* 135(1):153-156, 1987.

72. Brambilla I, Arlati S, Chiusa I, Micallef E: Technical aspects of oxygen saving devices, *Lung* 168 Suppl:816-819, 1990.

73. Lucas J: Ventilator care at home. In Lucas J, Golish JA, Sleeper G, O'Ryan JA, editors: *Home Respiratory Care,* Norwalk, 1988, Appleton & Lange.

74. Gilmartin ME: Long-term mechanical ventilation: patient selection and discharge planning, *Respir Care* 36(3):205-216, 1991.

75. Make BJ, Gilmartin ME: Mechanical ventilation in the home, *Crit Care Clin* 6(3):785-796, 1990.

76. O'Ryan JA: An overview of mechanical ventilation in the home, *Respir Mgmt* 17:27-36, 1987.

77. Gilmartin ME, Make BJ: Mechanical ventilation in the home: a new mandate, *Respir Care* 31(5):406-412, 1986.

78. Bach JR, Intintola P, Alba AS, Holland IE: The ventilator-assisted individual. Cost analysis of institutionalization vs rehabilitation and in-home management, *Chest* 101(1):26-30, 1992.

79. Sawicka EH, Loh L, Branthwaite MA: Domiciliary ventilatory support: an analysis of outcome, *Thorax* 43(1):31-35, 1988.

80. Giovannoni R: Chronic ventilator care from hospital to home, *Respir Ther* 14(4):29-33, 1984.

81. Goldberg AI, Frownfelter D: The ventilator-assisted individuals study, *Chest* 98(2):428-433, 1990.

82. Rosen RL, Bone RC: Economics of mechanical ventilation, *Clin Chest Med* 9(1):163-169, 1988.

83. Eigen H, Zander J: Home mechanical ventilation of pediatric patients. American Thoracic Society, *Am Rev Respir Dis* 141(1):258-259, 1990.

84. Frates RC, Splaingard ML, Smith EO, Harrison GM: Outcome of home mechanical ventilation in children, *J Pediatr* 106(5):850-856, 1985.

85. Gillis J, Tibballs J, McEniery J, et al: Ventilator-dependent children, *Med J Aust* 150(1):10-14, 1989.

86. Goldberg AI, Monahan CA: Home health care for children assisted by mechanical ventilation the physician's perspective, *J Pediatr* 114(3):378-383, 1989.

87. Mallory GB, Stillwell PC: The ventilator-dependent child issues in diagnosis and management, *Arch Phys Med Rehabil* 72(1):43-55, 1991.

88. Newald J: Home care of ventilator-dependent children urged, *Hospitals* 61(10):88, 1987.

89. Quint RD, Chesterman E, Crain LS, et al: Home care for ventilator-dependent children. Psychosocial impact on the family, *Am J Dis Child* 144:1238-1241, 1990.

90. Schreiner MS, Donar ME, Kettrick RG: Pediatric home mechanical ventilation, *Pediatr Clin North Am* 34(1):47-60, 1987.

91. Pierson DJ, George RB: Mechanical ventilation in the home: possibilities and prerequisites, *Respir Care* 31(4):266-270, 1986.

92. Niemer RJ: A program for nonhospital management of ventilator-dependent patients, *Respir Ther* 16(5):14-19, 1986.

93. Smith CE, Mayer LS, Parkhurst C, et al: Adaptation in families with a member requiring mechanical ventilation at home, *Heart & Lung* 20(4):349-356, 1991.

94. Thomas VM, Ellison K, Howell EV, Winters K: Caring for the person receiving ventilatory support at home: caregivers' needs and involvement, *Heart & Lung* 21(2):180-186, 1992.

95. O'Donohue WJ, Giovannoni RM, Goldberg AI, et al: Long-term mechanical ventilation. Guidelines for management in the home and at alternate community sites. Report of the Ad Hoc Committee, Respiratory Care Section, American College of Chest Physicians, *Chest* 90(1 Suppl) 1S-37S, 1986.

96. Make BJ: ACCP guidelines for mechanical ventilation in the home setting, *AARC Times* 1156-68, 1987.

97. American Association for Respiratory Care: Standards for the provision of care to ventilator-assisted patients in an alternative site, *AARC Times* 11:45-47, 1987.

98. Kacmarek RM, Spearman CB: Equipment used for ventilatory support in the home, *Respir Care* 31(4):310-328, 1986.

99. Emergency Care Research Institute: Portable ventilators, *Health Devices* 17(12):368, 1988.

100. Kacmarek RM, Stanek KS, McMahon KM, Wilson RS: Imposed work of breathing during synchronous intermittent mandatory ventilation provided by five home care ventilators, *Respir Care* 35(5):405-414, 1990.

101. American Association for Respiratory Care: Consensus statement on the essentials of mechanical ventilators-1992, *Respir Care* 37(9):1000-1008, 1992.

102. Gilmartin ME: Monitoring in the home and outpatient setting, in Kacmarek RM, Hess D, Stoller JK, editors: *Monitoring in Respiratory Care,* St Louis, 1993, Mosby.

103. Flasch M: Negative pressure ventilatory support in the home, *Respir Ther* 16(5):21-25, 1986.

104. Shneerson JM: Assisted ventilation. Non-invasive and domiciliary ventilation: negative pressure techniques, *Thorax* 46(2):131-135, 1991.

105. Splaingard ML, Frates RC, Jefferson LS, et al: Home negative pressure ventilation: report of 20 years of experience in patients with neuromuscular disease, *Arch Phys Med Rehabil* 66(4):239-242, 1985.

106. Shapiro SH, Macklem PT, Gray-Donald K, et al: A randomized clinical trial of negative pressure ventilation in severe chronic obstructive pulmonary disease: design and methods, *J Clin Epidemiol* 44(6):483-496, 1991.

107. Hill NS: Clinical applications of body ventilators. *Chest* 90(6):897-905, 1986.

108. Kerby GR, Mayer LS, Pingleton SK: Nocturnal positive pressure ventilation via nasal mask, *Am Rev Respir Dis* 135(3):738-740, 1987.

109. DiMarco AF, Connors AF, Altose MD: Management of chronic alveolar hypoventilation with nasal positive pressure breathing, *Chest* 92(5):952-954, 1987.

110. Ellis ER, Bye PT, Bruderer JW, Sullivan CE: Treatment of respiratory failure during sleep in patients with neuromuscular disease. Positive-pressure ventilation through a nose mask, *Am Rev Respir Dis* 135(1):148-152, 1987.

111. Bach JR, Penek J: Obstructive sleep apnea complicating negative-pressure ventilatory support in patients with chronic paralytic/restrictive ventilatory dysfunction, *Chest* 99(6):1386-1393, 1991.

112. Bach JR, Alba AS, Saporito LR: Intermittent positive pressure ventilation via the mouth as an alternative to tracheostomy for 257 ventilator users. *Chest* 103(1):174-82, 1993.

113. Branthwaite MA: Assisted ventilation. Non-invasive and domiciliary ventilation: positive pressure techniques, *Thorax* 46(3):208-212, 1991.

114. Bach JR, McDermott IG: Strapless oral-nasal interface for positive-pressure ventilation, *Arch Phys Med Rehabil* 71(11):910-913, 1990.

115. Hill NS, Eveloff SE, Carlisle CC, Goff SG: Efficacy of nocturnal nasal ventilation in patients with restrictive thoracic disease, *Am Rev Respir Dis* 145(2 Pt 1):365-371, 1992.

116. Waldhorn RE: Nocturnal nasal intermittent positive pressure ventilation with bi-level positive airway pressure (Bi-PAP) in respiratory failure, *Chest* 101(2):516-521, 1992.

117. Bach JR, Alba AS: Management of chronic alveolar hypoventilation by nasal ventilation, *Chest* 97(1):52-57, 1990.

118. Gay PC, Patel AM, Viggiano RW, Hubmayr RD: Nocturnal nasal ventilation for treatment of patients with hypercapnic respiratory failure, *Mayo Clin Proc* 66(7):695-703, 1991.

119. Leger P, Jennequin J, Gerard M, Robert D: Home positive pressure ventilation via nasal mask for patients with neuromuscular weakness or restrictive lung or chest-wall disease, *Respir Care* 34(2):73-79, 1989.

120. Segall D: Noninvasive nasal mask-assisted ventilation in respiratory failure of Duchenne muscular dystrophy, *Chest* 93(6):1298-1300, 1988.

121. Bach JR, O'Brien J, Krotenberg R, Alba AS: Management of end stage respiratory failure in Duchenne muscular dystrophy, *Muscle Nerve* 10(2):177-182, 1987.

122. Bach JR: Alternative methods of ventilatory support for the patient with ventilatory failure due to spinal cord injury, *J Am Paraplegia Soc* 14(4):158-174, 1991.

123. Bach JR, Alba AS: Noninvasive options for ventilatory support of the traumatic high level quadriplegic patient, *Chest* 98(3):613-619, 1990.

124. Guilleminault C, Stoohs R, Schneider H, et al: Central alveolar hypoventilation and sleep. Treatment by intermittent positive-pressure ventilation through nasal mask in an adult, *Chest* 96(5):1210-1212, 1989.

125. Bach JR, Alba AS, Bohatiuk G, et al: Mouth intermittent positive pressure ventilation in the management of postpolio respiratory insufficiency, *Chest* 91(6):859-864, 1987.

126. Carrey Z, Gottfried SB, Levy RD: Ventilatory muscle support in respiratory failure with nasal positive pressure ventilation, *Chest* 97(1):150-158, 1990.

127. Ellis ER, Grunstein RR, Chan S, et al: Noninvasive ventilatory support during sleep improves respiratory failure in kyphoscoliosis, *Chest* 94(4):811-815, 1988.

128. Rapoport DM, Sorkin B, Garay SM, Goldring RM: Reversal of the "Pickwickian syndrome" by long-term use of nocturnal nasal-airway pressure, *N Engl J Med* 307(15):931-933, 1982.

129. Elliott MW, Simonds AK, Carroll MP, et al: Domiciliary nocturnal nasal intermittent positive pressure ventilation in hypercapnic respiratory failure due to chronic obstructive lung disease: effects on sleep and quality of life, *Thorax* 47(5):342-348, 1992.

130. Ambrosino N, Nava S, Bertone P, et al: Physiologic evaluation of pressure support ventilation by nasal mask in patients with stable COPD, *Chest* 101(2):385-391, 1992.

131. Hodson ME, Madden BP, Steven MII, et al: Non-invasive mechanical ventilation for cystic fibrosis patients—a potential bridge to transplantation, *Eur Respir J* 4(5):524-527, 1991.

132. Piper AJ, Parker S, Torzillo PJ, et al: Nocturnal nasal IPPV stabilizes patients with cystic fibrosis and hypercapnic respiratory failure, *Chest* 102(3):846-850, 1992.

133. Carroll N, Branthwaite MA: Control of nocturnal hypoventilation by nasal intermittent positive pressure ventilation, *Thorax* 43(5):349-53, 1988.

134. Goldstein RS, De Rosie JA, Avendano MA, Dolmage TE: Influence of noninvasive positive pressure ventilation on inspiratory muscles, *Chest* 99(2):408-415, 1991.

135. Lucas J: Adjunctive respiratory modalities and techniques. In: Lucas J, Golish JA, Sleeper G, O'Ryan JA, editors: *Home Respiratory Care*. Norwalk: 1988, Appleton & Lange.

136. Grady KJ, Golish JA, Mehta AC: Sleep apnea. In: Lucas J, Golish JA, Sleeper G, O'Ryan JA, editors: *Home Respiratory Care*. Norwalk: 1988, Appleton & Lange.

137. Orlowski JP: Infant apnea monitoring. In: Lucas J, Golish JA, Sleeper G, O'Ryan JA, editors: *Home Respiratory Care*. Norwalk: 1988, Appleton & Lange.

138. American Association for Respiratory Care. Clinical practice guideline. Bland aerosol administration, *Respir Care* 38(11):1196-1200, 1993.

139. Conway JH, Fleming JS, Perring S, Holgate ST: Humidification as an adjunct to chest physiotherapy in aiding tracheobronchial clearance in patients with bronchiectasis, *Respir Med* 86(2):109-114, 1992.

140. Choy FN, Wilson DC, Willcox GS, Crocker KS: Experience with home aerosolized pentamidine treatment in patients with AIDS, *DICP* 24(6):592-594, 1990.

141. Green ST, Nathwani D, Christie PR, et al: Domiciliary nebulized pentamidine for secondary prophylaxis against Pneumocystis carinii pneumonia, *J R Soc Med* 83(1):18-19, 1990.

142. Update: universal precautions for prevention of transmission of human immunodeficiency virus, hepatitis B virus, and other bloodborne pathogens in health-care settings, *MMWR* 37(24):377-382, 387-388, 1988.

143. Thomas-Payne L: Respiratory reimbursement, *Home Care* (Respiratory Focus—Suppl)21-24, 1993.

144. American Association for Respiratory Care: Clinical practice guideline. Intermittent positive pressure breathing, *Respir Care* 38(11):1189-1195, 1993.

145. American Association for Respiratory Care: Clinical practice guideline. Use of positive airway pressure adjuncts to bronchial hygiene therapy, *Respir Care* 38(5):516-521, 1993.

146. Kimoff RJ, Cosio MG, McGregor M: Clinical features and treatment of obstructive sleep apnea, *Can Med Assoc J* 15;144(6):689-695, 1991.

147. Kryger MH: Management of obstructive sleep apnea, *Clin Chest Med* 13(3):481-492, 1992.

148. Mishoe SC: The diagnosis and treatment of sleep apnea syndrome, *Respir Care* 32:183-201, 1987.

149. Grady KJ, Golish JA, Mehta AC: Sleep apnea. In Lucas J, Golish JA, Sleeper G, O'Ryan JA, editors: *Home Respiratory Care*. Norwalk: 1988, Appleton & Lange.

150. Andersen AP, et al: Obstructive sleep apnea initiated by a lax epiglottis, *Chest* 91:621-623, 1990.

151. Stauffer JL, Fayter NA, MacLurg BJ: Conjunctivitis from nasal CPAP apparatus, *Chest* 86:802, 1989.

152. Strumpf DA, et al: Massive epistaxis from nasal CPAP therapy, *Chest* 95(5):1141, 1989.

153. Strumpf DA, Carlisle CC, Beadles SC, Milman RP: Alternative methods of humidification during use of nasal CPAP, *Respir Care* 35(3):217-221, 1990.

154. Sanders NH, Gruendl CA, Rogers RM: Patient compliance with nasal CPAP therapy for sleep apnea, *Chest* 90:330-333, 1986.

155. Sanders MH, Kern N: Obstructive sleep apnea treated by independently adjusted inspiratory and expiratory positive airway pressures via nasal mask. Physiologic and clinical implications, *Chest* 98(2):317-324, 1990.

156. Emergency Care Research Institute: Infant home apnea documentation monitors, *Health Devices* 21(10):339-373, 1992.

157. Emergency Care Research Institute: Issues in selecting and using apnea documentation systems, *Health Devices* 21(10):374-379, 1992.

158. McIntosh NA: Home monitoring in infants and children with obstructive apnea, *Otolaryngol Clin North Am* 23(4):713-725, 1990.

159. Southall DP: Home monitoring and its role in the sudden infant death syndrome, *Pediatrics* 72(1):133-138, 1983.

160. Hammond LJ, Caldwell S, Campbell PW: Cystic fibrosis, intravenous antibiotics and home therapy, *J Pediatr Home Care* 5(1):24-30, 1991.

161. Selecting infusion therapy services, *AIDS Patient Care* 3(1):12-14, 1989.

162. Giordano SP: Why aren't the respiratory care professional's services reimbursed?, *AARC Times* 11:53-57, 1987.

163. Larson K: DME referrals what's legal and what's not, *AARTimes* 10:28-31, 1986.

164. American Association for Respiratory Care: *Statement of principles on fraud and abuse in home care,* Dallas, undated, American Association for Respiratory Care.

165. Lantos JD, Kohrman AF: Ethical aspects of pediatric home care, *Pediatrics* 89(5 Pt 1):920-924, 1992.

APPENDIX 1

Temperature Correction of Barometric Reading

Temperature (°C)	730 mm Hg	740	750	760	770	780
15.0	1.78	1.81	1.83	1.86	1.88	1.91
16.0	1.90	1.93	1.96	1.98	2.01	2.03
17.0	2.02	2.05	2.08	2.10	2.13	2.16
18.0	2.14	2.17	2.20	2.23	2.26	2.29
19.0	2.26	2.29	2.32	2.35	2.38	2.41
20.0	2.38	2.41	2.44	2.47	2.51	2.54
21.0	2.50	2.53	2.56	2.60	2.63	2.67
22.0	2.61	2.65	2.69	2.72	2.76	2.79
23.0	2.73	2.77	2.81	2.84	2.88	2.92
24.0	2.85	2.89	2.93	2.97	3.01	3.05
25.0	2.97	3.01	3.05	3.09	3.13	3.17
26.0	3.09	3.13	3.17	3.21	3.26	3.30
27.0	3.20	3.25	3.29	3.34	3.38	3.42
28.0	3.32	3.37	3.41	3.46	3.51	3.55
29.0	3.44	3.49	3.54	3.58	3.63	3.68
30.0	3.56	3.61	3.66	3.71	3.75	3.80
31.0	3.68	3.73	3.78	3.83	3.88	3.93
32.0	3.79	3.85	3.90	3.95	4.00	4.05
33.0	3.91	3.97	4.02	4.07	4.13	4.18
34.0	4.03	4.09	4.14	4.20	4.25	4.31
35.0	4.15	4.21	4.26	4.32	4.38	4.43

From US epartment of Commerce, Weather Bureau: *Barometers and the measurement of atmospheric pressure,* Washington, DC, 1941, US Government Printing Office.

APPENDIX 2

Factors to Convert Gas Volumes From ATPS to STPD

Observed PB	15°	16°	17°	18°	19°	20°	21°	22°	23°	24°	25°	26°	27°	28°	29°	30°	31°	32°
700	0.855	851	847	842	838	834	829	825	821	816	812	807	802	797	793	788	783	778
702	857	853	849	845	840	836	832	827	823	818	814	809	805	800	795	790	785	780
704	860	856	852	847	843	839	834	830	825	821	816	812	807	802	797	792	787	783
706	862	858	854	850	845	841	837	832	828	823	819	814	810	804	800	795	790	785
708	865	861	856	852	848	843	839	834	830	825	821	816	812	807	802	797	792	787
710	867	863	859	855	850	846	842	837	833	828	824	819	814	809	804	799	795	790
712	870	866	861	857	853	848	844	839	836	830	826	821	817	812	807	802	797	792
714	872	868	864	859	855	851	846	842	837	833	828	824	819	814	809	804	799	794
716	875	871	866	862	858	853	849	844	840	835	831	826	822	816	812	807	802	797
718	877	873	869	864	860	856	851	847	842	838	833	828	824	819	814	809	804	799
720	880	876	871	867	863	858	854	849	845	840	836	831	826	821	816	812	807	802
722	882	878	874	869	865	861	856	852	847	843	838	833	829	824	819	814	809	804
724	885	880	876	872	867	863	858	854	849	845	840	835	831	826	821	816	811	806
726	887	883	879	874	870	866	861	856	852	847	843	838	833	829	825	818	813	808
728	890	886	881	877	872	868	863	859	854	850	845	840	836	831	826	821	816	811
730	892	888	884	879	875	870	866	861	857	852	847	843	838	833	828	823	818	813
732	895	891	886	882	877	873	868	864	859	854	850	845	840	836	831	825	820	815
734	897	893	889	884	880	875	871	866	862	857	852	847	843	838	833	828	823	818
736	900	895	891	887	882	878	873	869	864	859	855	850	845	840	835	830	825	820
738	902	898	894	889	885	880	876	871	866	862	857	852	848	843	838	833	828	822
740	905	900	896	892	887	883	878	874	869	864	860	855	850	845	840	835	830	825
742	907	903	898	894	890	885	881	876	871	867	862	857	852	847	842	837	832	827
744	910	906	901	897	892	888	883	878	874	869	864	859	855	850	845	840	834	829
746	912	908	903	899	895	890	886	881	876	872	867	862	857	852	847	842	837	832
748	915	910	906	901	897	892	888	883	879	874	869	864	860	854	850	845	839	834
750	917	913	908	904	900	895	890	886	881	876	872	867	862	857	852	847	842	837
752	920	915	911	906	902	897	893	888	883	879	874	869	864	859	854	849	844	839
754	922	918	913	909	904	900	895	891	886	881	876	872	867	862	857	852	846	841
756	925	920	916	911	907	902	898	893	888	883	879	874	869	864	859	854	849	844
758	927	923	918	914	909	905	900	896	891	886	881	876	872	866	861	856	851	846
760	930	925	921	916	912	907	902	898	893	888	883	879	874	869	864	859	854	848
762	932	928	923	919	914	910	905	900	896	891	886	881	876	871	866	861	856	851
764	934	930	926	921	916	912	907	903	898	893	888	884	879	874	869	864	858	853
766	937	933	928	925	919	915	910	905	900	896	891	886	881	876	871	866	861	855
768	940	935	931	926	922	917	912	908	903	898	893	888	883	878	873	868	863	858
770	942	938	933	928	924	919	915	910	905	901	896	891	886	881	876	871	865	860
772	945	940	936	931	926	922	917	912	908	903	898	893	888	883	878	873	868	862
774	947	943	938	933	929	924	920	915	910	905	901	896	891	886	880	875	870	865
776	950	945	941	936	931	927	922	917	912	908	903	898	893	888	883	878	872	867
778	952	948	943	938	934	929	924	920	915	910	905	900	895	890	885	880	875	869
780	955	950	945	941	936	932	927	922	917	912	908	903	898	892	887	882	877	872

$$\text{Factor} = \frac{[\text{PB}_{abs} \text{ corrected for } t_{amb} - \text{P}_{H_2O} \text{ at } t_{amb}] \times 0.359}{[t_{amb} + 273]}$$

APPENDIX 3

Factors to Convert Gas Volumes From STPD to BTPS at Given Barometric Pressues

Pressure	Factor	Pressure	Factor
740	1.245	760	1.211
742	1.241	762	1.208
744	1.238	764	1.203
746	1.235	766	1.200
748	1.232	768	1.196
750	1.227	770	1.193
752	1.224	772	1.190
754	1.221	774	1.188
756	1.217	776	1.183
758	1.214	778	1.181

$$\text{Factor} = \frac{863}{[PB_{amb} - 47]}$$

APPENDIX 4

Low-Temperature Characteristics of Selected Gases and Water

Substance	Critical temperature °C	°F	Critical pressure (atm)	Boiling point* °C	°F	Melting (freezing) point °C	°F
Acetylene	36.0	96.0	62.0	− 88.5	−119.2	− 81.8	−114.6
Air	−140.7	−221.0	37.2	−194.4	−317.9	—	—
Ammonia	132.4	270.3	111.5	− 33.4	− 28.1	− 77.7	−108.0
Carbon dioxide	31.1	87.9	73.0	− 78.5	−109.3	− 56.6	− 69.9
Cyclopropane	124.7	256.4	54.2	− 32.9	− 27.2	−127.5	−197.7
Freon-12	111.6	233.6	40.6	− 29.8	− 21.6	−158.0	−252.4
Freon-14	− 45.4	− 49.9	36.8	−128.0	−198.4	−184.0	−299.2
Helium	−267.9	−450.2	2.3	−268.9	−452.1	−272.2	−455.8
Hydrogen	−239.9	−399.8	12.8	−252.8	−423.0	−259.2	−434.5
Nitrogen	−147.1	−232.6	33.5	−195.8	−320.5	−209.9	−345.9
Nitrous oxide	36.5	97.7	71.8	− 88.5	−127.2	− 90.8	−131.6
Oxygen	−118.8	−181.1	49.7	−183.0	−297.3	−218.4	−361.8
Propane	95.6	206.2	43.0	− 42.2	− 43.7	−189.9	−305.8
Water	374.0	705.0	218.0	100.0	212.0	0.0	32.0

*Boiling point at 1 atmosphere (760 mm Hg) pressure.

Glossary

A

a/A ratio the ratio of arterial to alveolar oxygen partial pressures (PaO_2/PAO_2); a measure of the efficiency of oxygen transfer across the lung

AARC abbreviation for the American Association for Respiratory Care, the primary voluntary professional association for respiratory care practitioners

abduct to move a limb away from the body

absorbance the degree of absorption of light or other radiant energy by a medium through which the radiant energy passes

absorption the taking up of liquids or gases; particularly the passage of these substances through a body surface into body fluids or tissues

absorption atelectasis atelectasis due to the absorption of oxygen from obstructed or partially obstructed alveoli with high oxygen concentrations

A/C alternative abbreviation for assist/control ventilation; see *assist/control*

ACCP abbreviation for the American College of Chest Physicians

accreditation the process by which a private, nongovernmental agency recognizes that an institution or organization meets prespecified standards of quality; commonly applies to educational institutions or programs, and health care agencies such as hospitals and nursing homes

acetazolamide a carbonic anhydrase inhibitor with diuretic properties; inhibits formation of carbonic acid in the proximal tubules of the kidneys, thereby promoting elimination of sodium, potassium, bicarbonate and water; prolonged use can cause an alkaline diuresis leading to metabolic acidosis

acetylcholinesterase an enzyme that inactivates the neurotransmitter acetylcholine by hydrolyzing the substance to choline and acetate

acetylcysteine a mucolytic agent that lowers the viscosity of mucoid secretions by chemically disrupting the sulphydryl bonds of mucopolysaccharides

achalasia an abnormal condition characterized by the inability to relax smooth muscle sphincters, particularly those in the gastrointestinal tract; commonly refers to failure of the lower esophagus to relax during swallowing (achalasia cardia)

acid any substance that serves as a proton donor in a chemical reaction

acidemia a combining form meaning an 'increased hydrogen-ion concentration in the blood;' as applied to arterial blood denotes a pH less than 7.35

acidosis an abnormal physiologic process resulting in an increase in the hydrogen ion concentration in the body; may be caused by either an excess accumulation of an acid or the loss of base

acid-fast of or pertaining to a bacterial stain that does not decolorize easily when washed with an acid solution; also refers to certain bacteria (especially Mycobacteria) which retain red dyes after an acid wash

aciduria the presence of a greater than normal hydrogen ion concentration in the urine (normal urine pH ranges from 4.6 to 8.0, with an average value of 6.0)

acquired immune deficiency syndrome (AIDS) an immune disorder caused by infection with the human immunodeficiency virus (HIV); HIV directly attacks the T-lymphocytes and T-helper cells of the immune system, thereby compromising both cell-mediated and humoral (antibody) immunity

acromegaly a chronic metabolic condition characterized by a gradual, marked enlargement and elongation of the bones of the face, jaw, and extremities

acronym a word formed by the initial letters of each major part of a multiword term, e.g., "PEEP" is the acronym for positive end-expiratory pressure

ACTH abbreviation for adrenocorticotropic hormone, a pituitary hormone that stimulates the adrenal cortex

actinomycosis a chronic, systemic fungal disease caused by infection with organisms of the genus Actinomyces; most commonly affects the skin, but can involve the lungs and other organ systems

action potential a rapid reversal in the membrane potential occurring in certain nerve and muscle cells, caused by a change in the membrane permeability for sodium ions, which rapidly diffuse into the cell, thereby reversing its charge

actual damages compensation for actual injuries or losses such as medical expenses, lost wages, etc.

actuator that portion of a mechanical or electronic device that initiates a given action or process

ACV alternative abbreviation for assist/control ventilation; see *assist/control*

additive effect a form of drug interaction in which the effect of two drugs together equals the simple sum of their individual effects

Addison's disease a life-threatening condition caused by partial or complete failure of adrenocortical function, often resulting from autoimmune processes, infection (especially tubercular or fungal), neoplasm, or hemorrhage in the gland

adduct to move a limb toward the axis of the body

adenopathy any enlargement of a gland, especially a lymphatic gland

adenovirus any one of the 33 medium sized viruses of the Adenoviridae family, pathogenic to humans, that cause conjunctivitis, upper respiratory infection, or GI infection

ADH abbreviation for antidiuretic hormone, a hormone stored and released by the posterior lobe of the pituitary gland which stimulates the reabsorption of water by the renal tubular epithelial cells; due to mild vasopressor effects ADH is also called vasopressin

adhesion the physical property by which unlike substances can attract each other and hold together; also refers to the abnormal formation of fibrous tissues (resulting from inflammation or injury) that bind together body structures which are normally separate

adiabatic a process of gas compression or expansion in which in which no heat energy is added to or taken away from the gas during the process; rapid adiabatic compression causes a rapid increase in temperature; compare to *isothermal*

ADL abbreviation for activities of daily living, a quantifiable measure of an individual's ability to perform common tasks associated with independent functioning

adrenergic of or pertaining to the sympathetic nerve fibers of the autonomic nervous system that use epinephrine or epinephrine-like substances as neurotransmitters; any chemical or drug which mimics the effect of these neurotransmitters

adrenocorticosteroid (also corticosteroid) a broad term referring to any of the steroid hormones produced by the adrenal cortex, including their synthetic equivalents; major categories include the glucocorticoids (e.g., hydrocortisone),the mineralocorticoids (e.g., aldosterone) and the androgens

adult respiratory distress syndrome (ARDS) a pattern of clinical, physiologic and pathologic features characterizing the lung's response to a variety of injuries and resulting in diffuse damage to the alveolar-capillary membrane

advocacy taking a position in favor of a certain issue or person; in health care commonly refers to supporting the patient's needs over those of the institution or health care professional

aerobic living only in the presence of oxygen

aerobic exercise any physical activity that requires increased cardiac output and ventilation to meet the increased oxygen demands of the skeletal muscles

aerosol a suspension of solid or liquid particles in a gas

aerosol density (particulate) the number of aerosol particles per unit of carrier gas

aerosol density (weight) the actual weight of aerosol carried in a given volume of gas; two units of weight density are common: grams of aerosol per square meter (g/m^3) or milligrams of aerosol per liter (mg/L)

AFB abbreviation for acid-fast bacillus, especially Mycobacteria which retain red dyes after an acid wash

afferent carrying or conduction impulses toward the central nervous system; opposite of efferent

affidavit a written statement of facts given voluntarily under oath

affinity in pharmacology, the tendency a drug has to combine with a receptor; refer to *agonist*

afterload the load or resistance against which the ventricles must eject their volume of blood during contraction

agammaglobulinemia a rare disorder characterized by the absence of the serum immunoglobin, gamma globulin, associated with an increased susceptibility to infection

agglomeration the process of gathering together into a mass, as when many small aerosol particles come together to form a single large particle

agonist of or pertaining to a chemical substance or drug which has affinity and exerts a desired or expected effect (as opposed to an *antagonist*)

AHI abbreviation for the apnea-hypopnea index, used to quantify the severity of obstructive sleep apnea (OSA) and its response to treatment with CPAP

AIDS abbreviation for acquired immune deficiency syndrome

airborne transmission transmission of infectious organisms via dissemination of the infectious agent in the air, either by aerosol droplets, droplet nuclei or dust particles

airway conductance a measure of the ease with which gas flows through the respiratory tract; abbreviated as G, conductance is the reciprocal of airway resistance, i.e., $G \approx$ flow/change in pressure

airway resistance a measure of the impedance to ventilation caused by the movement of gas through the airways; abbreviated as Raw, airway resistance is computed as the change in pressure along a tube divided by the flow;

alar nasi the wing-like lateral projections of the nose

aldehyde any of a large category of organic compounds derived from a corresponding alcohol by the removal of two hydrogen atoms, as in the conversion of ethyl alcohol to acetaldehyde

aldosterone a corticosteroid produced by the adrenal cortex to regulate sodium and potassium balance in the blood

aldosteronism a condition characterized by hypersecretion of aldosterone, occurring as a primary disease of the adrenal cortex or, more often, as a secondary disorder in response to various extra-adrenal pathologic processes

algorithm a predetermined group of directions to solve a problem in a finite number of steps

aliquot a fractional portion of a liquid or solid substance

alkalemia a combining form meaning an 'decreased hydrogen-ion concentration in the blood;' as applied to arterial blood, denotes a pH greater less than 7.45

alkaloid any one of a large group of alkaline organic chemicals found in plants that exert powerful physiologic activity; examples include morphine, cocaine, nicotine, and atropine

alkalosis an abnormal physiologic process resulting in a decrease in the hydrogen ion concentration in the body; may be caused by either an excess accumulation of base or the loss of acid

allantois the ventral outgrowth of the hindgut of the early embryo; becomes a major component of the developing umbilical cord

allegation a written statement by a party to a suit concerning what the party expects to prove

allographic of or pertaining to a tissue graft or organ transplant between individuals of different genetic make-up

allopathic referring to the system of medicine whereby disease is treated by antagonistic therapy, such as an antibiotic to treat infection; more generally, the predominant system of medicine education in the US

alpha-1 antitrypsin a chemical substance that inhibits the action of the proteolytic enzyme trypsin; associated with a form of destructive emphysema

alphanumeric data composed of alphabetic and/or numeric characters

ALU abbreviation for Arithmetic Logic Unit, the segment of the CPU which carries out arithmetic and logic functions

alveolarization the process of alveolar development from epithelial tissue

ambient of or referring to the surrounding environmental conditions

ambulation the process of walking

amino acid one of a large class of organic compounds containing both an amino (NH_2^-) and carboxyl ($COOH^-$) group

amniocentesis the process of direct sampling and quantitative assessment of the amniotic fluid

amnion the innermost membrane enclosing the fetus and normally filled with amnionic fluid

ampere the basic unit of electrical current; equivalent to the amount of electrons flowing when one volt of electromotive force is applied to a circuit with one ohm of resistance

amyotrophic lateral sclerosis (ALS) a degenerative disease of the motor neurons, characterized by atrophy of the muscles of the hands, forearms, and legs spreading to involve most of the body

anaerobe a microorganism that grows and lives in the complete or almost complete absence of oxygen

anaerobic of or referring to the ability to live without oxygen

anaerobic threshold during exercise, the point where increased levels of lactic acid result in an increased CO_2 production and minute ventilation; the RQ equals or exceeds 1.0, indicating that CO_2 production equals or exceeds O_2 consumption; at this point metabolism becomes anaerobic, thereby decreasing energy production and increasing muscle fatigue

analog a representation of numerical quantities by an output signal which measures continuous physical variables (such as voltage, length, pressure, flow) proportionate to the input

analog-to-digital converter (ADC) an instrument measuring an analog signal and converting it to digital form, thus enabling the data to be fed to a computer

anaphylaxis an exaggerated hypersensitivity reaction to a previously encountered antigen

anastomosis a communication between two ducts or blood vessels that allows flow from one to another

anecdotal of or pertaining to a brief description of a prior event or incident

anemia an abnormal condition characterized by a reduction in the number of circulating red blood cells or the amount of normal hemoglobin available to carry oxygen

anesthesiology the science of anesthesia; using drugs or chemical substances to cause partial or complete loss of sensation, particularly pain

anesthetic a drug or chemical substance that causes partial or complete loss of sensation

aneurysm a localized dilatation of the wall of a blood vessel, usually caused by atherosclerosis and hypertension, or, less frequently, by trauma, infection, or a congenital weakness in the vessel wall

angina pectoris a paroxysmal attack of severe chest pain associated with coronary insufficiency; commonly radiates from the heart to the shoulders and arms

angiography the X-ray visualization of the internal anatomy of the heart and blood vessels after the intravascular introduction of radiopaque contrast medium

angiotensin a blood polypeptide formed by the action of renin and angiotensinogin; the active form (angiotensin II) causes vasoconstriction and stimulates aldosterone secretion by the adrenal cortex

anhydrous containing no water; dry

anion an ion that migrates to the anode (positive electrode) in an electrolytic solution; a negative ion

anion gap the difference in concentration between the major serum electrolyte cations and anions; used to help diagnose the cause of metabolic acidosis

ankylosing spondylitis a chronic inflammatory disease of unknown origin, first affecting the spine and adjacent structures, and commonly progressing to eventual fusion (ankylosis) of the involved joints

anode the electrode to which anions migrate in an electrolytic reation; the positive electrode

anomaly a broad term denoting any deviation from what is regarded as normal

anorexia lack or loss of appetite, resulting in the inability to eat

ANSI abbreviation for the American National Standards Institute, a private nongovernmental agency that establishes voluntary standards in a wide variety of technical fields, including medical instrumentation

antagonist in pharmacology, is a drug that has affinity but produces no effect; an antagonist can be competitive (forms reversible bond with receptor) or noncompetitive (forms irreversible bond)

antecubital fossa the triangular area at the bend of the elbow; frequently used as the site for venipuncture and brachial artery blood sampling

anterolateral situated in front and to one side or the other

anteroposterior from the front to the back of the body, commonly associated with the direction of the roentgenographic or X-ray beam (an "AP" exposure)

antiarrhythmic of or pertaining to a procedure or substance that prevents, alleviates, or corrects an abnormal cardiac rhythm

antibody a soluble protein synthesized by plasma cells in response to a specific antigen with which it interacts; in conjunction with the activation of complement, antibody production represents a key component of the humoral immunity

anticholinergic of or pertaining to a blockade of acetylcholine receptors that results in the inhibition of the transmission of parasympathetic nerve impulses

antigen a substance, usually a protein, that causes the formation of an antibody and reacts specifically with that antibody; see *antibody*

antiinflammatory of or pertaining to a substance or procedure that counteracts or reduces inflammation

antisepsis the destruction of pathogenic microorganisms existing in their vegetative state on living tissue

antiseptic a chemical solution capable of antisepsis

antitoxin an antibody capable of neutralizing a specific toxin, e.g., tetanus antitoxin

anxiolytic a drug or chemical agent capable of reducing anxiety, apprehension, or restlessness

AoA abbreviation for the Administration on Aging of the US Department of Health and Human Services, an agency which supports state and local efforts to address the health care, economic, and social concerns of older Americans

aortic regurgitation backflow of blood from the aorta into the left ventricle; indicates an incompetent valve

aPEEP abbreviation; see *auto-PEEP*

Apgar score the evaluation of an infant's physical condition, usually performed 1 minute, and again, 5 minutes after birth, based on a rating of five factors that reflect the infant's ability to adjust to extrauterine life

aphagia a condition characterized by the loss of the ability to swallow as a result of organic or psychologic causes

aphasia an abnormal neurologic condition in which language function is defective or absent because of an injury to certain areas of the cerebral cortex

apical of or pertaining to the summit or apex

apnea an absence of spontaneous breathing

apnea of prematurity a disorder of preterm infants, probably of CNS origin, characterized by frequent apneic pauses lasting more than 20 seconds, and often associated with cyanosis, pallor, hypotonia or bradycardia

apneustic breathing a pattern of respirations characterized by a prolonged inspiratory phase followed by expiratory apnea

apneustic center a localized collections of neurons in the pons located at the level of the area vestibularis that moderate the rhythmic activity of the medullary respiratory centers

application software a program which enables the computer to perform specific functions, such as word processing or data processing

aponeurosis a strong sheet of fibrous connective tissue that serves as a tendon to attach muscles to bone or as fascia to bind muscles together

APRV abbreviation for airway pressure release ventilation, a form of partial ventilatory support in which airway pressure is continually maintained above atmospheric during spontaneous breathing, interspersed with brief periods of pressure release to enhance ventilation.

arachidonic acid a naturally occurring fatty acid involved in the biosynthesis of certain prostaglandins and having a role in the inflammatory process

ARCF abbreviation for the American Respiratory Care Foundation, a philanthropic agency that promotes the field of respiratory care through grants and awards

archive to store data in such a way that supports retrieval, or the collection of data itself which is stored in this manner

ARDS acronym; see *adult respiratory distress syndrome*

arrhythmia any deviation from the normal pattern of the heartbeat

arteriography a method of radiologic visualization of arteries performed after a radiopaque contrast medium is introduced into the bloodstream or into a specific vessel by injection or through a catheter

arteriole one of the blood vessels of the smallest branch of the arterial circulation

arteriolized blood blood that has been fully oxygenated by passage through the lungs

artificial intelligence (AI) a synthetically created intellect which is capable of engaging in humanoid thought processes; includes the ability to absorb new data, understand new input, solve problems via logical reasoning, and especially, to "remember", to learn from past errors and experiences

asbestosis a restrictive lung disease caused by prolonged exposure to asbestosis fibers; associated with a high incidence of malignant lung tumors and pleural abnormalities

ascites an abnormal intraperitoneal accumulation of a fluid containing large amounts of protein and electrolytes

asepsis the absence of pathogenic microorganisms; the removal of pathogenic microorganisms or infected material

aspergillosis an infection caused by a fungus of the genus Aspergillus, capable of causing inflammatory, granulomatous lesions on or in any organ

asphyxia cessation of ventilation leading to acute hypoxia and hypercapnia

aspirate (verb) to withdrawn fluid by negative pressure; (noun) the fluid so withdrawn

aspiration the act of inhaling, especially in reference to the pathological aspiration of vomitus or material foreign to the respiratory tract (see *aspiration pneumonia*); also the process of withdrawing fluid by negative pressure

aspiration pneumonia an inflammatory condition of the lungs and bronchi caused by the inhalation of foreign material or vomitus containing acid gastric contents

assault any conduct which creates a reasonable apprehension of being touched in an injurious manner; no actual touching is required to prove assault

assist/control (A/C or ACV) continuous mandatory ventilation (CMV) in which the minimum breathing rate is predetermined by the ventilator controls, but the patient can initiate ventilation at a faster rate (patient or time-triggered ventilation)

ASTM abbreviation for the American Society for Testing and Materials, a nongovernmental agency that establishes performance standards for various equipment and materials

asymptomatic literally 'without symptoms'

asynchronous breathing an abnormal breathing pattern in which the rib cage and abdomen do not move outward together, indicating that the respiratory muscles are not working in synchrony; an early indicator of an excessive respiratory muscle load

asynchrony pertaining to ventilatory support, a situation in which interaction between the patient and machine is poorly coordinated, causing extra patient effort and discomfort

asystole the absence of a heartbeat, as distinguished from fibrillation, in which electric activity persists but contraction ceases

ATA abbreviation for atmospheric pressure absolute, a measure of pressure used in hyperbaric medicine; one ATA equals 760 torr or 101.32 kPa

atelectasis an abnormal condition characterized by the collapse of lung tissue, preventing the exchange of carbon dioxide and oxygen with the pulmonary capillary blood

atherosclerosis an arterial disorder characterized by the deposit of plaques of cholesterol, lipids and cellular debris in the inner layers of the walls of arteries

atomizer a device that produces an aerosol suspension of liquid particles without using baffles to control particle size

atopy a hereditary tendency to develop immediate allergic reactions, as in asthma, atopic dermatitis, or vasomotor rhinitis, because of the presence of an antibody

atrial myxoma a benign tumor that originates in the intratrial septum of the heart

atrial natriuretic hormone a hormone that inhibits sodium reabsorption by the kidneys, thus increasing sodium and water excretion in the urine

atrioventricular of or pertaining to the area between the atrial and ventricles of the heart

atrophy a wasting or diminution of size or physiologic activity of a part of the body because of disease or other influences, especially muscle tissue

ATS abbreviation for the American Thoracic Society

auditory pertaining to the sense of hearing

auscultation the act of listening for sounds within the body to evaluate the condition of the heart, lungs, pleura, intestines, or other organs or to detect the fetal heart sound

authoritarian of or pertaining to the principle of blind obedience of one to another

autoclave a apparatus that uses steam under pressure to sterilize articles and equipment

autogenous self-generating

autoimmune disease one of a large group of diseases characterized by the subversion or alteration of the function of the immune system of the body

autonomy the individual characteristic or right to self-determination

auto-PEEP abnormal and usually undetected residual pressure above atmospheric remaining in the alveoli at end-exhalation due to dynamic air trapping

autoregulation automatic control of a mechanical or physiologic system; necessitates both a sensing mechanism (to measure what is regulated) and a feedback 'loop' (to respond to changes)

autosomal inheritance a pattern of inheritance in which the transmission of a recessive gene on an autosome results in a carrier state if the person is herterozygous for the trait and in the affect state if the person is homozygous for the trait

avirulent the inability of a microorganism to cause a pathologic effect

axilla a pyramid-shaped space forming the underside of the shoulder between the upper part of the arm and the side of the chest; i.e., the 'armpit'

axillary of or pertaining to the axilla

azoospermia lack of sperm in the semen

azotemia the buildup of excess nitrogenous waste products in the blood, usually due to renal failure

B

Babinski's reflex dorsiflexion of the big toe with extension and fanning of the other toes elicited by firmly stroking the lateral aspect of the sole of the foot

backup a system for saving data should a computer failure occur (such as caused by power outages)

bacteremia the presence of bacteria in the blood

bacteriocidal destructive to bacteria

bacteriostatic tending to restrain bacterial growth

baffle a surface in a nebulizer designed specifically to cause impaction of large aerosol particles, causing either further fragmentation, or removal from the suspension via condensation back into the reservoir

bagassosis a self-limited lung disease caused by an allergic response to bagasse, the fungi-laden, dusty debris left after the syrup has been extracted from sugar cane

BAL abbreviation; see *bronchoalveolar lavage*

barbiturate any one of a group of organic compounds derived from barbituric acid which have the capacity to cause depression of the central nervous system; examples include amitol, phenobarbitol, and sodium pentothal

baroreceptor one of the pressure-sensitive nerve endings in the walls of the atria of the heart, the vena cava, the aortic arch, and the carotid sinus

barotrauma physical injury sustained as a result of exposure to ambient pressures above normal; commonly refers to pulmonary damage resulting from the application of positive pressure ventilation, such as pneumothorax, pneumomediastinum, and subcutaneous emphysema

base any substance that serves as a proton receptor in a chemical reaction

base excess (BE) the difference between the normal buffer base (NBB) and the actual buffer base (BB) in a whole blood sample, expressed in mEq/L; a normal BE is +/− 2 mEq/L

BASIC Beginners All-purpose Symbolic Instruction Code, an easily learned and simple to use programming language that uses mnemonic devices for commands (RUN, PRINT, etc) and possesses a wide variety of features

batch a set of data and directives processed by the computer as a single unit in one run

battery (legal) an unconsented actual touching that causes injury

baud rate a measurement of speed in telecommunications The measure is of each discrete signal element transmitted in one second Assuming each signal element is one bit, the number of bits transmitted per second is the baud rate

BCG vaccine an active immunizing agent against tuberculosis prepared from Bacille Calmette-Guerin

behavioral pertaining to or caused by human conduct (as opposed to structural or physiologic causes)

beneficiary one who benefits from; commonly used to refer to the recipient of social or health services provided by a public or private agency

benign not malignant or recurrent; characterized by mild symptoms or effect

bigeminy literally 'an association in pairs'; commonly refers to the cardiac arrhythmia characterized by paired premature ventricular contractions

bilirubin the orange-yellow pigment of bile, formed principally by the breakdown of hemoglobin in red blood cells after termination of their normal life span

binary a condition where one of only two alternatives must exist (on or off); a numerical system utilizing only the digits 1 and 0

biofeedback a process providing a person with visual or auditory information about the autonomic physiologic functions of his or her body, as blood pressure, muscle tension, and brain wave activity, usually through use of instrumentation

biopsy the procedure whereby tissues are excised for microscopic examination and diagnosis

BiPAP® a spontaneous breath mode of ventilatory support which allows separate regulation of the inspiratory and expiratory pressures

biphasic consisting of two phases

bit Binary digIT, a quantum of data in computer storage corresponding to a 1 or 0

board certified holding certification in a medical specialty; usually obtained by passing one or more examinations offered by a specialty society or credentialing agency

body humidity the absolute humidity in a volume of gas saturated at a body temperature of 37°C; equivalent to 43.8 mg/L

Bohr effect the impact of variations in blood pH on the affinity of hemoglobin for oxygen

boiling point the temperature at which the vapor pressure of a liquid equals the ambient pressure exerted on the liquid

BOMA abbreviation for the Board of Medical Advisors, the medical advisory group for the American Association for Respiratory Care

bore the internal diameter of a tube

botulism an often fatal form of food poisoning caused by an endotoxin produced by the bacillus Clostridium botulinum

BPF abbreviation; see *bronchopleural fistula*

brachial of or pertaining to the arm

brachocephalic trunk the short branch of the aortic arch giving rise to the right common carotid and right subclavian arteries; also called the innominate artery

brachytherapy treatment of malignant neoplasms by implanting radioactive materials directly into the tumor

bradycardia an abnormal condition characterized by a heart rate of less than 60 per minute

bradykinin a polypeptide cellular mediator responsible for provoking smooth muscle contraction

bradypnea an abnormally slow rate of breathing

breach of contract failure, without legal excuse, to carry out the terms of a legal agreement

breach of duty failure to complete an assignment that is legal and agreed upon

breathing exercises a broad category of physical activities designed to increase the strength and endurance of the respiratory muscles, and to promote their more efficient use

bribery, commercial the advantage which one competitor secures over fellow competitors by his secret and corrupt dealing with employees or agents of prospective purchasers

brief a written statement prepared by an attorney arguing a case in court; a brief contains a summary of the facts of the case, the pertinent acts to include those who had the right of control over the negligent actions

bronchiectasis an abnormal condition of the bronchial tree characterized by irreversible dilatation and destruction of the bronchial walls

bronchiolitis an acute infection of the lower respiratory tract causing expiratory wheezing, respiratory distress, inflamma-

tion, and obstruction of the bronchioles; bronchiolitis is usually caused by the respiratory syncytial virus (RSV) and is most common in infants under the age of two

bronchitis an acute or chronic inflammation of the mucous membranes of the tracheobronchial tree

bronchoalveolar lavage (BAL) the instillation and aspiration of fluids into the lungs in order to diagnose or treat certian conditions

bronchoconstriction narrowing of the bronchi due contraction of their smooth muscle

bronchodilation the reversal of bronchoconstriction, usually via sympathetic stimulation

bronchogenic carcinoma the most common malignant lung tumor originating in bronchi

bronchography an X-ray examination of the bronchi after they have been coated with a radiopaque substance

bronchophony the normal transmission of voice sounds from a large bronchus to the chest wall as heard by a stethoscope

bronchopleural fistula a direct communication between a bronchus and the pleural space; a common cause of pneumothorax

bronchorrhea the excessive discharge of respiratory tract secretions

bronchoscopy the visual examination of the tracheobronchial tree, using either a rigid, tubular metal bronchoscope or the narrower, flexible fiberoptic bronchoscope (FFB)

bronchospasm an abnormal contraction of the smooth muscle of the bronchi, resulting in an acute narrowing and obstruction

bronchovesicular breath sounds sharing the characteristics of those heard over the trachea (bronchial sounds) and those arising from the more distal alveolar region (vesicular sounds)

bruit an abnormal sound heard on auscultation of the heart or large vessels, caused by turbulence or obstruction

BTU abbreviation for British Thermal Unit, the fps unit of heat energy; a BTU is the amount of heat required to raise the temperature of 1 lb of water 1°F; one BTU equals 252 calories (cgs)

buccal of or pertaining to the inside of the cheek or the gum next to the cheek

buffer a chemical substance that, when added to a solution, minimizes fluctuations in pH

buffer system a chemical solution consisting of a weak acid and its salt, which has the ability to minimize changes in pH when adding acid or alkali

bulla a thin-walled blister of the skin, mucous membranes, or lung greater than one centimeter in diameter

BUN abbreviation for blood urea nitrogen, a major by-product of protein metabolism which is normally excreted by the kidneys

buoyancy the physical principle (responsible for floatation) whereby an object submersed in a liquid such as water appears to weigh less than in air

burden of proof the requirement of proving facts in dispute on an issue raised between the parties in a case

by-product a secondary, often unwanted product of a chemical reaction

byte a collection of eight data bits which function as one; one byte can represent a character, and several bytes together can represent a word

C

C a programming language for microcomputers developed by Bell Laboratories; a special version (called C++) deals mainly with object oriented programming (OOP)

CAAHEP abbreviation for the Commission on Accreditation of Allied Health Education Programs, an independent voluntary organization responsible for the accreditation of many allied health educational programs; CAAHEP collaborates with disciplinary review committees such as the Joint Review Committee for Respiratory Therapy Education (JRCRTE)

cachexia general ill health and malnutrition characterized by weakness and emaciation

canals of Lambert intercommunicating channels between terminal bronchioles and the alveoli which are about 30 μm in size and appear to remain open even when bronchiolar smooth muscle is contracted

candidiasis infection of the skin or mucous membranes caused chiefly by the yeastlike fungus Candida albicans; commonly referred to as 'thrush' when localized to the mouth and pharynx; can spread systemically in immunocompromised hosts

cannula any flexible tube that is inserted into the body

cannulation the insertion of a cannula into a body duct or cavity, as into the nose, trachea, bladder, or a blood vessel

capillary action a physical phenomenon whereby a liquid in a small tube tends to move upward, against the force of gravity; due to both adhesive and surface tension forces

capnography the process of obtaining a tracing of the proportion of carbon dioxide in expired air using a capnograph

capnometer an instrument used in anesthesia, respiratory physiology, and respiratory care to measure the proportion of carbon dioxide in expired air

carbamino compound a chemical compound consisting of carbon dioxide combined with one or more free amino groups (NH_2) of a protein molecule

carbonaceous containing a high proportion of carbon

carboxyhemoglobin a compound produced by the chemical combination of hemoglobin with carbon monoxide

carboxyhemoglobinemia a decrease in the oxygen carrying capacity of the blood due the saturation of hemoglobin with carbon monoxide instead of oxygen

carcinogenic of or pertaining to the ability to cause the development of a cancer

cardiac index a standardized measure of cardiac performance equal to a patient's cardiac output in L/min divided by the body surface area in square meters

cardiac tamponade compression of the heart due to the collection of blood, fluid or gas under pressure in the pericardium

cardiogenic originating in or caused by the heart; as in cardiogenic shock

cardiomegaly hypertrophy of the heart caused most frequently by pulmonary hypertension;also occurring in arteriovenous fistula, congenital aortic stenosis, ventricular septal defect, patent ductus arteriousus, and Paget's disease

cardiomyopathy any disease that affects the myocardium, as alcoholic cardiomyopathy

cardioversion the restoration of the heart's normal sinus rhythm by delivery of a synchronized electric shock through two metal paddles placed on the patient's chest

carotid sinus reflex the decrease in the heart rate as a reflex reaction from pressure on or within the carotid artery at the level of its bifurcation

cartilagenous of or pertaining to cartilage

case mix a weighted measure of the types and varieties of patient diagnoses handled by a hospital and used to determine third-party reimbursements

catabolism the destructive phase of metabolism whereby complex substances are broken down into simpler ones, with the concurrent release of energy

catecholamine any one of a group of sympathomimetic compounds composed of a catechol molecule and the aliphatic portion of an amine

catheterization the introduction of a catheter into a body cavity or organ to inject or remove a fluid

cathode the negative pole or electrode of an electrical source

cation an ion that migrates to the cathode (negative electrode) in an electrolytic solution; a positive ion

cationic of or pertaining to positive ions in solution

cavitary pertaining to a process resulting in cavitation, or the lesion so formed

cavitation the formation of cavities within the body, as those formed in the lung by tuberculosis

CBC abbreviation for complete blood count

CC abbreviation for chief complaint

CDC abbreviation for Centers for Disease Control

CD-ROM computer disk read-only memory; similar to audio disks which are read by laser, CD-ROMs are used for access to large unchanging reference databases

cellulitis an infection of the skin characterized most commonly by local heat, redness, pain, and swelling, and sometimes by fever, malaise, chills, and headache

Central Processing Unit (CPU) the primary component of the computer; the CPU houses the core memory, the control component to manage computer system operations, and the arithmetic and logic unit (ALU)

cephalad toward the head

cerebral aneurysm an abnormal localized dilatation of a cerebral artery, most commonly the result of congenital weakness of the media or muscle layer of the vessel wall

cerebral hemorrhage a hemorrhage from a blood vessel in the brain; sometimes called a cerebrovascular accident or CVA

cerebral palsy a motor function disorder caused by a permanent, nonprogressive brain defect or lesion present at birth or shortly thereafter

cerebrospinal pertaining to or involving the brain and the spinal cord

cerebrovascular of or pertaining to the vascular system of the brain

certification a voluntary process whereby a nongovernmental or private agency or association grants recognition to an individual who has met certain predetermined qualifications for recogniton in a given field of study or practice

certified pulmonary function technician (CPFT) an individual, qualified by education and/or experience, who has successfully completed the pulmonary function certification examination of the NBRC

certified respiratory therapy technician (CRTT) a respiratory therapy technician who has successfully completed the technician (entry-level) certification examination of the NBRC

cervical of or pertaining to the neck or the region of the neck

CHAMPUS abbreviation for Civilian Health and Medical Programs of the Uniformed Services

chelating agent a chemical substance that binds metallic ions

chemoreceptor a sensory nerve cell activated by changes in the chemical environment surrounding it, as the chemoreceptors in the carotid artery that are sensitive to the PCO_2 in the blood, signaling the respiratory center in the brain to increase or decrease ventilation

chemotaxis a cell response involving movement either toward or away from a chemical or humorla stimulus

chest physical therapy (CPT) a collection of therapeutic techniques designed to aid clearance of secretion, improve ventilation, and enhance the conditioning of the respiratory muscles; includes positioning techniques; chest percussion and vibration; directed coughing; and various breathing and conditioning exercises

Cheyne-Stokes breathing an abnormal breathing pattern characterized by alternating periods of apnea and periods of rising then falling tidal volumes

CHF abbreviation for congestive heart failure

chip a very small integrated circuit, generally a few centimeters in length, which can handle a large amount of data relative to its size

choanal atresia a congenital anomaly in which a bony or membranous occlusion blocks the passageway between the nose and pharynx

cholesterol an organic monohydric alcohol ($C_{27}H_{45}OH$) widely found in animal tissue

cholinergic of or pertaining to nerve fibers that elaborate acetylcholine at the myoneural junctions

chronotropism the effect of neural or humoral influences on the rate of cardiac contractions; a positive chronotropic effect increases the heart rate, while a negative chronotropic effect decreases the heart rate

civil action action brought to enforce, redress, or protect private rights, including all types of actions other than criminal proceedings

civil law the body of law which every particular nation, state or city establishes to provid civil or private rights and remedies

clearance removal; in aerosol therapy, the process whereby deposited particles are removed from the site of deposition, or the removal of still suspended particles in the exhaled air

clubbing bulbous swelling of the terminal phalanges of the fingers and toes, often associated with certain chronic lung diseases

CMN abbreviation for a certificate of medical necessity; the documentation needed for a patient to receive reimbursement for home O_2 therapy

CMV abbreviation for continuous mandatory ventilation; the application of pressure greater than atmospheric at the airway opening during every inspiration, used to support ventilation; during expiration, pressure returns to atmospheric; CMV may be applied in either the control or assist/control mode

CNS abbreviation for central nervous system

coalescence the growing together of two or more objects, as in the coalescence of water vapor molecules into water droplets

Coanda effect a phenomenon in hydrodynamics whereby a fluid in motion may be attracted or held to a wall

coarctation of the aorta a congenital cardiac anomaly characterized by a localized narrowing of the aorta, which results in increased pressure proximal to the defect and decreased pressure distal to it

COBOL COmmon Business Oriented Language, a high-level programming language used widely for handling business operations and data

coccidioidomycosis an infectious fungal disease caused by the inhalation of spores of the organism Coccidioidcs immitis, which is carried on windborne dust particles

coefficient of elastic expansion (EE) the volumetric expansion of a compressed gas cylinder's under hydrostatic test conditions, expressed in cubic centimeters

coercion compulsion; constraint; compelling by force or arms or threat; the force may be actual, direct, implied, or legal

cohesion the attractive force between like molecules

cohort a collection or sampling of individuals who share a common characteristic, as members of the same age or the same sex

coliform of or pertaining to the colon-aerogenes group, or the Escherichia coli species of microorganisms, constituting most of the intestinal flora in humans and other animals

collagen a protein consisting of bundles of tiny reticular fibrils, which combine to form the white glistening inelastic fibers of the tendons, the ligaments, and the fascia

colloid a state of matter in which large molecules or aggregate of molecules (between 1 and 100 μm) remain dispersed in another medium (like water) without precipitating; egg white, gelatin, and intracellular protoplasm are common examples of colloids

colonization the process by which microorganisms establish a presence and grow in or on the human body; does not necessarily indicate a pathological response

colorimetry measurement of the intensity of color in a fluid or substance

combustible flammable or apt to catch fire

combustion the process of burning; any rapid oxidation with the emission of heat

compensation payment of damages; giving an equivalent or substitute of equal value for a loss sustained

complainant one who applies to the courts for legal redress by filing a complaint; one who instigates prosecution or who prefers accusation against a suspected person

complaint the first document filed in court by the plaintiff to begin a suit

compliance the relative ease with which a body stretches or deforms; in pulmonary physiology, a measure of volume change

per unit pressure change under static conditions; the reciprocal of elastance

computerized tomography (CT) a tomographic method that employs a narrowly collimated beam of X-rays to image the body in cross-sectional slices

CON abbreviation for Certificate of Need, a verification made by a regulatory group that a major capital improvement, such as the addition of a wing to a hospital or the purchase of a MRI device, is needed

concave curved or rounded inward like a bowl

concentric of or pertaining to groups of circles having a common center, like a bull's-eye

concurrent tortfeasor one whose independent, negligent act(s) combined at one point in time to cause injury to a third party

conduction the transfer of heat by the direct interaction of atoms or molecules in a hot area that contact atoms or molecules in a cooler area

conductivity the ability of of myocardial tissue to propagate electrical impulses

congential present at birth, as a congenital anomaly or defect

congenital diaphragmatic hernia an abnormality in the development of the diaphragm resulting in a persistent opening between the abdominal and thoracic cavities; due to displacement of the abdominal contents into the thorax, this condition may impede lung growth and development on the affected side

conjugated protein a protein, such as hemoglobin, that has a characteristic chemical group other than amino acids as part of its structure; in hemoglobin, the globin portion represents the simple amino acid chain, while the four heme chains contain chemical groups other than amino acids

conjunctivitis inflammation of the conjunctiva, caused by bacterial or viral infection, allergy, or environmental factors

consolidation the process of becoming solid; especially applies to the loss of aeration of the terminal respiratory units due to fluid extravasation and the collection of exudate, as in certain forms of pneumonia

constriction a narrowing or squeezing together

constrictive pericarditis an inflammation of the pericardium (usually chronic) in which calcium and fibrous deposits surround the heart and restrict its normal filling

consumerism the philosophy (and popular movement) of promoting the consumers' interests over those of the seller; as applied to health care, the promotion of patient choice and decision-making in the selection of use of health care services

contact transmission transmission of infectious organisms between an infected individual and a host via direct contact, indirect contact, or droplet contact

continuing education educational activity designed to upgrade, enhance, or expand a professional's knowledge or skills which is conducted after completion of formal entry-level educational preparation

contractility the property of muscle tissue to shorten in response to a stimulus, usually electrical

contract, expressed an actual agreement between parties whose terms are stated orally or written, at the time the agreement is made

contract, implied a contract not created or evidenced by the explicit agreement of the parties, but inferred by the law, as a matter of reason and justice from their acts or conducts, making it a reasonable assumption that a contract existed between them by tacit understanding

contracture an abnormal, usually permanent condition of a joint, characterized by flexion and fixation and caused by atrophy and shortening of muscle fibers or by loss of the normal elasticity of the skin, as from the formation of extensive scar tissue over a joint

contraindication any circumstance that renders a particular treatment or treatment approach inadvisable or improper

control mode continuous mandatory ventilation (CMV) in which the frequency of breathing is determined by the ventilator according to a preset cycling pattern without initiation by the patient (time-triggered ventilatory support)

convalescence the period of recovery from an illness, operation, or injury

convex curved or rounded outward like the exterior of a sphere

convection heat transfer through the mixing of fluid molecules at different temperature states via thermal currents

convective of or pertaining to the process of heat transfer by convection

COPD abbreviation for chronic obstructive pulmonary disease; COPD is a broad term used to describe generalized airways obstruction that is not fully reversible with treatment; almost always a mixture of emphysema and chronic bronchitis, with, at times, elements of asthma

cor pulmonale right ventricular hypertrophy/failure and pulmonary hypertension due to certain parenchymal or vascular lung disorders

CORF abbreviation for Comprehensive Out-Patient Rehabilitation Facility; a Medicare-approved facility that provides a broad scope of ambulatory rehabilitation services as defined in section 933 of Public Law 96-499

corroborating that which confirms or supports with evidence

corticosteroid any one of the natural or the synthetic hormones associated with the adrenal cortex, which influences or controls key processes of the body, as carbohydrate and protein metabolism, electrolyte and water balance, and the function of the cardiovascular system and kidneys

costochondral of or pertaining to a rib and its cartilage

costophrenic pertaining to the ribs and diaphragm; especially the angle cormed by the lower ribs intersection with the diaphragmde

costovertebral of or relating to a rib and the vertebral column

countershock a highly-intensity, short duration electric shock applied to the heart, resulting in total depolarization

Coxsackievirus any of 30 serologically different RNA enteroviruses resembling the polio virus; coxsackieviruses primarily affect children and are associated with diseases such as herpangina; hand, foot and mouth disease; myocarditis; pericarditis; and aseptic meningitis

CPAP abbreviation for continuous positive airway pressure; a method of ventilatory support whereby the patient breathes spontaneous without mechanical assistance against threshold resistance, with pressure above atmospheric maintained at the airway throughout breathing

CPFT abbreviation for certified pulmonary function technician

CQI abbreviation for Continous Quality Improvement, a management strategy designed to enhance organization performance

creatinine a substance formed from the metabolism of creaine, commonly found in blood, urine, and muscle tissue

credentialing a broad term referring to the recognition of individuals who have met certain predetermined standards attesting to their occupational skill or competence; includes both licensure and certification

crepitus a dry crackling sound or sensation; may apply to breath sounds, i.e., 'a crepitant rale' or to the sensation felt when palpating an area of subcutaneous emphysema

cricothyrotomy an emergency incision into the larynx between the cricoid and thyroid cartilages, performed to open the airway in a person choking

critical pressure the pressure exerted by a vapor in an evacuated container at its critical temperature

critical temperature the highest temperature at which a substance can exist as a liquid, regardless of pressure

cross-training the process of providing health care professional with multiple skills in areas that span single disciplines, e.g., training a respiratory care practitioner to take chest X-rays

croup an infectious disorder of the upper airway occurring chiefly in infants and children which normally results in subglottic swelling and obstruction;

CRTT abbreviation for certified respiratory therapy technician

cryogenic producing extremely low temperatures

crystalloid of or pertaining to a solution in which ionic compounds serve as the solute

CSF abbreviation for cerebrospinal fluid

cuboidal of or pertaining to the shape of a cube

Cushing's disease a metabolic disorder characterized by the abnormally increased secretion of adrenocortical steroids caused by increased amounts of adrenocorticotropic hormone (ACTH) secreted by the pituitary, as by pituitary adenoma

CVA abbreviation for cerebrovascular accident

CVP abbreviation for central venous pressure, the blood pressure measured in or near the right atrium

CWP abbreviation for coal-workers' pneumoconiosis; CWP is due to chronic exposure to coal dust, which consists mainly of carbon; pathological changes are similar to silicosis

cyanide poisoning poisoning resulting from the ingestion or inhalation of cyanide

cyanosis bluish discoloration of the skin and mucous membranes caused by an excess of deoxygenated hemoglobin in the blood

cyanotic heart disease of or pertaining to anatomic congenital heart defects that cause large right-to-left shunting; such 'venous admixture' results in the characteristic cyanosis

cycling mechanism (ventilator) the means by which a ventilator ends the inspiratory phase of mechanical ventilation, either pressure, volume flow or time

cystic fibrosis an autosomal recessive disease characterized by pancreatic insufficiency, abnormally thick secretions from the exocrine glands, and an increased concentration of sodium and chloride in the sweat glands; known in Europe as mucoviscidosis

cystoscopy the direct visualization of the urinary tract by means of a cystoscope inserted in the urethra

cytochrome oxidase system the major intracellular pathway for oxidative metabolism and energy production

cytokine a chemical or humoral factor that influences cellular proliferation and immune responses; also called peptide regulatory factors

cytomegalovirus a member of a group of large species-specific herpes-type viruses with a wide variety of disease effects

cytologic of or pertaining to the cells

cytotoxic of or pertaining to chemical or biological substances that are lethal to living cells

D

damped referring to a analog waveform in which oscillations have a diminished (and erroneous) amplitude

data any information or arrangement of character set meant to represent information

database a group of related records and files on a direct access storage device, stored in such a way to allow appending, manipulating, and retrieving data

deadspace respired gas volume that does not participate in gas exchange; may be anatomic, alveolar or mechanical

deamidization freeing of the ammonia from an amide

debilitated weakness, especially to the extent of being unable to participate in care

debridement the removal of foreign material and dead tissue from an infected or traumatized area in order to expose healthy tissue

decongestant of or pertaining to a substance or procedure that eliminates or reduces congestion or swelling

decontamination the process whereby contaminants are removed from objects, usually by simple physical means, such as washing

decubitus ulcer an inflammation, sore, or ulcer in the skin over a bony prominence

defendant the person denying the party against whom relief or recovery is sought in an action or suit; also, the accused in a criminal case

defibrillation the termination of ventricular fibrillation by delivering a direct electric countershock to the patient's precordium

deglutition swallowing

demyelination the process of destruction or removal of the myelin sheath from a nerve or nerve fiber

denature as applied to sterilization and disinfection, to alter or break down a protein

density a measure of the mass per unit volume of a substance

dependent (gravity) being bottom-most relative to the earth's gravitational field

depolarization the reduction of a membrane potential to a less negative value; in cardiac fibers, this results in the release calcium ions into the myofibrils and activates the contractile process

deposition the testimony of a witness taken upon interrogatories, either oral or in writting

deponent one who testifies to the truth of certain facts; one whose deposition is given

dermatitis an inflammatory condition of the skin, characterized by erythema and pain or pruritus

desquamate a normal process in which the cornified layer of the epidermis is sloughed in fine scales; also refers to the loss of epithelial cells in general

determinant a causal factor

detoxify the process of removing toxic agents or poisons

dew point the temperature at which water vapor condenses to back to its liquid form

DHHS abbreviation for the federal Department of Health and Human Services

diabetic ketoacidosis an acute, life-threatening complication of uncontrolled diabetes mellitus in which urinary loss of water, potassium, ammonium, and sodium results in hypovolemia, electrolyte imbalance, extremely high blood glucose levels, and the breakdown of free fatty acids, causing a severe metabolic acidosis, often with coma

dialysis the process of separating colloids and crystalline substances in solution by the difference in their rate of diffusion through a semipermeable membrane

diaphoresis the secretion of sweat, especially the profuse secretion associated with an elevated body temperature, physical exertion, exposure to heat, and mental or emotional stress

diaphragmatic hernia the protrusion of part of the stomach through an opening in the diaphragm, most commonly an abnormally enlarged esophageal hiatus

DIC abbreviation for disseminated intravascular coagulation; DIC is a thrombohemorrhagic disorder that accompanies a variety of clinical conditions and involves activation of the clotting cascade, the generation of excess thrombin, intravascular coagulation, occlusion of capillaries and arterioles with fibrin, and tissue ischemia

dichrotic notch a notch on the descending limb of a pulse tracing; especially that seen in the tracing of arterial blood pressure due to closure of the mitral valve

didactic intended for instruction; commonly refers to classroom (as opposed to clinical) learning

diencephalon the division of the brain between the telencephalon and the mesencephalon

diffusion the physical process whereby atoms or molecules tend to move from a area of higher concentration or pressure to an area of lower concentration or pressure

diffusion coefficient the rate of diffusion of a gas; in cgs units, the diffusion coefficient is defined as the number of milliliters of a gas at 1 atmosphere of pressure that will diffuse a distance of 1 μm over a square centimeter surface area per minute

diffusion deposition the deposition of aerosol particle on a surface due to their random bombardment by carry gas molecules

diplegia bilateral paralysis of both sides of any part of the body or of like parts on the opposite sides of the body

diplopia double vision

dipole equal, opposing electrical charges

disability the lack of ability to perform normal mental or physical tasks; especially the loss of mental or physical powers due to injury or disease

disequilibrium a condition characterized by a lack of balance, either literally (as with dizziness) or figuratively, as in any disruption to a homeostatic system

disinfectant a chemical agent capable of destroying at least the vegetative phase of pathogenic microorganisms; there are five major categories of disinfectants used in clinical practice; the alcohols, the phenols and their derivatives, the halogens, the aldehydes, and the quaternary ammonium compounds.

disinfection the process of destroying at least the vegetative phase of pathogenic microorganisms by physical or chemical means

disposition one's attitude toward things or events

distensibility of or pertaining to the ease of inflation or compliance

distillation the condensation of a vapor obtained by heating a liquid; commonly used to separate out liquids with different boiling points as in the production of oxygen by fractional distillation

diuresis increased formation and secretion of urine

diuretic a chemical substance which causes diuresis

DME company a company that manufactures, sells, or rents durable medical equipment

DO$_2$ common abbreviation for delivery of oxygen to the tissues (the product of cardiac output time arterial oxygen content)

DOS abbreviation for disk operating system, a computer operating system allowing access to hard or floppy disks for data storage

DRG abbreviation for Diagnosis Related Group; a system of coding used by the Health Care Financing Administration to set prospective reimbursement schedules for Medicare patients according their diagnosis

due process of law law in its regular course of administration through courts of justice

duodenum the shortest, widest, and most fixed portion of the small intestine, taking an almost circular course from the pyloric valve of the stomach so that its termination is close to its starting point

duty a human action which is exactly conformable to the laws or moral obligations which require us to obey them

duty cycle during breathing, the ratio of inspiratory time to the total time for a complete breathing cycle

dysarthria difficult, poorly articulated speech, resulting from interference in the control over the muscles of speech, usually because of damage to a central or peripheral motor nerve

dysphagia difficulty in swallowing

dysphasia impaired speech

dysphonia same as *dysphasia;* impaired speech

dysplasia a combining form meaning '(condition of) abnormal development'; chondrodysplasia, epidermodysplasia, osteomyelodysplasia

dyspnea a subjective sensation of difficult or labored breathing

dysoxia an abnormal metabolic state in which the tissues are unable to properly utilize the oxygen made available to them

dysynchrony pertaining to ventilatory support, a situation in which interaction between the patient and machine is poorly coordinated, causing extra patient effort and discomfort

E

eccentric in mechanics, off-center, as a drive wheel with an off-center axle or shaft

ECG abbreviation for electrocardiogram

echocardiography a diagnostic procedure for studying the structure and motion of the heart

ECMO abbreviation for extrcorporeal membrane oxygenation; the procedure whereby venous blood is pumped outside the body to a heart-lung machine for oxygenation and returned to the body through an artery

eclampsia the gravest form of toxemia of pregnancy, characterized by grand mal convulsion, coma, hypertension, proteinuria, and edema

ectopic situated in an unusual place, away from its normal location; for example, an ectopic pregnancy is a pregnancy that occurs outside the uterus

edema a local or generalized condition due to the build up of excessive amounts of extracellular fluid and characterized by swelling

EDTA abbreviation for ethylenediaminotetraacetate, a chelating agent used in poisoning with lead or other heavy metals; also used in the treatment of hypercalcemia; overuse can cause hypocalcemia and respiratory and cardiac arrest

EE abbreviation for the coefficient of elastic expansion

effector that which produces an effect; that part of a mechanical or physiologic system which acts to create a specific condition or change

efferent carrying or conduction impulses away from the central nervous system; opposite of afferent

efficacy effectiveness; ability to produce the intended effect

efficacy (of a drug) the peak or maximum biological effect

effort-dependent of or pertaining to a test or procedure the accuracy or success of which depends on patient effort

effort-independent of or pertaining to a test or procedure the accuracy or success of which does not depend on patient effort

effusion the escape of fluid from blood vessels because of rupture or seepage, usually into a body cavity

egocentrism the tendency to be overly concerned with one's self

egophony the sound of normal voice tones as heard through the chest wall during auscultation

EGTA abbreviation for the esophageal gastric tube airway; a modification of the esophageal obturator airway (EOA) that includes a gastric tube which can be extended beyond the distal tip into the stomach in order to remove air or gastric contents

EIP abbreviation for end-inspiratory pause; a technique whereby a specific inflation volume is momentarily held at the end of inspiration during mechanical ventilation, for either therapeutic or diagnostic purposes

ejection fraction (EF) the ratio of cardiac stroke volume to end-diastolic volume

EKG abbreviation for electrocardiogram

elastance (also elasticity) the tendency of matter to resist a stretching force and recoil or return to its original size or form after deformation or expansion; the reciprocal of compliance

elastin a protein that forms the principal substance of yellow elastic tissue fibers

electrocardiography the process of obtaining a tracing of the electrical activity of the heart (an electrocardiogram) for purposes of identifying abnormalities

electrocautery the application of a needle or snare heated by electric current for the destruction of tissue, as for the removal of warts or polyps

electrolysis the process of applying an electrical current across an anode and cathode in a solution, usually to create or enhance a chemical reaction

electrolyte a chemical substance which dissociates into ions when placed into solution, thus becoming capable of conducting electricity

electromyography the recording and study of the electrical properties of muscle

electrooculogram a recording of the electrical activity of the eye muscles, indicating type and magnitude of eye movements

electrophysiology the recording and study of the electrical properties of living tissue

ELISA abbreviation for enzyme-linked immunosorbent assay, a test commonly used to detect the presence of antibodies to specific infectious agents, such as the HIV virus

embolectomy a surgical incision into an artery for the removal of an embolus or clot, performed as emergency treatment for arterial embolization

embolization the process by which an embolus forms and lodges in a branch of the vasculature

embolus a foreign object, a quantity of air or gas, a bit of tissue or tumor, or a piece of a thrombus that circulates in the bloodstream until it becomes lodged in a vessel

emetic of or pertaining to a substance that causes vomiting

emphysema a destructive process of the lung parenchyma leading to permanent enlargement of the distal airspaces; classified as either centrilobular (CLE), which mainly involves the respiratory bronchioles, or panlobular (PLE) which can involve the entire terminal respiratory unit

empirical ascertained or discovered by observation

empyema an accumulation of pus in a body cavity, especially the pleural space, as a result of bacterial infection, as pleurisy or tuberculosis

emulsification the process of mixing two or more substances which are not mutually soluble into a uniform dispersion; specifically applies to the breakdown of fat globules in the intestines via the action of bile acids

encode in data communications, the process of preparing a message for transmission

endobronchial within a bronchus

endocarditis inflammation of endocardium and the heart valves, as caused by a variety of diseases

endocrine system the network of ductless glands and other structure that elaborate and secrete hormones directly into the bloodstream, affecting the function of specific target organs

endogenous growing within or arising from the body

endorphin any one of the neuropeptides composed of many amino acids, elaborated by the pituitary gland and acting on the central and the peripheral nervous systems to reduce pain

endoscopy the visualization of the interior of organs and cavities of the body with an endoscope

endothelium the layer of squamous epithelial cells that lines the heart, the blood and the lymph vessels, and the serous cavities of the body

endotracheal within or through the trachea

enteric of or pertaining to the intestinal tract

Enterobacteriaceae a family of aerobic and anaerobic bacteria that includes both normal and pathogenic enteric microorganisms

enterocolitis an inflammation involving both the large and small intestines

entitlement a right or claim; alternatively the process of granting or providing a right, such as the right to adequate health care

enzyme an organic catalyst produced by living cells

EOA abbreviation for esophageal obturator airway; the EOA consists of a cuffed hollow tube tipped with a soft plastic obturator at its tip; the tube passes through a mask and has several holes in its upper portion; once passed into the esophagus, the cuff is inflated, thereby preventing aspiration and allowing ventilation with positive pressure

eosinophilia an increase in the number of eosinophils in the blood, accompanying many inflammatory conditions

EPAP abbreviation for expiratory positive airway pressure, or the application of positive pressure to the airway during expiration only (as opposed to continuous positive airway pressure)

epidemiology the study of the relationships among various factors and the distribution and frequency of diseases in the population

epigastric of or pertaining to the epigastrium

epigastrium the part of the abdomen in the upper zone between the right and left hypochondriac regions

epiglottitis an acute and often life-threatening infection of the upper airway which causes severe obstruction secondary to supraglottic swelling; caused primarily by *Haemophilus influenzae,* type B, and affecting mainly children under the age of five

epinephrine an adrenal hormone and synthetic adrenergic vasoconstrictor

epistaxis bleeding from the nose caused by local irritation of mucous membranes, violent sneezing, fragility of the mucous membrane or of the arterial walls, chronic infection, trauma, hypertension, leukemia, vitamin K deficiency, or most often, picking of the nose

epithelium the covering of the internal and external organs of the body, including the lining of vessels

Epstein-Barr virus the herpesvirus associated with infectious mononucleosis

equal pressure point (EPP) during forced exhalation, the point along an airway where the pressure inside its wall equals the intrapleural pressure; upstream beyond this point, the pleural pressure exceeds the pressure inside the airway, tending to promote bronchiolar collapse

equilibrate to bring into balance

equilibration the process of bringing into balance

eradicate to eliminate

ergometer an apparatus designed to measure the amount of work performed by an animal or human subject

erythema a redness of the skin due to capillary congestion; caused by injury, inflammation, or infection

erythema nodosum a hypersensitivity vasculitis characterized by tender red subcutaneous nodules on the shins and associated with strep infections, TB, and sarcoidosis

erythrocyte a red blood cell

erythrocythemia an increase in the number of erythrocytes circulating in the blood

erythrocytosis the process resulting in an abnormal increase in the number of circulating red cells

erythropoiesis the process of erythrocyte production involving the maturation of a nucleated precursor into a hemoglobin-filled, nucleus-free erythrocyte that is regulated by erythropoietin, a hormone produced by the kidney

esophageal opening pressure the oral pressure at which the esophagus distends and opens, allowing gas to insufflate the stomach; estimated to range from 20 to 25 cm H_2O

ethacrynic acid a potent diuretic

ethnicity racial origin

ethylene chlorohydrin a chemical substance toxic to living tissue that is formed when polyvinyl chloride reacts with ethylene oxide gas

ethylene oxide a gas used to sterilize surgical instruments and other supplies

EtO common abbreviation for ethylene oxide

eukaryotic of or pertaining to cells with true nuclei bounded by a nuclear membrane and capable of mitosis

evacuate to remove or withdraw from, especially to empty of air and create a vacuum

evaporation the change in state of a substance from its liquid to its gaseous form occurring below its boiling point

exacerbate to worsen

exacerbation a worsening of a condition, usually acutely

excitability a property of myocardial tissue, shared with other muscle and nerve tissues, and representing a responsiveness to stimulation caused by electrical, chemical, or mechanical factors in the cell or in its surrounding environment

exfoliate to fall off in layers

expectorant a chemical agent that promotes the expectoration of respiratory tract secretions, usually by increasing their production or by lowering their viscosity

expiratory reserve volume (ERV) the total amount of gas that can be exhaled from the lung following a quiet exhalation

expiratory resistance (retard) a modification of the expiratory phase of positive pressure ventilation in which a restricted orifice, or flow resistor, is used to slow the flow of exhaled gases from the patient

exponential a nonlinear relationship between two variables in which one varies with a power of the other, e.g., $x=y^2$

extracellular occurring outside a cell or cell tissue or in cavities or spaces between cell layers or groups of cells

extracorporeal something that is outside the body, as extracorporeal circulation in which venous blood is diverted outside the body to a heart-lung machine and returned to the body through a femoral or other artery

extrapolation to infer unknown data from known data, as to extrapolate a value existing between two known points on a curve

extrasystole cardiac contraction that is abnormal in timing or in origin of impulse with respect to the fundamental rhythm of the heart

extrathoracic outside the thorax

extrauterine occurring or located outside the uterus

extravasation a passage or escape into the tissues, usually of blood, serum or lymph

extrinsic allergic alveolitis an inflammatory form of interstitial pneumonia that results from a Type III or immune complex antigen-antibody reactions to certain organic dusts

extubate withdrawing a tube from an orifice or cavity of the body

exudate a fluid with a high protein content that escapes into the extracellular space; usually due to inflammation or infection

F

facultative not obligatory, having the ability to adapt to more than one condition, as a facultative anaerobe that can live with or without oxygen

false imprisonment the unlawful arrest or detention of a person without warrant, or by an illegal warrant, or by an illegally executed warrant

fasciculation a small involuntary muscular contraction visible under the skin

faucial of or pertaining to the fauces, the constricted opening leading from the mouth to the oropharynx and bounded by the soft palate, base of tongue, and the palatine arches

FDO$_2$ the fraction of oxygen delivered by a oxygen therapy device; same as FIO_2 (inspired oxygen fraction) for high flow systems, but always higher than FIO_2 for low flow systems

feedback that portion of the output of a dynamic system that is returned as input to control or vary the underlying process; in human communication, feedback represents a message returned by the receiver to the sender to help enhance meaning between the parties

fenestrated open like a window; from the Latin fenestra, meaning 'window'

fenestrated tracheotomy tube a double cannulated tracheotomy tube tube that has an opening in the posterior wall of the outer cannula above the cuff; removal of the inner cannula allows free breathing through the tube

fermentation the oxidative decomposition of substances via enzymes produced by microorganisms

fetid foul-smelling

FDA abbreviation for the Food and Drug Administration, the federal agency responsible for overseeing the testing and assuring the purity and effectiveness of drugs

FFB abbreviation for flexible fiberoptic bronchoscope

fibrinolysis a continual process of fibrin decomposition by fibrinolysin that is the normal mechanism for the removal of small fibrin clots

fibroplasia the formation of fibrous tissue

fibrosis synonym for fibroplasia

file a group of related records forming a data structure accessible by computer; also, a unit of disk storage for computer programs or data

filling density the ratio between the weight of liquid gas put into the cylinder and the weight of water the cylinder could contain if full; for example, the filling density for carbon dioxide is 68%

fissure a narrow cleft or slit

fistula any tubelike passageway between two organs or between an organ and the body surface

fixed acid a titratable, nonvolatile acid representing the byproduct of protein catabolism, examples include such as phosporic or sulfuric acid

flaccid weak or flabby; especially as applied to muscles lacking normal tone

flail chest a traumatic chest injury in which a portion of the rib cage becomes unstable due to multiple rib fractures or costochondral separation; typically, the flail region exhibits paradoxical movement during inspiration, contributing to a maldistribution of ventilation

flange a rim used to strengthen an object, to help guide it, to facilitate its attachment to another object

floppy disk a thin plastic disk, usually 5.25 or 3.5 inches in diameter, used for magnetic storage of computer files; also called a diskette

flow generator a ventilator which delivers a flow pattern that is independent of the patient's respiratory mechanics or effort

flowmeter a device operated by a needle valve that controls and measures gas flow, according to the principles of viscosity and density

flow restrictor a fixed orifice, constant pressure flow metering device

fluidics a branch of engineering in which hydrodynamic principles are incorporated into flow circuits for such purposes as switching, pressure and flow sensing, and amplification

FMG abbreviation for foreign medical graduate; a physician whose undergraduate medical education was not completed in the US

fomite nonliving material, such as bed linens or equipment, which may transmit pathogenic organisms

foramina pleural form of foramen, an opening in a membraneous structure or bone

forced expiration technique (FET) a modification of the normal cough sequence designed to facilitate clearance of bronchial secretions while minimizing the likelihood of bronchiolar collapse

for-profit designed to generate revenues in excess of expenditures for the benefit of owners or shareholders

FORTRAN FORmula TRANslator, a high-level programming language mainly for the execution of mathematical programs

fossa a hollow or depression, especially on the surface of the end of a bone, as the olecranon fossa or the coranoid fossa

fractional distillation the process of separating the components of a liquid mixture according to their boiling points via the application of heat; the primary commercial process used to produce oxygen

FRC abbreviation for functional residual capacity

fremitus a tremulous vibration of the chest wall that can be auscultated or palpated during physical examination

French scale a measurement scale used commonly to delineate the diameter of catheters; 1 French unit equals approximately 0.33 mm

Freon a trademark for a hydrocarbon gas commonly used as a refrigerant and propellant

FTE abbreviation for full-time equivalent, a unit corresponding to the number of hours per week (or month or year) worked by a normal full-time employee

fungicide an agent destructive to fungi

functional residual capacity (FRC) the total amount of gas left in the lungs after a resting expiration

function key special keys available on most computer keyboards that can be programmed to perform special or often used functions; often preceded by the letter F (F1, F2)

furosemide (Lasix) a rapid acting sulfonamide diuretic and antihypertensive agent; inhibits reabsorption of sodium and chloride in the loop of Henle, and the proximal and distal tubules; also enhances the excretion of potassium, calcium, hydrogen and bicarbonate ions; can cause hypokalemic metabolic alkalosis and hypocalcemic tetany

FVC abbreviation for forced vital capacity

G

galvanometer an instrument that measures the flow of electrical current by electromagnetic action

gastroenteritis inflammation of the stomach and intestines accompanying numerous GI disorders

gastrointestinal of or pertaining to the organs of the GI tract, from mouth to anus

gaw abbreviation for gram atomic weight; the atomic weight of an element expressed in grams

GDP abbreviation for gross dosmetic product, a measure of the total value of all goods and services produced in the United States in a given year

genitourinary referring to the genital and urinary systems of the body, either the organ structures or functions or both

gEq abbreviation for gram equivalence; the weight in grams of an ion that will combine with or replace one mole of hydrogen ions or one mole of electrons

gestation the period of development of the embryo and fetus from fertilization of the ovum to birth

globin the protein component of hemoglobin

glomerulonephritis an inflammation of the glomerulus of the kidney, characterized by proteinuria, hematuria, decreased urine production and edema

glomerulus the network of vascular tufts in the nephron responsible for filtration of plasma

glossopharyngeal of or pertaining to the tongue and pharynx

glucocorticoid an adrenocortical steroid hormone that increases glyconeogenesis, exerts an antiinflammatory effect, and influences many body functions

glutamine a nonessential amino acid found in many proteins in the body

glutaraldehyde a high level disinfectant solution that can also be used as a sterilant

goiter a hypertrophic thyroid gland associated with abnormal thyroid function

Goodpasture's syndrome a chronic relapsing pulmonary hemosiderosis, usually associated with glomerulonephritis and characterized by a cough with hemoptysis, dyspnea, anemia, and progressive renal failure

granulocytopenia an abnormal condition of the blood, characterized by a decrease in the total number of granulocytes

granuloma a circumscribed mass of cells (mainly histiocytes) normally associated with the presence of chronic infection or inflammation

granulomatous composed of or having the characteristics of a granuloma

gravida a combing form indicating number of pregnancies, e.g., gravida 2 indicates two pregnancies

Guillain-Barre syndrome an idiopathic, peripheral polyneuritis characterized by lower extremity weakness that progresses to the upper extremities and face; may lead to flaccid paraplegia and marked respiratory muscle weakness

gylcocalyx a film composed of polysaccharides and bacteria which forms on the surface of artificial devices such as tracheal airways; glycocalyx seems to protect the bacteria from antibiotics and phagocytosis by macrophages

gynecology the branch of medicine involved in the diagnosis and treatment of diseases of the female genital tract

H

Haldane effect the influence of hemoglobin saturation with oxygen on CO_2 dissociation

half-life in pharmacology, the time taken by the body to decrease a given concentration of a drug to half its initial level

hardcopy computer output which is physically represented on paper such as graphs or printed material

hard disk a magnetic disk for storing data which can store more data than a floppy disk and access that data much more quickly; also called a fixed disk

Hb common abbreviation for hemoglobin

HbA abbreviation for hemoglobin A, or normal adult hemoglobin

HbCO abbreviation for carboxyhemoglobin, hemoglobin saturated with carbon monoxide

HCFA abbreviation for the federal Health Care Financing Administration, the division of the Department of Health and Human Services responsible for Medicare funding

health a state of physical, mental, and social well-being

health education a process of planned learning opportunities designed to enable individuals to make informed decisions about and act to promote their health

health maintenance organization (HMO) an organized system providing a comprehensive range of health care services to a voluntarily enrolled consumer population; in return for a prepaid, fixed fee, the enrollee is guaranteed a defined set of benefits

health promotion that combination of educational, organization, economic and environmental support necessary for behavior conducive to health; includes both disease prevention and wellness activities

health services activities designed to maintain or improve health. Includes public health services (e.g., communicable disease control); environmental health services (e.g., air pollution control); and personal health services (e.g., diagnosis, treatment, and rehabilitation)

heat capacity the number of calories required to raise the temperature of 1 g of a substance 1°C (cgs) or 1 pound of a substance 1°F (fps); by definition, the heat capacity of water is 1 cal in the cgs system and 1 BTU in the fps system

heat-labile subject to damage or destruction by high temperatures

Heimlich maneuver an emergency procedure for dislodging a bolus of food or other obstruction from the trachea to prevent asphyxiation

hematocrit a measure of the packed cell blood volume, obtained by centrifugation of a blood sample

hematogenous originating or transported in the blood

hematology the branch of medicine involved in the study of blood morphology, physiology and pathology

hematopoiesis the normal formation and development of blood cells in the bone marrow

heme the pigmented iron-containing, nonprotein portion of the hemoglobin molecule

hemidiaphragm pertaining to the left or right dome of the diaphragm

hemithorax either the left or right side of the thorax

hemizygos vein a large vein of the lower left thoracic wall which empties into the azygos vein (trunk connecting the superior and inferior vena cavae)

hemorrhage the escape of blood from the vascular system

hemodialysis a procedure in which impurities or wastes are removed from the blood, used in treating renal insufficiency and various toxic conditions

hemodynamic monitoring the bedside collection of data on the performance of the cardiovascular system, including the assessment of both cardiac and vascular parameters

hemolysis rupture of the red blood cells

hemoptysis coughing up of blood from the respiratory tract

hemosiderosis an increased deposition of iron in a variety of tissues, usually in the form of hemosiderin, and usually without tissue damage

hemostasis the termination of bleeding by mechanic or chemical means or by the complex coagulation process of the body, consisting of vasoconstriction, platelet aggregation, and thrombin and fibrin synthesis

hemothorax an accumulation of blood and fluid in the pleural cavity, between the parietal and visceral pleura, usually the result of trauma

HEPA abbreviation for 'high efficiency particulate air,' usually applied to air filtration devices capable of 99.99% efficacy on particulate matter down to 0.3 μm in size

hepatomegaly abnormal enlargement of the liver

Hering-Breuer reflex a parasympathetic inflation reflex mediated via the lung's stretch receptors which appears to influence the duration of the expiratory pause occurring between breaths

herniation a protrusion of a body organ or portion of an organ through an abnormal opening in a membrane

herpes any inflammatory disease caused by a herpesvirus, especially herpes zoster or herpes simplex

heterogeneous not of uniform structure or composition

hexachlorophene a topical bacteriocide and detergent

HFJV abbreviation for high frequency jet ventilation, a mode of ventilatory support in which small pulses of pressurized gas are delivered through a catheter at rates between 100 and 200/min, as controlled by a pneumatic, electric, or mechanical valve assembly

HFO abbreviation for high frequency oscillation, a mode of ventilatory support characterized by extremely high rates (ranging up 3600/min), with 'tidal volumes' in the 1.5 to 3.0 mL/kg range, as controlled by an eccentric wheel-driven piston, an audio loudspeaker, or a rotating flow interrupter

HFPPV abbreviation for high frequency positive pressure ventilation, a mode of ventilatory support characterized by rates between 60 and 100/min, I:E ratios of 1:3 or less, and small tidal volumes, often approaching the anatomic deadspace

HHA abbreviation for home health agency; a public or private provider of home health care services, usually regulated by state departments of health; HHAs can provide a broad range of services, including the provision of home health aids, nursing care and rehabilitative personnel

HHb symbol for reduced (deoxygenated) hemoglobin

hiatal hernia the protrusion of any abdominal structure through the esophageal hiatus

hierarchical of or pertaining to an organizational structure

high frequency ventilation ventilatory support provided at rates significantly higher than normal breathing frequencies; see *HFPPV*, *HFJV*, and *HFO*

high level language a computer programming language such as BASIC, C, or PASCAL which can accommodate a variety of functions and is not dependent on the machine language of a computer The primary advantage of high level languages is that commands use forms of English words descriptive of the task they perform

hilum (also hilus) a depression in any organ where blood vessels and nerves enter or exit; especially as pertains to the 'root' of the lung

histoplasmosis an infection caused by inhalation of spores of the fungus *Histoplasma capsulatum*

histotoxic poisonous to cells

histotoxic hypoxia hypoxia due to chemical poisoning of the cells, as by cyanide, which occurs in the presence of normal oxygen delivery to the tissues

HIV abbreviation for the human immunodeficiency virus, the cause of AIDS

HME abbreviation for heat and moisture exchanger, a passive device used to humidify and warm the inpired air of patients receiving ventilatory support

HMO abbreviation for *health maintenance organization*

holistic of or pertaining to the whole; in health care, a philosophy whereby the person is viewed in totality as a mental, physical and emotional being interacting with the environment

home health care the provision of health services in the home setting to aged, disabled, sick or convalescent individuals who do not need institutional care

homeostasis a relative constancy in the internal environment of the body, naturally maintained by adaptive responses that promote healthy survival

homogeneous of uniform structure or composition

host (computer) the primary or controlling computer which directs the operations of a group of other computers; or a central information system or database which can be accessed by multiple users

humidity water in molecular vapor form; absolute humidity is a measure of the actual content or weight of water present in a given volume of air; relative humidity is the ratio of actual water vapor present in a gas to the capacity of the gas to hold the vapor at a given temperature

humoral of or pertaining to the body fluids; used especially to denote physiological activity occurring via chemical or biological mediators in the body fluids (as opposed to neurologic stimulation)

hydrolysis the chemical alteration or decomposition of a compound with water

hydrodynamics the branch of fluid physics involved in the study of fluids in motion

hydronium ion the hydrated form of the hydrogen ion (H_3O^+)

hydrostatic of or pertaining to the physics of static fluids (as opposed to hydrodynamics)

hydroxyl ion a radical alkaline compound containing an oxygen atom and a hydrogen atom (OH^-)

hygrometer an instrument for measuring relative humidity

hyperalimentation overfeeding or the ingestion or administration of a greater than optimal amount of nutrients in excess of the demands of the appetite

hyperbaric oxygenation the therapeutic application of oxygen at pressures greater than one atmosphere (1 atm or 760 torr)

hyperbasemia the abnormal presence of an excess of total buffer base in the blood; a base excess (BE) greater than 2.0

hyperbilirubinemia greater than normal amounts of the bile pigment bilirubin in the blood, often characterized by jaundice, anorexia, and malaise (normal blood levels for total bilirubin range from 0.2 to 0.9 mg/dL)

hypercalcemia greater than normal amounts of calcium in the blood, most often resulting from excessive bone resorption and release of calcium, as occurs in hyperparathyroidism, metastatic tumors of bone, Paget's disease, and osteoporosis (normal serum calcium levels range from 8.5 to 10.5 mg/L or 4.25 to 5.25 mEq/L)

hypercapnia the abnormal presence of excess amounts of carbon dioxide in the blood (in arterial blood, a PCO_2 greater than 45 torr)

hyperchloremia an excessive level of chloride in the blood (normal serum levels of chloride range between 96 and 105 mEq/L)

hyperextension a position of maximum extension

hyperinflation a condition of maximum inflation; as pertaining to artificial ventilatory support, the application of volumes greater than normal to reinflate collapsed alveoli

hyperkalemia greater than normal amounts of potassium in the blood (normal serum potassium concentrations range from 3.5 to 5.0 mEq/L)

hyperlucent extremely clear or transparent; as applied to X-rays, allowing easy X-rays penetration and thus appearing black on the negative film

hypernatremia greater than normal concentration of sodium in the blood, caused by excessive loss of water and electrolytes owing to polyuria, diarrhea, excessive sweating, or inadequate water intake (normal serum concentration of sodium range from 135 to 145 mEq/L)

hyperosmolarity a state of condition of abnormally increased osmolarity in the blood or body fluids (normal blood osmolarity ranges from 285 to 295 mOsm/L)

hyperoxia a condition of abnormally high oxygen tension in the blood

hyperoxygenation the application of oxygen concentrations in excess of those needed to maintain adequate oxygenation in order to prevent hypoxemia during certain procedures such as suctioning

hyperphosphatemia greater than normal concentration of phosphate ions in the blood (normal serum levels of phosphate range from (1.2 to 2.3 mEq/L, or 2.0 to 4.5 mg/dL, with higher values in children)

hyperplasia an increase in the size of a tissue or organ due to a growth in the number of cells present

hyperplastic of or pertaining to a condition of hyperplasia

hyperpnea deep breathing

hyperpyrexia an extremely elevated temperature sometimes occurring in acute infectious diseases, especially in young children

hyperreactivity a condition characterized by greater than normal response to stimuli

hyperreflexia a condition characterized by exaggerated reflex responses

hypersensitivity of or pertaining to a tendency of the immune system to exhibit an excessive or exaggerated response against environmental antigens that are not normally harmful

hypersomnolence a condition characterized by pathologically excessive drowsiness or sleep

hypertension persistently high blood pressure

hyperthyroidism a condition characterized by hyperactivity of the thyroid gland

hypertonic having a greater concentration of solute than another solution, hence exerting more osmotic pressure than that solution, as a hypertonic saline solution that contains more salt than is found in bodily fluids

hypertrophy an increase in the size of a tissue or organ due to a growth in the size of cells present

hyperventilation ventilation in excess of that necessary to meet metabolic needs; signified by a PCO_2 less than 35 torr in the arterial blood

hypervolemia an increase in the amount of extracellular fluid, particularly in the volume of circulating blood or its components

hypnotic a drug or chemical agent that induces sleep

hypobarism pertaining to the effects of exposure to pressures less than those normally encountered at sea level; often used to refer to high-altitude sickness

hypobasemia the abnormal presence of a deficit of total buffer base in the blood; a negative base excess (BE) greater than −2.0

hypocalcemia a deficiency of calcium in the serum that may be caused by hypoparathyroidism, vitamin D deficiency, kidney failure, acute pancreatitis, or inadequate plasma magnesium and protein (normal serum calcium levels range from 8.5 to 10.5 mg/L or 4.25 to 5.25 mEq/L)

hypocapnia the presence of lower than normal amounts of carbon dioxide in the blood (in arterial blood, a PCO_2 less than 35 torr)

hypochloremia a decrease in the chloride level in the blood serum below the normal range (normal serum levels of chloride range between 96 and 105 mEq/L)

hypoglycemia a less-than-normal amount of glucose in the blood, usually caused by administration of too much insulin, excessive secretion of insulin by the islet cells of the pancreas, or by dietary deficiency (normal blood glucose levels range from 70 to 110 mg/dL)

hypokalemia a condition in which an inadequate amount of potassium, the major intracellular cation, is found in the circulating bloodstream (normal serum potassium concentrations range from 3.5 to 5.0 mEq/L)

hyponatremia a less than normal concentration of sodium in the blood, caused by inadequate excretion of water or by excessive water in the circulating bloodstream (normal serum concentration of sodium range from 135 to 145 mEq/L)

hypoparathyroidism a condition of decreased parathyroid function

hypopharynx the lowest portion of the pharynx, just above the larynx (also called the laryngopharynx)

hypopnea shallow breathing

hypotension an abnormal condition in which the blood pressure is not adequate for normal perfusion and oxygenation of the tissues

hypothalamus a portion of the brain lying beneath the thalamus and at the base of the cerebrum; responsible for temperature regulation, certain behavioral functions, and the secretory activities of the pituitary gland

hypothermia an abnormal and dangerous condition in which the temperature of the body is below 32° C, usually owing to prolonged exposure to cold

hypothyroidism a condition characterized by decreased activity of the thyroid gland

hypotonia a condition characterized by decreased muscle tone or strength

hypoventilation ventilation less than that necessary to meet metabolic needs; signified by a PCO_2 greater than 45 torr in the arterial blood

hypovolemia an abnormally low circulating blood volume

hypoxemia an abnormal deficiency of oxygen in the arterial blood

hypoxia an abnormal condition in which the oxygen available to the body cells is inadequate to meet their metabolic needs

hysteresis the failure of two associated phenomena to coincide, as in the observed difference between the inflation and deflation volume-pressure curves of the lung

Hz symbol for Hertz, a physical terms meaning cycles per second

---

I _____

iatrogenic caused by treatment or diagnostic procedures

ICP abbreviation for intracranial pressure

idiopathic without known cause

IEEE abbreviation for the Institute of Electrical and Electronic Engineers a voluntary group responsible, in part, for developing standards related to electrical devices and equipment, including those used in respiratory care

I:E ratio the ratio of inspiratory to expiratory time during mechanical ventilation; by convention, the ratio is always reduced so that the numerator (inspiratory time) equals 1, e.g., 1:4 or 1:2.5

ileus an obstruction of the intestines, as an a dynamic ileus caused by immobility of the bowel, or a mechanical ileus in which the intestine is blocked by mechanical means

ILV abbreviation for independent lung ventilation, a mode of ventilation in which each lung receives a different level or type of support

immunocompromised immunodeficient

immunodeficient pertaining to conditions in which a patient's cellular or humoral immunity is inadequate and resistance to infection is decreased

immunofluorescence a technique used for the rapid identification of an antigen by exposing it to known antibodies tagged with the fluorescent dye fluorescein and observing the characteristic antigen-antibody reaction of precipitation

immunoglobin (immunoglobulin) any five structurally and antigenically distinct antibodies present in the serum and external secretions of the body, and formed in response to specific antigens

immunosuppressed of or pertaining to the purposeful administration of agents designed to interfere with the ability of the immune system to respond to antigenic stimulation

impairment a decrease in ability, either mental or physical

impedance (electrical) a form of electrical resistance observed in an alternating circuit expressed as the ratio of voltage applied to current produced

impedance (mechanical) the force opposing movement in a mechanical system; as applied to ventilatory mechanics, the sum of the resistive and elastic forces opposing inflation

IMV abbreviation for intermittent mandatory ventilation; periodic ventilation with positive pressure, with the patient breathing spontaneously between breaths. These periodic breaths may be either time-triggered (control mode IMV) or patient-triggered (synchronous intermittent mandatory ventilation, or SIMV)

inadvertent accidental or unintentional

incisura a cut, notch, indentation or depression; often used to refer to the dicrotic notch observed on the tracing of arterial blood pressure

incoherent unable to think or express one's thoughts in a clear manner

induration hardening of tissue, particularly the skin

indwelling located inside the body; common refers to invasive diagnostic or therapeutic devices

inert not taking part in chemical reactions; not pharmacologically active

infarction the development and formation of a localized area of tissue necrosis

infiltrate a fluid that passes through body tissues

influenza an acute, usually self-limiting infectious viral disorder that produces fever, myalgia, headache, and malaise

informed consent a general principle of law which states that health professionals have a duty to disclose what a reasonably prudent health professional in the medical community in the exercise of reasonable care would disclose to a patient as to whatever grave risks of injury might be incurred from a proposed course of treatment

infrared (light) electromagnetic radiation with wavelengths between 10^{-5} and 10^{-4} meters; infrared radiation is perceived as heat when it strikes the body

infrastructure pertaining to physical facilities and associated structures; e.g., buildings, parking decks, power generating stations

inguinal of or pertaining to the groin

inherent rhythmicity the unique ability of cardiac muscle to spontaneously originate an electrical impulse; also called automaticity

innominate without a name; commonly refers to the innominate artery, also called the brachiocephalic trunk

inoculum a substance introduced into the body to cause or to increase immunity to a specific disease or condition

inotropic pertaining to the force or energy of muscular contractions, particularly contractions of the heart muscle

input the data fed into a computer or program which is used to generate the output

insensible water loss the loss of body fluids by means other than through the urinary system, GI tract, or sweating; includes evaporative water loss through the lungs and skin

in-service education a program of education or training occurring at the work site and provided for employees, usually based on the needs of the employing institution

in situ in the natural or usual place

insomnia inability to sleep

inspiratory capacity (IC) the maximum amount of air that can be inhaled from the resting end-expiratory level or FRC; the sum of the tidal volume and inspiratory reserve volume

inspiratory reserve volume (IRV) the maximum volume of air that can be inhaled following a normal quiet inspiration

inspissated (of a fluid) thickened or hardened through the absorption or evaporation of the liquid portion, as can occur with respiratory secretion when the upper airway is bypassed

instill to introduce a fluid into a body cavity or passage

instruction (computer) a command which orders the computer to perform a specific task

insufflation blowing of a gas or powder into a tube, cavity, or organ to allow visual examination, to remove an obstruction, or to apply medication

integrated circuit (IC) a circuit residing on a small silicon chip within which all the electronic components of the entire circuit are contained

intent the design, resolve, or determination with which a person acts; the state of mind with which the act is done or omitted

intercartilaginous of or pertaining to the space between cartilages; especially the space between the costal cartilages

intercellular between or among cells

intercostal of or pertaining to the space between two ribs

interdisciplinary pertaining to the relationship between two or more disciplines

interface the means of connection between electronic devices or between an electronic device and a human

intermammary between the mammary glands or breasts

interosseous of or pertaining to the space between two bones

interpersonal between persons; usually refers to a communication context

interphase between phases; the metabolic stage in the cell cycle during which the cell is not dividing; also the 'dividing line' between two states of matter

interrogatories a set or series of written questions drawn up for the purpose of being addresses to a party, witness, or other person having information of interest in the case

interstitial of or pertaining to the interstitium

interstitium the extracellular space

interventricular of or pertaining to the space between the ventricles of the heart

intervertebral of or pertaining to the space between any two vertebrae, as the fibrocartilaginous discs

intra-abdominal within the abdomen

intraalveolar within the alveoli

intra-aortic balloon counterpulsation a circulatory support technique in which a balloon placed in the aorta is synchronously inflated during diastole in order to increase mean aortic pressures and coronary blood flow to the myocardium

intrabursal within the bursa; often used to refer to the synovial fluid 'sack'

intracardiac within the heart

intracellular within cells

intracranial with the cranium

intractable having no relief, as a symptom or disease that remains unrelieved despite the application of therapeutic measures

intramuscular within a muscle; used commonly to refer to an injection method whereby a hypodermic needle is introduced into a muscle to administer a medication

intraoperative within or during a surgical procedure

intrapartum of or pertaining to the period commencing from the onset of labor to the completion of the third stage of labor (expulsion of the placenta)

intrapersonal within one's self

intrapleural within the pleural 'space'

intrapulmonary within the lungs

intrathoracic within the thorax

intrauterine within the uterus

intravascular within a blood vessel or in the vascular fluid compartment

intravenous (IV) within a vein; usually describing a method for infusing fluids and drugs

intubation the passage of a tube into a body aperture; commonly refers to the insertion of an endotracheal tube within the trachea

in utero in the uterus

invasive characterized by a tendency to spread or infiltrate; also refers to the use of diagnostic or therapeutic methods requiring access to the inside of the body

in vitro (of a biological reaction) occurring in a laboratory apparatus

in vivo (of a biological reaction) occurring in a living organism

I/O abbreviation for intake and output; the recording of a patient's fluid intake and output; may also refers to computer input/output

iodophor an antiseptic or disinfectant that combines iodine with another agent

IPPB abbreviation for intermittent positive pressure breathing; the application of inspiratory positive pressure, usually with accompanying humidity or aerosol therapy, to a spontaneously breathing patient as a short-term treatment modality, usually for periods of time not exceeding 15 to 20 minutes

IPPV common abbreviation for intermittent positive pressure ventilation, a general term for ventilatory support using positive pressure

iridium a silvery-bluish metallic element, the radioactive form of which (Ir 192) is used in endobronchial radiotherapy

ischemia a localized reductions in perfusion to a body organ or part, often marked by pain and organ dysfunction, as in ischemic heart disease

ISO abbreviation for the International Standards Organization, a nongovernmental agency that sets standards for various technical equipment and procedures

isoelectric of or pertaining to a condition of electrical neutrality; also refers to the electric base line of an electrocardiogram

isoelectric point the pH at which an electrolytic compound is dissociated into an equal number of positively and negatively charged ion

isolation protocols infection control measures that combine barrier-type precautions (include handwashing, and the use of gloves masks and/or gowns) with the physical separation of infected patients in specific disease categories in order to disrupt transmission of pathogenic microorganisms

isomer a chemical compound with the exact same molecular formula as another, but with a different geometric structure

isopleth a line on a two dimensional x-y graph denoting the relationship to a third variable

isothermal a process of gas compression or expansion in which the gas temperature remains constant; heat energy must be either added (during expansion) or taken away (during compression) to maintain the energy equilibrium; compare to adiabatic

isotonic (of a solution) having the same concentration of solute as another solution, hence exerting the same amount of osmotic pressure as that solution, as an isotonic saline solution that contains an amount of salt equal to that found in the extracellular fluid

isovolumic having the same volume

IT abbreviation for implantation tested; as applied to invasive devices, indicates that the materials used have been been shown noxtoxic to living tissue

IV abbreviation; see *intravenous*

IVH abbreviation for intraventricular hemorrhage, a severe brain complication common in premature infants

J–K

jargon the special technical language and terms of a particular field or profession

jaundice a yellow discoloration of the skin, mucous membranes and eyes due to high tissue level of bilirubin

JCAHO abbreviation for the Joint Commission on Accreditation of Healthcare Organizations, a private, voluntary association that establishes standards for accrediting institutions and agencies responsible for health care delivery

Joule-Thompson effect a physical phenomenon in which the rapid expansion of a gas without the application of external work causes a substantial drop in the temperature of the gas; used in the liquifcation of air for the production of oxygen and nitrogen

JRCRTE abbreviation for the Joint Review Committee for Respiratory Therapy Education; the JRCRTE, in collaboration with the Commission on Accreditation of Allied Health Education Programs (CAAHEP) establishes standards for and oversees the accreditation of educational programs in respiratory care

juxtamedullary situated near the medulla

ketoacidosis a metabolic acidosis due to the accumulation of excess ketones in the body, resulting from faulty carbohydrate metabolism, as can occur in certain forms of diabetes

keyboard a device arranged like a typewriter for entering alphanumeric datain to a computer or program

kilobyte (Kb) a unit of computer data equal to 1024 bytes

kinetic energy the energy a body possesses by virtue of its motion

Korotkoff sound sounds heard during the taking of blood pressure using a sphygmomanometer and stethoscope

kyphoscoliosis an abnormal condition characterized by an anteroposterior and lateral curvature of the spine

kyphosis an abnormal condition of the vertebral column, characterized by increased anteroposterior convex curvature of the thoracic spine

L

lamina a thin layer or plate

lamina propria a layer of connective tissue that lies just under the epithelium of the mucous membrane

laminar pertaining to laminae or layers; specifically refers to a pattern of flow consisting of concentric layers of fluid flowing parallel to the tube wall at linear velocities that increase toward the center

laparotomy any surgical incision into the peritoneal cavity, usually performed under general or regional anesthesia, often on a exploratory basis

laptop a small personal computer that can be held on the lap, usually weighs less than 7 pounds; also sometimes called portable or notebook computer

laryngectomy a surgical removal of the larynx, performed to treat cancer of the larynx

laryngitis inflammation of the larynx

laryngoscope an endoscope for examining the larynx

laryngoscopy the process of viewing the larynx with a laryngoscope

laryngospasm an involuntary contraction of the laryngeal muscles resulting in complete or partial closure of the glottis

laryngotracheobronchitis an inflammation of the larynx, trachea, and large bronchi that can result in hoarseness, a nonproductive cough, and dyspnea

laryngotracheitis inflammation of the larynx and trachea

lassitude weariness, fatigue, or listlessness

latent heat of fusion the additional heat energy needed to effect the changeover of a substance from it solid to its liquid form

latent heat of vaporization the heat energy required to vaporize a liquid at its boiling point

lateral away from the body midline; situated on the side

lateral decubitus a side-lying position (either left or right)

lavage the washing or irrigation of an organ, such as the stomach or lung

LC circuit a direct current electrical circuit consisting of an inductance coil (L) and a capacitor (C) in series

LED abbreviation; see *light emitting diode*

legionellosis an acute bacterial pneumonia caused by infection with *Legionella pneumophila* and characterized by an influenza-like illness followed within a week by high fever, chills, muscle aches, and headache

length of stay (LOS) a measure pertaining to the number of elapsed days between a patient's admission and their discharge from an in-patient health care facility

lesion a general term referring to any injury or pathologic change in body tissue

lethicin a general term referring to one of a complex class of lipids derived from phosphatidic acid (also called phosphatidyl cholines); the lecithins represent a major lipid constituent of tissues

leukocyte a white blood cell, one of the formed elements of the circulating blood system

leukocytopenia an abnormal decrease in the white blood cells (usually fewer than 5000 cells per mm^3)

leukocytosis an abnormal increase in the number of circulating white blood cells

LGA abbreviation for large for gestational age; of or pertaining to newborn infants whose body weight falls above the 90th percentile for their gestational age

liability a legal obligation or responsibility

licensure the granting of permission by a competent authority (usually a governmental agency) to an organization or individual to engage in a specific practice or activity

lifespan the full scope or period of one's life

lifestyle the pattern of behavior characterizing one's way of living

ligate to tie off a blood vessel or duct with a suture or wire ligature performed to stop or prevent bleeding during surgery, to stop spontaneous or traumatic hemorrhage, or to prevent passage of material through a duct, as in tubal ligation or to treat varicosites

light-emitting diode (LED) an electronic component that emits light when exposed to current flow; used in instruments to display digital data

lingula a division of the left upper lobe of the lung corresponds developmentally to the right middle lobe

lipid any of a class of greasy organic substances insoluble in water but soluble in alcohol, chloroform, ether, and other solvents

lipoprotein a conjugated protein which lipids form an integral part of the molecule

liquefication the conversion of a substance into its liquid form; also called liquefaction

LFPPV-ECCO$_2$R acronym for low frequency positive pressure ventilation with extracorporeal carbon dioxide removal; a mode of ventilatory support designed to minimize the harmful effects of conventional mechanical ventilation

lobectomy a type of chest surgery in which a lobe of a lung is excised, performed to remove a malignant tumor and to treat uncontrolled bronchiectasis, trauma with hemorrhage, or intractable tuberculosis

lobule literally a small lobe; in pulmonary anatomy may refer to the primary lobule or terminal respiratory unit of the lung (also called the acinus), or the secondary lobule; the secondary lobule is the smallest gross anatomical unit of lung tissue set apart by true connective tissue septa, and corresponds correspond to clusters of from three to five primary lobules

logarithm a number system founded on exponential relationships using a base value such as 10 or e (the natural log)

longevity duration of life

long-term care the provision of medical, social, and/or personal care services on a recurring or continuing basis to persons with chronic physical or mental disorders

lordotic of or pertaining to a radiographic position in which the patient stands with his or her back toward the film and leans backward, such that only the shoulders, neck and head touch the film; this positions the X-ray beam at an angle ideal for viewing the lung apices without obstruction by the normally superimposed shadows of the clavicles

lumen a cavity within any organ or structure of the body, or a channel in a tube or catheter

lung abscess an inflammatory lesion resulting in necrosis of lung tissue and associated with one or more of the following: suppression of the cough reflex, aspiration of infected material, bronchial obstruction, pneumonias, ischemia, as with pulmonary infarction, or blood sepsis

lupus erythromatosus a chronic, superficial inflammation of the skin in which redish lesions or macules up to 3 to 4 cm in size spread over the body

LVEDP abbreviation for left ventricular end-diastolic pressure

lymphadenopathy of or pertaining to and disease of the lymph nodes; refers also to the visualization of enlarged lymph nodes on X-ray

lymphocytosis an increase in blood lymphocytes

lymphoid resembling lymph tissue

lymphokine one of the chemical factors produced and released by T-lymphocytes that attract macrophages to the site of infection or inflammation and prepare them for attack

lymphoma a neoplasm of lymphoid tissue that is usually malignant but, in rare cases, may be benign

lyse a combining form meaning 'to produce decomposition'

lysis of or pertaining to the process of decomposition

M

machine language binary code to which a computer directly responds; the lowest level of computer instructions

macro a collection of keystrokes or commands stored by the computer, usually within an application program; a macro can be "played back" to perform a repetitive task as often as needed

macrophage any phagocytic cell of the reticuloendothelial system

mainframe the largest of computers, sometimes filling several rooms; the storage capacity and operating speed of a mainframe computer is far greater than mini or microcomputers

mainstem of or pertaining to the first branching or generation of the tracheobronchial tree

malignant tending to become worse; as applied to tumors, having the property of metastasis

malposition literally 'bad position;' in an abnormal place, or not positioned where intended

manifold a pipe with many connections; in medical gas storage, a collection of gas cylinders linked together for purposes of bluk storage, and usually including at least one reserve bank and other safety systems, such as low pressure alarms

MAO abbreviation for monoamine oxidase, an enzyme that catalyzes the oxidation of amines

MAO inhibitor any of a chemically heterogeneous group of drugs used primarily in the treatment of depression or anxiety, and sometimes hypertension; MAO inhibitors may interact with a variety of foods and indirect acting adrenergics like ephedrine, causing severe hypertensive episodes

mass spectrometry an analytic method for assessing the concentration of gas mixtures based on their separation by molecular weight

mass storage an external (secondary) data storage device used by computers to store large volumes of data

maxillary of or pertaining to the maxilla, or upper jaw

maxillofacial of or pertaining to the upper jaw, nose and cheek

maximum inspiratory force (MIF) a measure of the output of the inspiratory muscles against a maximum stimulus, as measured in cm H_2O negative pressure; also known as the negative inspiratory force (NIF) or maximum inspiratory pressure (MIP or PImax)

MDC abbreviation for major diagnostic category, a grouping of DRGs used for diagnostic classification and reimbursement under Medicare; for example, major diagnostic category –4 includes disorders of the respiratory system

MDI abbreviation for metered dose inhaler, a pressurized cartridge used for self-administration of exact dosages of aerosolized drugs

meatus an opening or tunnel through any part of the body, as the meati formed by the turbinates or concha in the nasal cavity

mechanoreceptor any sensory nerve ending that responds to mechanical stimuli, as touch, pressure, sound, and muscular contractions

meconium a material that collects in the intestines of a fetus and forms the first stools of a newborn

medial situated or oriented towards the midline of the body

mediastinoscopy a diagnostic procedure whereby a device is inserted into the mediastinum for purposes of visualization or biopsy

mediastinum a portion of the thoracic cavity lying in the middle of the thorax (between the two pleural cavities) and containing the trachea, esophagus, heart, and great vessels of the circulatory system

medulla the most internal part of an organ or structure; e.g., medulla oblongata: the bulbous portion of the spinal cord just above the foramen magnum that contains the cardiac, respiratory and vasomotor 'centers'

megabyte (Mb) a unit of computer data equivalent to 1024 kilobytes, or approximately 1 million bytes

megahertz (MHz) a measure of the frequency of wave cycles; one million cycles per second

memory (computer) a device which can record data and store it for retrieval

menu a visual display of possible options and functions of a computer program from which a user can choose

MEP abbreviation for maximum expiratory pressure; a measure of the output of the expiratory muscles against a maximum stimulus, as measured in cm H_2O postive pressure

mesencephalon one of the three parts of the brain stem, lying just below the cerebrum and just above the pons

mesenteric of or pertaining to the mesentery, a broad fan-shaped fold of peritoneum connecting the jejunum and ileum with the dorsal wall of the abdomen

mesothelioma a rare malignant tumor of the mesothelium of the pleura or peritoneum, associated with earlier exposure to asbestos

mesothelium a layer of cells that lines the body cavities of the embryo and continues as a layer of squamous epithelial cells covering the serous membranes of the adult

metaphase the second of the four stages of nuclear division in mitosis and in each of the two divisions of meiosis, during which the chromosomes become arranged in the equatorial plane of the spindle to form the equatorial plate, with the centromeres attached to the spindle fibers in preparation for separation

metastasis the process by which tumor cells are spread to distant parts of the body

methemoglobin an abornmal form of hemoglobin in which the iron component has been oxidized from the ferrous to the ferric state

methemoglobinemia an abnormal condition characterized by high levels of methemoglobin in the blood and thus a reduction in oxygen carrying capacity; may be caused by nitrite poisoning or ingestion of an certain oxidizing agents or a genetic defect in the enzyme NADH methemoglobin reductase (an autosomal dominant trait)

methylene blue a bluish-green crystalline substance used as a histologic stain and as a laboratory indicator; also used to test the integrity of protective upper airway reflexes in patients being considered for extubation

methylxanthine a category of naturally occurring drug agents (including caffeine and theophylline) that exert a broad range of physiologic effects, including CNS and myocardial stimulation, smooth muscle relaxation, and diuresis; used commonly in respiratory care as bronchodilators or respiratory stimulants

METS abbreviation for the multiple equivalents of resting O_2 consumption, a indirect measure of physiologic work performed during exercise and strees testing

microaerosol an extremely fine aerosol of uniform and small particle size produced by sequential baffling and characterized by mass median diameters that are generally less than 1.0 μm

microampere (μA) a unit of electrical current equivalent to one millionth (10^{-6}) ampere (an ampere in the current produced by one volt applied across a resistance of one ohm)

microatelectasis localized or focal atelectasis that may note manifest itself on radiographic examination

microcomputer also called a personal computer (PC) or desktop computer; a small inexpensive computer which can fit on a table top and run complex programs for a variety of applications

microelectrode a miniature electrode, often small enough to be placed within a tissue cell

microembolization embolization due to extremely small bloodbourn particles, usually smaller than that visible with the naked eye

micrognathia underdevelopment of the jaw, especially the mandible

midaxillary of or pertaining to the imaginary line drawn vertically downward from the middle of the axilla

midclavicular of or pertaining to the imaginary line drawn vertically downward from the middle of the clavicle

midline an imaginary line that divides the body into right and left halves

midscapular of or pertaining to the imaginary line drawn vertically downward from the middle of the scapula

midsternal of or pertaining to the imaginary line vertically bisecting the sternum

milliequivalent (mEq) a quantitative amount of a reacting substance that has a specific chemical combining power; 1 mEq equals the gram atomic weight of a substance divided by its valence x 0.001

millimole a SI unit of matter equal to 1/1000 of a mole (a mole is any quantity of matter that contains 6.023 x 10^{23} atoms, molecules, or ions)

millivolt (mV) one-thousandth of a volt

minicomputer an intermediate sized more expensive computer with capabilities between those of a microcomputer and of a mainframe; often used in multiuser, multitasking environments

MIP abbreviation for maximum inspiratory pressure, the negative pressure generated during a maximally forced inspiratory effort against an obstruction to flow; also called negative inspiratory force (NIF) and PImax

mitochondria small rodlike, granular organelles within the cellular cytoplasm that function in cellular metabolism and respiration

mitosis the process whereby a cell normally replicate itself, forming two daughter cells, each with the same number of chromosomes as the parent cell

MLT abbreviation for minimal leak technique, a method for determining the cuff inflation volume on endotracheal tubes; during MLT, air is slowly injected into the cuff until the leak stops; once a seal is obtained, a small amount of air is removes, allowing a slight leak at peak inflation pressure

MMV abbreviation for mandatory minute ventilation a mode of ventilatory support; MMV ensures delivery of a preset minimum minute volume, with the patient allowed to breathe spontaneously

modem MOdulator-DEModulator, a device which uses modulation to convert a digital signal to an analog signal for transmission across a standard telephone line

mole the SI unit of matter equal containing 6.023 × 10^{23} atoms, molecules, or ions

monitor (computer) the video display screen with which the user observes the action of the computer, an output device

monoclonal antibody an antibody derived from specially produced cells called hybridomas

morbidity the state of being ill, in statistics, the ratio of those ill to those who are well

morphology the study of structures and forms in living things

morphometry the actual process of measuring the form of living things

mortality the number of deaths per unit population in any specific age group, disease category

mottling a condition of spotting with patches of color

mouse a hand held computer input device which a user can move to manipulate a screen cursor and select corresponding choices from the screen

MOV abbreviation for minimal occluding volume; the minimum endotracheal tube cuff pressure needed to prevent gas leakage during a positive pressure inspiration

MSVC abbreviation for maximum sustainable ventilatory capacity

mucociliary of or pertaining to ciliated mucosa

mucoid resembling mucus

mucokinesis the process of moving mucous, i.e., therapeutic methods designed to aid in removal of excess or abnormal secretion of the respiratory tract

mucolysis the breaking down of mucous; usually refers to chemical degradation of mucopolysaccharide by certain drug agents called mucolytics

mucolytic a drug agent capable of mucolysis

mucopolysaccharide any one of a group of polysaccharides containing hexosamine and being the chief constituent of normal mucous

mucoprotein a compound, present in all connective and supporting tissue, that contains polysaccharides combined with protein, and is relatively resistant to denaturation

mucopurulent characteristic of a combination of mucus and pus

mucosa a general terms referring to any mucous membrane

multicompetent of or pertaining to an individual skilled in more than one area or discipline, such as a respiratory care practitioner who is also skilled in basic radiography

multidisciplinary consisting of or involving more than one discipline

multifocal an action, such as the transmission of an electrical impulse, that arises from more than two foci

muscarinic of or pertaining to the effect of acetylcholine on the parasympathetic postganglionic effector sites; e.g., smooth muscle, cardiac muscle, exocrine glands

muscular dystrophy a general term applying to a group of hereditary disorders characterized by progressive degeneration of the skeletal muscles, resulting in severe muscle weakness

myalgia diffuse muscle pain, usually accompanied by malaise, occurring in many diseases

myasthenia gravis an abnormal condition characterized by the chronic fatigability and weakness of skeletal muscles, especially those of the face, throat and respiratory system, and arising as a result of a defect in the conduction of nerve impulses at the myoneural junction

mycelium a mass of interwoven, branched, threadlike filaments that make up most fungi

Mycobacteria acid-fast microorganisms belonging to the genus Mycobacterium

Mycoplasma a genus of ultramicroscopic pleomorphic organisms that lack rigid cell walls, grow on artificial media but do not retain the Gram stain, and are able to pass through bacterial filters; a causes of atypical pneumonia

mycoses any disease caused by fungi

myelosuppresive referring to any process that inhibits the production of blood cells and platelets in the bone marrow

myocarditis an inflammatory condition of the myocardium caused by viral, bacterial, or fungal infection, serum sickness, rheumatic fever, or chemical agents, or as a complication of a collagen disease

myocardial infarction occlusion of a coronary artery resulting in distal myocardial tissue necrosis, often accompanied by significant complications

myoneural of or pertaining to the junction between an efferent motor nerve and the muscle it innervates

myopathy an abnormal condition of skeletal muscle characterized by muscle weakness, wasting, and histologic changes within muscle tissue, as seen in any of the muscular dystrophies

myositis inflammation of muscle tissue, usually of the voluntary muscles

myxedema a severe form of hypothyroidism characterized by dry swelling and abnormal deposits of mucin in the tissues

myxoma a connective tissue neoplasm that often grows to enormous size

N

narcolepsy a idiopathic syndrome characterized by sudden sleep attacks

nasal flaring dilation of the alar nasi on inspiration; an early sign of an increase in ventilatory demands and the work of breathing, especially in infants

nasogastric of or pertaining the passageway from the nose to the stomach; usually applied to tubes or catheters placed in the stomach through the nose

nasotracheal of or pertaining the passageway from the nose to the trachea; usually applied to tubes or catheters placed in the trachea through the nose, such as a nasotracheal tube, or nasotracheal suctioning

NBRC abbreviation for the National Board for Respiratory Care, Inc., the national credentialing agency for respiratory care practitioners and pulmonary function technologists

nebulizer a device that produces an aerosol suspension of liquid particles in a gaseous medium using baffling to control particle size

necrosis local tissue death due to disease or injury

necrotizing pertaining to a process that produces necrosis

NEEP acronym; see *negative end-expiratory pressure*

negative end-expiratory pressure (NEEP) the application of subatmospheric pressure to the airway during the expiratory phase of positive pressure ventilation

negative feedback control mechanism a mechanical, electrical, or physiologic control mechanism in which feedback to a sensor or receptor evokes an opposite response from an effector mechanism, so that a balance in a parameter can be maintained

negligence the omission to do something which a reasonable person, guided by those ordinary considerations would do

negligence, contributory the act of doing something or failing to do something which results in the want of ordinary care on part of complaining party; this act or omission occurs concurrently with the defendant's negligence, and is the proximate cause of the plaintiff's harm

neonatal pertaining to the period between birth and 28 days of age

neoplasia the new and abnormal development of cells that may be benign or malignant

neoplasm an abnormal growth of new tissue, either benign or malignant

neoplastic of or pertaining to a neoplasm

neovascularization the formation of new blood vessels

nephron a structural and functional unit of the kidney, resembling a microscopic funnel with a long stem and two convoluted sections

nephrotoxic toxic or destructive to a kidney

network a system of one or more computers connected through communication lines to various terminals or computers

neuroeffector a chemical or electrical stimulus that causes nerve cell depolarization

neurogenic originating in the nervous system

neurologic of or pertaining to neurology or the nervous system

neuromuscular of or pertaining to the muscle and nerves

neuropathy any abnormal condition characterized by inflammation and degeneration of the peripheral nerves

neurosurgery any surgery involving the brain, spinal cord, or peripheral nerves

neurotoxic poisonous to the brain or central nervous system

neutral thermal environment an ambient enviroment that prevents or minimizes the loss of body heat

neutropenia an abnormal decrease in the number of neutrophils in the blood

neutrophil a polymorphonuclear granular leukocyte that stains well with neutral dyes; the circulating white blood cells essential for phagocytosis

nicotinic of or pertaining to the effect of acetylcholine at the parasympathetic and sympathetic ganglionic or somatic skeletal muscles receptor sites

NIPPV abbreviation for noninvasive positive pressure ventilation; positive pressure ventilation without endotracheal intubation or tracheotomy, usually via a form-fitting nasal mask

nitrite an ester or salt of nitrous acid, used as a vasodilator and antispasmodic, particularly in angina pectoris; common examples are amyl nitrite and sodium nitrite

nocturia excessive urination at night

nomogram a graphic representation of a numeric relationship

noncommunicable pertaining to diseases that cannot be contract-ed by contact between or among people or among people and animal vectors or inanimate objects; noninfectious

nonflammable not capable of combustion

noninvasive pertaining to a diagnostic or therapeutic technique that does not require the skin to be broken or a cavity or organ of the body to be entered, as obtaining a blood pressure reading by auscultation with a stethoscope and sphygmomanometer

nonjudgmental tending not to draw judgements about others

nonmotile not capable of movement; stationary

nonporous 'without pores;' impermeable to liquids or gases

nonresectable not removable by surgery

normocapnia a state characterized by a normal partial pressure of carbon dioxide in the arterial blood (35 to 45 torr)

normovolemic a state characterized by normal fluid volumes

nosocomial pertaining to or originating in a hospital, as a nosocomial infection

not-for-profit an activity in which any excess of expenses over revenue is reinvested into the operation, rather than being distributed to owners or shareholders; compare to *for-profit*

nuchal of or pertaining to the nape or back of the neck

nucleoprotein protein combined with a nucleic acid and originating in the cell nucleus

nucleotide any one of the compounds into which nucleic acid is split by the action of nuclease

O

O$_2$ER abbreviation for oxygen extraction ratio, the ratio of oxygen consumption to oxygen delivery

obligate ability to survive only in a certain environment; e.g., an obligate anaerobe

oblique slating; not perfectly vertical or horizontal

obliterate to remove or destroy

obstetrics the branch of medicine concerned with pregnancy and childbirth

obstructive sleep apnea (OSA) a condition in which five or more apneic periods (of at least 10 seconds each) occur per hour of sleep, and characterized by occlusion of the oropharyngeal airway with continued efforts to breath

obtunded insensitive to pain or other stimuli due to a reduced level of consciousness

obturator a device used to block a passage or a canal or to fill in a space, as the obturator used to inset a tracheostomy tube

ocular of or pertaining to the eye; also an eyepiece in any instrument

oliguria a diminished capacity to form and pass urine; for adults, generally defined as less than 500 mL/day

oncotic marked by or associated with swelling; often used as a synonym for osmotic forces

Ondine's Curse apnea caused by loss of automatic control of respiration (derived from the name of a fabled water nymph)

opacification the process of becoming opaque (less able to transmit light or penetrating radiation); used commonly to refer to the development of areas of increased density on the X-ray, as occurs in ARDS

operating system a group of programs which control when certain computer function will be executed, directs the operations of input/output devices, and controls access to available memory

opiate a narcotic drug that contains opium, derivatives of opium, or any of several synthetic chemicals with opium-like activity; morphine is the model in this category

opsonin an antibody or complement split product which, on attaching to foreign material, microorganism, or other antigen, enhances phagocytosis of that substance by leukocytes and other macrophages

optical scanning device an instrument which scans visual data and translates it into digital form for computer processing

orifice an entrance or outlet to a body cavity or tube

oropharynx the three anatomic divisions of the pharynx lying behind the oral cavity and midway between the naso- and laryngopharynx

orotracheal of or pertaining the passageway from the mouth to the trachea; usually applied to tubes or catheters placed in the trachea through the mouth, such as an orotracheal tube, or orotracheal suctioning

orthopnea an abnormal condition characterized by difficult breathing in any lying or recumbent position

orthostatic pertaining to or caused by standing upright, as with orthostatic hypotension

oscillator a mechanical or electrical device that creates regular and reciprocal waves or vibrations

oscillometric pertaining to the use of oscillations to measure physical quantities

OSA abbreviation for *obstructive sleep apnea*

OSHA abbreviation for the Occupational Safety and Health Administration, a branch of the US Department of Labor responsible regulation pertsining to on-the-job safety

osmolarity the osmotic pressure of a solution expressed in osmols or milliosmols per kilogram of the solution

osmotic pressure a measurable force produced by mobility of the solvent particles across a semipermeable membrane

osteoarthropathy any disease of the joints or bones

osteomylitis local or generalized infection of bone and bone marrow, usually caused by bacteria introduced by trauma or surgery, by direct extension from a nearby infection, or via the bloodstream

osteopathic referring to a system of medicine that combines conventional treatments with musculoskeletal manipulation; contrast with allopathic

osteoporosis a disorder characterized by abnormal rarefaction of bone, occurring most frequently in postmenopausal women, in sedentary or immobilized individuals, and in patients on long-term steroid therapy

otitis inflammation or infection of the ear, such as otitis media or otitis externa

otorhinolaryngologist a physician specializing in disorders of the ear, nose and throat

output data produced via a computer program from available input; for example, if a program is adds 4 to an input value, and the input is 5, the resulting output would be 9

overdistention a state of stretch or expansion beyond the normal limits

overhydration a state characterized by an excess of body fluids

overpressurization a condition of excessive pressure

OVP acronym for operational verification procedure, the process of verifying that equipment performs as expected or specified

oximeter a photoelectric device (usually noninvasive) used to determine the saturation of blood hemoglobin with oxygen

oximetry the process of determining the saturation of hemoglobin with oxygen with an oximeter

oxygen toxicity the pathological response of the body and its tissues resulting from long-term exposure to high partial pressure of oxygen; pulmonary manifestations include cellular changes causing congestion, inflammation, and edema

oxyhemoglobin the chemical combination resulting from the covalent bonding of oxygen to the ferrous iron pigment in hemoglobin

P-Q

$P_{0.1}$ the mouth pressure 100 miliseconds after the start of an occluded inspiration; a measure of the output of the respiratory center

P_{50} the partial pressure of oxygen at which hemoglobin is 50% saturated with oxygen, standardized to a pH of 7.40; used as a measure of hemoglobin affinity for oxygen; with a a normal value of 26.6 torr

PAC abbreviation for premature atrial contraction

PAWP abbreviation for pulmonary arterial wedge pressure (also called the pulmonary capillary wedge pressure (PCWP) or occluded pulmonary artery pressure PAo); reflects downstream pressure in the pulmonary circulation; under optimum conditions PAWP indicates left ventricular end-diastolic pressure (LVEDP), or left ventricular preload

palatine of or pertaining to the palate or roof of the mouth

pallor an unnatural paleness or absence of color in the skin

palmar of or pertaining to the palm

palpitation a pounding or racing of the heart

pancreatitis an inflammatory condition of the pancreas, either acute or chronic

pandemic (of a disease) occurring throughout the population of a country, a people, or the world

pantomime expression or communication using only body or facial movements

paradox something contrary to common sense, logic or experience

paradoxical breathing a pattern of breathing in which the abdomen is observed to move outward while the lower rib cage moves inward during inspiration; paradoxical breathing usually indicates an excessive respiratory muscle load, and may serves notice of impending respiratory failure

paranasal situated near or alongside the nose, as the paranasal sinuses

parasympathetic of or pertaining to the craniosacral component of the autonomic nervous system, consisting of the oculomotor, facial, glossopharyngeal, vagus, and pelvic nerves; any physiologic action mediated by or mimicking that of acetylcholine

parasympathomimetic denoting a pharmacologic agent that mimics the effects of stimulation of organs and structures by the parasympathetic nervous system by occupying cholinergic receptor sites and acting as an agonist or by increasing the release of the neurotransmitter acetylcholine

parenchyma the functional tissue of an organ (as opposed to the supporting or connecting tissue)

parenteral not in or through the digestive system

paresis slight or incomplete paralysis

paresthesia any subjective sensation, experienced as numbness, tingling, or a 'pins and needles' feeling

parietal of or pertaining to the outer wall of a cavity or organ

parotitis inflammation of infection of one or both parotid salivary glands

paroxysmal nocturnal dyspnea (PND) attacks of dyspnea commonly occurring at night, especially in the recumbent position, and associated with congestive heart failure and cardiac pulmonary edema

partial pressure the pressure exerted by a single gas in a gas mixture

partial thromboplastin time (PTT) a test for detecting coagulation defects of the intrinsic clotting system by adding activated partial thromboplastin to a sample of test plasma and comparing it to a control of normal plasma; normal is 60 to 80 seconds

parturition the process of giving birth

PASCAL an easy-to-learn, high level programming language (named after the 17th century French mathematician) which permits very structured precise programming

password a key or set of characters which a user can enter into a computer system in order to gain access to the system

patent open and unblocked, as a patent airway

pathogenic capable of producing disease

pathologic indicative of or caused by a disease

pathophysiology the study of the biologic and physical manifestations of disease as they correlate with the underlying abnormalities and physiologic disturbances

patient-physician privilege the right of patients to refuse to divulge or have divulged by their physician, the communications made between them and their physician

PAV abbreviation for proportional assist ventilation, a mode of ventilatory support in which the level of mechanical assistance varies with patient demand

PCIRV abbreviation for pressure controlled inverse ratio ventilation; equivalent to time-triggered, pressure-limited, time-cycled ventilation with I:E ratios greater than 1:1.

PCV abbreviation for pressure controlled ventilation; equivalent to time-triggered, pressure-limited, time-cycled ventilation

PCP abbreviation for *Pneumocystis carinii* pneumonia; caused by *Pneumocystis carinii* (probably a fungi), PCP causes an acute interstitial pneumonia with high mortality ($> 50\%$); PCP is most common among patients with an abnormal or altered immunologic status, particularly those suffering from AIDS; current treatment is with co-trimoxazole or pentamidine isethionate

PCWP abbreviation for pulmonary capillary wedge pressure; see *PAWP*

PDA abbreviation for patent ductus arteriosus, a common cardiovascular anomaly of infants in which the ductus arteriosus either fails to close or reopens after birth

peak expiratory flow rate (PEFR) the maximum flow achieved after forced exhalation from TLC

pectoriloquy the transmission of the sounds of speech through the chest wall

pectus carinatum chicken breasted; undo protrusion of the sternum

pectus excavatum funnel breasted; undo concavity of the sternum

pediatrics the branch of medicine concerned with the treatment and prevention of disorders of childhood

pedicle a stem or stalk; the boney process that projects posteriorly from each vertebra

pediculosis infestation with lice

PEEP acronym for *positive end-expiratory pressure*

pendelluft movement of gas from 'fast' to 'slow' filling spaces during breathing; alternatively, the ineffective movement of gas back and forth (accompanied by mediastinal shifting) between a healthy lung and one with a flail segment caused by a crushing chest injury

penetration as applied to aerosols, the maximum depth that suspended particles can be carried into the respiratory tract by the inhaled tidal air

penicillinase resistant a descriptive term applied to certain antibiotics resistant to the action of penicillinase, an enzyme produced by some bacteria which inactivates penicillin

percent body humidity (%BH) to the amount of water vapor in a volume of gas as the percent of the water in gas saturated at a body temperature of 37 °C (43.8 mg/L)

percutaneous through the skin

perfuse the passage of fluid (usually blood) through the body

peribronchial around the bronchi

pericarditis an inflammation of the pericardium associated with trauma, malignant neoplastic disease, infection, uremia, myocardial infarction, collagen disease, or idiopathic causes

pericardium a fibrous serous sac that surrounds the heart and the roots of the great vessels

peripheral any of a variety of devices which can be attached to a computer and directed by the CPU, including printers, display devices, external data storage, instrument interfaces and communication devices

perinatal of or pertaining to the time and process of giving birth to being born

perioperative of or pertaining to the period of time immediately before, during and after surgery

periosteum a fibrous vascular membrane covering the bones, except at their extremities

peritoneal dialysis a dialysis procedure in which the peritoneum is used as the diffusible membrane, with a dialysate fluid infused directly into the peritoneal cavity

peritubular around the tubules; specifically around the proximal or distal tubules of the nephron

permanent gas the gaseous phase of a substance with a critical temperature so low that it cannot be compressed into a liquid under ambient conditions

PERRLA acronym indication pupils equal, round, react to light, accomdation, e.g., a normal physical exam finding

pertussis an acute, highly contagious respiratory disease characterized by paroxysmal coughing that ends in a loud whooping inspiration

petechia a tiny purple or red spot that appear on the skin as a result of minute hemorrhages within the dermal or submucosal layers

petition a formal written request addressed to some governmental authority, usually a formal written application to a court requesting judicial action on a certain matter

P/F ratio a ratio of the arterial partial pressure of oxygen to the inspired fractional concentration of oxygen (PaO_2/FiO_2); a measure of the efficiency of oxygen transfer across the lung

phagocytosis the process by which certain cells engulf and dispose of microorganisms and cell debris

pharmacopeia a compendium containing descriptions, recipes, strengths, standards of purity, and dosage forms for selected drugs

pharyngitis inflammation or infection of the pharynx, usually causing symptoms of a sore throat

phonocardiography the analog recording of heart sounds, usually on a strip chart recorder; useful in the diagnosis of certain valvular abnormalities that produce heart murmurs

phospholipid one of a class of compounds, widely distributed in living cells, containing phosphoric acid, fatty acids, and a nitrogenous base

photodetector a device capable of detecting light

photoplethysmography the use of light waves to detect changes in the volume of an organ or tissue; pulse oximeters use the principle of photoplethysmography to measure the arterial pulse

physical plant the 'bricks and mortar' or building facilities that make up the physical presence of an institution

Pickwickian syndrome an abnormal condition characterized by severe obesity, decreased responsiveness to carbon dioxide, a restrictive pulmonary function pattern, hypersomnolence, and polycythemia

PIE abbreviation for pulmonary interstial emphysema, a form of pulmonary barotrauma due to air leakage into lung tissue

piezoelectric transducer a transducer capable of converting electrical energy in the physical energy of high frequency vibrations

PImax abbreviation for maximum inspiratory pressure, or the negative pressure generated during a maximally forced inspiratory effort against an obstruction to flow; also called maximum inspiratory force (MIF) and negative inspiratory force (NIF)

pK the negative log of the ionization constant of a solution; the buffering power of a buffer system is greatest when its pH and pK values are equal; pKa is the negative log of the acid component of a buffer system

placenta the highly vascular organ through which the fetus absorbs oxygen and vital nutrients, and excrete carbon dioxide and other waste products of metabolism

placenta abruptio (also abruptio placentae) separation of a normally implanted placenta in a pregnancy of 20 weeks or more duration or during labor but before delivery; a significant cause of maternal and fetal mortality

placenta previa an abnormal condition of pregnancy in which the placenta is implanted low in the uterus, such that it impinges or covers the internal os of the cervix

plaintiff a person who brings an action; a person who seeks remedial relief for an injury to his rights

plasma the watery, colorless fluid portion of the blood and lymph in which cellular elements are suspended

plasmapheresis a laboratory procedure in which the plasma proteins are separated by electrophoresis for identification and evaluation of the proportion of the various proteins

platypnea the opposite of orthopnea, i.e., an abnormal condition characterized by difficult breathing in the standing position, which is relieved in the lying or recumbent position

pleading the formal allegations by the parties of their respective claims and defenses

pleomorphic consisting of many distinct shapes

plethysmograph any instrument designed to measure and record variations in the volume of an organ or body part; the body plethysmograph measures changes in thoracic volume by measuring pressure changes in the box during breathing

plethysmography the process of measuring and recording variations in the volume of an organ or body part with a plethysmograph

pleural effusion the abnormal collection of fluid in the pleural space

pleural empyema a pleural effusion in which the fluid is purulent or contains pyogenic organisms

pleurisy a condition characterized by abnormal deposition of a fibrinous exudate on the pleural surface, usually as a complication of other disorders, such as pneumonia, pulmonary infarction, and pulmonary neoplasms

plexus a network of intersecting nerves or blood vessels

PMI abbreviation for point of maximum impulse

PND abbreviation for paroxysmal nocturnal dyspnea

pneumatocele a thin-walled, air-filled cyst occurring in lung tissue

pneumocardiography the recording of variations in cardiac function through sensors that monitor respiratory changes, such as pressure changes in the bronchi, or changes in thoracic dimensions

pneumocephalus a condition in which gas or air is inside the cranium

pneumography recording of respiratory movements on a graph

pneumoconiosis any disease of the lung caused by chronic inhalation of inorganic dusts, usually mineral dusts of occupational or environmental origin

pneumocyte (also pneumonocyte) a general term applied to the cells constituting the alveolar region of the lungs

pneumomediastinum a presence of air or gas in the mediastinal tissues, which may lead to pneumothorax or pneumopericardium

pneumonectomy the surgical removal of all or part of a lung

pneumonia an inflammatory process of the lung parenchyma, usually infectious in origin

pneumonitis inflammation of the lung

pneumopericardium a presence of air or gas in the pericardium

pneumoperitoneum a presence of air or gas in the peritoneal cavity; may occur as the result of disease, or may be induced for diagnostic visualization

pneumotachometer a transducer designed to measure the flow of respiratory gases, usually by measuring pressure differences across a tube of known resistance

pneumotachygraph an instrument that incorporates a pneumotachometer to recording variations in the flow of respiratory gases

pneumothorax the presence of air or gas in the pleural space of the thorax; if this air or gas is trapped under pressure, a tension pneumothorax exists

polarity having two poles; in physics, the distinction between a negatively and positively charged pole

polarographic of or pertaining to a device or instrument which employs the flow of electrical current between negatively and positively charged poles to measure a physical phenomenon

poliomyelitis an infectious disease caused by one of three small RNA viruses, which can impaired anterior horn cell and produce a clinical picture ranging from asymptomatic to severe paralysis

pollutant any unwanted substance that occurs in the environment

polycythemia an abnormal increase in the number of erythrocytes in the blood; termed secondary if attributable to defined causes other than direct stimulation of the bone marrow, such as occurs in chronic hypoxemia

polymorphonuclear having a nucleus with a number of lobules or segments connected by a fine thread

polymyositis inflammation of many muscles, usually accompanied by deformity, edema, insomnia, pain, sweating, and tension

polypeptide a chain of amino acids joined by peptide bonds

polyposis a condition characterized by numerous polyps

polyps small, tumor-like growths that project from the surface of a mucous membrane

polysaccharide a carbohydrate that contains three or more molecules of simple carbohydrates

polysomnography the measurement and recording of variations in airflow and diaphragmatic activity during sleep; used in the diagnosis of sleep apnea

pons the prominence on the ventral surface of the brainstem, between the medulla oblongata and the cerebral pedicules of the midbrain

pores of Kohn direct intercommunications between alveoli ranging in size from 5 to 15 μm in diameter

porphyrin an iron or magnesium-free pyrole derivative occurring in many plant and animal tissues

port a point of contact between an external device and a computer's CPU through which data can be transferred; parallel and serial ports are the most common

positive end-expiratory pressure (PEEP) the application and maintenance of pressure above atmospheric at the airway throughout the expiratory phase of positive pressure mechanical ventilation

posterolateral situated behind and to one side or the other

posteromedial situated behind and toward the middle

post-term of or pertaining to an infant born after 42 weeks gestation, regardless of weight

postural drainage the therapeutic use of patient positioning and gravity to facilitate the mobilization of respiratory tract secretions

potency in pharmacology, the biological activity of a drug per unit weight, or the amount a drug required to produce a given effect

potential energy the energy a body possesses by virtue of its position

potentiation a phenomenon in clinical pharmacology whereby the administration of a one drug increases the effect of another

potentiometer a voltage measuring device

power of attorney an instrument authorizing another to act as one's agent or attorney

PPD abbreviation for purified protein derivative, a material used in testing for tuberculin sensitivity

ppm abbreviation for parts per million, a common ratio measure for dilute solution or gas mixtures

PPO abbreviation for preferred provider organization, a health care service organization that negotiates special rates for its services with selected groups or organizations

precordium the external anterior anatomic region over the heart and lower thorax

precursor something that comes before or precedes; in chemistry and pharmacology, a substance from which another is formed or synthesized; in clinical diagnosis, a symptom or sign that precedes another

pre-eclampsia an abnormal condition of pregnancy characterized by the onset of acute hypertension after the 24th week of gestation, usually accompanied by proteinuria and edema

preload the initial stretch of myocardial fiber at end diastole

premium the sum paid for a contract, such as that for heath insurance

preoperative of or pertaining to the period of time preceding a surgical procedure

pressure generator a ventilator that delivers a pressure pattern which is independent of the patient's respiratory mechanics

pressure support ventilation (PSV) pressure limited assisted ventilation designed to augment a spontaneously generated breath; the patient has primary control over the frequency of breathing, the inspiratory time, and the inspiratory flow

pressure-time index (PTI) the ratio of the mean to maximum transdiaphragmatic pressure difference times the inspiratory duty cycle; a measure of load that correlates highly with oxygen consumption of the ventilatory muscles

pressure-time product the product of pressure over a time interval, usually pleural pressure times inspiratory time during breathing

preterm of or pertaining to an infant born prior to 38 weeks gestation, regardless of weight

preventative maintenance the regularly scheduled testing and service of in-use equipment, designed to prevent failure or malfunction

primary memory memory which can be accessed directly by a computer's CPU

printer any device that can convert computer output into printed form

printout hardcopy, printed output

procaryotic of or pertaining to plant-like microorganisms (including blue-green bacteria and true bacteria) whose cells have no true nucleus surrounded by a nuclear membrane

prognostic referring to a finding that is diagnostic or predictive

program (computer) a logical, sequential arrangement of instructions to a computer which correctly manipulate the input and generate the desired output

prolapsed cord an umbilical cord that protrudes beside or ahead of the presenting part of the fetus

prophylactic preventing the spread of disease; preventive

proprioceptor any sensory nerve ending, as those located in muscles, tendons, and joints, that responds to stimuli arising from movement or spatial position

prospective payment a system of health care cost reimbursement in which the amount paid to a provider is determined in advance and irrespective of actual costs incurred

prostaglandin one of several naturally occurring 20-carbon unsaturated fatty acids synthesized mainly in the seminal vesicles, kidneys and lungs; prostaglandin E1 and E2 cause relaxation of bronchial smooth muscle; prostaglandin F2a causes contraction of bronchial smooth muscle.

proteinaceous protein-like

proteolytic of or pertaining to any substance that promotes the breakdown of protein

prothrombin a plasm protein synthesized in the liver that, when exposed to thromboplastin and calcium, forms the thrombin component of a blood clot

prothrombin time (PT) a one-stage test for detecting certain plasma coagulation defects caused by deficiencies in factors V, VII, or X

protocol a written plan specifying the procedures to be followed in a given activity; as applied to electronic communications, a collection of rules which determine how two or more computers 'talk' to each other

pseudocolumnar literally, 'column-like;' used to describe a type of epithelial cell that appears columnar in shape

pseudostratified of or pertaining to an epithelial cell type that appear to be organized in layers, but in which each cell actually contacts the basement membrane

psig abbreviation for pounds per square inch-gauge, i.e., the pressure above atmospheric registered on a meter or gauge

PSV abbreviation for *pressure support ventilation*

PSVmax the pressure support level needed to provide tidal volumes of 10-15 mL/kg

psychosis any major medical disorder characterized by extreme derrangement of personality; e.g., severe depression, agitation, regressive behavior

psychosocial of or pertaining to the mental, emotional and social aspects of human existence or development

psychosomatic of or pertaining to the relationship between the emotional state or outlook of an individual (psyche) and the physical responses of the individual's body (soma)

PTI abbreviation; see *pressure-time index*

ptosis an abnormal condition of one or both upper eyelids in which the eyelid droops owing to a congenital or acquired weakness of the levator muscle or paralysis of the third cranial nerve

pulmonary alveolar proteinosis a chronic lung disease characterized by deposition of an eosinophilic proteinaceous material in the alveolar region which severely impairs gas exchange

pulmonary edema a condition in which excessive amounts of plasma enter the pulmonary interstitium and alveoli; usually accompanied by severe respiratory distress, tachypnea, and hypoxemia

pulmonary hemosiderosis a pulmonary disorder characterized by the deposition of abnormal quantities of hemosiderin (an insoluble form of ferric oxide) in the lung parenchyma

pulmonary hypertension a condition characterized by abnormally high pulmonary artery pressures, i.e., mean pulmonary artery pressures in excess of 22 mmHg

pulmonologist a medical doctor who specializes in the treatment of disorders of the respiratory system and holds certification in pulmonary diseases through the American Board of Internal Medicine

pulse deficit the discrepancy between the ventricular rate auscultated at the apex of the heart and the arterial rate of the radial pulse

pulse oximetry the noninvasive estimation of arterial oxyhemoglobin saturation based on the combined principles of photoplethysmography and spectrophotometry

pulse pressure the difference between the systolic and diastolic pressures, normally about 30 to 40 mmHg

pulsus alternans a pulse characterized by a regular alternation of weak and strong beats without changes in the length of the cycle

pulsus paradoxus an abnormal decrease in systolic pressure and pulse-wave amplitude during inspiration

purulent consisting of or containing pus

PVC abbreviation for premature ventricular contraction; also used as an abbreviation for polyvinyl chloride

pyogenic pus-producing

R

RAAS abbreviation for renin-angiotensin aldosterone system

racemic pertaining to a compound made up of optical isomers

radioaerosol an aerosol with particles that have been labeled with a radioactive isotope; used to assist researchers in analyzing pulmonary aerosol deposition and clearance

radiolucent of or pertaining to a substance or tissue that readily permits the passage of X-rays or other radiant energy; compare with radiopaque

radionecrosis the destruction of tissue by radiant energy

radiopaque of or pertaining to a substance or tissue that does not readily permit the passage of X-rays or other radiant energy; compare with radiolucent

rale discontinuous types of lung sound heard on auscultation of the chest, usually during inspiration; the term crackle is noe preferred

random access memory (RAM) a volatile memory storage system in which specific storage locations can be addressed directly, without the need for sequential searching

reabsorption the return of fluids or gases through a body surface and into body fluids or tissues

readaptation the process of relearning; commonly refers to the development of key coping skills after disability or injury

read only memory (ROM) unalterable computer memory from which data can be read but not written or modified; typically, ROM holds permanent sets of instructions such as those used repetitively by the system hardware; compare to *random access memory (RAM)*

reasonable man doctrine the standard which one must observe to avoid liability for negligence; includes the foreseeability of harm to an individual

rebreathe to inhale expired gas (high in carbon dioxide content)

rebreathed volume the volume of any breathing apparatus that results in previously expired gas being inhaled; equivalent to the mechanical deadspace

reconcentration the process of undergoing repeated concentration

recontamination the process by which articles previously contaminated and cleaned or sterilized become contaminate again

recredentialing the process by which an individual who already holds a credential in a given profession demonstrates ongoing competency by successfully completing current credentialing requirements

REDOX an acronym pertaining to any REDuction-OXidation chemical reaction

redress satisfaction or equitable relief for an injury sustained

reducing valve a device designed to reduce a source gas pressure

REE abbreviation for resting energy expenditure, a measure of caloric outlays at rest

referred pain pain occurring at a site distal to its origin

refractory pertaining to a disorder that is resistant to treatment

refractory period the period of time during the depolarization stage of the action potential in which cardiac tissue fibers cannot respond to additional electrical stimulation

registered pulmonary function technologist (RPFT) an individual, qualified by education and/or experience, and previously certified in pulmonary function technology, who has successfully completed the pulmonary function registry examination of the NBRC

registered respiratory therapist (RRT) a respiratory therapist who has successfully completed the registry (therapist) examination of the NBRC

regressive behavior an abnormal return to an earlier mental state characterized by inappropriate behavior

regulator a device designed to controls both the pressure and flow of a compressed gas

regurgitation 'backward flow;' refers commonly to the return of swallowed food back to the mouth or the backflow of blood through a defective valve

rehabilitation the restoration of the individual to the fullest medical, mental, emotional, social and vocational potential of which he/she is capable

rehabilitation (pulmonary) a multidisciplinary program designed to help stabilize or reverse both the physio- and psychopathology of pulmonary diseases and return patients to the highest possible functional capacity allowed

reliability pertaining to equipment, the consistency of fault-free operation, often measured as the mean time between failures; in statistic, the repeatability of a test or measure

remote referring to the components of a computer system which are not located in proximity to the CPU, such as devices connected via modem

repolarization the process by which the cell is restored to its resting potential.

resect to remove surgically

residual volume (RV) the volume of gas remaining in the lungs after a complete exhalation

res ipsa loquitur 'the thing speaks for itself;' rule of evidence whereby negligence of alleged wrongdoer may be inferred from the mere fact that the accident happened

resistance impedance to flow in a tube or conduit; quantified as ratio of the difference in pressure between the two points along a tube length divided by the volumetric flow of the fluid per unit time

respiratory alternans an abnormal breathing pattern in which the patient is observed to switch back and forth between mainly diaphragmatic and mainly intercostal muscle activity; indicative of end-stage respiratory muscle fatigue

Respiratory Index (RI) the ratio of the alveolar-arterial oxygen tension gradient to the arterial partial pressure of oxygen $(P(A-a)O_2/PaO_2)$; a measure of the efficiency of oxygen transfer across the lung

respiratory failure a condition in which the exchange of oxygen and/or carbon dioxide between the alveoli and the pulmonary capillaries is inadequate

respiratory insufficiency a condition in which breathing is accompanied by abnormal signs or symptoms, such as dyspnea or paradoxical breathing

respiratory therapist A graduate of a a CAAHEP/JRCRTE accredited school designed to qualify the graduate for the registry examination of the National Board for Respiratory Care (NBRC)

respiratory therapy technician A graduate of a CAAHEP/JRCRTE approved school designed to qualify the graduate for the technician (entry-level) certification examination of the NBRC

respirometer a device used to measure the volume of respired air or gas

respondeat superior 'let the master answer;' It means that the master is liable in certain cases for the wrongful acts of his servant; e.g., a doctor may be liable for the wrongful acts of his assistant; the doctrine is inapplicable where injury occurs while the servant is acting outside the legitimate scope of authority

response time a measure (usually in msec) of the speed with which a mechanical ventilator can respond to a patient's inspiratory effort and cycle into the inspiratory phase

resting potential a difference in charge, or negative electrical potential, that exists between the inside and outside of a nerve or cardiac tissue cell in the resting state due to concentration differences of potassium and sodium ions across the cell membrane

restrictive lung disease a broad category of disorders with widely variable etiologies, but all resulting in a reduction in lung volumes, particularly the inspiratory and vital capacities; categorized according to origin; i.e., skeletal/thoracic, neuromuscular, pleural, interstitial and alveolar

retention as applied to aerosol therapy, the proportion of particles deposited within the respiratory tract, either at a specific location or as a whole

retinopathy a noninflammatory eye disorder resulting from changes in the retinal blood vessels

retractions the visible indrawing of the soft tissues of chest wall between the bones

retrolental fibroplasia a formation of fibrous tissue behind the lens of the eye, resulting in blindness

retrosternal behind the sternum

rheostat a variable resistor that controls the flow of electrical current

rhinitis inflammation of the mucous membranes of the nose, usually accompanied by swelling of the mucosa and a nasal discharge.

rhinorrhea the free discharge of a thin nasal mucus

rhinovirus any of about 100 serologically distinct, small RNA viruses that cause about 40% of acute respiratory illnesses

rhonchi abnormal sounds heard on auscultation of a respiratory airway obstructed by thick secretions, muscular spasm, neoplasm, or external pressure

rigor mortis rigid stiffening af the body after death

rise-time the rate of increase in a parameter; in ventilatory support, the rate at which airway pressure rises duing early inspiration (a function of flow)

ROS abbreviation for review of symptoms, a component of the medical history

rostal toward the head, cephalad

RSV abbreviations for respiratory synctial virus

S

salicylate any of several widely prescribed drugs derived from salicylic acid

sarcoidosis a chronic disorder of unknown origin characterized by the formation of tubercles of nonecrotizing epithelioid tissue

sclera the tough white outer layer of the eye

scleroderma a relatively rare autoimmune disease that results in chronic thickening of the connective tissue, including that in the skin, heart, kidneys and lungs

sclerosis any condition characterized by hardening of tissue, especially that due to hyperplasia of connective tissue

scoliosis an abnormal lateral curvature of the spine

seminal vesicles the paired pouches that produce seminal fluid and certain hormones in the male; the seminal vesicles are connected to the posterior portion of the urinary bladder and continuous with to the ejaculatory duct

semipermeable a biological or synthetic membrane that permits the passage of molecules of solvent only but not solute

sensitivity a measure of the amount of negative pressure that must be generated by a patient in order to trigger a mechanical ventilator into the inspiratory phase; alternatively, the mechanism used to set or control this level; also called the trigger level

sensitivity (of a test) the ratio of true positive tests results to all patients having the condition being tested for

sensorium a general term referring to the relative state of a patient's consciousness or alertness

sepsis a general term connoting infection or contamination; more specifically used to denote the presence of pathogenic microorganisms or their toxins in the body

septicemia systemic infection in which pathogens are present in the circulating blood stream, having spread from an infection in any part of the body; also called *bacteremia*

septic shock shock due to bacteria in the blood stream (bacteremia), especially Gram-negative organisms associated with nosocomial infections

sequela any abnormal condition that follows and is the result of a disease, treatment, or injury, as paralysis following poliomyelitis, deafness following treatment with an ototoxic drug, or a scar following a laceration

serodiagnosis a diagnosis made via analysis of antigen-antibody reactions in the serum

serotonin a naturally occurring derivative of tryptophan found in platelets and in cells of the brain and the intestine; serotonin is a potent vasoconstrictor

serotype a classification of microorganism based on an analysis of its cellular antigens

serous of or pertaining to the serum; any tissue type that produces or contains serum

SGA abbreviation for small for gestational age; of or pertaining to newborn infants whose body weight falls below the 10th percentile for their gestational age

shock a condition in which perfusion to vital organs is inadequate to meet their metabolic needs; includes hypovolemic, cardiogenic, septic, anaphylactic, and neurogenic forms

shunt as applied in pulmonary medicine, a bypass between the venous (right) and arterial (left) sides of the circulation; if 'right-to-left,' dilution of arterial blood oxygen content occurs; if 'left-to-right,' oxygen content of thearterial blood is not affected, however, cardiac workload is significantly increased

Shy-Drager Syndrome a rare progresive neurologic disorder characterized by orthostatic hypotension, tremor, rigidity, ataxia and muscle wasting

side effect in pharmacology, any effect produced by a drug other than its desired effect

SIDS abbreviation for sudden infant death syndrome, commonly called crib death; the leading cause of death in infants less than one year old in the US

silicosis a lung disorder caused by continued, long-term exposure to the dust of an inorganic compound, silicon dioxide, which is found in sands, quartzes, and in many other stones; chronic silicosis is marked by widespread fibrotic nodular lesions in both lungs

SIMV abbreviation for synchronous intermittent mandatory ventilation

singultus hiccup

sinusitis an inflammation of one or more paranasal sinuses

sinusoidal of or pertaining to the shape of a sine wave

situs inversus lateral transposition of the organs of the abdomen and thorax; one of the features of Kartagener's syndrome

SNF abbreviation for skilled nursing facility

softkey a computer hardware key (usually on a keypad or instrument) which varies its function under control of a software application program

software programs or ROM-based instructions which control the computer

solenoid an electronically-powered actuator or switch

solubility coefficient (gas) the volume of that gas that can be dissolved in 1 mL of a given liquid at standard pressure and specified temperature

somnolence sleepiness

sonography the process of imaging deep structures of the body by measuring and recording the reflection of pulsed or continuous high-frequency sound waves

specific compliance the absolute compliance value of the lung divided by the lung volume at FRC and expressed in units of mL/cm H_2O/L

specifity (of a test) the ratio of true negative tests results to all patients not having the condition being tested for

spectrophotometry the measurement of color in a solution by determining the amount of light absorbed in the ultraviolet, infrared, or visible spectrum, widely used in clinical chemistry to calculate the concentration of substances in solution

sphygmomanometer an instrument for measuring the force of the pulse (from which the blood pressure is estimated)

spirometer a apparatus designed to measure and record lung volumes and flows

spirometry laboratory evaluation of lung function using a spirometer

splanchnic of or pertaining to the viscera

SpO$_2$ abbreviation for oxyhemoglobin saturation, as measured by pulse oximetry

sporicidal destructive to the spore form of bacteria

sporicide any agent effective in destroying spores, as compounds of chlorine and formaldehyde, and the gluteraldehydes

sporulation a type of reproduction that occurs in lower plants and animals, as fungi, algae, and protozoa, and involves the formation of spores by the spontaneous division of the cell into four or more daughter cells, each of which contains a portion of the original nucleus

spurious false

squamous appearing like plates or scales; a type of epithelial tissue

stability in aerosol therapy, a measure of the ability of an aerosol to remain in suspension over time

standard bicarbonate the plasma concentration of HCO$_3$ in mEq/L that would exist if the PCO$_2$ were normal (40 torr)

stasis a disorder in which the normal flow of a fluid through a vessel of the body is slowed or halted

status asthmaticus an acute, severe, and prolonged asthma attack that does not respond to normal treatment approaches

statute an act of the legislature declaring, commanding, or prohibiting something

statute of limitations a statute declaring that no suit shall be maintained nor any criminal charge be made unless brought about within a specified period of time after the right accrued

statutory imposed by legal authority

stenosis an abnormal condition characterized by the constriction or narrowing of an opening or passageway in a body structure

sterile free from any living microorganisms

sterilization the complete destruction of all microorganisms, usually by heat or chemical means

sternoclavicular of or pertaining to the sternum and clavicle

Stokes-Adams syncope episodes of syncope due to heart block

stopcock a valve capable of directing flow in a fluid circuit

strabismus deviation of the eye position from normal which is not under the voluntary control of the patient

stridor an abnormal, high-pitched, harsh inspiratory breath sound which is usually audible to the naked ear and caused by an obstruction in region of the larynx

structured query language (SQL) a high level programming language designed specifically for interrogating relational databases

stylet a thin metal probe used either to clean the hollow portion of a tube or catheter or to help provide support for insertion of these devices into the body

subatmospheric below atmospheric; used to describe pressures below ambient; see *hypobarism*

subcostal below the ribs

subcutaneous beneath the skin

subglottic below the glottis

sublingual beneath the tongue

submicronic of or pertaining to a particle (particularly colloid particles) less than 10^{-5} cm in size and not visible with a standard light microscope

submucosa beneath the mucosa

subphrenic below the diaphragm

sulfhemoglobin a form of hemoglobin containing an irreversibly bound sulfur molecule that prevents normal oxygen binding

supernumary greater than the normal number

suppurative producing pus

supraclavicular the area of the body above the clavicle, or collar bone

supraglottic above the glottis

suprasternal above the sternum

supraventricular above the ventricles

surveillance (bacteriologic) an ongoing process designed to ensure that infection control procedures are working; generally involves equipment processing quality control, sampling of in-use equipment, microbiological identification, and epidemiological investigation

suspension a dispersion of large particles suspended in a fluid medium; without physical agitation, the particles will eventually settle out

sustained maximal inspiration (SMI) a therapeutic breathing maneuver in which patients are coached to inspire from the resting expiratory level up to their inspiratory capacity (IC), with an end-inspiratory pause

sympathetic of or pertaining to the thoracolumbar component of the autonomic nervous system, for which norepinephrine serves as the the postganglionic neurotransmitter; also used to describe any physiologic action mediated by or mimicking that of norepinephrine or epinephrine; see adrenergic

sympathomimetic denoting a pharmacologic agent that mimics the effects of stimulation of organs and structures by the sympathetic nervous system by occupying adrenergic receptor sites and acting as an agonist or by increasing the release of the neurotransmitter norepinephrine at postganglionic nerve endings

synaptic cleft the space between two neurons or between a neuron and an effector organ

syncope temporary unconsciousness; fainting

synchronous intermittent mandatory ventilation (SIMV) periodic assisted ventilation with positive pressure, with the patient breathing spontaneously between breaths

synergistic acting together; more specifically, having the characteristics of synergism, the phenomenon whereby two agents acting together have an effect greater than their algebraic sum

syringomyelia a disorder characterized by the formation of abnormal fluid-filled cavities in the spinal cord

systemic of or pertaining to the body as a whole

TUV

tachycardia an abnormal condition in which the myocardium contracts regularly but at a rate greater than 100 beats per minute

tachyphylaxis a phenomenon in which the repeated administration of some drugs results in a marked decrease in effectiveness

tachypnea an abnormally rapid rate of breathing

tamponade stoppage of the flow of blood to an organ or a part of the body by pressure, as by a tampon or a pressure dressing applied to stop a hemorrhage or by the compression of a part by an accumulation of fluid, as in cardiac tamponade

tangent a line drawn perpendicular to a given point in a curve

target heart rate the heart rate achieved at 65% of a patient's maximum oxygen consumption during the exercise evaluation, used for aerobic conditioning

taxonomy an orderly classification, as a taxonomy of organisms

TDP abbreviation for therapist-driven protocol, a specification of actions that allow RCPs to independently initiate and adjust therapy, within guidelines previously established by medical staff

telecommunications data transmissions over communication lines between locations distant from one another

tempered moderated or mollified; modified or altered by the mixture of an additional ingredient; steel that has been hardened by heating and rapid cooling

term of or pertaining to an infant born between 38 to 42 weeks gestation

terminal a device (usually a keyboard and a video display) used to input data and receive output from a computer

tetany a condition characterized by cramps, convulsions, twitching of the muscles, and sharp flexion of the wrist and ankle joints

tetralogy of Fallot a congenital cardiac anomaly that consists of four defects; pulmonic stenosis, ventricular septal defect, malposition of the aorta to that it arises from the septal defect or the right ventricle, and right ventricular hypertrophy

therapeutic positioning application of gravity to achieve specific clinical objectives, including mobilization of secretions (postural drainage), improving the distribution of ventilation (dependent positioning), and relieving dyspnea (relaxation positioning)

thermistor an electronic thermometer the impedance of which varies with temperature; used for measuring changes in temperature or flow

thermophilic growing best under conditions of high temperature

thermostat an electrical or mechanical device that regulates and maintains a set temperature in a given system

thoracentesis the surgical perforation of the chest wall and pleural space with a needle for the aspiration of fluid for diagnostic or therapeutic purposes or for the removal of a specimen for biopsy

thoracotomy a surgical opening into the thoracic cavity

threshold potential the membrane potential or voltage difference in cardiac tissue fibers at which spontaneous depolarization occurs

threshold response pertaining to a physiologic action caused by the minimum stimulus needed to provoke it

thrill a fine palpable vibration felt accompanying a cardiac or vascular murmur

thrombocytopenia an abnormal condition in which the number of blood platelets is reduced, usually associated with neoplastic diseases or an immune response to a drug

thrombolysis the process by which thrombi are dissolved

thrombophlebitis inflammation of a vein, often accompanied by formation of a clot

thromboplastin a prothrombin activator crucial in the formation of thrombin and therefore essential in blood clotting

thrombosis an abnormal vascular condition in which thrombus develops within a blood vessel of the body

thrombus an aggregation of platelets, fibrin and cellular blood components that can cause obstruction of a blood vessel

tibial of or pertaining to the tibia

time constant a mathematical expression describing the relative efficacy of lung unit filling and emptying, and computed as the product of compliance times resistance, with a resulting measure in seconds

timesharing a multi-user computer system where a fast processor alternates between several programs or routines to accommodate several terminals in a manner that seems simultaneous

titrate to determine by titration

titration the determination of the activity of a given substance in solution by the addition of chemical reagents until an equilibrium or predefined endpoint is achieved

titratable pertaining to a base or acid whose activity can be ascertained by titration

tomography an X-ray technique that produces a film representing a detailed cross section of tissue structure at a predetermined depth

tonicity the relative degree of osmotic pressure exerted by a solution; physiologically, any other solution with a tonicity equivalent to a 0.9% solution of NaCl is called isotonic, one with greater tonicity is called hypertonic, and one with less hypotonic

torr a unit of pressure equivalent to 1/760 atmosphere at STPD.

tort a legal wrong committed upon a person or property independent of contract

tortfeasor a wrong doer; the individual who commits or is guilty of a tort

total buffer base (BB) the total quantity of all blood buffers capable of binding hydrogen ions, normally ranges from 48 to 52 mEq/L

total lung capacity (TLC) the total amount of gas in the lungs after a maximum inspiration

tourniquet a device applied around an extremity which is designed to compress blood vessels and thereby prevent blood flow to or from the distalarea

tracheitis any inflammatory condition of the trachea

tracheobronchial of or pertaining to the trachea and large bronchi

tracheobronchomegaly a rare congenital condition in which the size of the large airways are greatly enlarged

tracheoesophageal of or pertaining to the trachea and esophagus, as with a tracheoesophageal fistula

tracheomalacia softening of the tracheal cartilages

tracheostomy an opening through the neck into the trachea, through which an indwelling tube may be inserted

tracheotomy the procedure by which an incision is made into the trachea through the neck below the larynx, in order to gain access to the lower airways

tranducer a device capable of converting one form of energy into another, and commonly used for measurement of physical events; for example, a pressure transducer may convert the physical phenomenon of force per unit area into an analog electrical signal

transaction any human interaction; in human communication, denotes a two-way process, in which participants are mutually influenced by the interaction

transbronchial across the bronchi or bronchial wall, as a transbronchial biopsy

transcutaneous across the skin, as a transcutaneous PO_2 electrode

transect to sever or cut across, as in preparing a cross section of tissue

transfill to fill across; to fill a vessel from another vessel

transfusion the direct introduction of blood or blood products from another source into the blood stream

transmural across the wall; usually pertains to the pressure difference between inside and outside a vessel or conducting tube

transplacental across or through the placenta, specifically in reference to the exchange of nutrients, waste products, and other material between the developing fetus and the mother

transpulmonary across the lung; of or pertaining to the difference in a parameter (like pressure) between the alveoli and pleural space

transrespiratory across the respiratory system; of or pertaining to the difference in a parameter (like pressure) between the alveoli and body surface

transthoracic across the thorax; of or pertaining to the difference in a parameter (like pressure) between the pleural space and body surface

transudate a fluid passed through a membrane or squeezed through a tissue or into the space between the cells of a tissue

transudation the process of fluid passage through a membrane

transvenous through the veins, as with a transvenous pacemaker

treatment regimen a comprehensive plan of various treatments designed to combat a certain disease or disorder

Trendelenburg position a position in which the head is low and the body and legs are on an inclined plane

triage a classification of casualties of war and other disasters according to the gravity of injuries, urgency of treatment, and place for treatment

trigeminy occurring in groups of threes; used frequently to describe certain cardiac arrhythmias, especially three premature ventricular contractions in a row

triple point that combination of temperature and pressure that allows the solid, liquid, and vapor forms of a given substance to exist in equilibrium with one another

trismus a prolonged tonic spasm of the muscles of the jaw

TTOT abbreviation for trantracheal oxygen therapy

turgor the normal resiliency of the skin caused by the outward pressure of the cells and interstitial fluid

ulnar of or pertaining to the ulnar bone or the area around it

ultrasound sound waves that occur at frequency beyond that which humans can normally discern, i.e., over 20,000 vibrations per second

ultrasonography the diagnsotic use of ultrasound to provide visualization of internal organs and structures

ultrastructure anatomic structure smaller that visible with a standard light microscope

unifocal occurring or originating in one place

univariate consisting of a single variable

unperfused lacking blood flow

untoward unexpected or unplanned

uremia the presence of excessive amounts of urea and other nitrogenous waste products in the blood, as occurs in renal failure

urethritis an inflammatory condition of the urethra that is characterized by dysuria, usually the result of an infection of the bladder or kidneys

urinalysis a physical, microscopic, or chemical examination of urine

urticaria a pruritic skin eruption characterized by transient wheals of varying shapes and sizes well-defined erythematous margins and pale centers

USP abbreviation for the United States Pharmacopeia, an officially recognized compedium of drug uses, strengths and purity standards

uteroplacental insufficiency a general term describing any physiologic or anatomic abnormality of the placental system which impairs normal exchange across the placenta and threatens the viability of the fetus

uvulopalatopharyngoplasty a surgical procedure used in treating severe obstructive sleep apnea which involve shortening of the soft palate, and removal of the uvula and tonsils

vacuum an absence of pressure

vagolytic of or pertaining to an action or agent which antagonizes or blocks parasympathetic activity

vagotomy a cutting of certain branches of the vagus nerve, performed with gastric surgery, to reduce the amount of gastric acid secreted and lessen the chance of recurrence of gastric ulcer

vago-vagal reflex a reflex caused by stimulation of parasympathetic receptors in the airways that can result in laryngospasm, bronchoconstriction, hyperpnea, and bradycardia; often associated with mechanical stimulation, as during procedures such as tracheobronchial aspiration, intubation, or bronchoscopy

valance a number indicating the combining power of a chemical substance

validity the degree to which the results of a given test actually reveal what the test intends to measure

Valsalva maneuver any forced expiratory effort against a closed glottis, as when an individual holds the breath and tightens the muscles in a concerted, strenuous effort to move a heavy object or to change position in bed

Van der Waals forces the mutual attractive forces exerted between atoms or molecules in close proximity to each other

vaporization the process whereby matter in its liquid form is changed into its vapor or gaseous form

vaporizer a device which converts a liquid into a vapor; more specifically, an apparatus designed to increase ambient humidity using the principles of either evaporation or boiling

VAPS abbreviation for variable assist pressure support, a form of pressure support ventilation that assures a minimum tidal volume

venous admixture the mixing of venous blood with arterial blood, resulting in a decrease in the oxygen content of the latter; occurs in anatomic and physiologic shunting

V/Q imbalance any abnormal deviation in the distribution of ventilation to perfusion among the lung's alveolar-capillary units

vascularization the process by which body tissue becomes vascular and develops proliferating capillaries

vasculitis inflammation of the blood vessels

vasoconstriction a narrowing of the lumen of any blood vessel, especially the arterioles and the veins in the blood reservoirs of the skin and the abdominal viscera

vasodilation widening or distention of blood vessels, particularly arterioles, usually caused by nerve impulses or certain drugs that relax smooth muscle in the walls of the blood vessels

vasomotor pertaining to the nerves and muscles that control the caliber of the lumen of the blood vessels

vasopressin see *ADH* (antidiuretic hormone)

vasopressor of or pertaining to a process, condition or substance that causes the constriction of blood vessels

VCV acronym for volume controlled ventilation, a mode of ventilatory support in which volume (or flow x time) serves as the cycle variable

vectorborne transmission of infectious organisms from one host to another via an animal carrier, especially an insect

vehicle transmission the transmission of infectious organisms that occurs when a susceptible host is exposed to an infectious agent transmitted through contaminated food or water

venipuncture a technique in which a vein is punctured transcutaneously by a sharp rigid stylet or cannula carrying a flexible plastic catheter or by a steel needle attached to a syringe or catheter

venomotor pertaining to the nerves and muscles that control the caliber of the lumen of the capacitance veins

ventricular fibrillation sustained, chaotic depolarization of the ventricular myocardium resulting in discoordinated and ineffective contraction

ventrolateral positioned or located toward the back and side

venule any one of the small blood vessels that gather blood from the capillary plexuses and anastomose to form the veins

vertebrochondral between the vertebral column and costal cartilages

vertebrosternal between the vertebral column and sternum

vestibule a space or a cavity that serves as the entrance to a passageway, as the vestibule of the nose

virucidal destructive to viruses

virucide any agent that destroys or inactivates viruses

virulence the power of microorgansims to produce disease

viscera the internal organs enclosed within a body cavity, primarily the abdominal organs

viscosity the internal force that opposes the flow of a fluid, either liquids and gases

viscous resistance impedance to motion caused by frictional forces among molecules, especially in fluids

vital capacity (VC) the total amount of air that can be exhaled after a maximum inspiration; the sum of the inspiratory reserve volume, the tidal volume, and the expiratory reserve volume

VNA abbreviation for visiting nurses' association

vocational of or pertaining to work

volatile acid an acid which can be excreted in its gaseous form; physiologically, carbonic acid is a volatile acid; some 24,000 mM of CO_2 are eliminated from the body daily via normal ventilation

VQI abbreviation for ventilation-perfusion index, an estimate of the venous admixture or physiologic shunt occurring in the lungs

VT/TI the mean spontaneous inspiratory flow, used to assess respiratory drive

WXYZ

watt a unit of power, equivalent to work done at the rate of 1 joule per second

wellness a dynamic state of health in which an individual progresses toward a higher level of functioning, achieving an optimum balance between internal and external environment

word processor a computer program for handling text; includes text entry and display, editing, formatting, and printing of the final output

xanthine a nitrogenous byproduct of the metabolism of nucleoproteins

xiphisternal of or pertaining to junction of the xiphoid process with the body of the sternum

xiphoid of or pertaining to the xiphoid process of the sternum

zeolite a commercial name for inorganic sodium-aluminum silicate; due to its ability to absorb both gaseous nitrogen and water vapor from air, zeolite is used extensively in certain oxygen concentrators

Ziehl-Neelsen Test one of the most widely used methods of acid-fast staining, commonly used in the microscopic examination of a smear of sputum suspected of containing Mycobacterium tuberculosis

Z-79 an abbreviation for the Z-79 Committee of the American National Standards Institute; when appearing on endotracheal tubes, this abbreviation signifies that the tube meets the design standards established by this voluntary regualtory group

INDEX